Clinical Practice of the Dental Hygienist

Clinical Practice of the
Dental Hygienist

Clinical Practice of the Dental Hygienist

TWELFTH EDITION

Esther M. Wilkins, BS, RDH, DMD
Department of Periodontology
Tufts University School of Dental Medicine
Boston, Massachusetts

Charlotte J. Wyche, RDH, MS
Department of Periodontics and Oral Medicine
University of Michigan School of Dentistry
Ann Arbor, Michigan

Linda D. Boyd, RDH, RD, EdD
Forsyth School of Dental Hygiene
MCPHS University
Boston, Massachusetts

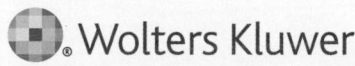 Wolters Kluwer

Philadelphia • Baltimore • New York • London
Buenos Aires • Hong Kong • Sydney • Tokyo

Senior Acquisitions Editor: Jonathan Joyce
Senior Product Development Editor: Amy Millholen
Editorial Assistant: Tish Rogers
Senior Marketing Manager: Leah Thomson
Senior Production Product Manager: Alicia Jackson
Design Coordinator: Holly McLaughlin
Manufacturing Coordinator: Margie Orzech
Prepress Vendor: S4Carlisle Publishing Services

Twelfth Edition
© 2017 Wolters Kluwer
Two Commerce Square
2001 Market Street
Philadelphia, PA 19103 USA
LWW.com

Printed in China

Library of Congress Cataloging-in-Publication Data
Wilkins, Esther M., author.
 Clinical practice of the dental hygienist / Esther M. Wilkins, Charlotte J. Wyche,
Linda D. Boyd. — 12th edition.
   p. ; cm.
 Includes bibliographical references and index.
 ISBN 978-1-4511-9311-4
 I. Wyche, Charlotte J., author. II. Boyd, Linda D., author. III. Title.
 [DNLM: 1. Dental Prophylaxis—Outlines. 2. Dental Hygienists—Outlines. WU 18.2]
 RK60.5
 617.6'01—dc23
                                                                    2015021080

Care has been taken to confirm the accuracy of the information presented and to describe generally accepted practices. However, the authors, editors, and publisher are not responsible for errors or omissions or for any consequences from application of the information in this book and make no warranty, expressed or implied, with respect to the currency, completeness, or accuracy of the contents of the publication. Application of the information in a particular situation remains the professional responsibility of the practitioner.

The authors, editors, and publisher have exerted every effort to ensure that drug selection and dosage set forth in this text are in accordance with current recommendations and practice at the time of publication. However, in view of ongoing research, changes in government regulations, and the constant flow of information relating to drug therapy and drug reactions, the reader is urged to check the package insert for each drug for any change in indications and dosage and for added warnings and precautions. This is particularly important when the recommended agent is a new or infrequently employed drug.

Some drugs and medical devices presented in the publication have Food and Drug Administration (FDA) clearance for limited use in restricted research settings. It is the responsibility of the health care provider to ascertain the FDA status of each drug or device planned for use in their clinical practice.

To purchase additional copies of this book, call our customer service department at (800) 638-3030 or fax orders to (301) 223-2320. International customers should call (301) 223-2300.

Visit Lippincott Williams & Wilkins on the Internet at LWW.com. Lippincott Williams & Wilkins customer service representatives are available from 8:30 am to 6 pm, EST.
10 9 8 7 6 5 4

DEDICATION

The twelfth edition of *Clinical Practice of the Dental Hygienist* is dedicated to all past and present students who have studied from the preceding editions. Gratitude is expressed to their teachers in the many different dental hygiene programs around the world, for their leadership in, and devotion to, dental hygiene education.

A very special recognition goes to the students of the first 10 classes in dental hygiene at the University of Washington in Seattle for whom the original "mimeographed" syllabus was created. They are remembered with much appreciation because their need for text study material made this book possible in the first place.

Esther M. Wilkins

To my great-aunt Victoria Tondrowski, who became a dental hygienist in 1926. Vickie taught dental hygiene at the University of Michigan for more than 30 years. When I was young, she talked about the women she worked with, taught with, respected and admired. As she spoke about them, she would always pause and say, "She's a dental hygienist, you know!" as if that credential conjured up the highest levels of awe and respect.

Charlotte J. Wyche

Gratitude to my husband, who has supported me tirelessly on my academic journey, and to my grandmother, Fay Nelson, who instilled a love of learning. Special thanks to my professional mentors who recognized my potential: Dr. John Chirgwin, Dr. Carole Palmer, and last, but never least, Dr. Esther Wilkins.

Linda D. Boyd

Contributors

Jessica August, RDH, MS
Instructor
Forsyth School of Dental Hygiene
MCPHS University
Boston, Massachusetts

Caren M. Barnes, RDH, BS, MS
Professor
Department of Dental Hygiene
University of Nebraska Medical Center College of Dentistry
Lincoln, Nebraska

Lisa Bennett-Johnson, RDH, MSDH
Adjunct Faculty
Forsyth School of Dental Hygiene
MCPHS University
Boston, Massachusetts

Sara L. Beres, RDH, BA, MS
Instructor
Department of Dental Hygiene
Sheridan College
Sheridan, Wyoming

Linda D. Boyd, RDH, RD, EdD
Dean & Professor
Forsyth School of Dental Hygiene
MCPHS University
Boston, Massachusetts

Ernestine R. Daniels, RDH, BS
Adjunct Instructor, Dental Programs
Department of Dental Hygiene
Florida State College at Jacksonville
Jacksonville, Florida

Elena M. Francisco, RDH, RDHAP, MSDH
Clinical Instructor (Retired)
Department of Dental Hygiene
University of the Pacific Arthur A. Dugoni School of Dentistry
San Francisco, California

Lori J. Giblin, RDH, MS
Assistant Professor
Forsyth School of Dental Hygiene
MCPHS University
Boston, Massachusetts

Janet M. Gruber, RDH, MPA
Associate Professor
Department of Dental Hygiene
Farmingdale State College of New York
Farmingdale, New York

Jane F. Halaris, RDH, MA
Adjunct Clinical Lecturer
Department of Periodontics and Oral Medicine
University of Michigan School of Dentistry
Ann Arbor, Michigan

Susan J. Jenkins, RDH, MS
Associate Professor
Forsyth School of Dental Hygiene
MCPHS University
Boston, Massachusetts

Janis G. Keating, RDH, MA
Professional Education Resources
Philips Sonicare
Lakewood, Colorado

Pamela S. Kennard, BSN, RDH, MA
Program Director
Department of Dental Hygiene
State College of Florida
Bradenton, Florida

Lisa M. LaSpina, RDH, MS
Assistant Professor
Forsyth School of Dental Hygiene
MCPHS University
Boston, Massachusetts

Allyson Ligor, RDH, BS
Community Programs Faculty
Dental Hygiene Department
Middlesex Community College
Lowell, Massachusetts

Judi S. Luxmore, RDH, BAS, MS
Clinical Associate Professor (Retired)
Department of Periodontology and Dental Hygiene
University of Detroit Mercy School of Dentistry
Detroit, Michigan

Christine Macarelli-Rogers, RDH, MS
Assistant Professor
Dental Hygiene Program
New York City College of Technology
Brooklyn, New York

Deborah S. Manne, RDH, RN, MSN, OCN
Adjunct Instructor
Department of Otolaryngology—Head and Neck Surgery
St. Louis University School of Medicine
St. Louis, Missouri

Stacy A. Matsuda, RDH, BS, MS
Clinical Instructor
Department of Periodontology
Oregon Health and Science University School of Dentistry
Portland, Oregon

Durinda J. Mattana, RDH, MS
Adjunct Clinical Lecturer
Department of Periodontology and Dental Hygiene
University of Detroit Mercy School of Dentistry
Detroit, Michigan

Jill Moore, RDH, BSDH, MHA
Dental Sealant Coordinator
Michigan Department of Health and Human Services
Lansing, Michigan

Luisa Nappo-Dattoma, RDH, RD, EdD
Associate Professor
Department of Dental Hygiene
Farmingdale State College
Farmingdale, New York

Debra November-Rider, RDH, MSDH
Adjunct Assistant Professor
Forsyth School of Dental Hygiene
MCPHS University
Boston, Massachusetts

Elizabeth Gorvin Onik, RDH, MEd
Instructor, Second-year Dental Hygiene Coordinator
Department of Dental Hygiene
San Juan College
Farmington, New Mexico

Kristeen Perry, RDH, MSDH
Assistant Professor
Forsyth School of Dental Hygiene
MCPHS University
Boston, Massachusetts

Lori Rainchuso, RDH, MS
Graduate Program Director, Associate Professor
Forsyth School of Dental Hygiene
MCPHS University
Boston, Massachusetts

Erin Relich, RDH, BSDH, MSA
Assistant Professor
Division of Periodontics and Oral Medicine
University of Detroit Mercy School of Dentistry
Detroit, Michigan

Pamela S. Ridilla, RDH, MS
Chair, Professor
School of Dental Sciences
Daytona State College
Daytona Beach, Florida

Dianne Smallidge, RDH, BS, MDH
Associate Professor
Forsyth School of Dental Hygiene
MCPHS University
Boston, Massachusetts

Robert Smethers, RDH, BASDH
Instructor
Forsyth School of Dental Hygiene
MCPHS University
Boston, Massachusetts

Katherine Soal, RDH, MSDH
Assistant Professor
Department of Dental Hygiene
Quinsigamond Community College
Worcester, Massachusetts

Tammy K. Swecker, BSDH, MEd
Associate Professor
Division of Dental Hygiene
Virginia Commonwealth University
Richmond, Virginia

Terri S. I. Tilliss, RDH, MS, MA, PhD
Professor
Department of Graduate Orthodontics
University of Colorado School of Dental Medicine
Aurora, Colorado

Marsha A. (Black) Voelker
Associate Professor, Junior Clinic Coordinator
Division of Dental Hygiene
University of Missouri—Kansas City School of Dentistry
Kansas City, Missouri

Dianna Weikel, RDH, MS
Associate Professor
Department of Oncology and Diagnostic Sciences
University of Maryland School of Dentistry
Baltimore, Maryland

Lisa Welch, RDH, BS, MSDH
Assistant Professor
Department of Dental Hygiene
Dixie State College
St. George, Utah

Esther M. Wilkins, BS, RDH, DMD
Department of Periodontology
Tufts University School of Dental Medicine
Boston, Massachusetts

Lane Wilson-Foreman, CDA, RDH, BS
Associate Professor
Department of Dental Health Programs
Tallahassee Community College
Tallahassee, Florida

Katherine A. Woods, PhD, MPH, RDH
Professor, Associate Degree Dental Hygiene Program
Department of Dental Hygiene
St. Petersburg College
St. Petersburg, Florida

Charlotte J. Wyche, RDH, MS
Adjunct Lecturer
Department of Periodontics and Oral Medicine
University of Michigan School of Dentistry
Ann Arbor, Michigan

Katherine A. Yee, RDH, BSDH, MPH
Dental Hygiene Degree Completion Recruitment &
    Admissions Coordinator, Adjunct Clinical Lecturer
Division of Periodontics and Oral Medicine
University of Michigan School of Dentistry
Ann Arbor, Michigan

Carolynn A. Zeitz, RDH, BS, RDA, MA
Clinical Associate Professor
Pediatric Dentistry
University of Detroit Mercy School of Dentistry
Detroit, Michigan

Reviewers

Sandra Curren, RDH, MS
First Year Lead Instructor and Clinic Coordinator
Dental Hygiene
Portland Community College
Portland, Oregon

Kathleen D'Ambrisi, RDH, MS
Program Director
Dental Hygiene
Community College of Baltimore County
Baltimore, Maryland

Susan Davide, RDH, MS, MSEd
Assistant Professor
Dental Hygiene
New York City College of Technology
Brooklyn, New York

Donna Davis, RDH, MEd
Director, Associate Professor
Dental Hygiene
Northeast Texas Community College
Mt. Pleasant, Texas

Leslie DeLong, RDH, MHA
Clinic Coordinator
Dental Hygiene
Lamar Institute of Technology
Beaumont, Texas

Ronda DeMattei, RDH, MSEd, PhD
Program Director
Dental Hygiene
Southern Illinois University
Carbondale, Illinois

Jeanie Dent, RDH, BA
Program Manager
Dental Hygiene
Brevard Community College
Cocoa, Florida

Gail Devlin, CRAII, CDR
Dental Program Chair
Everest College
North York, Ontario, Canada

Elizabeth Di Silvio, RDH, MEd
Associate Professor
Dental Hygiene
Northern Virginia Community College
Springfield, Virginia

Christine Dominick, MEd
Associate Dean, Professor
Forsyth School of Dental Hygiene
Massachusetts College of Pharmacy and Health Sciences
Worcester, Massachusetts

Debra Doxey, RDH, BS, MPH
Adjunct Assistant Professor
Dental Hygiene
Pasadena City College
Pasadena, California

Patricia Dray, RDH, MEd
First Year Dental Hygiene Coordinator
Dental Hygiene
Sheridan College
Sheridan, Wyoming

Cindy Drucks, MA, RDH, CDA
Associate Professor
Allied Dental Education
University of Medicine and Dentistry of New Jersey
Plains, New Jersey

Barbara Ebert, CDA, RDH, MA
Program Director
Dental Hygiene
Wallace State Community College
Hanceville, Alabama

Suzanne Edenfield, RDH, ASDH, BS, MHS, EdD
Department Head
Dental Hygiene
Savannah Technical College
Savannah, Georgia

Barbara Ellis, RDH, MA, BS, AAS
Instructor
Health Professions
Monroe Community College
Rochester, New York

Jennifer Fulk, RDH, BS, MEd
First Year Clinic Coordinator
Dental Hygiene
Guilford Technical Community College
Jamestown, North Carolina

Joy Gall, RDH, MBA
Program Director, Dental Hygiene
Dental Studies
Pima Community College
Tucson, Arizona

Deborah Graeff, RDH, MS
Professor
Dental Hygiene
Erie Community College
Williamsville, New York

Tammy Hale, RDH, BS
First Year Clinical Coordinator, Professor
Dental Hygiene
Collin College
McKinney, Texas

Kathleen Harlan, RDH, MS
Associate Professor
Dental Hygiene and Medical Imaging
Ferris State University
Big Rapids, Michigan

Linda Hecker, CDA, RDH, BS, MA
Director of Dental Hygiene
Rowan College at Burlington County
Pemberton, New Jersey

Emily Henderson, RDH, BS
Clinical Coordinator
Dental Hygiene
Collin College
McKinney, Texas

Mary J. Hoffman, RDH, BSDH
Co-Program Director
Dental Hygiene
Madison Area Technical College
Madison, Wisconsin

Joyce C. Hudson, RDH, MS
Dental Hygiene Program Chair
School of Health Sciences/Dental Hygiene
Ivy Tech Community College
Anderson, Indiana

Patricia Johnson, RDH, BSDH, MS
Professor Program Coordinator
Allied Health, Dental Hygiene
Tunxis Community College
Farmington, Connecticut

Mark G. Kacerik RDH, MS
Associate Professor
Dental Hygiene
University of New Haven
West Haven, Connecticut

Janet Kinney, RDH, MS
Director Division of Dental Hygiene,
Clinical Assistant Professor
Department of Periodontics and Oral Medicine
University of Michigan School of Dentistry
Ann Arbor, Michigan

Dina L. Korte, RDH, BSDH
Clinical Lecturer
Department of Periodontics and Oral Medicine
University of Michigan School of Dentistry
Ann Arbor, Michigan

Melisa McCannel, BS
Program Director
Dental Hygiene
Pima Medical Institute
Seattle, Washington

Debbie Moon, RDH, MA
Junior Clinic Coordinator
Dental Hygiene
Moreno Valley College
Moreno Valley, California

Christine Nielsen Nathe, RDH, MS
Professor and Program Director
Division of Dental Hygiene
University of New Mexico
Albuquerque, New Mexico

Betty Ann Pryzdial, BSc, RDH, PIP
Instructor
Vancouver College of Dental Hygiene
Vancouver, British Columbia, Canada

Pamela P. Quinn, RDH, BSE, MS
Program Director
Dental Hygiene
State University of New York
Canton, New York

Carolyn Ray, RDH, MEd
Professor
Dental Hygiene
University of Oklahoma College of Dentistry
Midwest City, Oklahoma

Mathias Schede, DDS
Clinical Assistant Professor
Oral Health Sciences
Vancouver College of Dental Hygiene
Vancouver, British Columbia, Canada

Emily Soler
Clinical Instructor
Clinical Department
Vancouver College of Dental Hygiene
Richmond, British Columbia, Canada

Tonette Steeb, BS
Clinic Coordinator, Instructor
Dental Hygiene
Diablo Valley College
Pleasant Hill, California

Sharon Struminger, RDH, MPS, MA
Professor
Dental Hygiene
Farmingdale State College
Farmingdale, New York

Barbara Tarwater, RDH, CDA, BASDH
Assistant Professor
Health Sciences
Pensacola Junior College
Pensacola, Florida

Kelly Tanner Williams, RDH, MSDH
Associate Professor
Dental Hygiene
Thomas Nelson Community College
Hampton, Virginia

Karen Wynn, RDH, MEd
Professor
Dental Hygiene
New Hampshire Technical Institute–Concord's Community
College
Concord, New Hampshire

Gail Yee, BA, DipDH
Clinical Instructor
Dental Hygiene
Vancouver College of Dental Hygiene
Vancouver, British Columbia, Canada

Preface

Dental hygienists are oral healthcare specialists with professional goals centered on the prevention and/or control of oral disease and the maintenance of oral and general health. As primary healthcare professionals, dental hygienists can apply their knowledge and skills in a wide variety of areas related to clinical practice, education, research, public health, and advocacy for health promotion and disease prevention. Dental hygienists collaborate with dentists and members of other health professions to provide oral health care that links with total body health care. New emphasis on the effect of oral health on systemic health challenges dental hygienists to widen their scope of practice.

OBJECTIVES

Objectives of the 12th edition include:

▶ To help prepare the beginning dental hygiene student to recognize the requirements of evidence based dental hygiene practice.

▶ To develop skills and knowledge for entry into the profession.

▶ To help when studying for Licensure Board examinations; the condensed outline form aids to make review easier.

▶ To update professional hygienists already in practice, and assist long-term practitioners to recognize the new responsibility to apply evidence-based scientific approaches to patient care.

THE TEXTBOOK PLAN

Highlights

Highlights of *Clinical Practice of the Dental Hygienist*, 12th edition, include the following:

▶ Color images have been added throughout.

▶ Chapter 1 includes a new section on the history of the dental hygiene profession and information on alternative practice and mid-level providers.

▶ A new major section on documentation as part of the process of care has been added.

▶ Chapter 8 has been moved to Section II Preparation for Dental Hygiene Practice.

▶ Chapter 26 has been updated to highlight a motivational interviewing approach to patient counseling.

▶ Risk assessment for oral disease has been added to Chapters 12, 19, and 27.

▶ Chapter 58 has been expanded with a focus on providing dental hygiene care in alternative practice settings.

Organization of the Textbook

As in past editions, sections of *Clinical Practice of the Dental Hygienist* are sequenced to conform to the Dental Hygiene Process of Care. There are nine sections in the 12th edition, six of which are specifically identified by name with the recognized components of the Process of Care. They are *assessment, dental hygiene diagnosis, care planning, implementation, evaluation, and documentation*.

The textbook opens with chapters devoted to an introduction to the profession of dental hygiene and chapters related to preparation for practice. They include infection control and ergonomic health for the clinical practitioner and patient. The final large section, Section IX, applies the process of care to patients with special needs.

The nine major sections are:

I. Orientation to Clinical Dental Hygiene Practice
II. Preparation for Dental Hygiene Practice
III. Documentation
IV. Assessment
V. Dental Hygiene Diagnosis and Care Planning
VI. Implementation: Prevention
VII. Implementation: Treatment
VIII. Evaluation
IX. Patients with Special Needs

Supplementary information is available in appendices:

I. American Dental Hygienists' Association Code of Ethics for Dental Hygienists
II. National Dental Hygienists' Association Code of Ethics
III. Canadian Dental Hygienists Association Dental Hygienists' Code of Ethics
IV. International Federation of Dental Hygienists' Code of Ethics

FEATURES OF THE NEW EDITION

All chapters have been updated, and many have been extensively revised. Each chapter includes the following features:

► Detailed **outline format** for the text makes it easier to study and locate information quickly. In this era of information growth related to new research and products available for professional clinical practice as well as teaching patients self-care, the condensation of printed material into outline form can provide busy, overloaded students with a new efficiency for learning.

► **Chapter outlines** at the opening of each chapter provide a preliminary review for readers before they start to concentrate on the meat of the chapter; the outline can help readers locate material within the chapter at any time.

► **Learning Objectives** at the beginning of each chapter guide the student in studying the chapter.

► **Key Words boxes** near the beginning of each chapter identify spelling and definition for the new vocabulary of the particular chapter. Each key word is listed in the index, so a quick reference to definitions in other chapters is possible.

► **Everyday Ethics boxes** ("EEs") provide students with the opportunity to become aware of and discuss clinical problems from real-life practice. Principles of ethical dental hygiene practice need to be brought into the curriculum at an early stage if students are to develop into ethical practitioners. This feature has been continued from previous editions because of expressed appreciation of teachers and students.

► **Factors to Teach the Patient** boxes help students to select topics from the chapter that need special emphasis while teaching patients self-care and responsibility for oral health for their own lifetime as well as that of their family and community.

► **Documentation** brings to full cycle the clinical care of a patient. Example documentation for a variety of patients, written using the SOAP notes format outlined in Chapter 9, can increase students' awareness of the necessary components and significance of such notes in the permanent record of each patient.

STUDENT WORKBOOK

A unique study guide, *Active Learning Workbook for Clinical Practice of the Dental Hygienist*, prepared by Charlotte J. Wyche for previous editions, has been recognized as a major contribution to student learning. The 12th edition workbook, revised to highlight new chapters and updated information from the textbook, also contains revised crossword and word search puzzles.

Everyday Ethics boxes in the workbook include individual learning, cooperative learning, or discovery activities designed to help the student reflect on or apply ethical theory-related "Questions for Consideration" found in the textbook. Activities and questions related to patient case scenarios, patient assessment summaries, and documentation of patient care provide an emphasis on case-based application of knowledge. New boxes in each chapter contain Medical Subject Heading (MeSH) terms to help students develop effective and efficient PubMed literature searches.

ADDITIONAL RESOURCES

Digital Connections

Clinical Practice of the Dental Hygienist, 12th edition, includes additional resources for both instructors and students that are available on the book's companion Web site at http://thepoint.lww.com/Wilkins12e.

Instructors

Approved adopting instructors will be given access to the following additional resources:

► Test generator
► PowerPoint presentations
► Lesson plans
► Image bank of all the images and tables in the book
► LMS (Learning Management System) course cartridges for Angel, Blackboard, and Moodle
► Answers to the exercises found in *Active Learning Workbook for Clinical Practice of the Dental Hygienist*, by Charlotte J. Wyche, Jane F. Halaris, and Esther M. Wilkins (book available for separate purchase)

Students

Students who have purchased *Clinical Practice of the Dental Hygienist*, 12th edition, have access to the following additional resources:

► Quiz bank
► Audio pronunciation glossary for select clinical terms
   See the inside front cover of this text for more details, including the code you will need to gain access to the Web site.

INDIVIDUALIZED REVIEW

PrepU for Wilkins' Clinical Practice of the Dental Hygienist is an adaptive, formative quizzing program that remediates to the book. PrepU helps students identify where they need to spend more study time and provides instructors with real-time data for maximizing class performance. (Available for separate purchase: visit www.lww.com for more information.)

ACKNOWLEDGMENTS

A textbook of the size and scope of *Clinical Practice of the Dental Hygienist* shows the work of many contributors. Comments and suggestions come from teachers, students, and practitioners from around the world, as the book has been translated into a variety of languages. Any suggestion, whether for one word or whole chapters, is welcomed and considered. It is hoped that this new edition will bring comments and requests as in the past.

Recognition for Our Contributors

We start with expressed recognition and appreciation to our listed contributors for their new or revised chapters. Each has spent much time for selective revision and to survey the literature for new material and references.

Other Appreciation

Appreciation is expressed to the following:

Marcia Williams of Santa Fe, New Mexico. Many illustrations for this and previous editions have been the work of our talented artist. Her personal interest and patience in preparing new drawings, revising previous ones, and adding color to enhance the line drawings are acknowledged with sincere gratitude.

Pamela Bretschneider, BA, MEd, PhD, of Framingham, Massachusetts. For her help with many chapters for computer searches for the new research provided over the entire 2 to 3 years while revision was in action—her generous assistance is greatly appreciated.

Anna Pattison, RDH, MS, of Los Angeles, California. For many thoughtful contributions and review of Chapter 48.

Elizabeth Ioakimidis of Boston, Massachusetts. For her help printing, scanning, pick up, and delivery of the chapter drafts for review and editing.

Our Readers. And, finally, an expression of appreciation goes to our readers over the years: students, teachers, and practicing dental hygienists. Send us your comments and suggestions. As stated in the first edition, it is hoped that through greater understanding of each patient's oral and general health needs, more complete and effective dental hygiene services can be rendered.

Esther M. Wilkins

Contents

SECTION V
DENTAL HYGIENE DIAGNOSIS
AND CARE PLANNING   393

Orientation to Clinical Dental Hygiene Practice

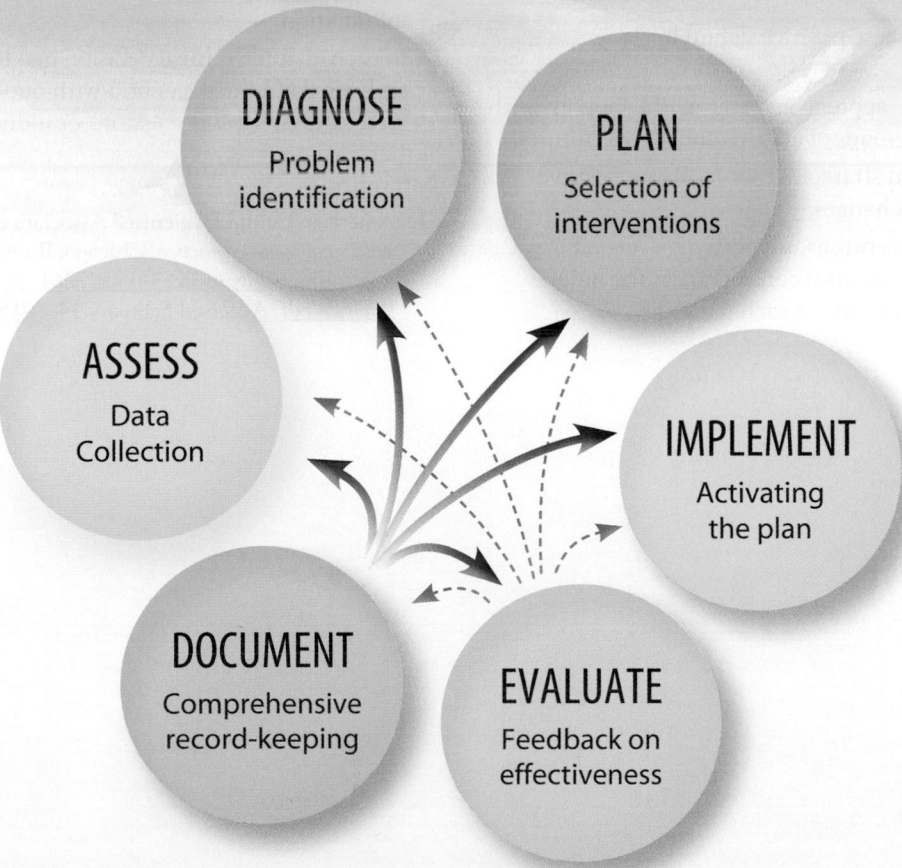

DIAGNOSE
Problem identification

PLAN
Selection of interventions

ASSESS
Data Collection

IMPLEMENT
Activating the plan

DOCUMENT
Comprehensive record-keeping

EVALUATE
Feedback on effectiveness

FIGURE I-1 The Dental Hygiene Process of Care.

INTRODUCTION FOR SECTION I

Professional dental hygiene practice is not defined solely by the clinical duties that are traditionally associated with private practice dental care settings. The professional roles, responsibilities, and ethical standards of the dental hygienist encompass both traditional clinical practice and alternative dental hygiene practice settings.

The dental hygienist is:

▶ An educated and licensed primary healthcare provider who fills numerous roles that contribute to better oral health.

▶ Concerned with the general health and well-being of both individual patients and population groups.

▶ Skilled in accessing, understanding, and analyzing the validity of current health information.

THE PROFESSIONAL DENTAL HYGIENIST

The professional dental hygienist is dedicated to:

▶ A dental hygiene process of care that meets standards for clinical dental hygiene practice.

▶ Ethical standards and core values outlined in professional Codes of Ethics to dental hygiene practice in every setting.

▶ Evidence-based, best-practice dental hygiene interventions.

▶ Communication approaches that build rapport with individuals and groups of all ages and across cultures.

▶ Patient education strategies that motivate positive health behavior changes.

▶ Healthcare interventions, supported by current research, which take into consideration the unique needs and requirements of each patient.

STANDARD OF CARE AND THE DENTAL HYGIENE PROCESS OF CARE

▶ The American Dental Hygienists' Association *Standards for Clinical Dental Hygiene Practice*[1] outlines criteria for competency in dental hygiene care, as illustrated by the components of the Dental Hygiene Process of Care.

▶ The Dental Hygiene Process of Care is the basis for providing preventive, educational, and therapeutic dental hygiene services that meet accepted standards of patient care.

▶ The process, illustrated by **Figure I-1**, as well as similar figures that are repeated on each section heading page, explains the series of interrelated steps that the dental hygienist follows to provide clinical patient care.

▶ The overall process is explained in Chapter 1. Each step in the process is described more completely throughout the sections of the textbook.

ETHICAL APPLICATIONS

▶ Basic ethical concepts are described in the introduction to each section of the textbook.

▶ Reference charts are included to summarize ethical information.

▶ In each chapter, ethical decision making is illustrated in an Everyday Ethics scenario with questions that can be used to guide class discussions or individual reflection.

Reference

1. American Dental Hygienists' Association. *Standards for clinical dental hygiene practice.* Chicago, IL: ADHA; 2008. http://www.adha.org/resources-docs/7261_Standards_Clinical_Practice.pdf. Accessed February 14, 2015.

The Professional Dental Hygienist

Esther M. Wilkins, BS, RDH, DMD, Charlotte J. Wyche, RDH, MS, and Linda D. Boyd, RDH, RD, EdD

CHAPTER OUTLINE

LEARNING OBJECTIVES

After studying this chapter, the student will be able to:

1. Identify and define key terms and concepts related to the professional dental hygienist.

2. Describe the scope of dental hygiene practice.

3. Identify and describe the components of the dental hygiene process of care.

4. Identify and apply components of the dental hygiene code of ethics.

5. Explain legal, ethical, and personal factors affecting dental hygiene practice.

6. Apply concepts in ethical decision making.

▶ The American Dental Hygienists' Association defines the professional dental hygienist[1] as *a primary care oral health professional* who:
- Has graduated from an accredited dental hygiene program in an institution of higher education.
- Is licensed in dental hygiene.
- Supports overall health through the promotion of optimal oral health.

▶ The cornerstone of dental hygiene practice has been the direct provision of education and clinical care to individual patients.

▶ Dental hygiene roles and responsibilities have developed and grown since early years.

▶ The term *dental hygiene care* denotes all integrated preventive, educational, and treatment services administered for a patient by a dental hygienist.

▶ The term is parallel to the commonly used term "dental care," which refers to the services provided by the dentist.

▶ Key words relating to dental hygienists and their practice are defined in Box 1-1.

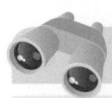

BOX 1-1   KEY WORDS AND ABBREVIATIONS: Professional Dental Hygienist

ADHA: American Dental Hygienists' Association.

ADHP: Advanced Dental Hygiene Practitioner. The dental-hygiene-based, alternative workforce model, proposed by the American Dental Hygienists' Association, would be a registered dental hygienist with additional training who could autonomously provide additional oral health services.

CDHA: Canadian Dental Hygienists' Association.

CEU: continuing education unit; 1 unit commonly refers to 1 clock hour of instruction.

Collaborative Practice of Dental Hygiene (Affiliated Practice): the science of the prevention and treatment of oral disease through the provision of educational, assessment, preventive, clinical, and other therapeutic services in a collaborative working relationship with a consulting dentist, with general supervision.

Competency: the skills, understanding, and professional values of an individual ready for beginning dental hygiene practice.

Continuing education: postlicensure short-term educational experiences for refresher, updating, and renewal; continuing education units may be required for relicensure.

Cotherapist: term used to describe the relationships between patient, dentist, and dental hygienist when coordinating the efforts to attain and maintain the oral health of the patient.

Dental hygiene care plan: the services within the framework of the total treatment plan to be carried out by the dental hygienist, patient, and caregiver.

Dental hygiene care: the science and practice of the prevention of oral diseases; the integrated preventive and treatment services administered for a patient by a dental hygienist.

Dental hygiene diagnosis: identification of an existing or a potential oral health problem that a dental hygienist is qualified and licensed to treat.

Dental hygiene process of care: an organized, systematic group of activities that provides the framework for delivering quality dental hygiene care.

Dental hygienist: oral health specialist whose primary concern is the maintenance of oral health and the prevention of oral disease (see also opening section of this chapter).

Dental Therapist: a mid-level oral health care provider with expanded training who provides direct patient care under an expanded scope of practice that includes the ability to diagnose and perform restorative services. Dental therapists provide safe, quality dental care in many countries around the world.

Dentistry: the diagnosis and treatment of diseases of the teeth, gums, and related structures of the mouth, including repair or replacement of defective teeth.

Direct Access: allows a dental hygienist to initiate dental hygiene treatment based on assessment of the patient's needs and without the specific authorization or presence of a dentist.

Health promotion: the process of enabling people to improve their health through self-care, mutual aid, and the creation of a healthy environment.

Health: state of physical, mental, and social well-being, not only the absence of disease.

Hygiene: the science of health and its preservation; a condition or practice, such as cleanliness, that is conducive to the preservation of health.

IFDH: International Federation of Dental Hygienists.

Interprofessional Collaborative Practice: comprehensive health care delivered by multiple health care providers with different professional backgrounds who work together with each other, the patient, the family and other caregivers to meet the patient's needs.

Intervention: an action taken by a dental hygienist to maintain or restore a patient's optimal oral health.

License by credential: acceptance for licensure by a regulatory body (state, province) based on evidence from a license obtained in another state with equivalent standards and requirements also called reciprocity, a mutual or cooperative exchange.

NDHA: National Dental Hygienists' Association.

Oral hygiene: procedures for preservation of health of the oral cavity; personal maintenance of cleanliness and other measures recommended by dental professionals.

OSHA: Occupational Safety and Health Administration. A U.S. government agency that helps employers protect their workers and reduce workplace deaths, injuries, and illnesses.

Primary healthcare: employs the techniques and agents to abort the onset of disease, to reverse the progress of the initial stages of disease, or to arrest the disease process before treatment becomes necessary.

Profession: occupation or calling that:
- requires specialized knowledge, methods, and skills
- requires preparation, from an institution of higher learning, in the scholarly, scientific, and historic principles underlying such methods and skills
- continuously enlarges its body of knowledge,
- functions autonomously in formulation of policy
- maintains high standards of achievement and conduct.

Members of a Profession:
- are committed to continuing study
- place service above personal gain
- provide practical services vital to human and social welfare.

Prognosis: a forecast of the probable course and outcome of the treatment of a condition or disease.

Supervision: term applied to a legal relationship between dentist and dental team members in practice. Each state practice act defines the type of supervision required for dental hygiene practice.

HISTORY OF THE DENTAL HYGIENE PROFESSION[2]

▶ In the early part of the 20th century, Dr. Alfred C. Fones, a dentist in Bridgeport Connecticut, realized that most children already had dental decay by the time they reached his dental chair.

▶ He trained his assistant, Irene Newman, to demonstrate the value of education and prevention to reduce dental disease.

▶ The name "dental hygienist" evolved because Fones felt that this term would create an association with the prevention, rather than treatment of oral disease.

▶ Box 1-2 provides a timeline of major events in the development of the profession of dental hygiene.

▶ Figure 1-1 illustrates how the appearance of the clinical dental hygienist has changed as the profession has changed and grown.

BOX 1-2

The Development of the Profession of Dental Hygiene: A Timeline

1910–1919
- ▷ Irene Newman, Dr. Fones assistant, became:
  - ▷ Licensed as the first dental hygienist.
  - ▷ The first president of an organized dental hygiene society in Connecticut.
- ▷ Graduates from the first dental hygiene school, created by Dr. Fones, began working in public schools.
- ▷ A dental hygienist was employed outside of a public school setting, in New Haven Hospital.

1920–1929
- ▷ Licensed dental hygienists began to practice in numerous states, including Hawaii.
- ▷ The ADHA:
  - ▷ Was incorporated in Detroit, Michigan, in 1927.
  - ▷ Began publication of the *Journal of the ADHA*.

1930–1939
- ▷ Dental hygienists continued working in schools, began making home visits, and most found positions in private dental practices.
- ▷ Transportation was provided to Forsyth Dental Infirmary from Boston Schools and children visiting the clinic received oral prophylaxis and oral health instruction from dental hygiene students.
- ▷ ADHA and American Dental Association recommended minimum high-school graduation as one requirement for dental hygiene licensure.
- ▷ University of Michigan offered the first baccalaureate degree in dental hygiene.

1940–1949
- ▷ ADHA recommended:
  - ▷ Changing a 1-year program to 2-year course of study for dental hygiene licensure.
  - ▷ The term "registered dental hygienist" as the official credential for the profession
- ▷ Minimum standards for dental hygiene programs adopted.
- ▷ Dr. Frank Lamons wrote the first dental hygienist oath, to be used in graduation exercises.
- ▷ Grand Rapids, Michigan, became the first city to add fluoride to its drinking water.

1950–1959	▷ All states granted licensure for dental hygienists.
	▷ Minimum education standards for dental hygiene education set and the accreditation process for dental hygiene programs began.
	▷ Sigma Phi Alpha, the dental hygiene honor society, was founded.
	▷ ADHA membership restrictions based on race, creed, or color removed.
	▷ The first edition of the *Clinical Practice of The Dental Hygienist* textbook by Esther M. Wilkins, BS, RDH, DMD was published in 1959.
1960–1969	▷ The first National Dental Hygiene Board Examination implemented.
	▷ The first Regional Board Examination (North East) given.
	▷ The first dental hygiene master's degree program began at Columbia University in New York.
	▷ ADHA bylaws amended to allow for male dental hygienist members.
1970–1979	▷ The first International Symposium on Dental Hygiene, organized and funded by the ADHA, held in Italy.
	▷ The Forsyth Experiment, a groundbreaking investigation, proved conclusively that appropriately trained dental hygienists are safely and cost effectively able to provide a defined set of restorative services.
	▷ Some state practice acts expand to include administration of local anesthesia by dental hygienists.
	▷ Continuing education guidelines drafted.
	▷ Dental hygienists began to serve on some state boards of dental examiners.
1980–1989	▷ Washington was the first state with unsupervised dental hygiene practice in hospitals, nursing homes, and other specified settings.
	▷ Colorado allowed unsupervised practice for dental hygienists in all settings.
	▷ ADHA advocated for baccalaureate as the minimum degree for entry into the dental hygiene profession.
	▷ On the basis of research about the transmission of blood-borne infectious diseases, dental hygiene clinicians began wearing gloves during all procedures.
1990–1999	▷ OSHA's rules on occupational exposure to blood-borne pathogens implemented; use of gloves and face masks during dental hygiene procedures became standard practice.
	▷ The *Dental Hygiene Process: Diagnosis and Care Planning* textbook published, establishing a standard for clinical dental hygiene practice.
	▷ The National Center for Dental Hygiene Research established.
	▷ New Mexico became the first state to allow:
	▷ Self-regulation of the profession by a dental hygiene committee.
	▷ Dental hygiene practice under a collaborative agreement with a dentist rather than supervision.
	▷ California created the Registered Dental Hygienist in Alternative Practice (RDHAP), allowing dental hygienists to provide unsupervised oral care to special populations in alternative settings.
2000–2010	▷ The U.S. Department of Health and Human Services published Oral Health in America: A Report of the Surgeon General, which highlights the relevance of oral health to general health.
	▷ U.S. Centers for Disease Control and Prevention published Guidelines for Infection Control in Dental Health Setting.
	▷ Development of the mid-level oral health provider explored.
	▷ The ADHA adopted policy to develop the ADHP.
	▷ DHATs began providing dental care on tribal land in Alaska.
	▷ Minnesota passed the first law in the United States, allowing dental hygienists to be further licensed as dental therapists using ADHP competencies.
	▷ Master-level dental hygiene programs increased in number.
	▷ Many states implemented "direct access" policies that allow dental hygienists in at least some settings to initiate dental hygiene care:
	▷ Based on their assessment of the patient's needs.
	▷ Without the specific authorization of a dentist.
2011–2020 and Beyond– Focus on the Future	▷ In 2013, ADHA celebrated 100 years of dental hygiene at the 90th ADHA Annual Session meeting in Boston.
	▷ Dental hygiene degree-completion programs and online education opportunities expand.
	▷ Opportunities for alternative setting and autonomy in dental hygiene practice expand.
	▷ The dental hygiene profession affirms and pursues its commitment to:
	▷ Optimal oral health as an essential component of general health.
	▷ Access to safe, effective, oral health services for all people.
	▷ Collaborative, interprofessional partnerships and coalitions for oral health.

Source: American Dental Hygienists' Association. *100: Celebrating a Century of Professional Pride.* Chicago, IL: ADHA; 2013:48.

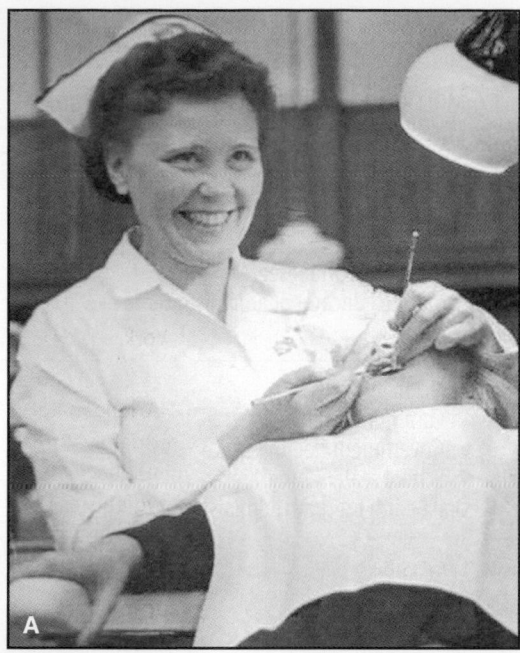

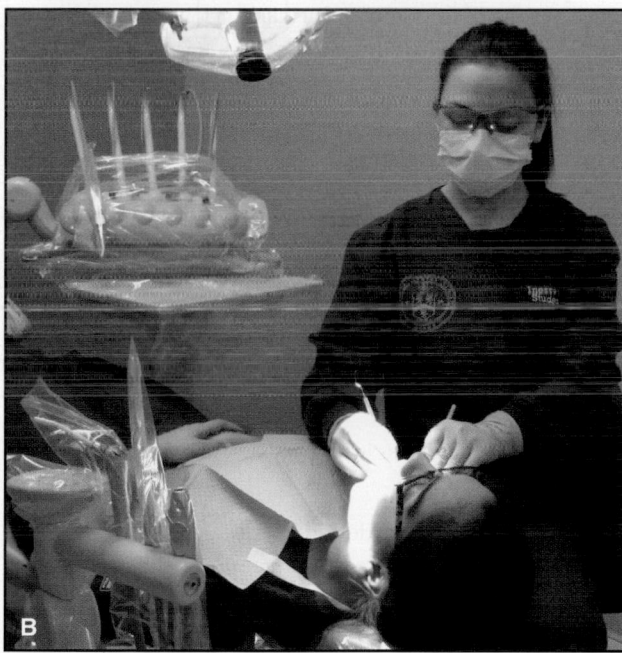

FIGURE 1-1 **There is more difference than just a uniform,** but over time the dental hygienist's commitment to safe and effective patient care remains. **A:** The dental hygienist providing patient care in the 1930s dressed in a starched white uniform and cap (as nurses also did) to indicate their commitment to cleanliness and good care. **B:** The dental hygienist of today protects self and patient from cross-infection by donning personal protective equipment (PPE) and surface barriers during patient care.

SCOPE OF DENTAL HYGIENE PRACTICE

▶ In the first textbook for dental hygienists, Dr. Alfred C. Fones, the "father of dental hygiene," emphasized education as the most important role in the practice of dental hygiene. He wrote:

> *It is primarily to this important work of public education that the dental hygienist is called. She must regard herself as the channel through which dentistry's knowledge of mouth hygiene is to be disseminated. The greatest service she can perform is the persistent education of the public in mouth hygiene and the allied branches of general hygiene.*[3]

▶ While the role of education is still primary, dental hygiene has changed and the scope of practice has developed and broadened from Dr. Fones' original concept.

I. Roles of the Dental Hygienist

▶ Various roles of licensed dental hygienists include the following:
  • Education
  • Assessment
  • Diagnosis
  • Prevention
  • Therapy
  • Research
  • Administration.

▶ Dental hygienists support oral health through their work in many settings including:
  • General and specialty dental practices.
  • Public health programs.
  • Research centers.
  • Professional education institutions.
  • Hospital and residential care facilities.
  • Federal programs, including the armed services.
  • The dental corporate industries.

▶ Within the wide span of dental hygiene practice areas, dental hygienists may serve in a variety of capacities.

▶ Areas of responsibility in this variety of roles are defined in Table 1-1.[4]

II. Supervision and Scope of Practice

▶ The professional dental hygienist is responsible to provide only those services allowed within the scope of practice outlined within the Dental Hygiene Practice Act of each state.[5]

▶ The type of supervision by a dentist required for delivery of dental hygiene services is also determined by individual practice acts in each state.

▶ Types of supervision commonly used for dental hygiene practice are defined in Box 1-3.[6–8]

▶ Many states have enacted collaborative practice legislative initiatives and adopted practice rules that allow dental hygienists to provide care autonomously for underserved populations in specifically designated public health settings.[9,10]

III. Types of Clinical Services

The clinical responsibilities of the dental hygienist are divided into preventive, educational, and therapeutic

TABLE 1-1	Professional Roles of the Dental Hygienist	
ROLE	**DESCRIPTION**	**EXAMPLE EMPLOYMENT SETTINGS AND POSITIONS**
Clinician	Provide direct patient care in collaboration with other health professionals	■ Private dental practices and community-based clinics ■ Hospitals and long-term care facilities ■ Schools
Corporate	Employment in a company that supports oral health through promotion of oral health products and services	■ Product sales and research ■ Corporate educator or administrator

Public health	Enhance access to care in community health programs funded by government or nonprofit organizations	■ Clinician in:
		  • Community clinics
		  • Government health service
		  • School sealant programs
		■ Oral health program administrator

Researcher	Conduct studies to test new procedures, products, or theories for accuracy and effectiveness	■ Universities ■ Corporations ■ Government agencies
Educator	Use educational theory and methodology to educate competent oral health professionals or provide continuing education for licensed providers	■ Dental hygiene program clinical or classroom instruction ■ Corporate educator
Administrator	Apply organizational skills, communicate objectives, identify and manage resources, evaluate and modify health or education programs	■ Program director in clinical, educational or corporate settings
Entrepreneur	Initiate or finance new oral health-related enterprises	■ Practice management or product development ■ Consulting ■ Independent clinical practice ■ Professional speaker or writer

Source: American Dental Hygienists' Association. Education and career: career paths. http://www.adha.org/ professional-roles. Accessed January 19, 2015.

services. Clinical and educational activities are inseparable and overlap as patient care is planned and accomplished.

▶ *Preventive services* are the methods employed by the clinician and/or patient to promote and maintain oral health.
  • Prevention is an essential component of dental hygiene practice.
  • The three categories of preventive services are defined in Box 1-4.
▶ *Educational services* are strategies developed for an individual or a group to elicit behaviors directed toward health.
  • Educational aspects of dental hygiene service permeate the entire patient care system.
  • The patient's understanding of dental hygiene procedures and personal oral care affects the success of both preventive and therapeutic services.
▶ *Therapeutic services* are clinical treatments designed to arrest or control disease and maintain oral tissues in health.
  • Dental hygiene treatment services are an integral part of the patient's overall treatment plan.

  • Scaling and root debridement, along with the steps in posttreatment care, are parts of the therapeutic phase in the treatment of periodontal infections.

IV. Patient Education

▶ Clinical services, both dental and dental hygiene, have limited long-range probability of success if the patient does not understand the need for cooperation in daily procedures of personal care and diet and for regular appointments for professional care.
▶ Educational and clinical services, therefore, are mutually dependent and inseparable in the total dental hygiene care of the patient.
▶ Scientific information about the prevention of oral diseases has been advancing steadily.
▶ The public has become increasingly aware of the need for dental hygiene care and the value of oral health instruction provided by the dental hygienist.

V. Dental Hygiene Specialties

▶ Entry-level dental hygiene programs prepare students for basic clinical dental hygiene practice.[11]

▶ Continuing education can help build skills in advanced periodontal instrumentation.

▶ Private practice orthodontics, pediatric dentistry, and periodontics clinics particularly value dental hygienists as partners in prevention.

▶ Some educational institutions offer dental hygiene bachelor's degree or degree completion programs.

▶ Bachelor and advanced degrees enhance the ability of dental hygienists to pursue opportunities outside of clinical practice.[11]

▶ Dental hygienists earn masters or doctoral degrees in a variety of sciences as well as:
  • Dental hygiene education.
  • Health behavior and education.
  • Public health and health policy.
  • Nutrition and dietetics.
  • Business and administration.
  • Law.

▶ A dental hygienist interested in specialty areas of practice can take advantage of many learning opportunities to enhance knowledge and skills.

▶ Many continuing education opportunities exist for learning in all areas of dental hygiene practice.

▶ In other special areas, short-term courses have been developed, such as instruction in the care of patients with disabilities.

▶ In-service training may be available in long-term care institutions, hospitals, and skilled nursing facilities.

▶ Other dental hygienists have learned to practice in a specialty through private study, special conferences, and personal experience.

VI. Alternative Practice Settings

▶ In 2014, 37 states allow dental hygienists to provide direct access care (Figure 1-2) in a variety of community settings including, but not limited to:[12]
  • Schools
  • Public health settings
  • Headstart settings
  • Nursing home facilities
  • Free clinics
  • Community centers.

▶ *Direct access* means the dental hygienist can treatment plan and initiate treatment based on patient assessment without specific authorization of the dentist.[12]
  • Each state practice act varies as to the scope of practice and level of supervision by a dentist.

▶ Dental hygiene care in alternative practice settings is further described in Chapter 58.

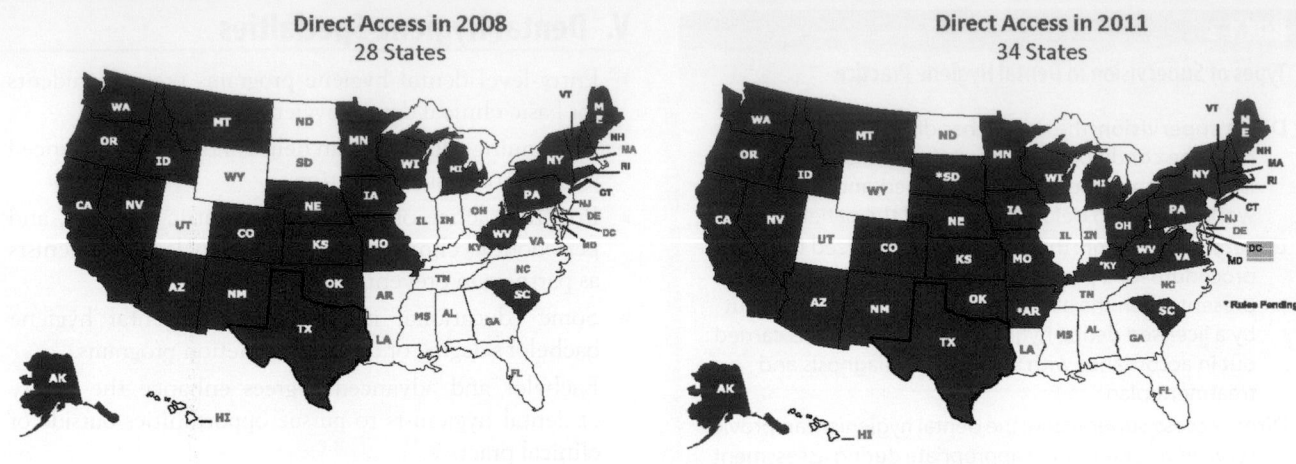

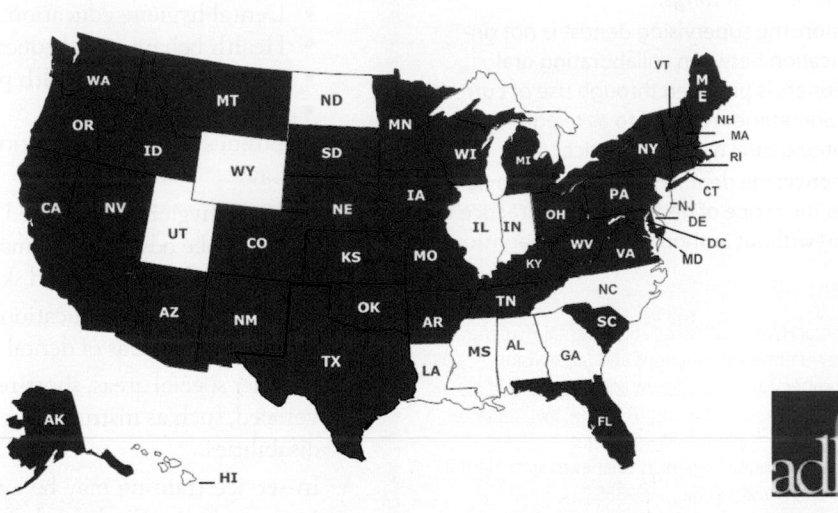

FIGURE 1-2 ADHA Direct Access. Maps of the United States to show the changes in the number of and location of states with Direct Access since 2008.

VII. Advanced Practice Dental Hygiene

▶ The current dental care model leaves many low-income individuals, at-risk populations, and those living in rural areas and inner cities without access to dental care.

▶ A number of mid-level dental provider models with a variety of names have emerged to address basic restorative and preventive care, particularly to children and in some states/countries to adults.

- Internationally, the dental therapist was first introduced in 1921 in New Zealand and is found in 53 countries.[13]

- In 1949, Forsyth Dental Infirmary began an experiment to train New Zealand-type dental nurses, but it was stopped because of pressure from the American Dental Association.[14]

- In 1971–1972, the Forsyth Experiment (more commonly known as the Rotunda Experiment) began training dental hygienists in basic restorative dentistry and local anesthesia.[15]

- From 1971 to 1976, University of Iowa and University of Kentucky both trained dental hygienists with advanced skills in restorative dentistry.[16]

- A Dental Health Aide Therapist (DHAT) was introduced in Tribal villages in Alaska in 2006.[17]

A. Advanced Dental Hygiene Practitioner or Advanced Dental Therapist

▶ A 2009 PEW Report[13] first recognized that creating new mid-level oral health care providers, such as the Advanced Dental Hygiene Practitioner (ADHP) proposed by the American Dental Hygienists' Association could enhance access to oral health services for underserved populations.

▶ In 2009, the state of Minnesota approved the development of the master's-level degree program for advanced dental therapists (ADT), which requires applicants to be licensed dental hygienists holding a bachelor's degree.[18–20]

▶ These providers are dual licensed as a dental hygienist and dental therapist in Minnesota to provide preventive and basic restorative dental services:
- Directly to underserved populations.[18–20]
- Via a collaborative management agreement with a supervising dentist.[18–20]

▶ Research regarding the safety and efficacy of mid-level dental providers is ongoing.[21–23]

▶ Currently, a variety of oral health stakeholder groups in many states are exploring proposals to create new workforce models that will increase access to quality oral health care for all individuals.[24–26]

▶ The Commission on Dental Accreditation has developed accreditation standards for dental therapy programs.[27]

B. Clinical Role of the Advanced Dental Therapist

▶ In addition to the traditional process of care performed by dental hygienist, the dental therapist has the following scope of practice[27]:
- Caries removal, placement, and finishing of composite/resin and amalgam restorations.
- Placement of space maintainers.
- Fabrication and placement of stainless steel crowns and temporary crowns.
- Pulpotomy.
- Pulp vitality testing.
- Simple extractions of erupted primary teeth.
- Other duties may be specified in the state's scope of practice.

▶ ADT practice under a collaborative agreement with a dentist and patients who need more advanced care are referred.

C. Impact of Advanced Dental Therapist

▶ The first dental therapists graduated in Minnesota in 2011.

▶ Initial impacts of this provider as part of the dental team include the following:[18]
- An increase in the number of patients served in mobile dental clinics, and community health centers, particularly the underserved and special populations.
- Reduction in waiting times for patients to receive services.
- Decreased travel time for patients because preventive and restorative care can be provided during the same appointment.
- Possible reduction in emergency room use for dental care.
- Increased productivity of the dental team.
- Improved patient satisfaction.

BOX 1-5

Four Competency Domains for Interprofessional Collaborative Practice

Values/Ethics for Interprofessional Practice: personal values and ethics that:
▷ Are patient centered with a community orientation.
▷ Grounded in a sense of shared purpose to support good health.
▷ Reflect a shared commitment to safe, efficient, effective systems of care.

Roles/Responsibilities: an understanding of how professional roles and responsibilities complement each other in delivering patient-centered care.

Interprofessional Communication: ability and openness to express:
▷ Knowledge and appreciation of the role and value of other health professions.
▷ Willingness to work together and share expertise across professional lines.

Teams and Teamwork: learning to:
▷ Become a part of a small complex system organized to share care that contributes to positive health outcomes.
▷ Share expertise, functioning, and accountability.
▷ Relinquish some professional autonomy to share decision making.

Source: The Interprofessional Education Collaborative Expert Panel. *Core Competencies for Interprofessional Collaborative Practice.* Washington, DC: Interprofessional Education Collaborative; 2011. http://www.aacn.nche.edu/education-resources/IPEC Report.pdf. Accessed January 19, 2014.

VIII. Interprofessional Collaborative Patient Care

▶ In many situations, dental hygienists provide clinical patient care as a member of a dental team.

▶ In a growing number of facilities, dental hygienists provide care in collaboration with an interprofessional team of healthcare providers to meet the needs of patients with complex medical problems.

▶ Four competency domains necessary for participating in interprofessional collaborative practice, developed by a group of medical and dental professional associations, are explained in Box 1-5.[28]

IX. Advocacy for Oral Health

▶ The professional dental hygienist is an active advocate for oral health in both personal and professional situations.

- The dental hygienist who is an advocate for oral health:
  - Influences legislators, health agencies, and other organizations to bring available resources together to improve access to care.
  - Analyzes barriers to change and helps develop mechanisms to effect change.
  - Implements and evaluates health policy and programs that promote health for individuals, families, or communities.
  - Promotes lifestyle changes that contribute to oral health.
- Examples of oral health advocacy activities include:
  - Joining other dental hygiene professionals to meet with legislators and public officials to encourage the inclusion of dental services in healthcare legislation.
  - Making public statements that support the oral health value of optimal fluoridation in community water systems when a community is considering defluoridation.

OBJECTIVES FOR PROFESSIONAL PRACTICE

I. Overall Goals

- Overall professional goals of the dental hygiene profession relate to health promotion and disease prevention.
- The goal of each dental hygienist is *to aid individuals and groups in attaining and maintaining optimum oral health*. Other professional objectives are related to this primary goal.
- A dental hygienist's self-assessment is essential to attain goals of perfection for service to each patient and community.
- Personal and professional goals are outlined and reviewed frequently in a plan for continued self-improvement.

II. Personal Goals

- Exemplify the highest degree of professional ethics and conduct.
- Demonstrate interpersonal relationships that assure oral health information is presented effectively.
- Apply a continuing process of self-evaluation throughout professional life.
- Recognize the need for lifelong learning to acquire updated knowledge through reading professional literature and enrolling in continuing education programs.
- Maintain membership and participate actively in the local, national, and international dental hygiene professional associations.

III. Clinical Practice Goals

- Apply evidence-based knowledge and understanding of the basic and clinical sciences to:
  - Recognition of oral conditions.
  - Prevention of oral diseases.
  - Clinical and instructional procedures.
- Recognize each patient as an individual and adapt clinical procedures, care planning, and interventions accordingly.
- Plan and carry out effectively the dental hygiene interventions essential to the total care program for each individual patient.
- Identify and care for the needs of patients who have unusual general health problems that affect dental hygiene procedures and instructions.
- Provide a complete and personalized instructional service to help each patient become motivated toward changes in oral health behavioral practices.
- Practice safe and efficient clinical routines for the application of standard precautions for infection control.

STANDARDS FOR CLINICAL DENTAL HYGIENE PRACTICE

- The primary purpose of standards for clinical practice is to guide dental hygiene practitioners in the development of a clinical relationship with their patients.[29]
- A secondary purpose is to educate the public, other healthcare providers, and policy makers about the profession of dental hygiene and the scope of dental hygiene practice.
- The six components of the dental hygiene process of care provide:
  - The foundation for clinical decision making and dental hygiene practice.
  - The framework for organizing the sections in this book.

DENTAL HYGIENE PROCESS OF CARE

- The dental hygiene process of care includes assessment, dental hygiene diagnosis, planning, implementation, evaluation, and documentation as illustrated in Figure 1-3.[29,30]
- The procedures of evaluation and documentation are integrated within each of the other components in the process.
- As a process, the procedures performed are continual in nature and may overlap or occur simultaneously.

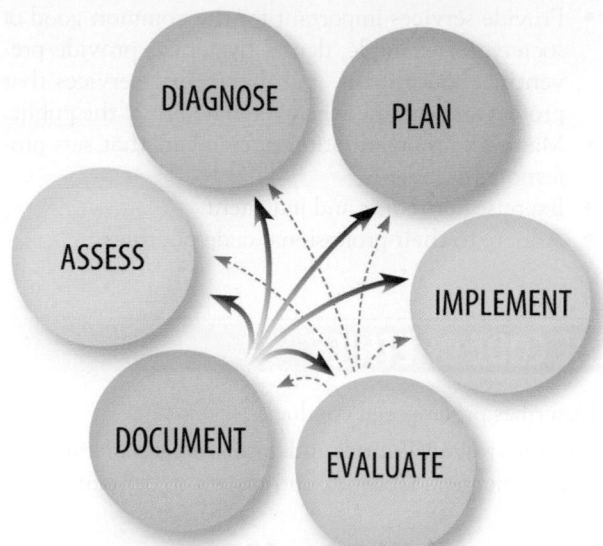

FIGURE 1-3 **The Six Interrelated Components of the Dental Hygiene Process of Care.** The steps in the process are followed one after another in a cycle, beginning with assessment. Evaluation and documentation are each linked to all of the other steps.

I. Purposes of the Dental Hygiene Process of Care

▶ To provide a framework within which individualized needs of a patient can be met.

▶ To identify the causative and risk factors of a condition that can be reduced, eliminated, or prevented through dental hygiene interventions.

II. Assessment

▶ The assessment phase is the first component of the dental hygiene process.

▶ This phase provides a foundation for patient care by collecting both subjective and objective data.

▶ Chapters 10–23 in this textbook are devoted to the assessment component of the dental hygiene process of care.

III. Dental Hygiene Diagnosis

▶ Dental hygiene diagnostic statements:
  • Employ the use of critical thinking to interpret assessment data, as indicated in Box 1-6.
  • Identify the health behaviors of each patient as well as the actual or potential oral health problems that dental hygienists are licensed to treat.
  • Provide the basis on which the dental hygiene care plan is designed, implemented, and evaluated.
  • Justify the treatment proposed to the patient.
  • Challenge the dental hygienist to assume responsibility for patient care and to move beyond a rote system of clinical practice.

▶ Sample dental hygiene diagnoses are provided in Box 1-7.

▶ Chapter 24, section on Dental Hygiene Diagnosis, provides more information.

IV. The Dental Hygiene Care Plan

▶ Dental hygiene care planning is the selection of strategies and interventions that meet the needs of the patient in attaining oral health.

▶ The dental hygiene care plan is presented:
  • To the dentist for integration with the comprehensive dental care plan.
  • To the patient to develop understanding of the interventions needed and appointment requirements.
  • To the patient to obtain informed consent for treatment.

▶ Chapters 24 and 25 describe care planning and provide a template for the development of a written dental hygiene care plan.

V. Implementation

▶ The implementation phase in the dental hygiene process of care is the activation of the care plan.

▶ Further discussion of the concepts and procedures associated with implementation of dental hygiene preventive and treatment interventions is presented in Chapters 26–46.

VI. Evaluation

▶ The evaluation phase determines whether the patient needs to be retreated, referred, or placed on a continuing care schedule.

▶ Evaluation of dental hygiene care is detailed in Chapter 47.

▶ Development of continuing care protocols is described in Chapter 48.

VII. Documentation

▶ The documentation of dental hygiene care:
  • Details all assessment data, diagnosis, care plan, treatments, patient education, and evaluation in a condensed, consistent format.
  • Represents a chronologic history of the patient's total care.

▶ Details for documentation are described in Chapter 9 and examples of documentation for a variety of dental hygiene interventions can be found at the end of each chapter.

DENTAL HYGIENE ETHICS

▶ The ethics of a profession provide the general standards of right and wrong that guide the behavior of the members in that profession.

▶ Key words relating to ethics and ethical principles are defined in Box 1-8.

▶ The members of a profession
  • Have extensive specialized education.
  • Possess an intellectual body of knowledge from study and research.

• Provide services important for the common good of society, for example, dental hygienists provide preventive, educational, and therapeutic services that protect and enhance the overall health of the public.
• Maintain an organization of members that sets professional standards.
• Exercise autonomy and judgment.
• Adhere to their professional code of ethics.

THE CODE OF ETHICS

▶ Describes professional conduct.
▶ Outlines responsibilities and duties of each member toward patients, colleagues, and society in general.

I. Purposes of the Code of Ethics

▶ To increase the awareness of, and sensitivity to, ethical situations in practice.
▶ To define a standard of conduct that will give each individual a strong sense of ethical consciousness in professional practice as well as in all phases of life.

II. Dental Hygiene Codes

▶ The Codes of the American Dental Hygienists' Association, the National Dental Hygienists' Association, the Canadian Dental Hygienists' Association, and the International Federation of Dental Hygienists can be read in Appendices I–IV at the end of this book.
▶ Each dental hygienist is responsible for the study and application of the codes of the particular associations in which memberships are held.

CORE VALUES

"Core values" are selected principles of ethical behavior that can be considered as the heart of the code of a profession.

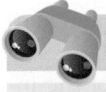

BOX 1-8	**KEY WORDS:** Ethics

Core values: basic values of a profession; guide to choices or actions by implying a preference for what is deemed to be acceptable in the profession.

Ethical dilemma: a problem that involves two morally correct choices or courses of action. There may not be a single answer and, depending on the choice, the outcomes can differ.

Ethical issue: a common problem wherein a solution is readily grounded in the governing practice act, recognized laws, or acceptable standards of care. Decisions involving ethical issues are generally more clearly defined than are dilemmas.

Ethics: a sense of moral obligation; a system of moral principles that governs the conduct of a professional group, planned by them for the common good of people; principles of morality.

Moral: a principle or habit with respect to right or wrong behavior.

Rights: expectations by the patient that correlate with the duties of a professional person when providing care.

Virtue: character trait; one must intend to act virtuously as a professional. Examples include honesty, compassion, care, and wisdom.

BOX 1-9

Core Values in Professional Dental Hygiene Practice

Individual Autonomy and Respect for Human Beings: the right to informed consent and respect for self-determination by persons with the ability to make a choice or decision. Autonomy exists for both the dental hygienist and the patient.

Confidentiality: the right of patients to privacy and the duty of dental hygienists to protect privileged communication.

Societal trust: maintaining a bond of trust in the relationships between the dental hygienist and patients, other professional persons, and the public.

Nonmaleficence: avoidance of harm to others; a core value.

Beneficence: the act of doing good.

Justice/fairness: fair treatment according to an equitable distribution of benefits and burdens; impartiality.

Veracity: a duty to tell the truth when information is disclosed to patients about treatment.

Source: American Dental Hygienists' Association. Bylaws and Code of Ethics. Chicago, Il :ADHA; Adopted June 23, 2014. http://www.adha.org/resources-docs/7611_Bylaws_and_Code_of_Ethics.pdf. Accessed April 6, 2015.

I. Core Values in Professional Practice

▶ The core values of the profession of dental hygiene are listed and defined in Box 1-9 and in the American Dental Hygienists' Association Code of Ethics (in Appendix I).

II. Personal Values

▶ Value development begins at an early age and is influenced by familial, social, and economic factors.

▶ Life experiences, grounded in previous successes and failures, serve as a foundation for professional virtues.

▶ Members of a health profession can benefit from periodic self-assessment of individual values, attitudes, and responsibilities.

III. The Patient First

▶ The responsibility to put the patient first is foremost.

▶ Dental hygienists are ethically, morally, and legally responsible to provide oral care for all patients without discrimination.

▶ Ethical decision making and professional behavior are reflected in every aspect of dental hygiene practice.

IV. Lifelong Learning: An Ethical Duty

▶ To ensure optimal care for each patient.

▶ To maintain competency.

▶ To learn scientific advances from new research.

▶ To provide evidence-based patient care.

▶ To apply consistent ethical reasoning.

▶ To ensure fulfillment of each patient's rights.

ETHICAL APPLICATIONS

A dental hygienist may be involved in a variety of moral, ethical, and legal situations as part of the daily routine. In ethics, a problem situation is considered either an *ethical issue* or an *ethical dilemma*.

I. Ethical Issue

▶ More clearly defined than a dilemma.

▶ A common problem wherein a solution is grounded in the governing practice act, recognized laws, or accepted standards of care based on the standard rules of practice.

II. Ethical Dilemma

▶ A problem that may involve two morally correct choices or courses of action.

▶ May not have a single answer and, depending on the choice, the outcomes can differ.

▶ To resolve a dilemma, the facts are gathered, ethical principles and theories are applied, and options are explored.

III. Steps in the Resolution of an Issue or a Dilemma

Four steps that can be used by the professional dental hygienist to resolve an ethical issue or dilemma in dental hygiene practice are presented in Box 1-10.

IV. Summary: The Final Decision

▶ Many factors can be used to solve a dilemma.

▶ All dental healthcare providers involved in the decision process can participate in a follow-up evaluation of the action taken.

▶ Questions to ask once a decision has been made, include:
  • Is the decision/action that is selected morally defensible?
  • Can the choice to solve the dilemma be defended?

▶ A professional dental hygienist may need to defend it to the patient, the dentist, members of the dental team, a state board, or even a court of law.

▶ Most importantly, the decision must be defensible based on standards of practice established for the dental hygiene profession.

BOX 1-10

Steps in the Resolution of an Ethical Issue or Dilemma

▷ Step 1 Dental Hygiene Situation
  ▷ Is this situation an ethical issue or a dilemma?
  ▷ What is the chief concern/problem?
  ▷ Summarize the history of the situation.
  ▷ List all the facts from all the people involved.
▷ Step 2 Individual Preferences
  ▷ What are the rights of the individuals involved?
  ▷ In a clinical case: has informed consent been obtained?
▷ Step 3 Choices *versus* Alternatives
  ▷ Which core values apply to this case?
  ▷ Describe the realistic alternatives that exist.
  ▷ Explain the benefits and disadvantages of all possible outcomes.
▷ Step 4 Case Parameters
  ▷ Does the "scope of practice" apply to the situation? If so, explain.
  ▷ What financial, legal, or cultural factors need consideration?
  ▷ Compare the anticipated action with acceptable professional standards.
  ▷ Is there a conflict of interest between the patient, dental providers, or other individuals?
  ▷ Is there a need for an outside source to be consulted?

V. Applications: Everyday Ethics

▶ Various ethical issues and dilemmas are presented throughout this book for discussion and consideration.

▶ The examples are found in special boxes called "Everyday Ethics" and usually appear at the end of the chapter where the problem may apply.

LEGAL FACTORS IN PRACTICE

▶ The law must be studied and respected by each dental hygienist practicing within the state, province, or country.

▶ Although the various practice acts have certain basic similarities, differences in scope and definition exist.

▶ Terminology varies, but each practice act regulates the patient services that may be delivered by the licensed dental hygienist. Changes to the practice act may be made from time to time.

▶ A frequent review of the practice acts and/or regulations will keep the dental health professional up to date.

PERSONAL FACTORS IN PRACTICE

▶ Each dental hygienist represents the entire profession to the patient or community.

▶ The dental hygienist's expressed or demonstrated attitudes toward dentistry, dental hygiene, and other health professions, as well as toward health services and preventive measures, will affect the subsequent attitude of the patient toward other dental hygienists and dental hygiene care in general.

▶ Members of health professions who exemplify the traits they hold as objectives for others enhance probability of positive response and cooperation from their patients.

▶ Many personal factors of general physical health, oral health, cleanliness, appearance, and mental health are to be considered. A few of these are included here.

▶ *General physical health*: Optimum physical health depends to a great extent on:
  • Well-planned, healthy diet, sufficient amount of sleep, adequate amount of recreation and exercise.
  • Routine examinations at least annually, including tests for hearing, sight, and certain communicable diseases.
  • Immunizations recommended for healthcare providers are listed in the Personal Protection for the Dental Team section of Chapter 5.

▶ *Oral health*: The maintenance of a clean, healthy mouth demonstrates by example that the dental hygienist follows the teachings of the dental and dental hygiene professions relative to prevention and control of oral disease.

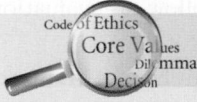 **EVERYDAY ETHICS**

The first term of the dental hygiene curriculum has just finished. The instructor asks for student volunteers to help at the college's health fair to provide basic routine brushing and flossing instructions for people who stop at the dental hygiene information table. Three students, Alice, Annette, and Josephine, sign up to volunteer for this community service. The day before the health fair, which takes place on a Saturday, Annette is asked to work in the dental office where she is employed part-time. Since she really needs the money, she decides not to attend

the health fair and instead goes to work without telling anyone.

Questions for Consideration

1. In general, would this situation be described as a professional issue or an ethical dilemma? Explain.

2. Discuss Annette's actions in terms of the core ethical values.

3. What aspects of the dental hygiene code of ethics can support her student colleague's choice of action?

▶ *Mental health*: The mental health of the dental hygienist is reflected in interpersonal relationships and the ability to inspire confidence through a display of professional and emotional maturity. Participation in professional and community activities can contribute to optimum mental health.

Factors To Teach The Patient

▷ The role of the dental hygienist as a cotherapist with each patient, with the dentist, and with members of other health professions.

▷ The moral and ethical nature of becoming a dental hygiene professional.

▷ The scope of service of the dental hygienist as defined by various practice acts.

▷ The interrelationship of instructional and clinical services in dental hygiene patient care.

▷ The patient's potential state of oral health and how it can be improved and maintained.

References

1. American Dental Hygienists' Association. *Policy Manual.* Chicago, IL: ADHA. https://www.adha.org/resources-docs/7614_Policy_Manual.pdf. Updated October 17, 2014. Accessed January 19, 2015.

2. American Dental Hygienists' Association. *100: Celebrating a Century of Professional Pride.* Chicago, IL: ADHA; 2013:48.

3. Fones AC, ed. *Mouth Hygiene.* 4th ed. Philadelphia, PA: Lea & Febiger; 1934:248.

4. American Dental Hygienists' Association. Education and career: career paths. http://www.adha.org/professional-roles. Accessed January 19, 2015.

5. American Dental Hygienists' Association. Advocacy: scope of practice. http://www.adha.org/scope-of-practice. Accessed January 19, 2015.

6. American Dental Hygienists' Association. Dental hygiene practice acts overview: permitted functions and supervision levels by state. 2013. http://www.adha.org/resources-docs/7511_Permitted_Services_Supervision_Levels_by_State.pdf. Accessed January 19, 2015.

7. Catlett A. A comparison of dental hygienists' salaries to state dental supervision levels. *J Dent Hyg.* 2014;88(6):380–385.

8. Summerfelt FF. Teledentistry-assisted, affiliated practice for dental hygienists: an innovative oral health workforce model. *J Dent Educ.* 2011;75(6):733–742.

9. American Dental Hygienists' Association. Stateline. http://www.adha.org/stateline. Accessed January 19, 2015.

10. American Dental Hygienists' Association. Advocacy: direct access. http://www.adha.org/direct-access. Accessed January 19, 2015.

11. Battrell A, Lynch A, Steinbach P, et al. Advancing education in dental hygiene. *J Evid Based Dent Pract.* 2014;14, Suppl:209–221.

12. American Dental Hygienists' Association. Direct Access States. 2014. http://www.adha.org/resources. Accessed February 4, 2015.

13. PEW Center on the States, National Academy for State Health Policy, WK Kellogg Foundation. *Help Wanted: A Policy Maker's Guide to New Dental Providers.* Washington, DC; 2009. http://www.pewtrusts.org/~/media/legacy/uploadedfiles/pcs_assets/2009/DentalReportHelpWantedpdf.pdf. Accessed April 4, 2015.

14. American Dental Association. Massachusetts dental nurse bill rescinded. *J Am Dent Assoc.* 1950;41:371.

15. Lobene RR. *The Forsyth Experiment: An Alternative System for Dental Care.* Cambridge, MA: Harvard University Press; 1979.

16. Nash DA, Nagel RJ. Confronting oral health disparities among American Indian/Alaska Native children: the pediatric oral health therapist. *Am J Public Health.* 2005;95(8):1325–1329.

17. Evaluation of the dental health aid therapist workforce model in Alaska. WK Kellogg Foundation, Rasmussen Foundation, Bethel Community Services Foundation. https://www.rti.org/pubs/alaskadhatprogramevaluationfinal102510.pdf. Accessed February 4, 2015.

18. Early impacts of dental therapists in Minnesota. Minnesota Department of Health, Minnesota Board of Dentistry. http://www.health.state.mn.us/divs/orhpc/workforce/dt/dtlegisrpt.pdf. Accessed February 1, 2015.

19. Gwozdek AE, Tetrick R, Shaefer HL. The origins of Minnesota's mid-level dental practitioner: alignment of problem, political and policy streams. *J Dent Hyg.* 2014;88(5):292–301.

20. American Dental Hygienists' Association. *The History of Introducing a New Provider in Minnesota.* Chicago, IL: American Dental Hygienists' Association; 2009:2. https://www.adha.org/resources-docs/75113_Minnesota_Story.pdf. Accessed January 19, 2015.

21. Mathu-Muju KR. Dental therapists provide technically competent clinical care when performing irreversible restorative procedures. *J Evid Based Dent Pract.* 2014;14(1):25–27.

22. Phillips E, Shaefer HL. Dental therapists: evidence of technical competence. *J Dent Res.* 2013;92(7, Suppl):11S–5S.

23. Bailit HL, Beazoglou TJ, DeVitto J, et al. Impact of dental therapists on productivity and finances: I. Literature review. *J Dent Educ.* 2012;76(8):1061–1067.

24. PEW Charitable Trusts. *Expanding the Dental Team: Increasing Access to Care in Public Settings.* Philadelphia, PA: PEW Charitable Trusts; 2014. http://www.pewtrusts.org/~/media/Assets/2014/06/27/Expanding_Dental_Case_Studies_Report.pdf. Accessed January 19, 2015.

25. American Association of Public Health Dentistry. Special issue: workforce development in dentistry: addressing access to care. *J Public Health Dent.* 2011;71 (Suppl 2):S1–S41.

26. Institute of Medicine. Board on Healthcare Services. *The U.S. Oral Health Workforce in the Coming Decade: Workshop Summary.* Washington, DC: National Academic Press; 2009. http://www.iom.edu/Reports/2009/OralHealthWorkforce.aspx. Accessed January 19, 2015.

27. Commission on Dental Accreditation. *Accreditation Standards for Dental Therapy Education Programs.* Chicago, IL: ADA; 2014. http://www.ada.org/~/media/CODA/apx7_proposed_dentaltherapy.ashx. Accessed February 2, 2015.

28. The Interprofessional Education Collaborative Expert Panel. *Core Competencies for Interprofessional Collaborative Practice*. Washington, DC: Interprofessional Education Collaborative; 2011. http://www.aacn.nche.edu/education-resources/IPECReport.pdf. Accessed January 19, 2014.

29. American Dental Hygienists' Association. *Standards for Clinical Dental Hygiene Practice*. Chicago, IL: ADHA; 2008. http://www.adha.org/resources-docs/7261_Standards_Clinical_Practice.pdf. Updated September, 2014. Accessed January 19, 2015.

30. Mueller-Joseph L, Petersen M. *Dental Hygiene Process: Diagnosis and Care Planning*. Albany, NY: Delmar; 1995:9–14.

ENHANCE YOUR UNDERSTANDING

thePoint® DIGITAL CONNECTIONS
(see the inside front cover for access information)
- **Audio glossary**
- **Quiz bank**

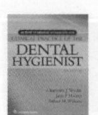

SUPPORT FOR LEARNING
(available separately; visit lww.com)
- *Active Learning Workbook for Clinical Practice of the Dental Hygienist, 12th Edition*

prepU INDIVIDUALIZED REVIEW
(available separately; visit lww.com)
- **Adaptive quizzing with *prepU for Wilkins' Clinical Practice of the Dental Hygienist***

Evidence-Based Dental Hygiene Practice

Charlotte J. Wyche, RDH, MS and Judi S. Luxmore, RDH, BAS, MS

CHAPTER OUTLINE

EVIDENCE-BASED PRACTICE
- I. Definition
- II. Purpose
- III. Need for Evidence-Based Practice
- IV. Evidence-Based Decision Making Process
- V. Skills Needed for Evidence-Based Dental Hygiene Practice

A SYSTEMATIC APPROACH
- I. Determine Clinical Issue
- II. Develop Researchable Question
- III. Search for Evidence
- IV. Analyze Evidence
- V. Apply Evidence
- VI. Evaluate Results

READING AND UNDERSTANDING RESEARCH
- I. Publication Types
- II. Research Approaches
- III. Research Types
- IV. Levels of Evidence

INTERNET-BASED HEALTH INFORMATION
- I. Computer/Internet Literacy
- II. Content Analysis

ETHICS IN RESEARCH
- I. Ethical Standards
- II. Ethical Research Involving Human Subjects
- III. Informed Consent for Research
- IV. Institutional Review Board

DOCUMENTATION

EVERYDAY ETHICS

FACTORS TO TEACH THE PATIENT

REFERENCES

LEARNING OBJECTIVES

After studying this chapter, the student will be able to:

1. Explain evidence-based dental hygiene practice and identify the skills needed to practice evidence-based dental hygiene care.

2. Discuss research approaches and connect research types to the strength of evidence each provides.

3. Describe a systematic approach to finding science-based information.

4. Describe skills needed for analyzing Internet-based health information.

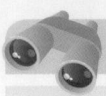

BOX 2-1   KEY WORDS: Evidence-Based Dental Hygiene Practice

Best practice: approach or intervention that has consistently shown results (outcomes) superior to those achieved with other means; used as a benchmark based on repeatable research over time on large diverse groups of people.

Biomedical database: organized collection of medically related journal articles, systematic reviews, research reports, theses, and/or dissertations typically in digital form.

Clinical significance: practical or observed difference expected in patient care outcomes following a clinical intervention; in research, a clinically observable difference rather than statistical difference.

Descriptive statistics: use of numbers to describe the main features or characteristics of a particular person, event, or group, determine the frequency with which something occurs, or categorize information.

Evidence: source of information used to support, determine, or demonstrate the truth of a statement.

Evidence-based dental hygiene (EBDH) practice: a scientific, research-supported approach to decide dental hygiene interventions for each patient.

Inferential statistics: numerical data designed to allow generalization from a sample to a population.

Levels of evidence: hierarchy for making clinical judgments for patient care based on types of research studies.

Medical subject headings (MeSH): National Library of Medicine (NLM)-controlled vocabulary; descriptors used to index articles in the MEDLINE database.

Outcome: end result that follows from an action.

Peer review: review of a journal article by a panel of experts prior to publication.

Reference citation: a number or other notation in the text of a manuscript that refers to the source of the information listed in a reference list.

Reliability: the ability of a measurement instrument or test to get the same results repeatedly.

Scientific evidence: Evidence repeatedly tested through research with valid and reliable methods.

Search engine: a computer program that uses key words or terms to locate documents or data from the World Wide Web or other Internet databases.

Statistical significance: identifies the extent to which the results are not due to chance; indicated in research by the "*p*-value" notation.

Tutorial: a method of transferring knowledge or instructions needed to complete a specific task, using an individual or small group interactive-type learning setting that seeks to teach by example; online tutorials are available on a variety of topics.

Validity: ability to measure what was intended.

Variable: factors in a research study that can be manipulated and measured.

    Independent (intervention) variable: treatment manipulated during the conduct of a study to produce an effect on the dependent variable, for example, type of toothbrush.

    Dependent (outcome) variable: patient factor on which manipulation of the treatment can have an effect—e.g., the amount of biofilm on a tooth following tooth brushing.

The main goal of clinical dental hygiene practice is to improve and maintain the oral health of the patient. Clinical questions and/or problems that arise on a daily basis require current and reliable information to identify best-practice treatment interventions and oral self-care recommendations that will improve the patient's health.

▶ The concepts of evidence-based practice will assist dental hygienists in formulating a plan for objective, effective, and scientifically sound interventions that meet patient needs and assure positive health outcomes.

▶ Key words related to evidence-based practice and research are found in Box 2-1.

EVIDENCE-BASED PRACTICE

I. Definition

▶ A formalized approach to clinical care in which the clinician, in consultation with the patient, uses the best scientific evidence available to make decisions about clinical interventions needed to optimize personal oral health.

▶ Evidence-based practice involves two fundamental principles:
  - Patient care decisions are based on patient needs and preferences as well as scientific evidence.
  - A hierarchy of weaker to stronger information sources, discussed more completely later in the chapter, provides a guide for clinical decision-making.

II. Purpose

▶ To answer clinical questions quickly and efficiently.

▶ To identify research-supported, best-practice interventions that contribute to positive patient outcomes.

▶ To ensure application of the most up-to-date practice interventions in the delivery of patient care.

III. Need for Evidence-Based Practice

Keeping current on evidence-based best practices is a commitment to excellence in patient care.[1] A professional dental hygienist understands the following concepts and embraces the role of the healthcare provider in evidence-based patient care.

- Patients have become more sophisticated about searching the Internet for health information. They:
  - Expect the clinician to know the latest developments in health care.
  - Value a practitioner who can discuss and help them evaluate the relevance, validity, and reliability of information obtained elsewhere.
  - Demand healthcare providers who are up-to-date with evidence-based information on the most current oral health practices, techniques, and products.
- Differences in practice procedures
  - Clinicians are not consistently knowledgeable about new therapies.
  - There may be inconsistencies between what is taught in dental hygiene schools and procedures tested by regional examination for licensure.
- Gap between current research knowledge and application into practice
  - A practitioner's limited personal journal collection, rather than an extensive range of scientific publications, may remain the dominant source for making treatment decisions.
  - Ability to access, or an individual's selection of, continuing education courses can affect the clinical practitioner's knowledge of current therapies.
  - Gap in knowledge of up-to-date care widens the longer clinicians have been out of school.
  - Evidence-based decision-making behaviors and research analysis skills may not be well understood by every dental professional.
- Information explosion management[2]
  - The amount of published research increases yearly.
  - Effective strategies to disseminate new evidence are limited by the large number of publications and by lag time between research completion and publication.
  - Clinicians' time to access a growing number of publications with new information is limited.

IV. Evidence-Based Decision-Making Process[3]

The evidence-based decision-making process for dental hygiene care is based on an interaction between four components, as illustrated in Figure 2-1.
- *Scientific evidence*. Review of relevant and current clinical research of high quality identifies best-practice treatment choices.
- *Patient preferences or values*. The patient's needs, wants, and expectations are considered, respected, and weighed (i.e., cultural, religious, capabilities).
- *Clinical/patient circumstances*. The unique and specific particulars of each patient are considered (i.e., age, health concerns, disease state).
- *Clinician's experience and judgment*. The clinical skill and experiences of the clinician enhance the ability to

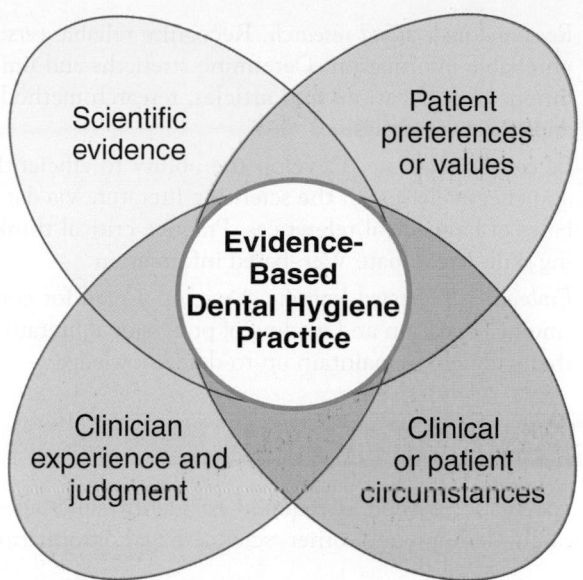

FIGURE 2-1 An Evidence-Based Decision-Making Model for Dental Hygiene Practice.

identify quickly the patient's health, risks, needs, and potential for various interventions.

V. Skills Needed for Evidence-Based Dental Hygiene Practice

A variety of skills are needed to implement evidence-based dental hygiene practice (EBDH) into everyday clinical practice. Finding evidence to support treatment and preventive interventions and recommendations requires the dental hygienist to:
- *Understand EBDH practice*. Study a tutorial (examples listed in Box 2-2) to learn more about the evidence-based decision-making process.
- *Follow a systematic approach*. Develop a step-by-step approach to asking questions related to clinical practice to ensure success.

BOX 2-2
Evidence-Based Tutorials and Learning Opportunities*

- University of North Carolina at Chapel Hill: http://www.hsl.unc.edu/Services/Tutorials/EBM/welcome.htm
- University of Illinois at Chicago: http://researchguides.uic.edu/ebm
- SUNY Downstate Medical Center: http://library.downstate.edu/EBM2/contents.htm
- University of Michigan: http://guides.lib.umich.edu/EBP
- The Cochrane Collaboration: http://www.cochrane.org/About%20us/Evidence-based%20health%20care/Webliography/Tutorials-tools
- PubMed Tutorial: http://www.nlm.nih.gov/bsd/disted/pubmedtutorial/cover.html

*Many other examples can be found by typing "Evidence-Based Tutorials" into an Internet search engine.

▶ *Read and understand research.* Recognize reliable *versus* unreliable information. Determine strengths and limitations of publications and articles, research methods, and statistical analysis.

▶ *Be computer literate.* Develop the ability to efficiently and effectively search the scientific literature via databases of biomedical references. Practice critical thinking skills to evaluate Web-based information.

▶ *Embrace self-directed learning.* Develop a plan for continuing education and reading of professional literature that will help to maintain up-to-date knowledge.

A SYSTEMATIC APPROACH

A systematic method is required to identify and select research findings and other science-based information related to a particular patient's oral and systemic health. Figure 2-2 illustrates a step-by-step procedure, explained later in the chapter, that will aid the practitioner in the development of these crucial skills.[3]

I. Determine Clinical Issue

▶ Asking the right question is fundamental, and critical, to the evidence-based decision-making process.

▶ Include important characteristics of the patient (i.e., age, gender).

II. Develop a Researchable Question

A good, researchable question includes four parts, referred to as PICO.[3] Examples of PICO questions related to dental hygiene practice can be found in Table 2-1.

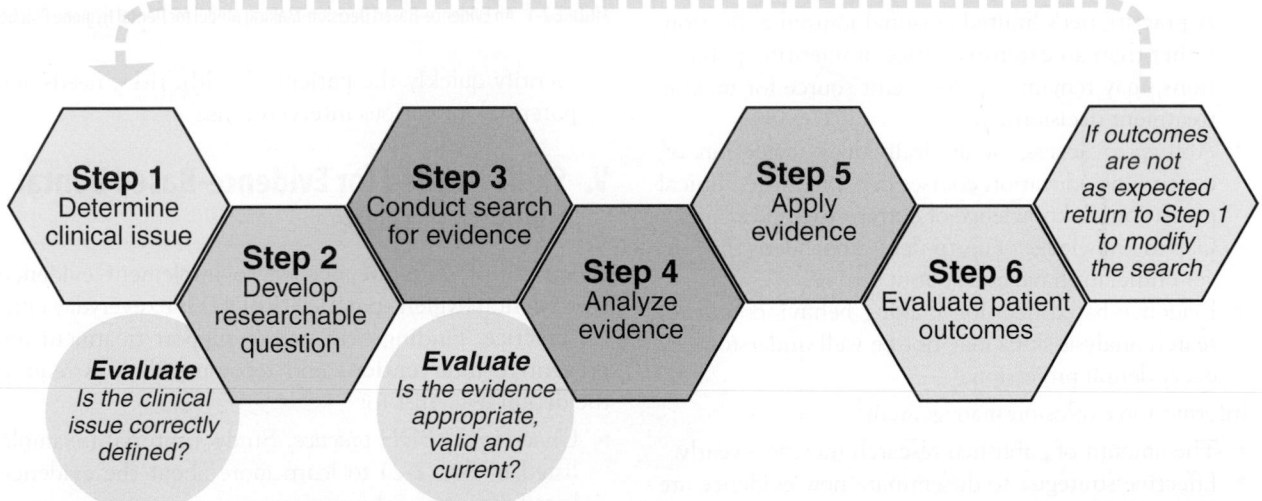

FIGURE 2-2 **Steps for a Systematic Approach to Evidence-Based Dental Hygiene Practice.** Evaluation is an ongoing and important component of the process.

TABLE 2-1	Example PICO Questions
SCENARIO	**PICO QUESTION**
Mrs. Winnie is a 79-year-old African American woman who presents for a routine maintenance appointment. Her health history identifies that she has arthritis. She states that because of limited wrist and hand mobility, she has been having trouble maneuvering a toothbrush to reach all surfaces of her teeth. Her friend told her about a new kind of toothbrush that has curved bristles that are able to brush both inner and outer surfaces of the teeth at the same time.	For a patient with limited hand/wrist movement, will a curved-bristle toothbrush be as effective at removing the biofilm from all surfaces of the teeth as a regular toothbrush is? ■ **Patient/problem:** Limited hand mobility ■ **Intervention:** Regular toothbrush ■ **Comparison:** Curved-bristle toothbrush ■ **Outcome:** Effective biofilm removal/healthy gingiva
Mrs. Arthur is an attractive 48-year-old mother of two who has come into the clinic for her regular checkup. She is very interested in whitening her teeth because her 30th high school reunion is coming up in 1 month. She has heard about various bleaching methods and is wondering which method would be right for her. She is on a limited budget, but is willing to pay the extra expense if an in-office treatment will get her teeth whiter.	For a patient who is dissatisfied with her tooth color, will using an over-the-counter bleaching system be as effective as an in-office bleaching? ■ **Patient/problem:** Wants teeth whitened ■ **Intervention:** In-office professional bleaching procedure ■ **Comparison:** At-home or over-the-counter bleaching system ■ **Outcome:** Lighter tooth color

NOTE: Research about comparative cost is done in addition to the literature search.

▶ *Patient problem or population (P):* What are the most important characteristics of the patient or population of interest?

▶ *Intervention (I):* Which main intervention, prognostic factor, or exposure is being considered?

▶ *Comparison (C):* What is the main alternative to compare with the intervention? The clinical question does not always need a specific comparison.

▶ *Outcome (O):* What is the desired outcome, accomplishment, measure, improvement, or effect?

III. Search for Evidence

Select appropriate resources and conduct a search for science-based information. Scientific articles can still be accessed in a traditional library, but more often, searches are accomplished on a computer using an appropriate search engine or database.

A. Finding Information

▶ An Internet search engine is designed to search for information on the World Wide Web.

▶ The search results are generally presented in a list of results (Websites or articles related to the topic) and are often called "hits."

▶ Use of popular general search engines, such as Google or the Wikipedia, may lead to some results, but:
  • Accuracy and unbiased sources of information can rarely be assured.
  • Only a fraction of all available resources are displayed.

▶ Web search engines can also provide access to more reliable sites that offer a variety of statistical data and medical information such as:
  • Government agencies
  • Professional associations
  • Independent organizations that offer a variety of statistical data and other information regarding medicine and health.

▶ Dedicated search engines and databases devoted to specific professional literature provide access to information from scholarly articles in biomedical and other health-related journals.

B. Biomedical Databases

▶ Some valid and reliable Internet databases for locating evidence-based information related to oral health and patient care are listed in Box 2-3.

C. The Medline Database

▶ Most complete database of biomedical and health-related journal articles.

▶ Provides access to articles from more than 5,500 professional and scientific journals and also the Cochrane Collaboration database.

BOX 2-3

Databases for Locating Biomedical Information

▷ **MEDLINE (PubMed),** http://www.ncbi.nlm.nih.gov/pubmed/: a service of the U.S. National Library of Medicine that includes over 16 million citations from MEDLINE and other life science journals for biomedical articles back to the 1950s; includes links to full-text articles and related resources.

▷ **CINAHL (Cumulative Index to Nursing and Allied Health Literature),** http://www.ebscohost.com/nursing/products/cinahl-databases/cinahl-complete/: a bibliographic database that includes abstracts of nursing and allied health articles.

▷ **Cochrane Library (The Cochrane Collaboration),** http://www.cochrane.org/: an international nonprofit and independent organization; produces and disseminates systematic reviews of healthcare interventions and promotes the search for evidence in the form of clinical trials and other studies of interventions.

▷ **ADA's EBD Website (The American Dental Association's Evidence-Based Dentistry),** http://ebd.ada.org: a dental informatics resource; provides practitioners with access to current scientific information that is easy to comprehend and that can be quickly reviewed at the point of care.

▷ **National Institutes of Health,** http://health.nih.gov: a searchable encyclopedia of health topics.

BOX 2-4

Medline Literature Search Techniques Using the PubMed Search Engine

▷ A text or key word search locates articles that have the relevant terms in the title, abstract, or body of an article.

▷ A medical subject heading (MeSH) search locates articles indexed in the database through the use of specific headings.

▷ A clinical queries search locates articles related to three specific clinical research categories: clinical studies, systematic reviews, and medical genetics.

▶ When a list of journal articles or the abstract for a specific article is displayed, PubMed also provides:
  • The complete citation in NLM format.
  • In some cases, a link to the full text of the article.
  • Links to access "related citations."

▶ Systematic and effective MEDLINE searches include:
  • A combination of three search techniques, described in Box 2-4.
  • Use of the "related citations" link.

▶ Checking the references listed in journal articles for additional relevant citations.

▶ Using a combination of search techniques results in more efficient and effective searches.[4,5]

D. The Cochrane Collaboration Database

▶ Global, independent network working to promote access to credible, unbiased health information for both practitioners and patients.

▶ Produces high-quality, systematic reviews (SRs) and other synthesized research evidence to support clinical decision-making.

▶ Each review article includes:
  • Complete scientifically written and well-supported analysis of search methods, data collection, and findings.
  • Plain language summary of results for non-healthcare providers.

▶ Has a searchable database for a large number of health-related topics, including oral and dental health.

IV. Analyze Evidence

▶ Analyze the evidence for validity (closeness to the truth and how well the studies answer the clinical question).[6]
  • Determine whether the report follows logical and complete steps of research process.
  • Determine whether the focus of study is similar to patient's concerns.
  • Examine results for accuracy and completeness.
  • Determine availability and affordability of treatment.

▶ Analyze the evidence for value (usefulness in clinical practice).[6]
  • Analyze the difference between statistical *versus* clinical significance.
  • Determine whether treatment outcomes are large enough to justify treatment.
  • Determine whether researchers have provided a critical argument for using results in clinical practice.

V. Apply Evidence

▶ Return to the patient and apply the evidence, guided by clinical expertise/experience and the patient's preferences.

▶ Consider potential results in association with the patient's needs and the clinician's ability to obtain results.

VI. Evaluate Results

▶ Determine whether:
  • The evidence-based decision-making process was successfully carried out.
  • Additional search strategies and information are needed.
  • A modification of original outcome goal is needed.

▶ Begin the process again if patient outcome is not successful.

READING AND UNDERSTANDING RESEARCH

The sources for obtaining scientific information are growing daily. Knowing how to determine the validity and

---

BOX 2-5

Questions to Ask When Considering the Validity of a Publication

▷ Who is sponsoring?
▷ Is there an editorial review board? Are the articles peer reviewed?
▷ What are the credentials of the contributors?
▷ Are there advertisements? How many?
▷ Are there good-quality production standards?
▷ Is manuscript preparation information included?
▷ What type of articles are included? (i.e., Informational? Opinion/editorial? Case reports? Scientific study?)

---

reliability of information is paramount for selecting successful patient care strategies and interventions. A checklist of questions to ask when considering the validity of a publication is found in Box 2-5.

I. Publication Types

▶ Textbooks
  • Good as background resources but, because of a drawn-out publication process, can become outdated quickly.

▶ Commercial-based journals/magazines
  • Often free, which means that they are based on product sponsorship.
  • Articles may be written by in-house staff members without professional credentials.
  • Most carry informational articles; however, some have articles summarizing recent research that contain reference citations, but may not include all available scientific studies.

▶ Professional journals
  • Produced by professional organizations. Membership dues payment is required, or receiving publications is a benefit of being a member.
  • Part or all of the publication is devoted to scientific studies. Most contain articles with supporting reference citations.

▶ Peer-reviewed (refereed) publications
  • Before publication of any scholarly article or research report in these journals, one or more dental hygiene experts or statisticians have critically examined all components of the manuscript. Peer-reviewed journals usually list all review board members and their credentials in each issue of the journal.
  • After receiving feedback from the reviewers, the article is not published until the author revises the manuscript to address significant concerns or answer questions expressed by the reviewers.
  • The purpose of this process is to help assure the validity and unbiased nature of the supporting review

of the literature, the research results, and the conclusions or recommendations put forth by the author.

II. Research Approaches

► Qualitative
  • Results are reported using a narrative; often uses quotations.
  • Systematic; subjective approach.
  • Uses numbers only to report demographic information.
► Quantitative
  • Results reported in numbers.
  • Data can be counted and analyzed by descriptive or inferential statistics.

III. Research Types

► Descriptive
  • Often, a first step in classifying and organizing information.
  • Asks "how often" or "to what extent" something occurs.
  • Helps identify relationships that can be further explored in subsequent studies.
  • Descriptive statistics are used to describe what exists, determine frequency of occurrences, and categorize information.
► Correlational
  • Looks at the relationship between two or more variables.
  • Determines the strength and type of relationships.
  • Variables are not manipulated; no cause and effect is determined.
  • Statistical analysis of findings helps determine linkages between variables.
► Experimental
  • Intervention variables are manipulated to discover the effect of one variable on another.
  • Contains a control group and randomly assigned subjects; provides an intervention to only the experimental group.
► Quasi-experimental
  • Designed to examine cause-and-effect relationships.
  • Has less control by the researcher than true experimental designs.
  • No control group, or subjects may not be randomly assigned.

IV. Levels of Evidence

The concept of "levels of evidence" is used to evaluate the strength (scientific rigor and quality) of scientific evidence and to provide a hierarchy for making clinical judgments related to patient care. Six levels (shown in Figure 2-3) are organized based on types of research.

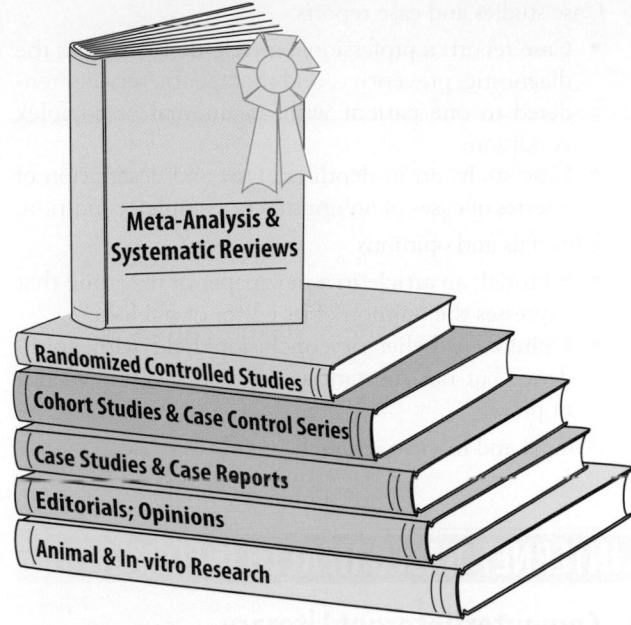

FIGURE 2-3 Levels of Evidence Pyramid. Source: SUNY Health Sciences. *Guide to Research Methods: The Evidence Pyramid* (last updated January 6, 2004). New York, NY: Evidence Based Medicine Course, SUNY (State University of New York) Downstate Medical Center; © 2014. http://library.downstate.edu/EBM2/2100.htm. Accessed October 21, 2010.

► The three highest levels of evidence provide the strongest basis for making clinical decisions; the less relevant research method types follow in descending order.
► The levels are often visualized as a pyramid because there are a smaller number of studies in the more clinically valuable top levels compared with the number of studies in the lower levels.
► Systematic reviews (SRs) and meta-analysis (MA): the highest level of evidence.
  • SR is a critical evaluation of all published studies that investigate a specific question by a group of experts using preestablished criteria to produce a summary of results.
  • MA is the statistical process used during a SR to combine data from various studies into one analysis.
► Randomized controlled double-blind studies (RCTs): the most rigorous clinical studies
  • RCT is a type of scientific experiment most commonly used in testing the efficacy or effectiveness of healthcare services or health technologies.
  • It eliminates selection bias, balancing both known and unknown factors, in the assignment of treatments.
► Cohort studies and case–control series
  • Cohort (follow-up or prospective): study in which the same subjects are followed over a period of time to observe the occurrence of a particular event.
  • Case–control (retrospective): study design in which persons with a disease of interest (cases) are compared with those without the disease (controls); researchers look back to identify possible causes.

▶ Case studies and case reports
  • Case report: a professional article that describes the diagnostic, preventive, and therapeutic services rendered to one patient with an unusual or complex condition.
  • Case study: an in-depth analysis and description of a series of cases of an unusual or complex condition.
▶ Editorials and opinions
  • Editorial: an article in a newspaper or magazine that expresses the opinion of its editor or publisher.
  • Opinion: a belief or conclusion held with confidence but not substantiated by positive knowledge or proof.
▶ Animal and in vitro research

INTERNET-BASED HEALTH INFORMATION

I. Computer/Internet Literacy

▶ The amount of online information is overwhelming.
▶ Finding valid and reliable information from an appropriate Website takes an understanding of both location and content.
▶ Skills using Internet search engines to find health information and analyze the content are enhanced by practice.

II. Content Analysis[7–9]

A. Choose the Correct Online Source for Reliable Information.

▶ Many popular search engines lead to newspaper and magazine articles or Websites that may not provide science-based, research-supported information.
▶ Reliable biomedical information is found in databases such as those listed in Box 2-3 or on government, professional association, or education Websites.

B. Determine the Purpose of the Site (e.g., to Educate, Entertain, or Market Products?).

▶ Be familiar with domain names and what they mean.
▶ .edu and .gov are considered reliable sites for educational and governmental information.
▶ .org indicates nonprofit organizations; understanding of the mission and purpose of the organization helps determine reliability.
▶ .com, .biz, and .net tend to be from less reliable special-interest groups or advertising.

C. Analyze the Information to Make Sure It Is Relevant.

▶ Topic covered in-depth
▶ Bibliography present

▶ References to other Websites included
▶ All points of view covered

D. Determine Who is Responsible for the Information (i.e., Author and Publisher).

▶ Author: credentials and contact information
▶ Publisher of the site: To locate the publisher, look at the site address (URL) and the Website's home page, under links such as "About Us" or "Our Mission," or at the bottom of the page.

E. Determine the Accuracy and Objectivity of the Site.

▶ Accuracy
  • Information similar to other sources (textbooks/journal articles)
  • Reference citations provided
▶ Objectivity
  • Conflicts of interest and/or bias apparent
  • All points of view discussed
  • Credentials of the author and publisher (to determine the underlying connection) provided

F. Note How Well the Site is Maintained.

▶ Up-to-date
  • Last update indicated
  • Publication date for specific information
▶ Quality control
  • Easy to navigate and find what is needed
  • Links current and working
  • No grammar and spelling errors

G. Put it All Together (Strengths and Weaknesses of the Website).

Weigh the appropriateness of all the aforementioned factors to determine whether the Website is worthwhile in relation to the topic and the clinical situation.

▶ In addition, accrediting organizations provide certification aimed at assuring accurate and objective health information on the Internet.
  • Health on the Net Foundation[10]
  • URAC Health Website Accreditation Program[11]
▶ Sites that display a symbol of accreditation from these organizations have met specific guidelines intended to assure the quality of health information they provide.

ETHICS IN RESEARCH[12]

▶ Ethics in research is about the responsibility of researchers to conduct nonbiased research, report accurate results, and protect the rights of individuals who participate as research subjects.

- Although many dental hygienists may not actively fulfill the role of a dental hygiene researcher, each can look for evidence that ethical principles were followed when reading the report of a research study.
- Basic ethical principles and decision-making guidelines are discussed in Chapter 1 and also in section introductions throughout this textbook.

I. Ethical Standards

The same ethical theories and ethical principles that guide professional interactions of the dental hygienist with patients, dental colleagues, other healthcare providers, and community members can also be applied to conducting research. Some examples are:

- Honesty
- Concepts of right and wrong or fairness
- Norms for conduct that distinguish between acceptable and unacceptable behavior and treatment.
- Reliance on a professional code of ethics or other guidelines to make decisions for addressing ethical issues and dilemmas.

II. Ethical Research Involving Human Subjects

Ethical standards in research are designed to protect individuals who participate as research subjects, with regard to their rights to:

- Self-determination
- Privacy
- Anonymity and confidentiality
- Fair treatment
- Protection from discomfort and harm
- Understand the risks and benefits of participating in the study
- Informed consent

III. Informed Consent for Research

- A standardized written consent form is signed by each individual who participates as a study subject.
- Discussion of informed consent is included within the research proposal and includes:
  - Complete and advanced information about the nature of a study and what the study participant can expect.
  - A statement of possible benefits and/or risks of the study.
  - A confidentiality statement assuring the participant of anonymity.

IV. Institutional Review Board

- Before conducting any research study, a federal mandate requires the institution in which the project is being implemented to evaluate the research proposal.
- The institutional review board (IRB) is a group of individuals within the institution who review research proposals submitted by researchers. The group can require modifications before approving research or disapprove research based on its review.
- The purpose of IRB review is to protect the rights and welfare of human subject volunteers in research.
- Published research articles often include a statement that IRB approval was received before conducting the study.

DOCUMENTATION

If current research findings from a journal article or other source are used to plan dental hygiene recommendations/interventions, the following factors are included in the patient's record:

- The PICO question used to search for information.
- Citations for references that support the recommendation/intervention.

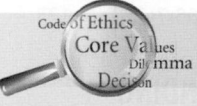

EVERYDAY ETHICS

After discussing a new surface disinfection product with Rick, a dental product representative, and conducting a review of the literature related to the efficacy and safety of the primary ingredient, Sondra, the dental hygienist, reports to the office manager that there is no scientific evidence that supports the claim that this product is as good as what they are already using for surface disinfection in their clinic. The office manager, who has been dating Rick for the last few months, is in charge of ordering all office supplies, orders the product anyway and tells Sondra that she selected it because the product is considerably less expensive than what they have been using. She supports her decision by restating the claims in the company's brochure related to the efficacy of the product.

Questions for Consideration

1. Explain why this situation is an ethical issue as well as an ethical dilemma for Sondra.

2. What is the chief concern/problem related to this situation? What are the long-term implications if Sondra is not able to resolve the situation?

3. What core values apply as Sondra considers alternatives for resolving this situation? What personal values might Sondra review as she considers alternative actions to pursue?

▶ Patient factors that may influence the recommendation/intervention.

▶ Timeline for evaluation of patient response to the recommendation/intervention.

▶ An example patient progress note is found in Box 2-6.

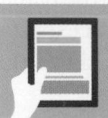

BOX 2-6
Example Documentation: Providing an Evidence-Based Recommendation

S – A patient with a history of arthritis and limited hand/wrist movement presents for routine continuing care appointment. She asks about using a new kind of curved-bristle toothbrush that her friend has told her about. Patient states that she knows where she can purchase this kind of brush and is interested in trying it out.

O – This patient's biofilm levels, particularly at gingival margins in the molar areas, have consistently been high.

A – Review of the literature (P = limited hand mobility, I = regular toothbrush, C = curved-bristle toothbrush, O = effective biofilm removal, healthy gingiva) found evidence that this kind of toothbrush can have successful clinical outcomes (Chava VK. An evaluation of the efficacy of a curved bristle and conventional toothbrush: A comparative clinical study. *J Periodontol.* 2000 May;71(5):785–9.)

P – Verbal and written instruction on basic technique for using the curved-bristle toothbrush provided for patients. Written instructions downloaded from Internet: http://www.dental.wa.gov.au/info/pamphlets/disability/Collis%20Curve%20toothbrush%20instructions%20for%20use%20.pdf

Next Step: Patient will bring the toothbrush at her next scheduled continuing care appointment in 3 months and her success in biofilm removal will be assessed.

Signed: _____, RDH

Date: _____

Factors To Teach The Patient

▷ A result from one study does not necessarily provide the best answer. The type of study, patient parameters, and other factors are taken into consideration before a decision is made about best-practice interventions.

▷ Research method, study design, source of information, and many other factors can affect the validity, reliability, and usefulness of health-related information.

▷ A statistical significance cited in a study does not mean that clinically it is the best decision for a patient.

References

1. Forrest JL, Overman PO. Keeping current. *J Dent Hyg.* 2013;87 (Suppl 1):33–40.

2. Aravamudhan K, Frantsve-Hawley J. American Dental Association's resources to support evidence-based dentistry. *J Evid Based Dent Pract.* 2009;9(3):139–144.

3. Forrest JL, Miller SA. Translating evidence-based decision making into practice: EBDM concepts and finding the evidence. *J Evid Based Dent Pract.* 2009;9:59–72.

4. Agoritsas T, Merglen A, Courvoisier DS, et al. Sensitivity and predictive value of 15 PubMed search strategies to answer clinical questions rated against full systematic reviews. *J Med Internet Res.* 2012;14(3):e85.

5. Richter RR, Austin TM. Using MeSH (medical subject headings) to enhance PubMed search strategies for evidence-based practice in physical therapy. *Phys Ther.* 2012;92(1):124–132.

6. Miller SA, Forrest JL. Translating evidence-based decision making into practice: appraising and applying the evidence. *J Evid Based Dent Pract.* 2009;9:164–182.

7. Cornell University Library. *Five Criteria for Evaluating Web Pages.* Ithaca, NY: Cornell University; June 28, 2010. http://olinuris.library.cornell.edu/ref/research/webcrit.html. Accessed March 12, 2014.

8. University of California at Berkeley. *Evaluating Web Pages: Techniques to Apply & Questions to Ask.* Berkeley, CA: University of California at Berkeley; May 08, 2012. http://www.lib.berkeley.edu/TeachingLib/Guides/Internet/Evaluate.html. Accessed March 12, 2014.

9. University of Michigan Library. *Criteria for Website Evaluation.* Ann Arbor, MI: University of Michigan; July 11, 2013. http://guides.lib.umich.edu/content.php?pid=30524. Accessed March 12, 2014.

10. Health on the Net Foundation. *HONCode Certification: What Is It?* Geneva: Health on the Net Foundation; June 13, 2013. http://www.hon.ch/HONcode/Pro/Visitor/visitor.html. Accessed March 12, 2014.

11. URAC. *Health Website Accreditation Program.* Washington, DC: URAC. https://www.urac.org/accreditation-and-measurement/accreditation-programs/all-programs/health-website/. Accessed March 12, 2014.

12. Aita M, Richer M. Essentials of research ethics for healthcare professionals. *Nurs Health Sci.* 2005;7(2):119–125.

ENHANCE YOUR UNDERSTANDING

thePoint° DIGITAL CONNECTIONS
(see the inside front cover for access information)

- **Audio glossary**
- **Quiz bank**

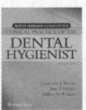

SUPPORT FOR LEARNING
(available separately; visit lww.com)

- *Active Learning Workbook for Clinical Practice of the Dental Hygienist, 12th Edition*

prepU INDIVIDUALIZED REVIEW
(available separately; visit lww.com)

- **Adaptive quizzing with *prepU for Wilkins' Clinical Practice of the Dental Hygienist***

Effective Health Communication

Charlotte J. Wyche, RDH, MS

LEARNING OBJECTIVES

After studying this chapter, the student will be able to:

1. Discuss the skills and attributes of effective health communication.

2. Explain how the patient's age, culture, and health literacy level affect health communication strategies.

3. Identify barriers to effective communication.

4. Identify communication theories relevant to effective health communication and motivational interviewing.

▶ Health communication is the use of communication strategies to enhance the ability to provide patient-centered health information, motivate positive changes in health behaviors, and achieve improved health outcomes.

▶ In the context of dental hygiene care, good communication skills help patients embrace healthy behaviors of all types that allow them to attain and maintain oral health.

▶ Key words related to health communication are found in Box 3-1.

TYPES OF COMMUNICATION

▶ Communication is a process that involves at least two, and sometimes multiple, individuals.

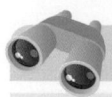 **BOX 3-1   KEY WORDS:** Health Communication

Affect: as used by mental health professionals, refers to an expressed or observed emotional response or lack of expression or emotional response (flat or restricted affect).

Aphasia: communication disorder caused by damage to certain parts of brain, making it difficult for an individual to read, write, express, or understand language.

Communication: a process of defining the meaning of a message shared between a sender and one or more intended recipients.

    Mass communication: communication from one source intended to reach a large group of individuals.

    Nonverbal communication: sending and receiving wordless messages; usually refers to body language, gestures, facial expressions, eye contact, and verbal elements such as rhythm and intonation.

    Verbal communication: sending and receiving messages using words; usually defined as spoken or written communication.

Culture: a learned set of beliefs, values, attitudes, convictions, and behaviors that are common to a group (especially an ethnic group) of people and usually passed down from generation to generation.

Cultural competence: a set of congruent attitudes, skills, behaviors, and policies that enable effective cross-cultural communication for delivery of oral health services.

Cultural sensitivity: making an effort to understand the language, culture, and behaviors of diverse individuals and groups.

Cultural rapport: actions that foster understanding, empathy, and enhanced communication between individuals with different cultural backgrounds.

Culturally effective oral healthcare: refers to a dynamic relationship between provider and patient resulting in culturally relevant and culturally specific oral healthcare recommendations; delivery of oral healthcare services in a way respectful of and responsive to the cultural norms and linguistic needs of individual patients.

Decoding: the reverse process of encoding; the receiver takes the words, gestures, or other signs to recreate the thought.

Dyadic: one-on-one communication between two people; in contrast to communication among a group or from one person toward a group of individuals.

Dysarthria: a motor/speech disorder that weakens or paralyzes the muscles of the face, mouth, larynx, and vocal cords, causing slurred, slow, and difficult to understand speech.

Encode: the translation of a thought into words, gestures, or other linguistic signs that will allow thoughts to be

expressed in some understandable way to another; encoding can be verbal or nonverbal, oral, visual, or tactile.

Feedback: the receiver's direct response to a communicated message.

Haptics: touch as a form or component of communication.

Health behaviors: routines, practices, or habits that have an effect on health status.

Kinesics: body language or physical movement.

Linguistic competence: providing culturally appropriate oral and written health information for persons with limited proficiency in English (or other dominant local language).

Mass media: method of communication using technology (such as print, television, or Internet) to reach a large, diverse audience.

Motivational interviewing: a patient-centered communication approach to changing health behaviors (see Chapter 26).

Neurolinguistics: the study of the causes and effects of language disorders and how to communicate with individuals with language disorders (such as aphasia).

Occulesics: eye behavior, such as direct or indirect eye contact, during communication.

Oral health disparities: significant differences in oral health status and/or access to oral health services between one population and another; populations affected by disparities include racial and ethnic minorities, the elderly, and persons with disabilities.

Plain language: verbal or written health information provided using simplified terminology, clear and to the point sentence structure, pictures, or any other method that can enhance understanding for patients with limited language proficiency or health literacy.

Pragmatics: study of the impact of language and how people use language.

Proxemics: the component or dimension of physical space or distance in the context of human communication.

Semantics: study of the meaning of language.

Social determinants of health: social, environmental, and physical circumstances that have an effect on health status; these conditions are shaped by the distribution of power, money, and resources at a global, national, or local level.

Stereotype: an attitude or a judgment (either positive or negative) made about people that is usually not based on personal experience but rather on what has been learned from other sources; seeing individuals from a population group as having no individuality as though all have the same characteristics.

Vocalic: a type of cue, such accent, loudness, tempo, pitch, cadence, and tone that occurs during verbal communication.

► The source, who has a desire to communicate some specific concept, encodes and then transmits a message to at least one receiver who decodes the message.

► This process can then reverse itself and the receiver becomes the sender of a return message that may or may not provide direct feedback to the original message that was sent.

► The effectiveness of the communication depends on how closely the encoding and the decoding match. Barriers to effective communication are discussed later in the chapter.

► All communication is either verbal or nonverbal. Each can be subdivided into vocal and nonvocal.

I. Verbal

► A form of communication based on language or words.
► Vocal communication is spoken language.
► Nonvocal communication is based on signs or signals that express language concepts, and include writing, braille, and sign language.

II. Nonverbal

► Messages expressed by body language or affective (expressive) display can influence or interfere with a healthcare provider's ability to communicate, perhaps even more than the verbal method used.

► Some nonverbal, nonvocal factors include:
• Body position (posture or use of social space)
• Movement of body parts such as hands or arms
• Eye movements and facial expression
• Appearance (grooming and dress).
► Nonverbal, vocal factors include:
• Vocal qualifiers (volume, pitch, tempo, and cadence)
• Vocal characterizers (crying, laughing).

III. Media Communication

► Media communication refers to the use of tools or technology to convey information.
► Media communication can be directed to:
• An individual recipient (written care plan provided for an individual patient)
• A wider, more diverse target audience (patient education brochures developed by a professional association or health information on the Internet).
► Public health efforts to enhance the health of populations are based on a community-based media approach to providing quality health information.
► Commercial media efforts, such as television commercials or magazine advertisements for various products, have an astonishing effect on the health-related choices made by targeted audiences.[1]

HEALTH COMMUNICATION

I. Objectives of Health Communication

► The ultimate goal of health communication is to persuade behavior change that will support optimum health.
► Healthy People 2020 health communication objectives[2] related to direct patient care include:
• Shared decision making between patients and providers
• Personalized, targeted, accurate, accessible, and actionable information, self-management tools, and resources
• Increase of health literacy skills.

II. Skills and Attributes of Effective Health Communicators

► Healthcare providers who most effectively deliver preventive interventions demonstrate the following during patient interactions[3]:
• Expertise and knowledge in health and prevention
• Understanding of learning/behavior change theories and principles of good communication
• Relationship building skills
• Interview and role modeling skills
• Assessment for readiness to change behaviors
• Attention to the patient's attitudes and beliefs
• Personal attributes of confidence and flexibility.
► A motivational interviewing approach to patient counseling, based on development and use of those skills, is presented in Chapter 26.
► The use of "plain language" in both verbal and written health communication can improve patients' response to health messages.[4]
► The use of plain language does not "dumb down" or "talk down" to the patient, but rather provides information in a clear and to the point manner, using words the patient can understand.
► The National Institute of Dental and Craniofacial Research website provides free plain language patient brochures on a variety of oral health topics. (Available from: https://catalog.nidcr.nih.gov/OrderPublications/.)

III. Attributes of Effective Health Information

Recommendations made by a health educator are more likely to be effective if the patient perceives the information to be[5]:

► Evidence-based, accurate, balanced, and reliable
► Consistent with information from other sources
► Culturally and linguistically appropriate
► Delivered in an easily understood and accessible way

TABLE 3-1	Barriers to Effective Health Communication
BARRIER	**DESCRIPTION**
Cultural	Differences in social norms or perceptions related to differences in gender, age, language, economic, or ethnic background
Interpersonal	Discomfort related to perceptions about the individual; appearance causes distraction; individuals do not see "eye to eye" or relate well to each other
Attitudinal	Lack of sensitivity or respect; over or underconfidence displayed by either patient or clinician
Physical	Distractions related to the physical environment; noise levels; face-to-face positioning not used
Physiological	Inability to hear, see, touch, or vocalize as required to communicate
Psychosociological	Emotional factors such as fear or pain cause distraction
Insufficient knowledge	Either the clinician is not well informed and cannot provide sufficient information or the patient has low health literacy and cannot understand the information provided
Lack of access to knowledge	Inability to access media or use technology to find information
Lack of interest	Patient is not ready to engage in health behavior change; clinician is experiencing "burn out" or disinterest in patient education
Information overload	Too much information on too many topics is provided at one time; no written reinforcement is provided
Poor communication skills	Either the patient or the clinician is not able to respond or provide feedback to messages received; clinician uses "jargon" or professional terminology that the patient does not understand

▶ Provided when the patient is most ready to receive it

▶ Repeated and reinforced over time.

IV. Barriers to Effective Health Communication

▶ It is rare that every message coded and transmitted by a sender is decoded and understood with complete accuracy by the receiver.

▶ Multiple factors that can affect the way health messages are understood are described in Table 3-1.

▶ Many of the factors listed in the table overlap in their description; more than one barrier may exist and have an effect on any attempt at communication.

▶ All of the factors listed can provide a barrier to communication in either direction between the clinician and the patient.

▶ Dental hygienists who strive to develop good listening skills enhance their ability to assess a patient's needs, and approach each individual with empathy and respect can go far toward overcoming the barriers to effective health communication.

V. Web-Based Health Messages

▶ There has been an explosion of web-based health-related websites and an increasing number of patients of all ages who access Internet-based health information.

▶ Patients bring information they find on the Internet to the attention of their healthcare providers.

▶ Healthcare providers are responsible to keep up-to-date on Internet sources of information in order to respond to questions patients may bring to a health education discussion.

▶ The dental hygienist can help patients determine reliability and credibility of websites as well as providing recommendations for high-quality resources for patients searching for additional information. (See Chapter 2, Internet-Based Health Information section.)

VI. Additional Factors that Influence Health Communication

▶ In addition to the communication skills of the caregiver and effectiveness of the health information, additional factors can affect:
  • The ability of healthcare providers to influence health behaviors
  • Whether or not patients and populations are able to take advantage of new knowledge provided by the health messages.

▶ These factors are discussed more completely in this chapter and include:
  • Health literacy of the patient or population receiving the health message.
  • The age and communication style preferences of individuals receiving information.

- The social and economic ability of the targeted individuals to take advantage of recommendations contained in the health messages.
- The cultural background and health-related cultural norms of the individual receiving the message.
- Cultural sensitivity and the ability to establish cultural rapport of individuals providing the health messages.

HEALTH LITERACY

▶ Health literacy is a set of cognitive and social skills that determine the ability of a patient to obtain, process, understand, and respond to health messages and be motivated to make health decisions that promote and maintain good health.[6]

▶ A large part of even an educated population may have low health literacy and often these are the patients with the highest treatment needs and the greatest barriers to receiving health information.

▶ Populations particularly vulnerable to low health literacy include:
- Older adults
- Immigrant populations
- Minority populations
- Individuals living below the poverty level.

▶ Low health literacy is associated with less use of healthcare services and resources and ultimately with poorer health outcomes.[7]

I. Health Learning Capacity

▶ The level of a patient's health literacy depends on not only the reading level but also the complex interaction of cognitive and psychosocial skills.[8]

▶ Individuals faced with complex health information need to be able or learn to[9]:
- Access services and navigate complex healthcare facilities and systems.
- Locate and be able to understand health information.
- Evaluate information for credibility and quality.
- Communicate with healthcare providers.
- Analyze relative risks and benefits of treatment recommendations.
- Evaluate test results.
- Calculate medication dosages.

▶ Skills that support health-learning capacity are listed in Table 3-2.

II. Assess and Address Health Literacy

To enhance communication with all patients regardless of oral health literacy level[10,11]:

▶ Assess health literacy level and provide an individualized approach for every patient.

▶ Ensure a clinic environment that is helpful and user friendly by providing clear directions, visible and

TABLE 3-2	Skills Necessary to Increase Health Literacy Capacity
DOMAINE	**SKILL SET**
Cognitive	■ Information (processing ability)
	■ Attention
	■ Short- and long-term memory capacity
	■ Reasoning ability
	■ Visual literacy (ability to understand graphs)
Combined cognitive/ psychosocial	■ Numeracy (mathematical ability)
	■ Computer literacy (and access)
	■ Information obtaining ability
	■ Verbal ability
	■ Reading
Psychosocial	■ Self-efficacy
	■ Communication ability
	■ Previous health-related experience

Source: Wolf MS, Wilson EA, Rapp DN, et al. Literacy and learning in health care. *Pediatrics.* 2009;124 (Suppl 3): S275–S281 and National Network of Libraries of Medicine. Health literacy: skills needed for health literacy. http://nnlm.gov/outreach/consumer/hlthlit.html#A3. Accessed September 26, 2014.

clearly written signs or universal symbols, and color-coded maps where necessary.

▶ Encourage patients to write down and bring questions about their oral health to each appointment.

▶ Provide health history, informed consent forms that are written in plain language. Provide help if required in completing forms.

▶ Build on the patient's current knowledge base to encourage healthy decision making.

▶ Provide written patient education materials that use plain, easily understandable language rather than materials that use professional jargon or provide complex explanations of patient conditions.

▶ Excellent "plain language" oral health patient education publications have been developed by the U.S. Department of Health and Human Services and are available for free on the National Institute of Dental and Craniofacial Research website (see Figure 3-1).

▶ Use visual aids such as drawings or photographs for education materials when appropriate (see Figure 3-2).

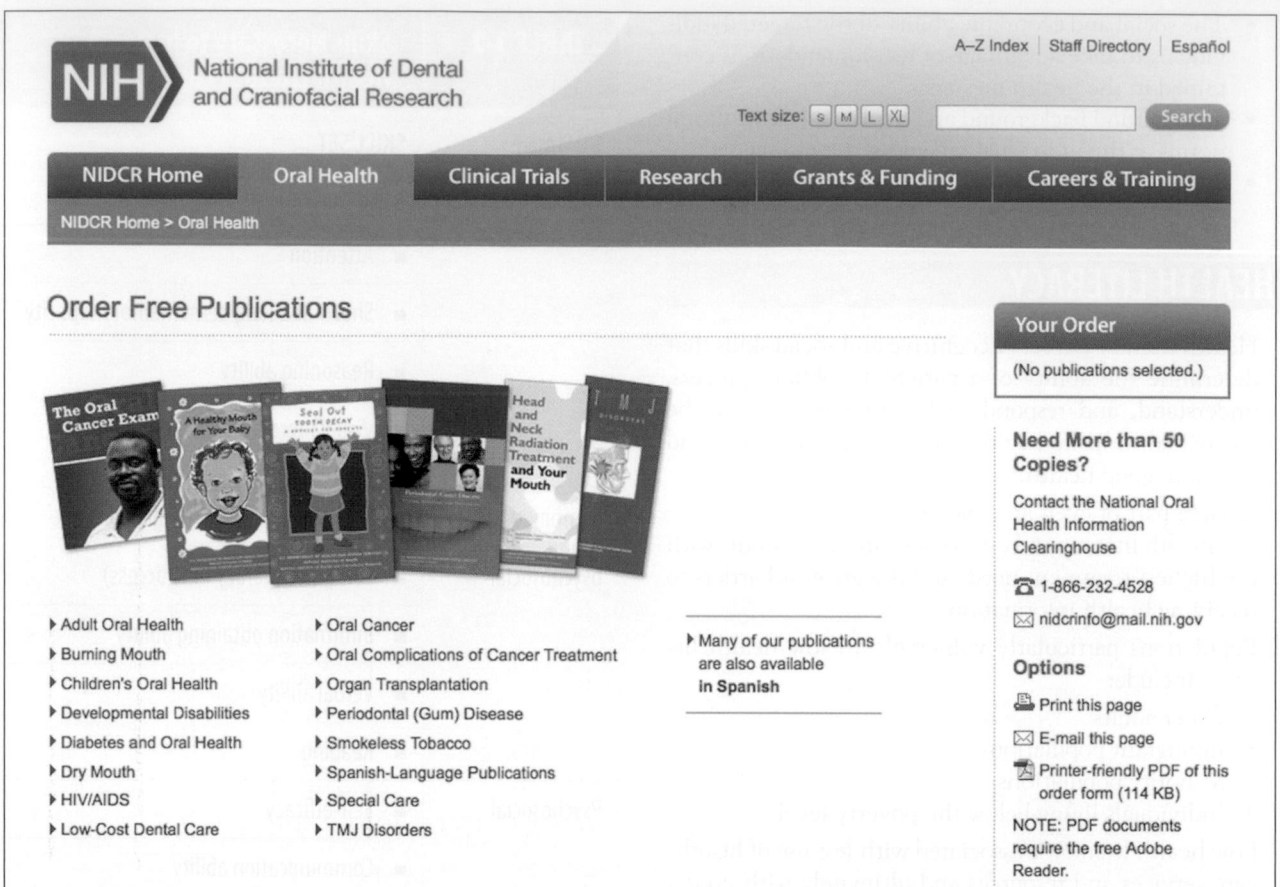

FIGURE 3-1 A variety of excellent "plain language" oral health patient education publications have been developed by the U.S Department of Health and Human Services, National Institutes of Health, and are available for free from the National Institute of Dental and Craniofacial Research website at: https://catalog.nidcr.nih.gov/OrderPublications/. Accessed October 23, 2014.

▶ Monitor to determine understanding of all forms and education materials. The "teach-back" method of asking patients to explain following instructions is a helpful approach.

COMMUNICATION ACROSS THE LIFESPAN

Irrespective of the patient's age, building rapport is the key to effective health communication. Tips for establishing rapport with patients of all ages are found in Box 3-2. Key points related to specific age groups are discussed in the subsequent sections.

I. Children and Adolescents

Complete information about the oral health needs of children and adolescents is found in Chapter 50. Some age-appropriate communication strategies are listed below.[12]

A. Infants (Birth to 12 Months)

Infants communicate primarily through their senses of touch, sight, and hearing. Techniques the clinician can use to communicate with an infant during a dental hygiene examination include:

▶ Interact playfully with a receptive infant by mimicking facial expressions, rocking, and talking softly or singing.

▶ Encourage an adult who is familiar with the infant to distract and comfort the child.

▶ Wait until the infant is calm to approach closely.

B. Toddlers and Preschoolers (Ages 1 to 2 and 3 to 5)

▶ Although dependent on adults for their care, most children appreciate and respond to being approached directly.

▶ Development of a sense of self enhances the need to assert independence and maintain control over any situation.

▶ Offer encouragement and gentle hints or engage in "parallel" actions to demonstrate, rather than directly assisting, to promote success in age-appropriate self-care tasks.

▶ Calmly distract or direct toward an alternative behavior to counter defiance or inappropriate behavior.

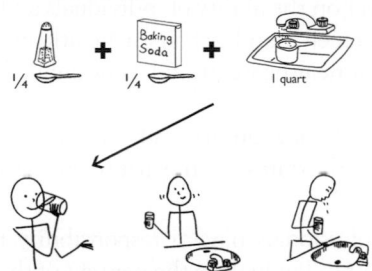
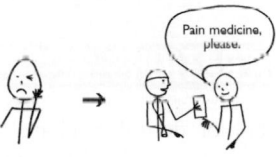

Tips for Mouth Problems

Sore Mouth, Sore Throat

- Rinse often with
  - ¼ teaspoon of salt and
  - ¼ teaspoon of baking soda in 1 quart (4 cups) of warm water
- Don't swallow.

¼   + Baking Soda +   1 quart

- Ask your cancer care team about medicine that can help with the pain.

Pain medicine, please.

FIGURE 3-2 This example, which uses drawings to provide patient education, is taken from the illustrated booklet *"Three Good Reasons to See a Dentist BEFORE Cancer Treatment."* **Illustrated patient education materials are appropriate for adults with reading skills at the second grade level or below and for children. This entire publication can be downloaded or ordered from the NIDCR website at:** https://catalog.nidcr.nih.gov/OrderPublications/. **Accessed October 23, 2014.**

BOX 3-2

Tips for Establishing Rapport with Patients of All Ages

▷ Listen more than talk, especially at the beginning of a conversation.

▷ Practice attentive listening rather than multitasking during conversations.

▷ Sit eye to eye with the patient rather than with the patient in a reclined position or standing/sitting taller than the patient does.

▷ Convey a nonjudgmental attitude, reinforce an atmosphere of respect and valuing of the individual, even if the behavior is not acceptable.

▷ Maintain a calm, unhurried demeanor.

▷ Use a normal tone of voice and vocabulary that is appropriate, but does not talk down, to the patient.

▷ Look for clues, share your thoughts and observations, and ask questions.

▷ Do not jump to conclusions.

▷ Link information to activities of daily living to help provide context for recommendations.

▶ To effectively control unwanted behavior, state specifically what the child is expected to do rather than criticize.

▶ Ask simple, specifically focused questions to help the child remember past experiences.

▶ To overcome the limited ability to process auditory information and short attention span, provide brief, truthful, and simple instructions and responses to questions.

▶ Toddlers are beginning to converse in short sentences, but if the adult becomes impatient or abrupt, the child may feel frustrated or ashamed and become unresponsive.

▶ Children of this age understand more than they are given credit for but often misinterpret language that is not familiar to them; therefore, serious discussions or use of certain words may distress them.

C. School-Age Children (6 Through 11)

▶ The ability is developing to understand serious events logically and comprehend impact on themselves.

▶ More aware of the needs of others but may be reluctant to state their own needs.

▶ The ability and desire to respond to simple questions can allow the dental hygienist to assess knowledge and misconceptions.

D. Adolescents (12 Through 21)

▶ Marked by intense and often extreme feelings about situations and persons in their world.

▶ Strongly independent and desire to have their viewpoint considered with respect.

▶ Tendency to withdraw or become hostile if they feel they are misunderstood.

▶ A straightforward approach that explains and then solicits input into a discussion on topics that interest the adolescent is most effective to build rapport and establish trust.

▶ Confidentiality laws, which vary from state to state, can help determine what behavior-related information the dental hygienist discusses with a parent or guardian. Anything that is an immediate safety issue (such as thoughts of suicide) is reported immediately.

▶ To develop a rapport and a trusting relationship with an adolescent patient:
  - Address the adolescent directly even when parent/guardian is present.
  - Ensure the adolescent has the opportunity to ask and answer questions independently (privately) as well as with parents/guardians.[13]

II. Older Adults [14,15]

Oral health issues related to aging are discussed in Chapter 53. Providing effective health education for aging patients who are experiencing a communication difficulty requires

---

BOX 3-3

Strategies for Effective Communication with Older Adults

▷ Identify each individual's communication barriers (such as cognitive impairments) and modify communication approach appropriately.
▷ Avoid patronizing "elderspeak" and respect the patient's level of competence and independence.
▷ Practice attentive listening.
▷ Face the patient and maintain eye contact; remove masks during conversations.
▷ Speak slowly, clearly, and loud enough for the patient to hear.
▷ Use simple, patient-appropriate language.
▷ Present one idea at a time.
▷ Use visual aids, teach-back techniques, and repetition of key messages.
▷ Provide written summary or follow-up for key messages.

---

respect for the needs of the individual and response to functional ability or limitations.

Strategies for communicating with older individuals experiencing communication difficulty are listed in Box 3-3.

A. Physical and Cognitive Changes

► Cognitive disabilities are more likely to be present as an individual ages and to interfere with understanding health-related information.

► Communication disorders such as dysarthria and aphasia are associated with conditions that are more common in an aging population.

► Sensory loss (particularly hearing loss) can provide challenges in interpersonal communication.

► Physiologic changes may occur in speech patterns, including voice tremor, pitch, loudness, and speaking rate.

B. Communication Predicament[15–17]

► Healthcare providers often use an inappropriate over-modification of speech and language when addressing older patients.

► *Accommodative speech* refers to use of a high-pitched tone of voice, a "sing song" cadence, and relatively simplistic language when addressing an older adult.

► The use of *terms of endearment* (honey, sweetie, dearie) and *diminutive* forms of a patient's name can reflect a lack of respect for the individual as an adult person.

► The use of plural pronouns ("Are we ready for our appointment?") can imply that the patient cannot act alone or make independent decisions.

► This "baby talk" or "elderspeak" approach to communication does not enhance comprehension and can be perceived as patronizing or demeaning.

SOCIAL AND ECONOMIC ASPECTS OF HEALTH COMMUNICATION

► Social and economic factors, sometimes referred to as "social determinants of health," are the circumstances in which people are born, grow up, live, work, play, and age.[18]

► These factors:
  • Have an effect on the ability of individuals and communities to receive and act upon health messages received from healthcare providers or public health media.
  • Are responsible for unfair and avoidable differences in health status seen within and between populations.[18,19]

► Oral health professionals have a responsibility to address the needs of individuals in the context of their environment and experience when providing oral health education.[19,20]

CULTURAL CONSIDERATIONS

Culturally sensitive delivery of dental hygiene services can make a positive difference in oral health outcomes.[21] A cultural awareness checklist is found in Box 3-4.

BOX 3-4

A Checklist to Enhance Cultural Awareness During Patient Care

▷ Examine and recognize any personal bias that may affect communication when working with patients from a different culture.
▷ Conduct all patient assessments with cultural sensitivity in mind.
▷ Assess to determine the patient's cultural identification and, if necessary, research to identify implications for dental hygiene practice.
▷ Determine language barriers, identify patient's preferred method of communication, and regularly double-check to assure comprehension.
▷ Identify religious and health-related beliefs, views, or misconceptions that may influence dental hygiene interventions.
▷ Identify and address cultural dietary considerations.
▷ Double-check verbal and nonverbal signs routinely to determine the level of the patient's trust of healthcare providers.

Source: Seibert PS, Stridh-Igo P, Zimmerman CG. A checklist to facilitate cultural awareness and sensitivity. *J Med Ethics.* 2002;28(3):143–146.

I. Culture and Health

A. Effects of Culture on Health Status

▶ The increasing diversity of ethnic/racial communities and linguistic groups in the United States presents a challenge to the delivery of oral health services.

▶ Health disparities related to racial, ethnic, and socioeconomic background exist in the healthcare system.[22]

▶ Ignoring culture can lead to negative health consequences and/or poor clinical outcomes because culture and language can influence:
  • Beliefs and behaviors related to health, healing, and wellness.
  • Perceptions of illness, diseases, and their causes.
  • Attitudes of patients toward accessing health services or attitudes toward healthcare providers.
  • Attitudes and behaviors of providers who may have learned a set of values that are different from those of their patients.

B. Culturally Effective Oral Care

▶ Culturally effective healthcare provides care for each patient responsive to diverse cultural health beliefs, practices, preferred languages, health literacy, and other communication needs.[23]

▶ Sensitivity to the effects of culture on health care delivery is critical to reducing health disparities and improving access to high-quality care.[24]

▶ Meeting each patient's individual oral care needs is the hallmark of dental hygiene practice.

▶ The ability to provide effective oral health education and dental hygiene services for culturally diverse patients requires the ability to assess, be sensitive to, and respect each patient's cultural differences.

▶ Culturally effective dental hygiene care respects each patient's health beliefs, practices, values, customs, and traditions in the plan for dental hygiene care.

II. Cross-Cultural Communication

▶ Communication with patients from other cultures is enhanced when the dental hygienist develops knowledge about and avoids stereotyping traditional behaviors and values of a patient's cultural group.

▶ Knowing general principles can enhance communication.

A. Nonverbal Communication

▶ Some culturally related differences in nonverbal communication are identified in Table 3-3.

▶ To communicate successfully the dental hygienist will:
  • Follow the patient's lead for touching or personal space.
  • Use hand and arm gestures with caution.
  • Be careful interpreting facial expressions.
  • Follow the patient's lead for making eye contact.

B. Language Proficiency

▶ Simplify language as much as possible without speaking down to the patient.

▶ Eliminate professional jargon.

▶ Use pictures, diagrams, and demonstrations to help increase understanding.

▶ Provide "plain language" health information or publications in the patient's primary language to reinforce and support compliance with oral health recommendations.

C. Using an Interpreter

▶ When the patient's skills in the dominant language are not sufficient to assure informed consent or compliance with recommendations, a professional interpreter can be used to enhance communication.

▶ Family members or friends are not the same as a professional interpreter.

▶ A professional interpreter will have proficiency in both languages as well as an ability to convey complex information completely and accurately. Informal interpreters are more likely to modify important information or interject their own opinions, beliefs, or prejudices.

▶ It is particularly inadvisable to ask children to interpret sensitive health information.

▶ Focus on and direct all communication to the patient, with pauses to allow the interpreter to translate.

D. Family Decision Making

▶ In many cultures, an individual's health problem is considered to be a family problem.

▶ Involvement of certain family members in the treatment planning process may be a key factor in assuring compliance with recommendations.

▶ Sensitivity is needed when family members or children, even older children, are involved in the discussion.

III. Attaining Cultural Competence

▶ Achieving cultural competence in providing healthcare is a process[25] that requires a commitment to cultural awareness, a motivation to engage in cultural encounters, and an ongoing acquisition of cultural knowledge and communication skills.

▶ The dental hygienist who strives to become adept at providing culturally effective care:
  • Values (and not simply tolerates) diversity.
  • Conducts honest self-assessment to determine how personal health beliefs, traditions, and biases influence ability to relate to culturally different individuals.
  • Actively acquires knowledge about patients' health beliefs, behaviors, and cultural norms.
  • Is nonjudgmental regarding cultural traditions and beliefs.

TABLE 3-3	Nonverbal Communication and Cross-Cultural Considerations
ATTRIBUTE	**EXPLANATION**
Facial expressions	■ Smiling, winking, and blinking may not signify the same intent in all cultures. ■ People from some cultures point at an object by shifting eyes or pursing lips because pointing with a hand or finger is inappropriate. ■ Expressions of pain and discomfort may differ among cultures or according to family experiences. Some cultures value stoicism while others seem to emote effusively.
Gestures	■ Hand signs can be interpreted in many ways among cultures. ■ Some commonly used gestures, such as the "OK" finger-thumb circle shape or the "thumbs-up" gesture have vulgar connotations for members of some cultures.
Head movements and physical postures	■ Head movement signs for "yes" and "no" vary greatly in some cultures. ■ Some cultures nod head (as in "yes") to indicate attention to or respect for the speaker—even if the answer to the question is not yes or if they do not understand what is being said. ■ Standing with hands on hips might indicate a challenge to members of some cultures. ■ Many cultures consider slouching or poor posture as a sign of disrespect. ■ Showing the bottom of the shoe (resting foot on top of knee while sitting) is considered impolite in some cultures.
Personal space and touching	■ Individuals from some cultures are accustomed to standing or sitting very close and sometimes touching, even during casual interactions; others may express alarm if the provider stands or sits too close. ■ A light touch, a brief kiss on the cheek, or warm handshake is common in some cultures, even among people who have just met or individuals of the same gender. ■ In some cultures, such physical contact may be extremely inappropriate. ■ In some cultures, touching or accepting an article with the left hand is considered unclean.
Eye contact	■ In some cultures making direct eye-to-eye contact is a sign of respect; in others, it is a sign of disrespect especially if done by a child or toward an authority figure such as a healthcare provider. ■ The "languid" or half-closed eyes of individuals from some cultures in not necessarily a sign of disrespect or inattention.

Source: Management for Health Sciences Electronic Resource Center. The Provider's guide to quality & culture: non-verbal communication. http://erc.msh.org/mainpage.cfm?file=4.6.0.htm&module=provider&language=English. Accessed September 26, 2014.

- Avoids stereotypes.
- Routinely adapts delivery of dental hygiene care in a way that reflects understanding of each patient's diversity and unique oral health needs.

IV. Cultural Competence and the Dental Hygiene Process of Care

Respect for each patient's cultural differences, healthcare practices, health beliefs, and values can be integrated into all areas of the dental hygiene process of care.[26]

A. Assessment

▶ The ability to collect accurate, complete assessment data is the key to providing dental hygiene interventions that meet patient needs.

▶ Culturally effective nonverbal communication and listening skills help build trust dand patient rapport that can facilitate the transfer of essential personal health information.

▶ Skillful, nonjudgmental questioning can help elicit cultural specific data such as health beliefs and values, as well as avoid misunderstandings about a patient's culturally related health practices.

▶ Asking permission before touching a patient during the extra- and intraoral examination procedures can avoid problems with cultural differences in personal space.

B. Diagnosis

▶ A dental hygiene diagnosis is predicated on a clear understanding of the patient's history, medical status, symptoms, and current treatment modalities.

▶ The culturally competent dental hygienist will prepare diagnostic statements that take into consideration:
  - Culture-specific health risks that are related to oral status.
  - Cultural practices that may impact the patient's oral health status.

C. Planning

▶ The dental hygiene care plan formulates oral health goals that meet the needs of each individual patient realistically.

▶ The goals identified in the plan are based on a synthesis of needs determined by the dental hygienist and those expressed by the patient.

▶ A culturally sensitive dental hygiene care plan respects and takes into consideration the patient's current health practices and beliefs.

▶ With the patient's input, the plan may be devised to accept, modify, or eliminate current culturally relevant healthcare practices.

▶ The plan is sensitive to the practices, products, or substances that the patient's culture prohibits, such as mouthrinses containing alcohol for patients in some cultures.

▶ A culturally and linguistically sensitive approach to communicating the dental hygiene care plan can facilitate informed consent for dental hygiene interventions.

D. Implementation

▶ Culturally appropriate communication can enhance the patient's cooperation during treatment.

▶ Knowledge of culturally determined expressions of pain and discomfort during treatment can help the dental hygienist determine appropriate pain control measures during treatment.

▶ Language-appropriate instructions before, during, and after each procedure can enhance patient compliance with treatment.

▶ "Plain language" oral health materials can enhance patient compliance with recommendations.

E. Evaluation

▶ A dental hygienist who is sensitive to cultural differences evaluates treatment success on the basis of goals determined in a previously prepared culturally relevant care plan.

▶ Feedback provided for the patient respects culturally diverse beliefs and values related to oral health.

▶ Self-evaluation regarding the cultural effectiveness of the practitioner's approach can provide insight for planning modifications to the patient's continuing care plan.

Interprofessional Communication

▶ Interprofessional collaboration is changing the way healthcare is delivered and resulting in positive healthcare outcomes.[27,28]

▶ Teamwork is a vital skill that relies on collaboration between a variety of healthcare providers who have responsibility for the often complex aspects of an individual patient's care.

▶ Sufficient and ongoing communication is a major factor in developing a collaborative practice workforce that strengthens healthcare systems, provides high-quality care, and supports positive patient outcomes.[27,29–30]

▶ Continuous efforts to enhance interprofessional communication are necessary to improve the quality of patient care.[30,31]

▶ The ability to communicate with other health professionals in a manner that supports a team approach to patient care requires competency in the following skills[29]:

• Select effective communication tools and techniques, including information systems and communication technologies.

• Organize and express information in a form that is easily understood by providers in other health disciplines.

• Demonstrate active listening; encourage others to share ideas and opinions.

• Provide timely, sensitive, and instructive feedback to other members of the team.

• Use respectful language when in a difficult situation or a professional conflict.

• Recognize how one's own communication style contributes to the interprofessional relationship.

• Consistently communicate the importance of teamwork in patient-centered care.

COMMUNICATION WITH CAREGIVERS

▶ Many patients with disabling conditions and also young children rely on someone else to help with or provide daily self-care regimens.

▶ In this situation, the dental hygienist communicates with the caregiver or parent as well as the patient.

▶ In a group conversation, keep the primary focus on the patient by maintaining eye contact and directing comments/questions to the patient, if appropriate, as well as the caregiver.

▶ Assess patient needs and caregiver relationships carefully to determine the extent of the caregiver's role in daily self-care.

▶ Encourage the caregiver to allow the patient to maintain as much independence as possible.

DOCUMENTATION

When documenting communication aspects of a patient visit, the following factors are included:

▶ Patient's age, gender, and ethnicity

▶ Factors or observations related to health literacy level

▶ Cultural characteristics that can affect communication or delivery of dental hygiene care

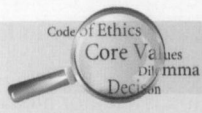

EVERYDAY ETHICS

Abelena Flores, a 65-year-old Mexican American female, presents to the clinic for the first time for her initial assessment appointment. Mrs. Flores speaks English moderately well, but Lisel, the dental hygienist, notices that she is not able to read the health history and seems to be confused during more complex explanations. Lisel offers to obtain a medical translator for the next appointment, but Mrs. Flores insists that her son, who speaks English and her son's new wife who does not speak English, will accompany her to help interpret and make decisions about the treatment plan Lisel will present to her at that visit. Lisel is concerned that the family members will not be knowledgeable enough to be able to explain the needed treatment so that informed consent can be obtained.

Lisel considers arranging for a friend who is a medical translator to be present without telling Mrs. Flores

beforehand. Lisel knows that her patient will not be charged for that service because the medical translator is a volunteer who has provided free translation services at the clinic in the past.

Questions for Consideration

1. Is this an ethical issue or an ethical dilemma for Lisel?

2. Explain which Core Values (Table II-1, Section II Introduction) Lisel will need to consider as she determines what action to take regarding the use of a translator during Mrs. Flores next appointment.

3. How might personal values related to Lisel's and Mrs. Flores' cultural differences affect Lisel's ethical duty in resolving this situation?

BOX 3-5

Example Documentation: Communication Aspects of a Patient Visit

S –Following an initial data collection appointment, a 65-year-old African American male presents for a second appointment to receive and discuss his complex treatment plan. Patient has significant hearing loss and does not use a hearing aid but reads lips during casual conversation. He prefers to ask complex questions and receive answers by writing on a notepad.

O –Written dental hygiene care plan and dental treatment plans have been developed and are ready to present for patient consent.

A –Patient understanding is necessary for documenting informed consent.

P –Sequential presentation of each written component of the dental hygiene care plan and dental treatment plan. Additional appointment time scheduled so all questions can be answered in writing, as the patient prefers. Following the presentation of each component of the plan, the patient was asked to summarize or restate in writing to demonstrate that he understood what was discussed. At the end of the discussion, the patient wrote on his note pad that all of his questions were answered. Treatment Consent form was signed and dated.

Next Step: Begin implementation of phase 1 of dental hygiene care plan.

Signed _____, RDH
Date _____

▶ Significant factors such as patient hearing loss, need to communicate with caregiver, use of an interpreter, and description of specific modifications made to accommodate those factors

▶ An example of documentation for communication aspects of a patient visit is found in Box 3-5.

Factors To Teach The Patient

▷ The dental hygienist's ability to provide good dental hygiene care is affected by the willingness and ability of the patient to communicate accurate and complete information about health status, needs, and concerns.

▷ The patient's motivation to follow oral health recommendations is affected by the rapport established and the trust developed between the patient and the clinician.

References

1. Zimmerman FJ, Shimoga SV. The effects of food advertising and cognitive load on food choices. *BMC Public Health.* 2014;14:342.

2. HealthyPeople.gov Website. Healthy People 2020 topics and objectives: health communication and health information technology. http://www.healthypeople.gov/2020/topicsobjectives2020/overview.aspx?topicId=18. Accessed September 30, 2014.

3. Burke LE, Fair J. Promoting prevention: skill sets and attributes of health care providers who deliver behavioral interventions. *J Cardiovasc Nurs.* 2003;18(4):256–266.

4. National Institute of Health. Plain language. http://www.nih.gov/clearcommunication/plainlanguage/index.htm. Accessed September 26, 2014.

5. U.S. Department of Health and Human Services. *Healthy People 2010: Objectives for Improving Health.* Vol 1, Part A, Focus Area 11-Health communication:11.3–11.22. 2nd ed. Washington, DC: U.S. Government Printing Office; 2000.

6. National Institute of Medicine. Health literacy: a prescription to end confusion. http://www.iom.edu/Reports/2004/Health-Literacy-A-Prescription-to-End-Confusion.aspx. Accessed September 26, 2014.

7. Berkman ND, Sheridan SL, Donahue KE, et al. Low health literacy and health outcomes: an updated systematic review. *Ann Intern Med.* 2011;155(2):97–107.

8. Wolf MS, Wilson EA, Rapp DN, et al. Literacy and learning in health care. *Pediatrics.* 2009;124 (Suppl 3):S275–S281.

9. National Network of Libraries of Medicine. Health literacy: skills needed for health literacy. http://nnlm.gov/outreach/consumer/hlthlit.html#A3. Accessed September 26, 2014.

10. Horowitz AM, Kleinman DV. Oral health literacy: the new imperative to better oral health. *Dent Clin North Am.* 2008;52(2):333–344, vi.

11. Horowitz AM, Kleinman DV. Creating a health literacy-based practice. *J Calif Dent Assoc.* 2012;40(4):331–340.

12. Deering C, Cody D. Communicating with children and adolescents. *Am J Nurs.* 2002;102(3):34–41.

13. Mappa P, Baverstock A, Finlay F, et al. Current practice with regard to 'seeing adolescents on their own' during outpatient consultations. *Int J Adolesc Med Health.* 2010;22(2):301–305.

14. Yorkston KM, Bourgeois MS, Baylor CR. Communication and aging. *Phys Med Rehabil Clin N Am.* 2010;21(2):309–319.

15. Stein PS, Aalboe JA, Savage MW, et al. Strategies for communicating with older dental patients. *J Am Dent Assoc.* 2014;145(2):159–164.

16. Brown A, Draper P. Accommodative speech and terms of endearment: elements of a language mode often experienced by older adults. *J Adv Nurs.* 2003;41(1):15–21.

17. Williams K, Kemper S, Hummert ML. Enhancing communication with older adults: overcoming elderspeak. *J Gerontol Nurs.* 2004;30(10):17–25.

18. World Health Organization. Social determinants of health: what are the social determinants of health? http://www.who.int/social_determinants/sdh_definition/en/. Accessed September 26, 2014.

19. Williams DM, Sheiham A, Watt RG. Oral health professionals and social determinants. *Br Dent J.* 2013;214(9):427.

20. Lee JY, Divaris K. The ethical imperative of addressing oral health disparities: a unifying framework. *J Dent Res.* 2014;93(3):224–230.

21. Rayman S, Almas K. Transcultural barriers and cultural competence in dental hygiene practice. *J Contemp Dent Pract.* 2007;8(4):43–51.

22. U.S. Department of Health and Human Services Agency for Healthcare Research and Quality Website. National Healthcare Disparities Report, 2013. Chapter 11: Priority Populations. http://www.ahrq.gov/research/findings/nhqrdr/nhdr13/chap11.html. Accessed September 26, 2014.

23. U.S. Department of Health and Human Services Office of Minority Health. National standards for culturally and linguistically appropriate services in health and health care. http://minorityhealth.hhs.gov/omh/browse.aspx?lvl=2&lvlid=53. Accessed September 26, 2014.

24. National Institutes of Health. Clear communication: cultural competency. http://www.nih.gov/clearcommunication/culturalcompetency.htm. Accessed September 26, 2014.

25. Campinha-Bacote J. The process of cultural competence in the delivery of healthcare services: a model of care. *J Transcult Nurs.* 2002;13(3):181–184.

26. Fitch P. Cultural competence and dental hygiene care delivery: integrating cultural care into the dental hygiene process of care. *J Dent Hyg.* 2004;78(1):11–21.

27. World Health Organization. *Framework for Action on Interprofessional Education & Collaborative Practice.* Geneva: World Health Organization; 2010. http://www.who.int/hrh/resources/framework_action/en/. Accessed September 28, 2014.

28. Zwarenstein M, Goldman J, Reeves S. Interprofessional collaboration: effects of practice-based interventions on professional practice and healthcare outcomes. *Cochrane Database Syst Rev.* 2009;(3):CD000072.

29. Interprofessional Education Collaborative Expert Panel. *Core Competencies for Interprofessional Collaborative Practice: Report of an Expert Panel.* Washington, DC: Interprofessional Education Collaborative; 2011. http://www.aacn.nche.edu/education-resources/ipecreport.pdf. Accessed September 28, 2014.

30. Kishimoto M, Noda M. The difficulties of interprofessional teamwork in diabetes care: a questionnaire survey *J Multidiscip Healthcare.* 2014;7:333–339.

31. Hepp SL, Suter E, Jackson K, et al. Using an interprofessional competency framework to examine collaborative practice. *J Interprof Care.* 2014;10:1–7.

ENHANCE YOUR UNDERSTANDING

 thePoint® DIGITAL CONNECTIONS
(see the inside front cover for access information)
- **Audio glossary**
- **Quiz bank**

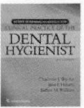 **SUPPORT FOR LEARNING**
(available separately; visit lww.com)
- ***Active Learning Workbook for Clinical Practice of the Dental Hygienist, 12th Edition***

prepU INDIVIDUALIZED REVIEW
(available separately; visit lww.com)
- **Adaptive quizzing with *prepU* for Wilkins' *Clinical Practice of the Dental Hygienist***

Preparation for Dental Hygiene Practice

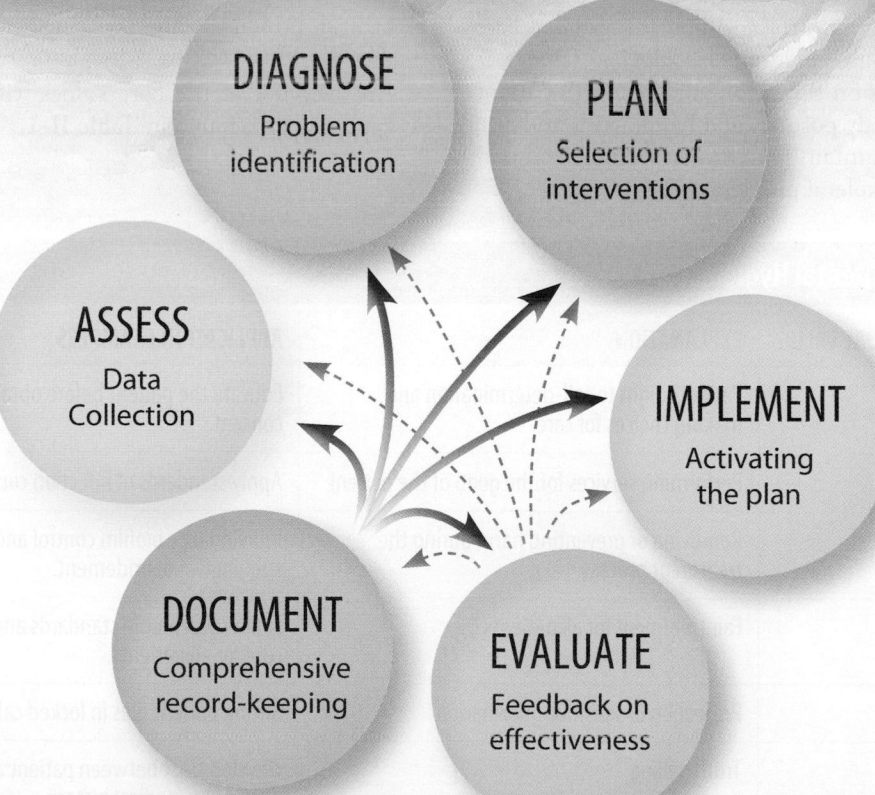

FIGURE II-1 The Dental Hygiene Process of Care.

INTRODUCTION FOR SECTION II

Preparation for dental hygiene care is centered on the use of standard precautions for infection control to ensure the comfort and safety of patients, dental personnel, and others who come in contact with the environment of the clinic or office.

▶ Health services facilities, including dental facilities, must be places for cure and prevention, not for increasing risk of disease or discomfort following inadequate precautionary measures and habits of the professional personnel.

▶ The responsibility of the entire team is to develop and maintain work practices for all appointments that will:

• Prevent direct or indirect cross-infection between dental personnel and patients and from one patient to another.

• Maintain comfort for both the patient and the oral health provider.

▶ Chapters in this section:

• Provide specific information about the chain of infection and the microorganisms that can be transmitted in the dental setting when standard precautions are not observed.

• Describe specific materials and procedures necessary for safe clinical practice. Appendix V is related to these chapters and contains the United States Centers for Disease Control and Prevention *Guidelines for Infection Control in Dental Health-Care Settings*.

• Place emphasis on the ergonomic factors of patient positioning, body posture, and hand, wrist, and arm positions to maintain practitioner comfort and prevent musculoskeletal problems.

THE DENTAL HYGIENE PROCESS OF CARE

Preparation for clinical practice does not form a specific step in the Dental Hygiene Process of Care (Figure II-1); however, practices described in this section protect the patient and the practitioner and are encompassed within all of the components of the process.

ETHICAL APPLICATIONS

▶ A dental hygienist may be involved in a variety of moral, ethical, and legal situations during all professional actions related to the process of care.

▶ A goal of preparation for dental hygiene practice is to increase awareness of, and sensitivity to, potential ethical situations.

▶ Basic core values and principles, as outlined in the various *Dental Hygiene Codes of Ethics* found in the Appendices, are applied in every phase of the dental hygiene appointment.

▶ Basic core values in dental hygiene are identified as selected principles of ethical behavior that can be considered integral to the code of the dental hygiene profession.

▶ Ethical principles contained in the codes clarify the standards of judgment that professionals will follow.

▶ Ethical principles are combined with philosophical theories when making a decision.

▶ An overview of the core values with definitions and applications is found in **Table II-1**.

TABLE II-1	Dental Hygiene Core Values	
ETHICAL PRINCIPLE/CORE VALUE	**EXPLANATION**	**APPLICATION EXAMPLES**
Autonomy	Patient's right to self-determination and making choices for care	Educate the patient before obtaining informed consent.
Beneficence	Performing services for the good of the patient	Apply standards of infection control for all patients.
Nonmaleficence	Removing or preventing harm during the treatment process	Individualize biofilm control and perform subgingival debridement.
Justice	Fair treatment for all patients	Follow acceptable standards and provide access to care for all patients.
Confidentiality	Protection of sensitive information	Secure patient files in locked cabinets.
Veracity	Truth-telling	Develop trust between patient and provider to obtain the medical history.
Fidelity	Keeping promises	Help a fearful patient be comfortable by using local anesthesia or nitrous oxide.

4

Infection Control: Transmissible Diseases

Katherine Soal, RDH, MSDH

CHAPTER OUTLINE

STANDARD PRECAUTIONS
I. Standard Precautions: Definition
II. Additional Transmission-Based Precautions

MICROORGANISMS OF THE ORAL CAVITY
I. Origin
II. Infection Potential
III. Cross-Contamination

THE INFECTIOUS PROCESS
I. Essential Features for Disease Transmission
II. Airborne Infection
III. Prevention of Transmission

PATHOGENS TRANSMISSIBLE FROM THE ORAL CAVITY

TUBERCULOSIS
I. Transmission
II. Clinical Management

HEPATITIS
I. Hepatitis B
II. Hepatitis C
III. Hepatitis D

HERPES VIRUS DISEASES
I. General Characteristics
II. Relation to Periodontal Infections
III. Clinical Management for Herpes

HUMAN PAPILLOMAVIRUS (HPV)

HIV/AIDS INFECTION
I. Transmission
II. Serological Tests

METHICILLIN-RESISTANT STAPHYLOCOCCUS AUREUS

DOCUMENTATION

EVERYDAY ETHICS

FACTORS TO TEACH THE PATIENT

REFERENCES

LEARNING OBJECTIVES

After studying this chapter, the student will be able to:

1. Apply the concept of standard precautions to the process of dental hygiene care.

2. Describe the infectious disease process and prevention of disease transmission.

3. Describe and identify transmissible diseases that may pose a risk to patients and dental healthcare personnel (DHCP).

4. Evaluate the oral healthcare needs of each patient with a transmissible disease.

For healthcare providers, infection and communicable disease can lead to illness, disability, and loss of work time. In addition, patients, family members, and community contacts can become exposed, may become ill, and lose productive time or suffer permanent aftereffects.

▶ In oral healthcare practice, the objective is to protect patients, dental personnel, and others who may become exposed to infectious agents in the environment of the office or clinic.

▶ Health services facilities, including dental facilities, are places for cure and prevention, not for dissemination of disease due to inadequate precautionary measures and habits of the professional personnel.

▶ The first responsibility of the entire dental team is to organize and maintain a system for the disinfection, sterilization, and care of instruments and equipment.

▶ The second step is to develop and maintain work practices for all appointments that will prevent direct or indirect cross-infections between dental personnel and patients and from one patient to another.

▶ Box 4-1 lists and defines terms that apply to the transmission of infectious agents.

STANDARD PRECAUTIONS

I. Definition[1]

▶ Represent a standard of care that protects healthcare providers and their patients from pathogens that can be spread by blood or any other body fluid, excretion, or secretion.

▶ Apply to all patients.

▶ Apply to contact with the following:
  • Blood
  • All body fluids, secretions, and excretions (except sweat), regardless of whether they contain blood
  • Nonintact (broken) skin
  • Mucous membranes.

II. Additional Transmission-Based Precautions

▶ Droplet precautions
  • Respiratory or mucous membrane contact transmitted through airborne droplets (sneezing, coughing).
  • Examples: *Mycobacterium tuberculosis*, influenza virus, chickenpox virus
▶ Contact precautions
  • Reduce risk of transmission of organisms and specific diseases by direct skin or indirect contact.
  • Examples: Vancomycin-resistant enterococci, Methicillin-resistant *Staphylococcus aureus* (MRSA)
▶ Airborne precautions
  • Reduce risk of airborne transmission of infectious agents by droplet nuclei.

  • Special air handling and ventilation required.
  • Examples: *Legionella pneumophila*, *Mycobacterium tuberculosis*
▶ Sharps precautions
  • Reduce risk of bloodborne pathogen transmission and infection by percutaneous sharps injury.
  • Examples: Hepatitis B virus (HBV) and hepatitis C virus (HCV), human immunodeficiency virus (HIV)

MICROORGANISMS OF THE ORAL CAVITY

I. Origin

▶ *In utero* the oral cavity is sterile, but after birth within a few hours to one day a simple oral flora develops.[2]

▶ Microorganisms are transmitted to the infant from the mother and other family members or caretakers.

▶ As the infant grows, there is continuing introduction of microorganisms that are normal for an adult oral cavity. The microbiota of the adult is very complex.[2]

▶ Many of the salivary bacteria come from the dorsum of the tongue, but some are from mucous membranes and gingival/periodontal tissues.

▶ High counts of total microorganisms are found in dental biofilm, periodontal pockets, and carious lesions.

II. Infection Potential

▶ Intact mucous membranes of the oral cavity provides some protection against infection.
  • Pathogenic (disease-producing), potentially pathogenic, or nonpathogenic microorganisms may be present in the oral cavity of each patient.
  • Patients may be carriers of certain diseases but show no signs or symptoms.
  • Pathogenic organisms may be transient.
▶ Inadvertent transmission to subsequent susceptible patients or to dental personnel may occur because of inappropriate work practices, such as:
  • Careless handwashing
  • Unhygienic personal habits
  • Inadequate sterilization and handling of sterile instruments and materials.

III. Cross-Contamination

▶ Spread of microorganisms from one source to another: person to person, or person to an inanimate object and then to another person.

▶ Recognition of the possible transfer of infection in a dental practice or clinic provides a basis for planning the system of disinfection, sterilization, and management of instruments and equipment.

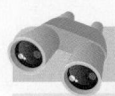 **BOX 4-1   KEY WORDS:** Disease Transmission

Aerosol: an artificially generated collection of particles suspended in air.

Microbial aerosol: suspension of particles in the air that consists partially or wholly of microorganisms; it may be capable of causing an infection.

Anergy: diminished reactivity to specific antigen(s); inability to react to skin-test antigen (even if person is infected with the organism tested) because of immunosuppression.

Antibody: a soluble protein molecule produced and secreted by body cells in response to an antigen; it is capable of binding to that specific antigen.

Antigen: a substance capable, under appropriate conditions, of inducing a specific immune response and of reacting with the products of that specific antibody.

Carrier: a person who harbors a specific infectious agent in the absence of discernible clinical disease and serves as a potential source of infection. The carrier state may be temporary, transient, or chronic.

Asymptomatic carrier: an individual who harbors pathogenic organisms without clinically recognizable symptoms; a carrier may infect those contacted.

CDC: United States Centers for Disease Control and Prevention, Department of Health and Human Services, Public Health Service, Atlanta, GA 30333. www.cdc.gov

CFU: colony-forming unit.

Communicable period of a disease: the time during which an infectious agent may be transferred directly or indirectly from an infected person to another person; the communicable period may include or overlap the Incubation period.

Droplet: diminutive drop, such as the particles of moisture expelled while coughing, sneezing, or speaking, that may carry infectious agents.

ELISA or EIA: an enzyme-linked immunosorbent assay; a laboratory test to detect antibody in the blood serum.

Western blot (WB): a laboratory test for antibody that is more specific than EIA and is used to validate seropositive reactions to the EIA.

Endemic: the constant presence of a disease or an infectious agent within a geographic area.

Epidemic: widespread occurrence of cases of an illness in a community or region; greater than the expected number of cases for the particular population.

Fomite or fomes: an inanimate object or material on which disease-producing agents (microorganisms) may be conveyed.

HCP: healthcare personnel; **DHCP:** dental healthcare personnel.

Healthcare-associated infection: an infection associated with or acquired during a medical or surgical intervention; replaces nosocomial, which is limited to an adverse infectious outcome occurring in a hospital.

Herpes Simplex 1 Skin-Related Viruses:

Herpes gladiatorum: infection transmitted by skin contact among wrestlers and other athletes. Incidence as high as 3% has been reported among high-school wrestlers.

Herpes barbae: herpes simplex spread over the bearded part of the face due to minor injuries of daily shaving or contamination from razor.

Heterotrophic: utilizing only organic material for nourishment.

Immunity: the resistance that a person has against disease; it may be natural or acquired.

Active immunity: immunity either naturally attained by infection, with or without clinical manifestations, or artificially acquired by inoculation of the agent in a killed, modified, or variant form; in response, the body produces its own antibodies; usually lasts for years.

Passive immunity: short-duration immunity either naturally attained by transplacental transfer from the mother or artificially acquired by inoculation of specific protective antibodies.

Incubation period: the time interval between the initial contact with an infectious agent and the appearance of the first clinical sign or symptom of the disease.

Infection: a state caused by the invasion, development, or multiplication of an infectious agent into the body.

Latent infection: persistent infection following a primary infection in which the causative agent remains inactive within certain cells.

Primary infection: first time; no pre-existing antibodies.

Recurrent infection: symptomatic reactivation of a latent infection.

Infectious agent: organism capable of producing an infection.

Jaundice: yellowness of skin, sclerae, mucous membranes, and excretions due to hyperbilirubinemia and deposition of bile pigments. Also called *icterus*.

Microbiota: the microscopic living organisms of a region.

Pandemic: widespread epidemic usually affecting the population of an extensive region, several countries, or sometimes the entire globe.

Parenteral: injection by a route other than the alimentary tract, such as subcutaneous, intramuscular, or intravenous.

Parotitis: inflammation of the parotid gland.

Pathogen: a virus, microorganism, or other substance that causes disease.

Opportunistic pathogen: capable of causing disease only when the host's resistance is lowered.

Percutaneous: by way of, or through, the skin.

Permucosal: by way of, or through, a mucous membrane.

Planktonic: microscopic organisms floating or swimming in a liquid environment.

Prion: abnormal infectious protein particle lacking nucleic acid that has been implicated as the cause of certain neurodegenerative diseases; an example is Creutzfeldt–Jacob disease.

Prodrome: early or premonitory symptom (adj: prodromal).

Replication: process by which viruses reproduce and multiply.

Retrovirus: virus with RNA as its core genetic material; requires the enzyme reverse transcriptase to convert its RNA into proviral DNA.

Risk population: group having an increased prevalence of infection, increased chances or likelihood of infection, and increased prevalence of disease carriers.

Serologic diagnosis: the identification of a disease by serum markers of that specific condition.

Seroconversion: after exposure to the etiologic agent of a disease, the blood changes from negative ("seronegative") to positive ("seropositive") for the serum marker for that disease; the time interval for conversion is specific for each disease.

Serum marker: a specific finding (such as an antibody or antigen) by laboratory blood analysis that identifies an existing disease state. May be referred to as a "titer."

Shedding (viral): presence of virus in body secretions, in excretions, or in body surface lesions with potential for transmission.

Standard precautions: an approach to infection control to protect healthcare providers and patients from pathogens that can be spread by blood or any other body fluid, secretion, or excretion (except sweat), regardless of whether they contain blood.

STD: sexually transmitted disease.

Surveillance (of disease): continuing scrutiny of all aspects of occurrence and spread of a disease that are pertinent to effective control.

Susceptible host: host not possessing resistance against an infectious agent.

Transmission (horizontal): passage of an infectious agent from one individual to another.

Vertical transmission: passage of an infectious agent from one generation to another by breast milk or across the placenta.

Vector: a carrier that transfers an infectious microorganism from one host to another.

Biologic vector: an arthropod, insect, or other living carrier in whose body the infecting organism multiplies before becoming infective to the recipient.

Vehicle: a substance or object that serves as an intermediate means by which an infectious agent is transported and introduced into a susceptible host through a suitable portal of entry.

Virion: complete virus particle made up of the *nucleoid* (the genetic material) and *capsid* (the shell of protein that protects the nucleoid).

Virulence: the degree of pathogenicity or disease-evoking power of an infectious agent.

Virus: a subcellular genetic entity capable of gaining entrance into a limited range of living cells and capable of replication only within such cells; a virus contains either DNA or RNA but not both. (DNA and RNA are defined in Box 4-2.)

Window period: the time between exposure resulting in infection and the presence of detectable serum antibody; antibody test is negative but infectious agent is transmissible during the window period.

THE INFECTIOUS PROCESS

I. Essential Features for Disease Transmission

A chain of events is required for the spread of an infectious agent. The six essential links are shown in Figure 4-1 and described here.

▶ An infectious agent, the invading organism such as:
  • Bacterium, virus, fungus, rickettsia, protozoa.
  • Each organism has its own specific reaction in an infected host.

▶ A *reservoir* where the invading organisms live and multiply. An infectious agent has its own essential environment, which may be inanimate matter, an insect, or human cells or blood.
  • For example, soil is the reservoir for *Clostridium tetani*, and humans are reservoirs for herpetic infections.

▶ A *port of exit* or mode of escape from the reservoir.
  • Organisms exit through various body systems, such as the respiratory tract, or through skin lesions.
  • Escape from the blood stream may be through skin abrasions, hypodermic needles, or dental procedures.

▶ A mode of transmission
  • May be direct, person to person, or indirect by way of an intermediate vehicle, such as contaminated hands or a hypodermic needle.
  • Transmission by a droplet may be direct from the respiratory tract of one person to the oral cavity of the receiving host.
  • Droplets may also pass indirectly to hands or inanimate objects to be transferred indirectly to the susceptible host.

▶ A port *of entry* or mode of entry of the infectious agent into the new host.
  • Modes of entry may be similar to modes of escape.
  • Examples: the respiratory tract, eyes, mucous membranes, needlestick, or a break in the skin.

▶ A *susceptible host* that does not have immunity to the invading infectious agent.
  • A heart valve may be defective because of a congenital or an acquired condition.
  • Example: a valve may be susceptible to infective endocarditis resulting from a bacteremia created during dental or dental hygiene instrumentation.

II. Airborne Infection

A. Dust-Borne Organisms

▶ *Clostridium tetani* (tetanus bacillus) and enteric bacteria are among the organisms that may travel in the dust brought in from outside and move in and about dental treatment areas.

▶ When doors are opened and closed and people pass in and out, dust is set into motion and can settle on instruments, other objects, or people.

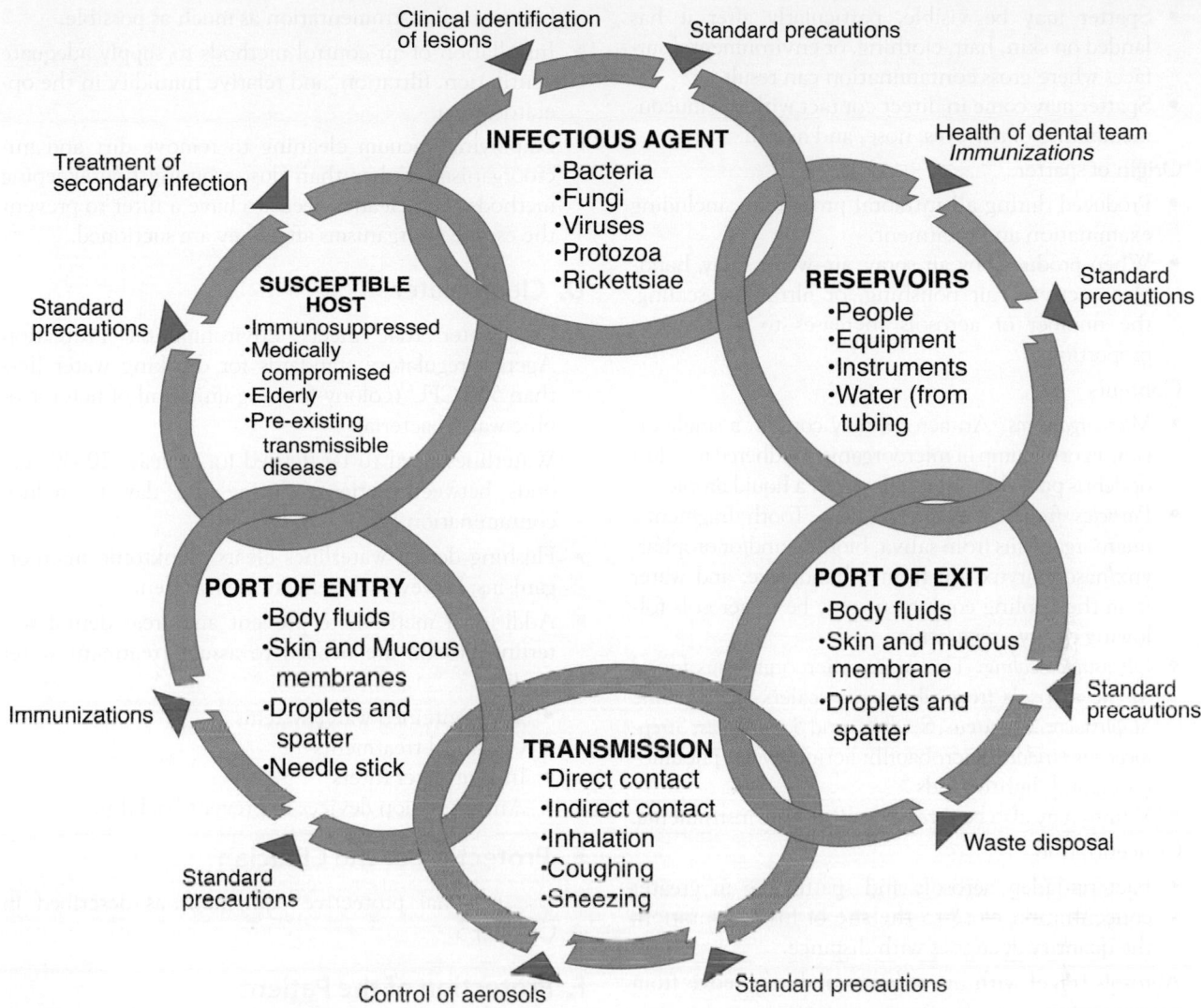

FIGURE 4-1 Interventions to Break the Chain of Disease Transmission. A break in the chain of six major links is required to stop the spread of an infectious agent. Standard precautions are applied to interrupt the chain.

▶ Infectious microorganisms can reach dust from the oral cavities of patients by way of large airborne particles produced by coughing, sneezing, and talking.

▶ Dust-borne organisms may be sources of contamination for dental instruments and hands of dental personnel.

▶ Surface disinfection of all equipment contacted during an appointment contributes to control of dust-borne pathogens.

▶ Procedures for surface disinfection are described in the Preparation of the Treatment Room section of Chapter 6.

B. Aerosol Production

Airborne particles are classified by size as either aerosols or spatter. They are constantly being produced.

▶ Aerosols
  • A particle of a true aerosol is less than 50 μm in diameter; nearly all are less than 5 μm.[3]

• Aerosols are biologic contaminants that occur in solid or liquid form, are invisible, and may remain suspended in air for long periods.

• Aerosol particles (sometimes called droplet nuclei) that are 5 μm or smaller may be breathed deep into the lungs.

• Larger particles get trapped higher in the respiratory tree.

• The tiny particles may contain respiratory disease–producing organisms or traces of mercury or amalgam that collect in the lung because they are not biodegradable.

C. Spatter

▶ Heavier, larger particles may remain airborne a relatively short time because of size and weight, then drop or spatter on objects, people, and the floor.

▶ Spatter is composed of particles greater than 50 μm in diameter that usually fall within 2 ft of origin.[3]

- Spatter may be visible, particularly after it has landed on skin, hair, clothing, or environmental surfaces where gross contamination can result.
- Spatter may come in direct contact with the mucous membranes of the eyes, nose, and mouth.
▶ Origin of spatter
  - Produced during all intraoral procedures, including examination and treatment.
  - When produced by air spray, air–water spray, handpiece activity, air polishing, or ultrasonic scaling, the number of aerosols increases to tremendous proportions.
▶ Contents
  - *Microorganisms*. An aerosol may contain a single organism or a clump of microorganisms adhered to a dust or debris particle contained within a liquid droplet.
  - *Particles from cavity preparation*. Tooth fragments; microorganisms from saliva, biofilm, and/or oropharynx/nasopharynx; oil from a handpiece; and water from the cooling equipment may be in aerosols following cavity preparation.
  - *Ultrasonic scaling*. The many microorganisms found in the aerosols from ultrasonic scalers may include *Staphylococcus aureus*, *S. albus*, and *S. pyogenes*; *Streptococcus viridans*; lactobacilli; actinomyces; pneumococci; and diphtheroids.[4]
  - Viruses may also be spread by ultrasonic instruments.
▶ Concentration
  - Bacteria-laden aerosols and spatter are in greater concentration close to the site of instrumentation; the quantity decreases with distance.
▶ Aerosols travel with air currents and may move from room to room.

III. Prevention of Transmission

A. Airborne Infection Can Be Controlled By:

▶ Elimination or limitation of the organisms at their source
▶ Interruption of transmission
▶ Protection of the potentially susceptible recipient
▶ Carefully monitored procedures for all patients with or without a known serious communicable disease.

B. Preprocedural Oral Hygiene Measures

▶ Biofilm removal: toothbrushing and flossing by the patient prior to beginning of appointment.
▶ Use of an antiseptic or antimicrobial mouthrinse to reduce the numbers of bacteria contained in aerosols.
  - Swish vigorously to force mouthrinse between teeth.
  - Hold in mouth before expectorating.

C. Interruption of Transmission

▶ Use a rubber dam and high-volume evacuation for sealants, and other procedures that produce aerosols.

▶ Use manual instrumentation as much as possible.
▶ Installation of air-control methods to supply adequate ventilation, filtration, and relative humidity in the operatory area.
▶ Employing vacuum cleaning to remove dirt and microorganisms rather than dust-arousing housekeeping methods. The cleaner needs to have a filter to prevent the escape of organisms after they are suctioned.

D. Clean Water

▶ Use water that meets Environmental Protection Agency regulatory standards for drinking water [less than 500 CFU (colony-forming units)/ml of heterotrophic water bacteria].
▶ Waterlines need to be flushed for at least 20–30 seconds between patients during the day to reduce contamination.[1]
▶ Flushing dental waterlines clears planktonic microorganisms; however, the effects are transient.
▶ Additional methods to prevent and treat dental waterline biofilm are needed to assure treatment water quality.[5]
  - Self-contained water systems
  - Chemical treatments
  - In-line water filters
  - Antiretraction devices to prevent backflow

E. Protection of the Clinician

▶ Use personal protective equipment as described in Chapter 5.

F. Protection of the Patient

▶ Use protective eyewear to prevent direct spatter and aerosols to the face and eyes.

G. Maintain Infection Control Protocols

PATHOGENS TRANSMISSIBLE FROM THE ORAL CAVITY

▶ Selected pathogens that may be transmitted by way of the oral cavity and their disease manifestations, mode of transfer, and incubation and communicability periods are provided in Table 4-1.
▶ Pathogens are often present within the oral cavity without producing oral signs or symptoms, a fact of particular importance to the total consideration of prevention of disease transmission.
▶ Tuberculosis (TB), viral hepatitis, herpetic infections, and acquired immunodeficiency syndrome (HIV/AIDS) are included in this chapter because of the special problems they create in personal and patient care.

TABLE 4-1	Infectious Diseases				
INFECTIOUS AGENT	**DISEASE OR CONDITION**	**ROUTE OR MODE OF TRANSMISSON**	**INCUBATION PERIOD**	**COMMUNICABLE PERIOD**	**VACCINE**
HIV	HIV infection (AIDS)	Blood and blood products (infected IV needles) Sexual contact Transplacental and perinatal	To detectable antibodies: <1 mo To disease diagnosis: <1–8 y or more	From asymptomatic through life	Vaccine in progress
HBV	Type B hepatitis "Serum" hepatitis	Blood Saliva and all body fluids Sexual contact Perinatal	60–150 d (average 90 d)	Carrier state: indefinite	Yes
HCV	Type C hepatitis	Percutaneous exposure to blood and blood products (infected IV needles) Transplacental and perinatal	2 wk–6 mo (average 6–9 wk)	1 wk before onset of symptoms, persists in most persons indefinitely Carrier state: indefinite	Vaccine in progress
Delta hepatitis virus (HDV) Delta agent	Delta hepatitis	Coinfection with HBV Blood Sexual contacts Perinatal	2–8 wk	All phases of active infection	HBV vaccine
Hepatitis E virus (HFV) ET-NANB	Type E hepatitis Enterically transmitted non-A, non-B	Fecal–oral Contaminated water Consumption of infected animals	15–60 d (average 40 d)	Unknown	No
Herpes simplex virus Type 1 (HSV-1) Type 2 (HSV-2)	Acute herpetic Gingivostomatitis Herpes labialis Ocular herpes Herpetic whitlow Genital herpes	Saliva Direct contact (lip, hand) Indirect contact (on objects, limited survival) Sexual contact	2–20 d (average 6 d)	Labialis: 1 d before lesions are crusted Acute stomatitis: 7 wk after recovery Viral shedding in saliva 1–4 d Asymptomatic infection: with viral shedding Reactivation period: with viral shedding	No
HPV	Genital warts Cervical cancer Anogenital cancer Oropharangeal cancer Recurrent respiratory papillomatosis	Sexual contact	2–3 mo	Contagious for life	Vaccine available for types 6,11,16,18
VZV (HHV-3)	Chicken pox Shingles (Herpes zoster)	Chicken pox: direct and indirect contact, airborne droplet Shingles: reactivation of HHV-3	10–21 d Average 14–16 d	1–5 d prior to onset of rash until all vesicles are crusted of vesicles	Yes

(continues)

TABLE 4-1	Infectious Diseases *(continued)*				
INFECTIOUS AGENT	**DISEASE OR CONDITION**	**ROUTE OR MODE OF TRANSMISSON**	**INCUBATION PERIOD**	**COMMUNICABLE PERIOD**	**VACCINE**
EBV HHV-4	Infectious Mononucleosis Oral hairy leukoplakia	Direct contact Saliva	4–6 wk	Prolonged Pharyngeal excretion up to 1 y after infection	No
CMV HHV-5	Neonatal CMV infection Cytomegaloviral disease	Perinatal Direct contact (most body secretions) Blood transfusion Organ transplantation Saliva	3–12 wk postpartum 2–4 wk after transfusion or transplant	Months to years	No
Mycobacterium tuberculosis	Tuberculosis	Droplet nuclei Sputum Saliva	3–8 wk Occasionally 12 wk Latency decades or indefinite	As long as viable bacilli are discharged in sputum	BCG (Bacille Calmette Guérin) has limited efficacy approx. 15 y
Corynebacterium diphtheriae	Diphtheria	Direct and indirect	2–5 d	4 wk if no treatment 3 d after antibiotic treatment started	Yes
Treponema pallidum	Syphilis Congenital syphilis	Direct contact Transplacental	10 d–3 mo (average 21 d)	Variable and indefinite 2–4 y	No
Neisseria gonorrhoeae	Gonorrhea Gonococcal pharyngitis	Direct contact Indirect (short survival of organisms)	2–5 d	May be subclinical and continue for months and years if untreated	No
Bordetella pertussis	Whooping cough Pertussis	Direct contact with discharges	up to 3wk (average 7–10 d)	Untreated: 3 wk after paroxysmal cough Treated: 5 d after antibiotic started	Yes
Mumps virus (paramyxovirus)	Infectious parotitis (mumps)	Direct contact (saliva) Airborne droplet	14–25 d (average 18 d)	From 1 wk before parotid swelling until 5 d after swelling	Yes
Poliovirus types 1, 2, 3	Poliomyelitis	Direct contact (saliva) Droplet Fecal–oral	7–14 d	As long as virus is secreted, most infectious 7–10 d before and after onset of symptoms	Yes
Influenza viruses (A, B, C)	Influenza	Nasal discharge Respiratory droplets	Average 7–67 hr Type A average 34 hr Type B average 14 hr	1 d before symptoms Peaks 1–2 d after Can last for 7 d	Yes
Measles virus (Morbillivirus)	Rubeola (measles)	Direct contact Saliva Airborne droplet	7–18 d (average 10d) to fever, 14 d to rash	Few days before fever to 4 d after rash appears	Yes

(continues)

TABLE 4-1	Infectious Diseases (*continued*)				
INFECTIOUS AGENT	**DISEASE OR CONDITION**	**ROUTE OR MODE OF TRANSMISSON**	**INCUBATION PERIOD**	**COMMUNICABLE PERIOD**	**VACCINE**
Rubella virus (Togavirus)	Rubella (German measles) Congenital rubella syndrome	Nasopharyngeal Secretions Direct contact Airborne droplets Maternal infection first trimester	13–20 d	From 1 wk before to 5 d after rash appears Highly communicable Infants shed virus for months after birth	Yes
Group A streptococci (beta-hemolytic) Streptococcus pyogenes	Streptococcal sore throat Scarlet fever Impetigo Erysipelas Cellulitis Toxic shock syndrome Wound infections	Respiratory droplets Direct contact	1-5 d (average 2 d)	14–21 d, untreated Many nasal oropharyngeal carriers	No
Staphylococcus aureus Staphylococcus epidermidis	Abscesses Boils (furuncle) Cellulitis Impetigo Bacterial pneumonia	Saliva Exudates Respiratory droplets Nasal discharge	4–10 d Variable and indefinite	While lesions drain and carrier state persists	No
Candida albicans	Candidiasis	Secretions Excretions (oral, skin, vaginal)	Variable 2–5 d for "thrush" in children	While lesions are present	No
Streptococcus pneumoniae	Pneumonia Pneumococcal pneumonia	Droplet Direct contact Indirect	1–3 d Not well determined	While virulent organisms are discharged	Yes

TUBERCULOSIS[6]

Mycobacterium tuberculosis, the etiologic agent in TB, is a resistant organism that requires special consideration when sterilization and disinfection methods are selected and administered. Clinical procedures are planned to prevent exposure and infection from this serious disease.

▶ Drug-resistant TB may occur when patients are noncompliant in their required extended drug therapy or if the medication is not available.

▶ Multidrug-resistant TB refers to resistance to at least two of the first-line drugs.

▶ Extensively drug-resistant TB refers to resistance to first-line drugs and at least one of three second-line drugs.[7]

▶ Additional information about TB is included in Chapter 66.

I. Transmission[6]

▶ Inhalation
  • TB is contracted when a vulnerable person inhales aerosolized droplet nuclei containing tubercle bacilli from sputum and saliva of an infected individual during coughing, sneezing, speaking, or singing (Figure 4-2).
  • Use of ultrasonic, air polishing, and other handpieces, and air–water spray creates aerosols that can carry the tubercle bacilli.
  • Droplet nuclei are small enough to pass through over 95% bacterial filtration efficiency required of standard surgical masks, and may remain suspended in the air for hours. Standard precautions may be insufficient to protect the DHCP from transmission of TB in the healthcare setting.
  • National Institute of Occupational Safety and Health recommend airborne isolation measures be used.[7]

▶ Factors affecting transmission of TB
  • The degree to which the infected person produces infectious droplets.
  • The amount and duration of exposure.
  • The susceptibility of the recipient.
  • Some patients are more contagious than are others.

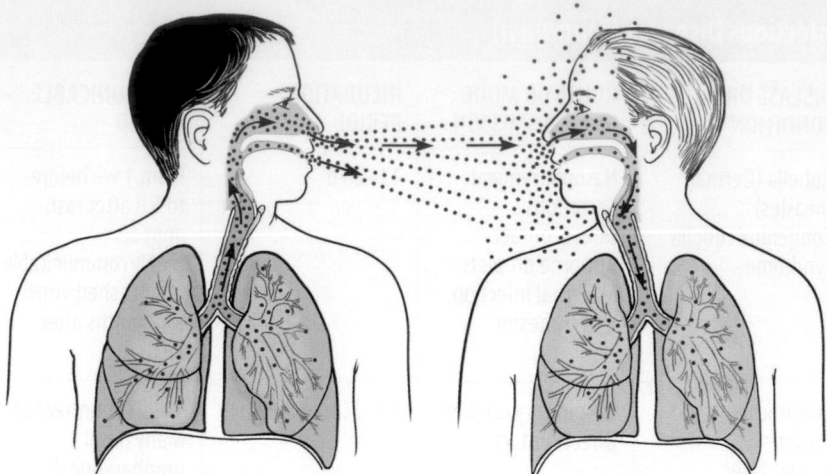

FIGURE 4-2 Droplet Nuclei. Many potentially pathogenic microorganisms are disseminated by aerosols and spatter. The primary mode of transmission of tubercle bacilli is by droplet nuclei breathed directly into the lung.

- Maximum communicability is usually just before the disease is diagnosed, when the person may have a severe cough and other respiratory symptoms.
▶ Areas of infection
  - Infection primarily of the lungs.
  - Extrapulmonary TB: the tubercle bacillus also infects lymph nodes, meninges (TB meningitis), kidneys, bone, skin, and the oral cavity.
  - Figure 66-5 (in Chapter 66) shows a TB ulcer of the tongue.

II. Clinical Management

Official recommendations from the Centers of Disease Control and Prevention (CDC)[7] include the following:
▶ Risk assessment conducted annually.
▶ DHCP: Screen all newly employed DHCP for latent TB infection and TB disease. A baseline two-step tuberculin skin test (TST), followed by annual TST is recommended.
▶ DHCP with persistent cough (more than 3 weeks) or other suggestive symptoms are referred promptly for medical evaluation.
▶ Medical history: Patients are routinely questioned about TB history and symptoms suggestive of TB infection; history is updated regularly.
▶ Referral: Patients with symptoms or history suggestive of TB are referred immediately for medical evaluation.
▶ A patient management guide is available in Chapter 66, Table 66-9.
▶ Urgent dental care: Patients suspected of active TB infection are treated only in a facility with an airborne isolation room.
▶ Respiratory protection with a minimum N95 disposable filtration mask is used when caring for a patient with active (or suspected active) TB.

▶ Separation of suspected or confirmed TB patients; patients are isolated in a separate area until referral to the appropriate facility can be made.

HEPATITIS

▶ Viruses with bloodborne route of transmission by contact with infected body fluids:
  - HBV, HCV, and Hepatitis D virus (HDV)
  - Chronic or carrier disease state may occur with HBV, HCV, and HDV
  - Directly impact the practice of dental hygiene and patient care
  - Table 4-2 lists terminology with abbreviations.

I. Hepatitis B[8]

Hepatitis B is a serious, endemic, worldwide disease. It can occur at any age. Immunization is necessary for newborns and at all ages.

A. Transmission

▶ Blood and other body fluids
  - Almost all body fluids including blood and blood products and saliva contain HBV.
  - No transmission of HBV infection due to saliva alone has been documented.
  - Transmission of HBV can occur from inanimate objects that have been exposed.
▶ Modes of transmission
  - Hepatitis B is transmitted through percutaneous and permucosal exposure.
  - Percutaneous including intravenous, intramuscular, and subcutaneous
  - Accidents with needlestick and other sharp instruments

TABLE 4-2	Viral Hepatitis: Abbreviations and their Significance	
ABBREVIATION	**TERM**	**SIGNIFICANCE**
HEPATITIS A		
HAV	Hepatitis A virus	Etiologic agent for Hepatitis A
Anti-HAV	Antibody to hepatitis A virus	Acute or resolved infection Protective immune response to infection
HEPATITIS B		
HBV	Hepatitis B virus (Dane particle)	Etiologic agent for Hepatitis B Current HBV infection
HBsAg	Hepatitis B surface antigen	Surface marker in acute disease and carrier state indicates infectivity
Anti-HBs	Antibody to Hepatitis Bs antigen	Indicates (1) *Active immunity* to HBV (past infection) (2) *Passive immunity* from HBIG (3) Immune response from HB vaccine
HBeAg	Hepatitis Be antigen	Presence indicated viral replication and high infectivity, found in both acute and chronic carrier states
Anti-HBe	Antibody to Hepatitis Be antigen	Seroconversion from e antigen to e antibody is a predictor of long-term clearance of HBV in patients
HBcAg	Hepatitis B core antigen	Nucleocapsid core of HBV
Anti-HBc	Hepatitis B core antibody	Indicates prior HBV infection
HEPATITIS C		
HCV	Hepatitis C virus	Etiologic agent for Hepatitis C Indicates acute disease and chronic state
Anti-HCV	Antibody to Hepatitis C virus	Does not indicate immunity in >50% of persons infected
HEPATITIS D		
HDV	Hepatitis delta virus	Etiologic agent for Hepatitis D Only infectious in presence of acute or chronic HBV infection
HDV-Ag	Delta antigen	Detectable during early acute HDV infection
Anti-HDV	Antibody to Hepatitis D virus	Indicates acute, resolved, or chronic infection
IMMUNE GLOBULINS		
IG	Immune globulin	Contains antibodies to HAV and low-titer HBV antibodies
HBIG	Hepatitis B immune globulin	Contains high-titer antibodies to HBV

- Exchanging contaminated needles, syringes, and other intravenous drug paraphernalia
- Sexual exposure
- Infection from blood transfusion and blood products: rare since donor and blood screening was instituted in 1985.
▶ Perinatal transmission
  - Maternal transmission of HBV to the fetus is efficient and not rare.

- HBV-infected mothers positive for both hepatitis Bs antigen (HBsAg) and hepatitis Be antigen (HBeAg): high risk for infant to be infected and become chronic carrier.
- Can lead to chronic liver disease or cancer of the liver later in life.
- Prevention of perinatal transmission:
  1. Screen all pregnant women for the presence of HBsAg.

2. Provide Hepatitis B vaccine and Hepatitis B immune globulin (HBIG) to infants born to HB-infected mothers within 12 hours of birth to protect them from infection.

▶ Carrier state or chronic Hepatitis B

- All HBsAg-positive persons are potentially infective. Chronically infected individuals vary in infectivity from high (HBeAg-positive, elevated (HBV-DNA) to moderate (anti-HBe-positive).
- A chronic carrier of HBV is an individual with the HBsAg-positive serological results in the blood on at least two occasions at least 6 months apart.
- A carrier state may also result following a subclinical undiagnosed exposure and may be unknown to the individual.

▶ Immunity

- Protective immunity follows infection if antibodies (anti-HBsAg) develop to the Hepatitis B surface antigen.
- The antibody may be present, although unknown, whether immunity was acquired following a subclinical, or otherwise unrecognized case of Hepatitis B.

B. Prevention

▶ HBVs cause serious illness, including acute and chronic hepatitis, cirrhosis, and liver cancer, sometimes leading to disability and death.

▶ Hepatitis B is a critical occupational hazard for dental personnel because of their close association with the potentially infected body fluids of patients.

▶ Every healthcare individual requires immunization so that the possibilities of disease acquisition and transmission can be minimized.

C. Preventive Methods

▶ Prenatal testing of all pregnant women for HBsAg to identify household contacts who need to be vaccinated.

▶ Universal immunization of infants and children to be accomplished during routine healthcare visits when vaccinations are usually administered. Hepatitis vaccine can be combined with other childhood immunizations to reduce the number of injections.

▶ Immunization of adolescents and adults, particularly those at high risk. Eventually, as the universal vaccination of children continues, adult requirements will be lessened.

▶ Enforce blood bank control measures.

- Screening of donors; reject individuals with history of viral hepatitis, drug addiction, recent transfusion or tattoo, and travelers from HBV endemic areas.
- Strict testing for all donated blood.

▶ Enforce use of disposable syringes and needles.

- For acupuncture, skin testing, parenteral inoculations, body piercing
- Education of public to expect certain standards.

D. Active Immunization: the Vaccines

▶ Effective Hepatitis B vaccines have been available since 1982 for preexposure and postexposure prophylaxis.

▶ All vaccines act to stimulate antibodies and convey immunity.

II. Hepatitis C[8]

A serologic test for antibody to HCV became available in 1991, and routine blood screening was implemented in 1992.

A. Transmission

▶ Hepatitis C is primarily transmitted parenterally and other modes similar to Hepatitis B.

▶ Transmission rarely occurs from mucous membrane exposures to blood, and no transmission has been documented from intact or nonintact skin exposures to blood.

▶ Environmental contamination with blood containing HCV is not a significant risk for transmission in the healthcare setting.

▶ Although infrequent, sexual transmission of HCV can occur especially among HIV-infected persons.

B. Prevention

▶ Education and behavior modification is essential since no vaccine is available for Hepatitis C.

▶ Strict attention to standard infection control procedures for all healthcare personnel.

▶ Measures recommended for Hepatitis B can be applied to Hepatitis C.

III. Hepatitis D[8]

The Hepatitis D virus, also called the delta agent, cannot cause infection except in the presence of HBV infection.

A. Transmission

▶ Delta infection is superimposed on HBsAg carriers.

▶ Occurs primarily in persons who have had multiple exposures to HBV, patients with hemophilia, and intravenous drug users.

▶ Transmission is similar to HBV; by direct exposure to contaminated blood and serous body fluids, contaminated needles and syringes, sexual contacts, and perinatal transfer.[9]

B. Prevention

▶ All measures to prevent Hepatitis B will prevent delta hepatitis because HDV is dependent on the presence of HBV.

▶ Immunization with Hepatitis B vaccine also protects the recipient from Hepatitis D infection.

HERPES VIRUS DISEASES

▶ Herpes viruses are endemic worldwide, with over 95% of the adult population infected.

▶ Each virus causes a wide variety of disease entities that are highly infectious.

▶ Herpes virus diseases are a significant public health problem because of the lack of effective therapeutics and vaccines.

▶ Of the many identified herpes viruses, the eight major types that are known to infect humans are listed in Table 4-3 with abbreviations and some of the infections they cause.

I. General Characteristics

▶ Herpes viruses produce diseases with latent, recurrent, and sometimes malignant tendencies.

- For example, herpes simplex virus type 2 (HSV-2) has been implicated in cervical cancer; herpes simplex virus type 1 (HSV-1) in oral cancer, and Epstein–Barr virus (EBV; HHV-4) has been implicated in various types of cancer.[10]

▶ Herpes viruses travel along sensory nerve pathways to specific ganglia where they may remain latent and become reactivated to produce recurrent infection after certain stimuli or when the body's immunity is significantly lowered.

- HSV-1 travels to the trigeminal ganglion (Figure 4-3).
- HSV-2 goes to the thoracic, lumbar, and sacral dorsal root ganglia.
- Varicella–zoster virus (VZV) travels to the sensory ganglia of the vagal, spinal, or cranial nerves.

▶ Immunosuppressed patients have more frequent and severe herpes infections.

▶ Herpes viruses are among the opportunistic organisms in HIV/AIDS.

II. Relation to Periodontal Infections[11]

▶ Human herpes viruses (HHVs) occur in periodontitis pockets with relatively high prevalence.

▶ Herpes virus-positive periodontitis lesions involving cytomegalovirus (CMV), EBV, and other herpes viruses have higher levels of periodontopathic bacteria. An association exists between active infection of CMV and EBV and dual infection with CMV and EBV and periodontitis.[11]

▶ HHV-1, HHV-6, HHV-7, and HHV-8 have also been detected in some periodontal lesions.[11]

▶ Infection with herpes viruses can suppress a patient's immunity. As a result, subgingival overgrowth of opportunistic periodontal pathogens can occur and periodontal disease symptoms can be more severe.

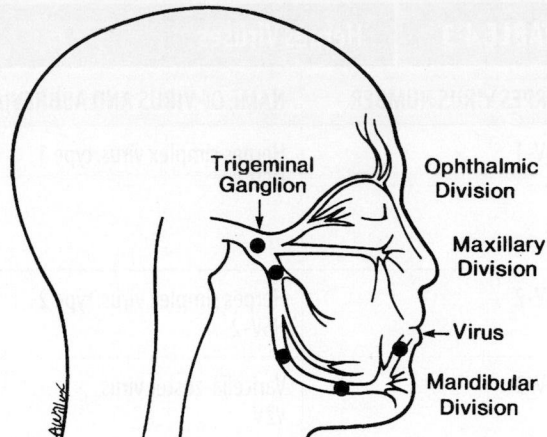

FIGURE 4-3 Latent Infection of Herpes Simplex Virus. Path of the virus traced from point of viral penetration on lip to establishment of latent infection in the trigeminal ganglion.

III. Clinical Management for Herpes[12]

▶ Terminology may be a problem, so such terms as "fever blisters" or "cold sores" need to be used to ensure patient understanding and reduce alarm.

▶ Postpone appointment with patient with active lesion.

▶ Explain the contagious nature of the disease:

- Limit personal contact with others while the lesion is active, especially saliva transfer.
- Stress the importance of meticulous hygiene.

▶ Prodromal stage can be the most transmissible to other patients and clinicians.

- Autoinoculation possible from instrumentation that can splash viruses to the patient's eye or extend the lesion to the nose.
- Irritation to the lesions can prolong the course and increase the severity of the infection.

A. HHV-1 (HSV-1)

Infection with HSV-1 is widespread, and it is estimated that up to 95% of adults have antibodies to the virus.

- Primary infection usually occurs in children but may occur at any age, and especially in the immunocompromised.[11]
- Antibodies (anti-HSV) are produced but do not guarantee immunity to recurrent herpes or to other herpesvirus infections.
- Sulcular epithelium can serve as a reservoir for the viruses. Anti-HSV is present in the gingival sulcus fluid. Trauma to the oral area during a dental or dental hygiene appointment may trigger a herpetic recurrence.

▶ Primary herpetic gingivostomatitis

- Many cases of primary infection with HSV-1 are asymptomatic or mild and isolated to marginal and attached gingiva.

TABLE 4-3	Herpes Viruses	
HERPES VIRUS NUMBER	**NAME OF VIRUS AND ABBREVIATION**	**INFECTIONS**
HHV-1	Herpes simplex virus, type 1 HSV-1	Herpetic gingivostomatitis Herpes labialis Herpetic whitlow Herpetic conjunctivitis
HHV-2	Herpes simplex virus, type 2 HSV-2	Genital herpes
HHV-3	Varicella-zoster virus VZV	Chicken pox Shingles
HHV-4	Epstein–Barr virus EBV	IM Oral hairy leukoplakia Burkitt's lymphoma Lymphoepithelial cysts of parotid gland Lymphatic cancers Nasophyarngeal cancers Periapical lesions Periodontal disease severity
HHV-5	Human cytomegalovirus CMV	Asymptomatic infections Severe Associated with periapical pathosis and increased severity of periodontal diseases along with EBV and HSV Immunosuppressed persons: CMV retinitis, neurologic deficiencies, pneumonia, encephalitis
HHV-6	Herpes lymphotropic virus (HLV) HPV-6A HPV-6B	HBV-6A lymphopoliferative disorders HBV-6B Roseola (*exanthem infantum*) Immune system suppression Seen in HIV-periodontitis with EBV
HHV-7	Human herpes virus 7 HHV-7	Primary infection in childhood Asymptomatic or Roseola-like macular cutaneous eruptions Infection may occur following bone marrow and solid organ transplants
HHV-8	Kaposi's sarcoma–related virus KSRV or KS	Development of KS

- Acute herpetic gingivostomatitis is the most common pattern of symptomatic primary herpetic infection.
- Full-blown herpetic gingivostomatitis presents with widespread oral ulcers that also may involve the pharyngeal areas.
- When clinical disease is evident, gingivostomatitis and pharyngitis are the most frequent manifestations, with fever, malaise, severe pain often interfering with the ability to eat, and lymphadenopathy for 2–7 days.
- Painful oral vesicular lesions may occur on the gingiva, mucosa, tongue, and lips.
- Manifestations may vary from mild to severely debilitating.

- A patient may be a subclinical carrier, and reactivation from the trigeminal ganglia (Figure 4-3) may be followed by asymptomatic excretion of the viruses in the saliva.
- Reactivation may also lead to herpetic ulcerations of the lip, the typical "cold sore."
▶ Herpes labialis (cold sore, fever blister)[13]
- Both HSV-1 and HSV-2 cause genital and oral facial infections that cannot be distinguished clinically, although they are antigenically different.
- HSV-1 is spread predominantly through infected lesions in oral and ocular areas, and is found in mucous membranes and skin above the waist.
- Recurrent HSV symptomatic lesions are common and may occur at or near the primary lesion at the

vermillion border of the lower lip. Triggers include trauma, stress, sunlight, illness, or any conditions that deplete the patient's immune system.[12]

- Dental and dental hygiene appointments with associated emotional stress and oral trauma involved may be triggers of HSV lesions.
- Six to 24 hours before the lesion appears, pain, burning, slight stinging, or sensations of localized warmth and erythema of the affected epithelium with slight swelling serve as a forewarning. A group of vesicles forms, eventually ruptures, and crusting follows; healing may take up to 10 days.
- Lesions are infectious; the shedding virus may lead to autoinfection of the eye, mucous membranes or fingers, and infection of other people.

▶ Herpetic whitlow
- Herpetic whitlow is the herpes simplex infection of the fingers that results from the virus entering through minor skin abrasions most frequently around a fingernail.
- Whitlow was common among DHCP before wearing gloves became a requirement; standard precautions have almost eliminated the incidence of whitlow among DHCP.

▶ Ocular/ophthalmic herpes
- Herpes simplex lesions in the eye can be a primary or recurrent infection of HSV-1 or HSV-2.
- Transmission can occur from splashing saliva or fluid from a vesicular lesion directly into an unprotected eye.
- Prevent ocular herpetic infection by using standard precautions and the use of proper personal protection including eye covering for both clinician and patient.

B. HHV-2 (HSV-2)[13]

▶ HSV-2 is commonly known as genital herpes, but it also occurs as an oral and perioral infection.

▶ *Neonatal herpes* is a serious disease that can cause delayed mental development, blindness, neurological problems, and death to the newborn infected during childbirth.
- Obstetricians may recommend delivery by cesarean section to women with active genital herpes to avoid transmission to the infant.

▶ Antiviral therapy can suppress HSV-2 lesions. The latency of the virus never can be eradicated.

C. HHV-3 (VZV)[9]

▶ Chickenpox (varicella) and shingles (herpes zoster) are caused by the same virus, the VZV.

▶ Chickenpox is the primary infection, with latency occurring.

▶ Reactivation may occur many years later in the form of herpes zoster or shingles.

▶ Chickenpox/Varicella infection
- Chickenpox is an extremely contagious childhood disease.
- Transmission occurs by respiratory droplets and direct skin contact with articles soiled by discharges from the vesicles and the respiratory tract.
- Chickenpox can be life threatening in children who are immunocompromised, such as those with HIV infection.
- Live attenuated vaccine has been available in the United States since 1995 and has reduced reported infections.
- Primarily a disease of children, chickenpox may occur in adults not previously exposed; adults have a more serious course of illness with more complications.

▶ Shingles/Zoster infection[9]
- Chickenpox leaves a lasting immunity, but the VZV remains latent in the dorsal root ganglia.
- Reactivation in adulthood may result from immunosuppression such as from drug therapy or HIV/AIDS infection, and in people with advanced neoplastic disease.
- Lifetime risk for herpes zoster is highest in the elderly and immunocompromised persons; prevalence increases with age.
- A live attenuated VZV vaccine, Zostavax, approved for use in adults 60 years of age and older, greatly reduces prevalence as well as morbidity and mortality of the disease.[9]

D. HHV-4 (EBV)[10]

The EBV is one of the most common human viruses; many cases may be asymptomatic. EBV has been associated with a variety of diseases (Table 4-3); it can remain latent and become reactivated, if the immune system is compromised.

▶ Infectious mononucleosis (IM)
- Mononucleosis is a symptomatic disease caused by infection with the EBV.
- Viruses can be excreted through the saliva even when the patient has no symptoms of disease; there may be a long period of communicability or a lasting carrier state.[10]
- Prevention: minimize contact with saliva by frequent handwashing, avoiding drinking from a common container; standard precautions by DHCP.

▶ Oral hairy leukoplakia
- EBV replicates within epithelial cells in oral hairy leukoplakia; it is considered a marker for immunosuppression.
- Oral hairy leukoplakia can be identified in HIV-infected individuals by the clinical appearance of white linear patches along the lateral border of the tongue.

E. HHV-5 (CMV)[14]

CMV infections are widespread with the most severe disease develops in infants infected *in utero* and in immunocompromised patients, including HIV/AIDS.

▶ Transmission
  - Respiratory droplets, especially among children. Children attending day care have a high prevalence of CMV infection.
  - Blood transfusion: cause of posttransfusion mononucleosis.
  - Posttransplant infection: for solid organs and bone marrow.
  - Sexual transmission through semen, vaginal fluid, or saliva.

▶ Neonatal transmission
  - Virus from the mother's primary or recurrent infection can infect the infant *in utero*, in the birth canal, or through breast milk.
  - CMV infection in a fetus may lead to a child that is premature, is anemic, or has mental disabilities, microcephaly, motor disabilities, deafness, or chronic liver disease.

▶ Prevention
  - Personal hygiene: handwashing.
  - Utilization of standard precautions by healthcare personnel.
  - Seropositivity of donor checked before organ transplant and other surgery.

F. HHV-6 Herpes Lymphotropic Virus (HLV)

▶ Widespread distribution among humans; prevalence of close to 90% by age 5 in the United States.[12]
▶ HHV-6 has been classified as HHV-6A and HHV-6B.[15]
▶ HHV-6A is generally associated with lymphopoliferative disorders and central nervous system disorders in immunocompromised patients.
▶ HHV-6B is related to *Roseola infantum*; the clinical infection presents in children ages 6 months to 2 years and produces a high fever and rash.
▶ Commonly isolated from saliva and transmitted by respiratory droplets.
▶ Primary infection is usually asymptomatic; latency in CD4 T lymphocytes HLV-6 persists indefinitely.
▶ HHV-6 can produce a variety of neurologic diseases, including encephalitis and febrile seizures.
▶ Reactivation depresses the immune system; depletes CD4 lymphocytes; may be a cofactor in HIV/AIDS progression.[15]
▶ Reactivation can also occur after bone marrow transplantation and solid organ transplants, and may be complicated by rejection of the transplant.

G. HHV-7 (HHV)

▶ Closely related to HHV-6, prevalent in the general population; reactivation of latent infection is common in immunocompromised persons.
▶ Primary infection, very common in childhood, is usually asymptomatic.
▶ Symptomatic disease causes roseola-like macular cutaneous eruption.
▶ Infection may occur following bone marrow and solid organ transplants.
▶ Periodontal connection: gingival tissue may serve as a reservoir for HHV-7; high prevalence of HHV-7 was detected in both periodontally diseased and in healthy gingival tissue.[11]

H. HHV-8 Kaposi's Sarcoma–related Herpesvirus (KSRV)

▶ Human herpesvirus-8 (HHV-8) seroprevalence among the general population in the United States is 1% to 5% and is much greater among men with male sexual partners (20% to 77%).[16]
▶ HHV-8 is found in saliva and genital secretions.[11]
▶ HHV-8 is associated with all forms of Kaposi's sarcoma (KS).
▶ KS is considered an AIDS-defining lesion. The overall incidence of KS has dropped significantly since effective antiretroviral therapy has become available.
▶ In persons with normal immune system, primary infection is usually asymptomatic.
▶ Associated symptoms occurring primarily in the immunocompromised patient include fever, rash, lymphadenopathy, bone marrow failures, and occasional rapid progression to KS.[16]

HUMAN PAPILLOMA VIRUS (HPV)[17]

▶ There are over 100 types of HPV and it is the most commonly transmitted infection.
▶ There are 40 types of HPV that may infect the genital areas of men and women. These HPV's can also infect the mouth and throat.
▶ Types 16 and 18 are oncogenic and cause 70% of cervical cancers; they are also associated with anogenital cancers in men and women, and some oropharyngeal cancers.
▶ Ninety percent of genital wart cases are caused by types 6 and 11.
▶ HPV testing
  - HPV testing is available for women undergoing cervical cancer screening.

- HPV prevention
  - A three-dose vaccination against the high risk HPV's 6, 11, 16, and 18 is available.
  - The CDC recommends vaccination for girls and boys aged 11 or 12, and for males and females aged 13–26 if they did not receive vaccination when they were younger.
  - Vaccination is also recommended for men who have sex with men and men with compromised immune systems through age 26 if they did not receive vaccination when they were younger.

HIV/AIDS INFECTION[18]

- AIDS is a severe pandemic disease caused by infection with the HIV.
- HIV was first recognized in 1981 as a cluster of diseases that were characterized by a loss of cellular immunity.
- The major types of HIV are HIV-1 and HIV-2. HIV-1 is more prevalent in the United States and Europe and has been extensively researched and is the primary focus of this chapter.
- HIV-2 was isolated in West Africa and later in Europe and North America and has been shown to have similar characteristics as HIV-1, although pathogenicity and transmission may be slightly lower.
- The HIV diseases are slow, progressive, often lethal diseases with the ability to persist within cells such as macrophages for long periods.
  - Manifestations of HIV range from mild abnormalities in immune response without apparent signs and symptoms to a variety of life-threatening infections and malignant conditions.

- Box 4-2 provides abbreviations and terminology relating to HIV-1 infection and AIDS.

I. Transmission[19]

- All bodily secretions of a patient with HIV infection contain HIV.
  - Only blood, semen, vaginal secretions, and breast milk contain sufficient amounts of the virion to transmit infection.
- *Blood transfusion* was a source of HIV infection before availability of serological testing (1985). In developing countries where testing is not available, transfusions still may be a significant source of HIV transmission and a problem for travelers.
- Modes of transmission
  - Sexual contact accounts for the majority of cases of transmission in adults.
  - Exposure to blood and blood products.
  - Perinatal (vertical transmission)
    - *In utero*: HIV can be effectively transmitted across the placenta.
    - During delivery: the passage through an infected birth canal.
    - Breast-feeding increases transmission risk.

II. Serological Tests[20]

- **Serological** tests for antibodies to HIV have been commercially available since 1985.
  - EIA or ELISA (enzyme-linked immunosorbent assay) is the most commonly used screening tests.
- Confirmatory testing includes the Western blot (WB) or indirect fluorescent antibody test.

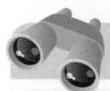

BOX 4-2   ABBREVIATIONS AND KEY WORDS FOR HIV/AIDS

AIDS: acquired immunodeficiency syndrome.

AZT (ZDV): zidovudine, retrovir; drug used for the treatment of HIV infection and AIDS; first antiviral drug approved by the United States Food and Drug Administration (FDA).

CD4+: T-helper lymphocyte; primary target cell for HIV infection; CD4+ count decreases with the severity of HIV-related illness.

DNA: deoxyribonucleic acid; a nucleic acid found in a cell nucleus; a carrier of genetic information.

HAART: highly active antiretroviral therapy containing several antiretroviral medications; the combination has been more effective than monotherapy in the treatment of HIV.

HIV: human immunodeficiency virus; causes AIDS.

HIV antibody: antibody to human immunodeficiency virus; antibody can be detected in the blood 6–8 weeks after infection.

IDU: injection-drug user.

KS: Kaposi's sarcoma; a malignant vascular tumor; an opportunistic neoplasm that may occur in people with HIV infection.

LAV: lymphadenopathy-associated virus; one of the former names for HIV.

MMWR: *Morbidity and Mortality Weekly Report*; publication of the United States Centers for Disease Control and Prevention (CDCP), Atlanta, GA.

OHL: oral hairy leukoplakia.

PCP: pneumocystis pneumonia; caused by *Pneumocystis jirovecii* an OI that occurs in people with HIV infection.

PGL: persistent generalized lymphadenopathy.

PWA: person with AIDS.

RNA: ribonucleic acid; a nucleic acid found in cytoplasm and in the nuclei of certain cells; RNA directs the synthesis of proteins and replaces DNA as a carrier of genetic codes in some viruses.

▶ The ELISA and WB cannot detect HIV infection during the acute phase and many infections are erroneously reported as negative.

▶ A new test HIV laboratory immunoassays (HIV IA) can detect acute HIV infection.

▶ Count of T-helper cells (CD4+) or percentage is the most used marker to evaluate the progression of HIV infection and to help clinicians make treatment decisions.

A. Clinical Course of HIV-1 Infection[21]

▶ Incubation period

- Detection of the antibody in the blood, or seroconversion, occurs within 6 weeks to 6 months after exposure to the HIV virus. The presence of the antibody indicates HIV infection.
- Viral production is high throughout all stages of the infection.
- Incubation period from establishment of infection to the appearance of symptoms of AIDS may be 15 years or longer.

▶ Acute seroconversion syndrome (primary HIV infection)

- CD4+ T lymphocytes more than 500.
- Within 2–3 weeks of infection, flulike symptoms varying from mild to profound may appear: symptoms may be vague so a diagnosis of HIV is not made.
- Detectable HIV antibody (anti-HIV) as a serum marker of the infection may be found.

▶ Early symptomatic HIV disease

- CD4+ T lymphocytes 200–500 cells; continued increase in viremia.
- Systemic symptoms are night sweats, weight loss, diarrhea, fever, malaise, general weakness.
- Opportunistic infections (OI) begin to occur.
- Oral lesions become more common; candidiasis may be predictive of the development of full-blown AIDS in untreated patients within 2 years.

▶ Late-stage disease: AIDS

- CD4+ cell count falls below 200.
- *Pneumocystis jirovecii* pneumonia (PCP) is a presenting feature with other AIDS-defining diseases.
- Presentation of full-blown AIDS is highly variable and is affected by the host's prior exposure to chronic infections and treatment.

▶ Symptoms: AIDS indicating conditions[21]

- CD4+ numbers decline.
- Approximately 16% of HIV-infected persons aged over 13 in the United States are unaware they are infected with HIV[22] and OI are often initial indicator of disease.
- OI become more frequent, extensive, and severe.
- AIDS–dementia complex occurs; often as progressive encephalopathy with significant neurologic dysfunction.

- TB infection: risk for progression from latent to active TB in HIV-infected individual is greater than in the general population.
- Constitutional disease: HIV wasting syndrome: long-term fever, severe weight loss, anemia, chronic diarrhea, and chronic weakness are all effects of loss of immune response and repeated opportunistic diseases.
- Neoplasms: several neoplasms, related to the underlying immunodeficiency, are common indicators of HIV-1 infection and AIDS including KS (HHV-8), primary B-cell lymphoma of the brain, non-Hodgkin's lymphoma, and cervical or rectal carcinoma.
- Untreated, the disease usually progresses to death in 1–3 years.

B. Oral Manifestations of HIV-1 Infection[23]

▶ Oral manifestations are significant indicators of HIV infection and markers of disease progression. The etiology of oral lesions associated with HIV/AIDS is listed in Table 4-4.

▶ Integrate with patient history for early recognition and referral for medical evaluation and testing.

▶ Early intervention is possible with drugs to slow down the process of the disease, prevent severe complications, and improve long-term quality of life.

- The advent of highly active antiretroviral therapy (HAART) has greatly changed the overall prevalence and patterns of oral manifestations of HIV disease.

Extraoral Examination

A careful extraoral assessment is essential at each appointment.

▶ Lymphadenopathy

- Palpation for enlarged lymph nodes is a routine part of every extraoral examination.
- Persistent generalized lymphadenopathy (PGL) is an early sign of HIV infection and a marker for AIDS progression.

▶ Skin lesions[23]

- KS is an AIDS-defining lesion, early lesions present as subtle purplish discolorations of the skin and oral mucosa and can be among the first signs of HIV infection. KS lesions can grow to considerable size and may be multiple in patients with advanced AIDS.
- Herpes simplex virus (HHV-1 and HHV-2) may present as recurrent herpes labialis; in patients with HIV/AIDS painful, deep blistering lesions, and fever may be manifest.
- Herpes zoster (HHV-3) or shingles lesions and blisters may appear on the head, face, and neck.
- HPV lesions generally occur intraorally but may manifest in the HIV patient as papillomatous lesions or mucosal tags in the labial commissures.

TABLE 4-4	Etiology of Oral Lesions Associated with HIV/AIDS	
FUNGAL INFECTIONS	**VIRAL INFECTIONS**	**BACTERIAL INFECTIONS**
Candida albicans *Candida glabrata* *Candida dubliniensis* Cryptococcosis Histoplasmosis Paracoccidiomycosis Penicilliosis Aspergilosis	Herpes simplex 1 (HHV-1) Herpes simplex 2 (HHV-2) Herpes zoster (HHV-3) Epstein–Barr (HHV-4) CMV (HHV-5) KS (HHV-8) Human papillomavirus (HPV)	*Mycobacterium tuberculosis* (TB) *Mycobacterium avium* Intracellulare Periodontal infections LGE Necrotizing ulcerative gingivitis (NUG) Necrotizing ulcerative periodontitis (NUP)

Intraoral Examination

▶ Fungal infections[23]

- *Candida albicans* is the most common species involved with oral fungal infections, but C. *glabrata* and C. *dubliniesis* may also be present.
- Oral candidiasis frequency and severity increases as HIV disease progresses.
- Candidiasis may be recognized by clinical examination, or the dentist may request the use of exfoliative cytology for definitive diagnosis.
- Although rare, other fungi such as cryptococcosis, histoplasmosis, paracoccidimycosis, penicilliosis, and aspergilosis may be the primary etiology of oral fungal infections.

▶ Viral infections[23]

- Herpes simplex virus (HHV-1 and HHV-2) may present intraorally as deep, painful, blistering lesions. Fever may be present.
- CMV (HHV-5) causes ulceration of oral mucosa and spread to the rest of gastrointestinal tract. Thought to be major cause of retinitis in HIV patients and may cause encephalitis.
- EBV (HHV-4) known to cause hairy leukoplakia. The "hairy" appearance is due to elongated filiform papillae.
- KS Virus (HHV-8) causes purple vascular lesions in the mouth.
- HPV causes papillomatous and sometimes pedunculated lesions of oral mucosa.
- Lesions tend to be more widespread, occur in atypical patterns, and may persist for months.

▶ Bacterial infections: gingival and periodontal infections

- Atypical gingival changes may be an initial indicator of undiagnosed HIV infection.
- Patients with HIV infection who maintain a high level of personal and professional oral care may present with healthier periodontal tissues.
- Periodontal infections associated with HIV infection tend to show more severe symptoms and to progress more rapidly.

- Linear gingival erythema (LGE)
  1. Presents as unusual of pattern of gingivitis with a distinctive band of erythema at the free gingival margin, extending 2–3 mm apically.
  2. LGE occurs independently of oral hygiene status, and does not respond as expected to improved personal biofilm control and periodontal therapy.
- Necrotizing ulcerative gingivitis (NUG) and periodontitis (NUP)
  1. Increased incidence of NUG with marked ulceration.
  2. NUG may progress to involve underlying bone and result in NUP, characterized by rapid attachment loss and severe tissue destruction.
  3. Deep pocketing rarely occurs, the extensive gingival and alveolar bone tissue destruction results in bone sequestrum.
  4. Attachment loss of more than 6 mm within a 6-month period is not uncommon.
- Mycobacterium TB[23]
  1. Mycobacterial infections are estimated to cause 13% of AIDS-related deaths.
  2. In advanced cases of HIV/AIDS extrapulmonary TB is more common and can manifest as oral lesions that may extend into paranasal sinuses.
  3. *Mycobacterium avium intracellulare* infection is rare but may cause oral lesions.
     - Recurrent apthous stomatitis
     - Intramucosal hemorrhages
     - Hyperpigmentation of oral mucosa
     - Necrotizing stomatitis occurs when NUG extends into adjacent soft tissues.

Dental Hygiene Management

▶ The dental hygienist may be the first to suspect HIV infection when oral manifestations and symptoms are recognized; referral for appropriate medical care is indicated.

▶ Dental healthcare professionals are ethically and legally obligated to treat HIV-infected patients of record and other patients seeking treatment. The patients are protected by the American with Disabilities Act.

▶ Assisting HIV-infected patients in maintaining their oral health can significantly improve their quality of life by reducing pain and susceptibility to other OI.

▶ Pain and oral manifestations may be caused by the disease or from adverse drug effects of HAART.

▶ Adverse effects of the primary antiretroviral medication Zidovudine (ZVD/AZT) are nausea and vomiting, which can be severe enough to contribute to dental caries and dental erosion.

▶ Emphasis on immaculate personal oral care and frequent professional periodontal therapy. Fluoride varnish needs to be included in the preventive oral hygiene program for all ages.

C. Prevention of HIV Infection[24,25]

▶ Until a vaccine is available, prevention depends to a large degree on community education for attitudinal and behavioral changes.

▶ Health education efforts need to be focused on awareness of risk, modes of transmission of the HIV, and preventive measures necessary to halt its transmission especially in high-risk groups.

▶ Dental personnel who are well informed with accurate, current information that can provide care for HIV-infected patients give support to community health programs.

Goals

▶ Primary prevention
  • The goal of primary prevention (for those not infected) is to lower the rate at which new cases of HIV infection appear.

• Programs for women, particularly of childbearing age; intravenous drug users who share needles; and teenagers are focused to reach the most vulnerable groups.

• HIV testing is required for all pregnant women and all newborns to control the increasing numbers of children with HIV infection.

• Provide routine testing for HIV as with other diseases.

▶ Secondary prevention
  • The goals of secondary prevention (for seropositive individuals) are to reduce the rate of transmission and to introduce treatment early.
  • Early intervention may postpone severe clinical manifestations of advanced illness.
  • A leading part of the program is to counsel the HIV-infected individuals to practice safe sex and to cooperate with the program to screen and counsel their sexual contacts and families.

Ongoing Programs

▶ Strict testing for blood donors and all tissue organ donors, as well as identification and counseling of recipients of blood transfusions before 1985 and their sexual partners. The incubation period has been shown to be much longer than was originally thought.

▶ With early diagnosis and medical intervention, people with HIV infection can be symptom free and healthy and can live longer than was possible earlier in the epidemic.

METHICILLIN-RESISTANT STAPHYLOCOCCUS AUREUS[26]

▶ *Staphylococcus aureus* is a common cause of infection.

▶ MRSA is a strain of *Staphylococcus aureus* resistant to many antibiotic therapies.

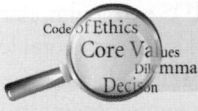

EVERYDAY ETHICS

Mr. Sands, a new patient to the dental hygiene clinic, had completed his admission history and basic examination at a previous appointment. He is assigned to Alison because she needs more credits for patients with heavy calculus. He is scheduled today for his personal instruction for home care, and scaling for the first quadrant.

When Alison starts to read the record before clinic opened, she learns that Mr. Sands has a history of Hepatitis C. She immediately makes up an excuse and asks Leah, her classmate in the clinic unit next to hers, to treat Mr. Sands, while she, Alison, attends to the two pediatric patients scheduled for sealants with Leah. Leah has already prepared for the appointment with the children and needs the four credits toward her sealants requirement, although she also needs credits for a patient with heavy calculus.

Questions for Consideration

1. Which of the dental hygiene Core Values (Table II-1, Section II Introduction) is Alison violating by her actions to avoid caring for this patient?

2. Is this an ethical dilemma or an ethical issue for Leah? How can Leah resolve the problem? What might be the consequences for both if Leah reports Alison's action to the instructor in charge? What if Alison does a similar thing in the future?

3. Using the "Steps in the Resolution of an Issue or a Dilemma" listed in Chapter 1, Box 1-10, determine a course of action that can help Leah resolve the problem.

BOX 4-3

Example Documentation: Patient with Recurrent Apthous Ulcers

S –28-year-old male presents for his regular periodontal maintenance appointment with chief complaint of large and frequently recurring apthous ulcers. Medical history indicates patient has been under care of his physician for 2 years and is being treated for HIV. He is currently taking Combivir (zidovudine + lamivudine) and Invirase (saquinivir) and reports his condition is well controlled with a CD4+ count of 700 and a low viral load. Patient states he has been keeping up with his homecare.

O –Extraoral examination reveals bilateral slightly enlarged lymph nodes. No fever is evident. Intraoral exam reveals several ulcerations of the oral mucosa ranging in size from 2 to 8 mm in diameter. The oropharynx is red with multiple white spots 2–3 mm in diameter. Saliva flow is difficult to stimulate. Oral hygiene: generalized light cervical biofilm. Gingival tissues: generally pink with isolated areas of slight marginal erythema around #6,7,26,27. Periodontal exam: slight BOP #6,7,26,27, probing depths 2–4 mm, no furcations involvement, no pathologic mobility. Radiographic exam: stable bone heights when compared to previous radiographs.

A –The patient is at increased risk for oral and/or systemic complications such as candidiasis, recurrent apthous ulcers, and moderate xerostomia.

P –Discussed etiology of candidiasis and apthous ulcers. Referred patient to his physician for evaluation and treatment of candidiasis and apthous ulcers. Discussed etiology and impacts of xerostomia. Advised patient to reduce frequency of sugar intake and take frequent sips of water. Oral hygiene reviewed and revised to address the areas of erythema and BOP #6,7,26,27. Regular periodontal maintenance was postponed until candidiasis and apthous ulcers have resolved

Signed: _____, RDH

Date: _____

▶ MRSA infections are difficult to treat and can be endemic in hospitals and institutions.

▶ It is associated with acute osteomyelitis, bacteremia, septicemia, cellulitis, conjunctivitis, pneumonia, and toxic shock syndrome.

▶ Infections are spread by direct contact and indirectly by skin scales, fomites, equipment, and the environment.

▶ The incubation period is 4–10 days and the person will remain infectious as long as the infection persists.

▶ Risk factors for acquisition of MRSA include prolonged hospital stay, intensive care, prolonged antimicrobial therapy, and surgical procedures.

DOCUMENTATION

Suggested documentation for the patient with an infectious disease includes the following:

▶ If the patient is under treatment for an infectious condition, note the patient's medication, its purpose, adverse effects, and effects on oral health.

▶ Record all consultations with specialists.

▶ When patient is not being treated, record referral and purpose.

▶ Record results of specific laboratory tests (CD4+ counts, neutrophil counts, and others) that potentially affect dental hygiene treatment; note those values at each appointment.

▶ Box 4-3 provides a sample Progress Note.

Factors To Teach The Patient

▷ Reasons for postponing an appointment when a herpes lesion ("fever blister" or "cold sore") is present on the lip.

▷ Importance of not touching or scratching the herpetic lesion because of self-infection to fingers or eyes.

▷ How the viruses can survive on objects and transfer infection to other people.

▷ How to help by keeping the medical history up to date by informing of additional exposures and immunizations to communicable diseases for self and family members.

▷ Importance of oral health to overall systemic health.

▷ Preparation for a dental or dental hygiene appointment by thorough mouth cleaning with toothbrush and dental floss to lower the bacterial count and thus lessen aerosol contamination in the treatment room.

References

1. Centers for Disease Control and Prevention. *Guidelines for Infection Control in Dental Health-Care Settings.* Atlanta, GA: Epidemiology Program Office; 2003:2–3. http://www.cdc.gov/mmwr/pdf/rr/rr5217.pdf. Accessed August 24, 2013.

2. Socransky SS, Manganiello SD. The oral microbiota of man from birth to senility. *J Periodontol.* 1971;42(8):485–494.

3. Harrel SK, Molinari J. Aerosols and splatter in dentistry: a brief review of the literature and infection control implications. *J Am Dent Assoc.* 2004;135(4):429–437.

4. Larato DC, Ruskin PF, Martin A. Effect of an ultrasonic scaler on bacterial counts in air. *J Periodontol.* 1967;38(6):550.

5. Centers for Disease Control and Prevention. *Guidelines for Infection Control in Dental Health-Care Settings.* Atlanta, GA: Epidemiology Program Office; 2003:28–29. http://www.cdc.gov/mmwr/pdf/rr/rr5217.pdf. Accessed August 24, 2013.

6. Hawker J, Begg N, Blair I, et al. Communicable disease control and health protection handbook. 3rd ed. Somerset, NJ: Wiley-Blackwell; 2012: 229–238.

7. Centers for Disease Control and Prevention. *Guidelines for Preventing the Transmission of Mycobacterium tuberculosis in Health-Care Settings.* Atlanta, GA: Coordinating Center for Health Information and Service; 2005:19–20. http://www.cdc.gov/mmwr/PDF/rr/rr5417.pdf. Accessed August 24, 2013.

8. Hawker J, Begg N, Blair I, et al. Communicable disease control and health protection handbook. 3rd ed. Somerset, NJ: Wiley-Blackwell; 2012: 127–137.

9. Centers for Disease Control and Prevention. *Epstein-Barr Virus and Infectious Mononucleosis.* Atlanta, GA: National Center for Immunization and Respiratory Diseases; 2006.http://www.cdc.gov/ncidod/diseases/ebv.htm.Accessed October 10, 2013.

10. Bilder L, Elimelech R, Machtei E. The prevalence of human herpes viruses in the saliva of chronic periodontitis patients compared to oral health providers and healthy controls. *Arch Virol.* 2013;158(6):1221–1226.

11. Centers for Disease Control and Prevention. Genital Herpes. Atlanta, GA: Division of STD Prevention. http://www.cdc.gov/std/Herpes/STDFact-herpes-detailed.htm. Accessed October 10, 2013.

12. Stoopler E, Kuperstein A, Sollecito T. How do I manage a patient with recurrent herpes simplex? *J Can Dent Assoc.* 2012;78:c154.

13. Centers for Disease Control and Prevention. *Herpes Zoster.* Atlanta, GA: Division of Viral Diseases; 2012. http://www.cdc.gov/shingles/hcp/clinical-overview.html. Accessed October 10, 2013.

14. Centers for Disease Control and Prevention. *Cytomegalovirus and Congenital CMV Infection.* Atlanta, GA: Division of Viral Diseases; 2010. http://www.cdc.gov/cmv/clinical/features.html. Accessed October 10, 2013.

15. Corti M, Villafane M, Trione N, et al. Human herpesvirus 6: report of emerging pathogen in five patients with HIV/AIDS and review of the literature. *Rev Soc Bras Med Trop.* 2011;44(4):522–525.

16. Panel on Opportunistic Infections in HIV-Infected Adults and Adolescents. Guidelines for the prevention and treatment of opportunistic infections in HIV-infected adults and adolescents: recommendations from the Centers for Disease Control and Prevention, the National Institutes of Health, and the HIV Medicine Association of the Infectious Diseases Society of America. http://aidsinfo.nih.gov/contentfiles/lvguidelines/adult_oi.pdf. Accessed October 10, 2013.

17. Centers for Disease Control and Prevention. *Genital HPV Infection Fact Sheet.* Atlanta, GA: Division of STD Prevention. http://www.cdc.gov/std/HPV/STDFact-HPV.htm. Accessed August 25, 2013.

18. Centers for Disease Control and Prevention. *HIV Basics.* Atlanta, GA: Division of STD Prevention; 2013. http://www.cdc.gov/hiv/basics/whatishiv.html. Accessed August 25, 2013.

19. Centers for Disease Control and Prevention. *HIV Transmission.* Atlanta, GA: Division of STD Prevention http://www.cdc.gov/hiv/basics/transmission.html. Accessed August 25, 2013.

20. Centers for Disease Control and Prevention. Detection of acute HIV infection in two evaluations of a new HIV diagnostic testing algorithm — United States, 2011–2013. MMWR; 2013:62(24);489–494. http://www.cdc.gov/mmwr/preview/mmwrhtml/mm6224a2.htm?s_cid=mm6224a2_e.

21. Hawker J, Begg N, Blair I, et al. Communicable disease control and health protection handbook. 3rd ed. Somerset, NJ: Wiley-Blackwell; 2012: 140–147.

22. Centers for Disease Control and Prevention. HIV Surveillance Report, 2013; vol. 25. http://www.cdc.gov/hiv/library/reports/surveillance/. Published February 2015. Accessed April 17, 2015.

23. Johnson NW. The mouth in HIV/AIDS: markers of disease status and management challenges for the dental profession. *Aust Dent J.* 2010;55 (Suppl 1):85–102.

24. Hawker J, Begg N, Blair I, et al. Communicable disease control and health protection handbook. 3rd ed. Somerset, NJ: Wiley-Blackwell; 2012: 145.

25. Centers for Disease Control and Prevention. Sexually transmitted diseases treatment guidelines. MMWR;59 (RR–12):69–78. http://www.cdc.gov/std/treatment/2010/STD-Treatment-2010-RR5912.pdf. Accessed August 25, 2013.

26. Hawker J, Begg N, Blair I, et al. Communicable disease control and health protection handbook. 3rd ed. Somerset, NJ: Wiley-Blackwell; 2012: 172–176.

ENHANCE YOUR UNDERSTANDING

thePoint® DIGITAL CONNECTIONS
(see the inside front cover for access information)

- **Audio glossary**
- **Quiz bank**

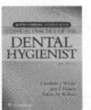

SUPPORT FOR LEARNING
(available separately; visit lww.com)

- *Active Learning Workbook for Clinical Practice of the Dental Hygienist, 12th Edition*

prepU INDIVIDUALIZED REVIEW
(available separately; visit lww.com)

- **Adaptive quizzing with *prepU for Wilkins'* Clinical Practice of the Dental Hygienist**

5

Exposure Control: Barriers for Patient and Clinician

Lori Giblin, RDH, MSDH

CHAPTER OUTLINE

LEARNING OBJECTIVES

After studying this chapter, the student will be able to:

1. Identify and define key terms and concepts related to exposure control, clinical barriers, and latex sensitivity.

2. Explain the rationale and techniques for exposure control.

3. Identify the criteria for selecting effective barriers.

4. Explain the rationale, mechanics, and guidelines for hand hygiene.

5. Identify and describe the clinical manifestations and management of latex sensitivity.

INFECTION CONTROL

▶ Exposure control refers to all procedures during clinical care necessary to provide top-level protection from exposure to infectious agents for members of the dental team and their patients.

▶ Dental healthcare personnel (DHCP) have a professional obligation to serve *all* patients with comprehensive oral care, including patients with known or unknown communicable diseases.

I. Standard Precautions

▶ The practice of *standard precautions* means that the body fluids of all patients are treated as if they were infectious.

- An organized system for exposure control is needed.
- A written exposure control plan is prepared to serve as a guide for the entire team.[1] The written plan can be the basis for training new personnel.
- Consistency between DHCPs is necessary to maintain standards of asepsis and to prevent cross-contamination.
- As new research and commercial products become available, and adopted for use, the written protocol is revised.
- Using the protocol and transferring the objectives and overall aims to the clinical setting are the responsibilities of each member of the dental team.
- Physical barriers and other requirements of the protocol provide safety for both the DHCP and the patients.

▶ Refer to Appendix IV to review specific recommendations from the U.S. Department of Health and Human Services.

▶ Selected terms for the application of exposure control and immunizations are defined in Box 5-1.

PERSONAL PROTECTION FOR THE DENTAL TEAM

The continuing health and productivity of DHCP depend to a large degree on the individuals' efforts to maintain themselves in a high standard of good health as expressed in the Personal Factors in Practice section of Chapter 1. Resistance to disease, if exposed, is enhanced in a person with top-level health habits.

▶ Loss of work time, personal suffering, long-term systemic effects, and even exclusion from continued practice are possible results from communicable disease infection.

▶ The only safe procedure is to practice defensively at all times, with specific precautions for personal protection.

▶ All clinical staff members need to be aware of the signs and symptoms of diseases that are occupational hazards for clinical dental and dental hygiene practitioners.

▶ Seek early diagnosis and treatment of a seemingly minor condition that could be the initial symptom of a more serious communicable disease.

I. Immunizations

Dental personnel in a hospital setting are subject to the rules and regulations for all hospital employees. Policies often require certain immunizations for new employees or proof of antibodies.

▶ In private dental practices, individual initiative is required to maintain standards of safety for all dental team members relative to immunizations.

▶ Immunizations recommended for healthcare workers include:

- Hepatitis B
- Influenza
- MMR (measles, mumps, rubella)
- Pertussis
- Varicella–zoster.

▶ General recommendations on immunizations are reviewed annually by the Advisory Committee on Immunization Practices.[2]

▶ At the time of employment, it is reasonable for a dentist employer to request a record of current immunizations, as well as specific tests, such as for tuberculosis.

▶ The needs differ in different climates, countries, and locations. Persons changing work location, or traveling for participation in dental hygiene programs, need to investigate specific precautions.

II. Maintain Records

▶ Records for personal immunizations are regularly updated.

▶ Obtain tests promptly when exposed to certain infectious diseases and seek prophylactic immunization as indicated and available.

▶ Keep confidential written records of immunizations, boosters, and reimmunizations; plan for regular follow-up.

▶ When the status of current immunizations is known, time is saved by not needing a susceptibility test before initiating passive immunizations when accidental exposure occurs.

CLINICAL ATTIRE

The clinical apparel of clinicians is vulnerable to contamination from splash, spatter, aerosols, and patient contact.

▶ Standard clothing, such as scrubs, and street clothes are not intended to protect against hazardous materials and are not considered protective clothing.[1]

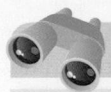 **BOX 5-1** | **KEY WORDS AND ABBREVIATIONS:** Exposure Control

Allergen: substance, protein or nonprotein, capable of inducing allergy or specific hypersensitivity; can enter the body by being inhaled, swallowed, touched, or injected.

Antimicrobial soap: a soap containing an active ingredient against skin microorganisms.

Atopy: clinical hypersensitivity state or allergy with a hereditary predisposition; includes hay fever, eczema, and asthma.

Barrier protection: refers to placing a physical barrier between the patient's body fluids (such as blood and saliva) and the healthcare personnel (HCP) to prevent disease transmission.

Barriers for HCP: include gloves, mask, protective eyewear, and protective clothing (gown).

Barriers for patient: include protective eyewear, head cover during surgeries, and rubber dam during restorative and sealant procedures.

Booster dose: amount of immunogen (vaccine, toxoid, or other antigen preparation), usually smaller than the original amount, injected at an appropriate interval after the primary immunization to sustain the immune response to that immunogen.

CDC: Centers for Disease Control and Prevention.

Exposure incident: a specific eye, mouth, mucous membrane, nonintact skin, or parenteral contact with blood or other potentially infectious material that results from the performance of one's usual professional duties.

Hand hygiene: a general term that applies to either handwashing, antiseptic handwash, antiseptic hand rub, or surgical hand antisepsis.

Hypoallergenic: property of a substance that indicates it does not create a hypersensitive reaction; may apply to various chemicals; not specified on manufacturer's labels.

Immunization: the process of rendering a subject immune to a particular disease by stimulation with a specific antigen to promote antibody formation in the body.

Inoculation: introduction of antigenic material or vaccine; more frequently used to refer to the introduction of material into a culture medium.

Latex allergy: an acquired hypersensitivity reaction to the proteins found in natural rubber latex (NRL).

Occupational exposure: reasonably anticipated skin, eye, mucous membrane, or parenteral contact with blood or other potentially infectious materials that may result from the performance of one's usual duties.

PPD: purified protein derivative for tuberculin intracutaneous skin test for tuberculosis; positive reaction means previous infection with *Mycobacterium tuberculosis.*

Rhinitis: inflammation of the mucous membrane of the nose; may result from infection by bacteria or virus, or may be a seasonal (hay fever) or nonseasonal allergic reaction.

Toxoid: toxin treated by heat or chemical agent to destroy its deleterious properties without destroying its ability to combine with, or stimulate the formation of, antitoxin; examples of toxoids used for active immunization are tetanus and diphtheria.

Tuberculin test (Mantoux): a test for the presence of active or inactive tuberculosis; a positive test is denoted by redness and induration at the injection site by 48–72 hours after injection.

Vaccination: process of introducing a vaccine into the body to produce immunity to a specific disease.

Vaccine: a suspension of attenuated or killed microorganisms administered for the prevention or treatment of an infectious disease.

▶ The recommended clinic attire is designed and cared for in a manner that protects exposure from infectious materials in splatter or aerosols and minimizes cross-contamination.

▶ Clinic attire and shoes are not to be worn outside the clinic practice setting.[1] When clinical attire is worn outside, contamination can be carried from, and brought into, the treatment area.

I. Protective Clothing

▶ Protective clothing, such as gowns or jackets, are designed to be worn over clinical attire to protect skin and prevent cross-contamination from blood and other potentially infectious materials.

▶ Gowns and jackets are expected to be clean and maintained as free as possible from contamination.

▶ The gown or jacket is closed at the neck and fastened in back.

▶ The fabric is disposable or reusable, stain and fluid resistant, can be washed commercially, and withstand washing with bleach.

▶ The garment must cover the knees when the patient is seated during treatment.

▶ Long sleeves with fitted cuffs permit protective gloves to extend over the cuffs.

▶ Gloved hands, prepared for patient treatment, are kept from touching objects or being placed in pockets.

▶ In addition, a washable or a disposable apron may be used over the gown or laboratory coat when clinical procedures involving blood, spatter, or aerosols are performed.

▶ If soaked or soiled by infectious materials, change protective clothing immediately.

▶ When protective clothing is removed, turn inside out to prevent exposure to infectious material

II. Hair and Head Covering

▶ Hair is worn off the shoulders and fastened back away from the face.

• Because the hair is exposed to contamination, an appropriate head cover is advised when using handpieces and ultrasonic or air-powder polishing instruments that create aerosols.

▶ Facial hair needs to be covered with a face mask and face shield.

USE OF FACE MASK: RESPIRATORY PROTECTION

Basic personal barrier protection is composed of face mask, protective eyewear, and gloves.

▶ The use of the face mask is described first because it needs to be positioned first when preparing for clinical care procedures.

▶ The protective eyewear is placed second. After that, hand hygiene[3] is performed before gloving.

I. Aerosols

▶ Dispersion of particles of debris, polishing agents, calculus, and water, all of which are contaminated by the patient's oral flora, occurs regularly during treatment procedures.

▶ Aerosols are created following the use of a handpiece, prophylaxis angle, or a power-driven ultrasonic scaler.

▶ Particles can spread on the face, protective eyewear, uniform, and on the barrier placed over the patient for protection from the spray.

II. Mask Efficiency

A. Criteria: Essential Characteristics (Box 5-2)

▶ *Filtration* (measured in BFE = bacterial filtration efficiency):

• The American Society for Testing and Materials uses a standard test method for evaluating the BFE of medical face masks. The BFE is a measurement of the masks resistance to bacteria.

• Use a surgical mask that will cover the nose and mouth with >95% BFE.[3]

BOX 5-2

Characteristics of an Ideal Mask

1. No contact with the wearer's nostrils or lips.
2. Has a high BFE rate.
3. Fits snugly around the entire edges of the mask.
4. No fogging of eyewear.
5. Convenient to put on and remove.
6. Made of material that does not irritate skin or induce allergic reaction.
7. Does not collapse during wear or when wet.

• Airborne droplets smaller than 3–5 μm in size can reach the alveoli of the lower respiratory track and may potentially cause infection.[4]

• Droplet nuclei (*Mycobacterium tuberculosis*) range from 0.5 to 1 μm and are a risk in healthcare settings.[5]

▶ *Fit*: Proper fit over face is vital to protect against inhaling droplet nuclei from aerosols.

▶ *Moisture absorption*: Soak through is an important factor. Lining needs to be impervious.

▶ *Comfort*: Degree of comfort encourages compliance in wearing.

B. Materials

▶ Various materials have been used for masks, including:
• Gauze and other cloth
• Plastic foam
• Fiberglass
• Synthetic fiber mat
• Paper

▶ Foam, paper, and cloth have been shown to be the least adequate filters of aerosols, whereas glass fiber and synthetic fiber mat were shown to be the most effective.[6,7]

▶ Particulate respirator mask (PRM)

• Use National Institute for Occupational Safety and Health (NIOSH) certified PRM (e.g., N95, N99, or N100), for potentially infectious patient (active tuberculosis) when ventilation is poor, and procedure likely to produce droplet spatter or aerosols of oral or respiratory fluids.[5]

• Heavy-duty mask designed with a tight fit.

III. Use of a Mask

▶ Adjust the mask and position eyewear before hand hygiene.

▶ Use a new mask for each patient.

• Change mask each hour during routine procedures or more frequently when it becomes wet.

▶ Keep the mask on after completing a procedure while still in the presence of aerosols.

• Particles 1–5 μm can remain suspended for hours and can be inhaled directly into terminal lung alveoli.[8]

• Removal of a mask in the treatment room immediately following the use of aerosol-producing procedures permits direct exposure to airborne organisms.

▶ Mask removal

• Grasp side elastic or tie strings to remove (Figure 5-1).

• Never handle the outside of a contaminated mask with gloved or bare hands. Never place the mask under the chin.

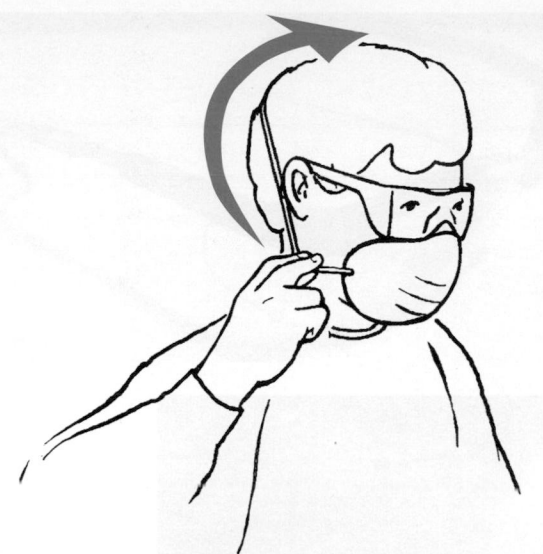

FIGURE 5-1 **Removal of Mask.** Handle only by the elastic or tie strings, carefully avoiding the contaminated mask.

USE OF PROTECTIVE EYEWEAR

Eye protection for the dental team members and patients is necessary to prevent physical injuries and infections of the eyes.

▶ Severe and disabling eye accidents and infections have been reported.[9-11]

▶ Eye involvement may lead to pain, discomfort, loss of work time, and, in certain instances, permanent injury.

▶ Accidents can occur at any time, and as with most accidents, they occur when least prepared for or expected.

▶ Eye infections can follow the accidental dropping of an instrument on the face or the splashing of various materials from a patient's oral cavity into the eye.

▶ Contamination can be introduced from saliva, biofilm, carious material, pieces of old restorative materials during cavity preparation, bacteria-laden calculus during scaling, and any other microorganisms contained in aerosols or spatter.

▶ Careful, deliberate techniques and instrument management, with evacuation and other procedures for the control of oral fluids, contribute to the prevention of accidents and infections of the eyes.

▶ All measures described for the prevention of airborne disease transmission by aerosols and spatter apply to eye protection.

▶ The most effective defense is the use of protective eyewear by all involved—dental team members and patients.

I. Indications for Use of Protective Eyewear

A. Dental Team Members

▶ Protective eyewear is worn for all procedures.

▶ Dental personnel who do not require corrective lens for vision wear protective eyewear with clear lens.

B. General Features of Acceptable Eyewear

▶ Sufficient eye coverage, with side shields, to protect around the eye.

▶ Shatterproof; made of strong, sturdy plastic.

▶ Lightweight.

▶ Flexible and with rounded smooth edges to prevent discomfort.

▶ Easily disinfected.
  • Smooth surface areas to prevent accumulation of infectious material.
  • Disinfectant used cannot damage or distort the frames or lens.

▶ A clear or lightly tinted lens, rather than a very dark lens, permits the dental team members to watch the patient's reactions and maintain contact and response.

▶ Desirable but not required: scratch resistant, antifog, and antistatic.

C. Types of Eyewear

Many styles, including regular eyeglass shapes and those described as follows, have been used.

▶ *Goggles:* Shielding on all sides of the glasses may give the best protection, provided they fit closely around the edges. Goggle-style coverage is necessary for protection during laboratory work.

▶ *Eyewear with side shields* (Figure 5-2A): A side shield can provide added protection. For the member of the dental team who depends on a prescription lens, separate side shields are available that can be connected to the bows.

▶ *Eyewear with curved frames* (Figure 5-2B): When the sides of the eyewear are curved back, they may provide a protection somewhat similar to that offered by those with the side shield.

▶ *Postmydriatic spectacles used by ophthalmologist:* Disposable glasses are available that are made of anti-UV flexible plastic (Figure 5-2C).

▶ *Dental loupes* (Figure 5-2D): Designed to protect the eyes and magnify the oral cavity. When they are designed with a light or flip-up, do not touch during clinical procedures.

▶ *Child-sized:* Child-sized sunglasses and children's play spectacles have been used.

D. Face Shield

▶ A clinician needs to wear a face shield over a regular mask when aerosol-producing handpiece, power scaler, or power polishing equipment is used.

E. Protective Eyewear for Patients

▶ Protective eyewear is essential for each patient at each appointment. A patient who has not been asked

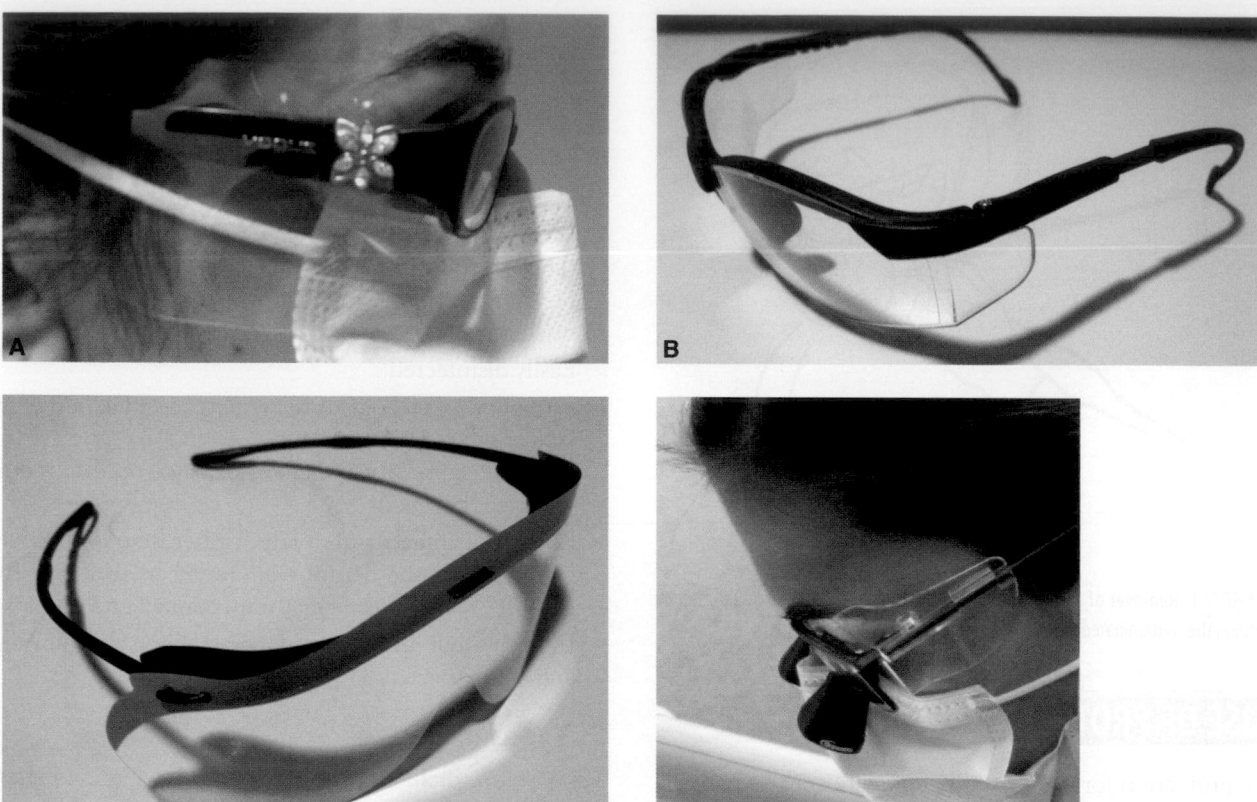

FIGURE 5-2 Protective Eyewear. Protective cover for both patient and clinician may be goggles-style (**A**) glasses with side shields, (**B**) safety glasses, (**C**) disposable eyewear, and (**D**) loupes.

to wear protective eyewear at previous appointments will appreciate a simple explanation of the reasons for doing so.

▶ Patients with their own prescription lenses may prefer to wear them, but for the safety of the patient's glasses, the use of the protective eyewear provided in the office or clinic may be advisable.

▶ Protection against glare. Certain patients may request tinted lenses or prefer to wear their own sunglasses when their eyes are especially sensitive to the dental light.

II. Suggestions for Clinical Application

A. Contact Lenses

▶ Dental team members and patients who wear contact lenses always need to wear protective eyewear over them during dental and dental hygiene procedures.

B. Care of Protective Eyewear

▶ Rinse eyewear under running water to remove abrasive particles. Rubbing an abrasive agent over the plastic lens can create scratches.

▶ Materials used for protective lens may be damaged by some disinfectants. Clean with detergent and rinse thoroughly. Air-dry.

▶ Check periodically for scratches on the lens, and replace appropriately.

C. Eye Wash Station

▶ Eye wash station equipment needs to be attached to a sink not used by clinicians for patient preparation.

▶ It must not be connected to the regular faucets unless the hot water source is turned off permanently.

HAND CARE

▶ In the infectious process of disease transmission, the hands may serve as a *means of transmission* of the blood, saliva, and dental biofilm from a patient.

▶ The hands, especially under the fingernails, may serve as a *reservoir* for microorganisms.

▶ *Skin breaks in the hands may serve as a port of entry* for potentially pathogenic microorganisms.

▶ By caring properly for the hands, using effective hand-hygiene procedures, and following the basic rules for gloving, primary cross-contamination can be controlled.

▶ A conscious effort is made to keep the gloved hands from touching objects other than the instruments and disinfected parts of the equipment prepared for the immediate patient.

I. Bacteriology of the Skin

▶ Resident bacteria

- Many relatively stable bacteria inhabit the surface epithelium or deeper areas in the ducts of skin glands or depths of hair follicles; ultimately, they are shed with the exfoliated surface cells, or with excretions of the skin glands.
- Resident bacteria tend to be less susceptible to destruction by disinfection procedures.

▶ Transient bacteria

- Transient bacteria reflect continuous contamination by routine contacts; some bacteria are pathogens.
- They may be washed away or, in the event that a skin break exists, may cause an autogenous infection.
- Most transients can be removed with soap and water by washing thoroughly or with 60–95% ethanol or isopropanol-based hand rubs as directed by manufacturer.

II. Hand Care

A. Fingernails

▶ Maintain clean, smoothly trimmed, short fingernails with well-cared-for cuticles to prevent breaks where microorganisms can enter.

▶ Effects of short nails:

- Make handwashing more effective because of fewer microorganisms harbored under the nails.[12]
- Prevent cuts from long nail in disposable gloves.
- Permit selection of a closer fit of glove; longer glove fingers may be required to protect nails.
- Allow greater dexterity during instrumentation.
- Decrease chance of patient discomfort.

B. Artificial Nails

▶ Artificial nails or extenders are associated with fungal and bacterial pathogens in hospital settings and not recommended for clincians.[13-16]

- Wearing rings and nail polish is not recommended because chipped nail polish and skin under the ring may harbor bacteria.[3,17]

C. Wristwatch and Jewelry

▶ Remove hand and wrist jewelry at the beginning of the day.

▶ Microorganisms can become lodged in crevices of rings, watchbands, and watches.

D. Gloves

▶ After handwashing, put on gloves. Never expose open skin lesions or abrasions to a patient's oral tissues and fluids.

▶ After glove removal, wash hands to remove microorganisms.

HAND-HYGIENE PRINCIPLES

I. Rationale

▶ Effective and frequent hand hygiene can reduce the overall bacterial flora of the skin and prevent the organisms acquired from a patient from becoming skin residents.

▶ It is impossible to sterilize the skin, but every attempt is made to reduce the bacterial flora to a minimum.

II. Purposes

Hand hygiene, including handwashing, hand antisepsis, or surgical hand antisepsis, is critical for reducing the bacterial flora of the hands. The chosen method is dependent on the procedure and the degree of contamination. An effective hand hygiene procedure can be expected to accomplish the following:

▶ Remove surface dirt and transient bacteria

▶ Dissolve the normal greasy film on the skin

▶ Rinse and remove all loosened debris and microorganisms.

III. Facilities

▶ Sink

- Use a sink with a foot pedal or electronic control for water flow to avoid contamination to/from faucet handles.
- For regular sink, turn on water at the beginning and leave on through the entire procedure. Turn faucets off with the towel after drying hands.
- Clean around brim of sink with disinfectant. The sink must be of sufficient size so that contact with the inside of the wash basin can be avoided. A sink cannot be sterilized and can become highly contaminated.
- Prevent contamination of clothing by not leaning against the sink.
- Use a separate area and sink reserved for instrument washing. Contaminated instruments must be removed from the treatment room before preparation for the next patient.

▶ Soap

- Use a liquid or foam soap.
- Apply from a foot- or knee-activated or electronically controlled dispenser to avoid contamination to and from a hand-operated dispenser or cake soap. Rinsing is a necessary part of the handwashing procedure.

▶ Scrub brushes

- Avoid overvigorous use of a brush to minimize skin abrasion. Skin irritation and abrasion can leave openings for additional cross-contamination.
- Disposable sponges are available commercially and may be preferred when a scrub brush is traumatic to the skin.

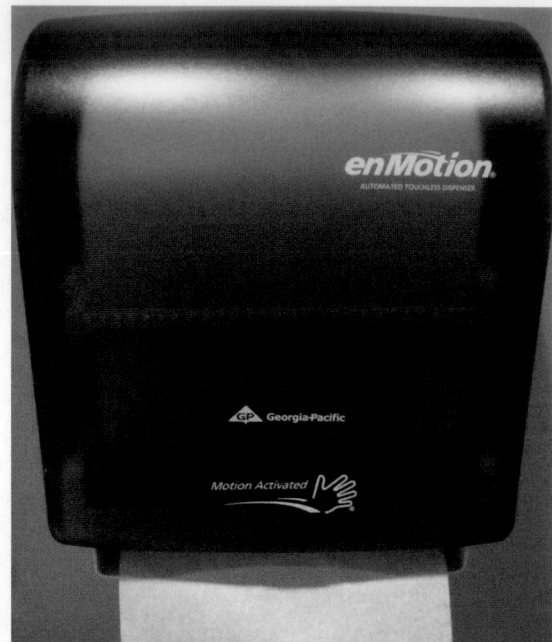

FIGURE 5-3 **Towel Dispenser.** Hands-free motion activated type of dispenser that requires no contact.

► Towels
  • Obtain disposable towel from a dispenser that requires no contact except with the towel itself, which hangs down (Figure 5-3) or a hands-free automatic dispenser.
  • Cloth towels are not recommended.

METHODS OF HAND HYGIENE

Hand hygiene is considered the most important single procedure for the prevention of cross-contamination (Box 5-3).

I. Indications

► Before and after treating each patient (before glove placement and after glove removal).
► Before regloving after removing gloves that are torn, cut, or punctured.
► After barehanded touching inanimate objects that may be contaminated with blood or saliva.
► When hands are visibly soiled.
► Before leaving the treatment room.

II. Descriptions[3]

A. Routine Handwash

Sufficient for routine dental examinations and nonsurgical dental procedures.
► Wet hands with water, apply liquid, nonantimicrobial soap (plain soap); avoid hot water.
► Rub hands together for at least 15 seconds; cover all surfaces of fingers, hands, and wrists.

► Interlace fingers and rub to cover all sides.
► Rinse under running water; dry thoroughly with disposable towels.
► Turn off faucet with the towel.

B. Antiseptic Handwash

► Water and antimicrobial liquid soap (e.g., chlorhexidine, iodine and iodophors, chloroxylenol [PCMX], triclosan).
► To remove or destroy transient microorganisms and reduce resident flora.
  1. Preliminary steps
    • Remove watch and jewelry from hands.
    • Fasten hair back securely.
    • Put on protective eyewear and mask before handwashing to prevent contamination of washed hands ready for gloving.
    • Use cool water.
  2. Handwashing procedure
    • Lather hands, wrists, and forearms quickly with liquid antimicrobial soap.
    • Rub all surfaces vigorously; interlace fingers and rub back and forth with pressure.
    • Rinse thoroughly, running the water from fingertips down the hands. Keep water running.
    • Repeat two more times. One lathering for 3 minutes is less effective than are three short latherings and three rinses in 30 seconds.
    • The latherings serve to loosen the debris and microorganisms and the rinsings wash them away.
    • Use paper towels for drying, taking care not to recontaminate.

C. Antiseptic Hand Rub

To remove or destroy transient microorganisms and reduce resident flora,
► Wash visibly soiled hands before use.
► Decontaminate hands with an (60–95% ethanol or isopropanol) alcohol-based hand rub.
► Apply the product (follow manufacturer's directions for amount to use) to the palm of one hand, and vigorously rub hands together.
► If hands are dry after 10–15 seconds, the amount used may need to be increased.

D. Surgical Antisepsis (Also Called Surgical Scrub)

► Water and antimicrobial liquid soap (e.g., chlorhexidine, iodine and iodophores, chloroxylenol [PCMX], triclosan).
► To remove or destroy transient microorganisms and reduce resident flora with a persistent or prolonged effect that inhibits proliferation or survival of microorganisms.

BOX 5-3

Hand Hygiene Methods and Indications[3]

Method	Agent	Purpose	Duration (minimum)	Indication
Routine handwash	Water and nonantimicrobial soap (e.g., plain soap)	Remove soil and transient microorganisms	15 seconds	Before and after treating each patient (e.g., before glove placement and after glove removal). After barehanded touching of inanimate objects likely to be contaminated by blood or saliva. Before leaving the dental operatory or the dental laboratory. When visibly soiled. Before regloving after removing gloves that are torn, cut, or punctured.
Antiseptic handwash	Water and antimicrobial soap (e.g., chlorhexidine, iodine and iodophors, chloroxylenol [PCMX], triclosan)	Remove or destroy transient microorganisms and reduce resident flora	15 seconds	
Antiseptic hand rub	Alcohol-based hand rub	Remove or destroy transient microorganisms and reduce resident flora	Rub hands until the agent is dry	
Surgical antisepsis	Water and antimicrobial soap (e.g., chlorhexidine, iodine and iodophors, chloroxylenol [PCMX], triclosan)	Remove or destroy transient microorganisms and reduce resident flora (persistent effect)	2–6 min	Before donning sterile surgeon's gloves for surgical procedures
	Water and non-antimicrobial soap (e.g., plain soap), followed by an alcohol-based surgical hand scrub product with persistent activity		Follow manufacturer instructions for surgical hand-scrub product with persistent activity	

Source: United States Department of Health and Human Services, Centers for Disease Control and Prevention Guidelines for infection control in dental health-care settings–2003. *MMWR.* 2003;52(RR–17):15,19.

▶ Each hospital or oral surgery clinic has rules and regulations for surgical antisepsis. These will be posted over the scrub sinks.

▶ A surgical antisepsis performed as the first one of the day will be 10 minutes and subsequent ones may be 3–5 minutes.

▶ Following treatment of a contagious or isolated patient, the procedure will take at least 5 minutes.

1. Preliminary steps
   - Remove watch and jewelry. Place hair and beard coverings and make sure hair is completely covered.
   - Put on protective eyewear and mask.
   - Open sterile brush package to have ready.
   - Wash hands and arms, using surgical liquid antimicrobial soap to remove gross surface dirt before using the scrub brush.
   - Lather vigorously with strong rubbing motions, 10 on each side of hands, wrists, and arms.

   - Interlace the fingers and thumbs to clean the proximal surfaces.
   - Rinse thoroughly from fingertips across hands and wrists. Hold hands higher than elbows throughout the procedure. Leave water running.
   - Use orangewood stick from the sterile package to clean nails. Rinse.

2. First hand
   - Lather the hands and arms and leave the lather on to increase the exposure time to the antimicrobial ingredient.
   - Apply surgical liquid antimicrobial soap, and begin the brush procedure. Scrub in an orderly sequence without returning to areas previously scrubbed.
   - First hand and arm.
   - Brush back and forth across nails and fingertips, passing the brush under the nails.

- Fingers and hand: use small circular strokes on all sides of the thumb and each finger, overlapping strokes for complete coverage.
- Continue to wrist. Apply more soap to maintain a good lather.
- When arm is completed, leave lather on.

3. Second hand
- Repeat on the other arm. Some systems require the use of a second sterile brush for the second hand. When this is so, discard the first brush into the proper container and obtain the second brush.
- At one-half of scrub time, rinse hands and arms thoroughly, first one and then the other, starting at the fingertips and letting water pass down over the arm.
- Lather and repeat.
- At the end of time (or counts), rinse thoroughly, each arm separately, from fingertips. Apply towel from fingertips to elbow without reapplying to hand area.
- Hold hands up and clasped together. Proceed to dressing area for gowning and gloving.

GLOVES AND GLOVING

Wearing gloves is a standard practice to protect both the patient and the clinician from cross-contamination.

I. Criteria for Selection of Treatment/ Examination Gloves

A. Safety Factors
▶ Effective barrier; evidence from manufacturer of quality control standards.
▶ Impermeable to patient's saliva, blood, and bacteria.
▶ Strength and durability to resist tears and punctures.
▶ Impervious to materials routinely used during clinical procedures.
▶ Nonirritating or harmful to skin; use nonlatex gloves when the patient or clinician is allergic.
▶ Length: glove cuff extends to provide coverage over cuff of long sleeve.

B. Ergonomic Choice Factors
▶ Fit hand well; no interference with motion.
▶ Tactile sense not decreased.
▶ No tight pull over palm or between thumb and index finger.

II. Types of Gloves
▶ Material
- Latex
- Nonlatex: neoprene, block copolymer, vinyl, *N*-nitrile

- For patient care
  - Nonsterile single-use examination/treatment: latex, nonlatex
  - Presterilized single-use surgical: latex, nonlatex
▶ Utility gloves
  - Heavy duty: latex, nonlatex (puncture resistant for clinic cleanup)
  - Plastic: Food handler's glove to wear as overglove

III. Procedures for Use of Gloves
▶ Mask and eyewear placement
  - Place mask and protective eyewear before hand hygiene and gloving.
  - Prevent the need for manipulating the mask around the face and hair after washing the hands.
▶ Pregloving hand hygiene
  - Use an antiseptic handwash or hand rub before gloving.
  - Hands must be dried thoroughly to control moisture inside glove and thus discourage growth of bacteria.
▶ Glove placement
  - Always glove and deglove in front of the patient; a patient may need assurance that gloves are new and used only for that appointment.
  - Place gloves over the cuff of long-sleeved clinic wear to provide complete protection of arms from exposure to contamination.
▶ Avoiding contamination
  - Keep gloved hands away from face, hair, clothing (pockets), telephone, patient records, clinician's stool, and all parts of the dental equipment that have not been predisinfected and covered with a barrier material.
▶ Torn, cut, or punctured glove
  - Remove immediately, wash hands thoroughly, and put on new gloves.
▶ Removal of gloves
  - Develop a procedure whereby gloves can be removed without contaminating the hands from the exposed external surfaces of the gloves.
  - Figure 5-4 illustrates one system for glove removal.
  - Wash hands promptly after glove removal. Organisms on the hands multiply rapidly inside the warm, moist environment of the glove, even when no external contamination has occurred.

IV. Factors Affecting Glove Integrity
▶ Length of time worn
  - New pair for each patient is the basic requirement.
  - Total time worn is no longer than 1 hour; when gloves develop a sticky surface, remove, wash hands, and reglove with a fresh pair.

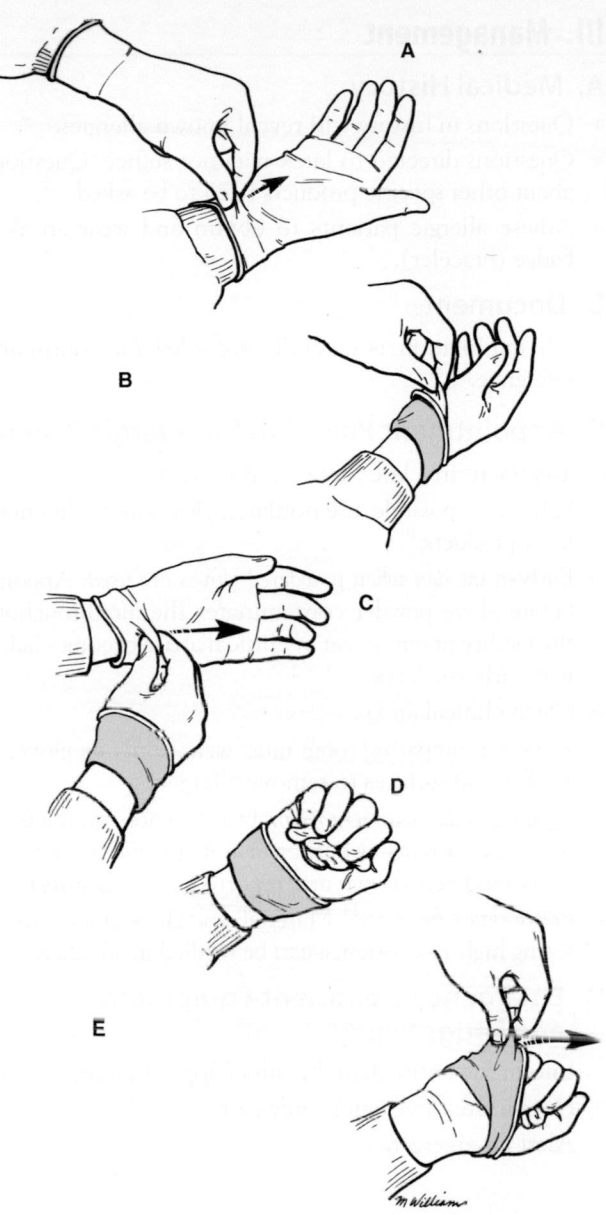

FIGURE 5-4 **Steps for Removal of Gloves. A:** Use left fingers to pinch right glove near edge to fold back. **B:** Fold edge back without contact with clean inside surface. **C:** Use right fingers to contact outside of left glove at the wrist to invert and remove. **D:** Bunch glove into the palm. **E:** With ungloved left hand, grasp inner noncontaminated portion of the right glove to peel it off, enclosing other glove as it is inverted.

- ▶ Complexity of the procedure
  - • Certain procedures are more likely to promote perforations, especially when sharp instruments must be changed frequently.
- ▶ Packaging of the gloves
  - • Gloves in a new package are tightly packed and can be torn when removed; must be handled carefully until pressure is relieved.
- ▶ Size of glove
  - • When too long, the extra material at the fingertips can get caught, torn, or in the way; picking up small objects is difficult, especially sharp instruments.

- ▶ Pressure of time
  - • Stress; working too fast increases the risk of glove damage.
- ▶ Storage of gloves
  - • Keep in cool, dark place; exposure to heat, sun, or fluorescent light increases potential for deterioration and perforations.
- ▶ Agents used
  - • Certain chemicals react with the glove material; for example, petroleum jelly, alcohol, and products made with alcohol tend to break down the glove integrity.
- ▶ Hazards from the hands
  - • Long fingernails and rings worn inside gloves.

LATEX HYPERSENSITIVITY

Patients and clinicians may have or may develop sensitivity to natural rubber latex (NRL). Symptoms of a hypersensitive reaction range from a dermatitis to a life-threatening anaphylactic shock. The only available treatment for latex allergy is avoiding all contact.

- ▶ Latex sensitivity is due to the protein allergens and to additives used when the commercial latex is prepared.
- ▶ Latex allergens occur in any equipment or product used that contains NRL.
- ▶ Gloves are the most frequently used item that contains latex.
- ▶ Equipment listed in Box 5-4 may contain NRL. However, many of the items are also made of alternative materials. When the label on a product does not list the contents, the manufacturer can be contacted to identify latex-free items.

BOX 5-4

Equipment That May Contain Latex

Bite blocks
Blood pressure cuff
Gloves
Goggles
Lead apron cover
Masks (elastic head band)
Mixing bowl
Nitrous oxide nosepiece and tubing rubber dam
O ring (on ultrasonic insert)
Orthodontic elastics
Rubber polishing cup
Stethoscope
Stopper in anesthesia carpule
Suction adapter

I. Clinical Manifestations

▶ Methods of exposure

- Direct exposure to latex products.
- Aeroallergen inhalation of the allergen when the powder (cornstarch) from the gloves becomes airborne.
- Mucosal contact.

▶ Type I hypersensitivity (immediate reaction)

- Urticaria: hives.
- Dermatitis: rash, itching.
- Nasal problems: sneezing, itchy nose, runny nose.
- Eyes: watery, itchy watery, itchy.
- Respiratory reaction: breathing difficulty, asthma-like wheezing, coughing.
- Drop in blood pressure: shock.
- Anaphylaxis.

▶ Type IV hypersensitivity (delayed reaction)

- Contact dermatitis develops 8 hours to 5 days after contact.[18]

II. Individuals at High Risk of Latex Sensitivity

▶ Have had frequent exposure to latex products

- Occupational exposure: Healthcare personnel (HCP) who wear latex gloves regularly for patient care or have worked in a rubber-manufacturing plant.
- Multiple medical surgeries or treatments requiring placement of rubber tubes or drains. Examples: genitourinary anomalies, spina bifida.

▶ Have other documented allergies

- Examples: food allergies (avocado, banana, kiwi fruit, chestnuts, papaya, peanuts).

III. Management

A. Medical History

▶ Questions in history will reveal known allergies.

▶ Questions directed to latex may not suffice. Questions about other specific products need to be asked.

▶ Advise allergic patients to obtain and wear an alert badge (bracelet).

B. Document

▶ All information is carefully recorded for continuing reference.

C. Appointment Planning for Allergic Patient

▶ Treatment in a latex-free environment.

▶ Whenever possible, use nonlatex gloves and other nonlatex products.[19]

▶ *Early in the day when powdered gloves are used*: Appoint before glove powder contaminates the air throughout the facility or outerwear of clinical attire becomes laden with airborne latex.

▶ Clean clinical areas:

- Person preparing room must wear nonlatex gloves.
- Wipe all surfaces to remove allergen.

▶ *No latex in the treatment room*: Use nonlatex products for high-risk patients (whether or not specific latex sensitivity has been known and reported in the history).

▶ *Prepare latex-free carts*[13]: Materials and gloves, for use when seeing high-risk patients, can be readied in advance.

D. Emergency Treatment Equipment and Drugs Ready

▶ Inform the entire dental team of appointment.

▶ Have a latex-free emergency cart available.[19]

▶ Alert for emergency.

EVERYDAY ETHICS

After Mr. Green's dental hygiene treatment is completed, the dentist, Dr. Root, is notified so that the final examination can be made. Dr. Root comes in shortly and sits down next to the patient. He browses through the notations made in the patient's chart and then picks up the mirror and explorer to proceed with a clinical examination. It is apparent that he has not washed his hands and may not even have put on a new pair of gloves since he left the other treatment room. A similar situation has happened occasionally before.

Questions for Consideration

1. Mabel, the dental hygienist, notes that the dentist did not change his gloves or wash his hands. Is Mable faced with an ethical dilemma or an ethical issue? Explain.

2. Read the nine "Standards of Professional Responsibility" in the ADHA Code of Ethics in Appendix I. Explain which of the standards are involved and how each is violated if Mable does not address this issue with Dr. Root.

3. Use the steps for making decisions in Chapter 1 Code of Ethics section to determine some actions that Mable might take to address this situation both immediately and long term.

DOCUMENTATION

Documentation needs to record the following:

▶ Irregularities related to personal protection that could have influenced the procedures of a routine appointment.

▶ How the special needs were taken care of for a patient with an allergy to latex.

▶ Information in medical alert that patient is sensitive to latex.

A sample progress note may be found in Box 5-5.

BOX 5-5
Example Documentation: Patient with a Latex Sensitivity

S –Initial appointment for new patient to our practice. She reports sensitivity to latex gloves.

O –History form and questions completed. Informed patient that the office is latex free. Radiographs taken, risk assessment, caries examination, and periodontal assessment. Pocket depths 5–6 mm in the area of #30–31 with bleeding on probing, all other areas 3 mm or less. Plaque score 30%.

A –Patient has a history of skin reactions when latex gloves are used. Careful attention to avoiding use of products containing latex. Localized moderate chronic periodontitis between #30 and #31.

P –Review of oral self-care with attention to optimal biofilm removal #30–31. Localized nonsurgical periodontal therapy with local anesthetic with prophylaxis full mouth. About 5% sodium fluoride varnish due to moderate caries risk.

Signed: _____, RDH Date: _____

Factors To Teach The Patient

▷ Need for the patient's complete history for the protection of both the patient and the professional person.

▷ Purposes for use of barriers (face mask, protective eyewear, and gloves) by the clinician for the benefit of the patient.

▷ Importance of eye protection.

▷ Significance of hand hygiene in the control of disease transmission (everywhere, not only dental office or clinic).

References

1. United States Department of Labor, Occupational Safety and Health Administration. 29 CFR Part 1910.1030. Occupational exposure to bloodborne pathogens; needlesticks and other sharps injuries; final rule. *Fed Regist.* 2001;66:5317–5325. As amended from and includes 29 CFR Part 1910.1030; Occupational exposure to bloodborne pathogens; final rule. *Fed Regist.* 1991;56:64174–64182.

2. United States Department of Health and Human Services, Centers for Disease Control and Prevention. Immunization of health-care personnel. *MMWR.* 2011;60(RR–07):1–45.

3. United States Department of Health and Human Services, Centers for Disease Control and Prevention guidelines for infection control in dental health-care settings–2003. *MMWR.* 2003;52(RR–17):15,19.

4. Gordon J, Ingalls T. Preventive medicine and epidemiology. *Prog Med Sci.* 1957;233:334–357.

5. United States Centers for Disease Control. Guidelines for preventing the transmission of *mycobacterium tuberculosis* in health-care facilities. *MMWR.* 1994;43(RR–13):1–132.

6. Micik RE, Miller RL, Leong AC. Studies on dental aerobiology: III. Efficacy of surgical masks in protecting dental personnel from airborne bacterial particles. *J Dent Res.* 1971;50(3):626–630.

7. Miller RL, Micik RE. Air pollution and its control in the dental office. *Dent Clin North Am.* 1978;22(3):453–476.

8. Wells WF. Aerodynamics of droplet nuclei. In: Wells WF, ed. *Airborne Contagion and Air Hygiene: An Ecological Study of Droplet Infections.* Cambridge, MA: Harvard University Press; 1955:13–19.

9. Cooley RL, Cottingham AJ, Abrams H, et al. Ocular injuries sustained in the dental office: methods of detection, treatment, and prevention. *J Am Dent Assoc.* 1978;97(6):985–988.

10. Wesson MD, Thornton JB. Eye protection and ocular complications in the dental office. *Gen Dent.* 1989;37:19.

11. Roberts-Harry TJ, Cass AE, Jagger JD. Ocular injury and infection in dental practice: a survey and a review of the literature. *Br Dent J.* 1991;170(1):20–22.

12. Allen AL, Organ RJ. Occult blood accumulation under the fingernails: a mechanism for the spread of blood-borne infection. *J Am Dent Assoc.* 1982;105(3):455–459.

13. Foca M, Jakob K, Whittier S, et al. Endemic *Pseudomonas aeruginosa* infection in a neonatal intensive care unit. *N Engl J Med.* 2000;343(10):695–700.

14. Moolenaar RL, Crutcher JM, San Joaquin VH, et al. A prolonged outbreak of *Pseudomonas aeruginosa* in a neonatal intensive care unit: did staff fingernails play a role in disease transmission? *Infect Control Hosp Epidemiol.* 2000;21(2):80–85.

15. Parry MF, Grant B, Yukna M, et al. Candida osteomyelitis and diskitis after spinal surgery: an outbreak that implicates artificial nail use. *Clin Infect Dis.* 2001;32(3):352–357.

16. Passaro DJ, Waring L, Armstrong R, et al. Postoperative *Serratia marcescens* wound infections traced to an out-of-hospital source. *J Infect Dis.* 1997;175(4):992–995.

17. Arrowsmith VA, Taylor R. Removal of nail polish and finger rings to prevent surgical infection. *Cochrane Database Syst Rev.* 2012;5:CD003325.

18. Muller BA. Minimizing latex exposure and allergy: how to avoid or reduce sensitization in the healthcare setting. *Postgrad Med.* 2003;113(4):91–97.

19. Centers for Disease Control, National Institute for Occupational Safety and Health. Alert: Preventing Allergic Reactions to Natural Rubber Latex in the Workplace, Cincinnati, OH: Public Health Service, U.S. Department of Health and Human Services: June 1997 Publication No. 97–135.

ENHANCE YOUR UNDERSTANDING

thePoint® DIGITAL CONNECTIONS
(see the inside front cover for access information)
- **Audio glossary**
- **Quiz bank**

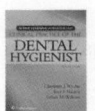

SUPPORT FOR LEARNING
(available separately; visit lww.com)
- *Active Learning Workbook for Clinical Practice of the Dental Hygienist, 12th Edition*

prepU INDIVIDUALIZED REVIEW
(available separately; visit lww.com)
- **Adaptive quizzing with *prepU for Wilkins' Clinical Practice of the Dental Hygienist***

6

Infection Control: Clinical Procedures

Lori Giblin, RDH, MSDH

CHAPTER OUTLINE

LEARNING OBJECTIVES

After studying this chapter, the student will be able to:

1. Describe the basic considerations for safe infection control practices.

2. Explain methods for cleaning and sterilizing instruments.

3. Describe procedures to prepare, clean, and disinfect the treatment area.

4. Explain process for managing hypodermic needles and occupational postexposure management.

5. List types of waste disposal and explain how each type is handled.

INFECTION CONTROL

The success of a planned system for control of disease transmission depends on the cooperative effort of each member of the dental health team.

▶ The aim is to provide the highest level of infection control possible and practical to ensure a safe environment for both patients and the clinical team.

▶ The presence of specific, disease-producing organisms is rarely known; therefore, application of protective, preventive procedures is needed before, during, and following *all* patient appointments.

▶ Definitions and abbreviations related to infection control are provided in Box 6-1.

I. Objectives

The following are guidelines necessary to prevent the transmission of infectious agents and eliminate cross-contamination:

▶ Reduction of available pathogenic microorganisms to a level at which the normal resistance mechanisms of the body can prevent infection.

▶ Elimination of cross-contamination by breaking the chain of infection (see Figure 4-1, Chapter 4).

▶ Application of standard precautions by treating each patient as if all human blood and bodily fluids are infectious.

II. Basic Considerations for Safe Practice

Basic factors involved in the conduct of safe practice include the following, to be described in this chapter:

▶ Treatment room features
▶ Instrument management
▶ Preparation for appointment
▶ Unit water lines
▶ Environmental surfaces
▶ Care of sterile instruments
▶ Patient preparation
▶ Summary of procedures for the prevention of disease transmission
▶ Disposal of waste

TREATMENT ROOM FEATURES

▶ When renovations or a new dental office or clinic are anticipated, plans can reflect the most advanced knowledge available relative to safety and disease control.

▶ A partial list of notable features is included here and illustrated in Figure 6-1. The objective is to have materials, shapes, and surface textures that facilitate the effective use of infection control measures.

I. Unit

▶ Designed for easy cleaning and disinfection, with smooth, uncluttered surfaces.

▶ Removable hoses that can be cleaned, disinfected, and covered.

▶ Syringes with autoclavable tips or fitted with disposable tips.

▶ Handpieces with antiretraction valves that can be autoclaved.

▶ Use of barrier covers where possible.

II. Dental Chair

▶ Foot-operated controls.

▶ Surface and seamless finish of easily cleaned plastic material that withstands chemical disinfection without damage or discoloring; cloth upholstery to be avoided.

III. Light

▶ Removable handle for sterilization or disposable barrier cover.

IV. Clinician's Chair

▶ Smooth, plastic seat cover that is easily disinfected and has a minimum of seams and creases.

▶ Set at correct height (before gloving) for individual clinician.

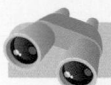

BOX 6-1 KEY WORDS AND ABBREVIATIONS: Infection Control

ADA: American Dental Association.

Antimicrobial agent: any agent that kills or suppresses the growth of microorganisms.

Antiseptic: a substance that prevents or arrests the growth or action of microorganisms either by inhibiting their activity or by destroying them; term used especially for preparations applied topically to living tissue.

Asepsis: free from contamination with microorganisms; includes sterile conditions in tissues and on materials, as obtained by exclusion, removing, or killing organisms.

Aseptic technique: procedures carried out in the absence of pathogenic microorganisms.

Bioburden: a microbiologic load; the number of contaminating organisms present on a surface before sterilization or disinfection.

Biofilm: the surface film that contains microorganisms and other biologic substances.

Biohazard: a substance that poses a biologic risk because it is contaminated with biomaterial that has a potential for transmitting infection.

Biologic indicator: a preparation of nonpathogenic microorganisms, usually bacterial spores, carried by an ampule or a specially impregnated paper enclosed within a package during sterilization and subsequently incubated to verify that sterilization has occurred.

Broad spectrum: indicates a range of activity of a drug or chemical substance against a wide variety of microorganisms.

Chain of asepsis: a procedure that avoids transfer of infection. The "chain" implies that each step, related to the previous one, continues to be carried out without contamination.

Chemical indicator: a color change stripe or other mark, often on autoclave tape or bag, used to monitor the process of sterilization; color change indicates that the package has been brought to a specific temperature, but color change is not an indicator of sterilization.

Contamination: introduction of microorganisms, blood, or other potentially infectious material or agent onto a surface or into tissue.

Decontamination: disinfection; use of physical or chemical means to remove, inactivate, or destroy pathogenic microorganisms on a surface or item to the extent that they are no longer capable of transmitting infectious disease; the surface or item is rendered safe for handling, use, or disposal.

Disinfectant: an agent, usually a chemical, but may be a physical agent, such as X-rays or ultraviolet light, that destroys microorganisms but may not kill bacterial spores; refers to substances applied to inanimate objects.

EPA: United States Environmental Protection Agency.

EPA registered: number on a label indicates that the product has the acceptance of EPA.

FDA: United States Food and Drug Administration regulates food, drugs, biologic products, medical devices, radiologic products.

Infection control: the selection and use of procedures and products to prevent the spread of infectious disease.

Infectious waste: contaminated with blood, saliva, or other substances; potentially or actually infected with pathogenic material; officially called "regulated" waste.

Invasive procedure: entry into tissues during which bleeding occurs or the potential for bleeding exists.

Healthcare-associated infection: an infection associated with or acquired during a medical or surgical intervention; replaces **nosocomial**, which is limited to an adverse infectious outcome occurring in a hospital.

OSAP: Organization for Safety and Asepsis Procedures Research Foundation.

OSHA: United States Occupational Safety and Health Administration, Department of Labor.

PEP: postexposure prophylaxis.

PPE: personal protective equipment.

Sanitation: the process by which the number of organisms on inanimate objects is reduced. It does not imply freedom from microorganisms and generally refers to a cleaning process.

Shelf life: stability of an item after it has been prepared; length of time a substance or preparation can be kept without changes occurring in its chemical structure or other properties.

Sporicide: substance that kills spores.

Sterilization: process by which all forms of life, including bacterial spores, are destroyed by physical or chemical means.

Synergism: the joint action of agents so that their combined effect is greater than the sum of their individual parts.

Waste

  Contaminated waste: items that have contacted blood or other body secretions.

  Hazardous waste: poses a risk to humans or the environment.

  Infectious waste: capable of causing an infectious disease.

  Regulated waste: liquid blood or saliva, sharps contaminated with blood or saliva, and nonsharp solid waste saturated with or caked with liquid or semisolid blood or saliva or tissue including teeth (OSHA).

  Toxic waste: capable of having a poisonous effect.

TREATMENT ROOM FEATURES

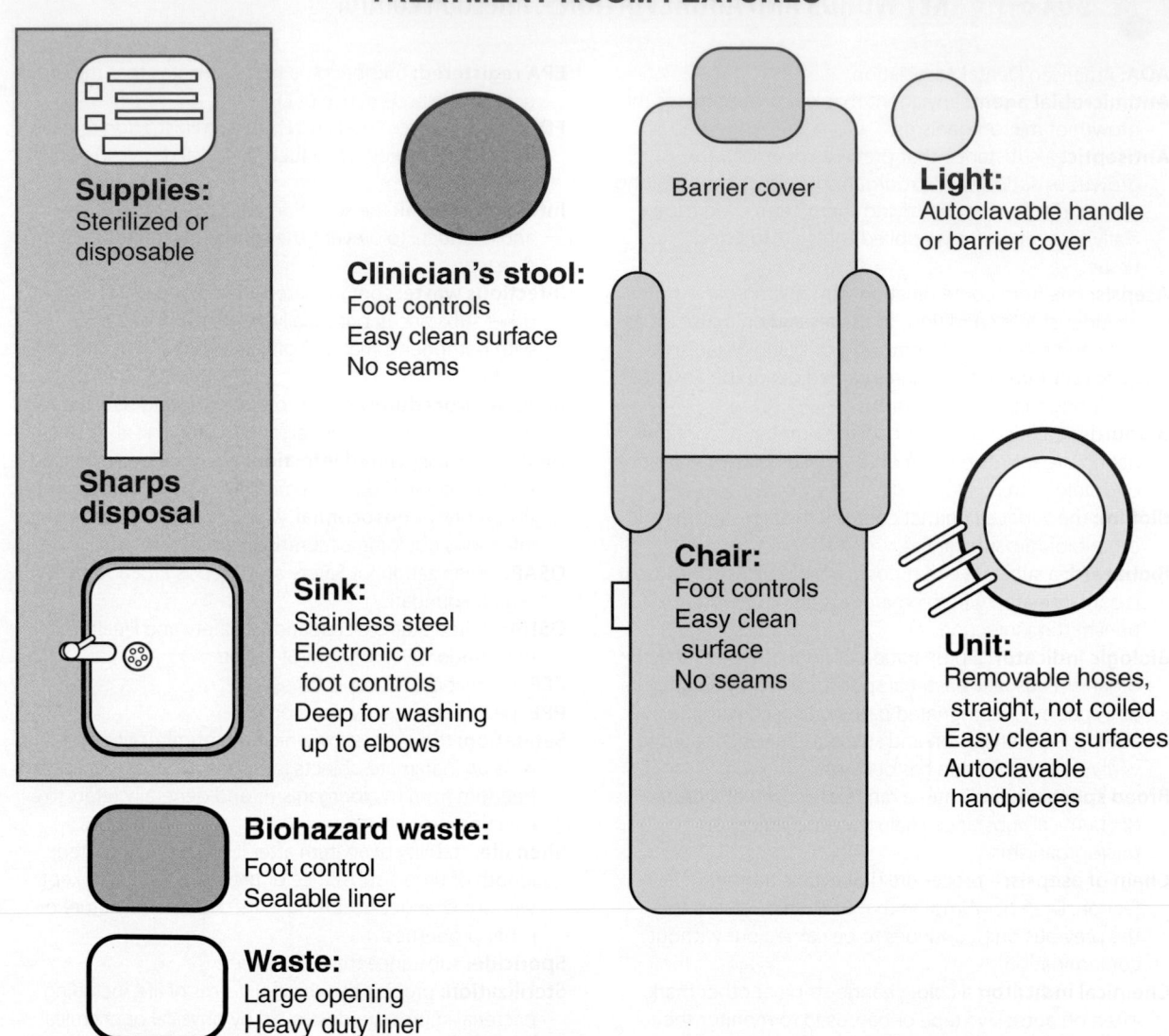

Supplies:
Sterilized or disposable

Sharps disposal

Clinician's stool:
Foot controls
Easy clean surface
No seams

Sink:
Stainless steel
Electronic or foot controls
Deep for washing up to elbows

Biohazard waste:
Foot control
Sealable liner

Waste:
Large opening
Heavy duty liner

Barrier cover

Light:
Autoclavable handle or barrier cover

Chair:
Foot controls
Easy clean surface
No seams

Unit:
Removable hoses, straight, not coiled
Easy clean surfaces
Autoclavable handpieces

Floor: Smooth, easy clean, nonabsorbent, no carpeting

FIGURE 6-1 **Optimal Treatment Room Features.**

V. Floor

▶ No cloth carpeting.
▶ Smooth floor covering, easily cleaned, nonabsorbent.

VI. Sink

▶ Smooth material (stainless steel).
▶ Wide and deep enough for effective handwashing without splashing or touching sides.
▶ Automatic water faucets and soap dispensers with electronic, "hand," "knee," or foot-operated controls.
▶ Separate room or area for contaminated instrument care.

VII. Supplies

▶ All sterilizable or disposable.

VIII. Waste

▶ Most waste is disposed with usual waste.
▶ Receptacle with opening large enough to prevent contact with sides when material is dropped in.
▶ Heavy-duty plastic bag liner to be sealed tightly for disposal.
▶ Separate sharps disposal.
▶ Small biohazard receptacle near treatment area to receive contaminated gauze 2 × 2s and other waste, for disposal in large waste container clearly marked for contaminated waste.

INSTRUMENT PROCESSING CENTER

The processing center for care, cleaning, packaging, sterilizing, and storing instruments is separated into respective areas, centrally located and apart from the treatment rooms.

▶ The successful practice of standard precautions to prevent cross-contamination depends on the development of, and strict adherence to, a planned program for instrument management.

▶ A good rule is to learn the most effective, safe system and then to follow it without exception.

▶ A specific routine is easier for the entire dental team to follow, and peer review is built in.

▶ The basic steps in the recirculation of instruments from the time an appointment procedure is completed until the instruments are sterilized and ready for use in a continuing clinical appointment are shown in the flowchart in Figure 6-2. Each of the steps is described in the following sections.

CLEANING PROCEDURES

The three basic methods for precleaning to remove any organic or inorganic debris from instruments before sterilization are using[1]:

▶ Washer/thermal disinfector

▶ Ultrasonic processing

▶ Manual scrubbing

I. Instrument Washer/Thermal Disinfector

▶ The *instrument washer* uses high-velocity hot water and a detergent to clean instruments.

• Some models are equipped to dry the instruments.

• Household dishwashers are different, and not appropriate for dental instruments.

▶ The *instrument washer/thermal disinfector* differs from the plain washer by having a higher degree of temperature, so that it disinfects as well as cleans the instruments (Figure 6-3A).

▶ Benefits from the use of washer/thermal disinfector and ultrasonic cleaning over manual scrubbing include the following[2]:

• Increased efficiency in obtaining a high degree of cleanliness for improved disinfection.

• Reduced danger to clinician from direct contact with potentially pathogenic microorganisms.

• Elimination of possible dissemination of microorganisms through release of aerosols and droplets, which can occur during the scrubbing process.

▶ Disinfection allows the instruments in cassettes to be handled with gloves while packaging.

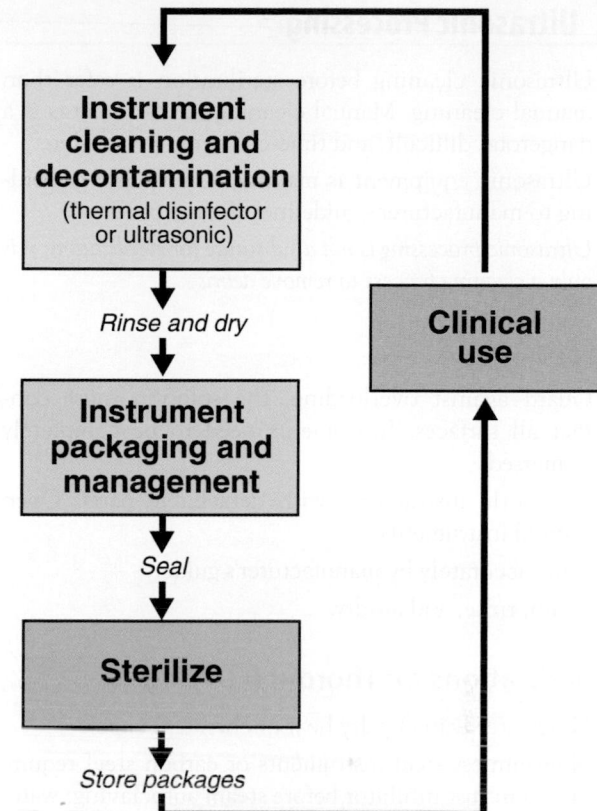

FIGURE 6-2 **Recirculation of Instruments.** Flowchart shows step-by-step process. At the completion of treatment, instruments are cleaned, packaged, sterilized, and stored. They are kept sealed until patient appointment begins.

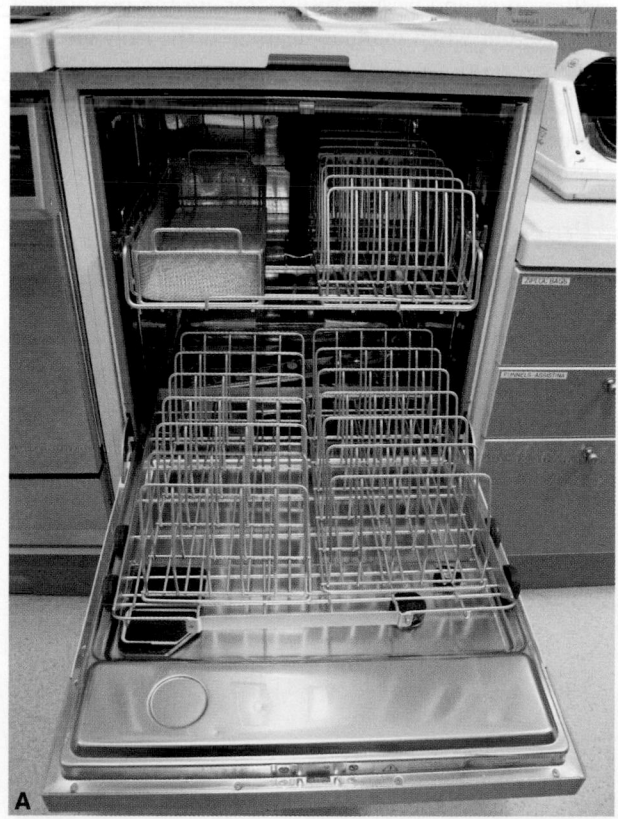

FIGURE 6-3A Instrument Washer.

II. Ultrasonic Processing

▶ Ultrasonic cleaning before sterilization is safer than manual cleaning. Manual cleaning of instruments is a dangerous, difficult, and time-consuming procedure.

▶ Ultrasonic equipment is maintained and used according to manufacturer's guidelines (Figure 6-3B).

▶ *Ultrasonic processing is not a substitute for sterilization; it is only a cleaning process to remove debris.*

A. Procedure

▶ Guard against overloading; the solution must contact all surfaces. Instruments need to be completely immersed.

▶ Dismantle instruments with detachable parts. Open jointed instruments.

▶ Time accurately by manufacturer's guide.

▶ Drain, rinse, and air-dry.

B. Indications for Thorough Drying

▶ When sterilizing by dry heat or chemical vapor.

▶ Nonstainless steel instruments or carbon steel require predip in rust inhibitor before steam autoclaving; water on instruments dilutes the antirust solution.

III. Manual Cleaning

▶ Ultrasonics and washer disinfector are the methods of choice, but when manual cleaning is the only alternative, precautions are needed.

▶ When instruments are not in a cassette, transfer forceps are needed for transferring contaminated instruments.

A. Procedure for Manual Scrubbing

▶ Wear heavy-duty gloves, protective eyewear, and mask.

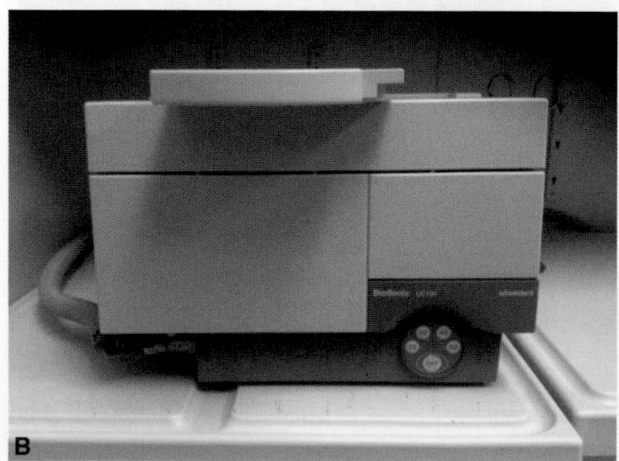

FIGURE 6-3B Ultrasonic Processor.

▶ Dismantle instruments with detachable parts. Open jointed instruments.

▶ Use detergent and scrub with a long-handled brush under running water; hold the instruments low in the sink. Scrubbing one instrument at a time minimizes risk of puncture injury.

▶ Brush with strokes away from the body; use care not to splash and contaminate the surrounding area.

▶ Rinse thoroughly.

▶ Air dry resting on paper towels (same reasons as those listed for ultrasonic processing).

B. Care of Brushes

▶ Color code instrument brushes to distinguish from hand-wash brushes.

▶ Soak and wash contaminated brushes in detergent; rinse thoroughly and sterilize.

INSTRUMENT PACKAGING AND MANAGEMENT SYSTEMS

I. Purposes

▶ To prevent contamination of newly sterilized instruments as soon as they are removed from the sterilizer.

▶ To provide a means of storing instruments to keep them organized in sets for individual appointment use and sterilized and ready for immediate use on opening.

II. Instrument Arrangement

▶ Each package is dated and marked for identification of contents: for example *Examination*.

▶ Clear packages that self-seal permit instrument identification without special labeling (Figure 6-3C).

▶ An efficient and safe mechanism to organize, process, and sterilize instruments.

▶ Instruments can be organized into tray systems, dental storage containers or cassettes customized based on various dental hygiene procedures such as an initial exam of an adult patient, child patient, or periodontal maintenance patient.

▶ They hold instruments and accessories in one unit and provide a sterile environment for instruments during treatment.

▶ After the treatment, they serve as packaging for the process of cleaning, disinfection, and sterilization.

▶ Containers or cassettes are wrapped with packaging material that allows penetration of the sterilization and maintains sterility during transport and storage.

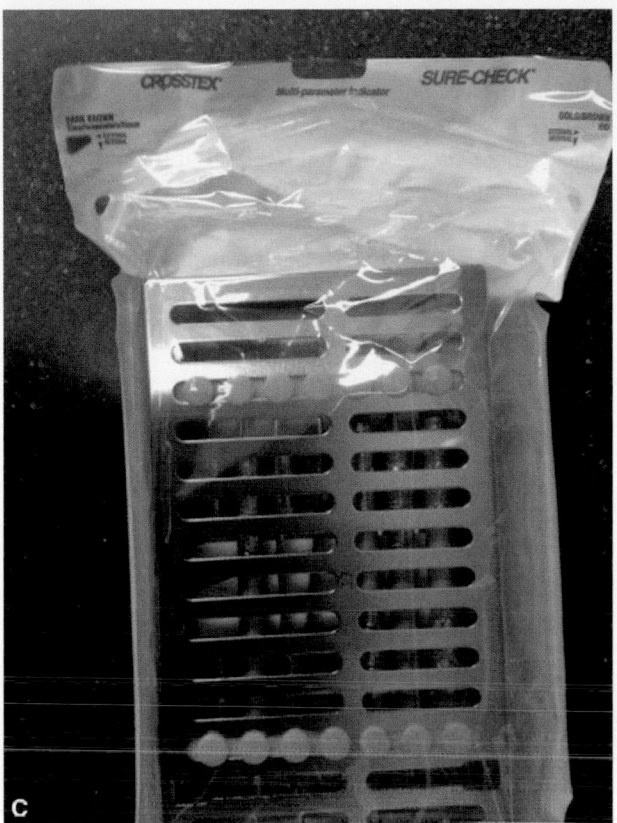

FIGURE 6-3C Instrument Cassette in a sterilization pouch.

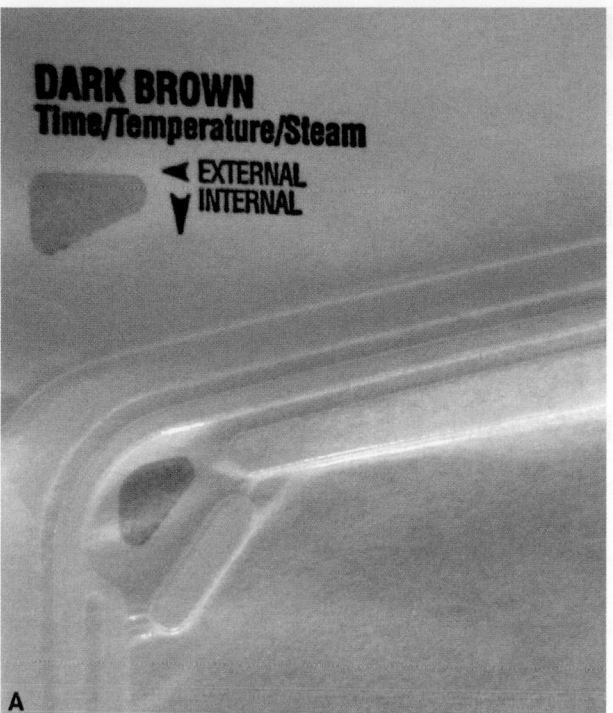

FIGURE 6-4A Built-In Chemical Indicator before Sterilization.

III. Preparation

▶ Cassettes are wrapped, and single instruments are packaged.

• Each method of sterilization has specific requirements, and the manufacturers' recommendations are followed.

• Sturdy wrapping is necessary to prevent punctures or tears that break the chain of asepsis and require a repeat of the process.

• The wrap permits the steam or chemical vapor to pass through the contents.

▶ Seal

• Pins, paper clips, or other types of metal fasteners are not used to seal packages because they provide holes for the entry of microorganisms.

• Chemical indicator tape is used unless the package is self-seal and the wrap has built-in indicators (Figure 6-4A) or (Figure 6-4B)

• The change of color means that the autoclave reached a designated temperature required for penetration but does not designate sterilization.

• When using indicator tape, distinct black stripes will appear. A lighter color change may be a warning signal that the autoclave function needs to be checked.

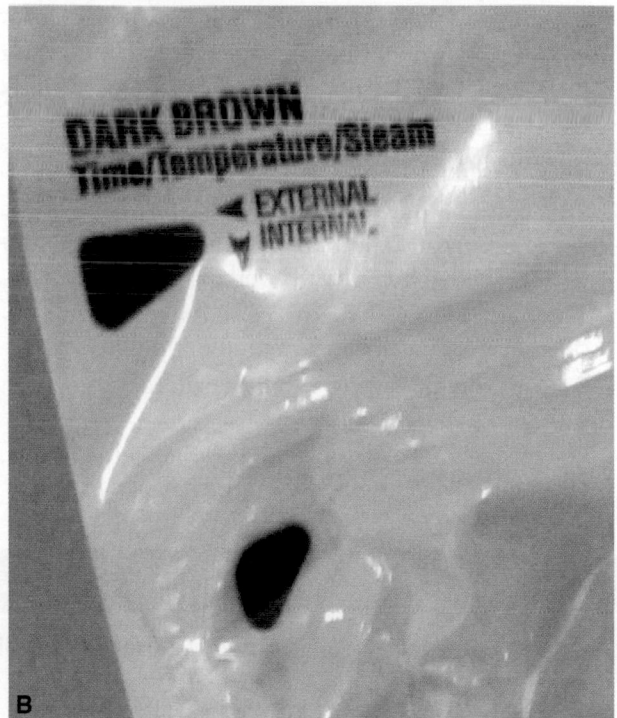

FIGURE 6-4B Built-In Chemical Indicator after Sterilization.

• The striped indicator tape is left on the sealed package and thereby serves to identify those packages ready for use. Packages are kept completely sealed until unwrapped in front of the patient.

STERILIZATION

I. Approved Methods

Sterilization is accomplished with equipment cleared by the Federal Drug Authority (FDA). Each of the methods listed here is described in the sections following. Table 6-1 summarizes the operating requirements of each:

▶ Steam under pressure (autoclave)

▶ Dry heat

▶ Chemical vapor.

II. Selection of Method

▶ Use sterilizing equipment in accord with the manufacturer's specifications.

▶ All materials and items cannot be treated by the same system of sterilization.

▶ The method for sterilization selected provides complete destruction of all microorganisms, viruses, and spores and yet must not damage the instruments and other materials.

▶ Incomplete sterilization frequently results from inadequate preparation of the materials to be sterilized (cleaning all debris, packaging), misuse of the equipment (overloading, timing, temperature selection), or inadequate maintenance.

III. Tests for Sterilization

▶ Sterilization is the process by which all forms of life are destroyed. That definition provides the rationale for testing whether a sterilizer is working properly.

▶ Three tests are used: an external and an internal chemical indicator and a biologic monitor.

▶ At least weekly testing is recommended; more often with heavy autoclave use.

▶ Equipment can be obtained for performing the testing, or commercial mail-in services are available.

▶ *External chemical indicator*: to seal the package and change color to show the autoclave temperature has been reached.

▶ *Internal chemical indicator*: color change assesses instrument exposure to temperature and steam for the required time.

▶ *Biologic monitor (spore testing)*: tests that the autoclave is functioning properly.

• The testing system requires the use of selected test microorganisms put through a regular cycle of sterilization and then cultured. When no growth occurs, the sterilizer has performed with maximum efficiency.

• *Microorganisms used*

1. Steam autoclave: *Geobacillus stearothermophilus* (formerly *Bacillus stearothermophilus*) vials, ampules, or strips.

2. Dry heat oven: *Bacillus atrophaeus* (formerly *Bacillus subtilis*) strips.

3. Chemical vapor: *Geobacillus stearothermophilus* (formerly *Bacillus stearothermophilus*) strips.

• *Procedures*

1. Manufacturer's directions determine the placement and location of bacterial indicators.[2] If there are not any instructions, the ampule, vial, or strip is placed in the center of a package, which in turn is placed in the middle of the load of packages to be sterilized.

2. After the cycle has been completed at the customary time and temperature, the ampule or strip is incubated. Ampules and vials show the color change associated with no living microorganisms, whereas the strip organisms are cultured and show no growth if the sterilizer has performed properly.

3. Table 6-2 lists indications for performing spore tests in dental settings. Records that are kept show dates and outcomes.

▶ Indications for spore testing[3]

• Once per week to verify proper use and functioning.

• Whenever a new type of packaging material or tray is used.

TABLE 6-1	Comparison of Methods for Sterilization	
	STERILIZING REQUIREMENT	
METHOD	*TIME (MIN)*	*TEMPERATURE*
Steam under pressure (autoclave)		
1. Gravity displacement	15–30	250°F (121°C)
2. Prevacuum	3.5–10	270°F (132°C)
Dry heat oven	120	320°F (160°C)
Unsaturated chemical vapor	20	270°F (132°C)

TABLE 6-2	Spore Testing	
WHEN	**WHY**
Once per week	To verify proper use and functioning
Whenever a new type of packaging material or tray is used	To ensure that the sterilizing agent is getting inside to the surface of the instruments
After training of new sterilization personnel	To verify proper use of the sterilizer
New sterilizer	To make sure unfamiliar operating instructions are being followed
After repair of a sterilizer	To make sure that the sterilizer is functioning properly
With every implantable device and hold device until results of test are known	Extra precaution for sterilization of item to be implanted into tissues
After any other change in the sterilizing procedure	To make sure change does not prevent sterilization

Source: United States Department of Health and Human Services, Centers for Disease Control and Prevention Guidelines for infection control in dental health-care settings–2003. *MMWR.* 2003;52(RR–17):27.

- After training new personnel to ensure proper use.
- During initial uses of a new sterilizer to make sure the directions are being followed.
- After sterilizer repair to check functioning.
- After any other change in the sterilizing procedure to make sure change does not prevent sterilization.
- Any load containing an implantable device and hold the device until results of the test are known.[4]

MOIST HEAT: STEAM UNDER PRESSURE

Destruction of microorganisms by heat takes place because of inactivation of essential cellular proteins or enzymes. Moist heat causes coagulation of protein.

I. Autoclave Types

▶ *Gravity displacement:* self-generation of steam forces out the air; steam enters to penetrate through the cassettes or packages

▶ *High-speed prevacuum:* pump removes the air from the chamber and allows faster penetration of the steam for sterilizing.

▶ A time/temperature comparison of the two autoclave systems is provided in Table 6-1.

II. Use

▶ Moist heat may be used for all materials except:
- Oils, waxes, and powders that are impervious to steam.
- Materials that cannot be subjected to high temperatures.

III. Principles of Action

▶ Sterilization is achieved by action of heat; pressure serves only to attain high temperature.

▶ Sterilization depends on the penetrating ability of steam.

▶ Air must be excluded; otherwise steam penetration and heat transfer are prevented.

▶ Space between objects is essential to ensure access for the steam.

▶ Air discharge occurs in a downward direction; load must be arranged for free passage of steam toward bottom of autoclave.

IV. Evaluation of Steam Under Pressure

▶ Advantages
- All microorganisms, spores, and viruses are destroyed quickly and efficiently.
- Wide variety of materials may be treated; most economical method of sterilization.

▶ Disadvantages
- May corrode carbon steel instruments if precautions are not taken.

DRY HEAT

The action of dry heat is oxidation.

I. Use

▶ Primarily for materials that cannot be safely sterilized with steam under pressure.

▶ For small metal instruments enclosed in special containers or that might be corroded or rusted by moisture.

II. Principles of Action: Dry Heat

▶ Sterilization is achieved by heat conducted from the exterior surface to the interior of the object; the penetration time varies among materials.

▶ Sterilization can result when the material is treated for a sufficient length of time at the required temperature; therefore, timing for sterilization must start when the entire contents of the sterilizer have reached the peak temperature needed for that load.

III. Operation

▶ Temperature
  • A temperature of 160°C (320°F) maintained for 2 hours; 170°C (340°F) for 1 hour. Timing starts after the desired temperature has been reached.
  • Penetration time: Heat penetration varies with different materials.
  • Nature and properties of various materials are considered.

▶ Care
  • Care is taken not to overheat because certain materials can be affected. Temperatures over 160°C (320°F) may destroy the sharp edges of cutting instruments.

IV. Evaluation of Dry Heat

▶ Advantages
  • Useful for materials that cannot be subjected to steam under pressure.
  • When maintained at correct temperature, this method is well suited for sharp instruments.
  • No corrosion compared with steam under pressure.

▶ Disadvantages
  • Long exposure time required; penetration slow and uneven.
  • High temperature critical to certain materials.

CHEMICAL VAPOR STERILIZER

▶ The unsaturated chemical vapor sterilizer is also called the Chemiclave or Harvey sterilizer.

▶ A combination of alcohols, formaldehyde, ketone, water, and acetone heated under pressure produces a gas that is effective as a sterilizing agent.

I. Use

Chemical vapor sterilization cannot be used for materials or objects that can be altered by the chemicals that make the vapor or that cannot withstand the high temperature. Examples are low-melting plastics, liquids, or heat-sensitive handpieces.

II. Principles of Action

Microbial and viral destruction results from the permeation of the heated formaldehyde and alcohol. Heavy, tightly wrapped, or sealed packages would not permit the penetration of the vapors.

III. Operation

▶ Temperature
  • From 132°C (270°F) with 20–40 pounds pressure in accord with the manufacturer's directions.

▶ Time
  • Minimum of 20 minutes after the correct temperature and pressure have been attained. Time is extended for a large load or a heavy wrap.

▶ Cooling at the completion of the cycle
  • Instruments are dry. Instruments need a short period for cooling.

IV. Care of Sterilizer

▶ Refilling depends on the amount of use and is needed at least every 30 cycles.

▶ In accord with manufacturer's instructions, the condensate tray is removed, the exhausted solution emptied, and the tray cleaned.

V. Evaluation of Chemical Vapor Sterilizer

▶ Advantages
  • Corrosion- and rust-free operation for carbon steel instruments.
  • Ability to sterilize in a relatively short total cycle.
  • Ease of operation and care of the equipment.

▶ Disadvantages
  • Adequate ventilation is needed; cannot use in a small room.
  • Slight odor, which is rarely objectionable.

CARE OF STERILE INSTRUMENTS

▶ Instruments stored without sealed wrappers are only momentarily sterile because of airborne contamination.

▶ Labeled, sterilized, and sealed packages are stored unopened in clean, dry cabinets or drawers.
  • All stored packages are dated and used in rotation.
  • Paper-wrapped packages are handled carefully to prevent tearing.

▶ Packages wrapped and sealed in paper may not need resterilizing for several months to 1 year.

▶ Plastic or nylon wrap with a tape or heat seal may be expected to remain sterile longer.

► The expected shelf life before resterilizing depends on the area surrounding the stored packages. A closed, protected area without exposure, such as a cabinet or drawer that can be disinfected routinely, is preferred for storage.

CHEMICAL DISINFECTANTS

► Chemical disinfectants are used in several forms, including:
- Surface disinfectants.
- Immersion disinfectants, immersion sterilants.
- Hand antimicrobials.
- Each variety has specific chemicals, dilutions, and directions for application.

I. Categories

► Disinfectants are categorized by their biocidal activity as high level, intermediate level, or low level.
► Biocidal activity refers to the ability of the chemical disinfectant to destroy or inactivate living organisms.
- *High-level disinfectants* inactivate spores and all forms of bacteria, fungi, and viruses. Applied at different time schedules, the high-level chemical is either a disinfectant or a sterilant.
- *Intermediate-level disinfectants* inactivate all forms of microorganisms but do not destroy spores.
- *Low-level disinfectants* inactivate vegetative bacteria and certain lipid-type viruses but do not destroy spores, tubercle bacilli, or nonlipid viruses.

II. Uses

► Environmental surfaces disinfection
- Following each appointment, the treatment area is cleaned and disinfected.
► Dental laboratory impressions and prostheses
- Impressions can be carriers of infectious material to a dental laboratory. Completed prostheses must be disinfected before delivery to a patient.

III. Principles of Action

► Disinfection is achieved by:
- Coagulation, precipitation, or oxidation of protein of microbial cells.
- Denaturation of the enzymes of the cells.
► Disinfection depends on the contact of the solution at the known effective concentration for the optimum period of time.
► Items are thoroughly cleaned and dried because action of the agent is altered by foreign matter and dilution.
► A solution has a specific shelf life, use life, and reuse life.
- Some may be altered by changes in pH, or the active ingredient may decrease in potency.
- Check manufacturer's directions.

IV. Criteria for Selection of a Chemical Agent

► Objective: to select a product that is effective in the control of microorganisms and practical to use.
- Properties of an ideal disinfectant are shown in Box 6-2.
► United States Environmental Protection Agency (EPA) approval.
- Use EPA-registered hospital disinfectant for low-level requirements.
- Use EPA-registered hospital disinfectant with a tuberculocidal claim for intermediate and high especially when there is visible blood or other potentially infectious material.
► Manufacturer's informational literature and container labels
- Provide facts about the product that ensure its effectiveness.
- When the label has insufficient information, the manufacturer is contacted and instructions are obtained.
► The criteria include at least the following: must be tuberculocidal, bactericidal, virucidal, and fungicidal.
► Label must state:
1. Effectiveness and stability expressed by
- *Shelf life*: the expiration date indicating the termination of effectiveness of the unopened container.

BOX 6-2

Properties of an Ideal Disinfectant

1. Broad spectrum	Wide antimicrobial spectrum
2. Fast acting	A rapid lethal action on all vegetative forms and spores of bacteria and fungi, protozoa, and viruses
3. Not affected by physical factors	Active in the presence of organic matter, such as blood, sputum, and feces
	Compatible with soaps, detergents, and other chemicals encountered in use
4. Nontoxic	
5. Surface compatibility	Will not corrode instruments and other metallic surfaces
	Will not cause the disintegration of cloth, rubber, plastics, or other materials
6. Residual effect on treated surfaces	
7. Easy to use	
8. Odorless	Inoffensive odor to facilitate routine use
9. Economical	Reasonable cost

Adapted from: Molinari JA, Harte JA. *Cottone's Practical Infection Control in Dentistry*. 3rd ed. Philadelphia: Lippincott Williams & Wilkins, 2009. Chapter 12, Environmental surface infection control: disposable barriers and chemical disinfection; p. 173.

- *Use life*: the life expectancy for the solution once it has been activated but not actually put to use with contaminated items.
- *Reuse life*: the amount of time a solution can be used and reused while being challenged with instruments that are wet or coated with bioburden.
2. Directions for activation (mixing proportions).
3. Type of container for storage and place (conditions such as heat and light).
4. Directions for use
   - Precleaning and drying of items to be submerged.
   - Time/temperature ratio.
5. Instructions for disposal of used solution.
6. Warnings
   - Toxic effects (on eyes, skin).
   - Specific directions for emergency care in the event of an accident (e.g., splash in eye).
   - Keep manufacturer's *Materials Safety Data Sheets* for reference.
▶ After the product has been selected, it is the responsibility of the dental personnel to use it as directed to obtain the best possible infection control.

PREPARATION OF THE TREATMENT ROOM

▶ The cleanliness and neatness of the treatment room reflect the character and conscientiousness of the dental personnel.
▶ The patient, with limited knowledge of dental science, may judge the ability of the dental personnel by the appearance of the office or clinic.

▶ Patients may inquire about sterilization and infection control.
▶ The patient's attitude is important, but more important is the relationship of cleanliness to the presence of microorganisms. The need is to provide clinical services in an environment that minimizes cross-contamination.
▶ The orderliness and immaculate cleanliness of the treatment rooms result from continuing care.
▶ An excellent test for the effects of care and any minor oversights is for each dental team member to sit in the dental chair occasionally and look around at what the patient sees from that vantage point.

I. Objective

Effective care of instruments and equipment contributes to the control of disease transmitted by way of environmental surfaces and the maintenance of the working efficiency of office equipment and instruments.

II. Preliminary Planning

▶ Preparation of the treatment room when time between appointments is limited requires an efficient procedural system.
▶ The classification of inanimate objects (Table 6-3) provides a guide for analysis.
▶ First, all surfaces and items that will be used or contacted during the appointment can be categorized and listed as critical, semicritical, or noncritical.
▶ The most logical and scientific sequence for preparation for the appointment can then be outlined.

TABLE 6-3	Classification of Inanimate Objects		
SURFACE CATEGORY	**DEFINITION**	**STERILIZATION/ DISINFECTION**	**EXAMPLES**
Critical	Penetrate soft tissue or bone	Sterilize or disposable	Needles Curets Explorers Probes
Semicritical	Touch intact mucous membrane, oral fluids Does not penetrate	Sterilize after each use High-level disinfection when sterilization cannot be used	Radiographic biteblock Ultrasonic handpiece Amalgam condenser Mirror
Noncritical	Do not touch mucous membranes (only contact unbroken epithelium)	Cleaning and tuberculocidal intermediate-level disinfection	Light handles Certain X-ray machine parts Safety eyewear
Environmental	No contact with patient surfaces (or only intact skin)	Cleaning and intermediate to low disinfection	Counter tops Equipment surfaces Housekeeping surface

▶ Hand *"Touch Contacts"*
- Only contacts essential to the service to be performed are made.
- Planning ahead to have materials ready so that cabinet knobs or drawer handles do not have to be contacted is an example.

▶ *Sterilizable items*
- Critical and semicritical items are sterilized or are disposable.

▶ *Disposable items*
- Disposable items are used wherever possible.

▶ *Items that may be covered*
- Barrier coverings prevent contamination from reaching surfaces.
- Covers for light handles, counter tops, X-ray machine parts, computer keyboard, and mouse are examples.
- Care is taken when removing the covers not to contaminate the object beneath.

▶ *Items that require chemical disinfection*
- Objects and surfaces that cannot be included in one of the preceding categories are treated with a chemical disinfectant.
- When the material is not compatible with the chemical action of the disinfectant, a disposable or coverable substitute, is needed.

III. Clean and Disinfect Environmental Surfaces[5–7]

A. Agent

▶ The effectiveness of the disinfection procedure is the result of two actions:
- The physical rubbing and removal of contaminated material.
- The chemical inactivation of the living microorganisms.

▶ Surface disinfectants are concentrated, premixed solutions, sprays, foams, impregnated wipes, and dissolved tablets.
- Pump sprays are considered the best method for delivering cleaning/disinfecting agents to contaminated surfaces because they penetrate into crevices without aerosols.
- Do not store gauze sponges in the solution because cotton fibers contained in gauze may shorten the effectiveness of disinfectants when stored in containers.[5]

B. Procedure

1. Wear heavy-duty household gloves and mask.
2. Use several large gauze sponges or paper towels. A disinfectant-soaked sponge in each hand can decrease the time of cleaning certain objects. Contaminated objects, such as tubings, can be held with one sponge while scrubbing with the other sponge.
3. Spraying of a disinfectant must be followed by vigorous scrubbing in order to remove the film of microorganisms.
4. Scrub the disinfectant over the entire surface, with attention to irregularities where contaminated material can aggregate.
5. Spray and leave the surfaces wet for the time stated on the manufacturers disinfectant.

Follow manufacturer's directions when using premoistened wipes.

IV. Unit Water Lines

▶ A biofilm of microorganisms can form on the inside of the water-line tubings during overnight standing.

▶ Tests have been conducted on tubings to handpieces, water syringes, and ultrasonic scalers. When the lines were flushed for 2 minutes, the microbial counts were reduced.[1]

▶ Contaminated water cannot be used for surgical purposes or during the irrigation of pocket areas because infective microorganisms can be introduced.

▶ If contaminated water is directed forcefully into a pocket, microorganisms can enter the tissue and infection or bacteremia can result.
- Procedure for clinical use is to flush all water lines at least 2 minutes at the beginning of each day.
- Run water through water tubing for 30 seconds before and 30 seconds after each patient appointment.

▶ Refer to Appendix IV for the recommendations from the U.S. Department of Health and Human Services.

PATIENT PREPARATION

▶ Oral procedures that require penetration of tissues, such as giving anesthesia by injection or scaling subgingival pocket surfaces, can introduce bacteria into the tissues and hence into the bloodstream.
- Organisms injected into the tissue could multiply and create an abscess. Natural resistance helps the body handle and destroy invading microorganisms, provided the numbers can be kept to a minimum.

▶ Practical procedures for the preparation of a patient include preprocedural oral hygiene measures and rinsing with an antimicrobial mouthrinse.

I. Preprocedural Oral Hygiene Measures

▶ Toothbrushing
- Demonstration of biofilm removal from the teeth, tongue, and gingiva contributes to lowering the microbial count before treatment procedures.

▶ Rinsing
  • The numbers of bacteria on the gingival or mucosal surfaces can be reduced by the use of a preprocedural antiseptic mouthrinse.[8]
  • The substantivity of 0.12% chlorhexidine provides a lowered bacterial count for more than 60 minutes. Preprocedural rinsing before injections is advised.

II. Application of a Surface Antiseptic

▶ *Before injection of anesthetic*[7]
  • As a needle is introduced into the mucosa for penetration to deeper tissues, microorganisms on the surface can be carried into the tissue.
  • A topical antiseptic applied before the injection can decrease the risk of introducing septic material into the soft tissue.[9]
▶ *Before scaling and other dental hygiene instrumentation*[8]
  • Instrumentation in a sulcus or pocket and around the gingival margin can create breaks in the tissue where bacteria can enter.
  • Subgingival instrumentation in a pocket with broken down sulcular epithelium contributes to the entrance of bacteria into the underlying tissues and bacteremia.[9,10]
  • Dry the surface and swab the area with a topical antiseptic before instrumentation. Use an antiseptic solution to irrigate the sulci and pockets carefully.

SUMMARY OF STANDARD PROCEDURES

Basic procedures for clinical management are listed here.

I. Patient Factors

▶ Prepare a comprehensive patient history. Refer patients suspected of carrying infectious disease for medical evaluation.
▶ Ask the patient to rinse with an antimicrobial mouthrinse to reduce the numbers of oral microorganisms.
▶ Provide protective eyewear.
▶ Avoid elective procedures for a patient who is suffering from a communicable condition, such as a respiratory infection, or who has an open lesion on or about the lips or oral tissues, for the benefit of all who would be subjected to exposure.

II. Clinic Preparation

▶ Run water through all water lines, including the air–water syringe, handpieces, and ultrasonic unit, for 2 minutes at the start of the day and for at least 30 seconds before and after each use during the day.

▶ Disinfect all environmental surfaces that may be "touch surfaces" during the appointment. Make an orderly sequence for surface cleaning and disinfection. Apply barrier covers as indicated.
▶ Sterilize instruments and all other equipment that can be sterilized by one of the methods for complete sterilization. Maintain closed sterilized packages until ready for use.

III. Factors for the Dental Team

▶ Have medical examinations; keep immunizations up to date; have appropriate testing on a periodic basis.
▶ Always use mask, protective eyewear, gloves, and a clean closed-front gown with fitted wrist cuffs.
▶ Utilize thorough hand hygiene and cleansing before putting on and after removing gloves.
▶ Develop habits that minimize contacts with switches and other parts of the dental unit, dental chair, light, and clinician's stool, and avoid all environmental contacts unrelated to the procedure at hand.

IV. Treatment Factors

A. Hypodermic Needles

▶ Use a safe recapping and disposal methods (Figure 38-7, Chapter 38) to prevent accidental penetration or self-inoculation.

B. Removable Oral Prostheses

▶ Gloves are worn to receive a prosthesis from a patient.
▶ Place the prosthesis in a disposable cup and cover with a disinfectant. Use a fresh solution of 0.05% iodophor in water, or a 1:5 dilution of 5% sodium hypochlorite.
▶ Clean by ultrasonics.

V. Posttreatment

▶ Use heavy puncture-resistant gloves to handle used instruments.
▶ Follow routines to disinfect, clean, and prepare the instruments for sterilization.
▶ Contaminated waste is secured in plastic disposal bags.
▶ Disinfect safety eyewear for patient and dental team members.

OCCUPATIONAL POSTEXPOSURE MANAGEMENT

Accidents happen even to the most skillful clinician. Accidental percutaneous (laceration, needle stick) or permucosal (splash to eye or mucosa) exposure to blood or other body fluids requires prompt action.

I. Significant Exposures

▶ Percutaneous or permucosal stick or wound with needle or sharp instrument contaminated with blood, saliva, or other body fluids.

▶ Contamination of any obviously open wound, nonintact skin, or mucous membrane with blood, saliva, or a combination.

▶ Exposure of patient's body fluids to unbroken skin is not considered a significant exposure.

II. Procedure Following Exposure

▶ Immediately wash the wound with soap and water; rinse well.

▶ Flush nose, mouth, eyes, or skin with clear water, saline, or a sterile irrigant.

▶ Report to designated official.

▶ Complete an incident report as required.

▶ Follow the required predetermined, posted procedures of the clinic, institution, or individual practice setting

III. Follow-Up

▶ Report signs and symptoms associated with infectious disease such as hepatitis or human immunodeficiency virus (HIV).

▶ Obtain medical evaluation of any illness involving fever, rash, and lymphadenopathy

▶ Pursue counseling and further testing.

DISPOSAL OF WASTE

Types of waste are defined in Box 6-1. Each type of waste requires special handling.

I. Regulations

▶ Investigate the regulations of each town or city sanitation division for rules concerning disposal of contaminated waste.

▶ Figure 6-5 illustrates the universal label required by the United States Occupational Safety and Health Administration (OSHA). The labels must be attached to containers used to store or transport hazardous waste materials.

II. Guidelines for Disposal of Waste

▶ Disposable materials, such as gloves, masks, wipes, paper drapes, or surface covers, that are contaminated with blood or body fluids are carefully handled and discarded in sturdy, impervious plastic bags to minimize human contact.

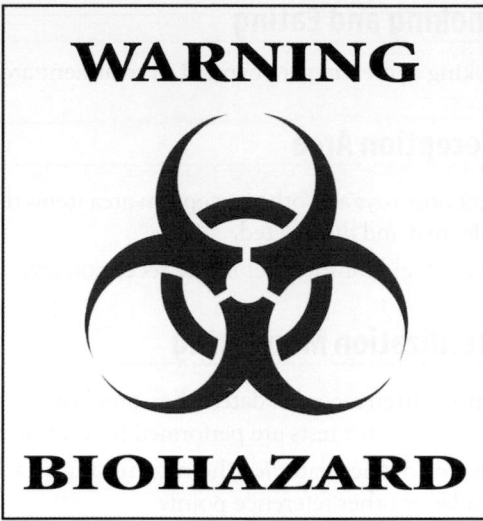

FIGURE 6-5 Universal Label for Hazardous Material. A hazard-warning label is fluorescent orange or orange-red with lettering or a symbol in a contrasting color. The label must be attached to containers used to store or transport waste. A label is not required for regulated waste that has been decontaminated (such as dental waste that has been autoclaved).

▶ Blood, suctioned fluids, or other liquid waste may be carefully poured into a drain that is connected to a sanitary sewer system in compliance with applicable local regulations.

▶ Sharp items, such as needles and scalpel blades, are placed intact into a puncture-resistant, leak-proof container.

▶ Human tissue and contaminated solid wastes can be disposed of according to the requirements established by local or state environmental regulatory agencies and published recommendations.

▶ Infectious medical waste, including tissues and culture media, are handled in a manner consistent with local regulations before disposal.

▶ Disposal methods for both liquid and solid chemicals vary with the type of chemical and local regulations governing waste-management practices.

SUPPLEMENTAL RECOMMENDATIONS

I. Cleaning the Face

▶ Check and clean the exposed parts of the face not covered by mask or protective eyewear, where spatter collects, as an aid to disease control as well as for general sanitation.

▶ In reality, cleaning the face several times each day and washing before eating is a logical procedure for personal hygiene and safety.

II. Smoking and Eating

▶ Smoking and eating are banned in treatment areas.

III. Reception Area

▶ Select only toys and other reception area items that can be cleaned and disinfected.

▶ Provide hand sanitizer gel in the reception area.

IV. Sterilization Monitoring

▶ Keep a written record of dates when processing tests and biologic monitor tests are performed for each sterilizer.

▶ Indicate advance dates for the next testing clearly on a calendar or other reference point.

▶ Perform tests made weekly on the same day to simplify remembering.

V. Office Policy Manual

▶ Include in the clinic or office policy manual outlines of procedures to follow for standard precautions.

▶ Addresses for sources of various materials can be kept in a special reference section of the manual.

▶ Emergency procedures to follow when accidentally exposed are defined clearly.

DOCUMENTATION

Documentation for a patient with concerns about infection control procedures would include:

▶ Name, record number, address, telephone (home and cell), e-mail.

▶ Medical history for history of hepatitis B virus (HBV), hepatitis C virus (HCV), or HIV; high-risk history associated with these diseases; patient consent to be tested for HBV, HCV, and HIV.

▶ HIV-positive patient: current medications and previously taken, if they were ineffective; most recent viral load, current CD4 if known.

▶ A sample progress note for a patient with concerns about infection control procedures can be reviewed in Box 6-3.

BOX 6-3

Example Documentation: Patient with Concerns about Infection Control

S –Patient presents for routine periodontal maintenance appointment. Patient asked how instruments were "cleaned" between patients.

O –Health history update indicates patient has been recently diagnosed as HIV positive.

A –She was concerned about an increased risk for opportunistic infections as well as the fact that her condition might increase risk for other patients seen in the office.

P –Explained that standard precautions and infection control procedures used during all patient treatment are designed to protect all patients from cross-contamination. Explained each set of instruments is sterilized utilizing steam under pressure (autoclave). Tests for sterilization are done for each cycle of instruments, in addition to weekly and monthly tests to ensure the autoclave is functioning properly. Opened all sterilized instrument kits in her presence.

Signed: _____, RDH
Date: _____

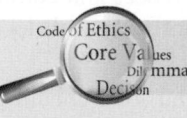

EVERYDAY ETHICS

Kimberly, the dental hygienist, is about to begin the patient examination when she notices that the indicator tape on the sterilizing cassette had not changed color. She excuses herself and finds out from the receptionist that a call to the repair service has been made because the autoclave has been shutting down before completion of the cycle. It is after 1:00 PM and patients are scheduled all afternoon.

Questions for Consideration

1. When proper sterile technique is not followed, what ethical principles and core values are involved? Describe Kimberly's duty to her patients.

2. Use the steps to decision making in Box 1-10 in Chapter 1 to determine possible solutions for this situation. Describe how each could be defended to the patient, the dentist, and other dental team members.

3. Which American Dental Hygienist Association professional roles (Table 1-1 in Chapter 1) does Kimberly serve in when she plans to make changes that ensure that this kind of situation does not happen again? Explain each role and how it applies for Kimberly.

Factors To Teach The Patient

▷ The meaning of "standard precautions" and what is included under the term; how these precautions protect the patient and the dental team members.

▷ The contribution of the accurately completed medical and dental personal history to the provision of the best, safest treatment possible.

▷ Methods for sterilization of instruments, including handpieces; how the autoclave or other sterilizer is tested daily or weekly.

▷ Facts about the normal oral flora and the factors that influence an increased number of bacteria on the tongue, mucosa, and in the dental biofilm on the teeth.

▷ Methods for personal daily control of the oral bacteria through biofilm control and tongue brushing.

▷ Reasons for preprocedural rinsing.

▷ Method for thorough rinsing.

References

1. United States Department of Health and Human Services, Centers for Disease Control and Prevention. Guidelines for infection control in dental health-care settings–2003. *MMWR.* 2003;52(RR 17):27.

2. Miller CH, Tan CM, Beiswanger MA, et al. Cleaning dental instruments: measuring the effectiveness of an instrument washer/disinfector. *Am J Dent.* 2000;13:39–43.

3. Miller CH. Use of spore test for quality assurance in infection control. *Am J Dent.* 2001;14:114.

4. Association of the Advancement of Medical Instrumentation, American National Standards Institute. *Steam Sterilization and Sterility Assurance Using Table-Top Sterilizers in Office-Based, Ambulatory-Care Medical, Surgical, and Dental Facilities.* ANSI/AAMI ST40-1998. Arlington, VA: Association for the Advancement of Medical Instrumentation; 1998.

5. Cottone JA, Terezhalmy GT, Molinari JA. *Practical Infection Control in Dentistry.* 2nd ed. Philadelphia, PA:Williams & Wilkins;1996:195.

6. Miller CH, Palenik CJ. *Infection Control and Management of Hazardous Materials for the Dental Team.* St Louis: Mosby; 2005.

7. OSAP's infection control in practice: demystifying disinfectants, August 2002 and OSAP's Monthly Focus #6, 1998. Organization for Safety and Asepsis Procedures. http://www.osap.org/?FAQ_Instrum_Disinf2. Accessed February 3, 2014.

8. Reddy S, Prasad MG, Kaul S, et al. Efficacy of 0.2% tempered chlorhexidine as a pre-procedural mouth rinse: a clinical study. *J Indian Soc Periodontol.* 2012;16(2):213–217.

9. Johnson SM, Saint John BE, Dine AP. Local anesthetics as antimicrobial agents: a review. *Surg Infect (Larchmt).* 2008;9(2):205–213.

10. Fine DH, Korik I, Furgang D, et al. Assessing preprocedural subgingival irrigation and rinsing with an antiseptic mouthrinse to reduce bacteremia. *J Am Dent Assoc.* 1996;127(5):641–642.

ENHANCE YOUR UNDERSTANDING

thePoint® DIGITAL CONNECTIONS
(see the inside front cover for access information)

- **Audio glossary**
- **Quiz bank**

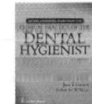

SUPPORT FOR LEARNING
(available separately; visit lww.com)

- *Active Learning Workbook for Clinical Practice of the Dental Hygienist, 12th Edition*

prepU INDIVIDUALIZED REVIEW
(available separately; visit lww.com)

- **Adaptive quizzing with *prepU for Wilkins' Clinical Practice of the Dental Hygienist***

7

Patient Reception and Ergonomic Practice

Jane F. Halaris, RDH, BS, MA and Esther M. Wilkins, BS, RDH, DMD

CHAPTER OUTLINE

LEARNING OBJECTIVES

After studying this chapter, the student will be able to:

1. Describe the rules of etiquette in relationship to patient reception and care.

2. Describe the components of ergonomic practice and relationship to career longevity.

3. Identify the range of working positions for a right-handed and left-handed clinician.

4. Describe the elements of a neutral working position (NWP).

5. Explain the musculoskeletal disorders and their causes and symptoms most often associated with the clinical practice of dental hygiene.

6. Explain the ergonomic risk factors of clinical dental hygiene practice.

The patient's presence in the office or clinic is an expression of confidence in the dentist and the dental hygienist. Confidence is inspired by the reputation for professional knowledge and skill, the appearance of the office, and the actions of the workers in it.

▶ The physical arrangement and interpersonal relationships provide the setting for specific services to be performed.

▶ The patient's well-being is the all-important consideration throughout the appointment.

▶ At the same time, the clinician must function effectively and efficiently in a manner that minimizes stress and fatigue to ensure personal health.

▶ Musculoskeletal disorders, repetitive stress injuries, and cumulative trauma disorders are common work-related conditions that require continuing preventive physical and mental energy on the part of each clinical dental hygienist.

▶ The science of ergonomics has provided information for the development of standards for human performance and workplace design that can maximize health, comfort, and efficiency for dental hygienists in clinical practice.

▶ Key words related to ergonomics, patient reception and care, and workplace design are defined in Box 7-1.

PREPARATION FOR THE PATIENT

I. Treatment Area

The requirements for preparation of the treatment area are *standard precautions* for all patients whether or not the presence of a communicable disease is known.

▶ *Environmental surfaces*: All contact areas are thoroughly disinfected or covered to control cross-contamination.

▶ *Instruments*: Sterile packaged instruments remain sealed until the start of the actual treatment.

▶ *Equipment*: Prepare and make ready other materials that will be used, such as for the determination of blood pressure and patient instruction. Anticipate specific needs for procedures being delivered.

▶ *Patient's dental chair*: Upright for current patient reception; chair arm up for access.

▶ *Clinician's chair*: Set at proper height for the entire day.

II. Records

▶ For the patient of record, the patient's medical and dental history for pertinent appointment information, updating, and assessment are reviewed.

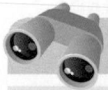

BOX 7-1 **KEY WORDS:** Chair Positioning and Ergonomic Practice

Body language: a set of nonverbal signals, including body movements, postures, gestures, and facial expressions, that gives expression to various physical, mental, and emotional states.

Body mechanics: the field of physiology that studies muscular actions and functions in the maintenance of the posture of the body.

Cumulative trauma disorder, work-related musculoskeletal disorder, repetitive strain injury, bioaccumulated stress: terms used to describe disorders of the musculoskeletal, autonomic, and peripheral nervous system caused by repeated, forceful, and awkward movements of the human body, as well as by exposure to mechanical stress, vibration, and cold temperatures. Often work related.

Ergonomics: study of human performance and workplace design to maximize health, comfort, and efficiency.

Kyphosis: naturally occurring curve in the thoracic region of spine that, when viewed from the side, is curved toward the back of the body.

Lordosis: naturally occurring curves in the cervical and lumbar regions of the spine that, when viewed from the side, are curved toward the front of the body.

Neutral working position: the position of the body in which the normal curvatures of the spine are maintained and the muscles and joints are naturally aligned.

Postural hypotension: also called orthostatic hypotension; a fall in blood pressure associated with dizziness, syncope, and blurred vision that occurs upon standing or when standing motionless in a fixed position.

Risk factor: anything that puts the clinician or the patient at risk or increases their risk of exposure to an identified hazard.

Safe work practice: any work practice that improves clinician and patient safety. This includes but is not limited to decreased physical demands, improved layout, environmental factors, and work process organization.

Stress: a physical, chemical, or emotional factor that causes physical or mental tension and may be a factor in disease causation or fatigue.

Supine: flat position with head and feet on the same level.

Trendelenburg: the modified supine position when the head is lower than the heart.

Work simplification: application to clinical procedure of time and motion studies, analysis of instruments and equipment, and body mechanics to provide the patient with a smooth, systematic, simplified approach for comprehensive dental hygiene therapy.

▶ Read previous appointment progress notes to focus the current treatment plan.

▶ Anticipate examination procedures and new record making for a new patient.

PATIENT RECEPTION

I. Introductions

▶ The dental assistant or the dentist may introduce the new patient to the dental hygienist, but more frequently, a self-introduction is in order.

▶ The patient is greeted by name, and the hygienist's name is clearly stated, for example, "Good morning, Mrs. Smith; I am Anna Jones, the dental hygienist."

▶ Procedure for introducing the patient to others:
  • A woman's name always precedes a gentleman's.
  • An older person's name precedes the younger person's (when of the same sex and when the difference in age is obvious).
  • In general, the patient's name precedes that of a member of the dental personnel.
  • An older patient is not called by the first name except at the patient's request.

II. Escort Patient to Dental Chair

▶ Invite patient to be seated and adjust the chair as needed.

▶ Assist the elderly, disabled, or very small children; guide into the chair (support the patient's arm when patient requests or accepts it).

▶ Assist with wheelchair. Bring wheelchair adjacent to the dental chair. Wheelchair procedures are described in the Wheelchair Transfer section in Chapter 57.

▶ Suggestions for helping the patient with a vision impairment may be found in Chapter 60.

▶ Place handbag in a safe place, if possible within the patient's view.

▶ Provide protective eyewear. When a patient removes personal corrective eyeglasses to substitute those provided, make sure the personal glasses are placed in their case in a safe place.

POSITION OF THE PATIENT

I. General Positions

Four body positions for delivery of care are shown in Figure 7-1.

A. Upright

▶ This is the initial position for patient reception from which chair adjustments are made.

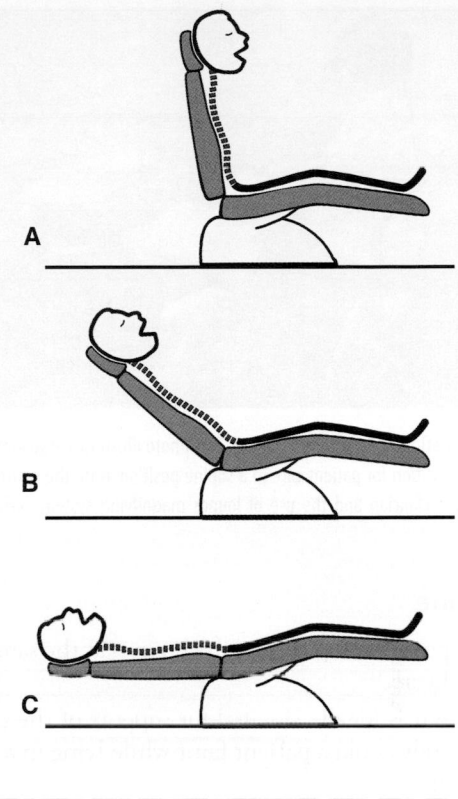

FIGURE 7-1 Basic Patient Positions. A: Upright. **B:** Semi-upright. **C:** Supine or horizontal with the brain on the same level as the heart. **D:** Trendelenburg, with the brain lower than the heart and the feet slightly elevated.

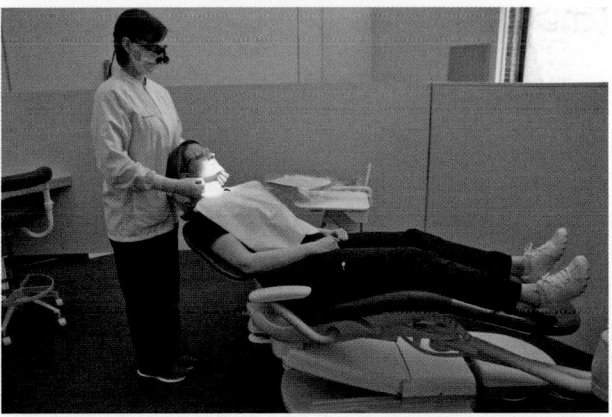

FIGURE 7-2 Patient in a Semi-Upright Position. This photograph illustrates ergonomic patient and clinician position for patient care in a semi-upright position when, the clinician stands to provide care for the patient who cannot be moved to the supine position.

B. Semi-Upright

▶ Patients with certain types of cardiovascular, respiratory, or vertigo problems may need this position.

▶ Figure 7-2 illustrates the patient and clinician using a semi-upright position during patient care.

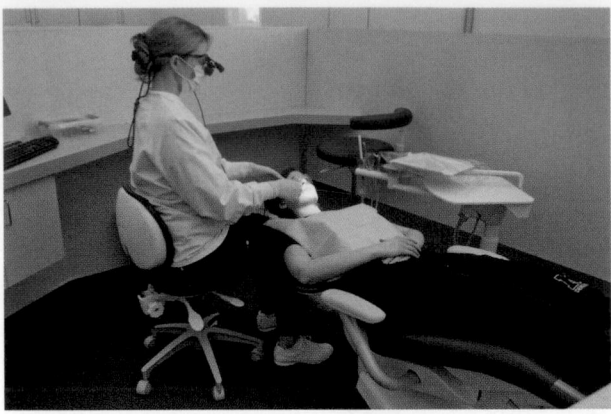

FIGURE 7-3 Patient in a Supine Position. This photo illustrates ergonomic patient and clinician position for patient care in a supine position. Note the neutral seating position of the clinician and the use of loupes magnifying system with attached headlamp.

C. Supine

- In a supine or flat position, the brain is at the same level as the heart.
- A patient is ideally situated for support of the circulation; rarely could a patient faint while lying in a supine position.
- The back of the chair is parallel to the floor.
- Position used most for treatment procedures.
- Figure 7-3 illustrates the patient and clinician while using the supine position.

D. Trendelenburg

- The patient is in the supine position and tipped back and down 10° to 15° so that the brain is lower than the heart.
- The back of the chair is less than parallel to the floor.

II. The Dental Chair

- A dental chair provides complete body support for the patient, which increases patient relaxation.
- A comfortable patient is more compliant and allows the procedure to be completed more efficiently.
- Seat and leg support moves as a unit; back and headrest move as a unit; both are power controlled.
- Has a thin back so that the chair may be lowered close to the clinician's elbow height.
- Chair base permits the chair to be lowered as needed for appropriate treatment position.
- Chair controls need to be available to both the assistant and clinician.

III. Use of Dental Chair

A. Prepositioning for Patient Reception

- Chair at low level; back upright.
- Chair arm raised on side of approach.

B. Adjustment Steps

- Patient is seated with back upright.
- Chair seat and foot portion are raised first to help the patient settle back.
- Lower back to the supine position for maxillary instrumentation and to a 20° angle with the floor for mandibular treatment.
- Request patient to slide up to rest the head at upper edge of the headrest or backrest and turn head to left or right as needed for visibility and access.
- Adjust chair height until patient's mouth is at the clinician's elbow height with shoulder relaxed (Figure 7-3).

C. Conclusion of Appointment

- Move instrument tray away and turn off light.
- Slowly raise back of chair and tilt chair forward.
- Request patient to remain seated in upright position briefly to avoid postural hypotension.

D. Contraindications for Supine Position

- Review patient history for indications of need for adaptation.
- Patient may request a position variation.
- Conditions that may contraindicate the supine position include congestive heart failure, vertigo, and respiratory conditions such as emphysema, severe asthma, or sinusitis.
- During the third trimester of pregnancy, some women may be uncomfortable. Chair positioning for the pregnant patient is described in Chapter 49.

POSITION OF THE CLINICIAN

- The clinician is in the neutral working position (NWP), with good access, light, and visibility, which in turn contribute to an efficient procedure.
- The patient is positioned so that a thorough, biologically oriented service may be performed conveniently and efficiently within a reasonable length of time.
- The positions of the patient and the clinician are interdependent.
- When clinician and patient positioning is considered, it is realistic to remember that the patient's position will be assumed for a relatively short time compared with that of the clinician.

NEUTRAL WORKING POSITION (NWP)

I. Objectives

Objectives concern the health of the clinician, the service to be performed, and the effect on the patient.

The preferred neutral position attempts to accomplish the following:

▶ Contribute to and preserve rather than detract from clinician's health and wellness.

▶ Contribute to ease and efficacy of performance that encourages patient cooperation.

▶ Allow endurance for prolonged periods of peak efficiency.

▶ Reduce potential for overexertion and injury from mental and physical stress and fatigue.

▶ Give the patient a sense of well-being, security, and confidence.

▶ Accommodate a patient with special needs.

II. The Effects of NWP

▶ NWP needs to be developed, practiced daily, and made habitual.

▶ Habitual neutral position will translate to all activities, outside of work as well. An internal environment can be created for on-going physical ease, comfort, safety, and activity.

▶ Without practicing the principles of neutral position on a regular daily basis, a clinician can experience discomfort, pain, and work-related stress disorders. The long-term result can be shortened or compromised career longevity with changes in daily life activities.

▶ Analysis and assessment of posture can give direction to corrections for treatment. A posture assessment instrument is available.[1]

III. Description of Neutral Seated Position[2,3]

▶ A neutral seated position is illustrated in Figure 7-4A.

▶ *Back*: in neutral alignment with natural spinal curves, including cervical lordosis, thoracic kyphosis, and lumbar lordosis.

▶ *Head*: on top of neutral spine with forward neck flexion between 15° and 20° or less.

▶ *Eyes*: directed downward to prevent neck and eye strain.

▶ *Shoulders*: relaxed and parallel with the hips and floor.

▶ *Elbows*: close to the body.

▶ *Forearms*: parallel with the floor.

▶ *Wrist*: forearm and wrist are in a straight line.

▶ *Hips*: slightly higher than knees.

▶ *Thighs*: full body weight distributed evenly on seat; comfortable space (about 3 inches) between edge of seat and back of knee.

▶ *Knees*: slightly apart.

▶ *Feet*: flat on the floor.

IV. Clinician/Patient Positioning

A. Distance

▶ Patient's oral cavity is adjusted to clinician's elbow height.

▶ Distance from clinician's eyes to the patient's oral cavity when the clinician is seated in neutral position will be within the range of 15–22 inches (Figure 7-4B).

▶ The distance is defined as the "working distance," which is a significant measurement when fitting magnification loupes for an individual clinician.

B. Selection

▶ NWP is combined with effective access to the patient for treatment procedures.

▶ Orientation of position of the clinician to patient can be compared to the hours of a clock around the patient's head with 12:00 O'clock at the top of the patient's head as shown in Figure 7-5.

▶ Clock hours correspond with clinician/patient relation associated with instrumentation in different areas of the patient's oral cavity.

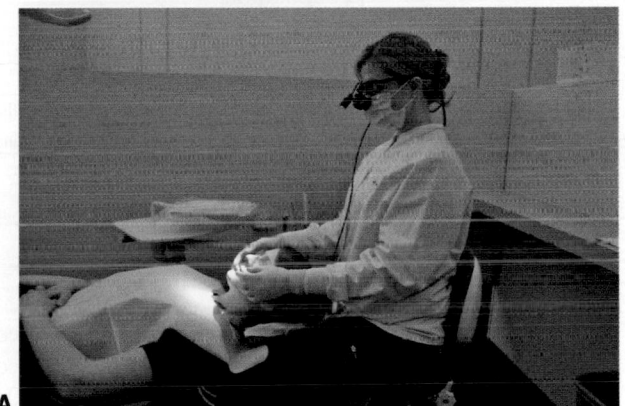

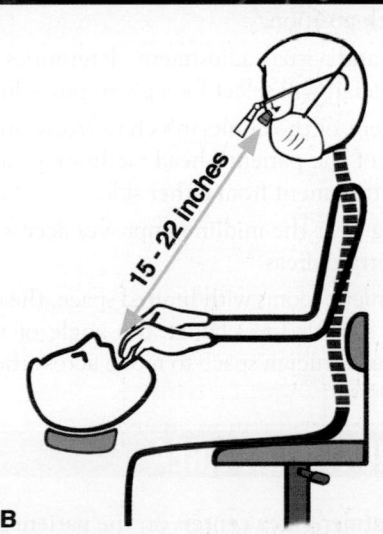

FIGURE 7-4 Clinician's Working Distance. A: Clinician in 12:00 working position and drawing. **B:** Clinician in 8:00 working position. Both illustrate acceptable positioning, which shows the patient at the clinician's elbow level and the oral cavity of the patient between 15 and 22 inches from the clinician's eyes.

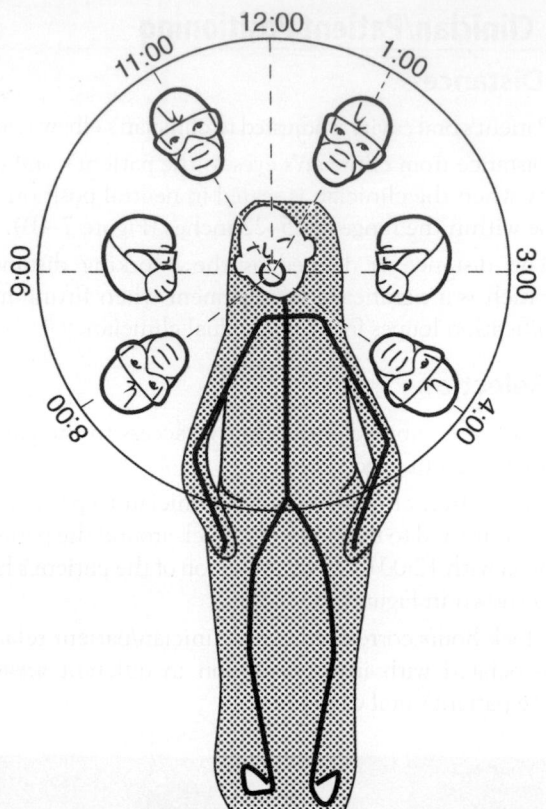

FIGURE 7-5 Range of Positions for Clinician. The patient's head is placed at the upper edge of the backrest or headrest for convenient access by the clinician during treatment. The range of positions is compared with the numbers on a clock.

C. Flexibility[2]

Orientation for the right-handed clinician is associated with the 8:00–12:00 o'clock position; for the left-handed clinician, orientation is associated with the 12:00–4:00 o'clock position.[3]

▶ Access and visual adjustment determines which side the clinician will select for a given procedure.

▶ Movement of the clinician's chair freely on wheels and turning of the patient's head facilitate positioning and patient treatment from either side.

▶ Crossing over the midline improves access and visibility in certain areas.

▶ In treatment rooms with limited space, the dental chair may be swiveled to change the angle of the chair to allow the clinician space to move across the midline.

THE TREATMENT AREA

▶ The treatment area centers on the patient's oral cavity.

▶ The entire "work area" refers to the dental chair with patient, the unit, and the instrument tray as they are positioned for the convenience and accessibility of the clinician and assistant for four-handed dental hygiene.

▶ For the clinician, the essentials for access and visibility for patient care are provided by the flexibility of movement of the clinician's stool and appropriate lighting, supplemented by the clinician's own visibility enhanced by wearing magnification loupes with head light.

I. The Clinician's Chair

▶ The chair is a significant adjunct to implement ergonomic practice.

▶ Optimal design provides adequate support and the opportunity and means to change body posture frequently during the workday as clinicians, patients, and procedures change.

▶ The clinician adjusts the chair to personal specifications.

A. Characteristics of an Acceptable Chair[4]

▶ *Base*: broad and heavy with five casters; a chair with five casters provides greater stability.

▶ *Seat design*:
  • *Traditional*:
    ◦ Size needs to support thighs without back of knees touching edge, seamless upholstery, padded firmly, with ability to tilt the seat; accommodates requirements for neutral seated position.
  • *Saddle chair*:
    ◦ This is a relatively new type of chair modeled after a riding saddle; promotes neutral spine position.

▶ *Armrests*: adjustable at a height that supports the forearm without raising shoulders.

▶ *Height*: adjustable for wide personal variability.

▶ *Back*: adjustable lumbar support to accommodate different positions, procedures, and clinicians.

▶ *Mobility*: completely mobile; built with free-rolling casters; not connected to other dental equipment; free movement around the patient's head for instrumentation from either side.

▶ *Adjustment*: multiple adjustments for different positions, procedures, and clinicians; mechanisms easy to learn and use.

▶ *Infection control friendly*: all surfaces able to withstand standard precautions regimen.

II. Vision: Lighting

▶ During treatment, visibility in the oral cavity is prerequisite to thoroughness without undue trauma to the tissues.

▶ With adequate light, efficiency increases, treatment time is decreased, and patient cooperation increases.

▶ Many lighting options are available. All need to be directed properly to the oral cavity for adequate visualization, optimal patient care, and clinician comfort and safety.

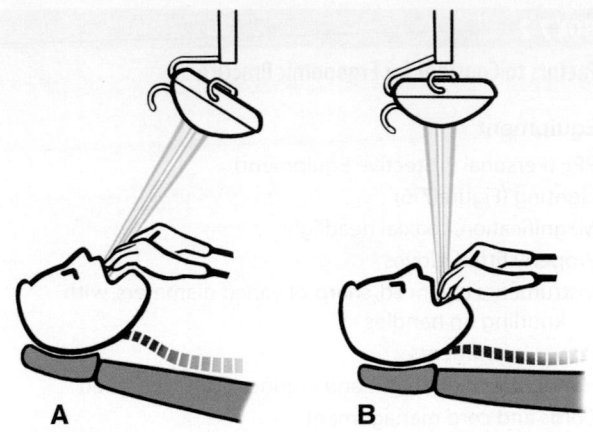

FIGURE 7-6 **Lighting.** Light does not obstruct clinician, allows clear illumination of the treatment area. **A:** Maxillary arch; chin up position; beam of light often between 60°→45° angle to floor. **B:** Mandibular arch; chin down position; beam of light nearly perpendicular to floor.

A. Dental Light: Suggested Features

▶ Is readily adjustable both vertically and horizontally.

▶ Beam of light is capable of being focused.

▶ Set within a comfortable arm's reach.

▶ Does not require awkward or forceful movement to position it for visualization.

B. Dental Light: Location

▶ *Attachment*
  • Unit attachment.
  • Ceiling-mounted light on a track is most versatile.

▶ *Dual lighting*
  • Advantages of the use of two clinic lights have been demonstrated with a supine patient position in a contoured chair.
  • One light directed from the front of the patient may be attached to the dental unit; the other light is mounted on a ceiling track.

▶ *Dental light: adjustment principles*
  • Light allows clear illumination of entire treatment area.
  • Figure 7-6 shows position of light for maxillary and mandibular treatment.

III. Vision: Magnification[5–7]

Magnification is needed to improve visualization, support NWP, and enhance treatment procedures.

A. Choice of Loupe Systems

▶ Fixed through the lens: customized for individuals:
  • Adjusted with the clinician's prescription as needed.
  • Magnifying lenses mounted directly into the lens.
  • Fixed interpupillary distance; angle of the lens not adjustable.
  • Not adjustable; enables the clinician to maintain correct posture.

▶ Front lens mounted without vertical adjustment
  • Prescription lenses are available.
  • Magnifying lenses mounted to a hinge on the frame; loupes can be adjusted up or down. Interpupillary distance can be adjusted; angle of lens not adjustable.

▶ Front lens mounted with vertical adjustment
  • Prescription lenses are available.
  • Magnifying lenses mounted to a hinge on the frame; loupes can be adjusted up or down.
  • Interpupillary distance can be adjusted; angle of lens can be adjusted.

▶ Loupes with coaxial headlight: improves visualization with targeted illumination.

B. Features

▶ Proper fit is essential to successful incorporation of magnification into the clinician's treatment environment.

▶ Proper fit is dependent on the clinician's working distance and neutral position.

▶ Clinicians need to research the differences to select best option.

IV. Handpieces

▶ Technology has provided handpieces that are ergonomically compatible with procedures clinicians provide.

▶ The best designs are small, light, and well-suited for the size of dental hygienist's hand.

A. Ergonomically Designed Handpieces

▶ Are lightweight, decreasing stress on hand and wrist.

▶ Fit in the contours of the clinician's hand and allow functional light grasp.

▶ Reduce fatigue and strain.

▶ Allow maneuverability.

▶ Provide power assist without strain.

▶ Produce less heat buildup.

▶ Are available in a cordless option.

V. Cords

A. Management

▶ Managing cords is a significant aspect of ergonomic practice.

▶ Cords are part of most dental units and are an integral part of delivery of care for every patient.

▶ Ultrasonics, air/water syringes, slow-speed handpieces, and all power-driven equipment requires cords connected to a power source.

▶ Improper management and inefficient design of the cords can increase drag on hand, wrist, and arm increasing risk of repetitive injury.

▶ Care is needed that cords can be sanitized, and are not dragging on the floor of the clinic.

B. Curly Cords

▶ Can cause excessive stretching and pulling by clinician.

▶ Associated with bending, reaching, and awkward postures to position for treatment.

▶ Increase the strain on hand, wrist, arm, and shoulder of clinician.

▶ Provide an ergonomic risk by increasing fatigue level and creating muscle imbalances.

▶ Straight cords may be generally easier to manage.

ERGONOMIC PRACTICE

I. Scope of Ergonomic Dental Hygiene

▶ Includes all practices that make work safe, decrease strain and fatigue, eliminate hazards, and improve work process affecting health and well-being of clinician and patient.

▶ Terminology related to ergonomics is included in Box 7-1.

▶ Box 7-2 lists items of the equipment, work layout, and work process organization that need attention during practice if physical occupational disorders are to be prevented.

II. Related Occupational Problems

▶ The physical challenges inherent in dental hygiene practice place the clinicians at risk for developing work-related musculoskeletal disorders.[8]

▶ Table 7-1 lists a variety of disorders that can occur among clinicians.

▶ Prevention of the slow developing conditions is a daily responsibility.

III. Ergonomic Risk Factors

▶ Prevention begins with the recognition of the risk factors that can point to potential body injury and more serious permanent musculoskeletal disorders.[9]

▶ Table 7-2 lists and defines significant risk factors and provides examples of various practices that can lead to musculoskeletal disorders.

SELF-CARE FOR THE DENTAL HYGIENIST

▶ Responsible self-care and attention to the risk factors of musculoskeletal disorders are central to ergonomic practice.

BOX 7-2

Factors to Consider for Ergonomic Practice

Equipment

PPE (Personal Protective Equipment)
Lighting (Figure 7-6)
Magnification, coaxial headlight
Properly fitted gloves
Instruments balanced, sharp, of varied diameters, with knurling on handles
Power instruments
Handpiece lightweight and ergonomically designed
Cords and cord management
Foot pedals
Suction
Air/water syringe

Work Layout

Uncluttered, easy access to patient, patient records, computer, radiographs
Counters clear with designated area for documentation
Instrument tray within arm's reach
Light fixture within arm's length, easy to move and adjust
Orderly tray setup with complete armamentarium for services to be delivered
Convenient treatment room setup and design for patient chair, air/water syringe, suction, cords, foot pedals

Work Process Organization

Clinician NWP
Use of magnification system supporting NWP
CPP (Clinician-Patient Positioning)
Light within easy arm's reach with clear illumination of treatment area
Access and management of suction and air/water syringe
Cords and cord maintenance

Instrumentation

Reach of tray
Order of instruments on tray
Consistent instrumentation sequence for all surfaces of sextants
Proper grasp and fulcrum technique for dominant hand
Proper grasp and fulcrum technique for nondominant hand
Sharp instruments
Correct working stroke for location and type of deposit
Inclusion of power instrumentation
Placement and access of foot pedals
Selective polishing
Placement and access to overgloves
Documentation procedure

TABLE 7-1	Musculoskeletal Disorders Affecting Dental Hygienists

With any symptoms or any ongoing discomfort, take action to find the source of the problem and how to relieve the symptom. Prevention is the best course of action. Early intervention will decrease the risk of a more involved condition or a more costly injury. If not addressed in a timely manner, any of these conditions could lead to a limited ability to practice or total disability.

CONDITION	CAUSES	SYMPTOMS
Carpal Tunnel Syndrome		
A symptomatic compression of the median nerve within the carpal tunnel (Figure 7-7)	Deviations of wrist from neutral. Pinch grasp with insufficient rest.	Numbness; tingling in the thumb, index, and middle fingers.
Thoracic Outlet Syndrome		
Painful disorder of the fingers, hand, and/or wrist from compression of the brachial nerve plexus and vessels between the neck and shoulder.	Tilting head forward. Hunched and/or rounded forward shoulders. Continuously reaching overhead.	Numbness, tingling, and/or pain in the hand or wrist.
Bursitis		
Inflammation of the bursa.	Areas of friction or impingement anywhere in the body, usually the shoulder.	Decreased range of motion. Aching.
Tendonitis		
Painful inflammation of the wrist resulting in strain.	Repeated wrist extension or palmar flexion.	Pain in the wrist, especially along the outer edges of the hand rather than through the center of the wrist.
Disc Herniation		
Displacement of the nucleus of the disc with resultant pressure on the spinal cord or peripheral nerves.	Prolonged, static postures of forward flexion, hyperextension, lateral bending, or rotation of the spine. Can present on cervical, thoracic, or lumbar areas of the spine.	Pain, numbness, tingling of the arm, fingers, lower back, hip, or leg

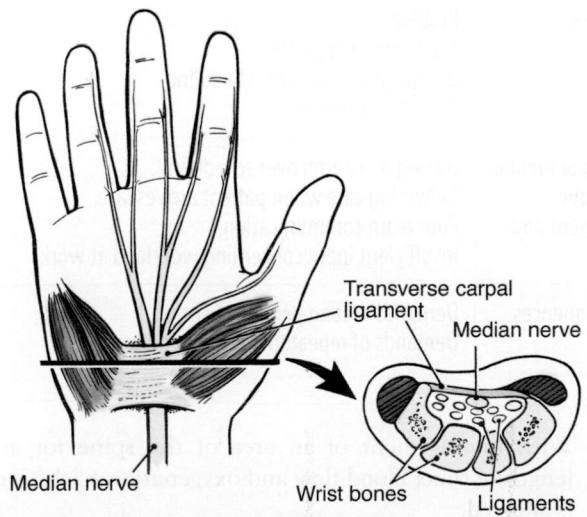

FIGURE 7-7 **Anatomy of the Wrist (palmar view).** Left, the median nerve passes through the transverse carpal tunnel of the wrist and branches to innervate the thumb, the index and middle fingers, and the medial aspect of the ring finger. Right, cross section of wrist shows the median nerve passing through the carpal tunnel. The tunnel is formed by the concave arch of the carpal (wrist) bones and roofed over by the transverse carpal ligament.

▶ Self-care is built on but not limited to all safe work practices that incorporate ergonomic principles for health and well-being. Self-care includes but is not limited to:
- *Physical fitness*: immunizations, healthy diet, adequate sleep, exercise.
- *Standard precautions*: personal protective equipment (PPE).
- *Clinical practice*: clinician/patient positioning (CPP), instrument selection and use, prevention of sharps injuries.
- *NWP*: in all activities, not only clinical practice.
- *Stress management*: reasonable patient scheduling; adequate breaks.

I. Daily Functional Movement Exercises

▶ In dental hygiene practice, it is necessary to give constant attention to maintaining a healthy spine.
- Achieving neutral work posture throughout the work day.

TABLE 7-2	Ergonomic Risk Factors	

Intensity (strength or concentration of exposure), **frequency** (how often is the exposure), and **duration** (length of time of exposure) are related to the detrimental effects of the risk factor. A combination of risk factors intensifies risk and increases potential for injury.

RISK FACTOR	DEFINITION	EXAMPLE
Prolonged awkward position	Body postures that deviate from the normal resting or neutral positions.	Twisting the torso during instrumentation. Arm raised when scaling.
Static positions long-term static load	Assuming and holding any position for a long period; stresses the body, accelerates fatigue and discomfort.	Bending neck for long periods. Retracting cheek with nondominant hand without stable fulcrum. Prolonged seated posture.
Repetition	Performing the same motion or series of motions continually or frequently.	Scaling and root planing. Probing. Exposing radiographs. Use of computer keyboard. Writing.
Force/grasp	Physical effort needed to lift, push, pull, grasp, and pinch items in the work environment. Often required to handle and control equipment and tools. Force increases as contact area decreases.	Manual instrumentation. Exposing radiographs.
Environmental	Can directly influence comfort and risk of injury.	Cold. Heat. Poor lighting. Noise.
Vibration	The physical exposure to rapidly oscillating tools or machinery.	Tools such as jackhammers. Additional research is needed to demonstrate effect power scaling and handpieces have on dental personnel.
Insufficient rest	Performing the same motion or series of motions continually or frequently without sufficient recovery time for muscles.	Scaling procedures. Probing. Exposing radiographs. Unreasonable patient scheduling. Insufficient breaks.
Stress	A physical, chemical, or emotional factor that causes bodily or mental tension and may be a factor in disease causation or fatigue. Involves clinician perception of control of work environment and psychosocial factors.	Having no control over scheduling. Delivering care when patient arrives late. Poor team communication. Insufficient input concerning workload at work.
Poor physical fitness	Decreased capacity for body to resist the negative consequences of physical demands of dental hygiene practice.	Demands of long periods of sitting. Demands of repeated instrumentation.

- Performing effective CPP, and practicing daily functional movement exercises will protect and encourage a healthy spine.
- A healthy spine requires that it be flexible. To accomplish a flexible spine, encourage movement in all directions so that no one area of the spine becomes overused, limiting its movement potential and affecting other areas of the spine.

- With impingement of an area of the spine for any length of time, blood flow and oxygenation to the area is affected.
- Chronic poor postural habits can lead to nerve impingement resulting in chronic pain and possible injury.
- Practicing daily functional movement exercises (Figure 7-8) for the spine and other joints in the practice setting and at home is a preventive strategy for all dental personnel.

A. Objectives of Exercises

With consistent practice, the following can be accomplished:

▶ Stretch, lengthen, and maintain the health of muscles.

▶ Support the structure of the natural curves of the spine.

▶ Stabilize range of motion of the joints.

▶ Maintain balance of musculoskeletal system.

▶ Maintain flexibility and comfort.

▶ Decrease stress of physical challenges on internal systems.

▶ Aid in development and maintenance of good postural work habits.

▶ Improve awareness to develop skill in creating necessary adjustments to maintain dynamic postural integrity.

▶ Foster ideal upright posture that translates to all functional movement.

▶ Retrain muscles and develop neuromuscular patterns for good postural habits that will transfer to all life activities.

▶ Develop a safe internal environment for injury prevention.

▶ Provide a structurally organized base upon which to build strength and conditioning.

B. Functional Movement Exercises

▶ Sequence designed specifically for dental personnel to:
- Create functional movement patterns.
- Gently stretch and lengthen muscles that have occupational demands.
- Encourage full range of motion for healthy joints.
- Support the natural curves of the spine.
- Exercises can be performed during clinical practice hours, at chair side between patients, in nonpatient areas of the office, and/or at home.
- Do movement exercises slowly and with awareness. Figure 7-8 describes and illustrates a series of functional movement exercises.
- Additional exercises are shown in the Prevention of Cumulative Trauma section in Chapter 39.

DOCUMENTATION

Documentation for a patient with requirements for a personalized dental chair positioning during instrumentation would include:

▶ Medical history notations indicating health history and current problem causing physical limitations or breathing difficulties.

▶ Potential emergency that could occur if patient is overstressed; need for preparation at future appointments.

▶ Notation for reference to length of appointment and time of day if needed.

▶ Example documentation using the SOAP format can be reviewed in Box 7-3.

BOX 7-3

Example Documentation: The Patient Who is Unable to Tolerate the Supine Position

S–Patient presents for routine 3 month periodontal maintenance appointment; however, she came in on crutches due to a broken hip in a recent car accident. The patient provided a letter from her orthopedic surgeon clearing her for dental treatment. She is undergoing physical therapy twice a week for the next month or longer. The patient reports moderate soreness of back, arms, legs, and neck. Chief complaint is having a "dirty mouth" due to time spent in hospital and rehab, combined with inability to keep arms raised to clean teeth. She requests that the chair remain in the upright position during treatment.

O–Examination showed limited opening of mouth, PI score 72%, compared with PI of 12% from last visit. Noted: moderate biofilm on maxillary and mandibular posterior teeth, supra gingival calculus in the mandibular anterior region; probing mostly within 3 mm range with a few bleeding spots.

A–The patient's current medical condition is preventing her from providing adequate self-care. Pain in arms and shoulders may be from use of crutches.

P–Adjusted chair per patient's request for most comfortable position. Limited opening and patient position caused difficulty in accessing dentition. Completed assessments only; patient requested appointment be stopped due to pain in back and legs. Advised patient to alert physician and physical therapist if increase in level, duration, or frequency of pain.

Next Step: Reappoint patient in 1 month for periodontal maintenance completion pending improved physical condition.

Signed _____, RDH

Date _____

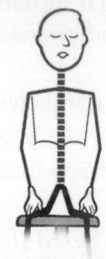

A. Sitting in neutral position, close eyes, do full diaphragm breathing. Allow abdomen to be full as lungs become full. Exhale with lips slightly parted.

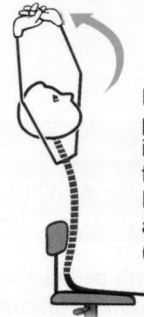

B. Standing or sitting in neutral position, stretch both arms up, interlace fingers, turn interlaced fingers so that palms are up. Look at hands and follow with eyes as you pull hands backward (spinal extension). Return to neutral.

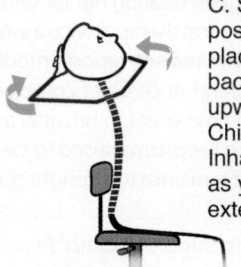

C. Standing or sitting in neutral position, interlace fingers and place on back of head; push elbows backward while slowly looking upward then slowly return to neutral. Chin moves up towards ceiling. Inhale as you look up and exhale as you return to neutral (thoracic extension).

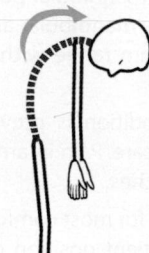

D. Standing in neutral position, slowly bend forward, rounding the back, gently bring the chin in the direction of the chest, letting the arms and hands hang down freely (spinal flexion).

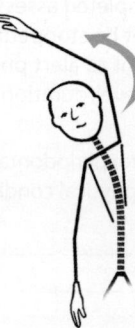

E. Standing in neutral position, raise left arm, palm facing toward midline; right arm hangs by side, palm facing hip. Bend trunk to the right and return to neutral. Right ribs flex and come closer together. Left ribs extend and move away from each other. Repeat on opposite side.

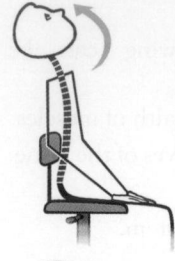

F. As chest moves forward and upward allow the head to move back (thoracic extension); chin moves in an upward direction. Inhale fully, count to five; exhale as you slowly return to neutral. Jaw remains relaxed.

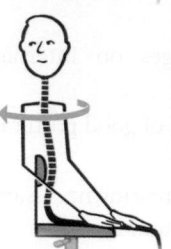

G. Sitting in neutral position, palms resting on thighs. Very gently look over right shoulder and allow right shoulder to move back as left shoulder moves forward (spinal rotation). Right palm will move along thigh back toward hip. Left palm will move forward along thigh toward knee. Repeat on opposite side.

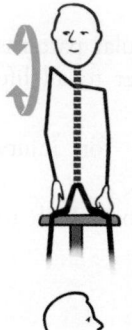

H. Shoulders relaxed in neutral position. Move right shoulder up toward right ear, backward and down. Do this movement in a clockwise direction 10 times and in a counter-clockwise direction 10 times. This movement should be done slowly and with awareness of movement of shoulder in all directions. Repeat on opposite side.

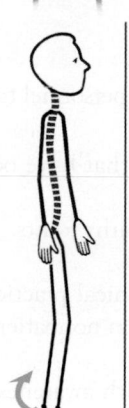

I. Standing, roll onto balls of feet, roll back onto heels of feet. Stand near wall for support.

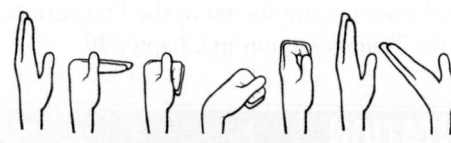

J. Tendon gliding exercise for fingers, hand and wrist. This is a fluid movement involving movement of wrist as you perform the sequence, left to right.

FIGURE 7-8 Functional Movement Exercises. Movements for each exercise are repeated in 10 unit cycles, seated or standing with weight supported evenly by both feet flat on the floor. The ideal plan is to perform some segments after each patient.

EVERYDAY ETHICS

After practicing for a few years as a dental hygienist, Delia has developed chronic pain in her neck, back, and hands. As a result, she knows that her instrumentation is affected and patients are not receiving definitive scaling at their appointments.

Questions for Consideration

1. What is Delia's ethical responsibility to herself in this situation? (Note: the *ADHA Code of Ethics for Dental Hygienists*, Section 7, Standards of Professional Responsibility, is found in Appendix I.)

2. Explain which core values (Table II-1 in the Section II Introduction) apply to Delia's ethical responsibility to her patients if her ability to perform dental hygiene treatment is compromised?

3. Explain which of the questions included in (Chapter 1, Box 1-10) for making ethical decisions might help direct Delia in determining actions she can take now to assure that her patients continue to receive the best possible dental hygiene care.

Factors To Teach The Patient

▷ How certain positions of the clinician are necessary for safe ergonomic practice and patient care.

▷ How patient cooperation makes it possible for the dental hygienist to practice with less stress and strain to prevent musculoskeletal discomfort and pain, and deliver better patient care.

References

1. Branson B, Simmer-Beck M. Personal assessment. *Dimens Dent Hyg.* 2009;7(4): 20–23.
2. Sanders MJ, Turcotte CM. Posture makes perfect. *Dimens Dent Hyg.* 2011;9(11):30–32, 35.
3. Brame JL. Seating, positioning, and lighting. *Dimens Dent Hyg.* 2008;6(9):36–37.
4. Jordre BD, Bly J. Prevent pain with the right operator stool. *Dimens Dent Hyg.* 2014;12(1):16–18.
5. Shah MA, Pellegrini JM. Magnification basics. *Dimens Dent Hyg.* 2010;8(11):36–38.
6. Maillet JP, Millar AM, Burke JM, et al. Effect of magnification loupes on dental hygiene student posture. *J Dent Educ.* 2008;72(1): 33–44.
7. Chang BJ. Ergonomic benefits of surgical telescope systems: selection guidelines. *J Calif Dent Assoc.* 2002:30(2):161–169.
8. Hayes MJ, Smith DR, Cockrell D. An international review of musculoskeletal disorders in the dental hygiene profession. *Int Dent J.* 2010;60(5);343–352.
9. Sanders MJ, Turcotte CM. Occupational stress in dental hygienists. *Work.* 2010;35(4):455–65.

 ## ENHANCE YOUR UNDERSTANDING

thePoint® **DIGITAL CONNECTIONS**
(see the inside front cover for access information)
- **Audio glossary**
- **Quiz bank**

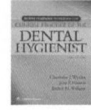 **SUPPORT FOR LEARNING**
(available separately; visit lww.com)
- *Active Learning Workbook for Clinical Practice of the Dental Hygienist, 12th Edition*

prepU INDIVIDUALIZED REVIEW
(available separately; visit lww.com)
- **Adaptive quizzing with *prepU for Wilkins' Clinical Practice of the Dental Hygienist***

Emergency Care

Lane W. Foreman, CDA, RDH, BS

LEARNING OBJECTIVES

After studying this chapter, the student will be able to:

1. Develop a plan to prevent and prepare for medical emergencies.

2. Identify signs and symptoms related to a possible emergency.

3. Define key words related to emergencies.

4. Describe stress minimization techniques.

5. Identify procedures for specific emergencies.

6. Incorporate documentation into the emergency plan.

EMERGENCY PREPAREDNESS

The public expects competence in emergency situations. This chapter is designed to help prevent emergencies from escalating into more serious conditions. The more emergency drills are practiced the more competent the dental team can become in managing an emergency. Emergencies in the dental office are rare, but the following measures can increase emergency preparedness:

▶ Periodic review of the literature to update drills is necessary for evidence-based response to emergency situations.

▶ Equipment well-maintained and is kept in a convenient place.

▶ Quick reference (posted chart) readily available.

▶ The principal objective of a "Quick Reference" is to include symptoms, equipment needed, and management of common emergencies.

▶ Key terms, definitions, and abbreviations are listed in Box 8-1 and Box 8-2.

PREVENTION OF EMERGENCIES

I. Attention to Prevention

Prevention of emergencies requires preparedness, alertness, and anticipation. The best way to prevent an emergency is to employ proper patient assessment techniques, including the following:

▶ Thorough medical history questionnaires updated at every appointment.

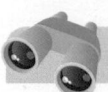 **BOX 8-1** | **KEY WORDS: Emergencies**

Angioneurotic edema: sudden and temporary appearance of large areas of painless swelling in the subcutaneous tissue or submucosa; a symptom related to allergy; also called angioedema.

Arrhythmia: variation from normal rhythm, especially the heartbeat.

Autoinjector: a syringe with a spring-loaded needle that delivers a preloaded dose of medication; often used for self-administration of epinephrine to relieve anaphylaxis.

Basic life support (BLS): the phase of emergency cardiac care that supports the ventilation and circulation of a victim of respiratory or cardiac arrest.

Cannula: a tube for insertion into a duct or cavity.
  Nasal cannula: a semicircle of plastic tubing with two plastic tips that fit into the patient's nostrils.

Cardiac arrest: sudden and often unexpected stoppage of heart action; circulation ceases and vital organs are deprived of oxygen.

Crepitation: dry crackling sound, such as that produced by the grating of the ends of a fractured bone.

Cricothyrotomy: incision through the skin and the cricothyroid membrane to secure a patent airway for emergency relief of upper airway obstruction.

Defibrillation: termination of atrial or ventricular fibrillation, usually accomplished by electric shock.

Defibrillator: an apparatus used to produce defibrillation by application of brief electric shock to the heart directly or through electrodes placed on the chest wall.

Dyspnea: labored or difficult breathing; indication of inadequate ventilation or of insufficient oxygen in the circulating blood.

Fibrillation: involuntary muscular contraction caused by spontaneous activation of single muscle cells or fibers.
  Ventricular fibrillation: a cardiac arrhythmia marked by fibrillary contractions of the ventricular muscle caused by rapid repetitive excitation of myocardial fibers

without coordinated ventricular contraction; a frequent cause of cardiac arrest.

Hypoxemia: deficient oxygenation of the blood; insufficient oxygenation of the blood eventually leads to **hypoxia**, which is diminished oxygen to body tissues.

Kussmaul breathing: loud, slow, labored breathing common to patients in diabetic coma.

Orthostatic hypotension: a drop in systolic and diastolic blood pressure due to change in body position, usually from lying back or sitting to a standing position. The resulting reduction in blood flow can cause temporary shortage of oxygen to the brain and a feeling of light-headedness or syncope.

Parenteral: not through the alimentary canal; administered by subcutaneous, intramuscular, or intravenous injection.

Pruritis: itching.

Recovery position: Patient is placed on one side with the top leg bent at the hip and knee to form a right angle. The arm closest to the floor is outstretched above the head so that it will stabilize the upper body, while the bent knee stabilizes the lower body.

Rescue breathing: a rescuer delivers a volume of 800–1200 ml with each ventilation; the exhaled air contains 16–17% oxygen, sufficient for the needs of the victim.

Syncope: temporary loss of consciousness caused by a sudden fall in blood pressure resulting in generalized cerebral ischemia; can have serious consequences, particularly in patients with a cardiovascular disease; commonly referred to as *fainting*.

Trendelenburg's position: the patient is supine with the heart higher than the head on a surface inclined downward about 45°.

Urticaria: vascular reaction of the skin with transient appearance of slightly elevated patches (wheals) that are redder or paler than the surrounding skin; may be accompanied by severe itching; also called *hives*.

Emergency Care Abbreviations

▷ **ACLS:** advanced cardiac life support
▷ **AED:** automated external defibrillator
▷ **AHA:** American Heart Association
▷ **ALS:** advanced life support
▷ **BLS:** basic life support
▷ **BCLS:** basic cardiac life support
▷ **CAD:** coronary artery disease
▷ **CPR:** cardiopulmonary resuscitation
▷ **ECC:** emergency cardiac care
▷ **ECG:** electrocardiogram
▷ **EMD:** emergency medical dispatcher
▷ **EMS:** emergency medical service
▷ **EMT:** emergency medical technician
▷ **EMT-P:** emergency medical technician paramedic

▶ Documentation of vital signs at each appointment to record baseline findings.

▶ Documentation of findings on Medical Alert Tags; wrist or ankle bracelet or necklace that provides information on patient's medical condition.

▶ Completion of a physical assessment begins with the first interaction with a patient.

▶ Incorporation of proper risk management and stress reduction protocols into the patient care plan.

▶ Careful review and update of the patient record before each appointment so that preparatory steps can be taken. Box 8-3 suggests a basic five-point plan for emergency prevention.

II. Factors Contributing to Emergencies

▶ Increased number of older patients in society with natural teeth and dental diseases that require invasive procedures.

▶ Many patients, especially older adults, are taking medications that may interact adversely with drugs used in dentistry.

▶ More complex dental procedures require longer appointments.

BOX 8-3

Five-Point Plan to Prevent Emergencies

▷ Use careful, routine patient assessment procedures.
▷ Document and update accurate, comprehensive patient records.
▷ Implement stress reduction protocols.
▷ Recognize early signs of emergency distress.
▷ Organize team management plan for emergency preparedness.

▶ Increased use of drugs in dentistry.
  • Anesthesia: local, general, conscious sedation.
  • Tranquilizers.
  • Pain medications (central nervous system depressants).
  • Antibiotics.

PATIENT ASSESSMENT

I. Assessment for Routine Treatment

A. First Contact

▶ Start with the first interaction with the patient.

▶ Note abnormalities of patient's voice on the telephone during appointment scheduling.

▶ Handwriting on medical history can indicate steadiness, ability to communicate, and education.

▶ Assess overall appearance and gait when patient enters the dental office or clinic.

▶ Document findings in the patient's record.

B. Parts of the Assessment

▶ Physical assessment (signs and symptoms).
▶ Comprehensive medical history.
▶ Vital signs.
▶ Extraoral and intraoral examination.
▶ Comprehensive documentation of findings.

C. Emergency Indicators

Changes in a patient's appearance on the day of an appointment may suggest indicators that encourage preparation for emergencies.

II. The Patient's Medical History

A. Update and Document Changes

▶ Review at each appointment.

▶ Discuss changes with dental team members who are providing treatment for the patient.

▶ A comprehensive medical history includes all the items listed in Tables 10-1 through 10-3 (in Chapter 10).

B. Use of Medical Alert Box

▶ Many dental offices utilize computerized patient records but some are limited to paper records.

▶ Folders are required for confidentiality and Health Insurance Portability and Accountability Act.

▶ Only the patient's name and/or record number may be included on the folder.

▶ The "Medical Alert Box" is usually located on the front page of the medical history to alert the dental team of information that may predispose a patient to a medical emergency before, during or postdental treatment. Significant items include:

- Physical conditions that may lead to an emergency.
- Diseases the patient has or previously had.
- Previous surgeries.
- Medical emergencies the patient experienced previously.
- Medications the patient has taken within the past 2 years.
- Allergies and adverse drug reactions.
- Previous adverse reactions to dental treatment.

III. Vital Signs

▶ Vital signs are essential to assess a patient's overall health status and to evaluate the severity of a medical emergency by comparison with baseline findings.

▶ A well-prepared dental team takes vital signs routinely to record baseline findings, not only during the earliest sign of emergency distress.

A. The Vital Signs

Pulse, blood pressure, respirations, temperature, height, weight, and the information from the patient's personal Medical Alert Tag (bracelet, necklace, or anklet) provide essential information.

B. Baseline Vital Signs

The vital signs taken at a routine appointment are considered baseline. The ranges of vital signs are described in Table 11-1, in Chapter 11.

C. During Emergency

During a medical emergency, the vital signs are compared to the baseline findings.

▶ *Compensating*: In most medical emergencies, patients will experience a "fight or flight" reaction, during which time they are said to be compensating. The vital signs are elevated above the baseline findings.

▶ *Decompensating*: When vital signs have fallen below baseline, the patient could be going into a state of shock.

▶ *Shock*: A state of lack of perfusion (saturation) of oxygenated blood to all cells of the brain and body. When brain cells are deprived of oxygenated blood, they cease to provide respiratory and circulatory function.

IV. Extraoral and Intraoral Examinations

Extraoral and intraoral examinations can provide significant clues to underlying disease processes that predispose a patient to a medical emergency. Thorough examinations are an integral part of the prevention of medical emergencies.

A. Extraoral

Blood disorders and endocrine disorders may be suspected or discovered from extraoral palpation, skin color changes, abnormalities of the eyes, and asymmetry of the face or neck.

B. Intraoral

Oral manifestations and lesions can be indications of many disease states, such as diabetes, anemia, leukemia, lupus erythematosus, or human immunodeficiency virus/acquired immune deficiency syndrome.

V. Recognition of Increased Risk Factors

The carefully prepared and regularly updated medical and personal history, with adequate follow-up consultation with the patient's physician for integration of dental and medical care, can prevent many emergencies by alerting dental personnel to the individual patient's needs and idiosyncrasies. Special needs may include:

▶ Specific physical conditions that may lead to an emergency, for example, genetic predispositions, seizures, diabetes.

▶ Diseases for which the patient is (or has been) under the care of a physician and the type of treatment, including medications.

▶ Allergies or drug reactions or interactions.

STRESS MINIMIZATION

▶ Stress and anxiety are the basis for many of the common emergencies that occur in a dental office or clinic.

▶ The clinic atmosphere and the warmth and sincerity of the personnel can help a patient feel accepted and secure.

▶ The apprehension and anxiety associated with dental treatment compounds the risk factors for medical emergencies.

I. Recognize the Patient with Stress Problems

▶ Apprehension about any dental procedure.

▶ Elderly patients are prone to medical emergencies, as they may have cardiovascular diseases or other conditions that have or have not been diagnosed.

▶ Essential medications: certain prescriptions are required to be taken on schedule or the patient is at risk for an emergency. The medications may cause adverse reactions that can lead to a medical emergency such as orthostatic hypotension.

II. Suggestions for Effective Communication

Any patient who is apprehensive or medically predisposed to emergencies can be provided with a stress reduction plan. Reduction of stress includes the development of patient rapport through effective communication between the dental team and the patient.

A. Actively Listen to a Patient's Fears

▶ Develop rapport so the patient senses the listener is empathetic and interested in alleviating the apprehension.

▶ Communicate with the patient about their fear of treatment. When a patient confides in a caregiver, trust is established and the patient is calmer.

▶ Patient trust in the care provider can be beneficial for emergency prevention.

B. Effects of Fear

Patients who try to repress their fears are more likely to hyperventilate or experience syncopal episodes.

III. Reduction of Stress

A. Appointment Scheduling[1]

▶ *New patient*: Initial appointment for consultation and assessment provides an opportunity to build rapport and to evaluate the patient's level of anxiety. Stress reduction can be built into treatment appointments.

▶ *Time of appointment*: Plan in accordance with personal health requirements.

▶ *Waiting time minimized*: First appointment in the morning prevents building of anxiety by waiting all day for the appointment. In addition, anxiety can be decreased by taking the patient into the treatment room immediately and starting treatment promptly.

▶ *Eating requirements*: Identify usual mealtime and ask about previous meal eaten to prevent or hypoglycemia.

▶ *Length of appointment*: Limited to the patient's tolerance.

B. Medication

▶ Premedication when indicated and prescribed by the physician or dentist.

▶ Pain control during treatment.

▶ Patient's own prescriptions. Patients subject to emergencies are instructed to bring their own prescribed medicines; for example, the patient with asthma or one who is subject to attacks of angina pectoris.

C. Posttreatment Care

▶ Postcare instructions for prevention and/or relief of discomfort.

▶ Place a follow-up telephone call to an anxious patient to make certain there were no postoperative complications.

EMERGENCY MATERIALS AND PREPARATION

▶ Organization is a key concept in emergency preparedness.

▶ The first steps in preparing for managing emergencies include setting up the emergency equipment and a systematic protocol.

▶ Group planning and individual acceptance of responsibility can provide the team with efficiency, composure, and freedom from fear at the time of crisis.

I. Communication: Telephone Numbers for Medical Aid

Telephone numbers can be posted near each extension from which outside calls can be made.

▶ Rescue squads with paramedics (fire, police, flying squad, or 911 in many cities in the United States).

▶ Ambulance service.

▶ Nearest hospital emergency department.

▶ Poison information center: 1-800-222-1222 in the United States.

▶ Physicians
  • Patient's physician is listed in the permanent record in a standard, convenient place.
  • Physicians available for emergency calls.

II. Equipment for Use in an Emergency

▶ Every dental office or clinic plans and sets up an emergency kit or cart,[1,2] and everyone in the office becomes familiar with its contents. The kit is kept in order, its contents replenished, and outdated materials replaced as needed.

▶ The emergency equipment is portable, well-maintained, and kept in a place readily accessible to all treatment rooms.

▶ Materials are plainly marked and kept separate from other office supplies.

▶ Materials included are selected to accomplish emergency treatment by current methods.

▶ The items included in the kit imply proper training in their use.

▶ Members of a team can add new items for the list in keeping with their training and abilities.

▶ Table 8-1, provides a typical list of essential emergency equipment items.

III. Care of Drugs

▶ All dental personnel become familiar with the emergency drugs maintained in the particular office or clinic.

TABLE 8-1	Equipment in an Emergency Kit or Cart
CATEGORY	**ESSENTIAL ITEMS**
Required equipment	■ Series E portable oxygen tank 　• Low-flow oxygen regulator 　• Nasal cannula 　• Simple face mask 　• Nonbreather mask 　• Bag-valve masks (adult and pediatric) 　• Demand valve resuscitator ■ Automated external defibrillator (AED) ■ Oro- and nasopharyngeal and airways 　• Sizes: pediatric to large adult 　• Water-soluble lubricant ■ Sphygmomanometer 　• Blood pressure cuffs: pediatric, adult regular and large adult ■ Magils forceps ■ Syringes: 2–3 ml luer lock-tip 21-gauge needles ■ Medical Emergency Report Forms ■ Criothyrotomy equipment* ■ Intravenous equipment*
Injectable drugs	■ Epinephrine via autoinjector ■ Diphenhydramine ■ Cortisone* ■ Glucagon* ■ Midazolam* ■ Atropine*
Non-injected drugs	■ Antiplatelet: aspirin ■ Respiratory stimulant: ammonia vaporoles ■ Bronchodilator: albuterol inhaler ■ Antihypoglycemic: glucose gel, glucagon paste ■ Vasodilator: nitroglycerine tablets, nitrolingual spray ■ Diphenhydramine tablets ■ Naloxone (Narcan): nasal spray
Supplementary equipment	■ Thermometer ■ Blood glucose meter, lancets, and test strips ■ Pen flashlight ■ Stopwatch ■ Razor (for hair removal for AED pads) ■ Scissors ■ Cotton pliers ■ Emesis basin ■ Blanket ■ Pillow ■ Inflatable splints ■ Backboard (12 × 24' for patients who cannot be moved for CPR) ■ Quick-activated cold packs ■ Betadine wipes ■ Sterile packages of gauze and adhesive tape 　• 2 × 2" 　• 4 × 4" 　• Rolled gauze (2" × 5')

*Administered only by personnel with advanced medical training.

▶ Only specially trained, experienced persons will administer injectable medications.

▶ The only drugs kept in the dental office are those that the dentist or emergency team are trained to use.[3]

A. Identification

▶ The purpose and method of administration of each drug is clearly identified on the container.

▶ The use of a compartmentalized clear plastic cabinet or box can be useful for this purpose because the labels and instructions can be seen from the outside and efficient selection can be made.

▶ The replacement date appears clearly on each item that has a limited shelf life.

▶ When narcotics are included in the list of drugs available for emergencies, they are stored in a secured location other than the emergency kit, and purchased in predosed amounts for specific emergency situations.

B. Record of Drugs

▶ Label each with information about shelf life and due date for replacement. Example: Nitroglycerin is replaced at 6 months.

▶ Check weekly to maintain emergency kit in workable order.

▶ A complete record of each available drug is kept. The following are recorded:
  • Name of drug
  • Dosage
  • Date purchased
  • Address of source if different from the usual local pharmacy
  • Itemized record, signed by the staff member responsible
  • Specific entry as each drug is used
  • Expiration dates checked at routine intervals
  • Instructions for disposal.

C. Disposal of Drugs

▶ Follow specific disposal instructions on the drug label or patient information sheet.

▶ Do not flush prescription drugs down the toilet.

▶ Take advantage of community drug take-back programs that allow the public to bring unused drugs to a central location for disposal.

IV. Medical Emergency Report Form

▶ Figure 8-1 shows an example of a form that can be used to record the essential information during an emergency.

▶ Such a form can be filed or scanned and stored in the computerized patient record control system to include in patient's permanent record.

▶ A pad of the forms on noncarbon replication paper is placed on a clipboard on the emergency cart.

▶ A copy of the emergency report is given to the emergency medical service (EMS) personnel to present to those in the emergency room at the hospital or other medical facility when the patient is admitted.

A. Purposes

▶ Organize data collected during the emergency.

▶ Serve as a time reference during the monitoring of vital signs.

▶ Prepare a record from which the medical personnel can interpret the patient's condition at the time of transfer from the dental facility.

B. Uses

▶ Evaluation for planning dental and dental hygiene appointments so future emergencies for the patient can be avoided.

▶ Provide a reference in the event legal questions arise. A well-kept record can be vital, and each emergency, however insignificant the incident may seem, is recorded.

V. Practice and Drill

A. Staff Instruction

▶ In an emergency situation, moments count and there is no time for fumbling or discussion.

▶ Each member of the clinic and office staff is thoroughly familiar with the location, purpose, effect, and application of each item of equipment and its source.

▶ Each staff member also knows the order of procedures in all types of emergencies (Figure 8-2), and can assume any role when needed.

B. Assignments

▶ *Preparation*: The assignment of specific responsibilities during an emergency is the result of planning by the whole team.

▶ *Substitutions*: Because a staff member may be absent from the scene at the time of an emergency, each person learns and practices the duties for all positions so that substitutions can be made and duties doubled with a minimum of discussion and no confusion.

▶ Figure 8-3 shows an example of a possible distribution of duties when three people are available to attend to the patient.

▶ *Advantages of assignments*
  • Organization efficiently uses personnel.
  • Sharing responsibility relieves pressure.
  • Duties can be carried out quietly, without excess discussion or attention from others in the clinic.
  • Necessary work gets done without duplication and without omissions.

Medical Emergency Report

| Patient's Name *Smith, Joe* | | Today's Date *10/27/20* | |

Description of incident: *Patient exhibited signs of anaphylaxis after exposure to latex gloves. Urticaria and pruritus were evident on arms, neck and chest. Signs of lip, tongue and laryngeal edema were exhibited with difficulty swallowing and breathing. Quickly explained to patient that he was having an allergic reaction. Patient was immediately given epinephrine (.3mg) via EpiPen autoinjector and EMS was summoned. 50mg of Benadryl and 100mg of Solu-Cortef were also administered IM. Oxygen was delivered by non-rebreather at 15 L/min. Within 5 minutes vital signs and symptoms improved. At 8 minutes vital signs were near baseline. Patient was released to EMS in 15 minutes and transported to the hospital.*

Time of onset		Time EMS summoned		Time EMS arrived		Time patient was released	
Stopwatch	Clock time	Stopwatch	Clock time	Stopwatch	Clock time	Stopwatch	Clock time
0:00 minutes	*10:30 am*	*0:10 minutes*	*10:30 am*	*13:00 minutes*	*10:43 am*	*15:00 minutes*	*10:45 am*

Patient released to: *EMS who transported patient to Tallahassee Memorial Regional Medical Center*

Cessation of breathing: Ø		Cessation of pulse: Ø		CPR initiated: Ø	
Stopwatch	Clock time	Stopwatch	Clock time	Stopwatch	Clock time
N/A	*N/A*	*N/A*	*N/A*	*N/A*	*N/A*

	Initial findings	Stopwatch times	Followup finding	Stopwatch times	Followup finding	Stopwatch times
Blood pressure	*90/60*	*2:15 minutes*	*110/80*	*5:15 minutes*	*120/80*	*8:15 minutes*
Pulse	*50 bpm*	*1:00 minutes*	*68 bpm*	*5:00 minutes*	*72 bpm*	*8:30 minutes*
Respirations	*10*	*1:30 minutes*	*12*	*5:30 minutes*	*16*	*8:00 minutes*
O₂ delivery method	*non-rebreather (15 L/min)*	*1:45 minutes*	*non-rebreather (15 L/min)*	*5:30 minutes*	*non-rebreather (15 L/min)*	*8:30 minutes*

Drugs administered	Route	Dosage	Stopwatch times
Epinephrine via EpiPen ®	*I.M. (Quad)*	*.3 mg*	*0:45*
Benadryl ®	*I.M. (Deltoid)*	*50 mg*	*1:15*
Solu-Cortef ®	*I.M. (Deltoid)*	*100 mg*	*1:30*

FIGURE 8-1 **Sample Medical Emergency Report.** The form is prepared in duplicate. One copy accompanies the patient to the emergency clinic, and the second copy is retained in the patient's dental record file.

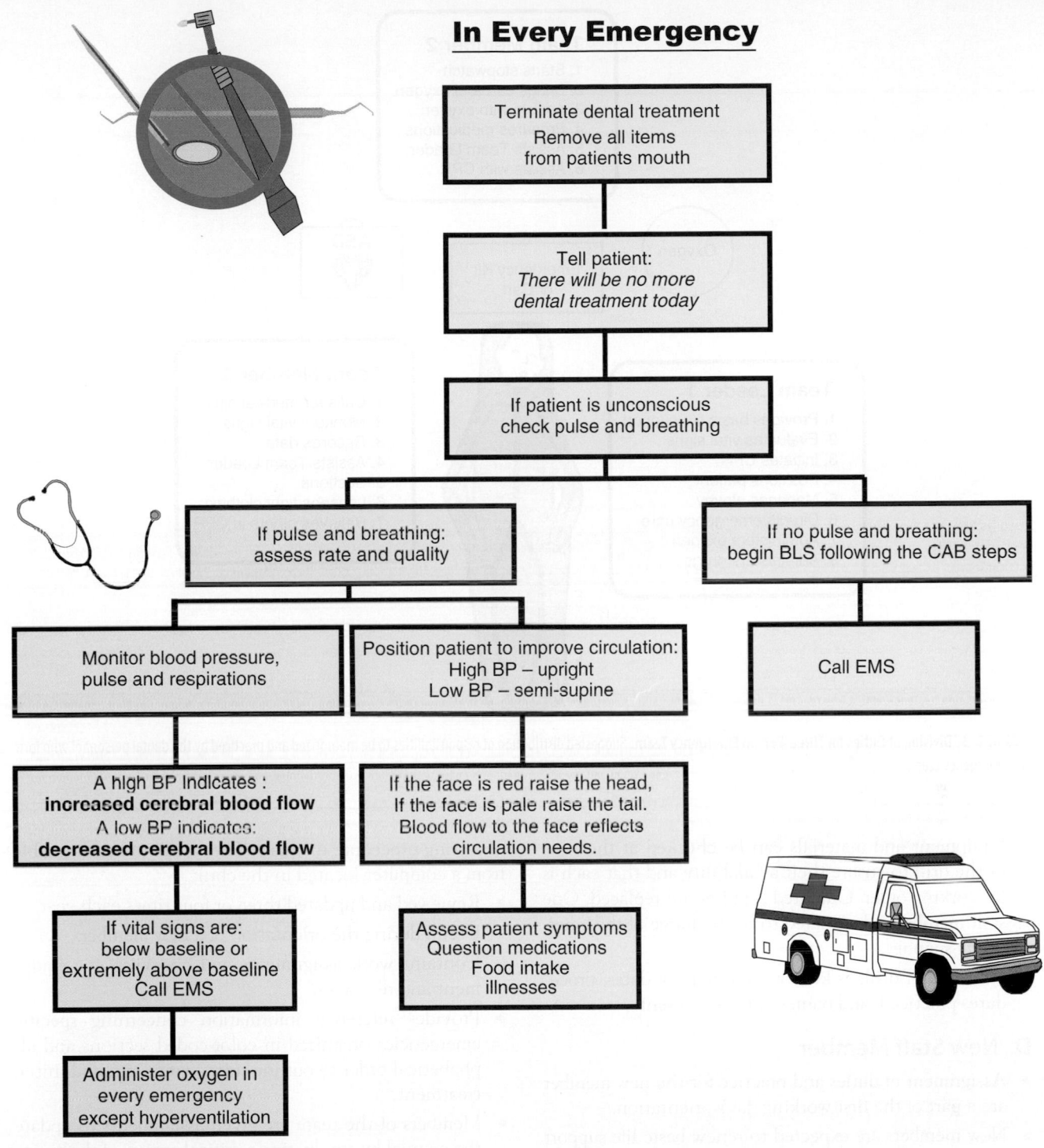

In Every Emergency

Terminate dental treatment
Remove all items
from patients mouth

↓

Tell patient:
*There will be no more
dental treatment today*

↓

If patient is unconscious
check pulse and breathing

↓

| If pulse and breathing: assess rate and quality | | If no pulse and breathing: begin BLS following the CAB steps |

If pulse and breathing:
assess rate and quality

If no pulse and breathing:
begin BLS following the CAB steps

Monitor blood pressure,
pulse and respirations

Position patient to improve circulation:
High BP – upright
Low BP – semi-supine

Call EMS

A high BP indicates :
increased cerebral blood flow
A low BP indicates:
decreased cerebral blood flow

If the face is red raise the head,
If the face is pale raise the tail.
Blood flow to the face reflects
circulation needs.

If vital signs are:
below baseline or
extremely above baseline
Call EMS

Assess patient symptoms
Question medications
Food intake
illnesses

Administer oxygen in
every emergency
except hyperventilation

FIGURE 8-2 Flowchart: In Every Emergency.

C. Drills

► Regular reviews and rehearsals for each type of emergency are conducted, preferably on a "surprise" basis, at least once a month.

► A specific emergency code call can be used when an intercom or other message system is available. Mentioning "code" in front of a number or phrase may panic the other patients; therefore, it is best to use only a number like "17."

► For each type of emergency, practice in the use of procedures, including oxygen administration, resuscitation, and airway maneuvers, as well as specific positioning of a patient for all emergencies, is indicated.

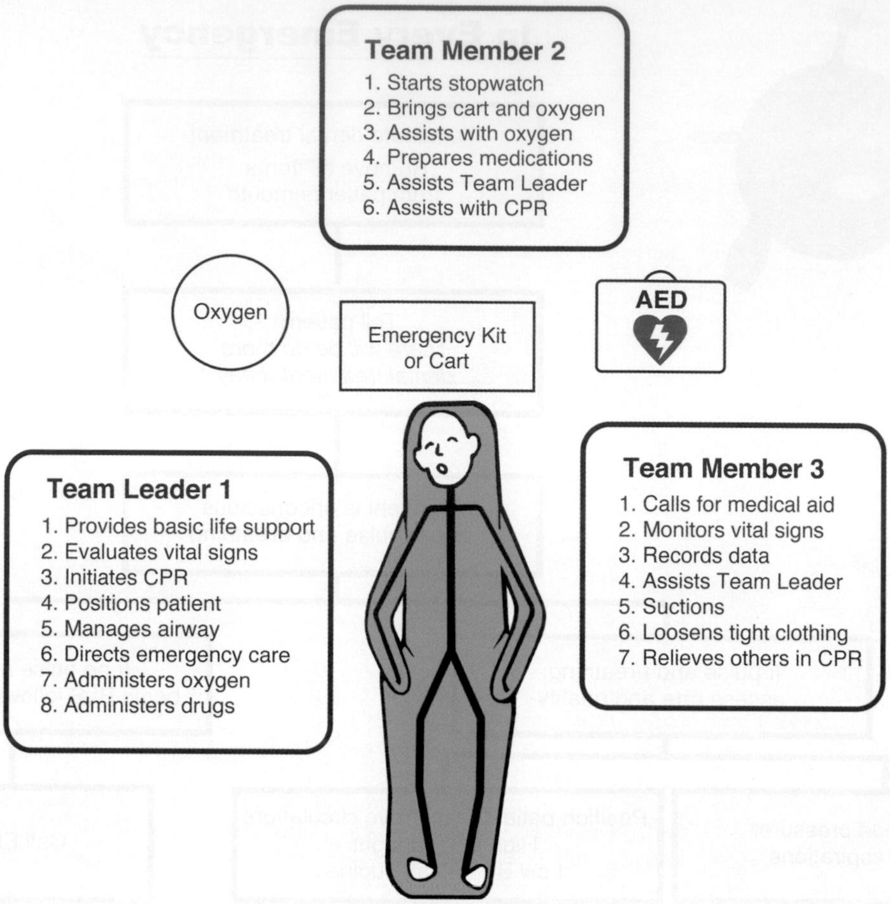

Team Member 2
1. Starts stopwatch
2. Brings cart and oxygen
3. Assists with oxygen
4. Prepares medications
5. Assists Team Leader
6. Assists with CPR

Oxygen

Emergency Kit
or Cart

AED

Team Leader 1
1. Provides basic life support
2. Evaluates vital signs
3. Initiates CPR
4. Positions patient
5. Manages airway
6. Directs emergency care
7. Administers oxygen
8. Administers drugs

Team Member 3
1. Calls for medical aid
2. Monitors vital signs
3. Records data
4. Assists Team Leader
5. Suctions
6. Loosens tight clothing
7. Relieves others in CPR

FIGURE 8-3 Division of Duties for Three-Person Emergency Team. Suggested distribution of responsibilities to be memorized and practiced by the dental personnel who form the emergency team.

▶ Equipment and materials can be checked at the time of the drill to ensure their availability and that each is in working order. Outdated supplies are replaced. One staff member is designated to be in charge of the emergency supplies.

▶ A record of drills is kept with a diary of dates, procedures practiced, and names of those present.

D. New Staff Member

▶ Assignment of duties and practice for the new member are a part of the first working day's orientation.

▶ New members are expected to renew basic life support (BLS)/cardiopulmonary resuscitation (CPR) certification by taking necessary refresher courses within a specified time. Most states require a renewal certificate for annual licensure.

▶ The Commission on Dental Accreditation has established standards that require all clinic personnel to be healthcare provider BLS/CPR certified.

E. Procedures Manual

A paper manual is a valuable study and work reference, but an electronic format is a currently accepted method of storing procedure manuals. They need to be accessable from a computer located in the clinic.

▶ Reviewed and updated three or four times each year.

▶ Useful during the orientation of a new member.

▶ Contains work assignments and checklists for equipment and resources.

▶ Provides reference information concerning specific emergencies organized in color-coded sections and alphabetical order to outline signs, symptoms, and initial treatment.

▶ Members of the team are given assignments to update the manual by conducting a critical review of the scientific literature for quality assurance and evidence-based, patient-centered care.

▶ All updates are referenced in the index of the manual.

BASIC LIFE SUPPORT CERTIFICATION

▶ Licensed dental hygienists are expected to maintain a current BLS/CPR certification.

▶ The American Heart Association (AHA) provides guidelines and training for healthcare professionals.

The *AHA BLS for Healthcare Providers Manual* is updated regularly to reflect the most current information and procedures to follow when responding to an emergency situation.

OXYGEN ADMINISTRATION

▶ High concentration of oxygen is contraindicated for chronic obstructive lung diseases, especially emphysema.
▶ Oxygen is also not indicated in the presence of hyperventilation because the patient is receiving increased amounts of oxygen in air inhaled and is in need of carbon dioxide.
▶ The use of oxygen is beneficial in all other emergencies.
▶ When the patient is not breathing, positive pressure oxygen (also known as demand valve resuscitator) delivery is needed.

I. Equipment

Oxygen delivery systems with indications, flow rate, and percentage of oxygen delivered are listed in Table 8-2. A portable oxygen delivery system is shown in Figure 8-4.

A. Parts

Oxygen resuscitation equipment consists of the following:
▶ An oxygen tank
▶ A reducing valve
▶ A flow meter
▶ Tubing
▶ Mask
▶ A positive pressure bag.

The *E* cylinder, which can provide oxygen for 30 minutes, is the minimum size recommended. Smaller tanks provide little oxygen for short periods only, and larger tanks are less portable.

B. Directions

Box 8-4 outlines the steps for operation of an oxygen tank. Clear, readable directions are permanently attached to the tank's portable carriage. Practice is a definite part of team drills.

II. Patient Breathing: Use Supplemental Oxygen

▶ Apply a full-face clear mask or a nasal cannula.
▶ Supplemental oxygen is started at 4 to 6 liters per minute.
▶ Monitor breathing; if breathing stops, proceed with positive pressure oxygen.

TABLE 8-2	Oxygen Delivery Systems		
DEVICE	**INDICATIONS**	**FLOW RATE (L/MIN)**	**OXYGEN DELIVERY (%)**
Cannula	For patient who is breathing and needs low levels of oxygen	2–6	25–40
Face mask	For patient who is breathing and needs moderate levels of oxygen: • When cannula is not tolerated • When more oxygen is desired • Patient is in shock	8–12	60
Nonrebreather mask	For patient who is breathing and needs high levels of oxygen: • Patient is in shock • When more oxygen is desired	10–15	60–90
Bag mask	When patient has stopped breathing; bag mask is used instead of mouth-to-mouth resuscitation	10–15	90–100
Demand valve resuscitation	Positive pressure delivery of oxygen on demand	Used by emergency medical technicians (EMTs) or others professionally trained	100

Laminate and affix to the oxygen tank.

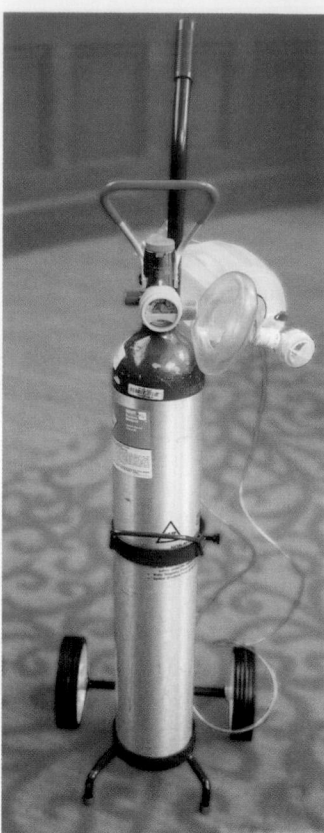

FIGURE 8-4 **Portable Oxygen Delivery System.** The portable unit is stored in an area immediately accessible to all treatment areas in the dental clinic. If a fixed oxygen delivery system is available in the treatment area, it can be used in an emergency situation.

III. Patient not Breathing: Use Positive Pressure

For persons not trained in the use of the bag-valve mask or positive pressure delivery, a mouth-to-mask procedure is used.

▶ Apply full-face clear mask so that a tight seal is formed. One dental team member may need to apply pressure to the facemask to maintain a complete seal.

▶ Adjust oxygen flow so that the positive pressure bag remains filled.

▶ Compress the bag manually, one ventilation every 5 to 6 seconds to provide 10 to 12 respirations per minute for an adult. For a child, 1 ventilation every 3 seconds.

▶ Watch chest rise. When the chest does not rise, recheck airway for obstruction. Proceed with airway obstruction management.

▶ *Call EMS.*

SPECIFIC EMERGENCIES

▶ Certain systemic disease conditions and physical injuries require specific treatment during an emergency.

BOX 8-4

Operation of Oxygen Tank

OPERATION OF OXYGEN TANK

To turn on:

▷ Attach oxygen delivery system to tank.

▷ Turn **key** on top of tank in *counter-clockwise direction* to open flow of oxygen.

▷ Read **Low Flow Regulator Knob turn in direction arrow indicates to increase or open**; many regulators are opposite of sink faucets and open clockwise instead of counterclockwise.

▷ Attach oxygen delivery system to patient.

To turn off:

▷ Remove oxygen delivery system from patient.

▷ Turn **key** on top of tank in *clockwise direction* to shut off flow of oxygen.

▷ Turn the **Low Flow Regulator Knob** in open position to bleed oxygen from the system.

▷ After bleeding, gently close the **Low Flow Regulator Knob.**

LAMINATE AND AFFIX TO THE OXYGEN TANK

To turn on:

▷ Attach oxygen delivery system to tank.

▷ Turn **key** on top of tank in counterclockwise direction to open flow of oxygen.

▷ Read **Low Flow Regulator Knob.**

▷ **To increase O_2 flow: turn the knob in the direction the arrow indicates.** (Many regulators are the opposite of sink faucets and open clockwise instead of counterclockwise.)

▷ Attach oxygen delivery system from patient.

To turn off:

▷ Remove oxygen delivery system from patient.

▷ Turn **key** on top of tank in *clockwise direction* to shut off flow of oxygen.

▷ Turn the **Low Flow Regulator Knob** to open position to bleed oxygen from the system.

▷ After bleeding, gently close the **Low Flow Regulator Knob.**

▶ In Tables 8-3 and 8-4, the *Emergency Reference Charts*, several conditions are listed with their symptoms and treatment procedures.

▶ Some of the same conditions have been described in detail in Section IX of this book.

DOCUMENTATION

All details about the patient, the treatments, reactions, healing, and comments by the patient provide crucial information in a medical emergency or posttreatment complication.

TABLE 8-3	Emergency Reference Chart: Medical Emergencies	
EMERGENCY	**SIGNS/SYMPTOMS**	**PROCEDURE**
All Cases Call EMS immediately if problem with: Breathing Unconsciousness Anaphylaxis Bleeding Poisoning Chest pain		I. Determine consciousness (tap and shout): yell for help. **If patient is unconscious: Call EMS and get AED** II. Conduct primary assessment: C. Circulation: check for pulse for 10 s, if none: Start compressions. A. Airway: open with head tilt-chin lift B. Breathing: (look, listen, feel) if none: Give 2 (1-s) breaths D. Defibrillate: 1 shock: then 5 cycles of CPR. **If patient is breathing and conscious:** III. Conduct secondary assessment: A. Evaluate level of consciousness. 1. Does patient know own name, location, date? 2. Use penlight to see if pupils react equally to light. 3. If conscious: check for equal hand strength by asking patient to squeeze your hands. 4. Position according to signs/symptoms. If face is red, raise the head. If face is pale, raise the tail. 5. Evaluate heart rate, blood pressure, respirations. B. Findings in patient record or medical alert bracelet 1. Disabilities, diseases, drugs, baseline vital signs: **Call EMS.**
Respiratory failure	Labored or weak respirations or cessation breathing Cyanosis or ashen-white with blood loss Pupils dilated Loss of consciousness	Position: semisupine if not breathing; upright if breathing. Check for and remove foreign material from mouth. Establish airway. **Begin CPR.** If patient does not spontaneously breathe: **Call EMS.** Monitor vital signs: blood pressure, pulse, respirations. Administer oxygen by nonrebreather mask if patient is already breathing.
Mild airway obstruction	Good air exchange, coughing, wheezing (patient can speak)	Sit patient up. Loosen tight collar, belt. No treatment; let patient cough.
Severe airway obstruction	Poor air exchange; noisy breathing; weak, ineffective cough; difficult respirations; gasping. Unable to speak, breathe, cough. Cyanosis, dilated pupils	Reassure patient. Treat for complete obstruction. **Conscious patient** Perform Heimlich maneuver. Patient becomes unconscious: Begin CPR. **Unconscious patient** **Call EMS.**
Hyperventilation syndrome	Light-headedness, giddiness Anxiety, confusion Dizziness Overbreathing (25–30 respirations/min) Feelings of suffocation Deep respirations Palpitations (heart pounds) Tingling or numbness in the extremities	Terminate oral procedure. Remove rubber dam and objects from mouth. Position upright. Immediately tell patient: "There will be no more dental treatment today." Loosen tight collar. Reassure patient. Explain overbreathing; request that each breath be held to a count of 10. Ask patient to breathe deeply (7–10 per min) into a paper bag adapted closely over nose and mouth. Never use a bag for a patient with diabetes or patients exhibiting signs of diabetic coma, e.g., fruity breath odor, Kussmaul breathing, lethargy, dry skin.

(continues)

TABLE 8-3	Emergency Reference Chart: Medical Emergencies (*continued*)

EMERGENCY	SIGNS/SYMPTOMS	PROCEDURE
Heart failure	Difficult or labored breathing Pulmonary congestion with cough and difficulty breathing May cough up pink sputum Rapid, weak pulse Dilated pupils May have chest pain	Place patient in upright position. **Call EMS.** Make patient comfortable: cover with blanket. Administer oxygen by nonrebreather mask. Reassure patient. BLS.
Cardiac arrest	Skin: ashen gray, cold, clammy No pulse No heart sounds No respirations Eyes fixed, with dilated pupils; no constriction with light Unconscious	**Call EMS.** Check oral cavity for debris or vomitus; leave dentures in place for a seal. **Begin CPR.**[4]
Asthma attack	Difficulty breathing, wheezing, (extreme cases—silence, indicating little to no air exchange) Cyanosis Dilated pupils Confusion due to lack of oxygen Chest pressure Sweating	Position patient upright with arms up and supported forward. Assist with patient's own bronchodilator. Administer supplemental oxygen by nasal cannula. Epinephrine if patient decompensates. Supplemental cortisone to patients on corticosteroid therapy. BLS—may need demand valve resuscitator if patient experiences respiratory depression. **Call EMS.**
Syncope (Fainting)	Pale gray face, anxiety Dilated pupils Weakness, giddiness, dizziness, faintness, nausea Profuse cold perspiration Rapid pulse at first, followed by slow pulse Shallow breathing Drop in blood pressure Loss of consciousness	Position: Trendelenburg. Open airway. Loosen tight collar, belt. Place cold, damp towel on forehead. Crush ammonia vaporole under patient's nose. Keep warm (blanket). Monitor vital signs: blood pressure, pulse, respirations. Keep airway open. Administer oxygen by nasal cannula. Keep in supine position 10 min after recovery to prevent nausea and dizziness. Reassure patient, especially during recovery.
Shock	Skin: pale, moist, clammy Rapid, shallow breathing Low blood pressure Weakness and/or restlessness Nausea, vomiting Thirst, if shock is from bleeding Eventual unconsciousness if untreated	Position: Trendelenburg Open airway. Keep quiet and warm. Monitor vital signs: blood pressure, respirations, pulse. Keep airway open. Administer oxygen by nonrebreather bag. If patient does not recover fully and/or vital signs not at baseline: **Call EMS.**

(continues)

TABLE 8-3	Emergency Reference Chart: Medical Emergencies (*continued*)	
EMERGENCY	**SIGNS/SYMPTOMS**	**PROCEDURE**
Stroke (cerebrovascular accident)	*Premonitory* Dizziness, vertigo Transient paresthesia or weakness Transient speech defects Serious Headache (with cerebral hemorrhage) Breathing labored, deep, slow Chills Paralysis one side of body Nausea, vomiting Convulsions Loss of consciousness (slow or sudden onset)	**Conscious patient** **Call EMS.** Turn patient on paralyzed side; semiupright. Loosen clothing about the throat. Reassure patient; keep calm, quiet. Monitor vital signs: blood pressure, pulse, respirations. Administer oxygen by nasal cannula. Clear airway; suction vomitus because the throat muscles may be paralyzed. **Unconscious patient** Position: supine. BLS. Cardiopulmonary resuscitation if indicated.
Cardiovascular diseases	Symptoms vary depending on cause	**For all patients** **Call EMS.** Be calm and reassure patient. Keep patient warm and quiet; restrict effort. Always administer oxygen when there is chest pain.
Angina pectoris	Sudden crushing, paroxysmal pain in substernal area Pain may radiate to shoulder, neck, arms Pallor, faintness Shallow breathing Anxiety, fear	Position: upright, as patient requests, for comfortable breathing. If patient has been diagnosed with angina and has own nitroglycerine: Place nitroglycerin sublingually only when the blood pressure is at or above baseline. Administer oxygen by nasal cannula. Reassure patient. Without prompt relief from nitroglycerin: **Call EMS.** Treat as a myocardial infarction.
Myocardial infarction (heart attack)	Sudden pain similar to angina pectoris, which may radiate, but of longer duration Pallor; cold, clammy skin Cyanosis Nausea Breathing difficulty Marked weakness Anxiety, fear Possible loss of consciousness	**Call EMS.** Position: with head up for comfortable breathing. Symptoms are not relieved with nitroglycerin. Encourage chew 1 adult (not enteric coated) or 2 low-dose "baby" aspirin if the patient has no allergy to aspirin.[5] Monitor vital signs: blood pressure, pulse, respirations. Administer oxygen by nonrebreather bag. Alleviate anxiety; reassure.
Adrenal crisis (cortisol mental deficiency)	Anxious, stressed Confusion Pain in abdomen, back, legs Muscle weakness Extreme fatigue Nausea, vomiting Lowered blood pressure Elevated pulse Loss of consciousness Coma	**Conscious patient** Terminate oral procedure. **Call EMS.** Request telephone call for medical assistance. Administer oxygen by nonrebreather mask. Monitor blood pressure and pulse. Place patient on stable side with legs slightly raised. **Unconscious patient** BLS. Try ammonia vaporole when cause is undecided. Administer oxygen. **EMS transport to hospital.**

(*continues*)

TABLE 8-3	Emergency Reference Chart: Medical Emergencies *(continued)*

EMERGENCY	SIGNS/SYMPTOMS	PROCEDURE
Insulin reaction (hyperinsulinism, hypoglycemia)	Sudden onset Skin: moist, cold, pale Confused, nervous, anxious Bounding pulse Salivation Normal to shallow respirations Convulsions (late)	**Conscious patient** Administer glucose gel. Observe patient for 1 h before dismissal. Determine time since previous meal, and arrange next appointment following food intake. **Unconscious patient** **Call EMS.** BLS. Position: supine. Maintain airway. Administer oxygen by nonrebreather bag. Monitor vital signs. Administer intramuscular glucagon or intravenous glucose.
Diabetic coma (ketoacidosis) (hyperglycemia)	Slow onset Skin: flushed and dry Breath: fruity odor Dry mouth, thirst Low blood pressure Weak, rapid pulse Exaggerated respirations (Kussmaul breathing)	**Conscious patient** **Call EMS.** Keep patient warm. Administer oxygen by nasal cannula. **Unconscious patient** BLS. Position: supine.
Seizure • Generalized tonic-clonic • Generalized absence	Coma Anxiety or depression Pale, may become cyanotic Muscular contractions Loss of consciousness Brief loss of consciousness Fixed posture Rhythmic twitching of eyelids, eyebrows, or head May be pale	**Call EMS.** Position supine: Do not attempt to move from dental chair. Make safe by placing movable equipment out of reach. Do not force anything between the teeth; a soft towel or large sponges may be placed while mouth is open. Open airway; monitor vital signs. Administer oxygen by nasal cannula or face mask. Allow patient to sleep during postconvulsive stage. EMS to determine need for transport to hospital. Take objects from patient's hands to prevent their being dropped.
Allergic reaction • Delayed (anaphylactic shock)	Skin Erythema (rash) Urticaria (wheals, itching) Angioedema (localized swelling of mucous membranes, lips, larynx, pharynx) Respiration Distress, dyspnea Wheezing Extension of angioedema to larynx: may have obstruction from swelling of vocal apparatus	Skin. Administer antihistamine. Respiration. Position: upright. Administer oxygen by nasal cannula. Epinephrine may be needed if breathing difficulty. If airway obstruction: Position: supine. Airway maintenance. Epinephrine (Epi-Pen).

(continues)

TABLE 8-3	Emergency Reference Chart: Medical Emergencies (*continued*)	
EMERGENCY	**SIGNS/SYMPTOMS**	**PROCEDURE**
• Immediate anaphylaxis	Skin Urticaria (wheals, itching) Flushing Nausea, abdominal cramps, vomiting, diarrhea Angioedema Swelling of lips, membranes, eyelids Laryngeal edema with difficulty swallowing Respiration distress Cough, wheezing Dyspnea, airway obstruction Cyanosis Cardiovascular collapse Profound drop in blood pressure Rapid, weak pulse Palpitations Dilation of pupils Loss of consciousness (sudden) Cardiac arrest	Rapid treatment needed. Administer epinephrine via autoinjector. **Call EMS.** Position: supine (except when dyspnea predominates). Administer oxygen by nonrebreather mask. BLS. Monitor vital signs. Cardiopulmonary resuscitation if airway obstructed.
Local anesthesia reactions • Psychogenic • Allergic (very rare) • Toxic overdose	Reaction to injection, not the anesthetic Syncope Hyperventilation syndrome Anaphylactic shock Allergic skin and mucous membrane reactions Bronchial asthma attack Effects of intravascular injection rather than increased quantity of drug more common Stimulation phase Anxious, restless, apprehensive, confused Rapid pulse and respirations Elevated blood pressure Tremors Convulsions Depressive phase follows stimulation phase Drowsiness, lethargy Shocklike symptoms: pallor, sweating Rapid, weak pulse and respirations Drop in blood pressure Respiratory depression or respiratory arrest Unconsciousness	Syncope. Hyperventilation. See earlier in this table. Mild reaction. Stop injection. Position: supine. Loosen tight clothing. Reassure patient. Monitor blood pressure, heart rate, respirations. Administer oxygen by nasal cannula. Severe reaction: **Call EMS.** BLS: maintain airway. Administer oxygen by nonrebreather mask. Continue to monitor vital signs. Cardiopulmonary resuscitation. Administration of anticonvulsant.

TABLE 8-4	Emergency Reference Chart: Traumatic Injuries	
EMERGENCY	**SIGNS/SYMPTOMS**	**PROCEDURE**
Hemorrhage	Prolonged bleeding Spurting blood: artery Oozing blood: vein	Compression over bleeding area 1. Apply gauze pack with direct pressure. 2. Bandage pack into place firmly where possible. 3. Elevate injury above the heart if possible. Severe bleeding: digital pressure on pressure point of supplying vessel. If shock symptoms: **Call EMS.**
	Bleeding from tooth socket	Pack with folded gauze; do not dab. Have patient bite down firmly. If bleeding does not stop, instruct patient to gently bite down on a damp tea bag and hold in place for 10 min.
	Bleeding of an extremity	**Call EMS.** Elevate the part: support with pillows. Apply tourniquet only when limb is amputated, mangled, or crushed.
	Nosebleed	Seat patient upright, head elevated. Tell patient to breathe through mouth. Apply cold application to nose. Press nostril on bleeding side for a few minutes. Advise patient not to blow the nose for an hour or more. If bleeding does not stop, wet cotton rolls with water and lubricate with water-soluble lubricant. Pack nostril. Instruct patient to breathe through the mouth. Leave packing in place until patient sees a physician.
Burns 1. First degree	Skin reddened Swelling Pain	*First- and second-degree burns.* Do not give food or liquids; anticipate nausea. Be alert for signs of shock.
2. Second degree	Skin reddened, blisters Swelling Wet surface Pain (more than third degree) Heightened sensitivity to touch	Do not apply ointment, grease, or bicarbonate of soda. Immerse in cool water to relieve pain; do not apply ice. Gently clean with a mild antiseptic. Dress lightly with a dry sterile bandage. Elevate burned part. **Call EMS.**
3. Third degree (full thickness)	Leathery look Insensitive to touch	**Call EMS.** Treat for shock. BLS: maintain airway. Check for other injuries. Wrap in clean sheet: EMS transport.
4. Chemical burn	Reddened, discolored	Immediate: copious irrigation with water for ½ h. Check directions on container from which the chemical came for antidote or other advice. Burn caused by an acid may be rinsed with bicarbonate of soda; burn caused by alkali may be rinsed in weak acid such as acetic (vinegar).

(*continues*)

TABLE 8-4	Emergency Reference Chart: Traumatic Injuries (*continued*)	
EMERGENCY	**SIGNS/SYMPTOMS**	**PROCEDURE**
Internal poisoning	Signs of corrosive burn around or in oral cavity Evidence of empty container or information from patient Nausea, vomiting, cramps	Call Poison Control Center: 1-800-222-1222. Be calm and supportive. BLS: airway maintenance. Artificial ventilation (inhaled poison). Record vital signs. Do *not* give water or milk or Ipecac unless instructed to do so by Poison Control Center. Avoid nonspecific and questionably effective antidotes, stimulants, sedatives, or other agents, which may do more harm. **Call EMS.**
Foreign body in eye	Tears Blinking	Wash hands. Ask patient to look down. Bring upper lid down over lower lid for a moment; move it upward. Turn down lower lid and examine: if particle is visible, remove with moistened cotton applicator. Use eye cup: wash out eye with plain water. When unsuccessful, seek medical attention: prevent patient from rubbing eye by placing gauze pack over eye and stabilizing with adhesive tape.
Chemical solution in eye	Tears Stinging	Irrigate promptly with copious amounts of water. Turn head so water flows away from inner aspect of the eye; continue for 15–20 min.
Dislocated jaw	Mouth is open: patient is unable to close	Stand in front of seated patient. Wrap thumbs in towels and place on occlusal surfaces of mandibular posterior teeth. Curve fingers and place under body of the mandible. Press down and back with thumbs, and at the same time pull up and forward with fingers (Figure 8-5) As joint slips into place, quickly move thumbs outward. Place bandage around head to support under chin.
Facial fracture	Pain, swelling Ecchymoses Deformity, limitation of movement Crepitation on manipulation Zygoma fracture: depression of cheek Mandibular fracture: abnormal occlusion	Place patient on side. BLS. Support with bandage around face, under chin, and tied on the top of the head. **Call EMS.**
Tooth forcibly displaced (avulsed tooth)	Swelling, bruises, or other signs of trauma depending on the type of accident	Instruct patient or parent to hold the tooth by the crown, and avoid touching the root(s). If the tooth is dirty, rinse it gently in cool water, but do not scrub it or remove tissue fragments from its root surface. Keep the tooth moist by placing it in milk to transport to dentist. Bring the tooth and the patient to dental office or clinic *immediately*. The longer the time lapse between avulsion and replantation, the poorer the prognosis.

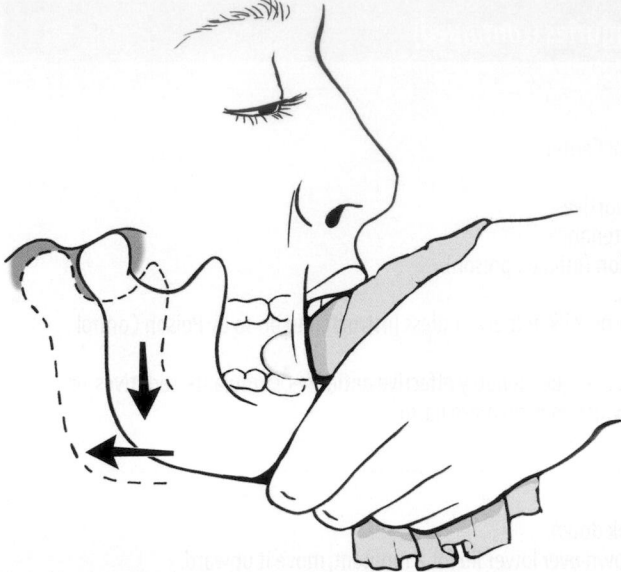

FIGURE 8-5 **Treatment for a Dislocated Mandible.** With thumbs wrapped in toweling and placed on the buccal cusps of the mandibular teeth, the fingers are curved under the body of the mandible. The jaw is pressed down and back with the thumbs while pulling up and forward with the fingers to permit the condyle to pass over the articular eminence into its normal position in the glenoid fossa. As the jaw slips into place, the thumbs are moved quickly aside.

I. Comprehensive Record Keeping

▶ All medical findings and changes.

▶ Treatments provided, including types and amounts of local anesthesia, general anesthesia, nitrous oxide, or other types of sedation.

▶ Regimens of medications prescribed for patients are crucial information should a medical emergency or a posttreatment complication occur.

II. Consults

In the patient's record, document telephone and written responses of consultations with physicians.

III. New Entries

▶ *Response to treatment*: Document a patient's reactions and responses to treatments, whether they are unremarkable or remarkable.

▶ *Previous appointment review*: Complete a comprehensive review of previous appointment documentation before providing additional treatment at sequential appointments.

BOX 8-5
Example Documentation: Emergency during Patient Treatment

S–Patient experienced blatant signs of anaphylaxis after exposure to latex gloves during a routine scaling appointment.

O–Patient presented with urticaria and pruritus on the arms, neck, and chest. Signs of lip, tongue, and laryngeal edema were exhibited with difficulty swallowing and breathing. Quickly informed the patient that he was experiencing an allergic reaction and needed an injection of epinephrine.

A–Findings indicate need for nonlatex gloves and caution during dental appointments especially when using new materials. At 8 minutes, the patient's vital signs were near baseline. Patient was released to EMS after 15 minutes to determine the extent of anaphylaxis. Patient was in stable condition.

P–Epinephrine was administered via EpiPen® and EMS was summoned. About 50 mg of Benadryl and 100 mg of Solu-Cortef were also administered intramuscularly. Oxygen was delivered by nonrebreather mask at 15 l/min. A Medical Emergency Report Form (Figure 8-1) was completed and given to EMS with one copy included in the patient's chart and the other sent to the patient's physician.

Signed _____, DDS or DMD Date _____

Signed _____, RDH Date _____

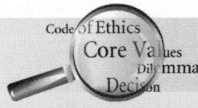

EVERYDAY ETHICS

A 12-year-old patient, Jonathan, had just received local anesthesia in Dr. Spar's treatment room in preparation for a restorative procedure. Suddenly Jonathan started to have a rhythmic twitching of the eyelids and appeared pale. Dr. Spar's assistant, Loraine, called the usual emergency alarm, and Elisa, the dental hygienist joined in the team protocol for medical emergencies.

In a few minutes, the generalized absence (petit mal) seizure was over and the patient was conscious with no other symptoms evident. Dr. Spar went about the dental procedure as if nothing had happened. Neither Loraine nor Dr. Spar made an entry in the record at the time. Elisa glanced over the patient's record and nothing she could find in the history showed that Jonathan had a

susceptibility to seizures. As Elisa went back to her own treatment room, she wondered if she needed to record the emergency or ask Dr. Spar about it.

Questions for Consideration

1. Which of the dental hygiene core values (Table II-1, Section II Introduction) apply in this situation? Explain the relationship.

2. Who needs to be informed of the event, and what potential ethical responsibilities are related to the patient?

3. What considerations for future treatment appointments are needed? From an ethical point of view, in what way were the patient's best interests compromised?

▶ *Current information*: Update information about the patient's health status as an integral part of the prevention of medical emergencies.

▶ *Emergency documentation*: Include a copy of the emergency Medical Emergency Report Form (Figure 8-1) that was completed during the emergency in the patient's permanent record.

▶ *Progress notes*: Box 8-5 contains an example progress note for an emergency that happens during an appointment.

Factors To Teach The Patient

▷ Stress minimization to prevent emergencies.
▷ Take medication prescribed by dentist at times indicated on the prescription.
▷ Schedule appointments when there is no waiting, first appointment of the morning or afternoon.
▷ Eat breakfast before morning appointment, or lunch before afternoon appointment unless instructed by the patient's physician not to eat before the appointment.
▷ If patient has prescription medications for emergency episodes, bring those medications to the appointment. Examples: nitroglycerin tablets for angina, asthma inhaler, glucagon for hypoglycemia.

References

1. Meiller TF, Wynn RL, McMullin AM, et al. *Dental Office Medical Emergencies*. 5th ed. Hudson, OH: Lexi-Comp; 2012: 9, 89.

2. Hass DA. Emergency drugs. *Dent Clin North Am*. 2002;46(4):815–830.

3. Malamed SF. *Medical Emergencies in the Dental Office*. 7th ed. St. Louis, MO: Mosby; 2014:39, 66.

4. Berg RA, Hemphill R, Abella BS, et al. Adult basic life support: 2010 American Heart Association Guidelines for cardiopulmonary resuscitation and emergency cardiovascular care. *Circulation*. 2010;122(Suppl 3):S685–S705.

5. Markenson D, Ferguson JD, Chameides L, et al. Part 17: first aid: 2010 American Heart Association and American Red Cross Guidelines for first aid. *Circulation*. 2010;122(18)(Suppl 3):S934–S946.

ENHANCE YOUR UNDERSTANDING

thePoint° DIGITAL CONNECTIONS
(see the inside front cover for access information)
- **Audio glossary**
- **Quiz bank**

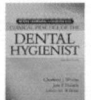

SUPPORT FOR LEARNING
(available separately; visit lww.com)
- *Active Learning Workbook for Clinical Practice of the Dental Hygienist, 12th Edition*

prepU INDIVIDUALIZED REVIEW
(available separately; visit lww.com)
- **Adaptive quizzing with *prepU for Wilkins' Clinical Practice of the Dental Hygienist***

SECTION

III

Documentation

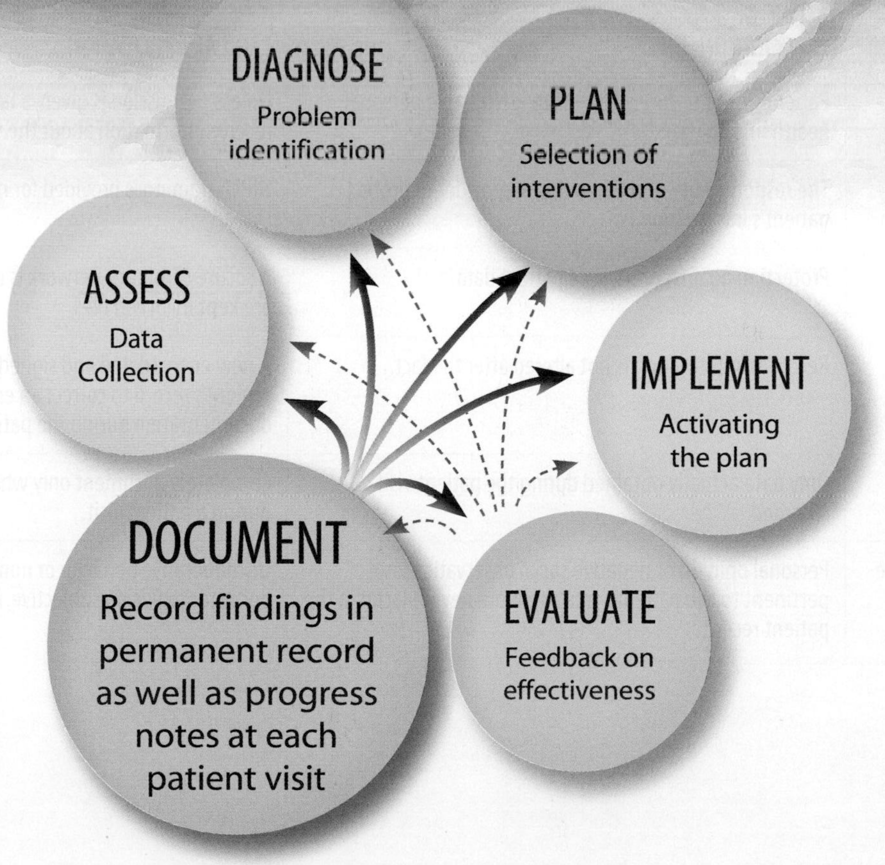

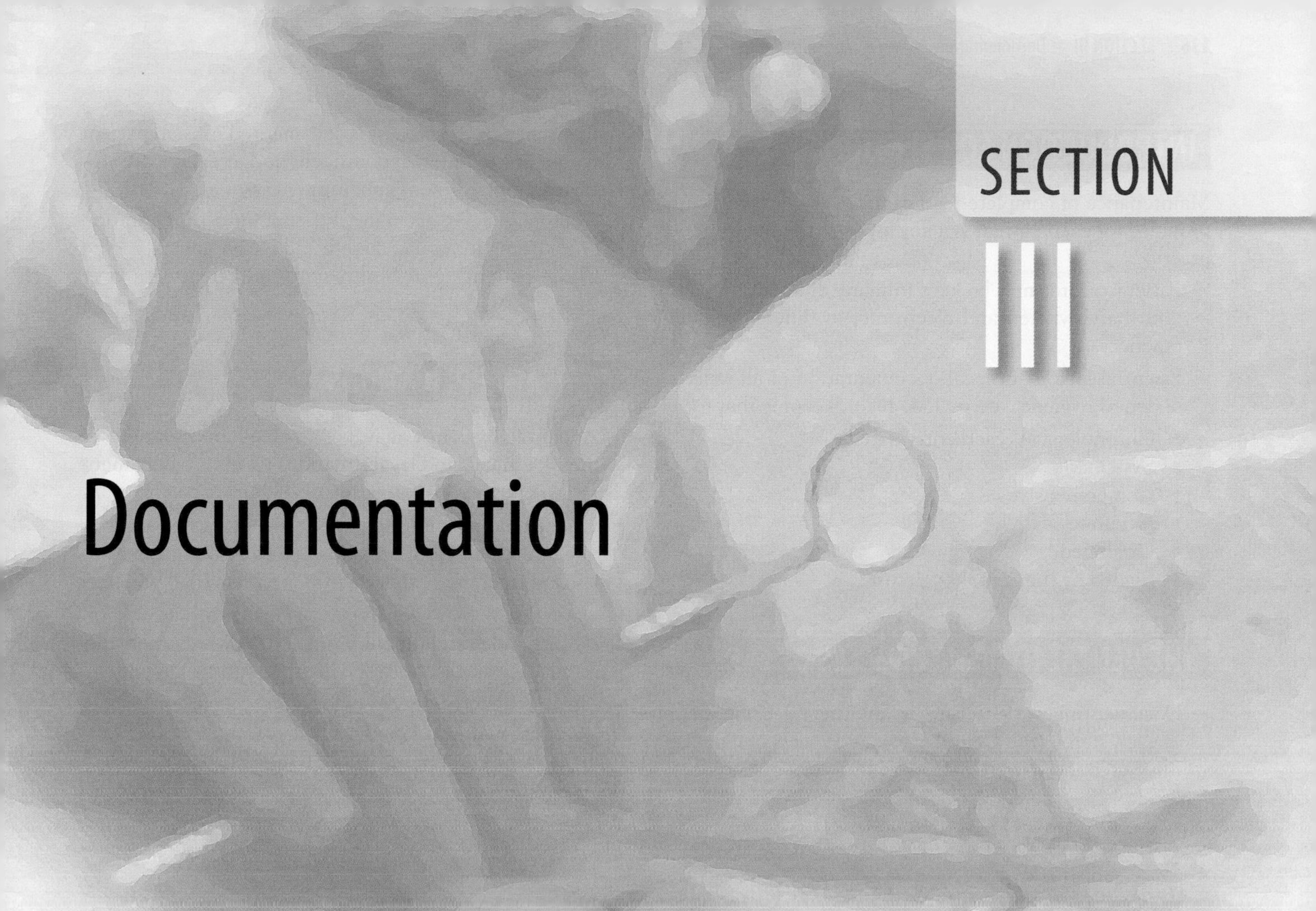

FIGURE III-1 The Dental Hygiene Process of Care.

INTRODUCTION FOR SECTION III

Maintenance of complete records for every aspect of care provided for each patient is a key aspect of dental hygiene practice.

▶ Patient records may be kept in many different formats, both hand-written and electronic, in different dental practices.

▶ Essential factors for legal documentation of all aspects of dental hygiene care include recordkeeping that is:

- Chronological (each entry dated),
- Systematic
- Comprehensive
- Accurate
- Unaltered
- Signed by the dental hygienist

THE DENTAL HYGIENE PROCESS OF CARE

▶ Documenting patient care is an integral component of each step in the Dental Hygiene Process of Care, as illustrated in **Figure III-1**.

▶ Every step in the process is documented in each patient record at the initial appointment and at every continuing care or treatment appointment.

▶ Comprehensive, accurate and concise documentation of each step forms a complete and chronological record of the patient's oral health status and treatment over time.

ETHICAL APPLICATIONS

▶ A dental hygienist may be involved in a variety of moral, ethical, and legal situations related to documentation of patient information during practice.

▶ Understanding that the patient record can be subpoenaed in the event of litigation is a basic tenant of ethical and legal risk management for professional practice.

▶ Knowledge of and adherence to Health Insurance Portability and Accountability Act (HIPAA) requirements for privacy and security of patient records is imperative.

▶ An overview of the key concepts in patient record keeping, with explanations and examples of ethical applications is found in **Table III-1**.

TABLE III-1	Essentials of Ethical Record Keeping	
CONCEPT	**EXPLANATION**	**ETHICAL APPLICATION**
Privacy	Patient's right to control access to identifiable personal health information.	Unless permission is given, a family member cannot receive information about the patient.
Confidentiality	The responsibility of the healthcare provider to protect patient's information.	HIPPA training is provided for new employees.
Security	Protection against unsecured patient data.	A secure computer network is used or paper records are kept in locked files.
Accuracy	Recorded information is not altered after the fact.	A new entry (dated and signed) is made in the patient's record to correct an error or omission in documentation during the patient appointment.
Authenticity	Only data actually obtained during the patient visit is recorded.	Completely document only what actually happened during a patient visit.
Impersonal/Objective	Personal opinion or negative social observations not pertinent to the patient's treatment are never placed in the patient record	Uncooperative behavior or non-compliance are documented using subjective, factual statements.

9

Documentation for Dental Hygiene Care

Charlotte J. Wyche, RDH, MS

CHAPTER OUTLINE

LEARNING OBJECTIVES

After studying this chapter, the student will be able to:

1. Identify and define key terms and concepts related to written and computerized dental records and charting.

2. Describe concepts related to ensuring confidentiality and privacy of patient information.

3. Compare three tooth-numbering systems.

4. Discuss the various components of a patient's permanent, comprehensive dental record.

5. Recognize and explain a systematic method for documenting patient visits.

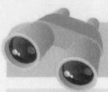

BOX 9-1   KEY WORDS: Records and Charting

Chart: a form or graphic used as a component of a patient's permanent health record.

Charting: the process of tabulating clinical information on a graphic form.

Encryption: translation of computerized data into a secret code; the most effective way to achieve data security; in order to read an encrypted file, the reader needs access to a secret key or password that enables changing the "cipher text" into plain text.

Forensic: pertaining to or used in legal proceedings.

Forensic dentistry (forensic odontology): application of dental knowledge and use of dental records or oral health data in legal proceedings, criminal investigations, or the identification of found human remains.

Malpractice: professional negligence; an act or an omission by a healthcare provider that causes injury to a patient; a deviation from acceptable standards of care.

Patient record: a written document that contains information identifying an individual patient, such as a patient's name, address, and phone number, as well as information

related to that particular patient's care, such as health history information, dental charting items, treatment dates, and treatment codes.

Electronic record: in a computerized database management system, a record is a complete set of information. Records are composed of electronic fields, each of which contains space for one item of information.

Sign: objective, observable evidence of an illness or disorder; a physical manifestation of a disorder that is apparent to a trained healthcare provider and sometimes to the patient.

Symptom: any change in the body or its function that is perceived by the patient; the subjective experience of a disease or disorder.

Triage: screening and classification of individuals in order to make optimal use of treatment resources; sorting and allocating relative priority for patient treatment needs.

Unique identifier: secret name and/or password used by an individual to access computerized information that is not available to others who do not have permission to access the information.

▶ Complete, accurate documentation of patient information and treatment provided, maintained in comprehensive records, and chartings is a basic requirement of providing patient care.

▶ Accurate record keeping is essential to a safe, thorough, and caring dental hygiene practice as well as clinical and ethical risk management.[1]

▶ Box 9-1 defines key terms related to patient records and charting.

THE PATIENT RECORD

I. Purposes and Characteristics

▶ Patient health records provide a means of communication between the members of the health team, as well as with their patients.

▶ Complete patient care records facilitate coordinated planning and continuity of care.

▶ Patient records serve as a basis for the evaluation of the quality of care and aid when a review is made of the effectiveness of patient care practices.

▶ Data from health records are utilized in research and education.

▶ Documentation in the patient's record is considered legal evidence in any legal or forensic situation.[2,3]

▶ Documentation in a patient record is:[2]
  • Authentic: genuine and undisputed reality.
  • Accurate and comprehensive.
  • Legible.
  • Objective.

▶ Patient record entries are:
  • Recorded promptly during or following treatment.
  • Recorded using clear, concise, subjective statements.
  • Dated.
  • Signed by the clinician.

II. Components of a Patient Record

▶ The format of patient record will vary among private dental practices and clinics.

▶ All information collected during the initial examination and during continuing patient appointments is an official part of the permanent records.[2,4,5]

▶ To meet the dental hygiene standard of care, all components of the dental hygiene process of care are addressed, including the dental hygiene care plan.[6]

▶ Required components of a complete and regularly updated patient record include:[2]
  • Medical history and vital signs
  • Dental history
  • Clinical assessment and diagnosis
  • Treatment recommendations and written treatment plan
  • Progress notes for each patient visit
  • Signed acknowledgment of confidentiality measures (see HIPAA section in this chapter).

▶ Additional components, required when applicable, include:[2]
  • Informed consent forms[7]
  • Radiographs and radiographic assessment
  • Periodontal risk assessment
  • Caries risk assessment

- Trauma and/or surgery anesthesia records
- Study models
- Oral photographs[8]
- Orthodontic records, if available
- Laboratory orders and test results
- Referral records and copies of consultation correspondence with dental specialists or medical practitioners.

▶ Each component of the patient record is marked with patient identification and/or demographic information.

III. The Handwritten Record

▶ Historically, dental healthcare personnel have maintained handwritten documentation of patient records.

▶ Handwritten records are recorded legibly and written in ink.

▶ Records have also been dictated into a machine to be typewritten into the permanent record later.

▶ Mistakes are corrected by placing a single line through the error, writing the correct information immediately after, and signing the entry.

▶ If a late entry is necessary, the new information:
- Follows the most recent entry in the patient record
- Is noted as a late entry
- Includes the date and time that the late entry was made.

▶ Systems may involve the completion of forms with topics and spaces to check off and spaces for writing descriptive information and/or prose-style summary.

▶ Strict infection control protocols are required to prevent contamination of paper records during patient care.

▶ For written records, a filing system is needed that provides accessibility to the health records by authorized personnel only.

IV. The Electronic Record

A. Characteristics[9]

▶ Computerized records have provided a faster, more convenient, and better organized mode of information gathering and preserving patient information.

▶ Data can be accessed from anywhere within the system by authorized personnel.

▶ A variety of custom software programs are available to include complete patient information, appointment schedules, medical alerts, and financial aspects of patient care.

▶ Systems may provide methods for documenting dental and periodontal assessments with automated, voice-activated recordings.

▶ Other systems permit printing hard copies for the patient when indicated.

▶ Computerized records require computer terminals where only authorized personnel can access required information.

▶ Computer monitors are directed away from the view of unauthorized persons.

▶ Infection control protocols include providing plastic barriers for computer keyboard and mouse, as well as disinfection of chairside monitors.

B. Features

Specially designed software and record storage systems can:

▶ Standardize terminology used for data entry.

▶ Improve efficiency and accountability; speed up entry of information and encourage entry of more comprehensive information.[10]

▶ Increase the legibility of information.

▶ Provide easier, faster access to clinical information.

▶ Enhance communication with patients and with consulting dental specialists or other multidisciplinary team members who may not be together at one clinical site.[10]

▶ Provide new ways of analyzing clinical information and outcomes of various clinical treatment approaches or treatment procedures.

▶ Maintain digital radiographs and photographs within the patient record.

THE HEALTH INSURANCE PORTABILITY AND ACCOUNTABILITY ACT

▶ The Health Insurance Portability and Accountability Act of 1996 (HIPAA) took effect for dental practices in the United States on April 14, 2003.

▶ The law provides federal privacy standards that protect patient records and other health-related information in an emerging electronic information environment.[11]

▶ The law applies to
- healthcare facilities
- healthcare insurance companies
- healthcare providers.

▶ Some states may have stricter laws that take precedence over the federal standards.

▶ Legislation is in place in Canada and some European countries to protect the privacy of personal information.[12,13]

▶ The current law is divided into two separate components that address:
- Privacy and the patient's ability to access their health information
- Security of patient information in healthcare settings.

I. The HIPAA Privacy Rule

▶ Establishes a national standard to protect individual's privacy and access to medical records and other health informaiton.[14]

▶ Patients have the right to:
- Receive a copy of personal health records.
- Ask to change incorrect or incomplete information.

- Receive reports on when, why, and with whom their health information is shared.
- Decide, in some cases (such as marketing), whether health information can be shared.
- Ask to be contacted regarding health information in a specific location or by a specific method such as telephone or mail.
- File a complaint with the provider, health insurer, or United States government regarding concerns about use of their health information.

▶ Healthcare facilities are responsible to:
- Develop required privacy and confidentiality forms.
- Adopt written privacy policies and educate staff about confidentiality of patient information.
- Appoint staff privacy officers and privacy contact persons.
- Provide patients with a Notice of Privacy Practices document at the beginning of their care and receive signed acknowledgment of receipt.
- Implement security measures, policies, and formal protocols that protect patient information.
- Conduct analysis of security risks and vulnerabilities.
- Establish sanctions for workforce members who fail to comply with policies.

▶ Healthcare providers are responsible to:
- Comply with protocols and practices that protect patient information and avoid inappropriate disclosure.

II. The HIPAA Security Rule

▶ Updated in 2013 to strengthen digital security standards and enhance enforcement.[5]
▶ Establishes a national set of security standards for protecting health information that is held or transferred in electronic form.[15]

▶ Comprises three separate standards:[5]
- Administrative safeguards: limitation of access to appropriate members in the workforce.
- Physical safeguards: use of storage systems and procedures that prevent access for unauthorized individuals.
- Technical safeguards: use of technology, such as coding and encryption, to control access to patient information.

DOCUMENTING THE EXTRA- AND INTRAORAL EXAMINATION

▶ A specific objective of the intra- and extraoral examination as a part of the total patient assessment is the recognition of deviations from normal that may be signs and symptoms of disease (see Chapter 12).
▶ The need for careful, thorough documentation of examination findings cannot be overemphasized.
▶ Concentration and attention to detail are necessary in order that each slight deviation from normal may be entered on the record.

TOOTH-NUMBERING SYSTEMS

Different systems are used in the various dental offices and clinics worldwide. The three most commonly used tooth designation systems are described here:

I. Continuous Numbers 1–32

This tooth-numbering method is referred to as the *Universal* or *ADA* system.[16] Figure 9-1 shows the crowns of the teeth with the corresponding numbers.

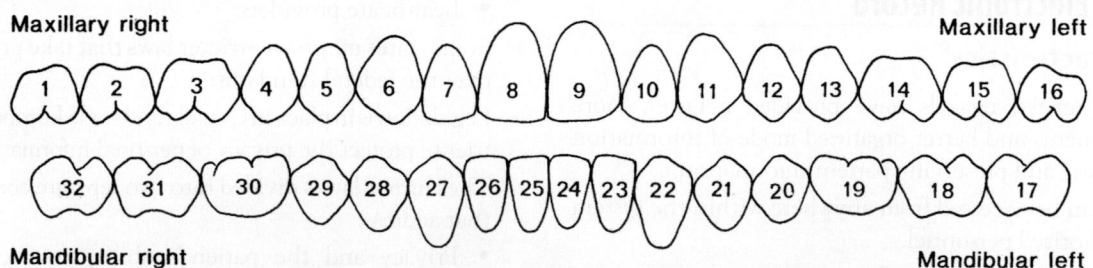

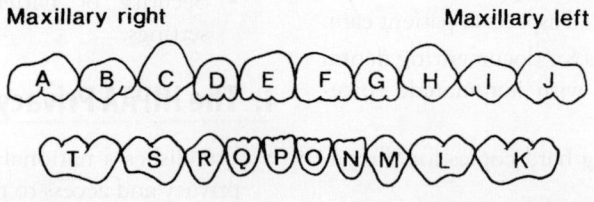

FIGURE 9-1 Universal Tooth Numbering (American Dental Association). *Above,* permanent dentition designated by numbers 1–32, starting at the maxillary right with 1 and following around to the maxillary left third molar (number 16) to the left mandibular third molar (number 17) and around to the right mandibular third molar (number 32). *Below,* primary teeth are designated by letters in the same sequence.

A. Permanent Teeth

▶ Start with the right maxillary third molar (number 1).

▶ Follow around the arch to the left maxillary third molar (16).

▶ Descend to the left mandibular third molar (17).

▶ Follow around to the right mandibular third molar (32).

B. Primary or Deciduous Teeth

▶ Use continuous upper case letters A–T in the same order as described for the permanent teeth.

▶ Right maxillary second molar (A) around to left maxillary second molar (J).

▶ Descend to left mandibular second molar (K) and around to the right mandibular second molar (T).

II. FDI Two Digit

The **Fédération Dentaire Internationale** (FDI) system (Figure 9-2) is also called the *International* system.[17,18]

A. Permanent Teeth

Each tooth is numbered by the quadrant (1–4) and by the tooth within the quadrant (1–8).

▶ Quadrant numbers

  1 = Maxillary right

  2 = Maxillary left

  3 = Mandibular left

  4 = Mandibular right

▶ *Tooth numbers within each quadrant*: Start with number 1 at the midline (central incisor) to number 8, third molar. Figure 9-2 shows each tooth number in the four quadrants.

▶ *Designation*: The digits are pronounced separately. For example, "two-five" (25) is the maxillary left second premolar, and "four-two" (42) is the mandibular right lateral incisor.

B. Primary or Deciduous Teeth

Each tooth is numbered by quadrant (5–8) to continue with the permanent quadrant numbers. The teeth are numbered within each quadrant (1–5).

▶ Quadrant numbers

  5 = Maxillary right

  6 = Maxillary left

  7 = Mandibular left

  8 = Mandibular right

▶ *Tooth numbers within each quadrant*: Number 1 is the central incisor, and number 5 is the second primary molar.

▶ *Designation*: The digits are pronounced separately. For example, "eight-three" (83) is the mandibular right primary canine, and "six-five" (65) is the maxillary left second primary molar.

III. Quadrant Numbers 1–8

Names to identify this method are the *Palmer System* or *Set-square*.[19]

A. Permanent Teeth

▶ Each tooth is designated using the numbers 1 (central incisor)–8 (third molar) in each quadrant.

▶ The appropriate quadrant for each tooth is designated using a specific pattern of vertical and horizontal lines as shown in Figure 9-3.

B. Primary or Deciduous Teeth

▶ Upper case letters A–E are used instead of the numbers.

PERMANENT TEETH

Q-1 Maxillary right								Q-2 Maxillary left							
18	17	16	15	14	13	12	11	21	22	23	24	25	26	27	28
48	47	46	45	44	43	42	41	31	32	33	34	35	36	37	38
Q-4 Mandibular right								Q-3 Mandibular left							

PRIMARY TEETH

Q-5 Maxillary right					Q-6 Maxillary left				
55	54	53	52	51	61	62	63	64	65
85	84	83	82	81	71	72	73	74	75
Q-8 Mandibular right					Q-7 Mandibular left				

FIGURE 9-2 International Tooth Numbering (FDI). Each quadrant is numbered 1–4, with number 1 on the maxillary right, number 2 on the maxillary left, number 3 on the mandibular left, and number 4 on the mandibular right. Each tooth in a quadrant is numbered 1–8 from the central incisor. Quadrants of the primary dentition are numbered from 5 through 8. It is a two-digit system.

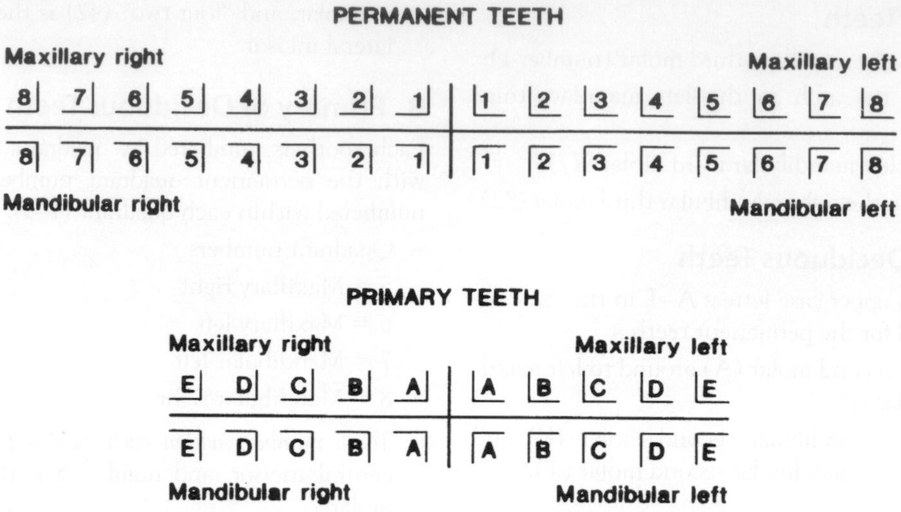

PERMANENT TEETH

Maxillary right									Maxillary left							
8	7	6	5	4	3	2	1		1	2	3	4	5	6	7	8
8	7	6	5	4	3	2	1		1	2	3	4	5	6	7	8

Mandibular right   Mandibular left

PRIMARY TEETH

Maxillary right					Maxillary left				
E	D	C	B	A	A	B	C	D	E
E	D	C	B	A	A	B	C	D	E

Mandibular right   Mandibular left

FIGURE 9-3 **Palmer System Tooth Numbering.** Each permanent tooth is designated by number 1–8, starting at the central incisor of each quadrant. Quadrants are designated by horizontal and vertical lines. Primary teeth are identified by the letters A–E, starting at the central incisor.

CHARTING

I. Purpose

The purpose of each type of charting is defined by its title:

▶ *Dental chart*: Includes diagrammatic representation of existing conditions of the teeth.

▶ *Periodontal chart*: Indicates clinical features of the periodontium.

▶ The use of separate chart forms to record the special features of periodontal and dental findings is preferable.

▶ Dental and periodontal charts are updated routinely on new forms with current dates to record changes in the patient's oral features over time.

▶ Neatness in the markings of symbols, drawings, and labels goes hand-in-hand with the accuracy of the examination itself.

▶ An accurate, detailed, and carefully recorded charting is used for:

• *Care planning*: The charting is a graphic representation of the existing condition of the patient's teeth and periodontium from which needed treatment procedures can be organized into a treatment plan.

• *Treatment*: During dental and dental hygiene appointments, the charting is useful for guiding specific procedures.

• *Evaluation*: The outcome and degree of treatment effects are determined by comparing the findings of the initially recorded examination with periodic follow-up examinations.

• *Protection*: In the event of misunderstanding by a patient, or if legal questions should arise, the records and chartings are evidence.

• *Identification*: In the event of emergency, accident, or disaster, a patient may be identified by the teeth for which a record has been maintained.

II. Forms Used for Charting

▶ Many variations of chart forms are in current use: some available commercially, and some designed by the individual practitioner to meet particular needs.

▶ Specifications for an adequate form include ample space to:

• Chart neatly, accurately, and completely

• Label as needed for clarity

• Record in a manner that can be interpreted by all who use it.

▶ *Anatomic drawings of the complete teeth*: Figure 9-4 provides a typical example of a form that may be used for periodontal and/or dental charting.

▶ *Geometric*: A diagrammatic representation that provides space to record findings for each tooth. Examples of geometric charting forms used to record a patient's disclosed biofilm for teaching personal disease control are shown in Figures 23-1 and 23-2 in Chapter 23.

III. Sequence for Charting

A. Basic Entries

▶ *Name, Birth date*.

▶ *Date of examination*: Every entry is dated.

▶ *Missing teeth*: When radiographs are available in advance, missing teeth can be charted before the clinic appointment. Whether dental or periodontal charting is completed first, marking the missing teeth will be necessary.

B. Systematic Procedure

▶ The use of a set routine is prerequisite to accomplishing a complete and accurate charting, not only for the tooth surface-to-surface pattern but also for the parts of the charting itself.

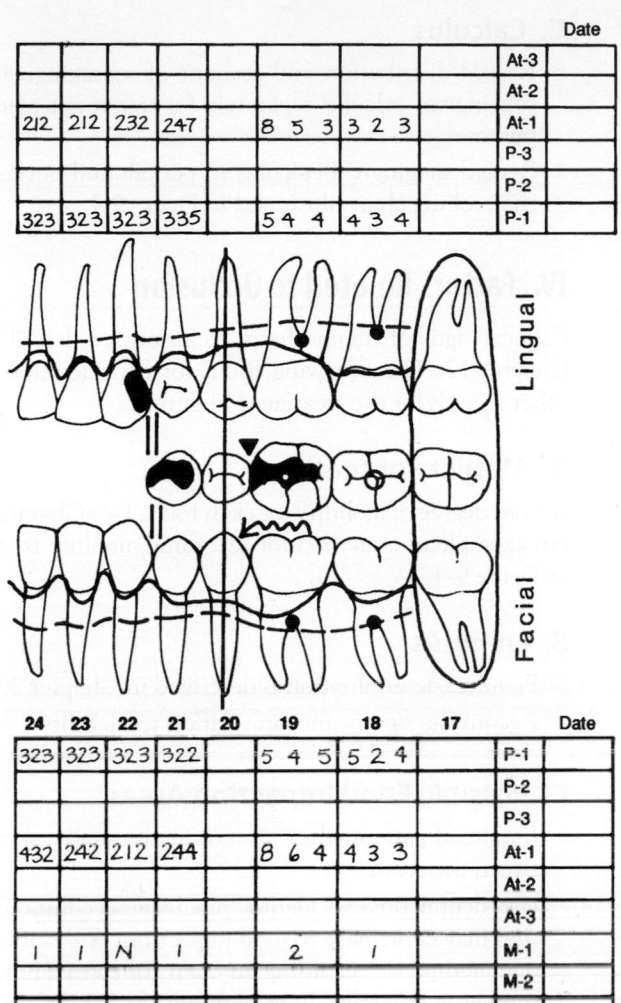

								Date	
							At-3		
							At-2		
212	212	232	247		8 5 3	3 2 3		At-1	
							P-3		
							P-2		
323	323	323	335		5 4 4	4 3 4		P-1	

Lingual

Facial

24	23	22	21	20	19	18	17	Date	
323	323	323	322		5 4 5	5 2 4		P-1	
								P-2	
								P-3	
432	242	212	244		8 6 4	4 3 3		At-1	
								At-2	
								At-3	
I	I	N	I		2	I		M-1	
								M-2	
								M-3	

Key

Missing Tooth: | or X
Unerupted or impacted: Encircle tooth
Drift and Migration: ∿∿
Open Contact: ||
Food Impaction: ↓ (at occlusal)

Periodontal Chart
Gingival Margin: Black line
Mucogingival Junction: Dashed line
Furca involved: ● (in furcation)
Probing depths: (mm) P-1, P-2, P-3
Clinical attachment level: (mm) At-1, At-2, At-3

Dental Chart
Dental Caries: red
Restorations: blue
Defective Restoration: circle with red
Overhang: ▼ (at occlusal)
Mobility: (+, N, 1, 2, 3) M-1, M-2, M-3
Fremitus: F-1 (recorded on maxillary only)

FIGURE 9-4   Periodontal and Dental Charting. Section of a charting (mandibular left quadrant) shows combined dental and periodontal charting. Dental caries and restorations are usually marked with colored pencils, such as blue for restorations and red for dental caries, on the anatomic crowns or roots. The gingival margin is clearly drawn to show areas of recession. Boxes at the apices of each tooth provide spaces for probing depths and clinical attachment level recordings, as well as for mobility notations.

▶ Charting all of one item for the entire mouth, rather than complete chartings of one tooth, helps to ensure accuracy.

• For example, in the dental charting, record all the restorations first.

• Then start again at the first tooth and chart all the deviations from normal.

• Charting all restorations and deviations for each tooth separately is less efficient.

C. Radiographic Charting

▶ The following may be charted from radiographs without the presence of the patient:

• Missing, unerupted, impacted teeth
• Endodontic restorations
• Overhanging margins of existing restorations
• Proximal surface carious lesions
• Other deviation from normal evident from the radiographs.

▶ Supplemental and confirmational observations and checks are made during the clinical examination with the patient. For example, when a carious lesion is suspected but not visible on the radiograph clinical examination is required.

D. Study Models

Study models are useful to record details related to occlusion (see Chapter 17).

PERIODONTAL RECORDS

▶ The patient's permanent records include the itemized findings of all the clinical and radiographic examinations.

▶ Prepare entries that are clear and easily understood by all who read them and use them in continuing treatment.

▶ Additions to the records are made to show the progress of treatment and comparative observations throughout the series of appointments.

▶ After the periodontium has been brought to a state of health, a continuing care plan is outlined.

▶ At each succeeding appointment, new and comparative records and chartings are made.

I. Clinical Observations of the Gingiva

Clinical observations are recorded either on the chart form or in the patient progress notes during each patient visit. Examine gingiva and record findings before disclosing agent is used for biofilm score.

A. Describe Gingiva

▶ Color, size, position, shape, consistency, and surface texture; extent of bleeding when probed; and areas where there is minimal attached gingiva (Table 18-1 in Chapter 18).

B. Describe Distribution of Gingival Changes

Localized or generalized; specify the areas of severest disease involvement. Use tooth numbers to identify adjacent gingival tissue.

II. Items to be Charted

▶ Missing teeth
▶ Location of bridges, pontics, and implants
▶ Gingival line (margin) and mucogingival lines (junctions)
▶ Probing depths (except around dental implants)
▶ Areas of suspected mucogingival involvement
▶ Furcation involvement
▶ Abnormal frenal attachments
▶ Mobility and fremitus of teeth.

III. Deposits

Deposits can be recorded on forms such as the one illustrated in Figure 9-4 or on dental index forms, which are illustrated in Chapter 23.

A. Stains

▶ *Extrinsic:* Record type of stain, color, distribution; specific location by tooth number; whether slight, moderate, or heavy.
▶ *Intrinsic:* Record separately from extrinsic and identify by type when known.

B. Soft Deposits

▶ *Food debris:* Distribution and amount. Record location by teeth when the biofilm control instruction requires special emphasis on a particular area.
▶ *Dental biofilm:*
  • Record direct observations with or without disclosing agent; include distribution and degree or amount.
  • Record biofilm film index or score as described in Chapter 23.

C. Calculus

▶ Record distribution and amount of supragingival and subgingival calculus separately for treatment planning purposes.
▶ Record subgingival calculus in periodontal pockets on the probing chart illustrated in Figure 9-4.

IV. Factors Related to Occlusion

Clinical signs of trauma from occlusion are described in Chapter 17. The following list is for consideration with other records for the treatment planning.

A. Mobility of Teeth

Record degree of mobility for each tooth (see Chapter 20). An example of a method for recording mobility is shown in Figure 9-4.

B. Fremitus

▶ Fremitus determination is described in Chapter 20
▶ Record the significance in relation to mobility.

C. Possible Food Impaction Areas

▶ Inquire of patient where fibrous foods usually catch between the teeth.
▶ Use dental floss to identify inadequate contact areas that may contribute to food impaction. An example of one method for recording an open contact is shown by the vertical parallel lines between teeth numbered 21 and 22 in Figure 9-4.

D. Occlusion-Related Habits

▶ Observe for evidence of, and question patient concerning, such parafunctional habits as bruxism or clenching.
▶ Note wear patterns and facets on study cast.
▶ Note attrition.

V. Radiographic Findings

▶ Specific notes are made to correlate the radiographic findings with the clinical observations just listed.
▶ Details of radiographic findings in periodontal disease are described in Chapter 20.
▶ The following are recorded in relation to the specific teeth involved:
  • Height of bone as related to the cementoenamel junction.
  • Horizontal or angular shape of remaining interdental bone.
  • Intact, broken, or missing crestal lamina dura.
  • Furcation involvement.
  • Widening of periodontal ligament space.
  • Overhanging fillings, large carious lesions, and other dental biofilm–retention factors.

VI. Severity of Periodontal Disease

▶ Determination of the severity of periodontal disease is based on analysis of gingival changes, periodontal probing recordings, sites of bleeding on probing, clinical attachment level, tooth mobility and fremitus, and the radiographic findings.

▶ A dental or dental hygiene diagnosis statement can be developed using the disease classifications outlined in Tables 19-1 and 19-2 in Chapter 19, as a reference.

DENTAL RECORDS

▶ The patient's permanent records include the itemized clinical and radiographic findings related to the teeth along with subjective symptoms reported by the patient.

▶ Information about conditions related to the teeth is included in Chapter 16.

▶ Occlusion and mobility of teeth are documented during the periodontal examination because the causes of mobility are related to the patient's periodontal status.

▶ After initial entries are recorded, new and comparative records and chartings are prepared at each periodic maintenance visit to show the progress of treatment.

▶ The need for meticulous examination and recording cannot be overemphasized.
  • Finding and recording a carious lesion may mean saving a tooth for the patient's lifetime.
  • Inadvertent neglect of a tooth may lead eventually to a need for endodontic therapy or even extraction.

I. The Anatomic Tooth Chart Form

Figure 9-4 is an example of a quadrant of dental charting using anatomic tooth drawings. When charting, clinical and radiographic findings are coordinated.

II. Items to Be Charted

A list of basic items to be charted includes:

▶ Missing teeth.

▶ Existing restorations. Note restorative materials so that the care plan can designate selective polishing agents that will not harm the surfaces of restorations.

▶ Fixed and removable prostheses.

▶ Dental sealants.

▶ Overhangs, open contacts, open margins, and other irregularities.

▶ Cavitated carious lesions and questionable demineralized noncavitated lesions.

▶ Inadequate contact areas and observed proximal surface roughness. Use dental floss. Fraying of dental floss as it is passed over a rough proximal surface may mean the defective margin of a restoration, a sharp cavity margin, or dental calculus.

▶ Pulp vitality. Record numbers in the permanent record. Chart forms sometimes include a specific place for the recording of such data.

▶ Tooth sensitivity. The patient may report hypersensitive areas. Record the tooth number and surface for reference during the treatment phase.

CARE PLAN RECORDS

▶ Along with a comprehensive dental treatment plan, a formal dental hygiene care plan that includes dental hygiene diagnostic statements and addresses the patient's risk factors is included in the patient's record.

▶ Chapter 25 provides more information about developing a written dental hygiene care plan.

▶ The initial care plan developed during an initial examination, as well as copies of updated plans are included as part of the comprehensive, permanent patient record.

INFORMED CONSENT

▶ Documentation of informed consent obtained before initiating treatment is an essential component of each patient's record.

▶ Information about obtaining and documenting informed consent is found in Chapter 25.

DOCUMENTATION OF PATIENT VISITS

I. Purpose

Documentation completed during or immediately following a patient visit, sometimes referred to as a progress note, is a chronologic history of treatment received by the patient during each appointment.

II. Essentials of Good Progress Notes

▶ Dental hygiene progress notes document all aspects of the dental hygiene process of care and records all interactions between the patient and the practice.[4]

▶ In addition to documentation about treatment rendered, essential components of a patient progress note are listed in Box 9-2.

▶ Each entry in the patient record is dated and signed by the clinician.

▶ The use of unique abbreviations that are not easily understood by others can cause clinical or legal problems. A selected list of standard abbreviations and symbols developed by the American Dental Association is found in Appendix VII.

▶ Information that is *never* in the patient record includes:
  • Speculation

BOX 9-2

Essential Components of a Patient Progress Note

▷ Purpose of the visit
▷ History review
▷ Assessment findings
▷ Description of treatment provided
▷ Drugs (including topical or local anesthetic) administered during treatment or prescribed by the dentist
▷ Self-care and other instructions provided
▷ Referrals, consultations with physician or dental specialist
▷ Laboratory tests ordered; results of laboratory tests
▷ Next visit appointments scheduled or recommended; appointment cancellations
▷ Details related to patient conversations, including telephone and e-mail
▷ Signature of clinician and date

• Derogatory statements
• Information about financial matters, professional disputes, legal actions, or risk-management protocol.

III. Systematic Documentation: The SOAP Approach

▶ A systematic, standardized approach to writing patient progress notes assures that no details are missing from the patient's record.

▶ Many clinicians develop their own systematic approach to make sure documentation is comprehensive.

▶ Several formalized documentation systems have been developed.

▶ One approach, which uses the acronym SOAP as a guide, is well accepted for use in the medical, and dental professions and recommended for use by the American Pediatric Dentistry Association.[2,5,20]

• S = Subjective
• O = Objective
• A = Assessment (or analysis)
• P = Procedures (provided or planned).

▶ Table 9-1 further defines the components of the SOAP acronym and provides examples of factors that are included in patient progress notes.

▶ Box 9-3 provides an example of documentation for a patient visit written using the SOAP format.

TABLE 9-1		Components of SOAP Documentation and Examples of Factors to Include in Progress Notes
DESCRIPTION		**EXAMPLES**
S	**Subjective** Characteristics stated by the patient or perceived by the clinician	▪ Patient's age ▪ Patient's gender ▪ Type of appointment scheduled ▪ Medical history findings provided by the patient ▪ Patient's chief complaint ▪ Patient's self-care regimen ▪ Social history
O	**Objective** Characteristics observed during examination	▪ Head and neck examination findings ▪ Periodontal exam findings; bleeding; soft tissue condition ▪ Hard tissue examination findings; current cavitated carious lesions and demineralized noncavitated lesions ▪ Radiographic findings ▪ Comparison of current findings with previous findings
A	**Assessment/Analysis** Identification of problems or patient needs	▪ Risk factors for oral disease ▪ Caries risk level ▪ Calculus level ▪ Current periodontal diagnosis/case type and status ▪ Periodontal disease risk level
P	**Procedures** Interventions performed or planned	▪ Dental hygiene interventions performed ▪ Medicaments or local anesthesia applied and to which teeth ▪ Consults with dentist or other health providers ▪ Self-care instructions ▪ Goals for patient improvement ▪ Pending/planned dental hygiene interventions

Source: Jacks ME, Blue C, Murphy D. Short- and long-term effects of training on dental hygiene faculty members' capacity to write SOAP notes. *J Dent Educ.* 2008;72(6):719–724.

EVERYDAY ETHICS

Mrs. Belvedere, the office manager in Dr. Grain's office, has online access to all electronic patient records from her computer at home. With Dr. Grain's permission, she often uses her home e-mail to contact patients and insurance companies regarding treatment plans, insurance coverage, or financial records. Patients receive HIPAA information about confidentiality and security of their information, but are not told that Mrs. Belvedere has access to their records at her home. Hanna, who is a new dental hygienist in the office, inadvertently finds out that sensitive patient information is being sent out from the same home e-mail account that is used by both Mrs. Belvedere's husband and her adult son. When Hanna approaches Dr. Grain about the potential breach in security of patient information, he seems unconcerned.

Questions for Consideration

1. What dental hygiene core values are being compromised if Hanna decides not to follow through to try to change the situation?

2. What standards of professional responsibility, identified in the American Dental Hygienists' Association code of ethics, apply in this situation?

3. Which essential record keeping concepts, as described in Table III-1 (Section III Introduction), can support Hanna as she decides how to approach Mrs. Belvedere and Dr. Grain to make changes in the way patient records and information are handled?

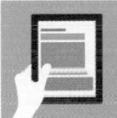

BOX 9-3

Example of Patient Care Documentation: Using the SOAP Format

S–Patient presents for reassessment of oral self-care 2 weeks following oral hygiene instruction. Patient states that he notices a reduction in biofilm following oral self-care instructions provided at the previous appointment.

O–Today's "Plaque Free Score" — 89%; sulcus bleeding index SBI score = 2.

A–"Plaque-Free Score" compared with previous score of 22%; SBI score compared with previous score of 5. Significant improvement in biofilm control noted in all areas except buccal surfaces of maxillary molars.

P–Patient congratulated on areas of success. Additional instruction provided specifically related to biofilm removal on posterior buccal and proximal tooth surfaces. Patient observed while brushing and flossing maxillary molar areas using a mirror. Next visit: 3 months re-evaluation.

Signed _____, RDH

Date _____.

▶ Additional documentation examples, each related to a clinical situation and formatted using the SOAP approach, can be reviewed near the end of each chapter of this book.

IV. Risk Reduction and Legal Considerations

▶ Malpractice allegations can, unfortunately, occur against even a dental hygienist who routinely meets every standard when providing dental hygiene care.

▶ Because litigation can occur years after the patient visit when the details and even the patient may have been forgotten, excellent comprehensive documentation in each patient record entry is the best protection for the clinician against allegations of wrongdoing.

Factors To Teach The Patient

▷ Interpretation of all recordings; meaning of all numbers used, such as for probing depths.

▷ The importance of making a complete study of the patient's oral problems before beginning treatment.

▷ Advantages of cooperation and patience in furnishing information that will help dental personnel to interpret observations accurately so that the correct diagnosis and appropriate treatment plan can be made.

▷ Assurance that all information received is completely confidential.

References

1. Collier A. The management of risk, Part 3: recording your way out of trouble. *Dent Update.* 2014;41(4):338–340.

2. American Academy of Pediatric Dentistry, Council on Clinical Affairs. *Guidelines on Record-Keeping.* Chicago, IL: American Academy of Pediatric Dentistry; 2012. http://www.aapd.org/media/Policies_Guidelines/G_Recordkeeping.pdf. Accessed September 16, 2014.

3. Dym H. Risk management techniques for the general dentist and specialist. *Dent Clin North Am.* 2008;52(3):563–577, ix.

4. American Association of Dental Boards. *Guidelines on the Dental Patient Record.* Chicago: American Association of Dental Boards; 2009:4–12.

5. Leeuw W. Maintaining proper dental records. *Dent Assist.* 2014;83(2):22–23,26–30,32–34.

6. American Dental Hygienists' Association. *Standards for Clinical Dental Hygiene Practice.* Chicago: American Dental Hygienists' Association; 2008:9.

7. Collier A. The management of risk. Part 2: good consent and communication. *Dent Update*. 2014;41(3):236–238, 241.

8. Wander P, Ireland RS. Dental photography in record keeping and litigation. *Br Dent J*. 2014;217(3):133–137.

9. Emmott L. Electronic dental records in dentistry. *J Am Coll Dent*. 2010;77(1):10–12.

10. Hudis S. Converting to electronic dental records. *J Am Coll Dent*. 2010;77(1):13–15.

11. U.S. Department of Health and Human Services. Health information privacy. http://www.hhs.gov/ocr/privacy/hipaa/administrative/index.html. Accessed September 16, 2014.

12. Office of the Privacy Commissioner of Canada. Privacy legislation in Canada. https://www.priv.gc.ca/resource/fs-fi/02_05_d_15_e.asp. Accessed September 16, 2014.

13. European Commission. Data Protection in the EU. http://ec.europa.eu/health/data_collection/data_protection/in_eu/index_en.htm. Accessed September 16, 2014.

14. U.S. Department of Health and Human Services. Health information privacy: summary of the HIPAA privacy rule. http://www.hhs.gov/ocr/privacy/hipaa/understanding/summary/index.html. Accessed September 16, 2014.

15. U.S. Department of Health and Human Services. Health information privacy: summary of the HIPAA security rule. http://www.hhs.gov/ocr/privacy/hipaa/understanding/srsummary.html. Accessed September 16, 2014.

16. American Dental Association. *System of Tooth Numbering and Radiograph Mounting*. Chicago, IL: American Dental Association; 1968, October. (historical reference).

17. Fédération Dentaire Internationale. Two-digit system of designating teeth. *Int Dent J*. 1971;21(1):104. (historical reference).

18. Türp JC, Alt KW. Designating teeth: the advantages of the FDI's two-digit system. *Quintessence Int*. 1995;26(7):501–504. (historical reference).

19. Palmer C. Palmer's dental notation. *Dent Cosmos*. 1891;33:194. (historical reference).

20. Rethman J. Clean up your records with SOAP. S (subjective findings), O (objective findings), A (assessment), P (plan). *Dent Today*. 1995;14(8):80.

 ## ENHANCE YOUR UNDERSTANDING

thePoint® DIGITAL CONNECTIONS
(see the inside front cover for access information)
- Audio glossary
- Quiz bank

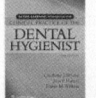 **SUPPORT FOR LEARNING**
(available separately; visit lww.com)
- *Active Learning Workbook for Clinical Practice of the Dental Hygienist, 12th Edition*

prepU INDIVIDUALIZED REVIEW
(available separately; visit lww.com)
- **Adaptive quizzing with *prepU* for *Wilkins' Clinical Practice of the Dental Hygienist***

SECTION IV

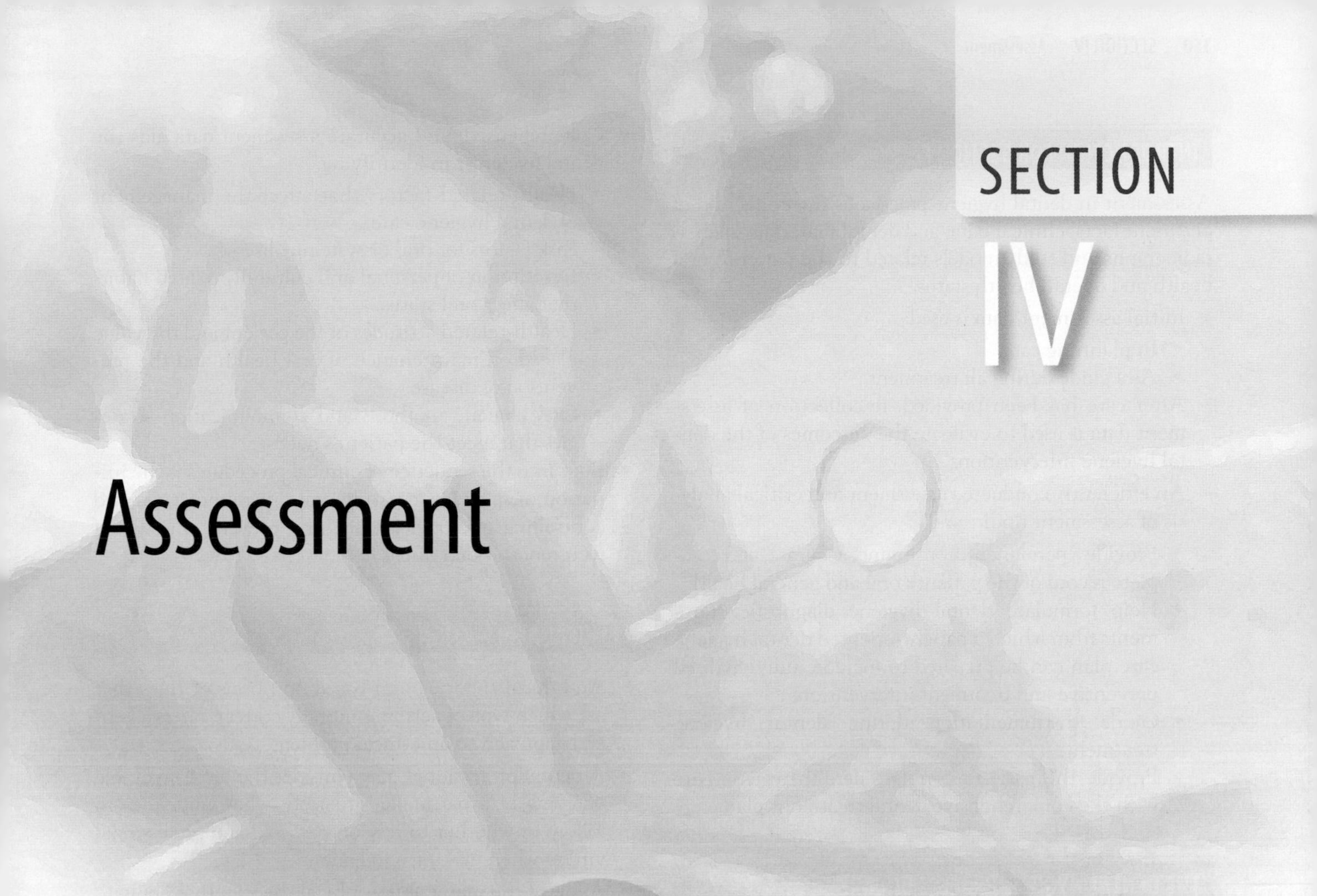

Assessment

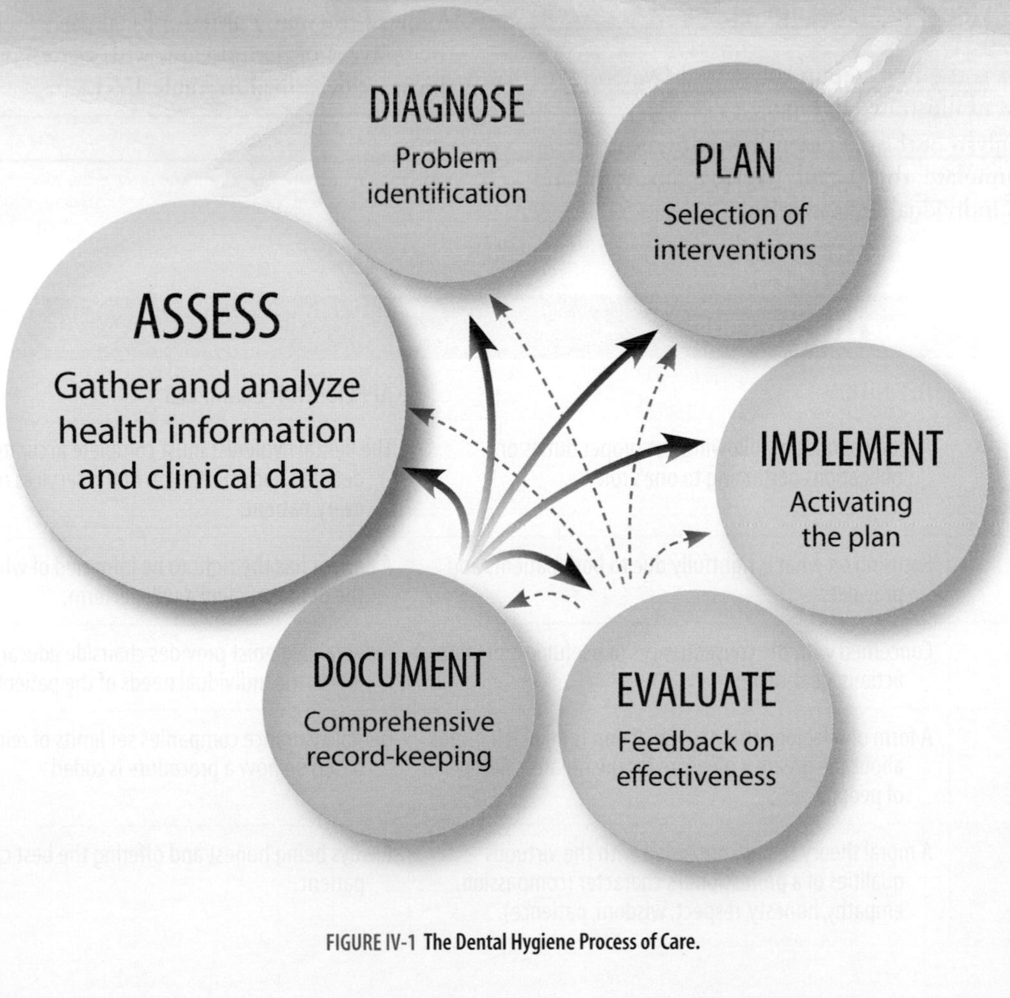

DIAGNOSE
Problem identification
PLAN
Selection of interventions
ASSESS
Gather and analyze health information and clinical data
IMPLEMENT
Activating the plan
DOCUMENT
Comprehensive record-keeping
EVALUATE
Feedback on effectiveness

FIGURE IV-1 The Dental Hygiene Process of Care.

INTRODUCTION FOR SECTION IV

Assessment in dental hygiene practice is the collection of pertinent facts, clinical data, and dental materials, such as radiographs and study models related to the patient's oral health and overall health status.

► Initial assessment data is used:
- In planning care.
- As a guide during all treatment.

► After care has been provided, re-collection of assessment data is used to evaluate the outcomes of the dental hygiene interventions.

► An efficiently conducted assessment and critical analysis of assessment findings:
- Provide a permanent, continuing, accurate, and complete record of the patient's oral and general health.
- Help formulate dental hygiene diagnostic statements from which a patient-oriented dental hygiene care plan can be prepared to include individualized preventive and treatment interventions.
- Guide instrumentation during dental hygiene treatment.
- Provide the basis to correlate dental hygiene care with the comprehensive dental treatment plan.

THE DENTAL HYGIENE PROCESS OF CARE

► Assessment is the first step in the dental hygiene process of care, as illustrated in **Figure IV-1**.

► Critical analysis of the data identifies patient problems used to formulate the dental hygiene diagnosis and develop an individualized care plan.

► Comprehensive and accurate assessment data aids the dental hygienist in identifying:
- Health-related factors that affect the management of dental hygiene care.
- Risk factors for oral or systemic disease.
- Description of personal and culturally related habits that affect oral status.
- Health-related attitudes of the patient and the value placed on maintenance of oral health and the prevention of disease.
- Oral hygiene methods and communication strategies that meet the patient's needs.

► Built into the sequence of clinical procedures is the initiation of steps for arresting oral disease processes and controlling etiologic factors, and prevent episodes of recurrence of oral disease.

ETHICAL APPLICATIONS

► An ethical theory, often based on norms or rules that ask which type of action is morally correct, offers a general approach to an ethical problem.

► A dental professional may consider the most favorable outcome of a particular situation, what guidelines to follow, or whether to rely on personal and professional virtues when making a judgment.

► A few of the many philosophical theories that apply to the delivery of dental care, with corresponding definitions, are described in **Table IV-1**.

TABLE IV-1	Some Ethical Theories	
THEORY	**DEFINITION**	**APPLICATION EXAMPLES**
Deontology	A study of rules by following the proper duties or obligations pertaining to one's role.	The dental hygienist must complete accurate and detailed documentation of the services rendered for every patient.
Rights Theory	Focusing on what is rightfully due to both patients and providers.	A patient has the right to be informed of what treatment the dental hygienist will perform.
Teleology	Concerned with the consequences or usefulness of one's actions, goal-driven.	A dental hygienist provides chairside education that meets the individual needs of the patient.
Utilitarianism	A form of teleology that says an action is good if it brings about the greatest pleasure for the greatest number of people.	Dental insurance companies set limits of reimbursement based on how a procedure is coded
Virtue Ethics	A moral theory that is concerned with the virtuous qualities of a professional's character (compassion, empathy, honesty, respect, wisdom, patience).	Always being honest and offering the best care to every patient.

10

Personal, Dental, and Medical Histories

Lisa Welch, RDH, MSDH and Charlotte J. Wyche, RDH, MS

CHAPTER OUTLINE

INTRODUCTION
I. Significance
II. Purposes of the History

HISTORY PREPARATION
I. Systems
II. Record Forms
III. Introduction to the Patient
IV. Limitations of a History

THE QUESTIONNAIRE
I. Types of Questions
II. Advantages of a Questionnaire
III. Disadvantages of a Questionnaire (If Used Alone Without a Follow-Up Interview)

THE INTERVIEW
I. Participants
II. Setting

III. Pointers for the Interview
IV. Interview Form
V. Advantages of the Interview
VI. Disadvantages of the Interview

ITEMS INCLUDED IN THE HISTORY
I. Personal History
II. Dental History
III. Medical History

IMMEDIATE APPLICATIONS OF PATIENT HISTORIES
I. Medical Consultation
II. Radiation
III. Prophylactic Premedication

PRETREATMENT ANTIBIOTIC PROPHYLAXIS
I. AHA Guidelines
II. Recommendations Based on Four Principles

III. Medical Conditions that Required Antibiotic Premedication Before Invasive Dental and Dental Hygiene Procedures
IV. Recommended Antibiotic Protocol

ASA DETERMINATION

REVIEW AND UPDATE OF HISTORY

DOCUMENTATION

EVERYDAY ETHICS

FACTORS TO TEACH THE PATIENT

REFERENCES

LEARNING OBJECTIVES

After studying this chapter, the student will be able to:

1. Relate and define key terms and concepts utilized in the creation of patient histories.

2. Explain the significance and purpose of accurate and complete patient personal, medical, and dental histories.

3. Compare and contrast the different methods available for the compilation of patient histories and the advantages and disadvantages of each.

4. Discuss how the components of patient histories relate directly to the application of patient care.

INTRODUCTION

For safe, evidence-based dental and dental hygiene care, a thorough patient health history is an essential part of the complete assessment. Key words relating to the preparation and use of the histories are defined in Box 10-1.

The history directs and guides steps to be taken in preparation for, during, and following appointments. Some important points about the patient history are listed here.

▶ The history is needed before oral examination procedures with periodontal probe and explorer are carried out.

▶ The use of instruments that would manipulate the soft tissue around the teeth is contraindicated until after it has been determined whether antibiotic premedication is required.

▶ When a question exists about the medical history as described by the patient, or when an unusual or abnormal condition is observed, consultation with the patient's primary care provider or referral for examination of the patient who does not have a primary care provider is required.

▶ Even emergency treatment must be postponed or kept to a minimum until the patient's medical status is determined.

I. Significance

The significance of taking a complete and accurate patient history cannot be overemphasized for the following reasons:

▶ Oral conditions reflect the general health of the patient; dental procedures may complicate or be complicated by existing pathologic or physiologic conditions elsewhere in the body.

▶ General health factors influence response to treatment, such as tissue healing, and thereby influence the outcomes that may be expected from oral care.

▶ The state of the patient's health is constantly changing. Therefore, the history must be updated continually.

II. Purposes of the History

Carefully prepared personal, medical, and dental histories are used in comprehensive patient care to:

▶ Provide information pertinent to the etiology and diagnosis of oral conditions and the total patient care plan.

▶ Reveal conditions that necessitate precautions, modifications, or adaptations during appointments to ensure dental and dental hygiene procedures will not harm the patient and to prevent emergency situations.

▶ Aid in the identification of possible unrecognized conditions for which the patient will be referred for further diagnosis and treatment.

▶ Permit appraisal of the general health and nutritional status, which, in turn, contributes to the prognosis of success in patient care and instruction.

▶ Give insight into emotional and psychological factors, attitudes, and prejudices that may affect present appointments as well as continuing care.

▶ Document records for reference and comparison over a series of appointments for periodic follow-up.

▶ Furnish evidence in legal matters if questions arise.[1]

▶ Identify cultural beliefs and practices that affect risk for oral disease.

▶ Determine ethnic/racial influences on risk factors for oral disease.

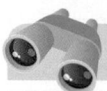

BOX 10-1 KEY WORDS: Personal, Medical, and Dental Histories

Allergy: state of abnormal and individual hypersensitivity acquired through exposure to a particular allergen.

Antibiotic premedication: provision of an effective antibiotic before invasive clinical procedures that can create a transient bacteremia, which, in turn, can cause IE or other serious infection.

Bacteremia: presence of microorganisms in the bloodstream.

Drug interaction: a change in the effect of one drug when a second drug is introduced concomitantly; the change may be desirable, adverse, or inconsequential.

Forensic: pertaining to or applied in legal proceedings.

Forensic dentistry: dentolegal science; the relation and application of dental facts to legal problems, as in using the teeth for identifying the dead.

Hematogenous: produced or derived from blood; disseminated through the bloodstream.

Immunocompromised: when the immune response is attenuated by administration of immunosuppressive

drugs, by irradiation, by malnutrition, or by certain disease processes.

Informed consent: a medicolegal document that holds providers responsible for ensuring that patients understand the risks and benefits of a procedure or medication before it is administered.

OTC: over-the-counter; nonprescription drug; pertains to distribution of drugs directly to the public without prescription.

PDR: *Physicians' Desk Reference*; contains current information about the actions, side effects, and interactions of drugs; a new edition is published annually.

Premedication: preliminary medication; may be for the purpose of allaying apprehension, preventing bacteremia, or otherwise facilitating the clinical procedure.

SBE: subacute bacterial endocarditis, now called infective endocarditis (IE).

HISTORY PREPARATION

The general methods in current use for obtaining a health history are the *interview*, the *questionnaire* (which may be paper or electronic), or a combination of the two. There are several systems for obtaining the history.

I. Systems

▶ Preappointment information

- Basic information obtained before the initial assessment appointment can save time and facilitate the process.
- A brief telephone screening interview or downloadable questionnaire can help determine potential medical problems, need for premedication or consultation with the patient's primary care provider, and identification of medically compromised or physically challenged patients for whom modifications in routine care may be needed.

▶ Self-history

- Because a self-history can be prepared at home, the history form can be provided online for the patient to download and complete, sent via e-mail, or mailed to the patient in advance of the first appointment.
- This kind of form might include some items that can be checked or circled, as in a questionnaire, and space to allow the patient to provide additional information.

▶ Complete history

- A complete patient history is made at the initial visit and is a combination of interview and questionnaire.
- At successive appointments, the complete history is reviewed with the patient and changes are considered when planning patient care.

II. Record Forms

▶ Basic history forms

- Forms are available commercially or from the American Dental Association (ADA) for a fee,[2] but many dentists and dental hygienists prefer to develop their own and have a form printed to their specifications.
- ADA and other organizations have basic history forms that have been translated into a variety of languages. Many are available on the Internet.

▶ An adequate basic history form will:

- Provide for conventional notation of important details in a logical sequence.
- Permit quick identification of special needs of a patient when the history is reviewed before each appointment.
- Allow ample space to record the patient's own words whenever possible in the interview method, or for self-expression by the patient on a questionnaire.

- Have space for notes concerning attitudes and knowledge as stated or displayed by the patient during the history-taking or other later appointments.
- Be provided, whenever possible, in a version that has been translated to the patient's primary or dominant language.

▶ Supplementary forms

- A secondary, more detailed questionnaire can be used to determine additional information for specialized topics.
- The basic questionnaire reveals whether the topic applies to the individual, and if the answer is positive, additional information is requested.
- *Example*: Simple questions on the basic questionnaire indicate the use of tobacco products. Completion of another questionnaire provides details about the type of tobacco used and frequency of use. Figure 34-2, Chapter 34, illustrates a tobacco use assessment form.

III. Introduction to the Patient

▶ Educate the patient about why the information requested in the history is essential before treatment can be undertaken.

▶ Convey the idea that oral health and general health are interrelated, without creating undue alarm concerning potential ill effects or harmful sequelae from required treatment.

▶ To build rapport, allow children to participate in their history preparation, but most of the information will need to be supplied by a parent or legal guardian. The signature of the responsible adult is required on the record.

IV. Limitations of a History

Many patients cannot or will not provide complete or, in certain cases, correct information when answering medical or dental history questions. Reasons for inaccuracy or incompleteness of information can include:

▶ Problems related to the method of obtaining the histories, how the questions are worded, or an inadvertent lack of neutrality in the attitude of the person gathering the history.

▶ Difficulty in comprehending a self-administered test because the patient cannot read, or has a language barrier.

▶ The location in which the questionnaire is completed, such as, a crowded reception area without sufficient privacy where other patients can see the form.

▶ The patient's limited knowledge and inability to understand the relationship between certain diseases or conditions and dental treatment. Information may seem irrelevant, so it is withheld.

▶ Reticence to discuss a health condition that may be embarrassing, such as history of infectious or communicable disease. The patient may fear refusal of treatment.

THE QUESTIONNAIRE

Positive findings on a questionnaire are explained further in a personal interview. A questionnaire by itself cannot be expected to satisfy the overall purposes of the history, but it can provide some basic personal history, dental history, and factual information in the medical history.

I. Types of Questions

The health questionnaires available from the ADA (adult questionnaire in Figure 10-1 and child questionnaire in Figure 10-2) provide useful examples of questions essential to patient evaluation.[2]

▶ *System oriented*
  • Direct questions to determine if the patient has had a disease. Often the questions are organized as a review of systems, for example, the digestive system, respiratory system, or urinary system.
  • The questions may contain references to specific organs, for example, the stomach, lungs, or kidneys.

▶ *Disease oriented*
  • A typical set of questions may start with "Do you have, or have you had, any of the following diseases or problems?"
  • A listing under that question contains such items as diabetes, asthma, or hypertension arranged alphabetically or grouped by systems or body organs.
  • Follow-up questions can determine dates of illness, severity, and outcome.

▶ *Symptom oriented*
  • In the absence of previous or current disease states, questions may lead to a suspicion of a condition, which, in turn, can provide an opportunity to recommend and encourage the patient to schedule an examination by a primary care provider.
  • Examples of the symptom-oriented questions are "Are you thirsty much of the time?" "Does your mouth frequently become dry?" or "Do you have to urinate more than six times a day?"
  • Positive answers could lead to tests for diabetes detection.

▶ *Culture oriented*
  Questions related to the patient's cultural background can help to:
  • Identify ethnic or gender-related increase in risk for systematic or oral disease.
  • Determine traditional culturally related health beliefs that may influence dental hygiene interventions or recommendations.

• Identify herbal preparations or other traditional medications used by the patient that may affect oral care or risk for disease.

II. Advantages of a Questionnaire

▶ Broad in scope; useful during the interview to identify positive answers that need additional clarification.
▶ Time saving.
▶ Consistent; all selected questions are included, and none is omitted because of time or other factors.
▶ Patient has time to think over the answers; not under pressure, nor under the eyes of the interviewer.
▶ Patient may write information that might not be expressed directly in an interview.
▶ Legal aspects of a written or an electronic record with the patient's signature.

III. Disadvantages of a Questionnaire (If Used Alone Without a Follow-Up Interview)

▶ Impersonal; no opportunity to develop rapport.
▶ Inflexible; no provision for additional questioning in areas of specific importance to an individual patient.

THE INTERVIEW

In long-range planning for the patient's health, much more is involved than asking questions and receiving answers. The rapport established at the time of the interview contributes to the continued cooperation of the patient.

I. Participants

▶ The interviewer is alone with the patient or parent of the child patient and, if necessary, a qualified professional translator/interpreter.
▶ The history is never to be taken in a reception area when other patients are present.

II. Setting

▶ A consultation room or office is preferred; move the patient away from the atmosphere of the treatment room, where thoughts may be on the services to be provided.
▶ The treatment room may be the only available place with privacy. If the treatment room is used for a patient interview:
  • Seat patient comfortably in upright position.
  • Turn off running water and dental light, and close the door (if possible).
  • Sit on clinician's chair to be at eye level and face-to-face with the patient.

Health History Form

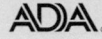

American Dental Association
www.ada.org

E-mail:	Today's Date:

As required by law, our office adheres to written policies and procedures to protect the privacy of information about you that we create, receive or maintain. Your answers are for our records only and will be kept confidential subject to applicable laws. Please note that you will be asked some questions about your responses to this questionnaire and there may be additional questions concerning your health. This information is vital to allow us to provide appropriate care for you. This office does not use this information to discriminate.

Name:			Home Phone: *Include area code*	Business/Cell Phone: *Include area code*
Last	First	Middle	( )	( )

Address:	City:	State:	Zip:
Mailing address			

Occupation:	Height:	Weight:	Date of birth:	Sex: M F

SS# or Patient ID:	Emergency Contact:	Relationship:	Home Phone:	Cell Phone:
			( )	( )
				Include area codes

If you are completing this form for another person, what is your relationship to that person?

Your Name | Relationship

Do you have any of the following diseases or problems: *(Check DK if you Don't Know the answer to the question)*

	Yes	No	DK
Active Tuberculosis	☐	☐	☐
Persistent cough greater than a 3 week duration	☐	☐	☐
Cough that produces blood	☐	☐	☐
Been exposed to anyone with tuberculosis	☐	☐	☐

If you answer yes to any of the 4 items above, please stop and return this form to the receptionist.

Dental Information *For the following questions, please mark (X) your responses to the following questions.*

	Yes	No	DK
Do your gums bleed when you brush or floss?	☐	☐	☐
Are your teeth sensitive to cold, hot, sweets or pressure?	☐	☐	☐
Does food or floss catch between your teeth?	☐	☐	☐
Is your mouth dry?	☐	☐	☐
Have you had any periodontal (gum) treatments?	☐	☐	☐
Have you ever had orthodontic (braces) treatment?	☐	☐	☐
Have you had any problems associated with previous dental treatment?	☐	☐	☐
Is your home water supply fluoridated?	☐	☐	☐
Do you drink bottled or filtered water?	☐	☐	☐
If yes, how often? Circle one: DAILY / WEEKLY / OCCASIONALLY			
Are you currently experiencing dental pain or discomfort?	☐	☐	☐

	Yes	No	DK
Do you have earaches or neck pains?	☐	☐	☐
Do you have any clicking, popping or discomfort in the jaw?	☐	☐	☐
Do you brux or grind your teeth?	☐	☐	☐
Do you have sores or ulcers in your mouth?	☐	☐	☐
Do you wear dentures or partials?	☐	☐	☐
Do you participate in active recreational activities?	☐	☐	☐
Have you ever had a serious injury to your head or mouth?	☐	☐	☐

Date of your last dental exam:
What was done at that time?

Date of last dental x-rays:

What is the reason for your dental visit today?

How do you feel about your smile?

Medical Information *Please mark (X) your response to indicate if you have or have not had any of the following diseases or problems.*

	Yes	No	DK
Are you now under the care of a physician?	☐	☐	☐

Physician Name:	Phone: *Include area code*
	( )

Address/City/State/Zip:

	Yes	No	DK
Are you in good health?	☐	☐	☐
Has there been any change in your general health within the past year?	☐	☐	☐

If yes, what condition is being treated?

Date of last physical exam:

	Yes	No	DK
Have you had a serious illness, operation or been hospitalized in the past 5 years?	☐	☐	☐

If yes, what was the illness or problem?

	Yes	No	DK
Are you taking or have you recently taken any prescription or over the counter medicine(s)?	☐	☐	☐

If so, please list all, including vitamins, natural or herbal preparations and/or diet supplements:

_____
_____
_____
_____

FIGURE 10-1 Adult Health History Form. (Copyright © 2010 American Dental Association. All rights reserved. Reprinted with permission).

Medical Information

Please mark (X) your response to indicate if you have or have not had any of the following diseases or problems.

	Yes	No	DK
(Check DK if you Don't Know the answer to the question)			
Do you wear contact lenses?	☐	☐	☐
Joint Replacement. Have you had an orthopedic total joint (hip, knee, elbow, finger) replacement?	☐	☐	☐
Date: _____ If yes, have you had any complications?_____			
Are you taking or scheduled to begin taking either of the medications, alendronate (Fosamax®) or risedronate (Actonel®) for osteoporosis or Paget's disease?	☐	☐	☐
Since 2001, were you treated or are you presently scheduled to begin treatment with the intravenous bisphosphonates (Aredia® or Zometa®) for bone pain, hypercalcemia or skeletal complications resulting from Paget's disease, multiple myeloma or metastatic cancer?	☐	☐	☐
Date Treatment began: _____			

	Yes	No	DK
Do you use controlled substances (drugs)?	☐	☐	☐
Do you use tobacco (smoking, snuff, chew, bidis)?	☐	☐	☐
If so, how interested are you in stopping?			
(Circle one) VERY / SOMEWHAT / NOT INTERESTED			
Do you drink alcoholic beverages?	☐	☐	☐
If yes, how much alcohol did you drink in the last 24 hours? _____			
If yes, how much do you typically drink In a week? _____			
WOMEN ONLY Are you:			
Pregnant?	☐	☐	☐
Number of weeks: _____			
Taking birth control pills or hormonal replacement?	☐	☐	☐
Nursing?	☐	☐	☐

Allergies - Are you allergic to or have you had a reaction to: To all **yes** responses, specify type of reaction.

	Yes	No	DK		Yes	No	DK
Local anesthetics_____	☐	☐	☐	Metals_____	☐	☐	☐
Aspirin _____	☐	☐	☐	Latex (rubber) _____	☐	☐	☐
Penicillin or other antibiotics_____	☐	☐	☐	Iodine _____	☐	☐	☐
Barbiturates, sedatives, or sleeping pills _____	☐	☐	☐	Hay fever/seasonal _____	☐	☐	☐
Sulfa drugs _____	☐	☐	☐	Animals_____	☐	☐	☐
Codeine or other narcotics _____	☐	☐	☐	Food_____	☐	☐	☐
				Other _____	☐	☐	☐

Please mark (X) your response to indicate if you have or have not had any of the following diseases or problems.

	Yes	No	DK		Yes	No	DK		Yes	No	DK
Artificial (prosthetic) heart valve	☐	☐	☐	Autoimmune disease	☐	☐	☐	Hepatitis, jaundice or			
Previous infective endocarditis	☐	☐	☐	Rheumatoid arthritis	☐	☐	☐	liver disease	☐	☐	☐
Damaged valves in transplanted heart	☐	☐	☐	Systemic lupus erythematosus.	☐	☐	☐	Epilepsy	☐	☐	☐
Congenital heart disease (CHD)				Asthma	☐	☐	☐	Fainting spells or seizures	☐	☐	☐
Unrepaired, cyanotic CHD	☐	☐	☐	Bronchitis	☐	☐	☐	Neurological disorders	☐	☐	☐
Repaired (completely) in last 6 months	☐	☐	☐	Emphysema	☐	☐	☐	If yes, specify:_____			
Repaired CHD with residual defects	☐	☐	☐	Sinus trouble	☐	☐	☐	Sleep disorder	☐	☐	☐
				Tuberculosis	☐	☐	☐	Mental health disorders	☐	☐	☐

Except for the conditions listed above, antibiotic prophylaxis is no longer recommended for any other form of CHD.

	Yes	No	DK		Yes	No	DK		Yes	No	DK		Yes	No	DK
								Cancer/Chemotherapy/				Specify:_____			
								Radiation Treatment	☐	☐	☐	Recurrent Infections	☐	☐	☐
Cardiovascular disease.	☐	☐	☐	Mitral valve prolapse	☐	☐	☐	Chest pain upon exertion	☐	☐	☐	Type of infection:_____			
Angina	☐	☐	☐	Pacemaker	☐	☐	☐	Chronic pain	☐	☐	☐	Kidney problems	☐	☐	☐
Arteriosclerosis	☐	☐	☐	Rheumatic fever	☐	☐	☐	Diabetes Type I or II	☐	☐	☐	Night sweats	☐	☐	☐
Congestive heart failure	☐	☐	☐	Rheumatic heart disease	☐	☐	☐	Eating disorder	☐	☐	☐	Osteoporosis	☐	☐	☐
Damaged heart valves	☐	☐	☐	Abnormal bleeding	☐	☐	☐	Malnutrition	☐	☐	☐	Persistent swollen glands			
Heart attack	☐	☐	☐	Anemia	☐	☐	☐	Gastrointestinal disease	☐	☐	☐	in neck	☐	☐	☐
Heart murmur	☐	☐	☐	Blood transfusion	☐	☐	☐	G.E. Reflux/persistent				Severe headaches/			
Low blood pressure	☐	☐	☐	If yes, date:_____				heartburn	☐	☐	☐	migraines	☐	☐	☐
High blood pressure	☐	☐	☐	Hemophilia	☐	☐	☐	Ulcers	☐	☐	☐	Severe or rapid weight loss	☐	☐	☐
Other congenital heart				AIDS or HIV infection	☐	☐	☐	Thyroid problems	☐	☐	☐	Sexually transmitted disease	☐	☐	☐
defects	☐	☐	☐	Arthritis	☐	☐	☐	Stroke	☐	☐	☐	Excessive urination	☐	☐	☐
								Glaucoma	☐	☐	☐				

	Yes	No	DK
Has a physician or previous dentist recommended that you take antibiotics prior to your dental treatment?	☐	☐	☐

Name of physician or dentist making recommendation: _____ Phone: _____

	Yes	No	DK
Do you have any disease, condition, or problem not listed above that you think I should know about?	☐	☐	☐
Please explain:			

NOTE: Both Doctor and patient are encouraged to discuss any and all relevant patient health issues prior to treatment.

I certify that I have read and understand the above and that the information given on this form is accurate. I understand the importance of a truthful health history and that my dentist and his/her staff will rely on this information for treating me. I acknowledge that my questions, if any, about inquiries set forth above have been answered to my satisfaction. I will not hold my dentist, or any other member of his/her staff, responsible for any action they take or do not take because of errors or omissions that I may have made in the completion of this form.

Signature of Patient/Legal Guardian: _____ Date: _____

FOR COMPLETION BY DENTIST

Comments:_____
_____
_____
_____

FIGURE 10-1 (*continued*).

Child Health/Dental History Form

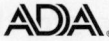

American Dental Association
www.ada.org

Patient's Name			Nickname	Date of Birth
LAST	FIRST	INITIAL		

Parent's/Guardian's Name	Relationship to Patient

Address			
PO OR MAILING ADDRESS	CITY	STATE	ZIP CODE

Phone		Sex M☐ F☐
Home	Work	

Have you (the parent/guardian) or the patient had any of the following diseases or problems? .... ☐ Yes ☐ No
1. Active Tuberculosis,   2. Persistent cough greater than a three-week duration,   3.Cough that produces blood?
If you answer yes to any of the three items above, please stop and return this form to the receptionist.

Has the child had any history of, or conditions related to, any of the following:

☐ Anemia	☐ Cancer	☐ Epilepsy	☐ HIV +/AIDS	☐ Mononucleosis	☐ Thyroid
☐ Arthritis	☐ Cerebral Palsy	☐ Fainting	☐ Immunizations	☐ Mumps	☐ Tobacco/Drug Use
☐ Asthma	☐ Chicken Pox	☐ Growth Problems	☐ Kidney	☐ Pregnancy (teens)	☐ Tuberculosis
☐ Bladder	☐ Chronic Sinusitis	☐ Hearing	☐ Latex allergy	☐ Rheumatic fever	☐ Venereal Disease
☐ Bleeding disorders	☐ Diabetes	☐ Heart	☐ Liver	☐ Seizures	☐ Other_____
☐ Bones/Joints	☐ Ear Aches	☐ Hepatitis	☐ Measles	☐ Sickle cell	

Please list the name and phone number of the child's physician:

Name of Physician _____ Phone _____

Child's History

                                                                                               Yes No

1. Is the child taking any prescription and/or over the counter medications or vitamin supplements at this time? .... 1. ☐ ☐
   If yes, please list: _____
2. Is the child allergic to any medications, i.e. penicillin, antibiotics, or other drugs? If yes, please explain: _____ 2. ☐ ☐
3. Is the child allergic to anything else, such as certain foods? If yes, please explain: _____ 3. ☐ ☐
4. How would you describe the child's eating habits? _____
5. Has the child ever had a serious illness? If yes, when: _____ Please describe: _____ 5. ☐ ☐
6. Has the child ever been hospitalized? .... 6. ☐ ☐
7. Does the child have a history of any other illnesses? If yes, please list: _____ 7. ☐ ☐
8. Has the child ever received a general anesthetic? .... 8. ☐ ☐
9. Does the child have any inherited problems? .... 9. ☐ ☐
10. Does the child have any speech difficulties? .... 10. ☐ ☐
11. Has the child ever had a blood transfusion? .... 11. ☐ ☐
12. Is the child physically, mentally, or emotionally impaired? .... 12. ☐ ☐
13. Does the child experience excessive bleeding when cut? .... 13. ☐ ☐
14. Is the child currently being treated for any illnesses? .... 14. ☐ ☐
15. In this the child's first visit to a dentist? If not the first visit, what was the date of the last dentist visit? Date........... 15. ☐ ☐
16. Has the child had any problem with dental treatment in the past? .... 16. ☐ ☐
17. Has the child ever had dental radiographs (x-rays) exposed? .... 17. ☐ ☐
18. Has the child ever suffered any injuries to the mouth, head or teeth? .... 18. ☐ ☐
19. Has the child had any problems with the eruption or shedding of teeth? .... 19. ☐ ☐
20. Has the child had any orthodontic treatment? .... 20. ☐ ☐
21. **What type of water does your child drink?** ☐ City water   ☐ Well water   ☐ Bottled water   ☐ Filtered water
22. **Does the child take fluoride supplements?** .... 22. ☐ ☐
23. **Is fluoride toothpaste used?** .... 23. ☐ ☐
24. How many times are the child's teeth brushed per day? _____ When are the teeth brushed? _____ 24. ☐ ☐
25. Does the child suck his/her thumb, fingers or pacifier? .... 25. ☐ ☐
26. At what age did the child stop bottle feeding? Age _____ Breast feeding? Age _____
27. Does child participate in active recreational activities? .... 27. ☐ ☐

NOTE: Both doctor and patient are encouraged to discuss any and all relevant patient health issues prior to treatment.
I certify that I have read and understand the above. I acknowledge that my questions, if any, about inquiries set forth above have been answered to my satisfaction. I will not hold my dentist, or any other member of his/her staff, responsible for any action they take or do not take because of errors or omissions that I may have made in the completion of this form.

Parent's/Guardian's Signature _____ Date _____

For completion by dentist
Comments _____
_____
_____
_____

For Office Use Only: ☐ Medical Alert ☐ Premedication ☐ Allergies ☐ Anesthesia   Reviewed by _____
Date _____

FIGURE 10-2 Child Health History Form. (Copyright © 2010 American Dental Association. All rights reserved. Reprinted with permission).

III. Pointers for the Interview

Interviewing involves communication between individuals. Communication implies the transmission or interchange of facts, attitudes, opinions, or thoughts, through words, gestures, or other means.

▶ Through tactful but direct questioning, communication can be successful, and the patient will provide the necessary information. Frequently, the patient is unaware of a health problem.

▶ The most effective attitude for the clinician to portray is one of friendly understanding, reassurance, and acceptance.

▶ Genuine interest and willingness to listen when a patient wishes to describe symptoms, complaints, or current health practices not only aids in establishing the rapport needed but also frequently provides insight into the patient's real attitudes and prejudices.

▶ By asking simple questions at first and more personal questions later after rapport has developed, the patient will be more relaxed and truthful in answering.

▶ Self-confidence and gentle efficiency on the part of the interviewer help give the patient a feeling of confidence.

▶ Skill is required because tact, ingenuity, judgment, and cultural sensitivity are taxed to the fullest in the attempt to obtain accurate and complete information from the patient.

▶ The culturally sensitive dental hygienist will be aware of nonverbal communication issues when interviewing a patient from a different culture (see Table 3-3 in Chapter 3).

IV. Interview Form

▶ The interviewer may use a structured form with places to check and fill in.

▶ Another method is to record on blank sheets from questions created from a guide list of essential topics.

▶ Either type of form can involve reference to the positive or negative answers on a previously completed questionnaire.

▶ Familiarity with the items on the history permits the interviewer to be direct and informal without reading from a fixed list of topics, a method that may lack the personal touch necessary to gain the patient's confidence.

▶ When appropriate, the patient's own words are recorded.

V. Advantages of the Interview

▶ Personal contact contributes to development of rapport for future appointments.

▶ Flexibility for individual needs; details obtained can be adapted for supplementary questioning.

VI. Disadvantages of the Interview

▶ Time consuming when not prefaced with questionnaire.

▶ Unless a list is consulted, items of importance may be omitted.

▶ Patient may be embarrassed to talk about personal conditions and may hold back significant information.

ITEMS INCLUDED IN THE HISTORY

Information obtained by means of the history is directly related to how the goals for patient care are established and will be accomplished. In Tables 10-1 through 10-3, items are listed with possible medications and other treatments the patient may have or has had, along with suggested considerations for appointment procedures.

▶ In specialized practices, objectives may require increased emphasis on certain aspects.

▶ The age group most frequently served will influence the focus of the history. *Example*: Parental history, prenatal, and postnatal information may take on particular significance for the treatment of a small child; in a pediatric dentistry practice, a special form could be devised to include all essential items.

▶ Insight and awareness shown while preparing the patient history depend on background knowledge of the manifestations of systemic diseases and the medications for various conditions.

▶ Objectives for the items to include in the various parts of the history are listed here.

I. Personal History (Table 10-1)

The basic objectives in gathering personal information about the patient are to:

▶ Collect data essential for appointment planning and business aspects.

▶ Identify need for approval for care of a minor patient and/or other legal requirements.

▶ Determine the need for consultation with the patient's primary care provider.

▶ Determine culturally appropriate communication measures.

II. Dental History (Table 10-2)

The dental history contributes to the care provider's knowledge of:

▶ The immediate problem, chief complaint, cause of present pain, or discomfort of any kind in the oral cavity.

TABLE 10-1	Items for the Personal History	
ITEMS TO RECORD IN PATIENT HISTORY	**RECORD NOTES**	**CONSIDERATIONS FOR APPOINTMENT PROCEDURES**
1. Name Addresses: residence and business Telephone numbers Gender Ethnic/racial category Marital status For child: name of parent or guardian For parent: age and sex of children	Accurate recording necessary for business aspects of dental practice	Aids in establishing rapport Instruction applicable to entire family Advice concerning fluorides for children Determine need for interpreter
2. Birth date	Whether of age or a minor Oral conditions related to age changes; diseases, healing, and other possible characteristics	Informed consent of parent or guardian necessary for care of minor or person with a mental handicap; signature is obtained Approach to patient instruction
3. Birthplace and residence in early years	Presence of fluoride in drinking water Food and eating patterns Conditions endemic to certain areas	Effects of fluoride on teeth Instruction in dietary needs adapted to cultural practices
4. Occupation: present and former Spouse's occupation For child: parent's occupation	May be a factor in etiology of certain diseases, dental stains, occlusal wear May affect diet, oral habits, general health	Instruction applied to specific needs Dexterity in use of self-care devices related to dexterity gained from occupation Influence on oral care of entire family For child: which parent will supervise and assist child in oral care
5. Physician	Name, address, and telephone number For consultation	Consultation indicated: • when disease symptoms are suspected but patient does not state • in an emergency • medication/premedication
6. Referred by and address	To whom to send referral acknowledgment and appreciation	Contribution to rapport with patient Patient referred by another patient may have concept of the office procedures

▶ Risk assessment forms, such as the American Association of Pediatric Dentistry Caries Risk Assessment Tool[3] and the American Dental Association Caries Risk Assessment forms[4,5] provide essential information for planning individualized dental hygiene interventions based on the patient's needs.

▶ The previous dental hygiene and dental care as described by the patient, including preventive care, periodontal treatments, and the extent of restorative and prosthetic replacement, as well as any adverse effects.

▶ The attitude of the patient toward oral health and care of the mouth as may be indicated by previous periodic dental and dental hygiene treatments and family history of oral care.

▶ The personal daily care exercised by the patient as evidence of knowledge of the purposes of continuing care and of the value placed on the teeth and their supporting structures.

▶ The patient's current beliefs and attitudes about health, illness, and oral health.

▶ Culturally related health practices that may impact the patient's oral health.

III. Medical History (Table 10-3)

Objectives of the medical history are to determine whether the patient has or has had any conditions in the following categories:

▶ *Conditions that may complicate certain kinds of dental and dental hygiene treatment*

Examples: Lowered resistance to infection; uncontrolled hypertension; or systemic disease that requires treatment before stressful dental procedures, particularly surgery, can be carried out.

▶ *Conditions or diseases that require special precautions or premedication before treatment*

TABLE 10-2	Items for the Dental History	
ITEMS TO RECORD IN THE HISTORY	**RECORD NOTES**	**CONSIDERATIONS FOR APPOINTMENT PROCEDURES**
1. Reason for present appointment	Chief complaint in patient's own words Pain or discomfort Onset, symptoms, duration of an acute condition	Need for immediate treatment Attitude toward dentistry and preventive care
2. Previous dental appointments	Date of last treatment Services performed Regularity	Patient knowledge concerning regular dental care Cooperation anticipated
3. Anesthetics used	Local, general Adverse reactions	Choice of anesthetic
4. Radiation history	Type, number, dates of dental and medical radiographs Therapeutic radiation Availability of dental radiographs from previous dentist Amount of exposure considered with exposure for medical purposes	Amount of exposure; limitations Patient's appreciation for need and use of radiographs
5. Family dental history	Parental tooth loss or maintenance	Attitude toward saving teeth and preventive dentistry Culturally related oral health beliefs and practices
6. Previous treatment	Type of treatment; frequency of maintenance appointments Whether referred to specialist	Attitude toward specialized care Previous familiarity with role of dental hygienist
a. Periodontal	History of acute infection (necrotizing ulcerative gingivitis) Surgery; posttreatment healing	Attitude toward self-care and disease control
b. Orthodontic	Age during treatment; completion date Previous problem Habit correction	For current treatment, consultation with orthodontist needed to determine instructions
c. Endodontic	Dates, etiology	Periodic recheck
d. Prosthodontic	Types of prostheses	Care of prostheses and abutment teeth
e. Other	Extent of restorations Tooth loss Implants	Understanding prevention
7. Injuries to face or teeth	Causes and extent Fractured teeth or jaws	Limitation of opening Special care during healing
8. Temporomandibular joint	History of injury, discomfort, disease, dislocation Previous treatment	Effect on opening; accessibility during instrumentation
9. Habits	Clenching, bruxism Mouth breathing Biting objects; fingernails, pipe stem, thread, other Cheek or lip biting Patient awareness of habits	Tension of patient Instruction relative to effects of habits

(continues)

TABLE 10-2	Items for the Dental History (*continued*)

ITEMS TO RECORD IN THE HISTORY	RECORD NOTES	CONSIDERATIONS FOR APPOINTMENT PROCEDURES
10. Tobacco use	Form of tobacco, amount used Frequency Knowledge of effects on oral tissues	Instruction concerning oral effects Tobacco cessation program Periodontal risk Dental stains; dentifrice selection
11. Fluorides	Systemic, topical, dates Residence during tooth development years Amount of fluoride in drinking water	Current preventive procedures and need for re-evaluation
12. Biofilm control procedures	Toothbrushing: current procedures type of brush (manual or powered) texture of filaments frequency of use age of brush; frequency of having a new brush Dentifrice name how selected; reason Additional cleansing devices and frequency of use dental floss water irrigation implants care Mouthrinse or other agents: frequency, purpose Source of instruction in care of oral cavity	Present practice and previous instruction New instruction needed; reception by patient Relation of techniques to prevention of dental caries and periodontal infections Supervision of child by parent: current practices Problems of habit change

TABLE 10-3	Items for the Medical History

ITEM TO RECORD IN HISTORY	RECORD NOTES	MEDICATIONS AND TREATMENT MODALITIES	CONSIDERATIONS FOR APPOINTMENT PROCEDURES
1. General health and appearance	Disabilities Overall impression of well-being Patient's appraisal of own health		Response, cooperation, and attitude to expect during appointments
2. Medical examination	Date of most recent examination Reason for the examination Tests performed; results Anticipated surgery	New prescriptions received Previous prescriptions continued	Verification with physician for added information Need for superior state of oral health in advance of surgery • When long recovery is expected and patient may miss maintenance appointments • Before transplant, heart surgery, or prosthesis
3. Major illnesses, hospitalizations, surgeries	Causes of illness Type and duration of treatment Anesthetics used Convalescence Course of healing: normal, not normal	Medications, treatments	Influence of illnesses on health and care of the oral cavity Anesthetic choice Expected outcome from gingival treatment
4. Age factors	Problems of health in different age groups Elderly: multiple disease entities; patient may need to bring the containers for identification of medications	See individual medical problem Update drug regimen at each appointment	Effects on dental and dental hygiene procedures and personal care

(continues)

| TABLE 10-3 | Items for the Medical History (*continued*) | | |

ITEM TO RECORD IN HISTORY	RECORD NOTES	MEDICATIONS AND TREATMENT MODALITIES	CONSIDERATIONS FOR APPOINTMENT PROCEDURES
5. Height and weight	Weight changes over past years or months Obesity Undernourishment Child growth pattern	Diet pills Substance abuse	Marked weight change may be a symptom of undiagnosed disease; suggest referral for medical examination Influence on dietary instructions for oral health
6. Medications prescribed by physician	Reasons: relation to dental care Frequency Patient's regularity of taking sugar content of liquid medicines, effect on dental caries (also true of over-the-counter [OTC] items) Previous history of bisphosphonate use	List all drugs by name Ask patient for drugs, medicine, injections, vitamins, patches, pills, capsules, to get a complete answer Dosage; route of administration	Consultation with physician concerning adjustments in dosage for dental or dental hygiene appointments Indications for premedication Side effects of drugs (e.g., increased risk of osteonecrosis with history of bisphosphonate use)
7. Self-medication	Type, frequency OTC preparations Substance abuse	Pain relievers Sleeping tablets Cough syrup Antacids Cathartics Vitamins Diet pills	Information not revealed by patient could complicate treatment Lack of interest in oral health, only pain relief Drug side effects
8. Family medical history	Predisposition to certain diseases (e.g., diabetes) History of diseases that occur in the family	Cultural beliefs about medications	May help patient seek medical examination when symptom suggests possible disease
9. Daily diet	Recommendations of patient's physicians, past and present Vitamin supplements Appetite Regularity of meals Food likes and dislikes	Vitamin supplements	Instructions to be given relative to oral health Prognosis for healing after treatment Need for dietary assessment and analysis
10. Alcohol consumption	Frequency Amount Substance abuse	Recovering alcoholic: May be taking disulfiram, avoid all alcohol-containing preparations including commercial mouthrinses	Excessive use: effect on anesthesia; increased healing time Poor nutritional state is common; lack of oral care Avoid alcohol-containing mouthrinse May result in poor patient cooperation
11. Allergies	Determine substances to which the patient is allergic • Latex • Anesthetics • Penicillin • Medicaments • Foods • Iodine	Antihistamines Inhalers Decongestants Steroids	Preparation for emergency Xerostomia Avoid use of substances to which the patient is allergic

(continues)

TABLE 10-3	Items for the Medical History (*continued*)		
ITEM TO RECORD IN HISTORY	**RECORD NOTES**	**MEDICATIONS AND TREATMENT MODALITIES**	**CONSIDERATIONS FOR APPOINTMENT PROCEDURES**
12. Arthritis	Joint pain Immobility Temporomandibular joint involvement	Aspirin Nonsteroidal anti-inflammatory drugs Corticosteroids Total joint replacements	Antibiotic premedication: consult physician if treated with chemotherapeutic agent Dental chair adjustment
13. Blood disorder	Type and duration of disease Leukemia: remission, thrombocytopenia	Vitamins Minerals: iron (iron-deficiency anemia) Folic acid supplement (macrocytic anemia) Antineoplastic drugs	Consultation with physician Need for high level of oral health Antibiotic premedication Immunosuppression Increased bleeding Oral lesions
14. Bleeding	Bleeding associated with previous dental appointments History of disorder with coagulation problem History of transfusions or other blood products Check use of aspirin and herbal supplements (relation to bleeding tendency) Laboratory tests for bleeding time, coagulation may be needed	Anticoagulant medication Hemophilia factor replacement	Emergency prevention through preappointment precautions May need to apply direct pressure or hemostatic agent after scaling Special measures for hemophilia
15. Cancer	Head and neck radiation effects on oral cavity, salivary glands Dental and dental hygiene therapy updated before start of surgery, radiation therapy, or immunosuppression Blood count before dental and dental hygiene therapy Previous history of bisphosphonate prescription	Radiation therapy Fluoride therapy: daily topical application Antineoplastic drugs, alkylating agents, antimetabolites, antibiotics, plant alkaloids, steroids	Bleeding; infection; poor healing response Avoid trauma to tissues Effect on oral radiographic survey: prevention of overexposure Dental caries: preventive measures Xerostomia: substitute saliva Increased risk of osteonecrosis with history of bisphosphonate use.
16. Cardiovascular diseases	Consultation with physician Refer for examination when patient seems unsure of problem	Cardiac glycosides Antiarrhythmics Antianginals Antihypertensives Anticoagulants	Minimize stress Premedication for stress Ensure medications have been taken Monitor vital signs
a. Congenital heart disease	Risk factors for Infective Endocarditis (IE) Type of problem		Antibiotic premedication may be required
b. Previous history of IE	Susceptibility to recurrence of IE Type of problem; date		Antibiotic premedication may be required

(continues)

TABLE 10-3	Items for the Medical History (*continued*)		
ITEM TO RECORD IN HISTORY	**RECORD NOTES**	**MEDICATIONS AND TREATMENT MODALITIES**	**CONSIDERATIONS FOR APPOINTMENT PROCEDURES**
c. Hypertension	Symptom of other disease state Monitor blood pressure for each appointment Anesthesia: consult with primary care provider about epinephrine use	Diuretics Antiadrenergic agents Vasodilators Angiotensin-converting enzyme inhibitors Calcium channel-blocking agent	Postural hypotension (raise dental chair slowly) Xerostomia: saliva substitute and fluoride rinse may be needed Gingival enlargement (drug side effect)
d. Angina pectoris	Prepare for symptoms; have ready amyl nitrite inhalant or nitroglycerin tablets or spray	Amyl nitrite, nitroglycerin, or other antianginal drugs	Allay fears and prevent stress Morning appointment
e. Heart diseases	History of disease symptoms of fatigue, shortness of breath, or cough Consult with physician	Glycosides (digitalis) Anticoagulants Antiarrhythmic drugs Pacemaker	Monitor vital signs Short, more frequent appointments Change dental chair slowly Patient with breathing problem (sleeps with two or more pillows) may need semi-upright position Bleeding tendency associated with anticoagulant Check use of ultrasonic (unshielded pacemaker)
f. Surgically corrected cardiovascular lesions	Type, date of surgery Consultation with physician Before surgical procedure, when possible: the patient needs complete oral evaluation and corrective dental work done, with motivation to high level of oral personal care daily	No tobacco use Anticoagulants Cyclosporine Nifedipine	Consult with primary care provider about antibiotic premedication Gingival bleeding can be expected Gingival enlargement
g. Cerebrovascular accident (stroke)	Date of onset; residual disabilities Speech, vision, mental function	No tobacco; low-salt diet Anticoagulants Antihypertensives Vasodilator Steroid Anticonvulsant	Gingival bleeding likely when anticoagulants are used Adapt procedures for physical disability
17. Communicable diseases	History of diseases; immunizations Present disease; communicability Residence or extended trips in countries with high endemic incidence of certain diseases Risk group factor	Immunizations Drug therapy for current infection	Appointment postponement
a. Hepatitis B	Jaundice history Clarification of type of hepatitis Laboratory clearance	Vaccine of hepatitis B virus	Precautions against percutaneous injury

(continues)

TABLE 10-3	Items for the Medical History (*continued*)		
ITEM TO RECORD IN HISTORY	**RECORD NOTES**	**MEDICATIONS AND TREATMENT MODALITIES**	**CONSIDERATIONS FOR APPOINTMENT PROCEDURES**
b. Tuberculosis	Active or passive Cough Duration of disease	Isoniazid Rifampin Pyrazinamide	Length of treatment; infectivity diminished after few months of treatment
c. Sexually transmitted infections (STIs)	May not obtain history of STIs Oral and pharyngeal lesions may be indicators of disease	Antibiotics	Infectiousness diminishes with antibiotic therapy for gonorrhea and syphilis Refer to physician and postpone treatment when lesions or other signs suggest infection Caution for risk from previously treated diseases
d. Herpes	Lesions can be transmitted readily	Nondefinitive; symptomatic and palliative treatment Acyclovir	Postpone routine care when oral lesions are present
e. HIV infection AIDS	Risk group identification Oral manifestations	Wide variety of opportunistic infections and complications require variety of drugs	Oral lesions Complete sterilization and barrier procedures as for all patients
18. Diabetes mellitus	Undiagnosed: excess thirst, appetite, and urination Family incidence: help in finding prediabetes or undiagnosed Severe advanced diabetes: complications (vision, kidney, cardiovascular, nervous system)	Insulin Diet control Hypoglycemics	Prepare for emergency; insulin; glucose gel Appointment time related to insulin therapy and mealtime Need frequent maintenance appointments Periodontal disease accelerated Referral for testing to identify undiagnosed diabetes
19. Ears	Deafness or degree of hearing impairment Infections, ringing, dizziness, balance	Treatment for infection Hearing aid	Adaptations for communication and biofilm control instruction
20. Endocrine	Age-group relations to certain conditions Growth, development Menstruation, menopause	Thyroid hormone supplement Antithyroid Estrogen/progestin Oral contraceptives Corticosteroids	Emphasis on high level of biofilm control Any patient taking steroids may need antibiotic premedication for appointments Monitor blood pressure
21. Epilepsy	Type, frequency of seizures precipitating factors Preparation for emergency seizure	Anticonvulsant Sedative	Minimize stress Medications make patient drowsy, less alert
22. Eyes	Disturbance of vision Purpose for corrective eyeglasses or contact lenses Manifestations of systemic disease	Eyedrops (e.g., glaucoma)	Protective eyewear during appointment Adaptations for communication with limited sight

(*continues*)

TABLE 10-3	Items for the Medical History (*continued*)		
ITEM TO RECORD IN HISTORY	**RECORD NOTES**	**MEDICATIONS AND TREATMENT MODALITIES**	**CONSIDERATIONS FOR APPOINTMENT PROCEDURES**
23. Gastrointestinal	Nature and treatment of the disease Diet restriction prescribed by physician	Antacids Antidiarrheals Laxatives Antispasmodics	Patient instruction in accord with prescribed diet and medication Xerostomia
24. Kidney	Renal disease; kidney stones Hemodialysis: hypertension, anemia, hepatitis carrier Transplant: hypertension, hepatitis	Salt restriction Many drugs are nephrotoxic Immunosuppressive drugs (cyclosporine)	Monitor blood pressure Bleeding tendency Poor healing Susceptibility to infection Limited stress tolerance
25. Liver	History of jaundice, hepatitis Impaired drug metabolism Cirrhosis: history of alcoholism	Nutritional emphasis Abstinence from alcohol	Laboratory test for hepatitis Bleeding problems
26. Mental, psychiatric	Emotional problems hinder oral care	Antipsychotic drugs Antianxiety drugs Tranquilizers Antidepressants Antiparkinsonism drugs	Limited stress tolerance Xerostomia (side effect) Avoid mouthrinse containing alcohol
27. Physical activity	Overall health consciousness	Good health habits Regular exercise	Contribute to cooperative attitude in maintaining oral health
28. Physical disabilities	Extent, cause, duration Type of treatment related to individual condition Consultation with physician or medical specialist	Pain reliever Muscle relaxant Anticonvulsant	Adjustment of physical arrangements Wheelchair accessibility and transfer Adaptations of techniques and instruction
29. Pregnancy	Month, parturition date Possible oral manifestations History of previous pregnancies Iron-deficiency anemia	Iron Folic acid Multivitamins	Adjust physical position for comfort Frequent appointments for maintaining high level of oral hygiene
30. Respiration	Breathing problems Persistent cough Cough up blood Chest pain Precipitation of asthmatic attack	Codeine cough syrup Antihistamine Bronchial dilator Expectorant Decongestant Steroid	Dental chair position Ultrasonic and air-powder polisher contraindicated Nitrous oxide contraindicated No aerosol agents

Examples: Increased osteonecrosis risk related to previous treatment with bisphosphonates; or antibiotic coverage for the patient at risk for infective endocarditis (IE).

▶ *Conditions under treatment by a physician that require medicating drugs that may influence or contraindicate certain procedures*

Examples: Anticoagulant therapy requires consultation with physician; antihypertensive drugs may alter the amount and/or choice of local anesthetic used.

▶ *Gender or ethnic/racial influences that increase risk for systemic and oral disease*

Example: American Indians and African Americans have increased risk for diabetes and a related increased risk for periodontal disease.

▶ *Allergic or untoward reactions*

Examples: Latex hypersensitivity; medication or material for which there was a previous adverse reaction.

▶ *Diseases and drugs with manifestations in the mouth*

Examples: Hematologic disorders; phenytoin-induced gingival overgrowth; infectious diseases such as herpesvirus.

▶ *Communicable diseases that endanger the dental personnel*

Examples: Active tuberculosis; viral hepatitis; herpes.

▶ *Physiologic state of the patient*

Examples: Pregnancy; puberty; menopause; birth control pills.

IMMEDIATE APPLICATIONS OF PATIENT HISTORIES

▶ Information from the histories influences all aspects of total patient care and dental hygiene care planning.

▶ Immediate evaluation of the histories is necessary before proceeding to complete the assessment.

▶ Together with information from all other parts of the diagnostic work-up, the patient histories are essential for the preparation of the dental hygiene care plan.

I. Medical Consultation

Dentist and primary care provider need to consult relative to the patient's current therapy and medications or to elements of the patient's past health status that could influence present dental treatment needs.[6]

▶ *Telephone or personal contact*
  • Immediate consultation may be needed so that urgent treatment may proceed.
  • Follow-up in writing either by electronic communication, fax, or mailed hard copy is essential because without legal record of the advice or decision, a misunderstanding could result.

▶ *Written request*
  • A letter of formal request is the preferred procedure for medical consultation. This may be e-mailed or faxed to the physician.
  • A prepared form can be developed with spaces for filling in the specific questions and with space in the lower half for the primary care provider to complete confidential information from the patient's medical record or to provide the necessary recommendations.

▶ *Referrals*
  • The patient is referred for medical examination when signs of a possible disease condition are apparent.
  • The patient is referred for laboratory tests when recent test results are not available or follow-up tests are needed.

II. Radiation

▶ When a patient is receiving radiation therapy or has had recent radiation for other purposes, a conference with the primary care provider or oncologist is recommended to discuss the quantity of radiation to be received from any necessary dental radiographs.

▶ It is the dental practitioners responsibility to utilize all available clinical, assessment, and health history information when contemplating the necessity of diagnostic radiographs in order to optimize care while minimizing radiation exposure.[7]

III. Prophylactic Premedication

▶ Selected patients at risk for IE receive antibiotic premedication before any oral tissue manipulation that could create a bacteremia.

▶ The patient history and the information in Box 10-2 are reviewed to identify a patient needing premedication in accordance with the recommendations of the American Heart Association (AHA) Guidelines.

▶ Routine use of antibiotic premedication is never indicated. Overuse of antibiotics can induce microbial resistance and, rarely, allergy or toxicity to the drug used.[8]

▶ The subgingival use of instruments (for example, periodontal probe or curet) is avoided until the level of risk has been assessed, the condition has been discussed with the patient's primary care provider, and the prescription has been obtained, and taken as directed.

▶ The oral antibiotic prescription is required one hour before instrumentation begins to assure the adequate blood concentration during and immediately following instrumentation.

▶ At-risk patients already taking an antibiotic for other health conditions may require additional antibiotic prophylaxis before dental and dental hygiene instrumentation. A different class of antibiotic is prescribed rather than to increase the dose of the current drug being taken.[8]

PRETREATMENT ANTIBIOTIC PROPHYLAXIS

I. AHA GUIDELINES

A. Brief Historical Review[9]

▶ The American Heart Association (AHA) has made recommendations for the prevention of IE for many years. The first document was published in 1955. There have been nine revisions since then including the latest one published in *Circulation* 2007 reviewed and updated on the AHA Website in 2014.[10,11]

B. Rationale for 2007 Revision and 2014 Review[10,11]

▶ Former guidelines were based more on expert opinion or individual case studies; the 2007 guidelines and 2014 review attempted to be more evidence based.

▶ Frequent exposure to random bacteremias resulting from daily activities are more likely to cause IE than treatment procedures performed at dental and dental hygiene appointments.

▶ Antibiotic prophylaxis may prevent a very small number of cases of IE, if any, in patients receiving a dental or dental hygiene treatment procedure.

▶ There are risks of antibiotic-associated adverse events that may exceed the benefit, if any, of antibiotic therapy.

▶ Maintenance of optimal oral health with daily biofilm removal may reduce the incidence of IE due to bacteremias caused by daily activities. Such prevention can be more significant than prophylactic antibiotics given occasionally for a dental or dental hygiene invasive treatment procedure.

▶ Literature reviews found no evidence-based method to decide exactly which procedures require prophylactic antibiotic premedication and which do not need it.

▶ Other factors that limit conducting controlled research are:

• Low incidence of IE.
• Wide variety of types of cardiac diseases.
• Wide variety of invasive dental procedures.
• Incidents when antibiotic premedication did not prevent IE following a dental invasive procedure.

II. Recommendations Based on Principles[10,11]

▶ Only an extremely small number of cases of IE might be prevented by antibiotic prophylaxis for dental procedures even if such prophylactic therapy were 100% effective.

▶ IE prophylaxis for dental procedures is recommended only for patients with underlying cardiac conditions associated with the highest risk of adverse outcomes from IE.

▶ For patients with these underlying cardiac conditions, prophylaxis is recommended for all dental procedures that involve manipulation of gingival tissue, the periapical region of teeth, or perforation of the oral mucosa.

▶ Prophylaxis is not recommended based solely on an increased lifetime risk of acquisition of IE.

III. Medical Conditions that Require Antibiotic Premedication Before Invasive Dental and Dental Hygiene Procedures

▶ Box 10-2 lists the cardiac conditions for which antibiotic prophylaxis is recommended.

▶ Box 10-3 lists the following:

• Dental and dental hygiene procedures for which endocarditis prophylaxis is recommended.
• Procedures for which prophylaxis is *not* needed.

▶ A codeveloped evidence-based guideline for the prevention of orthopedic implant infection in patients undergoing dental procedures was released in 2012 by the ADA and the American Academy of Orthopaedic Surgeons (AAOS) in response to a previous position paper published by the AAOS in 2010, which recommended antibiotic prophylaxis for all orthopedic implant patients undergoing any invasive procedure that may cause bacteremia.

▶ A 2014 systematic review found no direct evidence that dental procedures cause prosthetic joint implant infections.
  • Based on the 2014 systematic review, prophylactic antibiotics given prior to dental procedures are not recommended for patients with prosthetic joint implants.[12,13]
  • Consultation with the patient's primary care provider regarding the need for antibiotic prophylaxis for patients with prosthetic joints is recommended.

IV. Recommended Antibiotic Protocol

▶ Table 10-4 provides the recommended antibiotic prescriptions for prevention of cardiac endocarditis.

ASA DETERMINATION

With the completion of the patient histories, an overall estimate of medical risk of a patient can be made. American Society of Anesthesiologists (ASA) Physical Status Classification System[14,15] (Table 24-1, Chapter 24) describes six categories of physical status and provides examples of adaptations necessary for providing dental hygiene care for a patient in each category.

▶ **ASA I**: A patient without apparent systemic disease: a normal healthy patient.
▶ **ASA II**: A patient with mild systemic disease.
▶ **ASA III**: A patient with severe systemic disease that limits activity but is not incapacitating.

TABLE 10-4	Prophylactic Regimens for Dental, Oral, Respiratory Tract, or Esophageal Procedures		
		REGIMEN—SINGLE DOSE 30–60 MIN BEFORE PROCEDURE	
SITUATION	AGENT	ADULT	CHILD[a]
Standard general prophylaxis	Amoxicillin	2.0 g orally	50 mg/kg orally
Unable to take oral medications	Ampicillin or Cefazolin or celtriaxone	2.0 g IM or IV 1.0 g IM or IV	50 mg/kg IM or IV 50 mg/kg IM or IV
Allergic to penicillins or ampicillin—oral	Cephalexin[b] or Clindamycin or Azithromycin or Clarithromycin	2.0 g orally 600 mg orally 500 mg orally	50 mg/kg orally 20 mg/kg orally 15 mg/kg orally
Allergic to penicillins and unable to take oral medications	Cefazolin or ceftriaxone[b] or Clindamycin	1.0 g IM or IV 600 mg IM or IV	50 mg/kg IM or IV 25 mg/kg IM or IV

IM = intramuscularly; IV = intravenously.
[a]Total child dose never exceeds adult dose.
[b]Cephalosporins are not prescribed for individuals with immediate-type hypersensitivity reaction (urticaria, angioedema, or anaphylaxis) to penicillins or ampicillin.
Source: American Heart Association. *Endocarditis Prophylaxis Information.* Dallas, TX: American Heart Association. http://www.americanheart.org/presenter.jhtml?identifier=11086. Accessed January 20, 2011.

- ► **ASA IV**: A patient with an incapacitating systemic disease that is a constant threat to life.
- ► **ASA V**: A moribund patient not expected to survive 24 hours with or without care.

REVIEW AND UPDATE OF HISTORY

- ► Updating the patient's health history at each appointment is essential.
- ► Changes in health status revealed by interim medical examinations or evidenced by reported illness or hospitalizations are recorded and considered during continuing treatment.
- ► Post a wall plaque that states *"Please Advise Us of Any Change in Your Medical History Since Your Last Visit"* in an appropriate place in a dental office or clinic to remind patients about the importance of updating information at each appointment.
- ► Following a review of the previously recorded history, questions can be directed to the patient to compare the present condition with the previous one and to determine at least the following:
  - Interim illnesses; changes in health
  - Visits to physician; reasons and results
  - Laboratory tests performed and the results; blood, urine, or other analyses
  - Current medications
  - Changes in the oral soft tissues and the teeth observed by the patient.

DOCUMENTATION

- ► Date all records.
- ► All hard copy permanent records are written in ink.
- ► Electronic patient records are stored on a secure server on password-protected computers, with only office staff having access to the computers and passwords. All electronic charting documentation are signed electronically and saved in such a way that falsifications to patient records cannot be made.
- ► Provide a specific line on a health history form for the signature of the patient.[1,2] The completed history for a minor is signed by a parent or guardian. A signature is also needed on the informed consent form.
- ► Maintain all information obtained for a patient history in strictest privacy.
- ► For patients with special health problems that require premedication, use some type of coded tab on paper charts or pop up alert in electronic records to notify all

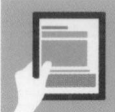

BOX 10-4

Example Documentation: Updating a Patient's Medical History

S–Forty-five-year-old patient presents for routine 6-month maintenance appointment. She is new to the office and reports she has always taken penicillin prior to her "cleaning" appointments. She completed and signed a new health history form. Her medical history indicates she has a heart murmur and she reports this is why she has been told to take penicillin before appointments. She became quite concerned about not premedicating with antibiotics.

O–The recommendations for antibiotic prophylaxis were reviewed with the patient and a consult with the primary care provider determined she was not a candidate for premedication. A full series of radiographs was taken and the clinical examination was completed. No dental caries noted. Pocket depths in the maxillary molar area ranges from 5 to 6 mm with bleeding on probing. No suppuration present. No mobility. Furcation involvement Grade II on ML and DL of #2, 3, 14, and 15. Plaque score 15%, primarily in maxillary molar areas.

A–Caries risk: low; periodontal risk: high; oral cancer risk: low. On the basis of the comprehensive periodontal examination and radiographic findings, she has localized moderate chronic periodontitis.

P–Oral self-care review of interdental brush for maxillary molar areas. Full mouth debridement with localized scaling and periodontal debridement on #2, 3, 14, and 15. One carpule: 2% lidocaine with 1:100,000 epinephrine for a posterior superior alveolar upper right and upper left. Selective polishing. 5% sodium fluoride varnish was applied. A 3-month periodontal maintenance interval was recommended.

Signed _____, RDH

Date _____

dental personnel to check the medical history before each appointment.

- ► Analyze the usefulness of items on the patient history form periodically, and plan for revision as scientific evidence reveals new information.
- ► Progress notes document regular update of forms completed and changes in personal, dental, or health history since last appointment.
- ► Box 10-4 provides an example of a progress note related to completion of personal, dental, and medical histories.

EVERYDAY ETHICS

Chris, the dental hygienist, was waiting for her new patient at 1:00 PM. All she knew was that Irina was 70 years old, from Russia, and could speak and understand English fairly well. Chris heard the front door to the office open and went out to greet her patient. The little lady was on the arm of a teenage boy who quickly helped Irina to a chair and turned to leave after saying to Chris (pointing to the patient) "Just back from hospital. They fixed her heart and told her to get her teeth cleaned to keep her healthy. Car not parked." Then to his grandmother "Back in an hour," before he rushed out.

Chris ushered Irina into the treatment room and helped her into the chair, then started the history questions with "What were you in the hospital for?" Irina grabs Chris' arm and firmly requests, "Want teeth cleaned." Chris attempts to explain why she is asking the questions about her health. Then she asks for her physician's name, and permission to call the physician to obtain the information. Irina points to her heart, but just becomes more agitated and keeps

repeating "Want teeth cleaned" and refuses to give approval to call her doctor. Chris is alarmed at the thought of providing care for this patient without complete information about her health history, but hates to waste the scheduled appointment time, given her well-filled schedule and the number of patients clamoring for appointments.

Questions for Consideration

1. Professionally and ethically, what are a dental hygienist's responsibilities to take time to help a patient understand the seriousness of an illness and the need for a complete personal, dental, and medical history before receiving dental treatment?

2. Provide an example of how each of the ethical theories (Table IV-1, Section IV Introduction) might apply as Chris determines how to resolve this issue?

3. Which of the dental hygiene core values apply as Chris determines what action to take?

Factors To Teach The Patient

▷ The need for obtaining the personal, medical, and dental history before performance of dental and dental hygiene procedures, and the need for keeping the histories up to date.

▷ The assurance that recorded histories are kept in strict professional confidence.

▷ The relationship between oral health and general physical health.

▷ The interrelationship of medical and dental care.

▷ All patients who require antibiotic premedication need special attention paid to (1) the importance of preventive dentistry, (2) the imperative need for regular dental care, and (3) the necessity for taking the prescribed prescription 1 hour before the appointment starts.

References

1. Collier A. The management of risk. Part 3: Recording your way out of trouble. *Dent Update.* 2014;41(4):338–340.

2. American Dental Association. *Medical History Form (5500).* Chicago: ADA Department of Salable Materials; 2007: 2pages.http://ebusiness.ada.org/productcatalog/product.aspx?ID=1158. Accessed April 11, 2015.

3. American Academy of Pediatric Dentistry, Council on Clinical Affairs. Policy on use of a caries-risk assessment tool (CAT) for infants, children, and adolescents. *Pediatr Dent.* 2008–2009;30(7, Suppl):29–33.

4. American Dental Association. *Caries Risk Assessment Form (age >6).* Chicago, IL: American Dental Association. http://www.ada.org/en/member-center/oral-health-topics/caries. Accessed April 11, 2015.

5. American Dental Association. *Caries Risk Assessment Form (age 0–6).* Chicago, IL: American Dental Association. http://www.ada.org/en/member-center/oral-health-topics/caries. Accessed April 11, 2015.

6. Chiodo GT, Rosenstein DI. Consultation between dentists and physicians. *Gen Dent.* 1984;32(1):19–22.

7. U.S. Department of Health and Human Services, U.S. Food and Drug Administration. Dental radiographic examinations: Recommendations for patient selection and limiting radiation exposure. http://www.fda.gov/radiation-emittingproducts/radiationemittingproductsandprocedures/medicalimaging/medicalx-rays/ucm116504.htm. Accessed April 11, 2015.

8. American Academy of Pediatric Dentistry. Guideline on antibiotic prophylaxis for dental patients at risk for infection (Originating Committee Clinical Affairs, Committee Review Council, Council on Clinical Affairs Adopted 1990 Revised 1991, 1997, 1999, 2002, 2005, 2007, 2008, 2011). http://www.aapd.org/media/Policies_Guidelines/G_AntibioticProphylaxis.pdf. Accessed July 13, 2014.

9. Pallasch TJ, Slots J. Antibiotic prophylaxis and the medically compromised patient. *Periodontology.* 2000;10:107–138.

10. Wilson W, Taubert KA, Gewitz M, et al. Prevention of infective endocarditis: guidelines from the American Heart Association: a guideline from the American Heart Association Rheumatic Fever, Endocarditis, and Kawasaki Disease Committee, Council on Cardiovascular Disease in the Young, and the Council on Clinical Cardiology, Council on Cardiovascular Surgery and Anesthesia, and the Quality Care and Outcomes Research Interdisciplinary Working Group. *Circulation.* 2007;116(15):1736–1754.

11. American Heart Association. Infective endocarditis. http://www.heart.org/HEARTORG/Conditions/CongenitalHeartDefects/TheImpactofCongenitalHeartDefects/Infective-Endocarditis_UCM_307108_Article.jsp. Accessed July 13, 2014.

12. American Academy of Orthopaedic Surgeons (AAOS) and American Dental Association (ADA) Clinical Practice Guideline Unit. Prevention of orthopaedic implant infection in patients undergoing dental procedures evidence-based guideline and evidence report. http://www.ada.org/sections/professionalResources/pdfs/PUDP_guideline.pdf. Accessed January 26, 2014.

13. Sollecito T, Abt E, Lockhart P, et al. The use of prophylactic antibiotics prior to dental procedures in patients with prosthetic joints: Evidence-based clinical practice guideline for dental practitioners — a report of the American Dental Association Council on Scientific Affairs. *JADA.* 2015;146(1):11–16.

14. American Society of Anesthesiologists. New classification of physical status. *Anesthesiology.* 1963;24(1):111.

ENHANCE YOUR UNDERSTANDING

thePoint® DIGITAL CONNECTIONS
(see the inside front cover for access information)
· **Audio glossary**
· **Quiz bank**

SUPPORT FOR LEARNING
(available separately; visit lww.com)
· *Active Learning Workbook for Clinical Practice of the Dental Hygienist, 12th Edition*

prepU INDIVIDUALIZED REVIEW
(available separately; visit lww.com)
· **Adaptive quizzing with *prepU for Wilkins' Clinical Practice of the Dental Hygienist***

11

Vital Signs

Lisa B. Johnson, RDH, MSDH, MPH and Esther M. Wilkins, RDH, DMD

CHAPTER OUTLINE

LEARNING OBJECTIVES

After studying this chapter, the student will be able to:

1. List and explain the vital signs and why proper assessment is key to identifying the patient's health status.

2. Demonstrate and explain the correct procedures for assessing the vital signs: temperature, respiration, radial pulse, and blood pressure.

3. Recognize and explain factors that may affect temperature, respiration, pulse, and blood pressure.

4. Describe and evaluate equipment used for assessing temperature and blood pressure.

5. Recognize normal vital signs across varied age groups.

INTRODUCTION

Determination of four vital signs—*body temperature, pulse, respiratory rates,* and *blood pressure*—is considered standard procedure in patient care. Table 11-1 summarizes the normal values of the four basic vital signs for infant through older adults.

I. Patient Preparation and Instruction

▶ Seat patient in upright position, at eye level for instruction.

▶ Explain the vital signs and obtain consent.

▶ Explain how vital signs can affect dental hygiene and dental treatment.

▶ During the process, explain each step as needed by the individual patient.

II. Dental Hygiene Care Planning

▶ Recording vital signs contributes to the proper systemic evaluation of a patient in conjunction with the complete medical history.

▶ Dental hygiene care planning and appointment sequencing are directly influenced by the findings.

▶ When vital signs are not within normal, advise the patient check with the physician.

▶ Referral for medical evaluation and treatment is indicated.

▶ Key words related to the vital signs are defined in Box 11-1.

BODY TEMPERATURE

While preparing the patient history and making the extraoral and intraoral examinations, the need for taking the temperature may become apparent, or the dentist may have requested the procedure in conjunction with current oral disease.

I. Indications for Taking the Temperature

▶ For the new patient's initial permanent record along with all vital signs.

▶ For complete examination during a continuing care appointment.

▶ When oral infection is known to be present.
  • Necrotizing ulcerative gingivitis or periodontitis.
  • Apical or periodontal abscess.
  • Acute pericoronitis.

▶ With other vital signs, prior to administration of local anesthetic.

▶ At any appointment when the patient reports illness or there is a suspected infection.
  • Protection of the health of the healthcare personnel and patients or families who may be exposed secondarily.
  • Special significance during epidemics when community exposures are at risk.
  • For patient's referral for medical care when indicated.

II. Maintenance of Body Temperature

▶ *Normal*
  • *Adults:* The normal average temperature is 98.6°F (37°C). The normal range is from 96 to 99.5°F (35.5 to 37.5°C).
  • *Older adults:* Over 70 years of age, the average temperature is slightly lower (96.8°F, 36.0°C).
  • *Children:* There is no appreciable difference between boys and girls. Average temperatures are as follows:
    • First year—99.1°F (37.3°C).
    • Fourth year—99.4°F (37.5°C).

TABLE 11-1	Resting Vital Sign Ranges Infant through Older Adult				
AGE (RANGE)	TEMPERATURE (°F)	PULSE (BPM)	RESPIRATION (RPM)	BLOOD PRESSURE (MM HG)	
				Systolic	Diastolic
1–12 mo	99.4–99.7	80–160	30–60	74–100	50–70
1–2 yr	99–99.7	80–130	24–40	80–112	50–80
4–5 yr	98.6–99	80–120	22–34	82–110	50–78
6–11 yr	98–98.6	75–110	18–30	84–120	54–80
Adolescent	97–99	60–90	12–20	94–120	62–80
Adult	97–99	60–100	12–20	90–120	60–80
Older adult (>60)	97–99	60–100	12–20	90–120	60–80

Children and adolescent blood pressure recommended by the USDHHS 4th Report on Diagnosis, Evaluation, and Treatment of Blood Pressure in Children and Adolescents.

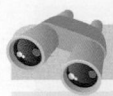

BOX 11-1   KEY WORDS: Vital Signs

Anoxia: oxygen deficiency; a reduction of oxygen in the tissues can lead to deep respirations, cyanosis, increased pulse rate, and impairment of coordination.

Apnea: temporary cessation of breathing; absence of spontaneous respirations.

Auscultation: listening for sounds produced within the body; may be performed directly or with a stethoscope.

Bradycardia: unusually slow heartbeat evidenced by slowing of the pulse rate.

Core temperature: the temperature of the deep tissues of the body; remains relatively constant; contrasts with body surface temperature, which rises and falls in response to environment.

Diastole: the phase of the cardiac cycle in which the heart relaxes between contractions and the two ventricles are dilated by the blood flowing into them; diastolic pressure is the lowest blood pressure.

Diurnal: pertaining to or occurring during the daytime or period of light.

Hypertension: systolic blood pressure of 140 mm Hg or greater and diastolic blood pressure of 90 mm Hg or greater.

Hypotension: systolic blood pressure of 90 mm Hg or lower and diastolic blood pressure of 60 mm Hg or lower.

Hyperthermia: higher-than-normal body temperature.

Hypothermia: lower-than-normal body temperature.

Korotkoff sounds: the sounds heard during the determination of blood pressure; sounds originating within the blood passing through the vessel or produced by vibratory motion of the arterial wall.

Normotensive: normal tension or tone; of or pertaining to having normal blood pressure.

Postural hypotension: a decrease in standing systolic blood pressure >10 mm Hg; associated with dizziness or fainting; more frequently seen in older patients with systolic hypertension and those taking certain prescription medications.

Pulse pressure: the difference between systolic and diastolic blood pressure; normally 40 mm Hg.

Pyrexia: an abnormal elevation of the body temperature above 37.0°C (98.6°F).

Stethoscope: instrument used to hear and amplify the sounds produced by the heart, lungs, and other internal organs.

Systole: the contraction, or period of contraction, of the heart, especially the ventricles, during which blood is forced into the aorta and the pulmonary artery; systolic pressure is the highest, or greatest, pressure.

Tachycardia: unusually fast heartbeat; at a rate greater than 100 BPM.

White-coat hypertension: elevated blood pressure as a result of feeling anxious in a medical environment.

- Fifth year—98.6°F (37°C).
- Twelfth year—98.0°F (36.7°C).

▶ *Temperature variations*
- *Fever (pyrexia):* Values over 99.5°F (37.5°C).
- *Hyperthermia:* Values over 105.8°F (41.0°C).
- *Hypothermia:* Values below 96.0°F (35.5°C).

▶ *Factors that alter body temperature*
- *Time of day:* Highest in late afternoon and early evening; lowest during sleep and early morning.
- *Temporary increase:* Exercise, hot drinks, smoking, or application of external heat.
- *Pathologic states:* Infection, dehydration, hyperthyroidism, myocardial infarction, or tissue injury from trauma.
- *Decrease:* Starvation, hemorrhage, or physiologic shock.

III. Methods of Determining Temperature[1–3]

A. Locations for Measurement

▶ *Oral:* most common site due to ease of access.
- Drinking hot or cold liquids just prior can affect results; wait at least 15 minutes before oral measurement is taken.
- Not recommended for infants, young children, unconscious, or highly behavioral patients.

▶ *Temporal artery (forehead):* measurements taken with electronic device; easily tolerated and results comparable to oral thermometers.

▶ *Ear:* with a tympanic device.

▶ *Medical/hospital applications:* also use axilla or rectum for assessment.

B. Types of Thermometers

▶ *Electronic thermometer* (Figure 11-1A)
- Cover with disposable protective sheath.
- Place under tongue; short time required.
- Read on the digital display.

▶ *Tympanic thermometer* (Figure 11-1B)
- Cover with protective sheath.
- Insert gently into ear canal.
- Short exposure (2–5 seconds) before record appears on digital unit.

▶ *Disposable paper (chemical) thermometer* (Figure 11-1C)
- Chemically treated paper for oral or axillary use; raised dots change color to reflect temperature.
- Single use is ideal when infection control is of concern; discard following use.

▶ *Temporal artery thermometer* (Figure 11-1D)
- Measures the temperature of the skin over the temporal artery on the head.

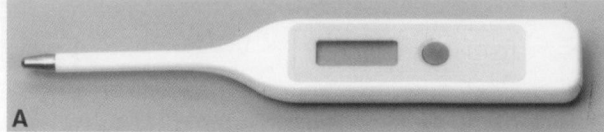

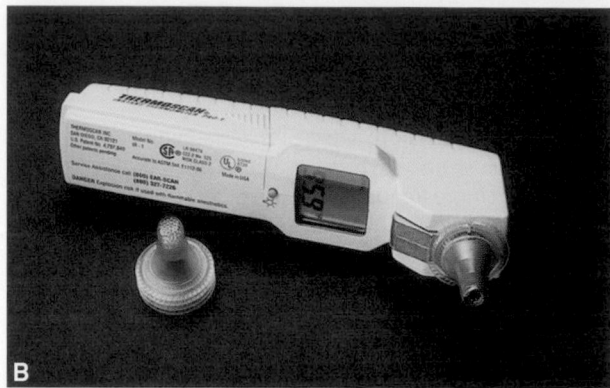

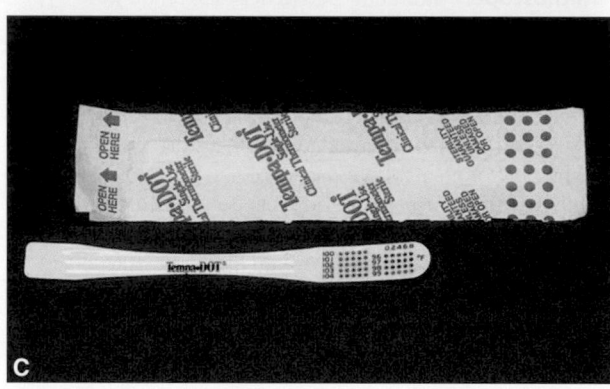

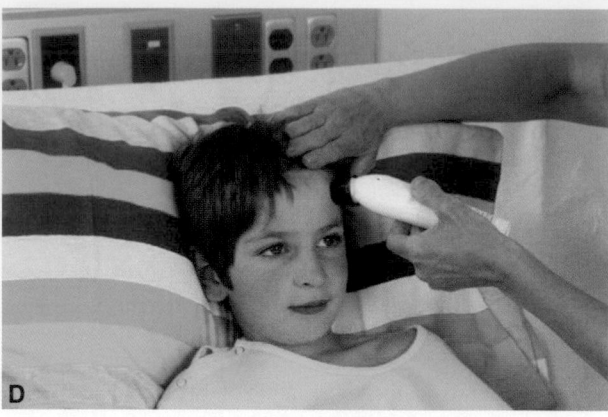

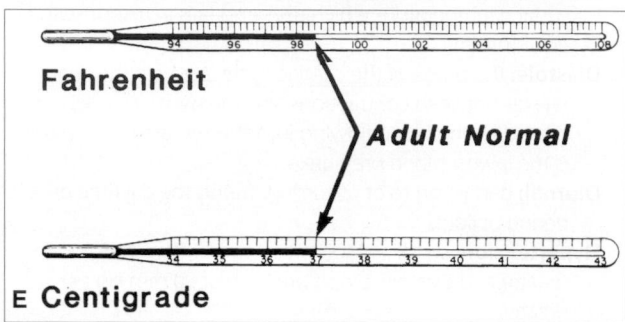

FIGURE 11-1 Types of Thermometers. A: Electronic thermometer. **B:** Tympanic membrane thermometer. **C:** Disposable paper thermometer; the dots change color to indicate temperature. **D:** Temporal artery thermometer. **E:** Mercury thermometer. (A, Reprinted from Springhouse. Nursing Procedures, 4th Ed. Lippincott Williams & Wilkins, 2006; B-D, Reprinted from Lynn P. Taylor's Clinical Nursing Skills, 3rd Ed. Philadelphia: Lippincott Williams & Wilkins; 2010; E, Reprinted from Kronenberger J, Woodson D. Clinical Medical Assisting, 4th Ed. Philadelphia: Lippincott Williams & Wilkins; 2012.)

- Place the scanner on the center of the forehead, midway between the eyebrow and hairline.
- Slide the thermometer across the forehead until the hairline is reached.
- Read the temperature on the display.
- Replace the protective cap.
- More accurate in infants than the tympanic thermometer.

▶ *Mercury in glass:* oral, blue tip; rectal, red tip (Figure 11-1E)
- No longer used due to risk of mercury exposure.[4]

IV. Care of Patient with Temperature Elevation

▶ *Temperature over 105.8°F (41°C)*
- Treat as a medical emergency.
- Transport to a hospital for medical care.

▶ *Temperature 99.6°F–105.8°F (37.6°C–41°C)*
- Check possible temporary causes, such as hot beverage or smoking; observe patient while repeating the determination.
- Review the dental and medical history.
- Postpone elective oral care when there are signs of respiratory infection or other possible communicable disease.

PULSE

▶ The pulse is the intermittent throbbing sensation felt when the fingers are pressed against an artery.

▶ It is the result of the alternate expansion and contraction of an artery as a wave of blood is forced out from the heart.

▶ The pulse rate or heart rate is the count of the heartbeats.

▶ Irregularities of strength, rhythm, and quality of the pulse are noted while counting the pulse rate.

I. Maintenance of Normal Pulse

A. Normal Pulse Rates

▶ *Adults:* There is no absolute normal. The adult range is 60–100 beats per minute (BPM), slightly higher for women than for men.

▶ *Children:* The pulse or heart rate falls steadily during childhood.

B. Factors that Influence Pulse Rate

An unusually fast heartbeat (over 100 BPM in an adult) is called *tachycardia*; an unusually slow heartbeat (below 50 BPM) is *bradycardia*.

▶ *Increased pulse*: Caused by exercise, stimulants, eating, strong emotions, extremes of heat and cold, and some forms of heart disease.

▶ *Decreased pulse*: Caused by sleep, depressants, fasting, quiet emotions, and low vitality from prolonged illness.

▶ *Emergency situations*: Listed in Tables 8-3 and 8-4, Chapter 8.

II. Procedure for Determining Pulse Rate

▶ *Sequence*
  • The pulse rate is obtained following the body temperature.

▶ *Sites*
  • The pulse may be felt at several points over the body.
  • *Radial pulse*: at the wrist (Figure 11-2).
  • Other sites convenient for use in a dental office or clinic are the *temporal* artery on the side of the head in front of the ear, or the *facial* artery at the border of the mandible.
  • *Carotid pulse*: used during cardiopulmonary resuscitation for an adult.
  • *Brachial pulse*: used for an infant (Figure 11-2).

▶ *Prepare the patient*
  1. Tell the patient what is to be done.
  2. Have the patient in a comfortable position with arm and hand supported, palm down.
  3. Locate the radial pulse on the thumb side of the wrist with the tips of the first three fingers (Figure 11-3). Do not use the thumb because it contains a pulse that may be confused with the patient's pulse.

▶ *Count and record*
  1. When the pulse is felt, exert light pressure and count for 1 clocked minute. Use the second hand of a watch or clock. Check with a repeat count when question rate or quality.
  2. While taking the pulse, observe the following:
     • Rhythm: regular, regularly irregular, irregularly irregular.
     • Volume and strength: full, strong, poor, weak, thready.
  3. Record the date, pulse rate as BPM, with other characteristics in patient's record. Document BPM reading prior to administering local anesthesia (see Chapter 38) when included in the care plan.
     • A pulse rate over 100 is considered abnormal for an adult and requires further investigation before proceeding with dental treatment.

RESPIRATION

▶ The function of respiration is to supply oxygen to the tissues and to eliminate carbon dioxide.

▶ Variations in normal respirations may be shown by such characteristics as the rate, rhythm, depth, and

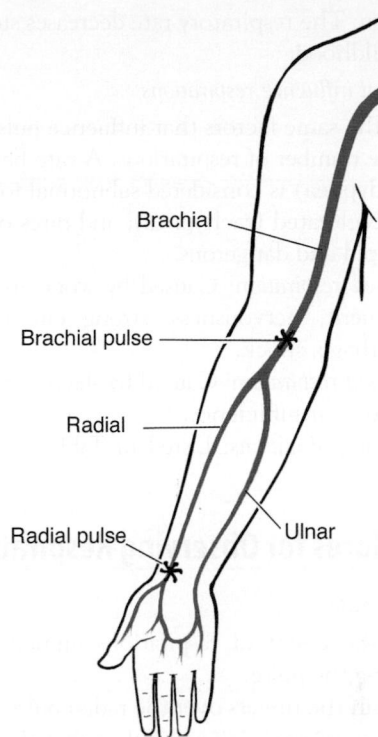

FIGURE 11-2 **Arteries of the Arm. Note the location of the radial pulse.** The brachial pulse may be felt just before the brachial artery branches into the radial and ulnar arteries.

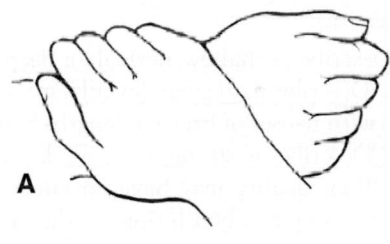

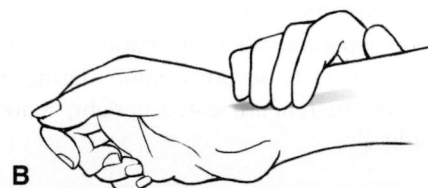

FIGURE 11-3 **Determination of Pulse Rate. A:** Correct position of hands. **B:** The tips of the clinician's first three fingers are placed over the radial pulse located on the thumb side of the ventral surface of the wrist.

quality and may be symptomatic of disease or emergency states.

I. Maintenance of Normal Respirations[2,5,6]

A respiration is one breath taken in and let out.

▶ *Normal respiratory rate*
  • *Adults*: The adult range is from 12 to 20 per minute, slightly higher for women.

- *Children*: The respiratory rate decreases steadily during childhood.

▶ *Factors that influence respirations*

Many of the same factors that influence pulse rate also influence the number of respirations. A rate below 12 per minute (bradypnea) is considered subnormal for an adult; over 28 is accelerated (tachypnea); and rates over 60 are extremely rapid and dangerous.

- *Increased respiration*: Caused by work and exercise, excitement, nervousness, strong emotions, pain, hemorrhage, shock.
- *Decreased respiration*: Caused by sleep, certain drugs, pulmonary insufficiency.
- *Emergency situations*: Listed in Tables 8-3 and 8-4, Chapter 8.

II. Procedures for Observing Respirations

▶ *Determine rate*

1. Make the count of respirations immediately after counting the pulse.
2. Maintain the fingers over the radial pulse.
3. Respirations must be counted so that the patient is not aware, as the rate may be voluntarily altered.
4. Count the number of times the chest rises in 1 clocked minute. It is not necessary to count both inspirations and expirations.

▶ *Factors to observe*

- *Depth*: Describe as shallow, normal, or deep.
- *Rhythm*: Describe as regular (evenly spaced) or irregular (with pauses of irregular lengths between).
- *Quality*: Describe as strong, easy, weak, or labored (noisy). Poor quality may have an effect on body color; for example, a bluish tinge of the face or nail beds may mean an insufficiency of oxygen.
- *Sounds*: Describe deviant sounds made during inspiration, expiration, or both.
- *Position of patient*: When the patient assumes an unusual position to secure comfort during breathing or prefers to remain seated upright, mark records accordingly.

▶ *Record*

Record all findings in the patient's record.

BLOOD PRESSURE[7]

I. Components of Blood Pressure

▶ *Blood pressure is the force exerted by the blood on the blood vessel walls.*

- When the left ventricle of the heart contracts, blood is forced out into the aorta and travels through the large arteries to the smaller arteries, arterioles, and capillaries. The vessels of the heart are shown in Figure 67-1 (Chapter 67).

- The pulsations extend from the heart through the arteries and disappear in the arterioles.
- During the course of the cardiac cycle, the blood pressure is changing constantly.

▶ *Systolic pressure*

Systolic pressure is the peak or the highest pressure. It is caused by ventricular contraction. The normal systolic pressure for an adult is less than 120 mm Hg.

▶ *Diastolic pressure*

Diastolic pressure is the lowest pressure. It is the effect of ventricular relaxation. The normal diastolic pressure for an adult is less than 80 mm Hg.

▶ *Pulse pressure*

The pulse pressure is the difference between the systolic and diastolic pressures.

II. Factors that Influence Blood Pressure

▶ *Maintenance of blood pressure*

Blood pressure depends on the following:

- Force of the heartbeat (energy of the heart).
- Peripheral resistance; condition of the arteries; changes in elasticity of vessels, which may occur with age and disease.
- Volume of blood in the circulatory system.

▶ *Factors that increase blood pressure*

- Exercise, eating, stimulants, and emotional disturbance.
- Use of oral contraceptives; blood pressure increases with age and length of use.

▶ *Factors that decrease blood pressure*

- Fasting, rest, depressants, and quiet emotions.
- Such emergencies as fainting, blood loss, shock (Tables 8-3 and 8-4, Chapter 8).

III. Equipment for Determining Blood Pressure[7]

A sphygmomanometer is made up of a pressure measuring device (manometer) and an inflatable cuff to wrap around the arm or under certain circumstances, the leg.

▶ *Mercury sphygmomanometer (analog)*

- Traditional system, but mercury, is a potential health hazard because of mercury spillage and is less commonly used.[7,8]
- Has shown to be more accurate and consistent than other types.

▶ *Aneroid sphygmomanometer (analog)*

- Compact, portable glass-enclosed gauge with needle for registration of blood pressure.
- Requires regular calibration to keep accurate.

▶ *Electronic sphygmomanometer (digital)*

- Automatic determination of blood pressure without use of stethoscope.
- Size: Choosing the correct size cuff (see Figure 11-4) is critical to accurate blood pressure results.

- The cuff needs to be long enough to encircle 80% of the arm and wide enough to encircle 40% of the arm at its midpoint. A longer, wider cuff is required for obese or muscular individuals and children require pediatric sized cuffs. Always refer to the recommended cuff sizes for accuracy of readings (Figure 11-5).

▶ *Wrist or finger devices*
- Considered to be less accurate and are not considered for professional use.[7]

▶ *Stethoscope*
- Consists of a diaphragm or cupped endpiece that transmits and sends sound through tubes to the earpieces.
- Used with mercury or aneroid-type analog sphygmomanometers.

IV. Procedure for Determining Blood Pressure

▶ *Prepare patient*
1. Tell patient briefly what is to be done. Detailed explanations need to be avoided because they may excite the patient and change the blood pressure.
2. Seat patient comfortably, with the arm slightly flexed, with palm up, and with the whole forearm supported on a level surface at the level of the heart.[9]
   - Arm above heart will result in a false low reading
   - Arm below heart level will result in false high reading
   - Improper cuff selection will result in false high or low depending on size.
3. Use either arm unless otherwise indicated, for example, handicap, history of vascular surgery or mastectomy would indicate arm on opposite side be used. Repeat blood pressure determinations need to be made on the same arm, because a variation in pressure may exist between arms.
4. Take pressure on bare arm, not over clothing. Loosen a tight sleeve.
5. Select cuff size as described in Figure 11-5.

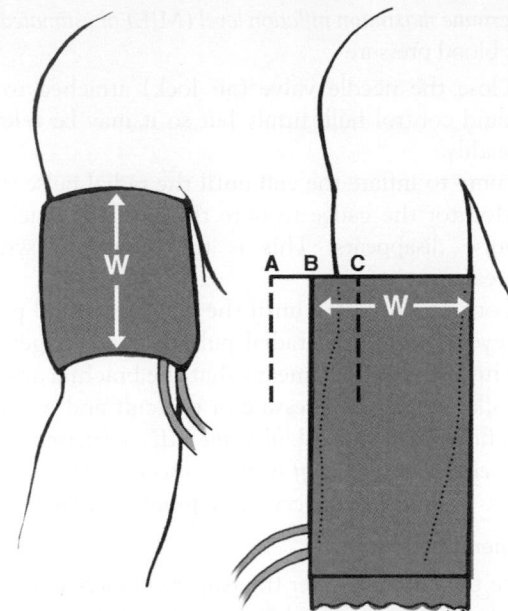

FIGURE 11-4 **A, B: Selection of Cuff Size.** The correct width (W) is 20% greater than the diameter of the arm where applied. **A:** Too wide. **B:** Correct width. **C:** Too narrow.

▶ *Apply cuff*
1. Apply the completely deflated cuff to the patient's arm, supported at the level of the heart. If the arm rests on the arm of a dental chair, lower than the heart, the diastolic pressure may show a small but significant increase.[7]
2. Place the portion of the cuff that contains the inflatable bladder directly over the brachial artery. The cuff may have an arrow to show the point that is placed over the artery. The lower edge of the cuff is placed 1 inch above the antecubital fossa (Figure 11-6). Fasten the cuff evenly and snugly.
3. Adjust the position of the gauge/dial so that is clearly visible and facing you.

▶ *Locate the radial pulse* (Figures 11-2 and 11-3)
1. Palpate 1 inch below the antecubital fossa to locate the brachial artery pulse (Figure 11-6).
2. Hold the fingers on the pulse.

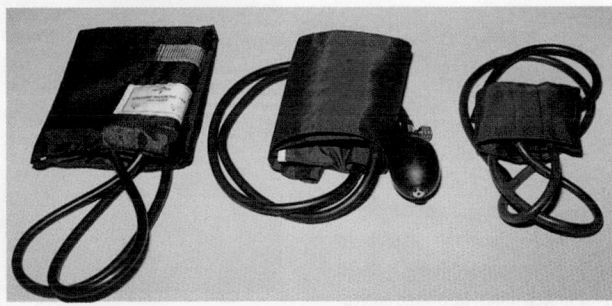

FIGURE 11-5 **Three Sizes of Blood Pressure Cuff.** Extra-large, regular, and pediatric cuff.

▶ *Determine maximum inflation level (MIL) or estimated systolic* blood pressure

1. Close the needle valve (air lock) attached to the hand control bulb firmly but so it may be released readily.

2. Pump to inflate the cuff until the radial pulse stops. Monitor the gauge to note the level at which the pulse disappears. This is the estimated systolic pressure.

3. Continue to pump until the gauge reads 30 points beyond where the radial pulse was no longer felt. This is the MIL. It means that the brachial artery is collapsed by the pressure of the cuff and no blood is flowing through. *Unless the MIL is determined, the level to which the cuff is inflated will be arbitrary. Excess pressure can be very uncomfortable for the patient.*[7]

▶ *Position the stethoscope*

Place the endpiece over the palpated brachial artery, 1 inch below the antecubital fossa, and slightly toward the

inner side of the arm (Figures 11-6 and 11-7). Hold lightly in place.

- Earpieces should be angled forward into the ear canal for proper auscultation (Figure 11- 8A, B).
- Bell or diaphragm end should be placed with light, steady, and complete contact with skin (Figure 11-7).
- Avoid contact with cuff to prevent extraneous sounds that may distract from Korotkof sounds.
- *Support patients arm at heart level* (see Figure 11-9). The position of the arm is critical to accuracy and can greatly influence readings. The upper arm raised above the heart can produce a false low reading and when placed below heart level will result in a false high reading.[7,9]

▶ *Deflate the cuff gradually*

1. Release the air lock slowly so that the dial drops very gradually and steadily, approximately two to three lines per second.

2. Listen for the first sound: systole ("tap tap"). This is the beginning of the flow of blood past the cuff. Note the number on the dial as the *systolic pressure*.

3. Continue to release the pressure slowly. The sound will continue, first becoming louder, then diminishing and becoming muffled, until finally disappearing. Note the number on the dial where the last distinct tap was heard. That number is the *diastolic pressure*.

4. Release further (about 10 points) until all sounds cease. That is the second diastolic point. In some clinics and hospitals, the last sound is taken as the diastolic pressure.

5. Let the rest of the air out rapidly.

▶ *Repeat for confirmation*

- Wait 30 seconds before inflating the cuff again.
- More than one reading is needed within a few minutes to determine an average and ensure a correct reading.

▶ *Record*

- Write date, arm used, and seated or standing.[10]
- Record blood pressure as a fraction, for example, 120/80.

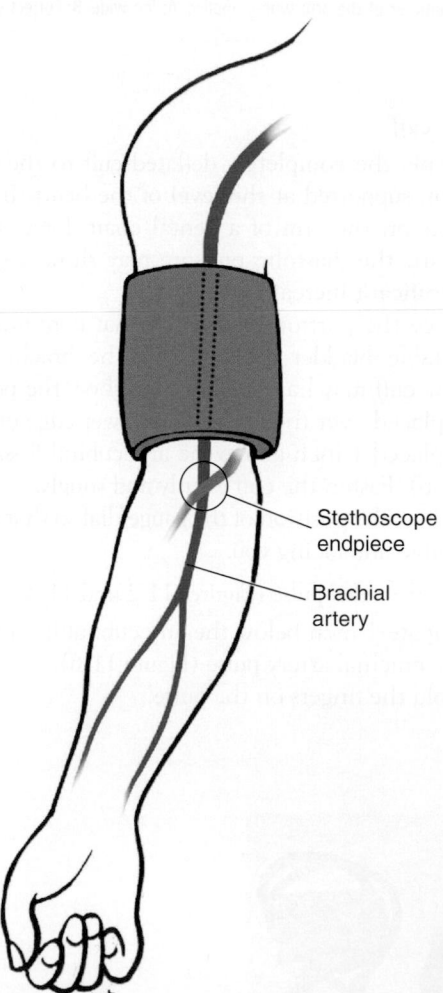

Stethoscope endpiece

Brachial artery

FIGURE 11-6 Blood Pressure Cuff in Position. The lower edge of the cuff is placed approximately 1 inch above the antecubital fossa. The stethoscope endpiece is placed over the palpated brachial artery pulse point approximately 1 inch below the antecubital fossa and slightly toward the inner side of the arm.

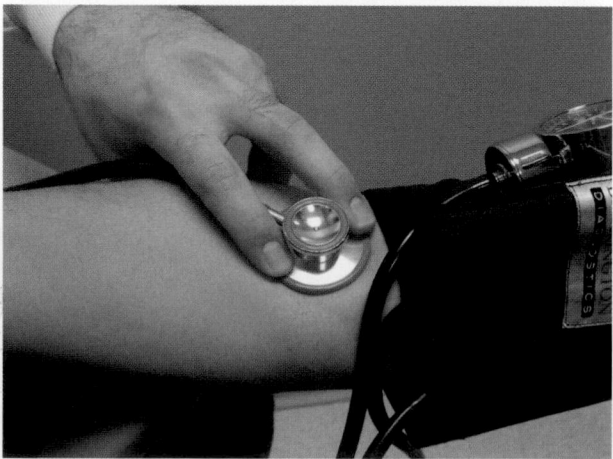

Figure 11-7 Forearm Properly Supported During Blood Pressure Assessment.

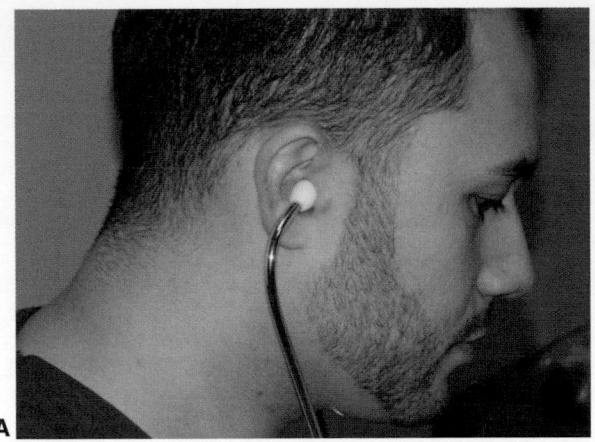
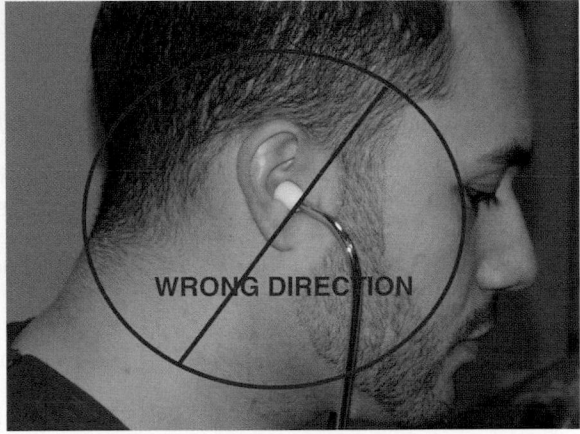

FIGURE 11-8 A: Proper placement of the earpieces for the stethoscope. **B:** Improper placement of the earpieces.

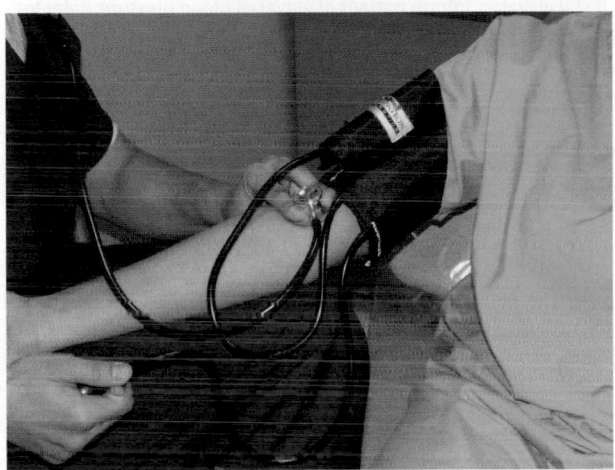

Figure 11-9 **Correct Stethoscope Endpiece Placement, Away from Cuff and in Contact with Skin.**

V. High Blood Pressure (Hypertension)

High blood pressure (HBP) or hypertension is a serious condition that affects nearly one out of every three individuals in the United States and is the leading cause of death in the United States.[11]

▶ Hypertension (HBP of >140/90 is associated with cardiovascular diseases, stroke, kidney failure, and premature death).[10,11]

▶ Contributing factors to hypertension include smoking, stress, obesity, alcohol and drug abuse, and life style.[11]

▶ Information about the patient's blood pressure is essential during dental and dental hygiene appointments because special adaptations may be needed.

▶ Blood pressure readings are recorded with the medical history and other assessment data.

▶ White-coat hypertension is more common in older adults and reported as frequent among centenarians.[11]

Readings taken at the start of an appointment can be significantly higher than at the end of treatment.[12]

▶ To establish a baseline reading and determine the need for patient referral for medical attention, more than one reading is advised. A comparison of the reading at the beginning of the appointment with one at the close of appointment when the patient is relaxed may be helpful.

▶ Screening for blood pressure in dental practices has been shown to be an effective health service for all ages since many patients are unaware that they have hypertension (see Table 11-2).

▶ Growing evidence indicates that primary hypertension is detectable and occurs commonly in young children and adolescents.[2]

• Children and adolescent blood pressure need to be matched to Guidelines in the USDHHS 4th Report on Diagnosis, Evaluation, and Treatment of Blood Pressure in Children and Adolescents.

• United States Department of Health and Human Services (USDHHS) guidelines use age, sex, and height percentile data to more accurately determine the presence or absence of hypertension in children and adolescents.[13]

▶ Cardiovascular diseases are described in Chapter 67. That information can be a helpful introduction and is recommended for reading in conjunction with this section on the techniques for obtaining blood pressure.

VI. Blood Pressure Follow-Up Criteria

▶ Dental personnel have an obligation to advise and *refer for further evaluation*.

▶ Diagnosis of hypertension would never be made or treatment started on the basis of an isolated reading.

▶ Vital signs should be recorded for all new patients, and pre- and postoperatively if medically compromised.

TABLE 11-2	Adult Blood Pressure Classifications[9,10,12,13]		
BLOOD PRESSURE CLASSIFICATION	SYSTOLIC (MM HG)	DIASTOLIC (MM HG)	RECOMMENDATIONS
Hypotension	<90	<60	Observe for possible light-headedness and syncope. If persistent, referral for evaluation is indicated.
Normal	<120	<80	Proceed as planned.
Prehypertension	120–139	80–89	Retake after 5 min. If still elevated, inform patient of prehypertension status. Recommend physician consult and encourage life style modifications (see Table 10-2).
Hypertension			
Stage 1	140–159	90–99	Retake after 5 min. If still elevated, inform patient of elevated blood pressure. Refer for physician consult. Employ stress reduction to routine dental treatment. Modify local anesthetic to 1:100,000 vasoconstrictor.
Stage 2	>160	>100	Retake after 5 min. If still elevated, inform patient of elevated blood pressure. Refer for urgent physician assessment. Delay dental treatment until hypertension is controlled.

Table 11-3	Lifestyle Modifications for Hypertension Management[9]	
MODIFICATION	RECOMMENDATION	APPROXIMATE REDUCTION IN SYSTOLIC BP RANGE
Weight loss	Normal body weight maintenance based on average body mass index	5–20 mm Hg/10 kg weight loss
Dietary approaches to stop hypertension (DASH)	A diet rich in fruits, vegetables, and low-fat dairy products with reduced saturated and total fat	8–14 mm Hg
Dietary sodium intake	Reduce Na intake to equal or less than 100 millimoles per day (2.4 g Na or 6 g NaCl)	2–8 mm Hg
Physical activity	Aerobic activity at least 30 min per day	4–9 mm Hg
Moderate alcohol consumption	Limit to no more than two drinks per day for most men and no more than one drink per day for women or lighter-weight individuals.[a]	2–4 mm Hg

[a]1 ounce or 20 ml ethanol, i.e., 24 oz beer, 10 oz wine, or 2 oz 80 proof whiskey.

▶ Rechecking within 1 year is recommended for persons at increased risk for hypertension, such as family history, weight gain, obesity, African American, use of oral contraceptives, smoking, and excessive alcohol consumption (see Tables 11-1 and 11-2).

▶ Lifestyle modifications are indicated for all levels of blood pressure classification[10] and HBP management

should follow current evidence-based management guidelines through collaborative efforts with the patients primary care provider.[14] Immediate consultation with a patient's primary care provider is indicated prior to dental or dental hygiene treatment when either reading is ≥180/110 (Tables 11-2 and 11-3).

EVERYDAY ETHICS

Gracie was having a very busy day and at 10:15 AM was already late for the 10:00 AM patient, Mr. McElroy, who had arrived early and was waiting in the reception area. While completing his history, to save time, she copied over the blood pressure recording from his previous appointment just 2 weeks ago. It had been 130/83, only slightly into the prehypertension level.

The appointment was planned for the maxillary left quadrant with anesthesia. After the scaling was complete and Mr. McElroy was climbing out of the dental chair, looking a bit unsteady as he stood up, he casually remarked: "I just remembered while you were working that my Doc gave me a new prescription—I suppose I should have told you before. But it is only one pill a day—for keeping the

blood pressure down. I don't have any trouble anyway, he just wanted to be sure."

Questions for Consideration

1. Explain how the principles of beneficence and maleficence apply to Gracie's actions with Mr. McElroy's examination and charting procedures.

2. How has Gracie placed the office at risk for a possible medical emergency given Mr. McElroy's physical status? Answer by describing the rights and duties of both the hygienist and the patient.

3. Who is responsible for ensuring that accurate documentation has been completed on all patients—from an ethical and a quality assurance perspective?

DOCUMENTATION[10]

Documentation in the permanent record of a patient with HBP would include the following:

▶ Carefully documented medical history with regular updates at each maintenance appointment.

▶ Reminder to help patient realize the importance of regularly taking prescribed medication.

▶ Prepared and documented blood pressure reading at each appointment especially when anesthesia is included in the care plan.

▶ Box 11-2 contains a sample progress note.

Factors To Teach The Patient

▷ How vital signs can influence dental and dental hygiene appointments.

▷ The importance of having a blood pressure determination at regular intervals.

▷ For the patient diagnosed as hypertensive, encourage regular continuing use of prescription drugs for control of HBP.

▷ Encourage healthy lifestyle changes such as tobacco cessation, drug and/or alcohol counseling, exercise, and healthy dietary habits (see Table 11-3)

BOX 11-2

Example Documentation: Vital Signs

S–Mrs. Patel apologized for arriving 5 minutes late and stated she had no concerns at the start of her dental appointment

O–Vital signs at 9:00 AM; pulse 64; respirations 12; BP (right arm) 190/88 seated

A–Hypertension stage 3 range

P–Advised Mrs. Patel her blood pressure is measuring at a high and an unsafe level for treatment. Blood pressure remained elevated when re-assessed 10 minutes later. Discussed hypertension range with dentist and referred patient to primary care physician for urgent follow-up. Delay maintenance appointment until hypertension under control. Follow-up later today by phone.

Signed _____, RDH

Date _____

References

1. Barnason S, Williams J, Proehl J, et al. Emergency nursing resource: non-invasive temperature measurement in the emergency department. *J Emerg Nurs.* 2012;38:523–530.

2. Institute for Clinical Systems Improvement (ICSI). Rapid response team. Health care protocol. Bloomington (MN): Institute for Clinical Systems Improvement (ICSI); 2011 Jul. 45 p.

3. Crawford D, Hicks B, Thompson M. Which thermometer? Factors influencing best choice for intermittent clinical temperature assessment. *J Med Eng Technol.* 2006;30:199–211.

4. MayoClinic. Thermometers: understand the options. http://www.mayoclinic.com/health/thermometers/MY01186/METHOD=print. Accessed September 2, 2013.

5. Fleming S, Thompson M, Stevens R, et al. Normal ranges of heart rate and respiratory rate in children from birth to 18 years of age: a systematic review of observational studies. *Lancet.* 2011;377:1011–1018.

6. National Institutes of Health. Vital signs: MedlinePlus Medical Encyclopedia. http://www.nlm.nih.gov/medlineplus/ency/article/002341.htm. Accessed September 2, 2013.

7. Pickering TG, Hall JE, Appel LJ, et al. Recommendations for blood pressure measurement in humans and experimental animals. Part 1: Blood pressure measurement in humans: a statement for professionals from the subcommittee of professional and public education of the American Heart Association council on high blood pressure research. *Hypertension*. 2005;45:142–161.

8. Herman WW, Konzelman Jr JL, Prisant LM. New national guidelines on hypertension: a summary for dentistry. *J Am Dent Assoc*. 2004;135:576–584.

9. Chobanian AV, Bakris GL, Black HR, et al. Seventh report of the Joint National Committee on prevention, detection, evaluation, and treatment of high blood pressure. *Hypertension*. 2003;42:1206–1252.

10. High Blood Pressure Fact Sheet | Data & Statistics | DHDSP | CDC. http://www.cdc.gov/dhdsp/data_statistics/fact_sheets/fs_bloodpressure.htm. Accessed January 21, 2014.

11. Aronow WS, Fleg JL, Pepine CJ, et al. ACCF/AHA 2011 expert consensus document on hypertension in the elderly: A Report of the American College of Cardiology Foundation Task Force on clinical expert consensus documents developed in collaboration with the American Academy of Neurology, American Geriatrics Society, American Society for Preventive Cardiology, American Society of Hypertension, American Society of Nephrology. *J Am Soc Hypertens*. 2011;5:259–352.

12. Bader JD, Bonito AJ, Shugars DA. A systematic review of cardiovascular effects of epinephrine on hypertensive dental patients. *Oral Surg Oral Med Oral Pathol Oral Radiol Endod*. 2002;93:647–653.

13. USDHHS, National Institutes of Health, National Heart, Lung and Blood Institute. *Fourth Report on Diagnosis, Evaluation and Treatment of Blood Pressure in Children and Adolescents*, May 2005, NIH Publication No. 05-5267. http://www.nhlbi.nih.gov/files/docs/resources/heart/hbp_ped.pdf. Accessed February 20, 2015.

14. James PA, Oparil S, Carter BL, et al. 2014 Evidence-based guideline for the management of high blood pressure in adults: report from the panel members appointed to the Eighth Joint National Committee (JNC 8). *JAMA*. 2014;311(5):507–520.

ENHANCE YOUR UNDERSTANDING

thePoint® DIGITAL CONNECTIONS
(see the inside front cover for access information)
- **Audio glossary**
- **Quiz bank**

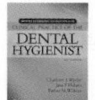

SUPPORT FOR LEARNING
(available separately; visit lww.com)
- *Active Learning Workbook for Clinical Practice of the Dental Hygienist, 12th Edition*

prepU INDIVIDUALIZED REVIEW
(available separately; visit lww.com)
- **Adaptive quizzing with *prepU for Wilkins' Clinical Practice of the Dental Hygienist***

12

Extraoral and Intraoral Examination

Lisa B. Johnson, RDH, MSDH, MPH

CHAPTER OUTLINE

**RATIONALE FOR THE EXTRAORAL/
INTRAORAL EXAMINATION**

COMPONENTS OF EXAMINATION
- I. Types of Examinations
- II. Methods for Examination
- III. Signs and Symptoms
- IV. Preparation for Examination

**ANATOMICAL LANDMARKS
OF THE ORAL CAVITY**
- I. Oral Mucosa

SEQUENCE OF EXAMINATION
- I. Extraoral Examination

- II. Intraoral Examination
- III. Documentation of Findings

MORPHOLOGIC CATEGORIES
- I. Elevated Lesions
- II. Depressed Lesions
- III. Flat Lesions
- IV. Other Descriptive Terms

ORAL CANCER
- I. Location
- II. Appearance of Early Cancer

**PROCEDURE FOR DETERMINING WHEN A
SUSPICIOUS LESION REQUIRES A BIOPSY**
- I. Exfoliative Cytology
- II. Spectroscopy
- III. Biopsy

DOCUMENTATION

EVERYDAY ETHICS

FACTORS TO TEACH THE PATIENT

REFERENCES

LEARNING OBJECTIVES

After studying this chapter, the student will be able to:

1. Explain the rationale for a comprehensive extra- and intraoral examination.

2. Explain the systematic sequence of the extra- and intraoral examination.

3. Identify normal hard and soft tissue anatomy of the head, neck, and oral cavity.

4. Describe and document physical characteristics (size, shape, color, texture, consistency) and morphological categories (elevated, flat, and depressed lesions) for notable findings.

5. Identify suspected conditions that require additional testing and referral for medical evaluation.

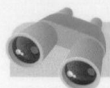

BOX 12-1   KEY WORDS: Extraoral/Intraoral Examination

Aphtha: a little white or reddish ulcer.

Crust: outer scablike layer of solid matter formed by drying of a body exudate or secretion.

Cyst: a closed, epithelial-lined sac, normal or pathologic, that contains fluid or other material.

Dorsal: back surface; opposite of ventral.

Epidermis: outermost and nonvascular layers of the skin composed of basal layer, spinous layer, granular layer, and horny layer.

Corium: the dermis or true skin just beneath the epidermis; well supplied with nerves and blood vessels.

Erosion: soft tissue slightly depressed lesion in which the epithelium above the basal layer is denuded.

Erythema: red area of variable size and shape; reaction to irritation, radiation, or injury.

Exophytic: growing outward.

Exostosis: a benign bony growth projecting from the surface of bone.

Fissure: a narrow slit or cleft in the epidermis where infected ulceration, inflammation, and pain can result.

Forensic: pertaining to or used in legal proceedings.

Idiopathic: of unknown etiology.

Induration: hardened; abnormally hard.

Lymphadenopathy: disease of the lymph nodes; regional lymph node enlargement.

Morphology: science that deals with form and structure.

Palpation: perceiving by sense of touch.

Papilla: small, nipple-shaped projection or elevation (papillary: adjective).

Patch: circumscribed flat lesion larger than a macule; differentiated from surrounding epidermis by color and/or texture.

Pedunculated: elevated lesion attached by a thin stalk.

Petechia: hemorrhagic nonraised spot of pinpoint to pinhead size.

Polyp: any growth or mass protruding from a mucous membrane.

Pseudomembrane: a loose membranous layer of exudate that contains microorganisms, precipitated fibrin, necrotic cells, and inflammatory cells produced during an inflammatory reaction on the surface of a tissue.

Punctate: marked with points or punctures differentiated from the surrounding surface by color, elevation, or texture.

Purulent: containing, forming, or discharging pus.

Rubefacient: reddening of the skin.

Scar: cicatrix; mark remaining after healing of a wound or healing following a surgical intervention.

Sclerosis: induration or hardening.

Sessile: elevated lesion with a broad base.

Temporomandibular disorder (TMD): a collective term that includes a wide range of disorders of the masticatory system characterized by one or more of the following: pain in the preauricular area, temporomandibular joint (TMJ), and muscles of mastication, with limitation or deviation in mandibular motion and TMJ sounds during mandibular function.

Torus: bony elevation or prominence usually located on the midline of the hard palate (torus palatinus) or the lingual surface of the mandible in the premolar area (torus mandibularis).

Trismus: motor disturbance of the trigeminal nerve, especially spasm of the masticatory muscles with difficulty in opening the mouth.

Ventral: inferior surface; opposite of dorsal.

Verruca: a wartlike growth.

RATIONALE FOR THE EXTRAORAL AND INTRAORAL EXAMINATION

The extraoral and intraoral examination is performed for early identification of abnormalities and pathologies, especially oral cancer.

Although an essential goal of the examination is to detect cancer of the mouth at the earliest possible stage, a thorough examination may also reveal signs of thyroid disorders, eating disorders, nutritional deficiencies, sexually transmitted diseases, and a host of systemic conditions.[1]

▶ Box 12-1 defines key terms used for extraoral and intraoral examination.

COMPONENTS OF EXAMINATION

▶ The standard of patient care is that the total patient is being treated, not only the oral cavity, and particularly not just the teeth and immediate surrounding tissues.

▶ The examination is all-inclusive to detect possible physical or psychological influences on the patient's oral health.

▶ Thorough examination is essential for each continuing care appointment so that the treatment for the control and prevention of oral diseases will be effective.

▶ Assessment of health-related risk factors such as:[1]
- Tobacco
- Alcohol use
- Cultural and genetic susceptibility
- Sun exposure and lack of use of sun protection
- Diet
- Certain surgeries such as organ or bone marrow transplant and subsequent long-term immunosuppressive medications increase the risk of cancer.[1]
- Sexual behaviors involving orogenital contact may increase risk of human papillomavirus (HPV) transmission and must also be considered within assessment.[1,2]

I. Types of Examinations

▶ *Complete*
- A complete examination includes a thorough summary of all the components of the assessment.
- The extraoral and intraoral examination is a component of a patient's complete assessment and is performed for all new patients and at each routine continuing care visit.

▶ *Screening*
- Screening implies a brief, preliminary examination, usually for a particular purpose such as pain relief or for initial patient assessment and triage to determine priorities for treatment.

▶ *Limited examination*
- A type of brief examination made for an emergency situation. It may be used in the management of an acute condition.

▶ *Follow-up*
- Brief follow-up examination to check healing following a treatment.

▶ *Continuing care/reevaluation*
- After a specific period of time following the completion of the care plan and the anticipated restoration to health.
- A continuing care examination is a complete reassessment from which a new dental hygiene diagnosis and care plan are derived.

II. Methods for Examination

The extraoral and intraoral examination is accomplished by various visual and tactile, manual, and instrumental methods. Patient position, optimum lighting, and effective retraction for accessibility and visibility contribute to the accuracy and completeness of the examination.

▶ *Visual examination*
- *Direct observation*: Visual observation is carried out in a systematic sequence to note surface appearance (color, contour, size) and to observe movement and other evidence of function.
- *Radiographic examination*: The use of radiographs can reveal deviations from normal not observable by direct vision.
- *Transillumination*: A strong light directed through a soft tissue or a tooth to enhance examination is useful for detecting irregularities of the teeth and locating calculus. Hold the mouth mirror to view from the lingual to see the translucency.

▶ *Palpation*
Palpation is examination using the sense of touch through tissue manipulation or pressure on an area with the gloved fingers of one hand or both.
- *Digital*: The use of a single finger. Example: Index finger applied to the lingual side of the mandible beneath the canine and premolar area to determine presence of a torus mandibularis.
- *Bidigital*: The use of finger and thumb of same hand. Example: palpation of the lips (Figure 12-1).
- *Bimanual*: The use of finger or fingers and thumb from each hand applied simultaneously in coordination. Example: index finger of one hand palpates on the floor of the mouth inside, while a finger or fingers from the other hand press on the same area from under the chin externally (Figure 12-2A and B).
- *Bilateral*: The two hands are used at the same time to examine corresponding structures on opposite sides of the body. Comparisons can be made. Example: fingers placed beneath the chin to palpate the submandibular lymph nodes (Figure 12-3B).

▶ *Instrumentation*
- Examination instruments, such as a periodontal probe and an explorer, are used for specific examination of the teeth and periodontal tissues. The uses of probe and explorer are described in Chapter 20.

▶ *Percussion*
- Percussion is the act of tapping a surface or tooth with the fingers or an instrument.
- Information about the status of health is determined either by the response of the patient or by the sound. When a tooth is known to be sensitive in any way, percussion needs to be avoided.

▶ *Electrical test*
- An electric pulp tester may be used to detect the presence or absence of vital pulp tissue.
- Methods for use of a pulp tester are described in Chapter 16.

▶ *Auscultation*
- Auscultation is the use of sound.
- Example: The sound of clicking of the temporomandibular joint when the jaw is opened and closed. Figure 12-4 shows examination of the temporomandibular joint.

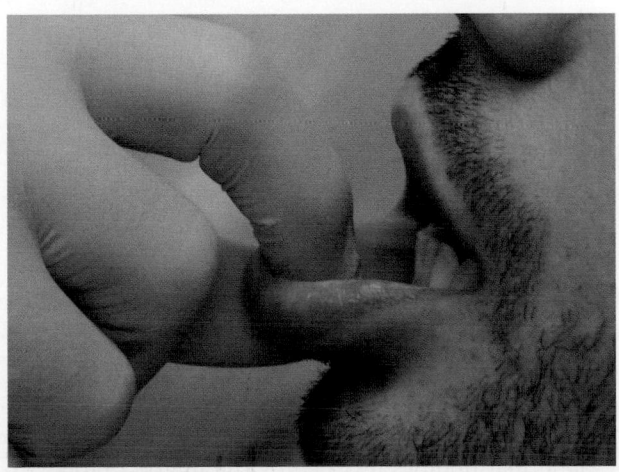

FIGURE 12-1 Bidigital Palpation. Palpation of the lip to illustrate the use of a finger and thumb of the same hand.

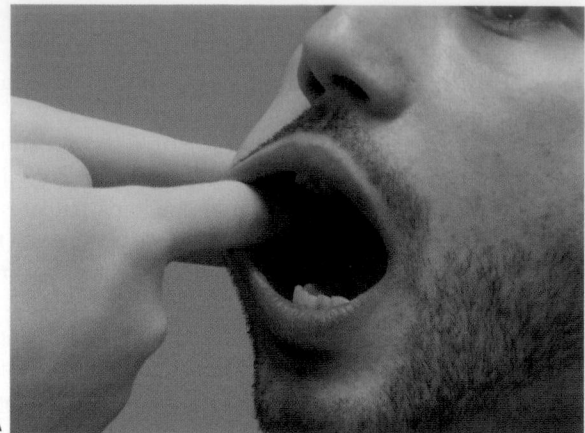

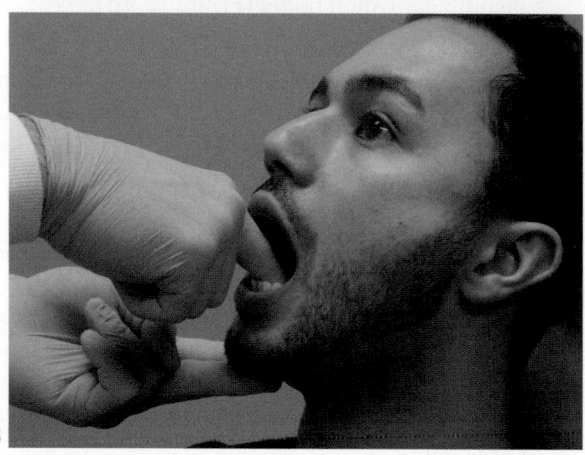

FIGURE 12-2 **Bimanual Palpation. A:** Examination of the buccal mucosa by simultaneous palpation on extraorally and intraorally. **B:** Examination of the floor of the mouth by simultaneous palpation with fingers of each hand in apposition.

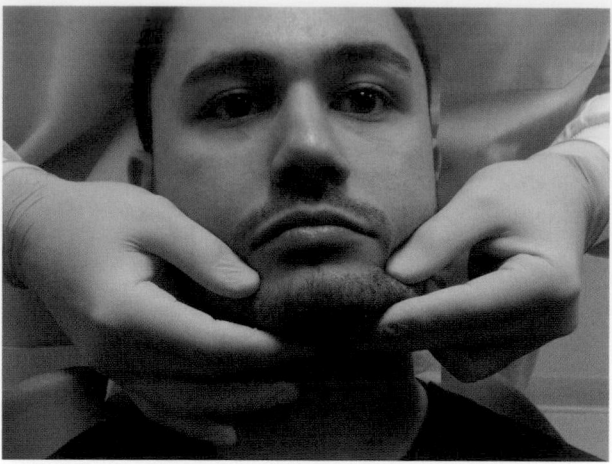

FIGURE 12-3 **Bilateral Palpation.** Bilateral palpation is used to examine corresponding structures on opposite sides of the body.

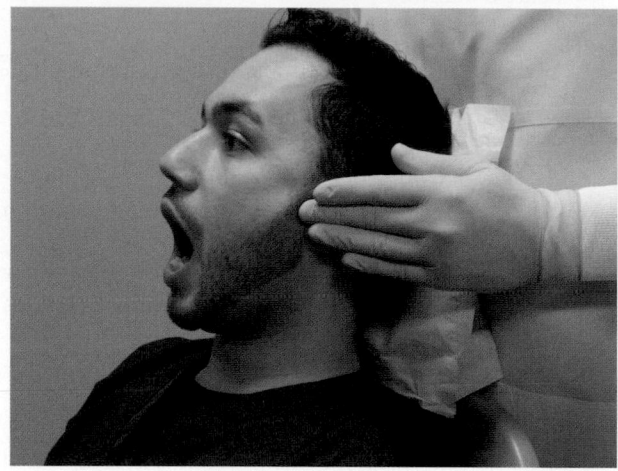

FIGURE 12-4 **Assessment of the Temporomandibular Joint.** The joint is palpated as the patient opens and closes the mouth.

III. Signs and Symptoms

▶ A specific objective for patient examination as a part of the complete assessment is the recognition of deviations from normal that may be signs or symptoms of disease.

▶ General signs and symptoms may occur in various disease conditions. Example: fever, or increase in body temperature accompanies most infections.

▶ A *pathognomonic* sign or symptom is unique to a particular disease and may be used to distinguish that condition from other diseases or conditions.

A. Signs

▶ A sign is any abnormality identified by a healthcare professional while examining a patient.

▶ A sign is an *objective symptom*. Examples of signs: observable changes such as color, shape, consistency, or abnormal findings revealed by the use of a probe, explorer, radiograph, or other instrument for disease detection.

B. Symptoms

▶ A symptom is any departure from normal that may be indicative of disease.

▶ It is a subjective abnormality that can be observed by the patient.

▶ Examples are pain, tenderness, and bleeding when toothbrushing as described by the patient.

IV. Preparation for Examination

▶ Review the patient's health histories and dental/medical record, including risk factors, radiographs, dental caries, periodontal, and oral cancer risk assessments.

▶ Examine radiographs on viewbox or in the computer.

▶ Explain the procedures to be performed and relevance of the procedures.

• Example: "I am going to perform an extra/intra oral examination to look for abnormalities that can affect your oral and overall health."

- Patient understanding the rational for an extraoral and intraoral examination is critical to acceptance and education.
- When a patient is wearing a scarf or other head/neck covering for cultural or religious purposes, the dental hygienist uses culturally sensitive communication skills (Chapter 3, Cultural Considerations section.).

ANATOMICAL LANDMARKS OF THE ORAL CAVITY

Familiarization with structures (Box 12-1, Figures 12-5 through 12-7) and normal anatomy is prerequisite to understanding abnormal presentations in the head and neck region.[1–3]

I. Oral Mucosa

The lining of the oral cavity, the oral mucosa, is a mucous membrane composed of connective tissue covered with stratified squamous epithelium. There are three divisions or categories of oral mucosa.

A. Masticatory Mucosa

▶ Covers the *gingiva* and *hard palate*, the areas most used during the mastication of food.
▶ Except for the free margin of the gingiva, the masticatory mucosa is firmly attached to underlying tissues.
▶ The normal epithelial covering is keratinized.

B. Lining Mucosa

▶ Covers the inner surfaces of the lips and cheeks, floor of the mouth, underside of the tongue, soft palate, and alveolar mucosa.
▶ These tissues are not firmly attached to underlying tissue.
▶ The epithelial covering is not keratinized.

C. Specialized Mucosa

▶ Covers the dorsum (upper surface) of the tongue.
▶ Composed of many papillae; some contain taste buds.
▶ The distribution of the four types of papillae is shown in Figure 12-5.
- *Filiform:* threadlike keratinized elevations that cover the dorsal surface of the tongue; they are the most numerous of the papillae.
- *Fungiform:* mushroom-shaped papillae interspersed among the filiform papillae on the tip and sides of the tongue, appear redder than the filiform papillae, and contain variable numbers of taste buds. The inset enlargement in Figure 12-5 shows the comparative shape and size of the filiform and fungiform papillae.
- *Circumvallate (vallate):* the 10 to 14 large round papillae arranged in a "V" between the body of the tongue and the base. Taste buds line the walls.
- *Foliate:* vertical grooves on the lateral posterior sides of the tongue; also contain taste buds.

SEQUENCE OF EXAMINATION

▶ Conducting an examination with routine order will minimize the possibility of excluding areas and overlooking details of importance. A systematic sequence improves efficiency, promotes professionalism, and inspires patient confidence.
▶ A recommended sequence for examination is outlined in Box 12-2 in which factors to consider during appointments are related to the actual observations made and recorded.
- This sequence is adapted from *Detecting Oral Cancer*, available from the National Institutes of Health and the National Cancer Institute.[4,5]
- In addition to proper sequence, familiarization of anatomical structures common to normal anatomy is critical to understanding abnormal findings (Table 12-1).[3]

I. Extraoral Examination

1. Observe patient during reception and seating to note physical characteristics and abnormalities, and make an overall appraisal.
2. Observe head, face, eyes, and neck, and evaluate the skin of the face and neck.
3. Request the patient remove prosthesis prior to performing the intraoral examination. Explain how this will improve the ability to inspect all areas of the mouth adequately.
4. Palpate the salivary glands and lymph nodes. Figure 12-8 shows the location of the major lymph nodes of the face, oral regions, and neck. Palpation is a significant component of the extra-/intraoral examination (Figure 12-9). Note any of the following symptoms or experiences:

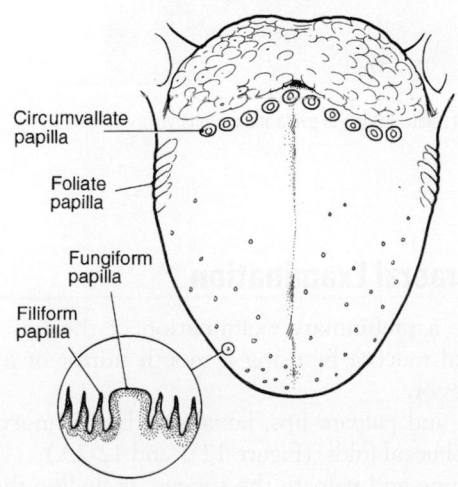

Circumvallate papilla

Foliate papilla

Fungiform papilla

Filiform papilla

FIGURE 12-5 Papillae of the Tongue.

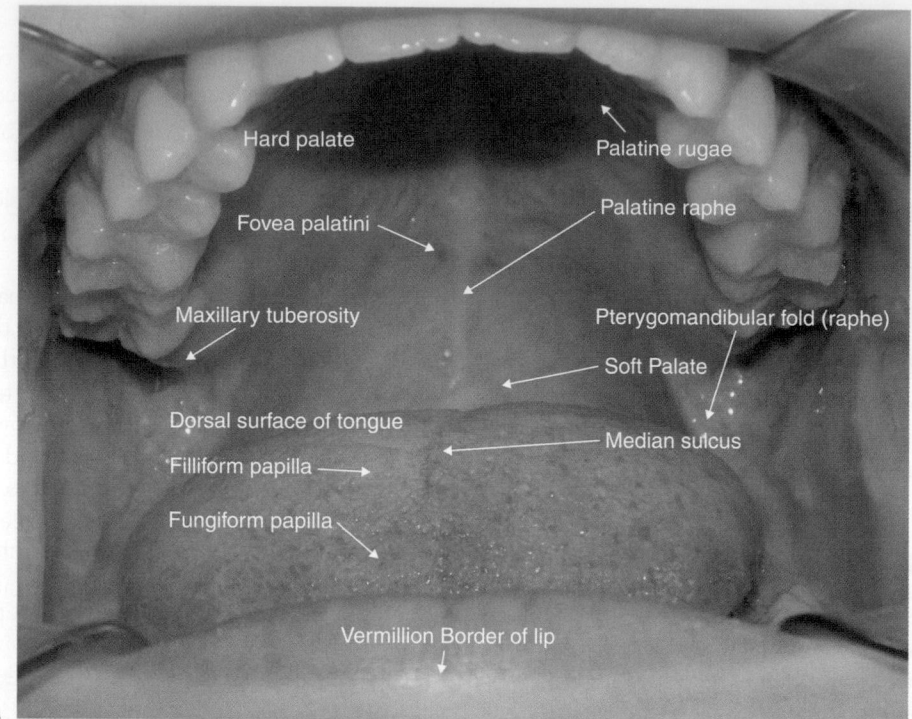

Hard palate

Palatine rugae

Fovea palatini

Palatine raphe

Maxillary tuberosity

Pterygomandibular fold (raphe)

Soft Palate

Dorsal surface of tongue

Median sulcus

Filliform papilla

Fungiform papilla

Vermillion Border of lip

A

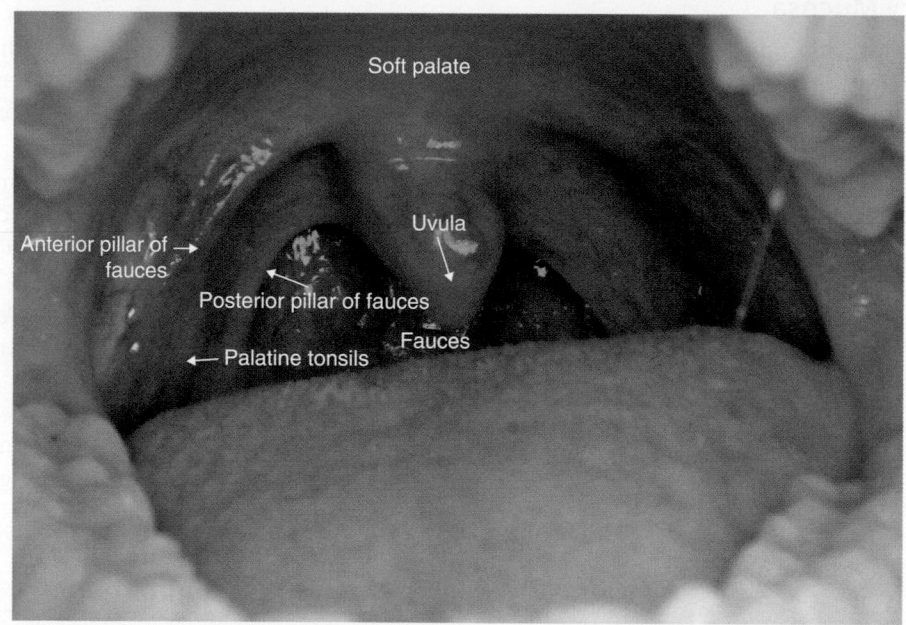

Soft palate

Uvula

Anterior pillar of fauces

Posterior pillar of fauces

Fauces

Palatine tonsils

B

FIGURE 12-6 **Anatomical Landmarks of the Oral Cavity-Dorsal Tongue View. A:** View of hard and soft palate. **B:** View of uvula and oro-pharynx.

- Pain or discomfort upon palpation and/or upon swallowing.
- Persistent difficulty swallowing in the absence of pain.
- Any recent noticeable lumps the patient may have experienced without pain.
- Persistent earache or hoarseness of voice.[6]

5. Observe mandibular movement and palpate the temporomandibular joint (Figure 12-4). Relate to items from questions in the medical/dental history.[7,8]

II. Intraoral Examination

1. Make a preliminary examination of the lips and intraoral mucosa by using a mouth mirror or a tongue depressor.
2. View and palpate lips, labial and buccal mucosa, and mucobuccal folds. (Figure 12-1 and 12-2A)
3. Examine and palpate the tongue, including the dorsal and ventral surfaces, lateral borders, and base. Retract

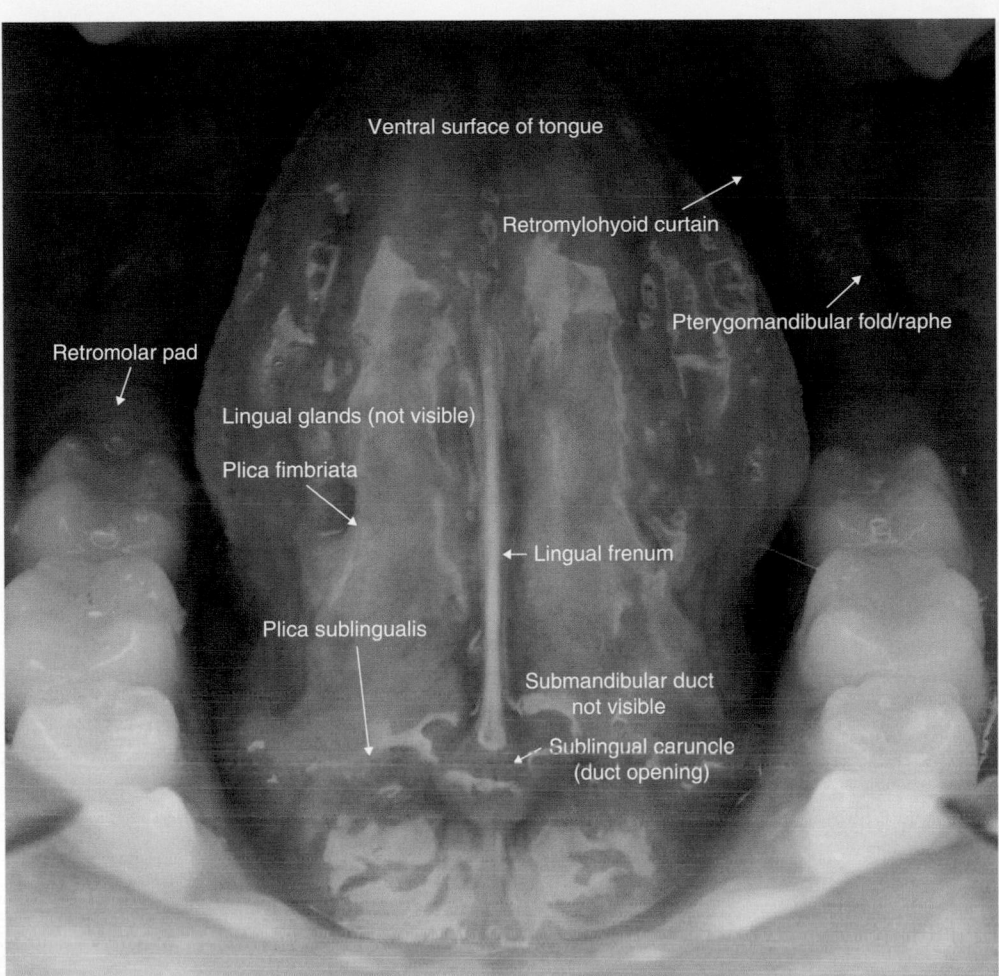

FIGURE 12-7 Anatomical Landmarks of the Oral Cavity-Ventral Tongue View.

to observe posterior third, first to one side then the other (Figure 12-10).

4. Observe mucosa of the floor of the mouth. Palpate the floor of the mouth (Figure 12-2B).

5. Examine the hard and soft palates, tonsillar areas, and pharynx (Figure 12-6 A and B). Use a mirror to observe the oropharynx, nasopharynx, and larynx.

6. Note amount and consistency of the saliva and evidence of dry mouth (xerostomia).

III. Documentation of Findings

A. History

Questions directed to the patient provide necessary information in the management of an oral lesion. Because alarming the patient must be avoided, judgment is needed for selecting the appropriate time to obtain the history of a lesion.

▶ Whether the lesion is known or not known to the patient; previous evaluation.

▶ If known, when first noticed; if recurrence, previous date.

▶ Duration, symptoms, changes in size and appearance.

B. Location and Extent

▶ When a lesion is first seen, its location is noted in relation to adjacent structures.

▶ Document a complete description of each finding including the location, extent, size, color, surface texture or configurations, consistency, morphology, and history.

▶ A printed diagram of parts of the oral cavity drawn into the record form can be a valuable aid for marking the location (Figure 12-11).[9]

▶ Descriptive words to define the location and extent include the following:

• *Localized*: Lesion limited to a small focal area.

• *Generalized*: Involves most of an area or segment.

• *Single lesion*: One lesion of a particular type with a distinct margin.

• *Multiple lesions*: More than one lesion of a particular type. Lesions may be:

• Separate: discrete, not running together; may be arranged in clusters.

• Coalescing: close to each other with margins that merge.

TABLE 12-1	Extraoral and Intraoral Examination	
SEQUENCE OF EXAMINATION	**OBSERVE**	**INDICATION AND INFLUENCES ON APPOINTMENTS**
1. Overall appraisal of patient	Posture, gait General health status; size Hair; scalp Breathing; state of fatigue Voice, cough, hoarseness	Response, cooperation, attitude toward treatment Length of appointment
2. Face	Expression: evidence of fear or apprehension Shape: twitching; paralysis Jaw movements during speech Injuries; signs of abuse	Need for alleviation of fears Evidence of upper respiratory or other infections Enlarged masseter muscle (related to bruxism)
3. Skin	Color, texture, blemishes Traumatic lesions Eruptions, swellings Growths, scars, moles	Relation to possible systemic conditions Need for supplementary history Biopsy or other treatment to recommend Influences on instruction in diet
4. Eyes	Size of pupils Color of sclera Eyeglasses (corrective) Protruding eyeballs	Dilated pupils or pinpoint may result from drugs, emergency state Eyeglasses essential during instruction Hyperthyroidism

5. Nodes (palpate) (Figure 12-8)
  a. Pre- and postauricular
  b. Occipital
  c. Submental; submandibular
  d. Cervical chain (Figure 12-9)
  e. Supraclavicular
	Adenopathy; lymphadenopathy
	Induration or pain
		Need for referral
		Medical consultation
		Ear infection
		Coordinate with intraoral examination

6. Glands (palpate)
  a. Parotid
  b. Submental
  c. Submandibular (Figure 12-3)
	Enlargement or pain
	Induration longer than 2 wk
		Referral for medical consult

7. Temporomandibular joint (palpate) (Figure 12-4)	Limitations or deviations of movement Tenderness; sensitivity Noises: clicking, popping, grating	Disorder of joint; limitation of opening Discomfort during appointment and during personal biofilm control

8. Lips
  a. Observe closed, then open
  b. Palpate (Figure 12-1)
	Color, texture, size
	Cracks, angular cheilosis
	Blisters, ulcers
	Traumatic lesions
	Irritation from lip-biting
	Limitation of opening; muscle elasticity; muscle tone
	Evidences of mouthbreathing
	Induration
		Need for further examination: referral
		Immediate need for postponement of appointment when a lesion may be communicable or could interfere with procedures
		Care during retraction
		Accessibility during intraoral procedures
		Patient instruction: dietary, special biofilm control for mouthbreather

9. Breath odor	Severity Relation to oral hygiene, gingival health	Possible relation to systemic condition Alcohol use history; special needs

(continues)

TABLE 12-1	Extraoral and Intraoral Examination	
SEQUENCE OF EXAMINATION	**OBSERVE**	**INDICATION AND INFLUENCES ON APPOINTMENTS**
10. Labial and buccal mucosa, left and right examined systematically 　a. Vestibule 　b. Mucobuccal folds 　c. Frena 　d. Opening of Stensen's duct 　e. Palpate cheeks (Figure 12-2A)	Color, size, texture, contour Abrasions, traumatic lesions, cheekbite Effects of tobacco use Ulcers, growths Moistness of surfaces Relation of frena to free gingiva Induration	Need for referral, biopsy, cytology Frena and other anatomic parts that need special adaptation for radiography or impression tray Avoid sensitive areas during retraction
11. Tongue 　a. Vestibule 　b. Dorsal (Figure 12-6A) 　c. Lateral borders 　d. Base of tongue (Figure 12-10) 　e. Deviation on extension	Shape: normal asymmetric Color, size, texture, consistency Fissures; papillae Coating Lesions: elevated, depressed, flat Induration	Need for referral, biopsy, cytology Need for instruction in tongue cleaning
12. Floor of mouth 　a. Ventral surface of tongue (Figure 12-7) 　b. Palpate (Figure 12-2B) 　c. Duct openings 　d. Mucosa, frena 　e. Tongue action	Varicosities Lesions: elevated, flat, depressed, traumatic Induration Limitation or freedom of movement of tongue Frena; tongue-tie	Large muscular tongue influences retraction, gag reflex, accessibility for instrumentation Film placement problems
13. Saliva	Quantity; quality (thick, ropy) Evidence of dry mouth; lip wetting Tongue coating	Reduced in certain diseases, by certain drugs Special dental caries control program Influence on instrumentation Need for saliva substitute
14. Hard palate (Figure 12-6A)	Height, contour, color Appearance of rugae Tori, growths, ulcers	Need for referral, biopsy, cytology Signs of tongue thrust, deviate swallow Influence on radiographic film placement
15. Soft palate, uvula (Figure 12-6B)	Color, size, shape Petechiae Ulcers, growths	Referral, biopsy, cytology Large uvula influences gag reflex
16. Tonsillar region, throat (Figure 12-6B)	Tonsils: size and shape Color, size, surface characteristics Lesions, trauma	Referral, biopsy, cytology Enlarged tonsils encourage gag reflex Throat infection, a sign for appointment postponement

C. Physical Characteristics

▶ *Size and shape*
- Record length and width in millimeters.
- The height of an elevated lesion may be significant.
- Use a probe to measure, as shown in Figure 12-12.

▶ *Color*
- Red, pink, white, and red and white are the most commonly seen.
- Other more rare lesions may be blue, purple, gray, yellow, black, or brown.

▶ *Surface texture*
- A lesion may have a smooth or an irregular surface.

- The texture may be papillary, verrucous or wartlike, fissured, corrugated, or crusted.
- Other descriptive terms are defined in Box 12-2 with the key words.

▶ *Consistency*
- Lesions may be soft, spongy, resilient, hard, or indurated.

MORPHOLOGIC CATEGORIES[10]

▶ Most lesions can be classified readily as *elevated*, *depressed*, or *flat* as they relate to the normal level of the skin or mucosa.

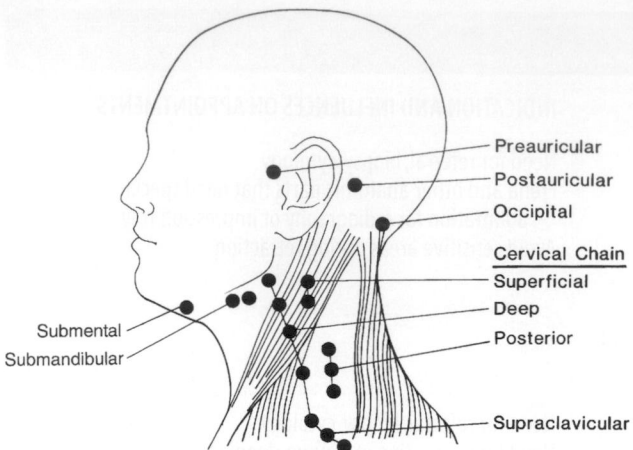

FIGURE 12-8 Lymph Nodes. The locations of the major lymph nodes into which the vessels of the facial and oral regions drain.

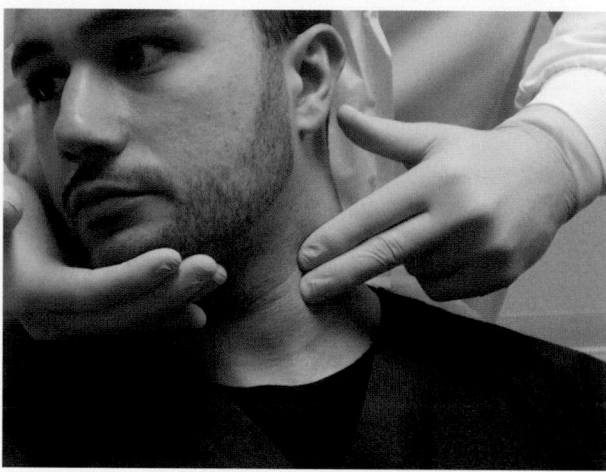

FIGURE 12-9 Cervical Node Palpation. Left anterior cervical lymph node chain is examined. Finger tips gently press and roll nodes along the length of the sternocleidomastoid muscle.

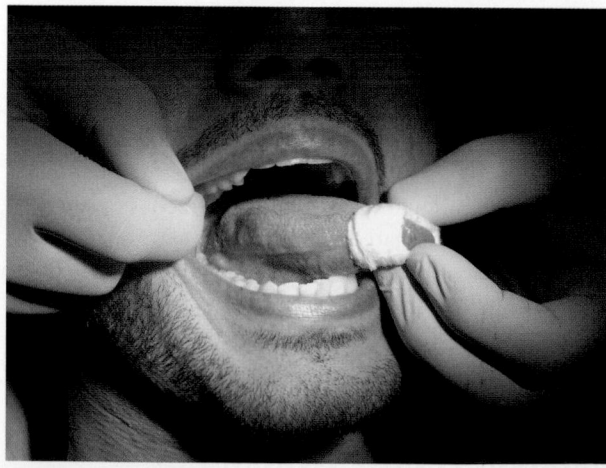

FIGURE 12-10 Examination of the Tongue. To observe the posterior third of the tongue and the attachment to the floor of the mouth, hold the tongue with a gauze sponge, retract the cheek, and move the tongue out, first to one side and then the other, as each section of the mucosa is carefully examined.

▶ Flowcharts Figures 12-13A elevated lesions, Figure 12-13B depressed lesions, and Figure 12-13C flat lesions break down the terms used for describing lesions in each category.

I. Elevated Lesions (Figure 12-13A)

An elevated lesion is above the plane of the skin or mucosa. Elevated lesions are considered *blisterform* or *nonblisterform*.

▶ Blisterform

Blisterform lesions contain fluid and are usually soft and translucent. They may be vesicles, pustules, or bullae.

- *Vesicle*: A vesicle is a small (1 cm or less in diameter), circumscribed lesion with a thin surface covering. It may contain serum or mucin and appear white.
- *Pustule*: A pustule may be more or less than 5 mm in diameter. It contains pus. Pus gives the pustule a yellowish color.
- *Bulla*: A bulla is large (more than 1 cm). It is filled with fluid, usually mucin or serum, but may contain blood. The color depends on the fluid content.

▶ Nonblisterform

Nonblisterform lesions are solid and do not contain fluid. They may be papules, nodules, tumors, or plaques. Papules, nodules, and tumors are also characterized by the base or attachment. As shown in Figure 12-14, the *pedunculated* lesion is attached by a narrow stalk or pedicle, whereas the *sessile* lesion has a base as wide as the lesion itself.

- *Papule*: A papule is a small (pinhead to 5 mm in diameter), solid lesion that may be pointed, rounded, or flat topped.
- *Nodule*: A nodule is larger than a papule (greater than 5 mm but less than 2 cm).
- *Tumor*: A tumor is 2 cm or greater in width. In this context, "tumor" means a general swelling or enlargement and does not refer to neoplasm, either benign or malignant.
- *Plaque*: A plaque is a slightly raised lesion with a broad, flat top. It is usually larger than 5 mm in diameter, with a "pasted on" appearance.

II. Depressed Lesions (Figure 12-13B)

A depressed lesion is below the level of the skin or mucosa. The outline may be regular or irregular, and there may be a flat or raised border around the depression. The depth can be described as superficial or deep. A deep lesion is greater than 3 mm deep.

▶ Ulcer

Most depressed lesions are ulcers and represent a loss of continuity of the epithelium. The center is often gray to yellow, surrounded by a red border. An ulcer may result from the rupture of an elevated lesion (vesicle, pustule, or bulla).

Draw outlines of abnormalities in proper locations
MUCOSAL ABNORMALITIES

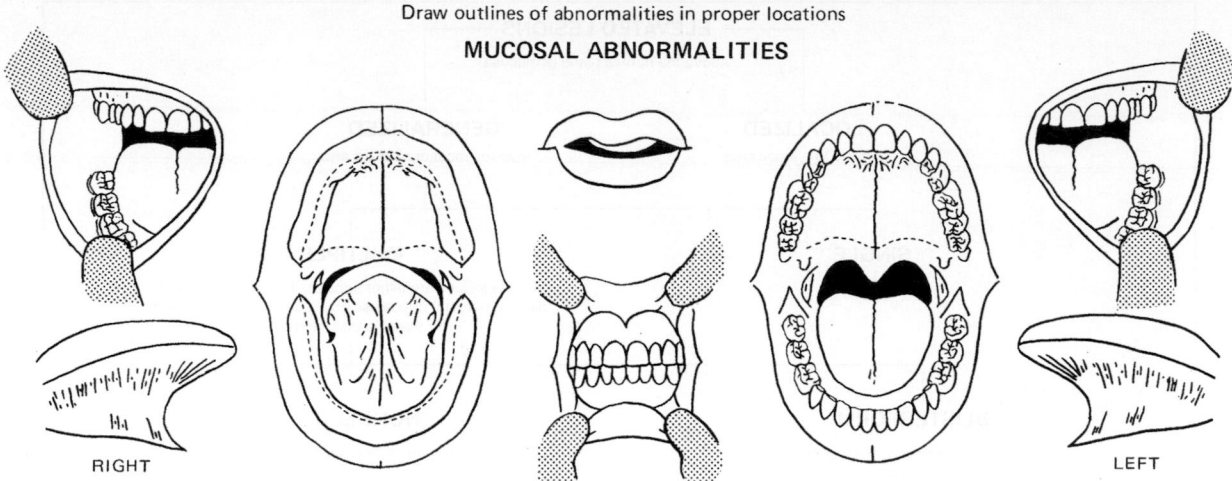

RIGHT   LEFT

FIGURE 12-11 Record Form for Clinical Findings. As part of a clinical examination record form, deviations from normal can be drawn to show the location and relative size. (Courtesy of the University of Southern California School of Dentistry.)

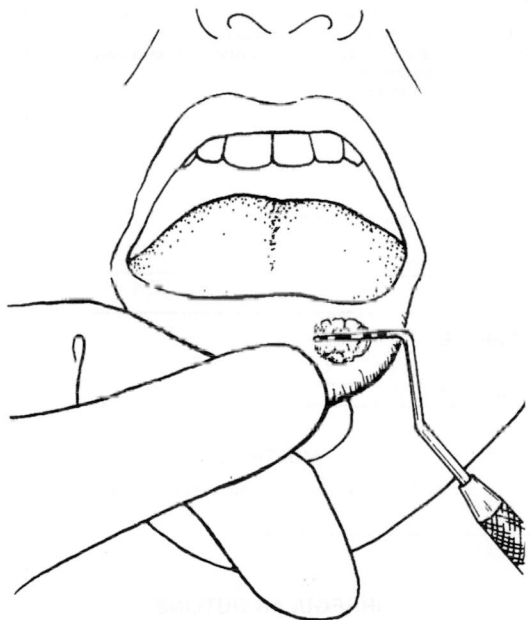

FIGURE 12-12 Use of a Probe to Measure a Lesion. In addition to the exact location, the width and length of a lesion is recorded. Using the probe provides a convenient method.

▶ Erosion

An erosion is a shallow, depressed lesion that does not extend through the epithelium to the underlying tissue.

III. Flat Lesions (Figure 12-13C)

A flat lesion is on the same level as the normal skin or oral mucosa. Flat lesions may occur as single or multiple lesions and have a regular or irregular form.

▶ A *macule* is a circumscribed area not elevated above the surrounding skin or mucosa.

• It may be identified by its color, which contrasts with the surrounding normal tissues.

IV. Other Descriptive Terms

▶ *Crust*: An outer layer, covering, or scab that may have formed from coagulation or drying of blood, serum, or pus, or a combination. A crust may form after a vesicle breaks; for example, the skin lesion of chicken pox is first a macule, then a papule, then a vesicle, and then a crust.

▶ *Erythema*: Red area of variable size and shape.

▶ *Exophytic*: Growing outward.

▶ *Indurated*: Hardened.

▶ *Papillary*: Resembling a small, nipple-shaped projection or elevation.

▶ *Petechiae*: Minute hemorrhagic spots of pinhead to pinpoint size.

▶ *Pseudomembrane*: A loose membranous layer of exudate containing organisms, precipitated fibrin, necrotic cells, and inflammatory cells produced during an inflammatory reaction on the surface of a tissue.

▶ *Polyp*: Any mass of tissue that projects outward or upward from the normal surface level.

▶ *Punctate*: Marked with points or dots differentiated from the surrounding surface by color, elevation, or texture.

▶ *Torus*: Bony elevation or prominence usually found on the midline of the hard palate (torus palatinus) and the lingual surface of the mandible (torus mandibularis) in the premolar area.

▶ *Verrucous* (verrucose): Rough, wartlike.

ORAL CANCER

▶ The oral cavity, pharynx larynx, paranasal sinuses and nasal cavity, and salivary glands are regions of the head and neck where cancer can begin.[11]

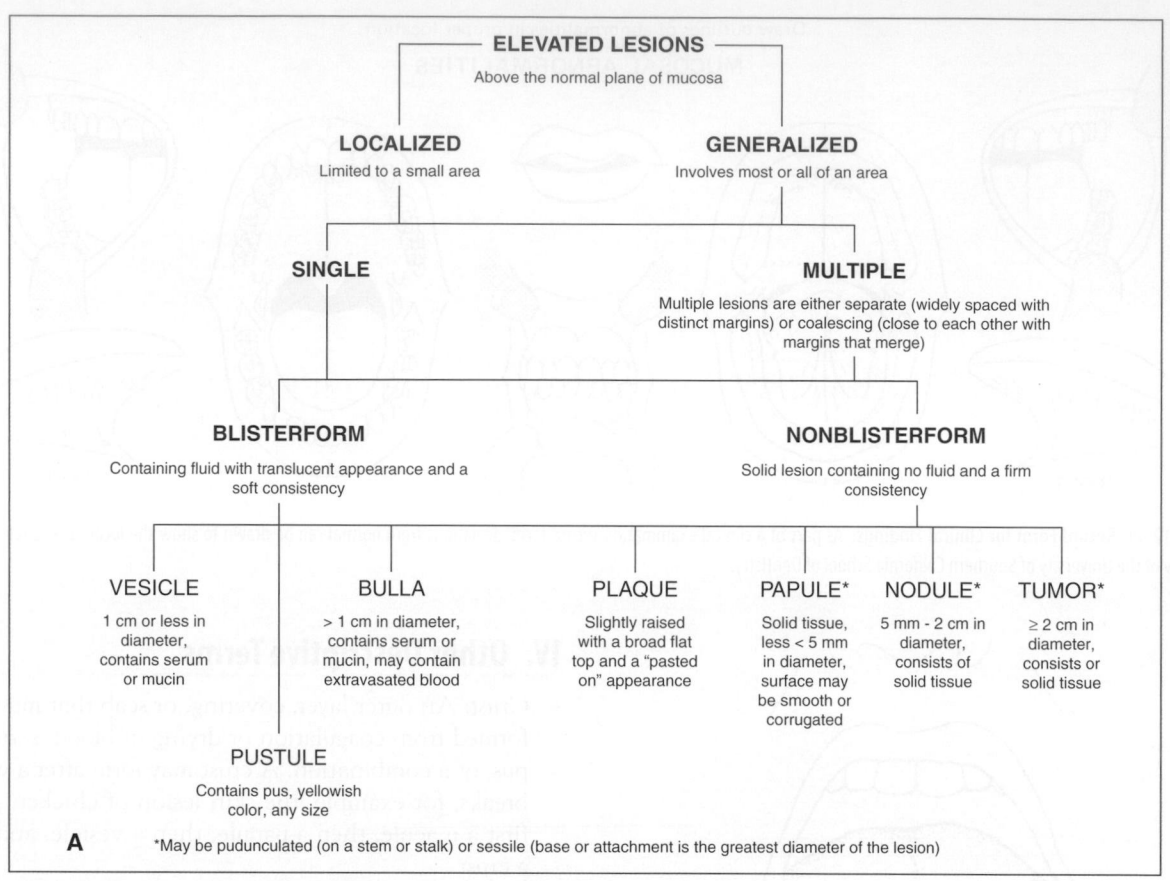

ELEVATED LESIONS
Above the normal plane of mucosa

LOCALIZED
Limited to a small area

GENERALIZED
Involves most or all of an area

SINGLE

MULTIPLE
Multiple lesions are either separate (widely spaced with distinct margins) or coalescing (close to each other with margins that merge)

BLISTERFORM
Containing fluid with translucent appearance and a soft consistency

NONBLISTERFORM
Solid lesion containing no fluid and a firm consistency

VESICLE
1 cm or less in diameter, contains serum or mucin

BULLA
> 1 cm in diameter, contains serum or mucin, may contain extravasated blood

PLAQUE
Slightly raised with a broad flat top and a "pasted on" appearance

PAPULE*
Solid tissue, less < 5 mm in diameter, surface may be smooth or corrugated

NODULE*
5 mm - 2 cm in diameter, consists of solid tissue

TUMOR*
≥ 2 cm in diameter, consists or solid tissue

PUSTULE
Contains pus, yellowish color, any size

A *May be pudunculated (on a stem or stalk) or sessile (base or attachment is the greatest diameter of the lesion)

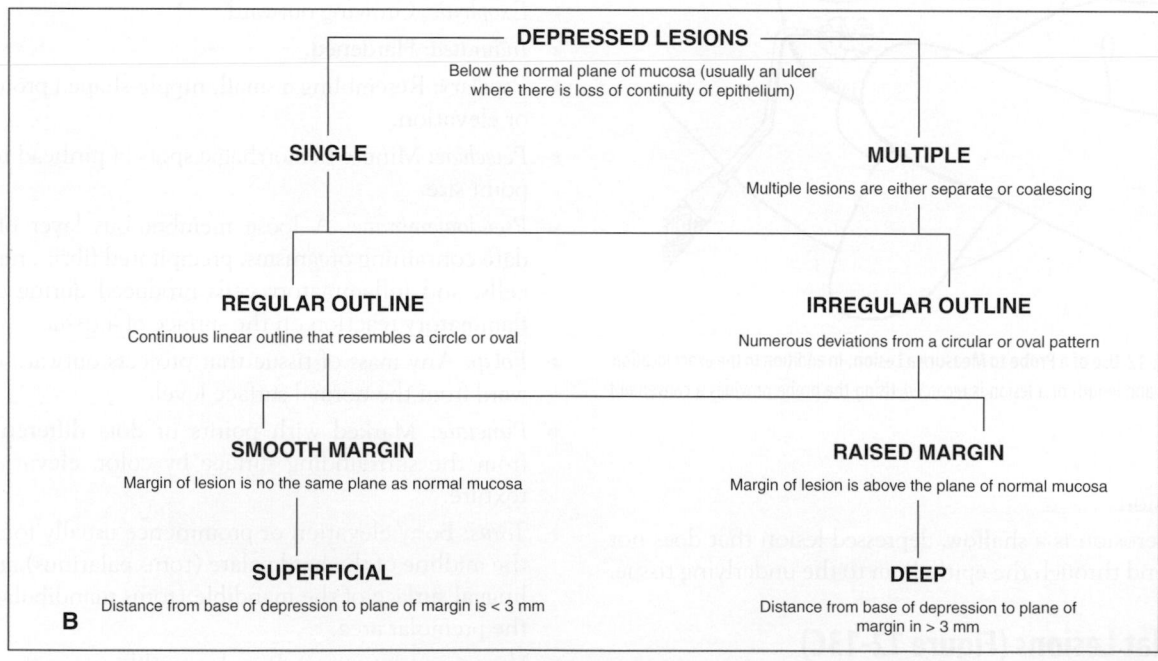

DEPRESSED LESIONS
Below the normal plane of mucosa (usually an ulcer where there is loss of continuity of epithelium)

SINGLE

MULTIPLE
Multiple lesions are either separate or coalescing

REGULAR OUTLINE
Continuous linear outline that resembles a circle or oval

IRREGULAR OUTLINE
Numerous deviations from a circular or oval pattern

SMOOTH MARGIN
Margin of lesion is no the same plane as normal mucosa

RAISED MARGIN
Margin of lesion is above the plane of normal mucosa

SUPERFICIAL
Distance from base of depression to plane of margin is < 3 mm

DEEP
Distance from base of depression to plane of margin in > 3 mm

B

FIGURE 12-13 A: Flow chart: description of elevated soft tissue lesions. Elevated lesions are blisterform or nonblisterform. **B:** Flow chart: description of depressed soft tissue lesions. Depressed lesions are below the normal plane of the mucosa, usually an ulcer where there is a loss of continuity of epithelium. **C:** Flow chart: description of flat soft tissue lesions. Flat lesions are on the level normal plane of the mucosa. (A–C reprinted with permission from McCann A. Describing soft tissue lesions of the oral cavity. *Dental Hygienist News.* 1992;5:9.)

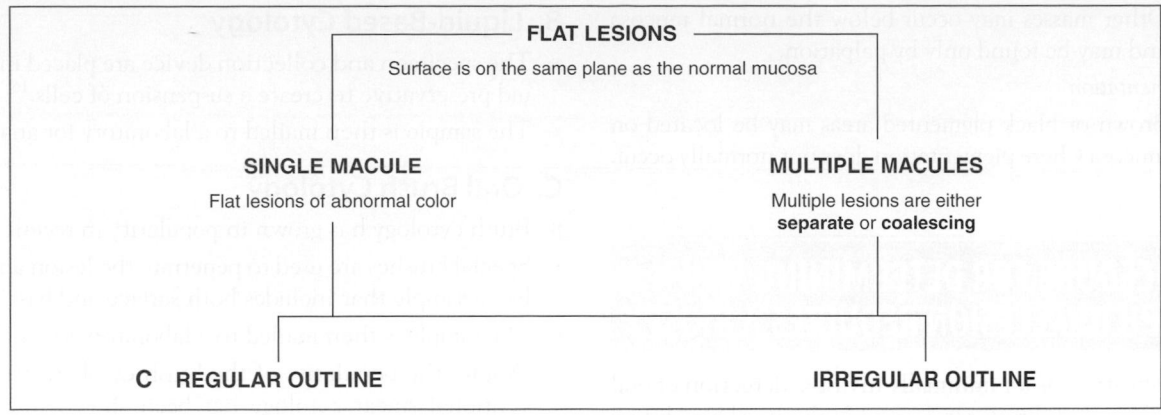

FLAT LESIONS
Surface is on the same plane as the normal mucosa

SINGLE MACULE
Flat lesions of abnormal color

MULTIPLE MACULES
Multiple lesions are either **separate** or **coalescing**

C   REGULAR OUTLINE

IRREGULAR OUTLINE

FIGURE 12-13 (*Continued*)

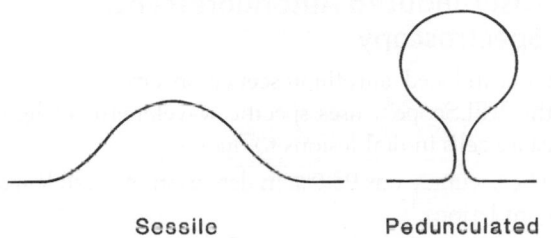

Sessile   Pedunculated

FIGURE 12-14 Attachment of Nonblisterform Lesions. The *sessile lesion has a base as wide as the lesion itself*; the pedunculated lesion is attached by a narrow stalk or pedicle.

- Cancers of the head and neck begin in the squamous cells that line moist, mucosal surfaces of the mouth, nose, and throat.[2,12]
- Salivary glands contain different types of cells that can also become cancerous.[2,12]

▶ Because the early lesions are generally symptomless, they may go unnoticed and unreported by the patient. Observation by the dentist or dental hygienist is the principal method for the detection of oral cancer.

▶ The first step is to examine the entire face, neck, and oral mucous membrane of each patient at the initial examination and at each continuing care appointment (Table 12-1).

▶ It is necessary to know how to conduct the oral examination, where oral cancer occurs most frequently, what an early cancerous lesion may look like, and what to do when such a lesion is found.

▶ In addition to the early lesions of oral cancers, the oral manifestations of neoplasms or abnormal growth of tissue, elsewhere in the body as well as the oral manifestations of chemotherapy, can be recognized.

▶ Most oral cancers are related to tobacco and/or excessive alcohol use.[1,11,13]

▶ Additional risk factors include infection with HPV-16 type, increased age >40, and sun exposure to the lips.[2]

▶ Increasing incidence of oral cancers in adults younger than 40 suggests all patients, regardless of age or risk factors, must be screened for oral cancer.[1,14]

I. Location

▶ The most common sites for oral cancer are the lateral borders of the tongue, floor of the mouth, the lips, and the soft palate complex.

II. Appearance of Early Cancer

Early oral cancer takes many forms and may resemble a variety of common oral lesions. All types need to be examined with suspicion. Five basic forms are listed here.

▶ *White areas*
- White areas vary from a filmy, barely visible change in the mucosa to heavy, thick, heaped-up areas of dry white keratinized tissue.
- Fissures, ulcers, or areas of induration in a white area are most indicative of malignancy.
- *Leukoplakia* is a white patch or plaque that cannot be scraped off or characterized as any other disease. It may be associated with physical or chemical agents and the use of tobacco.

▶ *Red areas*
- *Erythroplakia* is a term used to designate lesions of the oral mucosa that appear as bright red patches or plaques.
- Lesions appear red, of velvety consistency, and may coincide with small ulcers.
- *Erythroplakia is a rare oral precancerous lesion* that cannot be characterized as any specific disease.[12]

▶ *Ulcers*
- Ulcers may have flat or raised margins.
- Palpation may reveal induration.

▶ *Masses*
- Papillary masses, sometimes with ulcerated areas, occur as elevations above the surrounding tissues.

- Other masses may occur below the normal mucosa and may be found only by palpation.
▶ *Pigmentation*
  - Brown or black pigmented areas may be located on mucosa where pigmentation does not normally occur.

PROCEDURE FOR DETERMINING WHEN A SUSPICIOUS LESION REQUIRES A BIOSPY

▶ Diagnostic aids for minimally invasive detection of oral cancer include brush cytology and toluidine blue, diffuse tissue reflectance, and laser-induced autofluorescence.[15]

▶ Alternatively, as designated by the dentist, a lesion may be biopsied immediately and sent to a laboratory for evaluation. Biopsy confirmation is considered the gold standard outcome.

I. Exfoliative Cytology

▶ Exfoliative cytology is a minimally invasive approach to obtain a cell sample for diagnosis of a suspicious lesion.[16]

▶ Exfoliated cells and the cells beneath (basal cells) are removed by physical procedures such as surface scraping or brushing, rinses, or saliva specimens.[16,17]
  - A number of studies have been conducted to evaluate the different instruments used for obtaining cytology specimens.
  - Basic requirements include: easy to use, minimal patient discomfort, and collects enough cells for evaluation.[16]
  - Basal cells are necessary to collect ribonucleic acid to improve diagnostic accuracy.[16]
  - Except for candidiasis, treatment cannot be determined only by smear technique results. After a positive smear, a biopsy is needed for definitive diagnosis.

A. Cytological Smear

▶ The cytologic smear is a diagnostic aid in which surface cells of a suspicious lesion are removed for microscopic evaluation by noninvasive means such as a spatula or brush.

▶ Cytology is useful for identifying *Candida albicans* organisms in patients with suspected candidiasis (moniliasis).

▶ Limitations of smear technique include the following:
  - The smear detects only surface lesions.
  - It is difficult or impossible to scrape deep enough to obtain representative cells from a heavily keratinized lesion.
  - Because research has shown that the smear technique is not diagnostically reliable (there can be "false negatives," which turn out to be positive biopsies), a negative report cannot be considered conclusive.[16]

B. Liquid-Based Cytology

▶ The specimen and collection device are placed in a liquid preservative to create a suspension of cells.[16]

▶ The sample is then mailed to a laboratory for analysis.

C. Oral Brush Cytology

▶ Brush cytology has grown in popularity in recent years.

▶ Special brushes are used to penetrate the lesion and collect a sample that includes both surface and basal cells.

▶ The sample is then mailed to a laboratory for analysis.

▶ Despite the popularity of the brush cytology, the conventional smear cytology has been shown to have a higher specificity and be less expensive.[17]

II. Spectroscopy

A. Laser-Induced Autofluorescence Spectroscopy

▶ Laser-induced autofluorescence spectroscopy, such as the VELScope®, uses specific wavelengths of light to cause cells in oral lesions to fluoresce.

▶ The accuracy was 95.9% in detection of possible malignant lesions.[17]

▶ Limitation: Not effective for lesions on the lateral and dorsal tongue or vermillion border of the lip because normal mucosa in these areas has a fluorescent spectrum similar to malignant cells.

B. Diffuse Reflectance Spectroscopy

▶ Diffuse reflectance spectroscopy uses a fiber-optic probe to direct light to the suspicious lesion.

▶ Malignant cells scatter light differently than normal cells and this difference is measured.[17]

▶ This method is 96.5% accurate in identifying possible malignant lesions and the most accurate noninvasive method.[17]

III. Biopsy

▶ Biopsy is the removal and microscopic examination of a section of tissue or other material from the body for the purposes of diagnosis.
  - A biopsy is either *excisional*, when the entire lesion is removed, or *incisional*, when a representative section from the lesion is taken.
  - Considered the "gold standard" in oral cancer diagnosis.[18]

▶ *Indications for biopsy*
  - Any unusual oral lesion that cannot be identified with clinical certainty must be biopsied.
  - Any lesion that has not healed in 2 weeks is considered suspicious for malignancy until proven otherwise.
  - A persistent, thick, white, hyperkeratotic lesion and any mass (elevated or not) that does not break through the surface epithelium.

BOX 12-2
Anatomical Landmarks of the Oral Cavity

Refer to Figures 12-6A,B and 12-7

Lips	Lingual vein	Palatine tonsils
Vermillion border	Sublingual fold	Pharyngeal adenoid tonsils
Labial commissure	Plica fimbriata	Tonsillar pillars
Labial mucosa	Sublingual caruncle	Tongue:
Buccal mucosa	Median sulcus	Dorsal
Philtrum	Lingual tonsils	Ventral
Nasolabial groove	Lingual frenum	Lateral border
Fauces	Ankyloglossia	Filiform papilla
Oral pharynx	Marginal gingiva	Fungiform papilla
Vestibule	Attached gingiva	Folate papillae
Buccal vestibule	Free gingival groove	Circumvallate papilla
Buccinator muscle	Canine eminence	Lingual tonsils
Labial	Pterygomandibular raphe	Stensen's duct
Buccal	Parotid papilla	Maxillary tuberosity
Mucobuccal fold	Midpalatine raphe	Retromolar pad
Buccal frenum	Palatine rugae	Ramus of mandible
Labial frenum	Fovea palatine	Zygomatic arch
Exostosis	Torus palatinus	Mandibular tori
Whartons duct	Incisive papilla	Alveolar mucosa
	Uvula	Mylohyoid muscle

▶ *Pathology report*

If the laboratory report from the pathologist indicates Class III through Class V from a cytology smear, a biopsy is required.

- *Class I:* Normal.
- *Class II:* Atypical, but not suggestive of malignant cells.
- *Class III:* Uncertain (possible for cancer).
- *Class IV:* Probable for cancer.
- *Class V:* Positive for cancer.

DOCUMENTATION

Documentation in the permanent record of a patient who needed a biopsy (or smear) because of a questionable cancerous lesion will contain a minimum such as the following:

▶ Every detail of the oral examination and follow-up procedures with reports from consultants, laboratories, medical follow-up, and outcomes.

▶ Recommendations for the frequency of a complete oral examination, at future dental hygiene maintenance appointments.

▶ Review of all lifestyle habits that may provide a cause for such an oral lesion to appear in the first place with recommendations for specific preventive methods.

▶ A progress note representing the patient's first maintenance appointment following the incident of the biopsy and learning the lesion was not cancerous may be reviewed in Box 12-3.

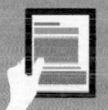

BOX 12-3
Example Documentation: Patient with an Oral Lesion

S–50-year-old female presents for routine preventive maintenance with no current concerns at today's appointment. When questioned during intraoral examination, patient recalls recently accidently biting her tongue.

O–Patient smokes 1 pack cigarettes daily/past 35 years and admits to drinking 1–2 beers nightly; left lateral border of tongue erythematous lesion 1 cm × 5 mm, flat.

A–High risk for oral cancer, erythematous lesion requires further evaluation.

P–Discuss concerns with patient regarding high risk behaviors of tobacco use and alcohol. Recommend 2-week follow-up for reevaluation of lesion and further referral if no improvement. Recommended and offered tobacco cessation information.

Signed _____, RDH

Date _____.

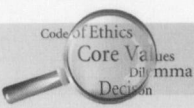

EVERYDAY ETHICS

Abby and Sylvia are the two part-time dental hygienists in Dr. Anthony's practice. They practice on different days at the office so rarely see each other except to attend local dental hygiene association meetings. Most patients know both hygienists and may be scheduled with either depending on available time.

Mr. Peters came in for his 3-month maintenance appointment carrying his unlit pipe as usual. This time his appointment was with Abby, and jokes were exchanged about the pipe. During the intraoral examination, Abby found a red lesion on the side of his tongue that was about 4 mm wide. She asked him if he had seen it and his answer was, "Oh yeah, Sylvia mentioned it when I was here last time." Abby glanced at the record and noted that his last date was over 4 months ago. Nothing could be found in the patient's dental record that mentioned any oral lesions.

Questions for Consideration

1. Which of the dental hygiene code values (Table II-1, in Section II Introduction) are involved here? How?

2. Consider the questions in Table VI, Section VI Introduction to help Abby decide which way to go to help Mr. Peters, and improve office policies.

3. Privately, Abby is upset, and she is determined that this needs to be discussed with both Sylvia and Dr. Anthony. Dr. Anthony has never specified a policy for this type of issue. Where and how can she approach them and what recommendations does she need to propose for an office policy?

Factors To Teach The Patient

▷ Reasons for a careful extraoral and intraoral examination at each maintenance appointment.
▷ Guidance and support on tobacco cessation and provide appropriate referral.
▷ How to conduct self-examination monthly to watch for changes in oral tissues and identify lesions that last longer than 2 weeks. Examination includes the face, neck, lips, gingiva, cheeks, tongue, palate, and throat. Any changes are reported to the dentist and the dental hygienist.
▷ General dietary and nutritional influences on the health of the oral tissues.
  ▷ Benefits of diet rich in fruits and vegetables.
▷ How the oral cavity tends to reflect the general health.
▷ The warning signs of oral cancer from the American Cancer Society[13] including the following:
  ▷ A swelling, lump, or growth anywhere, with or without pain.
  ▷ White scaly patches or red velvety areas.
  ▷ Any sore that does not heal promptly (within 2 weeks).
  ▷ Numbness or tingling.
  ▷ Excessive dryness or wetness.
  ▷ Prolonged hoarseness, sore throats, persistent coughing, or the feeling of a "lump in the throat."
  ▷ Difficulty with swallowing.
  ▷ Difficulty in opening the mouth.

References

1. Rethman MP, Carpenter W, Cohen EEW, et al. Evidence-based clinical recommendations regarding screening for oral squamous cell carcinomas. *J Am Dent Assoc.* 2010; 141(5):509–520.

2. Sciubba JJ. Oral cancer and its detection: history-taking and the diagnostic phase of management. *J Am Dent Assoc.* 2001;132(11, Suppl):12S–18S.

3. Council of Allied Dental Program Directors. Compendium of curriculum guidelines for allied dental education programs. http://www.adea.org/uploadedFiles/ADEA/Content_Conversion_Final/about_adea/governance/CompendiumofCurriculumGuidelinesforAlliedDentalEducationPrograms.pdf. Accessed February 9, 2013.

4. National Cancer Institute. Head and neck cancers. http://www.cancer.gov/cancertopics/factsheet/Sites-Types/head-and-neck. Accessed January 9, 2013.

5. The National Institute of Dental and Craniofacial Research. Detecting oral cancer: a guide for health care professionals. http://www.nidcr.nih.gov/oralhealth/topics/oralcancer/detectingoralcancer.htm. Accessed January 9, 2013.

6. Pinto A, Glick M. Management of patients with thyroid disease: oral health considerations. *J Am Dent Assoc.* 2002;133(7):849–858.

7. McNeil C, Mohl ND, Rugh JD, et al. Temporomandibular disorders: diagnosis, management, education, and research. *J Am Dent Assoc.* 1990;120(3):253–255,257.

8. Coakley MC. Temporomandibular joint dysfunction (TMJ): the role of the dental hygienist. *J Dent Hyg.* 1988;62(10):521–526.

9. The Oral Cancer Foundation. Referral-form-2013.pdf. http://oralcancerfoundation.org/events/pdf/Referral-form-2013.pdf. Accessed February 9, 2013.

10. McCann AL WR. A method for describing soft tissue lesions of the oral cavity. *Dent Hyg.* 1987;61(5):219–223.

11. The National Institute of Dental and Craniofacial Research. Oral cancer. http://www.nidcr.nih.gov/oralhealth/topics/oralcancer/. Accessed January 9, 2013.

12. Speight PM, Farthing PM, Bouquot JE. The pathology of oral cancer and precancer. *Curr Diagn Pathol.* 1996;3(3):165–176.

13. American Cancer Society. What are the key statistics about oral cavity and oropharyngeal cancers? http://www.cancer.org/cancer/oralcavityandoropharyngealcancer/detailedguide/oral-cavity-and-oropharyngeal-cancer-key-statistics. Accessed January 9, 2013.

14. Shiboski CH, Schmidt BL, Jordan RCK. Tongue and tonsil carcinoma: increasing trends in the U.S. population ages 20-44 years. *Cancer.* 2005;103(9):1843–1849.

15. Patton LL, Epstein JB, Kerr AR. Adjunctive techniques for oral cancer examination and lesion diagnosis a systematic review of the literature. *J Am Dent Assoc.* 2008;139(7):896–905.

16. Perez-Sayansm M, Somoza-Martin JM, Barros-Angueira F, et al. Exfoliative cytology for diagnosing oral cancer. *Biotech Histochem.* 2010;85(3):177–187.

17. Fuller C, Camilon R, Nguyen S, et al. Adjunctive diagnostic techniques for oral lesions of unknown malignant potential: systematic review with meta-analysis. *Head Neck.* 2015 May;37(5):755–62.

18. Kämmerer PW, Rahimi-Nedjat RK, Ziebart T, Bemsch A, Walter C, Al-Nawas B, Koch FP. A chemiluminescent light system in combination with toluidine blue to assess suspicious oral lesions-clinical evaluation and review of the literature. *Clin Oral Investig.* 2015 Mar;19(2):459–466.

ENHANCE YOUR UNDERSTANDING

the Point® DIGITAL CONNECTIONS
(see the inside front cover for access information)
- **Audio glossary**
- **Quiz bank**

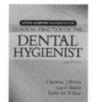

SUPPORT FOR LEARNING
(available separately; visit lww.com)
- *Active Learning Workbook for Clinical Practice of the Dental Hygienist, 12th Edition*

prepU INDIVIDUALIZED REVIEW
(available separately; visit lww.com)
- **Adaptive quizzing with *prepU for Wilkins' Clinical Practice of the Dental Hygienist***

13

Dental Radiographic Imaging

Janet M. Gruber, RDH, MPA

CHAPTER OUTLINE

LEARNING OBJECTIVES

After studying this chapter, the student will be able to:

1. Compare different imaging systems, and describe the advantages and disadvantages of each.

2. Describe factors that influence the finished radiograph.

3. Identify electrical components located in an X-ray unit's tube head and describe how radiographs are produced.

4. Explain clinician and patient radiation protection guidelines and published recommendations for patient selection and exposure.

5. Describe procedures for image receptor placement and X-ray beam alignment for various types of dental radiographic exposures.

Radiographic images are integral assessment components useful when planning comprehensive care for a patient. They provide the clinician with important diagnostic tools that can be used:

► To detect lesions, diseases, and other conditions of teeth and supporting structures.

► To localize foreign objects.

► To assess growth and development.

► To document changes in, and progress of, a condition over time.[1]

The dentist is responsible for determining the need for radiographs.

► Designation of the number and types of dental exposures is made selectively only after a review of the patient's health history and a complete clinical examination.[2]

► A history of oral and body exposures to radiation is recommended.

► Excessive dental exposure to low levels of ionizing radiation cannot be justified.[3]

The objective in radiography is to use procedures that expose the patient to the least possible amount of radiation to produce radiographs of the greatest interpretive value. The first consideration is to limit the number of exposures to those that have been deemed necessary.

This chapter provides a summary of terminology and fundamentals of:

► X-ray production

► Procedures for all image receptor exposures and traditional film processing

► Safety factors

► Analysis of the completed radiographs

► Suggestions for patient instruction.

Selected terms used in the study of radiography are listed and defined in Box 13-1. Box 13-2 provides a list of universally used abbreviations.

HOW X-RAYS ARE PRODUCED

X-ray energy is electromagnetic ionizing radiation of very short wavelengths, resulting from the bombardment of a target made of tungsten by highly accelerated electrons in a high vacuum. Electric and magnetic fields positioned at right angles to one another produce the electromagnetic energy.

The various types of energy in the electromagnetic spectrum have similar attributes. The properties of X-rays are listed in Box 13-3.

Essential to X-ray production are:

► A source of electrons

► A high voltage to accelerate the electrons

► A target to stop the electrons.

The parts of the tube and the circuits within the machine are designed to provide these elements.

I. The X-Ray Tube (Figure 13-1)

A. Protective Tube Housing

► A heavy metal enclosure houses the X-ray tube and reduces primary radiation to permissible exposure levels.

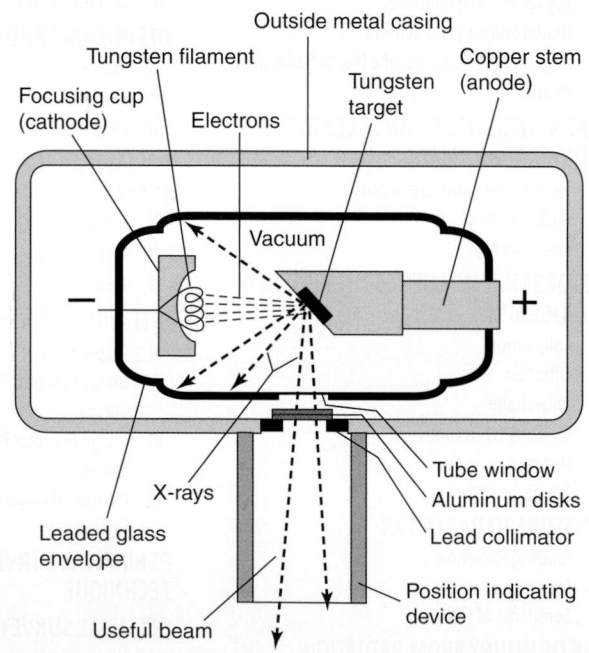

FIGURE 13-1 X-Ray Tube. High-speed electrons flowing from cathode to anode hit the tungsten target, and create X-ray photons. X-rays exit through the tube window and PID.

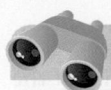

BOX 13-1   KEY WORDS: General Radiography Terms

Ammeter: an instrument for measuring electric current in amperes.

Attenuation: the process by which a beam of radiation is reduced in intensity when passing through some material; the combination of absorption and scattering processes leads to a decrease in flux density of the beam when projected through matter.

Cassette: a light-tight container in which X-ray image receptors are placed for exposure to X-radiation; usually backed with lead to reduce the effect of backscatter radiation; may be made of cardboard, plastic, or of metal with an exposure side of bakelite, aluminum, plastic, or magnesium and containing an intensifying screen(s).

Image receptors: traditional film and digital sensors used to capture and record a radiographic image.

Digital sensors: include CCD, CMOS, and PSP plates.

Impulse: the burst of radiation generated during a half cycle of alternating current (AC); film exposure time is measured in impulses.

Intensifying screen: a card or plastic sheet coated with fluorescent material positioned singly or in pairs in a cassette. When the cassette is exposed to X-radiation, the visible light from the fluorescent image on the screen adds to the latent image produced directly by X-radiation.

Irradiation: exposure to radiation; one speaks of radiation therapy and irradiation of a body part.

Latent image: the invisible change produced in an X-ray film emulsion by the action of X-radiation or light from which the visible image is subsequently developed and fixed chemically.

Paraclinical procedures: supplemental to chairside clinical procedures; includes processing of the films and mounting of radiographs for diagnostic and clinical use.

Penumbra: the secondary shadow that surrounds the periphery of the primary shadow; in radiography, it is the blurred margin of an image detail (geometric unsharpness).

Photoelectric effect: the ejection of bound electrons by an incident photon such that the whole energy of the

photon is absorbed and transitional or characteristic X-ray emissions are produced.

Photon: a finite bundle of energy of visible light or electromagnetic radiation.

PSP Plates: photostimuable phosphor plates. Image receptor used in digital imaging to capture and record a radiographic image.

Radiation: the emission and propagation of energy through space or a material medium in the form of waves or particles. Types of radiation are defined in Box 13-4.

Radiograph: a visible image on a radiation-sensitive film emulsion or a digitized image on a computer monitor after exposure of the image receptor to ionizing radiation that has passed through an area, region, or substance of interest.

Radiography: the art and science of making radiographs.

Radiologic health: the art and science of protecting human beings from injury by radiation, as well as of promoting better health through beneficial applications of radiation.

Radiology: that branch of science that deals with the use of radiant energy in the diagnosis and treatment of disease.

Radiolucency: the appearance of dark images on a radiograph as a result of the greater amount of radiation that penetrates low-density objects and reaches the image receptor.

Radiopacity: the appearance of light (white) images on a radiograph as a result of the greater amount of radiation that is absorbed by dense objects and does not reach the image receptor.

Rare earth: commonly used to refer to intensifying screens containing rare earth elements; it may also refer to a screen-film system used for X-ray imaging; the systems are considered "fast" exposure systems.

Rectification: conversion of alternating current (AC) to direct current (DC); a **rectifier** changes AC to DC.

Soma: the entire body with the exclusion of germ cells.
   Somatic: adj.

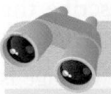

BOX 13-2   KEY WORDS: Abbreviations Used in Radiography

ALARA: as low as reasonably achievable
Gy: gray
HVL: half value layer
kVp: kilovolt peak
mA: milliampere
mAi: milliampere impulse
mAs: milliampere second
mGy: milligray
MPD: maximum permissible dose

mSv: millisievert
PID: position-indicating device
PSP: photostimuable phosphor plate
R: Roentgen
Rad: radiation-absorbed dose
Rem: Roentgen equivalent man
Sv: Sievert
XCP: extension cone paralleling

BOX 13-3

Properties of X-Rays

Characteristic
▷ Invisible
▷ No mass
▷ No weight

Travel
▷ In straight line; can be scattered
▷ At the speed of light

Wavelengths
▷ Have short wavelengths, high frequency
▷ Hard X-rays: short wavelengths, high penetration
▷ Soft X-rays: relatively longer wavelengths; relatively less penetrating; more likely to be absorbed into the tissue

Penetration
▷ Pass through matter, or
▷ Absorbed by matter, depending on atomic structure of matter

Causes
▷ Ionization
▷ Fluorescence of certain crystals
▷ Biologic changes in living cells

Produces
▷ A radiographic image

B. X-Ray Tube

► A highly evacuated leaded-glass tube composed of a cathode and an anode and surrounded by a specially refined oil with high insulating powers.

C. Cathode (–)

► Tungsten filament, which is a coiled wire heated to generate a cloud of electrons. It is a component of the low-voltage circuit.
► Molybdenum cup around the filament to focus the electrons toward the anode.

D. Anode (+)

► A tungsten target embedded in a copper stem, positioned at an angle to the electron beam.

E. Aperture

► The window through which the useful beam emerges from the tube; covered with a permanent seal of glass.

F. Aluminum Disks

► Thin (0.5-mm) sheets of aluminum placed over the aperture to filter out longer-wavelength X-rays.

G. Lead Diaphragm

► A lead collimator with a hole to restrict the size of the X-ray beam.

H. Position-Indicating Device (PID)

► Open-ended cylinder, or rectangle, that shapes and aims the X-ray beam.

II. Circuits

A circuit is the complete path over which an electrical current may flow. Two circuits are used to produce X-rays. Refer to Figure 13-2 to examine the electrical circuits in a dental X-ray machine. Two circuits used to produce X-rays are:

► Low-voltage filament circuit
► High-voltage cathode–anode circuit.

III. Transformers

A transformer increases or decreases the incoming voltage.
► *Autotransformer*
  • A voltage compensator that corrects minor variations in line voltage.
► *Filament step-down transformer*
  • Decreases the line voltage to approximately 3 volts to heat the filament and form the electron cloud.
► *High-voltage step-up transformer*
  • Increases the current from 110 V to 60 to 90 kVp (kilovoltage peak) to give electrons the required energy necessary to produce X-ray photons.

IV. Machine Control Devices

Machines vary, but, in general, when operating an X-ray machine, there are four factors to control: the power switch (to the electrical outlet), the kilovoltage, the milliamperage, and the time.

A. Voltage Control

Voltage is the unit of measurement used to describe the force that pushes an electric current through a circuit.
► *Circuit voltmeter*: Registers line voltage before voltage is stepped up by the transformer (with alternating current [AC], this is 110 V), or may register the kilovoltage that results after step-up.
► *kVp (selector)*: Used to change the line voltage to a selected kilovoltage (60–90 kVp).

B. Milliamperage Control

► *Ampere*: The unit of intensity of an electrical current produced by 1 V acting through a resistance of 1 Ω. A milliampere (mA) is 1/1,000 of an ampere.
► *Milliammeter*: Instrument used to select the actual current through the tube circuit during the time of exposure.

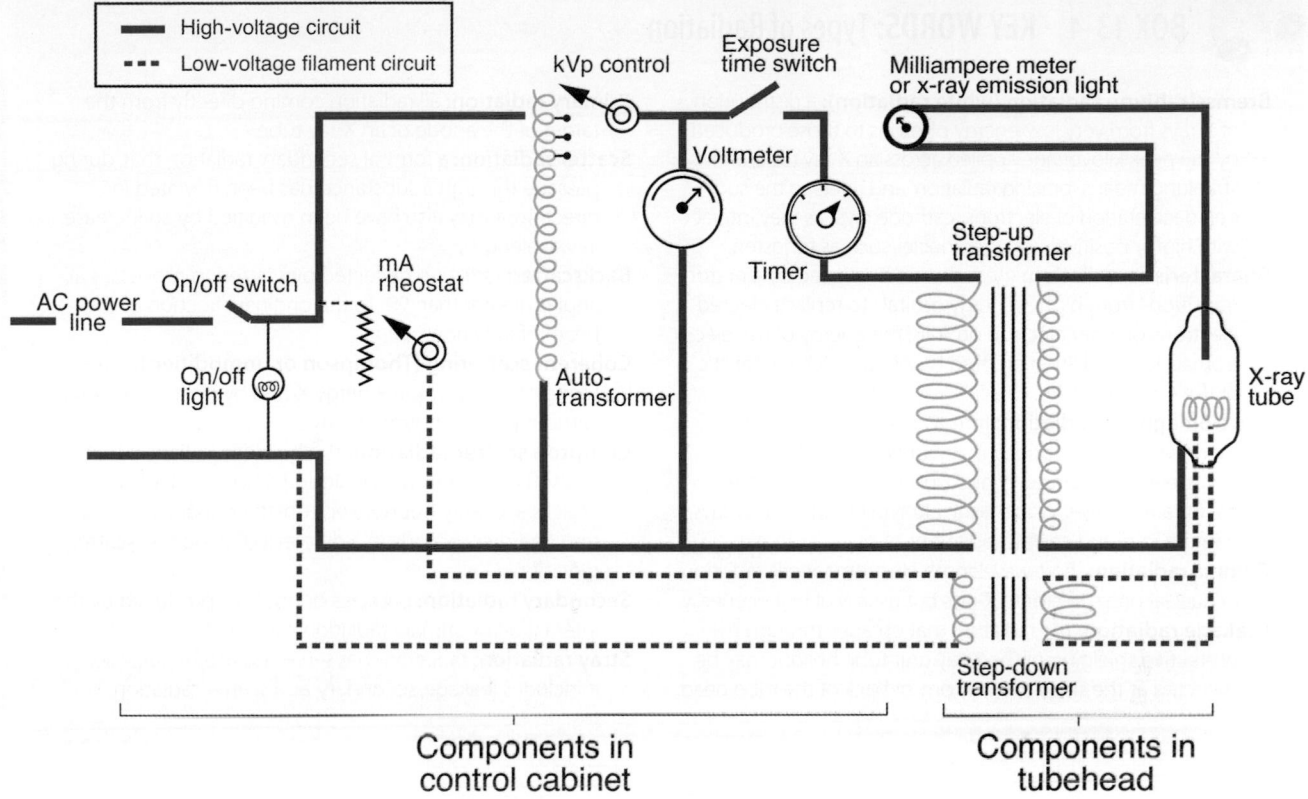

FIGURE 13-2 Dental X-Ray Machine Circuits. High- and low-voltage circuits in a dental X-ray machine demonstrating flow of electricity from the on/off switch to the X-ray tube head. (Adapted with permission from Olson SS. *Dental Radiography Laboratory Manual*. Philadelphia, PA: W.B. Saunders; 1995:40.)

C. Time Control

▶ *X-Ray timer*: A time switch mechanism used to control the length of the exposure time.

▶ *Time-delay switch*: Mechanism that applies power to the high-voltage circuit once the filament is heated.

▶ *Electronic timer*: Vacuum tube device; resets itself automatically to the last-used exposure time. The timer is calibrated in seconds or in impulses, with 60 *impulses* in each second (in a 60-cycle AC current).

V. Steps in the Production of X-rays

X-rays are produced when high-speed electrons are slowed down or stopped suddenly. The many types of radiation produced are defined in Box 13-4.

▶ Tungsten filament is heated, and a cloud of electrons is produced.

▶ Difference in electrical potential is developed between the anode and the cathode.

▶ Electrons traveling at a high speed are attracted to the anode from the cathode when the anode is charged positive and the cathode negative. When AC is used with a self-rectifying tube, the electrons are attracted back into the tungsten filament.

▶ Curvature of the molybdenum cup controls the direction of the electrons and causes them to be projected toward the focal spot.

▶ Reaction of the electrons as they strike the tungsten target results in loss of energy.

• Approximately 1% of the energy of electrons is converted to X-ray energy (greater percentage at higher kilovoltages).

• Approximately 99% of the energy is converted to heat and is dissipated through the copper anode and oil of the protective tube housing.

▶ *General (bremsstrahlung, or braking) radiation* occurs when speeding electrons stop, "brake," or slow down near the tungsten target in the anode.

• When an electron hits the nucleus of the tungsten atom, all of its kinetic energy is converted into a high-energy X-ray photon.

• When an electron comes close to but misses the nucleus, an X-ray photon of lower energy is created.

• General radiation produces X-rays of many different energies.

▶ *Characteristic radiation results*:

• When a bombarding electron, at 70 kVp or above, displaces an electron from a shell of the target atom, ionizing the atom.

• Another electron in an outer shell replaces the missing electron, causing a cascading effect.

• When the displaced electron is replaced, a photon is emitted, resulting in characteristic radiation.

• Characteristic radiation contributes approximately 10% to the useful beam.

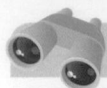

BOX 13-4 | KEY WORDS: Types of Radiation

Bremsstrahlung radiation (white radiation): a distribution of X-rays from very low-energy photons to those produced by the peak kilovoltage applied across an X-ray tube; Bremsstrahlung means "braking radiation" and refers to the sudden deceleration of electrons (cathode rays) as they interact with highly positively charged nuclei, such as tungsten.

Characteristic radiation: the radiation produced by electron transitions from higher energy orbitals to replace ejected electrons of inner electron orbitals; the energy of the electromagnetic radiation emitted is unique or "characteristic" of the emitting atom.

Electromagnetic radiation: forms of energy propagated by wave motion as photons; the radiations differ widely in wavelength, frequency, and photo energy; examples are infrared waves, visible light, ultraviolet radiation, X-rays, gamma rays, and cosmic radiation.

Gamma radiation: short-wavelength electromagnetic radiation of nuclear origin similar to X-rays but usually of higher energy.

Leakage radiation: the radiation that escapes through the protective shielding of the X-ray unit tube head; it may be detected at the sides, top, bottom, or back of the tube head.

Primary radiation: all radiation coming directly from the target of the anode of an X-ray tube.

Scatter radiation: a form of secondary radiation that, during passage through a substance, has been deviated in direction; it may also have been modified by an increase in wavelength.

Backscatter: radiation deflected by scattering processes at angles greater than 90° to the original direction of the beam of radiation.

Coherent scattering (Thompson or unmodified): scattering of relatively low-energy X-rays by elastic collisions without loss of photon energy.

Compton scatter radiation: the incident radiation that has sufficient energy to dislodge a bound electron but attacks a loosely bound electron; the remaining radiation energy proceeds in a different direction as scatter radiation.

Secondary radiation: particles or photons produced by the interaction of primary radiation with matter.

Stray radiation: radiation that serves no useful purpose; it includes leakage, secondary, and scatter radiation.

▶ X-rays leave the tube through the aperture to form the useful beam.

- *Useful beam:* The part of the primary radiation that is permitted to emerge from the tube head aperture and the accessory collimating devices.
- *Central beam* (central ray): The center of the beam of X-rays emitted from the tube.

DIGITAL RADIOGRAPHY

▶ Traditional film-based systems to record radiographic images have been in existence in dentistry since 1895.

▶ In the mid to late 1980s, the first direct digital imaging system was introduced and adopted by dental professionals.

▶ Digital systems include intraoral, panoramic, and cephalometric imaging. Terminology for digital radiography is listed and defined in Box 13-5.

I. Digital Imaging Principles

▶ Digital radiography requires conventional equipment to generate X-rays.

▶ The image is captured on sensors or plates of varying sizes, similar to conventional film.

▶ The information is then recorded as a digital image and displayed as pixels representing multiple shades of gray.

▶ The image is subsequently displayed on a computer monitor.

▶ The image can be enhanced and manipulated, by changing factors such as density and contrast, stored on the hard drive for future reference, and/or electronically sent to other professionals.[4–6]

II. Digital Imaging and Sensors

A. Direct Digital Imaging

▶ A corded or cordless charge-coupled device (CCD) or complementary-metal-oxide semiconductor (CMOS) sensor in a rigid case is used (Figure 13-3).

▶ Viewing of the image is possible within seconds of exposure.

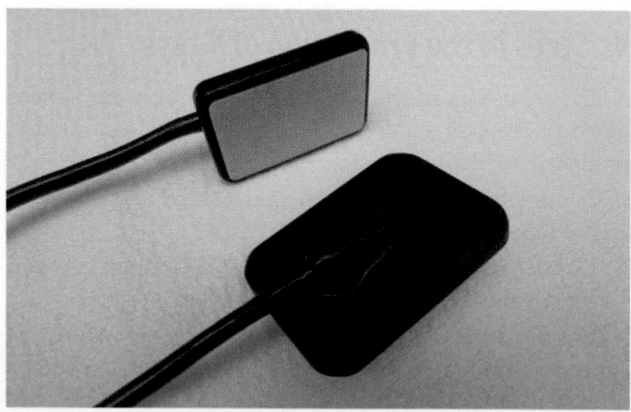

FIGURE 13-3 Direct Digital Sensors. Two sensor sizes are shown. CCD or CMOS sensors have integrated circuits made up of a grid of small transistor elements that convert X-rays to electrons in electron wells. Each element represents one pixel in the final image. This information is passed through a cable to the computer for processing.

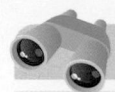

BOX 13-5 | KEY WORDS: Digital Radiography

Analog: continuous and variable representation of an image as opposed to digital, which is a binary representation (0's and 1's) of an image. An analog image will include all levels of clarity and will not be enhanced as the digital representation.

Charge-coupled device (CCD): a solid-state detector, used in corded intraoral sensors as an image receptor, that converts X-rays to electrons, which are stored in electron wells and then converted to a visible image.

Complementary-metal-oxide semiconductor (CMOS): a corded sensor that has the same characteristics as a CCD, except the individual pixels can be made smaller.

Digital radiography: a filmless imaging system; a method of capturing a radiographic image using a sensor, breaking it into small electronic pieces, and presenting and storing the image using a computer.

Digitize: to convert an image into a digital form that can be used by the computer using a grid of pixels.

Direct digital imaging: a filmless method of obtaining a digital image in which an intraoral sensor is directly exposed to X-rays and immediately displays an image, in digital form, on a computer monitor.

Indirect digital imaging: a method of obtaining a digital image in which a PSP plate is exposed to X-rays and captures an image. The image is then converted from analog to digital by use of a laser scanner and subsequently displayed on a computer monitor.

Photostimuable phosphor plate (PSP): a cordless sensor that converts X-radiation into stored energy. When the PSP is scanned by a laser, the stored energy is released as blue fluorescent light that is converted to digital data and displayed on a computer monitor.

Pixel: the smallest discrete component of an image or a picture on a screen that makes up the overall picture; usually dots arranged in rows and columns.

Sensor: a small detector that is placed intraorally to capture a radiographic image.

Storage phosphor imaging: a method of obtaining a digital image in which the image is recorded on phosphor-coated plates and then placed into an electronic processor where a laser scans the plate and produces an image on a computer screen.

B. Indirect Digital Imaging

▶ A cordless photostimuable phosphor (PSP) plate is used (Figure 13-4).

▶ Information on the PSP plate is read by a laser scanner.

▶ The digital image is displayed on a monitor.

▶ Traditional films can also be scanned as analog images and converted to digital.

III. Steps in the Production of a Digital Radiograph

▶ The sensor, direct or indirect (Figures 13-3 and 13-4), is encased in a plastic sleeve (Figure 13-5), held in a sensor holder and placed in the patient's mouth.

▶ When exposed to radiation, an electronic charge is produced on the surface of the sensor.

▶ With direct digital imaging: the image is immediately converted from analog form to digital form and displayed on the monitor (Figure 13-6).

▶ With indirect digital imaging: the PSP plates store the image until placed in a high-speed laser scanner, which converts the information into a digitized image and displays it on the monitor.

▶ The image can then be stored, manipulated, enhanced, retrieved, and transmitted.

▶ The CCD or CMOS (direct imaging) sensors can be reused immediately on the same patient, or unwrapped and sanitized, according to the manufacturer's recommendations.

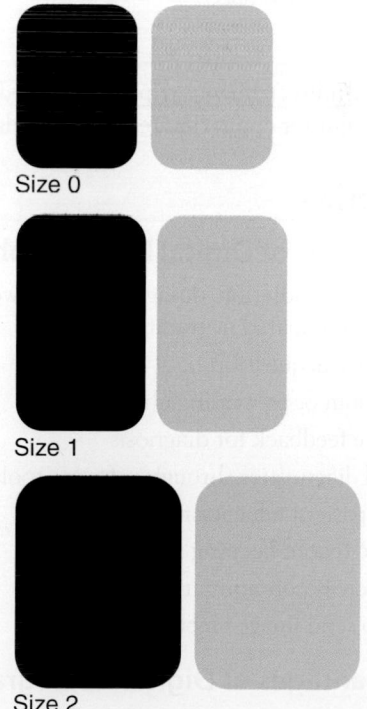

Size 0

Size 1

Size 2

FIGURE 13-4 Indirect Digital Sensors. The light blue exposure and black nonexposure sides of three sizes of PSP sensors are shown. PSP sensors are available in intraoral 0–4 sizes, as well as panoramic and cephalometric sizes. The light blue exposure side is covered with phosphor crystals that store X-ray exposure energy. When the sensor is placed in a laser scanner, the energy is released from the phosphor layer and converted to a digital image.

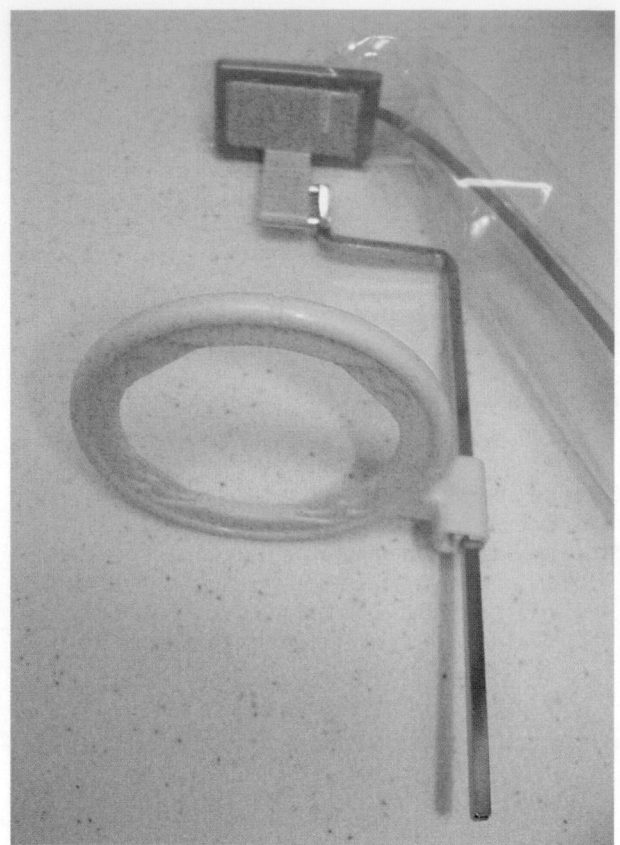

FIGURE 13-5 Sensor Holder in Plastic Sleeve. The sensor holder is encased in a plastic sleeve for infection control purposes.

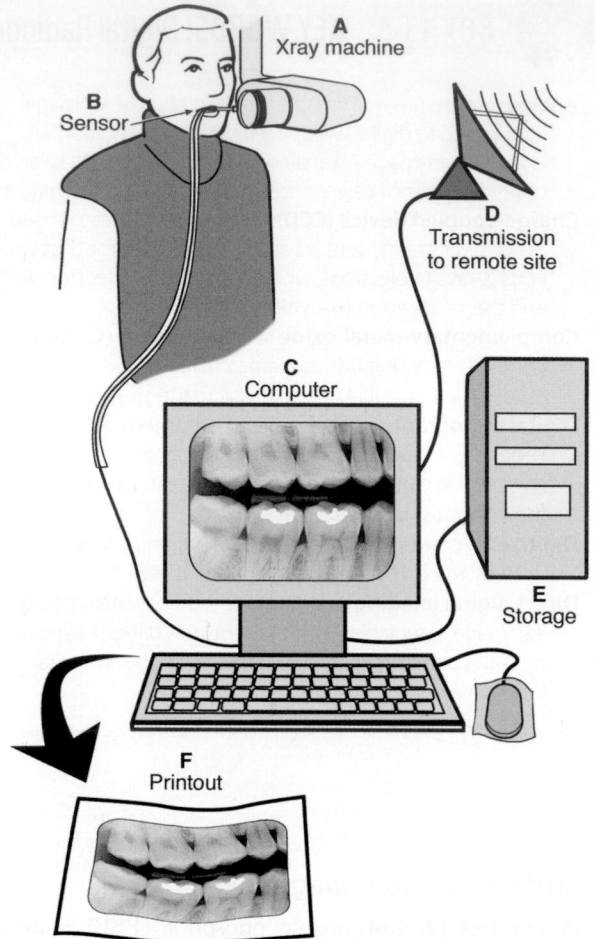

FIGURE 13-6 Direct Digital Imaging System. A: The image is exposed by an X-ray machine, **B:** captured on a CCD or CMOS sensor in the patient's mouth. **C:** The signal is transmitted via a cable to the computer, where it is digitized into multiple gray levels. The image is displayed on the computer's monitor, **D:** transmitted electronically to a remote site, **E:** stored on a file server, or **F:** printed on paper.

▶ The PSP (indirect imaging) plate is erased by a high-intensity light for approximately 30 seconds.

IV. Evaluation

A. Advantages of Digital Radiography

▶ Reduction of radiation dosage due to lower exposure time when compared to traditional film

▶ Faster image acquisition

▶ No darkroom or processing chemistry

▶ Immediate feedback for diagnosis

▶ Improved diagnostics through software tools

▶ Effective patient education tool

▶ Electronic record keeping

▶ Reduced cross-contamination

▶ Ability to send image electronically.

B. Disadvantages of Digital Radiography

▶ Initial setup expense

▶ Bulky direct imaging sensors may increase film placement errors

▶ Infection control of sensors: are covered by plastic sleeves as they cannot be heat sterilized

▶ Direct imaging sensors are fragile and expensive.

CHARACTERISTICS OF AN ACCEPTABLE RADIOGRAPHIC IMAGE

A *radiographic image* is the visible image on a radiation-sensitive film or a digitized image created by the computer.

▶ The image is produced after exposure to ionizing radiation that has passed through an area, or specifically for dentistry, through teeth or a part of the oral cavity.

▶ A *radiographic survey* refers to a series of radiographic images.

▶ Before making a radiographic image, it is necessary to know the characteristics that are expected to result in a radiograph of maximum diagnostic value. The basic essentials are:

• The appearance of the image itself
• The area covered
• The quality of the processed radiograph.

Table 13-1 provides a list of characteristics of an acceptable radiograph.

TABLE 13-1	Characteristics of an Acceptable Radiograph
CHARACTERISTIC	**APPEARANCE**
Image	All parts of teeth of interest are shown close to natural size, with minimal overlap and minimal distortion
Area covered	Sufficient tissue surrounding tooth for diagnostic purposes
Density	Proper density for diagnosis
Contrast	Proper contrast for diagnosis
Definition and sharpness	Clear outline of objects; minimal penumbra

I. Radiolucency and Radiopacity

▶ A radiographic image has gradations from white to black that are referred to as radiopaque or radiolucent.

▶ For example, a dense material, such as a metallic restoration, prevents the passage of X-rays and appears white on the processed radiograph.

▶ Soft tissue does not resist passage of X-rays and, thus, appears black to gray.

II. Radiopacity

The appearance of light (white) images on a radiograph is a result of the lesser amount of radiation that penetrates the structures and reaches the image receptor.

▶ A radiopaque structure inhibits the passage of X-rays.

Examples include:

- Enamel
- Dentin
- Metallic restorations
- Implants.

III. Radiolucency

The appearance of dark images on a radiograph is a result of the greater amount of radiation that penetrates the structures and reaches the image receptor.

▶ A *radiolucent* structure permits the passage of radiation with relatively little attenuation by absorption.

Examples include:

- Pulp
- Cysts
- Cavitated lesions
- Periodontal ligament.

FACTORS THAT INFLUENCE THE FINISHED RADIOGRAPH

As the beam leaves the X-ray tube (Figure 13-1):

▶ It is collimated, filtered, and allowed to travel a designated source–image receptor (or focal spot–image receptor) distance before reaching the image receptor of a selected speed.

▶ The quality or diagnostic usefulness of the finished radiograph, as well as the total exposure of the patient and clinician, are influenced by the *kilovoltage, milliampere seconds, time, collimation, filtration, target–receptor distance, object–receptor distance,* and *film speed,* as outlined in Box 13-6.

BOX 13-6

Factors that Influence the Radiographic Image

Kilovoltage Peak
▷ Affects contrast and density
▷ Low kVp yields high (short-scale) contrast
▷ High kVp yields low (long-scale) contrast

Milliamperage
▷ Affects density
▷ High mA yields high density
▷ Low mA yields low density

Time
▷ Affects density
▷ Long time yields high density
▷ Short time yields low density

Collimation
▷ Restricts and shapes the beam
▷ Not to exceed 2.75 inches or 7 cm at the patient's skin

Lead Diaphragm
▷ PID
▷ Rectangular
▷ Cylindrical

Filtration

Types
▷ Aluminum filters remove low-energy X-rays
▷ Rare earth filters remove low- and high-energy X-rays
 Methods of Filtration

Inherent
▷ Glass window
▷ Insulating oil
▷ Tube head seal

Added
▷ Aluminum disks
▷ 1.5 mm for 50–70 kVp
▷ 2.5 for above 70 kVp

Total Filtration

▷ Combination of inherent and added

Target–Film Distance

▷ Longer PID increases resolution of image
▷ Longer PID decreases scatter of radiation

Object–Film Distance

▷ Increased object–film distance achieves parallelism
▷ Decreased object–film distance decreases penumbra

Film Speed

▷ Faster-speed film decreases definition; image is more grainy

---

▶ Traditional film processing also directly influences the quality of the radiograph and indirectly the total exposure. Re-exposure would be necessary should the film be rendered inadequate during processing.

I. Collimation

▶ Collimation is the technique for controlling the size and shape of the beam of radiation emitted.
▶ A *collimator* is a diaphragm or system of diaphragms made of an absorbing material designed to define the dimensions and direction of a beam of radiation.

A. Purposes

▶ Eliminate peripheral or divergent radiation.
▶ Minimize exposure to patient's face.
▶ Minimize secondary radiation, which can fog the film and expose the bodies of patient and clinician.

B. Methods

▶ Lead diaphragm
  • Made of lead with a central aperture of the smallest practical diameter for making radiographic exposure.

  • Located between the aluminum filters in the tube head and the PID.
  • Recommended thickness of lead: 1/8 inch.
  • Recommended maximum size of aperture: to permit a diameter of the beam of radiation equal to 2.75 inches or 7 cm at the end of the PID next to the patient's face.
▶ Rectangular collimation
  • As shown in Figure 13-7.
  • When used, the size of the beam is greatly reduced and patient receives approximately 66% less radiation compared to round collimation.
  • The beam of radiation's diameter is approximately 50 mm × 38 mm at the skin.
  • The collimator is rotated to accommodate films positioned horizontally or vertically.
▶ Lead-lined cylindrical or rectangular PID
  • The PID is an open-ended cylinder, or rectangle, lined with lead, to reduce secondary radiation.

C. Relation to Techniques

▶ Dimensions of #2 size image receptors range in size and can be up to approximately 44.0 × 32.2 mm.
▶ Precise angulation techniques are required to eliminate "cone-cut" of image receptor, particularly when rectangular collimation is used.
▶ "Cone-cut" refers to an error of technique that results when the PID is not angled with the central ray centered on the image receptor being exposed.

II. Filtration

Filtration is the insertion of absorbers or filters for the preferential attenuation of radiation from a primary beam of X-radiation. Two different types of filters provide filtration in the dental X-ray machine.

A. Types of Filters

▶ *Aluminum filters* remove low-energy X-ray photons from the X-ray beam.

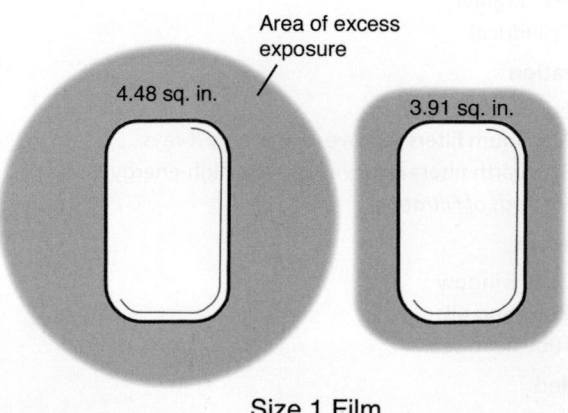

Area of excess exposure

4.48 sq. in.   3.91 sq. in.

Size 1 Film

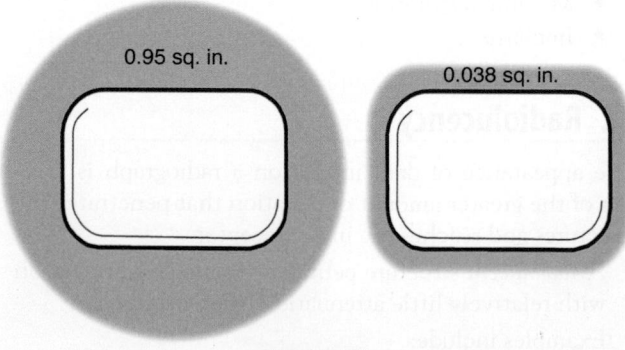

0.95 sq. in.   0.038 sq. in.

Size 2 Film

FIGURE 13-7 Cylindrical and Rectangular PID. The useless areas of radiation are greatly lessened when rectangular collimation is used. The patient can be spared exposure to excessive radiation. (Adapted from Shannon SA. Rectangular versus cylindrical collimation. *Dent Hyg.* 1987;61:173. Copyright © 1987 by the American Dental Hygienists' Association.)

▶ *Rare earth filters* selectively remove both low- and high-energy photons from the X-ray beam. Examples of rare earth filters include samarium, erbium, yttrium, niobium, gadolinium, terbium-activated gadolinium oxysulfide, and thulium-activated lanthanum oxybromide.

B. Purpose

▶ To minimize exposure of the patient's skin to unnecessary radiation.

C. Methods

▶ *Inherent filtration*: Includes the glass envelope encasing the X-ray tube and the glass window in the tube housing (Figure 13-1).

▶ *Added filtration*: Thin, pure, aluminum disks inserted between the lead diaphragm and the X-ray tube.

▶ *Total filtration*: The sum of inherent and added filtration. The recommended total is the equivalent of 0.5 mm (below 50 kVp), 1.5 mm (50–70 kVp), and 2.5 mm (above 70 kVp) of aluminum.

III. Kilovoltage

Kilovoltage is the potential difference of force that moves electrons between the negative cathode and the positive anode of an X-ray tube.

▶ When the kilovoltage is increased, the speed of electrons is increased and the resulting X-rays have a shorter wavelength and more penetrating power.

▶ kVp refers to the crest value (in kilovolts) of the potential difference of a pulsating generator. When only one-half of the wave is used, the value refers to the useful half of the cycle.

A. How kVp Affects the Radiographic Image

▶ *Affects the contrast*
  • Low kilovoltage produces high contrast, with sharp black–white differences in densities between adjacent areas but a small range of distinction between subject thicknesses recorded.
  • High kilovoltage produces low contrast, with a wide range of subject thicknesses recorded; greater range of densities from black to white (more gray tones), which provide more interpretive details.

▶ *Affects the density*
  • Increased kilovoltage results in increased density (other factors remaining constant).
  • To maintain the same image *density*, the milliampere seconds is decreased as the kVp is increased.

B. Advantages of High kVp

▶ Permits shorter exposure time.

▶ Reduces exposure to tissues lying in front of the image receptor.

▶ Facilitates the detection of bone changes.

C. Disadvantages of High kVp

▶ Increased radiation to tissues outside the edges of the image receptor.

▶ More internal scattered radiation at 90 kVp than at 70 kVp.

IV. Milliampere Seconds

A. Milliamperage

▶ The measure of the electron current passing through the X-ray tube.

▶ Regulates the heat of the filament, which determines the number of electrons available to bombard the target.

▶ As the milliamperage is increased, the density of the image is increased.

B. Quantity of Radiation

▶ Quantity of radiation is expressed in milliampere seconds (mAs) or milliampere impulses (mAi).

▶ Definition: mAs is the milliamperes multiplied by the exposure time in seconds; mAi is the milliamperes multiplied by the exposure time in impulses.

▶ Example: At 10 milliamperes for 1/2 second, the exposure of the image receptor would be 5 mAs. At 10 milliamperes for 15 impulses, the exposure of the image receptor would be 150 mAi.

V. Distance

Several distances are involved in X-ray exposure. The object–image receptor and the target–image receptor distances are considered for image receptor placement.

A. Object–Image Receptor Distance

▶ Refers to the distance between the object (teeth of interest) and the image receptor.

▶ With the paralleling technique and the use of an image receptor holder, the object–image receptor distance is greater than it is for the bisecting-angle technique.

▶ A collimated beam and increased source–image receptor distance compensate to maximize definition and resolution.

B. Target–Image Receptor Distance

▶ The PID on the X-ray machine is designed to indicate the direction of the X-ray beam and to serve as a guide in establishing desired target–surface and target–image receptor distances.

▶ Techniques using 8-, 12-, and 16-inch target–image receptor distances are common.

▶ The *source* is the *tungsten target*. The target–image receptor distance (sometimes called the source–image receptor distance) is the sum total of the distance from the tungsten target to the film. The PID lightly touches the face.

- Principles related to target–image receptor distance are as follows:
  - The intensity of the X-ray beam varies inversely as the square of the target–image receptor distance.
  - For example, if two image receptors requiring the same impulses were used, one at a 16-inch target–image receptor distance and one at an 8-inch distance, the image receptor at 16 inches would require four times the exposure (time) to maintain the same density in the finished radiograph.
  - The exposure decreases as the distance increases; when the distance is doubled, the radiation exposure to the patient is reduced to one fourth.
  - To maintain radiographic density when distance is increased, an increase in mAs, kVp, or time is required.

C. Advantages in the Use of a Long PID

- Increased definition.
- Decreased magnification.
- Decreased skin exposure owing to decreased scatter.

VI. Image Receptors

- Image receptors refer to both traditional film and digital sensors used to capture a radiographic image.
- With optimum filtration, collimation, fast film, and digital sensors, the skin dose to the face can be reduced significantly.
- Very slow-speed films have been discontinued, and the speed of traditional films has been increased.
- Digital imaging also requires a low exposure time.

A. Traditional Film Composition

A film is a thin, transparent sheet of cellulose acetate coated on both sides with an emulsion of gelatin and silver halide crystals.

- *Film base*: A flexible piece of polyester plastic that is used to provide support for the emulsion.
- *Halide crystals*: Silver bromide and silver iodide crystals are used in dental X-ray film. They are sensitive to radiation and light.
- *Emulsion*: A coating of gelatinous and nongelatinous materials attached to both sides of the film base that keeps the silver halide crystals evenly dispersed in a suspension.
- *Adhesive layer*: A thin layer of adhesive material that covers both sides of the film base and keeps the emulsion on the film base.

B. Traditional Film Packet

Sealed paper or plastic envelope that is small, light proof, and moisture resistant, containing an X-ray film (or two), black paper, and a thin sheet of lead foil.

- Two-film packet: useful for processing one film differently from the other to make diagnostic comparisons; for sending to specialist to whom patient may be referred; for legal evidence.

- Purpose of black paper: to protect against light.
- Purposes of lead foil backing: to prevent exposure of the film by scattered radiation that could enter from back of packet and to protect the patient's tissues lying in the path of the X-ray.

C. Traditional Film Speed

- Film speed or film emulsion speed refers to the sensitivity of the film to radiation exposure.
- The speed is the amount of exposure required to produce a certain image density.
- The smaller the grain size, the slower the film speed.
- The slower the film speed, the less grainy the resulting image.
- *Classification*: Films have been classified by the American National Standards Institute (ANSI) in cooperation with the American Dental Association (ADA).
- The ANSI/ADA Specification No. 22 designates six groups:
  - A–F speed groups.
  - A, B, and C, the slowest, are associated with excess radiation exposure and are no longer used.
  - D and E are the slowest of those still in use.
  - *Choice*: F-speed film is recommended for use with rectangular collimation for marked reduction in radiation exposure.

D. Digital Sensors

- In digital radiography, there are three types of receptors that replace traditional film:
  - CCD
  - CMOS
  - PSP plates.
- CCD and CMOS detectors are known as "direct imaging sensors." When exposed to X-ray energy, an image appears on a computer monitor within seconds.
- PSP plates are known as "indirect imaging sensors." When irradiated, an image is stored on them until scanned by a laser. The scanner then transmits the image to the computer.[2]
- CCD and CMOS sensors require radiation exposure times approximately 10–20% lower than "F"-speed film.
- PSP plate exposure times are similar to "F"-speed requirements.

EXPOSURE TO RADIATION

I. Ionizing Radiation

Ionizing radiation is electromagnetic radiation (e.g., *X-rays or gamma rays*) or particulate radiation (e.g., *electrons, neutrons, or protons*) capable of ionizing air directly or indirectly.

- The phenomenon of separation of electrons from molecules to change their chemical activity is called ionization.

▷ Quality of the radiation
▷ Chemical composition of the absorbing medium
▷ Sensitivity of tissues
▷ Total dose and dose rate
▷ Blood supply to the tissues
▷ Size of the area exposed
▷ Somatic versus genetic cells

▶ The organic and inorganic compounds that make up the human body may be altered by exposure to ionizing radiation.

▶ The biologic effects following irradiation are secondary effects in that they result from physical, chemical, and biologic action set in motion by the absorption of energy from radiation.

▶ Factors that would influence the biologic effects of radiation are outlined in Box 13-7.

▶ Radiation to *somatic* tissues will affect only the irradiated individual, whereas radiation to *genetic* tissues will affect offspring and possibly future generations.

II. Exposure

A. Types of Exposure

Exposure is a measure of the X-radiation to which a person or an object, or a part of either, is exposed at a certain place; this measure is based on its ability to produce ionization.

▶ *Threshold exposure*: The minimum exposure that produces a detectable degree of any given effect.

▶ *Entrance or surface exposure*: Exposure measured at the surface of an irradiated body, part, or object. It includes primary radiation and backscatter from the irradiated underlying tissue.

▶ *Skin exposure*: Exposure measured at the center of an irradiated skin surface area.

▶ *Erythema exposure*: The radiation necessary to produce a temporary redness of the skin.

B. Exposure Units

▶ The units of absorbed dose are expressed in joules/kilogram (1 rad = 0.01 J/kg).

▶ The units shown in Table 13-2 are the recommendations of the International Commission on Radiation Units and Measurements.[7]

▶ The unit of measurement is the *gray* (Gy). An absorbed dose of 1 Gy is equal to 1 J/kg; therefore, an absorbed dose of 1 Gy is equal to 100 rad.

▶ The unit of biologic equivalence is the *Sievert* (Sv). 1 Sv = 100 rem.

C. Dose

▶ The radiation dose is the amount of energy absorbed per unit mass of tissue at a site of interest. The kinds of doses are defined in Box 13-8.

D. Permissible Dose

The amount of radiation that may be received by an individual *within* a specified period without expectation of any significantly harmful result is called the *permissible dose*.

▶ Assumptions on which permissible doses are calculated include the following:

• No irradiation is beneficial.
• There is a dose below which no somatic cellular changes can be produced.
• Children are more susceptible than are older people.
• There is a dose below which, even though it is delivered before the end of the reproductive period, the probability of genetic effects is slight.

E. Radiation Hazard

▶ A condition under which persons might receive radiation in excess of the maximum permissible dose is considered a hazard.

▶ Exposure would be a risk in an area where X-ray equipment is being used or where radioactive materials are stored.

TABLE 13-2	Radiation Units		
DEFINITION	**S.I. UNIT**	**TRADITIONAL UNIT**	**EQUIVALENT**
Unit of radiation exposure	Coulomb per kilogram (C/kg)	Roentgen (R)	-2.58×10^{-4} C/kg = 1 R
Unit of absorbed dose	Gray (Gy)	Rad	1 Gy = 100 rad
Unit of dose equivalent	Sievert (Sv)	Rem	1 Sv = 100 rem
Unit of radioactivity	Becquerel (Bq)	Curie (Ci)	3.7×10^{10} Bq = 1 Ci

S.I. (System International) is from the French *Système* International d'Unités.

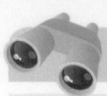

BOX 13-8 KEY WORDS AND ABBREVIATIONS: Types of Radiation Doses

Absorbed dose: the amount of energy imparted by ionizing radiation to a unit mass of irradiated material at a specific exposure point; the unit of absorbed dose is the gray (Gy).

Cumulative dose: the total dose resulting from repeated exposures to radiation of the same region or of the whole body.

Dose: the amount of energy absorbed per unit mass of tissue at a site of interest.

Dose equivalent: the product of absorbed dose and modifying factors, such as the quality factor, distribution factor, and any other necessary factors; different types of radiation cause differing biologic effects; the unit of dose equivalence is the Sievert (Sv).

Dose rate: rate of exposure.

Erythema dose: the minimum quantity of x or gamma radiation that produces the appearance of redness (erythema).

Exit dose: the absorbed dose delivered by a beam of radiation to the surface through which the beam emerges from an object.

Lethal dose: the amount of radiation that is, or could be, sufficient to cause the death of an organism.

LD 50–30: the dose of radiation that is lethal for 50% of a large population in a specified period of time, usually 30 days.

Maximum permissible dose: the maximum dose equivalent a person (or specified parts of that person) is allowed to receive in a stated period of time; the dose of radiation that would not be expected to produce any significant radiation effects in a lifetime.

Skin dose (surface absorbed dose): the absorbed dose delivered by a radiation beam and backscatter at the point where the central ray passes through the superficial layer of the object.

Threshold dose: the minimum dose that produces a detectable degree of any effect.

TABLE 13-3	Maximum Permissible Dose Equivalent Values (Mpd)^a to Whole Body, Gonads, Blood-Forming Organs, Lens of Eye		
AVERAGE WEEKLY EXPOSURE^b	**MAXIMUM 13-WK EXPOSURE**	**MAXIMUM YEARLY EXPOSURE**	**MAXIMUM ACCUMULATED EXPOSURE^c**
0.001 Sv	0.03 Sv	0.05 Sv	0.05(N−18)Sv
0.1 R	3 R	5 R	5(N−18)R^d

^{a}Exposure of persons for dental or medical purposes is not counted against their maximum permissible exposure limits.
^{b}Used only for the purpose of designating radiation barriers.
^{c}When the previous occupational history of an individual is not definitely known, it shall be assumed that the full dose permitted by the formula 5(N − 18) has already been received.
^{d}N = Age in years and is greater than 18. The unit for exposure is the roentgen (R) or Sievert (Sv).

F. National Council on Radiation Protection and Measurements

▶ Limits for dentists and dental personnel. See Table 13-3.

▶ Limits for patients: Exposure to radiation shall be kept to the minimum level consistent with clinical requirements for accurate diagnosis based on patient need.[8]

▶ Radiation exposures are kept as low as reasonably achievable (ALARA). This concept is accepted and enforced by all regulatory agencies.

III. Sensitivity of Cells

A. Factors Affecting Cell Sensitivity to Radiation

▶ *Cell differentiation*: Immature cells are most sensitive. Highly specialized cells are radioresistant.

▶ *Mitotic activity*: Rapidly reproducing cells are more sensitive; most sensitive when undergoing mitosis.

▶ *Cell metabolism*: Cells are more sensitive in periods of increased metabolism.

B. Radiosensitive and Radioresistant Tissues

▶ Radiosensitive: a cell that is sensitive to radiation.

▶ Radioresistant: a cell that is resistant to radiation.

▶ Radiation sensitivity of tissues and organs: the relative sensitivities are shown in Box 13-9.

C. Tissue Reaction

▶ *Latent period*: Lapse between the time of exposure and the time when effects are observed. (May be as long as 25 years or relatively shorter, as in the case of the production of a skin erythema.)

▶ *Cumulative effect*
  • Amount of reaction depends on dose; the reaction to radiation received in fractional doses is less than the reaction to one large dose.
  • Partial or total repair occurs as long as destruction is not complete.

BOX 13-9

Radiation Sensitivity of Tissues and Organs

High
▷ Bone marrow
▷ Reproductive cells
▷ Intestines
▷ Lymphoid tissue

Moderately High
▷ Oral mucosa
▷ Skin

Moderate
▷ Growing bone
▷ Growing cartilage
▷ Small vasculature
▷ Connective tissue

Moderately Low
▷ Salivary glands
▷ Mature bone
▷ Mature cartilage
▷ Thyroid gland tissue

Low
▷ Liver
▷ Optic lens
▷ Kidneys
▷ Muscle
▷ Nerve

- Some irreparable damage may be cumulative as, little by little, more radiation is added (e.g., hair loss, skin lesions, falling blood cell count).

RISK OF INJURY FROM RADIATION

▶ The risk of injury from dental diagnostic radiation is extremely low; however, the more radiation received, the higher the chance of cellular injuries.

▶ With each exposure to radiation, cellular damage is followed by repair.

▶ The effects of radiation exposure are cumulative, and any cellular changes not repaired result in damaged tissues.

▶ Most of the damage caused by dental diagnostic low-level radiation is repaired within the body cells.

I. Rules for Radiation Protection

▶ *Dental X-ray protection*, prepared by the National Council on Radiation Protection and Measurements,[9] provides specific information about radiation barriers, film speed group rating, film badge service sources, X-ray equipment data, and operating procedure regulations.

▶ To protect the clinician and patient from excessive radiation, attention is paid to unnecessary radiation that may result from retakes due to inadequate clinical procedures.

▶ Perfecting techniques contributes to the accomplishment of minimum exposure for maximum safety.

II. Protection of Clinician

A. Protection from Primary Radiation

▶ Stand behind a protective barrier.

▶ Avoid the useful beam of radiation.

▶ Never hand-hold the image receptor during exposure.

B. Protection from Leakage Radiation

▶ Do not hand-hold the tube housing or the PID of the machine during exposures.

▶ Test machine for leakage radiation.

▶ Wear monitoring device for testing exposure.

C. Protection from Secondary Radiation

The major sources of secondary radiation are the filter and the irradiated soft tissues of the patient. Other sources may be the leakage from the tube housing or scatter from furniture and walls contacted by the primary beam. Methods of protection are related to these sources.

Minimization of Total X-Radiation

▶ Use high-speed films and digital sensors.

▶ Have X-ray machines tested frequently for X-ray output and leakage.

▶ Replace older X-ray machines with modern equipment.

Collimation of Useful Beam

Use diaphragms and long PIDs to collimate the useful beam to an area no larger than 2.75 inches or 7 cm in diameter at the patient's skin. Rectangular collimation is shown to be more effective than round collimation (Figure 13-7).

Type of PID

Use a shielded cylinder that is rectangular, long, and open ended, or use some other form of rectangular collimation.

Position of Clinician While Making Exposures

▶ The correct position for the clinician is behind an appropriate radiation-resistant barrier wall, preferably with a leaded window to permit a view of the patient during exposures.

▶ When protective barrier shielding is not available, the clinician shall stand as far as practical from the patient, at least 6 ft (2 m) in the zone between 90° and 135° to the primary central ray, as shown in Figure 13-8.

▶ Safety increases with distance.

▶ *Exposure of the region of the central incisors*: Stand at a 45° to the path of the central ray. This position is approximately behind either the left or the right ear of the patient (Figure 13-8).

▶ *Exposure of other regions*: Stand behind the patient's head and at an angle of 45° to the path of the central ray of the X-ray beam.

D. Monitoring

The amount of X-radiation that reaches the dental personnel can be measured economically with a film badge. Badges can be obtained from one of several laboratories. The film badge is:

▶ Used to measure exposure of the wearer.

▶ Worn at waist level for 1, 2, or 4 weeks.

▶ Returned on a routine basis to the laboratory by mail and processed; its exposure is evaluated.

▶ Wearer is notified by mail of the exposure totals.

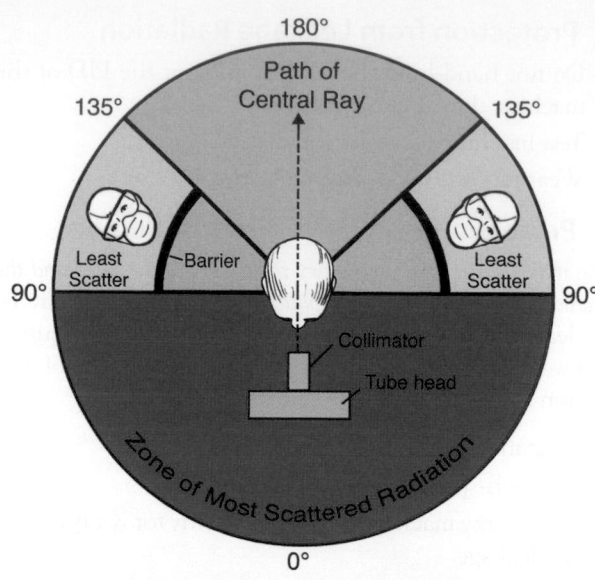

FIGURE 13-8 **Safe Position for Clinician.** While making an exposure, the clinician stands behind the patient's head, between 90° and 135° from the primary beam.

III. Protection of Patient

A. Image Receptors

▶ Use high-speed image receptors.

▶ Use the largest intraoral receptor that can be placed skillfully in the mouth. Maximum coverage is provided in this manner with one exposure.

▶ Two exposures may be required if smaller receptors are used to examine the same area.

• This factor is especially important when examining the mouths of children.

B. Collimation

▶ Use diaphragms and an open-ended, shielded (lead lined), rectangular PID to collimate the useful beam.

C. Filtration

▶ Use filtration of the useful beam to recommended levels.

D. Processing

▶ Process traditional films according to the manufacturer's directions with adherence to quality assurance guidelines. When a choice of two periods of development is offered, the exposure of the patient can be reduced if the longer development time is employed.

E. Total Exposure

▶ Do not expose the patient unnecessarily. Determine a valid reason for each exposure.

F. Patient Body Shields

▶ The use of leaded or lead-free alloy body shields and thyroid collars for each patient is required by law in

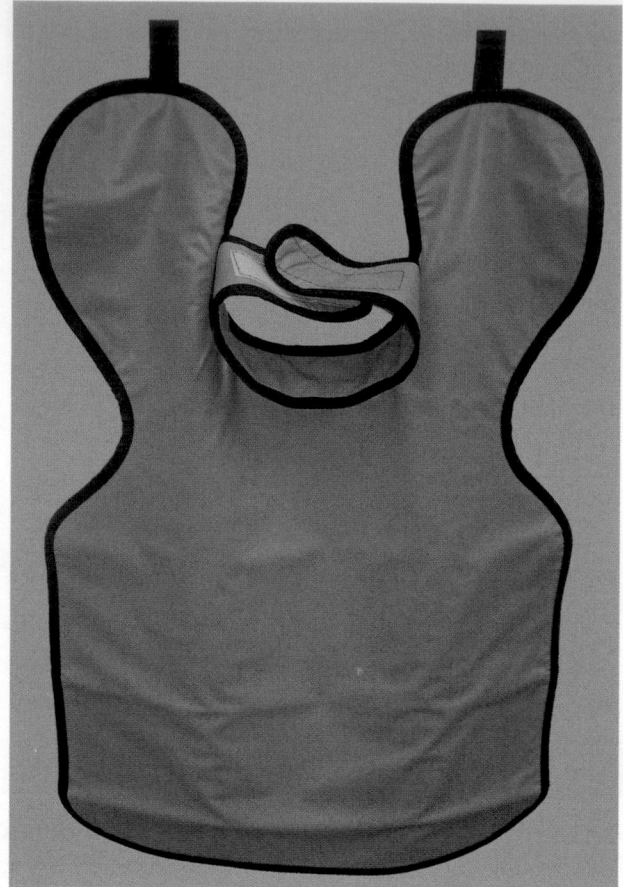

FIGURE 13-9 **Care of Leaded Apron.** The apron can be kept on hooks or a hanging device near the X-ray machine to prevent cracks and prolong the usefulness of the apron. The thyroid collar may be attached or a separate shield.

many states and countries. The purpose of the shield is to absorb scattered rays. An acceptable lead shield contains a minimum of 0.25 mm of lead thickness.

Protective Apron

▶ *Types*

• General body coverage with extensions over the shoulders and down over the gonadal area.

• Body coverage, with cervical thyroid collar attached.

• Body coverage, with added coverage for the patient's upper back for wear during panoramic radiography.

▶ *Care*

• Prevent cracks in leaded shields by hanging (Figure 13-9).

• Disinfect the apron and collar before and after each use.

Thyroid Cervical Collar

▶ Thyroid cancer can result from long-term exposure of the gland to X-rays.[9,10]

▶ The gland is completely covered during exposure to X-rays. Figure 13-10 shows the position of a thyroid collar over the neckline of a body apron.

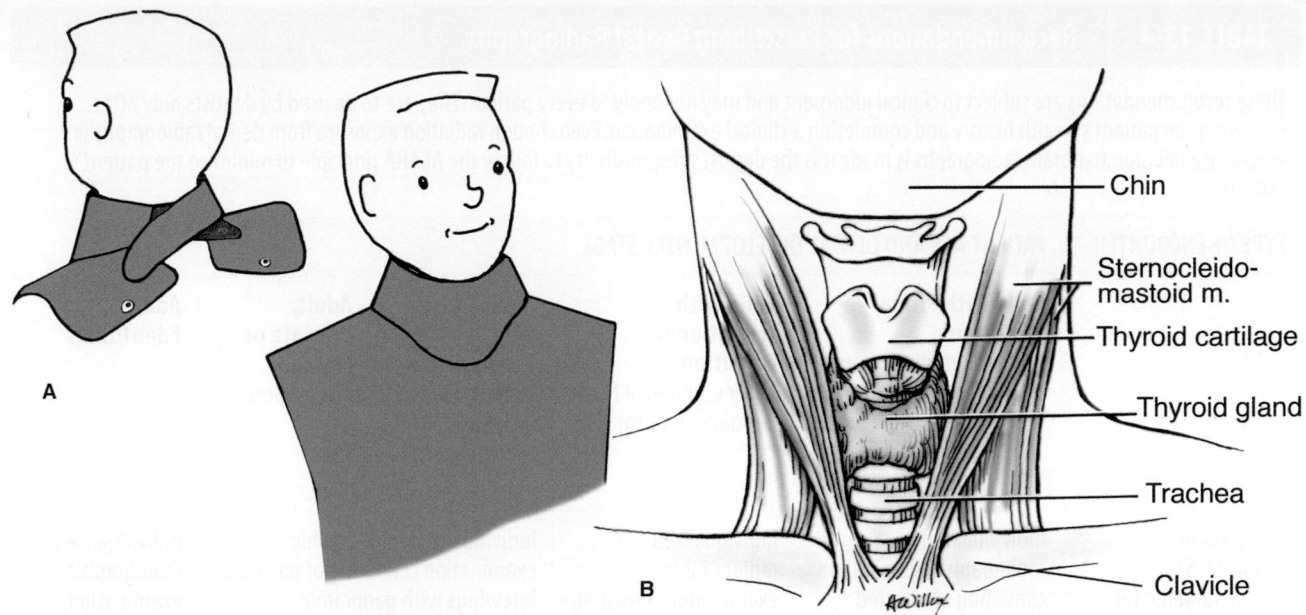

FIGURE 13-10 Thyroid Cervical Collar. A: Thyroid collar in position, covering the neck and overlapping the leaded apron used for general body coverage. Velcro tabs facilitate overlap fastening at back of neck. Collars are available in child and adult sizes. **B:** The thyroid gland is located over the trachea approximately halfway between the chin and the clavicles. Drawing shows anatomic relationship to the sternocleidomastoid muscle.

IV. Risk Reduction

A. Assessment for Need of Radiographs

▶ Review health history.

▶ Prepare or review radiation exposure history.

▶ Medical diagnostic or therapeutic radiation.

▶ Dates of dental surveys and availability of previous radiographs.

▶ Review clinical examination.

▶ Obtain dentist's prescription for number and type of radiographs. Refer to the *Guidelines for Prescribing Dental Radiographs* in Tables 13-4 and 13-5.[2]

B. Preparation of Clinic Facility: Infection Control Routine

▶ Standard precautions are followed for all radiographic equipment and materials.

▶ Use barrier single-use plastic covers for all surfaces to be contacted, including X-ray machine controls.

▶ Use disposable materials wherever possible.

▶ Wear gloves or overgloves for handling of all radiographic materials.

C. Preparation of Clinician

▶ Use full barrier protection that includes a cover-up gown, a mask, protective eyewear, and gloves.

▶ Apply standard precautions throughout the radiographic procedure.

D. Preparation of Patient

▶ Provide cup for holding removable dental prostheses

▶ For panoramic radiographs, request patient to remove oral and/or facial piercings and all other jewelry worn above the shoulders.

▶ Provide antiseptic mouthrinse to lower bacterial contamination of radiographs and aerosols.

E. Intraoral Examination

▶ To determine necessary adaptations during film placement.

Factors of Particular Interest

▶ Accessibility, determined by height and shape of palate, flexibility of muscles of orifice, floor of the mouth, possible gag reflex, and size of tongue.

▶ Position of teeth and edentulous areas.

▶ Apparent size of teeth.

▶ Unusual features, such as tori, sensitive areas of the mucous membranes.

F. Patient Cooperation: Prevention of Gagging

▶ Gagging may be the result of psychological or physiologic factors.

▶ May present some problem in the placement of all films for molar radiographs.

▶ May be initiated in the patient who ordinarily does not gag when techniques are carried out efficiently.

TABLE 13-4   Recommendations for Prescribing Dental Radiographs

These recommendations are subject to clinical judgment and may not apply to every patient. They are to be used by dentists only after reviewing the patient's health history and completing a clinical examination. Even though radiation exposure from dental radiographs is low, once a decision to obtain radiographs is made it is the dentist's responsibility to follow the ALARA principle to minimize the patient's exposure.

TYPE OF ENCOUNTER	PATIENT AGE AND DENTAL DEVELOPMENTAL STAGE				
	Child with Primary Dentition (prior to eruption of first permanent tooth)	**Child with Transitional Dentition** (after eruption of first permanent tooth)	**Adolescent with Permanent Dentition** (prior to eruption of third molars)	**Adult, Dentate or Partially Edentulous**	**Adult, Edentulous**
New patient (Table 13-5) being evaluated for oral diseases	Individualized radiographic examination consisting of selected periapical/occlusal views and/or posterior bitewings if proximal surfaces cannot be visualized or probed. Patients without evidence of disease and with open proximal contacts may not require a radiographic examination at this time.	Individualized radiographic examination consisting of posterior bitewings with panoramic examination or posterior bitewings and selected periapical images.	Individualized radiographic examination consisting of posterior bitewings with panoramic examination or posterior bitewings and selected periapical images. A full mouth intraoral radiographic examination is preferred when the patient has clinical evidence of generalized oral disease or a history of extensive dental treatment.		Individualized radiographic examination, based on clinical signs and symptoms.
Recall patient (Table 13-5) with clinical caries or at increased risk for caries[a]	Posterior bitewing examination at 6–12 mo intervals if proximal surfaces cannot be examined visually or with a probe.			Posterior bitewing examination at 6–18 mo intervals	Not applicable
Recall patient (Table 13-5) with no clinical caries and not at increased risk for caries[a]	Posterior bitewing examination at 12–24 mo intervals if proximal surfaces cannot be examined visually or with a probe		Posterior bitewing examination at 18–36 mo intervals	Posterior bitewing examination at 24–36 mo intervals	Not applicable
Recall patient (Table 13-5) with periodontal disease	Clinical judgment as to the need for and type of radiographic images for the evaluation of periodontal disease. Imaging may consist of, but is not limited to, selected bitewing and/or periapical images of areas where periodontal disease (other than nonspecific gingivitis) can be demonstrated clinically.				Not applicable
Patient (new and recall) for monitoring of dentofacial growth and development, and/or assessment of dental/skeletal relationships	Clinical judgment as to need for and type of radiographic images for evaluation and/or monitoring of dentofacial growth and development or assessment of dental and skeletal relationships	Clinical judgment as to need for and type of radiographic images for evaluation and/or monitoring of dentofacial growth and development, or assessment of dental and skeletal relationships. Panoramic or periapical examination to assess developing third molars.		Usually not indicated for monitoring of growth and development. Clinical judgment as to the need for and type of radiographic image for evaluation of dental and skeletal relationships.	

TABLE 13-4	Recommendations for Prescribing Dental Radiographs (*continued*)
TYPE OF ENCOUNTER	**PATIENT AGE AND DENTAL DEVELOPMENTAL STAGE**
Patient with other circumstances including, but not limited to, proposed or existing implants, other dental and craniofacial pathoses, restorative/endodontic needs, treated periodontal disease and caries remineralization	Clinical judgment as to need for and type of radiographic images for evaluation and/or monitoring of these conditions.

[a]Factors increasing risk for caries may be assessed using the ADA Caries Risk Assessment forms (0–6 years of age and over 6 years of age).
American Dental Association Council on Scientific Affairs, U.S. Department of Health and Human Services, U.S. Food and Drug Administration. Dental radiographic examinations: recommendations for patient selection and limiting radiation exposure. http://www.fda.gov/Radiation-EmittingProducts/RadiationEmittingProductsandProcedures/MedicalImaging/MedicalX-Rays/ucm116504.htm. Accessed August 20, 2013.

TABLE 13-5	Clinical Situations for Which Radiographs May Be Indicated Include, But Are Not Limited to:
A. POSITIVE HISTORICAL FINDINGS	**B. POSITIVE CLINICAL SIGNS/SYMPTOMS**
1. Previous periodontal or endodontic treatment 2. History of pain or trauma 3. Familial history of dental anomalies 4. Postoperative evaluation of healing 5. Remineralization monitoring 6. Presence of implants, previous implant-related pathosis or evaluation for implant placement	1. Clinical evidence of periodontal disease 2. Large or deep restorations 3. Deep carious lesions 4. Malposed or clinically impacted teeth 5. Swelling 6. Evidence of dental/facial trauma 7. Mobility of teeth 8. Sinus tract ("fistula") 9. Clinically suspected sinus pathosis 10. Growth abnormalities 11. Oral involvement in known or suspected systemic disease 12. Positive neurologic findings in the head and neck 13. Evidence of foreign objects 14. Pain and/or dysfunction of the temporomandibular joint 15. Facial asymmetry 16. Abutment teeth for fixed or removable partial prosthesis 17. Unexplained bleeding 18. Unexplained sensitivity of teeth 19. Unusual eruption, spacing or migration of teeth 20. Unusual tooth morphology, calcification or color 21. Unexplained absence of teeth 22. Clinical tooth erosion 23. Peri-implantitis

American Dental Association Council on Scientific Affairs, U.S. Department of Health and Human Services, U.S. Food and Drug Administration. Dental radiographic examinations: recommendations for patient selection and limiting radiation exposure. http://www.fda.gov/Radiation-EmittingProducts/RadiationEmittingProductsandProcedures/MedicalImaging/MedicalX-Rays/ucm116504.htm. Accessed August 20, 2013.

Causes of Gagging

▶ *Hypersensitive oral tissues*: Particularly common in posterior region of oral cavity.

▶ *Techniques*: Image receptor moved over the oral tissues or retained in the mouth longer than is necessary.

▶ *Anxiety and apprehension*

- Fear of unknown, and of the image receptor touching a sensitive area.
- Previous unpleasant experiences with radiographic techniques.

- Failure to comprehend the clinician's instructions.
- Lack of confidence in the clinician.

Preventive Procedures

▶ Inspire confidence in ability to perform the service.

▶ Alleviate anxiety; explain procedures carefully. Smile and display a positive attitude.

▶ Minimize tissue irritation.

- Ask patient to swallow before each image receptor placement.
- Expose anterior image receptors before posterior as placement is easier to tolerate.
- Place image receptor firmly and positively without sliding the film over the tissue, especially the palate.
- Rub a finger over the tissues where the image receptor placement is intended to desensitize the tissues.
- Instruct patient to breathe through nose with quick breaths.
- Use stick-on film cushions to make image receptor placement more comfortable.

▶ Use a premedicating agent prescribed by the dentist.

▶ Use a topical anesthetic.

PROCEDURES FOR IMAGE RECEPTOR PLACEMENT AND ANGULATION OF CENTRAL RAY

The image projected onto the radiograph is a shadow of the teeth and the surrounding structures. The dental radiographer follows as closely as possible the five principles of shadow casting, listed in Box 13-10, when exposing radiographs.

Basic intraoral procedures for periapical, bitewing, and occlusal radiographs are included in this chapter. The principles and uses of panoramic radiographs are also described.

Two fundamental periapical procedures are used in practice: the *paralleling* or right angle and the *bisecting angle*. The principles for image receptor placement are shown in Figure 13-11.

BOX 13-10

Principles of Shadow Casting

1. Place the image receptor as parallel as possible to the object.
2. Use as small an effective focal spot as practical.
3. Use as long a target–object distance as possible.
4. Use as short an object–image receptor distance as possible.
5. Aim the X-ray beam perpendicular to the image receptor.

Clinicians vary in their application of the principles of the two techniques. Basic to both the paralleling technique and the bisecting-angle technique are:

▶ The primary beam passes through the teeth of interest.

▶ The image receptor is placed in relation to the teeth so that all parts of the image are shown as close to their natural size and shape as possible.

▶ Dimensional distortion is minimized.

▶ The development of a systematic, comfortable, smooth procedure saves time and energy for both patient and clinician, and the clinician is able to:

- Increase the confidence of the patient.
- Allow for consistency in technique.
- Produce good-quality radiographs.
- Minimize the length of time the image receptor remains in the patient's mouth.

IMAGE RECEPTOR SELECTION FOR INTRAORAL SURVEYS

I. Periapical Surveys

A. Area Covered

▶ To obtain a view of the entire tooth and its periodontal supporting structures.

B. Traditional Film Sizes

▶ *Child size*: No. 0 (22 × 35 mm) for primary teeth and small mouths.

▶ *Anterior*: No. 1 (24 × 40 mm) for anterior regions where width of arch makes positioning of standard film difficult or impossible.

▶ *Standard*: No. 2 (31 × 41 mm) may be used for all positions.

▶ *Long bitewing*: No. 3 (27 × 54 mm) infrequently used as periapical film.

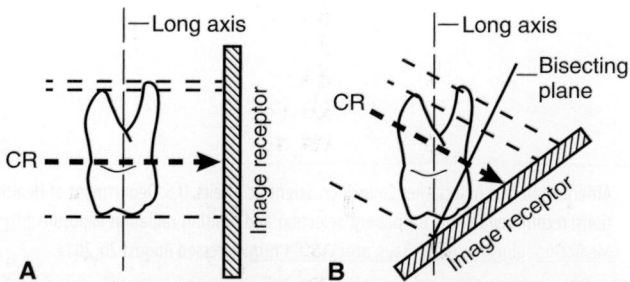

FIGURE 13-11 Comparison of Paralleling and Bisecting-Angle Techniques. A: Paralleling technique. The image receptor is parallel with the long axis of the tooth and the central ray (CR) is directed perpendicularly both to the image receptor and to the long axis of the tooth. **B:** Bisecting-angle technique. The central ray is directed perpendicularly to an imaginary line that bisects the angle formed by the image receptor and the long axis of the tooth.

C. Digital Sensor Sizes

▶ No. 0 for primary teeth and small mouths.
▶ No. 1 for anterior teeth where the width of the arch makes positioning of the size 2 sensor difficult or impossible.
▶ No. 2 may be used for all positions.
▶ No. 3 may be used for a long bitewing or periapical.

D. Number of Image Receptors Used in a Complete Survey

▶ Fourteen to 16 projections plus bitewings depending on:
  • The clinician's preferences.
  • The anatomy of the patient's mouth.
  • The size of the image receptors used.

II. Bitewing (Interproximal) Surveys

A. Area Covered

▶ *Horizontal bitewing radiographic images. To show:*
  • The crowns of the teeth and the alveolar crest in a dentition with normal to slight bone loss
  • Proximal surface root caries
  • Overhanging restorations.
▶ *Vertical bitewing radiographic images. To show:*
  • The crowns of the teeth and the alveolar bone level with moderate to severe bone loss
  • Proximal surface root caries
  • Overhanging restorations.

B. Image Receptors

Refer to Table 13-6 for film/sensor size and number guidelines.

The number and size of image receptors used for bitewing surveys are determined by:
▶ The size of the dental arch
▶ The number of teeth present
▶ Patient tolerance.

III. Occlusal Surveys

A. Purpose

▶ To show large areas of the maxilla, mandible, or floor of the mouth.

B. Image Receptors

▶ No. 4 for use in self-contained packet or in intraoral cassette.
▶ No. 2 for child or individual areas of adult.

DEFINITIONS AND PRINCIPLES

I. Planes

A. Sagittal or Median

▶ The plane that divides the body in the midline into right and left sides.

TABLE 13-6	Bitewing Film Surveys			
PATIENT	**RECEPTOR PLACEMENT**	**IMAGE RECEPTOR**[a]	**NUMBER OF IMAGE RECEPTORS**	**REGION**
Adult Posterior survey	Horizontal for dental caries Vertical for periodontal bone loss	2 or 3 2	4	Premolars and molars
Adult Anterior survey	Vertical	1 or 2	3	Centrals, laterals, canines
Child Survey: permanent dentition	Horizontal	2	2	Premolars and molars
Child Survey: mixed dentition	Horizontal	1 or 2	2	Premolars and/or primary molars and permanent molars
Child Survey: all primary teeth	Horizontal	0	2	Primary molars

[a]Film size is determined by size of dental arch and patient tolerance. Use largest film the patient will tolerate.

B. Occlusal

▶ The occlusal plane represents the mean curvature from the incisal edges of the central incisors to the tips of the occluding surfaces of the third molars.

▶ The occlusal plane of the premolars and first molar may be considered as the mean occlusal plane.

II. Angulation

A. Horizontal

▶ The angle at which the central ray of the useful beam is directed within a horizontal plane.

▶ Incorrect horizontal angulation results in *overlapping* or *superimposition* of parts of adjacent teeth in the radiograph and cone-cutting.

B. Vertical

The plane at which the central ray of the useful beam is directed within a vertical plane. Variations:

▶ Elongation: inadequate vertical angulation

▶ Foreshortening: excessive vertical angulation.

III. Long Axis of a Tooth

▶ The long axis can be represented by an imaginary line passing longitudinally through the center of the tooth.

▶ Because of marked variations in tooth position and root curvature, estimation of the long axis of a tooth is difficult.

PERIAPICAL SURVEY: PARALLELING TECHNIQUE

The paralleling technique is based on the principles that the image receptor is placed as parallel to the long axis of the tooth as the anatomy of the oral cavity permits, and the central ray is directed at right angles to the image receptor. Figure 13-11A shows the parallel relationship of the film or sensor with the long axis of the tooth and the right-angle direction of the central ray.

▶ *Maxillary projections:* The image receptor is placed toward the midline of the palate. Apicies missing due to shallow palate may require an increase in vertical angulation.

▶ *Mandibular projections:* The image receptor is placed close to the teeth of interest as long as parallelism is maintained.

▶ *Premolar projections:* The image receptor is placed toward the midline, as far forward as possible and closer to the opposite arch canine to capture the distal surface of the canine.[11]

I. Patient Position

▶ As long as the image receptor is parallel to the long axis of the tooth and the central ray is directed at right angles to the image receptor, the head may be in any position convenient to the clinician and comfortable for the patient.

▶ Slight modification of positioning may be needed for making radiographs in a supine position.

II. Image Receptor Placement

A. Image Receptor Position and Angulation of the Central Ray

▶ Instructions for image receptor placement and angulation are included in this section.

▶ Basic principles:
  • The principle for image receptor placement and angulation of the central ray.
  • Figures 13-12 and 13-13 show the image objective in the completed radiograph.

▶ *Horizontal angulation:* The central ray is directed at the center of the image receptor and through the interproximal area.

▶ *Vertical angulation:* The central ray is directed at a right angle to the image receptor.

B. Image Receptor Positioning Holders

▶ The use of an image receptor holder (film-positioning device) facilitates obtaining the correct angulation of the central ray.

▶ Lining up the PID with coordinating parts of the image receptor holder sets the correct vertical and horizontal angulation so that the central ray is perpendicular to the image receptor.

▶ Figure 13-14 shows an example of a disposable image receptor positioning device.

▶ *Purposes:* The use of a beam-guiding, field size-limiting, image receptor holding instrument provides:
  • Dose reduction.
  • Improved image quality.
  • Diagnostic radiographs without frequent retakes.
  • Improved infection control.

▶ *Characteristics:* An effective image receptor positioning device has characteristics such as the following:
  • Simple and adaptable to all positions.
  • Aids in reducing radiation exposure to patient.
  • Aids in alignment of X-ray beam.
  • Comfortable for the patient.
  • Minimal complexity for learning.
  • Disposable or conveniently sterilized.

▶ Types of film holders
  • Several types of image receptor holders are listed in Box 13-11.

Paralleling Technique
Maxillary

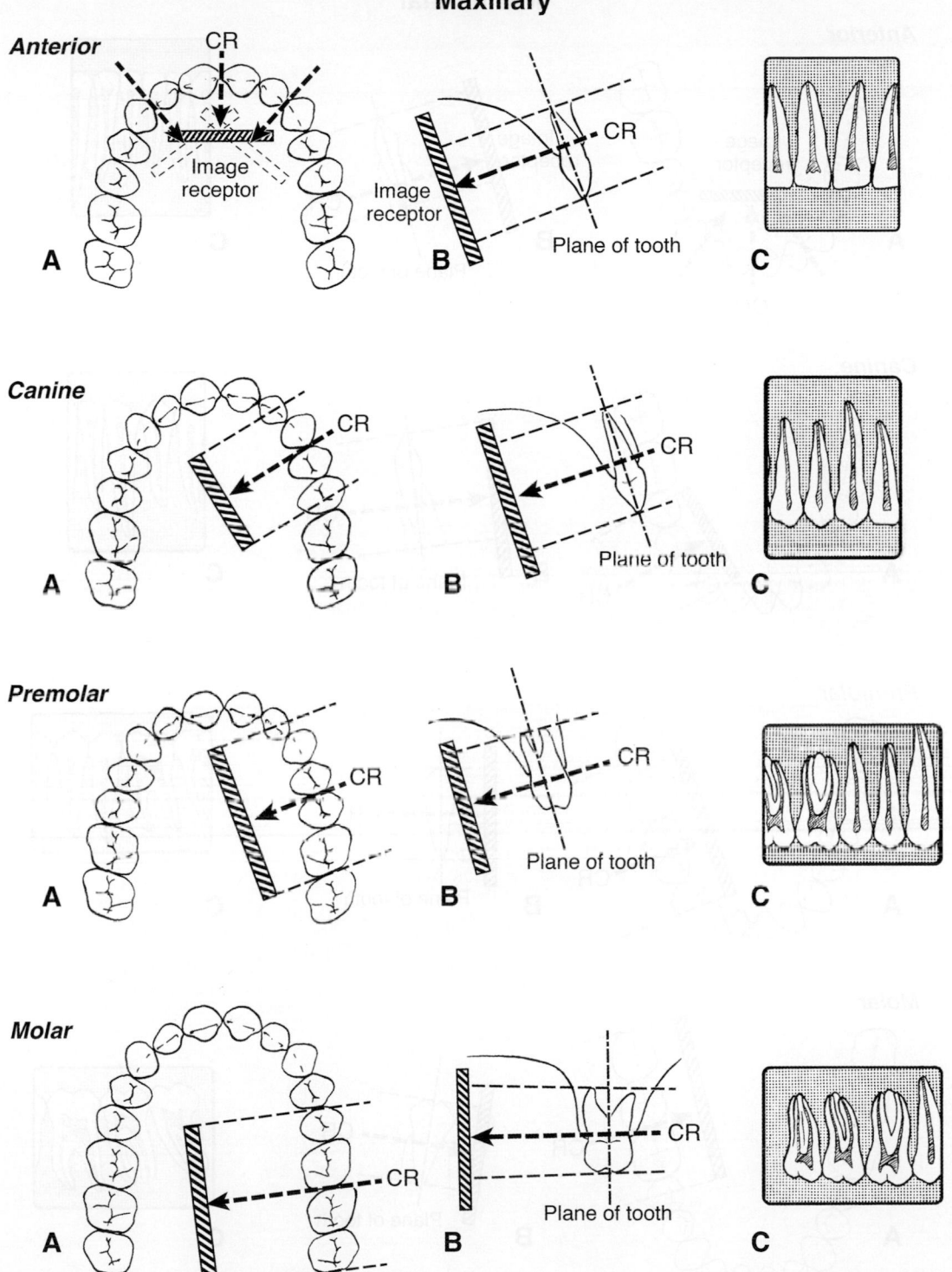

FIGURE 13-12 **Paralleling Technique, Maxillary Arch.** Image receptor positioning for the major maxillary positions. **A:** Horizontal angulation, with image receptor placed parallel to the long axes of the teeth; central ray directed parallel with a line through the interproximal space. **B:** Vertical angulation, with central ray directed at right angles to the image receptor. **C:** Image objective for the completed radiograph.

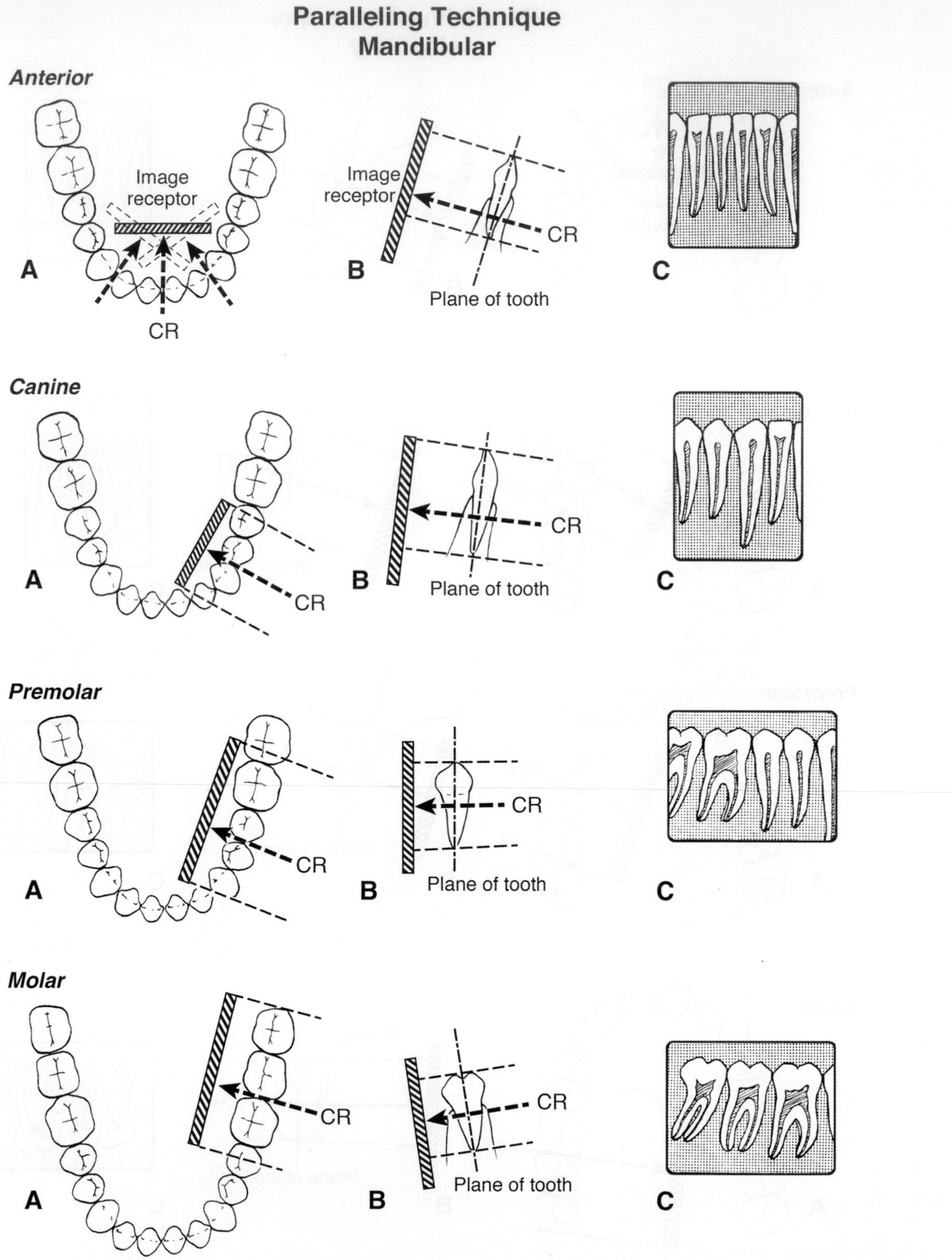
Paralleling Technique
Mandibular
Anterior
Image receptor
CR
A
Image receptor
CR
Plane of tooth
B
C
Canine
CR
A
CR
Plane of tooth
B
C
Premolar
CR
A
CR
Plane of tooth
B
C
Molar
CR
A
CR
Plane of tooth
B
C

FIGURE 13-13 **Paralleling Technique, Mandibular Arch.** Image receptor positioning for the major mandibular positions. **A:** Horizontal angulation, with image receptor placed parallel to the long axes of the teeth; central ray directed through the interproximal space. **B:** Vertical angulation, with central ray directed at right angles to the image receptor. **C:** Image objective for the completed radiograph.

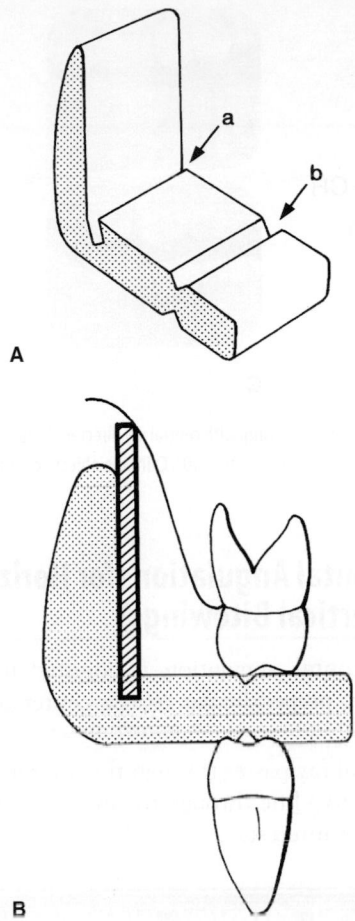

A

B

FIGURE 13-14 Styrofoam Disposable Film/PSP Holder. A: Empty holder to show: a, slot for insertion of the traditional film or PSP plate, and b, break-off point to shorten the bite surface for use in the mandibular posterior positions. B: Film/PSP plate placement for maxillary molar radiograph for patient with a high palatal vault.

► *Examples* of widely used types include the following:
  • Rinn X-C-P film and sensor holders. A plastic and stainless steel film holder with aiming devices that is used with the paralleling technique.

BOX 13-11

Image Receptor Positioning Devices

Bite blocks, plastic or foam
Stabe (Styrofoam disposable film/PSP plate holder)
Precision X-ray device
Snap-a-ray
X-C-P (extension cone paralleling)
B-A-I (bisecting-angle instrument)
V.I.P. (versatile intraoral positioner)
Hemostat with rubber bite block

Supplements

Removable denture for stabilization of film holder
Cotton roll to achieve parallelism

• Bite blocks vary depending on selected image receptor.
• Styrofoam disposable bite block for use with a traditional film or digital PSP plate when utilizing the paralleling or bisecting-angle techniques (Figure 13-14).

III. Paralleling Technique: Features

A. Accuracy

The paralleling technique gives a more accurate size and shape of dental structures with less distortion than when the bisecting-angle technique is used.

► In Figures 13-12 and 13-13, an accurate crown:root ratio is shown with facial and lingual aspects in proper relation to each other.
► Zygomatic bone can be shown in its normal position above the root apices of the molars and premolars.

B. Horizontal Ray Direction

No rays are directed toward the thyroid, whereas with the bisecting-angle technique, several maxillary radiographs require a relatively steep vertical angulation.

BITEWING SURVEY

I. Preparation

A. Patient Position

► *Traditional.* Sagittal plane perpendicular to the floor and occlusal plane parallel with the floor.
► *Patient in supine position:* The planes are reversed in their relation to the floor.

B. Vertical Angulation

► Set at +8° to +10° for horizontal or vertical bitewings (Figure 13-15B).

C. Patient Instruction

► Request patient to practice closing on posterior teeth before positioning image receptor for posterior bitewing and to practice edge-to-edge closure for anterior bitewing (Figure 17-4, in Chapter 17 shows edge-to-edge).

II. Image Receptor Placement: Horizontal Bitewing Survey

Figure 13-15 shows in diagram form the position of the horizontal molar bitewing image receptor in relation to the teeth, the horizontal and vertical angulation, and the image objective for both the premolar and the molar completed radiographs when standard image receptor is used.

► *Molar*
  • Standard image receptor in horizontal position.

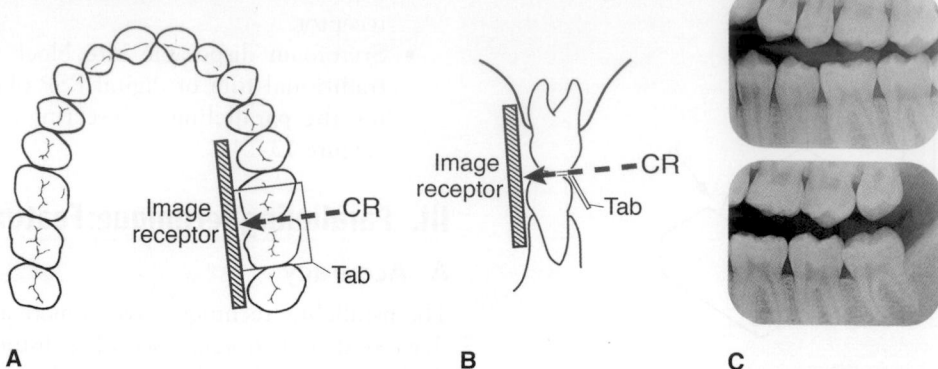

FIGURE 13-15 Horizontal Bitewing Radiograph. A: Image receptor position showing horizontal angulation for molar viewing, with central ray directed through the interproximal space to the center of the image receptor. Image receptor is centered over the second molar. **B:** Vertical angulation set at +8° to +10°. **C:** Image objective for molar (*above*) and premolar (*below*) regions.

- Center the image receptor on the second molar to ensure capturing the first and third molars on the radiograph (see Figure 13-15A).

▶ *Premolar*

- Standard image receptor in horizontal position.
- Center the film/sensor over the second premolar.
- Place the mesial border of image receptor at midline of the mandibular canine to include the distal surfaces of maxillary and mandibular canines and a clear view of both the first and second premolars.
- If using rigid sensors, move mesial portion of image receptor closer to the opposite arch canine to ensure canine visibility.

III. Image Receptor Placement: Vertical Bitewing Survey

▶ *Molar*

- Standard image receptor in vertical position.
- Center of the image receptor positioned over the middle of the second molar.
- Include at least the distal portion of both the maxillary and mandibular first molars and the mesial portion of the third molars, as illustrated in Figure 13-16.

▶ *Premolar*

- Standard image receptor in vertical position.
- Position the mesial border of image receptor at midline of the mandibular canine.
- Include the distal portion of maxillary and mandibular canines and a clear view of the first and second premolars.

▶ *Anterior*

- Center of image receptor at proximal space between the lateral and canine for the two canine/lateral bitewings.
- Center of image receptor at midline for central bitewing.

IV. Horizontal Angulation (for Horizontal and Vertical Bitewings)

▶ The horizontal angulation is adjusted to direct the central ray perpendicular to the center of the image receptor.

▶ The central ray passes through the interproximal space or parallel to a line through the interproximal spaces of the teeth of interest.

PERIAPICAL SURVEY: BISECTING-ANGLE TECHNIQUE

The bisecting-angle technique is based on the geometric principle that the central ray is directed perpendicularly to an imaginary line that is the bisector of the angle formed by the long axis of the tooth and the plane of the image receptor.

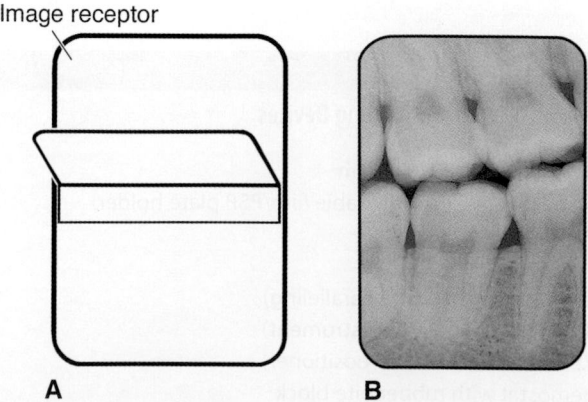

FIGURE 13-16 Vertical Bitewing Radiograph. A: Vertical bitewing image receptor with the tab positioned vertically over the center of the image receptor. **B:** Image objective of maxillary and mandibular molar regions. Image receptor is placed centered over the mandibular second molar.

▶ Figure 13-11B illustrates in diagram form the relationship of the long axis of the tooth, the image receptor, and the bisector of the angle formed by these two.

▶ Types of image receptors holders:

• *Rinn snap-a-ray*: A rigid plastic image receptor holder without a backing plate to prevent receptor bending, used in both posterior and anterior regions of the mouth. Useful in patients who cannot tolerate the receptor backing devices of a biteblock.

• *Rinn B-A-I film and sensor holders*: A plastic and stainless steel image receptor holder with an aiming device that is used with the bisecting-angle technique.

• *Styrofoam disposable holder*: A disposable bite block used with the bisecting-angle or paralleling technique.

OCCLUSAL SURVEY

The central midline films for maxillary and mandibular arches are described in this section. A variety of positions for the occlusal survey are possible, depending on the area to be examined.

I. Uses and Purposes

▶ To observe areas not shown on other image projections.

▶ To position image receptor when obtaining periapical image projections is impossible.

▶ To supplement the angulation provided by other image receptors for such conditions as fractures, impacted teeth, or salivary duct calculi.

II. Maxillary Midline Topographic Projection

A. Position of Patient's Head

▶ The line from the tragus of the ear to the ala of the nose is parallel with the floor.

B. Position of Film

▶ The exposure side of the image receptor is toward the palate.

▶ Posterior border of image receptor is brought back close to the third molar region. Image receptor is held between the teeth with edge-to-edge closure.

C. Angulation

▶ The PID is directed toward the bridge of the nose at a +65° angle.

III. Mandibular Topographic and Cross-Sectional Projection

A. Position of Patient's Head

▶ The head is tilted directly back.

B. Position of Image Receptor

▶ The exposure side is toward the floor of the mouth.

▶ The posterior border of the image receptor is in contact with the soft tissues of the retromolar area.

▶ The image receptor is held between the teeth in an edge-to-edge bite.

C. Angulation

▶ Topographical: Point PID at chin for incisal region: −55° angle.

▶ Cross-sectional: Direct PID under the chin for the floor of the mouth, perpendicular to the image receptor.

PANORAMIC RADIOGRAPHIC IMAGES

Panoramic radiography, or pantomography, refers to methods that produce continuous radiographs showing the maxillary and mandibular arches with adjacent structures on a single radiograph.

The panoramic radiograph is an option to a periapical survey, but it is not a substitute because of the loss of sharpness and detail. The principal advantages of panoramic images are:

▶ Broad coverage of facial bones and teeth.

▶ Low patient radiation dose.

▶ Convenience of the examination for the patient.

▶ Short time required to expose a panoramic image.

▶ Useful for patients who cannot open their mouths.

▶ Visibility for patient education.

I. Technique

A *panoramic radiograph is a radiographic projection that is positioned outside the mouth during X-ray exposure and is used to examine the maxillary and mandibular jaws on a single image.*

▶ The movement of the image receptor and tube head produces an image through the process known as tomography.

▶ The prefix *tomo* means section; tomography is a radiographic technique that depicts one layer or section of the body in focus while surrounding structures in other planes are blurred.

▶ In a panoramic tomograph, the attempt is to radiograph the maxillary and mandibular dentitions in focus on one image receptor.

▶ The image receptor and tube head rotate around the patient's head in opposite directions.

▶ The focal trough refers to a plane of tissue in focus during the exposure.

A. Patient Position

▶ Patient positioning depends on the panoramic unit and the patient's height, as they can be standing or sitting.

- Stabilize the head with a chin support or one of several types of head holders characteristic of each machine.
- Position the patient to ensure that the Frankfort plane (orbitale to tragus of the ear) is parallel to the floor and the midsagital plane perpendicular to the floor.
- Close the anterior teeth on the intraoral biteblock using the machine guide to ensure that the arch is not positioned too far back or forward.

B. Cassette

▶ Curved or flat.

▶ Rigid or flexible.

▶ Marked to denote left or right side of the patient.

▶ Contains calcium tungstate or preferably rare earth intensifying screens that provide for reduced radiation exposure to the patient.

II. Uses

▶ The numerous applications for panoramic radiographic images are outlined in Box 13-12.

▶ Routine use for patients seeking general oral care cannot be recommended as a substitute for a periapical survey as there is a loss of detail.

III. Limitations

▶ Loss of definition and detail compared with periapical radiographs.

▶ Distortion of structures and findings.

BOX 13-12

Uses for Panoramic Images

▷ Detection and diagnosis of oral pathologic lesions
▷ Evaluation of impacted teeth
▷ Examination of the extent of large lesions
▷ Survey for edentulous patients
▷ Detection of calcified carotid arteries: potential stroke victims
▷ Evaluation of growth and development for pedodontic patients
▷ Evaluation of teeth and jaw position for orthodontic patients
▷ Detection of fractured jaws and traumatic injuries
▷ When intraoral films are impossible
  Trismus
  Parkinson's disease
  Cerebral palsy
  Hyperactive gag reflex

▶ Proximal caries are usually not evident on radiographs, except for large cavitated lesions that can be seen by direct examination.

▶ Inadequate for examination of periodontal structures.

A. Inferiority of Definition and Detail

Causes of poor definition are:

▶ Use of intensifying screens.

▶ Increased object–image receptor distance.

▶ Movement of X-ray tube and image receptor.

B. Distortion

▶ Magnified images are produced because of increased distance between the image receptor and object.

▶ Overlapping

- In periapical techniques, each image receptor is angulated with the central ray so that when a tooth is out of line, adjustment is made to prevent overlapping.
- With panoramic technique, the head and teeth remain fixed, and the ray and image receptor are positioned only for the average.

IV. Procedures

Learning to use panoramic equipment is not difficult. Each machine has its own characteristics that can be learned readily from the manufacturer's instructions.

A. Patient Preparation

▶ Thyroid shield

- Cannot be used because of superimposition on the image.
- A special shield for panoramic radiography is available with coverage over the shoulders and partway or fully down the back.

B. Image Receptor

▶ Image receptor sizes are usually either 5 × 12 or 6 × 12 inches. Fast-speed film or digital sensors are used to minimize radiation.

C. Processing

▶ Regular processing solutions are used for traditional panoramic film. Special film holders for panoramic films are used during manual processing.

INFECTION CONTROL

I. Practice Policy

▶ Personnel of each office or clinic can determine a specific protocol appropriate to their facility and the type of processing used.

▶ A written policy is necessary for infection control during image receptor exposure, processing, and mounting and during management of the completed radiographs throughout clinical treatment appointments.[12]

II. Basic Procedures

Basic procedures are followed to prevent cross-contamination during transport to the digital laser scanner or darkroom and during use of manual and automatic processing equipment.[1,12] Steps are outlined in Boxes 13-13 and 13-14.

III. No-Touch Method for Films and PSP Plates

► With gloved hands and under appropriate safelight, pull open packets by their tabs or from their barrier envelopes as shown in Figure 13-17.

► Allow films/PSP plates to drop out into a cup, transport box, or onto the clean barrier-covered surface.

► Take care not to touch the films/PSP plates. Remove gloves, wash hands, and place films on hangers or into the automatic processor, being careful to touch the films by the edges only. Place PSP plates into the laser scanner.

► Dispose of waste properly.

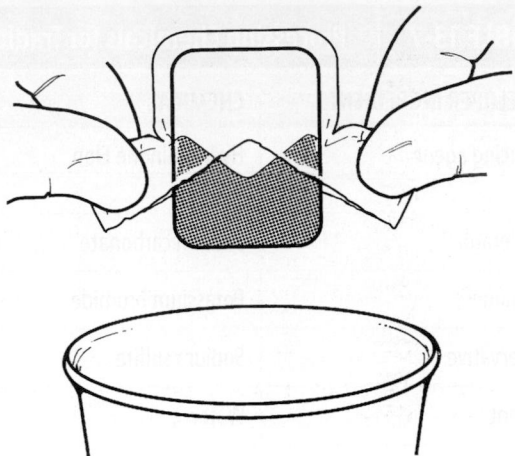

FIGURE 13-17　Plastic Film/PSP Plate Barrier. Opening plastic film/PSP plate barrier using the no-touch method. Plastic barriers placed over intraoral image receptors are used to protect image receptors from salivary contamination.

► Alternative no-touch method.
  • Wear overgloves over powder-free treatment gloves and remove them after dropping film/PSP plates into the cup.
  • Films/PSP plates are then processed while wearing powder-free treatment gloves.

BOX 13-13

Basic Infection Control Procedures

▷ Digital PSP plates and traditional films covered with contaminated saliva are confined to a disposable cup after exposure.

▷ Gloved hands fresh from contamination from the patients mouth do not come in contact with walls, doors, light switches, and other environmental surfaces when transporting a cup of contaminated exposed PSP plates to the scanner or traditional films to the dark room.

▷ The darkroom or laser scanner work area is prepared by the disinfection of all touch surfaces, and the counter is covered with clean paper.

▷ Processing procedures may reduce the bacterial counts, but the potential for cross-contamination still exists.

▷ Dispose of PSP plate and traditional film wrappers, cups, and contaminated gloves with contaminated waste. Lead foil is disposed of according to environmental waste guidelines.

BOX 13-14

Automatic Daylight Loader Film Processing Method

1. With powder-free regloved hands and exposed films in a paper cup, insert films in the daylight compartment.
2. Remove films from packets with the no-touch method, dropping films into a clean cup.
3. Remove gloves. Process films with ungloved hands, being careful to touch film by the edges only.
4. Remove ungloved hands from daylight loader. Don new gloves.
5. Disinfect daylight loader.

TRADITIONAL FILM PROCESSING

Film processing is the chemical transformation of the latent image, produced in a traditional film emulsion by exposure to radiation, into a stable image visible by transmitted light.

I. Standard Procedures

► Standardization of processing procedure goes hand-in-hand with standardized exposure techniques if consistently acceptable radiographs are to be prepared.

► Processing is treated as an exacting chemical procedure in which each step has specific objectives for the finished product.

► In Table 13-7, the developer and fixer ingredients are listed with the chemicals involved and their specific reactions.

II. Image Production

► Film emulsion contains crystals of silver halides (bromide and iodide).

► Development consists of selective reduction of affected silver halide salts to metallic silver grains.

► X-ray exposure changes the silver halides to silver and halide ions.

► Developer reacts with the halide ions, leaving only the metallic silver in an arrangement corresponding with the radiolucency and radiopacity of the tissue being exposed.

TABLE 13-7	Processing Chemicals for Traditional Film	
DEVELOPER INGREDIENTS	**CHEMICAL**	**ACTIVITY**
Reducing agent	Hydroquinone Elon	Converts exposed silver halide crystals to black metallic silver Generates gray tones in the image
Accelerator	Sodium carbonate	Swells the emulsion and provides an alkaline medium
Restrainers	Potassium bromide	Blocks the action of the reducing agent on the unexposed crystals
Preservative	Sodium sulfite	Slows the oxidation and breakdown of the developer
Solvent	Water	Mixes the chemicals
Fixer Ingredients		
Clearing agents	Ammonium thiosulfate or sodium thiosulfate	Removes all unexposed undeveloped silver halide crystals from emulsion
Acid or activator	Acetic acid Sulfuric acid	Stops development; neutralizes any remaining developer
Hardeners	Potassium alum	Toughens and shrinks the gelatin in the emulsion
Preservative	Sodium sulfite	Slows the oxidation of the fixer
Solvent	Water	Mixes the chemicals

- Fixation consists of selective removal of unaffected silver halide crystals.
- Fixer removes only those crystals of silver halide that were not exposed to radiation.
- Washing removes processing chemicals.
- End result is a *negative*, showing various degrees of lightness and darkness (microscopic grains of black metallic silver).

III. Darkroom Lighting

- Find and eliminate all possible light leaks.
- Conventional safelighting.
  - 15-watt bulb or less.
  - Positioned a minimum of 4 feet above the working surface.
  - Filter is selected according to film type.
- Light-emitting diode (LED) safelight.
  - Clusters of 20 red LEDs.
  - Twice as much visible light as conventional safelighting.

IV. Automated Processing

Automatic film processing refers to the use of equipment designed to transport film mechanically through a series of solutions under controlled conditions. Figure 13-18 illustrates the film being transported from the entry slot to the developer, fixer, water bath, dryer, and exit slot.

A. Advantages of Automated Processing

- Consistency of results.
- Conservation of time by dental personnel.
- Finished radiographs in 4–6 minutes.
- Radiographs available for immediate use.

B. Principles of Operation

- Rollers or tracks are used to carry traditional film through developing, fixing, washing, and drying. Some machines may process only standard intraoral films, whereas others may also accommodate extraoral sizes.
- Increased temperature decreases processing time.
- Frequent use and large film sizes require more solution and would therefore necessitate more frequent change of the solutions.

V. Manual Processing

The darkroom has three tanks of chemicals and water for processing by hand: the developing tank, fixing tank, and water bath. In most darkrooms, the developer is the left

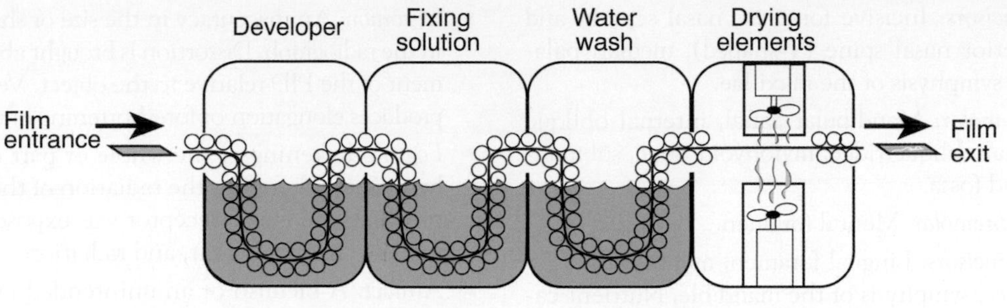

FIGURE 13-18 Automatic Processor. Diagram to show an automatic roller transport system that conveys traditional film over the rollers through the developer, fixer, water bath, and drying elements.

tank, the water bath is in the center tank, and the fixer is in the right tank. The fixer can be identified by a smell similar to vinegar.

A. Processing Temperature and Times

▶ The quality of the radiographic image depends greatly on the processing time and temperature, with optimal developing conditions for manual processing being 68°F for 5 minutes.

▶ Higher temperatures would produce films with excessive density; cooler temperatures, too little density. Follow manufacturer's directions for proper time and temperature.

B. Equipment and Steps for Manual Processing

▶ Check level and temperature of solutions with processing thermometer; stir solutions with stirring rods.

▶ Turn on safelights and turn off the white lights.

▶ Load films from the film packet or cassette onto hangers, making sure films are securely fastened.

▶ Immerse film in the developer; activate timer.

▶ When timer buzzes, rinse films in circulating water for 30 seconds.

▶ Immerse the films in the fixer for twice the clearing time.

▶ Wash the films in circulating water for 10 minutes.

▶ Dry films until they are no longer tacky.

C. Disposal of Liquid Chemicals

Fixer and developer are considered environmentally hazardous waste material and are disposed of according to governmental regulations.

ANALYSIS OF COMPLETED RADIOGRAPHS

The completed radiographs are mounted and examined at a viewbox with an adequate light source or a computer monitor. Interpretation of radiographs is difficult, and the determination of a pathologic condition requires keen evaluation. Attempting to base interpretation on inadequate, insufficient radiographs will result in guesswork rather than in an accurate, timely diagnosis.

I. Mounting

▶ If using traditional film, legibly mark the mount with the name of patient, age, date, name of dentist; printing is preferred.

▶ Handle radiographs only by the edges with clean, dry hands.

▶ Arrange radiographs in front of the viewbox on clean, dry paper.

▶ The embossed dot near the edge of the radiograph is the guide to mounting; the raised side of the dot is on the facial side.

▶ Identify individual radiographs by teeth and other anatomic landmarks.

▶ Approved mounting system is as follows: Looking at the teeth from outside the mouth, the teeth are viewed and mounted in the same manner as the approved tooth numbering system.

II. Anatomic Landmarks

A. Definition

An anatomic landmark is an anatomic structure, the image of which may serve as an aid in the localization and identification of the regions portrayed by a radiograph. The teeth are the primary landmarks.

B. Landmarks That May Be Seen in Individual Radiographs

▶ *Maxillary molar*: Maxillary sinus, zygomatic process, zygomatic (malar) bone, hamular process, coronoid process of the mandible, maxillary tuberosity, lateral pterygoid plate.

▶ *Maxillary premolar*: Maxillary sinus.

▶ *Maxillary canine*: Maxillary sinus, junction of the maxillary sinus and nasal fossa (Y-shaped, radiopaque).

▶ *Maxillary incisors:* Incisive foramen, nasal septum and fossae, anterior nasal spine (V-shaped), median palatine suture, symphysis of the maxillae.

▶ *Mandibular molar:* Mandibular canal, internal oblique line, external oblique ridge, mylohyoid ridge, submandibular gland fossa.

▶ *Mandibular premolar:* Mental foramen.

▶ *Mandibular incisors:* Lingual foramen, mental ridge, genial tubercles, symphysis of the mandible. Nutrient canals are seen most frequently in this radiograph.

III. Identification of Errors in Radiographs

Table 13-8 outlines the more common errors, their causes, and the keys to correction.

A. Causes

Errors may be related to any step in the entire procedure, including image receptor placement, angulation, exposure, processing, and care and handling of the image receptors.

B. Types

Errors appear as problems of improper density or contrast, incomplete or distorted images, fogging, artifacts, or stains.

▶ *Distortion:* An inaccuracy in the size or shape of an object in the radiograph. Distortion is brought about by misalignment of the PID relative to the object. Vertical distortion produces elongation or foreshortening of the object.

▶ *Fog:* A darkening of the whole or part of a radiograph by sources other than the radiation of the primary beam to which the image receptor was exposed. Types of fog include chemical, light, and radiation.

▶ *Artifact:* A blemish or an unintended radiographic image that can result from faulty manufacture, manipulation, exposure, or processing of an image receptor.

IV. Interpretation

Radiographs are used in conjunction with clinical assessment for a complete care program. Periodic radiographs permit continuing evaluation. As part of the permanent record, radiographs help to document the oral condition for comparison as well as for legal and forensic purposes.

The quality of the radiographs determines their value for diagnostic interpretation. Procedures for the preparation of radiographs are perfected so that the radiographs have maximum interpretability with minimum radiation exposure of the patient.

TABLE 13-8	Analysis of Radiographs: Causes of Errors	
	ERROR	**CAUSE: FACTORS IN CORRECTION**
Image	Elongation Foreshortening	Insufficient vertical angulation Excessive vertical angulation
	Superimposition (overlapping)	Incorrect horizontal angulation (central ray not directed through interproximal space)
	Partial image	Cone-cut (incorrect direction of central ray or incorrect image receptor placement) Incompletely immersed in processing tank Traditional film touched other film or side of tank during processing
	Blurred or double image	Patient, tube, or image receptor movement during exposure Image receptor exposed twice
	Stretched appearance of trabeculae or apices	Bent traditional film or PSP plate
	No image	Machine malfunction from time-switch to wall-plug Failure to turn on the machine Traditional film placed in fixer before developer
Density	Too dark	Excessive exposure for all image receptors For traditional film: Excessive developing Developer too warm Unsafe safelight Accidental exposure to white light

TABLE 13-8	Analysis of Radiographs: Causes of Errors (*continued*)	
	ERROR	**CAUSE: FACTORS IN CORRECTION**
	Too light	Insufficient exposure for all image receptors For traditional film: Insufficient development or excessive fixation Solutions too cool Use of old, contaminated, or poorly mixed solutions Film placement: tube side not placed toward teeth Film used beyond expiration date
Fog	Chemical fog	For traditional film: An imbalance or deterioration of processing solutions
	Light fog	For traditional film: An unintentional exposure to light to which the emulsion is sensitive, either before or during processing Unsafe safelight Darkroom leak Holding unprocessed films too close to the safelight too long Improper storage of unused traditional film
	Radiation fog	Traditional film exposed to scatter radiation before processing
Reticulation	(puckered or pebbly surface)	For traditional film: Sudden temperature changes during traditional film processing, particularly from warm solutions to very cold water
Artifacts	Dark lines	Bent or creased film or PSP plate Fingernail used to grasp traditional film or PSP plate For traditional film: static electricity when removed from wrapper with excessive force
	Herringbone pattern (light film)	Traditional film packet placed in mouth backward with foil next to teeth
Discoloration	Stains and spots	For traditional film: Unclean film hanger Spatterings of developer, fixer, dust Insufficient rinsing after developing before fixing Splashing dry negatives with water or solutions Air bubbles adhering to surface during processing (insufficient agitation) Overlap of film on film in tanks or while drying Paper wrapper stuck to film (film not dried when removed from patient's mouth)
	Stains at later date after storage of completed radiographs	For traditional film: Incomplete processing or rinsing Storage in too warm a place Storage near chemicals

A. Prerequisites for Interpretation

▶ *Mounting*: Mount traditional radiographs in an opaque mount to prevent light between each radiograph from creating glare and producing a blinding effect.

▶ *Viewbox*: Use an adequately lighted viewbox for traditional films. Dimmed room light improves visibility for contrasting radiolucent and radiopaque areas. Holding the radiographs up to view by window, room, or unit light is inadequate, and only gross interpretation can

be accomplished. When a viewbox is larger than the mount used, cover the edges to block out peripheral light.

▶ *Hand magnifying glass*: Examine traditional radiographs on a viewbox through a magnifying glass. A viewbox is available with a built-on magnifying glass.

▶ *Digital software tools*: Use magnifiers, manipulate brightness and contrast, invert image densities, etc. to enhance diagnostic capabilities.

B. Systematic Examination

▶ Observe one radiographic feature at a time. Examine all of the radiographs in a survey for that feature, rather than taking each radiograph separately to find everything. It is important to note comparisons for each change over the entire survey, and comparisons to past surveys if available.

▶ When examining a particular tooth, compare the appearance of that tooth in each radiograph in which it appears, including bitewings. At different angulations, different findings may become apparent.

C. Correlation with Clinical Examination

A description of radiographic examination of the teeth may be found in Chapter 16 and of the periodontal tissues in Chapter 20. Correlation of radiographic findings with the clinical examination, using probe and explorer, is basic to an understanding of the true oral condition of the patient.

OWNERSHIP

▶ Radiographs belong to the dental practice, even though they were paid for by the patient.

▶ Patient has a right to a copy of their records and their radiographs.

▶ If using traditional films, originals are kept by the dental practice and a duplicate series is to be given to the patient.

DOCUMENTATION

I. Radiation Exposure History

▶ Inquire whether the patient is receiving or has recently received radiation therapy. It may be necessary to minimize the number of exposures. A consultation with the patient's physician is recommended.

▶ Maintain an exposure log for each patient that indicates the date, number of exposures, kVp, mA, time, and area exposed.

II. Patient Care Progress Notes

Patient care progress notes include the following components:

▶ Patient complaint, if applicable, including:
  • Location of symptomatic area.
  • Duration and severity of symptoms.
▶ Clinical findings.
▶ Recommended diagnostic procedures.
  • Explain to patient necessity of radiographs for accurate diagnosis and treatment.
  • Patient has the right to refuse radiographs.
  • Obtain the patient's signature to a statement of refusal in the event a legal issue should arise.
▶ Type of radiographs (periapical or bitewing), number of exposures, and area(s) exposed.
▶ Box 13-15 provides example documentation for the patient who has received dental radiographs.

Box 13-15

Example Documentation: Assessment for Dental Radiographic Examination

S – Patient presents for routine maintenance appointment and complains about heat sensitivity related to tooth #10. The patient stated that he was hit in the mouth with a soccer ball approximately a year ago.

O – Last radiographs consisted of four Bitewings exposed 2 years ago. The most recent periapical radiograph of tooth #10, dated 3 years ago, reveals a healthy lamina dura and periodontal ligament space. The patient has several porcelain fused to metal crowns and large amalgam restorations in the posterior sextants. Teeth in the anterior sextants are natural and contain no restorative materials.

A – Discussed with the patient that #10 may have been traumatized and that a periapical pathology may exist. He has recently undergone numerous medical radiographs and requests minimal radiation exposure today.

P – After a complete clinical examination, and consultation with the patient, two premolar and two molar bitewing radiographs, along with one periapical film of #10 were exposed.

Next steps: Tooth #10 revealed a periapical pathology. The patient was referred to an endodontist for care.

Signed: _____, RDH

Date:_____

EVERYDAY ETHICS

Danielle, a recent dental hygiene graduate, is asked by her employer, Dr. Blum, to limit the number of gloves used to expose and process patients' traditional dental films due to cost constraints. Currently, she uses one pair to expose the patients' radiographs. She wears a second pair to process the exposed films in an automatic processor and uses a third pair to begin intraoral treatment for her patient. Dr. Blum would like her to wear the same gloves for all the aforementioned procedures. Danielle finds that method unacceptable.

Questions for Consideration

1. List ethical alternatives Danielle has for actions that take both patient safety and employer concerns into consideration. Is there another way to proceed, to limit the number of gloves used per patient?

2. Which core values (Table II-1 in the Section II Introduction) are involved as Danielle discussed those alternatives with her employer? Explain why the core values were chosen.

3. What ethical theory (Table IV-1 in the Section IV Introduction) can provide guidance as Danielle tries to resolve this issue? Explain the reason for your choice.

Factors To Teach The Patient

When the Patient Asks About the Safety of Radiation

▷ Patients ask questions about safety factors, and occasionally a patient may refuse to have any radiographs exposed. The patient can be reassured with confidence, instructed as to why radiographs are necessary at this time, and informed about how modern equipment and techniques are in accord with radiation standards.

▷ Adapt the answer to the patient. Certain patients have more fear; others have more knowledge about X-rays. The clinician who expresses confidence aids in allaying fears. Hesitation increases the patient's doubt.

▷ Radiographs are essential to diagnosis and treatment. Without the information provided, the clinician can only guess at conditions not visible clinically.

▷ The benefits resulting from the intelligent use of X-rays outweigh any possible negative effects.

▷ Modern X-ray machines are equipped for safety. Simple details about filtration, collimation, film speed, use of protective shields, and short exposure times can be explained.

Educational Features in Dental Radiographs

▷ Position of unerupted permanent teeth in relation to primary teeth.

▷ Detection of early cavitated carious lesions not visible by clinical examination.

▷ Effects of loss of teeth and the importance of having replacements.

▷ Periodontal changes and other pathologic conditions appropriate to an individual patient.

References

1. Iannucci JM, Howerton LJ. *Dental Radiography: Principles and Techniques.* 4th ed. St Louis, MO: Elsevier; 2012.

2. American Dental Association Council on Scientific Affairs, U.S. Department of Health and Human Services, U.S. Food and Drug Administration. Dental radiographic examinations: recommendations for patient selection and limiting radiation exposure. http://www.fda.gov/Radiation-EmittingProducts/RadiationEmitting ProductsandProcedures/MedicalImaging/MedicalX-Rays/ucm116504.htm. Accessed August 20, 2013.

3. United States National Research Council, (BEIR-V). *Health Effects of Exposure to Low Levels of Ionizing Radiation.* Washington, DC: National Academies Press; 1990.

4. Parks, ET. Digital radiographic imaging: is the dental practice ready? *JADA.* 2008;139(4):477–481.

5. White SC, Pharoah MJ. *Oral Radiology: Principles and Interpretation.* 6th ed. St. Louis, MO: Mosby; 2009:878–891.

6. van der Stelt, PF. Better imaging: the advances of digital radiography. *JADA.* 2008;139 (Suppl 3):7S–13S.

7. International Commission on Radiation Units and Measurements (ICRU). *Radiation Quantities and Units.* ICRU Report No. 33. Washington, DC: ICRU; 1980.

8. National Council on Radiation Protection and Measurements. *Radiation Protection in Dentistry.* NCRP Report No. 145. Washington, DC: NCRP; 2003.

9. White SC, Mallya SM. Update on the biological effects of ionizing radiation, relative dose factors and radiation hygiene. *Aust Dent J.* 2012;57 (Suppl 1):2–8.

10. Anjum M, Godward S, Williams D, et al. Dental x-rays and the risk of thyroid cancer: a case-control study. *Acta Oncol.* 2010;49(4):447–453.

11. Thomson EM. Reduce retakes. *Dimens Dent Hyg.* 2011;9(10):58–61.

12. Frommer HH, Stabulas-Savage JJ. *Radiology for the Dental Professional.* 9th ed. St. Louis, MO: Mosby; 2011.

ENHANCE YOUR UNDERSTANDING

the**Point** **DIGITAL CONNECTIONS**
(see the inside front cover for access information)
- **Audio glossary**
- **Quiz bank**

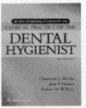

SUPPORT FOR LEARNING
(available separately; visit lww.com)
- ***Active Learning Workbook for Clinical Practice of the Dental Hygienist, 12th Edition***

prepU **INDIVIDUALIZED REVIEW**
(available separately; visit lww.com)
- **Adaptive quizzing with *prepU for Wilkins' Clinical Practice of the Dental Hygienist***

14

Study Models

Esther M. Wilkins, BS, RDH, DMD

CHAPTER OUTLINE

LEARNING OBJECTIVES

After studying this chapter, the student will be able to:

1. Define and describe impressions of the maxillary and mandibular dentitions.

2. Select and prepare equipment and dental materials needed to create acceptable impressions for the preparation of study models.

3. List the steps for making and finishing the final study models from the impressions.

4. Identify and explain the purposes and uses of study models in the clinical practice of dental hygiene.

As reproductions of the teeth, gingiva, and adjacent structures, study models can be useful adjuncts in the assessment and care of a patient. Accurate and esthetically acceptable models have a special use as visual aids for patient instruction.

The study models, radiographs, and clinical examination with recordings and chartings, together with the medical and dental histories, are utilized in the diagnosis, total care planning, treatment, and subsequent maintenance.

PURPOSES AND USES OF STUDY MODELS

▶ Serve as a permanent record of the patient's present condition.

▶ Give sharper delineation to and corroboration of the observations made during the oral examination.

▶ Observe normal conditions, the variations of and departures from the normal at the outset of treatment and, by comparison with subsequent periodic models, to compare and evaluate certain aspects of treatment.

▶ An effective visual aid to use when the oral conditions are explained and the dental and dental hygiene care plans are presented; to enable the patient to visualize and understand the need for the specific care outlined.

▶ Serve as a guide to clinical treatment procedures.

▶ Supplement clinical observations when the dental biofilm control program for the patient's daily self-care is explained.

▶ During dental charting of the teeth, to note missing teeth; anomalies of size, shape, or number; partial eruption; tooth positions, such as drifting, tilting, rotation, and open or closed contacts.

▶ During examination of the occlusion, to observe the static relations (Angle's classification, malrelations of groups of teeth, and malpositions of individual teeth) and other features, such as wear patterns and the effects of premature loss of teeth.

▶ During periodontal examination, to record anatomic features, such as the position, size, and shape of the gingiva and interdental papillae and the position of frena.

▶ Provide assistance during forensic examination along with radiographs.

STEPS IN THE PREPARATION OF STUDY MODELS

▶ Terms used to describe study models and their preparation are defined in Box 14-1. Procedures described in this chapter are as follows:

▶ Sequence of clinical procedures
- Assemble materials and equipment.
- Prepare the patient.
- Select and prepare the impression trays.
- Make the interocclusal record for occluding the maxillary and mandibular models.
- Make the mandibular impression.
- Make the maxillary impression.

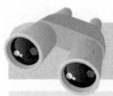

BOX 14-1 KEY WORDS: Study Models

Alginate: an impression material used for recording detail such as for study models.

Cast (model): a positive life-size reproduction of the teeth and adjacent tissues usually formed by pouring dental plaster or stone into a matrix or impression.

  Diagnostic or study model: used in the study of a patient's oral condition in preparation for treatment planning and patient instruction.

  Master model: used to fabricate a dental restoration or prosthesis.

Centric occlusion or habitual occlusion: the usual maximum intercuspation or contact of the teeth of the opposing arches.

Dental plaster: the beta form of calcium sulfate hemihydrate; a fibrous aggregate of fine crystals with capillary pores that are irregular in shape and porous in character; also referred to as plaster of Paris.

Dental stone: the alpha form of calcium sulfate hemihydrate with physical properties superior to those of the beta form (dental plaster); the alpha form consists of cleavage fragments and crystals in the form of rods and prisms and is therefore more dense than the beta form.

Impression: a negative imprint of an oral structure used to produce a positive replica of the structure; used to make models for a permanent record or in the production of a dental restoration or prosthesis; identified by the type of material used, such as hydrocolloid impression, alginate impression, or rubber base impression.

Interocclusal record: a registration of the positional relationship of the opposing teeth or dental arches made in a plastic material, such as a soft baseplate wax; also called the maxillomandibular relationship record or wax-bite.

Occlusal plane: the average plane established by the incisal and occlusal surfaces of the teeth; generally not actually a plane, but the planar mean of the curvature of those surfaces.

Polish: to make smooth and glossy usually by friction; the act or process of making a model smooth and glossy.

Prosthesis: an artificial replacement of an absent part of the human body; a therapeutic device to improve or alter function.

▶ Paraclinical procedures
  • Assemble materials and equipment.
  • Prepare the impression material for pouring.
  • Pour the models.
  • Trim and finish the models.
  • Polish the models.

CLINICAL PREPARATION

I. Assemble Materials and Equipment

▶ Patient bib, paper towels, and preprocedural mouthrinse.
▶ Impression trays
  • Perforated trays are generally used; small, medium, and large sizes are available.
  • Trays for use in the patient's mouth must be disposable or sterilized if metal.
▶ Mixing bowl
  • Clean, dry, flexible rubber with smooth, unscratched surface.
  • Reserve separate bowls for each dental material: one for impression material and another only for plaster or stone.
▶ Spatula
  • Clean, dry, stiff, with a smooth, rounded end that reaches every part of the bowl without scraping or cutting its surface.
▶ Saliva ejector
▶ Dental materials
  • Soft utility wax for preparation of tray rim (beading).
  • Impression material.
  • Soft baseplate wax for interocclusal record.
▶ Water thermometer.

II. Clinician Preparation

▶ Standard precautions are observed for all clinical procedures.
▶ A mask is worn when handling powder forms of dental materials to prevent inhalation.

III. Prepare the Patient

▶ History review
  • Review medical and dental histories for conditions that may require modifications such as respiratory concerns.
▶ Explain the procedure to be performed
  • The rationale and use of study models are explained to the patient.
  • The reaction of patients who have had previous impressions may range from indifference to dread,

and the conversation and approach can be individualized accordingly.
▶ Position the patient
  • Position the patient upright for maximum visibility and accessibility and to minimize gagging.
  • Stabilize the patient's head on the headrest.
▶ Removable prostheses
  • Provide a container with water in which the patient can place removable oral prostheses.
▶ Examine the oral cavity
  • Note facially displaced teeth, height of palate, undercut areas, and mandibular tori.
  • Note other anatomic features that may influence the size or preparation of the impression tray and the procedures to be carried out when making the impression.
▶ Free the mouth of debris
  • When excess debris is present, biofilm control instructions are initiated or reviewed.
  • Request patient remove debris and biofilm with a toothbrush.
▶ Provide preprocedural mouthrinse to:
  • Aid in the removal of debris and lessen the numbers of surface microorganisms.
  • Lower the mucin and surface tension; aids in preventing bubbles in the impression.
  • Provide a pleasant taste and feeling for the patient.
  • Distract an anxious patient while the trays are being prepared.
  • Explain purpose of vigorous swishing and rinsing procedure for several minutes to remove debris from interproximal areas.
▶ Dry the teeth
  • Use a cotton roll or compressed air stream to remove saliva from the teeth to prevent irregularities in the surface of the completed study model.
▶ Prevention of gagging
  • When the radiographic survey has been made before the study models, the clinician will have determined whether precautions to prevent gagging are needed.
  • With all patients a calm approach, an aura of confidence, a direct and efficient procedure, and a gentle handling of the patient's oral tissues will increase rapport and contribute to a satisfactory result.
  • The gag reflex is located on the posterior third of the tongue. It is necessary to keep impression materials from flowing onto that area.
  • Recommendations for prevention of gagging are summarized in Chapter 13.
▶ Technique considerations
  • Avoid excess impression material in the tray.
  • Seat the maxillary tray from posterior to anterior.
  • Instruct the patient to breathe deeply through the nose before the tray is inserted and after insertion; lean head forward.

THE INTEROCCLUSAL RECORD

I. Purposes

▶ Relates the maxillary and mandibular models correctly.
  • Many, if not most, models orient to each other readily in only one position.
  • When such problems as open bite, crossbite, edentulous areas, or end-to-end (or edge-to-edge) relations interfere with direct occlusion of the models, a bite registration is needed. The variety of tooth relations is shown in Chapter 17.
▶ Placed between the models during trimming and storage to prevent breakage of the model teeth.

II. Procedure

▶ Numerous materials are available to obtain registration, such as wax and quick setting materials.
▶ Manufacturer's instructions for use are followed.
▶ Request the patient practice opening and closing on the posterior teeth to ensure the habitual position can be obtained.
▶ Warm a piece of shaped soft baseplate wax or mix the bite registration material and place over the occlusal surfaces.
▶ Guide patient to close in habitual occlusion.
▶ Remove carefully to prevent distortion; chill wax in cold water. Disinfect.

PREPARATION OF IMPRESSION TRAYS[1]

I. Selection of Proper Size and Shape

▶ Width
  • Objective: to allow an adequate thickness of impression material on the facial and lingual surfaces of each tooth to provide strength and rigidity to the impression.
  • Tray flanges may be spread to accommodate for extra width in the molar regions, particularly lingual to the mandibular molars in the mylohyoid region.
  • When a tooth is in prominent labioversion, buccoversion, or linguoversion, a minimum thickness of 1/8 to 1/4 inch is suggested, but even then, the fragility of the impression material in that area is increased.
  • Tray: may appear in correct relation to the facial surfaces but may impinge on the lingual or palatal cusps of molars.
▶ Length
  • Objectives: To allow coverage of the retromolar area of the mandible and the tuberosity of the maxilla.

  • Anterior: plan for at least 1/4-inch clearance labial to the most protruded incisor without impingement on lingual or palatal gingiva.

II. Maxillary Tray Try-In

▶ Position of clinician
  • At side and toward the back of patient.
▶ Retraction
  • With index finger of nondominant hand, retract the patient's lip and cheek.
  • At the same time, use the side of the tray to distend the other side of the patient's mouth to gain entry (Figure 14-1).
▶ Insertion
  • With a slight rotary motion, insert the tray.
  • Orient the tray beneath the arch and center it by using the tray handle and the midline (usually between the central incisors and in line with the middle of the nose) as guides for positioning.
  • Bring the front of the tray to a position 1/4-inch labial to the most labially inclined incisor.
  • Seat the tray by bringing the posterior up before the anterior; retract the lip as the anterior is brought into place.
▶ Evaluation of the tray size
  • Lower the front of the tray while holding the posterior border of the impression tray in place (Figure 14-2).
  • Examine the relationship of the posterior border of the impression tray to the most posterior molars and the tuberosity areas to determine whether the coverage will be adequate.
  • Gently move the tray up and down to observe the relation to the facial surfaces of all teeth, malaligned teeth, protuberances, and other features and thus to assess the space for the impression material.

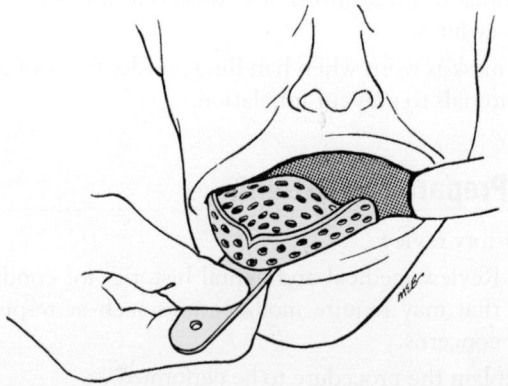

FIGURE 14-1 Maxillary Tray Insertion. The patient's lip and cheek are retracted with the fingers of the nondominant hand while the side of the tray is used to distend the other lip and cheek to gain entry. The tray is inserted with a rotary motion. The procedure for the mandibular tray is similar.

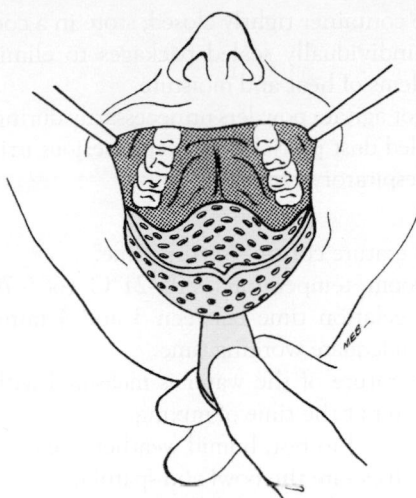

FIGURE 14-2 Selection of Impression Tray. Adequate coverage is determined as the posterior border of the tray is held in position while the front of the tray is lowered to observe the relationship of the posterior border to the maxillary tuberosity areas to be covered by the impression. The mandibular tray position is examined by lifting the tray to observe coverage of the retromolar areas.

III. Mandibular Tray Try-In

▶ Position of clinician
- At side front of patient.

▶ Retraction
- With index and middle fingers of nondominant hand, retract the patient's lip and cheek.
- At the same time, use the side of the tray to distend the side of the mouth to gain entry, similar to the procedure illustrated in Figure 14-1 for the maxillary tray.

▶ Insertion
- With a slight rotary motion, insert the tray.
- Orient the tray over the dental arch and center it by using the tray handle and the midline (usually between the central incisors and in line with the center of the chin) as guides for positioning.
- Bring the tray rim to about 1/4-inch anterior to the most labially positioned incisor; instruct the patient to raise the tongue to permit the lingual flange of the tray to pass by the lateral borders of the tongue without interference.
- As the tray is lowered, retract the cheeks in the posterior regions to make certain the buccal mucosa is not caught beneath the edge of the tray; hold the lip out to ascertain that there is clearance to the base of the vestibule.

▶ Evaluation of tray size
- Lift the tray handle while keeping the posterior border of the tray in position, similar to the procedure illustrated in Figure 14-2 for the maxilla, to determine whether the coverage will be adequate to include the retromolar areas posteriorly and to allow for 1/4-inch thickness of impression material laterally on the facial and lingual aspects of the teeth.

- Reselect larger or smaller trays as indicated and repeat try-in. When in doubt, use the larger rather than a smaller tray.
- Make note of tray sizes used in patient's permanent record for future reference.

IV. Application of Wax Rim Around Borders of Trays (Beading)

▶ Purposes
- Prevent the metal tray rims from causing discomfort to the soft tissues.
- Seat the vestibular periphery firmly into position with reduced pressure on the displaced tissues.
- Prevent penetration of the incisal or occlusal surfaces through the impression material and thus to prevent a defective model.
- Provide a slight undercut at the rim as an aid in the retention of the alginate in the tray during placement and removal.
- Create a posterior palatal seal to aid in preventing excess material from passing into the throat.

▶ Procedure
- Application of wax: attach a strip of soft utility wax firmly around the entire periphery of each tray (Figure 14-3).
- Mandibular tray: add extra layers from cuspid to cuspid labially, and notch the wax to fit about the labial frenum.
- Maxillary tray: add extra layers as needed to extend the tray into the vestibule above the anterior teeth, and notch the wax to fit about the labial frenum (Figure 14-4A).
- Apply extra thickness across the posterior palatal seal area.
- When a patient has a high palatal vault, apply extra wax to support the impression material in that area.

▶ Try-in: Try the rimmed trays in the mouth (Figure 14-4B); examine by retraction of the lips and cheeks and by use of a mouth mirror for lingual areas, hold the tray in position.

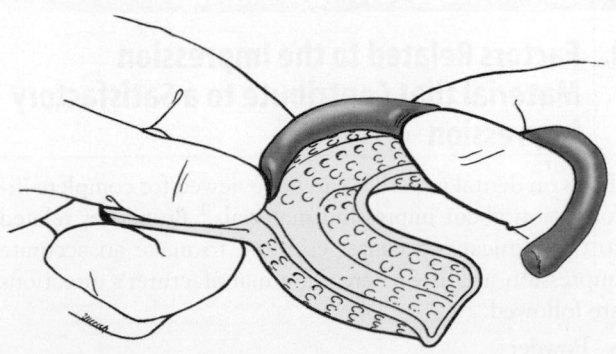

FIGURE 14-3 Beading the Tray. A strip of soft utility wax is applied around the periphery of each tray.

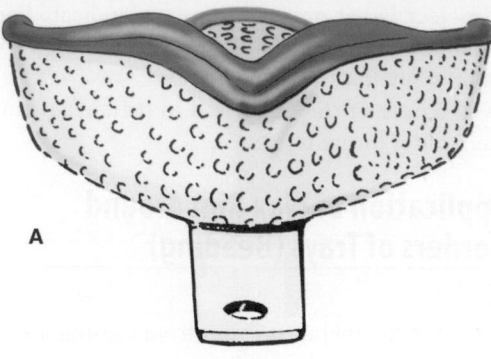

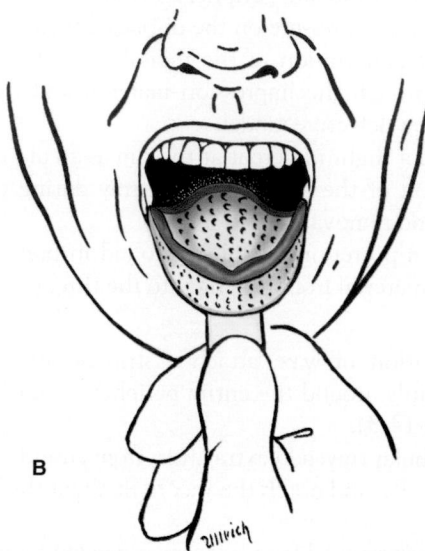

FIGURE 14-4 Check the Beading Wax. A: Tray with double layer of beading wax about the labial frenum. The extra wax extends the tray, protects the soft tissue from the metal rim, and provides a more complete impression of the area. **B:** Try-in after beading. The wax contacts all borders of the mucous membrane, displaces the soft tissue outward, and prevents the teeth from contacting the tray.

▶ Characteristics of the completed molding: When the tray is held firmly, all borders of the wax will contact the mucous membrane and displace the soft tissue outward and upward. The teeth do not touch the tray.

THE IMPRESSION MATERIAL[1]

I. Factors Related to the Impression Material that Contribute to a Satisfactory Impression

Texts on dental materials can be reviewed for complete information about impression materials.[1] Properties related to the clinical procedures essential to make an accurate impression are listed here. The manufacturer's directions are followed.

▶ Powder

The alginate material deteriorates on standing, particularly at high temperatures and humidity.

- Keep container tightly closed; store in a cool place.
- Use individually sealed packages to eliminate the problems of heat and moisture.
- Do not agitate powders unnecessarily during mixing. Inhaled dust particles can cause serious irritation to the respiratory system.

▶ Water
- Temperature controls setting time.
- At room temperature, 20°–21°C (68°–70°F), an ideal gelation time between 3 and 4 minutes provides adequate working time.
- Temperature of the water is measured with a thermometer at the time of mixing.
- For control in hot, humid weather, use cooler water and refrigerate the bowl and spatula.

▶ Strength and quality

The strength and quality of the finished impression depend on the following factors:
- Powder: water ratio accurately weighed and measured.
- Mixing time is 60 seconds for hand spatulation to homogenize, remove bubbles, and allow chemical reactions to proceed uniformly.
- Holding the impression material in position for an optimum period in accord with manufacturer's specifications. The elasticity of most alginates improves with time; therefore, a superior reproduction can be obtained by waiting. Distortion can result when the impression is left in the mouth too long.
- Certain impression materials have color-change properties for mixing time and setting time.

▶ Surface accuracy
- The model must be poured promptly to prevent loss of water from the impression. Permanent distortion can result.

II. Mixing the Impression Material

Follow manufacturer's specifications precisely for total time lapse for mixing and insertion.

▶ Place measured water 20°–21°C (68°–70°F), measured with a thermometer) in a clean, dry mixing bowl.

▶ Sprinkle measured powder (from individually sealed package or premeasured from large container) into the water.

▶ Quickly incorporate the powder and water using a clean, dry, stiff spatula.

III. Tray Preparation

The mandibular impression is made first to introduce the patient to the procedure in an area where discomfort or gagging may be the least likely.

▶ Working time
- The working time is 30 seconds.

- Filling the tray
  - Fill the tray from the posterior, being careful not to trap air bubbles.
  - Adapt the material to the tray thoroughly; press slightly through the perforations in the tray.
  - Do not overload; fill to a level just below the edge of the wax rim.
  - Wet index finger with cold water and pass lightly over the surface of the impression material.
  - Smooth the surface and make a slight indent where the teeth will insert.
- Excess material
  - Quickly gather the excess material from the bowl.
  - Bring the material on the spatula near to the patient to use for precoating the tooth surfaces.

THE MANDIBULAR IMPRESSION

I. Precoat Potential Areas of Air Entrapment

- The precoat prevents air bubbles in the finished impression.
- Take a small amount of impression material from the spatula onto the index finger.
- Apply quickly with a positive but light pressure to:
  - Undercut areas such as distal surfaces of teeth adjacent to edentulous areas
  - Cervical areas of erosion or abrasion
  - Gingival surfaces of fixed partial dentures
  - Vestibular areas, particularly anterior areas about the frena
  - Occlusal surfaces

II. Steps for Insertion of Tray

- Follow mandibular tray try-in. In summary, the procedure is as follows:
  - From 8 o'clock position (4 o'clock for left handed), retract lip and cheek outward with fingers of non-dominant hand.
  - Use side of tray to distend the other lip and cheek outward.
  - Rotate the tray into position and center it over the teeth.
  - Introduce the tray 1/4-inch anterior to the facial surface of the most anterior incisor.
  - Instruct patient to raise the tongue while the tray is lowered.
  - Retract cheeks and lip to clear the way for impression material to reach the base of the vestibule.
  - Seat the tray directly downward with a slight vibratory motion to aid in filling all crevices between the teeth.
- Instruct the patient to extrude the tongue briefly to mold the lingual borders of the impression.
  - Apply equal bilateral pressure firmly, holding the middle fingers over the premolar regions.

- Use the thumbs to support the mandible.
- When equal pressure can be maintained with one hand, place an index finger over the patient's premolar area on one side and the middle finger over the opposite side, with the thumb under the edge of the mandible for stabilization.
- Mold cheeks around the tray.
- When the impression tray is held with one hand or when assistance is available, slip the saliva ejector in over the tray and then remove it before the tray is removed.
- When the leftover material on the spatula has lost its surface stickiness (tackiness), hold the impression in position for 2 more clocked minutes.

III. The Completed Impression

- Removal of impression
  - Hold tray handle with thumb and fingers.
  - Retract cheek and lip with fingers and release the edge of the impression by depressing the buccal mucosa.
  - Do not rock the impression back and forth to release it because these movements may cause permanent distortion of the final impression.
  - Remove the impression with a gentle snap.
- Rinse the impression
  - Rinse under cool running water to remove saliva, blood, and bacteria.
  - Rinse carefully to prevent splashing contaminated saliva or blood over surroundings.
- Examine and evaluate the impression
  - Observe surface detail, proper extension over retromolar area, and peripheral roll (rounded border of the impression) generally.
- Repeat procedure when necessary
  - Correct mistakes rather than be satisfied with a substandard impression.
- Storage
  - Disinfect the impression.
  - Wrap mandibular impression in a wet towel while making the maxillary impression.

THE MAXILLARY IMPRESSION

I. Preparation

- Request patient rinse
  - To clear particles left from the mandibular impression and to relax the oral muscles.
- Examine the maxillary teeth
  - Examine for particles of mandibular impression material and remove. Request patient to use water to rinse for 2–3 minutes, swishing vigorously to remove particles from between teeth.

▶ Prepare the impression material
  • Fill the tray as described previously for the mandibular impression.
▶ Precoat undercut areas
  • Precoat undercut areas, vestibular areas, high palatal vault, tooth surfaces next to edentulous areas, and occlusal surfaces (see procedure for mandibular impression).

II. Steps for Insertion of Tray

▶ Follow maxillary tray try-in. In summary, the procedure is as follows:
  • From 11 o' clock position (1 o' clock if left handed), retract lip with fingers of nondominant hand.
  • Use side of tray to distend the lip and cheek.
  • Insert the tray with a rotary motion; center it over the teeth by using the small gap in the red wax border to relate to the labial frenum.
  • Introduce the material to the teeth so the wax rim is 1/4-inch facial to the most anterior incisor.
▶ Seat the tray from posterior to anterior to direct the impression material forward and thus prevent irritation to the soft palate area.
▶ Retract the lip and bring the tray to place with a slight vibratory motion to allow the material to flow into crevices and proximal areas.
▶ The middle finger of each hand is placed over the premolar region to support and guide the tray; the index fingers and thumbs hold the lip out.
▶ Request the patient to form a tight "O" with the lips to mold the impression material.
▶ Maintain equal pressure on each side of the tray throughout the setting. When assistance is available or if the pressure to hold the tray can be maintained with one hand, a saliva ejector can be inserted.
▶ When the leftover material on the spatula has lost its surface stickiness, hold the impression in place for 2 more minutes. Or use color guide when a color-change impression material is used.

III. The Completed Impression

▶ Remove impression
  • Hold the tray handle with the thumb and fingers of the dominant hand, and retract the opposite lip and cheek with the fingers of the other hand.
  • Elevate the cheek over the edge of the impression to break the seal, and remove the impression.
▶ Rinse
  • Rinse under cool running water to remove saliva, blood, and bacteria.
  • Rinse carefully to prevent creation of an aerosol and dissemination of bacteria.

▶ Examine
  • Examine surface detail and proper extension to include tuberosity areas and a complete reproduction of the height of the vestibule.
  • Excess unsupported impression material should be removed with a sharp knife so that when placed on a flat surface the impression does not become distorted.
▶ Repeat procedure when necessary
  • Repeat procedure rather than be satisfied with a substandard impression.

DISINFECTION OF IMPRESSIONS[2]

To prevent cross-contamination during laboratory procedures, impressions are disinfected in an approved disinfectant after rinsing. When impressions are to be sent to a laboratory, they are isolated in a package. A sealable plastic bag can be used.

▶ Apply standard precautions; wear protective gloves, eyewear, and mask to handle contaminated impressions.
▶ The impression can be sprayed or immersed in disinfectant with tuberculocidal activity.
▶ Place the impression in a plastic bag and seal tightly for the contact time recommended by the manufacturer.
▶ Discard disinfectant solution and rinse the impression under running water.

PARACLINICAL PROCEDURES

Supplemental to the chairside clinical procedures is the laboratory work involved in the production of the study models from the impressions. These duties may be the responsibility of the dental laboratory technician or other dental team member.

▶ *The most frequent error in the preparation of study models is a delay in pouring them.*
▶ Undue dehydration or water loss from the material causes permanent distortion, an uneven surface, and hence an inaccurate model.
▶ Regard for the sensitive properties of the dental materials, precision and practice in laboratory procedures, and pride in the production of neat, smooth, well-proportioned study models determine the finished product's appearance, usefulness, and accuracy.

I. Equipment and Materials

▶ Flexible rubber mixing bowl
▶ Wide blade stiff spatula
▶ Plaster knife
▶ Laboratory vibrator with protective covering
▶ Mechanical mixer

► Model-base formers and accessory items such as prefabricated base formers
► Dental materials
  • Baseplate wax (and wax spatula).
  • White dental stone.
► Water at room temperature, with measuring container.
► Ruler with millimeter markings.
► Model trimmer.

II. Preparation of the Impressions

► Rinse impressions under cool running water to remove residual disinfectant that may affect the plaster or stone surface after pouring:
  • Shake out excess water gently over the lab sink.
  • Spray impression with commercial debubblizer to reduce the surface tension to enhance the flow of the stone.
► When a rubber model-base form is not used, an artificial floor of the mouth for the mandibular model must be created to facilitate pouring and trimming of the model.
  • Trim the lingual impression all around so that the height is consistent from the occlusal and incisal surfaces to the base of the impression.
  • Mix a small portion of impression material.
  • Hold the mandibular impression upright in the nondominant hand, with the middle and ring fingers extended from under the tray into the tongue area.
  • Apply alginate over the fingers to form a flat bridge slightly above the lingual flanges of the impression; hold until the alginate sets.
  • Smooth the surface with a finger moistened with cool water.
  • When assisted at the chair, the floor of the mandibular impression can be made while the maxillary impression is being held for setting. There is usually sufficient alginate mixed with that for the maxillary impression to use for this purpose.

MIXING THE STONE

Texts on dental materials can be reviewed for complete information about gypsum products. Some pertinent properties are listed here as reference points.

► Dental stone
  • Sensitive to changes in the relative humidity of the atmosphere.
  • Store in airtight container; close soon after use; and do not let water enter the container.
  • Keep the spoon or scoop (used to remove the powder) clean and dry.
► Water
  • Controls the strength, rigidity, and hardness of the model.

• *Temperature*: Generally, cooler water decreases the setting time and warmer water increases it.
• *Quantity*: Follow manufacturer's proportions exactly. Increasing the water over the specifications prolongs the setting time and reduces the strength.
► Spatulation
  • Prolonged or very rapid mixing can hasten the chemical reaction and shorten the setting time.
  • Measure the water and powder by the manufacturer's specifications.
  • White stone is generally preferred for study models. Plaster produces a model more susceptible to breakage.
  • Ratio of 30–40 ml water to 100 g stone.
  • Place measured water (room temperature) in a clean, dry mixing bowl.
  • Sift in the powder gradually to prevent air trapping and to allow each particle to become wet.
  • Wait briefly until all powder is wet, and then vibrate to release large bubbles.
  • Use vacuum mixer (follow manufacturer's directions).
  • The result is a smooth, homogeneous, creamy mix.
► Information about gypsum products can be reviewed in textbooks about dental materials.

POURING THE MODEL

The finished model has two connected parts, the anatomic portion and the base or art portion (Figure 14-5).

I. Pouring the Anatomic Portion

► Shake water out of the impression and dry it with air.
► Hold the impression tray by the handle and press handle against the vibrator.
► With a small amount of stone mix on the end of the spatula, start at one posterior corner and allow the mix to flow through the impression. Use small amounts and vibrate continually.
  • Tip the impression so the material passes into the tooth indentations and flows slowly down the side, across the occlusal surface or the incisal edge, and up the other side of the impression of each tooth.
  • Air can be trapped when the process is hurried or when too large a quantity of mix is poured in at one time without attentive control of the flow.
► When all tooth indentations are covered, add larger amounts of mix to fill the impression slightly over the periphery. Vibrate.

II. One-Step Method for Forming the Base of the Model

► Fill rubber model-base form with the remainder of the mix, or form a mass of stone on a glass or ceramic slab or

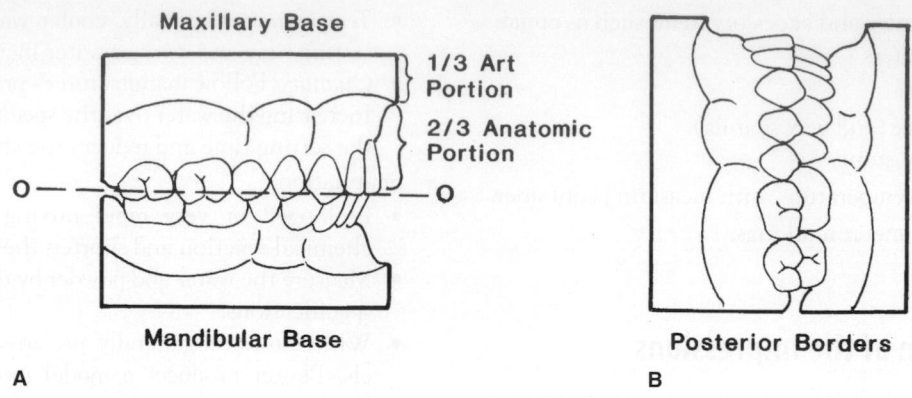

FIGURE 14-5 Finished Study Models. A: Proportions and planes. The art portion is one-third and the anatomic portion two-thirds of the total height of the model. Note parallelism of the maxillary and mandibular bases with the mean occlusal plane (0–0). **B:** Posterior borders are at right angles to the bases. When the maxillary and mandibular models are placed on their posterior borders, the teeth intercuspate exactly.

other nonabsorbent surface (waxed paper on a smooth surface). Add excess stone at the heel areas.

▶ Invert the poured impression onto the base.
  • Use a slight back-and-forth motion to secure the two parts together.
  • Avoid the common error of inverting the impression before the stone is firm. The mix can flow out of the impression.

▶ Adjust tray to proper position:
  • Occlusal plane (at premolars) should be parallel with the base of the model-base former or tabletop.
  • Midline (anterior as judged by handle of impression tray) centered at the midline of the model-base former.
  • Accommodate position so that a tooth in labioversion or buccoversion does not protrude over the trimming line of the art portion (Figure 14-5).

▶ Add stone on peripheral and heel areas to provide a smooth surface; remove excess so that wax periphery of the tray is visible. When excess stone above the edge of the tray rim is permitted to set, the tray is difficult to separate, and the use of a knife to carve the excess from the tray may damage the model.

▶ Final set occurs within 1 hour. Separate 1 hour after pouring to preserve the accuracy and prevent damage to the surface of the model.

III. Other Methods for Forming the Base of the Model

▶ Two-step or double-pour method
  • Both maxillary and mandibular impressions are poured and left upright (see the section Pouring the Anatomic Portion).
  • Stone is then prepared separately for the bases, and the model-base formers are filled or the mass is placed on the smooth nonabsorbent surface.

  • The impression is inverted and held on the surface of the new stone while the sides and periphery are shaped and smoothed.
  • An advantage to this method is that there is no danger of inverting the poured impression too soon.
  • If the model is turned before it starts to set, the unset stone can fall away from the occlusal and incisal portions and leave bubbles in critical areas.

▶ Boxing technique
  • Objective: to form a wall around the impression before pouring to provide a shape for the base as well as to prevent the need for inverting the poured impression.
  • A strip of utility (beading) wax is attached slightly below the periphery of the impression and completely around the impression.
  • Boxing wax or baseplate is applied around the strip of utility wax and attached to it by means of a warm spatula at a height that allows for proper thickness of the final model, about 1/2 inch.
  • Care must be taken not to displace the impression dimensionally or to touch the anatomic portions with the warm spatula.
  • Pouring is carried out as described previously.
  • Work-model formers with side walls to provide the boxing effect are available. Such a mold has a slot through the rubber where the handle of the impression tray can be inserted.

IV. Separation of the Impression and the Model

▶ Objective: to remove tray and impression material without breaking the teeth.

▶ When a model-base form is used, remove it first.

▶ Use the laboratory knife and cut away any excess stone that might interfere with removal of the model from the impression.

▶ Insert the knife between the stone and the impression tray starting in the anterior area and gently twist the laboratory knife to loosen and separate the model from the impression material. You may need to do this in posterior areas as well.

▶ The tray is lifted off in one upward motion. Lateral pressure may result in breaking teeth on the model.

▶ If the model will not release, soak the cast in cool water for 10 minutes and try the separation process again.

▶ Trimming is started promptly, or if delayed, the cast is thoroughly soaked in water before trimming.

TRIMMING THE MODELS

The exact proportions of the study models and the steps required to accomplish the trimming and finishing depend on several factors, including the measurements of the patient's dental arches, the positions of the teeth, and the preferences of the dentist. Development of a routine, systematic procedure for trimming can lead to the production of consistent, attractive, and useful diagnostic models.

I. Use of Model Trimmer

▶ Precision-type model trimmer.

▶ Angulators are available to fit on the table of the model trimmer to give average set angles for trimming the margins of the models (follow manufacturer directions).

▶ Use protective eyewear and mask while using a model trimmer. Goggles are indicated for laboratory procedures.

II. Characteristics of the Finished Models

Before the step-by-step description of the trimming procedures, observe Figure 14-5 for the overall proportions and planes of ideally finished study models. Figure 14-6 outlines the base shapes and Figure 14-7 shows the occlusal views of the maxillary and mandibular models.

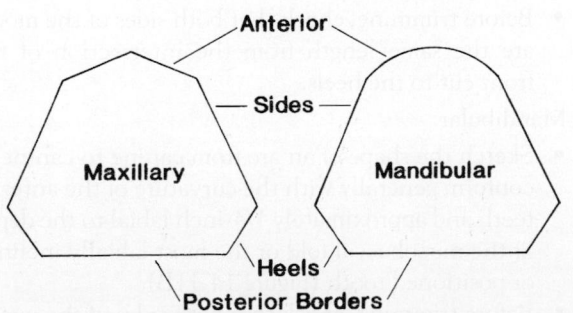

FIGURE 14-6 Base Shapes for Finished Study Models. Maxillary and mandibular models are trimmed at the labeled areas. See text for procedures.

III. Preliminary Steps to Trimming the Model

▶ Models must be wet; soak for 10–15 minutes.

▶ Remove bubbles of stone on or about the teeth with a small sharp instrument; use care not to scar the model.

▶ Level excess stone that is distal to the retromolar area and tuberosity so models may be occluded. Do not shorten the model anteriorly to posteriorly at this time.

▶ Trim models conservatively on the sides to make a smooth surface for marking.

IV. Trimming the Bases

▶ Objectives
  • To make bases parallel with the mean occlusal plane and to each other.
  • To make correct proportions for the height of the models; art portion one-third and anatomic portion two-thirds (Figure 14-5A).

▶ Mandibular model is trimmed first.
  Follow the following steps:

1. Measure the greatest height of the anatomic portion (usually this is from the tip of the canine to the depth of the vestibule) with a plastic ruler (Figure 14-8).
2. Divide by two to obtain the height of the art portion.
3. Add the measured height of the anatomic portion to the height of the art portion for the total height of the model.
4. Place the model teeth down on a flat surface and mark a line around the art portion at the height calculated in step 3. This line will be parallel with the occlusal plane (line O– –O in Figure 14-8). Trim the model at the line.

▶ Maxillary model base
  1. Measure the greatest depth of the anatomic portion (usually at the canine) and divide by two to obtain the height of the art portion.
  2. Relate the two models (use the wax bite if necessary) and place the mandibular base on the flat surface.
  3. Measure from the base of the mandibular model to the highest point of the maxillary anatomic portion (usually in the vestibule over the canine), and add this figure to the height of the maxillary art portion calculated in the aforementioned step 1.
  4. Set the compass at this measurement, and mark a line around the maxillary model at the total height. The line is parallel with the base of the mandibular model and with the mean occlusal plane.

V. Posterior Borders

1. *Select the longest model to trim first* by measuring from the incisors to points distal to the retromolar and tuberosity areas.
2. On the longest model, place the tip of the compass at the gingival border behind the midline anteriorly (usually this is between the central incisors) and mark an arc 1/4-inch distal to the tuberosity (if the maxillary

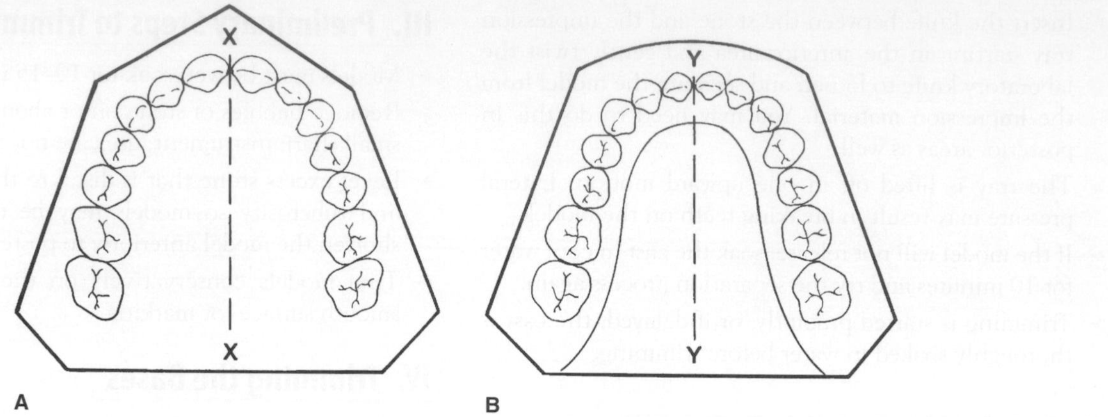

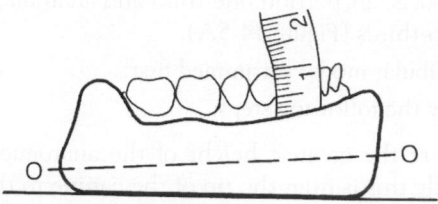

A   **B**

FIGURE 14-7 Occlusal Views of Finished models. A: Maxillary. **B:** Mandibular. The posterior border is perpendicular to the median line from the incisors through the palate (X–X) and the middle of the tongue (Y–Y). The tuberosity of the maxilla and the retromolar areas of the mandible are preserved.

FIGURE 14-8 Trimming the Base. Measure the anatomic portion at its greatest height, which is usually from the tip of the canine to the depth of the vestibule. Note ruler in position. One half of the measurement is the height of the art portion. The trimming line (0–0) is parallel with the mean occlusal plane. See text for details.

model) or retromolar area (if the mandibular model) on each side.

3. Intersect the arc with a line through the central grooves of the molars (Figure 14-9A).

4. Connect the two points across the back of the model (O– –O in Figure 14-9A). Check that this line is perpendicular to the median line from the incisors through the palate or the tongue (X–Y in Figure 14-9B).

5. With the base of the model flat on the model trimmer table, trim on the line marked for the posterior border.

6. For the shorter model, relate the two models with the wax bite and place flat on the base of the first trimmed model. Bring them carefully to the cutting surface of the model trimmer, and trim until the two posterior borders are even and parallel.

7. Check by placing the models on their posterior borders and bringing them together. They relate in their natural intercuspation (Figure 14-5B).

VI. Sides and Heels

▶ *Select the widest model to trim first*; models are usually widest at the molar region.

▶ Mark with a ruler two symmetrical lines 1/4-inch buccal from the buccal bony prominence at the premolar

regions and parallel with lines through the central grooves of the premolars (Figure 14-10A).

- Check that the lines form equal angles with the posterior border.
- Before trimming, make certain that the lines when cut would not remove any vestibular anatomy.
- Trim the sides with the base flat on the model trimmer table.

▶ Mark trimming lines for the heels; cuts are 1/4-inch wide and parallel with a line through the mesiodistal plane of the opposite canine (Figure 14-10B). Trim with base flat on the model trimmer table.

▶ Relate the opposite model with the wax bite, and trim the sides and heels to match the previously trimmed model.

VII. Anterior

The maxillary model is trimmed to a point, and the mandibular model is rounded (Figure 14-6).

▶ Maxillary

- A ruler can be used to draw guidelines for trimming on each side of the midline to the cuspid areas. Note the broken lines in Figure 14-11A. The lines need to be 1/4-inch labial to the depth of the mucobuccal fold (vestibule) or to the most labially inclined tooth.
- Before trimming, check that both sides of the model are the same length from the intersection of the front cut to the heels.

▶ Mandibular

- Sketch the shape of an arc from canine to canine to conform generally with the curvature of the anterior teeth and approximately 1/4-inch labial to the depth of the mucobuccal fold or the most labially inclined or positioned tooth (Figure 14-11B).
- Before trimming, check that both sides of the model are the same length from the intersection of the front cut to the heels.

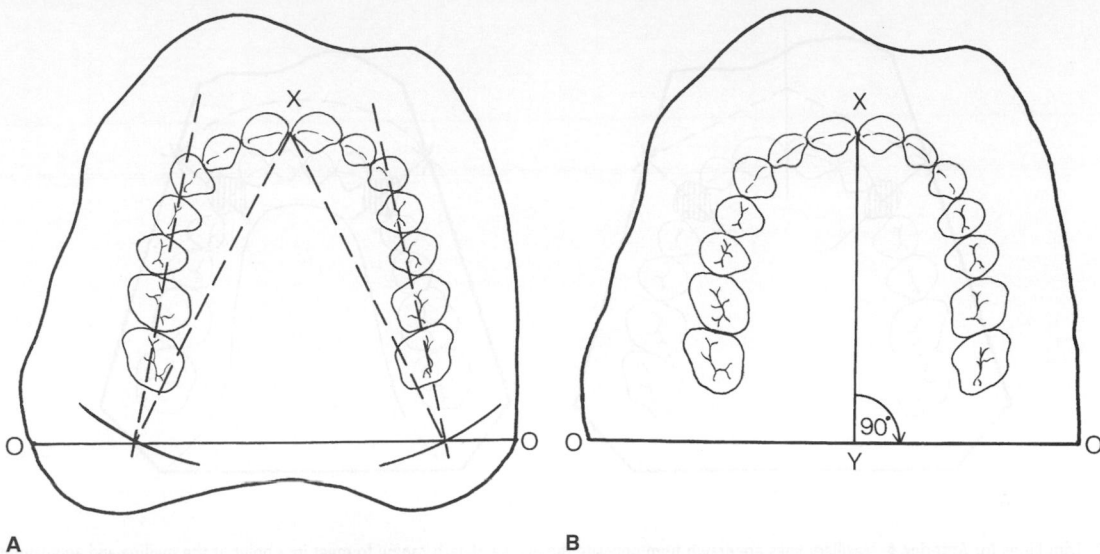

FIGURE 14-9 Trim Line for Posterior Borders. A: On the longest model use a compass to draw arcs from the anterior midline point (X) to 1/4-inch distal to the tuberosity (maxilla) or retromolar area (mandible). **B:** Intersect the arc with a line through the central grooves of the molars and connect the two points across the model (0–0).

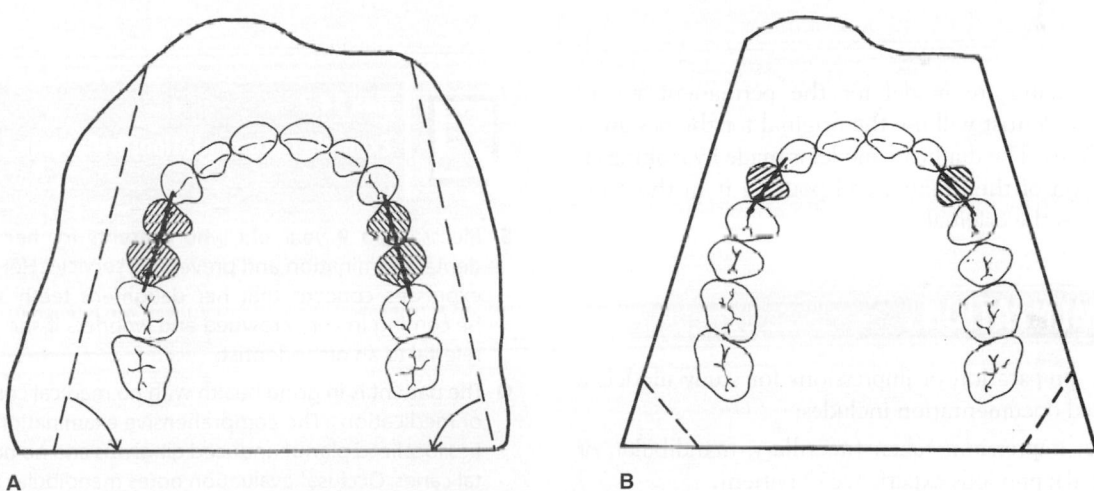

FIGURE 14-10 Trim Lines for Sides and Heels. A: On the widest model, trim lines for the sides are drawn parallel with lines through the central grooves of the premolars. The two symmetrical lines form equal angles with the posterior border of the model. **B:** Mark trim lines for heels 1/4-inch wide and parallel with lines through the mesiodistal plane of the opposite canine. The lines are symmetrical with each other and form equal angles with the posterior border.

VIII. Finishing and Polishing

▶ Trim rough edges and margins of both models and the lingual portion of the mandibular model to even off irregularities and make the depth of the vestibule visible. Remaining bubbles are removed.

▶ Use waterproof sandpaper and a plaster smoothing stone to remove marks left by the model trimmer on the art portion. Sandpaper is not used on the anatomic portion.

▶ Fill any holes in the wet models with stone applied with a spatula to the flat surfaces of the art portion or a camel's hair brush to the anatomic portion. Smooth off excess.

▶ Finish and polish
  • Allow models to dry thoroughly for 2–3 days.
  • Smooth the art portion with fine sandpaper.

  • Soak in heated soap solution for 30–60 minutes. An alternative is to use a commercial model luster spray or solution.
  • Buff models with chamois, cotton, or a soft cloth.

IX. Records and Storage of Models

▶ Label each model with the patient's name and the date. These may be inscribed into the posterior border of the model before soaping and polishing.

▶ Boxes of an appropriate size are available commercially for storage of one or more pairs of models.

▶ Record in the patient's permanent record the size of impression tray used to save time if follow-up models are needed.

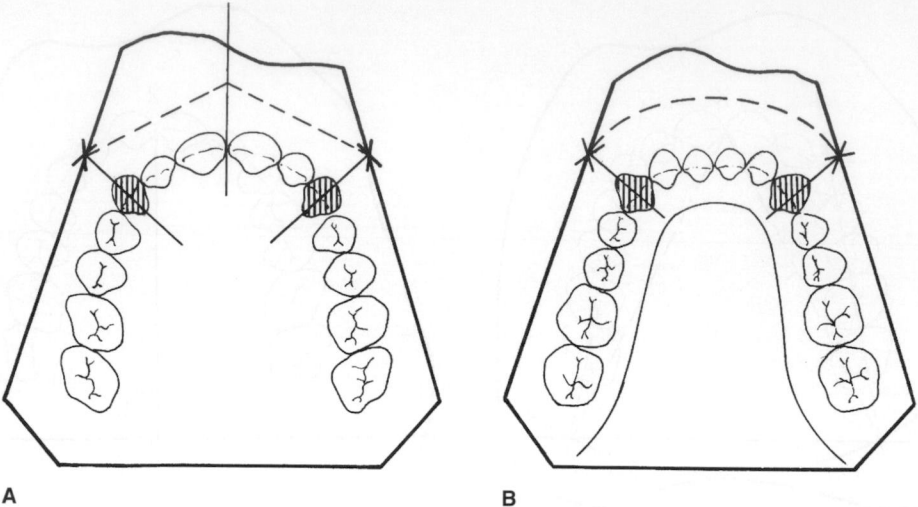

FIGURE 14-11 Trim Lines for Anterior. A: Maxillary lines are drawn from opposite the middle of each canine to meet in a point at the midline and approximately 1/4-inch labial to the most labially positioned tooth. **B:** Mandibular line forms an arc drawn from the middle of each canine approximately 1/4-inch labial to the most labially positioned tooth.

▶ Make a duplicate model for the permanent record when the dentist will use the original for the design of a prosthesis. The duplicate model is made by making an impression of the original and pouring it in the same manner as the original.

DOCUMENTATION

▶ For the preparation of impressions for study models a suggested documentation includes:
- Date; impressions taken (maxillary, mandibular, or partial); previous experience of patient.
- Patient positioning and special advice (e.g., relative to prevention of gagging).
- Materials used; trays: size, plastic or metal.
- Problems; patient comments; recommendations.

▶ Sample documentation note may be found in Box 14-2.

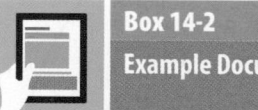

Box 14-2

Example Documentation: Orthodontic Consult

S–Melissa is a 9 year old who presents for her routine dental examination and preventive services. Her mother expresses concern that her daughter's teeth seem to be coming in very crowded and wonders if she needs a referral to an orthodontist.

O–The patient is in good health with no medical conditions or medications. The comprehensive examination identifies localized plaque-induced gingivitis and no new dental caries. Occlusal evaluation notes mandibular anterior teeth crowding and an open bite. Impressions for study models are indicated.

A–Small tray impression trays were used for alginate impressions. Patient tolerated procedure well. Oral self-care instruction, prophylaxis, and fluoride varnish completed.

P–Referral written for the orthodontist. Continuing care scheduled in 6 months.

Signed _____, RDH

Date: _____

EVERYDAY ETHICS

Everyone was rushing around the office trying to finish in time for lunch. Elena was asked to take the impressions for whitening trays for Mrs. Adams. As Elena places the maxillary tray, the patient begins to gag severely. Mrs. Lynch pushes Elena's arm out of the way and attempts to pull the tray out of her mouth. Elena calls for assistance while forcefully restraining Mrs. Lynch to keep the tray in until the impression material is set.

Questions for Consideration

1. Describe the ethical principle(s) that best describe(s) the actions of Elena.

2. By restraining the patient, were the patient's rights violated? Why or why not? Explain the rationale.

3. Professionally, what choices could Elena have exercised with Mrs. Lynch to improve the outcome?

Factors To Teach The Patient

▷ Importance and purposes of study models. Reasons for comparative models following treatment at a later date.

▷ Use the unidentified models of other patients to show effects of treatment or what can happen if the prescribed treatment is not carried out.

▷ Areas that present difficulty in the dental biofilm control program.

▷ Show anatomy of gingiva and teeth and demonstrate use of biofilm removal devices on the patient's own study models.

ENHANCE YOUR UNDERSTANDING

thePoint° **DIGITAL CONNECTIONS**
(see the inside front cover for access information)
- **Audio glossary**
- **Quiz bank**

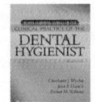

SUPPORT FOR LEARNING
(available separately; visit lww.com)
- *Active Learning Workbook for Clinical Practice of the Dental Hygienist, 12th Edition*

prepU   INDIVIDUALIZED REVIEW
(available separately; visit lww.com)
- *Adaptive quizzing with prepU for Wilkins' Clinical Practice of the Dental Hygienist*

References

1. Nandini VV, Venkatesh KV, Nair LC. Alginate impressions: a practical perspective. *J Conserv Dent.* 2008;11(1):37–41.

2. Dreesen K, Kellens A, Wevers M, et al. The influence of mixing methods and disinfectant on the physical properties of alginate impression materials. *Eur J Orthod.* 2013;35(3):381–387.

15

Dental Biofilm and Other Soft Deposits

Janis G Keating, RDH, MA, Allyson Ligor, RDH, MS, and Esther M. Wilkins, BS, RDH, DMD

CHAPTER OUTLINE

LEARNING OBJECTIVES

After studying this chapter, the student will be able to:

1. Define acquired pellicle and discuss the significance and role of the pellicle in the maintenance of oral health.

2. Describe the different stages in biofilm formation and identify the changes in biofilm microorganisms as biofilm matures.

3. Differentiate between the types of soft deposits.

4. Recognize the factors that influence biofilm accumulation.

5. Explain the location, composition, and properties of dental biofilm.

6. Design biofilm control strategies individualized to meet each patient's needs.

During clinical examination of the teeth and surrounding soft tissues, soft and hard deposits are assessed. The presence of dental biofilm is a primary risk factor for gingivitis, inflammatory periodontal diseases, and dental caries.

▶ Assessment is an integral aspect of the dental hygiene diagnosis. On the basis of assessment findings, an individualized preventive care plan can be formulated to meet the needs of the patient.

▶ Key words are defined in Box 15-1.

▶ The soft deposits are acquired pellicle, dental biofilm, materia alba, and food debris.

▶ The hard, calcified deposits on the teeth are dental calculus, which is described in Chapter 21.

▶ A comparison of types of dental deposits, with descriptions, is found in Table 15-1.

ACQUIRED PELLICLE

▶ The acquired pellicle is a thin acellular tenacious film formed of proteins, carbohydrates, and lipids.[1]

▶ Pellicle is uniquely positioned as the interface between the tooth surfaces and the oral environment. It forms over exposed tooth surfaces and prostheses.

▶ Pellicle thickness varies from 100 to 1,000 nm, depending on its location in the mouth; it is thickest near the gingival margin and areas undisturbed by the activities of chewing, swallowing, and speaking.[2]

I. Formation of the Pellicle[1]

▶ Within minutes after eruption or after all soft and hard deposits have been removed from the tooth surfaces

---

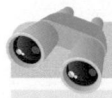

BOX 15-1   KEY WORDS: Dental Biofilm

Acellular: not made up of or containing cells.

Adsorption: attachment of one substance to the surface of another; the action of a substance in attracting and holding other materials or particles on its surface.

Aerobe: heterotrophic microorganism that can live and grow in the presence of free oxygen; some are obligate, others facultative; *adj.* aerobic.

Anaerobe: heterotrophic microorganism that lives and grows in complete (or almost complete) absence of oxygen; some are obligate, others facultative; *adj.* anaerobic.

Biofilm: dynamic, complex, multispecies communities of microorganisms that colonize the oral cavity. Unique characteristics allow biofilms to adapt to a variety of every changing environments; characteristics include: tenacious adherence to surfaces, protective EPS, three-dimensional structures with complex nutrient and communication pathways.

Calculogenic: adjective applied to dental biofilm that is conducive to the formation of calculus.

Cariogenic: adjective to indicate a conduciveness to the initiation of dental caries, such as a cariogenic biofilm or a cariogenic food.

EPS: extracellular polymeric substance are compounds secreted by microorganisms and form a matrix for biofilm.

Facultative: able to live under more than one specific set of environmental conditions; contrast with obligate.

Flora: the collective organisms of a given locale.

   Oral flora: the various bacteria and other microorganisms that inhabit the oral cavity. The mouth has an indigenous flora, meaning those organisms that are native to that area of the body. Certain organisms specifically reside in certain parts, for example, on the tongue, on the mucosa, or in the gingival sulcus.

Food impaction: the forceful wedging of food into the periodontium by occlusal forces.

Heterotrophic: not self-sustaining; feeding on others.

Infection: invasion and multiplication of a microorganism in body tissues.

Iatrogenic dentistry: adverse condition resulting from treatment by a dentist, i.e., over hanging restorations or open margin of a restoration.

Leukocyte: white blood corpuscle capable of amoeboid movement; functions to protect the body against infection and disease.

Materia alba: white or cream-colored "cheesy" mass that can collect over dental biofilm on unclean, neglected teeth; it is composed of food debris, mucin, bacteria sloughed epithelial cells.

Maturation: stage or process of attaining maximal development; become mature.

Microbiota: the microscopic living organisms of a region.

Microorganism: minute living organisms, usually microscopic; includes bacteria, rickettsiae, viruses, fungi, and protozoa.

Mycoplasma: pleomorphic, gram-negative bacteria that lack cell walls; many are regular oral cavity residents; some are pathogenic.

Obligate: ability to survive only in a particular environment; opposite of facultative.

Parasite: plant or animal that lives upon or within another living organism and draws its nourishment therefrom; may be obligate or facultative; *adj.* parasitic.

Pathogen: disease-producing agent or microorganism; *adj.* pathogenic.

Planktonic: free floating single bacteria such as in saliva gingival crevicular fluid.

Pleomorphism: assumption of various distinct forms by a single organism or within a species; *adj.* pleomorphic.

Polymeric: repeating molecular structures; in biofilms the polymers are glycoprotein polysaccharides.

TABLE 15-1	Tooth Deposits		
TOOTH DEPOSIT	**DESCRIPTION**	**DERIVATION**	**REMOVAL METHOD**
Acquired enamel pellicle	Translucent, homogeneous, thin, unstructured film covering and adherent to the surfaces of the teeth, restorations, calculus, and other surfaces.	Supragingival: saliva, oral mucosa, microorganism Subgingival: gingival crevicular fluid	Toothbrush and appropriate interdental aid such as floss.
Microbial (bacterial) biofilm Nonmineralized	Dense, organized bacterial communities embedded in EPS matrix adheres tenaciously to the teeth, calculus, prostheses, and other surfaces in the oral cavity.	Colonization of oral microorganisms	Toothbrush and appropriate interdental aid such as floss.
Materia alba Nonmineralized	Loosely adherent, unstructured, white or grayish-white mass of oral debris and bacteria that lies over dental biofilm	Incidental accumulation	Vigorous rinsing and water irrigation can remove materia alba.
Food debris Nonmineralized	Unstructured, loosely attached particulate matter	Food retention following eating	Self-cleansing activity of tongue and saliva. Rinsing vigorously removes debris. Toothbrushing, flossing, and other aids.
Calculus Mineralized	Calcified dental biofilm; hard, tenacious mass that forms on the clinical crowns of the natural teeth and on dentures and other oral appliances.	Biofilm mineralization	
a. Supragingival	Occurs coronal to the margin of the gingiva; is covered with dental biofilm.	Source of minerals is saliva	Manual instrumentation. Ultrasonic instrumentation.
b. Subgingival	Occurs apical to the margin of the gingiva; is covered with dental biofilm.	Source of minerals is gingival crevicular fluid	Manual instrumentation. Ultrasonic instrumentation.

(such as by rubber cup or air polishing), the pellicle begins to form and is fully formed within 30–90 minutes.[1,2]

▶ Composition: primarily glycoproteins that are selectively adsorbed by the hydroxyapatite of the tooth surface.

  • Protein components are derived from the saliva, oral mucosal cells, gingival crevicular fluid, and microorganisms.[3]

▶ Initial attachment of bacteria to the pellicle is by selective adherence of microorganisms that originate from the oral mucosa.

  • Innate characteristics of the pellicle determine the adhesive interactions that cause planktonic bacteria to aggregate and form clusters to initiate biofilm formation.

  • Salivary proteins have a high affinity for the hydroxyapatite tooth surface and initiate the process of pellicle formation.[3]

▶ The adsorbed material becomes a highly insoluble coating over teeth, existing calculus deposits, restorations, and partial or complete dentures.

II. Types of Pellicle[4]

A. Supragingival Pellicle

▶ The supragingival pellicle is clear, translucent, insoluble, and not readily visible until a disclosing agent has been applied.

▶ Pellicle can take on extrinsic stain and become gradations of brown, gray, or other colors, as described in Chapter 22.

- When stained with a disclosing agent, pellicle appears thin, with a pale staining that contrasts with the thicker, darker staining of dental biofilm.

B. Subgingival Pellicle

▶ Subgingival pellicle is continuous with the supragingival pellicle and can become embedded in tooth structure, particularly where the tooth surface is partially demineralized or rough from iatrogenic dentistry.

III. Significance of Pellicle[1]

The pellicle plays an important role in the maintenance of oral health as it protects, lubricates, and acts as a nidus of attachment for the bacteria and subsequent calculus on the tooth surfaces.

▶ Protective
- Pellicle appears to provide a barrier against acids; impacting remineralization and demineralization.

▶ Lubrication
- Pellicle keeps surfaces moist and prevents drying, which in turn enhances the efficiency of speech and mastication.

▶ Nidus for bacteria
- Pellicle participates in biofilm formation by aiding the adherence of microorganisms.

▶ Attachment of calculus
- One mode of calculus attachment is to the pellicle (see Chapter 21).

IV. Removal of Pellicle

▶ Pellicle is not resilient enough to withstand rigorous patient oral self-care.[5]

▶ Extrinsic factors that may interfere with pellicle formation and maturation include:[6]
- Abrasive toothpastes.
- Whitening products.
- Intake of acidic foods and beverages.

DENTAL BIOFILM

▶ Dental biofilm is a dynamic, structured community of microorganisms encapsulated in a self-produced extracellular polymeric substance (EPS) form a matrix around microcolonies.

▶ The matrix is composed of polysaccharides, proteins, and other compounds; it acts to protect the biofilm from the host's immune system and from antimicrobial and antibiotic agents.

▶ The microcolonies are separated by a network of open water channels that supply nutrients deep within the biofilm community.

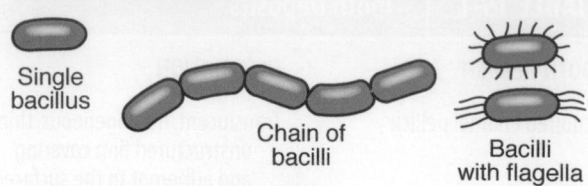

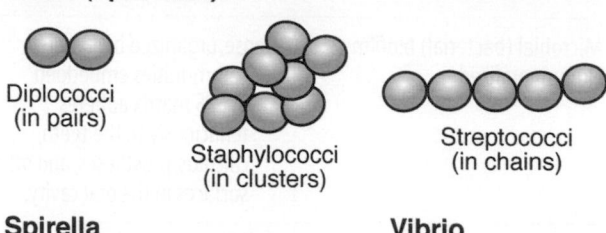

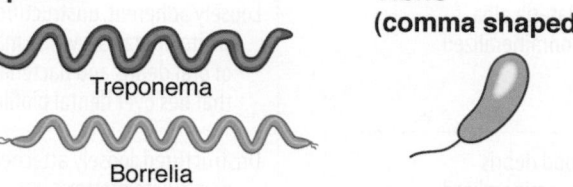

FIGURE 15-1 Bacteria Shapes: Cocci, Bacilli, Spiral. (Adapted from Sakai J. *Practical Pharmacology for the Pharmacy Technician.* Baltimore, MD: Lippincott Williams & Wilkins; 2008.)

▶ The three-dimensional structure of biofilms enhances their ability to communicate with each other, adapt, and respond to their environment.

▶ Dental biofilm adheres tenaciously to any inert or living moist surface; in the oral cavity, biofilms initially adhere to the pellicle on the teeth, existing calculus, fixed, and removable restorations.

▶ Biofilm communities also form on the oral mucosa, surfaces of the tongue, and tonsils; their presence especially on the tongue and tonsils may contribute to malodor.

▶ There are over 700 distinct bacterial species found in the oral cavity along with a variety of other microorganisms including viruses, protozoa, and yeast.[7] Morphologic forms of bacteria that are found within biofilms are shown in Figure 15-1.

I. Stages in the Formation of Biofilm[8]

▶ Biofilm formation does not occur randomly, but involves a series of complex interactions that are predictable and specific to oral biofilm development.

▶ Gene expression controls many of the growth and attachment capabilities and varies depending on species variety within a biofilm community.

A. Stage 1—Formation

▶ Biofilm formation begins with the initial attachment of planktonic bacterial cells to the pellicle on the tooth surface by the way of the bacteria's interactions with the pellicle (physicochemical).

▶ Initially the adherent cells are not yet "committed" to this process, and during this stage of adhesion, the process is reversible. When cells are disrupted (as would occur with oral self-care activities), they can dislodge from the surface to resume planktonic life and either be eliminated or begin the formation process elsewhere in the oral cavity.

B. Stage 2—Bacterial Multiplication and Colonization

▶ If the planktonic microorganisms are not removed, they will attach themselves more permanently using cell adhesion structures such as fimbriae, pili, flagella, and adhesion proteins.

▶ Microcolonies multiply in layers growing upward and outward, creating the three-dimensional aspect of biofilm structures.

▶ With increased size, colonies produce extracellular polymeric substance (EPS) to firmly attach in an irreversible manner; rough surfaces will result in more rapid irreversible attachment.

▶ Organisms that colonize within the first few hours are primarily gram-positive cocci and rods.

C. Stage 3—Matrix Formation

▶ Bacteria within the aggregate of cells continue to secrete EPS as bacteria multiply to form a matrix.

▶ Components of the EPS are:
   • Polysaccharides, glucans, and fructans or levans produced by certain bacteria within the community and from dietary sucrose.
   • The polysaccharides are sticky and cement the biofilm more firmly to the teeth.

▶ The EPS matrix anchors the bacteria together which increases its adherence to the tooth and other structures; in this way, the bacterial community is protected and continues to grow.

▶ The adhesion and stickiness of the EPS matrix make biofilm disruption challenging; ineffective toothbrushing will not adequately disrupt biofilm for this reason.

▶ The biofilm structure enhances its ability to survive, thrive, and adapt to ever-changing environments within the oral cavity both supragingivally and subgingivally.

▶ The adaptive characteristics, structure, and EPS of the biofilm limit the ability of antibiotic therapy to reduce the virulence of pathogenic bacteria found deep within the biofilm communities.[8]

D. Stage 4—Biofilm Growth

▶ This stage is characterized by further development of the biofilm architecture that enhances a cell-to-cell communication process:

   • The process is known as *quorum sensing*.
   • Activated by specific genes located on the surface of the bacterial cells within the biofilm.

▶ The mass and thickness of biofilm increases as a result of bacterial multiplication; left undisturbed bacteria continuously adhere to the biofilm community and surrounding surface area.

E. Stage 5—Maturation

▶ Bacterial colonies mature and release planktonic cells to spread and colonize other areas within the oral cavity.

▶ Bacteria can disperse as single cells or in clumps.

II. Changes in Biofilm Microorganisms

▶ Dental biofilm consists of a complex mixture of microorganisms in microcolonies. The microbial density is very high, and it increases as biofilm ages and matures.

▶ The potential for the development of dental caries and/or gingivitis increases with more microorganisms especially as the numbers of pathogenic outnumber non-pathogenic microorganisms.

▶ The pellicle, EPS, biofilm architecture, and resulting environment promote anaerobic gram-negative bacterial growth activity.

▶ With undisrupted biofilm or if the numbers of bacteria increase rapidly, the chance of potential disease activity such as dental caries, gingivitis, and eventually other inflammatory periodontal diseases increases.

▶ The changes in oral flora follow a pattern such as that shown in Figure 15-2 and vary by days of accumulation as described below.[9]

A. Days 1–2

▶ Early biofilm consists primarily of gram-positive cocci.

▶ Streptococci, which dominate the bacterial population, include *Streptococcus mutans* and *Streptococcus sanguis*.

B. Days 2–4

▶ The cocci still dominate, and increasing numbers of gram-positive filamentous form and slender rods join the surface of the cocci colonies.

▶ Gradually, the filamentous forms grow into the cocci layer and replace many of the cocci.

▶ People who form biofilm slowly will exhibit more cocci and fewer filamentous forms.

C. Days 4–7

▶ Filaments increase in numbers, and a mixed flora appears comprised of rods, filamentous forms, and fusobacteria.

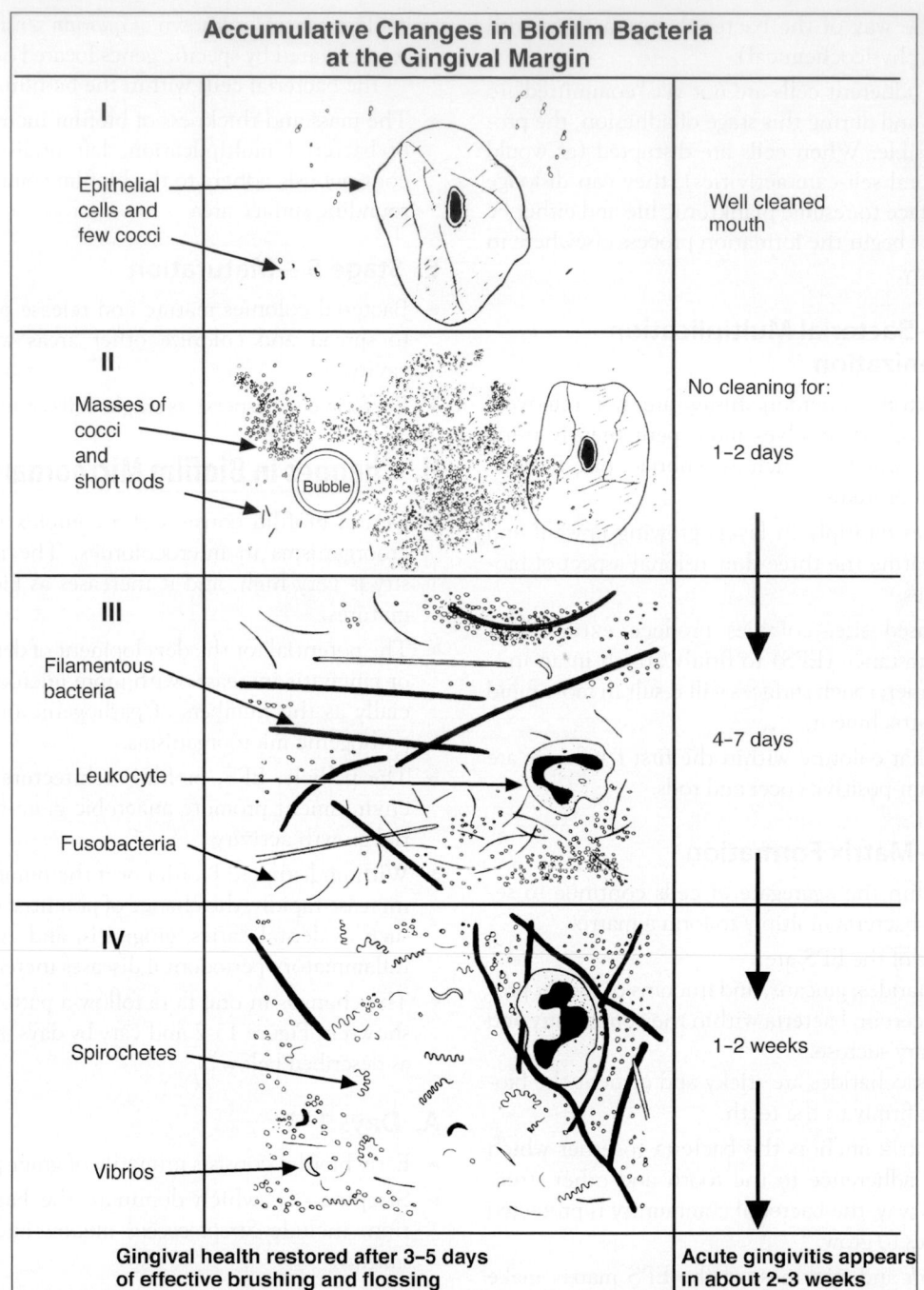

Accumulative Changes in Biofilm Bacteria at the Gingival Margin

I — Epithelial cells and few cocci — Well cleaned mouth

II — Masses of cocci and short rods / Bubble — No cleaning for: 1–2 days

III — Filamentous bacteria / Leukocyte / Fusobacteria — 4–7 days

IV — Spirochetes / Vibrios — 1–2 weeks

Gingival health restored after 3–5 days of effective brushing and flossing

Acute gingivitis appears in about 2–3 weeks

FIGURE 15-2 Biofilm Microorganisms. On the right are the time intervals from 1 day to 3 weeks. On the left are the changes in the biofilm content that take place as biofilm ages. As the numbers of microorganisms increase, the numbers of defense cells (leukocytes) also increase. (From Crawford JJ. Microbiology. In: Barton RE, Matteson SR, Richardson RE (eds.). *The Dental Assistant.* 6th ed. Philadelphia, PA: Lea & Febiger; 1988.)

▶ Biofilm near the gingival margin thickens as a more mature flora develops. Gram-negative spirochetes and vibrios proliferate.

▶ As biofilm spreads coronally, newer/younger biofilm is primarily coccal.

D. Days 7–14

▶ Vibrios and spirochetes appear, and the number of white blood cells increases.

▶ During this period, inflammation develops and can be observed in the gingival tissues.

E. Days 14–21

▶ In older biofilm, vibrios and spirochetes are prevalent, with fewer cocci and filamentous forms.

▶ Densely packed filamentous microorganisms can arrange themselves perpendicular to the tooth surface in a palisade.

▶ As biofilm matures and thickens, more gram-negative anaerobic organisms appear, which are protected by the biofilm architecture and environment.

▶ Gingivitis is evident clinically.

III. Experimental Gingivitis[9]

▶ Gingivitis develops in 2–3 weeks when biofilm is left undisturbed on the tooth surfaces.

▶ Most gingivitis is reversible, with mechanical biofilm disruption; healthy gingiva can return within a few days.

▶ An experimental gingivitis program to demonstrate the effect of biofilm can be conducted. The steps are outlined in Box 15-2.

SUPRAGINGIVAL AND SUBGINGIVAL DENTAL BIOFILM

I. Source

▶ Subgingival biofilm results from the apical proliferation and migration of supragingival biofilm.

▶ In the early stages of gingivitis and periodontitis, the supragingival biofilm is a strong influence on the accumulation and pathogenic features of the subgingival biofilm. Characteristics of supragingival and subgingival biofilms are listed in Table 15-2.

II. Microorganisms

▶ Recent technology innovations such as confocal scanning electron microscopy, epifluorescent microscopy, use of DNA probes, and gene amplification sequencing research studies have allowed for a more in-depth understanding of the science of biofilms.[10]

▶ The supragingival flora is predominantly gram-positive aerobic bacteria. Several species populate early "healthy" supragingival biofilm. Both Streptococcus and Actinomyces species are closely aligned with Lactobacillus and Candida species as this flora matures.

▶ Subgingival biofilm includes more predominantly gram-negative anaerobic and motile organisms of periodontal diseases. Actinomyces, *Tannerella forsythia*, *Fusobacterium nucleatum*, and a cluster of B-Cytophaga-Flavo bacterium-bacterodes have been identified.

▶ The study of biofilms has led to an identification of six groups of subgingival bacterial species in undisrupted aging biofilm.

  • Early colonizers, depicted as yellow and blue in Figure 15-3, transition to predominantly gram-negative organisms, depicted by orange- and red-colored complexes.

  • Older undisrupted biofilms consistently contain more of the orange and red species complexes (see Figure 15-3).[11,12]

III. Organization of Subgingival Biofilm

The biofilm architecture subgingivally arranges itself in layers:

▶ The initial layer is composed of Actinomyces that gives rise to an intermediate layer composed of spindle-shaped cells such as *F. nucleatum*, Tannerella, and *T. forsythia*. The top layer is composed of bacteroides clusters and spirochetes, which form a palisade-like lining.[10]

▶ Many gram-negative microorganisms and numerous white blood cells are loosely attached to the pocket epithelium.

▶ Virulent pathogenic organisms in this layer may be considered a focus for the advancement of periodontal infections.

▶ From this layer, microorganisms may invade the underlying connective tissue.

▶ Figure 15-4 shows bacteria within the connective tissue and on the bone surface.[13]

COMPOSITION OF DENTAL BIOFILM

▶ Microorganisms and EPS comprise 20% of the biofilm that are organic and inorganic solids. The other 80% is water.

▶ Composition differs among individuals and among tooth surfaces.

I. Inorganic Elements[14,15]

A. Calcium and Phosphorus

▶ Calcium, phosphorus, and magnesium are more concentrated in biofilm than in saliva.

▶ Saliva transports the minerals during the mineralization and demineralization processes.

TABLE 15-2	Characteristics of Supragingival and Subgingival Biofilm	
CHARACTERISTIC	**SUPRAGINGIVAL BIOFILM**	**SUBGINGIVAL BIOFILM**
Location	Coronal to the margin of the free gingiva	Apical to the margin of the free gingiva
Origin	Salivary glycoprotein forms acquired enamel pellicle Microorganisms from saliva are selectively attracted to pellicle	Downgrowth of bacteria from supragingival biofilm
Distribution	Starts on proximal surfaces and other protected areas Heaviest collection on areas not cleaned daily by patient Cervical third, especially facial Lingual mandibular molars Proximal surfaces Pit and fissure biofilm	Shallow pocket: similar to supragingival biofilm Undisturbed; held by pocket wall Attached biofilm covers calculus Unattached biofilm extends to the periodontal attachment
Adhesion	Firmly attached to acquired enamel pellicle, other bacteria, and tooth surfaces	Adheres to tooth surface, subgingival pellicle, and calculus
	Surface bacteria (unattached): loose; washed away by saliva or swallowed	Subgingival flora: loose, floating, motile organisms in deep pocket do not adhere; they are between adherent biofilm on tooth and the pocket epithelium
Retention	Rough surfaces of teeth, existing calculus, or restorations Malpositioned teeth Carious lesions	Pocket holds biofilm against tooth Overhanging margins of fillings that extend into pockets hold biofilm
Shape and size	Friction of tongue, cheeks, lips, limits shape and size Thickness: thicker at the cervical third and on proximal surfaces Healthy gingiva: thin biofilm, 15–20 cells thick Chronic gingivitis: thick biofilm, 100–300 cells thick	Molded by pocket wall to shape of the tooth surface Follows form created by subgingival calculus May become thicker as the diseased pocket wall becomes less tight
Structure	Adherent, densely packed microbial layer over acquired enamel pellicle on tooth surface Intermicrobial matrix Onset: small isolated colonies 2–5 d; colonies merge to form a covering of biofilm	Three layers (Figure 15-2) 1. Tooth-surface-attached biofilm: many gram-positive rods and cocci 2. Unattached biofilm in middle: many gram-negative, motile forms; spirochetes; leukocytes 3. Epithelium-attached biofilm: gram-negative, motile forms predominate; many leukocytes migrate through epithelium
Microorganisms	Early biofilm: primarily gram-positive cocci Older biofilm (3–4 d): increased numbers of filaments and fusiforms 4–9 d undisturbed: more complex flora with rods, filamentous forms 7–14 d: vibrios, spirochetes, more gram-negative organisms	Environment conducive to growth of anaerobic population Diseased pocket: primarily gram-negative, motile, spirochetes, rods
Sources of nutrients for bacterial proliferation	Saliva Ingested food Microorganisms metabolites	Tissue fluid (gingival crevicular fluid) Exudate Leukocytes
Significance	Etiology of Gingivitis Supragingival calculus Dental caries (Figure 15-6)	Etiology of Gingivitis Periodontal infections Subgingival calculus

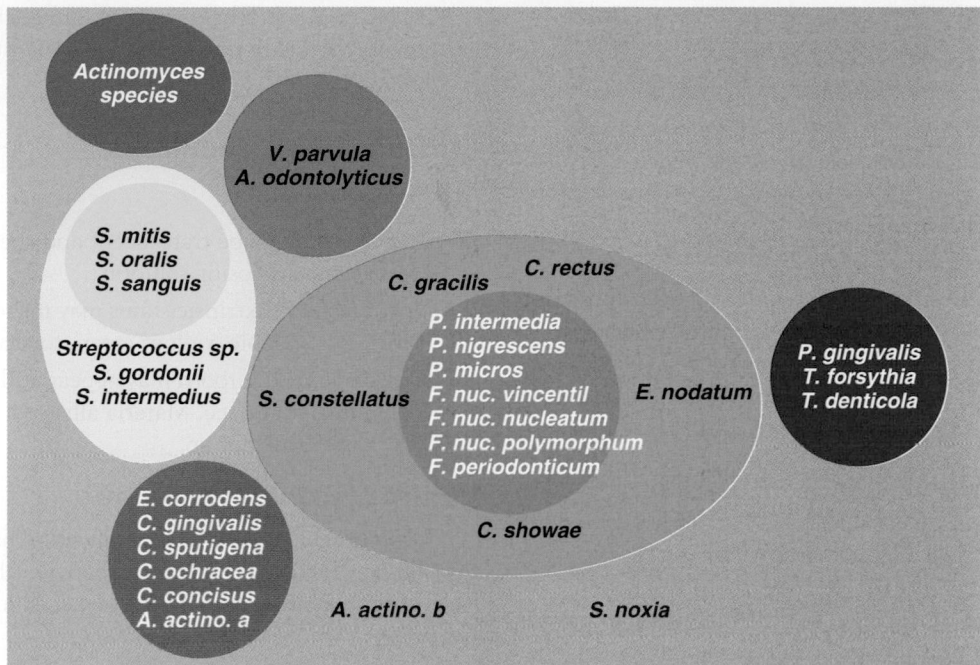

FIGURE 15-3 Diagram of the Subgingival Species Complexes. Diagram represents the relationships of the species within the subgingival complexes. The six groups differentiate the subgingival bacterial species in undisrupted aging biofilm. The yellow is early colonies and then progress to the orange then red colonies that are older undisrupted biofilm. (Source: Socransky SS, Haffajee AD, Cugini MA, et al. Microbial complexes in subgingival plaque. *J Clin Periodontol*. 1998;25(2):134–144, at 140.

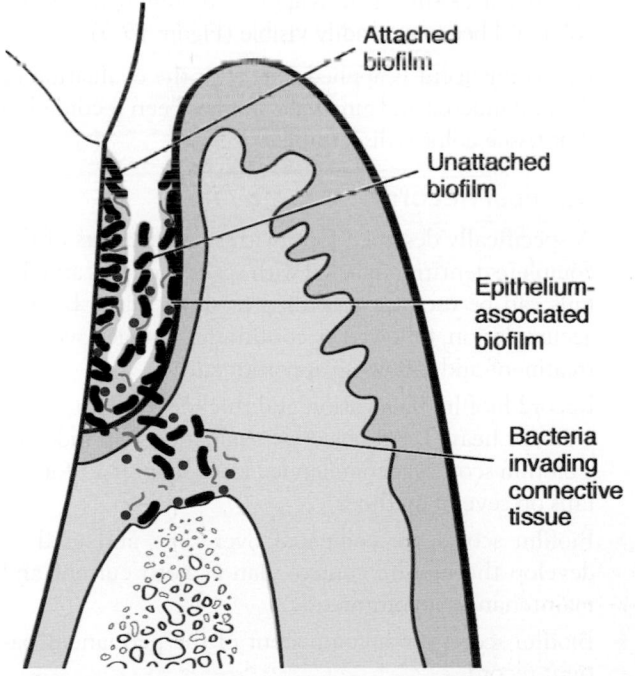

FIGURE 15-4 Bacterial Invasion. Diagram of a periodontal pocket shows attached and unattached biofilm bacteria within the pocket epithelium, in the connective tissue, and on the surface of the bone.

B. Fluoride

▶ The concentration of fluoride in biofilm is higher in the presence of fluoridated water and increases following professional topical applications of fluoride and the use of fluoride-containing dentifrices and mouthrinses.

II. Organic Elements

The organic EPS surrounds the microorganisms of biofilm and contains primarily carbohydrates and proteins, with small amounts of lipids.

A. Carbohydrates

▶ Carbohydrates include glucans such as dextran and fructans or levans formed by bacterial metabolism of dietary sucrose.

▶ Carbohydrates contribute to the adherence of microorganisms to each other and to the tooth, adding to biofilm's tenacious adherence to tooth surfaces.

B. Proteins

▶ The proteins of supragingival biofilm originate from the gingival sulcus fluid (crevicular fluid).

CLINICAL ASPECTS

I. Distribution of Biofilm

A. Location

▶ *Supragingival biofilm*: coronal to the gingival margin.

▶ *Gingival biofilm*: forms on the external surfaces of the oral epithelium and attached gingiva.

▶ *Subgingival biofilm*: located between the epithelial attachment and the gingival margin, within the sulcus or pocket.

▶ *Fissure biofilm*: develops in pits and fissures of the teeth.

B. By Surfaces

▶ *During formation*
- Supragingival biofilm formation begins at the gingival margin, particularly on proximal surfaces, and extends coronally when left undisturbed.
- It spreads over the gingival third and on toward the middle third of the crown.

▶ *Tooth surfaces involved*
- Biofilm is the heaviest on proximal surfaces and around the gingival third, associated with protected areas.
- Palatal surfaces of maxillary teeth may have the least biofilm due to the activity of the tongue during chewing, swallowing, and speaking.

C. Factors Influencing Biofilm Accumulation

▶ *Crowded teeth*: Dental biofilm accumulates readily around crowded mandibular anterior teeth as shown in Figure 15-5. With effective biofilm control, biofilm accumulation around crowded teeth is not greater than that around teeth in good alignment. Special accommodations such as using a toothbrush placed in a vertical position can remove thick biofilm on the lingual of the crowded mandibular anterior.

▶ *Rough surfaces*: Biofilm develops more rapidly on rough tooth surfaces, existing calculus, poorly contoured restorations, and removable appliances; thick dense deposits can be difficult to remove.

▶ *Occlusion*: Deposits may extend over an entire crown of a tooth that is unopposed, out of occlusion, or not actively used during mastication.

D. Removal of Biofilm

▶ Manual or power toothbrushing is the most universal daily mechanical disruption method.

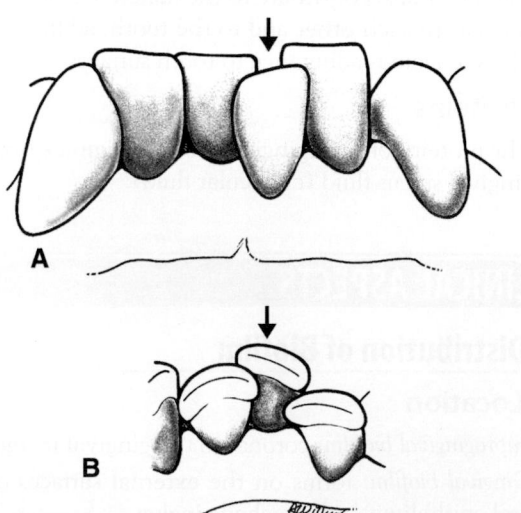

FIGURE 15-5 Biofilm Accumulation in Protected Areas. A: Crowded mandibular anterior teeth demonstrate dental biofilm after use of a disclosing agent. Thickest biofilm is on proximal surfaces and at cervical thirds of teeth; **B:** note central incisors with thick extensive biofilm on the less accessible protected surfaces.

▶ Daily flossing or other proximal surfaces biofilm disruption activities are necessary for the maintenance of optimal oral health.

II. Detection of Biofilm

A. Direct Vision

▶ *Thin biofilm:* May be translucent and therefore not visible without disclosing solution.

▶ *Stained biofilm:* Extrinsic stains may make biofilm more visible, for example, yellow, green, tobacco stains.

▶ *Thick biofilm:* The tooth may appear dull, dingy, with a matted furlike surface. Materia alba or food debris may collect over the biofilm.

B. Use of Explorer or Probe

▶ *Tactile examination:* When calcification has started, biofilm may feel slightly rough; otherwise, the surface may feel slippery from the coating of soft, slimy biofilm.

▶ *Removal of biofilm:* Biofilm may be detected by passing the side of the tip of a probe over the suspected tooth surface. When present, biofilm adheres to the probe tip.

C. Use of Disclosing Agent

▶ When a disclosing agent is applied, biofilm takes on the color and becomes readily visible (Figure 15-5).

▶ Disclosing agent is applied only after the evaluation of the oral mucosa and gingival color has been recorded so that tissue color is discernible.

D. Clinical Record

▶ A specifically designed form with several charts of the complete dentition labeled with space for dates and details can be used for recording to show initial biofilm accumulation, followed by continuing changes over the treatment and follow-up appointments.

▶ Record biofilm by location and thickness (slight, moderate, or heavy). For objective evaluations, an index or a biofilm score is recommended (see Chapter 23 for details on several methods).

▶ Biofilm scores are compared over time and used to develop the biofilm control plan at both current and maintenance appointments.

▶ Biofilm scores are a component of the permanent patient record.

SIGNIFICANCE OF DENTAL BIOFILM

▶ Microbial biofilm plays a major role in the initiation and progression of both dental caries and periodontal infections.

▶ Periodontal diseases and dental caries are infectious, transmissible diseases caused by pathogenic microorganisms found in oral biofilms.

▸ Biofilm is significant in the formation of dental calculus, which is essentially mineralized dental biofilm.

▸ Optimal oral hygiene depends on consistent daily dental biofilm disruption as complete removal of all biofilm is impossible.

▸ Accumulation of dental biofilm on the teeth, tongue, tonsils, and oral mucosa contributes to an unpleasant personal appearance as well as oral malodor.

DENTAL CARIES

▸ Dental caries is a disease of the dental calcified structures (enamel, dentin, and cementum) characterized by demineralization of the mineral components and dissolution of the organic matrix.

▸ Clinical characteristics and types of cavitated dental caries are described in Chapter 16.

▸ The process of dental caries is described in Chapter 27.

▸ The sequence of events leading to demineralization and dental caries is shown in Figure 15-6.

I. Cariogenic Microorganisms in Biofilm[16]

▸ Mutans streptococci (S. mutans and Streptococcus sobrinus, predominantly) and Lactobacilli acid-forming bacteria are the initial etiologic agents.

▸ Mutans streptococci initiate the caries process and Lactobacilli contributes to the progression of a carious lesion.

▸ Xerostomia (decreased salivary flow) and frequent fermentable carbohydrate exposure promote the growth of Streptococcus mutans and Lactobacilli, in dental biofilm.

▸ Biofilm architecture and EPS matrix of the biofilm community helps to maintain the caries causing acidic environment.[17]

II. The pH of Biofilm

▸ Acid formation begins *immediately* when the cariogenic substance is taken into the biofilm.

▸ The pH of the biofilm is lowered quickly, and 1–2 hours are required for the pH to return to a normal level, assuming the biofilm is left undisturbed.

▸ Biofilm pH before eating ranges from 6.2 to 7.0; it is lower in the caries-susceptible person and higher in the caries-resistant person.

▸ Immediately following sucrose intake into biofilm, a rapid drop in the pH of the biofilm occurs.[18]

▸ Critical pH for enamel demineralization averages 4.5–5.5. The critical pH for root surface demineralization is approximately 6.0–6.7, especially relevant for patients with multiple areas of recession and xerostomia.[19]

▸ The amount of demineralization depends on the length of time and frequency the pH is below critical level;

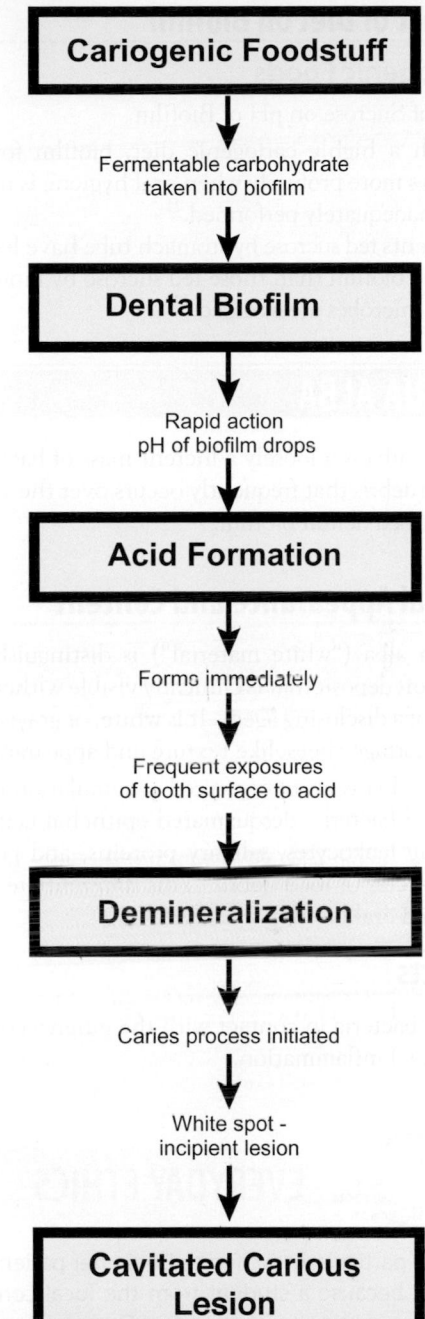

FIGURE 15-6 **Development of Dental Caries.** Flowchart shows the step-by-step action within the microbial biofilm on the tooth surface.

biofilm density and maturity are additional factors that affect the caries process.

▸ With each meal or snack that contains sucrose, the pH of the biofilm is lowered (Figure 35-5 in Chapter 35).

▸ Quantity of sucrose or carbohydrates eaten is less damaging than frequency, sucrose eaten with meals is less damaging than as snacks.[20]

▸ A discussion of dietary sucrose or carbohydrate consumption is part of a total dental caries assessment control program (see Chapter 35).

III. Effect of Diet on Biofilm

A. Cariogenic Foods

▶ Effect of Sucrose on pH of Biofilm

- With a highly cariogenic diet, biofilm forms and grows more profusely when oral hygiene is neglected or inadequately performed.[21]
- Patients fed sucrose by stomach tube have less acidogenic biofilm than those fed sucrose by mouth since oral microbes are avoided.[22]

MATERIA ALBA

▶ Materia alba is a loosely adherent mass of bacteria and cellular debris that frequently occurs over the surface of undisturbed dental biofilm.

I. Clinical Appearance and Content

▶ Materia alba ("white material") is distinguished as a bulky, soft deposit that is clinically visible without application of a disclosing agent. It is white, or grayish white, with a cottage cheeselike texture and appearance.

▶ Materia alba is an unorganized accumulation of living and dead bacteria, desquamated epithelial cells, disintegrating leukocytes, salivary proteins, and possibly a few particles of food debris. This differentiates it from organized oral biofilms

II. Effects

▶ Surface bacteria in contact with the gingiva contribute to gingival inflammation.

▶ Tooth surface demineralization and early noncavitated lesions can be seen under materia alba.

III. Prevention

▶ Materia alba can be removed with a water spray, oral irrigator, or tongue action, whereas only the surface organisms of biofilm can be removed.

▶ Clinical distinction of materia alba, food debris, and dental biofilm is necessary, but patient instruction for the removal of all three involves the same basic biofilm control procedures.

FOOD DEBRIS

▶ Loose food particles collect about the cervical third and proximal embrasures of the teeth.

▶ Cariogenic foods contribute to dental caries because liquefied carbohydrate diffuses rapidly into the biofilm and hence to the acid-forming bacteria.

▶ *Food impaction:* When there are open contact areas, mobility of teeth, or irregularities of occlusion such as plunger cusps, food may be forced between the teeth during mastication. This could result in vertical food impaction.

▶ Horizontal or lateral food impaction occurs in facial and lingual embrasures, particularly when the interdental papillae are reduced or missing.

▶ Food debris adds to a general unsanitary condition of the mouth. Some self-cleansing through the action of the tongue, lips, saliva, and related factors may take place.

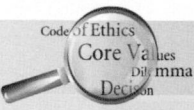

EVERYDAY ETHICS

Daria was particularly excited to begin her patient schedule today because a student from the local community college was coming to observe her. Daria had graduated from the same dental hygiene program 6 years earlier and had volunteered to participate in the program for students to observe practitioners.

Roland, a second-year student, presented promptly at the receptionist's window 15 minutes prior to the first patient. Daria was already busily preparing her treatment room, and she quickly introduced herself to the student. She invited Roland to ask her any questions but not in front of a patient. She said she would introduce him to the patient at the beginning of each appointment, and would request verbal approval from the patient for his presence; he would scrub up and assist. Roland was impressed with Daria's professionalism.

After the first appointment was completed, Roland asked Daria why she was still using the term "plaque"

during patient instruction instead of "biofilm" and why she didn't disclose the teeth before the providing education and selective polishing procedures. "Oh," Daria replied, "Is this something new you learned in school? I've only been to one continuing education course since I left school but I didn't hear anything about—what is it? Biofilm?"

Questions for Consideration

1. Role-play the dialogue that might take place regarding use of the term "plaque" versus "biofilm," which was a new concept for Daria.

2. Ethically, how is Daria violating/not violating any ethical principles relative to total patient care by not using disclosing agent to identify the biofilm? In what ways may terminology be important in practice?

3. Which of the dental hygiene core values (Table II-1, in Section II) are in action in this scenario? Describe how each one selected was in action.

▶ Debris removal by toothbrushing, and interproximal biofilm removal techniques constitutes a total biofilm control program. Cleansing of food debris from around fixed prostheses and orthodontic appliances is necessary to prevent disease.

DOCUMENTATION

The permanent records for each patient will include information for the soft deposits including:

▶ Clinical description of appearance of the teeth relative to the biofilm, materia alba, or food debris as indications of the personal oral care on a daily basis.

▶ Patient's understanding of biofilm and the significance of various deposits.

▶ Patient's description of the methods used daily: brush teeth, tongue, floss, rinse, and exactly what products are used at each mouthcare episode (such as in the morning after breakfast, chew xylitol gum after lunch, etc.).

A sample progress note for a patient's appointment may be reviewed in Box 15-3.

BOX 15-3

Example Documentation: Nonsurgical Periodontal Therapy Appointment for Patient with Inadequate Biofilm Removal

S –40-year-old female patient represents for third quadrant nonsurgical periodontal therapy (NSPT) with local anesthesia. Medical history includes an allergy to penicillin. There are no contradictions for treatment or anesthesia.

O –Update today indicates no changes to health history, allergies, or functions status. No changes in oral status indicated by assessment data. Only change is a biofilm score of greater than 60%, which has increased by 10% from last visit.

A –Discuss, review, and demonstrated proper oral self-care instructions and schedule final quadrant of NSPT with local anesthesia.

P –Medical history updated, intra- and extraoral examination performed, biofilm score using disclosing solution, assessed quadrants from last visit, and periodontal probed. Biofilm removal remains inadequate; discussed and showed her disclosed dentition where most proximal surfaces showed red and bleeding on probing. Demonstrated how to work the power toothbrush in between; she said she doesn't use her power brush much. When asked why, she shrugged and said it was a nuisance to care for it; tried to make some suggestions, with emphasis that it would help her gingiva get healthy sooner; I asked if this week she would use it and include all four quadrants, especially the next one we will do next (max. left) so we can see the difference from my scaling. She said she would try.

Next step: Schedule last quadrant of NSPT with local anesthesia.

Signed: _____, RDH

Date:_____

Factors To Teach The Patient

▷ Location, composition, and properties of dental biofilm, with emphasis on its role in dental caries and periodontal infections.

▷ The cause and prevention of dental caries.

▷ Effects of personal oral care procedures in the prevention of dental biofilm.

▷ Biofilm control procedures with special adaptations for individual needs.

▷ Sources of cariogenic foodstuff in the diet, with suggestions for control.

▷ Relationship of frequency of eating cariogenic foods to dental caries.

References

1. Siqueira WL, Custodio W, McDonald EE. New insights into the composition and functions of the acquired enamel pellicle. *J Dent Res.* 2012;91(12):1110–1118.

2. Hanning M. Ultrastructural investigation of pellicle morphogenesis at two different intraoral sites during a 24-h period. *Clin Oral Investig.* 1999;3:88–95.

3. Hanning M, Joiner A. The structure, function and properties of the acquired pellicle. *Monogr Oral Sci.* 2006;19:26–64.

4. Meckel AH. Formation and properties of organic films on teeth. *Arch Oral Biol.* 1965;10(4):585–598.

5. Kuroiwa M, Kodaka T, Kuroiwa M, et al. Acid resistance of human enamel by brushing with and without abrasive dentifrice. *J Biol Buccale.* 1992;20:175–180.

6. Hara AT, Zero DT. The caries environment: saliva, pellicle, diet, and hard tissue ultrastructure. *Dent Clin North Am.* 2010;54(3):455–467.

7. Aas JA, Paster BJ, Stokes LN, et al. Defining the normal bacterial flora of the oral cavity. *J Clin Microbiol.* 2005;43(11):5721–5732.

8. Stoodley P, Sauer K, Davies DG, et al. Biofilms as complex differentiated communities. *Annu Rev Microbiol.* 2002;56:187–209.

9. Löe H, Theilade E, Jensen SB. Experimental gingivitis in man. *J Periodontol.* 1965;36:177–187.

10. Zijnge V, van Leeuwen M, Degener J, et al. Oral biofilm architecture on natural teeth. *PLoS One.* 2010;5(2):e9321. http://www.plosone.org/article/info:doi/10.1371/journal.pone.0009321.

11. Socransky SS, Haffajee AD, Cugini MA, et al. Microbial complexes in subgingival plaque. *J Clin Periodontol.* 1998;25(2):134–144.

12. Socransky S, Haffajee A. Dental biofilms: difficult therapeutic target. *Periodontol 2000.* 2002;28:12–55.

13. Mandel ID. Relation of saliva and plaque to caries. *J Dent Res.* 1974;53(2):246–266.

14. Grøn P, Yao K, Spinelli M. A study of inorganic constituents in dental plaque. *J Dent Res.* 1969;48(5):799–805.

15. Van Houte J, Sansone C, Joshipura K, et al. Mutans streptococci and non-mutans streptococci acidogenic at low pH, and *in vitro* acidogenic potential of dental plaque in two different areas of the human dentition. *J Dent Res.* 1991;70(12):1503–1507.

16. Rosen S, Weisenstein PR. The effect of sugar solutions on pH of dental plaques from caries-susceptible and caries-free individuals. *J Dent Res.* 1965;44(5):845–849.

17. Koo H, Falsetta ML, Klein MI. The exopolysaccharide matrix: a virulence determinant of cariogenic biofilm. *J Dent Res.* 2013;92(12):1065–1073.

18. Hoppenbrouwers PM, Driessens FC, Borggreven JM. The mineral solubility of human tooth roots. *Arch Oral Biol.* 1987;32(5):319–322.

19. Gustafsson BE, Quensel CE, Lanke LS, et al. The Vipeholm dental caries study: the effect of different levels of carbohydrate intake on caries activity in 436 individuals observed for five years. *Acta Odontol Scand.* 1954;11(3–4):232–264.

20. Carlsson J, Egelberg J. Effect of diet on early plaque formation in man. *Odontol Revy.* 1965;16(1):112–125.

21. Littleton NW, Carter CH, Kelley RT. Studies of oral health in persons nourished by stomach tube. I. Changes in the pH of plaque material after the addition of sucrose. *J Am Dent Assoc.* 1967;74(1):119–123.

22. Egelberg J. Local effect of diet on plaque formation and development of gingivitis in dogs. III. Effect of frequency of meals and tube feeding. *Odontol Revy.* 1965;16(1):50–60.

ENHANCE YOUR UNDERSTANDING

thePoint **DIGITAL CONNECTIONS**
(see the inside front cover for access information)
- **Audio glossary**
- **Quiz bank**

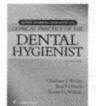

SUPPORT FOR LEARNING
(available separately; visit lww.com)
- *Active Learning Workbook for Clinical Practice of the Dental Hygienist, 12th Edition*

prepU **INDIVIDUALIZED REVIEW**
(available separately; visit lww.com)
- **Adaptive quizzing with *prepU for Wilkins' Clinical Practice of the Dental Hygienist***

16

The Teeth

Esther M. Wilkins, BS, RDH, DMD

CHAPTER OUTLINE

LEARNING OBJECTIVES

After studying this chapter, the student will be able to:

1. Identify the three divisions of the human dentition: primary teeth, mixed (transitional) dentition, and permanent teeth.

2. Recognize and explain the various developmental and noncarious dental lesions.

3. Describe types of dental injuries and tooth fractures that may occur.

4. List the G.V. Black classification of dental carious lesions as used for diagnosis, treatment planning, cavity preparations, and finished restorations.

5. Explain the initiation and development of early childhood caries (ECC).

6. Compare methods for determining the vitality of the pulp of a tooth.

7. Provide a list of the factors to be observed and recorded during a complete dental charting with a new patient.

Clinical examination and assessment of the teeth is essential before treatment to provide guidelines for treatment planning, instrumentation, instruction, and follow-up evaluation.

▶ In general, patients may be more concerned about their teeth than about the periodontium, the supporting structures that maintain the teeth in their positions.

▶ The concerns may be related to:
- Personal appearance
- Knowledge level, which may be greater about teeth than about the periodontium
- Sensitivity and pain associated with ailments of the teeth.

▶ Background study of dental anatomy, oral histology, and oral pathology is essential to this phase of clinical practice.

▶ Key words are defined in Box 16-1.

THE DENTITIONS

The three divisions are the primary dentition, the mixed (transitional) dentition, and the permanent dentition.

I. Primary Dentition

▶ Formation of the primary teeth begins in utero.

▶ The weeks in utero when each primary tooth begins to mineralize and the average months after birth when the enamel is completely formed before the date of eruption are listed in Table 50-4 in Chapter 50.

II. Mixed or Transitional Dentition

▶ The mixed or transitional dentition when primary teeth are being exfoliated and permanent teeth move

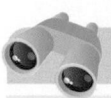

BOX 16-1 KEY WORDS: Teeth

Accessory root canal: a secondary canal extending from the pulp to the surface of the root; frequently found near the apex of a root but may occur higher and provide a connection to a periodontal pocket.

Amelogenesis imperfecta: disorder of production and development of enamel.

Avulsion: the tearing away or forcible separation of a structure or part. Tooth avulsion is the traumatic separation of a tooth from the alveolus.

Bruxism: an oral habit of grinding, clenching, or clamping the teeth; involuntary, rhythmic, or spasmodic movements outside the chewing range; may damage teeth and attachment apparatus.

Cariogenic: adj. conducive to dental caries.

Carious: adj. used to define a carious lesion.

Cementicle: a calcified spherical body, composed of cementum, lying free within the periodontal ligament, attached to the cementum or imbedded within the cementum.

Dental caries: disease of the mineralized structures of the teeth characterized by demineralization of the hard components and dissolution of the organic matrix.

Arrested caries: carious lesion that has become stationary and does not show a tendency to progress further; frequently has a hard surface and takes on a dark brown or reddish-brown color.

Primary caries: occurs on a surface not previously affected; also called initial caries; early lesion may be referred to as incipient caries.

Rampant caries: widespread formation of chalky white areas and incipient lesions that may increase in size over a comparatively short time.

Recurrent caries: occurs on a surface adjacent to a restoration; may be a continuation of the original lesion; also called secondary caries.

Dentition: the natural teeth in the dental arch.

Primary (deciduous) dentition: the first teeth; normally will be shed and replaced by permanent teeth.

Permanent dentition: the natural 32 teeth that serve throughout life.

Mixed dentition: combination of primary and permanent teeth between ages 6 and 12 when primary teeth are being replaced; starts with the eruption of the first permanent tooth.

Succedaneous: the permanent teeth that erupt into the positions of exfoliated primary teeth.

Edentulous: without teeth; referred to as partially edentulous when some, but not all, teeth are missing.

Electrolyte: a conductor; a substance that, in solution, dissociates into electrically charged particles (ions) and thus is capable of conducting an electric current.

Etiology: the science or study of the cause of a disease or disorder.

Exfoliation: loss of primary teeth following physiologic resorption of root structure.

Facet: a small flattened surface on a hard body, such as a tooth; a wear facet can result from attrition or repeated parafunctional contact.

Hypoplasia: incomplete development or underdevelopment of a tissue or organ.

Enamel hypoplasia: incomplete or defective formation of the enamel of either primary or permanent teeth. The result may be an irregularity of tooth form, color, or surface.

Idiopathic: denoting a condition of unknown cause.

Incipient: beginning; coming into existence.

pH: the symbol of hydrogen ion concentration expressed in numbers corresponding to the acidity or alkalinity of an aqueous solution; the range is from 14 (pure base) to 0 (pure acid); neutral is at 7.0.

Critical pH: the pH at which demineralization occurs; for enamel, pH 4.5–5.5; for cementum, pH 6.0–6.7.

Resorption: removal of bone or tooth structure; gradual dissolution of the mineralized tissue; may be internal or external; occurs during exfoliation of a primary tooth and from the pressure of orthodontic treatment.

in to take their places occurs between the ages of 6 and 12 years.

▶ Figure 16-1 illustrates the mixed dentition of a child approximately 6 years of age just as the first permanent molars are erupting.

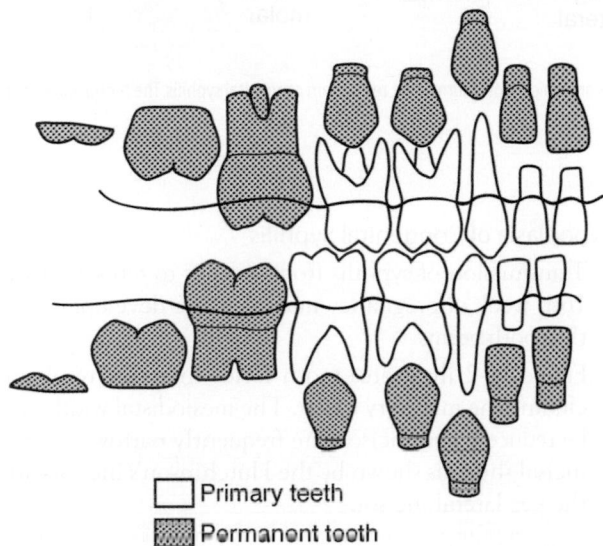

☐ Primary teeth
▨ Permanent tooth

FIGURE 16-1 Mixed Dentition at Approximately Age 6 Years. The average child has 20 primary teeth in place, and root resorption of the incisors has started as the developing permanent incisors move into position. The first permanent molars are partially erupted.

III. Permanent Dentition

▶ Mineralization of the permanent teeth starts at birth and continues into adolescence. The chronology of development and eruption of the permanent teeth is listed in Table 16-1.

▶ Roots normally are completed by 3 years after eruption.

DEVELOPMENTAL AND NONCARIOUS DENTAL LESIONS

I. Enamel Hypoplasia

Enamel hypoplasia is a defect that occurs as a result of a disturbance during formation of the enamel matrix.

A. Types and Etiology

Hereditary

Enamel is partly or wholly missing. An example is amelogenesis imperfecta, described in Chapter 22.

Systemic (Environmental)

Factors that may contribute to enamel hypoplasia during tooth development include:

▶ Severe nutritional deficiency, particularly rickets.

TABLE 16-1		Tooth Development and Eruption: Permanent Teeth			
		HARD TISSUE FORMATION BEGINS	ENAMEL COMPLETED (YEARS)	ERUPTION (YEARS)	ROOT COMPLETED (YEARS)
Maxillary	Central incisor	3–4 mo	4–5	7–8	10
	Lateral incisor	10 mo	4–5	8–9	11
	Canine	4–5 mo	6–7	11–12	13–15
	First premolar	1½–1¾ y	5–6	10–11	12–13
	Second premolar	2–2¼ y	6–7	10–12	12–14
	First molar	At birth	2½–3	6–7	9–10
	Second molar	2½–3 y	7–8	12–13	14–16
	Third molar	7–9 y	12–16	17–21	18–25
Mandibular	Central incisor	3–4 mo	4–5	6–7	9
	Lateral incisor	3–4 mo	4–5	7–8	10
	Canine	4–5 mo	6–7	9–10	12–14
	First premolar	1¾–2 yr	5–6	10–12	12–13
	Second premolar	2¼–2½ yr	6–7	11–12	13–14
	First molar	at birth	2½–3	6–7	9–10
	Second molar	2½–3 yr	7–8	11–13	14–15
	Third molar	8–10 yr	12–16	17–21	18–25

Source: Logan WH, Kronfield R. Development of the human jaws and surrounding structures from birth to age fifteen. *JADA*. 1933;35(20):379–424; Orban B. *Oral Histology and Embryology*. St. Louis, MO: Mosby; 1944. Schour I, McCall JO. Chronology of the human dentition. In Orban B (Ed). *Oral Histology and Embryology*. St Louis, MA: Mosby; 1944:240.

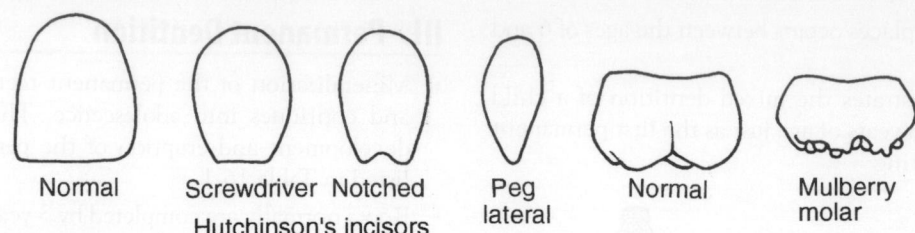

FIGURE 16-2 Crown Forms of Enamel Hypoplasia. Hutchinson's incisors and mulberry molars are typical crown forms that result from congenital syphilis. The central incisors are narrowed at the incisal third, and the lateral incisors may be conical or peg shaped.

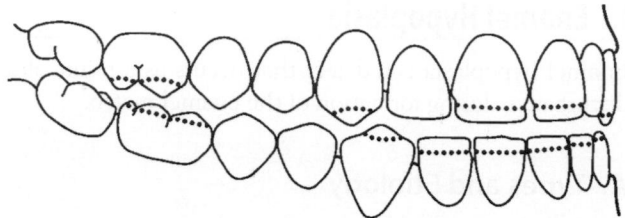

FIGURE 16-3 Enamel Hypoplasia. Chronologic hypoplasia, usually in the form of grooves or pits, appears in the enamel at a level corresponding with the stage of development of the teeth. For this patient, the disturbance in enamel development occurred at approximately 10 months of age.

- ▶ Fever-producing diseases, such as measles, chickenpox, and scarlet fever.
- ▶ Congenital syphilis: Hutchinsons's incisors and mulberry molars shown in Figure 16-2 are samples of the severe effects of congenital syphilis.
- ▶ Hypoparathyroidism.
- ▶ Birth injury or prematurity.
- ▶ Rh hemolytic disease.
- ▶ Fluorosis.

Local

A single tooth can be affected; trauma or a periapical inflammation about a primary tooth can injure the adjacent developing permanent tooth.

B. Appearance

Hereditary

The teeth may appear brown.

Systemic

Also called "chronologic hypoplasia" because the lesions are found in areas of the teeth where the enamel was forming during the systemic disturbance.

- ▶ *Single narrow zone* (smooth or pitted): Disturbance lasted a short period of time (Figure 16-3).
- ▶ *Multiple:* Disturbance to the ameloblast occurred over a period of time, or several times.
- ▶ *Teeth most frequently affected:* First molars, incisors, canines, because the disturbances generally occur during the first year when those teeth are mineralizing.

Hypoplasia of Congenital Syphilis

- ▶ Transmission of syphilis from mother to fetus after the 16th week of pregnancy may alter the development of the tooth germs.
- ▶ Figure 16-2 illustrates tooth forms that may result including the mulberry molar. The mesiodistal width may be reduced, and incisors are frequently narrowed at the incisal third, as shown by the Hutchinson's incisors and the peg lateral incisor.

Local Enamel Hypoplasia

A single tooth with a yellow or brown intrinsic stain.

II. Attrition

Attrition is the wearing away of a tooth as a result of tooth-to-tooth contact (Figure 16-4).

A. Occurrence

Location

May be found on occlusal, incisal, and proximal surfaces.

Age Factor

Effects of bruxism are cumulative over time so increases are associated with aging. Increases with age bruxism. More attrition is seen in men than in women of comparable age.

B. Etiology

Bruxism

Predisposing factors may be psychological, tension, or occlusal interferences.

Usage

Wear of surfaces on each other. Predisposing factors may be coarse foods, chewing tobacco, culturally related chewing habits, or abrasive dusts associated with certain occupations.

C. Appearance

Initial Lesion

Small polished facet on a cusp tip or ridge, or slight flattening of an incisal edge.

Advanced

Gradual reduction in cusp height; flattening of incisal or occlusal plane as shown in Figure 16-4.

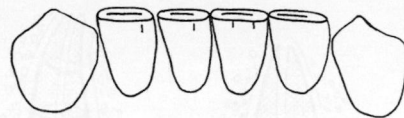

FIGURE 16-4 **Attrition.** Attrition of the incisal surfaces of mandibular anterior teeth has extended to expose the dentin. Dentin usually appears as a brown line or ring.

Staining of Exposed Dentin

Discoloration may occur; stain usually is brown.

Radiographic

The pulp chamber and canals may be narrowed and sometimes obliterated as a result of formation of secondary dentin.

III. Erosion

Erosion is the loss of tooth substance by a chemical process that does not involve known bacterial action.

A. Occurrence
Location

Facial or lingual surfaces, depending on cause.

Usually Involves Several Teeth

B. Etiology

The lesions are caused by some form of chemical dissolution.

Chronic Vomiting

Acid of chronic vomiting affects lingual surfaces, particularly anterior teeth.

▶ Pregnancy.
▶ Eating disorder, such as bulimia as described in Chapter 64.

Extrinsic

▶ *Industrial:* Workers' teeth can be exposed to atmospheric acids.
▶ *Dietary:* Facial surfaces are more frequently affected.
▶ Carbonated beverages.
▶ Lemons or other citrus fruit sucked frequently.

May Be Idiopathic (Unknown)

C. Appearance

▶ Smooth, shallow, hard, shiny (in contrast to dental caries, in which appearance is soft and discolored).
▶ Shape varies from shallow saucerlike depressions to deep wedge-shaped grooves; margins are not sharply demarcated.
▶ May progress to involve the dentin and stimulate secondary dentin.
▶ May occur in combination with dental caries, calculus, or dental restorations.[1]

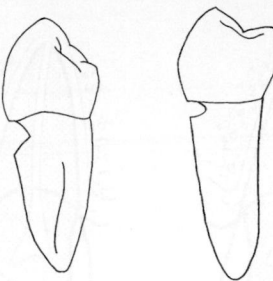

FIGURE 16-5 **Abrasion.** Profile view of the facial surface of mandibular premolars shows shape of abrasion on the root. Note that the area of abrasion undermines the enamel.

IV. Abrasion

Abrasion is the mechanical wearing away of tooth substance by forces other than mastication.

A. Occurrence

▶ Exposed root surfaces.
▶ At incisal edge or on occlusal surface.

B. Etiology

▶ The lesion originates from mechanical abrasion.
▶ The action of microorganisms is not essential for the development of abrasion. Dental caries may occur in the abraded area as a secondary lesion.
▶ *Abrasive agent:* A common cause is an abrasive dentifrice applied with vigorous horizontal toothbrushing. Figure 16-5 shows the effect on the root surface.
▶ *Occupational causes:* These include, for example, tacks held by carpenters and pins by dressmakers.
▶ A smoking or hookah pipe held between the teeth; may be held in the same place over many years.

C. Appearance

▶ V- or wedge shaped with hard, smooth, shiny surface and clearly defined margins.
▶ Except for incisal biting habits, the lesions occur initially on exposed cementum, then extend into the dentin.

FRACTURES OF THE TEETH

▶ Trauma to the face may involve fractured bones and teeth in addition to soft tissue injuries. Fractured jaw and methods of treatment are described in Chapter 8.
▶ Emergency care for a forcibly displaced tooth is found in Table 8-4, Chapter 8.

I. Causes of Tooth Fractures

▶ Automobile, bicycle, and diving accidents.

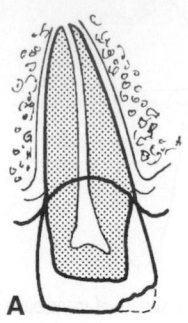 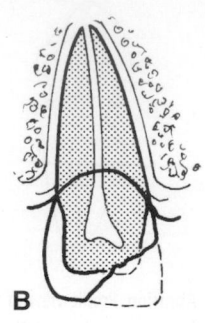 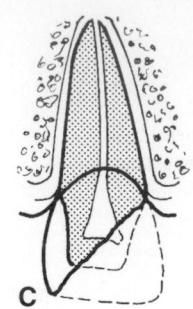 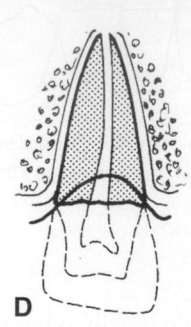 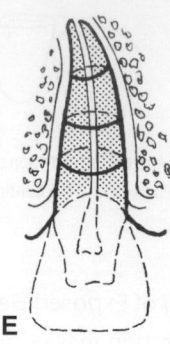

FIGURE 16-6 Fractures of Teeth. A: Enamel fracture. **B:** Crown fracture without pulpal involvement. **C:** Crown fracture with pulpal involvement. **D:** Fracture of crown and root near neck of tooth. **E:** Root fractures involving cementum, dentin, and the pulp may occur in the apical, middle, or coronal third of the root.

▶ Contact sports when mouth protectors are not worn.

▶ Blows incurred while fighting.

▶ Falls.

II. Description

A. Line of Fracture

▶ May be horizontal, diagonal, or vertical.

▶ Figure 16-6 illustrates fractures of a central incisor.

B. Radiographic Signs of Recent Trauma

▶ Widened periodontal ligament (PDL) space.

▶ Radiolucent fracture line.

▶ Radiopaque areas where fracture segments overlap.

▶ Tooth displacement.

III. Classification of Dental Injuries[2]

▶ Both primary and permanent dentitions are included.

• Fracture of enamel of tooth such as chipping and incomplete fractures (cracks).

• Fracture of crown of tooth without pulpal involvement.

• Fracture of crown with pulpal involvement.

• Fracture of root of tooth.

• Fracture of crown and root of tooth with or without pulpal involvement.

• Luxation (dislocation) of tooth: This category may involve concussion, subluxation, and luxation. Concussion means the tooth is sensitive to percussion but is not loosened or displaced. Loosening without displacement is subluxation, and loosening with displacement is luxation.

• Intrusion or extrusion of tooth: Intrusion into the alveolar bone is usually accompanied by fracture of the alveolar socket. Extrusion from the socket is a partial displacement.

• Avulsion of tooth: Avulsion is the complete displacement of the tooth out of its socket.

IV. Recommendations for Treatment

▶ Diagnosis and planning are necessary for satisfactory healing.

▶ Guidelines for treatment planning have been prepared by the *International Association of Dental Traumatology* and include[2]:

• Clinical diagnosis and immediate emergency treatment

• Radiographs to detect root fracture

• Location of tooth fragments

• Pulp testing

• Mobility; tenderness

• Follow-up for additional requirements.

DENTAL CARIES

The World Health Organization has defined dental caries as a "localized, posteruptive, pathologic process of external origin involving softening of the hard tooth tissue and proceeding to the formation of a cavity."[3] Dental caries is a preventable disease.

I. Development of Dental Caries

Requirements for the development of a carious lesion are microorganisms, fermentable carbohydrate, and a susceptible tooth surface. Figure 35-2 in Chapter 35 shows four overlapping circles to illustrate the essential factors in dental caries initiation.

▶ Dental biofilm may contain numerous types of acid-forming bacteria. *Streptococcus mutans* in the initiation and *lactobacillus* in the progression of the lesion have been specifically implicated.

▶ The role of dental biofilm and the many factors involved are described in Chapter 15.

II. Classification of Carious Lesions

A. G.V. Black's Classification[4]

▶ The standard method for classifying dental caries was developed by Dr. G.V. Black, a noted dental educator who divided the categories into classes according to surfaces of the teeth; each class is represented by a Roman numeral.

▶ The categories customarily are used for carious lesions, cavity preparations, and finished restorations. Figure 16-7 defines and illustrates the classifications.

B. Nomenclature by Surfaces

▶ *Simple cavity*: involves one tooth surface. Example: occlusal cavity.

▶ *Compound cavity*: involves two tooth surfaces. Example: mesio-occlusal cavity, referred to as an "M-O" cavity.

▶ *Complex cavity*: involves more than two tooth surfaces. Example: mesio-occlusal-distal, referred to as an "M-O-D" cavity.

CLASSIFICATION: LOCATION	APPEARANCE	METHOD OF EXAMINATION
Class I. Cavities in pits or fissures a. Occlusal surfaces of premolars and molars b. Facial and lingual surfaces of molars c. Lingual surfaces of maxillary incisors	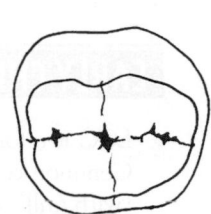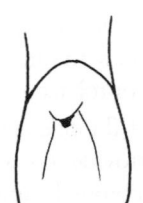	Direct or indirect visual Radiographs not useful
Class II. Cavities in proximal surfaces of premolars and molars	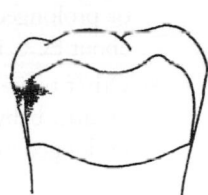	Early caries: by radiographs only Moderate caries not broken through from proximal to occlusal: Visual by color changes in tooth and loss of translucency Extensive caries involving occlusal: direct visual
Class III. Cavities in proximal surfaces of incisors and canines that do not involve the incisal angle	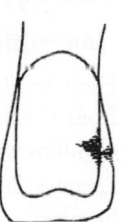	Early caries: by radiographs or transillumination Moderate caries not broken through to lingual or facial: 1. Visual by tooth color change 2. Radiograph Extensive caries; direct visual
Class IV. Cavities in proximal surfaces of incisors or canines that involve the incisal angle	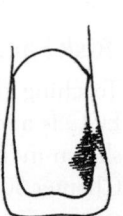	Visual Transillumination
Class V. Cavities in the cervical 1/3 of facial or lingual surfaces (not pit or fissure)	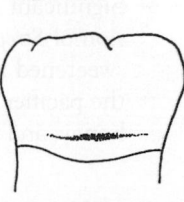	Direct visual: dry surface for vision Dull probe to distinguish demineralization: whether rough or hard and unbroken Areas may be sensitive to touch
Class VI. Cavities on incisal edges of anterior teeth and cusp tips of posterior teeth	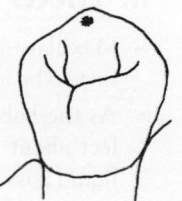	Direct visual May be discolored

FIGURE 16-7 Dental Caries: Classification of Cavities.

ENAMEL CARIES

I. Steps in the Formation of a Carious Lesion

A. Phase I: Incipient Lesion

▸ *Subsurface demineralization:* Acid products from cariogenic dental biofilm pass through microchannels (pores) from the surface of the enamel to the subsurface area in the dentin.

▸ *Visualization:* The area of demineralization is not visible by clinical observation during initial changes; a thin layer of enamel remains over the surface.

▸ *First clinical evidence:* White area spot lesion appears with no breakthrough to enamel surface; with time, area may turn brown from food, beverages, or tobacco use.

▸ *Remineralization:* Low concentrations of fluoride applied frequently during the early phase can provide sources for uptake by the demineralized zone. The porous demineralized area readily takes up fluoride from dentifrice, mouthrinse, fluoridated drinking water, and all possible sources.

▸ Figure 36-3 in Chapter 36 shows examples of levels of concentration of fluoride in surface enamel and in a white demineralized area.

B. Phase II: Untreated Incipient Lesion

▸ *Breakdown of enamel over the demineralized area:* Visible to observation and irregular to the gentle application of the side of an explorer tip or blunt probe.

▸ *Progression of carious lesion:* Follows general direction of enamel rods.

▸ *Spread of carious lesion:* Spreads at dentinoenamel junction; continues along the dentinal tubules (Figure 16-8).

II. Types of Dental Caries (Described by Location)

A. Pit and Fissure

▸ Caries begins in a minute fault in the enamel.

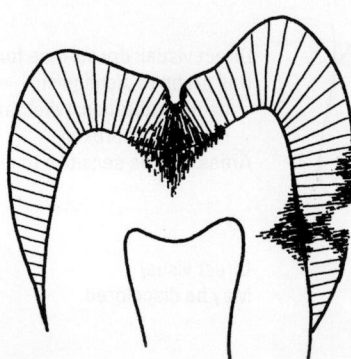

FIGURE 16-8 Dental Caries. Cones of dental caries in a pit and fissure and on a smooth tooth surface. Dental caries follows the general direction of the enamel rods, spreads at the dentinoenamel junction, and then continues along the dentinal tubules.

▸ Pit or fissure irregularity occurs where three or more lobes of the developing tooth join; closure of the enamel plates is imperfect. Examples: occlusal pits of molars and premolars.

B. Smooth Surface

▸ Caries begins in smooth surfaces where there is no pit, groove, or other defect.

▸ It occurs in areas where dental biofilm is protected from removal, such as proximal tooth surfaces, protected area near a contact, cervical thirds of teeth, and other difficult-to-clean areas.

EARLY CHILDHOOD CARIES (ECC)[5,6]

▸ ECC is a form of caries found in very young children. Common causes are the routine use of a nursing bottle (with milk or sweetened beverage) when going to sleep or prolonged at-will breast-feeding. More information about ECC is discussed in Chapter 50.

▸ Other names for the same condition are nursing bottle mouth, baby bottle syndrome, baby bottle caries, and prolonged nursing habit.

I. Etiology

A. Microbiology

▸ High levels of *Mutans streptococci* have been cultured from the saliva and dental biofilm from the teeth of children with ECC.[7,8]

▸ *Lactobacilli* also are found in large numbers in the biofilm.

B. Risk Factors

▸ Teaching the parents about the cause and effects of ECC is a significant part of anticipatory guidance, as shown in Table 49-3 in Chapter 49 and Table 50-7 in Chapter 50.

▸ Significant risk factors include maternal transmission of *Streptococcus mutans*, nursing bottle containing sweetened milk or other fluid sweetened with sucrose; the pacifier dipped or filled with a sweet agent, such as honey; and prolonged at-will breast-feeding.

II. Effects

▸ Maxillary anterior teeth and primary molars are the first to be affected (Figure 50-5 in Chapter 50).

▸ As the baby falls asleep, pools of sweet liquid can collect about the teeth. While the sucking is active, the liquid passes beyond the teeth.

▸ The nipple covers the mandibular anterior teeth; hence, they are rarely affected.

III. Recognition

▶ Children need to establish a dental home and have the first dental examination no later than 6 months after eruption of the first tooth and before the first birthday.[9]

▶ Demineralization may be noted along the cervical third of the maxillary anterior teeth. The source of the problem may be detected and preventive procedures initiated through parental counseling.

▶ At a later stage, the lesions appear dark brown. Eventually, the crowns may be destroyed to the gingival margin, abscesses may develop, and the child may suffer severe pain and discomfort (Figure 50-2 in Chapter 50).

ROOT CARIES

▶ Root caries is a soft, progressive lesion of cementum and dentin that involves bacterial infection and invasion. (see Figure 53-4 in Chapter 50). It is also called cemental caries, cervical caries, or radicular caries.

▶ The incidence of root caries increases with age, but not because of age. Gingival recession is necessary for root caries, and gingival recession is related to periodontal infections.

I. Steps in the Formation of a Root Surface Lesion

▶ Gingival recession exposes the cemental surface. Caries does not form in the root surface while periodontal fibers are still attached.

▶ Dental caries starts near the cementoenamel junction. Cementum is thin and is soon destroyed; dentin is invaded.

▶ Enamel is not involved when it is undermined. Root caries occurs in a mildly acidic environment. If the pH were lower, enamel would become carious.

▶ The critical pH for enamel is 4.5–5.0; for cementum, 6.0–6.7.[10]

▶ M. *streptococci* and *lactobacilli* are primary organisms associated with root caries. Antibody levels to S. *mutans* are elevated.[11,12]

II. Effects

▶ Low levels of root caries incidence has been shown to be directly related to the fluoride concentration in the drinking water.[13]

▶ Lifelong residence in a community with near-optimum levels of fluoride in the water was shown to be associated with an average 30% decrease in the incidence of root caries compared with that associated with lifelong residence in a nonfluoridated community.[14]

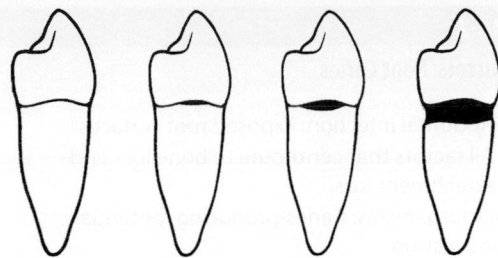

FIGURE 16-9 Root Caries. A root surface lesion starts near the cementoenamel junction after gingival recession has exposed the root surface. The lesion is progressive, undermines the enamel, and may eventually surround the cervical third of the cementum. (**Source:** Banting DW, Courtright PN. Distribution and natural history of carious lesions on the roots of the teeth. *Dent J.* 1975;41(1):45–9.)

III. Clinical Recognition

Cavitated lesions in root caries are described as soft, leathery, or hard.

▶ Soft, shallow, ill-defined lesion.

▶ Increases laterally to coalesce with other small lesions and eventually may extend completely around the tooth with undermining of the enamel (Figure 16-9).

▶ Yellowish, light brown, dark brown to black.

▶ Leathery in texture when explored (active lesion). Do not pick with a sharp explorer when remineralization is taking place; remineralization process can be arrested.

▶ Arrested root caries display cavitation and discoloration but are hard.

IV. Risk Factors for Root Caries

Risk factors are shown in Box 16-2. Prevention and control of root caries depend on control of risk factors.

CLINICAL EXAMINATION OF THE TEETH

I. Factors to Observe

▶ Table 16-2 lists factors to observe during the examination of the teeth and suggests relationships to appointment procedures.

▶ Careful identification of cavitated versus noncavitated lesions is essential to avoid exploring a remineralizing area.

▶ Information about hypoplasia, attrition, erosion, abrasion, and other tooth irregularities are recorded for the total patient history.

II. Recognition of Carious Lesions

A. Preparation

▶ Dry each tooth or group of teeth with compressed air; adjust mouth mirror for indirect light and vision.

BOX 16-2

Risk Factors: Root Caries

▷ Periodontal infection: Exposed root surfaces
  All factors that contribute to bone loss and attachment loss.
▷ Microorganisms: Caries-producing; potential transmission
▷ Local/behavioral
  Inadequate personal hygiene
  Dental biofilm accumulations
  Poor compliance
▷ Diet: Frequent use of cariogenic foods
▷ Low fluoride exposure
  Outside fluoridated community water supply
  Insufficient daily self-application (dentifrice, mouthrinse, frequency)
▷ Xerostomia
  Medications with side effects
  Radiation to head/neck
  Salivary gland dysfunction
▷ History of dental caries
  Many restorations: coronal and root
  Overhanging margins, open contact areas, and other biofilm traps
  Poor compliance for dental care
▷ Prosthetic devices
  Inadequate biofilm removal daily
  Overdentures, clasps, provide biofilm-retentive areas
▷ Tobacco use: sugar content of smokeless tobacco

▶ Carefully inspect each surface, first visually and then, only when necessary, gently with a blunt explorer to confirm visual findings (see Chapter 27).
▶ Avoid using a sharp explorer in a potentially remineralizing area.

B. Visual Examination

▶ Characteristic changes in the color and translucency of tooth structure may be observed.
▶ Changes noted can then be studied in the radiograph or documented for future review.
▶ Variations in color and translucency include the following:
  • Chalky white areas of demineralization.
  • Grayish-white discoloration of marginal ridges caused by dental caries of the proximal surface underneath.
  • Grayish-white color spreading from margins of restorations.
  • Dental caries may appear translucent in outer portions and white and opaque adjacent to an amalgam restoration.
  • Cavitated lesions may vary in color from yellowish-brown to dark brown.
  • Discoloration is generally less severe when dental caries progresses rapidly than when it progresses slowly.
  • Dull, flat white, opaque areas under direct light show loss of translucency, particularly of the enamel.
  • Dark shadow on a proximal surface may be shown by transillumination.
  • Transillumination is especially useful for anterior teeth and unrestored posterior teeth.

TABLE 16-2	Examination of the Teeth	
FEATURE	**TO OBSERVE**	**DENTAL HYGIENE IMPLICATION**
Morphology	Number of teeth (missing teeth verified by radiographic examination) Size, shape Arch form Position of individual teeth Injuries: fractures of the crown (root fractures observed in radiographs)	Selection and adaptation of instruments Areas prone to dental caries initiation, particularly difficult-to-reach areas during biofilm control Pulp test for vitality may be indicated
Development	Anomalies and developmental defects Pits and white spots	Distinguish hypoplasia and dental fluorosis from demineralization Identify pits for sealants
Eruption (Table 16-1)	Sequence of eruption: normal, irregular Unerupted teeth observed in radiographs	Care in using floss in the col area where the epithelium is usually less mature in young children Orthodontic needs Procedures for preservation of primary teeth
Deposits (Table 16-1) Food debris Biofilm Calculus Supragingival Subgingival	Overall evaluation of self-care and biofilm-control measures Relation of appearance of teeth to gingival health Extent and location of biofilm, debris, and calculus Calculus and the tooth surface pocket wall	Need for instruction and guidance Frequency of follow-up and maintenance appointments

FEATURE	TO OBSERVE	DENTAL HYGIENE IMPLICATION
Stains (See Chapter 21) Extrinsic Intrinsic	Extrinsic: colors relate to causes Intrinsic: dark, grayish Tobacco stain	Need for test for pulp vitality Stain removal procedures; selection of polishing agent Dentifrice recommendation Biofilm-control emphasis for biofilm-related stains Provide information concerning oral effects of tobacco use Tobacco cessation program (See Chapter 34)
Noncarious lesions	Attrition: primary and permanent Abrasion: physical agents that may be a cause Erosion	Evaluate causes and treat or counsel for prevention Dietary analysis Selection of nonabrasive dentifrice Habit evaluation
Exposed cementum	Relation to gingival recession, pocket formation Areas of narrow attached gingiva Hypersensitivity	Special care areas such as narrow attached gingiva Nonabrasive dentifrice advised Measures to prevent root-surface caries Care during instrumentation Indication for application of desensitizing agent
Dental caries	Areas of demineralization Stages of carious lesions Proximal lesions observed in radiographs Arrested caries Root caries	Charting Treatment plan Cavitated vs. noncavitated Preventive program for caries control, fluoride, dietary factors Follow up and frequency of maintenance
Restorations	Contour of restorations, overhangs Proximal contact Surface smoothness Staining	Chart and correct inadequate margins Selection of instruments and polishing agents Dentifrice selection to prevent discoloration
Factors related to occlusion	Health of supporting structures; observation of radiographs for signs of trauma from occlusion	Need for study of bruxism and other parafunctional habits
Tooth wear	Facets; worn-down cusp tips	Chart inadequate contacts for corrective measures
Proximal contacts	Use of floss to find open contact areas Areas of food retention	Use of floss by patient
Mobility	Degree; comparison of chartings Possible causes	Need for reduction of related inflammatory factors Dentist will identify and treat factors related to occlusal trauma
Classification	Position of teeth Angle's classification	Relationship to orthodontic treatment needs
Habits	Nail or object biting; lip or cheek biting Observe effects on lip, cheek, teeth Tongue thrust; reverse swallow	Guidance for habit correction when indicated
Edentulous areas	Radiographic evaluation for impacted, unerupted teeth, retained root tips, other deviations from normal	Alternative fulcrum selection during instrumentation Applied biofilm-control procedures for abutment teeth
Replacement for missing teeth Dentures partial dentures implants	Teeth and tissue that support a prosthesis Cleanliness of a prosthesis Factors that contribute to food and debris retention	Instruction in personal care of fixed and removable dentures; use of floss under fixed partial denture; other appropriate care
Saliva	Amount and consistency Dryness of mouth	Instruction for prevention of dental caries: more caries can be expected in a dry mouth Use of saliva substitute; fluoride

C. Exploratory Examination
Smooth Surface Caries
▶ *Technique*: Adapt the side of the tip of the probe or blunt explorer closely to the tooth surface (see Chapter 27). Examine for roughness versus smoothness and continuity of tooth surface versus breaks in continuity. *Do not use pressure or break the surface when exploring an area that may be remineralizing.*

▶ *Restorations*: Follow the margins of all restorations around with an explorer. Overhanging margins may or may not appear in the. Chart all irregularities of existing restorations.

Pit and Fissure Caries
▶ When a pit or fissure is discolored, it cannot be determined visually whether dental caries is present.

▶ When the objective is to identify pits and fissures for a sealant and the decision is made to place a sealant, the explorer can then be used to clean out debris in preparation for sealant placement.

▶ An obvious cavity does not need to be explored.

III. Radiographic Examination
▶ During the clinical examination, information revealed by radiographs is utilized for confirmation.

▶ Neither clinical nor radiographic examination is complete without the other. A few principal items to be seen in a radiographic examination of the teeth include: anomalies, impactions, fractures, internal and root resorption, and periapical radiolucencies.

▶ *Dental caries*: For coronal caries, use a horizontal bitewing survey; for root caries, use a vertical bitewing survey.

▶ Periodontal radiographic findings are described in Chapter 20 in the Radiographic Examination section. Vertical bitewing radiographs are needed for the evaluation of alveolar bone levels.

▶ Panoramic, extraoral, or occlusal radiographs are needed for detecting or defining anomalies and pathologic lesions outside the scope of periapical radiographs.

TESTING FOR PULP VITALITY

▶ Any tooth suspected of being nonvital needs to be tested for pulpal vitality or degree of vitality.

▶ The two basic types of pulp testing are thermal and electric.

▶ Diagnosis of vitality is made not only on the basis of a pulp test but also on consideration of all data from the patient history and clinical and radiographic examinations.

I. Causes of Loss of Vitality
▶ A tooth may become nonvital from bacterial causes, particularly invasion of the pulp from dental caries or periodontal diseases.

▶ Physical causes may be mechanical or thermal injuries. Examples of mechanical injuries are trauma, such as a blow, or iatrogenic dental procedures, such as cavity preparation or too-rapid orthodontic movement.

II. Observations that Suggest Loss of Vitality
A. Clinical
▶ Intrinsic discoloration of a tooth crown (Chapter 22).
▶ Fracture (part of the crown may be missing, Figure 16-6).
▶ Large carious lesion or large restoration.
▶ Fistula with opening into the oral cavity over the apical region of a tooth.

B. Radiographic
▶ Apical radiolucency, which may indicate a granuloma, cyst, or abscess.
▶ Bone loss with a widened periodontal ligament space extending to the apex.
▶ Fractured root.
▶ Large carious lesion or restoration that appears closely related to the pulp chamber.

III. Response to Pulp Testing
A. Rationale
▶ Pulp testing is based on the knowledge that a stimulus can create pain to which a patient will react. The pulp tester, therefore, determines the conduction of stimuli to the sensory receptors.

▶ The vitality of the pulp depends on its blood supply and not on its nerve supply. For that reason, a positive or negative pulp test may not always show the true condition of the pulp.

B. Factors that Influence a Patient's Response to a Pulp Test
▶ *Degree of pulpal degeneration or inflammation*: A necrotic pulp gives no response at all, whereas an acutely or chronically inflamed pulp responds at varying degrees between no response and full normal response.

▶ *Pain threshold*: The pain threshold is the lowest intensity of pain caused by a threshold stimulus. A threshold stimulus is the minimum stimulus necessary to induce patient response.

▶ *Reaction to pain*: May vary with a patient's attitude, age, sex, emotional security, fatigue, drugs used, as well as the size of the pulp and thickness of the dentin, particularly the amount of secondary dentin.

▶ *Nerve transmission blocks*: injuries or lesions of nerves, and anesthetics.

▶ *Adjacent metal*: restorations or continuous bridgework.

C. Responses

An electric tester reveals only whether a pulp is vital or nonvital. Using thermal testing may show the following:

▶ No response: necrotic pulp.

▶ Lingering pain after removal of stimulus: irreversible pulpitis.

▶ Pain subsides promptly: reversible pulpitis.

IV. Thermal Pulp Testing

Cold or hot stimuli may be used. For all methods, a control test is performed on a healthy tooth on the opposite side of the arch. Inform the patient in advance about the procedure and what to expect.

A. Cold Test

▶ *Materials*: Cold testing may be accomplished with an air blast, cold drink, ice stick, ethyl chloride in a spray or on a cotton swab, or a carbon dioxide dry-ice stick. Isolate the test teeth and dry with a gauze sponge.

▶ *Preparation of ice stick*: Small icicles may be prepared by freezing water in anesthetic needle covers.

▶ *Dry-ice stick*: Made from carbon dioxide and delivered using a special holder with a plunger.

B. Heat Test

▶ *Temporary stopping*: Warm temporary stopping (gutta-percha). Apply to a tooth dried with cotton sponge.

▶ *Water*: Warm to hot water. Isolate tooth and bathe in very warm water.

V. Electrical Pulp Tester

A. Types

▶ *Battery-operated*
  • Advantages: Hand held so a clinician can work alone; portable.
  • Disadvantage: Battery can run down. Some types have a light to indicate current in circuit.

▶ *Plug-in*
  • Advantage: More dependable than battery-operated.
  • Disadvantage: Not self-contained; requires an electrical outlet for a power source.

B. Precaution

▶ The application of an electrical current to a patient with a cardiac pacemaker or any electronic life-support device by the use of a pulp tester may interfere with the function of the life-support device and may constitute a serious health hazard.[15]

▶ A review of the patient history and consultation with the patient's cardiologist are necessary before application of a pulp tester.

C. Preparation and Use of Equipment

▶ Manufacturer's instructions are provided for each pulp tester and are followed carefully. When the tester rheostat is separate from the applicator tip, an assistant is needed.

▶ Consistency of procedures is essential to obtain consistent readings. The same pulp tester is used for a particular patient at continuing comparative tests. Notes in a patient's record can indicate specific directions for that patient.

D. General Procedures

▶ Assemble equipment.

▶ Explain briefly to the patient what is to be done, but avoid detailed description, which could create anxiety or apprehension.

▶ Dry the teeth to be tested to prevent the current from passing to the gingiva; isolate with cotton rolls and insert a saliva ejector, or use a rubber dam.

▶ Moisten the tip of the tester with a small amount of toothpaste. Another electrolyte (conductor) may be used if its consistency allows it to remain where placed and prevents it from flowing over the tooth surface.

▶ Instruct the patient to signal when a sensation is felt; suggest raising a hand or making a sound.

▶ Apply tester tip. The patient lightly holds the handle to complete the circuit.

▶ Apply first to at least one tooth other than the one in question, preferably an adjacent tooth and the same tooth on the contralateral side. Such a procedure determines a normal response for the patient.

▶ Place *without pressure* but with definite contact on sound tooth structure in a consistent location on the middle or gingival third. The middle third of the crown of a single-rooted tooth and the middle third of each cusp of a multirooted tooth are frequently used (Figure 16-10).

E. Readings

▶ Avoid contact with gingival or other soft tissues. A low-resistance circuit can be formed, thus allowing the circuit to by-pass the tooth.

▶ Avoid contact with metallic restorations. The metal is a more rapid conductor than tooth structure. When approximal restorations are in contact, the circuit can be transmitted across to the adjacent tooth. The reading obtained would then not pertain to the tooth in question (Figure 16-11). A nonconductive clear plastic matrix strip may be inserted to separate the two metallic restorations.

▶ Test each tooth at least twice. Average the readings.

▶ Record on patient's record the average number at which a minimal stimulus induced a response. Record for all teeth tested, not only the tooth in question.

F. Reasons for False-Negative Responses[16]

▶ Patient premedicated with analgesics, tranquilizers, narcotics, or alcohol.

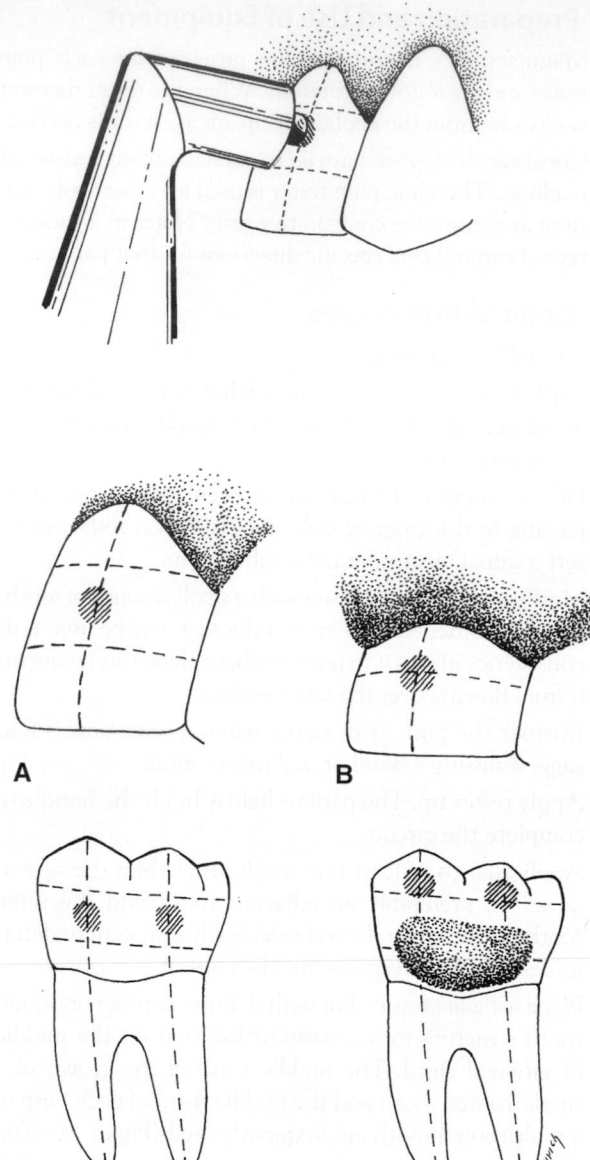

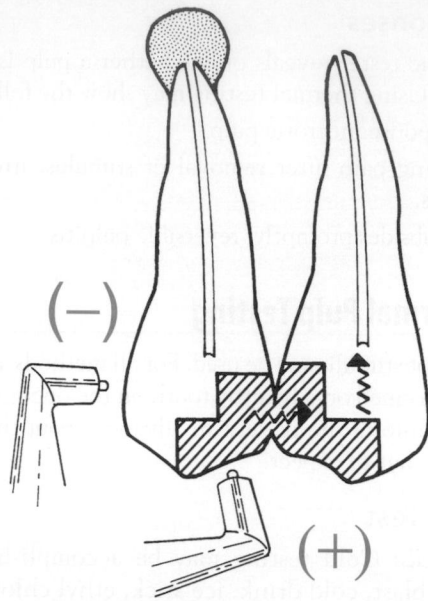

(−)

(+)

FIGURE 16-11 *Use of Pulp Tester.* False-positive response can result when the tester is placed on a metallic restoration. The current can be transmitted across a contact area to give a reading for the adjacent tooth rather than for the tooth in question. (**Source:** Antel J, Christie WJ. Electrical pulp testing. *J Can Dent Assoc.* 1979;45(11):597–600.)

A   **B**

C   **D**

FIGURE 16-10 Pulp Tester in Position. A: Correct contact point for tip of pulp tester is within the middle third of the crown. Avoid contact with gingiva or restorations. **B:** Adjustment of position of contact point because of gingival enlargement. **C:** Contact points on multirooted tooth. Place tip of pulp tester in the middle third over each root. **D:** Adjustment of position of contact points because of large Class V restoration.

▶ Recently traumatized tooth.
▶ Pulp canal narrow and calcified.
▶ Newly erupted tooth with incomplete closure at the apex; immature tooth.

SELF-CLEANSING MECHANISMS

The teeth, by their anatomy, alignment, and occlusion, function with the gingiva, tongue, cheeks, and saliva in a relationship called the self-cleansing mechanism of the oral cavity. A summary of the natural self-cleansing mechanisms during and following mastication is included here.

The following steps are described for food particles, but the same processes apply to any substances that enter the mouth and influence oral cleanliness and the formation of deposits on the teeth.

I. Food Enters the Mouth

Food is carried by the tongue, assisted by the lips and cheeks, to the occlusal surfaces for grinding.

▶ Salivary flow increases as a result of sensory reflex stimulation.
▶ Saliva begins lubrication of food and oral tissues.

II. The Teeth are Brought Together for Chewing

The food moves over the occlusal surfaces.

▶ Marginal ridges tend to force particles toward occlusal surfaces, away from the proximal region.
▶ Contact areas prevent interdental entrance.

III. Food is Forced out by Pressure of Bite

Food passes over the smooth facial and lingual surfaces.

▶ Embrasures provide spillways for the escape of particles.
▶ Cervical enamel ridges deflect particles away from the free gingiva onto the attached gingiva.
▶ Gingival crest prevents retention of particles by its position at a point below the height of contour of the cervical enamel ridge, by its knife-edge shape, and by its close adherence to the tooth surface.

▶ Interdental papilla fills the interproximal area and prevents particles from entering.

IV. Food Particles are Brought Back by the Tongue to the Occlusal Surfaces for Additional Chewing

The process is repeated until the food is ready for swallowing.

▶ Salivary flow continues to be stimulated by repeated masticatory movements.

▶ Saliva moistens food and oral mucosa and thus reduces the adhering capacity of the food.

V. Food Particles Remaining on the Teeth are Removed

▶ Tip of tongue explores and attempts to dislodge remaining particles.

▶ Lips and cheeks in conjunction with tongue aid in natural rinsing process by forcing saliva over and between the teeth.

▶ Saliva continues to flow in increased amounts during rinsing and swallowing of particles, then gradually returns to its normal flow.

DOCUMENTATION

The official permanent records of a patient who requires treatment of individual teeth needs at least the following included:

▶ Patient histories reviewed in total at least every year, but questioned at each maintenance appointment; complete oral radiographic survey with the initial examination and repeated at intervals in keeping with treatment planning.

▶ Emphasis in each entry of the patient's efforts in biofilm control and diet to lessen the potential for new dental caries activity.

▶ A sample progress note is included in Box 16-3.

BOX 16-3

Example Documentation: The Patient with Noncarious Tooth Lesions

S –87-year-old, male patient presents for new patient examination. He states, "My lower front teeth seem to be wearing away. And a month or so ago, I noticed some pieces chipped off my upper front tooth. In fact two of them are feeling kind of sharp." Further questioning revealed that his wife says he grinds his teeth at night and he states he often chews on a pencil while working on his daily crossword puzzle.

O –Generalized advanced attrition, and enamel fractures on 7, 8, and 9 charted on attached dental chart form.[a]

A –Patient needs referral for dental diagnosis and treatment plan.

P –Discussed risk to oral health status related to oral habits such as grinding and biting on hard objects. Answered patient questions about potential treatment options. Provided assurance that the dentist would thoroughly discuss the specific options best for the patient's particular circumstances. Referred to attending dentist for diagnosis and treatment planning.

Signed _____ , RDH

Date: _____ .

[a]Figure 9-4 in Chapter 9 provides an example of a dental chart form that can be used to chart noncarious lesions.

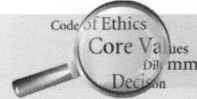

EVERYDAY ETHICS

Barbara, the dental hygienist, has just finished a thorough review of oral hygiene instruction with Mrs. Canavan when she is called out of the treatment room. In today's examination, Barbara had charted two possible carious lesions that will need to be restored. Barbara wanted Mrs. Canavan to realize all the things she could do to prevent dental caries. Her 9-year-old daughter, Millie, had several restorations today at her appointment with the dentist in another treatment room, had finished first, and was waiting for her mom.

When Barbara returned she could overhear Mrs. Canavan talking with her daughter and explaining how she got all the cavities. She described biofilm as painful and how "that's what happens when you eat a lot of candy and drink a lot of soft drinks instead of milk." Barbara stopped to watch quietly. Apparently Millie seemed to understand that it is the biofilm that causes all her cavities, but she was not getting accurate information on the mechanism of action. Mrs. Canavan seemed to be threatening her daughter.

Questions for Consideration

1. Which of the core values (Table II-1, in Section II Introduction) of dental hygiene are in effect in this situation? Would it be ethical for Barbara to join the conversation and attempt to clarify for both of them? How could she help them both understand the real prevention plan?

2. Describe the positive and negative effects that may occur if Barbara corrects the mother in front of the daughter, or instead, if she asks the daughter to go back to the reception room, and then tries to discuss daily biofilm removal and food selection again with Mrs. Canavan.

3. Explain how Barbara can use the questions in Table VI-1 (Section VI Introduction) to help Mrs. Canavan understand her daily personal care needs for prevention of carious lesions.

Factors To Teach The Patient

▷ The cause and process of enamel or root caries formation and development for the patient at risk.

▷ A description of the hardness of the enamel and of why a cavity in a tooth crown is sometimes larger in the dentin before there is evidence from the external surface.

▷ Why radiographs are needed to detect proximal incipient caries.

▷ Reasons for preservation of primary teeth.

▷ Frequency of complete oral examination in relation to a continuing preventive program.

▷ Preventive measures for control and prevention of tooth abrasion, such as dentifrice selection and correction of brush selection and use.

▷ Dietary factors related to erosion.

▷ Methods for prevention of dental caries, such as fluorides, biofilm prevention and control, and control of cariogenic foods in the diet.

▷ Methods for prevention of ECC. Nothing but plain water is used in bottles when putting the infant or child to bed. Avoid the use of a sweetener on a pacifier.

▷ Medicines or vitamin preparations made with heavy syrup (sucrose) have been shown to cause dental caries. Parents must learn to clean (rinse, not brush) children's teeth after sugar exposures.[17]

▷ Discuss accident prevention procedures, such as always wearing a mouthguard for contact sports and wearing seat belts.

References

1. Sognnaes RF, Wolcott RB, Xhonga FA. Dental erosion. 1. Erosion-like patterns occurring in association with other dental conditions. *J Am Dent Assoc.* 1972;84(3):571–576.

2. Andersson L, Andreasen JO, Day P, et al; and International Association of Dental Traumatology. International Association of Dental Traumatology guidelines for the management of traumatic dental injuries: 2. Avulsion of permanent teeth. *Dent Traumatol.* 2012;28(2):88–96.

3. World Health Organization. The World Oral Health Report 2003. Geneva: WHO; 2003. http://www.who.int/oral_health/publications/report03/en/. Accessed November 8, 2014.

4. Blackwell RE. G.V. Black's Operative Dentistry. Vol 2. 9th ed. Milwaukee, WI: Medico-Dental Publishing Co; 1955:1–4.

5. Leong PM, Gussy MG, Barrow SY, et al. A systematic review of risk factors during first year of life for early childhood caries. *Int J Paediatr Dent.* 2013;23(4):235–250.

6. Colak H, Dülgergil CT, Dalli M, et al. Early childhood caries update: a review of causes, diagnoses, and treatments. *J Nat Sci Biol Med.* 2013;4(1):29–38.

7. Kopycka-Kedzierawski DT. Maternal salivary bacterial challenge is associated with oral infection among children and predicts early childhood caries (ECC) incidence in a high-risk cohort of 36-month-old children. *J Evid Based Dent Pract.* 2014;14(3):147–148.

8. Holgerson PL, Vestman NR, Claesson R, et al. Oral microbial profile discriminates breast-fed from formula-fed infants. *J Pediatr Gastroenterol Nutr.* 2013;56(2):127–136.

9. American Academy of Pediatric Dentistry. Periodicity of examination, preventive dental services, anticipatory guidance, and oral treatment for infants, children, and adolescents. *Pediatr Dent.* 2013;36(6):118–125.

10. Hoppenbrouwers PM, Driessens FC, Borggreven JM. The mineral solubility of human tooth roots. *Arch Oral Biol.* 1987;32(5):319–322.

11. van Houte J, Lopman J, Kent R. The predominant cultivable flora of sound and carious human root surfaces. *J Dent Res.* 1994;73(11):1727–1734.

12. Zambon JJ, Kasprzak SA. The microbiology and histopathology of human root caries. *Am J Dent.* 1995;8(6):323–328.

13. Burt BA, Ismail AI, Eklund SA. Root caries in an optimally fluoridated and a high-fluoride community. *J Dent Res.* 1986;65(9):1154–1158.

14. Stamm JW, Banting DW, Imrey PB. Adult root caries survey of two similar communities with contrasting natural water fluoride levels. *J Am Dent Assoc.* 1990;120(2):143–149.

15. Roedig JJ, Shah J, Elayi CS, et al. Interference of cardiac pacemaker and implantable cardioverter-defibrillator activity during electronic dental device use. *J Am Dent Assoc.* 2010;141(5):521–526.

16. Peters DD, Baumgartner JC, Lorton L. Adult pulpal diagnosis. I. Evaluation of the positive and negative responses to cold and electrical pulp tests. *J Endod.* 1994;20(10):506–511.

17. Bigeard L. The role of medication and sugars in pediatric dental patients. *Dent Clin North Am.* 2000;44(3):443–456.

ENHANCE YOUR UNDERSTANDING

thePoint® DIGITAL CONNECTIONS
(see the inside front cover for access information)
- **Audio glossary**
- **Quiz bank**

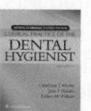

SUPPORT FOR LEARNING
(available separately; visit lww.com)
- *Active Learning Workbook for Clinical Practice of the Dental Hygienist, 12th Edition*

prepU INDIVIDUALIZED REVIEW
(available separately; visit lww.com)
- **Adaptive quizzing with *prepU* for *Wilkins' Clinical Practice of the Dental Hygienist***

17

The Occlusion

Esther M. Wilkins, BS, RDH, DMD

CHAPTER OUTLINE

LEARNING OBJECTIVES

After studying this chapter, the student will be able to:

1. Explain the basic principles of occlusion.

2. Classify occlusion on a patient or case study according to Angle's classification and describe the facial profile associated with each classification.

3. Describe functional and parafunctional contacts.

4. Give examples of parafunctional habits.

5. Discuss types of occlusal trauma and explain the effects on the oral structures.

Occlusion is the relationship of the teeth in the mandibular arch to those in the maxillary arch as they are brought together. Key words are defined in Box 17-1.

▶ The occlusion is examined and recorded as part of the oral examination.

▶ Recognizing a patient's occlusion and understanding the oral health problems of malocclusion can aid in the following:

• Providing information for the comprehensive assessment and planning dental hygiene care.
• Planning personalized instruction in relation to such factors as oral habits, masticatory efficiency, personal oral care procedures, and predisposing factors to dental and periodontal infections.
• Adapting techniques of instrumentation to malpositioned teeth or groups of teeth.
• Planning the frequency of maintenance appointments for professional care on the basis of deposit retention areas, particularly those that are difficult to reach in routine oral self-care.

• Providing recognition of malocclusion and identify patients needing orthodontic referral.

STATIC OCCLUSION

Static occlusal relationships are seen when the jaws are closed in centric occlusion. The static occlusion can be observed in occluded study casts and seen directly in the oral cavity when the lips and cheeks are retracted. Classification of malocclusion and the variations that occur with each category are described here.

I. Normal (Ideal) Occlusion

The ideal mechanical relationship between the teeth of the maxillary arch and the teeth of the mandibular arch is as follows:

▶ All teeth in the maxillary arch are in maximum contact with all teeth in the mandibular arch in a definite pattern.

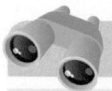

BOX 17-1   KEY WORDS: Occlusion

Ankylosis: union or consolidation of two similar or dissimilar hard tissues previously adjacent but not attached.
   Dental ankylosis: rigid fixation of a tooth to the surrounding alveolus as a result of ossification of the periodontal ligament; prevents eruption and orthodontic movement.

Centric occlusion: the maximum intercuspation or contact of the teeth of the opposing arches; also called habitual occlusion.

Centric relation: the most unstrained, retruded physiologic relation of the mandible to the maxilla from which lateral movements can be made.

Cephalometer: an orienting device for positioning the head for radiographic examination and measurement.

Cephalometric analysis: the process of evaluating dental and skeletal relationships by way of measurements obtained directly from the head or from cephalometric radiographs and tracings made from the radiographs.

Cephalostat: a head-holding instrument used to obtain cephalometric radiographs; head is held in a precisely defined position relative to the film and to the central ray of the X-ray source.

Diastema: a space between two adjacent teeth in the same arch.

Facet: a shiny, flat, worn spot on the surface of a tooth, frequently on the side of a cusp.

Occlusal guard: a removable dental appliance usually made of plastic that covers a dental arch and is designed to minimize the damaging effects of bruxism and other oral habits; also called bite guard, mouth guard, or night guard.

Occlusal prematurity: any contact of opposing teeth that occurs before the desirable intercuspation.

Orthodontic and dentofacial orthopedics: the specialty area of dentistry concerned with the diagnosis, supervision, guidance, and treatment of the growing and mature dentofacial structures; includes conditions that require movement of teeth and the treatment of malrelationships and malformations of the craniofacial complex.

Orthopedics: correction of abnormal form or relationship of bone structures; may be accomplished surgically (orthopedic surgery) or by the application of appliances to stimulate changes in the bone structure through natural physiologic response (orthopedic therapy); orthodontic therapy is orthopedic therapy.

Parafunctional: abnormal or deviated function, as in bruxism.

Pathologic migration: the movement of a tooth out of its natural position as a result of periodontal infection; contrasts with mesial migration, which is the physiologic process maintained by tooth proximal contacts in the normal dental arches.

Primate space: diastema or gap in the tooth row occasionally observed in the human primary dentition. It is characteristic of nearly all species of primates except man. The maxillary primate spaces accommodate the mandibular canines, and the mandibular primate spaces accommodate the maxillary canines when the teeth are in occlusion. As a reduction in the length of canines accompanied man's evolution, the canines no longer protruded beyond the occlusal level. The diastema (primate space) was no longer functional.

Tongue thrust: the infantile pattern of suckle-swallow movement in which the tongue is placed between the incisor teeth or alveolar ridges; may result in an anterior open bite, deformation of the jaws, and abnormal function.

Trauma from occlusion: injury to the periodontium that results from occlusal forces in excess of the reparative capacity of the attachment apparatus; also called occlusal traumatism.

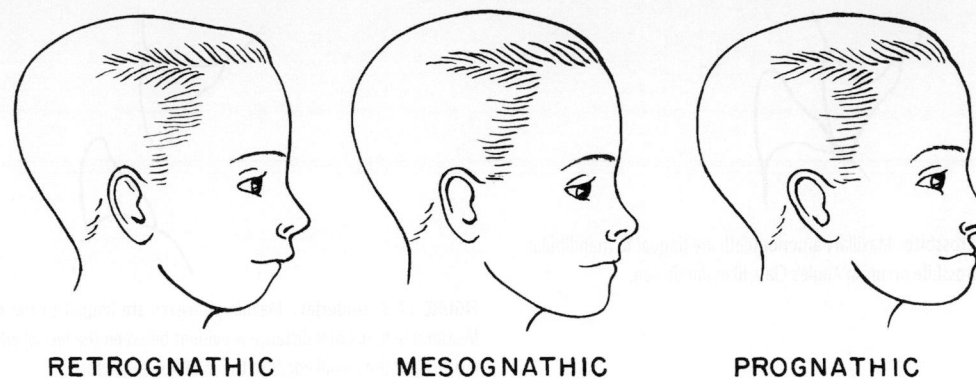

RETROGNATHIC   MESOGNATHIC   PROGNATHIC

FIGURE 17-1 **Types of Facial Profiles.**

▶ Maxillary teeth slightly overlap mandibular teeth on the facial surfaces.

II. Malocclusion

Any deviation from the physiologically acceptable relationship of the maxillary arch and/or teeth to the mandibular arch and/or teeth.

III. Types of Facial Profiles (Figure 17-1)

A. Mesognathic

Having slightly protruded jaws, which give the facial outline a relatively flat appearance (straight profile).

B. Retrognathic

Having a prominent maxilla and a mandible posterior to its normal relationship (convex profile).

C. Prognathic

Having a prominent, protruded mandible and normal (usually) maxilla (concave profile).

IV. Malrelations of Groups of Teeth

A. Crossbites

▶ *Posterior*: Maxillary or mandibular posterior teeth are either facial or lingual to their normal position. This condition may occur bilaterally or unilaterally (Figure 17-2).
▶ *Anterior*: Maxillary incisors are lingual to the mandibular incisors (Figure 17-3).

B. Edge-to-Edge Bite

Incisal surfaces of maxillary anterior teeth occlude with incisal surfaces of mandibular teeth instead of overlapping as in normal occlusion (Figure 17-4).

C. End-to-End Bite

Molars and premolars occlude cusp to cusp as viewed mesiodistally (Figure 17-5).

D. Open Bite

Lack of occlusal or incisal contact between certain maxillary and mandibular teeth because either or both have failed to reach the line of occlusion. The teeth cannot be brought together, and a space remains as a result of the arching of the line of occlusion (Figure 17-6).

E. Overjet

The horizontal distance between the labioincisal surfaces of the mandibular incisors and the linguoincisal surfaces of the maxillary incisors (Figure 17-7).

▶ One way to measure the amount of overjet is to place the tip of a probe on the labial surface of the mandibular incisor and, holding it horizontally against the incisal edge of the maxillary tooth, read the distance in millimeters.

F. Underjet

Maxillary teeth are lingual to mandibular teeth. Measurable horizontal distance between the labioincisal surfaces of the maxillary incisors and the linguoincisal surfaces of the mandibular incisors (Figure 17-8).

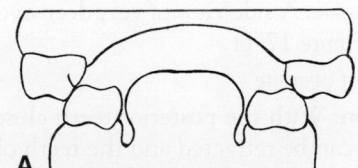   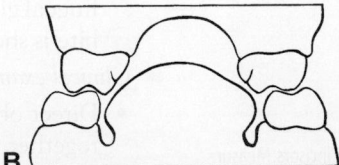   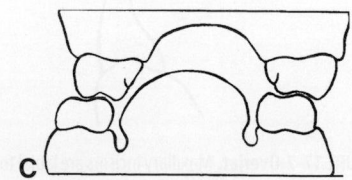

FIGURE 17-2 **Posterior Crossbite. A:** Mandibular teeth lingual to normal position. **B:** Mandibular teeth facial to normal position. **C:** Unilateral crossbite: right side, normal; left side, mandibular teeth facial to normal position.

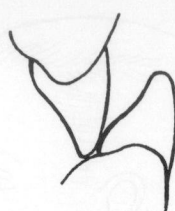

FIGURE 17-3 Anterior Crossbite. Maxillary anterior teeth are lingual to mandibular anterior teeth. Anterior crossbite occurs in Angle's Class III malocclusion.

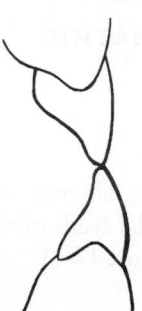

FIGURE 17-4 Edge-to-Edge Bite. Incisal surfaces occlude.

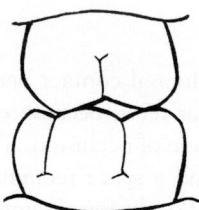

FIGURE 17-5 End-to-End Bite. Molars in cusp-to-cusp occlusion as viewed from the facial.

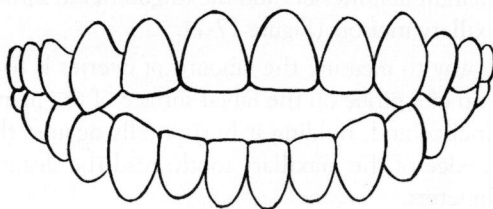

FIGURE 17-6 Open Bite. Lack of incisal contact. Posterior teeth in normal occlusion.

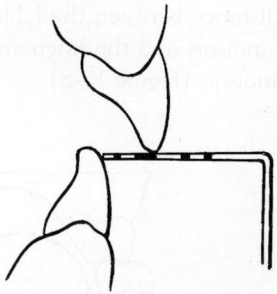

FIGURE 17-7 Overjet. Maxillary incisors are labial to the mandibular incisors. Measurable horizontal distance is evident between the incisal edge of the maxillary incisors and the incisal edge of the mandibular incisors. A periodontal probe can be used to measure for recording the distance.

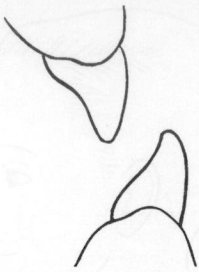

FIGURE 17-8 Underjet. Maxillary incisors are lingual to the mandibular incisors. Measurable horizontal distance is evident between the incisal edges of the maxillary incisors and the incisal edges of the mandibular incisors.

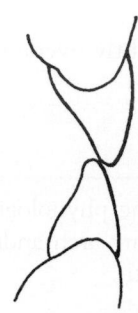

FIGURE 17-9 Normal Overbite. Profile view to show the position of the incisal edge of the maxillary tooth within the incisal third of the facial surface of the mandibular incisor.

G. Overbite

Overbite, or vertical overlap, is the vertical distance by which the maxillary incisors overlap the mandibular incisors.

▶ *Normal overbite:* An overbite is considered normal when the incisal edges of the maxillary teeth are within the incisal third of the mandibular teeth, as shown in Figure 17-9 in side view and in Figure 17-10A in anterior view.

▶ *Moderate overbite:* An overbite is considered moderate when the incisal edges of the maxillary teeth appear within the middle third of the mandibular teeth (Figure 17-10B).

▶ *Deep (severe) overbite*
  • Deep (severe): When the incisal edges of the maxillary teeth are within the cervical third of the mandibular teeth (Figure 17-10C).
  • Very deep: When in addition the incisal edges of the mandibular teeth are in contact with the maxillary lingual gingival tissue. A side view of very deep overbite is shown in Figure 17-11.

▶ *Clinical examination of overbite*
  • Direct observation: With the posterior teeth closed together, the lips can be retracted and the teeth observed, as in Figure 17-10. The degree of anterior overbite is judged by the position of the incisal edge of the maxillary teeth:

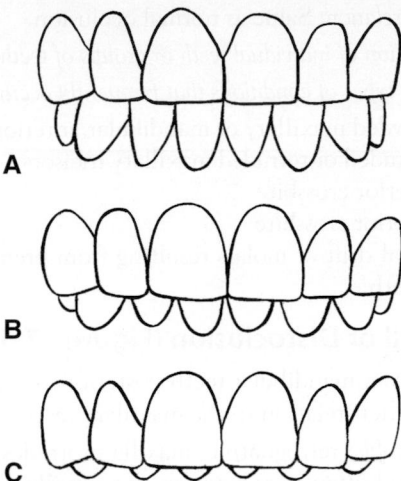

FIGURE 17-10 Overbite, Anterior View. A: Normal overbite: incisal edges of the maxillary teeth are within the incisal third of the facial surfaces of the mandibular teeth. **B:** Moderate overbite: incisal edges of maxillary teeth are within the middle third of the facial surfaces of the mandibular teeth. **C:** Severe overbite: the incisal edges of the maxillary teeth are within the cervical third of the facial of the mandibular teeth. When the incisal edges of the mandibular teeth are in contact with the maxillary lingual gingival tissue, the overbite is considered very severe. See the profile view in Figure 17-11.

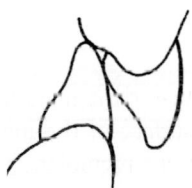

FIGURE 17-11 Deep (Severe) Anterior Overbite. Incisal edge of the maxillary tooth is at the level of the cervical third of the facial surface of the mandibular anterior tooth. See the facial view in Figure 17-10C.

- Mirror view: By placing a mouth mirror under the incisal edge of the maxillary teeth, one can sometimes see the mandibular teeth in contact with the maxillary palatal gingiva. When contact is not visible, an examination of the lingual gingiva may reveal teeth prints or at least enlargement and redness from the contact.

V. Malpositions of Individual Teeth

A. Labioversion

A tooth that has assumed a position labial to normal.

B. Linguoversion

Position lingual to normal.

C. Buccoversion

Position buccal to normal.

D. Supraversion

Elongated above the line of occlusion.

E. Torsiversion

Turned or rotated.

F. Infraversion

Depressed below the line of occlusion, for example, primary tooth that is submerged or ankylosed.

DETERMINATION OF THE CLASSIFICATION OF MALOCCLUSION

The determination of the classification of occlusion is based on the principles of Edward H. Angle, presented in the early 1900s. He defined normal occlusion as "the normal relations of the occlusal inclined planes of the teeth when the jaws are closed"[1] and based his system of classification on the relationship of the first permanent molars.

▶ Although authorities have since agreed that the maxillary first permanent molars do not occupy a fixed position in the dental arch, Angle's system serves to provide an acceptable basis for classification.

▶ A more comprehensive assessment of malocclusion is made by the orthodontist, who studies the relationship of the position of the teeth to the jaws, the face, and the skull.

▶ Three general classes of malocclusion are described in the following sections. These classes are designated by Roman numerals.

▶ Because the mandible is movable and the maxilla is stationary, the classes describe the relationship of the mandible to the maxilla. For example, in distoclusion (Class II) the mandible is distal, whereas in mesioclusion (Class III) the mandible is mesial to the maxilla, as compared to the normal position.

I. Normal (Ideal) Occlusion (Figure 17-12)

A. Facial Profile

Mesognathic (Figure 17-1).

B. Molar Relation

The mesiobuccal cusp of the maxillary first permanent molar occludes with the buccal groove of the mandibular first permanent molar.

C. Canine Relation

The maxillary permanent canine occludes with the distal half of the mandibular canine and the mesial half of the mandibular first premolar.

II. Malocclusion

A. Class I or Neutroclusion (Figure 17-12)

▶ *Facial profile:* Same as normal occlusion.

▶ *Molar relation:* Same as normal occlusion.

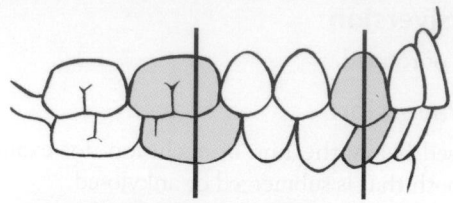

Normal (Ideal) Occlusion

Molar relationship: mesiobuccal cusp of maxillary first permanent molar occludes with the buccal groove of the mandibular first permanent molar.

Malocclusion

Class I: Neutroclusion.
Molar relationship: same as Normal, with malposition of individual teeth or groups of teeth.

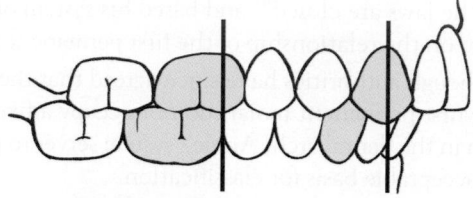

Class II: Distoclusion.
Molar relationship: buccal groove of the mandibular first permanent molar is distal to the mesiobuccal cusp of the maxillary first permanent molar by at least the width of a premolar.
Division 1: mandible is retruded and all maxillary incisors are protruded.

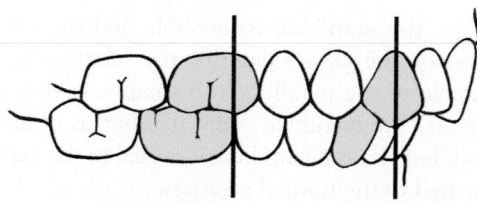

Class II: Distoclusion.
Division 2: mandible is retruded and one or more maxillary incisors are retruded.

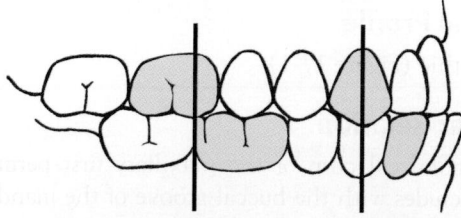

Class III: Mesioclusion.
Molar relationship: buccal groove of the mandibular first permanent molar is mesial to the mesiobuccal cusp of the maxillary first permanent molar by at least the width of a premolar.

FIGURE 17-12 Normal Occlusion and Classification of Malocclusion.

▶ *Canine relation:* Same as normal occlusion.

▶ *Malposition of individual teeth or groups of teeth.*

▶ *General types of conditions that frequently occur in Class I*
- Crowded maxillary or mandibular anterior teeth
- Protruded or retruded maxillary incisors
- Anterior crossbite
- Posterior crossbite
- Mesial drift of molars resulting from premature loss of teeth.

B. Class II or Distoclusion (Figure 17-12)

▶ *Description:* mandibular teeth posterior to normal position in their relation to the maxillary teeth.

▶ *Facial profile:* retrognathic; maxilla protrudes; lower lip is full and often rests between the maxillary and mandibular incisors; the mandible appears retruded or weak (Figure 17-1, retrognathic).

▶ *Molar relation*
- The buccal groove of the mandibular first permanent molar is distal to the mesiobuccal cusp of the maxillary first permanent molar by at least the width of a premolar.
- When the distance is less than the width of a premolar, the relation can be classified as *tendency toward Class II.*

▶ *Canine relation*
- The distal surface of the mandibular canine is distal to the mesial surface of the maxillary canine by at least the width of a premolar.
- When the distance is less than the width of a premolar, the relation can be classified as *tendency toward Class II.*

▶ *Class II, Division 1*
- Description: The mandible is retruded and all maxillary incisors are protruded.
- General types of conditions that frequently occur in Class II, Division 1 malocclusion: deep overbite, excessive overjet, abnormal muscle function (lips), short mandible, or short upper lip.

▶ *Class II, Division 2*
- Description: The mandible is retruded, and one or more maxillary incisors are retruded.
- General types of conditions that frequently occur in Class II, Division 2 malocclusion: Maxillary lateral incisors protrude while both central incisors retrude, crowded maxillary anterior teeth, or deep overbite.

▶ *Subdivision:* One side is Class I, and the other side is Class II (may be Division 1 or 2).

C. Class III or Mesioclusion (Figure 17-12)

▶ *Description:* Mandibular teeth are anterior to normal position in relation to maxillary teeth.

- *Facial profile*: prognathic; lower lip and mandible are prominent (Figure 17-1).
- *Molar relation*
  - The buccal groove of the mandibular first permanent molar is mesial to the mesiobuccal cusp of the maxillary first permanent molar by at least the width of a premolar.
  - When the distance is less than the width of a premolar, the relation can be classified as *tendency toward Class III*.
- *Canine relation*
  - The distal surface of the mandibular canine is mesial to the mesial surface of the maxillary canine by at least the width of a premolar.
  - When the distance is less than the width of a premolar, the relation can be classified as *tendency toward Class III*.
- *General types of conditions that occur in Class III malocclusion*
  - True Class III: Maxillary incisors are lingual to mandibular incisors in an anterior crossbite (Figure 17-3).
  - Maxillary and mandibular incisors are in edge-to-edge occlusion.
  - Mandibular incisors are very crowded but lingual to maxillary incisors.

OCCLUSION OF THE PRIMARY TEETH[2-5]

I. Normal (Ideal) Occlusion

A. Primary Canine Relation

Same as permanent dentition.

- *With primate space:*
  - Mandibular: between mandibular canine and first molar (Figure 17-13A).
  - Maxillary: between maxillary lateral incisor and canine (Figure 17-13B).
- *Without primate spaces*: closed arches.

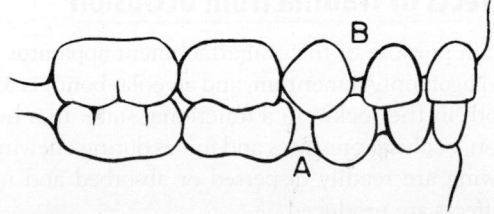

FIGURE 17-13 **Primary Teeth with Primate Spaces. A:** Mandibular primate space between the canine and the first molar. **B:** Maxillary primate space between the lateral incisor and the canine.

B. Second Primary Molar Relation

The mesiobuccal cusp of the maxillary second primary molar occludes with the buccal groove of the mandibular second primary molar.

- *Variations in distal surfaces relationships*: terminal step.
  - The distal surface of the mandibular primary molar is mesial to that of the maxillary, thereby forming a mesial step (Figure 17-14A).
  - Morphologic variation in molar size; maxillary and mandibular primary molars have approximately the same mesiodistal width.
- *Variation*: terminal plane.
  - The distal surfaces of the maxillary and mandibular primary molars are on the same vertical plane (Figure 17-14B).
  - The maxillary molar is narrower mesiodistally than the mandibular molar (occurs in many patients).
- *Effects on occlusion of first permanent molars*
  - Terminal step: First permanent molar erupts directly into proper occlusion (Figure 17-14A).
  - Terminal plane: First permanent molars erupt end to end. With mandibular primate space, early mesial shift of primary molars into the primate space occurs, and the permanent mandibular molar shifts into proper occlusion. Without primate spaces, late mesial shift of permanent mandibular molar into proper occlusion occurs, following exfoliation of second primary molar (Figure 17-14B).

II. Malocclusion of the Primary Teeth

Same as permanent dentition.

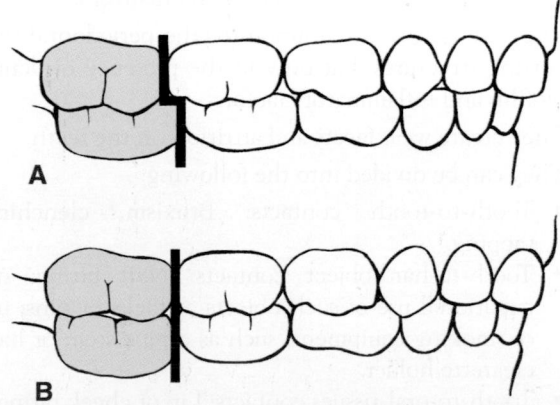

FIGURE 17-14 **Eruption Patterns of the First Permanent Molars. A:** Terminal step. The distal surface of the mandibular second primary molar is mesial to the distal surface of the maxillary primary molar. **B:** Terminal plane. The distal surfaces of the mandibular and maxillary second primary molars are on the same vertical plane; permanent molars erupt in end-to-end occlusion.

FUNCTIONAL OCCLUSION

In contrast to static occlusion, which pertains to the relationship of the teeth when the jaws are closed, functional occlusion consists of all contacts during chewing, swallowing, or other normal action. Functional occlusion is associated with performance:

▶ Pressures or forces created by the muscles of mastication are transmitted from the teeth, after contact, to the periodontium.

▶ Such forces are necessary to maintain the occlusal relationship of the teeth and guide the teeth during eruption.

▶ The forces are also necessary to provide functional stimulation for the preservation of the health of the attachment apparatus, namely, the periodontal ligament, the cementum, and the alveolar bone.

▶ Masticatory (chewing) effectiveness depends on the number and location of teeth.[6]

  • In a patient missing teeth, masticatory ability is significantly impaired if there are no molar teeth occluding.

  • In the older adult, loss of chewing ability may contribute to malnutrition and poor health.[6]

I. Types of Occlusal Contacts

A. Functional Contacts

Functional contacts are the normal contacts that are made between the maxillary teeth and the mandibular teeth during chewing and swallowing. Each contact is momentary, so the total contact time is only a few minutes each day.

B. Parafunctional Contacts

Parafunctional contacts are those made outside the normal range of function.

▶ They result from occlusal habits and neuroses.

▶ They are potentially injurious to the periodontal supporting structures, but only in the presence of dental biofilm and inflammatory factors.

▶ They create wear facets and attrition on the teeth.

▶ They can be divided into the following:

  • Tooth-to-tooth contacts: Bruxism, clenching, tapping.

  • Tooth-to-hard-object contacts: Nail biting; occupational use of such objects as tacks or pins; use of smoking equipment, such as a pipe stem or hard cigarette holder.

  • Tooth-to-oral-tissues contacts: Lip or cheek biting.

II. Proximal Contacts

Proximal contacts serve to stabilize the position of teeth in the dental arches and to prevent food impaction between the teeth. Attrition or wear of the teeth occurs at the proximal contacts.

A. Drifting

▶ When proximal contact is lost, teeth can drift into spaces created by missing teeth without replacement.

▶ There is a natural tendency for mesial migration of teeth toward the midline.

▶ In the absence of disease, the surrounding periodontal tissues adapt to repositioned teeth.

B. Pathologic Migration

▶ With destruction of the supporting structures of a tooth as a result of periodontal infection, and with a force to move a tooth weakened by disease and bone loss, migration of the tooth can result.

▶ Pathologic migration occurs when disease is present; in contrast, drifting is migration with a healthy periodontium.

TRAUMA FROM OCCLUSION

Periodontal tissue injury caused by repeated occlusal forces that exceed the physiologic limits of tissue tolerance is called *trauma from occlusion*. Other names are periodontal traumatism, occlusal traumatism, and periodontal trauma.

I. Types of Trauma from Occlusion

▶ Primary trauma from occlusion results when the following happens:

  • Excessive occlusal force is exerted on a tooth with normal bone support.

  • Example: the effect of a new restoration placed above the line of occlusion.

▶ Secondary trauma from occlusion occurs when the following happens:[7]

  • Excessive occlusal force is exerted on a tooth with bone loss and inadequate alveolar bone support.

  • The ability of the tooth to withstand occlusal forces is impaired.

  • A tooth has lost the support of the surrounding bone; even the pressures of what are usually considered normal occlusal forces may create lesions of trauma from occlusion.

II. Effects of Trauma from Occlusion

The main purpose of the oral attachment apparatus (periodontal ligament, cementum, and alveolar bone) is to keep the tooth in the socket in a functional state. In a healthy situation, occlusal pressures and forces during chewing and swallowing are readily dispersed or absorbed and no unusual effects are produced.

A. Excess Forces

▶ When the forces of occlusion are greater than can be tolerated by the attachment apparatus, damage can result.

▶ Circulatory disturbances, tissue destruction from crushing under pressure, bone resorption, and other pathologic processes are initiated.

B. Relation to Inflammatory Factors

▶ *Trauma from occlusion does not cause gingivitis, periodontitis, or pocket formation.* The steps in the development of inflammatory disease and pockets are outlined in Chapter 19.

▶ In the presence of inflammatory disease, the existing periodontal destruction may be aggravated or promoted by trauma from occlusion.

- However, secondary occlusal trauma is associated with the severity of attachment loss.[7]

III. Methods of Application of Excess Pressure

To understand the nature of the occlusal forces that can cause periodontal trauma from occlusion, it is helpful to recognize types of tooth contacts that can overburden a tooth or a group of teeth.

A. Individual Teeth that Touch Before Full Closure

The contact is premature and may put excessive force on an individual tooth.

B. Two or Only a Few Teeth in Contact During Movement of the Jaw

The teeth involved receive a disproportionate amount of force.

C. Initial Contacts on Inclined Planes of Cusps

Following the initial contact, when the teeth are brought together in a closed position, there may be excess pressure on the teeth where initial contact was made.

D. Heavy Forces Not in a Vertical or Axial Direction

▶ Normal occlusal relationships imply a direct cusp-to-fossa position during closure, with the force of occlusion in a vertical direction toward the tooth apex and parallel with the long axis.

▶ When pressures are exerted laterally or horizontally, excess force is placed on the periodontal attachment apparatus.

E. Increased Frequency, Intensity, and Duration of Contacts

In the presence of parafunctional habits, such as bruxism, clenching, tapping, or biting objects, many more than the usual number of tooth contacts are made each day, and the intensity and duration are altered.

IV. Recognition of Signs of Trauma From Occlusion

No one clinical or radiographic finding clearly defines the presence of trauma from occlusion. Diagnosis of the condition is complex. Clinical findings listed below are recorded for evaluation and correlation with the patient history and all other clinical determinations.

A. Clinical Findings Associated with Occlusal Trauma[8]

▶ Tooth mobility.

▶ Fremitus.

▶ Sensitivity of teeth to pressure, chewing, and/or percussion.

▶ Pathologic tooth migration.

▶ Wear facets or atypical incisal or occlusal wear.

▶ Chipped enamel or crown/root fractures.

▶ Open contacts related to food impaction.

▶ Neuromuscular disturbances in the muscles of mastication.

- In severe cases, muscle spasm can occur.

▶ Temporomandibular joint symptoms such as tenderness in the muscles of mastication.

B. Radiographic Findings[8]

Characteristics that may occur in trauma from occlusion include:

▶ Widened periodontal ligament spaces, particularly angular thickening (triangulation). This finding frequently occurs in conjunction with tooth mobility.

▶ Angular (vertical) bone loss in localized areas (see Figure 20-20, in Chapter 20).

▶ Root resorption.

▶ Furcation involvement.

▶ Thickened lamina dura. Although related to occlusal forces, thickened lamina dura cannot be considered a detrimental or destructive effect of trauma from occlusion. It may be a defense reaction to strengthen tooth support against occlusal forces. Thickened lamina dura is frequently associated with teeth that have undergone orthodontic treatment.

RECOMMENDATIONS FOR THE PATIENT WITH ORTHODONTIC NEEDS

▶ The American Association of Orthodontists recommends all children see an orthodontist by age of 7 for early identification of problems.[9]

▶ Observe the facial profile as the patient enters and is seated in the dental chair.

▶ Closing to centric relation can be performed most effectively by instructing the patient to curl the tongue

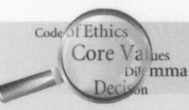

EVERYDAY ETHICS

Many of the first-year dental hygiene students struggled to learn the classifications of malocclusion and how to recognize them in their patients. The problem was often a locker room discussion item, and it was agreed that they noticed that the instructors didn't always look for the details of a patient's occlusion when the record was checked.

One clinic day Roxanne was confused, and she decided to write just anything down on the patient's chart. When the instructor came to check the oral examination, she questioned why Roxanne had the classification of the occlusion documented as a Class II Distoocclusion. Roxanne just shrugged her shoulders and said, "I don't know."

Questions for Consideration

1. Summarize the ethical concerns related to Roxanne's deciding to "just write down anything" rather than look up the information she needs to provide an accurate assessment of the patient's condition.

2. What legal issues might be connected with inaccurate documentation of information in the patient's permanent record? For an example, use a forensic examination team seeking help from a dental office record.

3. Discuss why this situation can be regarded as both an ethical issue and an ethical dilemma.

and to try to hold the tip of the tongue as far back as possible while closing.

▶ When a small child has difficulty in occluding, the clinician may firmly but gently press the cushions of the thumbs on the mucous membrane over the pterygomandibular raphe, holding the thumbs between the cheek and buccal surfaces of the teeth as the patient is requested to close.

▶ Educate parents and children on use of protective equipment to prevent and reduce the severity of orofacial trauma.[10]

- Prepare mouth guards for patients in contact sports such as football, lacrosse, field hockey, ice hockey, and wrestling.

▶ Study the occlusion of the patient with removable dentures with the dentures in and out of the mouth.

DOCUMENTATION

Documentation for the occlusion of every patient needs to include a minimum of the following:

▶ Basic classification of the occlusion with variations noted.

▶ Record occlusal habits including bruxism, clenching, or other parafunctional habits.

▶ Previous orthodontic treatment; dates, patient report of satisfaction.

▶ A progress note of a patient's appointment when seeking information about the need for orthodontic treatment may be read in Box 17-2.

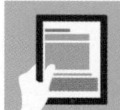

BOX 17-2

Example Documentation: Patient Needing Orthodontic Referral

S –9-year-old female patient, accompanied by her mother, presents for routine continuing care and oral examination. Chief complaint: Mother states, "Since the last time we saw you, I have notice that her teeth are all coming in crooked and her smile seems lopsided to me. Does she need to see an orthodontist?"

O –No changes in health history, no significant extraoral, intraoral, or radiographic findings. Good tissue health and low caries risk. Occlusion classification: Class II, Division 2 with retruded maxillary incisors, maxillary left lateral incisor and canine in buccoversion and rotated. Facial profile is normal.

A –Referral for orthodontic assessment is indicated.

P –Prophylaxis completed. Panoramic radiograph taken and a copy provided to the mother along with contact information for two local orthodontists who have treated our patients in the past. Discussed why her child's caries risk may be increased during orthodontic procedures and stressed the importance of maintaining the regular schedule of continuing care and dental hygiene appointments.

Signed: _____, RDH

Date: _____

Factors To Teach The Patient

▷ Interpretation of the *general* purposes of orthodontic care (function and esthetics) to patients referred by the dentist to an orthodontist.

▷ Dependence of masticatory efficiency on the occlusion of the teeth.

▷ Influence of masticatory efficiency on food selection in the diet.

▷ Influence of masticatory efficiency and diet on the nutritional status of the body and oral health.

▷ Interpretation of the dentist's suggestions for the correction of oral habits.

▷ The space-maintaining function of the primary teeth in prevention of malocclusion of permanent teeth.

▷ The role of malocclusion as a predisposing factor for dental biofilm retention in the formation of dental caries and periodontal infections.

▷ Dental biofilm removal methods for reducing dental calculus and soft deposit retention in areas where teeth are crowded, displaced, or otherwise not in normal occlusion.

▷ The relation of the occlusion and the position of the teeth to the patient's personal oral care procedures.

  ▷ Selection of the proper type of toothbrush.

  ▷ Application of thorough toothbrushing method or methods.

  ▷ Use of dental floss.

▷ Need for continuing care appointments related to malocclusion and while in the process of having orthodontic therapy.

References

1. Angle EH. *Malocclusion of the Teeth*. 7th ed. Philadelphia, PA: S.S. White Manufacturing; 1907:50–57.

2. Baume LJ. Physiological tooth migration and its significance for the development of the occlusion. I. The biogenetic course of the deciduous dentition. *J Dent Res*. 1950;29(2):123–132.

3. Baume LJ. Physiological tooth migration and its significance for the development of the occlusion. II. The biogenesis of the accessional dentition. *J Dent Res*. 1950;29(3):331–337.

4. Baume LJ. Physiological tooth migration and its significance for the development of the occlusion. III. The biogenesis of the successional dentition. *J Dent Res*. 1950;29(3):338–348.

5. Baume LJ. Physiological tooth migration and its significance for the development of the occlusion. IV. The biogenesis of overbite. *J Dent Res*. 1950;29(4):440–447.

6. Franco AL, de Andrade MF, Segalla JC, et al. New approaches to dental occlusion: a literature update. *Cranio*. 2012;30(2):136–143.

7. Branschofsky M, Beikler T, Schäfer R, et al. Secondary trauma from occlusion and periodontitis. *Quintessence Int*. 2011;42(6):515–522.

8. American Academy of Periodontology. Parameter on occlusal traumatism in patients with chronic periodontitis. *J Periodontol*. 2000;71(5, Suppl):873–875.

9. American Association of Orthodontists. Recommendation for orthodontic check-ups no later than age 7. http://www.olmortho.com/pdf/about-braces/PTWF_7yr_olds-MLMS-l.pdf. Accessed November 11, 2014.

10. American Academy on Pediatric Dentistry Clinical Affairs Committee, American Academy on Pediatric Dentistry Council on Clinical Affairs. Policy on prevention of sports-related orofacial injuries. *Pediatr Dent*. 2013;36(6):67–71. http://www.aapd.org/media/Policies_Guidelines/P_Sports.pdf. Accessed November 11, 2014.

ENHANCE YOUR UNDERSTANDING

thePoint° DIGITAL CONNECTIONS
(see the inside front cover for access information)

• **Audio glossary**
• **Quiz bank**

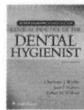

SUPPORT FOR LEARNING
(available separately; visit lww.com)

• *Active Learning Workbook for Clinical Practice of the Dental Hygienist, 12th Edition*

prepU INDIVIDUALIZED REVIEW
(available separately; visit lww.com)

• **Adaptive quizzing with *prepU* for Wilkins'** *Clinical Practice of the Dental Hygienist*

The Periodontium

Linda D. Boyd, RDH, RD, EdD and Esther M. Wilkins, BS, RDH, DMD

CHAPTER OUTLINE

LEARNING OBJECTIVES

After studying this chapter, the student will be able to:

1. Recognize normal periodontal tissues.

2. Know the clinical features of the periodontal tissues examined during a complete periodontal examination.

3. Describe the characteristics of healthy gingiva.

4. Compare and contrast the characteristics of gingiva in health and disease.

5. Describe characteristics of healthy gingiva following periodontal surgery.

The goal of successful periodontal treatment is to bring the diseased periodontal and peri-implant tissues to a state of health that can be maintained by the patient. To accomplish this goal, the first steps include:

▶ Recognizing normal, healthy tissue by clinical observation and evaluation with a periodontal probe.

▶ Educating and monitoring the patient's daily oral self-care as a necessary adjunct to professional care.

▶ Applying periodontal and preventive care knowledge to the treatment and supervision of the patient until health is attained.

A description of the clinical features of the periodontal tissues in health and disease is included in this chapter. Information on the clinical features and care of peri-implant tissues is discussed in Chapter 33. Key words are defined in Box 18-1.

THE TEETH

▶ Clinical crown

The part of the tooth above the attached periodontal tissues. It can be considered the part of the tooth where clinical treatment procedures are applied (Figure 18-1).

▶ Clinical root

The part of the tooth below the base of the gingival sulcus or periodontal pocket. It is the part of the root to which periodontal fibers are attached.

▶ Anatomic crown

The part of the tooth covered by enamel.

▶ Anatomic root

The part of the tooth covered by cementum.

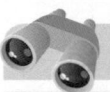

BOX 18-1 | KEY WORDS AND ABBREVIATIONS: The Periodontium

Attachment apparatus: the cementum, periodontal ligament (PDL), and the alveolar bone.

Clinical attachment level (CAL): the probing depth measured from a fixed point like the cementoenamel junction (CEJ).

Desmosome: cell junction; consists of a dense plate near the cell surface that relates to a similar structure on an adjacent cell, between which are thin layers of extracellular material.

Diastema: a space between two natural adjacent teeth.

Epithelium: specialized single layer (simple) or multiple (stratified) layers of cells that form on the surface of skin, mucosa, or serous membranes.

　Oral epithelium: the tissue serving as a liner for the intraoral mucosal surfaces.

　Squamous epithelium: composed of a layer of flat, scale-like cells; or may be stratified.

Fibroblast: fiber-producing cell of the connective tissue; a flattened, irregularly branched cell with a large oval nucleus that is responsible in part for the production and remodeling of the extracellular matrix.

Fibrosis: a fibrotic change of the mucous membrane, especially the gingiva, because of chronic inflammation; fibrotic gingiva may appear outwardly healthy, thus masking underlying disease.

GCF (Gingival Crevicular Fluid): fluid secreted from the gingival crevice or sulcus around the tooth.

Hemidesmosome: half of a desmosome that forms a site of attachment between junctional epithelial cells and the tooth surface.

Hyperkeratosis: abnormal thickening of the keratin layer (stratum corneum) of the epithelium.

Hyperplasia: abnormal increase in volume of a tissue or organ caused by formation and growth of new normal cells.

Hypertrophy: increase in size of tissue or organ caused by an increase in size of its constituent cells.

Keratinization: development of a horny layer of flattened epithelial cells containing keratin.

Marker: identifier; symptoms or signs by which a particular condition can be recognized; for example, clinical and microbiologic markers are used to identify gingival and periodontal infections.

Mastication: act of chewing.

MGJ (Mucogingival Junction): the line where mucosa from the cheeks or floor of the mouth and attached gingiva come together.

Nonkeratinized mucosa: lining mucosa in which the stratified squamous epithelial cells retain their nuclei and cytoplasm.

Periodontium: tissues surrounding and supporting the teeth are divided into two sections the gingival unit, composed of the free and attached gingiva and the alveolar mucosa, and the attachment apparatus, which includes the cementum, PDL, and alveolar process.

Probing depth: the distance from the gingival margin to the location of the periodontal probe tip inserted for gentle probing to the attachment.

Pus: a fluid product of inflammation that contains leukocytes, degenerated tissue elements, tissue fluids, and microorganisms.

Sharpey's fibers: penetrating connective tissue fibers by which the tooth is attached to the adjacent alveolar bone; the fiber bundles penetrate cementum on one side and alveolar bone on the other.

Stippling: the pitted, orange-peel appearance frequently seen on the surface of the attached gingiva.

Suppuration: formation of pus.

Taste bud: receptor of taste on tongue and oropharynx; goblet-shaped cells oriented at right angles to the surface of the epithelium.

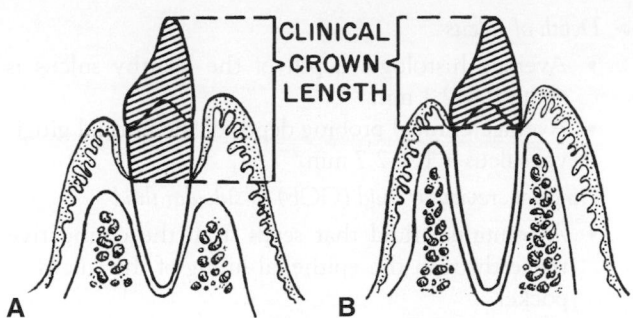

FIGURE 18-1 Clinical Crown. The part of the tooth that is above the attached periodontal tissue. **A:** When the periodontal pocket depth is increased, the clinical crown extends to a position at which the clinical crown length is greater than the clinical root length. The clinical root is the part of the tooth with attached periodontal tissues. **B:** When the clinical attachment level is at the CEJ, the clinical crown and the anatomic crown are the same.

THE NORMAL PERIODONTIUM

The periodontium is the functional unit of tissues surrounding and supporting the tooth. It is made up of two parts: the *gingiva*, which protects the underlying tissues, and the attachment apparatus, consisting of the *periodontal ligament (PDL)*, *cementum, alveolar bone.*[1]

I. Gingiva

▶ The part of the masticatory mucosa surrounding the necks of the teeth and attached to the teeth and alveolar bone.

▶ The gingiva is made up of the following:

• Free gingiva
• Attached gingiva
• Interdental gingiva or interdental papilla.

A. Free Gingiva (Marginal Gingiva)

In health, the free gingiva is closely adapted around each tooth. It connects with the attached gingiva at the free gingival groove and attaches to the tooth at the coronal portion of the junctional epithelium (JE) as shown in Figures 18-2 and 18-3.

▶ Free gingival groove

• The free gingival groove is a shallow linear groove demarcating the free from the attached gingiva. In health, about one-third of the teeth may show a visible gingival groove.

• In the absence of inflammation and pocket formation, the gingival groove runs slightly parallel with and about 0.5–1.5 mm from the gingival margin.[2]

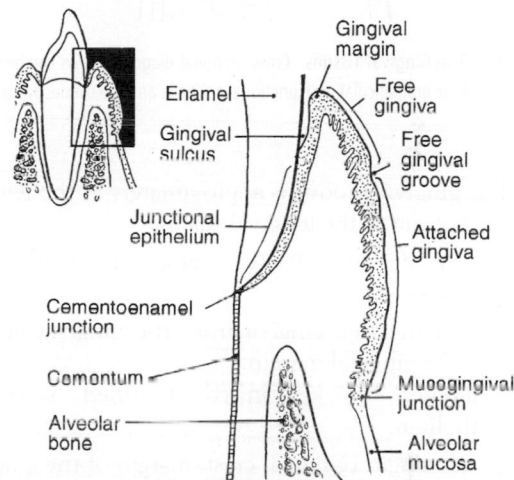

FIGURE 18-2 Parts of the Gingiva. Cross-sectional diagram shows the parts of the gingiva and adjacent tissues of a partially erupted tooth. Note that the JE is on the enamel.

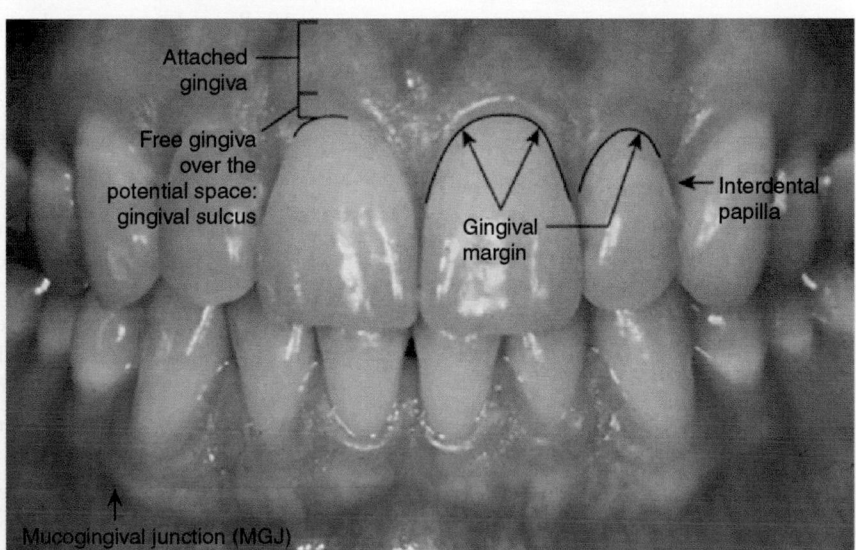

FIGURE 18-3 Picture of Gingival Tissues. Gingiva surrounds each tooth forming a characteristic scalloped shape gingival margin. Interproximal papillae fill the spaces between most teeth. The potential space between the free gingiva and the tooth can be accessed with a periodontal probe. The attached gingiva is the gingiva that is firmly attached to the underlying bone. The mucogingival junction (MGJ) where the attached gingiva and alveolar mucosa meet. (Reprinted from Scheid R, Weiss G. Woelfel's Dental Anatomy: Its Relevance to Dentistry, 8th Ed. Philadelphia: Lippincott Williams & Wilkins; 2011.)

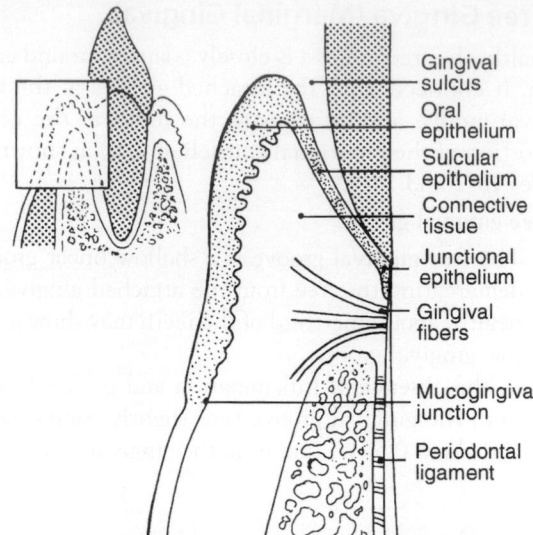

Gingival sulcus
Oral epithelium
Sulcular epithelium
Connective tissue
Junctional epithelium
Gingival fibers
Mucogingival junction
Periodontal ligament

FIGURE 18-4 The Gingival Tissues. Cross-sectional diagram shows the histologic relationships of the oral, sulcular, and junctional epithelia and the connective tissue.

- The gingival groove is approximately at the level of the bottom of the gingival sulcus.
- ▶ Oral epithelium (outer gingival epithelium, Figure 18-4)
  - Covers the free gingiva from the gingival groove over the gingival margin.
  - Composed of keratinized stratified squamous epithelium.
- ▶ Gingival margin (gingival crest, margin of the gingiva, or free margin, Figures 18-2 and 18-3)
  - This is the edge of the gingiva nearest the incisal or occlusal surface.
  - The gingival margin is about 0.08–2.1 mm coronal to the cementoenamel junction (CEJ) in health.[2]
  - Marks the opening of the gingival sulcus.

B. Gingival Sulcus (Crevice)

▶ *Location*

The crevice or space between the free gingiva and the tooth.

▶ *Boundaries* (Figure 18-4)
  - *Inner*: adjacent to the tooth surface and may be enamel, cementum, or part of each, depending on the position of the JE.
  - *Outer*: sulcular epithelium.
  - *Base*: coronal margin of the attached tissues and forms the base of the sulcus or pocket.

▶ *Sulcular epithelium*
  - The continuation of the oral epithelium from the free gingiva.
  - Nonkeratinized.[1]
  - Plays a crucial role in sealing off the oral environment from the periodontal tissues.

▶ *Depth of sulcus*
  - Average histologic depth of the healthy sulcus is about 0.8–2.1 mm.[2]
  - Average clinical probing depth of the normal gingival sulcus is 1.3–2.7 mm.[2]

▶ *Gingival crevicular fluid (GCF) or sulcular fluid*
  - A serumlike fluid that seeps from the connective tissue through the epithelial lining of the sulcus or pocket.
  - Flow rate is slight to none in a normal sulcus; GCF flow rate reflect changes in permeability of the tissue due to inflammation.[3]
  - It is part of the local defense mechanism and is able to transport many substances, including endotoxins, enzymes, antibodies, and certain systemically administered drugs.
  - Possible use as a diagnostic aid for periodontal disease activity because the composition changes in the presence of inflammation.[3]

C. Junctional Epithelium (JE)

▶ *Description*
  - Stratified squamous nonkeritinized epithelium made up of two strata (layers), one adjacent to the connective tissue and one facing the tooth surface.
  - The JE is continuous with the sulcular epithelium and completely encircles the tooth to form a tight seal.
  - JE cells have wider fluid-filled intercellular spaces that contain polymorphonuclear leukocytes and monocytes that pass into the gingival sulcus to manage the constant microbial challenge.[4]

▶ *Size*
  - The JE may be up to 15 or 30 cells in thickness where it joins the sulcular epithelium and tapers down to 1 or 3 cells in thickness at the apical end.[4]
  - The length ranges from 0.25 to 1.35 mm.

▶ *Position*
  - As the tooth erupts, the attachment is on the enamel; during eruption, the epithelium migrates toward the CEJ (Figure 18-5).
  - At full eruption, the attachment is usually on the cementum, where it becomes firmly attached (Figure 18-5D).
  - With wear of the tooth on the incisal or occlusal surface and with periodontal infections, the attachment migrates along the root surface (Figure 18-5E).

▶ *Relation of crest of Alveolar Bone to the Attached Gingival Tissue*
  - The distance between the base of the attachment and the crest of the alveolar bone is approximately 1.0–1.5 mm.
  - This distance is maintained in disease when the epithelium moves along the root surface and bone loss occurs.

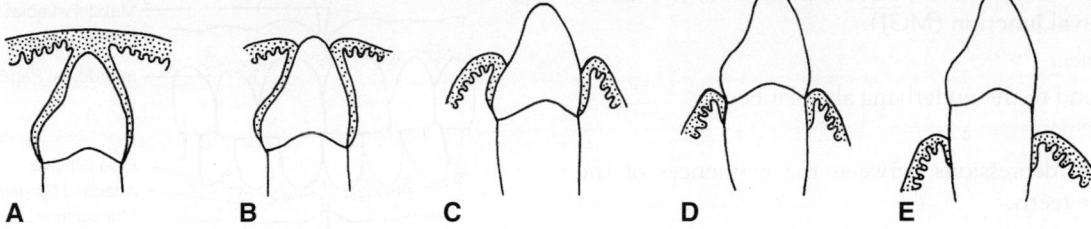

FIGURE 18-5 Tooth Eruption and the Gingiva. A: Before eruption, the oral epithelium covers the tooth. **B:** As the tooth emerges, the reduced epithelium joins the oral epithelium as the gingival sulcus is formed. **C:** Partial eruption with the JE along the enamel. **D:** Eruption complete, with JE at the CEJ. **E:** From disease or other cause, the attachment migrates along the root surface, exposing the cementum.

▶ *Epithelial attachment to the tooth surface*
- The attachment between the tooth and tissue is accomplished by hemidesmosomes and the basal lamina of the JE.

D. Interdental Gingiva (Interdental Papilla)

▶ *Location*
- In health, the interdental gingiva occupies the interproximal area between two adjacent teeth that are in contact (see Figure 18-3).
- The tip and lateral borders are continuous with the free gingiva, whereas other parts are attached gingiva.
- An interproximal area is also called an *embrasure*.

▶ *Papillary height may be classified as follows:*
- Type I embrasure: the tip of the interdental papilla is under the contact of adjacent teeth at the most coronal aspect of the CEJ.
- Type II embrasure: the tip of the interdental papilla is apical to the CEJ, but coronal to the height of the facial CEJ.
- Type III embrasure: complete loss of the interdental papilla due to extensive recession as shown in Figure 29-1 in Chapter 29.[5]

▶ *Shape*
- *Varies with spacing or overlapping of the teeth*: The interdental gingiva may be flat or saddle shaped when there are wide spaces between teeth, or it may be tapered and narrow when teeth are crowded or overlapped.
- *Between anterior teeth*: pointed, pyramidal.
- *Between posterior teeth*
  - Flatter than anterior papillae because of wider teeth, wider contact areas, and flattened interdental bone.
  - Two papillae, one facial and one lingual, connected by a col, are found when teeth are in contact.

▶ *Col*
- A col is the depression under the contact area between a lingual or palatal and facial papilla that conforms to the proximal contact area as shown in Figure 18-6.
- The center of the col area is not usually keratinized and thus is more susceptible to infection. Most periodontal infection begins in the col area.

E. Attached Gingiva

▶ *Extent*
- The attached gingiva is continuous with the oral epithelium of the free gingiva and is covered with keratinized stratified squamous epithelium.
- Maxillary palatal gingiva is continuous with the palatal mucosa.
- Attached gingiva of the mandibular facial and lingual gingiva and maxillary facial gingiva is

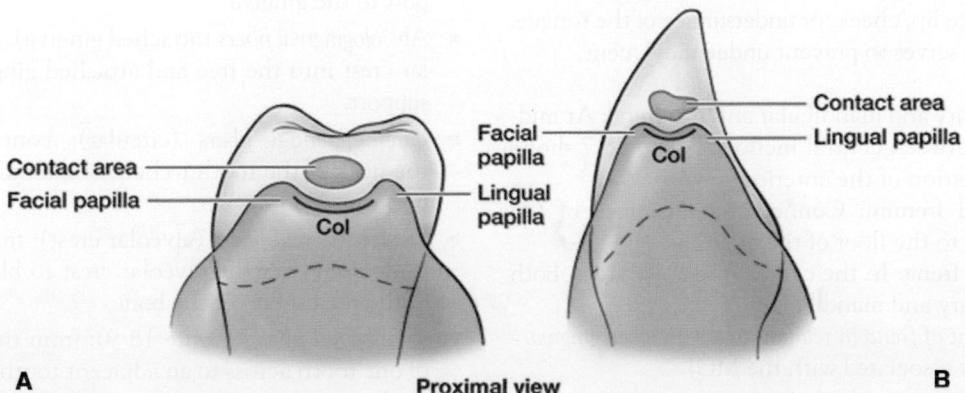

Contact area — Facial papilla — Col — Lingual papilla — Facial papilla — Col — Contact area — Lingual papilla

A   **Proximal view**   **B**

FIGURE 18-6 Col. A col is the depression between the lingual or palatal and the facial papillae under the contact area. **A:** Mesial of mandibular molar to show wide col area. **B:** Mesial of mandibular incisor to show a narrow col. The col deepens when gingival enlargement occurs. (Reprinted from Nield-Gehrig J, Willmann D. Foundations of Periodontics for the Dental Hygienist. Philadelphia: Lippincott Williams & Wilkins; 2011.)

demarcated from the alveolar mucosa by the muco-gingival junction (MGJ).

▶ *Attachment*

Firmly bound to the underlying alveolar bone.

▶ *Shape*

Follows the depressions between the eminences of the roots of the teeth.

F. Mucogingival Junction (MGJ)

▶ *Appearance*

- The MGJ appears as a line that marks the connection between the attached gingiva and alveolar mucosa.
- In the anterior area the MGJ is scalloped, but it is fairly straight in posterior areas.
- A contrast can be seen between the pink of the keratinized, stippled, attached gingiva, and more vascular alveolar mucosa that is a deeper reddish-pink.

▶ *Location*

- A mucogingival line is found on the facial surface of both arches and on the lingual surface of the mandibular arch.
- There is no alveolar mucosa on the palate. The palatal tissue is firmly attached to the bone of the roof of the mouth.
- In Figure 18-3 and Figure 18-7, the mandibular MGJ is where the attached gingiva and the alveolar mucosa meet.

G. Alveolar Mucosa

▶ *Description*

- Movable tissue loosely attached to the underlying bone.
- It has a smooth, shiny surface with nonkeratinized, thin epithelium. Underlying capillaries may be seen through the epithelium.

▶ *Frena (singular: Frenum or Frenulum)*

- *Description:* A frenum is a narrow fold of mucous membrane connecting more fixed tissue to movable mucosa, for example, from the attached gingiva at the MGJ to the lip, cheek, or undersurface of the tongue. A frenum serves to prevent undue movement.
- *Locations*
  - Maxillary and mandibular anterior frena: At midlines between central incisors. Figure 18-7 shows the location of the anterior frena.
  - Lingual frenum: Connects undersurface of the tongue to the floor of the mouth.
  - Buccal frena: In the canine–premolar areas, both maxillary and mandibular.
- *Attachment of frena in relation to the attached gingiva*
  - Closely associated with the MGJ.
  - When the attached gingiva is narrow or missing, the frena may pull on the free gingiva and

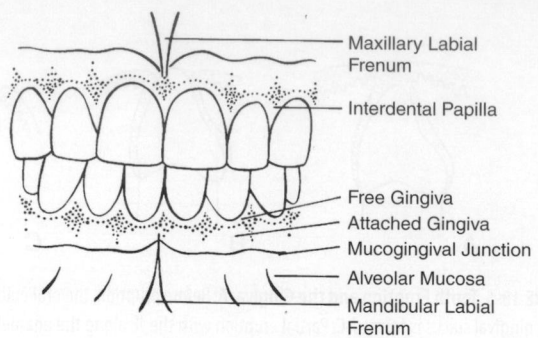

FIGURE 18-7 **Parts of the Gingiva.** The MGJ for each arch is shown in relation to the attached gingiva, alveolar mucosa, and labial anterior frena.

displace it laterally. A "tension test" is used to locate frenal attachments and check the adequacy of the attached gingiva (Chapter 20).

II. Periodontal Ligament (PDL)

- The PDL is the fibrous connective tissue that surrounds and attaches the alveolar bone to the cementum.
- It is composed of cells and an extracellular compartment.[1]
  - Cells include osteoblasts, osteoclasts, fibroblasts, epithelial cells, and cementoblasts.
  - The extracellular compartment contains collagen fiber bundles in a ground substance.
- The fibers are inserted into the cementum on one side and the alveolar bone on the other are called *Sharpey's fibers*.
- The two general groups of fibers are the *gingival groups* (around the cervical area within the gingival tissues) and the *principal fiber groups* (surrounding the root).[1]

A. Gingival Fiber Groups (Figure 18-8)

- *Dentogingival fibers* (free gingiva): from the cementum in the cervical region into the free gingiva to give support to the gingiva.
- *Alveologingival fibers* (attached gingiva): from the alveolar crest into the free and attached gingiva to provide support.
- *Circumferential fibers* (circular): continuous around the neck of the tooth to help to maintain the tooth in position.
- *Dentoperiosteal fibers* (alveolar crest): from the cervical cementum over the alveolar crest to blend with fibers of the periosteum of the bone.
- *Transseptal fibers* (Figure 18-9): from the cervical area of one tooth across to an adjacent tooth (on the mesial or distal only) to provide resistance to separation of teeth.

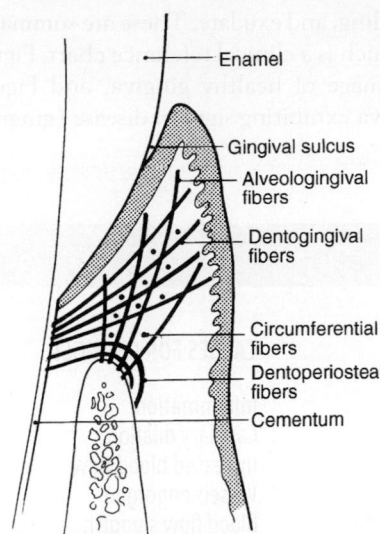

FIGURE 18-8 Gingival Fiber Groups. Cross section of the gingiva shows the relation of the gingival fiber groups to the gingival sulcus, free gingiva, cementum, and alveolar bone.

B. Principal Fiber Groups (Figure 18-9)

The five principal groups of collagen fibers are named for their location on the root and for their direction. They are also called the dentoalveolar fiber groups.

▶ *Apical fibers:* from the root apex to adjacent surrounding bone to resist vertical forces.

▶ *Oblique fibers:* from the root above the apical fibers obliquely toward the occlusal to resist vertical and unexpected strong forces.

▶ *Horizontal fibers:* from the cementum in the middle of each root to adjacent alveolar bone to resist tipping of the tooth.

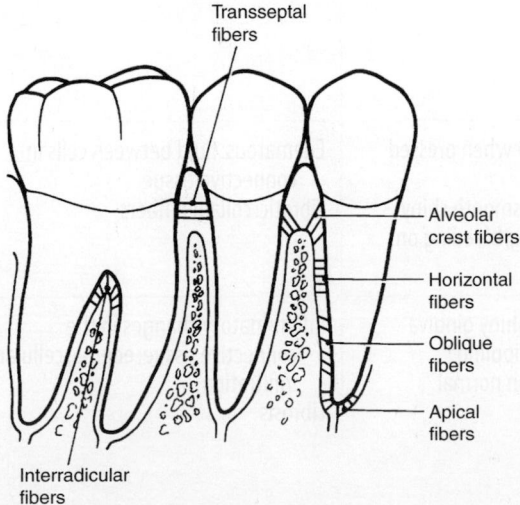

FIGURE 18-9 Principal Fiber Groups of the Periodontium. The five principal groups (apical, oblique, horizontal, alveolar crest, and interradicular) are shown. The transseptal fibers of the gingival fiber groups are also shown as they span across from the cervical area of one tooth to the neighboring tooth.

▶ *Alveolar crest fibers:* from the alveolar crest to the cementum just below the CEJ to resist intrusive forces.

▶ *Interradicular fibers:* from cementum between the roots of multirooted teeth to the adjacent bone to resist vertical and lateral forces.

III. Cementum

The cementum is a thin layer of calcified connective tissue that covers the tooth from the CEJ to, and around, the apical foramen.

A. Functions

▶ To seal the tubules of the root dentin.

▶ To provide attachment for the periodontal fiber groups.

B. Characteristics

▶ Thickness is 15–150 μm about the apex; 30–60 μm about the cervical area.[2]

▶ Two types of cementum[1]:

• *Primary cementum* (or acellular cementum) is on the cervical half to two-thirds of the root and serves as a place for attachment of the PDL fibers.

• *Secondary cementum* (cellular cementum) is on the apical half or third of the root and serves as a repair tissue to fill defects.

▶ Relationship of enamel and cementum at the cervical area is shown in Figure 18-10.

• In 10% of the instances, they do not meet and there can be a small area of exposed dentin; in 30%, they meet edge to edge; and in 60%, the cementum overlaps the enamel.[2]

IV. Alveolar Bone

▶ The alveolar bone consists of the lamina dura, which surrounds the tooth socket, and supporting bone.

▶ When teeth are lost, the alveolar bone is resorbed.

▶ The bone functions to support the teeth and provide attachment for the PDL fibers.

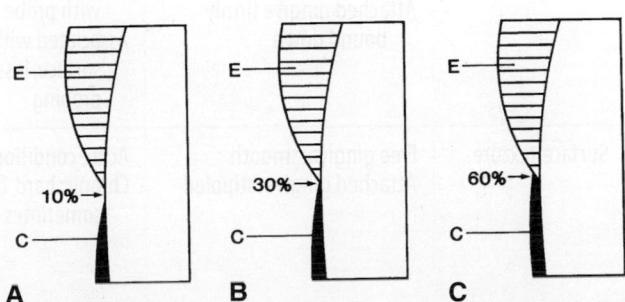

FIGURE 18-10 Relationship of Enamel and Cementum. The possible relationships of the enamel and the cementum of the CEJ. **A:** The cementum and the enamel do not meet, and there is a small zone of dentin exposed in 10% of teeth. **B:** The cementum meets the enamel in approximately 30% of teeth. **C:** The cementum overlaps the enamel in about 60% of teeth.

THE GINGIVAL DESCRIPTION

The examination of the gingiva includes evaluation of color, size, shape, consistency, surface texture, position, MGJs, bleeding, and exudate. These are summarized in Table 18-1, which is a clinical reference chart. Figure 18-11A shows an image of healthy gingiva, and Figure 18-11B shows gingiva exhibiting signs of disease (gingivitis).

TABLE 18-1	Examination of the Gingival Clinical Markers		
	APPEARANCE IN HEALTH	**CHANGES IN DISEASE CLINICAL APPEARANCE**	**CAUSES FOR CHANGES**
Color	Uniformly pale pink or coral pink Variations in pigmentation related to complexion, race	Acute: bright red Chronic: bluish pink, bluish red Attached gingiva: color change may extend to the mucogingival line	Inflammation Capillary dilation Increased blood flow Vessels engorged Blood flow sluggish Venous return impaired Anoxemia Increased fibrosis Deepening of pocket, mucogingival involvement
Size	Not enlarged Fits snugly around the tooth	Enlarged	Edematous: inflammatory fluid, cellular exudate, vascular engorgement, hemorrhage Fibrotic: new collagen fibers
Shape (contour)	Marginal gingiva: flat, knife-edged, follows a curved line about the tooth Papillae: • normal contact: papilla is pointed and pyramidal; fills the interproximal area • space (diastema) between teeth; gingiva is flat or saddle shaped	Marginal gingiva: rounded rolled Papillae: bulbous, flattened, blunted cratered	Inflammatory changes: edematous or fibrous Bulbous with gingival enlargement Cratered in necrotizing ulcerative gingivitis
Consistency	Firm Attached gingiva firmly bound down	Soft, spongy: dents readily when pressed with probe Associated with red color, smooth shiny surface, loss of stippling, bleeding on probing	Edematous: fluid between cells in connective tissue Fibrotic: collagen fibers
Surface texture	Free gingiva: smooth Attached gingiva: stippled	Acute condition: smooth, shiny gingiva Chronic: hard, firm, with stippling, sometimes heavier than normal	Inflammatory changes in the connective tissue; edema, cellular infiltration Fibrosis

TABLE 18-1	Examination of the Gingival Clinical Markers (*continued*)		
	APPEARANCE IN HEALTH	**CHANGES IN DISEASE CLINICAL APPEARANCE**	**CAUSES FOR CHANGES**
Position of gingival margin	Fully erupted tooth: margin is 1–2 mm above CEJ, at or slightly below the enamel contour	Enlarged gingiva: margin is higher on the tooth, above normal, pocket deepened Recession: margin is more apical; root surface is exposed	Edematous or fibrotic JE has migrated along the root; gingival margin follows
Position of junctional epithelium (JE)	During eruption along the enamel surface (Figure 18-7) Fully erupted tooth: the JE is at the CEJ	Position determined by the use of probe, is on the root surface	Apical migration of the epithelium along the root
Mucogingival junctions (MGJs)	Make clear demarcation between the pink, stippled, attached gingiva and the darker alveolar mucosa with smooth shiny surface	No attached gingiva: • Color changes may extend full height of the gingiva; mucogingival line obliterated • Probing reveals that the bottom of the pocket extends into the alveolar mucosa • Frenal pull may displace the gingival margin from the tooth	Apical migration of the JE Attached gingiva decreases with pocket deepening Inflammation extends into alveolar mucosa
Bleeding	No spontaneous bleeding or upon probing	Spontaneous bleeding Bleeding on probing: bleeding near margin in acute condition; bleeding deep in pocket in chronic condition	Degeneration of the sulcular epithelium with the formation of pocket epithelium Blood vessels engorged Tissue edematous
Exudate	No exudate expressed on pressure	White fluid, pus, visible on digital pressure Amount not related to pocket depth	Inflammation in the connective tissue Excessive accumulation of white blood cells with serum and tissue makes up the exudate (pus)

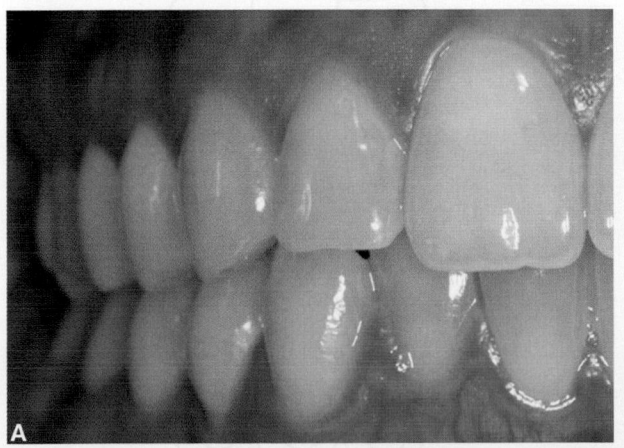
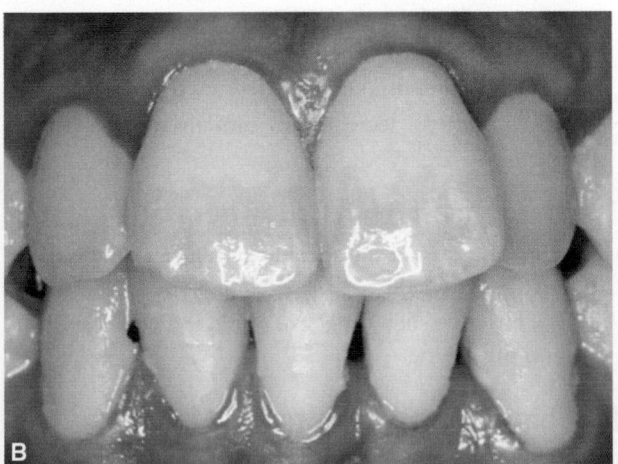

FIGURE 18-11 **Signs of Health. A:** Health: Coral pink color, stippling is evident, gingival margins are knife-edged, and interdental papilla are pointed. **Signs of disease. B:** Pinkish-red color, loss of stippling, redness and enlargement of gingival margin, and interdental papilla are slightly bulbous in maxillary areas. (Reprinted from Nield-Gehrig J, Weiss G. Fundamentals of Periodontal Instrumentation and Advanced Root Instrumentation, 7th Ed. Philadelphia: Lippincott Williams & Wilkins; 2012.)

I. Color

A. Signs of Health

► *Pale pink*: Darker in people with darker complexions due to melanin pigmentation.

► *Factors influencing color*
  • Vascular supply.
  • Thickness of epithelium.
  • Degree of keratinization.
  • Physiologic pigmentation: melanin pigmentation occurs frequently in African Americans, Asians, Indians, and Caucasians of Mediterranean countries.

B. Changes in Disease

► *In chronic inflammation*: dark red, bluish red, magenta, or deep blue.

► *In acute inflammation*: bright red.

► *Extent*: deep involvement can be expected when diffuse color changes extend into the attached gingiva, or from the marginal gingiva to the MGJ, or through into alveolar mucosa.

II. Size

A. Signs of Health

► *Free gingiva*: flat, not enlarged; fits snugly around the tooth.

► *Attached gingiva*
  • Width of attached gingiva varies among patients and among teeth for an individual, from 1 to 9 mm.
  • Wider in maxilla than mandible; broadest zone related to incisors, narrowest at the canine and premolar regions.

B. Changes in Disease

► *Free gingiva and papillae*:
  • Become enlarged.
  • May be localized or limited to specific areas or generalized throughout the gingiva.
  • The col deepens as the papillae increase in size.

► *Attached gingiva*: decreases in amount as the pocket deepens.

C. Enlargement from Drug Therapy

► Certain drugs used for specific systemic therapy cause gingival enlargement as a side effect.
  • Examples of such drugs are phenytoin, cyclosporine, and nifedipine.

III. Shape (Form or Contour)

A. Signs of Health

► *Free gingiva*
  • Follows a curved line around each tooth; may be straighter along wide molar surfaces.

  • The margin is knife edged or slightly rounded on facial and lingual gingiva; closely adapted to the tooth surface.

► *Papillae*
  • Teeth with contact area. Facial and lingual gingiva are pointed or slightly rounded papillae with a col area under the contact.
  • Spaced teeth (with diastemata). Interdental gingiva is flat or saddle-shaped.

B. Changes in Disease

► *Free gingiva*: rounded or rolled.

► *Papillae*: blunted, flattened, bulbous, cratered (Figure 18-12).

► *"McCall's festoon"*: an enlargement of the marginal gingiva with the formation of a lifesaver-like gingival prominence. Frequently, the total gingiva is very

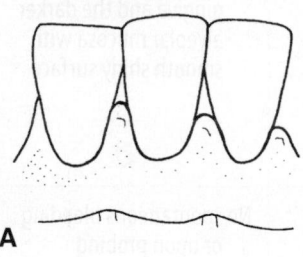

A

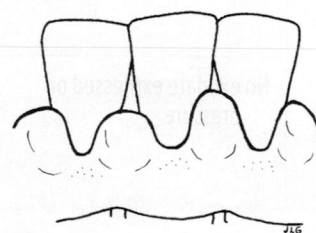

B

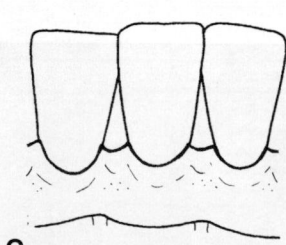

C

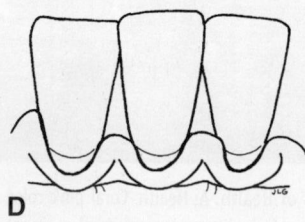

D

FIGURE 18-12 Gingival Shape or Contour. A: Blunted papillae. **B:** Bulbous papillae. **C:** Cratered papillae. **D:** Rolled, lifesaver-shaped "McCall's festoons."

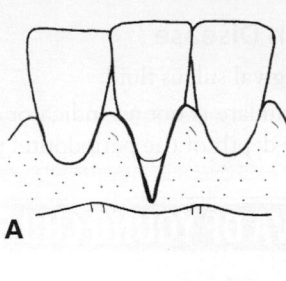

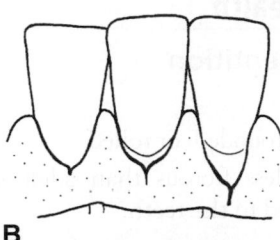

FIGURE 18-13 **Gingival Clefts. A:** V-shaped Stillman's cleft. **B:** Slitlike Stillman's clefts of varying degrees of severity in relation to the MGJ.

narrow, with associated apparent recession, as shown in Figure 18-12D.

► "Stillman's cleft" (Figure 18-13)
  • A localized recession may be V-shaped, apostrophe shaped, or form a slitlike indentation. It may extend several millimeters toward the MGJ or even to or through the junction.

► Floss cleft: A cleft created by incorrect floss positioning appears as a vertical linear or V-shaped fissure in the marginal gingiva and can result in bone loss if not corrected.[6]
  • Usually occurs at one side of an interdental papilla.
  • The injury can develop when dental floss is curved repeatedly in an incomplete "C" around the line angle so the floss is pressed across the gingiva.

IV. Consistency

A. Signs of Health

► Firm when palpated with the side of a blunt instrument (probe).
► Attached gingiva is bound down firmly to the underlying bone.

B. Changes in Disease

► *To determine consistency:* Gently press side of probe on free gingiva. Soft, spongy gingiva dents readily; firm, hard tissue resists.
► *Soft, spongy gingiva:* Related to acute stages of inflammation with increased infiltration of fluid and inflammatory elements.
  • The tissue appears red, may be smooth and shiny with loss of stippling.
  • Has marginal enlargement, and bleeds readily on probing.
► *Firm, hard gingiva:* Related to chronic inflammation with increased fibrosis.

  • The tissue may appear pink and well stippled.
  • Bleeding, when probed, usually occurs only in the deeper part of a pocket, not near the margin.
► *Retraction of the margin away from the tooth:* Normally, the free gingiva fits snugly about the tooth.
  • When the margin tends to hang slightly away or is readily displaced with a light air blast.
  • The gingival fibers that support the margin have been destroyed (Figure 18-8).

V. Surface Texture

A. Signs of Health

► *Free gingiva:* smooth.
  • *Attached gingiva:* stippled (minutely "pebbled" or "orange peel" surface).
  • *Interdental gingiva:* the free gingiva is smooth; the center portion of each papilla is stippled.

B. Changes in Disease

► *Inflammatory changes:* may be loss of stippling, with smooth, shiny surface.
► *Hyperkeratosis:* may result in a leathery, hard, or nodular surface.
► *Chronic disease:* tissue may be hard and fibrotic, with a normal pink color and normal or deep stippling.

VI. Position

► The *actual* position of the gingiva is the level of the attached periodontal tissue. It is not directly visible but can be determined by probing.
► The *apparent* position of the gingiva is the level of the gingival margin or crest of the free gingiva that is seen by direct observation.

A. Signs of Health

For the fully erupted tooth in an adult, the apparent position of the gingival margin is normally at the level of, or slightly below, the enamel contour or prominence of the cervical third of a tooth.

B. Changes in Disease

► *Effect of gingival enlargement:* When the gingiva is enlarged, the gingival margin may be high on the enamel, partly or nearly covering the anatomic crown.
► *Effect of gingival recession*
  • Definition: Recession is the exposure of root surface that results from the apical migration of the JE (Figure 18-14).
  • Actual recession: The actual recession is measured from the CEJ to the attachment.
  • Visible recession: Exposed root surface visible on clinical examination from the gingival margin to the CEJ.
  • Localized recession (Figure 18-15): A localized recession may be narrow or wide, and deep or shallow.

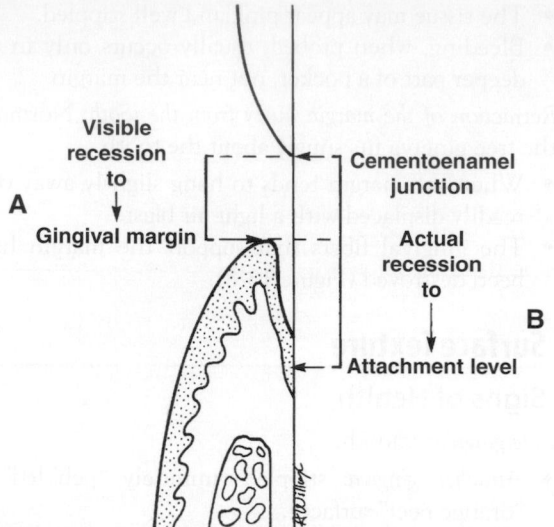

FIGURE 18-14 Gingival Recession. A: Clinically visible recession of the gingival margin with root surface apparent to the eye. **B:** The actual recession exposes the root surface as the periodontal attachment migrates along the root surface.

The root surface is denuded, and the visible recession may extend to or through the MGJ.

• Measurement: Both actual and visible recession can be measured with a probe from the CEJ. Total recession is the distance from the CEJ to the bottom of the sulcus.

VII. Bleeding

A. Signs of Health

▶ Healthy tissue does not bleed during periodontal probing.

B. Changes in Disease

▶ Sulcular epithelium becomes a diseased *pocket epithelium*.

▶ The ulcerated pocket wall bleeds spontaneously or during periodontal probing.

VIII. Exudate

A. Signs of Health

There is no exudate except slight gingival crevicular fluid (GCF). GCF cannot be seen by direct observation.

B. Changes in Disease

▶ Increased gingival sulcus fluid.

▶ Amount of exudate is not an indicator of the extent of disease or the depth of the periodontal pockets.

THE GINGIVA OF YOUNG CHILDREN

I. Signs of Health

A. Primary Dentition

▶ *Color*: pink.

▶ *Shape*: thick, rounded, or rolled.

▶ *Consistency*: less fibrous than adult gingiva; not as tightly adapted to the teeth.

▶ *Surface texture*: may or may not have stippling; in children with healthy gingiva, stippling may be present in less than 50%.[7]

▶ *Attached gingiva*: width of attached gingiva in children is typically between 4 and 5 mm.[8]

▶ *Interdental gingiva*

• Anterior: the maxillary midline diastema is present in the primary dentition in 97% of cases[9] and is considered normal; the papillae in areas of diastemae are flat or saddle shaped.

• Posterior: col between facial and lingual papillae when teeth are in contact (Figure 18-6).

B. Mixed Dentition

▶ Constant state of change related to exfoliation and eruption.

▶ Free gingiva may appear rolled or rounded, slightly reddened, shiny, and with a lack of firmness.

▶ The gingiva covers a varying portion of the anatomic crown, depending on the stage of eruption (Figure 18-5).

II. Changes in Disease

▶ A comprehensive periodontal examination is conducted at dental visits for early diagnosis of periodontal disease according to the Academy of Periodontology.[10]

▶ The British Society of Periodontology and the British Society of Paediatric Dentistry recommend the use

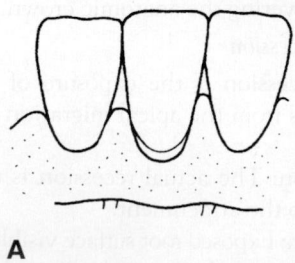
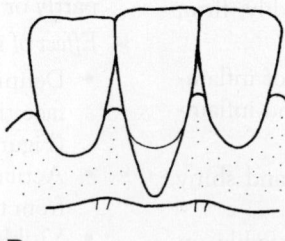
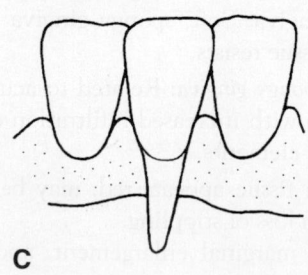

FIGURE 18-15 Localized Recession. A single tooth may show narrow or wide, deep or shallow recession. **A:** Wide, shallow. **B:** Wide, deep, with narrow attached gingiva. **C:** Narrow, deep, with missing attached gingiva.

of the Simplified Basic Periodontal Examination for screening of children and adolescents.[11]

▶ Gingivitis occurs frequently in children but is usually reversible with improved oral self-care without leaving permanent damage.

▶ Mucogingival problems occur in children. The recognition of deficiencies of attached gingiva has particular significance for the child who will need orthodontic treatment.[8]

THE GINGIVA AFTER PERIODONTAL SURGERY

I. Pocket Reduction Surgery

▶ The characteristics of "normal healthy gingiva" take on different dimensions for the patient who has completed treatment for pockets, bone loss, and other signs of a periodontal infection.

▶ The JE may be apical to the CEJ (see Figure 18-16).

▶ After healing, the sulcus depths may be within normal range and no bleeding occurs when probed.

▶ With each periodontal maintenance appointment, a thorough, careful examination is necessary to control factors that may permit recurrence of disease.

II. Gingival Grafting Surgery

▶ Depending on the exact surgery performed, examination shows changes from the initial evaluation.

  • For example, where the initial examination showed a deficiency of attached gingiva with frenal pull, mucogingival surgery may have created new attached gingiva.

III. Implant Surgery

▶ Gingiva around the implant should have the same color and consistency as gingiva surrounding a natural tooth (see Chapter 33).

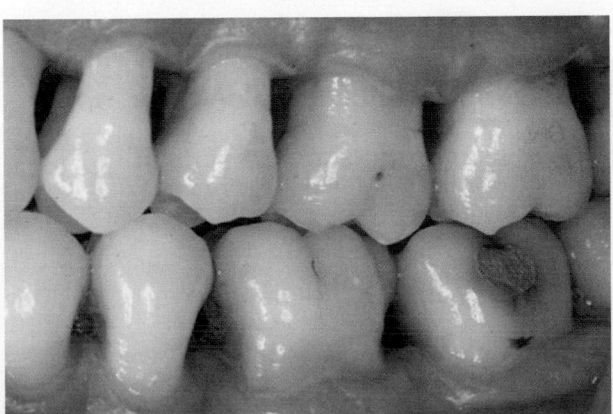

FIGURE 18-16 **Gingiva After Pocket Reduction Periodontal Surgery.** The gingival margin is significantly apical to CEJ leading to exposure of the root surface and root concavities. The embrasures (space) between teeth is no longer filled by the papillae. (Reprinted from Nield-Gehrig J. Fundamentals of Periodontal Instrumentation and Advanced Root Instrumentation, 7th Ed. Philadelphia: Lippincott Williams & Wilkins; 2012.)

▶ Contour of the gingiva will depend on the placement of the implant, but may result in open embrasures interproximally like those seen after pocket reduction surgery.

DOCUMENTATION

The permanent records of a patient who received treatment for a gingival or periodontal condition would have a minimum of the following:

▶ Health history with routine follow-up recorded for each visitation.

▶ Initial charting and descriptive material to show disease symptoms with information to show need for and actual treatment carried out by a series of progress notes defining each appointment with changes identified resulting from specific treatment.

▶ Individual instruction with biofilm scores from disclosing agent applications. Any personal care products recommended, their demonstration, and report of use by the patient. Record of improvements in gingival health noted over the series of appointments.

▶ Patient's own comments related to health change, habits changed, dietary changes, all successes, along with an agreement to a recommended plan for a periodontal maintenance program.

▶ A progress note for an individual patient appointment may be read in Box 18-2.

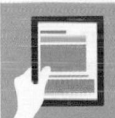

BOX 18-2

Example Documentation: Description of the Periodontium

S –55 year-old Hispanic female presents for continuing care appointment with chief complaint of bleeding when she brushes her teeth.

O –Gingival description: Color: normal pigmentation, dark reddish inflammation along all areas of free gingival margin. Size: general slight enlargement of interdental papilla. Shape: bulbous areas in maxillary anterior. Consistency: generally soft and spongy, shiny surface, generalized bleeding on probing. Probing depths generally 3-4 mm. Biofilm score: 50%.

A –Diagnosis is plaque-induced gingivitis.

P –Oral biofilm was disclosed and patient demonstrated toothbrushing and flossing technique. Review of modified Bass technique was provided to assist in accessing biofilm along gingival margins. Floss technique was good, but the patient needs to be more consistent in performing it daily. Treatment goals are: (1) brush 2x/day, (2) flossing daily, and (3) reduce bleeding on probing by 20%. Subgingival debridement and prophylaxis completed. About 5% sodium fluoride varnish applied. Next visit: 6 month continuing care.

Signed: _____, RDH

Date: _____

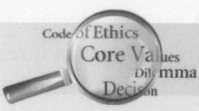

EVERYDAY ETHICS

Britain and Nicholas were first-year dental hygiene students just beginning to practice on each other as student partners in the preclinic program. Today their clinical practice was to provide the description of each other's gingiva; the next session would be learning to use the probe for the pocket/sulcus examination. Nicholas told her his "gums bled when he brushed." As she began, the gingiva seemed soft and loose, but Britain was not sure she understood what is "normal" when she remembered that her instructor had referred to a "range" of normal.

Britain decided to focus on and document the areas that looked pink with pointed papillae in the interproximal areas. She carefully recorded this information with great detail and then signaled for her instructor to verify the findings. When the instructor reviewed the examination, she was pleased with Britain's thoroughness. The instructor provided positive feedback and quickly moved on to the next pair of students. Britain began to feel uneasy that she hadn't pointed out the gingival tissues that she thought were possibly inflamed.

Questions for Consideration

1. Which of the core values (Table II-1, Section II Introduction) have application in this scenario? How and why?

2. Indicate how Nicholas is the center of this dilemma from both the perspective of Britain, a student, and the clinical instructor who finds out from another faculty member who had worked with Britain and Nicholas at an earlier clinical practice session for study cast impressions, that she thinks Nicholas has definite signs of periodontal disease and could use advise about the care he needs.

3. Ethically, what alternatives or actions can Britain take at this time to address the "uneasy" feeling she has about Nicholas' gingival status?

Factors To Teach The Patient

▷ Characteristics of normal healthy gingiva.
▷ The significance of bleeding; healthy tissue does not bleed.
▷ Relationship of findings during a gingival examination to the personal daily care procedures for infection control.
▷ The special attention needed for an area of gingival recession to prevent abrasion, inflammation, and further involvement.
▷ How the method of brushing, stiffness of toothbrush filaments, abrasiveness of a dentifrice, and pressure applied during brushing can be factors in gingival recession.

References

1. Nanci A, Bosshardt DD. Structure of periodontal tissues in health and disease. *Periodontol 2000.* 2006;40:11–28.

2. Ainamo J, Löe H. Anatomical characteristics of gingiva: a clinical and microscopic study of the free and attached gingiva. *J Periodontol.* 1966;37(1):5–13.

3. Gupta G. Gingival crevicular fluid as a periodontal diagnostic indicator-II: inflammatory mediators, host-response modifiers and chair side diagnostic aids. *J Med Life.* 2013;6(1):7–13.

4. Bosshardt DD, Lang NP. The junctional epithelium: from health to disease. *J Dent Res.* 2005;84(1):9–20.

5. Nordland WP, Tarnow DP. A classification system for loss of papillary height. *J Periodontol.* 1998;69(10):1124–1126.

6. Hallmon WW, Waldrop TC, Houston GD, et al. Flossing clefts: clinical and histologic observations. *J Periodontol.* 1986;57(8):501–504.

7. Bimstein E, Peretz B, Holan G. Prevalence of gingival stippling in children. *J Clin Pediatr Dent.* 2003;27(2):163–165.

8. Maynard JG Jr, Ochsenbein C. Mucogingival problems, prevalence and therapy in children. *J Periodontol.* 1975;46(9):543–552.

9. Gkantidis N, Kolokitha OE, Topouzelis N. Management of maxillary midline diastema with emphasis on etiology. *J Clin Pediatr Dent.* 2008;32(4):265–272.

10. Califano JV, Research, Science and Therapy Committee American Academy of Periodontology. Position paper: periodontal diseases of children and adolescents. *J Periodontol.* 2003;74(11):1696–1704.

11. Cole E, Ray-Chaudhuri A, Vaidyanathan M, et al. Simplified basic periodontal examination (BPE) in children and adolescents: a guide for general dental practitioners. *Dent Update.* 2014;41(4):328–330, 332–334, 337.

ENHANCE YOUR UNDERSTANDING

thePoint° DIGITAL CONNECTIONS
(see the inside front cover for access information)
- Audio glossary
- Quiz bank

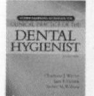

SUPPORT FOR LEARNING
(available separately; visit lww.com)
- *Active Learning Workbook for Clinical Practice of the Dental Hygienist, 12th Edition*

prepU INDIVIDUALIZED REVIEW
(available separately; visit lww.com)
- Adaptive quizzing with *prepU for Wilkins' Clinical Practice of the Dental Hygienist*

19

Periodontal Disease Development

Linda D. Boyd, RDH, RD, EdD and Esther M. Wilkins, BS, RDH, DMD

CHAPTER OUTLINE

LEARNING OBJECTIVES

After studying this chapter, the student will be able to:

1. List and describe the modifiable and nonmodifiable risk factors for periodontal disease.

2. Explain the signs and symptoms of periodontal disease.

3. Define the stages of development for periodontal lesions.

4. Compare and contrast the different classifications of periodontal disease.

5. Describe the dental hygienist's role in educating the patient about management of modifiable risk factors for periodontal disease.

The periodontium gives support needed to maintain the teeth in function (Figure 19-1).

▶ Periodontal diseases are infectious communicable diseases initiated by microorganisms in the dental biofilm which collects on the teeth when oral self-care is inadequate.

▶ Terminology for this chapter is available in Box 19-1.

PERIODONTAL-SYSTEMIC DISEASE CONNECTION

▶ There has been significant research on the association between periodontal infections and a number of systemic diseases and conditions in recent years including[1]:

• Cardiovascular disease
• Adverse pregnancy outcomes, including premature low birth weight babies
• Respiratory disease
• Chronic kidney disease
• Rheumatoid arthritis
• Obesity
• Cognitive impairment
• Osteoporosis
• Diabetes mellitus

▶ Despite the association, periodontal disease has not been shown to *cause* systemic disease.

▶ The mechanism for the association is not yet clear, but infection and/or inflammation are common elements of all the diseases and conditions.[2]

▶ The association between periodontal infection and various systemtic diseases/conditions makes it critical for early identification, treatment, and management of periodontal disease (infection) by dental hygiene professionals.

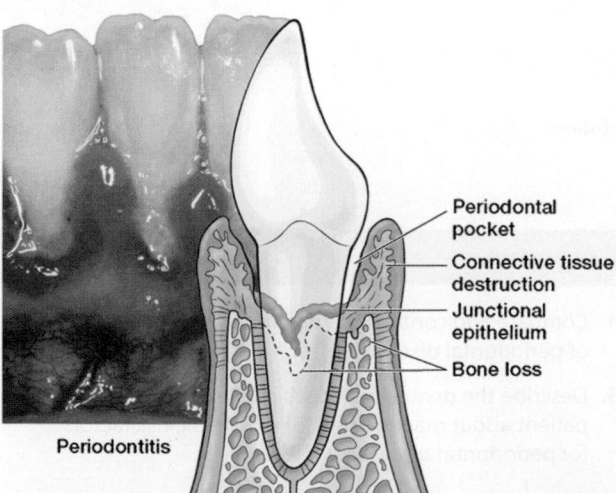

Periodontal pocket
Connective tissue destruction
Junctional epithelium
Bone loss

Periodontitis

FIGURE 19-1 Clinical Changes in Periodontitis. Periodontitis is characterized by inflammation within the supporting tissues of the teeth, progressive destruction of the periodontal ligament, and loss of supporting alveolar bone. (Reprinted from Nield-Gehrig J, Willmann D. Foundations of Periodontics for the Dental Hygienist, 3rd Ed. Philadelphia: Lippincott Williams & Wilkins; 2011.)

RISK ASSESSMENT

I. Types of Factors Involved

Complicating and risk factors for disease development may be etiologic, predisposing, or contributing. They are delineated as follows:

▶ *Etiologic factor*: the actual cause of a disease or condition.

▶ *Predisposing factor*: renders a person susceptible to a disease or condition.

▶ *Contributing factor*: lends assistance to, supplements, or adds to a condition or disease.

▶ *Risk factor*: increases the probability that disease will occur.

▶ Etiologic, predisposing, and contributing factors may be local or systemic, defined as follows:

• *Local factor*: a factor in the immediate environment of the oral cavity or specifically in the environment of the teeth and periodontium.

• *Systemic factor*: a factor that results from or is influenced by a general physical or mental disease or condition.

II. Risk Assessment Tools

▶ Risk assessment identifies the level of likelihood for developing periodontal disease and is an integral part of individualizing preventive strategies and periodontal treatment.[3,4]

▶ Risk assessment may reduce the need for more advanced periodontal therapy and improve patient outcomes to reduce oral healthcare costs.[3]

▶ Examples of periodontal risk assessment (PRA) tools:

• Periodontal risk calculator (PRC) is a web-based risk assessment tool that uses known factors such as smoking history, diagnosis of diabetes, and periodontal history and status to predict risk for periodontal disease and has shown a high level of accuracy in a 15-year study.[5,6]

• A *gum disease risk assessment test* is available on the American Academy of Periodontology (AAP) website www.perio.org for patients to use to assess risk.

• A Periodontal Risk Assessment (PRA) tool based on tooth loss, genetic, and systemic conditions and periodontal status can also be located on the internet www.perio-tools.com/pra/en/.[7]

▶ Risk assessment can be used to educate the patient about the level of risk and the factors that can be modified. The patient can use the tools to manage their personal disease risk.

ETIOLOGY OF PERIODONTAL DISEASE

▶ Microorganisms in the form of biofilm are the primary etiologic agents of periodontal disease/infection (see Figure 15-3 in Chapter 15).

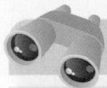

BOX 19-1   KEY WORDS AND ABBREVIATIONS: Periodontal Disease Development

AAP: American Academy of Periodontology is a professional organization for periodontists who specialize in diagnosis and treatment of periodontal disease.

Cicatrix: the fibrous tissue left after the healing of a wound; cicatricial: adj.

Collagen: white fibers of the connective tissue.

Collagenase: enzyme that catalyzes the degradation (hydrolysis) of collagen.

Desquamation: shedding of the outer epithelial layer of the stratified squamous epithelium of skin or mucosa.

Diastema: a space or an abnormal opening; as a dental term, it is a space between two adjacent teeth in the same dental arch.

Edema: an accumulation of excessive fluid in cells, tissues, or a serous cavity.

Enzyme: a protein secreted by body cells that acts as a catalyst to induce chemical changes in other substances but remains unchanged itself.

Food impaction: forceful wedging of food into the periodontium by occlusal forces.

Gingivitis: inflammation of the gingival tissues.

Iatrogenic: resulting from treatment by a professional person.

Infiltration: the diffusion or accumulation in a tissue or cells of substances not normal to it or in amounts in excess of normal.

Lesion: any pathologic or traumatic discontinuity of tissue or loss of function of a part; broad term including wounds, sores, ulcers, tumors, and any other tissue damage.

Nonsurgical periodontal therapy (NSPT): includes dental biofilm removal and biofilm control (by patient); supragingival and subgingival scaling; root planing; and the adjunctive use of chemotherapeutic agents for control of bacterial infection, desensitizing hypersensitive exposed root surfaces, and dental caries prevention as related to the health of the periodontium.

Periodontitis: inflammation in the periodontium affecting gingival tissues, periodontal ligament, cementum, and supporting bone.

Permeable: permitting passage of a fluid.

PRC: Periodontal risk calculator is a web-based periodontal risk assessment tool.

Refractory: not readily responsive to treatment.

Toxin: a poison; protein produced by certain animals, higher plants, and pathogenic bacteria.

Bacterial toxin: poison produced by bacteria; includes exotoxins, endotoxins, and toxic enzymes.

Xerostomia: dryness of the mouth from a lack of normal secretions.

- The type of organisms shift to gram-negative anaerobic species including *Porphyromonas gingivalis* and *Tannerella forsythia* (previously known as *Bacteroides forsythus*) with the initiation of periodontal disease.[8]
- *Aggregatibacter Actinomycetemcomitans* (Previously *Actinobacillus Actinomycetemcomitans*) has been associated with aggressive forms of periodontal disease.[8]
- Motile rods and spirochetes are prominent in diseased pockets versus healthy subgingival sulci.

RISK FACTORS FOR PERIODONTAL DISEASES

▶ Identification of risk factors for periodontal diseases can provide significant insight into assessment and care planning for an individual patient.

▶ The various periodontal pathogenic microorganisms do not affect all people with the same degree of severity. It is clear that host factors play a significant role.[8–10]

I. Modifiable Risk Factors

Modifiable risk factors include the following:

A. Tobacco Use (see Chapter 34)

▶ The evidence provides strong support for the risk of developing periodontal disease and attachment loss as a result of smoking (see Figure 19-2).[10]

▶ The odds for developing periodontal disease in people who smoke ranges from 3 to 7 times higher than in nonsmokers.[10]

▶ More than 40% of cases of periodontitis are a result of cigarette smoking.[8]

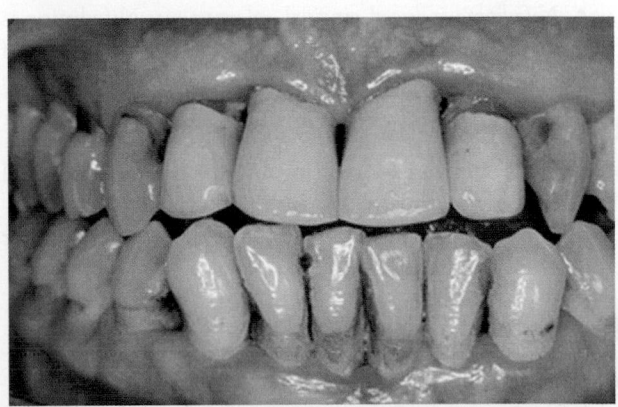

FIGURE 19-2 Attachment (Bone Loss) in Smoker. A 58-year-old female, cigarette smoker of 20 pack years with advanced periodontitis. Note that clinical signs of inflammation, such as marginal redness, are minimal. The teeth are discolored due to nicotine deposits. (Reprinted from Nield-Gehrig J, Willmann D. Foundations of Periodontics for the Dental Hygienist, 3rd Ed. Philadelphia: Lippincott Williams & Wilkins; 2011.)

- ▶ Periodontal treatment may be less effective in smokers than in those who do not smoke.
- ▶ Users of smokeless tobacco products experience oral effects, including predisposition to oral cancer. Periodontal lesions with severe recession and clinical attachment loss (CAL) occur where the quid is held.[11]

B. Diabetes Mellitus (see Chapter 69)

- ▶ Periodontal disease and diabetes mellitus have a bidirectional relationship, meaning a patient who does not control blood glucose is more likely to have more severe periodontal disease.
- ▶ Poor control of blood glucose (glycemic control) increases the risk of developing periodontal disease and results in poor outcomes to treatment.[10]
- ▶ As a result of the increase in diabetes in the US population, there is an increase in prevalence of periodontitis in children and adolescents with Type 1 diabetes mellitus.[8]
- ▶ Research suggests management of periodontal infection results in improvement in control of blood glucose.[8,10]

C. Psychosocial Factors[10]

- ▶ Some research suggests individuals under stress are more likely to have CAL and alveolar bone loss.
  - However, stress is not recognized as an independent risk factor for periodontal disease.

D. Medications[8]

- ▶ Medications for specific systemic conditions can lead to gingival enlargement.[8] The enlarged tissue encourages dental biofilm retention and complicate removal, thus increasing the potential for periodontal infections.
  - *Phenytoin-induced gingival enlargement:* Phenytoin is a drug used to control seizures (see Figure 19-3).
  - *Cyclosporine-induced gingival enlargement:* Cyclosporine is an immunosuppressant drug used for patients with organ transplants to prevent rejection.
  - *Nifedipine-induced gingival enlargement:* Nifedipine is a calcium-channel blocker used in the treatment of angina and ventricular arrhythmias.

E. Other Potential Risk Factors

- ▶ There is evidence for relationships between periodontal health and nutrition, alcohol, and socioeconomic status, but more research is needed to determine whether they are risk factors.[10]

II. Nonmodifiable Risk Factors

A. Genetic Predisposition

- ▶ From 33% to 39% of the risk for periodontal disease is related to genetic factors.[8]
- ▶ Genetic testing is likely to become more cost effective and will benefit patients and dental providers in targeting those at risk for enhanced prevention.

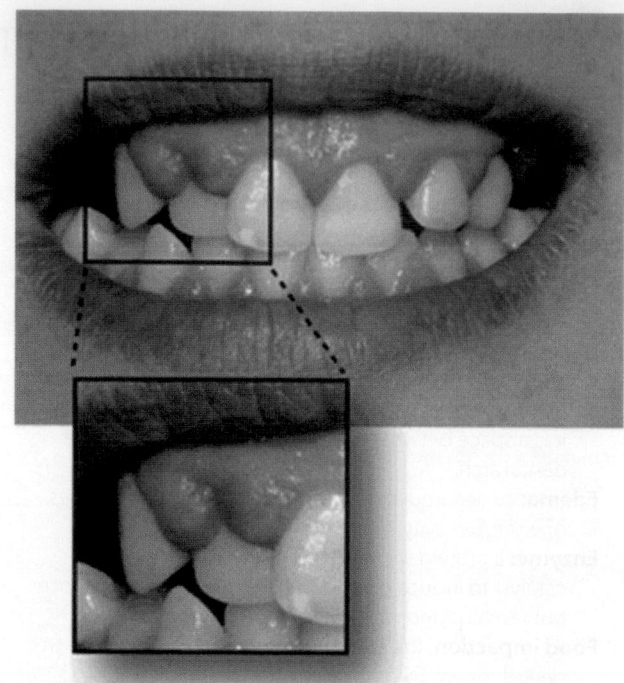

FIGURE 19-3 Gingival Hyperplasia in Patient Treated with Phenytoin. (Reprinted from Whalen K. Pharmacology, 6th Ed. Philadelphia: Lippincott Williams & Wilkins; 2014.)

B. Host Response

- ▶ Alterations in the immune response may result in periodontal damage and an increase in inflammation after a bacterial challenge.[9,10]
- ▶ Overly active neutrophils may be responsible for the tissue destruction seen in periodontal infection.[10]

C. Osteoporosis

- ▶ Many risk factors for osteoporosis are also risk factors for periodontitis, including cigarette smoking, nutritional deficiencies, glucocorticosteroid use, and immune dysfunction.
- ▶ Greater alveolar bone loss in patients with osteoporosis.[10]

D. Other Systemic Conditions

- ▶ Conditions associated with deficiencies in the immune system, such as Down syndrome, are related to periodontal disease.[10]

III. Local Factors

- ▶ Although dental biofilm is the primary etiologic factor in the development of inflammatory gingival and periodontal diseases, a variety of other factors predispose some patients to the retention of bacterial deposits and hence to the development of disease in the soft tissues.
- ▶ Retentive areas may be associated with rough surfaces of teeth and restorations, tooth contour and position, and gingival size, shape, and position.

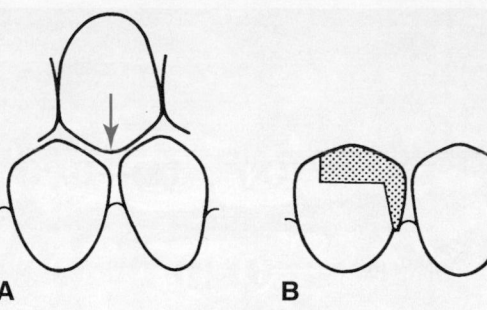

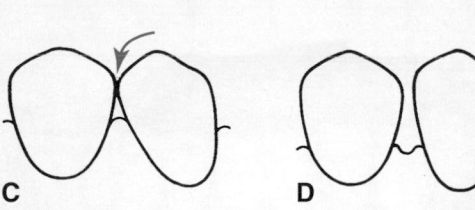

FIGURE 19-4 Effect of Tooth Position. A: Food impaction area, shown by plunger cusp (with arrow) directing pressure between lower teeth with open contact area. **B:** Inadequate restoration without proximal contact and with overhang. **C:** Tipped tooth leaving irregular marginal ridge relation. **D:** Natural open contact (diastema) with saddle-shaped gingival margin.

▶ Iatrogenic causes, that is, factors created by professionals during patient treatment or neglect of proper treatment, can be significant.

▶ Factors, such as mastication, saliva, the tongue, cheeks, lips, oral habits, and personal biofilm control procedures, contribute to retention.

A. Dental Factors

▶ Tooth surface irregularities

Pellicle and biofilm microorganisms attach to defective or rough surfaces, including the following:

* Pits, grooves, cracks
* Calculus
* Exposed altered cementum with irregularities
* Demineralization and cavitated dental caries
* Iatrogenic factors such as rough or grooved surfaces left after scaling or inadequately contoured and polished dental restorations (Figure 19-4B)

▶ Tooth contour

Altered shape may interfere with oral self-cleansing mechanisms (see Chapter 16).

* *Congenital abnormalities*: extra or missing cusps or bell-shaped crown with prominent facial and lingual contours that tend to provide deeper retentive areas in the cervical third.
* Teeth with flattened proximal surfaces have faulty contact with adjacent teeth, thus permitting debris to wedge between.
* Occlusal and incisal surfaces altered by attrition interrupt normal excursion of food during chewing. Marginal ridges have worn down.
* Areas of erosion and abrasion.
* Carious lesions.
* Heavy calculus deposits; biofilm retained on rough surface.
* Overcontoured, undercontoured, or overhanging restorations (see Figure 19-5).

▶ Tooth position

1. *Malocclusion*: Irregular alignment of a single tooth or groups of teeth leaves areas conducive

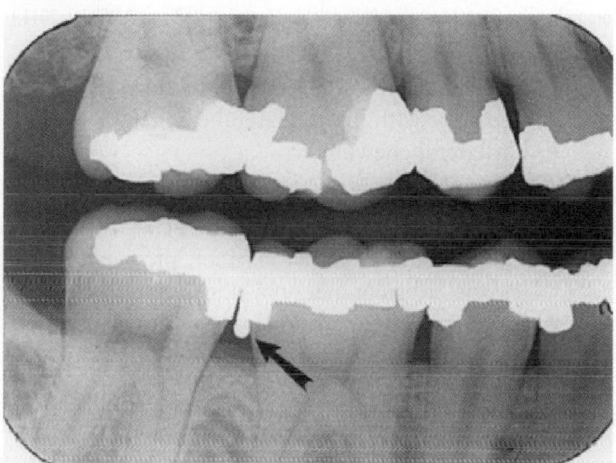

FIGURE 19-5 Restoration with an Overhang. The distal surface of the mandibular first molar in this radiograph has a faulty restoration that creates a food trap and harbors biofilm. (Reprinted from Nield-Gehrig J, Willmann D. Foundations of Periodontics for the Dental Hygienist, 3rd Ed. Philadelphia: Lippincott Williams & Wilkins; 2011.)

to collection of microorganisms for biofilm formation.

* Crowded or overlapped
* Rotated
* Deep anterior overbite (Figure 17-11, Chapter 17).
  * Mandibular teeth force food particles against maxillary lingual surface.
  * Lingual inclination of mandibular teeth allows maxillary teeth to force food particles against mandibular facial gingiva.

2. Tooth adjacent to edentulous area may be inclined or migrated; contact missing.

3. Opposing tooth missing; tooth may extrude beyond the line of occlusion.

4. *Related to eruption*
   * Incomplete eruption: the teeth do not erupt into the line of occlusion.
   * Partially erupted impacted third molar.

5. Lack of function or the use of teeth eliminates or decreases effectiveness of natural cleansing:
   * Lack of opposing teeth
   * Open bite (see Figure 19-6)

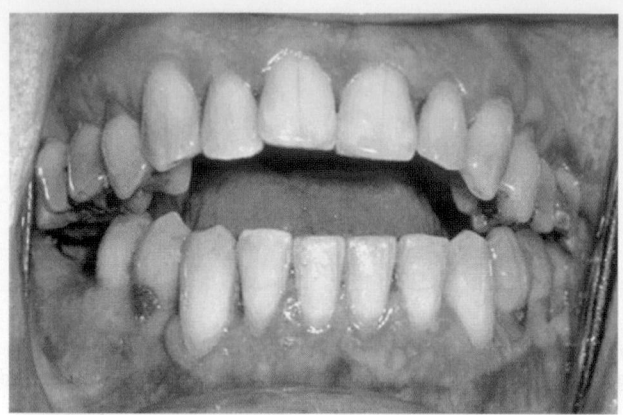

FIGURE 19-6 **Anterior Open Bite.** (Reprinted from Lippincott Williams & Wilkins' Comprehensive Dental Assisting. Philadelphia: Lippincott Williams & Wilkins; 2011.)

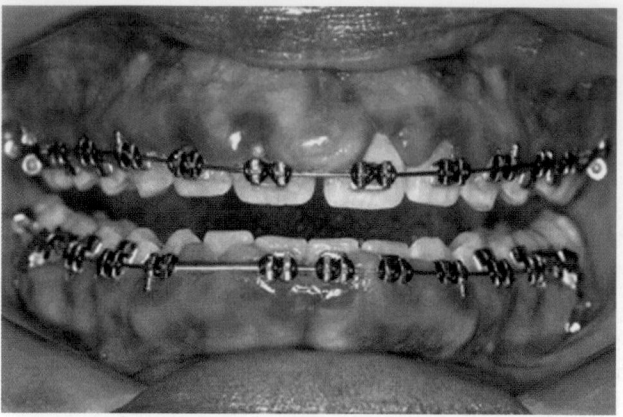

FIGURE 19-7 **Orthodontic Appliances as a Predisposing Factor for Periodontal Disease.** Infrequent oral self-care and biofilm accumulation results in periodontitis in this individual with orthodontic appliances. (Reprinted from Nield-Gehrig J, Willmann D. Foundations of Periodontics for the Dental Hygienist, 3rd Ed. Philadelphia: Lippincott Williams & Wilkins; 2011.)

- Marked maxillary anterior protrusion
- Crossbite with limited lateral excursion
- Unilateral chewing.

6. *Food impaction*
- Created by the combined effect of tooth contour, missing proximal contact, proximal carious lesions, irregular marginal ridge relationship.
- Inclination related to loss of adjacent tooth, and a plunger cusp from the opposite arch (Figure 19-4A).

7. *Defective contact area*
- Restoration margin is faulty, and the contact area is missing, improperly located, or unnaturally wide (Figure 19-4B).
- Inclined tooth with irregular marginal ridge relation (Figure 19-4C).

▶ Dental appliances and prostheses
- Orthodontic appliances provide retentive areas (see Figure 19-7).
- Fixed partial denture with deficient margin of an abutment tooth or an unusually shaped pontic.
- Removable partial denture with inadequately adapted clasps.

B. Gingival Factors

▶ *Position*
- Deviations from normal provide retentive areas for biofilm.
- *Receded*: depressed area is left at cementoenamel junction.
- *Enlarged*: extended to or over the height of contour.
- Reduced height of interdental papilla leaves open interdental area.
- Tissue flap over occlusal surface of erupting tooth.
- Periodontal pocket.
- Shape of pocket conducive to dental biofilm collection.
- Depth of pocket not accessible to toothbrush and cleaning aids.
- Calculus provides rough retentive surface.

▶ *Size and contour*
- Deviation of shape of enlarged gingiva: rolled, bulbous, cratered.
- Combination with presence of irregular restorations or dental prosthesis can result in marked biofilm retention.

▶ *Effect of Mouth Breathing*
- Dehydration of oral tissues in anterior region leads to changes in size, shape, surface texture, and consistency.

C. Other Factors

A variety of factors may predispose or contribute to the progression of periodontal infections. Some of the items listed here may have an indirect effect, whereas others have a direct effect on the oral tissues.

▶ Personal oral self-care
- *Neglect*: This can lead to generalized dental biofilm accumulation and disease promotion.
- *Faulty biofilm control techniques*: Incorrect use of brush, abrasive dentifrice, and the effects of other harmful, detrimental procedures are described in Chapter 28.
- *Awareness of oral cleanliness*: Cleansing habits, including both self-cleansing mechanisms and mechanical biofilm removal, depend in part on an individual's perception and feeling of debris through taste and tongue activity.

▶ Diet and eating habits
- Soft foods tend to adhere more than fibrous, firm foods.
- Cariogenic food selection.
- Masticatory deficiencies limit diet selection. Missing teeth, ill-fitting partial dentures, and various occlusal deficiencies alter diet selection and eating habits.

PATHOGENESIS OF PERIODONTAL DISEASES

Pathogenesis refers to the process by which a disease develops and progresses. The primary etiology of periodontal disease is bacteria that initiate an inflammatory process.

▶ The inflammatory process is very complex and influenced by patient and environmental factors.

I. Acute Inflammatory Response

▶ When the immune response is working effectively, the presence of biofilm results in gingival inflammation with no breakdown of tissue.[8]

▶ Activation of the local acute inflammatory response begins the process of lesion development.

II. Development of Gingival and Periodontal Infection

The stages of development of gingivitis and periodontitis are divided into the *initial lesion*, *early lesion*, *established lesion*, and *advanced lesion*.[12] With an accumulation of dental biofilm on the cervical tooth surface adjacent to the gingival margin, an inflammatory reaction is initiated, and the immune system responds.

A. The Initial Lesion

▶ Inflammatory response to dental biofilm
- Occurs within 2–4 days in response to bacterial accumulation.
- Migration and infiltration of white blood cells into the junctional epithelium and gingival sulcus result from the natural body response to infectious agents.
- Increased flow of gingival crevicular fluid.
- Early breakdown of collagen of the supporting gingival fiber groups (Figure 18-8 in Chapter 18).
- Fluid fills the spaces in the connective tissue.

▶ Clinical appearance
- No clinical evidence of change may appear in the earliest phases.
- Slight marginal redness with enlargement due to the fluid collection follows as the infection develops.

B. The Early Lesion

▶ Increased inflammatory response
- Dental biofilm becomes older and thicker (7–14 days; time reflects individual differences).
- Infiltration of fluid, lymphocytes, and neutrophils with a few plasma cells into the connective tissue.
- Breakdown of collagen fiber support to the gingival margin.
- *Epithelium proliferates*: Epithelial extensions and rete ridges are formed.

▶ Clinical appearance
- Early signs of gingivitis become apparent with slight gingival enlargement; will become an established lesion if undisturbed.
- Early gingivitis is reversible when biofilm is controlled and inflammation is reduced. Healthy tissue may be restored.
- Susceptibility of individuals varies; time before lesion becomes established varies.

C. The Established Lesion

▶ Progression from the early lesion
- Fluid and leukocyte migration into tissues and sulcus increase; plasma cells are related to areas of chronic inflammation.
- Formation of *pocket epithelium*.
  1. Proliferation of the junctional and sulcular epithelium continues in an attempt to wall out the inflammation.
  2. Pocket epithelium is more permeable; areas of ulceration of the lining epithelium develop.
  3. Early pocket formation with bleeding on probing.
- Collagen destruction continues; connective tissue fiber support is lost.
- Progression to early periodontal lesion may occur or the established lesion may remain stable for extended periods of time.

▶ Clinical appearance
- Clear evidence of inflammation is present with marginal redness, bleeding on probing, and spongy marginal gingiva.
- Later, chronic fibrosis develops.

D. The Advanced Lesion

▶ *Extension of inflammation*
- Bacteria from supragingival biofilm enter the sulcus and provide the source for subgingival biofilm.
- Biofilm microorganisms produce irritants.
- *Alveolar bone destruction* results from the host immune response to the bacteria causing a cascade of events to stimulate osteoclast activity.[9]

▶ *Progressive destruction of connective tissue*
- Connective tissue fibers below the junctional epithelium are destroyed; the epithelium migrates along the root surface.
- Coronal portion of junctional epithelium becomes detached.
- Exposed cementum where Sharpey's fibers were attached becomes altered by the host response to the bacterial challenge.
- Diseased cementum contains a thin superficial layer of endotoxins from the bacterial breakdown.
- Without treatment, loss of attachment results with an increase in pocket depth.

► *Characteristics of the advanced lesion*
  • Pocket formation, mobility, bone loss; all signs of periodontitis.
  • Persistence of the chronic inflammatory process; plasma cells predominate.
  • Junctional epithelium continues to migrate; lesion extends through connective tissue.
  • Periods of inactivity alternating with periods of activity can be expected.

GINGIVAL AND PERIODONTAL POCKETS

► It is the presence or absence of infection that distinguishes a pocket from a sulcus and the level of attachment on the tooth that distinguishes a gingival pocket from a periodontal pocket.

► A pocket has an *inner wall (the tooth surface)* and an *outer wall (the sulcular epithelium or pocket epithelium)* of the free gingiva. The two walls meet at the base of the pocket.
  • The base of the pocket is the coronal margin of the attached periodontal tissues.
  • Histologically, the base of a healthy sulcus is the coronal border of the junctional epithelium, whereas the base of a pocket (diseased sulcus) may be at the coronal border of the connective tissue attachment.

► *Substances found in a pocket*
  • Communication of the opening of the pocket with the oral cavity provides an opportunity for dental biofilm to collect.
  • The deeper the pocket, the more difficult it is to clean by toothbrushing or other biofilm control devices.

► The following may be found in a pocket:
  • *Microorganisms and their products*: enzymes, endotoxins, and other metabolic products.
  • Gingival crevicular fluid.
  • Desquamated epithelial cells.
  • Leukocytes, the numbers of which increase with increased inflammation in the tissues.
  • Purulent exudate made up of living and broken down leukocytes, living and dead microorganisms, and serum.

► Pockets are divided into *gingival* and *periodontal* types to clarify the degree of anatomic involvement.

► Periodontal pockets are further categorized by their position in relation to the alveolar bone, that is, whether their pocket base is suprabony or intrabony (Figure 19-8).

I. Gingival Pocket or Pseudopocket

► *Definition*: A pocket formed by gingival enlargement without apical migration of the junctional epithelium (Figure 19-8B).

► The margin of the gingiva has moved toward the incisal or occlusal without the deeper periodontal structures becoming involved.

► The tooth wall of the pocket is enamel.

► During eruption, the base of the sulcus is at various levels along the enamel. The base of the sulcus of a fully erupted tooth is near the cementoenamel junction.

► All gingival pockets are suprabony, that is, the base of the pocket is coronal to the crest of the alveolar bone.

II. Periodontal Pocket

► *Definition*: A pocket formed as a result of disease or degeneration causing apical migration of the junctional epithelium along the cementum.

► The periodontal deeper structures (attachment apparatus) are involved, that is, the cementum, periodontal ligament, and bone.

► The tooth wall of the pocket is cementum or partly cementum and partly enamel.

► The base of the pocket is on cementum at the level of attached periodontal tissue.

► Periodontal pockets may be suprabony or intrabony.
  • *Suprabony*: Pocket in which the base of the pocket is coronal to the crest of the alveolar bone (Figures 19-8 A, B, and C).
  • *Intrabony*: Pocket in which the base of the pocket is below or apical to the crest of the alveolar bone (Figure 19-8D). "Intra" means located within the bone. The term "infrabony" is used in some texts. "Infra" means under or beneath.

III. Tooth Surface Irregularities

► Supragingival tooth surface irregularities are detected by drying the surface and observing under adequate direct or indirect light; an explorer is used as needed.

► Subgingival examination is dependent, for the most part, on tactile and auditory sensitivity transmitted by a probe or an explorer.

► Causes of surface roughness on the enamel surface include the following:
  • Structural defects: cracks and grooves.
  • Demineralization; cavitated dental caries.
  • Calculus deposits and heavy stain deposits.
  • Erosion, abrasion.
  • Pits and irregularities from hypoplasia.

► *Root surface* irregularities
  • Diseased altered cementum
  • Cemental resorption
  • Root caries
  • Abrasion
  • Calculus
  • Deficient or overhanging filling (see Figure 19-5)
  • Grooves from previous improper instrumentation.

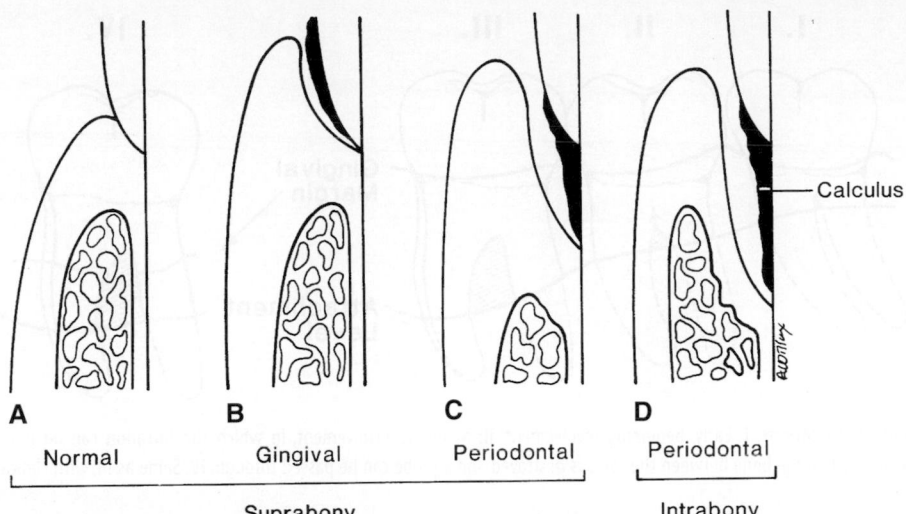

FIGURE 19-8 Types of Periodontal Pockets. A: Normal relationship of the gingival tissue and the cementoenamel junction in a fully erupted tooth. **B:** Gingival pocket showing attachment at the cementoenamel junction and the pocket formed by enlarged gingival tissue. There is no bone loss. **C:** Periodontal pocket showing attachment on cementum with root surface exposed. Gingival tissue has enlarged. **D:** Periodontal intrabony pocket with the bottom of the pocket within the bone. See the text for further description of each type of pocket.

▶ Irregularities at the cementoenamel junction
  • The relationships of enamel and cementum at the cementoenamel junction are shown in Figure 18-10 in Chapter 18.

COMPLICATIONS RESULTING FROM PERIODONTAL DISEASE PROGRESSION

I. Furcation Involvement

Furcation involvement means that the clinical attachment level and bone loss have extended into the furcation area between the roots of a multirooted tooth (see the Glickman furcation grades in Chapter 20 and Figure 19-9).

▶ Presence of furcation involvement increases the risk of tooth loss.[13]
  • It is difficult to adequately remove biofilm and calculus from the furcation area (see Figure 19-10) for both the dental hygienist and the patient who makes it challenging to manage the inflammation and infection in this area.

A. Clinical Observations

▶ When the gingiva over the furcation has not receded, the following may be seen:
  • The furcation is covered by the periodontal pocket wall.
  • No differences in color, size, or other tissue changes may exist to differentiate the area from adjacent gingiva, but when color changes do exist, they provide clues to guide further examination.
  • A radiolucency in the furcation area may be noted on the radiographs.

▶ When the gingiva over a molar furcation is receded, the root division may be seen directly (Figure 19-9, Grade IV).

B. Detection

A suggested procedure for probing furcation areas is described in Chapter 20.

II. Mucogingival Involvement

A pocket that extends to or beyond the mucogingival junction and into the alveolar mucosa is described as *mucogingival involvement* (see Figure 19-11). There is no attached gingiva in the area, and a probe can pass through the pocket and beyond the mucogingival junction into the alveolar mucosa.

A. Significance of Attached Gingiva

▶ Functions of attached gingiva
  • Give support to the marginal gingiva.
  • Withstand the frictional stresses of mastication and toothbrushing.
  • Provide attachment or a solid base for the movable alveolar mucosa for the action of the cheeks, lips, and tongue.

▶ Barrier to passage of inflammation
  • The junctional epithelium (epithelial attachment) acts as a barrier to keep infection outside the body.
  • With destruction of the connective tissue and periodontal ligament fibers under the junctional epithelium, the epithelium migrates along the root.
  • In mucogingival involvement, the bottom of the pocket extends into the alveolar mucosa. There, the unconfined inflammation can spread more rapidly in the loose connective tissue.

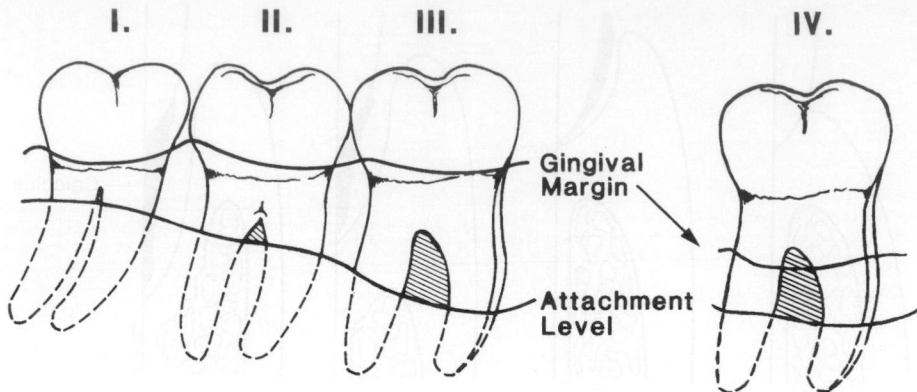

FIGURE 19-9 Classification of Furcations. I: Early, beginning involvement. **II:** Moderate involvement, in which the furcation can be probed but not through and through. **III:** Severe involvement, when the bone between the roots is destroyed and a probe can be passed through. **IV:** Same as III, with clinical exposure resulting from gingival recession.

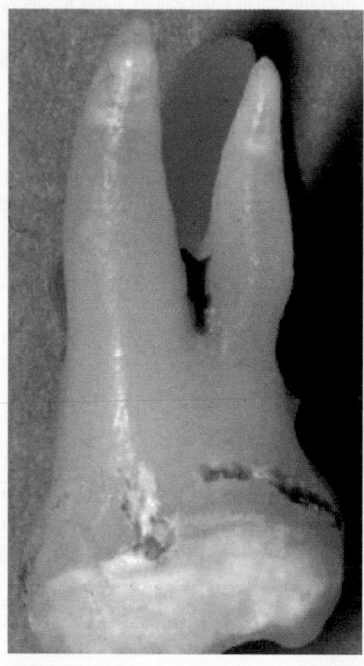

FIGURE 19-10 Calculus in the Furcation Area and Root Depressions. This extracted molar has mineralized deposits (calculus) in the furcation. Once disease progresses into the furcation area, access for removal becomes difficult. (Reprinted from Weiss G, Scheid R. Woelfel's Dental Anatomy, 9th Ed. Philadelphia: Lippincott Williams & Wilkins; 2016.)

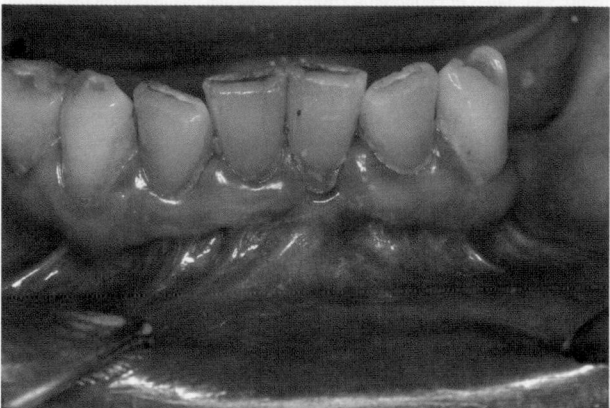

FIGURE 19-11 Mucogingival Defect. A mucogingival defect is suspected at tooth #24, which has a very narrow zone of keratinized gingiva. (Reprinted from Scheid R. Woelfel's Dental Anatomy, 7th Ed. Philadelphia: Lippincott Williams & Wilkins; 2007.)

B. Clinical Observations

▶ Color changes, tension test, and probe measurements are used during assessment of the mucogingival areas (see Chapter 20).

▶ *Width of attached gingiva:* A narrow zone of gingiva from gingival margin to mucogingival junction is more susceptible to developing mucogingival involvement because there is less attached gingiva for support.

▶ *Base of pocket at mucogingival junction:*

- When the attached gingiva measures 1–2 mm and there is no bleeding on probing or marginal inflammation, it is recorded and reevaluated at each

continuing care or periodontal maintenance appointment (see Figure 19-12A and Figure 19-12B).

- Long-term, longitudinal studies have shown that in the absence of inflammation, areas with a narrow band of attached gingiva can be maintained for long periods.[14]

- A patient with such an area needs specific instruction in biofilm control procedures for preventive maintenance.

▶ When an area of minimal attached gingiva (1–2 mm) is placed under stress by restorative, prosthetic, or orthodontic treatment procedures, the patient is referred to the periodontist for evaluation for the need for gingival or connective tissue grafting.

C. Classification

▶ Mucogingival deformities and conditions are included in the 1999 Classification of Gingival and Periodontal Diseases and Conditions: Periodontal Disease (Table 19-1) and is included in the diagnosis.[15]

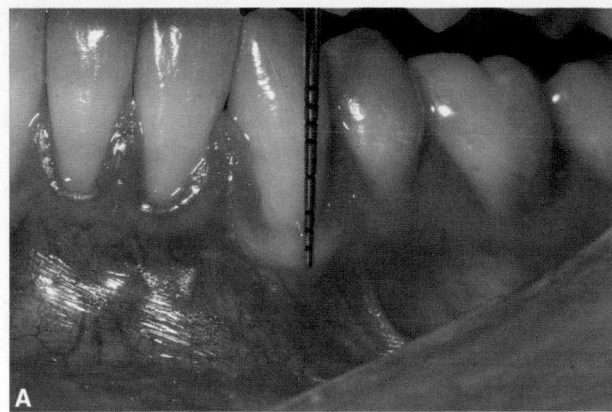

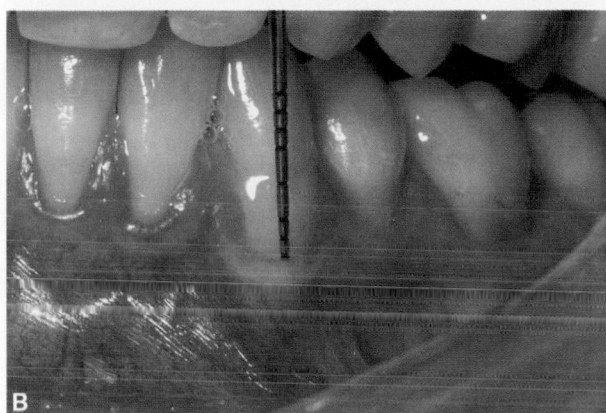

FIGURE 19-12 Measuring for a Mucogingival Defect. A: The width of keratinized gingiva is measured at 2 mm. **B:** The probe depth is measured at less than 2 mm (only 1 mm), indicating no mucogingival defect. If the probe depth reached or exceeded the mucogingival junction (exceeded the width of keratinized gingiva), there would be no attached gingiva, and a mucogingival defect would be present. (Reprinted from Scheid R. Woelfel's Dental Anatomy, 7th Ed. Philadelphia: Lippincott Williams & Wilkins; 2007.)

THE RECOGNITION OF GINGIVAL AND PERIODONTAL INFECTIONS

I. The Clinical Examination

The recognition of normal gingiva, gingival infections, and deeper periodontal involvement depends on a systematic, step-by-step examination.

▶ It is necessary to know the *extent* of the disease:
  • *Gingival infections* are confined to the gingiva.
  • *Periodontal infections* include all parts of the periodontium, namely, the gingiva, periodontal ligament, bone, and cementum.

▶ A basic examination performed to recognize the signs and effects of inflammation includes information about at least the following markers:
  • Gingival tissue changes (color, size, shape, surface texture, position)
  • Mucogingival involvement (adequate width of attached gingiva)

  • Probing depths; pocket formation (attachment levels)
  • Bleeding and exudate
  • Furcation involvement
  • Dental biofilm and calculus present
  • Mobility of teeth
  • Radiographic evidence.

II. Signs and Symptoms

▶ Patients may or may not have specific symptoms to report because periodontal infections are insidious in development.

▶ Symptoms the patient notices or feels may include:
  • Bleeding gingiva only while brushing.
  • Bleeding with drooling at night.
  • On occasion, spontaneous bleeding of the gingiva.

▶ Other possible symptoms the patient may notice include:
  • Sensitivity to hot and cold
  • Tenderness or discomfort while eating or pain after eating
  • Food retained between the teeth
  • Unpleasant mouth odors
  • Chronic bad taste
  • A feeling that the teeth are loose.
Most of these are symptoms of advanced disease.

III. Causes of Tissue Changes

▶ Disease changes produce alterations in color, size, position, shape, consistency, surface texture, bleeding readiness, and exudate production.

▶ To understand the changes that take place in the gingival tissues during the transition from health to disease, the clinician must understand:
  • The role of biofilm in the development of disease.
  • The inflammatory response initiated by the body.

▶ When the products of the biofilm microorganisms cause breakdown of the intercellular substances of the sulcular epithelium, injurious agents can pass into the connective tissue, where an inflammatory response is initiated.

▶ An inflammatory response means there is increased blood flow, increased permeability of capillaries, and increased collection of defense cells and tissue fluid.

▶ The changes produce the tissue alterations, such as in color, size, shape, and consistency, that are described in the following section.

IV. Descriptive Terminology

The severity and distribution of changes in the gingiva can be noted during the examination. When a deviation from normal affects a single area, it can be designated by the number of the adjacent tooth and the surface of the tissue involved, namely, facial, lingual, mesial, or distal.

A. Severity

▶ Severity is expressed according to the quantity of CAL; see Chapter 20 for more information:[16,17]
- Slight or mild = 1–2 mm CAL
- Moderate = 3–4 mm CAL
- Severe or advanced = >5 mm CAL

B. Distribution or Extent

Terms used for describing distribution are as follows:

▶ *Localized*: The gingiva is involved about a single tooth or a specific group of teeth (<30% of teeth involved).

▶ *Generalized*: The gingiva is involved about all or nearly all of the teeth throughout the mouth (>30% of teeth involved).

▶ *Marginal*: A change that is confined to the free or marginal gingiva. This is specified as either localized or generalized.

▶ *Papillary*: A change that involves a papilla but not the rest of the free gingiva around a tooth. A papillary change may be localized or generalized.

▶ *Diffuse*: Spread out, dispersed; affects gingival margin, attached gingiva, and interdental papillae; may extend into alveolar mucosa. A diffuse condition is more frequently localized, rarely generalized.

TABLE 19-1	Classification of Gingival and Periodontal Diseases and Conditions: Gingival Diseases

I. Gingival diseases
  A. Dental plaque-induced gingival diseases[a]
    1. Gingivitis associated with dental plaque only
      a. Without other local contributing factors
      b. With local contributing factors
    2. Gingival diseases modified by systemic factors
      a. Associated with the endocrine system
        1. Puberty-associated gingivitis
        2. Menstrual cycle–associated gingivitis
        3. Pregnancy associated
          a. Gingivitis
          b. Pyogenic granuloma
        4. Diabetes mellitus–associated gingivitis
      b. Associated with blood dyscrasias
        1. Leukemia-associated gingivitis
        2. Other
    3. Gingival diseases modified by medications
      a. Drug-influenced gingival diseases
        1. Drug-influenced gingival enlargements
        2. Drug-influenced gingivitis
          a. Oral contraceptive–associated gingivitis
          b. Other
    4. Gingival diseases modified by malnutrition
      a. Ascorbic acid–deficiency gingivitis
      b. Other
  B. Nonplaque-induced gingival lesions
    1. Gingival diseases of specific bacterial origin
      a. *Neisseria gonorrhea*–associated lesions
      b. *Treponema pallidum*–associated lesions
      c. Streptococcal species–associated lesions
      d. Other
    2. Gingival diseases of viral origin
      a. Herpesvirus infections
        1. Primary herpetic gingivostomatitis
        2. Recurrent oral herpes
        3. Varicella zoster infections
      b. Other

    3. Gingival diseases of fungal origin
      a. *Candida*-species infections
        1. Generalized gingival candidosis
      b. Linear gingival erythema
      c. Histoplasmosis
      d. Other
    4. Gingival lesions of genetic origin
      a. Hereditary gingival fibromatosis
      b. Other
    5. Gingival manifestations of systemic conditions
      a. Mucocutaneous disorders
        1. Lichen planus
        2. Pemphigoid
        3. Pemphigus vulgaris
        4. Erythema multiforme
        5. Lupus erythematosus
        6. Drug induced
        7. Other
      b. Allergic reactions
        1. Dental restorative materials
          a. Mercury
          b. Nickel
          c. Acrylic
          d. Other
        2. Reactions attributable to
          a. Toothpastes/dentifrices
          b. Mouthrinses/mouthwashes
          c. Chewing gum additives
          d. Foods and additives
        3. Other
    6. Traumatic lesions (factitious, iatrogenic, accidental)
      a. Chemical injury
      b. Physical injury
      c. Thermal injury
    7. Foreign body reactions
    8. Not otherwise specified (NOS)

[a]Can occur on a periodontium with no attachment loss or on a periodontium with attachment loss that is not progressing.

Source: Armitage GC. Development of a classification system for periodontal diseases and conditions. *Ann Periodontol*. 1999;4(1):1–6.

TABLE 19-2	Classification of Gingival and Periodontal Diseases and Conditions: Periodontal Diseases

II. Chronic periodontitis
   A. Localized
   B. Generalized
III. Aggressive periodontitis
   A. Localized
   B. Generalized
IV. Periodontitis as a manifestation of systemic diseases
   A. Associated with hematological disorders
      1. Acquired neutropenia
      2. Leukemia
      3. Other
   B. Associated with genetic disorders
      1. Familial and cyclic neutropenia
      2. Down's syndrome
      3. Leukocyte adhesion deficiency syndromes
      4. Papillon–Lefévre syndrome
      5. Chediak–Higashi syndrome
      6. Histiocytosis syndromes
      7. Glycogen storage disease
      8. Infantile genetic agranulocytosis
      9. Cohen's syndrome
      10. Ehlers–Danlos syndrome (Types IV and VIII)
      11. Hypophosphatasia
      12. Other
   C. Not otherwise specified (NOS)
V. Necrotizing periodontal diseases
   A. Necrotizing ulcerative gingivitis
   B. Necrotizing ulcerative periodontitis
VI. Abscesses of the periodontium
   A. Gingival abscess
   B. Periodontal abscess
   C. Pericoronal abscess
VII. Periodontitis associated with endodontic lesions
   A. Combined periodontic–endodontic lesions

VIII. Developmental or acquired deformities and conditions
   A. Localized tooth-related factors that modify or predispose to plaque-induced gingival diseases or periodontitis
      1. Tooth anatomic factors
      2. Dental restorations/appliances
      3. Root fractures
      4. Cervical root resorption and cemental tears
   B. Mucogingival deformities and conditions around teeth
      1. Gingival/soft tissue recession
         a. Facial or lingual surfaces
         b. Interproximal (papillary)
      2. Lack of keratinized gingiva
      3. Decreased vestibular depth
      4. Aberrant frenum/muscle position
      5. Gingival excess
         a. Pseudopocket
         b. Inconsistent gingival margin
         c. Excessive gingival display
         d. Gingival enlargement
      6. Abnormal color
   C. Mucogingival deformities and conditions on edentulous ridges
      1. Vertical and/or horizontal ridge deficiency
      2. Lack of gingiva/keratinized tissue
      3. Gingival/soft tissue enlargement
      4. Aberrant frenum/muscle position
      5. Decreased vestibular depth
      6. Abnormal color
   D. Occlusal trauma
      1. Primary occlusal trauma
      2. Secondary occlusal trauma

Source: Armitage GC. Development of a classification system for periodontal diseases and conditions. *Ann Periodontol.* 1999;4(1);1–6.

V. Early Recognition of Tissue Changes

▶ Marked changes, such as moderate-to-severe generalized redness, enlargement, sponginess, deep pockets, and definite mobility, are relatively easy to detect even with limited experience, provided there is good light and accessibility for vision.

▶ In contrast, when changes are subtle, localized about one or a few teeth, and of a lesser degree of severity, more skillful application of knowledge is needed.

▶ *Risk assessment along with early recognition and treatment of* gingival and periodontal infections results in the following[3]:

   • Prevention of disease progression and more complex surgical treatment.

   • Response to nonsurgical periodontal therapy (NSPT) is more predictable, resulting in the ability to restore and maintain a healthy periodontium.

DETERMINATION OF PERIODONTAL CLASSIFICATION

▶ The patient history, risk assessment, clinical examination, radiographs, and other data from the assessment are put together to determine the initial diagnosis, which may range from gingivitis to advanced periodontitis.

EVERYDAY ETHICS

Basic records for Gloria, who was new to the office, were completed at a previous appointment. On her medical history form, Gloria had written "early diabetes" but did not supply the name and phone number of her current physician and said that she would bring it the next time. There were no radiographs taken at the initial appointment because Gloria said she had full X-rays taken less than a year ago and she would request them from her previous dentist. As she rushed out of the office, Gloria made her dental hygiene appointment for one week later during her lunch hour from work.

Gloria arrived late for her scheduled appointment and said she had to be back at work in less than 1 hour. Tina, the dental hygienist, asked if she had eaten and she hadn't; Tina hesitated knowing that a basic rule about patients with diabetes is to make sure that they have eaten prior to the dental appointment. The care plan for Gloria included four quadrants of NSPT with local anesthesia because of the significant amount of calculus and bleeding on probing, but Gloria refused the anesthesia. She also stated that her dental hygiene maintenance appointment needs to take one hour for the whole mouth as it had with the dental hygienist at her previous dental office.

In Tina's judgment treatment cannot be provided for the following reasons: (1) the radiographs had not yet arrived from the other dentist; (2) Dr. Nedham had not been in the office to approve the treatment plan; and (3) the short time the patient was allowing for Tina to complete NSPT was inadequate. Tina told Gloria that the appointment needed to be rescheduled for another day, but Gloria insisted her dental hygiene maintenance care be completed at this appointment.

Questions for Consideration

1. Which of the dental hygiene core values have application in this scenario? Explain how each of the ones selected apply.

2. Is this situation either an ethical issue or a dilemma for Tina? Explain your answer.

3. Use the questions in Table VI-1, Section VI Introduction to determine what different actions Tina could have taken at this appointment and to plan what she can do next regarding future planning for Gloria's dental hygiene care.

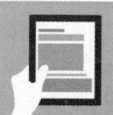

BOX 19-2

Example Documentation: Patient with Periodontal Disease

S –A 58-year-old male presents with chief complaint of painful bleeding gums. On the medical history the patient reports having Type 2 diabetes and hypertension. The patient takes Metformin and Cardizem. Patient indicates he smokes 1 pack/day and has smoked since he was 13 years old. He reports both his mother and father lost all their teeth because of gum disease.

O –Extraoral/intraoral findings were normal. Blood pressure: 120/80. Full mouth series of radiographs taken and reviewed. No new dental caries. A comprehensive periodontal examination reveals generalized 5–6 mm pocket depths with localized bleeding on probing. Radiograph reveals 3–4 mm of clinical attachment loss. No mobility with localized Grade I furcations involvement on the meso-lingual and disto-lingual of maxillary molars. The gingiva is pink and fibrotic with bulbous interdental papillae throughout. Generalized heavy supragingival and subgingival calculus. Dental biofilm score 40%.

A –The diagnosis is generalized moderate chronic periodontitis. Recommended patient return for four appointments of NSPT using local anesthesia followed by a re-evaluation in 4–6 weeks.

P –Patient education about the risk factors for periodontal disease present including biofilm, genetic history of periodontal disease, diabetes, and tobacco use. The patient is interested in tobacco cessation and was referred to the state quit line and his primary care provider. Oral self-care was reviewed with a soft toothbrush and floss. The patient had a difficult time manipulating the floss, so he was given floss picks to try and seemed to do well and like them. Next visit: Begin NSPT maxillary right quadrant and review oral self-care. Follow-up about progress on tobacco cessation.

Signed _____, RDH

Date _____

► Except in cases of advanced periodontitis, the need for additional treatment after initial non-surgical periodontal therapy (NSPT) is difficult to predict.
  • Re-evaluation following initial NSPT is built into the care plan.
  • At the outset, the patient is given a clear understanding of the purpose of such a re-evaluation.
► The classification of gingival and periodontal diseases is included in Tables 19-1 and 19-2.

DOCUMENTATION

Documentation for a patient with need for periodontal therapy includes at least the following in the patient's permanent record along with radiographs, physician's approvals for therapy, and other correspondence of record.

► Initially a complete history: medical, dental, former periodontal therapy, current symptoms and current complaint or problem, and clinical examination with charting of periodontal findings and of the teeth; summary of prognosis and diagnosis.

► At each appointment a complete record of treatment accomplished, and patient instruction, oral findings, and changes on the way to health.

► A sample progress note may be reviewed in Box 19-2.

Factors To Teach The Patient

▷ Educate the patient about the connections between periodontal disease and systemic disease related to the patient's medical history.
▷ Describe the risk factors that put the patient at risk for periodontal disease and assist the patient in identifying ways to manage the modifiable risk factors.
▷ Explain what a normal sulcus is versus a diseased periodontal pocket.
▷ Explain the need for a comprehensive periodontal examination to assess the extent and severity of disease.
▷ Clarify the need for adequate oral self-care and continuing care to prevent or manage periodontal disease (infection).

References

1. Linden GJ, Lyons A, Scannapieco FA. Periodontal systemic associations: review of the evidence. *J Periodontol.* 2013;84(4, Suppl):S8–S19.
2. Van Dyke TE, van Winkelhoff AJ. Infection and inflammatory mechanisms. *J Periodontol.* 2013;84(4, Suppl):S1–S7.
3. Douglass CW. Risk assessment and management of periodontal disease. *J Am Dent Assoc.* 2006;137, Suppl:27S–32S.
4. American Academy of Periodontology. American Academy of Periodontology statement on risk assessment. *J Periodontol.* 2008;79(2):202.
5. Page RC, Krall EA, Martin J, et al. Validity and accuracy of a risk calculator in predicting periodontal disease. *J Am Dent Assoc.* 2002;133(5):569–576.
6. Page RC, Martin J, Krall EA, et al. Longitudinal validation of a risk calculator for periodontal disease. *J Clin Periodontol.* 2003;30(9):819–827.
7. Lang NP, Tonetti MS. Periodontal risk assessment (PRA) for patients in supportive periodontal therapy (SPT). *Oral Health Prev Dent.* 2003;1(1):7–16.
8. Dentino A, Lee S, Mailhot J, et al. Principles of periodontology. *Periodontol 2000.* 2013;61(1):16–53.
9. Armitage GC, Robertson PB. The biology, prevention, diagnosis and treatment of periodontal diseases: scientific advances in the United States. *J Am Dent Assoc.* 2009;140 (Suppl 1):36S–43S.
10. Van Dyke TE, Sheilesh D. Risk factors for periodontitis. *J Int Acad Periodontol.* 2005;7(1):3–7.
11. Anand PS, Kamath KP, Bansal A, et al. Comparison of periodontal destruction patterns among patients with and without the habit of smokeless tobacco use—a retrospective study. *J Periodontal Res.* 2013;48(5):623–631.
12. Page RC, Schroeder HE. Pathogenesis of inflammatory periodontal disease. A summary of current work. *Lab Invest.* 1976;34(3):235–249.
13. Huynh-Ba G, Kuonen P, Hofer D, et al. The effect of periodontal therapy on the survival rate and incidence of complications of multirooted teeth with furcation involvement after an observation period of at least 5 years: a systematic review. *J Clin Periodontol.* 2009;36(2):164–176.
14. Freedman AL, Green K, Salkin LM, et al. An 18-year longitudinal study of untreated mucogingival defects. *J Periodontol.* 1999;70(10):1174–1176.
15. Armitage GC. Development of a classification system for periodontal diseases and conditions. *Ann Periodontol.* 1999;4(1):1–6.
16. Flemmig TF. Periodontitis. *Ann Periodontol.* 1999;4(1):32–38.
17. Armitage GC. Periodontal diagnoses and classification of periodontal diseases. *Periodontol 2000.* 2004;34:9–21.

ENHANCE YOUR UNDERSTANDING

thePoint® DIGITAL CONNECTIONS
(see the inside front cover for access information)
• **Audio glossary**
• **Quiz bank**

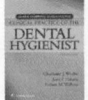

SUPPORT FOR LEARNING
(available separately; visit lww.com)
• *Active Learning Workbook for Clinical Practice of the Dental Hygienist, 12th Edition*

prepU INDIVIDUALIZED REVIEW
(available separately; visit lww.com)
• **Adaptive quizzing with *prepU for Wilkins' Clinical Practice of the Dental Hygienist***

20

Periodontal Examination

Linda D. Boyd, RDH, RD, EdD and Esther M. Wilkins, BS, RDH, DMD

CHAPTER OUTLINE

LEARNING OBJECTIVES

After studying this chapter, the student will be able to:

1. Describe the components of a comprehensive periodontal examination.

2. List the instruments used for a periodontal examination.

3. Explain the technique for use of the periodontal probe and explorers.

4. Explain how procedure for the comprehensive examination will be described to the patient.

BASIC INSTRUMENTS FOR EXAMINATION

▶ Parts of the dental and periodontal clinical examinations are made by direct visual observation, whereas other parts require *tactile* examination using a probe and/or an explorer.

• These two types of instruments, assisted by a mouth mirror, are key instruments in patient examination and assessment. Considerable skill is required for accurate and efficient probing and exploring.

▶ Cassette arrangements for all patients with permanent teeth need a basic setup composed of at least a mouth mirror, probes including a furcation probe, a plastic probe when dental implants are present, and a subgingival explorer.

▶ General principles of instrumentation are described in Chapter 39. Box 20-1 contains definitions for key words associated with this chapter.

THE MOUTH MIRROR

I. Description

A. Parts

The mirror has three parts: the handle, shank, and working end, which is the mounted mirror or mirror head.

B. Types of Mirror Surfaces

▶ *Plane (flat)*: may produce a double image.

▶ *Concave*: magnifying.

▶ *Front surface*: the reflecting surface is on the front of the lens rather than on the back as with plane or magnifying mirrors. The front surface eliminates "ghost" images. Also available is a double-sided mirror head.

C. Diameters

▶ Mirror diameters vary from 5/8 to 1 1/4 inches. In addition, special examination mirrors are available in 1½- to 2-inch diameters.

D. Attachments

▶ Mirrors may be threaded plain stem or cone socket joined to a handle.

▶ Because mirrors tend to become scratched, replacement of the working end is possible without purchasing new handles.

E. Handles

▶ Thicker handles contribute to a more ergonomically comfortable grasp and greater control.

▶ Light weight handles help decrease fatigue.

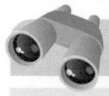

BOX 20-1   KEY WORDS: Periodontal Examination

Calibration: determination of the accuracy of an instrument by measurement of its variation from a standard.

Clinical attachment level (CAL): Probing depth (PD) as measured from the cementoenamel junction (CEJ) (or other fixed point) to the location of the probe tip at the coronal level of attached periodontal tissues.

Explorer: an instrument with a fine flexible, sharp point used for examination of the surfaces of the teeth to detect irregularities.

Fremitus: a vibration perceptible by palpation.

Periodontometer: instrument used to measure mobility.

Periodontal Probe: instrument with a rounded tip calibrated in millimeter increments to facilitate measurement of the pocket depth.

Probing depth (PD): the distance from the gingival margin (GM) to the location of the periodontal probe tip at the base of the sulcus.

Tactile: pertaining to the touch.

Tactile discrimination: the ability to distinguish relative degrees of roughness and smoothness, for example, on a tooth surface, using an explorer or a periodontal probe; also called tactile sensitivity.

Tension test: application of tension at the mucogingival junction (MGJ) by retracting cheek, lip, and tongue to tighten the alveolar mucosa and test for the presence of attached gingiva; area of missing attached gingiva is revealed when the alveolar mucosa and frena are connected directly to the free gingiva.

F. Disposable Mirrors

▶ Plastic mirrors can be useful for screening or other short examination procedures.

▶ Take-home mirrors for patient instruction. Patient may observe lingual and posterior aspects where biofilm may be difficult to remove.

II. Purposes and Uses

A mouth mirror is used to provide indirect vision, indirect illumination, transillumination, and retraction.

A. Indirect Vision

▶ Needed for all surfaces where direct vision is not possible.

▶ Examples are the distal surfaces of posterior teeth and lingual surfaces of anterior teeth.

B. Indirect Illumination

▶ Reflection of light from the dental overhead light or headlamp worn by the clinician to any area of the oral cavity can be accomplished by adapting the mirror.

C. Transillumination

▶ Transillumination refers to reflection of light through the teeth.

▶ Mirror is held to reflect light from the lingual aspect while the teeth are examined from the facial.

▶ Mirror is held for indirect vision on the lingual while light from the overhead dental light passes through the teeth. Translucency of enamel can be seen clearly, whereas dental caries or calculus deposits appear opaque.

D. Retraction

▶ The mirror is used to protect or prevent interference by the cheeks, tongue, or lips.

III. Procedure for Use

A. Grasp and Rest

▶ Use modified pen grasp with finger rest on a tooth surface near the working area.

▶ Provides stability and control.

▶ Assists in retraction of lips and cheek.

▶ Exercises for gaining skill in control of instruments are described in Chapter 39.

B. Retraction

▶ Use a thin layer of water-based lubricant on dry or cracked lips and corners of mouth.

▶ Adjust the mirror position so the angles of the mouth are protected from the undue pressure of the shank of the mirror.

▶ Insert and remove mirror carefully to avoid hitting the teeth because this can be uncomfortable for the patient.

C. Maintain Clear Vision

▶ Warm mirror with water; rub along buccal mucosa to coat mirror with thin transparent film of saliva.

▶ Request patient breathe through the nose to prevent condensation of moisture on the mirror.

IV. Care of Mirrors

▶ Examine carefully the mirror face after ultrasonic cleaning before sterilization to ensure removal of debris around back, shank, and rim of reflecting surface.

▶ Handle carefully during sterilization procedures to prevent other instruments from scratching the reflecting surface.

▶ Consult manufacturer's specifications for sterilizing or disinfecting procedures that may cloud the mirror, particularly the front surface type.

▶ Discard scratched mirrors.

AIR–WATER SYRINGE

I. Purposes and Uses

With appropriate, timely application of air to clear saliva and debris and/or dry the tooth surfaces, the following can be accomplished:

A. Improve and Facilitate Examination Procedures

▶ Make a thorough, more accurate examination.

▶ Dry supragingival calculus to facilitate exploring and scaling.
  • Small deposits may be light in color and not visible until they are dried.
  • Dried calculus appears chalky and presents a contrast to tooth color.

▶ Deflect the free gingival margin (GM) for observation into the subgingival area. Subgingival calculus usually appears darker than supragingival calculus.

▶ Identify areas of demineralization and carious lesions easier.

▶ Recognize location and condition of restorations, particularly tooth-color restorations.

B. Improve Visibility of the Treatment Area During Instrumentation

▶ Dry area for finger rest to provide stability during instrumentation.

▶ Facilitate positive effective scaling techniques.

▶ Minimize appointment time.

▶ Evaluate complete removal of supragingival calculus.

C. Prepare Teeth and/or Gingiva for Certain Procedures

▶ Examples are to dry surfaces for:
- Application of caries-preventive agents when indicated.
- Preparation to make impression for study model.
- Application of topical anesthetic.

II. Compressed Air Syringe

A. Description

▶ *Air source*: Air compressor with tubing attachment to syringe.

▶ *Air tip*: Has angled working end that can be turned for maxillary or mandibular application. Tip needs to be disposable or removable for sterilization.

B. Procedure for Use

▶ Use palm grasp around the handle of the syringe; place thumb on release lever or on button to activate air.

▶ Test the air flow before using in the mouth so the strength of flow can be controlled.

▶ Make controlled, relatively short, gentle applications of air.

▶ Supplement air drying with use of saliva ejector and folded gauze sponge placed in vestibule.

C. Precautions

▶ Avoid sharp blasts of air on sensitive cervical areas of teeth or open carious lesions. Such areas may be dried by blotting with a gauze sponge or cotton roll to avoid patient discomfort.

▶ Avoid forceful application of air, which can direct saliva and debris out of the oral cavity, contaminate the working area and clinician, and create aerosols.

▶ Air directed toward the posterior region of the patient's mouth may cause coughing.

▶ Avoid startling the patient; give a warning when air is to be applied.

EXPLORERS

I. General Purposes and Uses

An explorer is used for the following:

A. Detect, by Tactile Sense, the Texture and Character of the Tooth Surfaces

▶ For calculus defects or irregularities in the surfaces and margins of restorations, and other irregularities not apparent to direct observation.

▶ An explorer is used to confirm direct observation. Avoid use of an explorer on white spot lesions (demineralized tooth surfaces that can be remineralized).

B. Define the Extent of Instrumentation Needed and Guide Techniques

▶ For scaling and root planing.

▶ Removing an overhanging filling.

C. Evaluate the Completeness of Treatment

▶ For periodontal nonsurgical treatment as shown by the smooth tooth surface.

▶ For removal of an overhanging filling by the smooth margins of the restoration.

II. Description

A. Working End

▶ Slender, wirelike, metal *tip* that is circular in cross section and tapers to a fine sharp *point*.

▶ Design
- *Single*: A single instrument may be universal and adaptable to any tooth surface, or it may be designed for specific groups of surfaces. In Figure 20-1, Nos. 2 through 7, 17, 18, 20, and 23 are single instruments.
- *Paired*: Paired instruments are mirror images of each other, curved to provide access to contralateral tooth

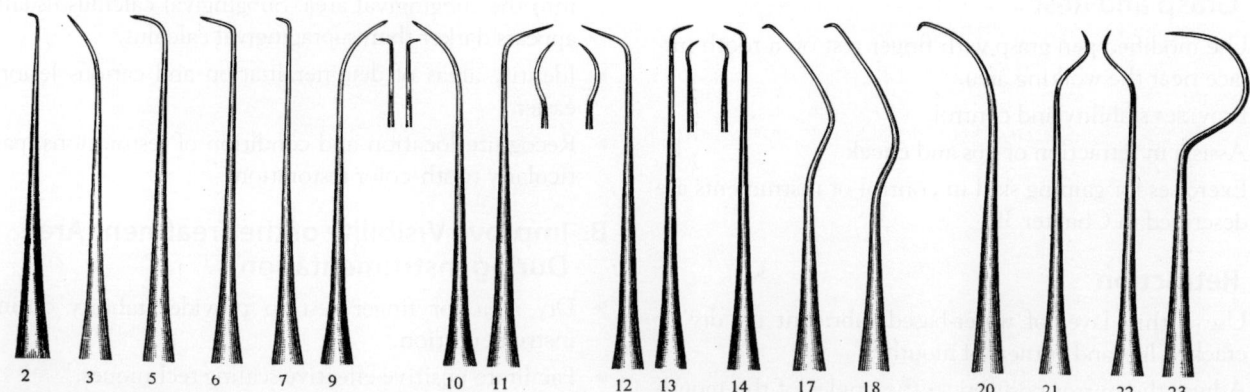

FIGURE 20-1 Explorers. This series from Nos. 2 through 23 shows standard shapes of explorer tips. Nos. 2 through 7, 17, 18, 20, and 23 are single instruments. Nos. 9 and 10, 11 and 12, 13 and 14, and 21 and 22 are paired instruments. (Courtesy of the S.S. White Company, Philadelphia, PA.)

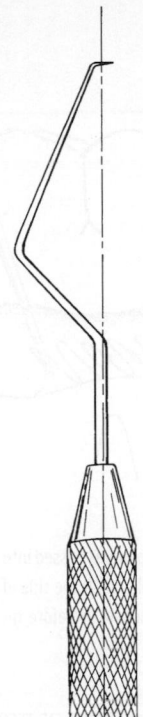

FIGURE 20-2 Balanced Explorer Design. With the middle of the tip centered over the long axis of the handle (shown by broken line from tip), the explorer can be positioned in a sulcus or pocket with ease and does not cause trauma to the gingival tissue. Shown is the balanced TU-17 explorer.

surfaces. In Figure 20-1, Nos. 9 and 10, 11 and 12, 13 and 14, and 21 and 22 are paired.

- *Design of a balanced instrument:* Middle of the working end is centered over the long axis of the handle (Figure 20-2).

B. Shank

- *Straight, curved, or angulated:* Whether a shank is straight, curved, or angulated depends on the use and adaptation for which the explorer was designed.
  - In Figure 20-1, compare the straight shanks of Nos. 2, 5, 6, 7, 13, and 14 with the others in the series, which are not straight.
  - A curved shank may facilitate application of the instrument to proximal surfaces, particularly of posterior teeth.
- *Flexibility:* The slender, wirelike explorers have a degree of flexibility that contributes to increased tactile sensitivity for the clinician.

C. Handle

- *Weight:* For increased tactile sensitivity, a lightweight handle is more effective.
- *Diameter:* A wider diameter with serrations for friction while grasping can prevent finger cramping from too tight a grasp. With a lighter grasp, tactile sensitivity is increased.

D. Construction

- *Single-ended:* A single-ended instrument has one working end on a separate handle.
- *Double-ended:* A double-ended instrument has two working ends, one on each end of a common handle.
  - Most paired instruments are available double ended.
  - Other double-ended instruments combine two single instruments, for example, two unpaired explorers or an explorer with a probe.

III. Preparation of Explorers

- Sharpen and retaper a dull explorer tip.
- With the explorer tip sharp and tapered, the following can be expected:
  - Increased tactile sensitivity with less pressure required.
  - Prevention of unnecessary trauma to the gingival tissue, because less pressure allows greater control.
  - Decreased instrumentation time with increased patient comfort.

IV. Specific Explorers and Their Uses

- A variety of explorers is available, as shown by the examples in Figure 20-1.
- The function of each type is related to its adaptability to specific surfaces of teeth at particular angulations.
  - Certain explorers are used for detection of occlusal dental caries such as No. 23.
  - Others are designed to be adapted to examine proximal surfaces for calculus or dental caries.
  - Certain ones are designed for subgingival use, such as ODU 11/12, whereas others cannot be adapted subgingivally without inflicting damage to the sulcular epithelium.

A. Explorers for Deep Pockets and Inside Furcations

- Several explorers designed for very deep pockets and inside furcation areas are in current use.
- Examples: Orban 20; TU-17; No. 3 (shown in Figure 20-1); ODU 11/12 designed like Gracey 11/12 curet.

B. Subgingival Explorer: The Pocket Explorer

- *Shape:* The pocket explorer has an angulated shank with a short tip (Figure 20-2). The tip can be measured to ensure that it is less than 2 mm. A longer tip cannot be adapted to the line angles of narrow roots.
- *Features for subgingival root examination*
  - Back of tip can be applied directly to the attached periodontal tissue at the base of the pocket without lacerating, as shown in Figure 20-3.
  - The short tip can be adapted to rounded tooth surfaces and line angles.

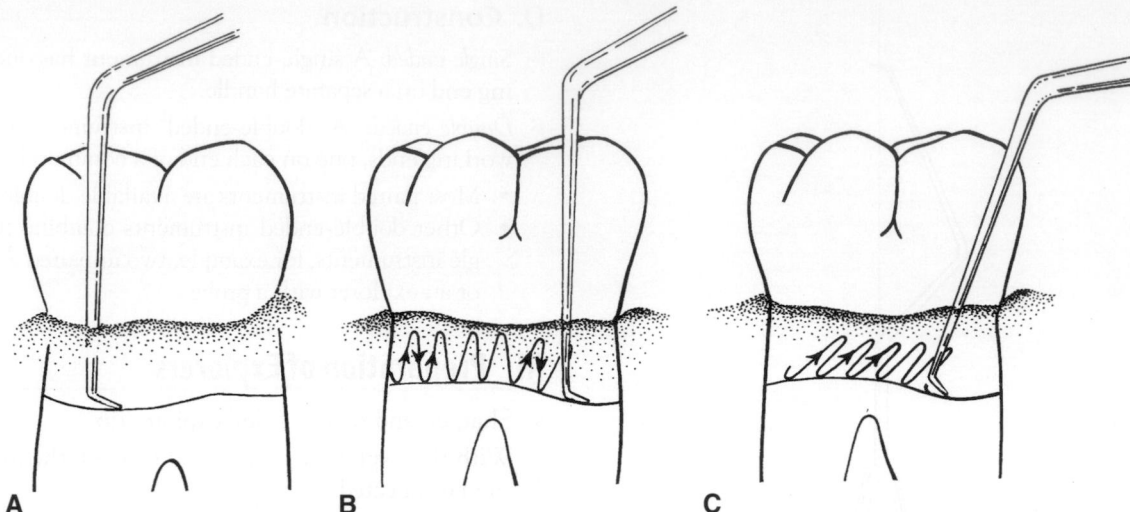

FIGURE 20-3 Use of Subgingival Explorer. A: The lower shank (next to tip) is held parallel with the long axis of the tooth. The explorer is passed into the pocket and lowered until the back of the working tip meets resistance from the attached periodontal tissue at the base of the pocket. **B:** Vertical walking stroke. With the side of the tip in contact with the tooth surface at all times, the explorer is moved over the surface. **C:** Diagonal walking stroke. Complete exploration of the surface is needed; therefore, groups of strokes are overlapped.

- Narrow short tip can be adapted at the base where the pocket narrows without undue displacement of the pocket soft tissue wall.
▶ *Supragingival use of No. TU-17:* It may be adapted to all surfaces and is especially useful for proximal surface examination. It is not adaptable to pits and fissures.

C. Sickle or Shepherd's Hook (No. 23 in Figure 20-1)

▶ *Use:* examining pits and fissures and supragingival smooth surfaces; examining surfaces and margins of restorations and sealants.
▶ *Adaptability*
  - Difficult to apply to proximal surfaces because the wide hook may contact an adjacent tooth and the straight long section of the tip can pass over a small proximal carious lesion.
  - Not adaptable for deep subgingival exploration. When the point is directed to the base of a pocket, trauma to the attachment area can result.

D. Pigtail or Cowhorn (Nos. 21 and 22 in Figure 20-1)

▶ *Use:* proximal surfaces for calculus, dental caries, or margins of restorations.
▶ *Adaptability:* as paired, curved tips, they are applied to opposite tooth surfaces.

BASIC PROCEDURES FOR USE OF EXPLORERS

▶ Development of ability to use an explorer and a probe is achieved first by learning the anatomic features of each

tooth surface and the types of irregularities that may be encountered on the surfaces.
▶ The second step is repeated practice of techniques for application of the instruments.
▶ The objective is to adapt the instruments in a routine manner that relays consistent comparative information about the nature of the tooth surface.
▶ Concentration, patience, attention to detail, and alertness to each irregularity, however small it may seem, are necessary.

I. Use of Sensory Stimuli

▶ Both explorers and probes can transmit tactile stimuli from tooth surfaces to the fingers.
▶ A fine explorer usually gives a more acute sense of tactile discrimination to small irregularities than does a thicker explorer.
▶ Periodontal probes vary in diameter; the narrow types may provide greater sensitivity.

II. Tooth Surface Irregularities

▶ Three basic tactile sensations can be distinguished when probing or exploring.
▶ These may be grouped as:
  - Normal tooth surface.
  - Irregularities created by excess or elevations in the surface.
  - Irregularities caused by depressions in the tooth surface.

Examples of these are listed below.

A. Normal

▶ *Tooth structure:* the smooth surface of enamel and root surface; anatomic configurations, such as cingula or furcations.

▶ *Restored surfaces*: smooth surfaces of metal (gold, amalgam) versus the feeling of composite; smooth margin of a restoration.

B. Irregularities: Increases or Elevations in Tooth Surface

▶ *Deposits*: calculus.

▶ *Anomalies*: enamel pearl.

▶ *Restorations*: overcontoured, irregular margins (overhangs).

C. Irregularities: Depressions, Grooves

▶ *Tooth surface*: demineralized or carious lesion, abrasion, erosion, pits such as those caused by enamel hypoplasia, areas of cemental resorption on the root surface.

▶ *Restorations*: deficient margin, rough surface.

III. Types of Stimuli

During exploring and probing, distinction of irregularities can be made through auditory and tactile means.

A. Tactile

▶ Tactile sensations pass through the instrument to the fingers and hand and to the brain for registration and action.

▶ Tactile sensations, for example, may be the result of catching on an overcontoured restoration, dropping into a carious lesion, encountering an elevated deposit, or simply passing over a rough surface.

B. Auditory

▶ As an explorer or a probe moves over the surface of enamel, cementum, a metallic restoration, a plastic restoration, or any irregularity of tooth structure or restoration, a difference in texture is apparent. With each contact, sound may be created.

▶ The clean smooth enamel is quiet; the rough cementum or calculus is scratchy or noisy. Sometimes a metallic restoration may "squeak" or have a metallic "ring." With experience, differentiations can be detected.

EXPLORERS: SUPRAGINGIVAL PROCEDURES

I. Use of Vision

▶ Supragingival exploration for defects of the tooth surface differs from subgingival in that when a surface is dried, much of the actual exploration is performed to confirm visual observation.

▶ The exceptions are the proximal areas near and around contact areas that cannot be directly observed.

▶ Unnecessary exploration can be avoided with adequate light and air, proper retraction, and use of a mouth mirror.

• For example, dried supragingival calculus can generally be seen as either chalky white or brownish-yellow in contrast to tooth color.

II. Facial and Lingual Surfaces

▶ Adapt the tip so the side of the point is always on the tooth surface.

▶ Move the instrument in short walking strokes over the surface being examined, or direct the side of the tip gently over a suspected carious lesion.

▶ An intact surface where remineralization can be going on must not be vigorously explored. Careful noninvasive examination can be made using the side of the tip of a probe gently to test whether the demineralized area has slight roughness. As described in Chapter 27, picking or scratching the surface can result in cavitation which requires restoration.

III. Proximal Surfaces

▶ Lead with the tip onto a proximal surface, rolling the handle between the fingers to ensure adaptation around the line angle. Keep the side of the point of the explorer in contact with the tooth surface at all times.

▶ Explore under the proximal contact area when there is recession of the papilla and the area is exposed. Overlap strokes from facial and lingual surfaces to ensure full coverage.

EXPLORERS: SUBGINGIVAL PROCEDURES

I. Essentials for Detection of Tooth Surface Irregularities

▶ Light grasp.

▶ Consistent finger rest with light pressure.

▶ Keep the side of the explorer tip in contact with the tooth.

▶ Light touch as the instrument is moved over the tooth surface.

II. Steps for Use of the Subgingival Explorer (Figure 20-3)

1. With the tip in contact with the tooth supragingivally, hold the lower shank (the part of the shank that is next to the tip) parallel with the long axis of the tooth.
2. Gently slide the tip under the GM into the sulcus or pocket.
3. Keep the lateral border of the point in contact with the tooth at all times to prevent unnecessary trauma to the pocket or sulcular epithelium. Adapt the tip closely to the tooth surface by applying the side of the point.
4. Slide the explorer tip over the tooth surface to the base of the pocket until, with the back of the tip, the

resistance of the soft tissue of the attached periodontal tissue is felt (Figure 20-3A).

5. Calculus deposits may obstruct direct passage of the instrument to the base of the pocket. Lift the tip slightly away from the tooth surface and explore over the deposit to proceed to the base of the pocket.

6. Use a "walking" stroke (Figure 20-3B).

7. Lead with the tip. Move it ahead as the instrument progresses.

8. Length of stroke depends on the depth of a pocket.
   - Shallow sulcus: The stroke may extend the entire depth.
   - Deep pocket: Controlled strokes 2- to 3-mm long can allow improved adaptation of the instrument.
   - Explore a deep pocket in sections. First explore the apical area next to the base of the pocket, then move up to a higher section.

9. Do not remove the explorer from the pocket for each stroke on a particular surface because
   - Trauma to the GM caused by repeated withdrawal and reinsertion can cause the patient posttreatment discomfort.
   - Concentration on the texture of the tooth surface is interrupted.

10. Proximal surface.
   - Lead with tip of instrument; do not "back into" an area.

11. Continue the strokes around the line angle. Roll the instrument handle between the fingers to keep the tip closely adapted as the tooth contour changes.

12. Continue strokes under the contact area. Overlap strokes from facial and lingual aspects for full coverage.

PERIODONTAL PROBE

- Early in the patient examination, the patient's periodontal disease status is determined. The probe determinations provide major information for determining disease status of the periodontal tissues.

- Treatment planning varies depending on whether the condition is gingivitis, which may be reversible, or periodontitis with periodontal pockets, bone loss, and root surface involvement, which require more extensive therapy.

I. Types of Probes

- Two general types of probes available are the traditional or standard manual probes and the controlled force or automated probes.

- Standard or traditional probes include the following:
  - Probes with colored markings in millimeter increments from 1 to 3 (see Figure 20-4).

- Plastic probes for assessing the health of dental implants.
- Probes specifically designed to assess furcation areas with and without colored millimeter markings, such as the Nabers probe (see Figure 20-5).

- Automated probes were developed and researched in an attempt to overcome the problems in obtaining consistent readings with traditional probes.

II. Purposes and Uses

A probe is used for the following purposes:

A. Assess the Periodontal Status for Preparation of a Treatment Plan

- Classify the disease as gingivitis or periodontitis by determining whether bone loss has occurred and whether the pockets are gingival or periodontal.
  - A systematic screening method can be used such as the periodontal screening record (PSR). The PSR is described in Chapter 23.

- Determine the extent of inflammation in conjunction with the overall gingival examination. Bleeding on probing (BOP) is an early sign of inflammation in the gingiva.

B. Make a Sulcus and Pocket Survey

- Examine the shape, topography, and dimensions of sulci and pockets.
- Measure and record probing depths (PDs).
- Evaluate tooth-surface pocket wall.
- Chart calculus location and severity.
- Record other root surface irregularities discerned by the probe.

C. Determine Clinical Attachment Level (CAL)

- Determination of the CAL is described later in this chapter (see Figure 20-13).

D. Conduct Mucogingival Examination

- Determine relationship of GM, attachment level, mucogingival junction (MGJ), and frena (Figure 18-7, in Chapter 18).

E. Make Other Gingival Determinations

- Evaluate bleeding on probing (BOP) and prepare a gingival bleeding index.
- Measure gingival recession.
- Determine the consistency of the gingival tissue.

F. Guide Treatment

- Summarize gingival characteristics, including PD, bleeding, and consistency (all determined using a probe), to provide a basis for patient instruction as part of the total treatment.

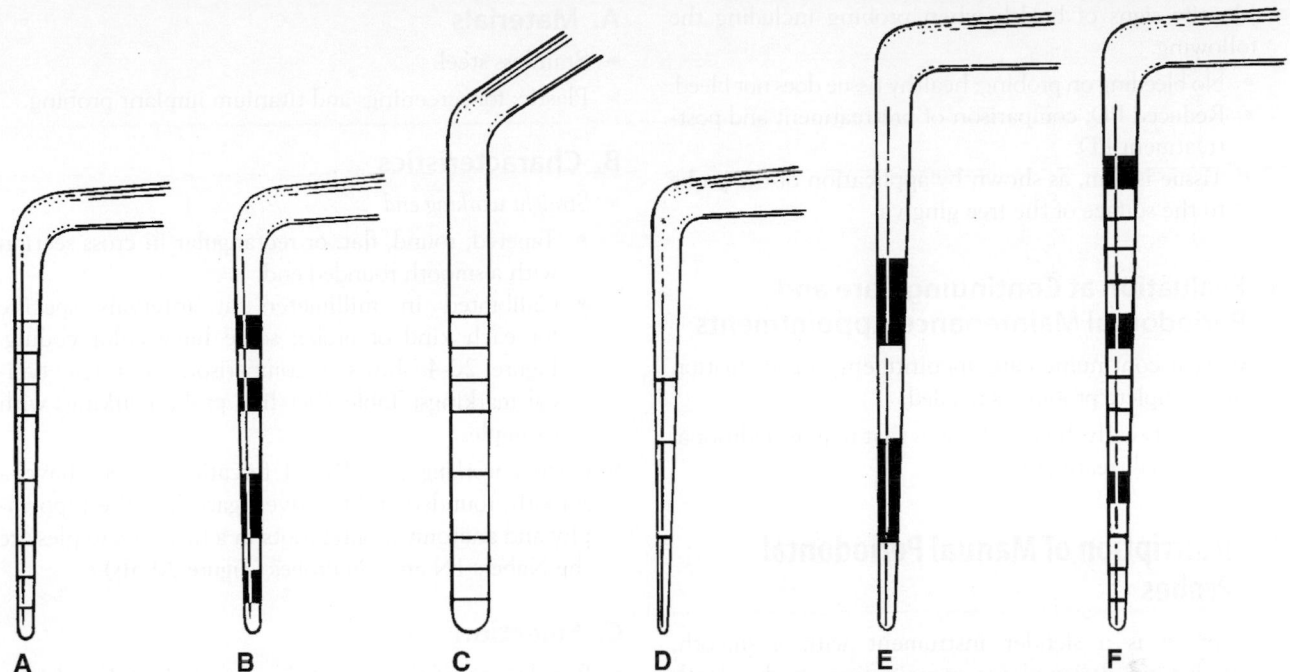

FIGURE 20-4 Examples of Probes. Names and calibrated markings shown are **A:** Williams (1-1-1-2-2-1-1-1), **B:** Williams, color-coded, **C:** Goldman-Fox (1-1-1-2-2-1-1-1), **D:** Michigan O (3-3-2), **E:** Hu-Friedy or Marquis color-coded (3-3-3-3 or 3-3-2-3), and **F:** Hu-Friedy UNC 15 (each millimeter to 15), color coded at 5-10-15. See Table 20-1 for additional data on probes.

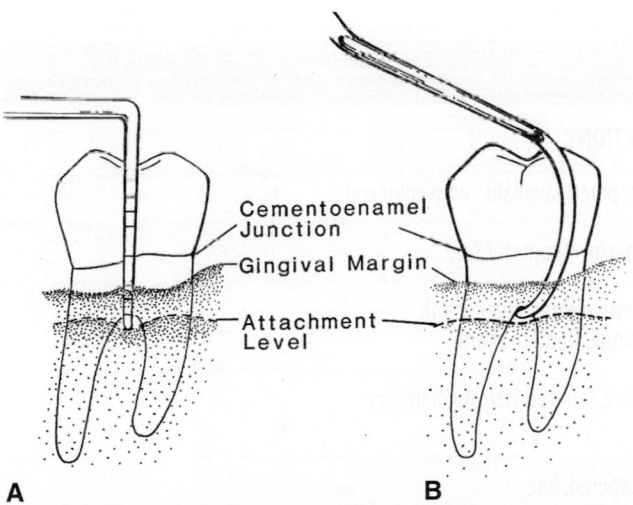

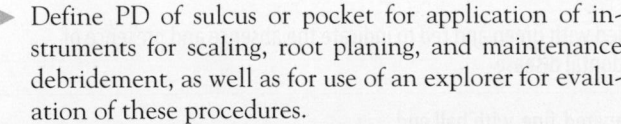

FIGURE 20-5 Furcation Examination. A: Limited access of a straight probe to examine a furcation. Williams probe inserted into bifurcation in area of gingival recession shows PD of 3 mm. **B:** Naber's furcation probe used to examine the topography of the furcation area.

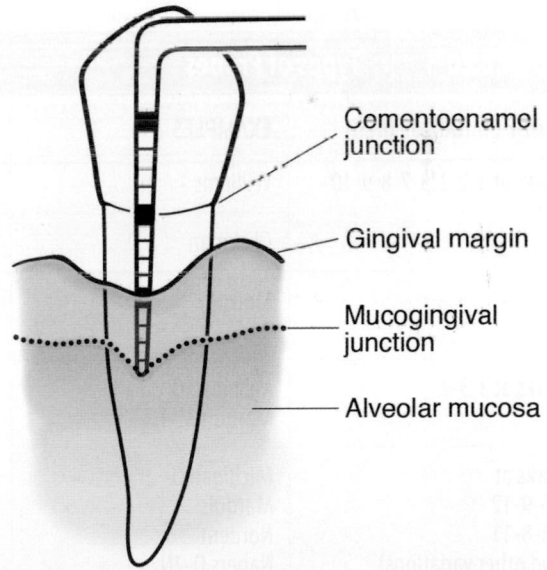

FIGURE 20-6 Mucogingival Examination. Probe in position for measuring PD where attached gingiva is missing. The absence of attached gingiva permits the probe to pass through the MGJ into the alveolar mucosa.

▶ Define PD of sulcus or pocket for application of instruments for scaling, root planing, and maintenance debridement, as well as for use of an explorer for evaluation of these procedures.

▶ Detect anatomic configuration of roots, subgingival deposits, and root irregularities that complicate instrumentation. For this, the probe is used in conjunction with the explorer.

G. Evaluate Success and Completeness of Treatment

▶ Evaluate posttreatment tissue response to professional treatment on an immediate, short-term basis, as well as at periodic maintenance examinations.

▶ Evaluate patient's oral self-care.

▶ Identify signs of health when probing including the following:
  - No bleeding on probing; healthy tissue does not bleed.
  - Reduced PD; comparison of pretreatment and post-treatment PD.
  - Tissue is firm, as shown by application of the probe to the surface of the free gingiva.

H. Evaluation at Continuing Care and Periodontal Maintenance Appointments

▶ At each continuing care appointment, a reevaluation with complete probing is needed.
▶ To identify early disease changes that require additional professional treatment.

III. Description of Manual Periodontal Probes

▶ A probe is a slender instrument with a smooth, rounded tip designed for examination of the depth and topography of a gingival sulcus or periodontal pocket.
▶ A probe has three parts: the handle, the angled shank, and the working end, which is the probe itself.

A. Materials

▶ Stainless steel.
▶ Plastic: for screenings and titanium implant probing.

B. Characteristics

▶ *Straight working end*
  - Tapered, round, flat, or rectangular in cross section with a smooth rounded end.
  - Calibrated in millimeters at intervals specific for each kind of probe; some have color coding. Figure 20-4 shows a comparison of a few typical markings; Table 20-1 lists probe markings with examples.
▶ *Curved working end:* Paired furcation probes have a smooth, rounded end for investigation of the topography and anatomy around roots in a furca. Examples are the Nabers 1N and 2N probes (Figure 20-5B).

C. Selection

▶ Regular use of the same type of periodontal probe results in greater consistency of readings.
▶ Analysis of a periodontal probe and comparison with other probes are recommended. Important features to be considered in probe selection are:

TABLE 20-1	Types of Probes	
PROBE MARKINGS (MM)	**EXAMPLES**	**DESCRIPTION**
Marks at 1-2-3-5-7-8-9-10	Williams	Round, tapered (available with color code)
	Glickman	Round, narrow diameter, fine
	Merritt B	Round, with longer lower shank Round, single bend to shank
Marks at 3-3-2	Michigan O Marquis M-1	Round, fine, tapered, narrow diameter
Marks at 3-6-9-12 3-6-8-11 (and other variations)	Michigan O Marquis Nordent Nabers Q-2N	Round, tapered, fine Color coded
Marks at each mm to 15	UNC 15	Round Color-coded at 5-10-15
Marks at 3-5-7-10	Perioscreen®	Round Color coded with green and red to indicate the absence and presence of periodontal disease
Marks at 3.5-5.5-8.5-11.5	WHO Probe (World Health Organization) (Figure 23-7)	Round, tapered, fine, with ball end Color coded
No marks	Nabers 1N, 2N	Curved, with curved shank for furcation examination

- *Adaptability*: The probe needs to be adaptable around the complete circumference of each tooth, both posterior and anterior, so that no millimeter area of the sulcus can be neglected. Flat probes require more attention to adaptation and are useful primarily on facial and lingual surfaces.
- *Markings*: Markings need to be easy to read so pocket depth (PD) can be readily identified and measured, and no disease area is overlooked. Color coding contributes to readability.

GUIDE TO PROBING

A pocket is a diseased gingival sulcus. The use of a probe is the only accurate, dependable method to locate, assess, and measure sulci and pockets.

I. Pocket Characteristics

- ▶ A pocket is measured from the base of the pocket (top of attached periodontal tissue) to the gingival margin (GM). Figure 20-7 shows two PDs beneath GMs that are at the same level.
- ▶ The pocket (or sulcus) is continuous around the entire tooth and the entire pocket or sulcus needs to be measured. "Spot" probing is inadequate for a thorough assessment for diagnosis and treatment planning.
- ▶ The depth varies around an individual tooth; PD rarely measures the same all around a tooth or even around one surface of a tooth.
  - The level of attached tissue assumes a varying position around the tooth.
  - The GM varies in its position on the tooth.
- ▶ Proximal surfaces are approached by entering from both the facial and lingual aspects of a tooth.

- Gingival and periodontal infections begin in the col area more frequently than in other areas (col area, Figure 18-6 in Chapter 18).
- PD may be deepest directly under the contact area because of crater formation in the alveolar bone (Figure 20-8).

▶ Anatomic features of the tooth surface wall of the pocket influence the direction of probing. Examples are concave surfaces, anomalies, shape of cervical third, and position of furcations.

II. Evaluation of Tooth Surface

- ▶ During the movement of the probe, calculus, and tooth surface irregularities can be felt and evaluated.
- ▶ The information obtained is used to plan the scaling and root planing appointments.

III. Factors that Affect Probe Determinations

- ▶ The general objectives of probing are accuracy and consistency so recordings are dependable for comparison

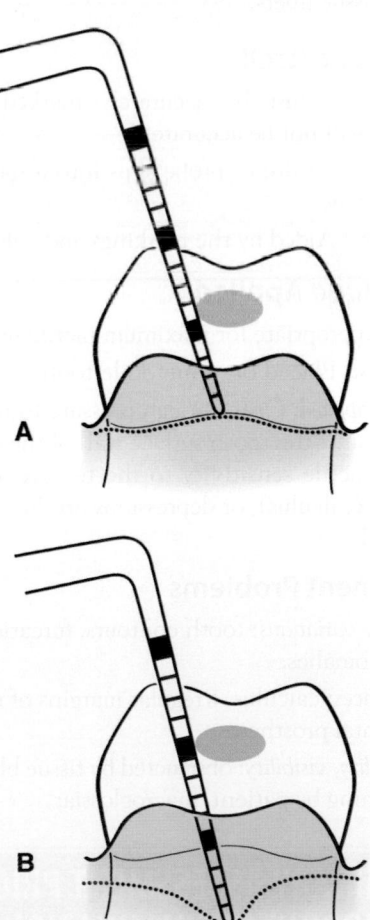

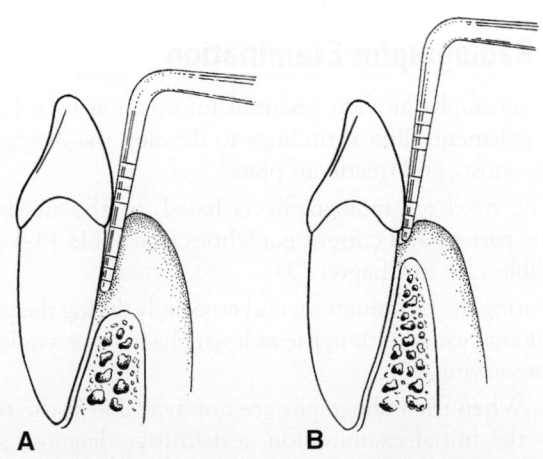

FIGURE 20-7 PD. A pocket is measured from the GM to the attached periodontal tissue. Shown is the contrast of probe measurements with GMs at the same level. **A:** Deep periodontal pocket (7 mm) with apical migration of attachment. **B:** Shallow sulcus (2 mm) with the attachment near the CEJ.

FIGURE 20-8 **Proximal Surface Probing. A:** Probe must be applied more than half way across from facial to overlap with probing from the lingual. **B:** Probe in area of crater formation. Probing is often deeper on the proximal surface under the contact area than on the facial or lingual surfaces.

with future probings as well as with colleagues in practice together.

▶ At the same time, patient discomfort and trauma to the tissues must be minimized.

▶ Probing is influenced by many factors, such as those described in the following topics.

A. Severity and Extent of Periodontal Disease

▶ With application of light pressure and a secure finger or hand rest, the probe is inserted under the GM, held against the tooth as it is passed along the tooth surface to the attached tissue level.

▶ Diseased tissue offers less resistance, so that with increased severity of inflammation, the probe inserts to a deeper level.[1]

- *Normal healthy tissue*: The probe is at the base of the sulcus or crevice, at the coronal end of the junctional epithelium.
- *Gingivitis and early periodontitis*: The probe tip is within the junctional epithelium.
- *Advanced periodontitis*: The probe tip passes through the junctional epithelium to reach attached connective tissue fibers.

B. The Probe Itself

▶ *Calibration*: Must be accurately marked; otherwise, readings will not be accurate.

▶ *Thickness*: A thinner probe slips into a narrow pocket more readily.

▶ *Readability*: Aided by the markings and color coding.

C. Technique Applied

▶ *Grasp*: Appropriate for maximum tactile sensitivity.

▶ *Finger rest*: Placed on nonmobile tooth.

▶ *Pressure applied*: Only enough pressure to maintain the probe against the tooth surface wall of the pocket is required. Tactile sensitivity to the texture, deposits, elevations (calculus), or depressions on the tooth surface is needed.

D. Placement Problems

▶ *Anatomic variations*: tooth contours, furcations, contact areas, anomalies.

▶ *Interferences*: calculus, irregular margins of restorations, fixed dental prostheses.

▶ *Accessibility, visibility*: obstructed by tissue bleeding, limited opening by patient, macroglossia.

PRELIMINARY ASSESSMENT PRIOR TO PERIODONTAL EXAMINATION[2]

I. Medical History

▶ A thorough medical history is taken and reviewed to identify issues that may affect treatment and outcomes.

▶ Patients at risk of bacteremia must receive prophylactic antibiotic premedication before examination or instrumentation (see Chapter 10).

II. Dental and Psychosocial History

▶ Document the dental history including oral self-care habits, previous dental history, and chief complaint.

▶ Psychosocial history may include information such as marital status, living situation, financial situation, work habits, diet, substance use, stress, and oral health literacy.

- Psychosocial factors are taken into consideration when planning treatment and setting treatment goals.

III. Vital Signs

▶ Vital signs are taken at each new patient appointment, at follow-up appointments for those with hypertension, and for treatment requiring local anesthesia (see Chapter 11).

IV. Extraoral/Intraoral Examination

▶ An extraoral/intraoral examination should be done at each examination appointment (see Chapter 12).

V. Risk Assessment

▶ The American Academy of Periodontology suggests risk assessment is becoming increasingly important in treatment planning and needs to be included in comprehensive dental and periodontal examinations.[3]

▶ Risk assessment for dental caries, periodontal disease, and oral cancer are conducted (see Chapters 27, 19, and 12 for information on risk assessment tools).

▶ Additional risk assessment for factors such as diabetes (see Chapter 69) or tobacco use (Chapter 34) may be performed based on individual patient needs.

VI. Radiographic Examination

▶ Radiographs provide essential information to aid and supplement clinical findings to develop the diagnosis, prognosis, and treatment plan.[4]

▶ The need for radiographs is based on the needs of the patient and current guidelines (see Table 13-4 and Table 13-5 in Chapter 13).

▶ During the examination, and especially during the periodontal examination, the radiographs must be available for viewing.

- When the radiographs are not available at the time the initial examination, a definitive diagnosis and treatment plan cannot be completed.
- The need for radiographs free from errors in technique and viewed with magnification on an adequately lighted viewbox or on the computer is essential.

▶ Selection of radiographs: For observing evidence of periodontal involvement, *periapical* radiographs are needed.

  • *Horizontal bitewing* radiographs do not show the complete periodontal tissues that extend around the roots. When bone loss is moderate to severe, the crest of the bone may be seen in a *vertical bitewing* survey (see Figure 13-16 in Chapter 13), which is necessary during the periodontal maintenance phase.

VII. Dental Examination

▶ The dental examination includes documentation of missing teeth, caries, restorations, tooth position, parafunctional habits, and occlusion (see Chapters 16 and 17).

VIII. Hard and Soft Deposits

The location of biofilm and calculus is documented (see Chapters 15 and 21).

A. Supragingival Calculus

▶ *Distribution*

Supragingival calculus is generally localized and most commonly confined to the lingual surfaces of the mandibular anterior teeth and the facial surfaces of the maxillary first and second molars, opposite the openings to the salivary ducts.

▶ *Amount*

Indicate a subjective measurement of slight, moderate, and heavy.

B. Subgingival Calculus

▶ *Distribution*

Subgingival calculus can be either localized or generalized. Record in relation to pocket PD on a chart or form to show exact locations.

▶ *Amount*

Indicate a subjective measurement of slight, moderate, heavy.

PARAMETERS OF CARE FOR THE PERIODONTAL EXAMINATION

I. Periodontal Probing Procedure

A. Periodontal Probe Insertion

▶ Grasp probe with modified pen grasp.

▶ Establish finger rest on a neighboring tooth, preferably in the same dental arch.

▶ Hold side of instrument tip flat against the tooth near the gingival margin (GM). The cervical third of a primary tooth is more convex (Figure 20-9).

▶ Gently slide the tip under the GM.

  • *Healthy or firm fibrotic tissue*: Insertion is more difficult because of the close adaptation of the tissue

to the tooth surface; underlying gingival fibers are strong and tight.

  • *Spongy, soft tissue*: GM is loose and flabby because of the destruction of underlying gingival fibers. Probe inserts readily, and bleeding can be expected on gentle probing.

B. Advance Probe to Base of Pocket

▶ Hold side of probe tip flat against the tooth surface; probe is parallel with long axis of the tooth for vertical insertion. The shape of the crown can make it difficult to maintain this angulation (Figure 20-9).

▶ Slide the probe along the tooth surface vertically down to the base of the sulcus or pocket.

  • Maintain contact of the side of the tip of the probe with the tooth.

  • *Gingival pocket*: Side of probe is on enamel.

  • *Periodontal pocket*: Side of probe is on the cemental or dentinal surface when inserted to a level below the cementoenamel junction (CEJ).

  • As the probe is passed down the side of the tooth, roughness may be felt, which may be calculus. Evaluation of the topography and nature of the tooth surface is essential to instrumentation.

  • When obstruction by a hard bulky calculus deposit is encountered, lift the probe away from the tooth and follow over the edge of the calculus until the probe can move vertically into the pocket again.

  • The base of the sulcus or pocket feels soft and elastic (compared with the hard tooth surface and calculus deposits).

  • With slight pressure, the tension of the attached periodontal tissue at the base of the pocket can be felt.

▶ Use only the pressure needed to detect by tactile means the level of the attached tissue, whether junctional epithelium or deep connective tissue fibers. A light pressure of 10 g and no more than 20 g is recommended.[5]

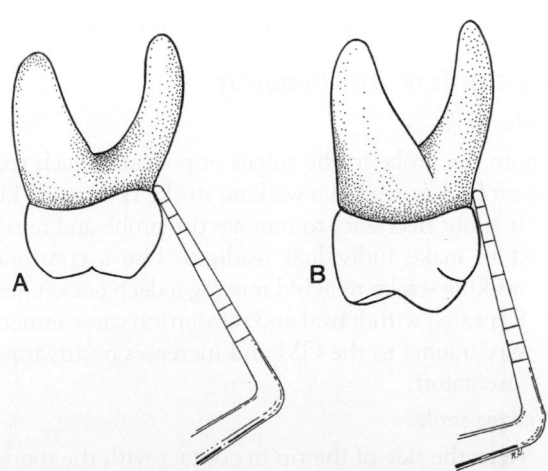

FIGURE 20-9 Primary and Permanent Maxillary Molars. A: Accentuated convexity of the cervical third and widespread roots of the primary molar complicate probe placement. Probe may encounter the root. **B:** Permanent tooth with less convexity of the cervical third and roots that are less widely spread.

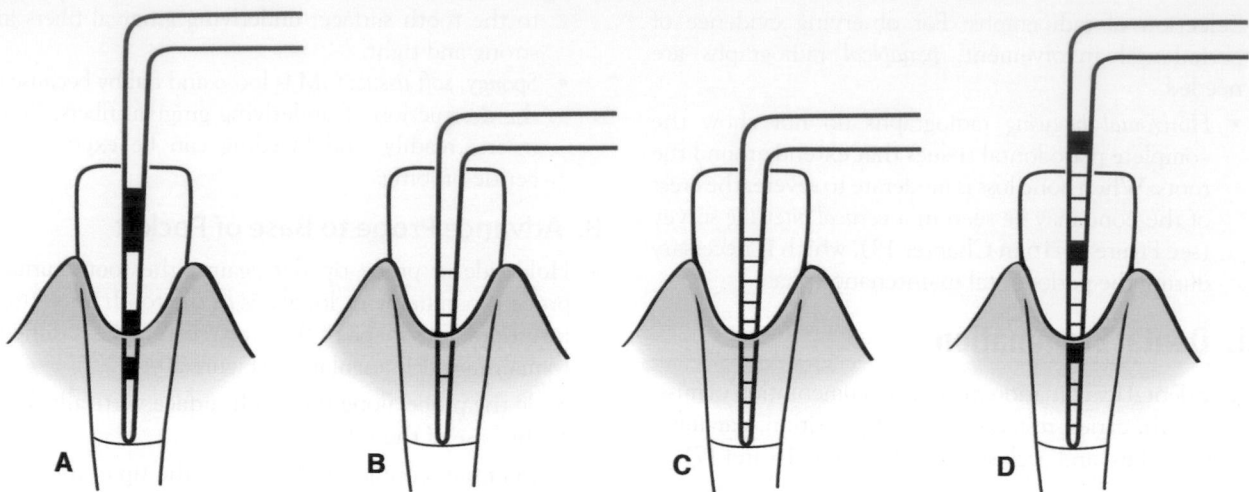

FIGURE 20-10 Comparison of Probe Readings. Measurement of same 5-mm pocket with four different probes. **A:** Color-coded, **B:** Michigan O, and **C:** Williams. **D:** Hu-Friedy UNC 15.

▶ Position the probe for reading.

- Bring the probe to position as nearly parallel with the long axis of the tooth as possible for reading the depth.
- Interference of the contact area does not permit placing the probe parallel for the measurement directly beneath the contact area. Hold the side of the shank of the probe against the contact to minimize the angle (Figure 20-8).

C. Reading the Probe Measurement

▶ Measurement for a PD is made from the GM to the attached periodontal tissue or base of the sulcus or pocket.

▶ A comparison of pocket measurement using probes with different calibrations is shown in Figure 20-10.

▶ When the GM appears at a level between probe marks, round up to the higher marking on the probe for the final measurement.

▶ Dry the area being probed to improve visibility.

D. Circumferential Probing

▶ *Probe stroke*

Maintain the probe in the sulcus or pocket of each tooth as the probe is moved in a walking stroke (Figure 20-11).

- It is not necessary to remove the probe and reinsert it to make individual readings. Use a continuous walking stroke to avoid missing a deep pocket area.
- Repeated withdrawal and reinsertion cause unnecessary trauma to the GM and increases posttreatment discomfort.

▶ *Walking stroke*

- Keep the side of the tip in contact with the tooth at the base of the pocket.
- Slide the probe up (coronally) about 1–2 mm and back to the attachment in a "touch … touch … touch …" rhythm (Figure 20-11).

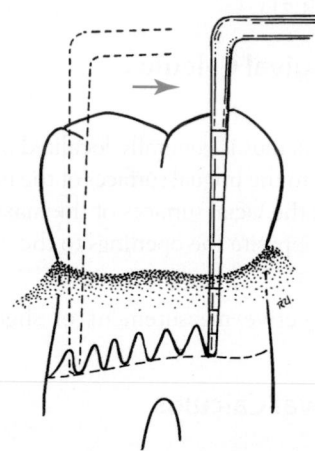

FIGURE 20-11 Probe Walking Stroke. The side of the tip of the probe is held in contact with the tooth. From the base of the pocket, the probe is moved up and down in 1- to 2-mm strokes as it is advanced in 1-mm steps. The attached periodontal tissue at the base of the pocket is contacted on each down stroke to identify PD in each area.

- Observe probe measurement at the GM at each location.
- Advance millimeter by millimeter along the facial and lingual surfaces into the proximal areas.

E. Adaptation of Probe for Individual Teeth

▶ *Molars and premolars*

- Orient the probe at the distal line angle for both facial and lingual application.
- Insert the probe at the distal line angle and probe in a distal direction; adapt the probe around the line angle; probe across the distal surface until the side of the probe contacts the contact area, then slant the probe to continue under the contact area to the midline of the proximal surface in the col area (Figure 20-8).
- Note the PD and slide the probe back to the distal line angle. Proceed in the mesial direction around the mesial line angle and across the mesial surface.

- When the side of the probe touches the contact area, the probe is slanted to continue measurements to the midline of the col area on the mesial surface.
- ► *Anterior teeth*
  - Initial insertion may be at the distal line angle or from the midline of the facial or lingual surfaces.
  - Proceed around the distal line angle and across the distal surface; reinsert and probe the other half of the tooth.
- ► *Proximal surfaces*
  - Continue the walking stroke around each line angle and onto the proximal surface.
  - Roll the instrument handle between the fingers to keep the side of the probe tip adapted to the tooth surface at line angles and as the tooth contour varies.
  - Continue the strokes under the contact area. Overlap strokes from facial surface with strokes from lingual surface to ensure full coverage (Figure 20-8). *Make sure that the col area under each contact has been thoroughly examined.*

F. Recording of Probing Measurements

- ► Six measurements are recorded for each tooth, three from the facial, and three from the lingual or palatal as shown in Figure 20-12.
- ► For each of the six areas, the deepest probing measurement is recorded.
- ► Two recordings each are made for proximal areas: Numbers 3 and 6 for the mesial, and 1 and 4 for the distal in Figure 20-12. Frequently the deepest probing will be in the col, directly under the contact area.
- ► Additional recordings may be needed for furcations, mucogingival involvements, or other special areas.
- ► Recordings of PDs are part of the total periodontal charting.
- ► Figure 9-4 (Chapter 9) illustrates a typical chart form in which boxes are provided for recording PD, CAL, and mobility for each tooth.

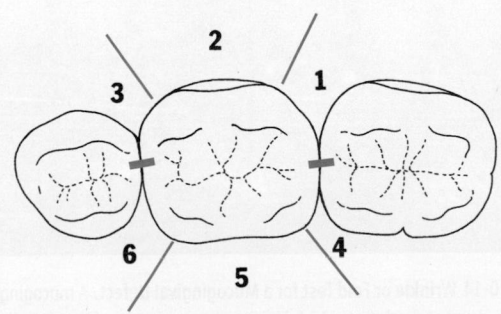

FIGURE 20-12 Recording Periodontal PDs. The pocket/sulcus is measured completely around each tooth. Record the deepest measurement for each of the six areas around the tooth. Areas 1, 3, 4, and 6 extend from the line angle to under the contact area.

G. Sources of Error in Periodontal Probing[6]

- ► Resistance of tissues that is affected by the level of inflammation in the tissues.
- ► Calculus.
- ► Diameter and/or variations in standardization of the probe marks.
- ► Clinician errors in angulation and/or insertion.
- ► Probing pressure or force.

II. Clinical Attachment Level

- ► Attachment level refers to the position of the periodontal attached tissues at the base of a sulcus or pocket.
- ► It is measured from a fixed point to the attachment, whereas the PD is measured from a changeable point (the crest of the free gingiva) to the attachment (Figure 20-13A).

A. Rationale

- ► Stability of attachment is a characteristic of health.
- ► A loss of clinical attachment is a primary clinical feature of periodontitis as the junctional epithelium migrates toward the apex.[7]
- ► When periodontal disease is active, pocket formation and migration of the attachment along the cemental surface continue.
- ► Evaluation can be made of the outcome of periodontal treatment and the stability of the attachment during maintenance examinations.

B. Procedure

- ► *Selecting a fixed point*
  - CEJ is used unless it cannot be detected because of abrasion or a restoration.
  - Margin of a permanent restoration.
- ► *Measuring in the presence of visible recession*
  - CEJ is visible directly.
  - Measure from the CEJ to the GM (Figure 20-13B).
  - The CAL is calculated by *addition* of the pocket depth to the GM to CEJ distance (PD + GM = CAL).
- ► *Measuring when the CEJ is covered by the gingiva margin*
  - Slide the probe along the tooth surface into the pocket until the CEJ is felt (Figure 20-13C). This is the CEJ to GM measurement.
  - *Subtract* the distance from the CEJ to GM from the total PD to the attachment (PD − GM = CAL).
- ► *Measuring when the GM is level with the CEJ*
  - With the GM at the CEJ, that measurement is the same as the PD.
  - The PD *equals* the CAL when the GM is level with the CEJ (Figure 20-13D).

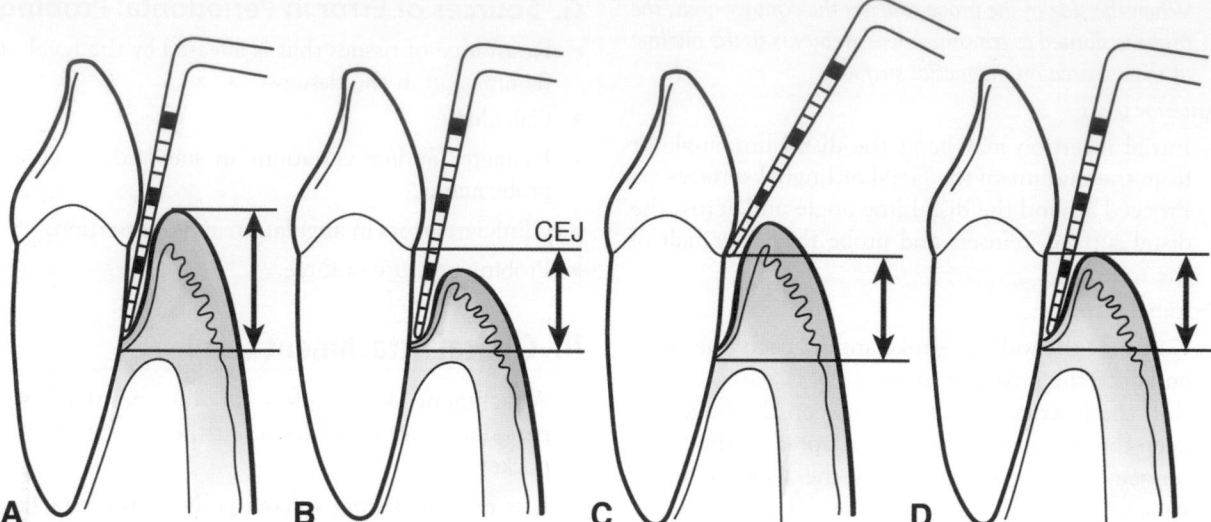

FIGURE 20-13 **Clinical Attachment Level (CAL). A:** Pocket Depth: is measured from the GM to the attached periodontal tissue. **B:** CAL in the presence of gingival recession is measured directly from the CEJ to the attached tissue. **C:** CAL when the GM covers the CEJ: first the CEJ is located as shown, and then the distance to the CEJ is measured and subtracted from the PD. **D:** The CAL is equal to the PD when the GM is at the level of the CEJ.

III. Mucogingival Examination

A. Methods for Identifying MGJ

▶ *Purposes*
  • To detect adequacy of the width of the attached gingiva.
  • To locate frenal attachments and their proximity to the free gingiva.
  • To identify promptly the MGJ.

▶ *Tension test procedure*
  • *Facial*
    1. Retract cheeks and lips laterally by grasping the lips with the thumbs and index fingers.
    2. Move the lips and cheeks up and down and back and forth, creating tension between the attached gingiva and mucosa to make the MGJ visible.
    3. Follow around from the molar areas on the right to molar areas on the left, both maxillary and mandibular. Observe frenal attachments.

▶ *Lingual (mandible)*
  1. Hold a mouth mirror to tense the mucosa of the floor of the mouth, gently retracting the side of the tongue, so that the MGJ is clearly visible.
  2. Request patient move the tongue to the left, to the right, and up to touch the palate.

▶ *Fold (or Wrinkle) test procedure*
  • Retract the lip gently, but not to the point of tension between the attached gingiva and buccal mucosa.
  • The periodontal probe is oriented horizontal to the MGJ and gentle pressure is used to fold or wrinkle the mucosa toward the GM (see Figure 20-14).[8]
  • This test can be used if the MGJ cannot be easily visualized with the tension test method.

B. Measurement of Width of Attached Gingiva

▶ Place the probe (no pressure) on the external surface of the gingiva and measure from the MGJ to the GM to determine the total width of the gingiva (Figure 20-15A).
▶ Measure PD (Figure 20-15B).
▶ Calculate the width of attached gingiva by *subtracting* the PD from the total width of the gingiva.
▶ Record findings.

B. Areas at Risk for Mucogingival Conditions[9]

▶ Area(s) of recession with little keratinized gingiva and the base of the sulcus or pocket is near the MGJ.

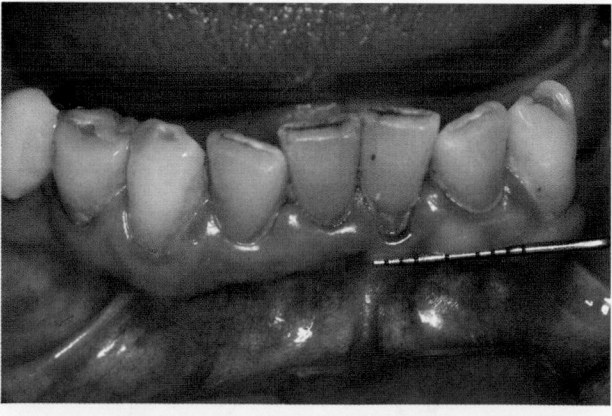

FIGURE 20-14 **Wrinkle or Fold Test for a Mucogingival Defect.** A mucogingival defect is suspected at tooth #24, which has a very narrow zone of keratinized gingiva. The periodontal probe is positioned at the MGJ and gently moved coronally against the mucosa. Blanching or wrinkling of the mucosa at the GM indicates no attached gingiva. (Reprinted from Scheid R. Woelfel's Dental Anatomy, 7th Ed. Philadelphia: Lippincott Williams & Wilkins; 2007.)

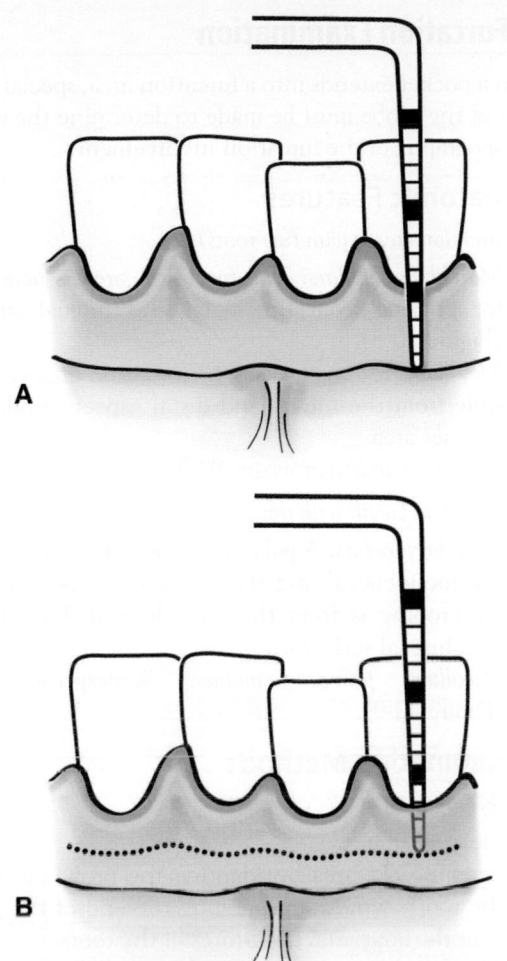

FIGURE 20-15 Measuring Attached Gingiva. A: Measure the total gingiva by laying the probe over the surface of the gingiva and measuring from the free margin to the MGJ. **B:** Measure the PD. Dotted line represents the base of the pocket. Subtract the PD (**B**) from the total gingiva (**A**) to obtain the width of attached gingiva. The area illustrated shows 2 mm of attached gingiva.

▶ When a pocket extends to or beyond the MGJ, the probe may pass through into the alveolar mucosa when probing the pocket (Figure 20-6).

▶ Absent or narrow attached (keratinized) gingiva.

▶ Anatomic differences such as tooth position and frenum insertions.

IV. Mobility Examination

▶ Because of the nature and function of the periodontal ligament, teeth have a slight normal mobility.

▶ Mobility can be considered abnormal or pathologic when it exceeds normal.

▶ Increased mobility can be a clinical sign of periodontal trauma from occlusion as described in Chapter 17.

A. Procedure for Determination of Mobility

1. Position the patient for clear visibility with good light.

2. Stabilize the head: Request the patient place the head against the headrest. Motion of the head, lips, or cheek can interfere with an accurate evaluation of tooth movement.

3. Use two single-ended metal instruments with wide blunt ends, held with a modified pen grasp. The use of wooden tongue depressors or plastic mirror handles are not recommended because of their flexibility. Testing with the fingers without the metal instruments can be misleading because the soft tissue of the fingertips can move and give an illusion of tooth movement.

4. Apply specific, firm finger rests (fulcrums): A standardized finger rest pressure contributes increased consistency to the determinations. The teeth may be dried with air or gauze to prevent slipping of the instruments or the finger on the finger rest.

5. Apply the blunt ends of the instruments to opposite sides of a tooth, and rock the tooth to test horizontal mobility. Keep both instrument ends on the tooth as pressure is applied first from one side and then the other.

6. Test vertical mobility (depression of the tooth into its socket) by applying pressure with one of the mirror handles to the occlusal or incisal surface.

7. Move from tooth to tooth in a systematic order.

B. Record Degree of Movement

The most widely used method to assess tooth mobility is the Miller Index first described in 1938.[10]

▶ *Scale*

The N, 1, 2, 3 or I, II, III are frequently used, sometimes with a plus sign (+) to indicate mobility between numbers.

▶ *Recording*

Although subjective, interpretation may be considered as follows[3]:

N = normal, physiologic

1 = slight mobility, greater than normal

2 = moderate mobility, greater than 1 mm displacement

3 = severe mobility, moves vertically and is depressible in the tooth socket.

▶ *The letter N means normal mobility*

All teeth that have a periodontal ligament have normal mobility. No tooth has zero mobility except in a condition, such as ankylosis, in which there is no periodontal ligament.

▶ *Chart form*

A chart form such as Figure 9-4 in Chapter 9 can provide for a place to record mobility. Preferably more than one space can be available so comparative readings can be recorded at successive maintenance appointments.

V. Fremitus

A. Definition

▶ Fremitus means palpable vibration or movement.

▶ In dentistry, fremitus refers to the vibratory patterns of the teeth. A tooth with fremitus has excess contact, possibly related to a premature contact. Usually, the tooth also demonstrates some degree of mobility because the excess contact forces the tooth to move.

▶ The test is used in conjunction with occlusal analysis and adjustment.

▶ Because fremitus depends on tooth contact, determination is made only on the maxillary teeth.

B. Procedure for Determination of Fremitus

1. Seat the patient upright with the head stabilized against the headrest; the occlusal biting plane is parallel with the floor.
2. Gently place the index finger on each maxillary tooth at about the cervical third (Figure 20-16).
3. Request the patient to close the back teeth together in a functional occlusion (see Chapter 17) and tap up and down repeatedly.[11]
4. Start with the most posterior maxillary tooth on one side, and move the index finger tooth by tooth around the arch.
5. Record by tooth number the teeth where vibration is felt and the teeth where actual movement is noted. The degree recorded may be subjective, but the following range has been suggested:

N = normal (without vibration or movement).
+ = One-degree fremitus; only slight vibration can be felt.
+ + = Two-degree fremitus; the tooth is clearly palpable but movement is barely visible.
+ + + = Three-degree fremitus; movement is clearly observed visually.

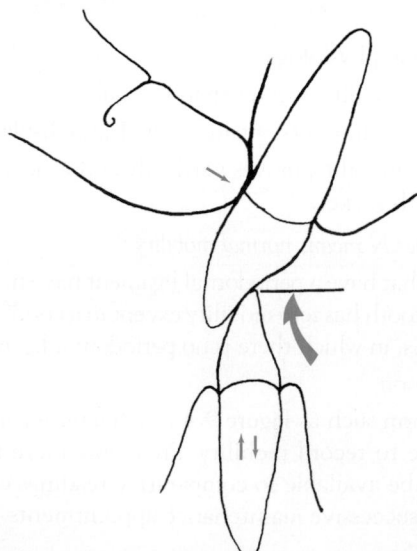

FIGURE 20-16 Fremitus. With the patient seated upright and the head stabilized against the headrest, an index finger is placed firmly over the cervical third of each maxillary tooth in succession starting with the most posterior tooth on one side and moving around the arch. The patient is asked to click the posterior teeth.

VI. Furcation Examination

When a pocket extends into a furcation area, special adaptation of the probe must be made to determine the extent and topography of the furcation involvement.

A. Anatomic Features

▶ *Bifurcation (teeth with two roots)*
1. *Mandibular molars:* The furcation area is accessible for probing from the facial and lingual surfaces (Figure 20-5).
2. *Maxillary first premolars:* The furcation area is accessible from the mesial and distal aspects, under the contact area.
3. *Primary mandibular molar:* Widespread roots.

▶ *Trifurcation (teeth with three roots)*
1. *Maxillary molars:* A palatal root and two buccal roots, the mesiobuccal and the distobuccal roots. Access for probing is from the mesiolingual, buccal, and distolingual surfaces.
2. *Maxillary primary molars:* Widespread roots (Figure 20-9).

B. Examination Methods

▶ *Early furcation*
1. Measure PD.
2. Examine the area by adapting the probe closely to the tooth surface and moving the end of the probe over the anatomic curvatures of the roots.
3. Check radiograph for signs of furcation involvement (Figure 20-17).

▶ *Points of access*
1. Measure PDs at points of access for each bifurcation or trifurcation area.
2. Position of GM will vary. Figure 20-5A shows apparent recession and 3-mm pocket at the level of the bifurcation.

▶ *Use of furcation probe*

The use of a furcation probe, such as a Nabers 1N or 2N, is preferred to assess the extent of furcation involvement over standard periodontal probes for accuracy (Figure 20-5B).[12]

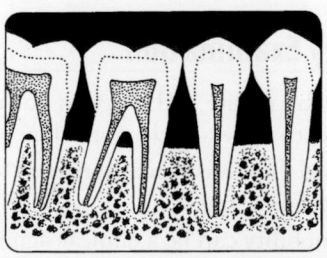

FIGURE 20-17 Horizontal Bone Loss (1). Bone level in periodontal disease is more than 1–1.5 mm from the CEJ. When bone loss is horizontal, the crest of the alveolar bone is parallel with a line between the CEJs of adjacent teeth. Note early furcation involvement in the second molar and moderate furcation involvement in the first molar.

▶ *Furcations grades*

Furcation involvement is usually classified by the amount of bone destroyed in the furcation area. The most common classification is the Glickman furcation grades (Figure 19-9 in Chapter 19) and include:[13]

- *Grade I*: early, beginning involvement. A probe can enter the concavity of the furcation but the bone between the roots (interradicular) is intact.
- *Grade II*: moderate involvement. Bone has been destroyed to an extent that permits Naber's probe to enter the furcation area between the roots but not extend all the way through to the opposite side.
- *Grade III*: severe involvement. A probe can be passed between the roots through the entire furcation.
- *Grade IV*: Same as Grade III, with exposure resulting from gingival recession, especially after periodontal therapy.

▶ *Complications*

Anatomic variations that complicate furcation examination are fused roots; anomalies, such as extra roots; or low or high furcations.

RADIOGRAPHIC CHANGES IN PERIODONTAL INFECTIONS

I. Bone Level

A. Normal Bone Level

The crest of the interdental bone appears from 1.0 to 1.5 mm from the CEJ (Figure 20-18).

B. Bone Level in Periodontal Disease

The height of the bone is lowered progressively as the inflammation is extended and bone is destroyed.

II. Shape of Remaining Bone

A. Horizontal Bone Loss

▶ When the crest of the bone is parallel with a line between the CEJs of two adjacent teeth, the term "*horizontal bone loss*" is used (Figures 20-17 and 20-19).

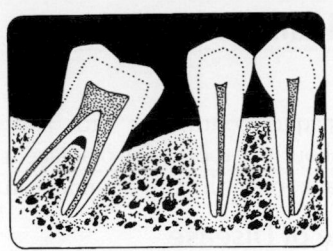

FIGURE 20-19 Horizontal Bone Loss (2). Second molar has drifted mesially into the space created when the first molar was removed. Note that the level of the crestal bone is parallel with a line between the CEJs of the second premolar and the tipped second molar.

▶ When inflammation is the sole destructive factor, the bone loss usually appears horizontal.

▶ When the amount of remaining bone is fairly evenly distributed throughout the dentition, the condition may be described as *generalized horizontal bone loss*. It may be designated either by millimeters from the position of the normal bone level or by percentage.

▶ When bone loss is confined to specific areas, the condition is described as *localized* horizontal bone loss.

B. Angular or Vertical Bone Loss

▶ Reduction in height of crestal bone that is irregular; the bone level is not parallel with a line joining the adjacent CEJs. Note in Figure 20-20 that the V-shaped mesial bone loss on the mesial of the first molar has lost its white lining of lamina dura. It is a true "vertical" or "angular" bone loss possibly related to trauma from occlusion. Contrast this area with the molar in Figure 20-19 where the lamina dura is an intact clear white line. The V-shaped area in this radiograph shows a tipped tooth due to extraction of the adjacent supporting tooth. No trauma or disease was involved.

▶ Angular bone loss is more commonly *localized*; rarely generalized.

▶ When inflammation and trauma from occlusion are combined in causing the destruction and irregular shape of the bone, the bone may appear with "angular defects" or with "vertical bone loss."

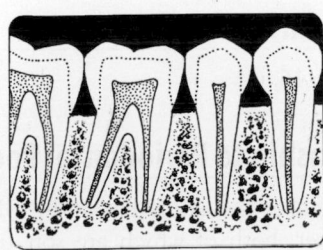

FIGURE 20-18 Normal Bone Level. Drawing of a radiograph to show normal bone level, 1–1.5 mm from the CEJ.

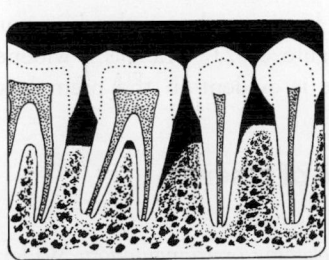

FIGURE 20-20 Angular or Vertical Bone Loss; Mesial of the First Molar. The level of the crestal bone between the second premolar and the first molar is not parallel with a line between the CEJs of the same teeth.

III. Crestal Lamina Dura

A. Normal

White, radiopaque; continuous with and connects the lamina dura about the roots of two adjacent teeth; covers the interdental bone of the two premolars in Figure 20-18.

B. Evidence of Disease

The crestal lamina dura is indistinct, irregular, radiolucent, fuzzy (Figure 20-20, mesial of first molar).

IV. Furcation Involvement

A. Normal

Bone fills the area between the roots (Figure 20-18).

B. Evidence of Disease

▶ Radiolucent area in the furcation.

▶ Early furcation involvement shown in the second molar in Figure 20-17, may appear as a small radiolucent black area or as a slight thickening of the periodontal ligament space. It can be confirmed by clinical assessment with a Naber's probe.

▶ Furcation involvement of maxillary molars may become more advanced before radiographic evidence is seen. Superimposition of the palatal root may mask a small area of involvement.

▶ When the height of the interdental bone in the radiograph is at the level of the furcation, it can be used as an approximate guide to possible furcation involvement.[14]

▶ Maxillary first premolar furcation involvement cannot be seen in a radiograph with correct vertical and horizontal angulation because the roots are superimposed.

V. Periodontal Ligament Space

A. Normal

▶ The periodontal ligament is connective tissue and, hence, appears as a fine black radiolucent line next to the root surface.

▶ On its outer side is the lamina dura, the bone that lines the tooth socket and appears radiopaque.

▶ A normal ligament shows clearly around the molar roots in Figure 20-21, whereas a widened black ligament space is evident in the premolars of the same radiograph.

B. Evidence of Disease

Widening or thickening.

▶ *Angular thickening or triangulation*: Widened only near the coronal third, near the crest of the interdental bone.

▶ *Complete periodontal ligament thickened along an entire side of a root to the apex, or around the root*

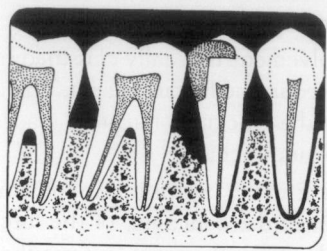

FIGURE 20-21 **Periodontal Ligament Space.** First and second molars have a normal periodontal ligament space, which appears as a fine black line about the roots. The first premolar shows thickening of the ligament space about the entire root, and the second premolar has thickening only about the mesial surface of the root.

(Figure 20-21): When viewed at different angulations (in the various radiographs of a complete survey), the ligament space may reveal varying thicknesses, thus showing the disease involvement is not consistent around the entire root or that other structures are superimposed.

OTHER RADIOGRAPHIC FINDINGS

▶ Any other radiographic findings related directly or indirectly to periodontal involvement and contributing factors are noted in the record.

▶ Certain findings have a direct relation to dental hygiene care and instruction, particularly local factors that contribute to food impaction or biofilm retention.

I. Calculus

▶ Gross deposits, primarily those on proximal surfaces, may be seen in radiographs.

▶ Radiographs have very limited value for calculus detection so clinical assessment with an explorer is needed to determine the location and extent of the deposit.

II. Overhanging Restorations

▶ Some proximal overhanging margins may be seen on radiographs (see Figure 19-5 in Chapter 19).

▶ The use of an explorer is necessary to detect irregular margins and to examine all proximal margins that do not reveal irregularities in the radiographs.

III. Dental Caries

▶ See Chapter 16.

IV. Relationship to Periodontal Pockets

▶ Because a pocket is measured from the GM to the base of the pocket, both of which are soft tissue, pockets cannot be seen on a radiograph. Probing is necessary to identify pocket depth.

EVERYDAY ETHICS

Mrs. Claren, a neat-appearing lady in her 50s, was new to the practice. After a careful review of the medical history, Brittany, the dental hygienist, completed the comprehensive periodontal examination. The PDs were generally 3–4 mm with localized 5 mm measurements. Brittany noted BOP in posterior areas with moderate subgingival calculus.

When Brittany finished the examination and sat the patient upright to discuss the findings, the patient said, "You aren't cleaning my teeth. What is it you are doing?" Brittany realized the patient may never have had a complete periodontal examination and was unaware of her localized moderate chronic periodontitis.

Questions for Consideration

1. Which of the dental hygiene core values in Section II, Introduction (Table II-1) come into play in this scenario with Brittany and Mrs. Claren? Think of each of the core values in relation to a first-time patient compared with a long-time patient.

2. Review the legal and ethical concepts described in Table V-1, Section V Introduction to consider how they may be of help to Brittany as she thinks over how to answer Mrs. Claren. Make a list of explanations Brittany might use.

3. Is Brittany's role simply to explain office policy to a new patient or is informed consent the priority here?

DOCUMENTATION

Documentation in the permanent record for a patient with a gingival or periodontal condition needs to include a minimum of the following:

▶ Findings by clinical observation and the use of a periodontal probe: sulcus and PDs, attachment levels, status of furcations, leading to the dental hygiene diagnosis.

▶ Mobility, fremitus, occlusal problems, and other findings that will tie the complete oral plan for dental hygiene care into the overall major treatment plan for dental care by a dentist.

▶ A sample progress note documenting a dental hygiene appointment is found in Box 20-2.

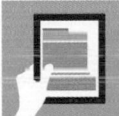

BOX 20-2
Example Documentation: Periodontal Examination Findings

S –Mr. Jones presents to the dental office for his first visit. He just moved to Boston a few months ago and needs a routine examination and "cleaning." He does not report any concerns about his mouth at this time. Mr. Jones reports he just had a physical examination with his new physician and was diagnosed with prediabetes and was put on metformin. His A1c was 6.5. He lives alone and eats out once or twice a day. He reports brushing daily, but he says he will not floss so don't lecture him about it.

O –His vital signs are normal, with a BP of 120/79. Extraoral examination/intraoral examination were normal. No full mouth series of radiographs in 5 years and his risk assessment indicated he was at high caries and periodontal risk. Comprehensive examination findings included a broken filling DO-#30 and a broken mesiolingual (ML) cusp on #31. He has generalized 5–6 mm pocket depths with BOP in all posterior areas with marginal inflammation. Grade I furcations noted ML and DL of #2, 3, 14, and 15. No mobility. Adequate attached gingiva in all areas.

A –The periodontal diagnosis is generalized moderate chronic periodontitis. High caries and periodontal risk.

Slight-to-moderate localized subgingival calculus. Plaque score 60%.

P –Patient education for oral self-care included refinement of modified Stillman brushing technique in posterior areas along with introduction of floss picks for interdental care. Patient demonstrated both home care aids. Education about periodontal disease and association with diabetes was discussed along with his diagnosis and need for nonsurgical periodontal therapy (NSPT) by quadrant with local anesthesia in posterior areas. The patient was shocked by the findings because he has been having "cleanings" every 6 months at his previous dental office, but he indicated he had never had all the "measuring" done before. He was very thankful to learn about the association between diabetes and periodontal disease. He seemed highly motivated to improve his oral health. The dentist also discussed the need for a crown on #31 and replacement of the filling on #30 once the NSPT was complete. Next visit: NSPT maxillary right quadrant with local anesthesia and review of oral self-care.

Signed _____, RDH

Date _____

Factors To Teach The Patient

▷ The need for a comprehensive examination to ensure treatment is planned to meet all of the patient's needs.

▷ The value of the various components of the comprehensive examination in assessing the patient's oral health. Examples are the complete radiographic survey, probing 360° around each tooth, and exploring each subgingival tooth surface.

▷ Why bleeding can occur when probing. Healthy tissue does not bleed.

▷ Relation of PD measurements to normal sulci.

▷ Significance of the periodontal findings, such as mobility, furcation involvement, or inadequate attached gingiva.

References

1. Listgarten MA. Periodontal probing: what does it mean? *J Clin Periodontol.* 1980;7(3):165–176.

2. American Academy of Periodontology. Parameter on comprehensive periodontal examination. *J Periodontol.* 2000;71(5, Suppl):847–848.

3. American Academy of Periodontology. American academy of periodontology statement on risk assessment. *J Periodontol.* 2008;79(2):202.

4. Corbet EF, Ho DK, Lai SM. Radiographs in periodontal disease diagnosis and management. *Aust Dent J.* 2009;(54, Suppl 1):S27–S43.

5. Larsen C, Barendregt DS, Slot DE, et al. Probing pressure, a highly undervalued unit of measure in periodontal probing: a systematic review on its effect on probing pocket depth. *J Clin Periodontol.* 2009;36(4):315–322.

6. Andrade R, Espinoza M, Gómez EM, et al. Intra- and inter-examiner reproducibility of manual probing depth. *Braz Oral Res.* 2012;26(1):57–63.

7. Flemmig TF. Periodontitis. *Ann Periodontol.* 1999;4(1):32–38.

8. Guglielmoni P, Promsudthi A, Tatakis DN, et al. Intra- and inter-examiner reproducibility in keratinized tissue width assessment with 3 methods for mucogingival junction determination. *J Periodontol.* 2001;72(2):134–139.

9. American Academy of Periodontology. Parameters of mucogingival conditions. *J Periodontol.* 2000;71 (Suppl):861–862.

10. Laster L, Laudenbach KW, Stoller NH. An evaluation of clinical tooth mobility measurements. *J Periodontol.* 1975;46(10):603–607.

11. Davies SJ, Gray RJ, Linden GJ, et al. Occlusal considerations in periodontics. *Br Dent J.* 2001;191(11):597–604.

12. Eickholz P, Kim TS. Reproducibility and validity of the assessment of clinical furcation parameters as related to different probes. *J Periodontol.* 1998;69(3):328–336.

13. Al-Shammari KF, Kazor CE, Wang HL. Molar root anatomy and management of furcation defects. *J Clin Periodontol.* 2001;28(8):730–740.

14. Grover V, Malhotra R, Kapoor A, et al. Correlation of the interdental and the interradicular bone loss: a radiovisuographic analysis. *J Indian Soc Periodontol.* 2014;18(4):482–487.

ENHANCE YOUR UNDERSTANDING

thePoint° DIGITAL CONNECTIONS
(see the inside front cover for access information)

• **Audio glossary**

• **Quiz bank**

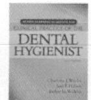

SUPPORT FOR LEARNING
(available separately; visit lww.com)

• *Active Learning Workbook for Clinical Practice of the Dental Hygienist, 12th Edition*

prepU INDIVIDUALIZED REVIEW

(available separately; visit lww.com)

• **Adaptive quizzing with *prepU for Wilkins' Clinical Practice of the Dental Hygienist***

21

Calculus

Esther M. Wilkins, BS, RDH, DMD

CHAPTER OUTLINE

LEARNING OBJECTIVES

After studying this chapter, the student will be able to:

1. Describe the characteristics and common location of supragingival calculus and how it is detected clinically.

2. Describe the clinical and radiographic characteristics of subgingival calculus and the use of an explorer or a periodontal probe to identify locations.

3. List and compare modes of attachment of supra- and subgingival calculus to the tooth.

4. Explain the methods to prevent calculus formation.

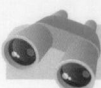

BOX 21-1 | KEY WORDS: Calculus

Amorphous: without definite shape or visible differentiation in structure.

Apatite: crystalline mineral component of bones and teeth that contains calcium and phosphate.

Dental calculus: also referred to as "tartar," calculus is dental biofilm that has been mineralized primarily with calcium and phosphorus and occur on the teeth and prosthetic appliances worn in the mouth.

Denture calculus: mineralized dental biofilm that occurs on a dental prosthesis.

Ectopic: out of place; arising or produced at an abnormal site or in a tissue where it is not normally found.

Ectopic oral calcification: examples are pulp stones, denticles, and salivary calculi.

Germfree: free of microorganisms; a germ-free animal in research is reared under completely sterile conditions.

Lamallae: thin concentric layers of bone or surrounding a central canal.

Matrix: intercellular or intermicrobial substance of a tissue, or the tissue from which a structure develops, gains support, and is held together.

Mineralization: addition of mineral elements, such as calcium and phosphorus, to the body or a part thereof with resulting hardening of the tissue.

Nidus: nucleus, focus, point of origin.

Pyrophosphate: inhibitor of calcification that occurs in parotid saliva of humans in variable amounts; anticalculus component of "tartar-control" dentifrices.

Saturated: holding all of a substance (solute) that can be dissolved in the solution.

Supersaturated: a solution containing more of an ingredient that can be held in solution permanently.

Dental calculus is dental biofilm mineralized by crystals of calcium phosphate mineral salts between previously living microorganisms.

► The calculus is covered with a layer of nonmineralized dental biofilm containing live bacteria.

► The hard, tenacious mass forms on the clinical crowns of natural teeth, dental implants, dentures, and other dental prostheses.

► Terms and key words associated with calculus are defined in Box 21-1.

► Comprehensive understanding of the characteristics, origin, development, and methods of prevention of calculus is essential to patient examination, assessment, treatment, and instruction.

► For successful treatment and prevention, the patient needs to know:
  • The interrelationship between biofilm, calculus, and oral health.
  • The need for complete removal of calculus.
  • The reasons for the meticulous manner in which scaling procedures must be carried out.

OBJECTIVES FOR DENTAL HYGIENE PRACTICE

► A major objective in nonsurgical periodontal therapy is to prepare the teeth, through definitive biofilm and calculus removal, to have biologically acceptable smooth surfaces, to facilitate healing and prevent recurrence of periodontal inflammatory diseases.

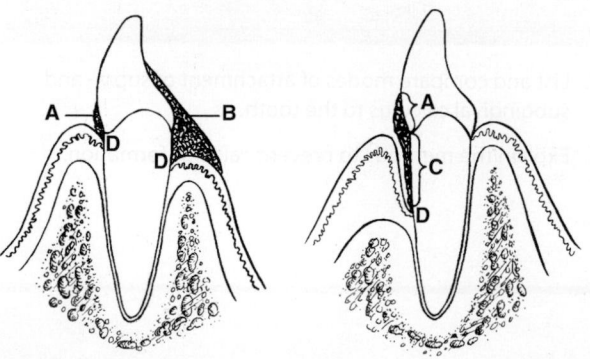

FIGURE 21-1 **Dental Calculus. A:** Supragingival calculus on cervical third of a mandibular anterior tooth extends slightly subgingivally. **B:** Supragingival calculus over crown, exposed root surface, and the margin of the gingiva. **C:** Subgingival calculus along root to the bottom of a periodontal pocket. **D:** Bottom of pocket.

CLASSIFICATION AND DISTRIBUTION OF CALCULUS

► Dental calculus is classified by its location on a tooth surface as related to the adjacent free gingival margin, that is, *supragingival* and *subgingival* calculus as shown in Figure 21-1.

► A comparison of supragingival and subgingival calculus is presented in Table 21-1.

I. Supragingival Calculus

A. Location

► On clinical crowns coronal to the margin of the gingiva (see Figure 18-1 in Chapter 18).

► On implants, complete and partial dentures.

B. Distribution: Most Frequent Sites

► On the lingual surfaces of mandibular anterior teeth and the facial surfaces of maxillary first and second molars, opposite the openings of the ducts of the submandibular and parotid salivary glands.

TABLE 21-1	Clinical Characteristics of Dental Calculus	
CHARACTERISTIC	**SUPRAGINGIVAL CALCULUS**	**SUBGINGIVAL CALCULUS**
Color	White, creamy yellow, or gray May be stained by tobacco, food, tea, or coffee Slight deposits may be invisible until dried with compressed air	Light to dark brown, dark green, or black Stains derived from blood pigments from diseased pocket
Shape	Amorphous, bulky Gross deposits may ■ Form interproximal bridge between adjacent teeth (Figure 21-2) ■ Extend over the margin of the gingiva Shape of calculus mass is determined by the anatomy of the teeth, contour of gingival margin, and pressure of the tongue, lips, cheeks	Flattened to conform with pressure from the pocket wall Combination of the following calculus formations occur ■ Crusty, spiny, or nodular ■ Ledge or ringlike ■ Thin, smooth veneers ■ Finger- and fernlike ■ Individual calculus islands
Consistency and texture	Moderately hard Newer deposits less dense and hard Porous surface covered with nonmineralized biofilm	Brittle, flintlike Harder and more dense than supragingival calculus Newest deposits near bottom of pocket are less dense and hard Surface covered with dental biofilm
Size and quantity	Quantity has direct relationship to ■ Personal oral care procedures and biofilm control measures ■ Physical character of diet ■ Individual tendencies ■ Function and use of the teeth Increased amount in tobacco smokers	Related to pocket depth Increased amount with age because of accumulation Quantity is related to personal care, diet, and individual tendency as it is with supragingival Subgingival is primarily related to the development and progression of periodontal infection
Distribution on individual tooth	Coronal to margin of gingiva May cover a large portion of the visible clinical crown, or may form fine thin line near gingival margin	Apical to margin of gingiva Extends to bottom of the pocket and follows contour of soft tissue attachment With gingival recession, subgingival calculus may become supragingival and become covered with typical supragingival calculus
Distribution on teeth	Symmetrical arrangement on teeth except when influenced by ■ Malpositioned teeth ■ Unilateral hypofunction ■ Inconsistent personal care ■ Abrasion from food Occurs with or without associated subgingival deposits Location related to openings of the salivary gland ducts: ■ Facial surface of maxillary molars ■ Lingual surface of mandibular anterior teeth	Heaviest on proximal surfaces, lightest on facial surfaces Occurs with or without associated supragingival deposits

Source: Everett FG, Potter GR. Morphology of submarginal calculus. *J Periodontol.* 1959;30(1):27–31.

▶ Figure 21-2 shows heavy supragingival calculus forming a continuous "bridge" across several teeth.

▶ On the crowns of teeth out of occlusion; nonfunctioning teeth; or teeth that are neglected during daily biofilm removal (toothbrushing, flossing, or other personal care).

▶ On surfaces of dentures, dental prostheses, and tongue piercings' barbells.

II. Subgingival Calculus

A. Location

▶ On the clinical crown apical to the margin of the gingiva and extending nearly to the clinical attachment on the root surface.

▶ On dental implants.

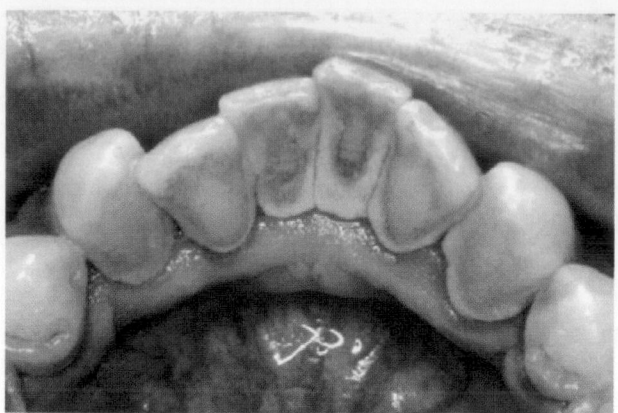

FIGURE 21-2 Supragingival Calculus. Heavy calculus deposits on the lingual surfaces of the mandibular anterior teeth. These deposits are so large that they interfere with the patient's oral self-care efforts. In addition, calculus deposits harbor living bacteria that are in constant contact with the gingival tissue. (Reprinted from Nield-Gehrig J, Willmann D. Foundations of Periodontics for the Dental Hygienist, 3rd Ed. Philadelphia: Lippincott Williams & Wilkins; 2011.)

B. Distribution

▶ May be generalized or localized on single teeth or a group of teeth.

▶ Heaviest deposits are related to areas most difficult for the patient to access during personal oral biofilm removal procedures.

▶ Figure 21-3 illustrates subgingival calculus on an extracted molar and premolar.
  • The calculus typically will form at the cemento-enamel junction (CEJ) as recession and pocket formation continue.
  • The color of subgingival calculus comes from exposure to the products of blood and blood breakdown products.

COMPOSITION

▶ Calculus is made up of inorganic and organic components and water.

▶ The percentages vary depending on the age, hardness of a deposit, and location from which the sample for analysis is taken.

▶ Mature calculus usually contains inorganic components; the rest is organic components and water.

▶ The chemical content of supragingival and subgingival calculus is similar.[1–3]

I. Inorganic Content

A. Major Inorganic Components

▶ The main components are calcium (Ca), phosphorus (P), carbonate (CO_3), sodium (Na), magnesium (Mg), and potassium (K).

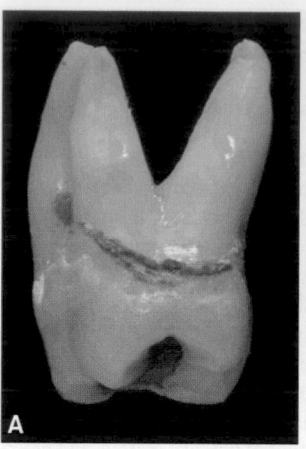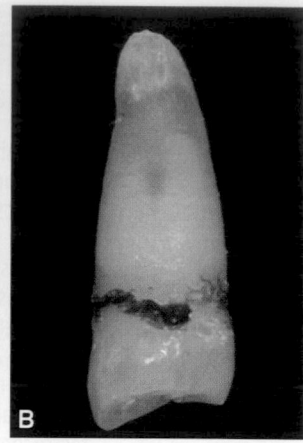

FIGURE 21-3 Subgingival Calculus on Extracted Teeth. A: On a maxillary first molar, calculus that formed in the subgingival environment is dark brown because elements of blood were incorporated during calcification. Additionally, some of the bacteria that are formed in calculus produce pigment. It can be seen here on surfaces where it most commonly forms and is often missed during periodontal instrumentation: near the CEJ, at line angles, in grooves (the concavity just coronal to the buccal furcation) and furcations. **B:** Calculus at and apical to the CEJ on a premolar. (Reprinted from Weiss G, Scheid R. Woelfel's Dental Anatomy, 9th Ed. Philadelphia: Lippincott Williams & Wilkins; 2016.)

B. Trace Elements

▶ Trace elements include chlorine (Cl), zinc (Zn), strontium (Sr), bromine (Br), copper (Cu), manganese (Mn), tungsten (W), gold (Au), aluminum (Al), silicon (Si), iron (Fe), and fluorine (F).

C. Fluoride in Calculus

▶ The concentration of fluoride in calculus varies depending on the patient's exposure to fluoride.

▶ Teeth receive fluoride from fluoridated drinking water, topical applications,[4] dentifrices,[5,6] or any form in contact with the external surface of the calculus.

D. Crystals

▶ At least two-thirds of the inorganic content of calculus is crystalline, principally apatite.

▶ The predominant form is hydroxyapatite, which is the same crystal present in enamel, dentin, cementum, and bone.

▶ Calculus also contains varying amounts of brushite, whitlockite, and octacalcium phosphate.[7]

E. Calculus Compared with Teeth and Bone

▶ Dental enamel is the most highly mineralized tissue in the body and contains 95–97% inorganic salts; dentin contains 65% and cementum and bone contain 45–70%.[8]

▶ Mature calculus has approximately 70–80% inorganic content.[9]

▶ A comparison of calculus with the tooth parts provides insight into the effects of instrumentation, the difficulty of distinguishing calculus from cementum or dentin when scaling subgingivally, and the modes of attachment of calculus to the tooth surface.

II. Organic Content

▶ The organic proportion of calculus consists of various types of microorganisms, desquamated epithelial cells, leukocytes, and mucin from the saliva.

▶ Substances identified in the organic matrix include lipids such as free fatty acids and phospholipids, and a protein portion.[10]

CALCULUS FORMATION[9,10]

Calculus results from the deposition of minerals into a biofilm organic matrix. Calculus formation occurs in three basic steps: *pellicle formation, biofilm formation,* and *mineralization*. Mineralization of supragingival and subgingival calculus is essentially the same, although the source of the elements for mineralization is not the same.

I. Pellicle Formation

▶ The pellicle, or cuticle, is composed of mucoproteins from the saliva and is an acellular material (see Chapter 15).

▶ The pellicle begins to form within minutes after all deposits have been removed from the tooth surface.

II. Biofilm Maturation

▶ Microorganisms settle in the pellicle layer.

▶ Colonies are formed. In early calculus, the colonies consist primarily of cocci and rod-shaped organisms. By the fifth day, the biofilm is mostly made up of filamentous organisms.

▶ The colonies grow together to form a cohesive biofilm layer.

III. Mineralization

A. Early Calculus Formation

▶ Mineralization foci (centers) form.

▶ Undisturbed, within 24–72 hours, more and more mineralization centers develop close to the underlying tooth surface. Eventually, the centers grow large enough to touch and unite.

▶ Mineralization first occurs within the intermicrobial matrix. The filamentous microorganisms provide the matrix for the deposition of minerals.

▶ As the deposit ages, mineralization within the bodies of the bacteria occurs.

B. Germ-free Animal Studies

▶ A calculus-like deposit has been observed on the teeth of germ-free animals that have no biofilm.[11-13]

▶ It may indicate other organic substances, such as the pellicle, mineralize.

▶ The pellicle is between the dental biofilm and the tooth surface. Since the attachment of calculus is very strong, it is likely the pellicle must mineralize to create such a firm bond.

C. Sources of Minerals

▶ *Supragingival calculus*: The source of elements for supragingival calculus is the saliva.

▶ *Subgingival calculus*: The gingival crevicular fluid and the inflammatory exudate supply the minerals for the subgingival deposits. Because the amount of GCF and exudate increases with increases in inflammation, more minerals are available for mineralization of subgingival biofilm.

D. Crystal Formation[10]

▶ Mineralization consists of crystal formation, namely, hydroxyapatite, octacalcium phosphate, whitlockite, and brushite, each with a characteristic developmental pattern.

▶ The crystals form in the intercellular matrix and on the surface of bacteria and finally within the bacteria.[14,15]

E. Mechanism of Mineralization[10]

▶ The mineralization process is considered the same for both supragingival and subgingival calculus.

▶ Calculus formation is affected by factors such as salivary flow, salivary supersaturation with calcium phosphate salts, and inhibitors and promoters of calculus formation.[10]

  • Calculus inhibitors include pyrophosphate and zinc salts.[10,16]

  • Calculus promotors include urea and silicon. Rice-based diets can be higher in silicon and contribute to greater calculus formation.[10]

▶ The difference between supragingival and subgingival calculus crystal is the calcium-to-phosphorus ratio is lower in supragingival calculus.[10]

  • Heavy calculus formers have higher salivary levels of calcium and phosphorus than do light calculus formers.

IV. Structure of Calculus

A. Layers

▶ Calculus forms in layers that are more or less parallel with the tooth surface.

▶ The layers are separated by lines that appear to be pellicle deposited over the previously formed calculus, and as mineralization progressed, the pellicle became imbedded.

▶ The lines between the layers of calculus can be called "incremental lines." They form around the tooth in supragingival calculus, but they form irregularly from crown to apex on the root surface in subgingival calculus. The lines are evidence calculus grows or increases by apposition of new layers.

B. Surface

▶ The surface of a calculus mass is rough and can be detected by the use of an explorer or a probe.

C. Outer Layer

▶ The outer layer of subgingival calculus is partly calcified.

▶ On the surface is a thick, mat-like, soft layer of dental biofilm.

▶ The outer surface of the biofilm on the subgingival calculus is in contact with the diseased pocket epithelial lining where it cannot be removed with daily oral self-care.

D. Types of calculus deposits[9]

▶ Crusty, spiny, or nodular deposits

▶ Ledge or ring formation

▶ Thin, smooth veneers

▶ Finger- and fern-like formations

▶ Individual calculus islands or spots

▶ Supragingival on subgingival deposits.

V. Formation Time

▶ Formation time means the average number of days required for the primary soft deposit to change to the mature mineralized stage.

▶ The average time is about 12 days, within a range from 10 days for rapid calculus formers to 20 days for slow calculus formers.[14] Mineralization can begin as early as 24–48 hours when a patient's personal daily oral hygiene is inadequate.

▶ Formation time depends on individual tendency, but it is strongly influenced by the roughness of the tooth surface.

▶ Estimation of the approximate formation time for an individual can be helpful when planning instruction and counseling as well as treatment planning for professional care and frequency of maintenance appointments.

ATTACHMENT OF CALCULUS[17]

▶ The ease or difficulty of calculus removal can be related to the manner of attachment of the calculus to the tooth surface.

▶ Several modes of attachment have been observed by conventional histologic techniques and electron microscopy. On any one tooth and in any one area, more than one mode of attachment may be found.

▶ When studying the attachment types, the character of the hard, smooth enamel surface and that of the rough, porous, cemental surface can be compared.

▶ Three general modes of attachment are described below.[17]

I. Attachment by Means of an Acquired Pellicle

▶ The pellicle is a thin, acellular, homogeneous layer positioned between the calculus and tooth surface.

▶ Calculus attachment is superficial because no interlocking or penetration occurs and calculus can be easily removed.

▶ Pellicle attachment occurs most frequently on enamel and newly scaled and planed root surfaces.

II. Attachment to Minute Irregularities in the Tooth Surface by Mechanical Locking into Undercuts

▶ Dentin irregularities include cracks, lamellae, and carious defects.

▶ Cemental irregularities include tiny spaces left at previous locations of Sharpey's fibers, resorption lacunae, root gouging from improper scaling, and cemental tears.

▶ Difficult to be certain all calculus is removed when it is attached by this method because calculus becomes locked into the irregularities.

III. Attachment by Direct Contact Between Calcified Intercellular Matrix and the Tooth Surface

▶ Interlocking of inorganic apatite crystals of the enamel and cementum with the mineralizing dental biofilm (calculus).

▶ Research suggests this mode of attachment results in a portion of the calculus that is prone to fracture during removed, but it may leave calculus crystals attached to the tooth surface.[17]

• These remaining calculus calcium phosphate crystals may serve as a nidus for biofilm formation.

SIGNIFICANCE OF DENTAL CALCULUS

There has been a long-standing debate over whether subgingival calculus has a role in periodontal disease.[9,16]

▶ Despite the debate, the disease-producing bacteria held in the rough surface of the calculus perpetuate the inflamed state supragingivally for gingivitis and subgingivally close to the pocket lining epithelium to promote periodontitis.[17]

▶ The cornerstone of nonsurgical periodontal therapy is the control of biofilm deposits by the patient on a daily basis, supplemented by definitive professional calculus removal, to reduce or eliminate gingival inflammation and bleeding on probing.

I. Relation to Dental Biofilm

▶ Subgingival biofilm develops as a result of downgrowth of supragingival biofilm.

▶ Subgingival biofilm contains pathogenic bacteria that cause inflammation and destruction in the soft tissue and lead to loss of attachment to the tooth surface and development and deepening of the pocket.

II. Relation to Attachment Loss and Pocket Formation

▶ Subgingival calculus is covered by masses of live biofilm bacteria.

• With its rough surface, permeable structure, and porosity, calculus acts as a reservoir for endotoxins and tissue breakdown products.

• The bacterial mass is in contact with the diseased pocket epithelium and promotes gingivitis and periodontitis.

• Irritation to the pocket lining stimulates greater flow of gingival sulcus fluid, which contains minerals for subgingival calculus formation.

▶ Calculus is a predisposing factor in pocket development in that it provides a haven for the collection of bacterial masses on the rough surface of the calculus deposit.

CLINICAL CHARACTERISTICS

▶ Identification of calculus prior to removal depends on knowledge of its appearance, consistency, and distribution.

▶ Appointment planning, selection of instruments, and techniques depend on understanding the texture, morphology, and mode of attachment of calculus. Table 21-1 lists a summary of clinical characteristics.

I. Supragingival Examination

A. Direct Examination

Supragingival deposits may be seen directly or indirectly, using a mouth mirror.

B. Use of Compressed Air

▶ Small amounts of calculus may be invisible when they are wet with saliva.

▶ With light and drying with air, small deposits usually can be seen.

II. Subgingival Examination

A. Visual Examination

▶ Dark edge of calculus may be seen at or just beneath the gingival margin.

▶ Gentle air blast can deflect the margin from the tooth for observation into the pocket.

▶ Using transillumination, a dark, opaque, shadow-like area seen on a proximal tooth surface may be subgingival calculus. Without calculus, stain, or thick soft deposit, the enamel is translucent.

B. Gingival Tissue Color Change

▶ Dark calculus may reflect through a thin margin and suggest the presence of subgingival calculus.

C. Tactile Examination

▶ *Probe*: While probing for sulcus/pocket characteristics, a rough subgingival tooth surface can be felt when calculus is present.

▶ *Explorer*: A fine subgingival explorer is needed that can be adapted close to the root surface all the way to the bottom of a pocket. Figure 20-3 in Chapter 20 shows the use of the subgingival explorer.

▶ Each subgingival area is explored carefully to the bottom of the pocket, completely around each tooth.

D. Radiographic Examination

▶ Radiographic examination is not useful for calculus detection except for proximal surfaces (see Figure 21-4A and B).

▶ Thick, highly mineralized calculus may be detected on proximal tooth surfaces except when there is overlapping.

E. Dental Endoscopy

▶ The use of the dental endoscopy in deep pockets and furcations can detect otherwise undetectable calculus, especially burnished or veneer-type calculus.[18]

PREVENTION OF CALCULUS

▶ Risk factors related to calculus formation are similar to those for dental biofilm formation and relate to biofilm removal during the patient's personal daily oral self-care.

▶ Patients at risk for calculus formation need personalized oral self-care education.

▶ There are several methods for managing and minimizing calculus formation including effective daily biofilm removal, professional clinical nonsurgical periodontal therapy, and chemotherapeutic agents such as pyrophosphates (antitartar) and triclosan (antimicrobial).[10]

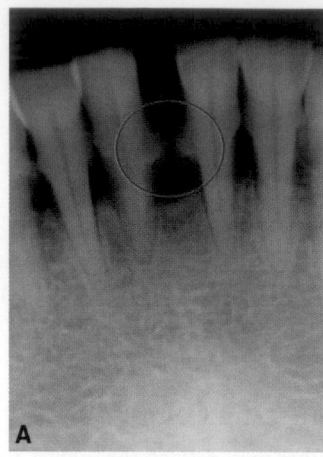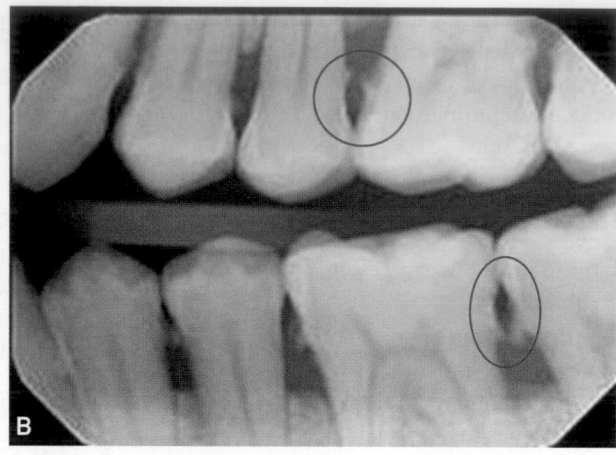

FIGURE 21-4 **Subgingival Calculus in Radiographs. A:** Heavy supra- and subgingival proximal calculus is shown on the mandibular anterior teeth (#24–25). **B:** The bitewing radiographs show heavy ledgers or spines of subgingival calculus in the proximal areas of premolar and molar areas.

I. Personal Dental Biofilm Control

A. Objective

▶ Removal of dental biofilm by appropriately selected brushing, interdental care, and supplementary methods is a major factor in the control of dental calculus reformation.

B. Instruction

▶ The patient needs to understand the necessity for individual daily biofilm removal and be motivated to spend time each day.

▶ Patient education includes:
   • Identification and hands-on demonstration of the oral hygiene aids appropriate for the patient's needs.
   • Follow-up at continuing care appointments to commend the patient's successes and review and refine techniques as necessary.
   • Identification of dietary behaviors that may be enhancing biofilm growth such as sugar-sweetened beverages and sugary snacks between meals.

C. Regular Professional Supervision

▶ Professional maintenance appointments on a regular basis can supplement the personal care.

II. Professional Removal of Calculus

▶ Thorough removal of calculus provides a smooth tooth surface in an environment conducive to gingival healing.

▶ The smooth surfaces can be easier for the patient to maintain.

▶ With emphasis on good oral hygiene and routine professional removal, low levels of supragingival and subgingival calculus can be maintained on a long-term basis.[19]

III. Anticalculus Dentifrice and Mouthrinse

A. Objective

▶ Calculus-control dentifrices currently available aim to inhibit calculus crystal growth, which in turn can lessen the amount of calculus deposited on the teeth.

▶ The dentifrices do not have an effect on existing calculus deposits and are offered as a preventive measure against the formation of new supragingival calculus.

▶ For a patient who cannot control supragingival calculus, and hence cannot achieve optimum gingival tissue health, an anticalculus dentifrice may provide motivation, as well as be a supplement to mechanical biofilm removal efforts.[20]

B. Chemotherapeutic Anticalculus Agents

▶ Agents used in "tartar-control" mouthrinses or dentifrices are mineralization inhibitors.
   • Examples include pyrophosphates, zinc citrate or zinc chloride, and triclosan.[10,16]

▶ Soft tissue irritation or dentinal hypersensitivity may contraindicate their use in selected patients.

DOCUMENTATION

The permanent record of the patient subject to formation of calculus needs to include a minimum of the following:

▶ Calculus deposits are described in the initial examination record: charted to show location for reference during the clinical removal and during teaching personal care for prevention.

▶ The extent of supragingival and subgingival deposits (slight, moderate, or heavy) is designated for diagnosis, treatment planning, and for reference during instrumentation.

EVERYDAY ETHICS

Coronal polishing for dental assistants legislation had just been passed at the state level. Certified dental assistants (CDA) were now eligible to take a short course and then begin polishing procedures for a patient after the dentist or the dental hygienist removes all calculus deposits. Mindy, the CDA in the office, completed the course and was ready to polish. As the hygienist in the office, Hilary was basically unaffected by the change in the dental practice act and continued to treat her patients in all aspects of the preventive protocol.

However, Dr. Bell found that additional services could be offered to his patients at the time of their restorative appointment by removing the calculus and then having Mindy finish with the polish. One day, as Hilary was on her way to find Dr. Bell to check her patient, she saw Mindy

using a curet to remove what she stated as "slight subgingival deposits that didn't come off with the rubber cup."

Questions for Consideration

1. Which of the dental hygiene core values (Table II-1 in Section II, Introduction) enter into the actions of this scenario? Explain the relationship of each of the selected ones.

2. Would you consider what the hygienist observed the dental assistant doing as an ethical issue or a dilemma? Explain your answer.

3. If Dr. Bell dismisses the fact that Mindy was using instruments to remove calculus, what choices of action could Hilary pursue?

▶ Personal patient care procedures demonstrated; preventive measures discussed; and frequency of continuing care appointments recommended.

▶ A sample patient progress note may be reviewed in Box 21-2.

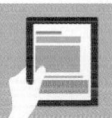

BOX 21-2
Example Documentation: Patient with Calculus

S –Female patient, aged 24, presents for routine maintenance appointment. Chief complaint: "For the last few weeks, I have had an irritated gum around the tongue-side of my lower left wisdom tooth and sometimes there is bleeding in that area when I brush. I think it is because I am left handed and I have a hard time turning the brush to reach that area."

O –Generalized pocket depths of < 3 mm with no bleeding on probing except #17, which had a distal pocket depth of 5 mm and a significant ledge of subgingival calculus on the distal and lingual surfaces.

A –It is possible that residual calculus remained in that area after her last dental hygiene appointment, and removing it will resolve the issue.

P –Prophylaxis completed with subgingival debridement full mouth, calculus removed from lingual and distal surfaces of tooth #17 and distal surface of #16 and #32. Educated patient regarding the etiology and significance of dental calculus build-up. Patient instruction related to turning the toothbrush head to reach below the margin of the gingiva on the lingual and distal surfaces of all last molars. Floss instruction for distal surfaces of last molars using tufted dental floss.

Next step: Reappoint in 2 weeks to reevaluate.

Signed _____, RDH

Date _____

Factors To Teach The Patient

▷ Optimal oral hygiene and frequent professional care for complete scaling are consistent with low levels of supragingival and subgingival calculus.

▷ What calculus is and how it forms from dental biofilm.

▷ The effect of calculus on the health of the periodontal tissues and, therefore, on the general health of the oral cavity.

▷ Properties of calculus that explain the need for detailed, meticulous scaling procedures.

▷ Reasons for producing a calculus-free smooth tooth surface during scaling.

▷ Biofilm control measures that the patient can carry out to minimize calculus deposits.

▷ What to expect from use of an anticalculus dentifrice.

▷ Select products with an American Dental Association Seal of Acceptance.

References

1. Mandel ID. Biochemical aspects of calculus formation. I. Comparative studies of plaque in heavy and light calculus formers. *J Periodontal Res*. 1974;9(1):10–17.

2. Glock GE, Murray MM. Chemical investigation of salivary calculus. *J Dent Res*. 1938;17:257.

3. Mandel ID, Levy BM. Studies on salivary calculus. I. Histochemical and chemical investigations of supra- and subgingival calculus. *Oral Surg Oral Med Oral Pathol*. 1957;10(8):874–884.

4. Schait A, Mühlemann HR. Fluoride uptake by calculus following topical application of fluorides. *Helv Odont Acta*. 1971;15(2):132–133.

5. Kinoshita S, Schait A, Schroeder HE, et al. Origin of fluoride in early dental calculus. *Helv Odont Acta*. 1965;9(2):141–147.

6. Mühlemann HR, Schait A, Schroeder HE. Salivary origin of fluorine in calcified dental plaques. *Helv Odont Acta.* 1964;8:128.

7. Gron P, Van Campen GJ, Lindstrom I. Human dental calculus. Inorganic chemical and crystallographic composition. *Arch Oral Biol.* 1967;12(7):829–837.

8. Palmer LC, Newcomb CJ, Kaltz SR, et al. Biomimetic systems for hydroxyapatite mineralization inspired by bone and enamel. *Chem Rev.* 2008;108(11):4754–4783.

9. Roberts-Harry EA, Clerehugh V. Subgingival calculus: where are we now? A comparative review. *J Dent.* 2000;28(2):93–102.

10. Jin Y, Yip HK. Supragingival calculus: formation and control. *Critc Rev Oral Biol Med.* 2002;13(5);426–441.

11. Fitzgerald RJ, McDaniel EG. Dental calculus in the germ-free rat. *Arch Oral Biol.* 1960;2:239–240.

12. Gustafsson BE, Krasse B. Dental calculus in germfree rats. *Acta Odontol Scand.* 1962;20(2):135–142.

13. Theilade J, Fitzgerald RJ, Scott DB, et al. Electron microscopic observations of dental calculus in germfree and conventional rats. *Arch Oral Biol.* 1964;9:97–100.

14. Gonzales F, Sognnaes RF. Electron microscopy of dental calculus. *Science.* 1960;131:156–158.

15. Zander HA, Hazen SP, Scott DB. Mineralization of dental calculus. *Proc Soc Exp Biol Med.* 1960;103:257–260.

16. White DJ. Dental calculus: recent insights into occurrence, formation, prevention, removal and oral health effects of supragingival and subgingival deposits. *Eur J Oral Sci.* 1997;105(5 Pt 2):508–522.

17. Rohanizadeh R, Legeros RZ. Ultrastructural study of calculus-enamel and calculus-root interfaces. *Arch Oral Biol.* 2005;50(1):89–96.

18. Osborn JB, Lenton PA, Lunos SA, et al. Endoscopic vs. tactile evaluation of subgingival calculus. *J Dent Hyg.* 2014;88(4):229–236.

19. Schätzle M, Faddy MJ, Cullinan MP, et al. The clinical course of chronic periodontitis. V. Predictive factors in periodontal disease. *J Clin Periodontol.* 2009;36(5):365–371.

20. Riley P, Lamont T. Triclosan/copolymer containing toothpastes for oral health. *Cochrane Database Syst Rev.* 2013;12:CD010514.

ENHANCE YOUR UNDERSTANDING

thePoint° DIGITAL CONNECTIONS
(see the inside front cover for access information)

- **Audio glossary**
- **Quiz bank**

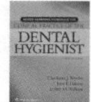

SUPPORT FOR LEARNING
(available separately; visit lww.com)

- ***Active Learning Workbook for Clinical Practice of the Dental Hygienist, 12th Edition***

prepU INDIVIDUALIZED REVIEW
(available separately; visit lww.com)

- **Adaptive quizzing with *prepU for Wilkins' Clinical Practice of the Dental Hygienist***

22

Dental Stains and Discolorations

Elizabeth G. Onik, RDH, MEd

CHAPTER OUTLINE

SIGNIFICANCE
I. Classification of Stains
II. Recognition and Identification
III. Application of Procedures for Stain Removal

EXTRINSIC STAINS
I. Yellow Stain
II. Green Stain
III. Black-Line Stain
IV. Tobacco Stain

V. Brown Stains
VI. Orange and Red Stains
VII. Metallic Stains

ENDOGENOUS INTRINSIC STAINS
I. Pulpless or Traumatized Teeth
II. Disturbances in Tooth Development
III. Drug-Induced Stains and Discolorations
IV. Other Systemic Causes

EXOGENOUS INTRINSIC STAINS
I. Restorative Materials
II. Endodontic Therapy
III. Stain in Dentin
IV. Local Causes

DOCUMENTATION
EVERYDAY ETHICS
FACTORS TO TEACH THE PATIENT
REFERENCES

LEARNING OBJECTIVES

After studying this chapter, the student will be able to:

1. Recognize and identify extrinsic and intrinsic dental stains and discolorations.

2. Differentiate between exogenous and endogenous stains.

3. Educate patients regarding the etiology and/or prevention of dental stains.

4. Determine appropriate clinical approaches for stain removal and/or tooth whitening.

Discolorations of the teeth and restorations occur in three general ways[1]:

▶ Adheres directly to the surfaces

▶ Contained within calculus and soft deposits

▶ Incorporated within the tooth structure or the restorative material.

Instructional and clinical procedures apply to all three. The first two types may be removed by scaling or polishing. Certain stains may be prevented by the patient's routine personal care and dietary habits.

SIGNIFICANCE

▶ The significance of stains is primarily the appearance or cosmetic effect.

▶ In general, any detrimental effect on the teeth or gingival tissues is related to the dental biofilm or calculus in which the stain occurs.

▶ Thick deposits of stain conceivably can provide a rough surface on which dental biofilm can collect and irritate the adjacent gingiva.

▶ Certain stains provide a means of evaluating oral cleanliness and the patient's habits of personal care.

▶ Key words that relate to dental stains and discolorations are defined in Box 22-1.

I. Classification of Stains

A. Classified by Location

▶ *Extrinsic*: Extrinsic stains occur on the external surface of the tooth and may be removed by procedures of toothbrushing, scaling, and/or polishing.

▶ *Intrinsic*: Intrinsic stains occur within the tooth surface and cannot be removed by scaling or polishing. Intrinsic stains may be improved by certain whitening procedures.

B. Classified by Source

▶ *Exogenous*: Exogenous stains develop or originate from sources outside the tooth. Exogenous stains may be extrinsic and stay on the outer surface of the tooth or

intrinsic and become incorporated within the tooth structure.

▶ *Endogenous*: Endogenous stains develop or originate from within the tooth. Endogenous stains are always intrinsic and usually are discolorations of the dentin reflected through the enamel.

II. Recognition and Identification

More than one type of stain may occur and more than one etiologic factor may cause the stains and discolorations of an individual's dentition. A differential diagnosis may be needed in order to plan whether an appropriate intervention is indicated.

A. Medical and Dental History

▶ Developmental complications, medications, use of tobacco, and fluoride histories all contribute necessary information.

▶ Accurately prepared medical, dental and social histories, and ethnic practices can provide information to supplement clinical observations.

B. Food Diary

▶ Assessment of a patient's food diary may aid in identifying certain contributing factors.

  • Examples of staining from beverages include tea and coffee.

C. Oral Hygiene Habits

▶ The history of personal biofilm removal with the type and frequency of use of toothbrush, floss, and other supplemental materials and devices may help explain the presence of certain stains.

▶ The state of oral hygiene and oral cleanliness is significant to the occurrence of dental stains.

III. Application of Procedures for Stain Removal

A. Stains Occurring Directly on the Tooth Surface

▶ Stains directly associated with the biofilm or pellicle on the surface of the enamel or exposed cementum are

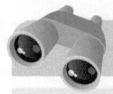

BOX 22-1 **KEY WORDS:** Dental Stains and Discolorations

Amelogenesis imperfecta: imperfect formation of enamel; hereditary condition in which the ameloblasts fail to lay down the enamel matrix properly or at all.

Chlorophyll: green plant pigment essential to photosynthesis.

Chromogenic: producing color or pigment.

Chronologic: arranged in order of time.

Dentinogenesis imperfecta: hereditary disorder of dentin formation in which the odontoblasts lay down

an abnormal matrix; can occur in both primary and permanent dentitions.

Endogenous: produced within or caused by factors within.

Exogenous: originating outside or caused by factors outside.

Extrinsic: derived from or situated on the outside; external.

Hypoplasia: incomplete development or underdevelopment of an organ or a tissue.

Intrinsic: situated entirely within.

removed as much as possible during toothbrushing by the patient.

▶ Certain stains can be removed by scaling, whereas others require scaling and/or polishing (see Chapter 45).

▶ When stains are tenacious, excessive polishing is avoided. As mild an abrasive agent as possible is used. Precautions are taken to prevent the following:
 • Abrasion of the tooth surface or gingival margin
 • Removal of a layer of fluoride-rich tooth surface
 • Overheating with a power-driven polisher.

B. Stains Incorporated Within Tooth Deposits

▶ When stain is included within the substance of a soft deposit or calculus, it is removed with the deposit.

C. Stains Incorporated Within the Tooth

▶ When stain is intrinsic, whether exogenous or endogenous, it cannot be removed by scaling or polishing. Evaluation for possible whitening procedures may be considered. (See Chapter 46.)

EXTRINSIC STAINS

The most frequently observed stains, yellow, green, black line, and tobacco, are described first; descriptions of the less common orange, red, and metallic stains follow.

I. Yellow Stain

A. Clinical Features

▶ Dull, yellowish discoloration of dental biofilm is illustrated in Figure 22-1.

B. Distribution on Tooth Surfaces

▶ Yellow stain can be generalized or localized.

C. Occurrence

▶ Common to all ages.

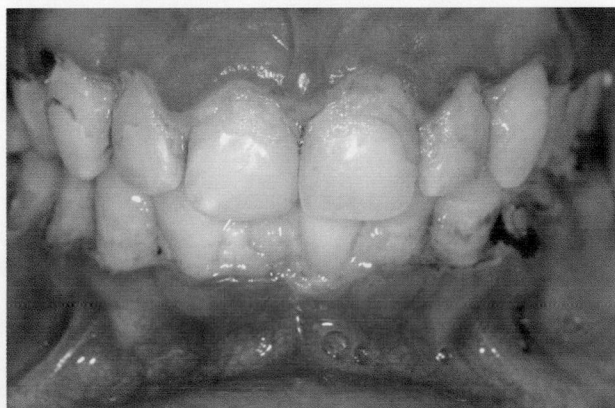

FIGURE 22-1. Yellow Stain. Generalized, dull, yellowish discoloration of dental biofilm. (Photograph used by permission of Dr. Ali Seyedain, University of Pittsburgh.)

▶ More evident when personal oral care procedures are neglected.

D. Etiology

▶ Usually dietary sources.

II. Green Stain

A. Clinical Features

▶ Light or yellowish green to very dark green.

▶ Embedded in dental biofilm.

▶ Occurs in three general forms:
 • Small curved line following contour of facial gingival margin.
 • Smeared irregularly, may even cover entire facial surface.
 • Streaked, following grooves or lines in enamel.

▶ The stain is frequently superimposed by soft yellow or gray debris (materia alba and food debris).

▶ Dark green may become embedded in surface enamel and be observed as an exogenous intrinsic stain when superficial layers of deposit are removed.

▶ Enamel under stain is sometimes demineralized as a result of cariogenic biofilm. The rough demineralized surface encourages biofilm retention, demineralization, and recurrence of green stain.

B. Distribution on Tooth Surfaces

▶ Primarily facial; often extends to proximal.

▶ Most frequently facial gingival third of maxillary anterior teeth.

C. Composition

▶ Chromogenic bacteria and fungi.

▶ Decomposed hemoglobin.

▶ Inorganic elements include calcium, potassium, sodium, silicon, magnesium, phosphorus, and other elements in small amounts.[2]

D. Occurrence

▶ May occur at any age; primarily found in childhood.

▶ Collects on both permanent and primary teeth.

E. Recurrence

▶ Recurrence depends on fastidiousness of personal care procedures.

F. Etiology

▶ Green stain results from poor oral hygiene, dental biofilm retention, chromogenic bacteria, and gingival hemorrhage.

▶ Chromogenic bacteria or fungi are retained and nourished in dental biofilm where the green stain is produced.

▶ Blood pigments from hemoglobin are decomposed by bacteria.

G. Clinical Approach

▶ Do not scale the area. Often, an area of demineralized tooth structure underlies the stain and soft deposits.

▶ Ask the patient to remove the soft deposits with a toothbrush during a dental biofilm control lesson. Initiate a daily fluoride remineralization program.

H. Other Green Stains

▶ In addition to the clinical entity known as "green stain" that was just described, dental biofilm and acquired pellicle may become stained a green color by a variety of substances.

▶ Differential distinction may be determined by questioning the patient or from items in the medical or dental histories. Green discoloration may result from the following:
  • Chlorophyll preparations
  • Metallic dusts of industry
  • Certain drugs. The stain from smoking marijuana may appear grayish-green.

III. Black-Line Stain

▶ Black-line stain is a highly retentive black or dark brown calculus-like stain that forms along the gingival third near the gingival margin. It may occur on primary or permanent teeth.

A. Other Names

▶ Pigmented dental biofilm, brown stain, black stain.

B. Clinical Features

▶ Continuous or interrupted fine line, 1 mm wide (average), no appreciable thickness.

▶ May be a wider band or even occupy entire gingival third in severe cases (rare).

▶ Follows contour of gingival margin about 1 mm from margin.

▶ Usually separated from gingival margin by clear white line of unstained enamel.

▶ Appears black at bases of pits and fissures.

▶ Heavy deposits slightly elevated from the tooth surface may be detected by the gentle application of an explorer. Black-line stain has been compared to a calculus deposit.

▶ Gingiva is firm, with little or no tendency to bleed.

▶ Teeth are frequently clean and shiny, with a tendency to lower incidence of dental caries.[3]

C. Distribution on Tooth Surfaces

▶ Facial and lingual surfaces; follows contour of gingival margin onto proximal surfaces.

▶ Rarely on facial surface of maxillary anterior teeth.

▶ Most frequently: lingual and proximal surfaces of maxillary posterior teeth.

D. Composition and Formation[4,5]

▶ Black-line stain, like calculus, is composed of microorganisms embedded in an intermicrobial substance.

▶ The microorganisms are primarily gram-positive rods, with smaller percentages of cocci.

▶ The composition of black-line stain is different from the composition of supragingival calculus, in which cocci predominate.

▶ Attachment of black-line stain to the tooth is by a pellicle-like structure.

▶ Mineralization in black-line stain is similar to the formation of calculus.

E. Occurrence

▶ All ages; more common in childhood.

▶ More common in female patients.

▶ Frequently found in clean mouths.

F. Recurrence

▶ Black-line stain tends to form again despite regular personal care.

▶ Quantity may be less when biofilm control procedures are meticulous.

G. Predisposing Factors

▶ No definitive etiology.[3]

IV. Tobacco Stain[1]

A. Clinical Features

▶ Light brown to dark leathery brown or black (see Figure 22-2).

▶ Shape
  • Diffuse staining of dental biofilm.

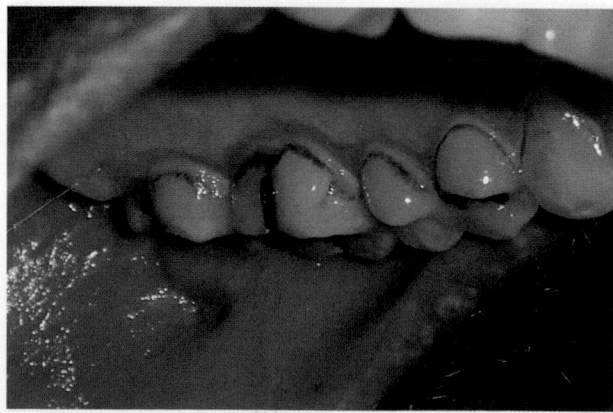

FIGURE 22-2. Tobacco Stain. Dark brown band following contour of gingival crest. (Photograph used by permission of Dr. Julius Manz, San Juan College, NM.)

- Narrow band that follows contour of gingival crest, slightly above the crest.
  - Wide, firm, tar-like band may cover cervical third and extend to central third of crown.
- Incorporated in calculus deposit.
- Heavy deposits (particularly from smokeless tobacco) may penetrate the enamel and become exogenous intrinsic.

B. Distribution on Tooth Surface

- Cervical third, primarily. Lingual surfaces, most frequently.
- Any surface, including pits and fissures.

C. Composition

- Tar and products of combustion.
- Brown pigment from smokeless tobacco.

D. Predisposing Factors

- Smoking or chewing tobacco, or use of hookah to inhale tobacco. The quantity of stain is not necessarily proportional to the amount of tobacco used.
- Personal oral care procedures: increased deposits occur with neglect.
- Extent of dental biofilm and calculus available for adherence.

V. Brown Stains

A. Brown Pellicle

- The acquired pellicle is smooth and structureless and recurs readily after removal (Figure 22-3).[6]
- The pellicle can take on stains of various colors that result from chemical alteration of the pellicle.[7]

B. Stannous Fluoride[8,9]

- Light brown, sometimes yellowish, stain forms on the teeth in the pellicle after repeated use of some stannous fluoride products.

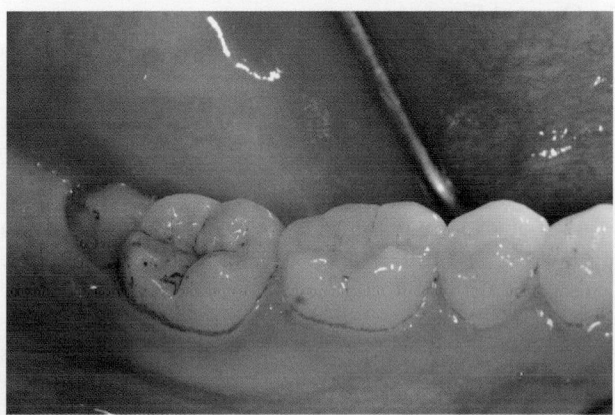

FIGURE 22-3. Brown Stain. Most likely cause by pigmented foods or drinks. (Photograph used by permission of Dr. Ali Seyedain, University of Pittsburgh.)

- The brown stain results from the formation of stannous sulfide or brown tin oxide from the reaction of the tin ion in the fluoride compound.

C. Pigmented Foods

- Tea, coffee, soy sauce, and other foods are often implicated in the formation of a brownish-stained pellicle.
- As with other brown pellicle stains, less stain occurs when the personal oral hygiene and biofilm control are excellent.

D. Anti-Biofilm Agents[10,11]

- Chlorhexidine and alexidine are used in mouthrinses and are effective against biofilm formation.
- A brownish stain on the tooth surfaces may result, usually more pronounced on proximal and other surfaces less accessible to routine biofilm control procedures.
- The stain also tends to form more rapidly on exposed roots than on enamel. Tooth staining has been considered a significant side effect.
- Clinical implications: Avoid use of these antimicrobials if enamel defects, porous restorations, or open margins are present. Stain may not be removable from these surfaces.

E. Betel Leaf[12]

- Betel leaf chewing is common among people of all ages in eastern countries. Betel has a caries-inhibiting effect.
- The discoloration imparted to the teeth is a dark mahogany brown, sometimes almost black. It may become thick and hard, with partly smooth and partly rough surfaces.
- Microscopically, the black deposit consists of microorganisms and mineralized material with a laminated pattern characteristic of subgingival calculus. It can be removed by gentle scaling.

F. Swimmer's Stain[13]

- Frequent exposure to pools disinfected with chlorine or bromine can cause yellowish or dark brown stains on the facial surfaces of maxillary and mandibular incisor teeth.

VI. Orange and Red Stains

A. Clinical Appearance

- Orange or red stains appear at the cervical third.

B. Distribution on Tooth Surfaces

- More frequently on anterior than on posterior teeth.

C. Occurrence

- Rare (red more rare than orange).

D. Etiology

▶ Chromogenic bacteria.

VII. Metallic Stains[1]

A. Metals or Metallic Salts from Metal-Containing Dust of Industry

▶ Clinical appearance/examples of colors on teeth:
  • Copper or brass: green or bluish-green.
  • Iron: brown to greenish-brown.
  • Nickel: green.
  • Cadmium: yellow or golden brown.
▶ Distribution on tooth surfaces
  • Primarily anterior; may occur on any teeth.
  • Cervical third more commonly affected.
▶ Manner of formation
  • Industrial worker inhales dust through mouth, bringing metallic substance in contact with teeth.
  • Metal imparts color to biofilm.
  • Occasionally, stain may penetrate tooth substance and become exogenous intrinsic stain.
▶ Prevention
  • Workers need to be advised to wear a mask while working.

B. Metallic Substances Contained in Drugs

▶ Clinical appearance/examples of colors on teeth:
  • Iron: black (iron sulfide) or brown.
  • Manganese (from potassium permanganate): black.
▶ Distribution on tooth surfaces
  • Generalized, may occur on all.
▶ Manner of formation
  • Drug enters biofilm substance, imparts color to biofilm and calculus.
  • Pigment from drug may attach directly to tooth enamel.
▶ Prevention
  • Use a medication through a straw or in tablet or capsule form to prevent direct contact with the teeth.

ENDOGENOUS INTRINSIC STAINS

I. Pulpless or Traumatized Teeth

Not all pulpless teeth discolor. Improved endodontic procedures have contributed to the prevention of discolorations. However, traumatized teeth that have not been treated endodontically often discolor.

A. Clinical Appearance

▶ A wide range of colors exists; stains may be light yellow-brown, slate gray, reddish-brown, dark brown, bluish-black, or black. Others have an orange or greenish tinge.

B. Etiology

▶ Blood and other pulp tissue elements may be available for breakdown as a result of hemorrhages in the pulp chamber, root canal treatment, or necrosis and decomposition of the pulp tissue.
▶ Pigments from the decomposed hemoglobin and pulp tissue penetrate and discolor the dentinal tubules.

II. Disturbances in Tooth Development[14]

Stains incorporated within the tooth structure may be related to the period of tooth development. Defective tooth development may result from factors of genetic abnormality or environmental influences during tooth development.

A. Hereditary: Genetic

▶ *Amelogenesis imperfecta*: The enamel is partially or completely missing because of a generalized disturbance of the ameloblasts. Teeth are yellowish-brown or gray-brown.
▶ *Dentinogenesis imperfecta* ("*Opalescent dentin*"): The dentin is abnormal as a result of disturbances in the odontoblastic layer during development. The teeth appear translucent or opalescent and vary in color from gray to bluish-brown.

B. Enamel Hypoplasia

▶ *Generalized hypoplasia* (chronologic hypoplasia resulting from ameloblastic disturbance of short duration): Teeth erupt with white spots or with pits. Over a long period, the white spots may become discolored from food pigments or other substances taken into the mouth.
▶ *Local hypoplasia* (affects single tooth): For example, individual white spots caused by trauma to a primary tooth interferes with development of permanent tooth resulting in "Turner's tooth." White spots may become stained as in generalized hypoplasia.

C. Dental Fluorosis

▶ Dental fluorosis was originally called "brown stain." Later, Dr. Frederick S. McKay, who studied the condition and described it in the dental literature, named it "mottled enamel."
▶ Etiology
  • Enamel hypomineralization results from ingestion of excessive fluoride ion from any source during the period of mineralization. The enamel alterations are a result of toxic damage to the ameloblasts.
  • When the teeth erupt, they have white spots or areas that may later become discolored from oral pigments and appear light to dark brown in color.
  • Severe effects of excess fluoride during development may produce cracks or pitting; the discoloration

concentrates in these. This condition and appearance led to the name mottled enamel.

- Classification
  - Dean provided the original definitions for five grades of fluorosis (Table 23-2 in Chapter 23). They ranged from "questionable" (a few white flecks or spots) to "severe" (marked brown staining and pitting of the enamel surfaces).[15]
  - More specific classifications have been developed for clinical and research purposes, such as the tooth surface index of fluorosis[16,17] (Table 23-3 in Chapter 23).

III. Drug-Induced Stains and Discolorations[18]

A. Tetracyclines

- Tetracycline antibiotics, used widely for combating many types of infections, have an affinity for mineralized tissues (Figure 46-3 in Chapter 46).
  - Are absorbed by the bones and teeth.
  - Can be transferred through the placenta and enter fetal circulation.
- Discoloration of the teeth of a child can result when the drug is administered to the mother during the third trimester of pregnancy or to the child in infancy and early childhood.
- Color of teeth may be light green to dark yellow, or a gray-brown, with or without banding.
- The discoloration depends on the dosage, the length of time the drug was used, and the type of tetracycline. After eruption, the teeth may fluoresce under ultraviolet light, but that property is lost with age and exposure.
- Discoloration may be generalized or limited to specific parts of individual teeth that were developing at the time of administration of the antibiotic.
- Refer to the timing of tooth development for primary teeth (Table 50-4 in Chapter 50) and permanent teeth (Table 16-1 in Chapter 16) to assess the impact of drug administration on tooth discoloration.
- The patient's medical history at that age may reveal the illness for which the antibiotic was prescribed.

B. Cipro and Minocycline

- Use of these antibiotics can result in a greenish discoloration of teeth.[18]

IV. Other Systemic Causes

- Several types of tooth discolorations may result from blood-borne pigments.
- Pigments circulating in the blood are transmitted to the dentin from the capillaries of the pulp. For example, prolonged jaundice early in life can impart a yellow or greenish discoloration to the teeth.
- Erythroblastosis fetalis (Rh incompatibility) may leave a green, brown, or blue hue to the teeth.

EXOGENOUS INTRINSIC STAINS

- When intrinsic stains come from an outside source, not from within the tooth, the stain is called exogenous intrinsic.
- Extrinsic stains, such as tobacco, tea, coffee, wine, and green stains, can become intrinsic (see Figure 22-4).
- Restorative materials cause staining of teeth, as described in the following section.
- Tooth-color restorations may become stained from extrinsic staining sources.

I. Restorative Materials

A. Silver Amalgam

- Silver amalgam can impart a gray to black discoloration to the tooth structure around a restoration.
- Metallic ions migrate from the amalgam restoration into the enamel and dentin.
- Silver, tin, and mercury ions eventually contact debris at the junction of the tooth and the restoration and form sulfides, which are products of corrosion.

B. Copper Amalgam

- Copper amalgam used for filling primary teeth may impart a bluish-green color.

II. Endodontic Therapy

Materials used during endodontic therapy can cause intrinsic staining.

- Silver nitrate: bluish-black.
- Volatile oils: yellowish-brown.
- Strong iodine: brown.
- Aureomycin: yellow.
- Silver-containing root canal sealer: black.

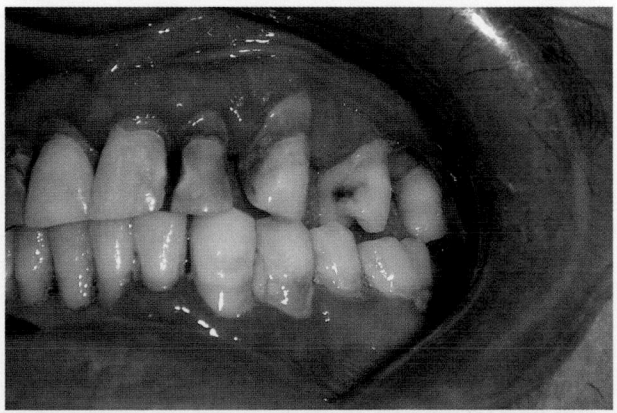

FIGURE 22-4. Intrinsic Stain. Most likely exogenous; likely from an outside source such as tobacco or food and became intrinsic over time. Areas of cervical erosion and recession allow yellow color of underlying dentin to be exposed and become further stained. (Photograph used by permission of Dr. Julius Manz, San Juan College, NM.)

III. Stain in Dentin

▶ Discoloration resulting from a carious lesion is an example.

▶ Arrested decay or secondary dentin can present as black stain on severely decayed teeth. The surface is hard and glossy, and stain cannot be removed.

IV. Other Local Causes

▶ Low pH. The degree and type of tooth discoloration are influenced by both the low pH and the food color rather than dietary pigment alone.[19]

▶ Enamel erosion is the loss of hard tissue by chemical means such as acidic foods (including carbonated drinks), eating disorders (bulimia), and acid reflux disease.

  • Resulting thinner enamel allows the yellow color of the underlying dentin to show through and cause the teeth to appear duller grey or yellow (Figure 22-4).

  • Age-related erosion is not supported by the literature; erosion a pathologic process.[20]

  • Whitening products are ineffective and contraindicated for erosion.

▶ Attrition of occlusal surfaces can result in loss of enamel, allowing a yellow outline of dentin to show through.

DOCUMENTATION

The permanent record of a patient with staining on the teeth contains explanations in the record about the type of stains, location, and other information of a descriptive nature.

▶ Record color, type, extent, and location of stains with the patient's examination and assessment.

▶ Make additions to the dental history as information is gained concerning the origin of stains such as those related to tooth development, systemic disease, occupations, or medications.

▶ A sample documentation of stain may be found in Box 22-2.

BOX 22-2

Example Documentation: Patient with Dental Stain

S –A 54-year-old female presents for lower left quadrant scaling/planing as indicated in her DH Care Plan. She states that she had difficulty with new brushing technique demonstrated at her last visit. She continues to smoke 1 pack of cigarettes/day.

O –No changes in medical history. BP 131/85; patient took Atenalol today. Generalized heavy extrinsic tobacco stain especially on mandibular anterior lingual surfaces. Plaque-free index is 60%, an improvement of 10%, but still poor.

A –Oral hygiene is poor. Likelihood of continued stain buildup and risk for periodontal complications is increased because of high tobacco use.

P –Scaled and root planed lower left quadrant and removed extrinsic tobacco stain using beaver tail insert of cavitron. Spent 15 minutes reviewing tobacco stain control methods. Reviewed use of power brush and introduced a Tobacco Cessation Plan. She did not act interested. Congratulated patient for returning for this appointment, despite her nervousness.

Next Steps: Review patient's reaction to stain removal today; review recommendations for stain control. Review tobacco cessation steps.

Signed _____, RDH

Date _____

EVERYDAY ETHICS

Daniel returned to the dental office of Dr. Windum after 3 years of working on the East Coast. At the age of 32, Daniel was exhibiting signs of early periodontitis with gingival inflammation and increased subgingival calculus. Ruthie, the dental hygienist, immediately began talking to Daniel about biofilm and suggesting improvements for his personal daily brushing and flossing to change his personal care of his gingival tissues. After she completed a quadrant of scaling with local anesthesia, she suggested that rinsing with chlorhexidine after brushing before going to bed would help the healing.

Dr. Windum confirmed Ruthie's recommendation and wrote the prescription. Daniel left the office only to call a few days later to complain about the "awful brown stain on his teeth and horrible taste of the mouthrinse." He further indicated that he had stopped using the product and wanted to come in and have the stain removed immediately.

Questions for Consideration

1. Which of the dental hygiene core values (in Section II, Introduction, Table II-1) have application in this scenario? How does each core value selected enter the picture?

2. Daniel seems more concerned about the tooth staining and flavor of the chlorhexidine rinse than about the health of his gingival tissues while Ruthie's concerns are for improving his gingival health. What ethical principles may be in effect here?

3. Using the questions in Table VI-1 (in Section VI, Introduction), help Ruthie work out a favorable response explaining her choice of therapy for her patient's poor gingival health.

Factors To Teach The Patient

▷ Etiology of individual's dental stains and discolorations.
▷ Personal care procedures that can aid in the prevention or reduction of stains.
▷ Advantages of starting a smoking cessation program.
▷ Reasons for not using an abrasive dentifrice with vigorous brushing strokes to lessen or remove stain accumulation.
▷ The need to avoid tobacco, coffee, tea, and other beverages or foods that can stain tooth structures or new restorations.
▷ Reasons for the difficulty of removing certain extrinsic stains during scaling and polishing.
▷ Effect of tetracyclines on developing teeth. Need to avoid use during pregnancy and by children to age 12.

References

1. Watts A, Addy M. Tooth discoloration and staining: a review of the literature. *Br Dent J*. 2001;190:309–316.
2. Shay DE, Haddox JH, Richmond JL. An inorganic qualitative and quantitative analysis of green stain. *J Am Dent Assoc*. 1955;50(2):156–160.
3. Żyła T, Kawala B, Antoszewska-Smith J, et al. Black stain and dental caries: a review of the literature. *Biomed Res Int*. 2015;2015:469392.
4. Theilade J, Slots J, Fejerskov O. The ultrastructure of black stain on human primary teeth. *Scand J Dent Res*. 1973;81(7):528–532.
5. Slots J. The microflora of black stain on human primary teeth. *Scand J Dent Res*. 1974;82(7):484–490.
6. Meckel AH. The formation and properties of organic films on teeth. *Arch Oral Biol*. 1965;10(4):585–598.
7. Eriksen HM, Nordbø H. Extrinsic discoloration of teeth. *J Clin Periodontol*. 1978;5(4):229–236.
8. Horowitz HS, Chamberlin SR. Pigmentation of teeth following topical applications of stannous fluoride in a nonfluoridated area. *J Public Health Dent*. 1971;31(1):32–37.
9. Leverett DH, McHugh WD, Jensen OE. Dental caries and staining after twenty-eight months of rinsing with stannous fluoride or sodium fluoride. *J Dent Res*. 1986;65(3):424–427.
10. Flötra L, Gjermo P, Rölla G, et al. Side effects of chlorhexidine mouth washes. *Scand J Dent Res*. 1971;79(2):119–125.
11. Formicola AJ, Deasy MJ, Johnson DH, et al. Tooth staining effects of an alexidine mouthwash. *J Periodontol*. 1979; 50(4):207–211.
12. Reichart PA, Lenz H, König H, et al. The black layer on the teeth of betel chewers: a light microscopic, microradiographic, and electronmicroscopic study. *J Oral Pathol*. 1985;14(6):466–475.
13. Escartin J, Arnedo A, Pinto V, et al. A study of dental staining among competitive swimmers. *Community Dent Oral Epidemiol*. 2000;28:10–17.
14. Langlais RP, Miller CS. *Color Atlas of Common Oral Diseases*. 3rd ed. Philadelphia, PA: Lippincott Williams & Wilkins; 2003:242.
15. Dean HT. Investigation of physiological effects by epidemiological method. In: Moulton FR, ed. *Fluorine and Dental Health*. Washington, DC: American Association for the Advancement of Science; 1942.
16. Thylstrup A, Fejerskov O. Clinical appearance of dental fluorosis in permanent teeth in relation to histologic changes. *Community Dent Oral Epidemiol*. 1978;6(6):315–328.
17. Horowitz HS, Driscoll WS, Meyers RJ, et al. A new method for assessing the prevalence of dental fluorosis—the Tooth Surface Index of Fluorosis. *J Am Dent Assoc*. 1984; 109(1):37–41.
18. Kumar A, Kumar V, Singh J, et al. Drug-induced discoloration of teeth: an updated review. *Clin Pediatr*. 2012; 51(2):181–185.
19. Azer SS, Hague AL, Johnston WM. Effect of pH on tooth discoloration from food colorant *in vitro*. *J Dent*. 2010;38 (Suppl 2):e106–e109.
20. Ashcroft AT, Joiner A. Tooth cleaning and tooth wear: a review. *Proc Inst Mech Eng Part J J Eng Tribol*. 2010;224(6): 539–549.
21. Ashcroft AT, Joiner A. Tooth cleaning and tooth wear: a review. *Proc Inst Mech Eng Part J J Eng Tribol*. 2010;224(6): 539–549.

ENHANCE YOUR UNDERSTANDING

thePoint® DIGITAL CONNECTIONS
(see the inside front cover for access information)
- **Audio glossary**
- **Quiz bank**

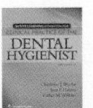
SUPPORT FOR LEARNING
(available separately; visit lww.com)
- ***Active Learning Workbook for Clinical Practice of the Dental Hygienist, 12th Edition***

prepU INDIVIDUALIZED REVIEW
(available separately; visit lww.com)
- **Adaptive quizzing with *prepU for Wilkins' Clinical Practice of the Dental Hygienist***

23

Indices and Scoring Methods

Charlotte J. Wyche, RDH, MS

CHAPTER OUTLINE

LEARNING OBJECTIVES

After studying this chapter, the student will be able to:

1. Identify and define key terms and concepts related to dental indices and scoring methods.

2. Identify the purpose, criteria for measurement, scoring methods, range of scores, and reference or interpretation scales for a variety of dental indices.

3. Select and calculate dental indices for a use in a specific patient or community situation.

This chapter provides an introduction to scoring methods used by clinicians, researchers, and community practitioners to evaluate indicators of oral health status. It is not possible to explain all of the many dental indices that have been used in a variety of settings, but several well-known and widely used indices and scoring methods are described in this chapter. Box 23-1 defines related terminology.

TYPES OF SCORING METHODS

Indices and scoring methods are used in clinical practice and by community programs to determine and record the oral health status of individuals and groups.

I. Individual Assessment Score

A. Purpose

In clinical practice, an index, a biofilm record, or a scoring system for an individual patient can be used for education, motivation, and evaluation.

▶ The effects of personal disease control efforts, the progress of healing following professional treatments, and the maintenance of health over time can be monitored.

▶ An example is the biofilm-free score, in which the dental hygienist is able to measure the effects of a patient's personal daily care efforts.

B. Uses

▶ To provide individual assessment to help a patient recognize an oral problem.

▶ To reveal the degree of effectiveness of oral hygiene practices.

▶ To motivate the patient during preventive and professional care for the elimination and control of oral disease.

▶ To evaluate the success of individual oral self-care and professional treatment over a period of time by comparing index scores.

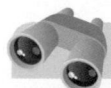

BOX 23-1 KEY WORDS: Indices and Scoring Methods

Calibration: agreement with a set standard of performance; determination of accuracy and consistency between examiners to standardize procedures and gain reliability of recorded findings. Examiners who collect dental index data for epidemiological research or community health assessment are trained to measure the index in exactly the same way each time.

Community oral health assessment: a multifaceted process of identifying factors that affect the oral health status of a selected population.

Data: pieces of information collected using measurements and/or counts.

Data collection: the process of gathering information (through the use of tools such as dental indices).

Determinant: a factor that can influence the outcome of some process. Health determinants include physical and social factors that influence the health outcomes of an individual or in a community.

Epidemiology: the study of the relationships of various factors that determine the frequency and distribution of diseases in the human community; study of health and disease in populations.

Incidence: the rate at which a certain event occurs, as the number of new cases of a specific disease occurring during a certain period of time.

Index: a graduated, numeric scale with upper and lower limits; scores on the scale correspond to a specific criterion for individuals or populations; *pl.* indices or indexes.

Dental index: describes oral status by expressing clinical observations as numeric values.

Indicator: a factor that typically characterizes a disease or health condition; a factor measured and analyzed to describe health status. Dental indices described in this chapter measure oral health indicators.

Pilot study: a trial run of a planned study using a small sample to pretest an instrument, survey, or questionnaire.

Placebo: an inactive substance or preparation with no intrinsic therapeutic value given to satisfy a patient's symbolic need for drug therapy; used in controlled research studies in a form identical in appearance to the material being tested.

Prevalence: the total number of cases of a specific disease or condition in existence in a given population at a certain time.

Ramfjord index teeth: teeth used for epidemiologic studies of periodontal diseases: the maxillary right and mandibular left first molars, maxillary left and mandibular right first premolars, and maxillary left and mandibular right central incisors.

Reliability: ability of an index or a test procedure to measure consistently at different times and under a variety of conditions; reproducibility; consistency.

Sample: a portion or subset of an entire population.

Screening: assessment of many individuals to disclose certain characteristics or diseases in a population.

Individual screening: brief assessment for initial evaluation and classification of need for additional examination and treatment planning.

Status: refers to the state or condition of an individual or population.

Surveillance: the ongoing systematic collection, analysis, and interpretation of outcome-specific data for use in planning, implementing, and evaluating the effect of public health programs and practices.

Validity: ability of an index or a test procedure to measure what it is intended to measure.

II. Clinical Trial

A. Purpose

A clinical trial is planned to determine the effect of an agent or a procedure on the prevention, progression, or control of a disease.

▶ The trial is conducted by comparing an experimental group with a control group that is similar to the experimental group in every way except for the variable being studied.

▶ Examples of indices used for clinical trials are the biofilm index[1] and the patient hygiene performance (PHP).[2]

B. Uses

▶ To determine baseline data before experimental factors are introduced.

▶ To measure the effectiveness of specific agents for the prevention, control, or treatment of oral conditions.

▶ To measure the effectiveness of mechanical devices for personal care, such as toothbrushes, interdental cleaning devices, or irrigators.

III. Epidemiologic Survey

A. Purpose

The word *epidemiology* denotes the study of disease characteristics of populations rather than individuals. Epidemiologic surveys provide information on the trends and patterns of oral health and disease in populations.

▶ An example is the DMFT (decayed, missing, and filled teeth) index[3] to determine the extent of dental caries.

B. Uses

▶ To determine the prevalence and incidence of a particular condition occurring within a given population.

▶ To provide baseline data on indicators that show existing dental health status in populations.

  • The Surgeon General's Report on *Oral Health in America* used epidemiologic data to identify oral health disparities in certain populations.[4]

▶ To provide data to support recommendations for public health interventions to improve the health status of populations, such as those provided in the United States *Healthy People 2020* document.[5]

IV. Community Surveillance

A. Purpose

Community surveillance of oral health indicators and determinants can be accomplished at many levels.

▶ Government agencies, local community-based service-providing agencies, and professional associations are examples of groups that collect data to determine oral health status by conducting oral health screenings.

▶ Information from community-wide oral screenings can be used when planning local community-based oral health services or education.

▶ An example of a system designed to be used by a community-based group is the Association of State and Territorial Dental Directors' (ASTDD) Basic Screening Survey (BSS).[6]

B. Uses

▶ To assess the needs of a community.

▶ To help plan community-based health promotion/disease prevention programs.

▶ To compare the effects or evaluate the results of community-based programs.

INDICES

An index is a way of expressing clinical observations by using numbers. The use of numbers can provide standardized information to make observations of a health condition consistent and less subjective than a word description of that condition.

I. Descriptive Categories of Indices

A. General Categories

▶ *Simple index:* measures the presence or absence of a condition. An example is the Biofilm Index that measures the presence of dental biofilm without evaluating its effect on the gingiva.

▶ *Cumulative index:* measures all the evidence of a condition, past and present. An example is the DMFT index for dental caries.

B. Types of Simple and Cumulative Indices

▶ *Irreversible:* measures conditions that will not change. An example is an index that measures dental caries experience.

▶ *Reversible:* measures conditions that can be changed. Examples are indices that measure dental biofilm.

II. Selection Criteria

A useful and effective index:

▶ is simple to use and calculate.

▶ requires minimal equipment and expense.

▶ uses a minimal amount of time to complete.

▶ does not cause patient discomfort nor is otherwise unacceptable to a patient.

▶ has clear-cut criteria that are readily understandable.

▶ is as free as possible from subjective interpretation.

▶ is reproducible by the same examiner or different examiners.

▶ is amenable to statistical analysis; has validity and reliability.

ORAL HYGIENE STATUS (BIOFILM, DEBRIS, CALCULUS)

Indices that measure oral hygiene status can be used in a clinical setting to educate and motivate an individual patient. When data are collected in a community setting, such as a nursing home, the findings can help determine how daily oral care is being provided and monitor the results of oral hygiene education programs.

I. Biofilm Index

This index was historically known as plaque index (Pl I).[1,7]

A. Purpose

To assess the thickness of biofilm at the gingival area.

B. Selection of Teeth

The entire dentition or selected teeth can be evaluated.

▶ *Areas examined*: Examine four gingival areas (distal, facial, mesial, and lingual) systematically for each tooth.

▶ *Modified procedures*: Examine only the facial, mesial, and lingual areas. Assign double score to the mesial reading, and divide the total by 4.

C. Procedure

▶ Dry the teeth and examine visually using adequate light, mouth mirror, and probe or explorer.

▶ Evaluate dental biofilm on the cervical third; pay no attention to biofilm that has extended to the middle or incisal thirds of the tooth.

▶ Use probe to test the surface when no biofilm is visible. Pass the probe or explorer across the tooth surface in the cervical third and near the entrance to the sulcus. When no biofilm adheres to the probe tip, the area is scored 0. When biofilm adheres, a score of 1 is assigned.

▶ Use a disclosing agent, if necessary, to assist evaluation for the 0–1 scores. When the Pl I is used in conjunction with the gingival index (GI), the GI is completed first because the disclosing agent masks the gingival characteristics.

▶ Include biofilm on the surface of calculus and on dental restorations in the cervical third in the evaluation.

▶ *Criteria*

BIOFILM INDEX

SCORE	CRITERIA
0	No biofilm.
1	A film of biofilm adhering to the free gingival margin and adjacent area of the tooth. The biofilm may be recognized only after application of disclosing agent or by running the explorer across the tooth surface.
2	Moderate accumulation of soft deposits within the gingival pocket that can be seen with the naked eye or on the tooth and gingival margin.
3	Abundance of soft matter within the gingival pocket and/or on the tooth and gingival margin.

D. Scoring

▶ *Pl I for area*
  • Each area of a tooth (distal, facial, mesial, lingual, or palatal) is assigned a score from 0 to 3.

▶ *Pl I for a tooth*
  • Scores for each area are totaled and divided by 4.

▶ *Pl I for groups of teeth*
  • Scores for individual teeth may be grouped and totaled and divided by the number of teeth. For instance, a Pl I may be determined for specific teeth or groups of teeth. The right side of the dentition may be compared with the left.

▶ *Pl I for the individual*
  • Add the scores for each tooth and divide by the number of teeth examined. The Pl I score ranges from 0 to 3.

▶ *Suggested range of scores for patient reference*

RATING	SCORES
Excellent	0
Good	0.1–0.9
Fair	1.0–1.9
Poor	2.0–3.0

▶ *Pl I for a group*
  • Add the scores for each member of a group and divide by the number of individuals.

II. Biofilm Control Record

This index was previously known as the plaque control record.[8]

A. Purpose

To record the presence of dental biofilm on individual tooth surfaces to permit the patient to visualize progress while learning biofilm control.

B. Selection of Teeth and Surfaces

▶ All teeth are included. Missing teeth are identified on the record form by a single thick horizontal line.

▶ Four surfaces are recorded: facial, lingual, mesial, and distal.

▶ Six areas may be recorded. The mesial and distal segments of the diagram may be divided to provide space to record proximal surfaces from the facial separately from the lingual or palatal surfaces (Figure 23-1).[9]

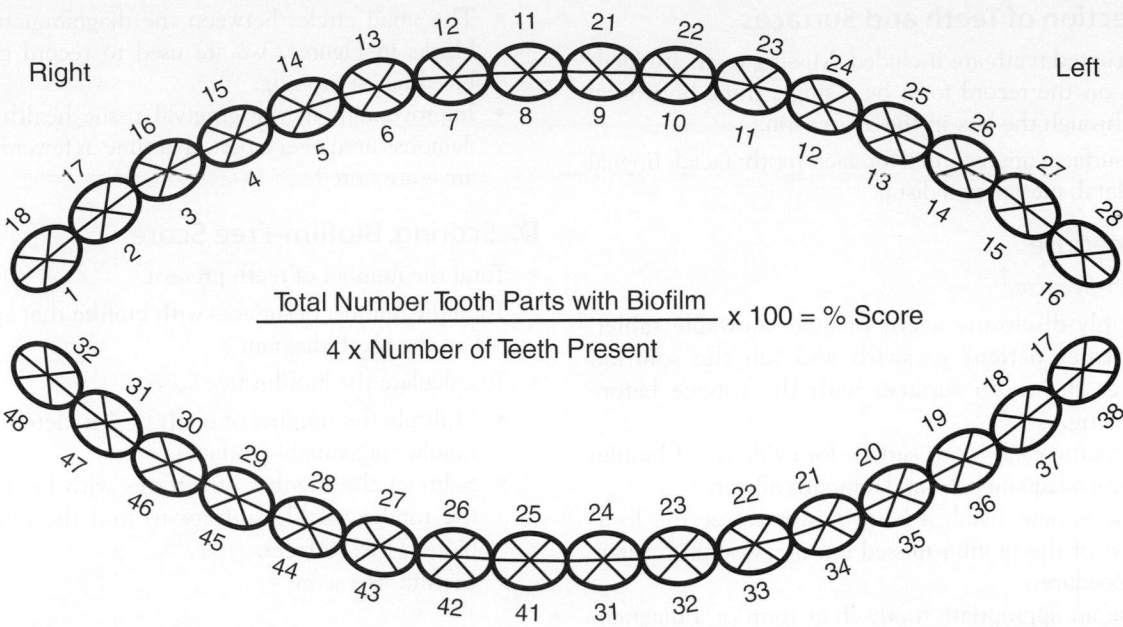

Right   Left

$$\frac{\text{Total Number Tooth Parts with Biofilm}}{4 \times \text{Number of Teeth Present}} \times 100 = \% \text{ Score}$$

FIGURE 23-1 Biofilm Control Record. Diagrammatic representation of the teeth includes spaces to record biofilm on six areas of each tooth. The facial surfaces are on the outer portion and the lingual and palatal surfaces are on the inner portion of the arches. Teeth are numbered by the American Dental Association (ADA) system on the inside and by the FDI system on the outside. (*Source*: Adapted with permission from Ramfjord SP, Ash MM. *Periodontology and Periodontics.* Philadelphia, PA: WB Saunders Co; 1979:273. and from O'Leary TJ, Drake RB, Naylor JE. The plaque control record. *J Periodontal* 1972;43:38.)

C. Procedure

▶ Apply disclosing agent or give a chewable tablet. Instruct patient to swish and rub the solution over the tooth surfaces with the tongue before rinsing.

▶ Examine each tooth surface for dental biofilm at the gingival margin. No attempt is made to differentiate quantity of biofilm.

▶ Record by making a dash or coloring in the appropriate spaces on the diagram (Figure 23-1) to indicate biofilm on facial, lingual, palatal, mesial, and/or distal surfaces.

D. Scoring

▶ Total the number of teeth present; multiply by 4 to obtain the number of available surfaces. Count the number of surfaces with biofilm.

▶ Multiply the number of biofilm-stained surfaces by 100 and divide by the total number of available surfaces to derive the percentage of surfaces with biofilm.

▶ Compare scores over subsequent appointments as the patient learns and practices biofilm control. Ten percent or less biofilm-stained surfaces can be considered a good goal, but if the biofilm is regularly left in the same areas, special instruction is indicated.

Calculation: Example for Biofilm Control Record
- Individual findings: 26 teeth scored; 8 surfaces with biofilm
- Multiply the number of teeth by 4: 26 × 4 = 104 surfaces

- Percent with biofilm =

$$\frac{\text{Number of surfaces with biofilm} \times 100}{\text{Number of available tooth surfaces}} = \frac{8 \times 100}{104}$$
$$= \frac{800}{104}$$
$$= 7.6\%$$

Interpretation
- Although 0% is ideal, less than 10% biofilm-stained surfaces has been suggested as a guideline in periodontal therapy. After initial therapy and when the patient has reached a 10% level of biofilm control or better, necessary additional periodontal and restorative procedures may be initiated.[8] In comparison, a similar evaluation using a biofilm-free score would mean that a goal of 90% or better biofilm-free surfaces would have to be reached before the surgical phase of treatment could be undertaken.

III. Biofilm-Free Score

This index was historically called the plaque-free score.[10]

A. Purpose

To determine the location, number, and percentage of biofilm-free surfaces for individual motivation and instruction. Interdental bleeding can also be documented.

B. Selection of Teeth and Surfaces

▶ All erupted teeth are included. Missing teeth are identified on the record form by a single thick horizontal line through the box in the chart form.

▶ Four surfaces are recorded for each tooth: facial, lingual or palatal, mesial, and distal.

C. Procedure

▶ *Biofilm-free score*

• Apply disclosing agent or give chewable tablet. Instruct patient to swish and rub the solution over the tooth surfaces with the tongue before rinsing.

• Examine each tooth surface for evidence of biofilm using adequate light and a mouth mirror.

• The patient needs a hand mirror to see the location of the biofilm missed during personal hygiene procedures.

• Use an appropriate tooth chart form or a diagrammatic form, such as that shown in Figure 23-2. Red ink for recording the biofilm is suggested when a red disclosing agent is used to help the patient associate the location of the biofilm in the mouth with the recording.

▶ *Papillary bleeding on probing*

• The small circles between the diagrammatic tooth blocks in Figure 23-2 are used to record proximal bleeding on probing.

• Improvement in the gingival tissue health will be demonstrated over a period of time as fewer bleeding areas are noted.

D. Scoring: Biofilm-Free Score

▶ Total the number of teeth present.

▶ Total the number of surfaces with biofilm that appear in red on the tooth diagram

▶ To calculate the biofilm-free score

• Multiply the number of teeth by 4 to determine the number of available surfaces.

• Subtract the number of surfaces with biofilm from the total available surfaces to find the number of biofilm-free surfaces.

• Biofilm-free score =

$$\frac{\text{Number of biofilm-free surface} \times 100}{\text{Number of available surfaces}}$$

$$= \text{Percentage of biofilm-free surfaces}$$

▶ Evaluate biofilm-free score: Ideally, 100% is the goal. When a patient maintains a percentage under 85%,

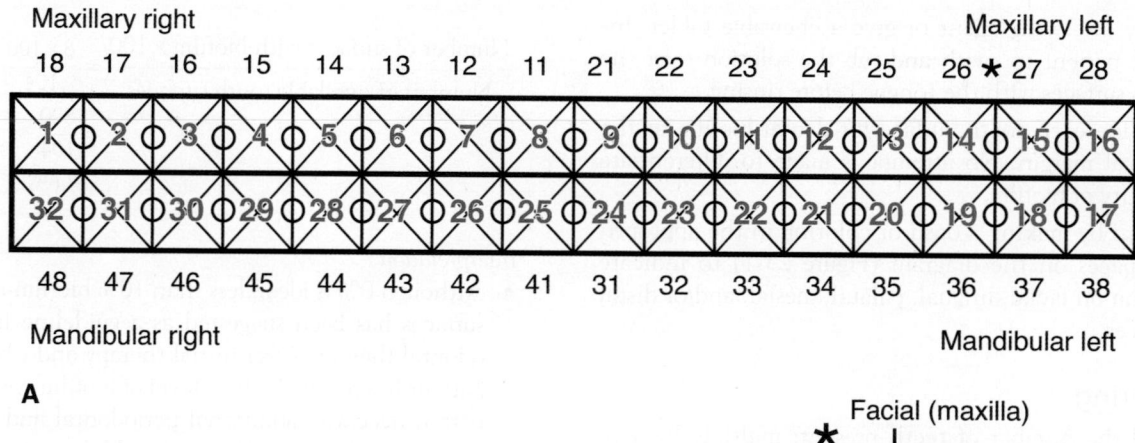

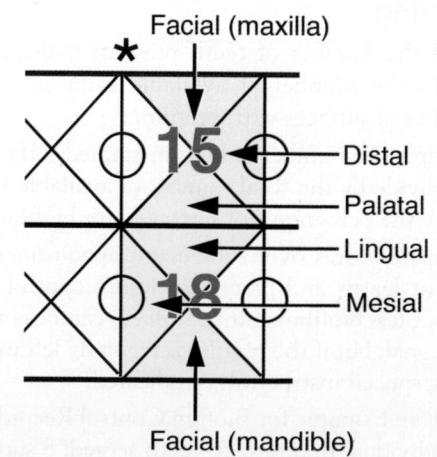

FIGURE 23-2 **Biofilm-Free Score. A:** Diagrammatic representation of the teeth used to record biofilm and papillary bleeding. **B:** Enlargement of one section of the diagram shows tooth surfaces. Teeth are numbered by the ADA system inside each block and by the FDI system outside each block. (*Source:* Adapted with permission from Grant DA, Stern IB, Listgarten MA. *Periodontics.* 6th ed. St. Louis, MO: Mosby; 1988:613.)

check individual surfaces to determine whether biofilm is usually left in the same areas. To prevent the development of specific areas of periodontal infection, remedial instruction in the areas usually missed is indicated.

▶ *Calculation:* Example for Biofilm-Free Score
- Individual findings: 24 teeth scored and 37 surfaces with biofilm.
- Multiply the number of teeth by 4: 24 × 4 = 96 available surfaces.
- Subtract the number of surfaces with biofilm from total available surfaces: 96 − 37 = 59 biofilm-free surfaces.
- Percentage of biofilm-free surfaces =

$$\frac{59 \times 100}{96} = 61.5\%$$

▶ *Interpretation*
- On the basis of the ideal 100%, 61.5% is poor. More personal daily oral care instruction is indicated.

E. Scoring: Papillary Bleeding on Probing

▶ Total the number of small circles marked for bleeding. A patient with 32 teeth has 30 interdental areas. The mesial or distal surface of a tooth adjacent to an edentulous area is probed and counted.

▶ Evaluate total interdental bleeding. In health, bleeding on probing does not occur.

IV. Patient Hygiene Performance (PHP)[2]

A. Purpose

To assess the extent of biofilm and debris over a tooth surface. Debris is defined for the PHP as soft foreign material consisting of dental biofilm, materia alba, and food debris loosely attached to tooth surfaces.

B. Selection of Teeth and Surfaces

▶ Teeth examined

MAXILLARY	MANDIBULAR
No. 3 (16)*	No. 19 (36)
Right first molar	Left first molar
No. 8 (11)	No. 24 (31)
Right central incisor	Left central incisor
No. 14 (26)	No. 30 (46)
Left first molar	Right first molar

*Fédération Dentaire Internationale (FDI) system tooth numbers are in parentheses.

▶ Substitutions
- When a first molar is missing, is less than three-fourths erupted, has a full crown, or is broken down, the second molar is used.

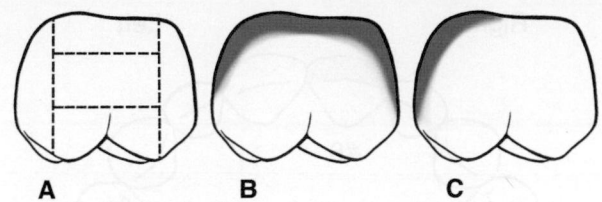

FIGURE 23-3 PHP. A: Oral debris is assessed by dividing a tooth into 5 subdivisions, each of which is scored 1 when debris is shown to be present after use of a disclosing agent. **B:** Example of debris score of 3. Shaded portion represents debris stained by disclosing agent. **C:** Example of debris score of 1. (*Source:* Podshadley AG, Haley JV. A method for evaluating oral hygiene performance. *Public Health Rep.* 1968;83(3):259–264.)

- The third molar is used when the second is missing.
- The adjacent central incisor is used for a missing incisor.

▶ Surfaces
- The facial surfaces of incisors and maxillary molars and the lingual surfaces of mandibular molars are examined.

C. Procedure

Apply disclosing agent. Instruct the patient to swish for 30 seconds and expectorate, but not rinse.

▶ Examination is made using a mouth mirror.

▶ Each tooth surface to be evaluated is subdivided (mentally) into five sections (Figure 23-3A) as follows:
- Vertically: Three divisions—mesial, middle, and distal.
- Horizontally: The middle third is subdivided into gingival, middle, and occlusal or incisal thirds.

▶ Each of the five subdivisions is scored for the presence of stained debris as follows:

PHP	
SCORE	CRITERIA
0	No debris (or questionable).
1	Debris definitely present.
M	When all three molars or both incisors are missing.
S	When a substitute tooth is used.

D. Scoring

▶ *Debris score for individual tooth*
- Add the scores for each of the five subdivisions. The scores range from 0 to 5. Examples are shown in Figures 23-3B and C.

▶ *PHP for the individual*
- Total the scores for the individual teeth and divide by the number of teeth examined. The PHP ranges from 0 to 5.

▶ *Suggested range of scores for evaluation*

RATING	SCORES
Excellent	0 (no debris)
Good	0.1–1.7
Fair	1.8–3.4
Poor	3.5–5.0

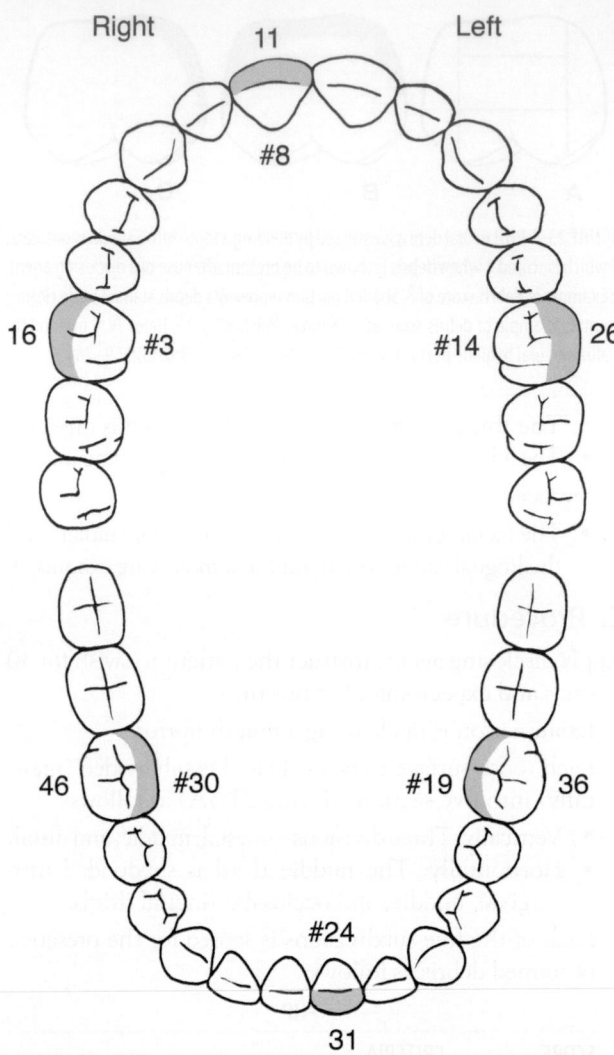

FIGURE 23-4 OHI-S. Six tooth surfaces are scored as follows: facial surfaces of maxillary molars and of the maxillary right and mandibular left central incisors, and the lingual surfaces of mandibular molars. Teeth are numbered by the ADA system on the lingual surface and by the FDI system on the facial surface.

Calculation: Example for an Individual

TOOTH	DEBRIS SCORE
No. 3 (16)	5
No. 8 (11)	3
No. 14 (26)	4
No. 19 (36)	5
No. 24 (31)	2
No. 30 (46)	3
Total	**22**

$$\frac{\text{Total debris score}}{\text{Number of teeth scored}} = \frac{22}{6} = 3.66$$

▸ *Interpretation*
  • According to the suggested range of scores, this patient with a PHP of 3.66 would be classified as exhibiting poor hygiene performance.

▸ *PHP for a group*
  • To obtain the average PHP score for a group or population, total the individual scores and divide by the number of people examined.

V. Simplified Oral Hygiene Index (OHI-S)[11,12]

A. Purpose

To assess oral cleanliness by estimating the tooth surfaces covered with debris and/or calculus.

B. Components

The OHI-S has two components, the simplified debris index (DI-S) and the simplified calculus index (CI-S). The two scores may be used separately or may be combined for the OHI-S.

C. Selection of Teeth and Surfaces

▸ *Identify the six specific teeth* (See Figure 23-4)
  • *Posterior:* The facial surfaces of the maxillary molars and the lingual surfaces of the mandibular molars are scored. Although usually the first molars are examined, the first fully erupted molar distal to each second premolar is used if the first molar is missing.
  • *Anterior:* The facial surfaces of the maxillary right and the mandibular left central incisors are scored. When either is missing, the adjacent central incisor is scored.

▸ *Extent*
  • Either the facial or lingual surfaces of the selected teeth are scored, including the proximal surfaces to the contact areas.

D. Procedure

▸ *Qualification:* At least two of the six possible surfaces are examined to calculate an individual score.

▸ *Record six debris scores*
  • Definition of oral debris: Oral debris is soft foreign matter, such as dental biofilm, material alba, and food debris on the surfaces of the teeth.

▸ *Examination:* Run the side of the tip of a probe or an explorer across the tooth surface to estimate the surface area covered by debris.

▸ *Criteria* (Figure 23-5 and Debris Index table on next page)

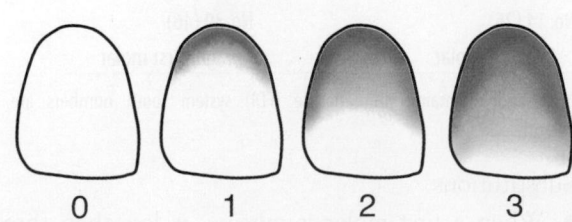

FIGURE 23-5 OHI-S. For the debris index, six teeth (Figure 23-3) are scored. Scoring of 0–3 is based on tooth surfaces covered by debris as shown.

DEBRIS INDEX (DI-S)

SCORE	CRITERIA
0	No debris or stain present.
1	Soft debris covering not more than one-third of the tooth surface being examined, or presence of extrinsic stains without debris, regardless of surface area covered.
2	Soft debris covering more than one-third but not more than two-thirds of the exposed tooth surface.
3	Soft debris covering more than two-thirds of the exposed tooth surface.

▶ *Record six calculus scores*
- *Definition of calculus*: Dental calculus is a hard deposit of inorganic salts composed primarily of calcium carbonate and phosphate mixed with debris, microorganisms, and desquamated epithelial cells.

▶ *Examination*: Use an explorer to estimate surface area covered by supragingival calculus deposits. Identify subgingival deposits by exploring and/or probing. Record only definite deposits of hard calculus.
- *Criteria*: Location and tooth surface areas scored are illustrated in Figure 23-6.

CALCULUS INDEX (CI-S)

SCORE	CRITERIA
0	No calculus present.
1	Supragingival calculus covering not more than one-third of the exposed tooth surface being examined.
2	Supragingival calculus covering more than one-third but not more than two-thirds of the exposed tooth surface, or the presence of individual flecks of subgingival calculus around the cervical portion of the tooth.
3	Supragingival calculus covering more than two-thirds of the exposed tooth surface or a continuous heavy band of subgingival calculus around the cervical portion of the tooth.

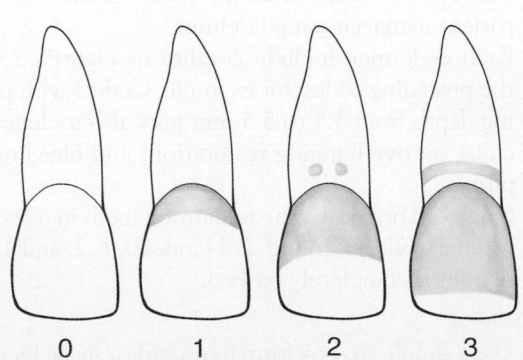

0   1   2   3

FIGURE 23-6 OHI-S. For the calculus index, six teeth (Figure 23-3) are scored. Scoring of 0–3 is based on location and tooth surface area with calculus as shown. Note slight subgingival calculus recorded as 2 and more extensive subgingival calculus as 3.

E. Scoring

▶ *OHI-S individual score*
▶ Determine separate DI-S and CI-S.
- Divide each total score by the number of teeth scored (6).
- DI-S and CI-S values range from 0 to 3.
▶ Calculate the OHI-S.
- Combine the DI-S and CI-S.
- OHI-S value ranges from 0 to 6.
▶ *Suggested range of scores for evaluation*[12]

INDIVIDUAL DI-S AND CI-S

RATING	SCORES
Excellent	0
Good	0.1–0.6
Fair	0.7–1.8
Poor	1.9–3.0

OHI-S (COMBINED DI-S AND CI-S)

RATING	SCORES
Excellent	0
Good	0.1–1.2
Fair	1.3–3.0
Poor	3.1–6.0

Calculation: Example for an Individual

TOOTH	DI S	CI-S SCORE
No. 3 (16)	2	2
No. 8 (11)	1	0
No. 14 (26)	3	2
No. 19 (36)	3	2
No. 24 (31)	2	1
No. 30 (46)	2	2
Total	13	9

$$\text{DI - S} = \frac{\text{Total debris score}}{\text{Number of teeth scored}} = \frac{13}{6} = 2.17$$

$$\text{CI - S} = \frac{\text{Total calculus scores}}{\text{Number of teeth scored}} = \frac{9}{6} = 1.50$$

$$\text{OHI - S} = \text{DI - S} + \text{CI - S} = 2.17 + 1.50 = 3.67$$

▶ *Interpretation*
- According to the suggested range of scores, the score for this individual (3.67) indicates a poor oral hygiene status.

▶ *OHI-S group score*
- Compute the average of the individual scores by totaling the scores and dividing by the number of individuals.

GINGIVAL AND PERIODONTAL HEALTH

Measurements for gingival and periodontal indices have varied over the years. Two indices, not completely described here, are of historic interest.

▶ The papillary-marginal-attached index, attributed to Schour and Massler[13] and later revised by Massler,[14] was used to assess the extent of gingival changes in large groups for epidemiologic studies.

▶ The periodontal index (PI) of Russell,[15] another acclaimed contribution to the study of disease incidence, was a complex index that accounts for both gingival and periodontal changes. Its aim was to survey large populations.

▶ For patient instruction and motivation, several bleeding indices and scoring methods have been developed.

▶ Bleeding on gentle probing or flossing is an early sign of gingival inflammation and precedes color changes and enlargement of gingival tissues.[16,17]

▶ Bleeding on probing is an indicator of the progression of periodontal disease so, testing for bleeding has become a significant procedure for assessment prior to treatment planning, after therapy to show the effects of treatment, and at maintenance appointments to determine continued control of gingival inflammation.

I. Periodontal Screening and Recording (PSR)[18,19]

A. Purpose

To assess the state of periodontal health of an individual patient.

▶ A modified form of the original community periodontal index of treatment needs (CPITN) index.[20]

▶ Designed to indicate periodontal status in a rapid and effective manner and motivate the patient to seek necessary complete periodontal assessment and treatment.

▶ Used as a screening procedure to determine the need for comprehensive periodontal evaluation.

B. Selection of Teeth

The dentition is divided into sextants. Each tooth is examined. Posterior sextants begin distal to the canines.

C. Procedure

▶ *Instrument*: Probe originally designed for World Health Organization (WHO) surveys (Figure 23-7), with markings at intervals from tip: 3.5, 5.5, 8.5, and 11.5 mm.

▶ Color coded between 3.5 and 5.5 mm.

▶ *Working tip*: A ball 0.5 mm in diameter. The functions of the ball are to aid in the detection of calculus, rough overhanging margins of restorations, and other tooth surface irregularities and to facilitate assessment at the probing depth and reduce risk of overmeasurement.

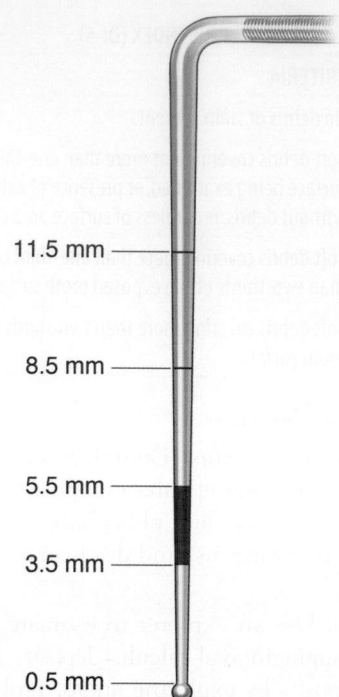

11.5 mm

8.5 mm

5.5 mm

3.5 mm

0.5 mm

FIGURE 23-7 WHO Periodontal Probe. The specially designed WHO probe measures 3.5-, 5.5-, 8.5-, and 11.5-mm intervals. This probe is used to make determinations for the PSR and the CPI. (*Source*: Fédération Dentaire Internationale. A simplified periodontal examination for dental practices. Based on the Community Periodontal Index of Treatment Needs—CPITN. *Aust Dent J.* 1985;30(5):368–370.)

▶ *Probe application*
- Insert probe gently into a sulcus until resistance is felt.
- Apply a circumferential walking step to probe systematically about each tooth through each sextant.
- Observe color-coded area of the probe for prompt identification of probing depths.
- Each sextant receives one code number corresponding to the deepest position of the color-coded portion of the probe.

▶ *Criteria*
- Five codes and an asterisk are used. Figure 23-8 shows the clinical findings, code significance, and patient management guidelines.
- Each code may include conditions identified with the preceding codes; for example, Code 3 with probing depth from 3.5 to 5.5 mm may also include calculus, an overhanging restoration, and bleeding on probing.
- One need not probe the remaining teeth in a sextant when a Code 4 is found. For Codes 0, 1, 2, and 3, the sextant is completely probed.

▶ *Recording*
- Use a simple six-box form to provide a space for each sextant. The form can be made into peel-off stickers or a rubber stamp to facilitate recording in the patient's permanent record.

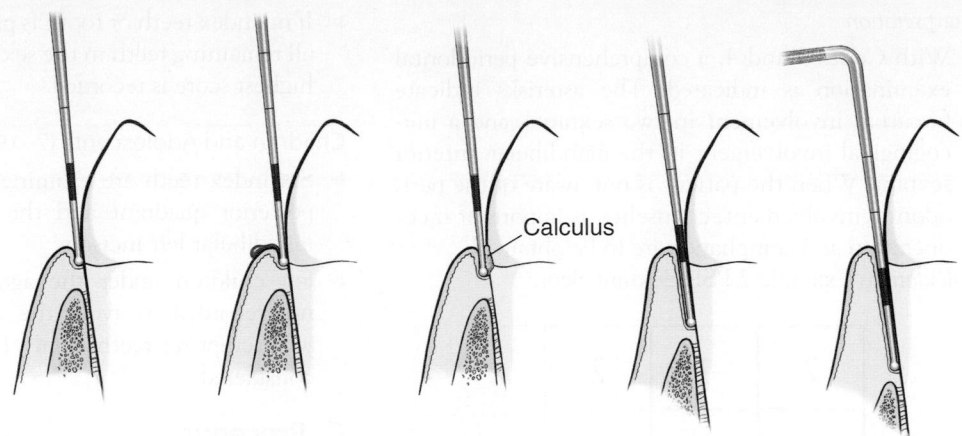

PSR and CPI sextant scores	Code 0	Code 1	Code 2	Code 3	Code 4
CPI description	• Entire black band of the probe is visible	• Entire black band of the probe is visible, but bleeding is present after gentle probin	• Entire black band is visible, but calculus is present • Bleeding may or may not be present.	• 4 to 5 mm pocket depth • Black band on probe partially hidden by gingival margin	• 6 mm or greater pocket depth • Black band of probe completely hidden by gingival margin
PSR sextant code description	• Colored area of probe completely visible • No calculus, defective restoration margins or bleeding	• Colored area of probe completely visible • No calculus or defective restoration margins • Bleeding after gentle probing	• Colored area of probe completely visible • Supra or subgingival rough surface or calculus • Defective restoration margins	• Colored area of probe only partially visible • Calculus, defective restorations, and bleeding may or may not be present	• Colored area of probe completely disappears (probing depth of 5.5 mm or greater)
PSR management guidelines	• Biofilm control instruction • Preventive care	• Biofilm control instruction • Preventive care	• Biofilm control instruction • Complete preventive care • Calculus removal • Correction of defective restoration margins	• Comprehensive periodontal assessment and treatment plan is indicated	• Comprehensive periodontal assessment and treatment plan is indicated

FIGURE 23-8 Community Periodontal Index (CPI) and Periodontal Screening Record (PSR) Codes. (*Source:* World Health Organization. *Oral Health Surveys: Basic Methods.* 4th ed. Geneva: WHO; 1997:27, 38 and the American Academy of Periodontology.[18])

• One score is marked for each sextant; the highest code observed is recorded. When indicated, an asterisk is added to the score in the individual space with the sextant code number.

D. Scoring

▶ *Follow-up patient management*

Patients are classified into assessment and treatment planning needs by the highest coded score of their PSR.

Calculation: Example 1: PSR Sextant Score

4*	2	3
3	2*	4*

▶ *Interpretation*
  • With Codes 3 and 4, a comprehensive periodontal examination is indicated. The asterisks indicate furcation involvement in two sextants, and a mucogingival involvement in the mandibular anterior sextant. When the patient is not aware of the periodontal involvement, counseling is important if cooperation and compliance are to be obtained.
▶ *Calculation*: Example 2 PSR Sextant Score

2	1	2
2	1*	2*

▶ *Interpretation*
  • An overall Code 2 can indicate calculus and overhanging restorations that can be removed. All restorations are checked for recurrent dental caries. Appointments for instruction in dental biofilm control are of primary concern.
    • In this example, the asterisks in two sextants indicate a notable clinical feature such as minimal attached gingiva.

II. Community Periodontal Index (CPI)[21]

A. Purpose

To screen and monitor the periodontal status of populations.

▶ Originally developed as the CPITN index that included a code to indicate an individual and group-summary recording of treatment needs. However, because of changes in management of periodontal disease, the treatment needs portion of the index has been eliminated.
▶ One component of a complete oral health survey[21] designed by the WHO that includes the assessment of many oral health indicators including mucosal lesions, dental caries, fluorosis, prosthetic status, and dentofacial anomalies.
▶ Later modified to form the PSR index for scoring individual patients.

B. Selection of Teeth

▶ The dentition is divided into sextants for recording on the assessment form.
▶ Posterior sextants begin distal to canines.

Adults (20 years and older)

▶ A sextant is examined only if there are two or more teeth present that are not indicated for extraction.
▶ Ten index teeth are examined.
▶ The first and second molars in each posterior sextant. If one is missing, no replacement is selected and the score for the remaining molar is recorded.
▶ The maxillary right central incisor and mandibular left central incisor.

▶ If no index teeth or tooth is present in the sextant, then all remaining teeth in the sextant are examined and the highest score is recorded.

Children and Adolescents (7–19 years of age)

▶ Six index teeth are examined; the first molar in each posterior quadrant and the maxillary right and the mandibular left incisors.
▶ For children under the age of 15, pocket depth is not recorded to avoid the deepened sulci associated with erupting teeth. Only bleeding and calculus are considered.

C. Procedure

▶ *Instrument*: A specially designed probe is used to record both the CPI and PSR. The probe is described in Figure 23-7.
▶ *Criteria*: CPI score.
  • Five codes are used to record bleeding, calculus, and pocket depth. Criteria for the CPI codes are similar to the criteria for the PSR, as illustrated in Figure 23-8 and the table below.

COMMUNITY PERIODONTAL INDEX (CPI)

CODE	CRITERIA
0	Healthy periodontal tissues.
1	Bleeding after gentle probing; entire colored band of probe is visible.
2	Supragingival or subgingival calculus present; entire colored band of probe is visible.
3	4- to 5-mm pocket; colored band of probe is partially obscured.
4	6 mm or deeper; colored band on the probe is not visible.

▶ *Criteria*: Loss of attachment (LOA) code.
  • In conjunction with the CPI, the WHO probe is also used to record LOA. The five LOA codes used are illustrated in Figure 23-9. LOA is not recorded for individuals less than 15 years of age.

LOA CODE	CRITERIA
0	0–3 mm LOA
1	4–5 mm LOA
2	6–8 mm LOA
3	9–11 mm LOA
4	12 mm or greater LOA

III. Sulcus Bleeding Index (SBI)[16]

A. Purpose

To locate areas of gingival sulcus bleeding and color changes in order to recognize and record the presence of early (initial) inflammatory gingival disease.

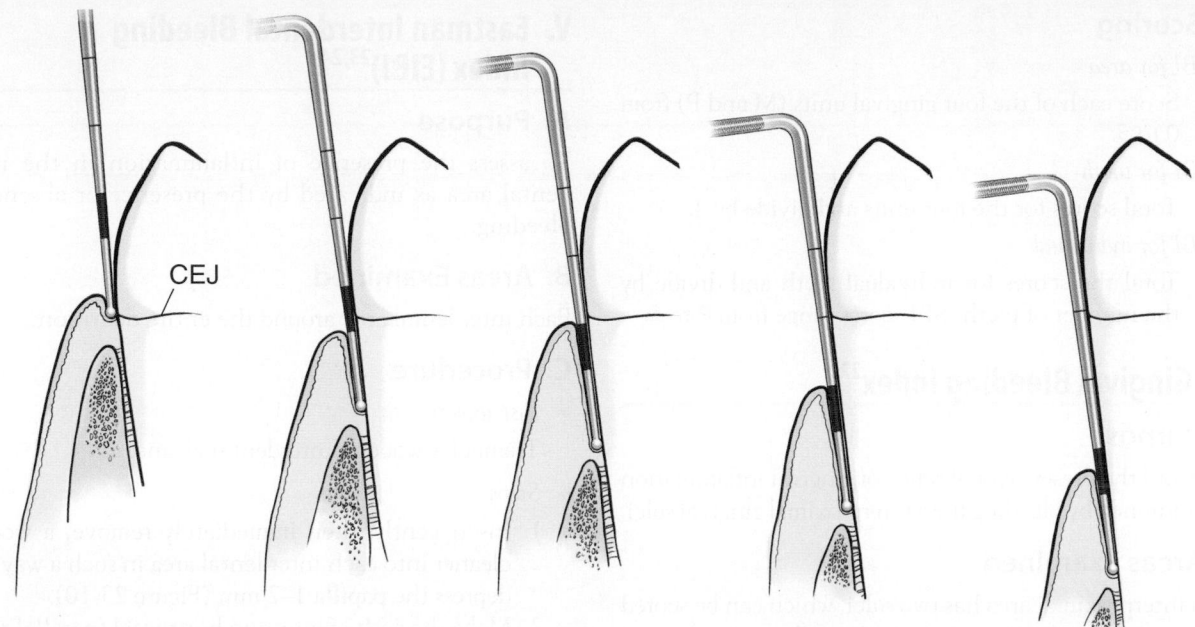

Code 0	Code 1	Code 2	Code 3	Code 4
• 0 to 3 mm loss of attachment • Cementoenamel junction (CEJ) is covered by gingival margin and CPI score is 0 to 3. If CEJ is visible, or if CPI score is 4, LOA codes 1 to 4 are used.	• 3.5 to 5.5 mm loss of attachment • CEJ is within the black band on the probe	• 6 to 8 mm loss of attachment CEJ is between the top of the black band and the 8.5 mm mark on the probe	• 9 to 11 mm loss of attachment • CEJ is between the 8.5 mm and 11.5 mm marks on the probe	• 12 mm or greater loss of attachment • CEJ is beyond the highest (11.5 mm) marks on the probe

FIGURE 23-9 Loss of Attachement (LOA) Codes. (*Source*: World Health Organization. *Oral Health Surveys: Basic Methods*. 4th ed. Geneva: WHO; 1997:27, 39.)

B. Areas Examined

Four gingival units are scored systematically for each tooth: the labial and lingual marginal gingiva (M units), and the mesial and distal papillary gingiva (P units).

C. Procedure

▶ Use standardized lighting while probing each of the four areas.

▶ Walk the probe to the base of the sulcus, holding it parallel with the long axis of the tooth for M units, and directed toward the col area for P units.

▶ Wait 30 seconds after probing before scoring apparently healthy gingival units.

▶ Dry the gingiva gently if necessary to observe color changes clearly.

▶ *Criteria*

SULCULAR BLEEDING INDEX (SBI)

CODE	CRITERIA
0	Healthy appearance of P and M, no bleeding on sulcus probing.
1	Apparently healthy P and M showing no change in color and no swelling, but bleeding from sulcus on probing.
2	Bleeding on probing and change of color caused by inflammation. No swelling or macroscopic edema.
3	Bleeding on probing and change in color and slight edematous swelling.
4	• Bleeding on probing and change in color and obvious swelling or • Bleeding on probing and obvious swelling.
5	Bleeding on probing and spontaneous bleeding and change in color, marked swelling with or without ulceration.

D. Scoring

▶ *SBI for area*
  • Score each of the four gingival units (M and P) from 0 to 5.
▶ *SBI for tooth*
  • Total scores for the four units and divide by 4.
▶ *SBI for individual*
  • Total the scores for individual teeth and divide by the number of teeth. SBI scores range from 0 to 5.

IV. Gingival Bleeding Index[22]

A. Purpose

To record the presence or absence of gingival inflammation as determined by bleeding from interproximal gingival sulci.

B. Areas Examined

Each interproximal area has two sulci, which can be scored as one interdental unit or scored separately.

▶ Certain areas may be excluded from scoring because of accessibility, tooth position, diastemata, or other factors, and if exclusions are made, a consistent procedure is followed for an individual and for a group if a study is to be made.

▶ A full complement of teeth has 30 proximal areas. In the original studies, third molars were excluded, and 26 interdental units were recorded.[23]

C. Procedure

▶ *Instrument*
  • Unwaxed dental floss is used. Floss has the advantages of being readily available and disposable
▶ *Steps*
  1. Pass the floss interproximally first on one side of the papilla and then on the other.
  2. Curve the floss around the adjacent tooth, and bring the floss below the gingival margin.
  3. Move the floss up and down for one stroke, with care not to lacerate the gingiva. Adapt finger rests to provide controlled, consistent pressure.
  4. Use a new length of clean floss for each area.
  5. Retract for visibility of bleeding from both facial and lingual aspects.
  6. Allow 30 seconds for reinspection of an area that does not show blood immediately either in the area or on the floss.
▶ *Criteria*
  • Bleeding indicates the presence of disease. No attempt is made to quantify the severity of bleeding.

D. Scoring

The numbers of bleeding areas and scorable units are recorded. Patient participation in observing and recording over a series of appointments can increase motivation.

V. Eastman Interdental Bleeding Index (EIBI)[23,24]

A. Purpose

To assess the presence of inflammation in the interdental area as indicated by the presence or absence of bleeding.

B. Areas Examined

Each interdental area around the entire dentition.

C. Procedure

▶ *Instrument*
  Triangular wooden interdental cleaner.

▶ *Steps*
  1. Insert gently, then immediately remove, a wooden cleaner into each interdental area in such a way as to depress the papilla 1–2 mm (Figure 23-10).
  2. Make the path of insertion horizontal (parallel to the occlusal surface), taking care not to angle the point in an apical direction.
  3. Insert and remove four times; move to next interproximal area.
  4. Record the presence or absence of bleeding within 15 seconds for each area.

D. Scoring

▶ *Number of bleeding sites*
  • The number may be totaled for an individual score for comparison with scores over a series of appointments.

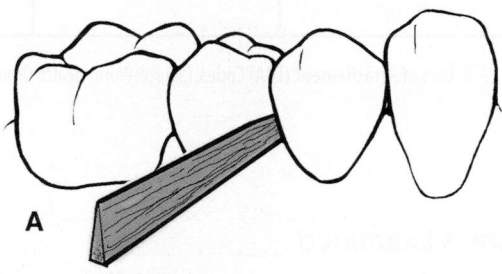
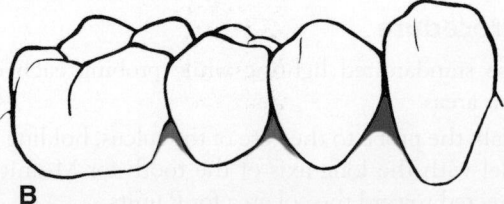

FIGURE 23-10 Eastman Interdental Bleeding Index (EIBI). The test for interdental bleeding is made by inserting a wooden interdental cleaner into each interdental space. **A:** Wooden interdental cleaner inserted in a horizontal path, parallel with the occlusal surfaces. **B:** The presence or absence of bleeding is noted within a quadrant 15 seconds after final insertion. Bleeding indicates the presence of inflammation.

Percentage scores

• Index is expressed as a percentage of the total number of sites evaluated. Calculations can be made for total mouth, quadrants, or maxillary versus mandibular.

Calculation example

• An adult with a complete dentition has 15 maxillary and 15 mandibular interproximal areas. The EIBI revealed 13 areas of bleeding. To calculate percentage:

$$\frac{\text{Number of bleeding areas}}{\text{Total number of areas}} \times 100 = \text{Percent bleeding area}$$

$$\frac{13}{30} \times 100 = 43\%$$

VI. Gingival Index (GI)[7]

A. Purpose

To assess the severity of gingivitis based on color, consistency, and bleeding on probing.

B. Selection of Teeth and Gingival Areas

A GI may be determined for selected teeth or for the entire dentition.

Areas examined

• Four gingival areas (distal, facial, mesial, and lingual) are examined systematically for each tooth.

Modified procedure

• The distal examination for each tooth can be omitted. The score for the mesial area is doubled, and the total score for each tooth is divided by 4.

C. Procedure

▶ Dry the teeth and gingiva; under adequate light, use a mouth mirror and probe.

▶ Use the probe to press on the gingiva to determine the degree of firmness.

▶ Slide the probe along the soft tissue wall near the entrance to the gingival sulcus to evaluate bleeding (Figure 23-11).

▶ *Criteria*

GI CODE	CRITERIA
0	Normal gingiva.
1	Mild inflammation—slight change in color, slight edema. *No bleeding* on probing.
2	Moderate inflammation—redness, edema, and glazing. *Bleeding* on probing.
3	Severe inflammation–marked redness and edema. Ulceration. Tendency to *spontaneous bleeding*.

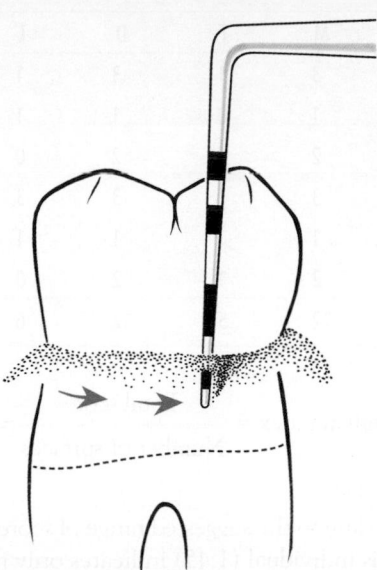

FIGURE 23-11 Gingival Index (GI). Probe stroke for bleeding evaluation. The broken line represents the level of attachment of the periodontal tissues. The probe is inserted a few millimeters and moved along the soft tissue pocket wall with light pressure in a circumferential direction. The stroke shown here is in contrast with the walking stroke used for probing depth evaluation and measurement.

D. Scoring

▶ *GI for area*

• Each of the four gingival surfaces (distal, facial, mesial, and lingual) is given a score of 0–3.

▶ *GI for a tooth*

• Scores for each area are totaled and divided by 4.

▶ *GI for groups of teeth*

• Scores for individual teeth may be grouped and totaled, and divided by the number of teeth. A GI may be determined for specific teeth, group of teeth, quadrant, or side of mouth.

▶ *GI for the individual*

• Scores for each tooth are added up and divided by the number of teeth examined. Scores range from 0 to 3.

▶ *Suggested range of scores for patient reference*

RATING	SCORES
Excellent (healthy tissue)	0
Good	0.1–1.0
Fair	1.1–2.0
Poor	2.1–3.0

▶ *Calculation:* Example for an Individual

• Using six teeth for an example of screening; teeth selected are known as the Ramfjord index teeth.[25]

TOOTH NO.	M	F	D	L	
3 (16)	3	1	3	1	
9 (21)	1	0	1	1	
12 (24)	2	1	2	0	
19 (36)	3	1	3	3	
25 (41)	1	1	1	1	
28 (44)	2	1	2	0	
Total	12	5	12	6	= 35

$$\text{Gingival index} = \frac{\text{Total score}}{\text{Number of surfaces}} = \frac{35}{24} = 1.45$$

▶ *Interpretation*
- According to the suggested range of scores, the score for this individual (1.45) indicates only fair gingival health (moderate inflammation).
- The ratings for each gingival area or surface can be used to help the patient compare gingival changes and improve oral hygiene procedures.

▶ *GI for a group*
- Add the individual GI scores and divide by the number of individuals examined.

DENTAL CARIES EXPERIENCE

Dental caries experience data are most useful when measuring the prevalence of dental disease in groups rather than individuals. The population scores can document such information as the number of persons in any age group who are affected by dental caries, the number of teeth that need treatment, or the proportion of teeth that have been treated.

I. Permanent Dentition: Decayed, Missing, and Filled Teeth (DMFT) or Surfaces (DMFS)[3,26]

A. Purpose

To determine total dental caries experience, past and present, by recording either the number of affected teeth or tooth surfaces.

B. Selection of Teeth and Surfaces

▶ The DMFT is based on 28 teeth.
▶ The DMFS is based on surfaces of 28 teeth; 128 surfaces.
- 16 posterior teeth × 5 surfaces (facial, lingual, mesial, distal, and occlusal) = 80 surfaces.
- 12 anterior teeth × 4 surfaces (facial, lingual, mesial, and distal) = 48 surfaces.
- Teeth missing due to dental caries are recorded using 5 surfaces for posterior and 4 surfaces for anterior teeth.

▶ Teeth not counted.
- Third molars.
- Unerupted teeth. A tooth is considered erupted when any part projects through the gingiva. Certain types of research may require differentiation between clinical emergence, partial eruption, and full eruption.
- Congenitally missing and supernumerary teeth.
- Teeth removed for reasons other than dental caries, such as an impaction or during orthodontic treatment.
- Teeth restored for reasons other than dental caries, such as trauma (fracture), cosmetic purposes, or use as a bridge abutment.
- Primary tooth retained with the permanent successor erupted. The permanent tooth is evaluated because a primary tooth is never included in this index.

C. Procedures

▶ *Examination*
- Examine each tooth in a systematic sequence.
- Observe teeth by visual means as much as possible.
- Use adequate light.
- Review the stages of dental caries in Chapter 27.

▶ *Criteria for recording*[26]
- Each tooth is recorded once when using the DMFT index.
- Five surfaces for posterior teeth and 4 surfaces for anterior teeth are recorded when using the DMFS index.
- DMF indices use a dichotomous scale (present or absent) to record decay.

DMF RATING	CRITERIA
Decayed (D)	Visible dental caries is present or both dental caries and a restoration are present.
Missing (M)	A tooth extracted because of dental caries or when it is carious, nonrestorable, and indicated for extraction.
Filled (F)	Any permanent or temporary restoration is present or a defective restoration without evidence of dental caries is present.

D. Scoring

▶ *Individual DMF*
- Total each component separately.
  Total D + M + F = DMF
- *Example*: An individual presents with dental caries on the mesial and occlusal surfaces of a posterior tooth and caries on the mesial surface of an anterior tooth. A molar tooth and an anterior tooth are missing because of dental caries, and there is an amalgam restoration on the mesial–distal–occlusal surfaces of a posterior tooth.
  DMFT = 2 + 2 + 1 = 5
  DMFS = 3 + 9 + 3 = 15

▶ A DMF score may have different interpretations. For example, an individual with a DMF score of 15 who has experienced regular dental care may have a distribution such as D = 0, M = 0, F = 15.

▶ *Group DMF*
- Total the DMFs for each individual examined.
- Divide the total DMFs by the number of individuals in the group.

▶ *Calculation:*
- *Example:* A population of 20 individuals with individual DMF scores of 0,0,0,0,2,2,3,3,3,4,9,9,9,10,10,10,11,11,12, and 16 equals a group total DMF of 124.

$$\frac{124}{20} = 6.2 = \text{the average DMF for the group}$$

- This DMF average represents accumulated dental caries experience for the group.

▶ The differences in caries experience between two groups of individuals within this population are notable and influence interpretation of the results. For the first 10 individuals, the group average is $\frac{17}{10} = 1.7$, and for the second 10 individuals the average DMF is $\frac{107}{10} = 10.7$.

▶ Scores for these two groups can be presented separately because of the wide difference.

▶ Average DMF scores can also be presented by age group.

▶ *Specific treatment needs of a group*
- To calculate the percentage of DMF teeth that need to be restored, divide the total D component by the total DMF.

▶ *Calculation:*
- *Example 1:* To calculate the *percent of DMF teeth* that need to be restored, divide the total D component by the total number of DMF teeth.
  D = 175, M = 55, F = 18
  Total DMFT = 248

$$\frac{D}{DMF} = \frac{175}{248} = 0.70 \text{ or } 70\% \text{ of the teeth need restorations}$$

- *Example 2:* The same type of calculations can be used to determine the *percent of all teeth* missing in a group of individuals.
  20 individuals have 28 × 20 = 560 permanent teeth.
  D = 175, M = 55, F = 18

$$\frac{M}{\text{Total \# of teeth}} = \frac{55}{560} = 0.098 \text{ or nearly } 10\% \text{ of all}$$

their teeth lost because of dental caries.

II. Primary Dentition: Decayed, Indicated for Extraction, and Filled (df and def)[27]

A. Purpose

To determine the dental caries experience for the primary teeth present in the oral cavity by evaluating teeth or surfaces.

B. Selection of Teeth or Surfaces

▶ deft or dft: 20 teeth evaluated.

▶ defs or dfs: 88 surfaces evaluated.
- *Posterior teeth:* Each has five surfaces: facial, lingual or palatal, mesial, distal, and occlusal. (8 teeth × 5 surfaces = 40 surfaces.)
- *Anterior teeth:* Each has four surfaces: facial, lingual or palatal, mesial, and distal. (12 teeth × 4 surfaces = 48 surfaces.)

▶ Teeth not counted
- Missing teeth, including unerupted and congenitally missing.
- Supernumerary teeth.
- Teeth restored for reasons other than dental caries are not counted as f.

C. Procedure

▶ *Instruments and examination*
Same as for DMF.

▶ *Criteria*

DECAYED, INDICATED FOR EXTRACTION, FILLED (df AND def)

RATING	CRITERIA
d	Primary teeth (or surfaces) with dental caries but not restored.
e	Primary teeth (or number of surfaces) that are indicated for extraction because of dental caries.
f	Primary teeth (or surfaces) restored with an amalgam, composite, or temporary filling. Each tooth (or surface) is scored only once. A tooth with recurrent caries around a restoration receives a "d" score.

▶ *Difference between deft/defs and dft/dfs*
- In the deft and defs, both "d" and "e" are used to describe teeth with dental caries. Thus, d and e are sometimes combined, and the index becomes the dft or dfs.

D. Scoring

▶ *Calculation:*
- *Example 1:* Individual def A 2½-year-old child has 18 teeth. Teeth A (55) and J (65) are unerupted. There is no sign of dental caries in teeth M (73), N (72), O (71), P (81), Q (82), and R (83). All other teeth have two carious surfaces each, except tooth B (54), which is broken down to the gum line.
  Summary:
  Total number of teeth = 18
  Number of "d" teeth = 11
  Number of "e" teeth = 1
  Number of "f" teeth = 0
  def = d + e + f = 11 + 1 + 0 = 12

▶ *Interpretation*
- Twelve of 18 teeth (67%) with carious lesions indicates a serious need for dental treatment and a caries management program for the child.

▶ *Calculation*: Example 2: individual dfs

  • Using the same 2½-year-old child to calculate dfs: Eleven teeth each have two carious surfaces: $11 \times 2 = 22$ carious surfaces

Tooth B has $1 \times 5 = 5$ carious surfaces

Total dfs: $d + f = 27 + 0 = 27$

▶ *Interpretation*

  • The child has 48 total anterior surfaces (12 teeth × 4 surfaces) and 30 total posterior surfaces (6 teeth × 5 surfaces) to total 78 surfaces.

$$\frac{dfs}{\text{Number of surfaces}} = \frac{27}{78}$$

$$= 0.34 \text{ or } 34\% \text{ of the surfaces in need of dental treatment}$$

E. Mixed Dentition

A DMFT or DMFS and a deft or defs are never combined or added together.

III. Primary Dentition: Decayed, Missing, and Filled (dmf)[27]

A. Purpose

To determine dental caries experience for children. Only primary teeth are evaluated.

B. Selection of Teeth or Surfaces

▶ dmft: 12 teeth evaluated (8 primary molars; 4 primary canines).

▶ dmfs: 56 surfaces evaluated.

  • *Primary molars*: 8×5 surfaces each $= 40$
  • *Primary canines*: 4×4 surfaces each $= 16$

▶ Each tooth is counted only once. When both dental caries and a restoration are present, the tooth or surface is scored as "d."

C. Procedure

▶ Instruments and examination are the same as for DMF.

▶ Criteria for dmft or dmfs

dmf RATING	CRITERIA
d	Primary molars and canines (or surfaces) that are carious.
m	Primary molars and canines (or surfaces) that are missing. A primary molar or canine is presumed missing because of dental caries when it has been lost before normal exfoliation.
f	Primary molars and canines (or surfaces) that have a restoration but are without caries.

D. Scoring

▶ *Calculation*: Example 1: individual dmf

• A 7-year-old boy has all primary molars and canines present. Examination reveals two carious surfaces on one molar tooth, one missing canine tooth, and one two-surface amalgam filling on a molar tooth:

dmft $= 1 + 1 + 1 = 3$

dmfs $= 2 + 4 + 2 = 8$

E. Mixed Dentition

Permanent and primary teeth are evaluated separately. A DMFT or DMFS and a dmf or dmfs are never added together.

IV. Early Childhood Caries (ECC and S-ECC)[28]

A. Purpose

To provide case definitions that determine dental caries experience of children 5 years of age or younger.

B. Selection of Teeth or Surfaces

Each surface (mesial, distal, facial, lingual, and occlusal) of each tooth visible in the child's mouth is evaluated. Only primary teeth are scored.

C. Procedure

▶ Visual examination of all surfaces of each erupted tooth.

▶ Criteria for case definition are included in Table 23-1.

D. Scoring

▶ A designation of ECC or S-ECC (severe early childhood caries) for a particular individual relates the age of the child with the status of DMFT surfaces observed.

▶ Community-based surveys identify the percentage of a population with ECC and/or S-ECC.

V. Root Caries Index (RCI)[29]

A. Purpose

To determine total root caries experience for individuals and groups and provide a direct, simple method for recording and making comparisons.

B. Selection of Teeth

▶ Up to four surfaces (mesial, distal, facial, and lingual/palatal) are counted for each tooth.

▶ Only surfaces with visible gingival recession are counted.

▶ Teeth with multiple roots and extreme recession, though rare, could present with two or three lesions on the same surface. In this case, the most severe lesion is selected for recording and each surface is counted only once.

C. Procedure

▶ *Examination*

  • Use adequate retraction and light to examine each tooth. Visible recession is shown in Figure 18-16,

TABLE 23-1	**ECC Case Definition**			
AGE	**BIRTH TO 3 YEARS (0–35 MONTHS)**	**3–4 YEARS (36–47 MONTHS)**	**4–5 YEARS (48–59 MONTHS)**	**5–6 YEARS (60–71 MONTHS)**
ECC	1 or more teeth with decayed (either cavitated or noncavitated), missing, or filled surfaces			
S-ECC	■ 1 or more teeth with decay (either cavitated or noncavitated) or fillings present on smooth surface enamel OR ■ 1 or more teeth missing due to caries	■ 1 or more cavitated or filled smooth surfaces in primary maxillary anterior teeth ■ 1 or more missing teeth due to caries OR ■ dmfs[a] score ≥4	■ 1 or more cavitated or filled smooth surfaces in primary maxillary anterior teeth ■ 1 or more missing teeth due to caries OR ■ dmfs[a] score ≥5	■ 1 or more cavitated or filled smooth surfaces in primary maxillary anterior teeth ■ 1 or more missing teeth due to caries OR ■ dmfs[a] score ≥6

[a]dmfs = total number of decayed missing and filled surfaces.
Source: Drury TF, Horowitz AM, Ismail AI, et al. Diagnosing and reporting early childhood caries for research purposes. *J Public Health Dent.* 1999;59(3):192–197.

Chapter 18. An example of root caries is shown in Figure 27-2 in Chapter 27.

- Apply current knowledge of the stages of dental caries to prevent damage to remineralizing areas during examination. Only cavitated lesions are recorded.

▶ *Record a rating for each root surface.*

RCI RATING	CRITERIA
No R	Root surface with a covered cementoenamel junction and no visible recession (R = recession).
R – D	Root surface with recession present and root caries present (D = decay).
R – F	Root surface with recession present and the surface is restored (F = filled).
R – N	Root surface with recession, but no caries or restoration is present.
M	The tooth is missing.

D. Scoring

▶ *Calculation*: Formula

$$\frac{[R-D]+[R-F]}{[R-D]+[R-F]+[R-N]} \times 100 = RCI$$

▶ *Calculation*: Example individual RCI
- A man, aged 70, presents with 23 natural teeth (23 × 4 = 92 surfaces). Clinical examination reveals:
R – D = 26
R – F = 8
R – N = 58

$$RCI = \frac{26+8}{26+8+58} = \frac{37}{92} \times 100 = 36.9\%$$

▶ *Interpretation*
- A score of 36.9% means that of all tooth surfaces with visible gingival recession, 36.9% have a history of root caries (cavitated or restored) carious lesions.

▶ *Group or community RCI*
- The R – D, R – F, and R – N scores for all individuals in the group are added together and the RCI formula is calculated using the total scores.

DENTAL FLUOROSIS

Dental indices such as the Thylstrup–Fejerskov index,[30] the fluorosis risk index,[31] and the developmental defects of dental enamel index[32,33] have been used to investigate the effects of fluoride concentration on dental enamel. The two indices described here are the most commonly used for community-based assessment.

I. Dean's Fluorosis Index[34]

A. Purpose

To measure the prevalence and severity of dental fluorosis.

- Originally developed in the 1930s and refined in 1942 to relate the severity of hypomineralization of dental enamel to concentration of fluoride in the water supply.
- Considered less sensitive than some other measures of fluorosis, but still recommended for use in community studies.

B. Selection of Teeth

The smooth surface enamel of all teeth is examined.

C. Procedure

Each tooth is visually examined for signs of fluorosis and assigned a numerical score using the descriptive categories listed in Table 23-2.

TABLE 23-2	Scoring System for Dean's Fluorosis Index	
CATEGORY	**DESCRIPTION**	**NUMERICAL SCORE**
Normal	Smooth, creamy white tooth surface	0
Questionable	Slight changes from normal transparency	1
Very mild	Small, scattered opaque areas; less than 25% of tooth surface	2
Mild	Opaque areas; less than 50% of tooth surface	3
Moderate	Significant opaque and/or worn areas; may have brown stains	4
Severe	Widespread, significant hypoplasia, pitting, brown staining, worn areas, and/or a corroded appearance	5

Source: Dean HT. The investigation of physiological effect by the epidemiological method. In: Moulton FR, ed. *Fluorine and Dental Health*. Washington, DC: American Association for the Advancement of Science; 1942:23–71.

D. Scoring

▶ An individual fluorosis score is assigned using the highest numerical score recorded for two or more teeth.

▶ Community levels of fluorosis are indicated by the percentage of individuals in the sample or population that receive scores in each category.

II. Tooth Surface Index of Fluorosis (TSIF)[35]

A. Purpose

▶ To measure the prevalence and severity of dental fluorosis.

▶ More sensitive than Dean's index in identifying the mildest signs of fluorosis.

B. Selection of Teeth

The smooth surface enamel, cusp tips, and incisal edges of all teeth are examined.

C. Procedure

Each tooth is examined visually and assigned a numerical score using the criteria in Table 23-3.

D. Scoring

TSIF data are presented as a distribution citing the percent of the population with each numerical score, rather than as mean scores for the entire group.

TABLE 23-3	Scoring System for TSIF	
DESCRIPTION		**NUMERICAL SCORE**
No evidence of fluorosis		0
Areas with parchment-white color; less than 1/3 of visible tooth surface; includes fluorosis confined to anterior incisal edges and posterior cusp tips		1
Parchment-white color on at least 1/3 but less than 2/3 of visible tooth surface		2
Parchment-white color on at least 2/3 of visible tooth surface		3
Staining (from light to very dark brown) in conjunction with parchment white areas as described above in levels 1, 2, or 3		4
Discrete stained and rough pitted areas, but no staining on intact enamel surfaces		5
Discrete pitting plus staining of intact enamel surfaces		6
Confluent pitting over large areas of tooth surface; anatomy of tooth may be altered; dark-brown stain usually present		7

Source: Horowitz HS, Driscoll WS, Meyers RJ, et al. A new method for assessing the prevalence of dental fluorosis—the tooth surface index of Fluorosis. *J Am Dent Assoc.* 1984;109(1):37–41.

COMMUNITY-BASED ORAL HEALTH SURVEILLANCE

Community oral health screenings can be performed at every level; local, national, and worldwide. Data collected by such screenings are useful for monitoring health status and determining population access to or need for oral health services.

I. WHO Basic Screening Survey (BSS)[21]

The World Health Organization (WHO) screening survey includes the CPI and the LOA indices previously described in this chapter.

A. Purpose

To collect comprehensive data on oral health status and dental treatment needs of a population. This system is suitable for surveying both adults and children.

B. Tissues/Areas Examined

Survey categories include the following:

▶ Orofacial (intraoral and extraoral) lesions and anomalies

▶ Temporomandibular joint status

▶ Periodontal status

▶ Dentition status and treatment need

▶ Prosthetic status and need

▶ Need for immediate care/referral.

C. Procedures

▶ Standardized assessment form with boxes for data entry identifies the codes and descriptive criteria for each data collection category.

▶ Standardized codes facilitate computerized data entry and analysis.

▶ Photographs in the training manual provide examples of criteria for each code.

D. Scoring

▶ Data can be analyzed by survey team or arrangements can be made for data entry forms to be analyzed by the WHO.

II. Association of State and Territorial Dental Directors (ASTDD) Basic Screening Survey (BSS)[6]

A. Purpose

▶ *Developed by the Association of State and Territorial Dental Directors (ASTDD) to provide oral screening for adult, school age, and/or preschool populations.*

• Data levels are consistent with monitoring the United States Public Health Service national health objectives.

• Data collected can easily be compared with data collected by other communities and states using the data collection techniques.

▶ *The system was designed to be used by screeners with or without dental background because:*

• Sometimes nondental personnel have better access to some population groups.

• Some communities have little access to dental public health professionals.

B. Selection of Teeth

All teeth are examined, but each individual patient receives one score for each category.

C. Procedure

▶ Oral screening can be combined with an optional questionnaire that collects additional data on demographics and access to dental care.

▶ Screeners are trained and calibrated. They record oral findings using photographs and detailed descriptions of associated criteria.

D. Scoring

▶ Table 23-4 outlines the scoring criteria and categories recorded for preschool and school children.

▶ Table 23-5 lists the scoring criteria and categories recorded for older adults.

▶ Data from each indicator can be compiled and expressed in frequency graphs or tables as a percentage of the population that exhibits a specific category trait.

DOCUMENTATION

Factors related to dental indices to document in the patient records include:

▶ Name of the index or indices used

▶ Score calculated for the index

▶ Objective statement that provides an interpretation of the index score

▶ Follow-up instructions provided to the patient

▶ An example of documentation for use of a dental index appears in Box 23-2.

TABLE 23-4	ASTDD BSS Scoring Criteria: Preschool and School Children		
CRITERIA	**SCORE**	**PRESCHOOLERS**	**SCHOOL CHILDREN**
Untreated caries (≥½ mm discontinuity in tooth surface)	0 = No untreated caries 1 = Untreated caries	√	√
Treated decay (amalgam, composite, or temporary filling)	0 = No treated decay 1 = Treated decay	√	√
ECC (3 years old with one or more 6 maxillary anterior teeth that were ever decayed, filled, or missing due to caries)	0 = No ECC 1 = ECC	√	
Sealants on permanent molars	0 = No sealants 1 = Sealants		√
Treatment urgency	0 = No obvious problem (routine dental care indicated) 1 = Early dental care (within two wks) 2 = Urgent care (as soon as possible—presents with pain, swelling, etc.)	√	√

A √ mark indicates that the oral condition category is scored in that particular age group. Some categories (i.e., sealants) are not scored in all age groups.

Source: Association of State and Territorial Dental Directors. *Basic Screening Surveys: An Approach to Monitoring Community Oral Health: Preschool and School Children*. Sparks, NV: ASTDD; 2008:36.

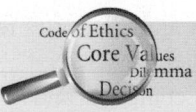

EVERYDAY ETHICS

Susanna began practicing in the team clinic at the dental school and found the work to be very challenging. As a hygienist, she was not only providing preventive treatment for patients but was also responsible for data collection for several research projects. Suddenly, the importance of understanding and calculating the various indices became critical. In particular, Susanna found herself reviewing the procedures for the OHI-S, bleeding indices, and the DMFT.

Susanna had always enjoyed her clinical interactions with patients, but now scoring and recording information on each and every tooth was beginning to cause her some stress. Generally Susanna practiced without an assistant and found it difficult to do both examining and recording. Near the end of one day when she was organizing the day's work for Dr. Lowe's caries study, she discovered that she had omitted several surfaces in one quadrant. This was the patient's final visit to the dental school. Susanna contemplated what to do when she realized the data were missing.

Questions for Consideration

1. Discuss how American Dental Hygienists' Association's roles for dental hygienists (Chapter 1) apply to Suzanna's daily duties.

2. Can Susanna "defend" her actions to Dr. Lowe by submitting the data she does have on the patient? Explain your rationale.

3. Which of the core values (Table II-1, Section II Introduction) or principles of ethical behavior come into play in collecting research data such as described in this scenario?

TABLE 23-5	ASTDD BSS Scoring Criteria: Older Adults
CRITERIA	**SCORE**
Removable upper denture	0 = No 1 = Yes
If yes Do you wear upper denture when eating?	0 = No 1 = Yes
Removable lower denture	0 = No 1 = Yes
If yes Do you wear lower denture when eating?	0 = No 1 = Yes
Number of upper natural teeth (include root fragments)	Range 0–16
Number of lower natural teeth (include root fragments)	Range 0–16
Root fragments	0 = No 1 = Yes 9 = Edentulous
Untreated decay	0 = No 1 = Yes 9 = Edentulous
Need for periodontal care	0 = No 1 = Yes 9 = Edentulous
Suspicious soft tissue lesions	0 = No 1 = Yes 9 = Edentulous
Treatment urgency	0 = no obvious problem—next scheduled visit 1 = Early care—within next several weeks 2 = Urgent care—within next week—pain or infection.

Source: Association of State and Territorial Dental Directors. *Basic Screening Surveys: An Approach to Monitoring Community Oral Health:Older Adults*. Sparks, NV: ASTDD; 2010:40–41.

BOX 23-2

Example Documentation: Use of a Dental Index During Patient Assessment

S –Patient presents for reassessment of biofilm and bleeding levels 14 days following oral hygiene instructions that were provided during the previous appointment.

O –Biofilm-free score = 89% compared to previous score of 22%; SBI score = 2 compared to previous score of 5.

A –Significant improvement noted in scores except on maxillary facial surfaces.

P –Patient congratulated on areas of success. Additional instruction provided specifically related to biofilm removal on posterior facial and proximal tooth surfaces. Patient observed while brushing and flossing maxillary molar areas using a mirror.

Next Step: 3 months re-evaluation.

Signed _____, RDH

Date _____

Factors To Teach Patient or Members of the Community

▷ How an index is used and calculated, and what the scores mean.

▷ Purpose for the selection of the particular index being used.

▷ Correlation of index scores with current oral health practices and procedures.

▷ Procedures to follow to improve index scores and bring the oral tissues to health.

References

NOTE: Many of the citations below may seem not to be current or even completely out-of-date, however the reader will note that most are "classic" references, which refer to the development and first use of the index.

1. Silness J, Loe H. Periodontal disease in pregnancy. II. Correlation between oral hygiene and periodontal condition. *Acta Odontol Scand*. 1964;22:121–135.

2. Podshadley AG, Haley JV. A method for evaluating oral hygiene performance. *Public Health Rep*. 1968;83(3):259–264.

3. Klein H, Palmer CE, Knutson JW. Studies on dental caries. I. Dental status and dental needs of elementary school children. *Public Health Rep*. 1938;53(19):751–765.

4. United States Department of Health and Human Services. *Oral Health in America: A Report of the Surgeon General*. Rockville, MD: U.S. Department of Health and Human Services, National Institute of Dental and Craniofacial Research, National Institutes of Health; 2000:63–89.

5. United States Department of Health and Human Services. *Healthy People 2020: Topics and Objectives: Oral Health*. Washington, DC: U.S. Department of Health and Human

Services; 2010. http://www.healthypeople.gov/2020/topics-objectives/topic/oral-health. Accessed May 19, 2015.

6. Association of State and Territorial Dental Directors. *Basic Screening Surveys*. Reno, NV: ASTDD; 2014. http://www.astdd.org/basic-screening-survey-tool/. Accessed March 19, 2014.

7. Löe H. The gingival index, the plaque index and the retention index systems. *J Periodontol*. 1967;38(6, Suppl):610–616.

8. O'Leary TJ, Drake RB, Naylor JE. The plaque control record. *J Periodontol*. 1972;43(1):38.

9. Ramfjord SP, Ash MM. *Periodontology and Periodontics*. Philadelphia, PA: WB Saunders Co; 1979:273.

10. Grant DA, Stern IB, Everett FG. *Periodontics*. 5th ed. St. Louis, MO: Mosby; 1979:529–531.

11. Greene JC, Vermillion JR. The simplified oral hygiene index. *J Am Dent Assoc*. 1964;68:7–13.

12. Greene JC. The Oral Hygiene Index—development and uses. *J Periodontol*. 1967;38(6, Suppl):625–637.

13. Schour I, Massler M. Prevalence of gingivitis in young adults. *J Dent Res*. 1948;27(6):733. Abstract #33 in IADR scientific proceedings.

14. Massler M. The P-M-A index for the assessment of gingivitis. *J Periodontol*. 1967;38(6, Suppl):592–601.

15. Russell AL. A system of classification and scoring for prevalence surveys of periodontal disease. *J Dent Res*. 1956;35(3):350–359.

16. Mühlemann HR, Son, S. Gingival sulcus bleeding—a leading symptom in initial gingivitis. *Helv Odontol Acta*. 1971;15(2):107–113.

17. Meitner SW, Zander HA, Iker HP, et al. Identification of inflamed gingival surfaces. *J Clin Periodontol*. 1979;6(2):93–97.

18. American Academy of Periodontology. Parameter on comprehensive periodontal examination. *J Periodontol*. 2000;71(5, Suppl):847–848.

19. Khocht A, Zohn H, Deasy M, et al. Assessment of periodontal status with PSR and traditional clinical periodontal examination. *J Am Dent Assoc*. 1995;126(12):1658–1665.

20. Ainamo J, Barmes D, Beagrie G, et al. Development of the World Health Organization (WHO) community periodontal index of treatment needs (CPITN). *Int Dent J*. 1982;32(3):281–291.

21. World Health Organization. *Oral Health Surveys: Basic Methods*. Geneva: WHO; 1997:26–39.

22. Carter HG, Barnes GP. The gingival bleeding index. *J Periodontol*. 1974;45(11):801–805.

23. Abrams K, Caton J, Polson A. Histologic comparisons of interproximal gingival tissues related to the presence or absence of bleeding. *J Periodontol*. 1984;55(11):629–632.

24. Caton JG, Polson, AM. The interdental bleeding index: a simplified procedure for monitoring gingival health. *Compend Contin Educ Dent*. 1985;6(2):88, 90–92.

25. Ramfjord SP. Indices for prevalence and incidence of periodontal disease. *J Periodontol*. 1959;30:51–59.

26. United States Department of Health and Human Services, Public Health Service, National Institutes of Health. *Oral Health Surveys of the National Institute of Dental Research, Diagnostic Criteria and Procedures*. Bethesda, MD: National Institute of Dental Research; 1991. NIH Publication No. 91-2870.

27. Gruebbel AO. A measurement of dental caries prevalence and treatment service for deciduous teeth. *J Dent Res*. 1944;23:163–168.

28. Drury TF, Horowitz AM, Ismail AI, et al. Diagnosing and reporting early childhood caries for research purposes. *J Public Health Dent*. 1999;59(3):192–197.

29. Katz RV. Assessing root caries in populations: the evolution of the root caries index. *J Public Health Dent*. 1980;40(1):7–16.

30. Thylstrup A, Fejerskov O. Clinical appearance of dental fluorosis in permanent teeth in relation to histologic changes. *Community Dent Oral Epidemiol*. 1978;6(6):315–328.

31. Pendrys DG. The fluorosis risk index: a method for investigating risk factors. *J Public Health Dent*. 1990;50(5):291–298.

32. Fédération Dentaire Internationale. An epidemiological index of developmental defects of dental enamel (DDE Index). Commission on Oral Health, Research and Epidemiology. *Int Dent J*. 1982;32(2):159–167.

33. Clarkson J, O'Mullane, D. A modified DDE index for use in epidemiological studies of enamel defects. *J Dent Res*. 1989;68(3):445–450.

34. Dean HT. The investigation of physiological effect by the epidemiological method. In: Moulton FR, ed. *Fluorine and Dental Health*. Washington, DC: American Association for the Advancement of Science; 1942:23–71.

35. Horowitz HS, Driscoll WS, Meyers RJ, et al. A new method for assessing the prevalence of dental fluorosis—the tooth surface index of fluorosis. *J Am Dent Assoc*. 1984;109(1):37–41.

 ENHANCE YOUR UNDERSTANDING

thePoint® **DIGITAL CONNECTIONS**
(see the inside front cover for access information)
- **Audio glossary**
- **Quiz bank**

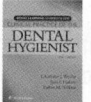 **SUPPORT FOR LEARNING**
(available separately; visit lww.com)
- *Active Learning Workbook for Clinical Practice of the Dental Hygienist, 12th Edition*

prepU **INDIVIDUALIZED REVIEW**
(available separately; visit lww.com)
- **Adaptive quizzing with *prepU for Wilkins' Clinical Practice of the Dental Hygienist***

SECTION

V

Dental Hygiene Diagnosis and Care Planning

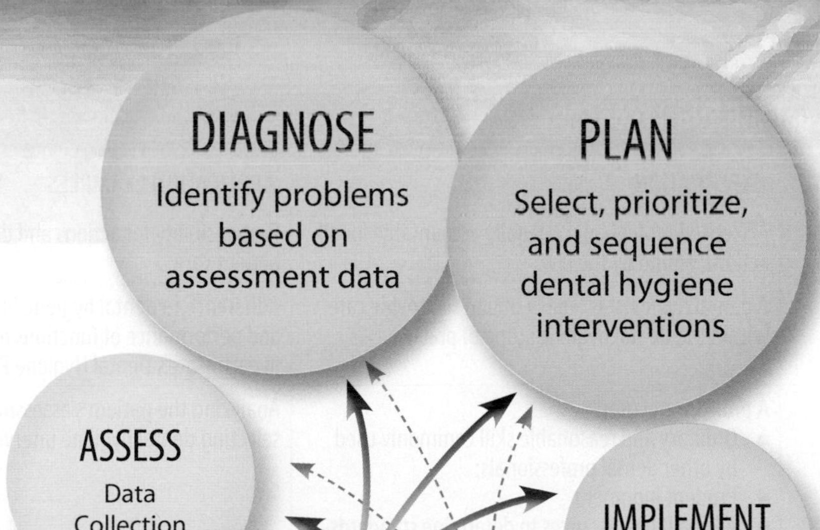
DIAGNOSE
Identify problems based on assessment data
PLAN
Select, prioritize, and sequence dental hygiene interventions
ASSESS
Data Collection
IMPLEMENT
Activating the plan
DOCUMENT
Comprehensive record-keeping
EVALUATE
Feedback on effectiveness

FIGURE V-1 The Dental Hygiene Process of Care.

INTRODUCTION FOR SECTION V

After the initial assessment is completed as described in Section IV, the data are assembled, sequenced, and analyzed in preparation for planning dental hygiene treatment and education interventions that help the patient acquire and maintain optimum oral health.

THE DENTAL HYGIENE PROCESS OF CARE

Figure V-1 on the previous page shows the position of diagnosis and care planning in the total Dental Hygiene Process of Care.

▶ Dental hygiene diagnosis statements:
  • Analyze patient assessment data to identify significant oral hygiene problems.
  • Focus attention on behavioral aspects as well as deviations from normal oral health.
▶ The formal, written dental hygiene care plan, integrated with the total treatment plan for the patient, is used to:
  • Identify dental hygiene interventions based on diagnostic statements that define patient needs.
  • Educate the patient.
  • Secure informed consent for treatment.
  • Communicate planned dental hygiene interventions with other oral care team members.

ETHICAL APPLICATIONS

▶ Basic concepts of healthcare law apply to all dental hygiene professionals.
▶ The dental hygiene practice acts of each state or province govern the scope of dental hygiene functions and the criteria for licensure.
▶ The potential for an ethical situation arises anytime a dental hygienist interacts with:
  • A patient.
  • Members of the dental or interprofessional healthcare team.
  • Other individuals involved in the special needs of the patient, such as family and caregivers.
▶ A dental hygienist who provides ethical patient care:
  • Is cognizant of the respect each patient deserves.
  • Maintains communication among all parties responsible for dental and dental hygiene treatment.
  • Attains knowledge of current standards of care and legal scope of practice.
  • Possesses the ability to assess and justify the reporting of unacceptable practices.
  • Selected legal concepts and suggestions for application are described in Table V-1.

TABLE V-1	Legal and Ethical Concepts	
LEGAL CONCEPT	**EXPLANATION**	**APPLICATION EXAMPLES**
Professional liability	A licensed professional is legally accountable for all actions; bound by the law.	Responsibility for actions and decisions made during patient care.
Scope of practice	A dental hygienist is legally bound to provide care within the dental hygiene scope of practice.	Adherence to dental hygiene licensure requirements and performance of functions defined as legal within in each state's Dental Hygiene Practice Act.
Standard of care	A professional uses: ■ Ordinary and reasonable skill commonly used by other dental professionals; ■ Prudent judgment ■ All available resources to determine standards of practice.	Analyzing the patient's assessment data before selecting dental hygiene interventions.
Informed consent	Voluntary affirmation by a patient to allow examination or treatment by authorized dental hygienist or other member of the dental team.	An ongoing process of communication and education about oral health treatment options, not only a printed form to sign.
Negligence/malpractice	Failure to perform professional duties according to the accepted standard of care.	Failure to inform and refer a patient when concerns outside the scope of dental hygiene practice exist.

Planning for Dental Hygiene Care

Charlotte J. Wyche, RDH, MS

CHAPTER OUTLINE

LEARNING OBJECTIVES

After studying this chapter, the student will be able to:

1. Identify and define key terms and concepts related to planning dental hygiene care.

2. Identify and explain assessment findings and individual patient factors that affect patient care.

3. Identify additional factors that can influence planning for dental hygiene care.

4. Apply the evidence-based decision-making process to determine patient care recommendations.

▶ Four basic steps[1] to be considered when planning patient care are:
  - Collect and analyze assessment information.
  - Establish the diagnosis.
  - Select treatment and education interventions.
  - Develop a formal plan for care.
▶ In the dental hygiene process of care (Figure 1-3, Chapter 1), the dental hygiene diagnosis is the result of analysis and synthesis of assessment data and the application of clinical judgment and critical thinking skills.
▶ Then, using an evidence-based approach, a dental hygiene care plan and appointment sequence are formalized.
▶ Terms and key words used in conjunction with these steps are defined in Box 24-1.

ASSESSMENT FINDINGS

Clinical assessment findings play a key role in the development of the dental hygiene diagnosis and dental hygiene care plan.

I. The Chief Complaint

▶ The patient's statement regarding the reason for seeking dental and dental hygiene care.
▶ A significant concern expressed by the patient, such as pain, is addressed before initiating dental hygiene treatment.

II. Risk Factors

▶ Risk factors increase the patient's potential for diminished oral health status.
▶ Anticipatory guidance through preventive education and counseling is an essential component of the care plan for a patient exhibiting one or more risk factors.

A. Risk Factors for Periodontal Infections or Poor Response to Periodontal Therapy[2,3]

▶ Behavioral factors (inadequate biofilm removal, diet, noncompliance with dental hygiene recommendations)
▶ Tobacco use

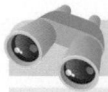

BOX 24-1 KEY WORDS AND ABBREVIATIONS: Planning for Dental Hygiene Care

ADLs (Activities of daily living): a measure of the ability to carry out the basic tasks needed for self-care.
  IADLs (Instrumental activities of daily living): a measure of the ability to perform more of the complex tasks necessary to function in our society; tasks that require a combination of physical and cognitive ability.
Anticipatory guidance: patient education and oral hygiene instructions that anticipate potential oral and systemic health problems associated with risk factors identified during patient assessment.
ASA: American Society of Anesthesiologists; originally developed the ASA Classifications to determine modifications necessary to provide general anesthetic to patients during surgical procedures.
Assessment: the critical analysis and evaluation or judgment of a particular condition, situation, or other subject of appraisal.
Chief complaint: the patient's concern as stated during the initial health history preparation; may be the reason for seeking professional care; a complaint such as pain or discomfort may require emergency dental diagnosis.
Compromised therapy: initial therapy and continued periodontal maintenance provided as the therapeutic end point in cases where the severity and extent of the disease or the age and health of the patient preclude optimal results of periodontal therapy.
Definitive care: complete care; end point at which all treatment required at the time has been completed.
Diagnose: to identify or recognize a disease or problem.
Diagnosis: a statement of the problem; a concise technical description of the cause, nature, or manifestations of a

condition, situation, or problem; identification of a disease or deviation from normal condition by recognition of characteristic signs and symptoms.
  Dental hygiene diagnosis: identification of an existing or a potential oral health problem that a dental hygienist is qualified and licensed to treat.
  Differential diagnosis: identification of which one of several diseases or conditions may be producing the symptoms.
Evidence-based care: providing oral care based on relevant, scientifically sound research.
OSCAR: a mnemonic that stands for Oral, Systemic, Capability, Autonomy, and Reality. Developed by the American Academy of Oral Medicine to provide a convenient, systematic approach to identifying dental, medical/pharmacologic, functional, ethical, and fiscal factors that need to be evaluated and weighed when planning treatment for geriatric individuals or those with disabilities.
Prognosis: prediction of outcome; a forecast of the probable course and outcome of a disease and the prospects of recovery as expected by the nature of the specific condition and the symptoms of the case.
  Dental hygiene prognosis: a judgment regarding the results (outcomes) expected to be achieved from oral treatment provided by a dental hygienist.
Risk factor: an attribute or exposure that increases the probability of disease, such as an aspect of personal behavior, environmental exposure, or an inherited characteristic associated with health-related conditions.
  Modifiable risk factor: a determinant that can be modified by intervention, thereby reducing the probability of disease.

▶ Systemic conditions (diabetes, decreased immune factors, osteoporosis, osteopenia)

▶ Hormonal considerations (pregnancy, menopause)

▶ Genetic factors

▶ Nutritional status[4]

▶ Iatrogenic factors (overhangs, open contacts, residual calculus)[5]

B. Periodontal Disease as a Risk Factor for Systemic Conditions

Current research suggests the presence of periodontal infection is associated with a variety of systemic conditions, including:

▶ Cardiovascular disease[6–8]

▶ Diabetes mellitus[6]

▶ Metabolic syndrome (a cluster of health conditions that increase risk for heart disease and diabetes)[7]

▶ Respiratory disease (especially pneumonia)[6–8]

▶ Infective endocarditis[6]

▶ Adverse pregnancy outcome[9,10]

▶ Osteoporosis[11]

C. Risk Factors for Dental Caries

▶ The current best-practice, evidence-based approach for management of dental caries is by identifying and addressing risk factors.[12]

▶ Risk factors for dental caries include[13–15]:
  • Behavioral factors (inadequate biofilm removal)
  • Dietary factors (frequent use of cariogenic foods/beverages)
  • Low fluoride
  • Tooth morphology and position (deep occlusal pits and fissures, exposed root surfaces, rotated positioning)
  • Xerostomia
  • Personal and family history of dental caries/restorative dentistry
  • Developmental factors (modifications of dental enamel)
  • Genetic factors (immune response)

C. Risk Factors for Oral Cancer[16,17]

▶ Tobacco use of any kind

▶ Heavy alcohol use

▶ Excessive sun exposure (lips and face)

▶ Exposure to the human papillomavirus

▶ Genetic susceptibility

III. Patient's Overall Health Status

A. Physical Status

▶ The extent of the patient's medical, physical, and psychological risk determines modifications necessary during treatment.

▶ Examples of systematic approaches used to assess physical status include:
  • The American Society of Anesthesiologists' (ASA) classification system (Table 24-1).[18]
  • The Oral, Systemic, Capability, Autonomy, and Reality (OSCAR) Planning Guide (Table 24-2).[19]

B. Tobacco Use

▶ Tobacco in all forms affects oral status and dental hygiene treatment outcomes.

▶ Information on planning dental hygiene interventions for the patient who uses tobacco is discussed in Chapter 34.

IV. Oral Healthcare Knowledge Level of the Patient

▶ Before planning individualized patient care, an attempt is made to assess the patient's oral health knowledge level.

▶ From that baseline, planned educational interventions can build on current knowledge rather than provide information too far above or below the patient's current understanding.

V. The Patient's Self-Care Ability

▶ The patient's ability to manipulate a toothbrush and floss and to comply with suggested oral care regimens will determine the success of planned interventions.

▶ Patients with disabilities or physical limitations will require modification to ensure adequate daily oral biofilm removal.

▶ An activities of daily living (ADL) classification level, described in Table 24-3, provides a guide to determine whether adaptive aids or caregiver training for personal oral care procedures are necessary.

THE PERIODONTAL DIAGNOSIS AND RISK LEVEL

Planning for the number and length of appointments in a treatment sequence is influenced by:

▶ Both the dental and dental hygiene periodontal diagnosis.[20]

▶ The patient's periodontal risk factors[20] (see the Risk Factors section).

I. Current Periodontal Status

A description of past and current periodontal conditions, as well as risk factors affecting the progress of disease, determine a patient's current periodontal status.

TABLE 24-1	ASA Physical Status Classification System		
ASA CLASSIFICATION		**EXAMPLES OF PHYSICAL OR PSYCHOSOCIAL MANIFESTATIONS**	**DENTAL HYGIENE TREATMENT CONSIDERATIONS**
ASA I	Without systemic disease; a normal, healthy patient with little or no dental anxiety	Able to walk one flight of stairs with no distress ADL/IADL level = 0	No modifications necessary
ASA II	Mild systemic disease or extreme dental anxiety	Needs to stop after walking one flight of stairs because of distress Well-controlled chronic conditions Upper respiratory infections Healthy pregnant woman Allergies ADL/IADL level = 1	Minimal risk; minor modifications to treatment and/or patient education may be necessary
ASA III	Systemic disease that limits activity but is not incapacitating	Needs to stop en route walking one flight of stairs Chronic cardiovascular conditions Controlled insulin-dependent diabetes Chronic pulmonary diseases Elevated blood pressure ADL/IADL level = 2 or 3	Elective treatment is not contraindicated, but serious consideration of treatment and/or patient/caregiver education modifications may be necessary
ASA IV	Incapacitating disease that is a constant threat to life	Unable to walk up one flight of stairs Unstable cardiovascular conditions Extremely elevated blood pressure Uncontrolled epilepsy Uncontrolled insulin-dependent diabetes	Conservative, noninvasive management of emergency dental conditions; more complex dental intervention may require hospitalization during treatment; caregiver training for daily oral care may be necessary
ASA V	Patient is moribund and not expected to survive	End-stage renal, hepatic, infectious disease, or terminal cancer	Only palliative treatment is delivered; caregiver training for daily oral care may be necessary

Source: American Society of Anesthesiologists. ASA physical status classification system. http://www.asahq.org/resources/clinical-information/asa-physical-status-classification-system. Accessed January 21, 2015.

TABLE 24-2	Treatment Planning with OSCAR
ISSUE	**FACTORS OF CONCERN**
A systematic approach to identifying factors to evaluate when planning dental hygiene care.	
Oral	Teeth, restorations, prostheses, periodontium, pulpal status, oral mucosa, occlusion, saliva, tongue, alveolar bone
Systemic	Normative age changes, medical diagnoses, pharmacologic agents, interdisciplinary communication
Capability	Functional ability, self-care, caregivers, oral hygiene, transportation to appointments, mobility within the dental office
Autonomy	Decision-making ability, dependence on alternative or supplemental decision makers
Reality	Prioritization of oral health, financial ability or limitations, significance of anticipated life span

Reprinted with permission from: Ship JA, Mohammad AR, eds. *Clinician's Guide to Oral Health in Geriatric Patients*. Baltimore, MD: American Academy of Oral Medicine; 1999:21.

TABLE 24-3	Measures of Patient Functioning[a]	
EXAMPLES OF ADLS	**EXAMPLES OF IADLS**	**LEVELS**
Brushing Flossing Applying interdental aids Feeding Ambulation (walking) Bathing Continence Communication Dressing Toileting Transfer (from bed to toilet) Grooming	Maintaining self-care regimens Ability to make and keep dental appointments Writing Cooking Shopping Climbing stairs Managing medication Reading Cleaning Using telephone	**Level 0** Ability to perform the task without assistance **Level 1** Ability to perform the task with some human assistance; may need a device or mechanical aid but or still independent **Level 2** Ability to perform the task with partial assistance **Level 3** Requires full assistance to perform the task; totally dependent

[a]This scale provides a simple means of summarizing a person's ability to carry out the basic tasks needed for self-care.

II. Classification of Periodontal Disease

The extent, severity, and chronic or aggressive nature of the patient's periodontal disease can be characterized as listed in Table 24-4.

For purpose of determining the sequences and number of appointments required for initial nonsurgical periodontal therapy, it is useful to divide the periodontal diagnosis the following classifications:

Type 1: Gingival Disease

Inflammation of the gingiva characterized by changes in color, form, size, position of margin, with bleeding on probing and no attachment loss.

Type 2: Early Periodontitis

Progression of inflammation into the deeper periodontal structures with slight bone loss and connective tissue attachment; subgingival calculus and measurable pocket depth with bleeding on probing.

Type 3: Moderate Periodontitis

A more advanced state of periodontal disease, with increased destruction of the periodontal structures, increased probing depths with bleeding, noticeable loss of bony support with early to moderate furcation invasions; mobility and fremitus.

Type 4: Advanced Periodontitis

Further progression of periodontal inflammation with increased probing depths with bleeding, major loss of bony support, furcation invasions, and possible evidence of trauma from occlusion with increased tooth mobility and fremitus, and other signs and symptoms.

III. Parameters of Care

▶ Clinical diagnosis, therapeutic goals, treatment considerations, and outcomes assessment for periodontal disease are outlined in the periodontal Parameters of Care.[21]

▶ Planning considerations are graded by the severity of infection. Examples are listed in Table 24-4.

DENTAL CARIES RISK LEVEL

▶ Treatment for dental caries is provided by the dentist; however, the plan for dental hygiene care includes interventions aimed at managing risk factors for dental caries.[22]

▶ Protocols and treatment guidelines for caries management based on risk factors are found in:
- Chapter 27, Table 27-1 (for adults).
- Chapter 50, Table 50-6 (for children 0–5).

THE DENTAL HYGIENE DIAGNOSIS

I. Basis for Diagnosis

▶ Patient interview data (chief complaint, identification of oral problems, and comprehensive personal/social, medical, and dental health histories).

▶ Physical assessment data (vital signs, extraoral and intraoral tissue examination, and dental and periodontal chartings).

▶ Treatment or education needs that may be addressed by providing oral care services within the dental hygienist's legal scope of practice.

▶ Treatment needs that may be addressed by consultation with another licensed healthcare professional.

TABLE 24-4	Parameters of Care		
CLINICAL DIAGNOSIS	**THERAPEUTIC GOALS**	**TREATMENT CONSIDERATIONS**	
Biofilm-induced gingivitis	■ To establish gingival health through elimination of etiologic factors	**Dental treatment plan** ■ The dental treatment plan may indicate surgical correction of gingival deformities.	**Dental hygiene care plan** ■ Customized patient education ■ Supra- and subgingival debridement ■ Antimicrobial agents, and correction of biofilm-retentive factors
Chronic periodontitis ■ With slight to moderate loss of periodontal support	■ To arrest progression of disease and prevent recurrence ■ To preserve health, comfort, and function	**Dental treatment plan** ■ If resolution of the condition does not occur, consider periodontal surgery	**Dental hygiene care plan** ■ Elimination and control of systemic and local risk factors ■ Biofilm control ■ Supra- and subgingival scaling and root planing ■ Adjunctive antimicrobial agents
Chronic periodontitis ■ With advanced loss of periodontal support	■ To alter or eliminate microbial etiology and contributing risk factors ■ To arrest the progression of disease	**Dental treatment plan** ■ May include regeneration of periodontal attachment following the completion and evaluation of initial therapy	**Dental hygiene care plan** ■ Initial therapy as described above **Compromised therapy** ■ Severity/extent of disease, or the age/health of the patient preclude optimal results ■ Initial therapy and continued periodontal maintenance become the endpoint
Periodontal maintenance	■ To minimize the recurrence and progression of the disease ■ To reduce the incidence of tooth loss		**Dental hygiene care plan** ■ Comparison of clinical data to previous baseline measurements ■ Assessment of personal oral hygiene status and compliance with maintenance intervals ■ Oral hygiene reinstruction or modification ■ Counseling on control of risk factors
Acute periodontal diseases include ■ Gingival abscess ■ Periodontal abscess ■ Necrotizing diseases ■ Herpetic gingivostomatitis ■ Pericoronitis ■ Periodontal-endodontic lesions	■ To eliminate acute signs and symptoms of the condition as soon as possible	**Dental treatment plan** ■ Treatment considerations depend on the presenting condition	**Dental hygiene care plan** ■ Collaborate with the attending dentist to prioritize treatment for the immediate need

CLINICAL DIAGNOSIS	THERAPEUTIC GOALS	TREATMENT CONSIDERATIONS	
Aggressive periodontitis	■ To alter or eliminate microbial etiology and contributing risk factors ■ To arrest or slow the progression of the disease	**Dental treatment plan** ■ General medical evaluation and consultation ■ Microbial identification ■ Antibiotic sensitivity testing ■ Alternative antimicrobial agents or delivery systems ■ Evaluation/counseling of family members	**Dental hygiene care plan** ■ Care parameters planned for chronic periodontitis
Mucogingival conditions ■ Deviations from normal anatomic relationship between gingival margin and mucogingival junction	■ To maintain and restore function and esthetics	**Dental treatment plan** ■ May include surgical treatment	**Dental hygiene care plan** ■ Careful comparison of baseline and follow-up findings, control of inflammation through biofilm control, scaling and root planing, and/or antimicrobial agents

Source: American Academy of Periodontology. Parameters of care. *J Periodontol.* 2000;71(5, Suppl):i–ii, 847–883.

II. Diagnostic Statements

▶ Provide the basis for planning interventions within the scope of dental hygiene practice.

▶ Reflect expected outcomes of dental hygiene interventions.

▶ Identify patient responses changeable by dental hygiene interventions.

▶ Exclude diagnoses that require treatments legally defined as dental practice.

▶ For examples of dental hygiene diagnostic statements, see Table 25-2, in Chapter 25.

III. Diagnostic Models

▶ Medical and dental models of diagnosis classify diagnostic statements according to disease processes.

▶ In contrast, diagnostic models for dental hygiene[23-27] have been developed that, like nursing models, encompass a broader focus to:
  • Address health functioning and behaviors.
  • Describe actual or potential health problems that dental hygienists are educated and licensed to treat.

▶ The dental hygiene diagnosis models, described in Table 24-5, provide direction and a scientific basis from which to determine dental hygiene interventions and formulate patient care plans.

THE DENTAL HYGIENE PROGNOSIS

▶ Prognosis is:
  • A look ahead to an anticipated outcome or end point expected from the dental hygiene intervention selected for an individual patient.
  • Expressed in general terms for either an individual tooth or the overall prognosis for the patient's teeth.
  • Based on treatment and self-care behavior goals set by the clinician with the patient during the planning phase of care.

▶ Examples of potential outcomes from dental hygiene interventions in a three-part care plan are listed in Chapter 25.

I. Criteria for Various Prognoses

The criteria for various prognoses are listed in Box 24-2.

II. Factors that Determine Prognosis

▶ Assessment data regarding current disease status

▶ The patient's risk factors

▶ The patient's commitment to personal care and preventive regimens

▶ Interventions with the potential to reverse a patient's oral problem

TABLE 24-5	Diagnostic Models used in Planning Dental Hygiene Care
MODEL NAME	**DIAGNOSTIC STATEMENTS**
Dental hygiene diagnostic model[23]	Developed by following six steps that form the process of diagnostic decision making: 1. Initial review 2. Hypothesis formation 3. Inquiry strategy 4. Problem synthesis 5. Diagnostic decision making 6. Learning from the process Recorded in patient treatment records using the notation "DHDX" and accompanied by a treatment plan or treatment goal statement
The human needs model[24]	Based on whether specific criteria defining eight human needs are met or unmet by the patient's current oral health status Written by outlining goals to be obtained for resolving each observed deficit
The dental hygiene process model[25]	Identify patient's problem in terms of response rather than need and state the possible etiology Classified into several categories, which include general systemic, soft tissue, periodontal, oral hygiene, and dental categories Written by stating the problem and the etiologic factor joined by the phrase "related to"
The oral health-related quality of life model[26]	Diagnostic statements for individuals/populations are based on the assessment of domains related to health/preclinical disease; biological/physiological disease; and the broad-based sequelae to disease, such as symptom status, function status, health perceptions, and overall quality of life Dental hygiene actions are formulated for each domain, incorporating a multidisciplinary approach to care

BOX 24-2

Criteria for Various Prognoses

Prognosis following periodontal therapy is determined by the presence of one or more of the following factors.

Good

▷ Adequate control of etiologic factors
▷ Adequate patient self-care ability
▷ Adequate periodontal support

Fair

▷ Adequate control of etiologic factors
▷ Adequate patient self-care ability
▷ Less than 25% attachment loss
▷ Class I or less furcation involvement

Poor

▷ Greater than 50% attachment loss with Class II furcation
▷ Patient self-care difficult due to location and depth of furcation

Questionable

▷ Greater than 50% attachment loss with poor crown-to-root ratio
▷ Poor root form: instrumentation access
▷ Inaccessible Class II furcation or Class III furcation
▷ Greater than 2+ mobility
▷ Significant root proximity

Hopeless

▷ Inadequate attachment to maintain the tooth

Source: McGuire, MK. Prognosis vs outcome: predicting tooth survival. *Compend Contin Educ Dent.* 2000;21:217–220, 222, 224.

▶ Treatment alternatives selected
▶ Evidence from the scientific literature.

ADDITIONAL CONSIDERATIONS

I. Role of the Patient

A. Purpose

The willingness and/or ability of the patient to participate in reducing risk factors and changing oral health behaviors will be the key to reaching goals set during planning.

B. Procedure

▶ Determine the patient's level of understanding of dental diseases, risk factors, and oral health behaviors.
▶ Determine the patient's physical ability to manipulate recommended oral care aids.
▶ Determine lifestyle factors that impact the patient's ability to comply with oral health recommendations.
▶ Educate patients regarding the importance of their role in eliminating modifiable risk factors, setting oral health goals and complying with recommendations.

II. Tissue Conditioning

Preparation or conditioning of the gingival tissue for scaling can be of particular significance when:

▶ There is spongy, soft tissue that bleeds on slight provocation.

▶ The area is generally septic from dental biofilm and debris accumulation.

A. Purpose

Anticipated outcomes of a tissue-conditioning program include:

▶ Gingival healing
- Tissues become less edematous.
- Bleeding is minimized.
- Scaling procedures are facilitated.

▶ Reduced bacterial accumulation
- Less likelihood that bacteremias will be produced during scaling.
- Contamination is reduced in the aerosols produced.

▶ Learning by the patient

While conditioning the tissue for scaling, the patient can do the following:
- Practice oral health behaviors
- Experience the benefits of a clean mouth
- Form lifetime habits for continued maintenance.

B. Procedure

▶ Initiate a pretreatment program of daily biofilm removal.

▶ Recommend daily use of an antibacterial rinse after thorough brushing and flossing before going to bed.

▶ Select affected quadrants for scaling only after patient cooperation has been demonstrated.

III. Preprocedural Antimicrobial Rinsing

Preprocedural removal of dental biofilm will lower bacterial count in aerosols and decrease potential for bacteremia.

▶ The first choice is patient brushing and flossing.

▶ Vigorous rinsing with antibacterial mouthwash will reduce bacteria in aerosols.[28,29]

IV. Pain and Anxiety Control

A. Purpose

▶ Control of discomfort during treatment procedures.

▶ More consistent patient compliance with recommended interventions and need to return for additional scheduled appointments.

B. Procedures

▶ When there is a patient complaint of pain or discomfort, treat those areas first unless tissue conditioning is required.

▶ Treat either the quadrant with the fewest teeth or the least severe periodontal infection first to ensure the following:
- Make the first scaling less complicated.
- Help orient an anxious patient to clinical procedures.

▶ Patient posttreatment discomfort is minimized to select a maxillary and mandibular quadrant on the same side when two quadrants are to be treated at the same appointment.

▶ The need for anesthesia is determined by:
- The patient's previous pain control experiences
- Severity of the periodontal infection
- Depth of pockets
- Consistency and distribution of calculus
- Potential patient discomfort during scaling
- Sensitivity of the patient's tissues.

V. Dental Hygiene Care During Dental Therapy

A. Purpose

When restorative, prosthetic, or orthodontic, treatment extends over a long period of time, periodic appointments with the dental hygienist are needed for monitoring the continued success of the patient's self-care.

B. Procedure

Dental hygiene care provided during extended dental therapy follows the dental hygiene process of care and includes:

▶ Gingival tissue assessment

▶ Probing to determine bleeding

▶ Biofilm check with disclosing agent

▶ Reinforcement of daily oral care measures

▶ Scaling and root planing to remove calculus

▶ Additional instruction for care of new prostheses

▶ Motivational encouragement.

VI. Four-Handed Dental Hygiene

A. Purpose

Planning patient care while practicing with a dental assistant increases the dental hygienist's efficiency through the use of:

▶ Flexible scheduling.

▶ Two treatment chairs in an overlapping time frame.

▶ Assistance with patient management.

B. Procedure

A well-trained dental hygiene assistant can be delegated duties such as:

▶ Patient reception and seating

▶ Medical history update before confirmation of findings by the dental hygienist

▶ Radiographs (following individual state certification guidelines)

▶ Reinforcement of oral hygiene instruction

▶ Chairside assistance during dental hygiene treatment

▶ Cleanup/disinfection of the treatment room in preparation for the next patient.

EVIDENCE-BASED SELECTION OF DENTAL HYGIENE INTERVENTIONS

▶ Dental hygiene interventions are planned using scientific evidence of efficacy and efficiency.

▶ Selecting interventions based on evidence from the professional literature can improve opportunities for achieving successful outcomes from dental hygiene treatment.

▶ The patient can benefit when the dental hygienist has developed skills in accessing and evaluating the scientific literature.

THE WRITTEN DENTAL HYGIENE CARE PLAN

Chapter 25 outlines specific procedures for preparation and documentation of a formal written dental hygiene care plan.

DOCUMENTATION

▶ All assessment findings are documented before developing a formal written, care plan.

▶ When patient records are not computerized, all entries are recorded in ink.

▶ All entries are dated and signed by the dental hygiene clinician.

▶ Standardized abbreviations, such as those found in Appendix VIII, are used to document all information; misunderstandings can lead to legal involvement.

▶ A suggested format for documenting a formal, written dental hygiene care plan is found in Chapter 25 (Figure 25-1).

▶ Example documentation for an assessment appointment prior to development of a dental hygiene care plan is found in Box 24-3.

BOX 24-3

Example Documentation: Assessment Before Developing a Dental Hygiene Care Plan

S –A 35-year-old Asian female patient presents for initial new patient visit. Patient states no dental concerns.

O –Completed assessment data collected and documented, including vital signs, medical, social and dental histories, intraoral and extraoral examination findings, and dental radiographs, in preparation for developing a formal written dental hygiene care plan. All findings documented on the appropriate assessment forms.

A –Analysis of assessment findings and risk factors will be prepared prior to development of a final care plan.

P –Briefly discussed assessment findings and their relevance to the care plan that will be prepared. Told patient the dentist and dental hygienist together would complete both a comprehensive dental hygiene care plan and dental treatment plan. Explained that the plan would take into consideration all of the examination findings and assessment of risk factors for oral disease that were identified during this assessment appointment. Patient had no questions at this point. Appointment scheduled in two weeks.

Next steps: completed plan for both dental and dental hygiene treatment will be presented to patient at next appointment, scheduled in 2 weeks.

Signed _____, RDH

Date _____.

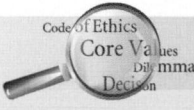

EVERYDAY ETHICS

Victoria, the dental hygienist, is discussing the assessment findings for her patient, Mr. Rush, with the rest of the dental team. Mr. Rush has stated that he has already been told at his general dental practice that he has extensive active periodontal disease. He was referred to this practice because he wants all of the most compromised teeth extracted and dental implants placed.

Mr. Rush has a number of risk factors, including poorly controlled diabetes and smoking. Because his dental insurance is running out in 3 months, everyone is in a hurry to get the treatment started, and the potential for a poor prognosis has not been discussed. In fact, Victoria's concerns about the patient's risk factors are being pushed aside.

Question for Consideration

1. Is this an ethical issue or an ethical dilemma?

2. What is Victoria's obligation (duty) to make sure that Mr. Rush understands how his risk factors compromise the prognosis of his treatment plan? What action can Victoria take if her concerns continue to be ignored and treatment progresses without interventions that address the risk factors involved in Mr. Rush's case?

3. How can Victoria proceed to obtain informed consent from Mr. Rush and ensure that his rights to optimal care are maintained?

Factors To Teach The Patient

▷ A clear explanation of how assessment data are used in planning dental hygiene care.

▷ The importance of using scientific evidence of success in the selection of patient-specific therapeutic and preventive interventions.

▷ Why disease control measures are learned before and in conjunction with scaling.

▷ Facts of oral disease prevention and oral health promotion relevant to the patient's current level of healthcare knowledge and individual risk factors.

▷ The long-term positive effects of comprehensive continuing care.

References

1. Newsome P, Smales R, Yip K. Oral diagnosis and treatment planning, Part 1: introduction. *Br Dent J.* 2012;213(1):15–19.

2. National Institute of Dental and Craniofacial Research. Periodontal (gum) disease: cause, symptoms, and treatment. http://www.nidcr.nih.gov/OralHealth/Topics/GumDiseases/PeriodontalGumDisease.htm#riskFactors. Accessed January 21, 2015.

3. Tatakis DN, Kumar PS. Etiology and pathogenesis of periodontal diseases. *Dent Clin North Am.* 2005;49(3):491–516.

4. Schifferle RE. Nutrition and periodontal disease. *Dent Clin North Am.* 2005;49(3):595–610.

5. Matthews DC, Tabesh M. Detection of localized tooth-related factors that predispose to periodontal infections. *Periodontol 2000.* 2004;34:136–150.

6. Chrysanthakopoulos NA, Chrysanthakopoulos PA. Association between indices of clinically-defined periodontitis and self-reported history of systemic medical conditions. *J Investig Clin Dent.* 2014. http://onlinelibrary.wiley.com/doi/10.1111/jicd.12119/pdf. Accessed May 20, 2015.

7. Linden GJ, Lyons A, Scannapieco FA. Periodontal systemic associations: review of the evidence. *J Clin Periodontol.* 2013;40 (Suppl 14):S8–S19.

8. Ahmed U, Tanwir F. Association of periodontal pathogenesis and cardiovascular diseases: a literature review. *Oral Health Prev Dent.* 2015;13(1):21–27.

9. Usin MM, Menso J, Rodríguez VI, et al. Association between maternal periodontitis and preterm and/or low birth weight infants in normal pregnancies. *J Matern Fetal Neonatal Med.* 2014. http://informahealthcare.com/doi/full/10.3109/14767058.2014.987751. Accessed May 20, 2015.

10. Ha JE, Jun JK, Ko HJ, et al. Association between periodontitis and preeclampsia in never-smokers: a prospective study. *J Clin Periodontol.* 2014;41(9):869–874.

11. Pereira FM, Rodrigues VP, de Oliveira AE, et al. Association between periodontal changes and osteoporosis in postmenopausal women. *Climacteric.* 2015;18:311–315.

12. Hurlbutt M, Young DA. A best practices approach to caries management. *J Evid Based Dent Pract.* 2014;14 (Suppl):77–86.

13. Kutsch VK. Dental caries: an updated medical model of risk assessment. *J Prosthet Dent.* 2014;111(4):280–285.

14. Yip K, Smales R. Oral diagnosis and treatment planning, Part 2: dental caries and assessment of risk. *Br Dent J.* 2012;213(2):59–66.

15. Jenson L, Budnez AW, Featherstone JD, et al. Clinical protocols for caries management by risk assessment. *J Calif Dent Assoc.* 2007;35(10):714–723.

16. Ram H, Sarkar J, Kumar H, et al. Oral cancer: risk factors and molecular pathogenesis. *J Maxillofac Oral Surg.* 2011;10(2):132–137.

17. Mayo Clinic. Mouth cancer: risk factors. http://www.mayoclinic.org/diseases-conditions/mouth-cancer/basics/risk-factors/CON-20026516. Accessed January 21, 2015.

18. American Society of Anesthesiologists. ASA physical status classification system. http://www.asahq.org/resources/clinical-information/asa-physical-status-classification-system. Accessed January 21, 2015.

19. Ship JA, Mohammed AR, eds. The Clinician's Guide to Oral Health in Geriatric Patients. Baltimore, MD: American Academy of Oral Medicine; 1999.

20. Corbet EF. Oral diagnosis and treatment planning, Part 3: periodontal disease and assessment of risk. *Br Dent J.* 2012;213(3):111–121.

21. American Academy of Periodontology. Parameters of care. *J Periodontol.* 2000;71(5, Suppl):i–ii, 847–883.

22. Yip K, Smales R. Oral diagnosis and treatment planning, Part 5: preventive and treatment planning for dental caries. *Br Dent J.* 2012;213(5):211–220.

23. Gurenlian JR. Recording the dental hygiene diagnosis. *Access.* 1994;8:15.

24. Darby ML, Walsh MM. Application of the human needs conceptual model to dental hygiene practice. *J Dent Hyg.* 2000;74(3):230–237.

25. Mueller-Joseph L, Petersen M. Dental Hygiene Process: Diagnosis and Care Planning. Albany, NY: Delmar; 1995.

26. Williams KB, Gadbury-Amyot CC, Bray KK, et al. Oral health-related quality of life: a model for dental hygiene. *J Dent Hyg.* 1998;72(2):19–26.

27. Keselyak NT, Gadbury-Amyot CC. Application of an oral health-related quality of life model to the dental hygiene curriculum. *J Dent Educ.* 2001;65(3):253–261.

28. Gupta G, Mitra D, Ashok KP, et al. Efficacy of preprocedural mouth rinsing in reducing aerosol contamination produced by ultrasonic scaler: a pilot study. *J Periodontol.* 2014;85(4):562–568.

29. Shetty SK, Sharath K, Shenoy S, et al. Compare the efficacy of two commercially available mouthrinses in reducing viable bacterial count in dental aerosol produced during ultrasonic scaling when used as a preprocedural rinse. *J Contemp Dent Pract.* 2013;14(5):848–851.

ENHANCE YOUR UNDERSTANDING

thePoint° DIGITAL CONNECTIONS
(see the inside front cover for access information)
- Audio glossary
- Quiz bank

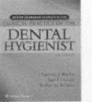

SUPPORT FOR LEARNING
(available separately; visit lww.com)
- *Active Learning Workbook for Clinical Practice of the Dental Hygienist, 12th Edition*

prepU INDIVIDUALIZED REVIEW
(available separately; visit lww.com)
- Adaptive quizzing with *prepU for Wilkins' Clinical Practice of the Dental Hygienist*

The Dental Hygiene Care Plan

Charlotte J. Wyche, RDH, MS

CHAPTER OUTLINE

LEARNING OBJECTIVES

After studying this chapter, the student will be able to:

1. Identify and define key terms and concepts related to the written dental hygiene care plan.

2. Identify the components of a dental hygiene care plan.

3. Write dental hygiene diagnostic statements based on assessment findings.

4. Prepare a written dental hygiene care plan.

5. Apply procedures for discussing a care plan with the dentist and the patient.

6. Identify and apply procedures for obtaining informed consent.

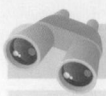

BOX 25-1   KEY WORDS: Planning Dental Hygiene Care

Consent: voluntary agreement to an action proposed by another.

Informed consent: a patient's voluntary agreement to a treatment plan after details of the proposed treatment have been presented and comprehended by the patient.

Informed refusal: a patient's decision to refuse recommended treatment after all options, potential risks, and potential benefits have been thoroughly explained.

Intervention: to happen or take place between other events; to intervene, as with a specific treatment.

Prioritize: to arrange in order of importance.

Sequence: a continuous or related series of things (such as dental hygiene interventions) following in a certain order or succession.

Total treatment plan: sequential outline of the essential services and procedures that are carried out by the dentist, the dental hygienist, and the patient to eliminate disease and restore the oral cavity to health and normal function.

Dental hygiene care plan: the services within the framework of the total treatment plan to be carried out by the dental hygienist.

PREPARATION OF A DENTAL HYGIENE CARE PLAN

▶ A formal written dental hygiene care plan is an essential part of the integrated components of the dental hygiene process of care.

▶ Terms and key words related to the dental hygiene care plan are defined in Box 25-1.

▶ Dental hygiene care is planned to address the needs of the entire oral cavity.

▶ The care plan is based on assessment of factors that influence the oral environment, including the:
  • Oral mucosa.
  • Teeth.
  • Periodontal supporting structures.
  • Patient's individual health factors.

▶ A care plan that integrates a basic three-part plan to care for all of the patient's dental hygiene needs has a major influence on the future oral health of the patient.

I. Description

The written care plan is a prioritized sequence of evidence-based dental hygiene interventions that are:

▶ Predicated on the dental hygiene diagnosis.

▶ Composed of integrated plans for the care and control of periodontal disease, dental caries control, management of risk factors, and other preventive interventions.

▶ Integrated into a total treatment plan that encompasses the patient's restorative and surgical needs, as listed in Table 25-1.

▶ Contained within the scope of dental hygiene practice as defined by each practice act.

II. Rationale

A written dental hygiene care plan will help to:

▶ Focus on individualized patient needs and risk factors when selecting dental hygiene interventions.

▶ Prioritize the sequence of planned treatment and education.

▶ Provide a checklist to ensure that all planned interventions are accomplished.

III. Objectives

A well-prepared dental hygiene care plan includes the following:

▶ Plans care for patient needs based on assessment data collected.

▶ Is flexible and realistic.

▶ Contains treatment and education goals to address problems and risk factors identified during the assessment phase.

▶ Provides interventions and recommendations based on current scientific evidence.

IV. Parts of a Care Plan

A. Periodontal/Gingival Health

▶ The primary objective of the dental hygiene plan for periodontal therapy is to restore and maintain health of the periodontal tissues.

▶ Attention is paid to interventions that can reduce:
  • Individualized risk factors for developing periodontal disease.
  • Potential complications related to associations between systemic disease and periodontal disease.

B. Dental Caries Control

▶ The plan for caries control, based on an individualized assessment of caries risk, includes:
  • A remineralization program.
  • Fluorides.
  • Dental sealants.
  • Dietary control of fermentable carbohydrates.

▶ Even when the patient's caries risk level is low, the plan includes:
  • A minimum frequency of professional oral examinations to monitor risk factors.
  • Preventive recommendations such as daily use of fluoride toothpaste.

TABLE 25-1	Components of a Master Treatment Plan	
PHASE	**PROCEDURES**	**INCLUDED IN THE DENTAL HYGIENE CARE PLAN**
Preliminary phase	■ Assessment data collection ■ Emergency care (pain, biopsy)	√
Phase I therapy	■ Dental biofilm control ■ Introduction of additional preventive measures (diet changes, fluorides, mouthguard) ■ Calculus removal ■ Correction of restorative and prosthetic irritants (biofilm traps, overhangs) ■ Restorative caries control	√ √ √
Outcomes evaluation of phase I	■ Probing depths ■ Clinical signs of inflammation ■ Dental biofilm control ■ Patient's participation	√ √ √ √
Phase II surgical	■ Periodontal ■ Endodontic ■ Implant placement	
Phase III restorative	■ Final restorations ■ Fixed/removable prostheses	
Evaluation of overall outcomes	■ Periodontal response to restorations/implants ■ Other response to restorations	√
Phase IV maintenance	■ Appointments for continuing care and supervision ■ Refining biofilm control techniques	√ √

C. Other

A plan for preventive care starts with the patient's personal daily oral biofilm control.

Additional interventions in an individual care plan can include:

▸ Interventions to eliminate modifiable risk factors for oral disease, such as tobacco cessation counseling.
▸ Desensitizing exposed dentin.
▸ Resolving halitosis.
▸ And much, much more.

COMPONENTS OF A WRITTEN CARE PLAN

▸ A dental hygiene care plan may be written using a variety of formats.
▸ Software for electronic, computerized patient records includes a treatment plan function that can be used to develop a dental hygiene care plan.
▸ Figure 25-1 is a suggested template for a patient-specific care plan that follows the dental hygiene process of care.

▸ The recommended components of a written care plan are described in this section.

I. Demographic Data

▸ Patient name, date of birth (age), and gender.
▸ A designation of initial or maintenance therapy.
▸ The name of the student or clinician who prepared the written plan.
▸ The date the written plan was prepared.
▸ Notation of the patient's chief complaint or statement indicating the patient's reason for presenting for treatment.

II. Assessment Findings and Risk Factors

This section of the plan contains a thorough, summarized description of significant findings.

A. Medical History

▸ Systemic diseases and conditions: current and past
▸ Medications
▸ Overall health status
▸ Functional assessment

Patient Specific Dental Hygiene Care Plan

Patient name _____ Age ____ Gender: M ☐ F ☐   Initial therapy ☐

Provider name _____ Date _____   Maintenance ☐

Chief complaint: Re-evaluation ☐

Assessment Findings

Medical history	At Risk For
Systemic disease	
Other conditions	
Medications	
ASA classification	
ADL/IADL level	
Social and dental history	
Treatment history	
Dental knowledge	
Health behaviors	
Cultural factors	
Dental examination	
Extraoral examination	
Intraoral examination	
Teeth/restorations	
Periodontal examination	

Periodontal Diagnosis and Status:	Caries Management Risk Assessment (CAMBRA) level: Low ☐ Moderate ☐ High ☐ Extreme ☐

Dental Hygiene Diagnosis

Problem	Related to (Risk Factors and Etiology)
Extraoral	
Intraoral	
Restorative/caries risk	
Periodontal status or risk	
Systemic health	
Self-care ability	

FIGURE 25-1 **Patient-Specific Dental Hygiene Care Plan.** The written care plan includes a summary of assessment findings, the dental hygiene diagnosis, planned dental hygiene interventions, expected outcomes, and an appointment plan that sequences treatment procedures and education interventions for each appointment. (Modified from a care plan model, based on the *Dental Hygiene Process of Care*, that was originally provided by Dr. Laura Mueller-Joseph.)

Planned Interventions
(to arrest or control disease and regenerate, restore or maintain health)

Clinical	Education/Counseling	Oral Hygiene Instruction/Home Care

Expected Outcomes

Goals	Evaluation Methods	Time Frame
1		
2		
3		
4		

Appointment Plan
(sequence of planned interventions)

Appt #	Plan for Treatment and Services		Plan for Education, Counseling and Oral Hygiene Instruction
		Quadrant	
1			
2			
3			
4			

Re-evaluation Findings

Re-treat ☐   Refer ☐   Continuing care interval _____

Description of post-treatment outcomes:

FIGURE 25-1 (*continued*)

B. Social and Dental History

▶ Treatment history

▶ Oral health knowledge and behaviors

▶ Cultural factors

C. Clinical Examination

▶ Extraoral and intraoral

▶ Soft and hard tissue

D. Link to Risk Factors

▶ Risk for increased oral disease

▶ Increased risk of systemic disease due to oral infection

▶ Potential for compromised treatment outcomes

III. Periodontal Diagnosis and Status

▶ The periodontal diagnosis formulated in collaboration with the dentist is included in the dental hygiene care plan.

▶ Guidelines for noting the periodontal diagnosis and parameters of care, useful for planning dental hygiene treatment interventions, are found in Chapter 24 and in Table 24-4.

IV. Caries Risk Status

▶ A caries risk assessment tool (CAMBRA) that provides guidelines for identifying caries risk status and selecting dental hygiene interventions based on risk factor assessment, is detailed in Table 27-1 for adult patients and for children 0–5 years old in Table 50-6.

▶ Understanding of a patient's individualized risks for dental caries can guide the plan for:

• Oral health education and counseling

• Selection of treatment interventions, such as dental sealants or fluoride recommendations to enhance remineralization.

V. Diagnostic Statements

Table 25-2 contains examples of dental hygiene diagnostic statements that:

▶ Link observed or potential oral health problems identified during the patient assessment to probable etiology or risk factors.

▶ Relate to problems and solutions that can be addressed within the dental hygiene scope of practice.

VI. Planned Interventions

Dental hygiene interventions are measures applied to regenerate, restore, or maintain oral health are specific to the individual patient's assessment findings and include:

▶ Clinical treatments, such as scaling, root planing, and debridement, selected for the purpose of arresting or controlling existing disease.

▶ Preventive measures, such as dental sealants, that maintain tooth integrity.

▶ Education and counseling in such topics as etiology and progression of oral disease and elimination of risk factors.

▶ Individualized oral hygiene instructions and personal daily oral care regimens based on patient needs and abilities.

VII. Expected Outcomes

A plan for treatment or personal oral care outcomes, created in consultation with the patient, contains:

▶ At least one goal for each oral health problem identified in the dental hygiene diagnosis.

▶ A realistic time frame for measuring success.

VIII. Evaluation Methods

▶ Evaluation of clinical outcomes is discussed more completely in Chapter 47.

TABLE 25-2	Examples of Dental Hygiene Diagnostic Statements
PROBLEM	**RISK FACTORS AND ETIOLOGY**
Hypersensitivity	**Related to:** Exposed cementum/gingival recession
Gingival bleeding	**Related to:** Biofilm accumulation causing inflammation
Increased caries risk (CAMBRA level = extreme)	**Related to:** Previous history of dental caries and consumption of sugar-sweetened beverages frequently throughout each day
Biofilm control record score = fair to poor score	**Related to:** Limited ability to perform oral self-care tasks (activities of daily living level 3)

▶ Evaluation methods identified in the dental hygiene care plan:
  • Include assessment data collection and comparison with initial assessment findings.
  • Clearly identify how progress toward each goal will be measured.
▶ An example of an evaluation method that could be identified in the written care plan is the use of periodontal probing to determine reduction in pocket depths.

IX. The Appointment Plan

An appointment plan for multiple appointments:
▶ Outlines interventions sequenced in order of clinical performance.
▶ Can be adapted at each appointment to respond to new information or an immediate need of the patient.
▶ Properly prioritized and sequenced treatment and education interventions will be:
  • More comfortable for the patient.
  • More effective in reaching planned oral health goals.

X. Re-evaluation

At the re-evaluation appointment:
▶ New assessment data are collected and analyzed.
▶ A determination is made regarding whether expected outcomes of the care plan have been met.
▶ Continuing care appointment interval is determined.

SEQUENCING AND PRIORITIZING PATIENT CARE

I. Objectives

Reasons for preparing a well-sequenced dental hygiene care plan are:

A. To Provide Evidence-Based, Individualized Patient Care

▶ Determined by analysis of assessment data.
▶ Based on documented evidence of success.
▶ Enhanced by the clinician's ability to assess the value of information available in the scientific literature.

B. To Eliminate or Control Etiologic and Predisposing Disease Factors

▶ The principal etiologic agents in both dental caries and periodontal and gingival diseases are the microorganisms of dental biofilm.
▶ Dental hygiene interventions can modify a variety of risk factors that predispose the patient to oral disease.

C. To Eliminate the Signs and Symptoms of Disease

Measures to eliminate signs of infection such as gingival bleeding and probing depths are included in the care plan.

D. To Promote Oral Health and Prevent Recurrence of Disease

Methods used to achieve optimum oral health include:
▶ Education on the etiology of oral disease.
▶ Counseling on prevention measures and elimination of risk factors.
▶ Instruction and supervision in daily self-care techniques.
▶ Encouragement of regularly scheduled maintenance follow-up for dental hygiene care.

II. Factors Affecting Sequence of Care

Treatment sequence defines the order in which the parts of an individual appointment are to be carried out. Sequence planning involves:
▶ Identification of overall treatment and education patterns appropriate for an individual patient's needs.
▶ Outline of a series of appointments, with specific services, treatment procedures, and educational interventions included.

The sequence of care for an individual patient is determined by numerous factors.

A. Urgency

Discomfort or pain that requires first attention could apply to:
▶ An area of the gingiva that is particularly difficult to clean because of inaccessibility.
▶ An area with a periodontal abscess or with necrotizing ulcerative gingivitis (NUG).

B. Existing Etiologic Factors

In patients with gingival or periodontal infection or risk for dental caries, success of the treatment depends on thorough, daily biofilm removal. Biofilm control measures are introduced and success is evaluated before additional dental hygiene interventions will be effective.

C. Severity and Extent of the Condition

The number and length of appointments and the sequencing of procedures planned are affected by the severity of the condition. Findings that indicate the severity of gingival or periodontal infection include:
▶ Changes in color, size, shape, or consistency of the gingiva.
▶ Probing depths.
▶ Bleeding on probing.
▶ Mobility of the teeth.

▶ Clinical and radiographic signs of attachment or bone loss.

D. Individual Patient Requirements

Items from a particular patient's history that may require adaptation in appointment length, spacing, or sequencing when planning dental hygiene care include:

▶ Antibiotic premedication
  - Current recommended standard prophylactic regimens and a list of conditions that require antibiotic premedication are found in Chapter 10.
  - Because bacteremia can occur, initial instruction and practice of biofilm-removing procedures are carried out while the patient is premedicated.
  - Efficient use of appointment time and/or spacing of appointment dates will avoid unnecessary extra antibiotic coverage.

▶ Systemic diseases
  - Chronic disease will influence the content and length of appointments.
  - The associations between periodontitis and systemic conditions influence patient counseling.

▶ Physical disability
  - Physical limitations, such as those described in Chapter 59, will require adaptation of the appointment plan.

▶ Other considerations
  - An outline for continuing care appointments can be found in Chapter 48.
  - A treatment sequence for a patient with NUG is found in the Necrotizing Periodontal Diseases section of Chapter 42.
  - A suggested approach for motivating patient health behavior change is found in Chapter 26.

PRESENTING THE DENTAL HYGIENE CARE PLAN

Before treatment is begun, the care plan is discussed with the dentist and explained to the patient.

I. Presenting the Plan to the Dentist

A. Purpose

▶ To integrate the dental hygiene care plan into the patient's total treatment plan.
▶ To provide a coordinated dental and dental hygiene statement to the patient regarding oral health needs.

B. Procedure

▶ Follow sequence on the patient's written care plan.
▶ Summarize demographic data.
▶ Summarize major systemic and dental health assessment findings.

▶ Summarize risk factors.
▶ Indicate planned intervention strategies, goals, and expected outcomes.
▶ Outline planned appointment sequence and services to be provided.
▶ Be prepared to give detail and answer questions.

II. Explaining the Plan to the Patient

▶ A clinician with good verbal communication skills and the ability to build a trusting relationship can influence patient acceptance of treatment needs and compliance with recommendations.[1]
▶ Use of an intraoral camera during presentation of the plan for care provides visual documentation of need for oral health interventions.
▶ Using a motivational interviewing approach (Chapter 26) while discussing the plan can help determine and respond to the patient's readiness to change health behaviors that increase risk for oral disease.

A. Purpose

▶ To provide the patient with information needed to give informed consent for treatment.
▶ To reinforce the patient's role in setting and reaching oral health goals outlined in the plan.

B. Procedure

▶ Position the patient in an upright position, face to face with clinician.
▶ Use terminology that is appropriate to the patient's level of understanding.
▶ Educate the patient regarding systemic and dental health assessment findings and their link to oral disease.
▶ Educate the patient regarding planned interventions, appointment sequence, dental hygiene services, and expected outcomes.
▶ Present information using visual aids such as the patient's own radiographs, dental models, drawings or pictures, videotapes, brochures, or an intraoral camera.
▶ Engage the patient in planning and setting goals.
▶ Be prepared to give detail and answer questions.
▶ Obtained signed informed consent.

INFORMED CONSENT

▶ It is every patient's right to possess knowledge that will:
  - Aid the patient in making optimal decisions.
  - Allow shared decision making with the oral care provider while treatment is being planned.
▶ Adequate documentation of informed consent in the patient's record includes evidence that the patient has received the information listed in Box 25-2.[2]

Box 25-2

Criteria for Adequate Content in Informed Consent

▷ Complete description of the procedure including:
  ▷ Rationale for treatment
  ▷ Duration of treatment and
  ▷ Effects of patient's current medical status on treatment.
▷ Risks and limitations of the proposed treatment including probability of risk occurring.
▷ Benefits of the treatment including prognosis.
▷ Alternative treatments available including no treatment and the consequences of no treatment.
▷ Purpose of treatment.
▷ Demonstration of the opportunity to ask questions.
▷ Permission to deliberate if needed.
▷ Demonstration of consent (patient signature).

Glick A, Taylor D, Valenza JA, et al. Assessing the content, presentation, and readability of dental informed consents. *J Dent Educ.* 2010;74(8):849–861.

BOX 25-3

Informed Consent

Information to Disclose

▷ *Diagnosis*: description of patient's problem(s)
▷ *Treatment*: nature and rationale for the proposed treatment(s)
▷ *Alternatives*: viable alternatives to the proposed treatment(s)
▷ *Consequences*: risks and benefits of all proposed treatment alternatives, including physical and psychological effects, costs, and potential resulting problems
▷ *Prognosis*: expected outcome with treatment(s), with alternative treatment(s), and without treatment

Principles of Informing

▷ Assess the patient's ability to give informed consent.
▷ Simplify the terminology so that the patient can understand.
▷ Encourage the patient and family to ask questions.
▷ Continue to assess the patient's understanding and re-educate as often as necessary.
▷ Document all relevant factors and include the signed form in patient record.

▶ Informed consent is a legal concept that can exist even without a written document.

▶ Informed consent can be lacking even when a document has been signed if the patient has not had the opportunity to comprehend and evaluate the risks and benefits of the suggested treatment.

▶ "Implied consent," granted by the patient's presence in the dental chair, only applies to nontreatment procedures, such as data collection, and treatment planning.

I. Informed Consent Procedures

▶ Box 25-3 provides information for obtaining informed consent.

▶ The patient is informed of all treatment options available and consents to follow the recommendations in the agreed-upon care plan.

▶ Patients do not always remember the information they received during informed consent; therefore, written documentation of all information provided for the patient is essential.[3]

▶ When potential risks, complications, or failure are associated with therapy, it is necessary to obtain consent in writing prior to beginning treatment.

▶ Informed consent includes recommendations for referral to other healthcare providers as necessary.[4]

▶ If necessary, use forms written in simpler terms, larger print, or the patient's primary language.

▶ Create a duplicate copy for the patient to take home.

EVERYDAY ETHICS

Ellen is responsible for explaining two alternative treatment plans to Mrs. Kwan, who is new to the practice. Mrs. Kwan needs to decide between several extractions, which would require crown and bridge or implant replacement, or the treatment of periodontally involved teeth with poor prognosis. The decision must be made today if she is to begin treatment early next week, when there are several open appointments available.

English is not Mrs. Kwan's first language, and no one in the practice speaks her language. Ellen has explained the information carefully, using pictures and patient-appropriate words, and she has gone over both treatment alternatives several times. When Ellen asks Mrs. Kwan to summarize her understanding of the care plan she just nods her head, smiles, and says, "I'll sign whatever you say."

Questions for Consideration

1. Does it appear that Mrs. Kwan understands her treatment alternatives and is informed sufficiently to give consent? What alternatives can Ellen consider so that informed consent is ensured?

2. Does Ellen have an ethical responsibility, as the knowledgeable professional, to select the choice of treatments as Mrs. Kwan requests? Why or why not?

3. In what ways does the pressure of making a timely decision reflect an inappropriate approach to meeting Mrs. Kwan's needs?

II. Informed Refusal

The patient's right to autonomy in making decisions regarding oral treatment requires that practitioners respect a patient's decision to refuse treatment.[5] Refusal of care as well as any recommended treatment options are documented in the patient's permanent record. Depending on the state practice act, this may or may not protect clinicians who provide treatment that does not meet the standard of care from legal action.

III. Additional Considerations

▶ Cultural differences of individual patients require special effort to obtain informed consent. Careful exploration of language skills, and potentially conflicting health beliefs and values can enhance communication.[6,7]

▶ Age or disability-related cognitive impairment may require consultation with a caregiver or legal guardian as well as the patient.[8]

DOCUMENTATION

▶ A written dental hygiene care plan documents all information related to each component of the formal plan as described in this chapter and illustrated in Figure 25-1.

▶ Example documentation for a patient appointment to explain the dental hygiene care plan and obtain informed consent is found in Box 25-4.

BOX 25-4

Example Documentation: Presentation of Care Plan and Informed Consent for Dental Hygiene Care

S –A 35-year-old female patient presents 2 weeks following assessment data collection appointment. Patient expects to discuss the formal written dental hygiene care plan related to periodontal therapy and quadrant scaling and root planing.

O –No changes in patient's health history or other relevant assessment findings since previous appointment for data collection. Written care plan and treatment plan completed and available.

A –Patient appeared engaged in the discussion and eager to begin treatment.

P –Explained all assessment findings and risk factors, discussed dental hygiene diagnosis statement, planned interventions, and expected outcomes of treatment. Responded to numerous questions related to the rationale for scheduling multiple treatment appointments. Patient stated that all questions had been answered, then signed/dated the informed consent form. Copy of signed care plan was given to patient and a copy was placed in the patient record.

Next step: Begin treatment as described for appointment #1 on the care plan form.

Signed _____, RDH

Date _____

Factors To Teach The Patient

▷ Why a dental hygiene care plan is made.
▷ Why patient input into the final care plan is important.
▷ Which parts of the plan are to be carried out by the patient.
▷ How the roles of patient and members of the dental team are interrelated in eliminating the patient's oral problems.
▷ The patient's rights and responsibilities regarding informed consent.

References

1. Goldie G. Enhance verbal skills to get patients to accept what they need. *Contemp Oral Hyg.* 2002;2:14.

2. Glick A, Taylor D, Valenza JA, et al. Assessing the content, presentation, and readability of dental informed consents. *J Dent Educ.* 2010;74(8):849–861.

3. Ferrús-Torres E, Valmaseda-Castellón E, Berini-Aytés L, et al. Informed consent in oral surgery: the value of written information. *J Oral Maxillofac Surg.* 2011;69(1):54–58.

4. Greenwell H; Committee on Research, Science, and Therapy, and The American Academy of Periodontology. Position paper: guidelines for periodontal therapy. *J Periodontol.* 2001;72(11):1624–1628.

5. Greco PM. Informed consent or informed refusal? *Am J Orthod Dentofacial Orthop.* 2013;143(5):598.

6. Chettih M. Turning the lens inward: cultural competence and providers' values in health care decision making. *Gerontologist.* 2012;52(6):739–747.

7. Fitch P. Cultural competence and dental hygiene care delivery: integrating cultural care into the dental hygiene process of care. *J Dent Hyg.* 2004;78(1):11–21.

8. Conti A, Delbon P, Laffranchi L, et al. Consent in dentistry: ethical and deontological issues. *J Med Ethics.* 2013;39(1): 59–61.

ENHANCE YOUR UNDERSTANDING

the Point® DIGITAL CONNECTIONS
(see the inside front cover for access information)
• **Audio glossary**
• **Quiz bank**

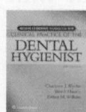

SUPPORT FOR LEARNING
(available separately; visit lww.com)
• *Active Learning Workbook for Clinical Practice of the Dental Hygienist, 12th Edition*

prepU INDIVIDUALIZED REVIEW
(available separately; visit lww.com)
• **Adaptive quizzing with *prepU* for Wilkins'** *Clinical Practice of the Dental Hygienist*

SECTION

VI

Implementation: Prevention

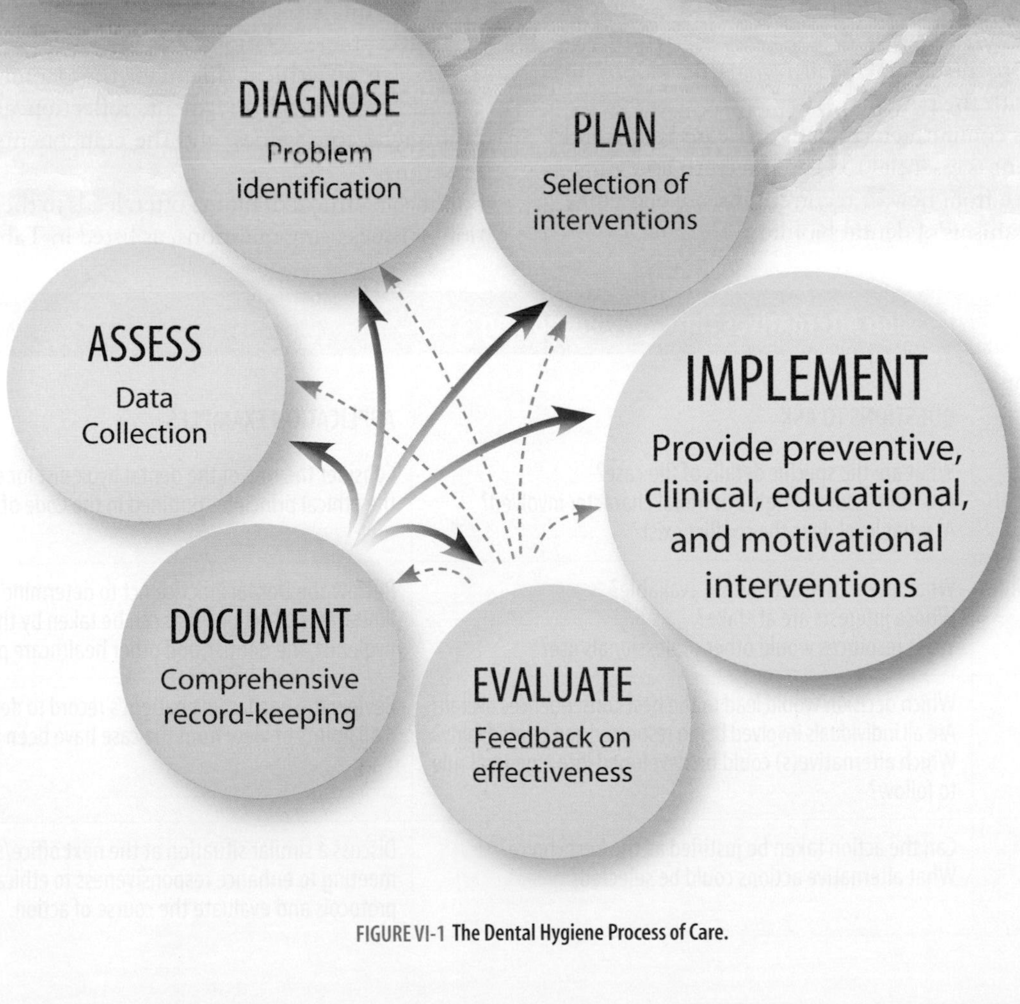

DIAGNOSE
Problem identification
PLAN
Selection of interventions
ASSESS
Data Collection
IMPLEMENT
Provide preventive, clinical, educational, and motivational interventions
DOCUMENT
Comprehensive record-keeping
EVALUATE
Feedback on effectiveness

FIGURE VI-1 The Dental Hygiene Process of Care.

INTRODUCTION FOR SECTION VI

The aim of health promotion and disease prevention is to help each patient accept responsibility for lifelong health practices and daily oral self-care regimens that prevent oral disease.

▶ Implementation of the prevention care plan is a significant component of both the dental hygiene care plan and the total treatment plan.

▶ The influence of oral health on total body health may be a new concept for many patients.

▶ In the sequence of patient treatment, introduction to preventive measures occurs first, before treatment interventions are implemented.

THE DENTAL HYGIENE PROCESS OF CARE

▶ The implementation phase of the Dental Hygiene Process of Care, illustrated in **Figure VI-1**, is about providing the dental hygiene interventions identified in a patient's dental hygiene care plan.

▶ Dental hygiene patient education and counseling interventions are:

  • The basis for oral health promotion and disease prevention.

  • Selected using individualized patient assessment data.

  • Designed to meet oral health goals developed in concert with the patient.

▶ The patient's commitment to daily self-care before and after treatment is essential to keep the teeth and gingival tissues free from new or recurrent disease caused by the microorganisms of dental biofilm.

▶ The dental hygienist has the responsibility to:

  • Consider each patient's current oral health practices, cultural factors, physical abilities, and life circumstances when implementing the preventive care plan.

  • Implement dental hygiene interventions for each patient that attain and maintain oral health and contribute to systemic health.

  • Educate about oral disease and prevention modalities based on individualized patient needs.

  • Identify an approach that will motivate each patient to accept and adhere to recommended preventive procedures and self-care protocols.

ETHICAL APPLICATIONS

▶ When complex ethical issues and dilemmas arise in the dental setting, the ethically competent dental hygienist can:

  • Understand how the patient feels.

  • View a concern from various perspectives.

  • Determine who is responsible.

  • Document and share clear, concise, and objective evidence.

  • Communicate clearly with all parties involved in the situation.

  • Act within acceptable moral standards to determine an acceptable decision.

▶ To resolve an ethical dilemma, the dental hygienist can use professional judgment, reflection about dental hygiene core values, and the components of moral reasoning.

▶ Solving an ethical dilemma often leads to the examination of issues using questions, as listed in **Table VI-1**.

TABLE VI-1	Decision Alternatives Through Questioning	
ETHICAL DECISION CONCEPT	**QUESTIONS TO ASK**	**APPLICATION EXAMPLES**
Recognize conflict	What are the specific details of the case? Are there issues of rights or moral character involved? At what level does the conflict exist?	Consider the role of the dental hygienist for each of the ethical principles outlined in the Code of Ethics.
Accumulate possible options	What alternative actions are available? Whose interests are at stake? What resources would other professionals use?	Review the Dental Practice Act to determine limitations of actions that can be taken by the dental hygienist, the dentist, and other healthcare providers.
Evaluate the alternatives	Which decision would lead to the best consequences overall? Are all individuals involved being respected and treated fairly? Which alternative(s) could be developed into a general rule to follow?	Review the entries in a patient's record to determine if all points of view from the case have been included.
Reflect on the decision	Can the action taken be justified as the best choice? What alternative actions could be selected?	Discuss a similar situation at the next office/staff meeting to enhance responsiveness to ethical protocols and evaluate the course of action.

26

Preventive Counseling and Behavior Change

Marsha A. Voelker, CDA, RDH, MS

LEARNING OBJECTIVES

After studying this chapter, the student will be able to:

1. Explain the steps in a preventive program, identify the need to conduct preventive counseling and describe the proper setting.

2. Describe the importance of partnering with the patient to come up with a plan for change.

3. Describe and explain the methods of motivational interviewing (MI).

4. Describe how to recognize and explore the patient's ambivalence and describe techniques to elicit and recognize change talk.

5. Understand and explain various plans to strengthen the patient's commitment for change.

The dental hygienist is a primary care provider of preventive services. A specialist in oral health care, the dental hygienist is involved at all levels of prevention.

▶ Within the process of dental hygiene care, the needs of a patient are assessed from the histories and clinical findings. Then a dental hygiene diagnosis is made, and the care plan is outlined.

▶ When planning the sequence of treatment for the patient, initiation of preventive measures precedes clinical services except in an emergency.

▶ Oral health can only be attained and maintained if the patient learns and practices proper daily self-care.

▶ Box 26-1 defines key terms related to health promotion and disease prevention for the individual patient.

STEPS IN A PREVENTIVE PROGRAM

Each patient needs a preventive care plan. To plan and carry out a program takes a collaborative effort by the patient and members of the dental team.

I. Assess the Patient's Needs

▶ Review all information from the histories, radiographic data, clinical examinations, and chartings.

▶ Identify the presence and severity of infection and the risk factors for systemic and oral disease.

▶ Utilize indices to rate the extent of the need and provide a baseline for continuing comparisons.

▶ For most patients, a dental biofilm score can be helpful to show the patient the extent of bacterial accumulation.

▶ A discussion of caries and periodontal risk factors will illustrate the dental concerns to the patient.

▶ The patient's use of oral aids (toothbrushing, flossing, interproximal aids) are assessed for proper technique.

▶ Factors to consider during assessment:
  • Explore what will work for the patient to make needed changes.
  • Determine the patient's motivation and confidence to make changes.
  • Consider what the patient values. The cultural values and beliefs can either promote or block the patient's efforts to make an oral health change.

II. Plan for Interventions

▶ Apply information about the patient, such as educational level, occupation, socioeconomic background, cultural influences, and attitudes regarding oral care.

▶ Determine the current personal oral care procedures carried out by the patient and the frequency.

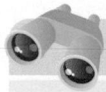

BOX 26-1   **KEY WORDS:** Health Promotion and Disease Prevention

Affirmation: to validate or confirm; commending a patient's efforts toward change.

Ambivalence: simultaneous conflict or uncertainty toward making a change.

Autonomy: individual's right to make their own decisions.

Behavior: manner in which an individual acts or manages themselves.

Behavior change: transition in the way a patient acts or manages themselves.

Change talk: any self-expressed language that is an argument for change.

Communication: verbal or nonverbal interaction or interchange.

Communication style: attitude and approach to assisting patients, a way of talking with them that describes the clinician's relationship with the patient.

Compliance: extent to which a person's health behaviors coincide with dental/medical counseling.

Elicit: to draw forth or bring out.

Evaluation: assessment of changes in patient's behavior or oral health status.

Evocation: eliciting or drawing out from patient through open-ended questions.

Explore: to investigate.

Learning: acquiring knowledge or skills though study, instruction, or experience.

Listening: to make an attempt to hear what someone is saying.

Active listening: a listening style of maintaining focus and remaining engaged with what the patient is saying and reacting by demonstrating you are listening and have understood the patient either through reflection of the main points or summarizing what has been said.

Passive listening: listening without reacting and not being focused or engaged in what the patient is saying.

Preventive counseling: professional guidance and support to assist a patient with acting ahead regarding oral health though the utilization of MI methods.

Motivation: internal driving force that prompts an individual to act to satisfy a need or desire or to accomplish a particular goal.

Motivational interviewing (MI): is a person-centered, goal-directed method of communication for eliciting and strengthening intrinsic motivation for positive change.

MI Spirit: the underlying perspective with which one practices MI.

Noncompliance: failure to carry out a prescribed health-care plan, for example, failure to take medications as prescribed.

Sustain talk: the individuals own arguments for not changing.

▶ Note factors that may affect the patient's dexterity when using oral cleaning devices. This information is helpful when the clinician is determining the appropriate oral health aid options to provide the patient.

▶ Recognize the influence of age, physical limitations, and cognitive disabilities. Determine whether another person (parent or other caregiver) is needed to carry out the necessary procedures.

▶ Discuss procedures needed and develop goals both short- and long-term goals with the patient.

▶ Discuss with the patient the expected oral health clinical outcomes.

III. Implement the Plan

▶ Initiate preventive counseling to help the patient become aware of oral health problems. This includes learning and practicing more effective health behaviors.

▶ Explore what oral aids and preventive measures the patient utilizes daily and motivation for oral self-care.

▶ Show methods for self-evaluation.

▶ Explore the patient's diet in relation to caries risk or periodontal conditions.

▶ Introduce tobacco cessation when indicated.

▶ Change takes time and preventive counseling needs to be revisited at each appointment.

IV. Perform Clinical Preventive Services

▶ Scaling for complete calculus and biofilm removal.

▶ Application of caries-preventive agents: such as fluoride (Chapter 35) and/or dental sealants (Chapter 27).

V. Evaluate Progressive Changes

▶ Have the patient demonstrate procedures for oral self-care to determine a need for modifications in technique.

▶ Record a dental biofilm score at each appointment and compare previous recordings with the patient.

▶ At appropriate intervals, probe to note improvement in tissue quality, bleeding on probing, and probing depths.

▶ If necessary, provide preventive counseling to explore why the patient's goals have not been met.

VI. Plan Short- and Long-term Continuing Care

▶ Determine appropriate maintenance intervals.

▶ Re-evaluate to monitor continuance of preventive practices.

▶ Provide supplemental care for the patient who does not respond to basic therapy.

PATIENT COUNSELING

▶ Personalized preventive counseling contributes to the knowledge, values, and practices of the individual. Then through the individual, these ideas can be passed on to the family and the community.

▶ Periodontal infections and dental caries can be prevented or controlled, and, therefore, teeth preserved throughout the lifetime of the individual.

▶ First, attention is given to the intra- and extraoral examination to recognize possible pathology requiring exfoliative cytology and/or biopsy.

▶ For most patients, major attention is placed on prevention and control of dental caries and/or periodontal infection.

▶ Other preventive measures involving oral trauma need to be brought to the patient's attention, such as mouth protectors for contact sports and accidents that lead to children's fractured anterior teeth.

▶ Knowledge and belief in health facts are not enough. Benefits result only when a partnership between the clinician and patient is established and patient autonomy is taken into consideration.

I. When to Conduct

▶ Preventive counseling is conducted after the clinician has completed the patient assessment.

▶ When having a conversation regarding preventive strategies, clinicians need to remember the patient is the decision maker and is key to making a sustainable behavior change.

▶ Preventive counseling is provided at each appointment to follow-up on the goals, both short- and long-term, established at the previous appointment.

▶ By revisiting goals at each appointment, the clinician is aware of how the patient is progressing toward the established oral health change. An example is provided in Box 26-2.

▶ Clinicians need to recognize that health behavior changes do not happen at one preventive counseling session.

▶ Patient education may take multiple sessions before progress is made toward change. An example would be patients who are smokers, due to the addictive nature of nicotine.

II. The Setting for Preventive Counseling

▶ Usually preventive counseling will take place in the dental hygiene treatment room with the patient placed in an upright position in the dental chair.

▶ The most effective counseling approach is with the clinician sitting face-to-face with the patient in a neutral position and maintaining eye contact.

BOX 26-2

Example of Revisiting Patient Progress at Subsequent Appointments

▷ The patient's long-term goal is to floss seven days a week and short-term goal is to begin flossing at least three days a week. The patient shows up for the three-month continuing care appointment and has only begun flossing two times a week.

▷ Clinician provides affirmation about the progress the patient has made by flossing twice a week.
  ▷ The clinician elicits to explore the possible obstacles the patient may have encountered and what ideas the patient has to overcome those obstacles.
  ▷ The clinician may find out that the type of floss is breaking a lot when flossing or not getting into the embrasure space well.

▷ Therefore, the clinician will need to explore and elicit from the patient what other options may work to be successful.

▶ Face-to-face positioning style allows the patient to recognize the clinician is attentive, focused, and listening as well as builds a trusting relationship.

▶ Providing the appropriate setting for the clinician to explore the patient's ideas and thoughts toward an oral health behavior change is needed to maintain patient autonomy.

PATIENT MOTIVATION AND BEHAVIOR CHANGE

▶ Control and management of oral health conditions are dependent upon the self-care and compliance of the patient.[1]

▶ Traditionally, behavior change in the dental field has been approached in a prescriptive, authoritative manner where the clinician provides the information and shows the patient what to do.[2]

▶ However, research has concluded changes needed to prevent further disease do not happen only by providing knowledge or information to a patient.[2–7]

▶ Many health behavior change theories (Health Belief Model and Transtheoretical Model) have provided important perspectives on the factors to promote change and maintenance.

I. Health Behavior Change Model

▶ Developed in 1950s in an effort to explain unsuccessful attempt of patients to participate in programs to prevent or detect disease.[8,9]

▶ Later the model expanded to include patients' responses to symptoms and behavior response to diagnose illness and compliance with medical regimens.[8,9]

TABLE 26-1	Key Concepts of the Health Behavior Model
Perceived susceptibility	Chances of getting a condition
Perceived severity	Seriousness of the disease and the effects
Perceived benefits	Effectiveness of the recommend action to reduce risk
Perceived barriers	Tangible and psychological costs of the recommend action
Cues to action	Strategies to motivate readiness
Self-efficacy	Confidence in the ability to take action

▶ The model is utilized to explain change and maintenance of health behavior and a guiding framework for health behavior interventions.

▶ Table 26-1 provides the key concepts of the health behavior model.

II. Transtheoretical Model

▶ The transtheoretical model suggests health behavior change involves progress through six stages of change.[9–12]

▶ Table 26-2 provides the six stages of change.

III. Motivation for Health Behavior Change

▶ Different theories have identified the following as important for clinicians to understand regarding behavioral change: various signs to change, six stages

TABLE 26-2	Transtheoretical Model—The Six Stages of Change
Precontemplation	Patient not intending to take action in future
Contemplation	Patient intends to change in next 6 mos
Preparation	Patient intends to take action in immediate future
Action	Patient made modifications to life style within the past 6 mos
Maintenance	Patient working to prevent relapse
Termination	Patient have no temptation and 100% self-efficacy

of change, self-efficacy, social support, and decisional processes.[9,10]

▶ All the various theories focus attention on the need to enhance a patient's motivation toward change. Therefore, the development of an effective approach for overcoming resistance to change was established, which is Motivational Interviewing (MI).[11]

MOTIVATIONAL INTERVIEWING (MI)[13]

▶ MI and brief motivational interviewing (BMI) are person-centered, goal-directed methods of communication for eliciting and strengthening intrinsic motivation for positive change.

▶ MI has been applied successfully within many health professions. This includes tobacco cessation, diabetic control, and eating behavior control, which all impact oral health.[2,14–21]

▶ BMI[13,22] during a dental hygiene appointment assists the clinician to:
  • Effectively elicit the patient's own understanding of current oral health status and ideas about needed behavior change.
  • Avoid pushing the clinicians own ideals for behavior change onto the patient.

▶ BMI is utilized in a healthcare or dental setting when MI is conducted in a brief amount of time, such as 5–10 minutes.[2,14,15,19,22]

▶ Table 26-3 lists the basic components of the MI approach to changing a patient's health behaviors.

I. Elements of the "MI Spirit"

▶ The "spirit of MI" is how a clinician relates to the patient through communication and interactions.

▶ Four interrelated elements of the spirit of MI can be easily remembered using the acronym PACE: partnership, acceptance, compassion, and evocation.

A. Partnership[23]

▶ Establish a positive interpersonal environment that encourages change but is not intimidating.

▶ Avoid the trap of communicating based entirely on professional expertise.

▶ Understand patients as individuals and attempt to see the world from their perspective.

▶ Patients are experts on themselves; it is more effective to elicit the patient's own ideas for change than to impose personal ideals or push expertise and knowledge.

B. Acceptance[23]

▶ The spirit of MI is an attitude of acceptance of what the patient brings.

▶ However, to accept a person does not mean to approve of the patient's actions and maintaining the status quo.

▶ There are four patient-centered conditions that convey acceptance.
  1. *Absolute worth*[23]
     • Honor the patient's worth and potential as a human being.
     • Respect the patient as an individual who has worth in their own right.
  2. *Accurate empathy*[23]
     • Empathy is not sympathy. The empathetic clinician demonstrates an active interest in understanding the patient's perspective.
  3. *Autonomy support*[13,23]
     • Autonomy is the patient's irrevocable right to choose and make an educated decision without being coerced, persuaded, or pressured.
     • The spirit of MI honors, respects, and provides support for a patient's autonomy.
     • Allows for patients to have complete independence to choose for themselves.
  4. *Affirmation*[13,23]
     • Affirmation instills hope and belief that the patient can indeed change and the recognition provides support and encouragement to the patient.

C. Compassion[23]

▶ Compassion is commitment to promoting the welfare and prioritizing the needs of the patient.

TABLE 26-3	Basic Components of MI

SPIRIT OF MI ELEMENTS (PACE)	GUIDING PRINCIPLES (RULE)	IMPLEMENTATION PROCESS

■ Partnership
■ Acceptance
  • Absolute worth
  • Accurate empathy
  • Autonomy support
  • Affirmation
■ Compassion
■ Evocation
	■ Resist righting reflex
	■ Understand the patient's motivation
	■ Listen to the patient
	■ Empower the patient
		■ Engaging
		■ Focusing
		■ Evoking
		■ Planning

▶ The clinician is addressing the patient's best interest and needs and not the clinician's agenda.

▶ A compassionate spirit can assist with establishing trust with the patient.

D. Evocation[13,23]

▶ Commitment to elicit patients' assessment of their own strengths, thoughts, ideas, and resources is necessary for successful preventive counseling and behavior change.

▶ Patients provide a lot of information to the clinician about what will work for them in order to achieve their oral health goals through evocation.

▶ The overall spirit of MI begins with the premise that patients already have within them much of what is needed.

▶ The task of the clinician is to elicit and draw the motivation for change out of the patient.

II. Guiding Principles[13]

▶ MI has four guiding principles that assist the clinician in maintaining a rapport with the patient.

▶ The four principles can be remembered with the acronym RULE: resist–understand–listen–empower.

A. Resist Righting Reflex[13]

▶ Clinicians often have a desire to help and fix what is wrong and take the "expert role."

▶ This approach loses focus on the patient's ideas, experiences, and obstacles to overcome due to the clinician who is busy pouring knowledge out onto the patient.

▶ This urge to correct the patient's problem is often an automatic or reflexive habit.

▶ The reflexive nature of the clinician response can create a negative effect because patients tend to resist persuasion, especially when they are ambivalent about change.

▶ Instead, to establish and maintain the MI spirit of partnership, it is necessary to explore by eliciting the patient's own motivation and ideas for change.

B. Understand the Patient's Motivation[13]

▶ Determine the patient's own reasons for change rather than focusing on the clinician's perspective about why the patient needs to make the change.

▶ Be interested in the patient's own concerns, values, and motivations.

▶ Utilize MI to evoke and explore the patient's own perception about their current situation and motivations for change.

▶ Help the patient voice their own arguments for behavior change.

C. Listen to the Patient[13]

▶ All patients love a good listener and a truly good listener will forgo their own agenda in the interest of giving full attention to understanding the patient.

▶ The expectation of a clinician typically has been to know all the answers and give them to the patient.

▶ Patients have ideas about how to make the change.

▶ Actively listening requires more than the clinician asking questions.

▶ Listening involves the clinician demonstrating an empathetic interest in making sure to understand the patient.

▶ A good listener does not direct or instruct, agree or disagree, persuade or advise, warn or analyze what a patient says. There is no agenda to achieve other than understanding the world of the patient.

D. Empower the Patient[13]

▶ Patient empowerment is about supporting the patient's right to autonomy.

▶ Outcomes of behavior change increase when patients take an active interest and role in their own health care.

▶ Encourage patients by exploring how they can make a difference in their oral health and by listening and understanding the patient's own ideas for change.

▶ Patients are more likely to take steps toward change when they are included in the discussion and take an active role in the decision making.

III. Processes of MI[23]

▶ The four processes of MI form the flow of how clinicians use MI to direct patient behavior change.

▶ The flow of the four processes throughout a conversation with a patient will overlap and repeat. These processes are like stair steps illustrated in Figure 26-1 in which each process builds upon the other yet continues as the foundation.

▶ Box 26-3 provides a checklist of questions to help the clinician gauge the success of their MI approach at each step.

MI IMPLEMENTATION

I. Information Exchange[13]

▶ To provide information to a patient, begin by asking permission.

▶ Asking permission to provide information indicates respect and increases the willingness of the patient to hear what the clinician has to say.

A. Ask Permission[13,23]

▶ There are two approaches a clinician utilizes to ask the patient's permission to provide further detail or additional information.

▶ The clinician can:
  • Relay information when a patient asks the clinician for that information.

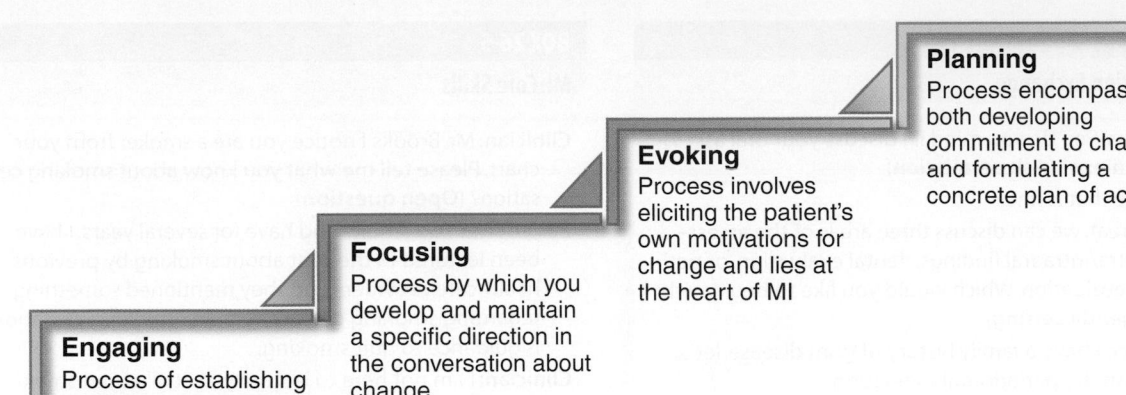

FIGURE 26-1 **Four Processes of Motivational Interview.**

BOX 26-3

Clinician Checklist of the Four Processes of MI[23]

Engaging

▷ How comfortable is the patient in talking to me (clinician)?

▷ Do I understand the patient's perspective and concerns?

▷ Does this feel like a collaborative partnership?

Focusing

▷ Are we (clinician and patient) working together for a common purpose?

▷ What goals for change does the patient have?

▷ Does this conversation feel more like dancing or a wrestling match?

Evoking

▷ What are the patient's own reasons for change?

▷ Is the reluctance for change about confidence or importance?

▷ What change talk am I hearing?

▷ Is the righting reflex pulling me (the clinician) to be the one arguing for change, instead of the patient?

Planning

▷ What would be a reasonable next step toward change?

▷ Am I remembering to evoke rather than prescribe a plan for the patient?

▷ Am I offering needed information or advice with permission when appropriate?

▷ Am I eliciting the patient's ideas for making the change?

- Directly ask permission to provide information even when the patient has not directly requested the information.

▶ For example, "I would like to discuss with you the assessment pertaining to your oral health; do you mind if I take a few minutes to go over my findings and address any concerns you may have?"

▶ Box 26-4 on the next page provides an example of information exchange utilizing asking permission.

B. Elicit Provide Elicit[13]

A strategy for easy exchange of information that maintains patient autonomy is the elicit-provide-elicit (EPE) approach.

▶ Three general functions of eliciting are:
- Asking permission.
- Exploring the patient's prior knowledge.
- Determining the patient's interest in the information that may be provided by the clinician.

▶ An exploration of the patient's prior knowledge is necessary.
- This avoids the "expert trap" so patients are not told things they already know.
- It also allows the clinician to fill in any variances or gaps in the patient's knowledge.

▶ Querying interest allows the clinician to determine:
- What the patient would like to know most.
- Provide the information that increases attention and receptiveness.
- Increase patient compliance.[10]

▶ Box 26-4 also provides an example utilizing the EPE strategy of information change.

II. Agenda Setting[13,23]

▶ Agenda setting is a brief discussion in which the patient is given as much decision-making freedom as possible to set the agenda for what information and recommendations the clinician provides and for when the information is provided.

▶ An agenda setting approach provides the patient with a list of topics regarding the oral health and to choose which topic to discuss first.

▶ For example, "Mrs. Smith there are three areas we can discuss regarding the assessment findings, which are extraoral/

BOX 26-4

MI: Information Exchange

Clinician: Mrs. Poe do you mind if I discuss your oral assessment findings? (**Ask permission**)

Patient: Sure that is fine.

Clinician: Great, we can discuss three areas of the assessment: Extra/intraoral findings, dental evaluation, or periodontal evaluation. Which would you like to begin with first? (**Agenda setting**)

Patient: Since I have a family history of gum disease, let's begin with the periodontal evaluation.

Clinician: Since you have a family history of gum disease, tell me what you know about gum disease? (**Elicit**)

Patient: My grandparents both wear dentures and father has a couple missing teeth due to losing teeth to bone loss. Gum disease involves the loss of bone.

Clinician: Yes that is correct gum disease also known as periodontal disease involves the loss of bone. What do you know about the various types of periodontal disease? (**Elicit**)

Patient: Nothing, I didn't realize there were different types. Can you tell me more about the kinds and how they relate to my current oral health?

Clinician: Sure I will be happy to elaborate (pulls out a chart illustrating the various stages). Gingivitis is reversible and inflammation of the gums, slight periodontitis includes slight bone loss and recession, moderate periodontitis (beginning of bone loss between the roots of the teeth and mobility), and severe periodontitis. Currently you have slight periodontitis due to the recession and slight bone loss revealed in the radiographs in conjunction with the probe readings taken today. (**Provide**) What are your thoughts about the information provided? (**Elicit**)

BOX 26-5

MI: Core Skills

Clinician: Mr. Brooks I notice you are a smoker from your chart. Please tell me what you know about smoking cessation? (**Open question**)

Patient: Yes I do smoke and have for several years. I have been lectured in the past about smoking by previous healthcare providers and they mentioned something regarding smoking cessation. I think smoking cessation is guidance to quit smoking.

Clinician: I am not here to lecture you at all about smoking Mr. Brooks, but I am here to assist you with ways to quit when you are ready. Seems you have tried to quit before since you are familiar with the smoking cessation program to guide smokers on alternatives ways to quit. (**Reflection**) What further information have you received regarding smoking cessation? (**Open question**)

Patient: Well they told me there are medications and patches that could be used to assist with quitting. I have tried going cold turkey in the past. I need something to assist me with decreasing the amount of cigarettes per day. Cold turkey does not work because it was just too much to handle with all the stress and I need something that will help me quit but slowly.

Clinician: I commend you on your efforts in the past to quit smoking and it seems you have really given thought to quitting based on what you are telling me your past experience. (**Affirmation**) You realize going cold turkey was not the best route and you need a way to decrease the amount of nicotine daily. More of a gradual way to quit smoking. (**Summary**)

intraoral evaluation, dental evaluation, and periodontal evaluation. Which area would you like to discuss first?"

▶ There may be areas the dental hygienist is concerned about; however, if the clinician decides the topic of conversation without consulting the patient, an opportunity to learn what behavior change the patient may be most ready to discuss is lost.

▶ Respect for the patient's autonomy to choose what topics to discuss will increase the patient's willingness to listen.

III. Core Skills[13,23]

▶ The core skills for MI are better known by the acronym OARS:

- **O**pen-ended questions
- **A**ffirmations
- **R**eflective listening
- **S**ummary.

▶ Box 26-5 provides an example of a brief patient conversation that illustrate MI core skills.

A. Open-Ended versus Closed Questions[13,23]

▶ A skillful blend of open-ended questions and reflective listening is essential in the MI approach to patient counseling.

▶ Open-ended questions permit the patient to think about the response. This may yield information and insight about topics the clinician may have missed.

▶ This style of questioning invites conversation focused in a particular direction and provides insight into the patient's values, understanding of the oral health status, as well as the ability to change.

▶ Examples of open-ended questions include:

- "What brings you here today?"
- "How do you hope your life might be like in 5 years?"
- "What do you know about cavities?"

▶ Box 26-5 provides an example of a patient conversation that begins with an open-ended question.

▶ Closed questions, while good for gathering specific types of information, tend to limit the person's options for responding. An example: "Do you smoke?"

▶ Closed questions can disguise themselves as an open question.

- An example would be "So what are you hoping to do: quit or cut down?"
- This type is termed a "leading" question and does not allow the patient the option to elaborate nor provide patient autonomy.

B. Affirmations[23]

▸ Affirmations emphasize the positive attributes, particularly concerning strengths the patient has expressed in regard to making a behavior change.

▸ Affirmations help encourage and support a patient.

▸ Affirmations are genuine and contain a reflection of what is true regarding the patient.

▸ Patients are more likely to spend time with, trust, listen to, and be open with a healthcare provider who they perceive recognizes and affirms their strengths.

▸ Affirmations decrease or reduce defensiveness.

▸ Encourage self-affirmation by asking the patient to describe strengths and past successes. This type of self-affirming has shown to facilitate openness.[24,25]

▸ Good affirmations center on the word "you." Using statements beginning with "I" will focus more on the clinician than on the patient.

▸ Example of an affirmation statement: "Your intention was good even though it didn't turn out as you would like."

▸ An example of a patient conversation that includes affirmation is found in Box 26-5.

C. Reflective Listening[13,23]

▸ Reflective listening (reflection) is a response to what the patient is conveying with a statement or summary that is more than repeating verbatim what the patient has said.

▸ This allows the patient to know the clinician is hearing and understanding.

▸ Two categories for reflections are simple reflection and complex reflection.

▸ Simple reflection is slightly rephrasing the content that was relayed to you by the patient.

▸ Box 26-6 provides an example of a simple reflection.

▸ Complex reflection:
  - Adds meaning or emphasis to what the patient said.
  - Makes a guess about the unspoken content or what might come next.

BOX 26-6

MI: Reflective Listening— Simple Reflection

Patient: I know that what you're trying to do is help me, but I'm just not going to do that!

Clinician: On the one hand, you know that there are some real problems here, and on the other, what I suggested is just not acceptable to you.

BOX 26-7

MI: Reflective Listening—Complex Reflection

Patient: You're probably going to give me a laundry list of ways to take care of my mouth that I need to stick to, and tell me I have to get some of these interproximal brushes, superfloss, power toothbrush, and a bunch of other products. I don't have time for all that!

Clinician: If I were to tell you a whole lot of things that you have to do, it would immobilize you even further. It's ironic, isn't it? When you feel like you are being forced to do something, it actually prevents you from doing what you want to do.

- Tend to move the conversation forward.
- Box 26-7 provides an example of a complex reflection.

D. Summarizing[13,23]

Summarizing information provided by the patient:

▸ Pulls together several items or ideas that a patient has provided.

▸ Is affirming because it implies the clinician remembers what the patient said and wants to understand.

▸ Assists the patient to reflect and think about the various experiences they communicated.

EXPLORING AMBIVALENCE[13,23]

▸ Patients often experience very divided feelings about changing health behaviors.

▸ On one hand, they may appreciate and value knowledge and recommendations the dental hygienist provides about how to attain and maintain their oral health.

▸ On the other hand, they often have very mixed feelings about how successful they could be at implementing the recommendations the care provider has suggested.

▸ The most effective way to explore and respond to a patient's ambivalence is by using the OARS core skills discussed in the previous section of this chapter.

I. Sustain Talk versus Change Talk[13,23]

▸ Listening carefully to the patient and responding appropriately is an important MI skill.

▸ Conversations with a patient may balance between sustain talk and change talk.

▸ A patient who is happy about current health-related behaviors will exhibit more discussion about maintaining the status quo (sustain talk) than someone who is ready to change.

▸ The skillful clinician who hears only sustain talk can use MI techniques to determine what information the patient is interested in receiving about oral health status and explore ambivalence.

- During patient conversations, the clinician may hear change talk, through patient statements that seem preparatory or mobilizing toward changing behaviors.
- When this occurs, the clinician can move to reflecting the change talk and eliciting a plan for change.
- Responding to both sustain talk and change talk, a clinician can use the MI process (OARS) to explore the patient's ambivalence toward change and to understand the issues that may be inhibiting their desire, motivation, or ability to change behaviors.

II. Decisional Balance[23]

A. The Balancing Act

- Decisional balance is the point at which a patient is determining whether the benefits outweigh the risks of the current behavior.
- The clinician can use this as an opportunity to explore and elicit more information from the patient about the pros and cons for making or not making the change.
- The key to success in this process is for the clinician to take a neutral position and provide a balanced way for the patient to explore the pros and cons of a behavior change.[25]
- The clinician's role is to elicit the patient's perception of:
  - Advantages of maintaining current behavior.
  - Disadvantages of maintaining the current behavior.
  - Advantages of making the change.
  - Disadvantages of making the change.
- The approach is very helpful when a patient seems to be uncertain about making a change.

B. Pro/Con Matrix

- Use of a pro/con matrix, illustrated in Figure 26-2, can also be beneficial in exploring decisional balance.
- The clinician can reflect and ask "What else?" at each interval during the patient's listing of pros and cons of making the change.
- When the decisional balance matrix has been completed, the clinician will focus on key items regarding the change of the behavior and provide a summary.

Pro/Con Matrix	Pros	Cons
If I don't change	A	B
If I do change	D	C

FIGURE 26-2 Decisional Balance: Pro and Con Matrix.

BOX 26-8

MI: Pro/Con Matrix

Clinician: What are the pros for not preventing cavities?

Patient: There are none really, but I really do like my soda and it provides me with the caffeine needed to stay alert after being up all night studying.

Clinician: So soda is your caffeine supply. (Reflection) What are the cons if you don't change?

Patient: I will continue to spend money on cavities. I want to keep my teeth and have them for a long time. Maintaining good oral health is important, but I don't know if I can quit my soda habit completely. I could make modifications with my snacks.

Clinician: You value your oral health and are willing to make modifications in your diet to prevent cavities. However, soda you are not willing to give up. (Reflection)

Patient: Yes, I would lose my caffeine source, so I would fall asleep during my classes and not be able to study the hours I need for my classes.

Clinician: I see, your performance of school would decrease due to lack of caffeine source. What are the cons for making the change? (Reflection, Open-ended Question)

Patient: None really except if I give up soda maybe lack of sleep. But maybe I could manage my time better and go to sleep at an earlier time.

Clinician: It is obvious you have no desire to quit drinking soda at this time. What are the pros if you do make the change? (Reflection, Open-ended Question)

Patient: I would not have to spend money on repairing my teeth. I really would like to keep my teeth. I could substitute fruit or vegetable for a candy bar when craving a snack. Maybe reduce the amount of soda or change to diet to reduce the sugar intake.

Clinician: It seems that you have good understanding regarding how you can prevent cavities and know it is important to maintain good oral health. You want to have your teeth for a long time, but you feel it will be hard for you to give up soda completely. However, you mentioned substituting fruit or vegetables for snacks instead of candy or substitute sugar-free candy instead. (Affirmation, Summary)

- Box 26-8 provides an example of the pro/con matrix in a conversation with a patient.

III. Readiness Ruler[23]

- A readiness ruler, illustrated in Figure 26-3, provides a visual aid during a discussion and is useful if the clinician is not sure how important, confident, or motivated the patient is toward making the behavior change.
- Example questions to ask when using the ruler are:
  - "How important is it to make this change?"
  - "On a scale of 1–10, where 1 means not motivated and 10 means extremely motivated, how motivated are you in making this change?"

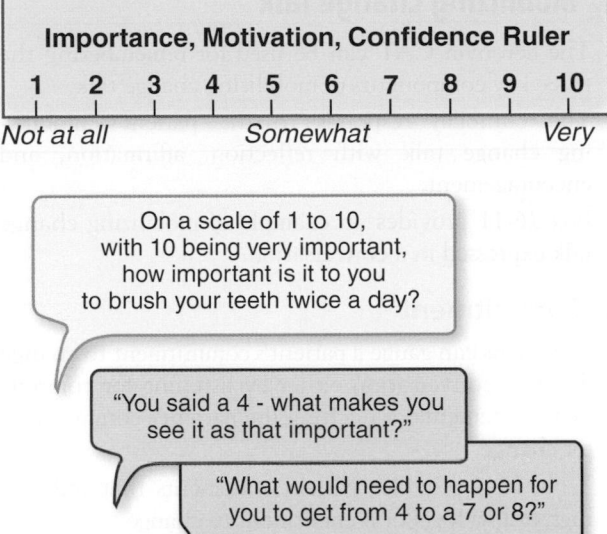

FIGURE 26-3 **Readiness for Change Ruler.** The utilization of this ruler will assist the clinician with eliciting the patient's importance, motivation, or confidence in making the change.

▶ Use of a ruler can not only tell the clinician about the patient's motivation, confidence, or importance for the change, but also the readiness ruler can elicit change talk.

▶ For example: A patient states they are a 5 on the scale from 1 to 10, the clinician responds, "So you are a 5? Why not a 3 or 4?"

▶ This approach can encourage the patient to explain why the behavior being discussed is important enough to designate it a 5 on the scale.

▶ Then the clinician can ask, "What are some ways for you to get to a 6 or 7?" to elicit the patient's ideas and potential strategies for making the change. Box 26-9 provides an example of the use of the readiness ruler.

ELICITING AND RECOGNIZING CHANGE TALK[13,23]

▶ During a conversation with a patient, the clinician needs to be able to elicit and recognize when change talk is exhibited.

▶ When change talk is heard in a conversation with the patient, the clinician provides reflection statements that incorporates and summarizes the change talk.

▶ Boxes 26-10 and 26-11 provide examples of a conversation between a patient who is making change talk and a clinician who reflects and summarizes the patient's change talk.

BOX 26-9

MI: Readiness Ruler

Clinician: On a scale of 1–10, where 1 means not confident and 10 means extremely confident, how confident are you in quitting smoking?
Patient: I'd say a 5.
Clinician: You are a 5, why not a 3 or 4?
Patient: Because I have tried in the past and have been successful, but at the same time I have some obstacles to overcome.
Clinician: You have learned from your past what works for you and you know the obstacles you have to overcome. What are some ways for you to get to a 6 or 7?

BOX 26-10

MI: Change Talk—Preparatory Change Talk

Patient: I know there are medications and patches that could be used to assist with quitting. I have tried in the past going cold turkey. (**Desire**) I need something to assist me with decreasing the amount of cigarettes per day. (**Need**) Cold turkey does not work because it was just too much to handle with all the stress and I need something that will help me quit but slowly. I can quit if I go slowly and have the support. (**Ability**)
Clinician: Seems you have really given thought to being successful in quitting based on your past experience. You realize going cold turkey was not the best route and you need away to decrease the amount of nicotine daily. More of a gradual way to quit smoking.
Patient: Yes I can quit with assistance and guidance. I really want to quit because I would like to be around for my wife and kids. (**Reason**) Plus I need to get in better health. (**Need**)

BOX 26-11

MI: Change Talk—Mobilizing Change Talk

Clinician: You value your health and family. You know you can quit smoking if you have something to assist with quitting. You mentioned using patches or medications in assisting.
Patient: Yes I have already researched the cost and the effectiveness of the patches and medications, plus chewing gums for quitting smoking. I intend to begin with the patches (**Commitment**), which I have already purchased (**Action toward**). I have scheduled an appointment with my physician to discuss which medication would be best that will not interfere with my heart medications. (**Taking steps**)

I. Preparatory Change Talk[13,23]

▶ Skillful application of MI can allow the clinician to elicit further information about the patient's desire, ability, reasons, and needs for making the behavior change.

▶ It is important for the clinician to be actively listening for the themes present in preparatory change talk and reflect those statements back to the patient when they occur in conversation.

▶ Some examples of change talk during a patient/clinician conversation are found in Box 26-10.

▶ The DARN acronym (desire, ability, reasons, need) is useful for remembering the four components of preparatory change talk that initiate the behavior change process.

A. Desire[13,23]

▶ During patient conversations, listen for words associated with desire for change.

▶ Examples of patient statements that the clinician may hear are "I want to…, I would like…, or I wish…"

▶ When eliciting change talk the clinician can pose questions that encourage the patient to express a desire for change.

▶ An example question for eliciting desire is: "How would you like for things to change?"

B. Ability[13,23]

▶ The theme of ability in change talk displays what a patient is thinking about regarding their capability or potential to make a change.

▶ Statements may be expressed during a conversation to demonstrate ability would include words like "can" or "could."

▶ Statements the clinician can use to elicit ability change talk are:
  • "What would you be willing to do?"
  • "What are some ideas you have for how to change?"

C. Reasons[13,23]

▶ This form of change talk expresses the patient's specific rationale or personal reasons for making a certain change.

▶ Examples of statements a clinician can use to elicit the patient's reasons for making a change are:
  • "What might be the good things about making this change?"
  • "What would be the downside of changing how things are now?"

D. Need[13,23]

▶ Need is expressed by patients when they recognize the urgency or begin to understand that they must make a change.

▶ Words associated with need change talk are "must," "have to," "got to," "should," "ought," or "need to."

▶ Example questions for eliciting the need to change are:
  • "What needs to happen?"
  • "How important is it for you to make this change?"[1]

II. Mobilizing Change Talk[13]

▶ The acronym CAT can be used for remembering the three key components of mobilizing change talk.

▶ The clinician responds to the patient's mobilizing change talk with reflection, affirmation, and encouragement.

▶ Box 26-11 provides an example of mobilizing change talk expressed in a conversation.

A. Commitment[13]

▶ Clinicians can gauge a patient's commitment to change during a conversation either by listening for commitment statements or eliciting the patient's commitment for change.

▶ Table 26-4 provides patient statements that indicate high or low level of commitment to change.

B. Action Toward[13]

▶ Clinicians may encounter change talk that indicates action toward change, and these types of statements mean the patient has taken some step toward change.

▶ For example, the patient might say: "I have bought dental floss." or "I have purchased a power toothbrush."

C. Taking Steps[13]

▶ Patients express steps they have already taken in making the change.

▶ For example, "I just began flossing twice a week" or "I have just started eating healthy snacks between meals instead of a candy bar."

▶ An example eliciting question is, "What have you done to make this change?"

STRENGTHENING COMMITMENT (THE PLAN)[13,23]

▶ The goal when having a conversation with a patient about making health behavior change is to have the patient come up with a plan to make the change.

TABLE 26-4	Patient Statements Indicating Commitment	
LOW-LEVEL COMMITMENT	**HIGH-LEVEL COMMITMENT**	
I will think about it	I will	
I'll consider it	I promise	
I plan to	I guarantee	
I hope to	I am ready to	
I will try to	I intend to	

▶ The signs a patient may be ready to proceed to a plan are:
- An increase in change talk.
- Talk about taking steps toward the change.
- Diminished sustain talk.
- Questions about making the change.

▶ It is important that the patient provide the solutions for change and the clinician allow the patient to develop the solutions that will work best for them.

▶ Patients are more successful and committed to a plan if their own ideas and needs are incorporated.

▶ The clinician utilizes the same MI techniques (OARS) when having a conversation regarding the patient's plan.

▶ After the patient articulates the plan, the clinician can summarize the patient's plan and follow-up with a commitment question.

▶ Box 26-12 provides a conversation with a patient that leads to a plan.

▶ There are three scenarios when it comes to planning.

I. Clear Plan[23]

▶ The first planning scenario is when the patient knows what they want or need to do.

▶ If the patient has decided on clear plan for change and they know how they will accomplish it, there is no need to explore other paths.

▶ Even when there is a clear plan, elicit the patient's thoughts about obstacles or unanticipated difficulties that may arise with the plan. In addition, discuss ideas the patient has about how to overcome these obstacles in order to be successful.

II. Several Clear Options[23]

▶ The second planning scenario is when the patient has determined there is more than one clear plan for working toward the goal.

▶ Through agenda setting, the clinician can help the patient prioritize and choose among the various plans.

III. Brainstorming[23]

▶ The last category of planning is when a patient has neither a clear plan nor an obvious set of options to choose from for making the desired behavior change.

▶ The patient is developing a plan from scratch.

▶ The conversation with the patient is a brainstorming-type session from which the clinician elicits ideas the patient has about making the change.

▶ The clinician utilizes agenda setting to determine what the patient would like to pursue initially from the ideas established.

BOX 26-12

MI: The Plan

Clinician: Mrs. Poe you have quit in the past and now you have some options to assist you with quitting. You know cold turkey did not work well in the past attempt to quit, but you seem to be highly interested in using the nicotine patch and gum supplements for your next quit attempt. (**Summary**)

Patient: Yes after discussing the various options, I am going to get the nicotine patches and gum to assist me with quitting. I really think this option will be more successful for me.

Clinician: Any thoughts on when you will begin the process of quitting? (**Eliciting**)

Patient: Well I am under a bit of stress right now and the holidays are coming up. Maybe January 1st.

Clinician: Seems smoking is a stress reliever for you and you would like to wait four months before beginning the smoking cessation program. (**Reflection**)

Patient: Yes smoking is a stress reliever and really all I am doing is trying to go slowly with quitting, so I am going to go out and get the patches and gum and begin on Monday with decreasing the amount I smoke a day. (**Change talk**) I can do other things to relieve my stress by walking or jogging, which I already do daily. I just will increase it when I feel more stressed. (**Change talk**)

Clinician: You have some alternative ways to relieve your stress that is not different from your daily routine now. Your plan is to begin with the patches and gum on Monday and slowly decrease the amount of cigarettes you smoke. Seems you want to be completely off of cigarettes by January 1. When you feel more stress you will extend your exercise time. (**Summary—the plan**)

Patient: Yes that is the plan.

Clinician: Great, I will make a note in your chart and follow-up with you at your next periodontal maintenance appointment.

MI WITH PEDIATRIC PATIENTS AND CAREGIVERS[26–28]

▶ MI can be utilized with pediatric patients and parents or other caregivers.

▶ The same core skills are utilized to explore ambivalence or elicit change talk.

▶ The age and self-care ability of the child determines whether the conversation regarding preventive behavior change is directed toward the child or the caregiver.

▶ Box 26-13 provides an example conversation utilizing MI with a pediatric patient and caregiver.

BOX 26-13

MI: The Pediatric Patient and Caregiver

Background: Jimmy is 8 years old and has been seeing the dentist since age one. Mom is with Jimmy today for his six-month visit. No past history of cavities. It is time for Jimmy to have some bitewings today, which mom has approved. The radiographs reveal Jimmy has proximal lesions on teeth #3, 14, 19, and 30 and incipient lesions present on several other teeth. Use of disclosing solution reveals a biofilm score of 80%.

Clinician: Jimmy what do you know about cavities? **(Eliciting)**

Patient: All I know about cavities is there are bugs that eat away at your tooth if you don't brush and eat too much sugar.

Clinician: Jimmy yes if you don't take care of teeth and eat properly teeth can become decayed. **(Affirmation, reflective listening)** Remember when the dentist was doing his examination and he mentioned there were a few areas where there were cavities? **(Closed question)**

Patient: Yes, does that mean I have teeth that have decayed?

Clinician: Yes Jimmy you do have areas of decay. May I bring your mom back to discuss what was found today when the dentist did his exam? **(Asking permission)**

Patient: Sure.

Clinician: (Brings mom back to discuss findings) Mrs. Jones the dentist found cavities during Jimmy's examination today that were not there six months ago. Are you aware of any changes in Jimmy's diet? **(Eliciting)**

Mrs. Jones (Mom): Well I have noticed he does consume a lot of Gatorade and Kool Aid between meals. He has an occasional snickers bar at least once a week, but he brushes twice a day for two minutes.

Clinician: Seems he enjoys Gatorade and Kool Aid and Jimmy I commend you on your brushing habits. **(Affirmation)** Jimmy and I reviewed his brushing technique today to ensure he was effectively getting all the plaque off when he brushes. What do you think may be contributing to his recent decay? **(Eliciting, Open-ended Question)**

MOTIVATIONAL TRAINING AND COACHING

► MI workshops alone will usually have little effect on the clinician's proficiency or changing practice.[15,22]

► In order to become proficient with MI, it is recommended to take introductory and advanced MI courses or workshops where feedback is provided through MI practice and coaching.[23,29]

► Ultimately, the skills of MI are learned through the feedback and coaching that is rendered and this can only be done by observed practice.

► Therefore, skill development is an ongoing process and MI must coincide with classroom, practice, and coaching in order to be properly trained.[23,29]

► There is additional information located on the MI Network of Trainers website (www.motivationalinterviewing.org), with additional information regarding trainings across the nation clinicians may attend as well as many other resources pertaining to MI.[30]

DOCUMENTATION

Routine documentation for a MI session includes a minimum of the following information.

► Assessment findings and areas of concern (disease status and risk).

► Patient's stage of readiness for making a change.

► Patient's motivation for change.

► The outcome of the conversation with the patient regarding the area(s) of concern such as:

• Knowledge and understanding of their disease status and risk.

• What the patient would like to address first.

• What has worked in the past or not worked.

• How they plan to make the change.

• Short- and long-term goals for making the change.

• When they plan to begin to make the change.

► A documentation example is found in Box 26-14.

BOX 26-14

Example Documentation: MI Session During a Patient Appointment

S –A 30-year-old Caucasian male presents for 3-month continuing care visit. Previous assessment indicates high intake of sugar sweetened beverages. Previous entries in patient record indicate on-going recommendations for limiting intake of sugar sweetened beverages. Patient states today that he sips 3–5 cans of cola-type beverage during the day and evening. He indicates he knows the beverages are what "cause my cavities" and that he would like to change his behavior so he wouldn't "get any more cavities," but that his motivation for behavior change on the readiness ruler is "about a 2."

O –Previous history of significant smooth surface decay, and today's examination indicates two new cavitated lesions on anterior facial surfaces, which were documented on the patient's dental chart.

A –Patient has knowledge of the cause of dental decay, but expresses ambivalence to change that can correct the problem.

P –Used MI approach and the pro/con matrix to help the patient explore his ambivalence to behavior change and to explore factors that might affect his ability to change behavior and stop continually drinking sugar sweetened beverages. He will continue to explore other ways he can cut down and might begin drinking bottle water with sugar-free flavoring.

Next Steps: Continue to use MI approach to provide follow-up discussion and encouragement during patient's visit for restorative treatment in 2 weeks and at his next dental hygiene appointment in 3 months.

Signed _____, RDH

Date _____

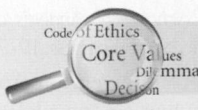

EVERYDAY ETHICS

Jeremy, now 15 years old, has been a patient of Tressa, the dental hygienist, since he was 3 years old. Jeremy had undergone extensive restorative work as a young child. He had collided on a swing set with an older sibling, which resulted in trauma to both maxillary and mandibular incisors and permanent tooth buds. Jeremy had received a "fair plus" on his oral homecare report card at the last few visits. However, this time when Tressa went to greet him in the waiting room, Jeremy's mother asked her to "really get on him" about brushing his teeth every day.

During her oral assessment, Tressa noted extremely heavy biofilm on all teeth, generalized bleeding on probing, staining on the anterior restorations, and a distinctly unpleasant odor. "Jeremy," she lectured, "you must take better care of your teeth! Your breath smells really bad. And you are jeopardizing all of that expensive dental work your parents have paid for." Turning very red, Jeremy pulled his cap over his eyes, crossed his arms, and refused to reply. As she continued to provide preventive counseling, Jeremy was clearly not paying attention and Tessa became annoyed. She commented that she was going to speak to his mother about his poor attitude.

In a final attempt to turn his attention to prevention, Tressa showed Jeremy intraoral photographs she taken that morning of a patient with extreme periodontal disease. "Is that what you want to look like?" she asked.

Questions for Consideration

1. Describe how Tressa's approach to prevention violates Jeremy's autonomy, even though he is technically still a child and in spite of his mother's request.

2. Explain why showing Jeremy another patient's intraoral photographs violates ethical standards of dental hygiene practice.

3. What core values and ethical principles can guide Tressa as she reflects on her communication style and develops an alternative approach to prevention that is both ethical and effective?

Factors To Teach The Patient

▷ Discuss the relationship between preventive measures and clinical services.

▷ Discuss preventive measures and suggested care plan options pertaining to the clinical assessment findings.

▷ Elicit what the patient knows about periodontal disease or their risk for caries and have a discussion utilizing the MI methods regarding possible changes the patient can pursue.

▷ Discuss Self-assessment and alternative methods (disclosing agent) for determining the health of gingiva.

▷ Determine the patient's self-care technique (e.g., toothbrushing power or manual, flossing, etc.) and provide suggestions if need to modified technique to be effective.

▷ Provide the patient with various options regarding preventive measures for the disease status to choose that will be effective.

▷ Elicit from the patient's short- and long-term goals pertaining to what the patient would like to achieve regarding disease status and overall self-care.

References

1. Gao X, Lo EC, Kot SC, et al. Motivational interviewing in improving oral health: a systemic review of randomized controlled trials. *J Periodontol.* 2014;85(3):426–437. http://www.joponline.org/doi/abs/10.1902/jop.2013.130205.

2. Bray KK, Catley D, Voelker MA, et al. Motivational interviewing in dental hygiene education: curriculum modification and evaluation. *J Dent Educ.* 2013;77(12):1662–1669.

3. Croffoot C, Krust Bray K, Black MA, et al. Evaluating the effects of coaching to improve motivational interviewing skills of dental hygiene students. *J Dent Hyg.* 2010;84(2):57–64.

4. Kalsbeek H, Truin GJ, Poorterman JH, et al. Trends in periodontal status and oral hygiene habits in Dutch adults between 1983 and 1995. *Community Dent Oral Epidemiol.* 2000;28(2):112–118.

5. Ronis DL, Lang WP, Farghaly MM, et al. Tooth brushing, flossing, and preventive dental visits by Detroit-area residents in relation to demographic and socioeconomic factors. *J Public Health Dent.* 1993;53(3):138–145.

6. Smedslund G, Berg RC, Hammerstrøm KT, et al. Motivational interviewing for substance abuse. *Cochrane Database Syst Rev.* 2011;(5):CD008063.

7. Yevlahova D, Satur J. Models for individual oral health promotion and their effectiveness: a systematic review. *Aust Dent J.* 2009;54(3):190–197. doi:10.1111/j.1834-7819.2009.01118.x.

8. Glanz K, Lewis FM, Rimer BK. *Health Behavior and Health Education.* 2nd ed. San Francisco, CA: Jossey-Bass; 1997:41–59.

9. Emmons KM, Rollnick S. Motivational interviewing in health care settings: opportunities and limitations. *Am J Prev Med.* 2001;20(1):68–74.

10. Prochaska JO, Velicer WF. The transtheoretical model of health behavior change. *Am J Health Promot.* 1997;12(1):38–48.

11. Wilson GT, Schlam TR. The transtheoretical model and motivational interviewing in the treatment of eating and weight disorders. *Clin Psychol Rev.* 2004;24(3):361–378.

12. Bundy C. Changing behaviour: using motivational interviewing techniques. *J R Soc Med.* 2004;97 (Suppl 44):43–47.

13. Rollnick S, Miller WR, Butler CC. *Motivational Interviewing in Health Care: Helping Patients Change Behavior.* New York, NY: The Guilford Press; 2008:3–107.

14. Rubak S, Sandbaek A, Lauritzen T, et al. Motivational interviewing: a systematic review and meta-analysis. *Br J Gen Pract.* 2005;55(513):305–312.

15. Lundahl BW, Kunz C, Brownell C, et al. A meta-analysis of motivational interviewing: twenty-five years of empirical studies. *Res Social Work Prac.* 2010;20(2): 137–159.

16. Lundahl B, Moleni T, Burke BL, et al. Motivational interviewing in medical care settings: a systematic review and meta-analysis of randomized controlled trials. *Patient Educ Couns.* 2013;93(2):157–168.

17. Hettema J, Steele J, Miller WR. Motivational interviewing. *Annu Rev Clin Psychol.* 2005;1:91–111.

18. Soria R, Legido A, Escolano C, et al. A randomised controlled trial of motivational interviewing for smoking cessation. *Br J Gen Pract.* 2006;56(531):768–774.

19. Koeber A, Crawford J, O'Connell K. The effects of teaching dental students brief motivational interviewing for smoking cessation counseling: a pilot study. *J Dent Educ.* 2003;67(4):439–447.

20. Hettema JE, Hendricks PS. Motivational interviewing for smoking cessation: a meta-analytic review. *J Consult Clin Psychol.* 2010;78(6):868–884.

21. Martins RK, McNeil DW. Review of motivational interviewing in promoting health behaviors. *Clin Psychol Rev.* 2009;29:283–293.

22. Rollnick S, Heather N. Negotiating behavior change in medical settings: the development of brief motivational interviewing. *J Mental Health.* 1992;1(1):25–38.

23. Miller WR, Rollnick S. *Motivational Interviewing: Helping People Change.* 3rd ed. New York, NY: The Guilford Press; 2013:3–292.

24. Critcher CR, Dunning D, Armor DA. When self-affirmations reduce defensiveness: timing is key. *Pers Soc Psychol Bull.* 2010;36(7):947–959.

25. Janis IL, Mann L. *Decision Making: A Psychological Analysis of Conflict, Choice and Commitment.* New York, NY: Free Press; 1977.

26. Skaret E, Weinstein P, Kvale G, et al. An intervention program to reduce dental avoidance behaviour among adolescents: a pilot study. *Eur J Paediatr Dent.* 2003;4:191–196.

27. Weinstein P, Harrison R, Benton T. Motivating parents to prevent caries in their young children: one-year findings. *J Am Dent Assoc.* 2004;135(6):731–738.

28. Weinstein P, Harrison R, Benton T. Motivating mothers to prevent caries: confirming the beneficial effect of counseling. *J Am Dent Assoc.* 2006;137:789–793.

29. Miller WR, Yahne CE, Moyers TB, et al. A randomized trial of methods to help clinicians learn motivational interviewing. *J Consult Clin Psychol.* 2004;72:1050–1062.

30. Motivational Interviewing Network of Trainers. MINT excellence in motivational interviewing: MI Training and Resources. http://www.motivationalinterviewing.org/. Accessed May 15, 2015.

ENHANCE YOUR UNDERSTANDING

thePoint® **DIGITAL CONNECTIONS**
(see the inside front cover for access information)
- Audio glossary
- Quiz bank

SUPPORT FOR LEARNING
(available separately; visit lww.com)
- *Active Learning Workbook for Clinical Practice of the Dental Hygienist, 12th Edition*

 prepU **INDIVIDUALIZED REVIEW**
(available separately; visit lww.com)
- Adaptive quizzing with *prepU for Wilkins' Clinical Practice of the Dental Hygienist*

27

Protocols for Prevention and Control of Dental Caries

Elena Francisco, RDH, MSDH

LEARNING OBJECTIVES

After studying this chapter, the student will be able to:

1. Describe the dental caries disease process.

2. Identify factors contributing to demineralization and remineralization.

3. Distinguish each step in caries management.

4. Evaluate each patient for individual risk for caries disease.

5. Apply caries risk status in developing individualized caries management protocols and carefully document.

THE DENTAL CARIES PROCESS

Dental caries is an infectious, transmissible disease. It is also preventable. When a caries infection occurs in the oral cavity, strategies exist to control the disease, reverse it in its early stages, and prevent further infection. Dental hygienists have new information from current research to share with their patients to increase their understanding of the dental caries process and disease prevention.

- On the tooth surface, a constant process of demineralization and remineralization is ongoing.
- This process takes place throughout the life of the tooth.
- Protocols exist to address caries disease prevention and management at the various stages of lesion development; the goal being to halt and control the disease process.
- The basic caries process starts with certain acidogenic bacteria in dental biofilm acting to metabolize the fermentable carbohydrates ingested by the patient.[1]
- Acids are formed that in turn act to demineralize the enamel, cementum, and/or dentin and lead to cavity formation.
- Figure 35-4 (Chapter 35) shows the interrelation of the microorganisms, tooth, salivary factors, and cariogenic foods in the caries process.
- Terminology to describe dental caries is defined in Box 27-1.

I. Acidogenic Bacteria

- Specific bacteria in the biofilm on the tooth surfaces metabolize acid from the fermentable carbohydrates ingested by the individual.
- Although there are many acid-forming bacteria present, two groups of bacteria predominate in the caries process: the *mutans streptococci* (including both *Streptococcus mutans* and *Streptococcus sobrinus*) and the *Lactobacillus* species. *Bifidobacteria* are also associated with childhood caries.[2]
- *Mutans streptococci* are infectious organisms that colonize the teeth and help to form the dental biofilm through their ability to create a sticky environment for survival and multiplication.
- *Mutans streptococci* and *Bifidobacteria* are most active during the initial stages of demineralization and cavity formation, whereas the lactobacilli are more active during the progression of the cavity.
- Permanent colonization of a child's teeth with *mutans streptococci* can take place soon after tooth eruption. Transmission of the acid-forming organisms is usually from close family members, particularly the mother.[3]

II. Role of Fermentable Carbohydrates[4]

- Commonly consumed fermentable carbohydrates include sucrose, glucose, fructose, and cooked starch.

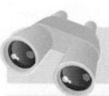

BOX 27-1 **KEY WORDS AND ABBREVIATIONS:** Dental Caries

Acidogenic bacteria: bacteria in dental biofilm capable of metabolizing fermentable carbohydrates into acids.

Buffer: a substance that by its presence in solution is capable of neutralizing alkali or acid.

CAMBRA (Caries Assessment and Management by Risk Assessment): procedure to assess risk for future dental caries development and identify approaches to managing caries risk.

CRA (Caries risk assessment): procedure to predict future dental caries development before the clinical onset of the disease.

Cariology: science and study of dental caries.

Cavitation: process in the formation of cavities; final stage in the caries process.

Cavity: a hole; the final stage of demineralization and breakdown of tooth structure. The classification of cavities by tooth surfaces and anatomic location is defined in Figure 16-4, Chapter 16.

Demineralization: major stage in the dental caries process in which minerals, primarily calcium and phosphorous, are removed from tooth structure by acids formed by acidogenic bacteria, primarily *mutans streptococci* and lactobacilli.

Dental caries: infectious disease of teeth caused by acidogenic bacteria with dissolution of enamel and dentin (coronal caries) and cementum and dentin (root caries).

Arrested caries: after remineralization, the caries process is halted; the area usually becomes discolored with a brownish tinge, darker with age or in a tobacco user.

Cavitated carious lesion: advanced lesion with break through the tooth surface; contrast with *noncavitated carious lesion*, when a dull probe passed over a white demineralized area detects no roughness or breakthrough.

Rampant caries: rapidly progressive caries occurring in many teeth simultaneously; also called acute caries in contrast to chronic caries (slow developing).

Secondary caries: carious lesions at the margin of an existing restoration; also called recurrent caries.

Remineralization: healing process in which minerals are redeposited in the demineralized tooth structure; accomplished by the protective factors of the saliva and the action of fluoride to inhibit demineralization and interfere with the enzymatic requirements of bacteria.

White spot lesion: early stage of the caries process when demineralization causes a change in the enamel to appear chalky white.

▶ Acids produced during the metabolic processes include acetic, lactic, formic, and proprionic.

▶ *Frequent* ingestion of fermentable carbohydrates can have a strong influence on the amount of acid produced and the extent of tooth destruction.

III. Acid Production[5]

▶ The acid formed passes freely into the tiny diffusion channels between the enamel rods or into the exposed root surfaces.

▶ Acids can dissolve the enamel crystals into calcium and phosphate ions.

▶ The subsurface initial carious lesion is formed as shown in Figure 36-3 (Chapter 36). It is observed clinically as a white area.

IV. Demineralization[4,5]

The process of demineralization and remineralization are natural processes as the fluids in the oral cavity constantly strive to maintain equilibrium.

▶ Demineralization is the process by which the minerals of the tooth structure are dissolved into solution by the organic acids produced from the fermentable carbohydrate by the acidogenic bacteria.

▶ With repeated bathing of the tooth surface with the acids produced in the course of a day, the tooth demineralization can outpace the remineralization process. The end product of this activity is the cavitated carious lesion.

▶ Smooth surface caries and pit and fissure carious lesions can result when cariogenic nutrients are available.

V. Remineralization[4,5]

Remineralization is the process of moving minerals back into the subsurface of the enamel. Saliva provides protective factors to promote remineralization.

A. Saliva

▶ Protective factors of the healthy saliva can balance or reverse the destruction of the tooth structure.

▶ Saliva has many properties and functions:
  • Buffer the acids.
  • Supply minerals to replace calcium and phosphate ions dissolved from the tooth during demineralization.

▶ Low saliva flow (xerostomia) reduces buffering capacity and aids in the demineralization process.

▶ Maintaining a neutral or basic saliva pH is necessary to maximize remineralization. Critical pH is addressed in Chapter 16.

▶ Exposure to topical fluoride can increase available salivary levels of fluoride. Fluoride accumulation in saliva comes from many sources, including water,

dentifrice, mouthrinse, and professionally applied therapies.

B. Fluoride Mechanisms of Action

▶ *Inhibits demineralization*: Fluoride available in biofilm and saliva can flow into the enamel diffusion channels and root surface and attach in the form of hydrogen fluoride (HF) as the oral environment attempts to achieve equilibrium.[1]

▶ *Enhances remineralization*: Sufficient saliva is integral in this process.
  • The buffering properties of saliva can neutralize acid pH.
  • This change in pH can reverse the equilibrium, driving calcium, phosphate, and fluoride into the tooth surface.[1]
  • The resulting fluorapatite bond is stronger than the hydroxyapatite bonds, resulting in a stronger tooth surface.

▶ Inhibits bacterial growth:
  • In the biofilm, the HF diffuses through the cell membrane of acidogenic bacteria.
  • Fluoride ions interfere with the essential enzyme activity within the bacterial cell wall.[1]

DENTAL CARIES DIAGNOSIS AND DETECTION[6]

▶ Formerly the term "dental caries" referred only to the destructive lesion of the tooth structure that penetrated the tooth surface and created a cavity.
  • Dental caries made its way through enamel and into dentin (see Figure 16-8, Chapter 16) or through the cementum and into the dentin (root caries).

▶ When unrestored, dental caries continues into the pulp, result in a toothache, and requires a root canal treatment or extraction.

▶ Currently, dental caries is treated as an infection, the *end stage* of the infection is the hole or cavity that requires therapy for restoration.

▶ The diagnosis of dental caries as an infection has transformed the detection of *cavities needing to be filled* to identification of each stage of the disease.

▶ Early diagnosis and detection of carious lesions while still in the subsurface, incipient, or noncavitated state allows the clinician to educate the patient, provide strategies, and provide preventive treatments that can reverse the lesion.

I. Prerequisites for Carious Lesion Detection[7]

▶ Adequate lighting.
▶ Sharp eyes or loupes.
▶ Blunt probes: no sharp explorers. Remineralizing surfaces must not be explored or altered in any way.

▶ Air–water explored for viewing teeth wet and dry.

▶ Current diagnostic bitewing radiographs can be useful to detect proximal carious lesions, but generally do not detect early, remineralizable lesions. *Vertical bitewings* are most effective for root caries detection.

II. The Stages of Dental Carious Lesion Development

A. Initial Infection: Invisible Lesion

Mutans streptococci and other acidogenic bacteria affect the tooth surface by:

▶ Clinging to the smooth tooth surface.

▶ Creating a biofilm.

▶ Producing acid from available fermentable carbohydrate.

▶ Acids produced diffuse through the microchannels between the enamel rods, dissolves the tooth minerals, and create the subsurface lesion (see Figure 16-8, Chapter 16).

B. White Area Lesion: Early Stage

▶ Examination: Run *blunt* probe gently over the surface. Blowing air under a bright light can show the white area of subsurface demineralization.

▶ Appearance: dull.

▶ Surface: smooth.

▶ Examine carefully: surface *must* not be broken or scratched.

▶ Picking or scratching a mineralizing surface can prevent further remineralization.[8,9]

▶ Remineralization process starts with buffering properties of saliva, including calcium, phosphate, and fluoride availability.

C. White Area: Later Stage (White Spot Lesion)

▶ Examination: Run blunt probe gently over the surface with no pressure.

▶ Appearance: dull.

▶ Surface: will be slightly rough, indicating beginning breakdown: Do not explore the surface (Figure 27-1).

▶ Remineralization may still be effective and allowed to continue.

D. Cavitated Lesion

▶ *Visual examination*
  - Open lesion can be observed directly (Figure 27-2).
  - Open lesion has no intact tooth structure over the surface.
  - Gentle air blast may be sufficient to clear loose biofilm and debris for direct vision.

▶ *Instrument examination*
  - Avoid picking or scratching a surface. Bacteria can be spread from a lesion to an uninfected tooth surface.

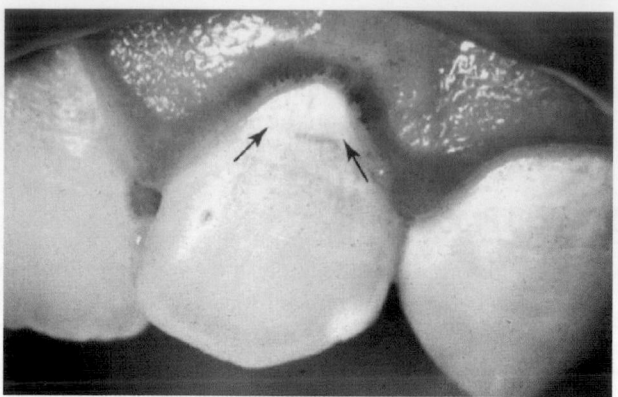

FIGURE 27-1 Smooth surface demineralization appearing as chalky white area (at arrows) seen in the cervical third of a maxillary lateral incisor is evidence of the first stages of dental caries. If this demineralization continued and did not reverse itself (through excellent oral hygiene, diet, and use of topical fluoride), this area could develop a cavitation that would need to be restored. Also notice the inflammation of the adjacent gingiva (gingivitis), which is also caused by bacterial biofilm. (Reprinted from Weiss G, Scheid R. Woelfel's Dental Anatomy, 9e. Philadelphia: Lippincott Williams & Wilkins; 2016.)

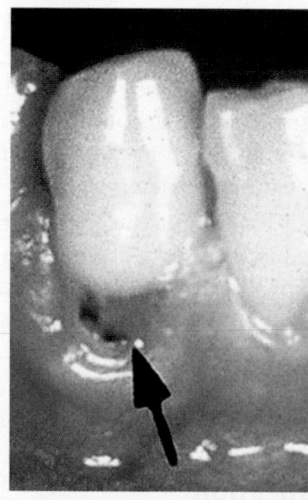

FIGURE 27-2 Root caries (arrow) on an area of exposed cementum after gingival recession. (Reprinted from Scheid R, Weiss G. Woelfel's Dental Anatomy. Philadelphia: Lippincott Williams & Wilkins; 2011.)

  - Probe or explorer not needed if visual examination of the occlusal, facial, palatal, or lingual identifies an open lesion.
  - Small proximal caries at the contact area needs radiograph for confirmation of depth.

▶ *Radiographic examination*
  - Horizontal bitewing views: primarily proximal surface lesion detection (see Figure 27-3).
  - Vertical bitewing views: for root caries detection, especially on periodontally involved individuals.
  - Early caries not extending into dentin: radiographs cannot reveal true depth because of tooth density.
  - Large open lesions do not need radiographic examination for detection, only for extension to pulpal involvement.
  - The dental hygienist can detect carious lesions. Typically a dentist diagnoses caries and plans appropriate intervention.

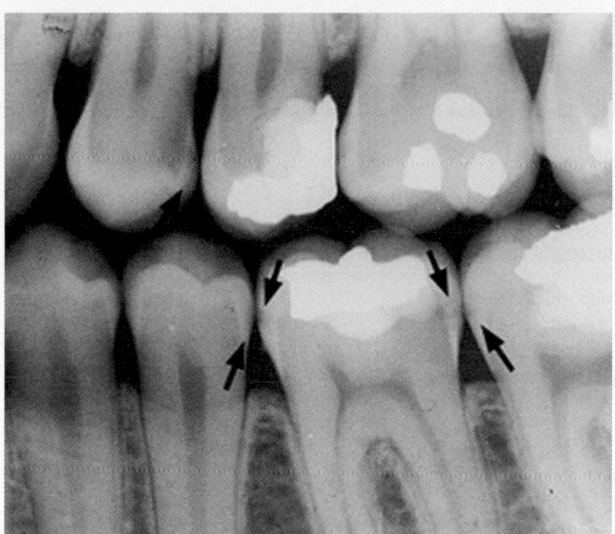

FIGURE 27-3 Radiographic image of several class II carious lesions (arrows). (Reprinted from Lippincott Williams & Wilkins' Comprehensive Dental Assisting. Philadelphia: Lippincott Williams & Wilkins; 2011.)

III. History of Dental Caries Management

▶ In the early half of the 20th century, the history of dental caries management included placing restorations, removing diseased teeth, and providing prosthetic replacements.

▶ Reductions in caries incidence of 40–60% since 1945 in the United States were observed for those fortunate enough to live in communities with community water fluoridation.[4]

▶ As the 20th century progressed, a drop in dental caries prevalence was generally related to the widespread home use of fluoride dentifrices and mouthrinses as well as professional topical applications of solutions, gels, and varnishes.

▶ In the early 21st century, studies showed caries prevalence has remained the same and even increased in some populations in the United States as a result of lack of access to care.[10]

▶ Dental caries is still a major problem in the health and welfare of adults, adolescents, and children.

ASSESSING CARIES RISK

I. Current Principles of Caries Management

A. Determine Current Status of Dentition, Including Restored and Unrestored Surfaces

Charting includes the following (see Table 16-2, Chapter 16):

▶ Existing restorations, including sealants.

▶ Cavitated carious lesions (final stage of caries disease process).

▶ Secondary (recurrent) carious lesions.

▶ Sealants in need of repair.

▶ White spot lesions (demineralized areas) which can benefit from remineralization.

▶ Radiographically detectable carious lesions.

B. Determine Areas that Require Restoration

▶ Active carious lesions are charted by the dental hygienist.

▶ Dentist will determine restorative interventions

C. Determine Areas that Require Remineralization

▶ Outline appropriate strategies for patient.

D. Define Steps for Remineralization Program

▶ Explain needs and discuss process of remineralization with patient.

▶ Apply principles of motivational interviewing to assess patient understanding and gain patient acceptance.

▶ Prepare and explain risk assessment for the individual.

▶ With the patient, select and demonstrate individualized oral self-care procedures.

▶ Plan for evaluation and revaluation at continuing care appointments.

II. Risk Factors

▶ Risk factors are habits, behaviors, lifestyles, or conditions that, when present, increase the probability of a disease occurring.

▶ The risk factors in Table 27-1 apply primarily to adult and teenage patients. Tables 50-5 (Chapter 50) lists the risk factors selected especially for the oral health of the child.

▶ Caries management begins with the risk factor assessment. This allows the clinician to provide individualized recommendations.

III. Caries Risk Assessment

Several caries risk assessment tools exist to aid in the systematic collect of data.

A. Purposes and Uses of Individual Patient Risk Assessment[11]

▶ Using the patient's own list of risk factors can be a significant educational experience for the patient.

▶ Discuss existing individual oral conditions with the patient.

▶ Provide factual information about the development and transmissibility of cariogenic bacteria.

▶ Relate the patient's cavitated carious and white spot lesions to behavioral and lifestyle habits that will need to change to improve the balance between remineralization and demineralization.

TABLE 27-1	CAMBRA

RISK FACTORS AND MANAGEMENT GUIDELINES FOR PATIENTS AGE 6 AND OLDER

MANAGEMENT GUIDELINES	CAMBRA RISK LEVEL			
	LOW RISK	MODERATE RISK	HIGH RISK[a]	EXTREME RISK[b]
Risk factors	The number and extent or severity of risk factors are taken into consideration to determine an individual caries risk level for each patient.			
Social history	Dentally aware. Regularly scheduled dental visits. Low caries rate in family members.	Low knowledge of dental disease. Irregular or nonexistent dental visits. Family history of caries and generally poor oral health. Personal history of recreational drug use.		
Medical history	No serious medical problems. No or few medications. Normal salivary flow. No physical problems or handicaps.	Medically compromised. Disabled/handicapped. Xerostomia (side effect of medications or systemic disease). Radiation therapy.		
Use of fluoride	Drinks/cooks with fluoridated water. Lived in a fluoridated community as a child. Uses fluoride dentifrice and/or fluoride mouthrinse regularly.	Does not drink fluoridated water. Did not live in a fluoridated community as a child. Irregular or nonexistent use of fluoridated dentifrice or fluoride rinses. Irregular personal oral care habits.		
Dietary habits	Infrequent fermentable carbohydrate intake. Rarely snacks between meals. Avoids acidic beverages between meals. Uses xylitol gum or mints between meals	Frequent sugar intake. Snacks frequently. Not familiar with USDA MyPlate. Uses chewing tobacco frequently.		
Clinical/oral	Regular brushing at least 2 times daily. Daily interdental cleansing. No prostheses, orthodontics, or other special care requirement. Good hand dexterity; no handicap. Low biofilm scores.	History of previous caries experience. Current cavitated lesions. Noncavitated (white) lesions. Multiple restorations. Unsealed deep pits and fissures. Exposed root surfaces; previously restored root surfaces.		
Bitewing radiographs vertical bitewings for root caries	Every 24–36 mo	Every 18–24 mo	Every 6–18 mo	Every 6 mo until no cavitated lesions are observed.
Frequency of caries recall examination	Every 6 mo	Every 4–6 mo	Every 3–4 mo	Every 3 mo
Chemotherapeutic management	OTC fluoride dentifrice Optional NaF varnish if root exposure or sensitivity	OTC fluoride toothpaste 0.05% NaF rinse daily Initial 1–2 application of NaF varnish, plus application at 4–6 mo recall	Fluoride varnish every 3–4 mo 1.1% NaF toothpaste used 2× daily 0.05% NaF rinse 2× daily	Fluoride varnish every 3 mo 1.1% NaF toothpaste used 2× daily 0.05% NaF rinse 2× daily
		Xylitol gum or candy 4× daily Optional: calcium phosphate topical paste if excessive root exposure	Initial 1–3 applications of NaF varnish, plus application at 3–4 mo recall Chlorhexidine rinse one minute daily for 1 wk each month Xylitol gum or candy 4× daily Optional: calcium phosphate topical paste	Initial 1–3 applications of NaF varnish, plus application at 3 mo recall Chlorhexidine rinse one minute daily for 1 wk each month Xylitol gum or candy 4× daily Acid-neutralizing rinses as needed if mouth feels dry Required: calcium phosphate topical paste 2× daily
Sealants	Optional	Recommended	Recommended	Recommended

[a]Patients with one or more cavitated lesions are assigned a *high* risk level.

[b]When xerostomia is present in addition to cavitated lesions, the *extreme* risk level is assigned.

Adapted with permission from Jenson L, Budnez AW, Featherstone JD, et al. Clinical protocols for caries management by risk assessment. *J Calif Dent Assoc.* 2007;35(10):714–723.

- Apply principles of motivational interviewing to encourage patient to initiate caries preventive strategies to family and other closely related individuals.
- Be a guide for the management of a caries prevention plan to reverse demineralizing lesions.

B. Identify and Evaluate Risk Factors[11]

- Information collected during patient medical, dental, and social history interview, includes:
  - Medications that promote dry mouth.
  - Systemic factors that affect oral health.
  - Patient *perception of need* may be seen in past dental experiences, family, and cultural influences.
  - *Value placed on oral health* can be detected by understanding the patient's perspective on appearance, cost, and personal time involved.
  - *Past dental experience* as shown by primary prevention (sealants), secondary prevention (restorations), and tertiary prevention (extractions and replacement of teeth).
  - *Fluoride history* in the form of home water fluoridation and availability of community water supply fluoridation throughout life.
  - Other exposures to fluoride, including dentifrice use over the years and professional application.
  - *Success in changing habits*, such as the person who was a tobacco user but was able to cease use completely can be very indicative of the patient's ability to reduce or eliminate caries-producing habits.
- Patient-centered interview
  - Briefly introduce a checklist to show current daily care and fluoride history.
  - A motivational interviewing approach can encourage the patient to look at current habits as causes of oral problems.
- Food diary
  - For an analysis of sugar exposures, see Figure 35-7 (Chapter 35).
  - Food diary form is illustrated in Figure 35-5, Chapter 35.

C. Application

- Preparation of an individualized approach with emphasis on remineralization of early, noncavitated lesions can lay the groundwork for a successful program.
- Most patients will learn very little about the seriousness of their problem if handed a checklist of things to be done every day.
- Participation in the process can inform the patient (and parents) of the needs and ways of coping with change.
- The list of questions in Box 27-2 can help a patient check off the factors that apply to personal lifestyle and oral health habits.

BOX 27-2

Patient's Checklist

ORAL HEALTH CHECK SHEET

Name: _____ Date: _____

PLEASE CHECK "YES" OR "NO" OR FILL IN OTHER

	Yes	No	Other (please write)
1. Fluoride in your drinking water as a small child?			
2. Fluoride in your drinking water where you live now?			
3. Use toothpaste with fluoride in it now? Favorite kind? _____			
4. Brush at least twice each day?			
5. Use dental floss every day?			
6. Wear orthodontic appliances?			
7. Use sugar-free chewing gum when you chew gum?			
8. Have dry mouth most of the time?			
9. Sip on beverages other than water throughout the day? Mostly what?_____			
10. Snack frequently? Mostly what?_____			

IV. Systemic Disease Factors

▶ Identify diseases, conditions, and medications that contribute or may cause dry mouth (xerostomia).

▶ Medically or nutritionally compromised patients may be at increased risk for dental caries and need additional preventive measures.

PLANNING CARE[11]

▶ The dental hygienist is challenged to select a management strategy to meet the needs of each individual patient.

▶ The care plan will not only need to provide for treatment of existing nonreversible carious lesions but also provide a framework for changes in personal care previously unrecognized by the patient to prevent development of new lesions.

▶ A plan for care is individualized depending on the disease risk level, physical and cognitive abilities, and patient or parent desire to change.

▶ A variety of patients present for dental hygiene care.

- On the one side will be the patient with no current new dental caries, but a few simple questions may reveal a patient with irregular habits of diet and personal oral care that could lead to serious problems later.

- At the opposite extreme is the need for early recognition of uncontrolled disease that presents as cavitated lesions in need of dental restorative care.

I. Recommendations for Specific Caries Risk Levels

A. The Patient with Low Caries Risk

▶ Primary prevention remains a top priority, as changes in habits may increase caries risk.

▶ Provide the patient with positive feedback and education so oral, periodontal, and dental health can be maintained.

▶ Review with the patient the existing habits that categorize them at *low caries risk*, such as good oral daily biofilm removal, healthy snacking habits, and daily exposure to fluoride.

▶ Recommend routine continuing care appointments.

B. The Patient with Moderate Caries Risk

▶ This patient exhibits factors that increase their risk for developing dental carious lesions.

▶ Provide the patient with positive feedback and support for the protective factors they currently exhibit, such as fluoride use, healthy snacking habits, or sugar-free chewing gum use.

▶ Work with the patient to guide them to reduce risk factors, such as acidic beverages, frequent fermentable carbohydrate snacks, improved daily biofilm removal.

- Discuss addition of caries-preventive foods to diet, such as nuts, sugar-free yogurt, cheese.[12]

- Allowing the patient to help choose behavior changes increases compliance.

▶ Increasing protective factors can be accomplished by the dental hygienist especially sealant placement and fluoride application.

▶ Recommend appropriate continuing care schedule.

C. The Patient with High Caries Risk

▶ The patient at high risk for caries displays *active carious* lesions, has a *recent history of restoration* to repair carious lesions, or may have *medications or systemic factors* that cause severe dry mouth.

▶ The nidus of infection needs to be addressed and active lesions restored.

▶ Bacterial infection can be reduced and controlled with fluoride application, daily biofilm removal, and antimicrobial therapy.

▶ Evaluation and strategies for reducing existing risk factors are addressed.

▶ Strategies for increasing protective factors are an important part of this discussion.

▶ Recommend appropriate continuing care schedule. Assess caries risk at regular intervals. Review current habits and address as needed.

D. Caries Management Protocols

▶ Table 27-1 gives examples of recommendations for preventive, maintenance, and therapeutic interventions to manage and lower caries risk.

▶ Some recommended products and protocols require a prescription while others are available to the patient over-the-counter (OTC).

A PROTOCOL FOR REMINERALIZATION[5]

▶ A first approach to treating dental caries as an infectious disease is to eliminate as many of the causative factors as possible.

▶ Of primary importance is daily removal of the acid-forming bacteria and the fermentable carbohydrates that allow the harmful bacteria to survive and multiply.

▶ When appropriate, advise close personal contacts and caregivers to have their own teeth checked and cavitated carious lesions restored.

I. Remove the Nidus of Infection

A. Restoration of All Carious Lesions

▶ Dental caries is a multifactorial disease. It is necessary to know the source of the infection prior to making treatment decisions.

▶ Dental carious lesions contain large numbers of acidogenic bacteria, especially *mutans streptococci* and lactobacilli. Cavitated carious lesions need to be restored or bacteria from within the lesion will remain a source of infection.

▶ Well-placed restorations with well-sealed margins will help lower the bacterial counts in the oral cavity.

▶ Restorative materials containing fluoride are recommended wherever possible.

▶ Properly placed sealants close off the pits and fissures where microorganisms can live, multiply, and contribute to carious lesion development. Microorganisms cannot survive under a properly placed sealant.

▶ Family members can continue to harbor cariogenic microorganisms.
  • Having close family members address and reduce their caries risk will further reduce individual exposure to these pathogens.

II. Initiate Daily Preventive Measures

A. Personal Fluoride Use

▶ Use fluoridated water; fill personal drinking bottles from faucets giving fluoridated water.

▶ Fluoride-containing dentifrice 2–3 times per day with brushing at least 3 minutes.

▶ Alcohol-free fluoride mouthrinse daily; may recommend daily gel tray.

▶ Use 1.1% neutral sodium fluoride dentifrice before bed with no further eating or drinking.

B. Dietary Modifications

▶ Eliminate fermentable carbohydrate exposures between meals and at the ends of meals.

▶ Select snacks from nonfermentable carbohydrate foods; avoid sweetened beverages.

C. Chew Sugar-Free Gum at Ends of Meals

▶ Use sugar-free chewing gum, with xylitol.[11,13]

▶ Xylitol reduces levels of *mutans streptococci* and promotes remineralization.

III. Professional and Prescribed Applications

▶ Caries management for high caries risk patients may include rinsing with 0.12% chlorhexidine, once a day with 10 ml for 1 minute 1 week each month.[11]

▶ Chlorhexidine is highly effective against mutans streptococcus infections.

▶ Neutral sodium fluoride 1.1% dentifrice applied twice daily for the 3 weeks following chlorhexidine short-term rinse.[12]

▶ Fluoride varnish applications at dental hygiene appointments.[11]

CONTINUING CARE

Managing dental caries means the clinician evaluates patient compliance at regular intervals. Continuing care planning begins prior to dismissing the patient.

I. Prior to Continuing Care Appointment

▶ Review the individualized caries management strategies with the patient.

▶ Follow-up with the patient through telephone and e-mail messages during the first month. This can help to show the concern of the dental hygienist for the patient and the oral health problems.

▶ Customized continuing care intervals needs to established to target the patient's highest risk factor for oral disease.
  • For instance, if caries disease risk is higher than risk of periodontal disease, a shorter maintenance interval may be prudent.

▶ Customize maintenance care appointments to monitor, educate, and apply preventive and therapeutic measures as necessary to manage or reduce caries risk.

▶ Motivational interviewing principles apply when evaluating all oral conditions at continuing care appointments.

II. Continuing Care Procedure

Continuing care appointments include the following:

▶ Biofilm control check: Use disclosing agent and record the biofilm score. Address oral care issues.

▶ Clinical detection for demineralization areas, need for sealants, and poor margins on restorations.

▶ Radiographs are never routine. Radiographs are prescribed only when specifically indicated by level of risk and clinical findings.

▶ Discuss details of the continuation of the remineralization program.

▶ Reassess patient compliance with fluoride therapy.

▶ Need for repeat short-term antimicrobial therapy as determined by current caries risk level. Patients with high caries risk who are on chlorhexidine therapy are seen for continuing care visits every 3 months until risk is reduced. Intervals of longer than 4 months may never be optimal for these patients, as bacterial challenges can occur at any time.

▶ Appropriate professional fluoride application.[11]

DOCUMENTATION

Caries risk assessment and risk level are documented at each continuing care visit. The principles of CAMBRA allow the clinician to evaluate and document patient

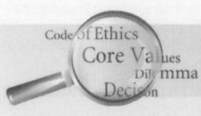

EVERYDAY ETHICS

Sophie and Helen were two sisters who had been Dr. Newbury's patients for the past 30 years. Now in their 70s, they were experiencing new concerns with restorations and crowns that showed signs of occlusal wear and recurrent caries. Many margins of amalgam restorations had catches with the explorer upon examination.

Ken, the dental hygienist, continued to stress the importance of more frequent continuing care visits, but Sophie curtly reminded him that she "has been coming to the dentist since before he was born!" Ken suspected they did not want to hear about crowns that should be replaced or make decisions about the restorations that needed replacement.

A progress note in Helen's chart read, "the patient was not open to new homecare education techniques or interested in a proposed treatment plan to replace amalgam restorations in teeth 15, 18, 19, 30, and 31."

Questions for Consideration

1. What ethical principles and dental hygiene Core Values are involved as Ken thinks about how to help these patients understand the need for treatment that they have stated they do not want?

2. Does the entry in the patient's chart provide sufficient information to document informed refusal? Why or why not? Explain your rationale using legal and ethical concepts in Table V-1 in Section V Introduction.

3. Consult the Decision Alternatives Through Questioning steps Table VI-1 in Section VI Introduction to determine at least two alternative approaches Ken might pursue in order to deliver a professional standard of care for these patients without compromising their rights.

progress including the determination of caries risk and patient compliance with previously prescribed protocols. Also integral to CAMBRA are minimally invasive therapies to control active caries and save enamel structure. These restorative procedures can be planned by the dentist as part of the caries management plan.

Thorough documentation includes assessment results, all discussion with the patient, instruction given, and patient response at each appointment.

▶ Initial planning: Record all instruction and survey report from the analysis of risk factors.

▶ Note specific oral care and dietary changes recommended and follow-up successes noted.

▶ Note any phone or e-mail follow-up messages.

▶ At continuing care, note patient comments on individual efforts, likes and dislikes, successes, and changes that can be made to improve success.

▶ Evaluation of teeth and periodontal tissues with probing and visual examinations.

▶ A sample of documentation can be found in Box 27-3.

BOX 27-3

Example Documentation: Patient with High Caries Risk

S –Admits drinking in the afternoon while studying. Chews lots of gum containing sugar. Brushes twice daily, but admits to flossing only a couple of times a week. Snacks frequently.

O –Resting pH—7.2; CRA—moderate. Moderate generalized biofilm in embrasures on disclosing with plaque-free score of 50%.

A –Increased risk for dental caries.

P –Recommended patient drink soda only during meals and sip fluoridated water while studying, chew sugar-free or xylitol gum, and use 1.1% sodium fluoride gel or paste daily. Discussed alternatives to flossing. Demonstrated interdental brushes. Pt. liked interdental brushes and said he would try to use them daily while studying. Reassess at 6 month continuing care visit.

Signed _____, RDH

Date _____

Factors To Teach The Patient

▷ What causes cavities and how they develop.

▷ Early dental caries is not a cavity: explain to the patient what demineralization means.

▷ How remineralization can be helped by using fluoride toothpaste and drinking fluoridated water daily.

▷ Use of appropriate fluoride based on risk for dental caries is necessary throughout life.

References

1. Featherstone JD. The science and practice of caries prevention. *J Am Dent Assoc.* 2000;131(7):887–899.

2. Palmer CA, Kent R Jr, Loo CY, et al. Diet and caries-associated bacteria in severe early childhood caries. *J Dent Res.* 2010;89(11):1224–1229.

3. Caufield PW, Cutter GR, Dasanayake AP. Initial acquisition of *mutans streptococci* by infants: evidence for a discrete window of infectivity. *J Dent Res*. 1993;72(1):37–45.

4. Featherstone JD. Prevention and reversal of dental caries: role of low-level fluoride. *Community Dent Oral Epidemiol*. 1999;27(1):31–40.

5. González-Cabezas C. The chemistry of caries: remineralization and demineralization events with direct clinical relevance. *Dent Clin North Am*. 2010;54:469–478.

6. Pitts NB. Clinical diagnosis of dental caries: a European perspective. *J Dent Educ*. 2001;65(10):972–978.

7. Kidd EA. Caries management. *Dent Clin North Am*. 1999;43(4):743–764.

8. van Dorp CS, Exterkate RA, ten Cate JM. The effect of dental probing on subsequent enamel demineralization. *ASDC J Dent Child*. 1988;55(5):343–347.

9. Warren JJ, Levy SM, Wefel JS. Explorer probing of root caries lesions: an *in vitro* study. *Spec Care Dentist*. 2003;23(1):18–21.

10. Beltrán-Aguilar EO, Barker LK, Canto MT, et al. Surveillance for dental caries, dental sealants, tooth retention, edentulism, and enamel fluorosis—United States, 1988–1994 and 1999–2002. *MMWR Surveill Summ*. 2005;54(3):1–43.

11. Jenson L, Budenz AW, Featherstsone JDB, et al. Clinical protocols for caries management by risk assessment. *J Calif Dent Assoc*. 2007;35(10):714–723.

12. Sönmez IS, Aras S. Effects of white cheese and sugarless yoghurt on dental plaque acidogenicity. *Caries Res*. 2007;41:208–211.

13. Hayes C. The effect of non-cariogenic sweeteners on the prevention of dental caries: a review of the evidence. *J Dent Educ*. 2001;65(10):1106–1109.

ENHANCE YOUR UNDERSTANDING

thePoint® DIGITAL CONNECTIONS
(see the inside front cover for access information)
- **Audio glossary**
- **Quiz bank**

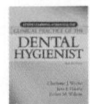

SUPPORT FOR LEARNING
(available separately; visit lww.com)
- *Active Learning Workbook for Clinical Practice of the Dental Hygienist, 12th Edition*

prepU INDIVIDUALIZED REVIEW
(available separately; visit lww.com)
- **Adaptive quizzing with *prepU for Wilkins' Clinical Practice of the Dental Hygienist***

28

Oral Infection Control: Toothbrushes and Toothbrushing

Christine Macarelli-Rogers, RDH, MS and Karen A. Raposa, RDH, MBA

CHAPTER OUTLINE

LEARNING OBJECTIVES

After studying this chapter, the student will be able to:

1. Identify characteristics of effective manual and power toothbrushes.

2. Differentiate between the different manual toothbrushing methods including limitations and benefits of each.

3. Describe the different motions of action for powered toothbrushes.

4. Identify the basis for powered toothbrush selection.

5. Describe tongue cleaning and its effect on reducing dental biofilm.

6. Identify negative effects improper toothbrushing can have on hard and soft tissues.

INTRODUCTION

▶ The personal oral healthcare plan for prevention interventions is determined by assessing each patient's oral health needs, dental caries risk factors, periodontal infection risk factors, and the patient's ability to perform self-care procedures.

▶ The dental hygienist has a professional ethical obligation to review current research and select appropriate methods and oral care devices that meets the needs of each patient or parent/caregiver.

▶ An objective for the dental hygienist is to teach and motivate each patient and the caregiver to maintain the oral cavity in a clean healthy state.

▶ Personal daily care requires the following sequence of procedures at least two times each day:
- Use dental floss first to remove biofilm from proximal surfaces and debris that may have collected in the interproximal embrasures.
- Flossing before brushing allows access of the proximal tooth surfaces and interdental gingiva to fluoride and other agents in the toothpaste for dental caries prevention and gingival health.
- Toothbrushing follows flossing to remove the adhering biofilm from tooth surfaces and to apply preventive agents to the gingival tissues and teeth.
- A final step in oral cleanliness and health is to clean the tongue.

▶ The toothbrush has been the principal instrument in general use for oral care and is a necessary part of oral disease control. Many different designs of both manual and power toothbrushes have been manufactured and promoted. Uses of the toothbrush include the following:
- Dental biofilm removal
- Application of preventive agents
- Contribute to halitosis control
- Sanitation of oral cavity.

▶ Patients who have not previously received professional advice concerning the best brush for their particular oral conditions may have used brushes selected on the following criteria:
- Cost
- Availability
- Advertising claims
- Family tradition
- Habit.

▶ Because of the variety of brushes currently available, and the constant development of new brushes, dental professionals need to maintain a high level of knowledge on these products to advise patients appropriately.

▶ Key words relating to toothbrushes are listed in Box 28-1 with their definitions.

DEVELOPMENT OF TOOTHBRUSHES

▶ Crudely contrived toothpicks, presumably used for relief from food impaction, are believed to be the earliest implements devised for the care of the teeth.

▶ Excavations in Mesopotamia uncovered elaborate gold toothpicks used by the Sumerians about 3000 B.C.

▶ The earliest record of the "chewstick," which has been considered the primitive toothbrush, dates back in the Chinese literature to about 1600 B.C. The care of the mouth was associated with religious training and ritual: the Buddhists had a "toothstick," and the Mohammedans used the "miswak" or "siwak." Chewsticks, made from various types of woods by crushing an end and spreading the fibers in a brush-like manner, are still used in several regions of the world.[1]

▶ The *Ebers Papyrus*, compiled about 1500 B.C. and dating probably to about 4000 B.C., contained reference to oral conditions similar to periodontal diseases and to preparations used as mouthwashes and dentifrices. The writings of Hippocrates (about 300 B.C.) include descriptions of diseased gums related to calculus and of complex preparations for the treatment of unhealthy mouths.[1–4]

I. Early Toothbrushes

▶ It is believed the first tooth brush made of hog's bristles was mentioned in the early Chinese literature.

▶ Pierre Fauchard in 1728 in *Le Chirurgien Dentiste* described many aspects of oral health. He condemned the toothbrush made of horse's hair because it was rough and destructive to the teeth and advised the use of sponges or herb roots.

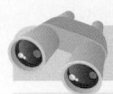

BOX 28-1   KEY WORDS: Toothbrushes

Abrasion (gingiva): lesion of the gingiva that results from mechanical removal of the surface epithelium.

Abrasion (tooth): loss of tooth structure produced by a mechanical cause (such as a hard-bristled toothbrush used with excessive pressure and an abrasive dentifrice); abrasion contrasts with erosion, which involves a chemical process.

Angled: a nylon filament that is placed in the brush head at an angle.

Bristle: individual short, stiff, natural hair of an animal; historically, toothbrush bristles were taken from a hog or wild boar, but current toothbrush bristles are made of nylon and are called filaments.

End-rounded: characteristic shape of each toothbrush filament; a special manufacturing process removes all sharp edges and provides smooth, rounded ends to prevent injury to gingiva or tooth structure during use.

Filament: individual synthetic fiber; a single element of a tuft fixed into a toothbrush head.

Mechanical biofilm control: oral hygiene methods for removal of dental biofilm from tooth surfaces using a toothbrush and selected devices for interdental cleaning;

contrasts with chemotherapeutic biofilm control in which an antimicrobial agent is used.

Power toothbrush: a brush driven by electricity or battery; also called power-assisted, automatic, electric, or mechanical (in contrast with manual toothbrush).

Sonic: a term used to describe a power toothbrush that operates in the audible range of human hearing.

Stiffness: the reaction force exerted per unit area of the brush during deflection; the term stiffness is used interchangeably with firmness of toothbrush bristles or filaments; the stiffness depends primarily on the length and diameter of the filaments.

Sulcular brushing: a method in which the end-round filament tips are directed into the gingival sulcus at approximately 45° for the purpose of loosening and removing dental biofilm from both the gingival sulcus and the tooth surface just below the gingival margin.

Toothbrush head: the part of the toothbrush composed of the tufts and the stock (extension of the handle where the tufts are attached).

Tuft: a cluster of bristles or filaments secured together in one hole in the head of a toothbrush.

▶ Fauchard recommended scaling of teeth and developed instruments and splints for loose teeth, as well as dentifrices and mouthwashes.

▶ One of the earlier toothbrushes made in England was produced by William Addis about 1780.

 • By the early 19th century, craftsmen in various European countries constructed handles of gold, ivory, or ebony in which replaceable brush heads could be fitted.

 • The first patent for a toothbrush in the United States was issued to H. N. Wadsworth in the middle of the 19th century.

▶ Many new varieties of toothbrushes were developed around 1,900, when celluloid was available for the manufacture of toothbrush handles.

 • In 1919, the American Academy of Periodontology defined specifications for toothbrush design and brushing methods in an attempt to standardize professional recommendations.[5]

▶ Nylon came into use in toothbrush construction in 1938.

 • World War II prevented Chinese export of wild boar bristles so synthetic materials were substituted for natural bristles.

 • Since then, synthetic materials have been improved and manufacturers' specifications standardized.

 • Most toothbrushes are made exclusively of synthetic materials.

▶ Power toothbrushes, although developed earlier, were not actively promoted until the 1960s.

II. Early Brushing Methods

▶ Historically, the purpose of brushing was to provide *massage* to increase the disease resistance of the gingival tissue.

 • Massage or friction from a hard-bristled brush was believed to *increase keratinization*, which, in turn, resulted in the resistance to bacterial invasion.[5]

▶ As quoted in Box 28-2, Koecker described, in 1842, a "new" method for daily care of teeth.[6] This early work proved to be a forerunner of contemporary oral care.

BOX 28-2

Historical Perspective on Proper Toothbrushing Instruction

Koecker, in 1842,[6] wrote that after the dentist has scaled off the tartar, the patient will clean the teeth every morning and after every meal with a hard brush and an astringent powder. For the inner surfaces, he recommended a conical-shaped brush of fine hog's bristles. For the outer surfaces, he believed in an oblong brush made of the "best white horsehair." He instructed the patient to press hard against the gums so the bristles go between the teeth and "between the edges of the gums and the roots of the teeth. The pressure of the brush is to be applied in the direction from the crowns of the teeth towards the roots, so that the mucus, which adheres to the roots under the edges of the gums, may be completely detached, and after that, removed by the friction in a direction towards the grinding surfaces."

MANUAL TOOTHBRUSHES

I. Characteristics of an Effective Toothbrush[7]

▶ Conforms to individual patient requirements in size, shape, and texture.

▶ Easily and efficiently manipulated.

▶ Readily cleaned and aerated; impervious to moisture.

▶ Durable and inexpensive.

▶ Functional properties of flexibility, softness, and diameter of the bristles or filaments, and of strength, rigidity, and lightness of the handle.

▶ End-rounded filaments.

▶ Designed for utility, efficiency, and cleanliness.

II. General Description

A. Parts (Figure 28-1)

▶ *Handle*: the part grasped in the hand during toothbrushing.

▶ *Head*: the working end; consists of tufts of bristles or filaments and the stock where the tufts are secured.

▶ *Shank*: the section that connects the head and the handle.

B. Dimensions

▶ *Total brush length*: about 15–19 cm (6–7.5 inches); junior and child sizes are shorter.

▶ *Head*: large enough to accommodate the tufts.

• Length of brushing plane, 25.4–31.8 mm (1–11/4 inches); width, 7.9–9.5 mm (5/16–3/8 inch).

• Bristle or filament height, 11 mm (7/16 inch).

III. Handle

A. Composition

▶ *Manufacturing specifications*: Most often a single type of plastic, or a combination of polymers.

▶ *Properties*: Combines durability, imperviousness to moisture, pleasing appearance, low cost, and sufficient maneuverability.

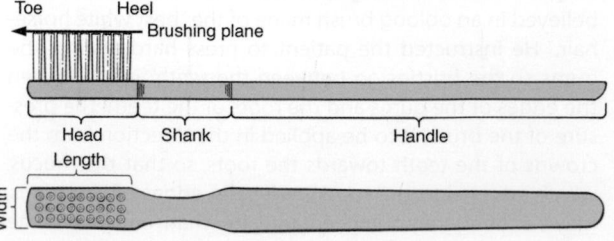

FIGURE 28-1 Parts of a Toothbrush.

B. Shape

▶ *Preferred characteristics*

• Easy to grasp.

• Does not slip or rotate during use.

• No sharp corners or projections.

• Lightweight, consistent with strength.

▶ *Variations*

• A twist, curve, offset, or angle in the shank with or without thumb rests may assist the patient in adaptation of the brush to difficult-to-reach areas.

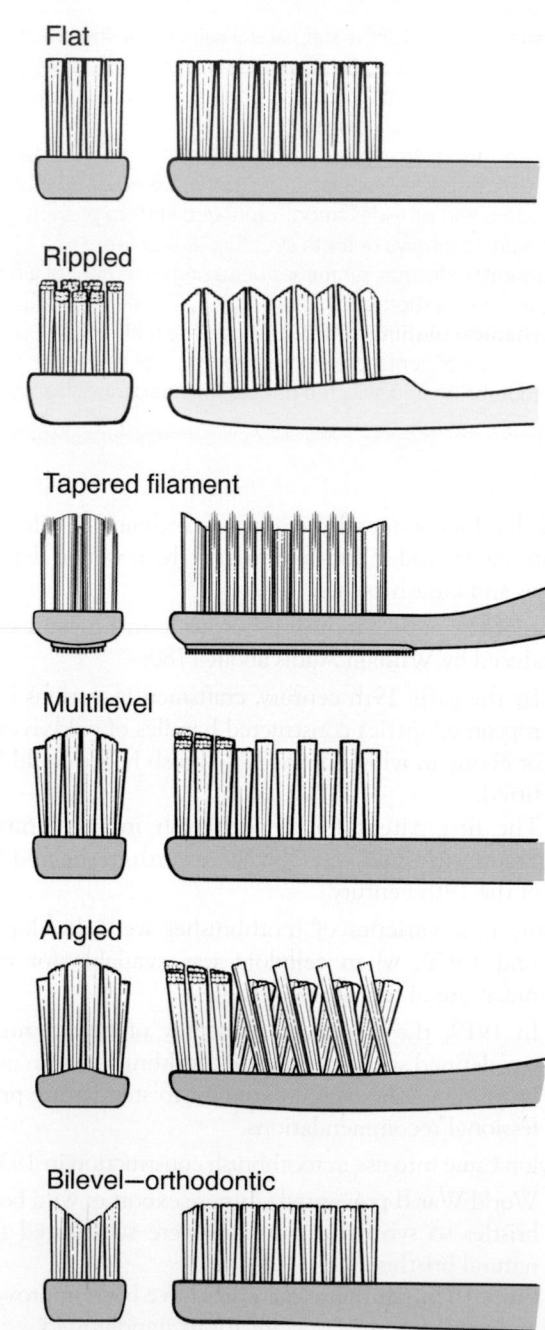

Flat

Rippled

Tapered filament

Multilevel

Angled

Bilevel—orthodontic

FIGURE 28-2 Manual Brush Trim Profiles. A variety of filament profiles are available. In addition to the classic flat planed brush, other trims include the rippled, tapered filaments, bilevel, multilevel, and angled. Brushes for use over orthodontic appliances are made with various bilevel shapes.

- A handle of larger diameter may be useful for patients with limited dexterity, such as children, aging patients, and those with a disability.

IV. Brush Head

A. Design

▶ *Length*: May be 5–12 tufts long and 3–4 rows wide.

▶ *Spacing*: Tufts that are widely spaced allow for easy cleaning. Those closely spaced allow the filaments to support each other.

▶ *Arrangement*: Tufts may be of a consistent shape on the brush head or varied as shown in Figure 28-2.

B. Brushing Plane (Profile)

▶ *Trim*: Variously shaped filament profiles.

▶ *Length*: Range from filaments of equal lengths (flat planes) to those with variable lengths, such as rippled, tapered, bilevel, multilevel, and angled (Figure 28-2).

▶ *Properties*: Soft and end-rounded for safety to oral soft tissues and tooth structure.

▶ *Efficiency in biofilm removal*: Efficiency for cleaning the hard-to-reach areas, such as extension onto proximal surfaces, malpositioned teeth, or exposed root surfaces, depends on individual patient abilities and understanding.

V. Bristles and Filaments

▶ Most current toothbrushes have nylon filaments.

- Natural bristles are relatively unsanitary, and their physical qualifications cannot be standardized.

- A comparison of natural bristles and synthetic filaments is reviewed in Table 28-1.

▶ Many manufacturers of synthetic filaments continue to refer to filaments as "bristles" when communicating with consumers on the toothbrush package and in advertising.

- Dental professionals need to be aware that most manufacturers of toothbrushes today produce brushes using "synthetic filaments" but still refer to these as "bristles."

▶ Companies that produce a toothbrush with "natural bristles" will distinguish themselves by using the word "natural" in the product description.

A. Factors Influencing Stiffness

The stiffness depends on the diameter and length of the filament. Brushes designated as soft, medium, or hard are not comparatively consistent between manufacturers.

▶ *Diameter*: Thinner filaments are softer and more resilient.

▶ *Length*: Shorter filaments are stiffer and have less flexibility.

▶ *Number of filaments in a tuft*: Increased density of filaments and tufts give added support to adjacent filaments, thus increasing the feeling of stiffness.

▶ *Angle of filaments*: Angled filaments may be more flexible and less stiff than straight filaments of equal length and diameter; there is no straight end-line force applied as with the straight filament.

B. End-Rounding

▶ *Process of end-rounding*: Each nylon filament is sealed and rounded by heat treatment. The quality of end-rounding varies depending on manufacturers.[8] Natural bristles cannot be end-rounded.

TABLE 28-1	Comparison of Natural Bristles and Synthetic Filaments	
	NATURAL BRISTLES	**FILAMENTS**
Source	Historically made from hair of hog or wild boar	Synthetic, plastic materials, primarily nylon
Uniformity	No uniformity of texture. Diameter or wearing properties depending upon the breed of animal, geographical location, and season in which the bristles were gathered	Uniformity controlled during manufacturing
Diameter	Varies depending on portion of bristle taken, age, and life of animal	Range from extra soft at 0.075 mm (0.003 inch) to hard at 0.3 mm (0.012 inch)
End shape	Deficient, irregular, frequently open ended	End-rounded to ensure fewer traumas. There is a direct relation between gingival damage and the absence of end-rounding[8,9]; Figure 28-3 shows examples of nonrounded and end-rounded filaments[10]
Advantages and disadvantages	■ Cannot be standardized ■ Wear rapidly and irregularly ■ Hollow ends allow microorganisms and debris to collect inside	■ Rinse clean, dry rapidly ■ Durable and maintain longer ■ End-rounded and closed, repel debris and water ■ More resistant to accumulation of microorganisms

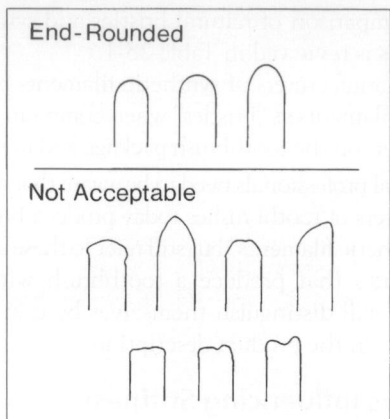

FIGURE 28-3 End-Rounded Filaments. Examples of the shape of acceptable end-rounding and of those that are not acceptable are shown. (Adapted from: Silverstone LM, Featherstone MJ. A scanning electron microscope study of the end rounding of bristles in eight toothbrush types. *Quintessence Int.* 1988;19(2):87–107 and Checchi L, Minguzzi S, Franchi M, et al. Toothbrush filaments end-rounding: stereomicroscope analysis. *J Clin Periodontol.* 2001;28(4):360–364.)

▸ *Effect:* A direct relation exists between gingival damage and the absence of end-rounding.[9,10]
▸ *Examples:* Figure 28-3 shows examples of nonrounded and end-rounded filaments.

TOOTHBRUSH SELECTION FOR THE PATIENT

I. Influencing Factors

Factors influencing the selection of the proper manual or power toothbrush for an individual patient include the following:

A. Patient
▸ Ability of the patient to use the brush and remove dental biofilm from tooth surfaces without damage to the soft tissue or tooth structure.
▸ Manual dexterity of the patient.
▸ The age of the patient and the differences in the dentition and dexterity.

B. Gingiva
▸ Status of gingival and periodontal health.
▸ Anatomic configurations of the gingiva.

C. Position of Teeth
Displaced teeth require variations in brush placement:
▸ Crowded teeth
▸ Open contacts.

D. Compliance
▸ Patient preference may dictate which method and which brush is recommended.

▸ Patient may have preferences and may resist change.
▸ Patient may lack motivation, ability, or willingness to follow the prescribed procedure.

E. Method Selected
Professional personnel may prefer to instruct patients in certain methods and with certain brushes.

II. Toothbrush Size and Shape
▸ Brush head selection is dependent on the patient's ability to maneuver and adapt the brush correctly to all facial, lingual, palatal, and occlusal surfaces for dental biofilm removal.
▸ Multilevel brush heads have been shown to be beneficial and were developed on the basis of their ability to improve cleaning performance and to reach critical sites easier (i.e., interproximal and at the gingival margin).[11]

III. Soft Nylon Brush

The following are suggested as advantages for the appropriate use of a soft end-rounded brush.
▸ More effective in cleaning the cervical areas, both proximal and marginal.
▸ Less traumatic to the gingival tissue; therefore, patients can brush the cervical areas without fear of discomfort or soft tissue laceration.
▸ Can be directed into the sulcus for sulcular brushing and into interproximal areas for partially cleaning of the proximal surfaces.
▸ Applicable around fixed orthodontic appliances or fixation appliances used to treat a fractured jaw.
▸ Tooth abrasion and/or gingival recession can be prevented or may be less severe in an overvigorous brusher.
▸ More effective for sensitive gingiva in such conditions such as necrotizing ulcerative gingivitis or severe gingivitis, or during healing stages following scaling and debridement or periodontal surgery.
▸ Small size is ideal for a young child as a first brush on primary teeth.

GUIDELINES FOR MANUAL TOOTHBRUSHING

▸ Comprehensive toothbrushing instruction for a patient involves teaching what, when, where, and how.
▸ In addition to description of specific toothbrushing methods, the succeeding sections consider the grasp of the brush, the sequence and amount of brushing, the areas of limited access, and supplementary brushing for the occlusal surfaces and the tongue.
▸ The possible detrimental effects from improper toothbrushing and variations for special conditions are described.

I. Grasp of Brush

A. Objectives

▶ Grasp and manipulate the brush for successful removal of dental biofilm.

▶ Provide patients with specific instruction in how to hold and place the brush.

▶ Remove dental biofilm that has been colored with a disclosing agent to show the tenaciousness of the biofilm and the need for controlled pressure.

▶ Using a light, comfortable grasp, the following can be expected:

- Control of the brush during all movements.
- Effective positioning at the beginning of each brushing stroke, follow-through during the complete stroke, and repositioning for the next stroke.
- Sensitivity to the amount of pressure applied.

B. Procedure

▶ Grasp toothbrush handle in the palm of the hand with thumb against the shank.

- Near enough to the head of the brush so it can be controlled effectively.
- Not so close to the head of the brush that manipulation of the brush is hindered or fingers can touch the anterior teeth when reaching the brush head to molar regions.

▶ Position filaments in the proper direction for placement on the teeth; direction depends on the brushing method to be used.

▶ Adapt grasp for the various positions of the brush head on the teeth throughout the procedure; adjust to permit unrestricted movement of the wrist and arm.

▶ Apply appropriate pressure for removal of the dental biofilm. Too much pressure, however, bends the filaments and curves them away from the area where brushing is needed.

II. Sequence

▶ The procedure in brushing, for any method, needs to ensure complete coverage for each tooth surface.

▶ Divide the mouth into quadrants.

▶ Start brushing from a molar region of one arch around to the midline facial then lingual.

▶ Use brush in vertical position for narrow anterior teeth.

▶ Repeat in the opposing arch.

▶ Each brush placement will overlap the previous one for thorough coverage as shown in Figure 28-4.

▶ Encourage the patient to begin by brushing one of the areas of greatest individual need as shown by disclosing agent.

- Areas most frequently missed.
- Areas most difficult for brush placement and/or manipulation, such as the right side for the right-handed brusher or the left side for the left-handed brusher.

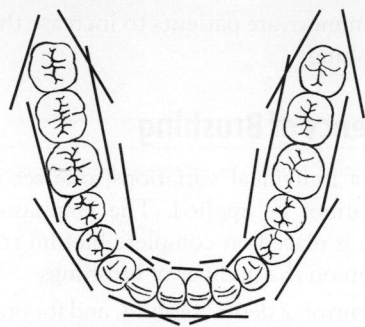

FIGURE 28-4 Brushing Positions. Each brush position, as represented by a black line, will overlap the previous position. Note placement at canines, where the distal aspect of the canine is brushed with the premolars and the mesial aspect is brushed with the incisors. Short lines on the lingual anterior aspect indicate brush placed vertically. The maxillary teeth require a similar number of brushing positions.

▶ Suggest the sequence be varied at least once each day so that the same areas are not always brushed last when time may be limited and biofilm removal may be less complete.

III. Amount of Brushing

▶ The main consideration is the removal of the dental biofilm. For infection control, dental biofilm needs to be removed from all surfaces of all teeth as completely as possible daily.

▶ The number of strokes and length of time spent depend on the patient's ability and efficiency in accomplishing the task.

A. The Count System

To ensure thorough coverage with an even distribution in the amount of brushing and to help the patient concentrate on the performance, a system of counting can be useful.

▶ Count the number of strokes in each area (or 5 or 10, whichever is most appropriate for the particular patient) for modified Stillman or other method in which a stroke is used.

▶ Count slowly to 10 for each brush position while brush is vibrated and filament ends are held in position for the Bass, Charters, or other vibratory method.

B. The Clock System

Some patients brush thoroughly while watching a clock or an egg timer for 3 or 4 minutes. Timed procedures cannot guarantee thorough coverage, because single areas that are most accessible may get more brushing time.

C. Combination

For many patients, the use of the "count" system in combination with the "clock" system produces the most complete removal of dental biofilm.

D. Built-in Timers

▶ Many power toothbrushes have built-in timers that signal lapsed time.

▶ Signals may be set for 30 seconds, 1 or 2 minutes.

▶ Timers can motivate patients to increase the total time spent brushing.

IV. Frequency of Brushing

▶ Because of individual variations, one set rule for frequency cannot be applied. The emphasis in patient education is placed on complete biofilm removal daily rather than on the number of brushings.

▶ For the control of dental biofilm, and for oral sanitation and halitosis control, at least two brushings, accompanied by appropriate interdental care, are recommended as a *minimum* for each day.

▶ The longer the bacteria remain undisturbed, the greater the pathogenic potential of the biofilm bacteria.

▶ A clean mouth before going to sleep is encouraged. Bacteria thrive in the dark, warm, moist climate of the oral environment.

▶ Patients who use a chewable fluoride tablet, mouthrinse, or gel application before going to bed need to complete their biofilm removal before fluoride application.

METHODS FOR MANUAL TOOTHBRUSHING

▶ Most toothbrushing methods can be classified based on the position and motion of the brush.

▶ Some of these methods are recorded for descriptive, comparative, or historic purposes only and are not currently recommended. A few may have been shown to be detrimental.

▶ Methods include the following:
  • Sulcular: Bass
  • Roll: Rolling stroke, modified Stillman
  • Vibratory: Stillman, Charters, Bass
  • Circular: Fones
  • Vertical: Leonard
  • Horizontal
  • Physiologic: Smith
  • Scrub-brush

THE BASS METHOD: SULCULAR BRUSHING

The Bass method is widely accepted as an effective method for dental biofilm removal adjacent to and directly beneath the gingival margin. The areas at the gingival margin and in the col are the most significant in the control of gingival and periodontal infections.

I. Purposes and Indications

▶ For all patients for dental biofilm removal adjacent to and directly beneath the gingival margin.

▶ For open embrasures, cervical areas beneath the height of contour of the enamel, and exposed root surfaces.

▶ For the patient who has had periodontal surgery.

▶ For adaptation to abutment teeth, under the gingival border of a fixed partial denture.

II. Procedure

A. Position the Brush

▶ Direct the filaments apically (up for maxillary, down for mandibular teeth).

▶ First position the sides of the filaments parallel with the long axis of the tooth (Figure 28-5A).

▶ From that position, turn the brush head toward the gingival margin to make approximately a 45° angle to the long axis of the tooth (Figure 28-6B).

▶ Direct the filament tips into the gingival sulcus (Figure 28-5A and B).

B. Strokes

▶ Press lightly so the filament tips enter the gingival sulci and embrasures and cover the gingival margin. Do not bend the filaments with excess pressure.

▶ Vibrate the brush back and forth with very short strokes without disengaging the tips of the filaments from the sulci.

▶ Count at least 10 vibrations.

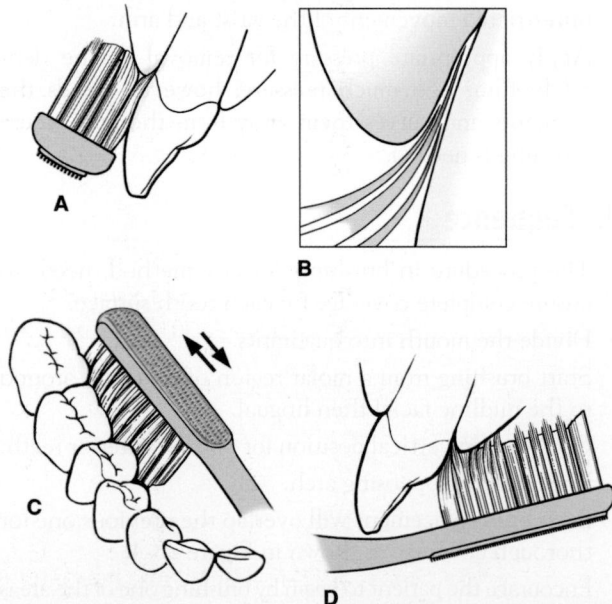

FIGURE 28-5 Sulcular Brushing. A: Filament tips are directed into the gingival sulcus at approximately 45° to the long axis of the tooth. **B:** Brushes designed with tapered filaments reach below the gingival margin with ease. **C:** Brush in position for lingual surfaces of mandibular posterior teeth. **D:** Position for palatal surface of maxillary anterior teeth.

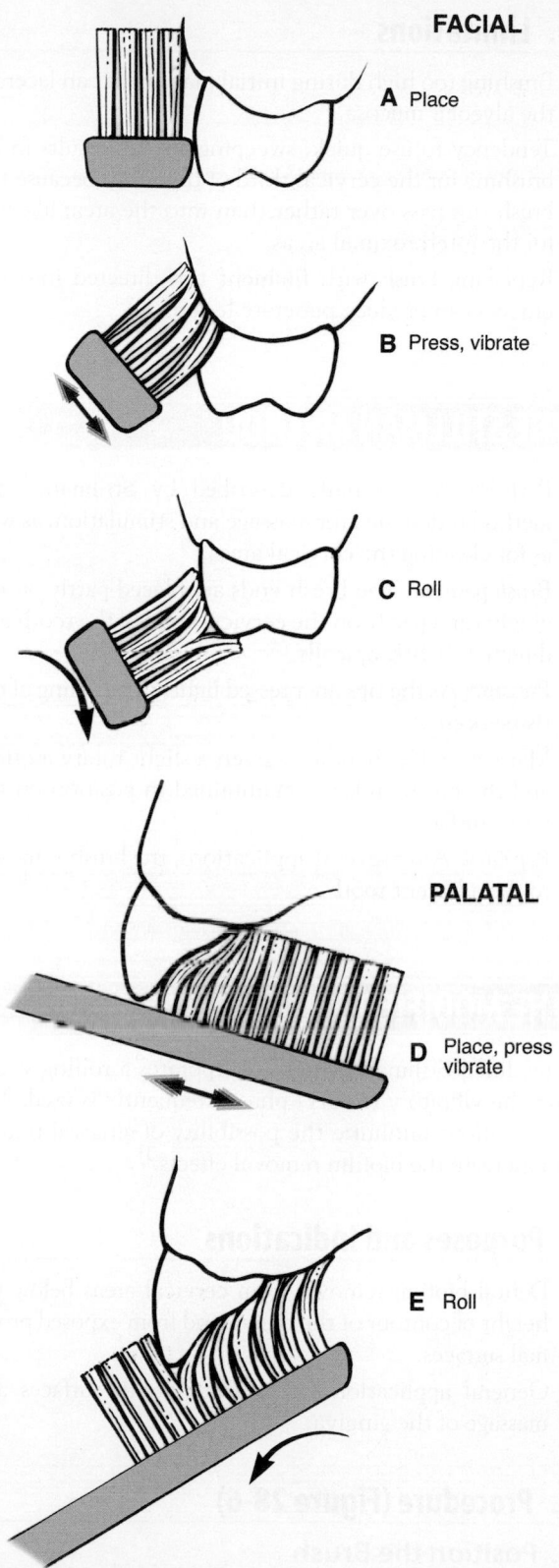

FACIAL

A Place

B Press, vibrate

C Roll

PALATAL

D Place, press vibrate

E Roll

FIGURE 28-6 Modified Stillman Method of Brushing. A: Initial brush placement with sides of bristles or filaments against the attached gingiva. **B:** The brush is pressed and angled, then vibrated. **C:** Vibrating is continued as the brush is rolled slowly over the crown. **D:** Maxillary anterior lingual placement with the brush applied the long way. **E:** Vibrating continues as the brush is rolled over the crown and interdental areas. Placement is similar for the lingual surfaces of the mandibular anterior teeth. The roll or rolling stroke brushing method has the same brush positions.

C. Reposition the Brush

Apply the brush to the next group of two or three teeth. Take care to overlap placement, as shown in Figure 28-4.

D. Repeat Stroke

The entire stroke (steps A–C) is repeated at each position around the maxillary and mandibular arches, both facially and lingually.

E. Position Brush for Lingual and Palatal Anterior Surfaces (Figure 28-5D)

Hold the brush the long narrow way for the anterior components. The filaments are kept straight and directed into the sulci.[12]

III. Limitations

▶ An overeager brusher may convert the previously mentioned "very short strokes" into a vigorous scrub that can cause injury to the gingival margin.

▶ Dexterity requirement may be difficult for certain patients. Because a 45° angle can be difficult to visualize, emphasis is on placing the tips of the filaments into the sulcus.

▶ Rolling stroke procedure may precede the sulcular brushing when a patient believes it helps to clean the teeth. The two methods are performed separately rather than trying to combine them in what has been referred to as a "modified Bass."

▶ The procedure of rolling the brush down over the crown after the vibratory part of the sulcular brush stroke has several disadvantages:

- Too often the brush is hastily and carelessly replaced into the sulcus position, or the opposite is true, and considerable time is consumed in the attempt to replace the brush carefully.
- Gingival margin injury by the constant replacement of the brush can result.
- The patient may tend to roll the brush down over the crown prematurely, thereby accomplishing very little sulcular brushing.

THE ROLL OR ROLLING STROKE METHOD

I. Purposes and Indications

▶ Removing biofilm, materia alba, and food debris from the teeth without emphasis on gingival sulcus.

- Used for children with relatively healthy gingiva and normal tissue contour, or when a sulcular technique may seem difficult for the patient of any age to master.
- Intended for general cleaning in conjunction with the use of a vibratory technique (Bass, Charters, Stillman).

▶ Useful for preparatory instruction (first lesson) for modified Stillman method because the initial brush placement is the same.

▶ Can be particularly helpful when there is a question about the patient's ability to master and practice a more complex method.

II. Procedure[4,13]

A. Position the Brush

▶ *Filaments*: Direct filaments apically (up for maxillary, down for mandibular teeth).

▶ *Place side of brush on the attached gingiva*: The filaments are directed apically. When the plastic portion of the brush head is level with the occlusal or incisal plane, generally the brush is at the proper height, as shown in Figure 28-6A.

B. Strokes

▶ *Press to flex the filaments*: The sides of the filaments are pressed lightly against the gingiva. The gingiva will blanch.

▶ *Roll the brush slowly over the teeth*: As the brush is rolled, the wrist is turned slightly. The filaments remain flexed and follow the contours of the teeth, thereby permitting cleaning of the cervical areas. Some filaments may reach interdentally.

C. Replace and Repeat Five Times or More

▶ *Repeat the entire stroke*: The entire stroke (steps A and B) is repeated at least five times for each tooth or group of teeth.

▶ *Rotate the wrist*: When the brush is removed and repositioned, the wrist is rotated.

▶ *Stretch the cheek*: The brush is moved away from the teeth, and the cheek is stretched facially with the back of the brush head. Care is taken not to drag the filament tips over the gingival margin when the brush is returned to the initial position (Figure 28-6A).

D. Overlap Strokes

When moving the brush to an adjacent position, overlap the brush position, as shown in Figure 28-4.

E. Position Brush for Anterior Lingual or Palatal Surfaces

▶ Use the brush the long, narrow way.

▶ Hook the heel of the brush on the incisal edge (Figure 28-6D).

▶ Press (down for maxillary, up for mandibular) until the filaments lie flat against the teeth and gingiva.

▶ Press and roll (curve up for mandibular, down for maxillary teeth).

▶ Replace and repeat five times for each brush width.

III. Limitations

▶ Brushing too high during initial placement can lacerate the alveolar mucosa.

▶ Tendency to use quick, sweeping strokes results in no brushing for the cervical third of the tooth because the brush tips pass over rather than into the area; likewise for the interproximal areas.

▶ Replacing brush with filament tips directed into the gingiva can produce punctate lesions.

THE STILLMAN METHOD

▶ *Purpose*: As originally described by Stillman,[14] the method is designed for massage and stimulation, as well as for cleaning the cervical areas.

▶ *Brush position*: The brush ends are placed partly on the gingiva and partly on the cervical areas of the tooth and directed slightly apically.

▶ *Pressure*: As the tips are pressed lightly, blanching of the tissue occurs.

▶ *Movement*: The handle is given a slight rotary motion, and the brush ends are maintained in position on the tooth surface.

▶ *Repeated*: After several applications, the brush is moved to the adjacent tooth.

THE MODIFIED STILLMAN METHOD

A modified Stillman, which incorporates a rolling stroke after the vibratory (rotary) phase, frequently is used. The modifications minimize the possibility of gingival trauma and increase the biofilm removal effects.[15]

I. Purposes and Indications

▶ Dental biofilm removal from cervical areas below the height of contour of the crown and from exposed proximal surfaces.

▶ General application for cleaning tooth surfaces and massage of the gingiva.

II. Procedure (Figure 28-6)

A. Position the Brush

▶ *Filaments*: Direct filaments apically (up for maxillary, down for mandibular teeth).

▶ *Place side of brush on the attached gingiva*: The filaments are directed apically. When the plastic portion of the brush head is level with the occlusal or incisal plane, generally the brush is at the proper height, as shown in Figure 28-6A.

B. Strokes

▶ *Press to flex the filaments*: The sides of the filaments are pressed lightly against the gingiva. The gingiva will blanch.

▶ *Angle the filaments*: Turn the handle by rotating the wrist so that the filaments are directed at an angle of approximately 45° with the long axis of the tooth.

▶ *Activate the brush*: Use a slight rotary motion. Maintain light pressure on the filaments, and keep the tips of the filaments in position with constant contact. Count to 10 slowly as the brush is vibrated by a rotary motion of the handle.

▶ *Roll and vibrate the brush*: Turn the wrist and work the vibrating brush slowly down over the gingiva and tooth. Make some of the filaments reach interdentally.

C. Replace Brush for Repeat Stroke

Reposition the brush by rotating the wrist. Avoid dragging the filaments back over the free gingival margin by holding the brush out, slightly away from the tooth.

D. Repeat Stroke Five Times or More

The entire stroke (steps A–C) is repeated at least five times for each tooth or group of teeth. When moving the brush to an adjacent position, overlap the brush position, as shown in Figure 28-4.

E. Position Brush for Anterior Lingual and Palatal Surfaces

▶ Position the brush the long, narrow way for the anterior components, as described for the rolling stroke technique and shown in Figure 28-6D and E.

▶ Press and vibrate, roll, and repeat.

III. Limitations

▶ Careful placement of a brush with end-rounded filaments is necessary to prevent tissue laceration. Light pressure is needed.

▶ Patient may try to move the brush into the rolling stroke too quickly, and the vibratory aspect may be ineffective for biofilm removal at the gingival margin.

THE CHARTERS METHOD

▶ *History*: During his long and productive dental career, Dr. W. J. Charters emphasized the importance of prevention.

▶ *Purpose*: The interproximal toothbrushing method he taught had as its objectives cleanliness through removal of the "film and mucin" from the proximal surfaces and gingival massage through mechanical stimulation.

▶ *Brush position*: Among his many published papers, Charters described two brush positions, one at a right angle to the long axis of the tooth[16] and another at a 45-degree angle with the tips of the bristles toward the occlusal plane. The right-angle position might have been intended primarily for patients with interdental periodontal tissue loss, where access permitted the bristles to enter the embrasure.

▶ *Method*: For either brush position, the instructions were to force the tips into the interproximal area.

▶ *Pressure*: "With the bristles between the teeth, as much pressure as possible is exerted, giving the brush several slight rotary or vibratory movements. This causes the sides of the bristles to come in contact with the gum margin, producing an ideal massage."[17]

▶ *Bristle position*: The classic periodontal textbooks[18] have described the Charters method with the bristles directed toward the occlusal plane at a 45-degree angle with the long axis of the tooth.

I. Purposes and Indications

▶ Loosen debris and dental biofilm.

▶ Massage and stimulate marginal and interdental gingiva.

▶ Aid in biofilm removal from proximal tooth surfaces when interproximal tissue is missing, for example, following periodontal surgery.

▶ Adapt to cervical areas below the height of contour of the crown and to exposed root surfaces.

▶ Remove dental biofilm from abutment teeth and under the gingival border of a fixed partial denture (bridge) or from the undersurface of a sanitary bridge.

II. Procedure[16]

A. Apply Rolling Stroke Procedure

Instruct in a basic rolling stroke for general cleaning to be accomplished first.

B. Position the Brush

▶ Hold brush (outside the oral cavity) with filaments directed toward the occlusal or incisal plane of the teeth to be brushed.

▶ Point tips down for application to the maxillary and up for application to the mandibular arch.

▶ Insert the brush held in the direction it will be used.

▶ Place the sides of the filaments against the enamel with the brush tips toward the occlusal or incisal plane.

▶ Angle the filaments at approximately 45° to the occlusal or incisal plane.

▶ Slide the brush to a position at the junction of the free gingival margin and the tooth surface (Figure 28-7B).

▶ Note contrast with position for the Stillman method (Figure 28-7A).

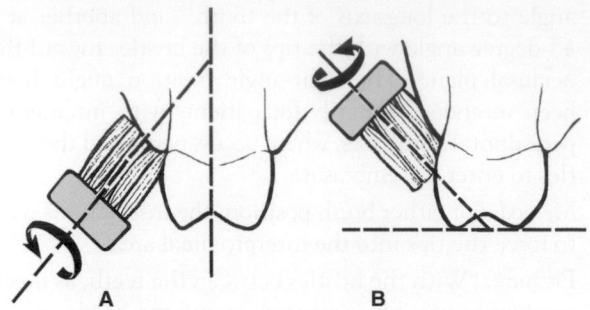

FIGURE 28-7 Stillman and Charters Methods Compared. A: Stillman: The brush is angled at approximately 45° to the long axis of the tooth. **B:** Charters: The brush is angled at approximately 45° to the occlusal plane, with brush tips directed toward the occlusal or incisal surfaces.

C. Strokes

- ▶ Press lightly to flex the filaments and force the tips between the teeth.
- ▶ Press the sides of the filaments against the gingival margin.
- ▶ Vibrate the brush gently but firmly, keeping the tips of the filaments in contact with the tooth surface.
- ▶ Count to 10 slowly as the brush is vibrated with a rotary motion of the handle.

D. Reposition the Brush and Repeat

Repeat steps B and C, as described, several times in each position around the dental arches.

E. Overlap Strokes

When moving the brush to an adjacent position, overlap the brush position, as shown in Figure 28-4.

F. Position Brush for Anterior Lingual and Palatal Surfaces

Because the Charters brush position is difficult to accomplish on the lingual surfaces, a modified Stillman technique is frequently advised. When the Charters method is preferred, the positions are as follows:

- ▶ *Posterior*
  - With brush tips pointed toward the occlusal surfaces, extend the brush handle across the incisal edge of the canine of the opposing side to be brushed.
  - Place the sides of the toe-end filaments against the distal surface of the most posterior tooth and subsequently at each embrasure.
  - Press and vibrate.
- ▶ *Anterior*
  - With brush handle parallel with the long axis of the tooth, place the sides of the toe-end filaments over the interproximal embrasure.
  - Press and vibrate.

G. Application of Brush for Fixed Partial Denture

When placing the brush, check to ensure the filament tips are directed under the gingival border of the pontic.

III. Limitations

- ▶ Brush ends do not engage the gingival sulcus to remove subgingival bacterial accumulations.
- ▶ In some areas, the correct brush placement is limited or impossible; modifications become necessary, consequently adding to the complexity of the procedure.
- ▶ Requirements in digital dexterity are high.

OTHER TOOTHBRUSHING METHODS

- ▶ The rolling stroke, modified Stillman, and Bass are the methods used most often for patient instruction either directly or as guidelines with variations.
- ▶ Other methods that have been used are included here. The technique and intent of some of the methods overlap.
- ▶ Assessment before special instruction may reveal a mixture of techniques may be in use by a patient.

I. Historical Methods

- ▶ Circular: Fones method (Table 28-2 and Figure 28-8)
- ▶ Vertical: Leonard method (Table 28-2)
- ▶ Physiologic: Smith's method (Table 28-2).

II. Methods Considered Detrimental

A. Horizontal

- ▶ An unlimited sweep with a horizontal scrubbing motion bears pressure on teeth that are most facially inclined or prominent.
- ▶ With the use of an abrasive dentifrice, such brushing may produce tooth abrasion.
- ▶ Because the interdental areas are not touched by this method, dental biofilm can remain undisturbed on proximal surfaces.

B. Scrub-Brush

- ▶ A scrub-brush procedure consists of vigorously combined horizontal, vertical, and circular strokes, with some vibratory motions for certain areas.
- ▶ Without caution, vigorous scrubbing can encourage gingival recession and, with a dentifrice of sufficient abrasiveness, can create areas of tooth abrasion.

POWER TOOTHBRUSHES

Power brushes are also known as power-assisted, automatic, mechanical, or electric brushes. The American Dental Association Council on Scientific Affairs evaluates power brushes for the reduction of dental biofilm and gingivitis.[24]

TABLE 28-2	Historical Toothbrushing Methods		
METHOD	**FONES**	**LEONARD**	**SMITH**
Alternate description	Circular	Vertical	Physiologic
History	Advocated by Alfred C. Fones	As described by Hirschfeld,[19] the up-and-down stroke was employed when teeth were cleaned with a primitive crude twig toothbrush.	Described by Smith[20] and advocated later by Bell.[21] Based on the principle that the toothbrush follows a physiologic pathway and traverses over the tissues in a "natural" masticating act.
Type of brush	A soft brush with 0.006–0.008-inch filament diameter	A soft brush with 0.006–0.008-inch filament diameter	A soft brush with "small tufts of fine bristles arranged in four parallel rows and trimmed to an even length."
Stroke	In abbreviated form, the technique described by Dr. Fones includes the following:[22] 1. With the teeth closed, place the brush inside the cheek over the last maxillary molar, lightly contacting the gingiva. 2. Use a fast, wide, circular motion with light pressure sweeping from the maxillary to the mandibular gingiva. 3. Bring anterior teeth in edge-to-edge contact holding lip out when necessary to make continuous circular strokes. 4. Lingual and palatal tooth surfaces require an in-and-out stroke. Brush sweeps across palate and back and forth to the molars on the mandibular arch (see Figure 28-8).	Paraphrased, Leonard's method is described as follows:[23] 1. With the teeth edge to edge, place the brush filaments against the teeth at right angles to the long axes of the teeth. 2. Brush vigorously with light pressure and mostly up-and-down strokes with a slight rotation or circular motion after striking the gingival margin with force. 3. Use enough pressure to force the filaments into the embrasures, but not enough to damage the brush. 4. The upper and lower teeth are not brushed in the same series of strokes. The teeth are placed edge to edge to keep the brush from slipping over the occlusal or incisal surfaces.	Direct the brush down over the lower teeth onto the gingiva and upward over the teeth for the maxillary. It is also suggested that a few gentle horizontal strokes be used to clean the portion of the sulci directly over the bifurcations of the roots.
Recommendations	An easy-to-learn first technique for young children.	Use when maxillary and mandibular teeth are to be brushed separately surfaces.	
Limitations	Possibly detrimental for adults, particularly when used by a vigorous brusher.		

I. Effectiveness

A. Evolution

▶ Current power brushes move at speeds and motions that cannot be duplicated by manual brushes.

▶ Power toothbrushes have evolved through time due to improved designs and features.

▶ Power toothbrushes of the 1960–1980 era mimicked the motions of manual brushing.

B. Power Versus Manual

▶ Research showed equivalence for power and manual brushes in biofilm removal and reduction of gingivitis.[25,26]

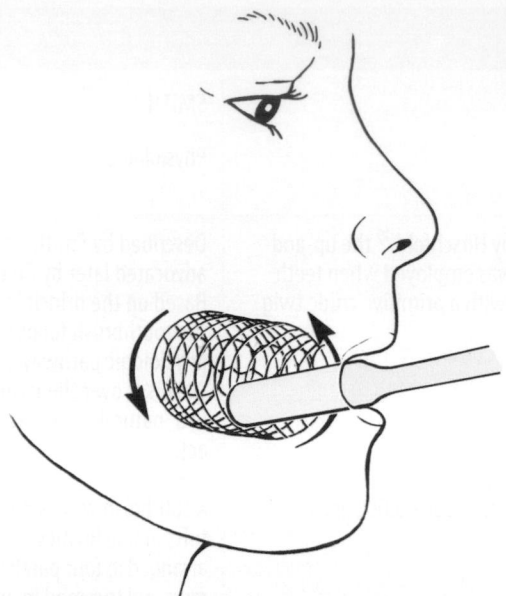

FIGURE 28-8 Fones Method of Brushing. With the teeth closed, a circular motion extends from the maxillary gingiva to the mandibular gingiva using a light pressure.

▶ Rotating oscillating action toothbrushes have been shown to be the most effective powered toothbrush for reducing plaque and gingivitis.[27,28]
  • Rotating oscillating action toothbrushes have been shown to be more effective in removing plaque and reducing gingivitis than manual toothbrushes.[28]
▶ Some patients may demonstrate better plaque removal with a manual toothbrush; therefore, patient education must be based on the individual's needs.
▶ The safety of power brushes as compared to manual has been well established.[29–32]

II. Purposes and Indications

A. General Application

▶ Recommended for physically able patients with ineffective manual biofilm removal techniques.
▶ To facilitate mechanical removal of dental biofilm and food debris from the teeth and the gingiva.
▶ Reduce calculus and stain buildup.[32]

B. Patients with Oral Health Challenges

Power brushes can be useful for many patients, including:

▶ Those with a history of failed attempts at more traditional biofilm removal methods.
▶ Those undergoing orthodontic treatment.
▶ Those undergoing complex restorative and prosthodontic treatment.
▶ Those with dental implants.
▶ Aggressive brushers: tendency to use less pressure when using a power brush than with a manual brush.[33–35]

  • Many models of powerbrushes will shut off automatically if too much pressure is applied during brushing, which can be a benefit for those who with tendency to apply too much pressure.
▶ Patients with disabilities or limited dexterity.
▶ The large handles of power brushes can be of benefit.
▶ Handle weight needs to be considered for these patients.
▶ Patients unable to brush.
▶ A power brush may be readily used by a parent or caregiver.

III. Description

A. Motion

There is great variety in the manner in which power brushes move, for example:

▶ The entire brush head moves as a unit in one type of motion.
▶ Groups of tufts on the same brush head may move differently.
▶ The entire brush head moves as a unit, but in different, yet simultaneous motions.
▶ Different-shaped brush heads move separately, and in different, yet simultaneous motions.
▶ A synopsis of the types of motions of power brushes is seen in Table 28-3.

TABLE 28-3	Power Toothbrush Motions
MOTION	**DESCRIPTION**
Rotational	Moves in a 360° circular motion.
Counter-rotational	Each tuft of filaments moves in a rotational motion; each tuft moves counter-directional to the adjacent tuft.
Oscillating	Rotates from center to the left, then to the right; degree of rotation varies from 25° to 55°.
Pulsating	When brush head is on the tooth, direct pulsations toward the interproximal.
Cradle or twist	Side to side with an arc.
Side to side	Side-to-side perpendicular to the long axis of the brush handle.
Translating	Up-and-down parallel to the long axis of the brush handle.
Combination	Combination of simultaneous yet different type of movement.
Ultrasonic	Brush head vibrates at ultrasonic frequency (>250 kHz).

B. Speeds

▶ Vary from low to high.

▶ Generally, power brushes with replaceable batteries move slower than those with rechargeable batteries.

▶ Movement varies from 3,800 to 40,000 movements per minute depending on the manufacturer and type.

C. Brush Head Design

▶ *Adult*: The variety of shapes is illustrated in Figure 28-9. They may be small and round, conical, or like traditional manual heads. Trim profiles include flat, bilevel, rippled, or angled.

▶ *Child*: A child's power brush head can be specially designed to accommodate a smaller mouth and the development of the dentition, as shown in Figure 28-10.

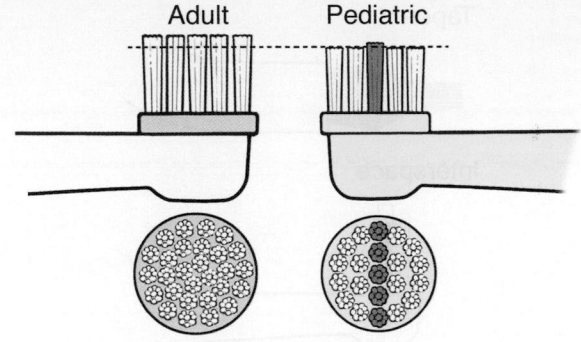

FIGURE 28-10 Child Power Brush Profile. Power brushes for children could necessitate smaller head sizes and shorter filaments to allow for distal reach in tight posterior areas. Raised blue filaments allow for better access to occlusal pits and fissures.

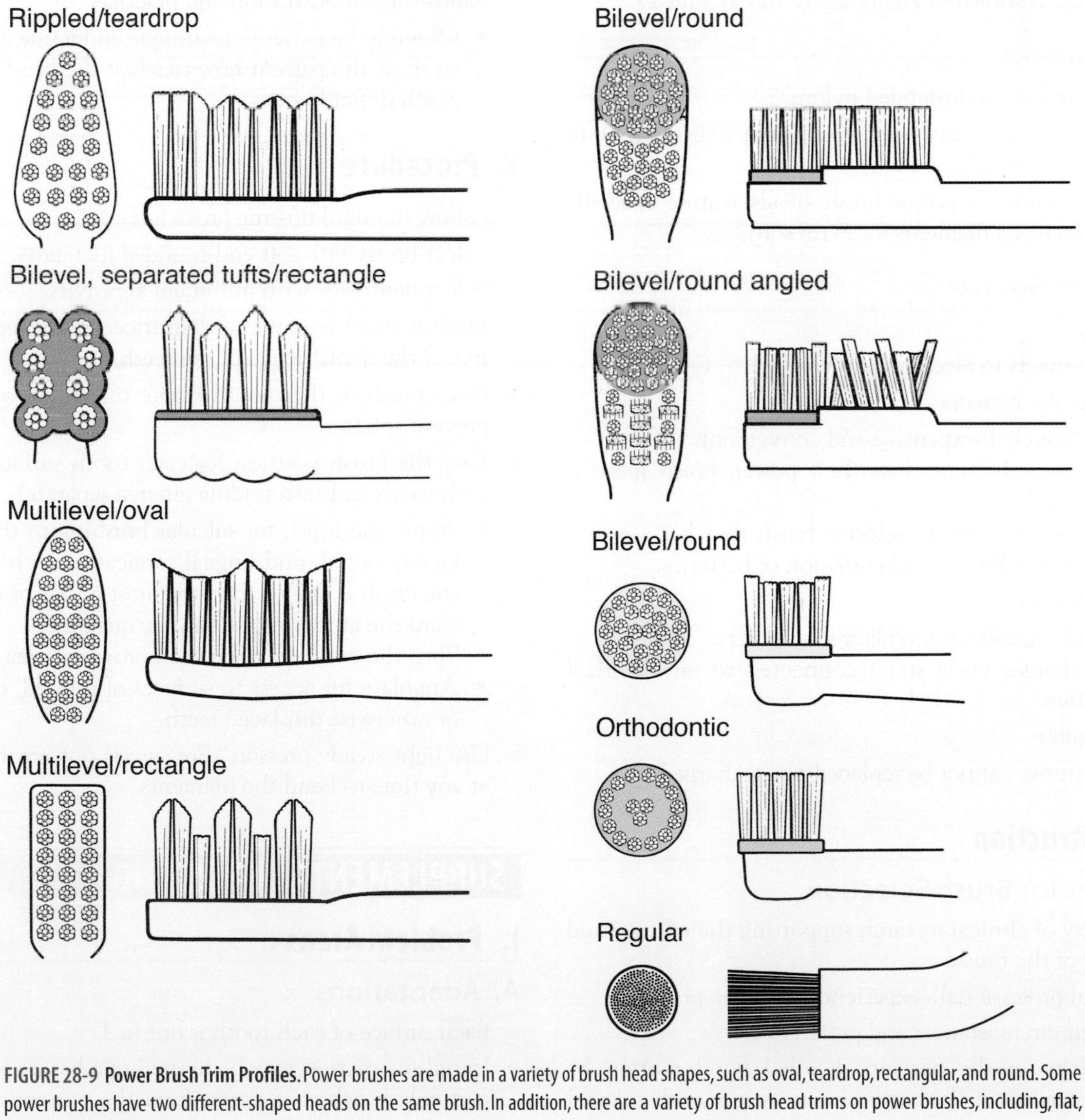

Rippled/teardrop

Bilevel/round

Bilevel, separated tufts/rectangle

Bilevel/round angled

Multilevel/oval

Bilevel/round

Multilevel/rectangle

Orthodontic

Regular

FIGURE 28-9 Power Brush Trim Profiles. Power brushes are made in a variety of brush head shapes, such as oval, teardrop, rectangular, and round. Some power brushes have two different-shaped heads on the same brush. In addition, there are a variety of brush head trims on power brushes, including, flat, bilevel, and multilevel.

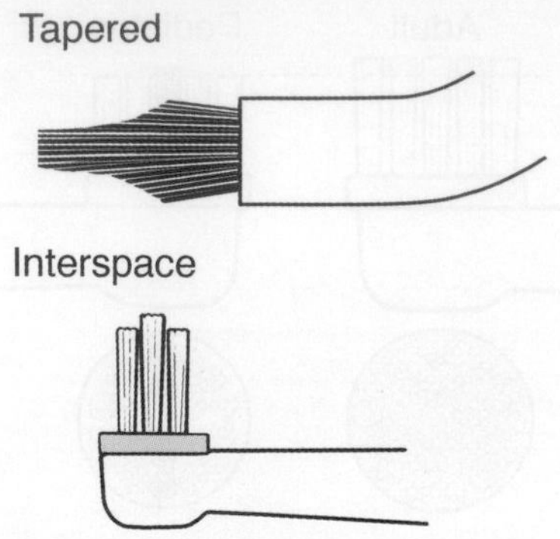

Tapered

Interspace

FIGURE 28-11 Interdental Power Brush Trim Profiles. Some power brushes offer brush heads especially for interdental and proximal surface dental biofilm removal and difficult-access areas such as around implants, orthodontic appliances, and exposed furcations.

▶ *Interdental*: The interdental brush heads pictured in Figure 28-11 are designed to fit a standard power brush handle and are similar in shape to manual interdental brushes, as shown in Figure 29-10 in Chapter 29.

D. Filaments

▶ Made of soft, end-rounded nylon.
▶ Diameters: from extra soft, 0.075 mm (0.003 inch), to soft, 0.15 mm (0.006 inch).
▶ Some children's power brush heads feature specially manufactured filaments for extra softness.

E. Power Source

▶ *Direct*
  • Connects to electrical outlet.
▶ *Replaceable batteries*
  • Relatively inexpensive and convenient.
  • As most batteries lose their power, brush speed is reduced.
  • Advise patients to select a brush that has a watertight handle to avoid corrosion of batteries.
▶ *Rechargeable*
  • Rechargeable, nonreplaceable battery.
  • Recharges via a stand connected to an electrical outlet.
▶ *Disposable*
  • Batteries cannot be replaced nor recharged.

IV. Instruction

A. Basis for Brush Selection

▶ Quality of clinical research supporting the efficacy and safety of the brush.
▶ Dental professional's experience with the product.
▶ Patient circumstances and preferences.
▶ Dexterity of the patient: detailed hand motion by patient is not a key requirement as it is with manual brushes.

▶ Brush head and batteries that can be replaced for maximum efficiency.
▶ Features that include a timer and pressure sensor.
▶ Patient affordability.
  • Battery-operated models are often less expensive and may be a good way for the patient to try out a powerbrush before investing in a more expensive rechargeable model.

B. Preparation for Instructing Patient

▶ Review manufacturer's instructions as they can differ.
▶ The dental hygienist needs to become familiar with the product before providing patient education.

C. Hands-on Instruction

▶ Provide a demonstration model of the brush and a video of the brushing instructions, when available.
▶ Teach the patient that the use of a power brush requires practice.
▶ Have patient bring toothbrush to appointment for hands-on demonstration and practice.
  • Observe the patient's technique and refine as needed to show the patient how to adapt the brush head to reach difficult areas.

V. Procedure

▶ Follow standard flossing procedure.
▶ Select brush with soft end-rounded filaments.
▶ Select dentifrice with minimum abrasivity.
▶ Place a small amount of dentifrice on the brush and spread the dentifrice over the teeth.
▶ Place brush in the mouth before turning power on to prevent splatter.
▶ Vary the brush position for each tooth surface. Brush each tooth and surrounding gingiva separately.
  • Apply the brush for sulcular brushing to the distal, facial, mesial, and lingual surfaces of each tooth as the brush is moved from the most posterior teeth toward the anterior, quadrant by quadrant.
  • Turn the brush to reach each proximal area.
  • Angulate for access to surfaces of rotated, crowded, or otherwise displaced teeth.
▶ Use light steady pressure. Pressure is not great enough at any time to bend the filaments.

SUPPLEMENTAL BRUSHING

I. Problem Areas

A. Adaptations

▶ Each surface of each tooth is brushed.
▶ Initial instruction may be limited to a basic procedure, particularly when it varies from the patient's present procedures.

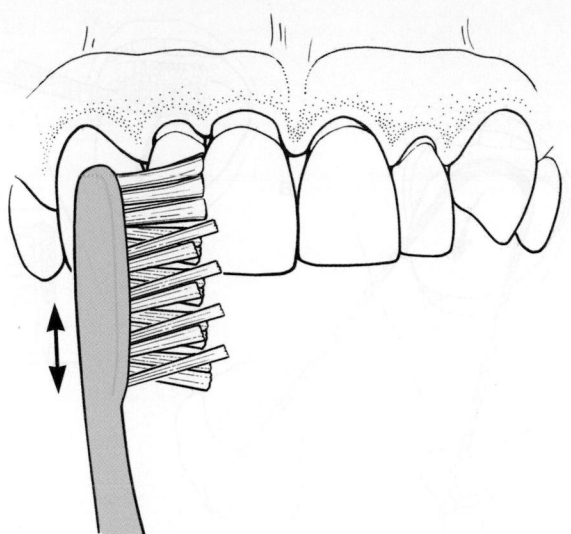

FIGURE 28-12 Brush in Vertical Position. For overlapped teeth, open embrasures, and selected areas of recession, the dental biofilm on proximal tooth surfaces can be removed with the brush held in a vertical position.

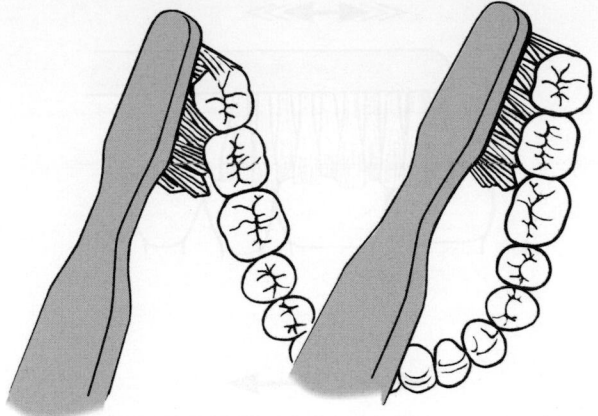

FIGURE 28-13 Brushing Problems. Brush placement to remove biofilm from the distal surfaces of the most posterior teeth. The distobuccal surface is approached by stretching the cheek; the distolingual surface is approached by directing the brush across from the canine of the opposite side.

▶ At succeeding lessons, the special hard-to-get areas can be reviewed.

▶ Suggestions are made and demonstrated for brush adaptation for areas missed.

B. Areas for Special Attention

▶ Facially displaced teeth, especially canines and premolars, where the zone of attached gingiva on the facial may be minimal and where toothbrush abrasion may occur.

▶ Inclined teeth, for example, lingual surfaces of mandibular molars that are inclined lingually.

▶ Exposed root surfaces; cemental and dentinal surfaces.

▶ Overlapped teeth or wide embrasures, which require use of vertical brush position (Figure 28-12).

▶ Surfaces of teeth next to edentulous areas.

▶ Exposed furcation areas.

▶ Right canine and lateral incisor, both maxillary and mandibular, which are commonly missed by right-handed brushers; the opposite is true for left-handed brushers.

▶ Distal surfaces of most posterior teeth (Figure 28-13). At best, the brush may reach only the distal line angles. Supplementation with dental floss or textured dental floss is needed for the distal surface (Figures 29-4G and 29-7).

II. Occlusal Brushing

A. Objectives

▶ Loosen biofilm microorganisms packed in pits and fissures.

▶ Remove biofilm deposits from occlusal surfaces of teeth out of occlusion or not used during mastication.

▶ Remove biofilm from the margins of restorations.

▶ Clean pits and fissures to prepare for sealants.

B. Procedure

▶ Place brush on occlusal surfaces of molar teeth with filament tips pointed into the occlusal pits at a right angle.

▶ Position the handle parallel with the occlusal surface.

▶ Extend the toe of the brush to cover the distal grooves of the most posterior tooth (Figure 28-14A).

▶ Strokes: Two acceptable strokes are suggested.

• Vibrate the brush in a slight circular movement while maintaining the filament tips on the occlusal surface throughout a count of 10. Press moderately so filaments do not bend but go straight into the pits and fissures (Figure 28-14C).

• Force the filaments against the occlusal surface with sharp, quick strokes; lift the brush off each time to dislodge debris; repeat 10 times.

▶ Move brush to premolar area, overlapping previous brush position.

C. Precaution

Long scrubbing strokes from anterior to posterior on an occlusal surface may contact only the prominent parts of the cusps (Figure 28-14B).

III. Tongue Cleaning

Total mouth cleanliness includes tongue care.

A. Microorganisms of the Tongue

▶ Main foci for oral microorganisms are:

• Dorsum of tongue
• Gingival sulci and pockets
• Dental biofilm on all teeth.

▶ Microorganisms in saliva are principally from the tongue.

▶ The microflora of the tongue is not constant, but changes frequently.[36]

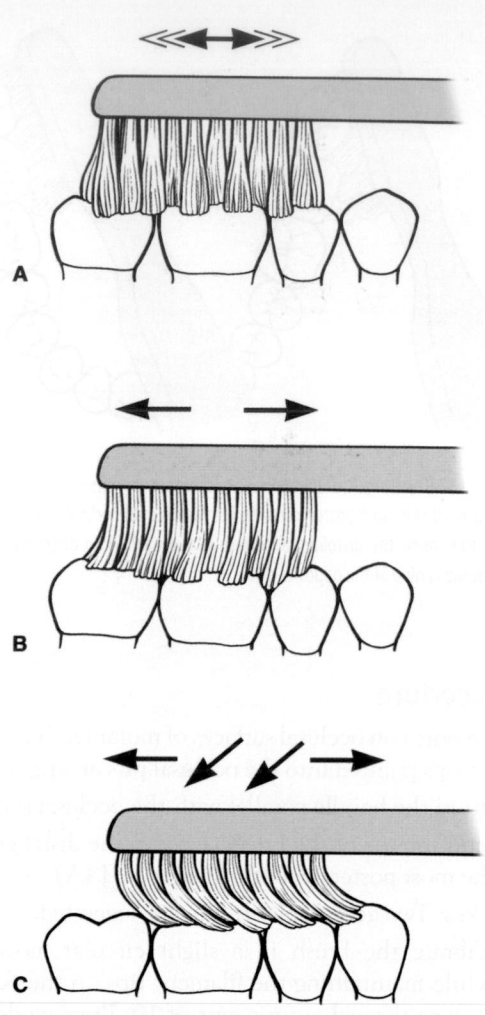

FIGURE 28-14 **Occlusal Brushing. A:** Vibrating brush with light pressure while maintaining filament tips on the occlusal surface permits tips to work their way into pits and fissures. **B:** Long horizontal strokes contact only the cusp tips. **C:** Excess pressure curves the filaments so that tips cannot get into the pits and fissures.

B. Purpose of Cleaning the Tongue

▶ Slows dental biofilm formation and total biofilm accumulation.

▶ Reduces number of microorganisms.

▶ Reduces potential for halitosis.

▶ Contributes to overall cleanliness.

▶ Improvements for the patient who has xerostomia, a coated tongue, deep fissures, or who uses tobacco products.

C. Anatomic Features of Tongue Conducive to Debris Retention

▶ *Surface papillae:* Numerous filiform papillae extend as minute projections, whereas fungiform papillae are not as high and create elevations and depressions that entrap debris and microorganisms (Figure 12-5, Chapter 12).

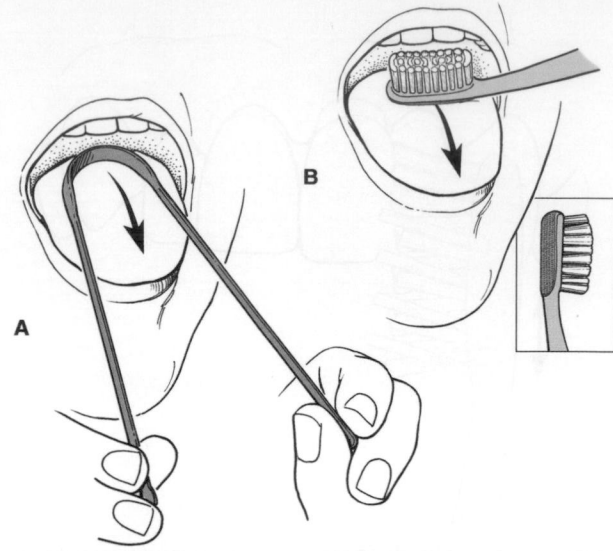

FIGURE 28-15 **Tongue Cleaners. A:** A variety of plastic or flexible metal cleaners are available to clean the dorsal surface of the tongue. **B:** An example of a toothbrush with a rubber tongue cleaner behind the brush head. The cleaner is pressed over the tongue with a light but firm stroke.

▶ *Fissured tongue:* Fissures may be several millimeters deep and retain debris.

D. Brushing Procedure

1. Hold the brush handle at a right angle to the midline of the tongue and direct the brush tips toward the throat.

2. With the tongue extruded, the sides of the filaments are placed on the posterior part of the tongue surface.

3. With light pressure, draw the brush forward and over the tip of the tongue. Repeat three or four times. Do not scrub the papillae.

4. A power brush can only be used for tongue cleaning when the switch is in the "off" position.

E. Tongue Cleaner

Tongue cleaners may be made of plastic, rubber, stainless steel, or other flexible metal. They are curved or raised, textured pads wide enough to fit over the tongue surface without hitting the teeth.

▶ *Types*
  • Curved with a single handle
  • Curved with two ends to hold (Figure 28-15A)
  • Raised, textured rubber pad on the back side of the brush head (Figure 28-15B).

▶ *Procedure*
  • Place the cleaner toward the most posterior area of the dorsal surface (Figure 28-15).
  • Press with a light but firm stroke, and pull forward.

- Repeat several times, covering the entire surface of the tongue.
- Wash the tongue cleaner under running water.

TOOTHBRUSHING FOR SPECIAL CONDITIONS

Even when an unusual oral condition develops, a patient is encouraged to brush wherever possible to reduce the possibility of infection and promote healing. Prolonged omission of biofilm removal is never indicated. Examples of conditions that may require a temporary departure from personal care routines are included here.

I. Acute Oral Inflammatory or Traumatic Lesions

When an acute oral condition precludes normal brushing, instruct the patient to:

▶ Brush all areas of the mouth not affected.
▶ Rinse with a warm, mild saline solution to encourage healing and debris removal.
▶ Resume regular biofilm control measures on the affected area as soon as possible.

II. Following Periodontal Surgery

Provide specific instructions concerning brushing while sutures and/or a dressing are in place.

▶ Brush the occlusal surfaces of the teeth and use light strokes over the dressing.
▶ Avoid direct, vigorous brushing to prevent displacement of a dressing.
▶ Brush other teeth and gingiva, not involved in the surgery, as usual.
▶ Additional instructions appear in Table 43-2 in Chapter 43.

III. Acute Stage of Necrotizing Ulcerative Gingivitis

▶ Lack of oral cleanliness can be a major contributing factor (see Chapter 42).
▶ Oral tissues are sensitive to touch during the acute stage, and toothbrushing therefore is neglected.
▶ Careful brush placement and an extra soft brush are indicated to avoid trauma.

IV. Following Dental Extraction

▶ Brush all teeth and gingiva except the surgical wound area.
▶ Clean the teeth adjacent to the extraction site the day following surgery.

▶ Brush areas not involved in the surgery as usual to reduce biofilm and promote healing.
▶ Detailed instructions for pre- and postsurgery are found in Chapter 55.

V. Following Dental Restorations

▶ Patients tend to avoid brushing a new crown, implant, newly placed fixed partial denture, or other prosthesis.
▶ Specific instructions are provided at the time of insertion with review at continuing care appointment.

EFFECTS OF TOOTHBRUSHING

I. The Gingiva

▶ Trauma occurs most frequently on the facial surfaces over prominent teeth in the dental arch.
▶ Lesions are frequently found over canines and premolars.
▶ Lesions occur most often immediately following initial instruction in the use of a new method of brushing; patient may be overzealous or may have misunderstood correct brush placement.
▶ Examination of patient's gingiva within a few days after instruction may be indicated.

A. Acute Alterations

Acute lesions are usually lacerations or ulcerations. The severity of the lesion may depend on the frequency and extent of brushing, as well as on the stiffness of the filaments and the force applied.

▶ Appearance
- Scuffed epithelial surface with denuded underlying connective tissue.
- Punctate lesions that appear as red pinpoint spots.
- Diffuse redness and denuded attached gingiva.

▶ Precipitating factors
- Horizontal or vertical scrub toothbrushing method.
- Excess pressure applied using firm palm grasp of handle.[37]
- Use of abrasive dentifrice.[38]
- Overvigorous placement and application of the toothbrush.
- Penetration of gingiva by filament ends.
- Use of a toothbrush with frayed, broken bristles or filaments.
- Application of filaments beyond attached gingiva.

B. Chronic Alterations

▶ Changes in gingival contour
- Appearance
  1. Rolled, bulbous, hard, firm marginal gingiva, in "piled up" or festoon shape ("McCall's festoon," Figure 18-12 in Chapter 18).

2. Gingival cleft, which is a narrow groove or slit that extends from the crest of the gingiva to the attached gingiva ("Stillman's cleft," Figure 18-13 in Chapter 18).
  • Location
    1. May appear only on the facial gingiva, because of the vigor with which toothbrush is used.
    2. Frequently gingival trauma is inversely related to the right-or left-handedness of the patient.
    3. Areas most often involved are around canines or teeth in labioversion or buccoversion.
▶ Gingival recession
  • *Appearance*: Margin has moved apically and root surface is exposed.
  • *Predisposing factors*
    1. Anatomic: Narrow band of attached gingiva and thin facial bone over teeth malposed in labioversion.
    2. Toothbrushing habits: Vigorous brushing with abrasive dentifrice.
▶ Suggested corrective measures
  • Recommend use of a soft toothbrush with end-rounded filaments.
  • Correct the patient's toothbrushing method; demonstrate a toothbrushing method better suited to the oral condition.

II. Dental Abrasion

Appearance: Wedge-shaped indentations with smooth, shiny surfaces, as seen in Figure 16-5 in Chapter 16.

A. Definition

▶ Abrasion is the wearing away of tooth structure that results from a repetitive mechanical habit.
▶ Incorrect toothbrushing, especially with an abrasive dentifrice is the most common cause.

B. Location

▶ Primarily on facial surfaces, especially of canines, premolars, and sometimes first molars, or, on any tooth in buccoversion or labioversion, those most available to the pressure of the toothbrush.
▶ Canines are susceptible because of their prominence on the curvature of the dental arches.
▶ Most abraded areas are on the cervical areas of exposed root surfaces, but occasionally they may occur on the enamel.
▶ When adjacent teeth are involved, the lesions appear in a linear pattern across the quadrant or sextant.

C. Contributing Factors

▶ Brushing with abrasive agent in the dentifrice.
▶ Horizontal brushing with excessive pressure.
▶ Form of filament ends: abrasion is less frequent when filaments are end-rounded.
▶ Prominence of the tooth surface labially or buccally.

D. Corrective Measures

▶ Explain the problem to the patient to ensure full cooperation.
▶ Advise use of a toothbrush with end-rounded filaments.
▶ Change the toothbrushing procedure.
▶ Recommend a less abrasive dentifrice.
▶ Use a smaller amount of dentifrice.
  • Start brushing in the area of the dentition where the most biofilm and calculus are noted.
  • Avoid applying the dentifrice vigorously to the same tooth surfaces.

III. Bacteremia

Evidence suggests toothbrushing and scaling can produce a detectable bacteremia.[39–41]

▶ The incidence and magnitude of bacteremia after scaling is significantly higher in patients with periodontitis than in gingivitis and healthy patients.[40]
▶ There is no definitive data on the relative risks of using manual or electric toothbrushes in patients who are predisposed to infective endocarditis.
▶ The mere fact that bacterial endocarditis can be produced through toothbrushing makes the need for maintaining proper oral hygiene a priority.[41]

CARE OF TOOTHBRUSHES

When discussing the type and features of the brush selected for an individual patient, the number of brushes needed and the frequency of replacement is included. An ideal time to teach cleaning and daily care of brushes would be after a practice session.

The condition of a brush depends on many factors, including the amount and manner of use, the type of care, and the quality of the brush at the start.

I. Supply of Brushes

▶ Recommend at least two brushes for home use and a third in a portable container for use at work, school, or travel.
▶ Purchase of brushes needs to be staggered so that all brushes are not new at the same time and, more importantly, so that they are all not old at the same time, thereby resulting in less than optimum maintenance of the gingival condition.

II. Brush Replacement

▶ Frequent replacement recommended; at least every 2–3 months.
▶ Brushes need to be replaced before filaments become splayed or frayed or lose resiliency. Duration of a brush is influenced by many factors, including frequency and method of use.

▶ Brush contamination occurs with use.[42,43] Contamination has the potential for causing systemic or localized infection.

▶ Patients who are debilitated, immunosuppressed, have a known infection, or are about to undergo surgery for any reason can be advised to disinfect their brushes or use disposable brushes.[43]

III. Cleaning Toothbrushes

▶ Clean thoroughly after each use.

▶ Hold brush head under strong stream of warm water from faucet to force particles, dentifrice, and bacteria from between the filaments.

▶ Tap the handle on edge of sink to remove remaining particles.

▶ Use one toothbrush to clean another brush; filaments can be worked between those of the other brush to remove resistant debris.

▶ Rinse completely and tap out excess water.

IV. Brush Storage

▶ Brushes need to be kept in open air with head in an upright position, apart from contact with other brushes, particularly those of another person to avoid cross contamination.

▶ Portable brush container needs sufficient holes to give air temporarily until the brush can be completely exposed for drying. A closed container encourages bacterial growth.

DOCUMENTATION

In the permanent record, the documentation for initial instruction will include the following:

▶ Type of toothbrush patient has used to date: manual versus power.

▶ Recommended changes in type of brush or method of use.

▶ Identify needs or changes in the soft tissue and teeth from a "plaque score" using a disclosing agent.

▶ Record areas patient has difficulty reaching with suggestions for follow-up.

▶ Tongue cleaning method instructed.

▶ Box 28-3 shows a sample documentation for toothbrush selection and toothbrushing method.

BOX 28-3

Example Documentation: Toothbrush Selection and Toothbrushing Method

S –A 30-year-old male presents for his 6-month preventive appointment with a chief complaint of gums bleeding during toothbrushing. Patient has a negative medical history and reports taking no medications. Patient reports brushing 1× day with a hard manual toothbrush and uses a back and forth "scrubbing" method.

O–Intraoral assessment reveals generalized moderate edema, marginal erythema, and moderate bleeding on probing. Moderate plaque is noted along the gingival margin of posterior teeth. Ulcerations and denuded gingiva noted, particularly on left side maxillary facial and mandibular molar lingual surfaces. Biofilm-free score 63%.

A –Acute tissue trauma related to use of hard toothbrush and scrubbing method.

P–Oral Self-Care—Oral self-care instructions given using a soft toothbrush, recommend twice daily using the modified Stillman method. Flossers were introduced to patient for removal of interdental plaque biofilm. Patient demonstrated modified Stillman method intraorally with some challenges on the lingual of mandibular molars. Patient demonstrated successfully the use of flossers. Patient committed to try the following behavior modifications: increase frequency of brushing from 1 to 2×'s a day, and floss at least 4×'s a week. Increase biofilm-free score to 85% at re-evaluation appointment. Next Visit—6–8 weeks re-evaluation of gingival condition, plaque-free score, evaluate biofilm removal, and assess patient's toothbrushing and flossing technique. Modify as needed. Determine appropriate continue care visit for patient.

Signed _____, RDH
Date _____

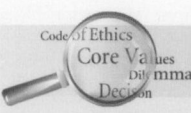

EVERYDAY ETHICS

Karen, a long-standing patient of the dental office, presents for her six-month continuing care visit. She has always been consistent with her preventive appointments and has a history of maintaining good oral self-care. A medical history update indicates that that Karen was recently diagnosed with rheumatoid arthritis. The condition is affecting her hands, limiting her dexterity and tactile sensitivity. She reports moderate joint pain especially in the morning hours. She presents with a chief complaint to Jennifer, the dental hygienist, "my gums bleed when I brush. I am worried something is wrong."

The oral examination indicates generalized moderate marginal biofilm and moderate bleeding on probing. It is clear that her oral health status has declined since her last continuing care appointment. Jennifer is new to the practice and running behind schedule so she decided to skip the oral hygiene instructions.

Questions for Consideration

1. Which core ethical values did Jennifer violate with regard to patient education? Explain how each applies to this scenario.

2. How could the information on the patient's health history been used to provide a patient-centered approach to oral self-care?

3. Given the client's physical challenges, list intervention strategies that could have been recommended to assist her with maintaining optimal oral health (e.g., toothbrush, interdental aids). Explain the rationale for each in relation to the Dental Hygiene Standard of Care (see Chapter 1)

4. What would be the best continuing care interval for Karen (2 months, 3 months, 6 months, or yearly)? How can you find evidence to support your choice?

Factors To Teach The Patient

▷ The effect of dental biofilm formation on the teeth and gingiva.
▷ Rationale for thorough removal of dental biofilm from the teeth daily, especially before going to sleep.
▷ The type of brush: manual, power, or both, recommended to maintain optimal oral health for a particular patient.
▷ Individualized hands-on instruction using an appropriate manual or power brushing method.
▷ Proper care and maintenance of manual and power brushes.
▷ Indications for and use of a tongue cleaner.

References

1. Hirschfeld I. *The Toothbrush: Its Use and Abuse.* Brooklyn, NY: Dental Items of Interest; 1939:1–27.

2. McCauley HB. Toothbrushes, toothbrush materials and design. *J Am Dent Assoc.* 1946;33:283–293.

3. Weinberger BW. *An Introduction to the History of Dentistry.* St. Louis, MO: Mosby; 1948:140–144.

4. American Academy of Periodontology. Committee report: the tooth brush and methods of cleaning the teeth. *Dent Items Int.* 1920;42:193.

5. Alexander JF. Toothbrushes and toothbrushing. In: Menaker L, ed. *The Biologic Basis of Dental Caries.* Hagerstown, MD: Harper & Row; 1980:482–496.

6. Koecker L. *Principles of Dental Surgery.* Baltimore, MD: American Society of Dental Surgeons; 1842, Chapter III: *exhibiting a new method of treating the diseases of the teeth and gums:*155–156.

7. American Dental Association, Council on Dental Therapeutics. *Accepted Dental Therapeutics.* 40th ed. Chicago, IL: American Dental Association; 1984:386–387.

8. Checchi L, Minguzzi S, Franchi M, et al. Toothbrush filaments end-rounding: stereomicroscope analysis. *J Clin Periodontol.* 2001;28(4):360–371.

9. Breitenmoser J, Mörmann W, Mühlemann HR. Damaging effects of toothbrush bristle end form on gingiva. *J Periodontol.* 1979;50(4):212–216.

10. Silverstone LM, Featherstone MJ. A scanning electron microscope study of the end rounding of bristles in eight toothbrush types. *Quintessence Int.* 1988;19(2):3–23.

11. Stiller S, Bosma MLP, Shi X, et al. Interproximal access efficacy of three manual toothbrushes with extended, x-angled or flat multitufted bristles. *Int J Dent Hyg.* 2010;8(3):244–248.

12. Bass CC. An effective method of personal oral hygiene. *J La State Med Soc.* 1954;106(3):57–73.

13. Hard D. Oral prophylaxis. In: Bunting RW, ed. *Oral Hygiene.* 3rd ed. Philadelphia, PA: Lea & Febiger; 1957:280–283.

14. Stillman PR. A philosophy of the treatment of periodontal disease. *Dent Digest.* 1932;38(9):314.

15. Hirschfeld I. *The Toothbrush: Its Use and Abuse.* Brooklyn, NY: Dental Items of Interest; 1939:380.

16. Charters WJ. Home care of the mouth. I. Proper home care of the mouth. *J Periodontol.* 1948;19:136–139.

17. Charters WJ. Eliminating mouth infections with the toothbrush and other stimulating instruments. *Dent Digest.* 1932;38:130.

18. Miller SC. *Textbook of Periodontia.* 3rd ed. Philadelphia, PA: The Blakiston Co; 1950:327–328.

19. Hirschfeld I. *The Toothbrush: Its Use and Abuse.* Brooklyn, NY: Dental Items of Interest; 1939:369–371.

20. Smith TS. Anatomic and physiologic conditions governing the use of the toothbrush. *J Am Dent Assoc.* 1940;27:874–878.

21. Bell DG. Home care of the mouth. III. Teaching home care to the patient. *J Periodontal Res.* 1948;19(4):140–143.

22. Fones AC. *Mouth Hygiene.* 4th ed. Philadelphia, PA: Lea & Febiger; 1934:299–306.

23. Leonard HJ. Conservative treatment of periodontoclasia. *J Am Dent Assoc.* 1939;26:1308–1315.

24. American Dental Association, Council on Scientific Affairs. *ADA Acceptance Program Guidelines for Toothbrushes.* Chicago, IL: American Dental Association. [about 10 screens]. http://www.ada.org/~/media/ADA/Science%20and%20Research/Files/guide_toothbrushes.ashx. Updated April 2012. Accessed November 30, 2014.

25. McKendrick AJW, Barbenel LM, McHugh WD. A two-year comparison of hand and electric toothbrushes. *J Periodontal Res.* 1968;3(3):224–231.

26. Frandsen A. Mechanical oral hygiene practices: state-of-the-science review. In: Löe H, Kleinman DV, eds. *Dental Plaque Control Measures and Oral Hygiene Practices.* Oxford: IRL Press; 1986:93–116.

27. Forrest JL, Miller SA. Manual versus powered toothbrushes: a summary of the Cochrane Oral Health Group's Systematic Review, Part II. *J Dent Hyg.* 2004;78:349–354.

28. Heanue M, Deacon SA, Deery C, et al. Manual versus powered toothbrushing for oral health. *Aust Dent J.* 2005;50(2):123–124.

29. Ho HP, Niederman R. Effectiveness of the Sonicare sonic toothbrush on reduction of plaque, gingivitis, probing pocket depth, and subgingival bacteria in adolescent orthodontic clients. *J Clin Dent.* 1997;8(1): Spec No 5–19.

30. Warren PR, Ray TS, Cugini M, et al. A practice-based study of a power toothbrush: assessment of effectiveness and acceptance. *J Am Dent Assoc.* 2000;131(3):389–394.

31. Danser MM, Timmerman MF, Ijzerman Y, et al. A comparison of electric toothbrushes in their potential to cause gingival abrasion of oral soft tissues. *Am J Dent.* 1998;11:S35–S39.

32. Sharma NC, Galustians HJ, Qaqish J, et al. The effect of two power toothbrushes on calculus and stain formation. *Am J Dent.* 2002;15(2):71–76.

33. van der Weijden GA, Timmerman MF, Reijerse E, et al. Toothbrushing force in relation to plaque removal. *J Clin Periodontol.* 1996;23(8):724–729.

34. Heasman P, Wilson Z, Macgregor I, et al. Comparative study of electric and manual toothbrushes in patients with fixed orthodontic appliances. *Am J Orthod Dentofacial Orthop.* 1998;114(1):45–49.

35. Boyd RL, McLey L, Zahradnik R. Clinical and laboratory evaluation of powered electric toothbrushes: in vivo determination of average force for use of manual and powered toothbrushes. *J Clin Dent.* 1997;8 (Special Issue):72–75.

36. van der Weijden GA, van der Velden U. Fluctuation of the microbiota of the tongue in humans. *J Clin Periodontol.* 1991;18:26–29.

37. Niemi ML, Ainamo J, Etemadzadeh H. The effect of toothbrush grip on gingival abrasion and plaque removal during toothbrushing. *J Clin Periodontol.* 1987;14:19–21.

38. Niemi M, Sandholm L, Ainamo J. Frequency of gingival lesions after standardized brushing as related to stiffness of toothbrush and abrasiveness of dentifrice. *J Clin Periodontol.* 1984;11(4):254–261.

39. Kinane DF, Riggio MP, Walker KF, et al. Bacteraemia following periodontal procedures. *J Clin Periodontol.* 2005;32(7):708–713.

40. Forner L, Larsen T, Kilian M, et al. Incidence of bacteremia after chewing, toothbrushing and scaling in individuals with periodontal inflammation. *J Clin Periodontol.* 2006;33(6):401–407.

41. Hartzell JD, Torres D, Kim P, et al. Incidence of bacteremia after routine tooth brushing. *Am J Med Sci.* 2005;329(4):178–180.

42. Glass RT. The infected toothbrush, the infected denture, and transmission of disease: a review. *Compend Contin Educ Dent.* 1992;13(7):592–598.

43. Müller HP, Lange DE, Müller RF. Actinobacillus actinomycetemcomitans contamination of toothbrushes from patients harbouring the organism. *J Clin Periodontol.* 1989;16(6):388–390.

ENHANCE YOUR UNDERSTANDING

the Point® DIGITAL CONNECTIONS
(see the inside front cover for access information)

- **Audio glossary**
- **Quiz bank**

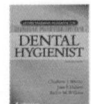

SUPPORT FOR LEARNING
(available separately; visit lww.com)

- *Active Learning Workbook for Clinical Practice of the Dental Hygienist, 12th Edition*

prepU INDIVIDUALIZED REVIEW
(available separately; visit lww.com)

- **Adaptive quizzing with *prepU* for Wilkins'** *Clinical Practice of the Dental Hygienist*

29

Oral Infection Control: Interdental Care

Esther M. Wilkins, BS, RDH, DMD and Deborah M. Lyle, RDH, BS, MS

CHAPTER OUTLINE

LEARNING OBJECTIVES

After studying this chapter, the student will be able to:

1. Review the anatomy of the interdental area and explain why toothbrushing alone cannot remove biofilm adequately for prevention of periodontal infection.

2. Describe types of dental floss and outline steps for use of floss for biofilm removal from proximal tooth surfaces.

3. Develop a list of the types and purposes of various floss aids and provide a rationale for the choice of the best ones to meet a specific patient's needs.

4. Compare types of interdental brushes and explain why they may be more effective than floss for some patients.

5. Demonstrate and recommend other devices for biofilm removal including toothpick in holder, wooden interdental cleaner, interdental rubber tip, and water irrigation.

▶ Toothbrushing cannot accomplish biofilm removal for the proximal tooth surfaces and adjacent gingiva to the same degree that it does for the facial, lingual, and palatal aspects. Interdental biofilm control, therefore, is essential to complete the patient's oral self-care program.

▶ Objectives and procedures for removal of dental biofilm from proximal tooth surfaces are included in this chapter.

▶ Key words are defined in Box 29-1.

▶ When the preventive treatment plan is outlined for an individual, assessment is made of the oral condition, the problem areas, and the overall prognosis for improvement or maintenance of gingival health.

  • Measures for interdental biofilm control are selected to complement biofilm control by toothbrushing.

THE INTERDENTAL AREA

▶ The three types of gingival embrasures are illustrated in Figure 29-1.

▶ In health, the interdental gingiva fills the interproximal area and under the contact of the adjacent teeth in a Type I embrasure.

▶ When the interdental papilla is missing or reduced in height, which is common as a result of periodontal infection, the shape of the interdental gingiva changes, and open Type II or Type III embrasures may be seen.

▶ Figure 29-2 shows a Type II embrasure from the proximal surface with the col and from the facial surface.

I. Anatomy of the Interdental Area

A review of the gingival and dental anatomy of the interdental area can give meaning to and clarify the role and purpose of the various devices available for interdental care.

A. Posterior Teeth

▶ Between adjacent posterior teeth are two papillae, one facial and one lingual or palatal.

▶ The papillae are connected by a col, a depressed concave area that follows the shape of the apical border of the contact area (Figure 29-2).

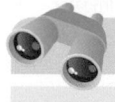

BOX 29-1   KEY WORDS: Interdental Care

Col: the depression in the gingival tissue under a contact area between the lingual (palatal) papilla and the facial papilla.

Embrasure: V-shaped spillway space next to the contact area of adjacent teeth, narrowest at the contact and widening toward the facial, lingual (palatal), and occlusal contacts.

Floss cleft: a cleft in the gingival margin usually at a mesial or distal line angle of a tooth where dental floss was repeatedly applied incorrectly. The lining of the cleft can be completely lined with epithelium.

Floss cut: unintentional incision at the gingival margin due to incorrect positioning and placement of dental floss.

Hydrotherapy: the use of forced intermittent or steady stream of water for a cleansing or therapeutic purpose.

Interproximal space: the triangular region bounded by the proximal surfaces of contacting teeth and the alveolar bone between the teeth, which forms the base of the triangle; the space is normally filled with the interdental papilla; also called the interdental area.

Irrigant: substance used for irrigation.

Irrigation: flushing of a specific area or site with a stream of fluid; application of a continuous or pulsated stream of fluid to a part of the body for a cleansing or therapeutic purpose.

  Supragingival irrigation: the point of delivery of the irrigation is at, or coronal to, the free gingival margin.

  Marginal irrigation: the point of delivery of the irrigation is angled at, or placed apically to, the gingival margin.

  Subgingival irrigation: the point of the delivery of the irrigation is placed in the sulcus or pocket and may reach the base of the pocket depending on its probing depth.

Keratinized epithelium: outer, protective surface of stratified squamous epithelium; covers the masticatory mucosa; interdental col area is not normally keratinized.

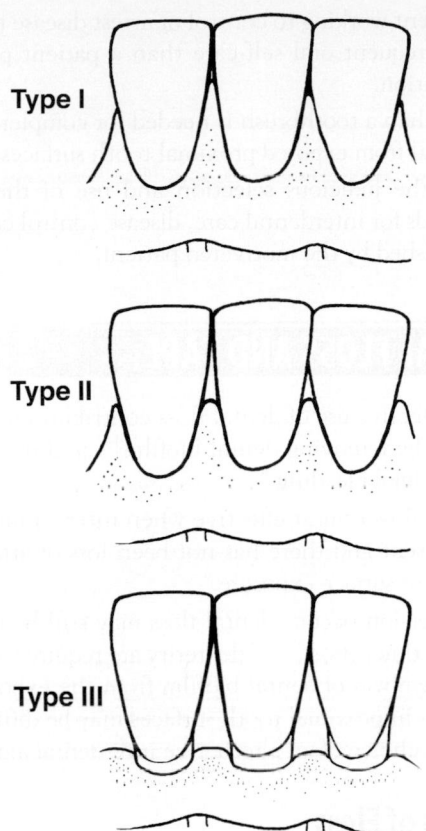

FIGURE 29-1 Types of Gingival Embrasures. Type I, interdental papilla fills the gingival embrasure. Type II, with slight-to-moderate recession of the interdental papilla. Type III, with extensive recession or complete loss of the interdental papilla.

B. Anterior Teeth

▶ Between anterior teeth in contact is a single papilla with a pyramidal shape.

▶ Tip of the papilla may form a small col under the contact area (Figure 29-2).

C. Epithelium

▶ The epithelium covering a col is usually thin and not keratinized.

▶ Col epithelium is protected and is less resistant to infection than keratinized surfaces.

▶ Inflammation in the papilla leads to enlargement; with increased inflammatory cells and edema, the col becomes deeper.

▶ The col area is inaccessible for ordinary toothbrushing; microorganisms are harbored in the concave center.

▶ Most gingival disease starts in the col area.

▶ The incidence of gingivitis is greatest in the interdental tissues.[1]

II. Proximal Tooth Surfaces

▶ With bacterial infection and loss of gingival attachment, the interdental papillae are reduced in height.

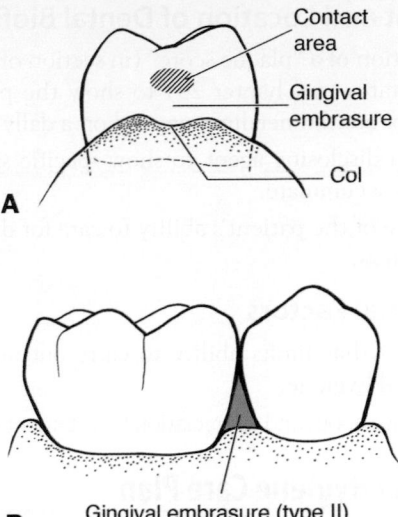

FIGURE 29-2 Type II Gingival Embrasure. A: Embrasure shown from the proximal surface with the col. **B:** Facial view, with gingival embrasure shown in blue.

▶ Proximal tooth surfaces become exposed.

▶ Dental biofilm can accumulate.

▶ Irregularities of tooth position, such as rotation or overlapping, and deviations related to malocclusion or tooth loss may be present.

▶ Easy access for removal of bacterial deposits by the individual is prevented.

▶ Root surface morphology of the proximal surfaces is typical for each tooth type.

▶ Concavities and grooves are predisposed to bacterial accumulations.[2,3]

▶ With advanced periodontitis, furcation areas of maxillary first premolars and molars open onto the proximal surfaces.

PLANNING INTERDENTAL CARE

I. Patient Assessment

A. History of Personal Oral Care

▶ Type of toothbrush, dental floss, and other interdental devices currently used.

▶ Frequency and time spent.

▶ Estimate of the patient's apparent priorities on personal oral self-care.

B. Dental and Gingival Anatomy

▶ Position of teeth.

▶ Types and shapes of embrasures: variation throughout the dentition.

▶ Probing depths: classification of the periodontal condition.

▶ Prostheses present: special interdental care required for fixed and removable prostheses.

▶ Areas where toothbrush cannot reach.

C. Extent and Location of Dental Biofilm

▶ Preparation of a "plaque score" (in section on Oral Hygiene Status in Chapter 23) to show the patient the extent of biofilm needing removal on a daily basis.

▶ Use of a disclosing agent to show specific sites where biofilms accumulate.

▶ Evidence of the patient's ability to care for difficult-to-access areas.

D. Personal Factors

▶ Disability that limits ability to carry out needed personal oral hygiene.

▶ Knowledge about and appreciation for interdental oral care.

II. Dental Hygiene Care Plan

A. Objectives

▶ Utilize motivational interviewing (Chapter 26) to select appropriate interdental aids to help the patient reach optimum oral cleanliness and health.

▶ Educate the patient on the oral care aids selected.

▶ Motivate the patient to accept responsibility for daily personal care.

B. Initial Care Plan

▶ At first, the simplest procedures are selected for the patient's convenience and ease of learning based on the patient's current knowledge, preferences, and oral self-care habits.

▶ Minimum frequency: thoroughly twice daily.

▶ Keep the daily oral self-care regimen at a realistic level with respect to the time the patient is able or willing to spend.

▶ As the values the patient places on oral health increase over time, and as the preventive maintenance program becomes a priority in the patient's lifelong self-care health goals, a more refined program can be introduced.

SELECTIVE INTERDENTAL BIOFILM REMOVAL

I. Relation to Toothbrushing

▶ Vibratory and sulcular toothbrushing, such as that performed with the Charters, Stillman, and Bass methods, can be successful to some degree in removing dental biofilm near the line angles of the facial and lingual or palatal embrasures.

▶ Brush in vertical position is effective for additional access around line angles onto the proximal surfaces (Figure 28-12 in Chapter 28).

II. Selection of Interdental Aids

▶ Dependent on oral health, disease status, and the risk for future recurrence.

▶ A patient working to control or arrest disease may need more frequent oral self-care than a patient practicing prevention.

▶ More than a toothbrush is needed for complete biofilm removal from exposed proximal tooth surfaces.

▶ With the judicious selection and use of the various methods for interdental care, disease control can be accomplished by the motivated patient.

DENTAL FLOSS AND TAPE

▶ The effective use of dental floss contributes to gingival health by removing dental biofilm[4–7] and reducing interproximal bleeding.[8]

▶ Dental floss is most effective when interdental papillae are present and there has not been loss of attachment with root surface exposure.[9]

▶ As recession occurs, dental floss may still be used, but greater time, effort, and dexterity are required and complete removal of dental biofilm from the exposed concavities in proximal tooth surfaces may be difficult and require choice of an alternative interdental aid.

I. Types of Floss

▶ Research has shown no difference in the effectiveness of waxed or unwaxed floss for biofilm removal.[4,6,10–12]

▶ Biofilm removal depends on how floss is applied. For optimal patient compliance, the patient may use a preferred type.[4,13]

A. Materials

▶ *Silk*: Historically, floss was made of silk fibers loosely twisted together to form a strand and waxed for proximal surface cleaning.

▶ *Nylon*: Nylon multifilaments, waxed or unwaxed, have been widely used in circular (floss) or flat (tape) form for biofilm removal from proximal tooth surfaces.

▶ *Polytetrafluoroethylene (PTFE)*: Monofilament PTFE is used for proximal tooth surface biofilm removal.

B. Features of Waxed Floss

▶ Smooth surface provided by the wax coating helps the floss slide through the contact area.

▶ Ease in sliding the floss between the teeth may minimize tissue trauma.

▶ Wax gives strength and durability during application to minimize breakage.

C. Features of Unwaxed Floss

▶ Thinner floss may be helpful when contact areas are tight; however, forcing the floss through may break the floss.

▶ Pressure against a tooth surface spreads the nylon fibers and gives a wider surface for biofilm removal.

▶ Sharper thin edge requires special attention to prevent injury to the gingival tissue when guiding floss through a tight contact area or when moving floss on the tooth surface in an apical direction.

▶ Squeaking sound effect when floss moves over a clean tooth surface may provide a motivation for patient thoroughness.

▶ Unwaxed floss, which can fray when rubbed over an irregular tooth surface, rough surface of a restoration, or calculus deposit, might cause the patient to become aggravated and discouraged, thereby resulting in lost motivation to floss regularly.

▶ Floss that is tightly wound around fingers tends to cut, hurt, and cause discomfort. This problem is as likely with wide dental tape or with waxed floss or tape.

D. Features of PTFE

▶ Monofilament type resists breakage or shredding when passed over irregular tooth surface, restoration, or calculus deposit.

▶ Reduces the force required to pass the floss through the contact which may improve patient compliance with regular flossing and reduce tissue injury or trauma.[14]

E. Enhancements

▶ Color and flavor have been added to dental floss.

▶ Therapeutic agents that have been added include fluoride and whitening agents. Limited research has been published relative to their effectiveness.

II. Procedure

▶ When dental floss is applied with firm pressure to a flat or convex proximal tooth surface, biofilm can be removed.

▶ Older biofilm is tenacious and may require several strokes for removal.

▶ When floss is placed over a concave surface, contact is not possible (Figure 29-3A), and supplementary devices are needed to remove a bacterial deposit completely.

A. When to Floss

For most patients, the best results can be obtained by using dental floss before toothbrushing. The following reasons may apply:

▶ When proximal tooth surfaces are flossed first and biofilm is removed, the fluoride from a dentifrice used while brushing reaches the proximal surfaces for prevention of dental caries.

▶ When brushing is accomplished first, flossing may not be carried out.

• The mouth feels clean; the need for flossing may not be appreciated.

• Time may be short and flossing may be postponed.

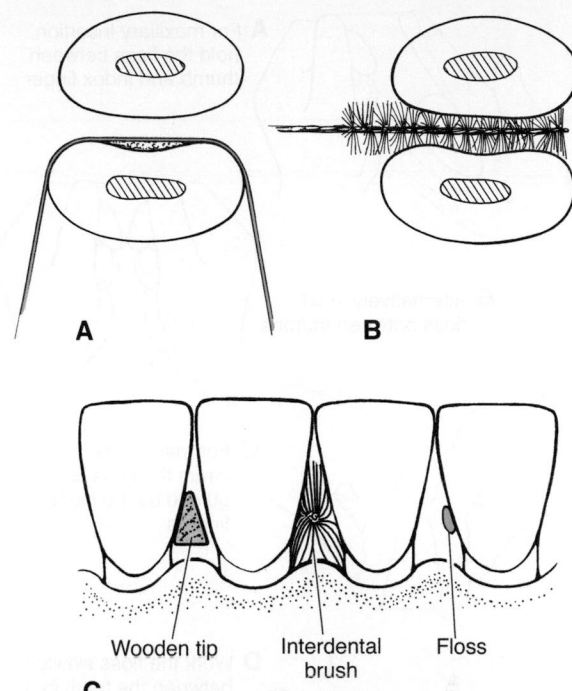

FIGURE 29-3 Interdental Care. A: Floss positioned on the mesial surface of a maxillary first premolar shows the inability of the floss to remove dental biofilm on a concave proximal tooth surface. **B:** The use of an interdental brush in the same interproximal area to show how the proximal surfaces can be cleaned free of dental biofilm. **C:** Comparison of the access of a wooden tip, an interdental brush, and a piece of dental floss to an open interdental area.

B. Floss Preparation

▶ Figure 29-4 outlines the flossing steps described in detail here in this section.

▶ Hold a 12- to 15-inch length of floss with the thumb and index finger of each hand; grasp firmly with only half inch of floss between the fingertips. The ends of the floss may be tucked into the palm and held by the ring and little finger, or the floss may be wrapped around the middle fingers (Figure 29-4A–C).

▶ A circle of floss may be made by tying the ends together; the circle may be rotated as the floss is used (Figure 29-5).[15]

C. Application

▶ *Maxillary teeth:* Direct the floss upward by holding the floss over two thumbs or a thumb and an index finger as shown in Figure 29-4A and B. Rest a side of a finger on teeth of the opposite side of the maxillary arch to provide balance and a fulcrum.

▶ *Mandibular teeth:* Direct the floss down by holding the two index fingers on top of the strand. One index finger holds the floss on the lingual aspect and the other on the facial aspect (Figure 29-4C). The side of the finger on the lingual side is held on the teeth of the opposite side of the mouth to serve as a fulcrum or rest.

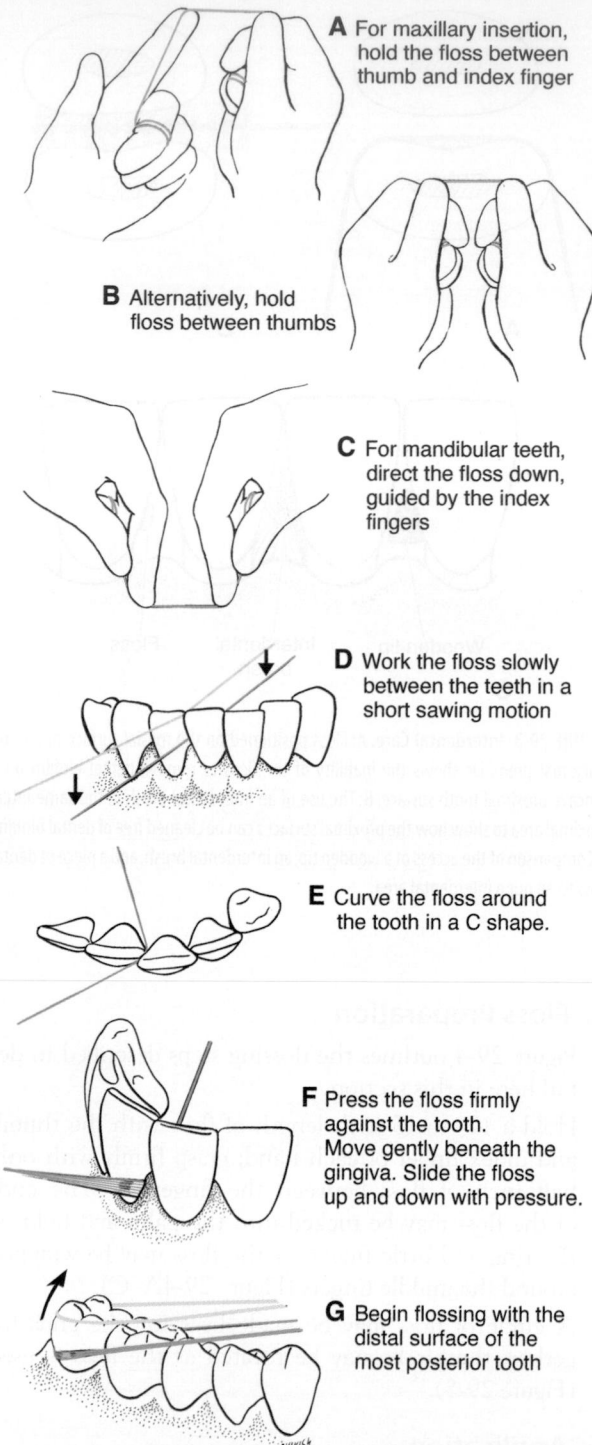

A For maxillary insertion, hold the floss between thumb and index finger

B Alternatively, hold floss between thumbs

C For mandibular teeth, direct the floss down, guided by the index fingers

D Work the floss slowly between the teeth in a short sawing motion

E Curve the floss around the tooth in a C shape.

F Press the floss firmly against the tooth. Move gently beneath the gingiva. Slide the floss up and down with pressure.

G Begin flossing with the distal surface of the most posterior tooth

Figure 29-4 Use of Dental Floss. For maxillary insertion, hold the floss between the thumb and index finger **A:** or between thumbs **B:** Grasp the floss firmly. Allow only 1/2-inch length between fingers. **C:** For the mandibular teeth, direct the floss down, guided by the index fingers. **D:** Work the floss slowly between the teeth in a short sawing motion. Avoid snapping through the contact area. **E:** Curve the floss around the tooth in a C-shape. Hold the floss toward the mesial for cleaning the distal surfaces and toward the distal for cleaning the mesial surfaces. **F:** Press the floss firmly against the tooth. Move gently beneath the gingiva until tissue resistance is felt. Slide the floss horizontally and vertically with pressure to remove biofilm. **G:** Begin flossing with the distal surface of the most posterior tooth, and work systematically around the arch.

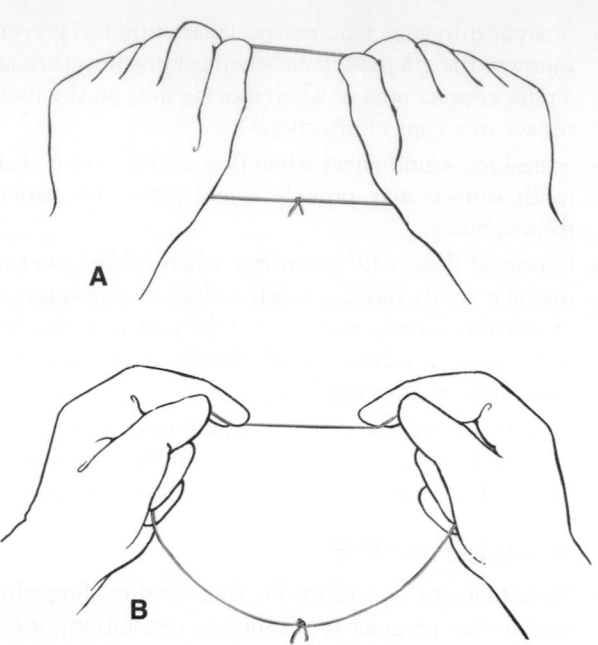

A

B

FIGURE 29-5 Circle of Floss. The ends of the floss are tied together for convenient holding. A child may be able to manage floss better with this technique. **A:** Floss held for maxillary teeth. **B:** Floss held for mandibular teeth.

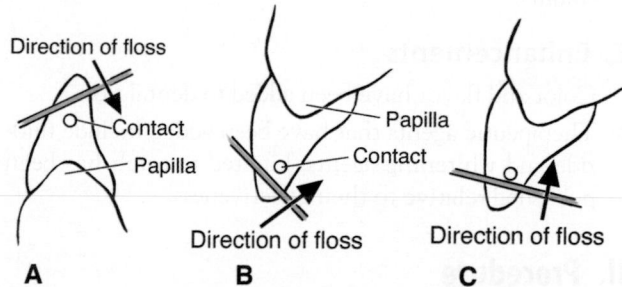

Direction of floss

Contact

Papilla

Papilla

Contact

Direction of floss

Direction of floss

A   **B**   **C**

FIGURE 29-6 Insertion of Floss. Hold floss in a diagonal or oblique position over the teeth where the floss will be inserted. Arrows indicate the direction of movement of the floss. **A:** Floss held for mandibular insertion. **B:** Floss held for maxillary insertion. **C:** Floss held incorrectly. When floss is held horizontally, the possibility for damage to the papilla is greater.

D. Insertion

▶ Hold floss firmly in a diagonal or oblique position (Figure 29-6).

▶ Guide the floss past each contact area with a gentle back and forth or sawing motion (Figure 29-4D).

▶ Control floss to prevent snapping through the contact area into the gingival tissue.

E. Cleaning Stroke

▶ Clean adjacent teeth separately; for the distal aspect, curve the floss mesially, and for the mesial aspect, curve the floss distally, around the tooth (Figure 29-4E and F).

▶ Pass the floss below the gingival margin, curve to adapt the floss around the tooth, press, and slide up and down over the tooth surface. Repeat.

▶ Loop the floss over the distal surfaces of the most posterior teeth in each quadrant and the teeth next to edentulous areas (Figure 29-4G). Hold firmly against the tooth and move the floss in an up-and-down motion.

F. Additional Suggestions

▶ Slide the floss to a new, unused portion for succeeding proximal tooth surfaces.

▶ Floss may be doubled to provide a wider rubbing surface.

▶ When a dentifrice is used with the floss, dental tape may be better than floss in retaining the dentifrice against the tooth.

III. Precautions

A. Pressure in Col Area

▶ The col area is not keratinized and is vulnerable to bacterial invasion.

▶ Biofilm control of the area is of great importance because most gingival and periodontal infection begins in the col area.

▶ Too great a pressure with floss one or more times daily, particularly very fine floss that tends to cut more easily than thicker floss, can be destructive to the attachment.

▶ Excess pressure of the floss against the attachment is particularly significant in children in whom teeth are in the process of eruption and the junctional epithelium is less firmly attached.

B. Prevention of Floss Cuts and Floss Clefts

▶ *Location*: Floss cuts or clefts occur primarily on facial and lingual or palatal surfaces directly beside or in the middle of an interdental papilla. They appear as straight-line cuts from the gingival margin and may result in a floss cleft (Figure 18-13B in Chapter 18).[16]

▶ *Causes*
  ● Using a piece of floss that is too long between the fingers when held for insertion.
  ● Snapping the floss through the contact area.
  ● Not curving the floss about the teeth; holding floss straight across the papilla.
  ● Not using a rest to prevent undue pressure.

TUFTED DENTAL FLOSS

I. Description

Tufted dental floss is also called a floss/yarn combination. Regular dental floss is alternated with a thickened tufted portion. Two variations are available commercially.

▶ *Single, precut lengths*

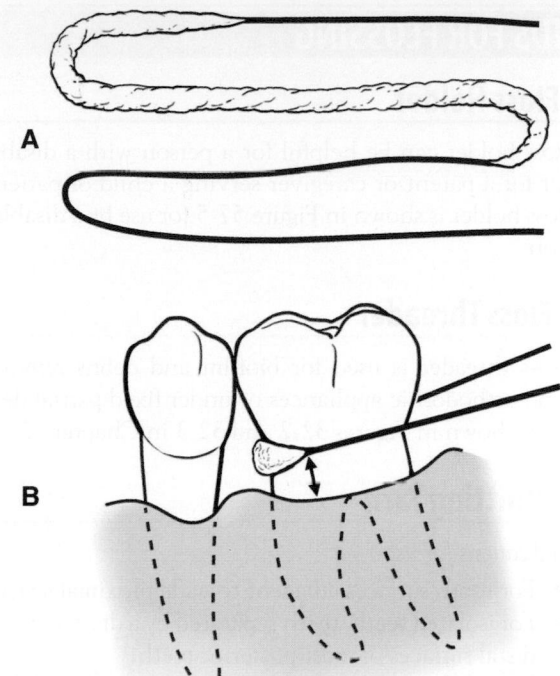

FIGURE 29-7 Tufted Dental Floss. The floss/yarn combination may be "Super Floss" (A) in a precut length with a tufted portion and a 3-inch stiffened end for insertion under a fixed prosthesis, (B) shows how the tufted part of the floss might be used interproximally to remove biofilm.

● Available in a 2-foot length composed of a 5-inch tufted portion adjacent to a 3-inch stiffened end for inserting under a fixed appliance or orthodontic attachment (Figure 29-7A).
● Example: Super Floss®.[17]

II. Indications for Use

▶ Biofilm removal from tooth surfaces adjacent to wide embrasures where interdental papillae have been lost.

▶ Biofilm removal from mesial and distal abutments and under pontic of a fixed partial denture, implant, or orthodontic appliance. The stiff end of Super Floss® is inserted like a floss threader (see Figure 32-3).

III. Procedure

A. Individual Surface of Tooth or Implant

Curve floss and/or tufted portion around the tooth or implant in a "C" to remove dental biofilm. Move floss vertically and horizontally (Figure 29-7B).

B. Fixed Partial Denture

Thread tufted floss over pontic and apply to distal surface of the mesial abutment and mesial surface of the distal abutment (Figure 32-3 in Chapter 32).

AIDS FOR FLOSSING

I. Floss Holder

A floss holder can be helpful for a person with a disability or for a parent or caregiver serving a child or patient. A floss holder is shown in Figure 57-5 for use by a disabled person.

II. Floss Threader

A floss threader is used for biofilm and debris removal around orthodontic appliances or under fixed partial dentures as shown in Figures 32-2 and 32-3 in Chapter 32.

III. Knitting Yarn

▶ Indications for use
- For tooth surfaces adjacent to wide proximal spaces.
- For isolated teeth, teeth separated by a diastema, and distal surfaces of most posterior teeth.
- For mesial and distal abutments of fixed partial dentures and under pontics, use a floss threader.

▶ Procedure
- Select about 8–10 inches of 3- or 4-ply smooth synthetic yarn.
- Fold yarn double. Loop through about 8 inches of dental floss; tie floss with one overhand knot.
- Insert floss through the contact area. Draw the yarn into the embrasure (Figure 29-8).
- Clean adjacent teeth separately with a facial-lingual, back-and-forth stroke. Hold the ends of the yarn distally and then around mesially.
- For specific areas where a papilla may be high or access is not otherwise sufficient for the wide yarn, use the dental floss end of the combination.
- Apply dentifrice and rub surface with the yarn back and forth, up and down.
- For closed contacts, use a floss threader (see Figure 32-2 in Chapter 32).

IV. Gauze Strip

▶ Uses
- For proximal surfaces of widely spaced teeth.
- For surfaces of teeth next to edentulous areas.
- For outer mesial and distal surfaces of abutment teeth of a fixed partial denture.
- For areas under posterior cantilevered section of a fixed appliance, such as the distal portion of a denture supported by implants.

▶ Procedure
- Cut 1-inch gauze bandage into a 6- to 8-inch length, and fold in thirds or down the center.
- Position the fold of the gauze on the cervical area next to the gingival crest and work back and forth several times; hold ends in a distal direction to clean

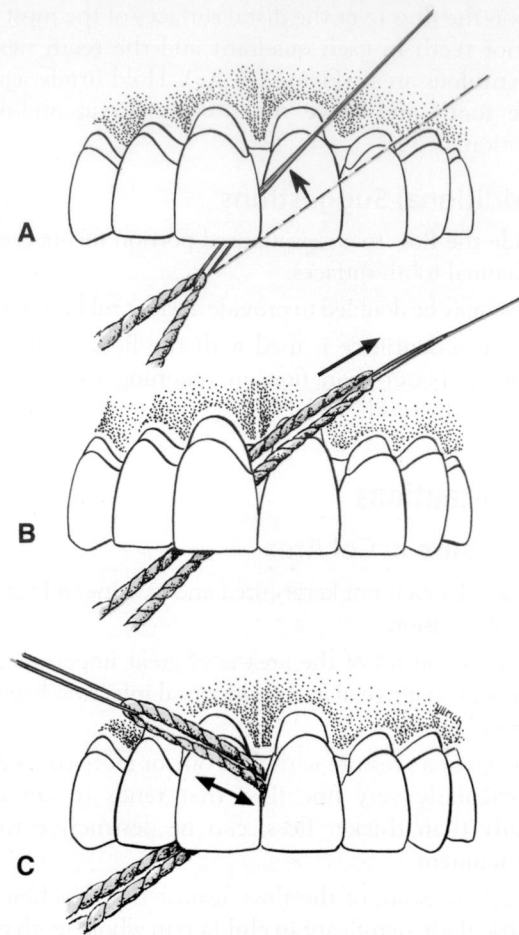

FIGURE 29-8 Knitting Yarn. A: Yarn is looped through dental floss, and the floss is drawn through the contact area in the usual manner, shown by the arrow. **B:** Yarn is drawn through the embrasure. **C:** Yarn is positioned against the surface of the tooth for biofilm removal. When tooth contact is missing and space permits, the yarn is used without floss.

a mesial surface, and in a mesial direction to clean a distal surface (Figure 29-9).

INTERDENTAL BRUSHES

I. Types

A. Small Insert Brushes with Reusable Handle

▶ Soft nylon filaments are twisted into a fine stainless steel wire for insertion into a handle with an angulated shank (Figure 29-10A). Select brush with plastic-coated wire.

▶ The small tapered or cylindrical brush heads are of varying sizes approximately 12–15 mm (1/2 inch) in length, with a diameter of 3–5 mm (1/8–1/4 inch).

B. Brush with Plastic Handle

▶ Soft nylon filaments are twisted into a fine stainless steel wire.

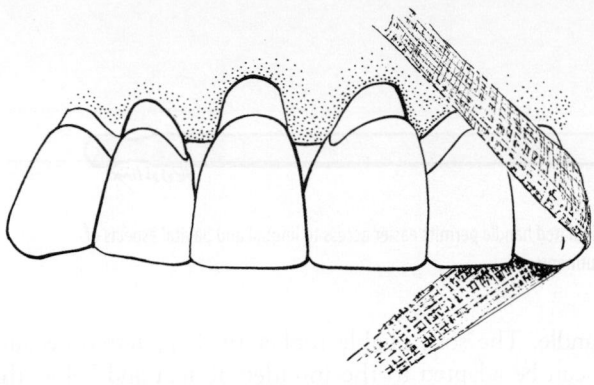

FIGURE 29-9 **Gauze Strip.** A 6- or 8-inch length of 1-inch bandage is folded in thirds and placed around a tooth adjacent to an edentulous area, a tooth with interdental spacing, or the distal surface of the most posterior tooth. A shoe-shine stroke is used to clean the dental biofilm from the surface.

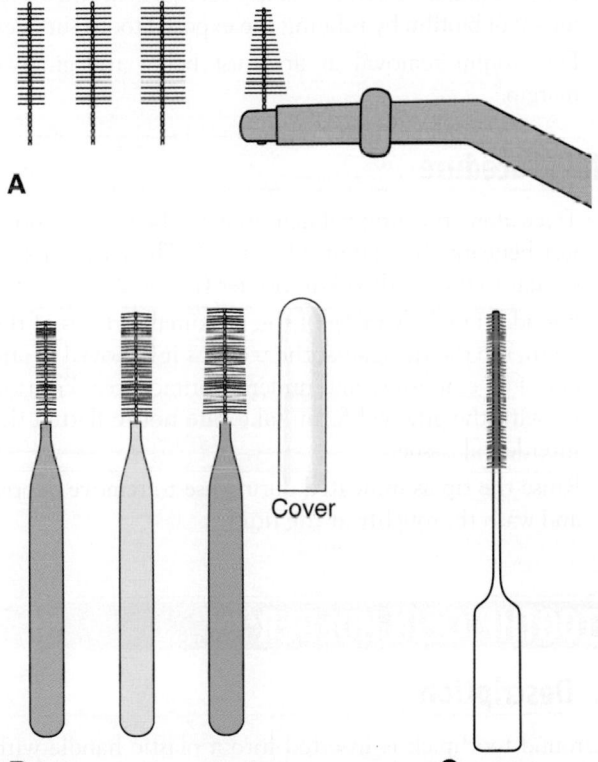

FIGURE 29-10 **Single-tuft and Interdental Brushes. A:** Insert brushes for a reusable handle with an angulated shank. **B:** Reusable interdental brush with filaments twisted onto a fine wire that ends in a handle and cover. **C:** Disposable interdental brush with handle.

- The wire is continuous with the handle, which is approximately 35–45 mm (1½–1¾ inches) in length (Figure 29-10A).
- Travel brushes are also available (Figure 29-10B) and may be more convenient for patients.
▶ The very short, soft filaments form a narrow brush approximately 30–35 mm (1¼–1½ inches) in length and 5–8 mm (1/4–5/16 inches) in diameter (Figure 29-10A and B).

C. Soft-picks[18]

▶ Similar to an interdental brush, but do not have a wire or bristles. The soft-pick has small elastomeric fingers that are perpendicular to a plastic core (Figure 29-10C).
▶ The soft-pick is effective at biofilm removal and reducing gingival inflammation.

II. Indications for Use

When sufficient space is available for the insertion of an interdental brush without excess force, the following applications are indicated:

A. For Removal of Dental Biofilm and Debris

▶ Proximal tooth surfaces adjacent to open embrasures, orthodontic appliances, fixed prostheses, dental implants, periodontal splints, and space maintainers, and other areas that are hard to reach with a regular toothbrush.
▶ Concave proximal surfaces where dental floss and other interdental aids cannot reach (Figure 29-3A). Floss will not access a concave surface, whereas the interproximal brush can reach and cleanse (Figure 29-3B).[1,19]
  • In patients with open embrasures and moderate to severe attachment loss, the interdental brush is more effective than floss.[19]
▶ Exposed Class IV furcations (Figure 19-9 in Chapter 19).

B. For Application of Chemotherapeutic Agents

▶ Fluoride dentifrice, gel, and/or mouthrinse for prevention of dental caries, particularly root surface caries, and for surfaces adjacent to any prosthesis.
▶ Antibacterial agents for control of dental biofilm and the prevention of gingivitis.
▶ Desensitizing agents.

III. Procedure

▶ Select brush of appropriate diameter.
▶ Moisten the brush and insert at an angle in keeping with gingival form; brush in and out.
▶ For wide embrasures, it will be important to remember to apply pressure against the proximal root surfaces to remove the biofilm thoroughly.
  • Insert the interdental brush as shown in Figure 29-3B and C.
  • Apply pressure toward the mesial proximal surface to remove biofilm.
  • Then apply pressure toward the distal proximal surface and remove the surface biofilm.

IV. Care of Brushes

▶ Clean brush during use to remove debris and biofilm by holding under actively running water.

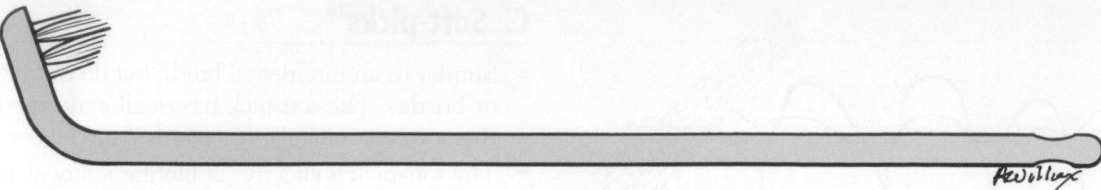

FIGURE 29-11 **Single-tuft Brush with Bent Shank.** Adaptation of brush with angulated handle permits easier access to lingual and palatal aspects of the natural teeth, as well as to orthodontic appliances, prostheses, and implant abutments.

▶ Clean thoroughly after use and dry in open air.

▶ Discard before the filaments become deformed or loosened.

SINGLE-TUFT BRUSH (END-TUFT, UNITUFT)

I. Description

The single tuft, or group of small tufts, may be 3–6 mm in diameter and may be flat or tapered (Figure 28-9). The handle may be straight or contra angled.

II. Indications for Use

▶ *For open interproximal areas*

▶ *For fixed dental prostheses*

- The single-tuft brush may be adaptable around and under a fixed partial denture, pontic, orthodontic appliance, precision attachment, or implant abutment.

▶ *For difficult-to-reach areas*

- The lingual surfaces of the mandibular molars, abutment teeth, the distal surfaces of the most posterior teeth, and teeth that are crowded are examples of areas where an end-tuft brush may be of value.

- The shank may be bent for easy adaptation (Figure 29-11).

III. Procedure

▶ Direct the tip of the tuft into the interproximal area and along the gingival margin; go around the distal surfaces from lingual and facial of the most distal teeth in all four quadrants.

▶ Combine a rotating motion with intermittent pressure especially in the interproximal areas to reach as much of the proximal surfaces as possible.

▶ Use a sulcular brushing stroke.

INTERDENTAL TIP

I. Composition and Design

Conical or pyramidal flexible rubber tip is attached to the end of the handle of a toothbrush or is on a special plastic handle. The soft, pliable rubber tip is preferred because it can be adapted to the interdental area and below the gingival margin without causing damage to the epithelial lining.

II. Indications for Use

▶ For cleaning debris from the interdental area and for removal of biofilm by rubbing the exposed tooth surfaces.

▶ For biofilm removal at and just below the gingival margin.

III. Procedure

▶ Trace along the gingival margin with the tip positioned just beneath the margin (1–2 mm). The adaptation is similar to the toothpick in holder (Figure 29-12).

▶ For additional cleaning of the proximal surfaces of the teeth, rub the tip against the teeth as it is moved in and out of an embrasure and under a contact area. Position tip with the gingival form; take care not to flatten the interdental tissue.

▶ Rinse the tip as indicated during use to remove debris, and wash thoroughly at the finish.

TOOTHPICK IN HOLDER[20]

I. Description

A round toothpick is inserted into a plastic handle with contra-angled ends for adaptation to the tooth surface at

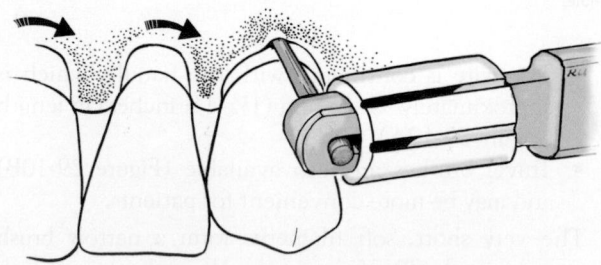

FIGURE 29-12 **Toothpick in Holder for Dental Biofilm at Gingival Margin.** The tip is placed at or just below the gingival margin. Trace the margin around each tooth.

the gingival margin for biofilm removal. The device also is called a Perio-Aid®.

II. Indications for Use

A. Patient with Periodontitis

For biofilm removal at and just under the gingival margin, for interdental cleaning, particularly for concave proximal tooth surfaces, and for exposed furcation area.

B. Orthodontic Patient

For biofilm removal at gingival margin above appliances.

III. Procedure

A. Prepare Instrument

▶ Insert round tapered toothpick into the end of the holder. One type of holder has angulated ends for use in various positions.

▶ Twist the toothpick firmly into place. Break off the long end cleanly so that sharp edges do not scratch the inner cheek or the tongue during use.

B. Application

▶ Apply toothpick at the gingival margin. Apply just under the gingival margin at a slant, with moderate pressure; trace the gingival margin around each tooth to remove biofilm.

▶ To remove biofilm just below the gingival margin, apply the end at less than 45°, maintain the tip on the tooth surface, and follow around the sulcus or pocket (Figure 29-12).

▶ Use a tip that has become soft and slightly frayed from use as a small cleaning "brush" to rub on tooth surfaces where biofilm has collected.

▶ For hypersensitive spots, usually at the cervical third of a tooth, the patient can use the tip daily to massage dentifrice for desensitization on the sensitive area.

▶ When a contact is inadequate and the patient indicates that floss or toothpicks are required to relieve pressure from impacted food, dental attention may be needed. The area is charted or otherwise brought to the attention of the dentist.

WOODEN INTERDENTAL CLEANER

I. Description

The wooden cleaner is a 2-inch-long device made of basswood or birch wood. It is triangular in cross section, as shown in Figure 29-13.

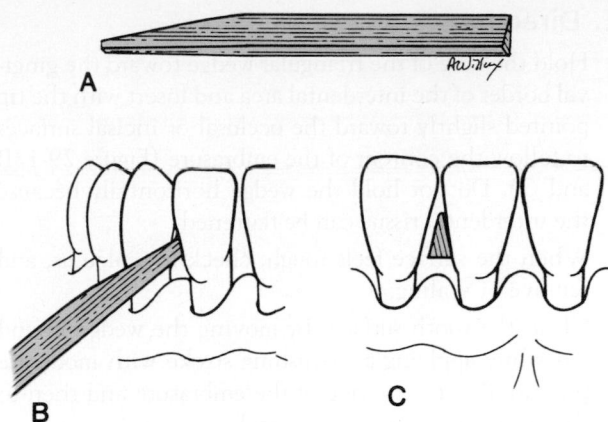

FIGURE 29-13 Wooden Interdental Cleaner. A: The 2-inch wooden triangular cleaner. **B:** Application on the proximal surface of a tooth with a Type III embrasure. The base of the triangle is on the gingival side. **C:** The side of the triangle is rubbed in and out against the proximal surface to remove dental biofilm.

II. Indications for Use

▶ *Application*

- For cleaning proximal tooth surfaces where the tooth surfaces are exposed and interdental gingiva are missing. Space must be adequate otherwise the gingival tissue can be traumatized.[21]

▶ *Advantages*[21]

- Ease of use.
- Transport easily and can be used throughout the day.

▶ *Limitation*

- As with most interdental devices, the wooden cleaner is advised only for the patient who follows instructions carefully.
- The wooden interdental cleaner cannot access exposed root concavities and irregularities to adequately remove dental biofilm.
- Difficult to use in posterior areas and from the lingual aspect of the teeth.[21]
- A fresh cleaner is advised for each arch or quadrant because the wood may become splayed.

III. Procedure

A. Fulcrum (Rest)

▶ First teach the patient to use a rest by placing the hand on the cheek or chin or by placing a finger on the gingiva convenient to the place where the tip will be applied. This precaution helps prevent insertion of the wedge with too much pressure.

B. Preparation

▶ Soften the wood by placing the pointed end in the mouth and moistening with saliva.

C. Directions

▶ Hold the base of the triangular wedge toward the gingival border of the interdental area and insert with the tip pointed slightly toward the occlusal or incisal surfaces to follow the contour of the embrasure (Figure 29-13B and C). Do not hold the wedge horizontally because the interdental tissue can be flattened.

▶ When the surface feels rough, check for calculus, and remove by scaling.

▶ Clean the tooth surfaces by moving the wedge in and out while applying a burnishing stroke with moderate pressure first to one side of the embrasure and then to the other, about four strokes each.

▶ Discard the cleaner as soon as the first signs of splaying are evident.

ORAL IRRIGATION

I. Description

▶ Irrigation is the targeted application of a pulsated or steady stream of water or other irrigant for preventive or therapeutic purposes.
  • The purpose of irrigation is to reduce the bacteria and inflammatory mediators that lead to the initiation or progression of periodontal infections.
  • For the patient, irrigation can be a part of routine self-care.

▶ Mechanical devices, including toothbrushes and interdental aids, can accomplish dental biofilm removal supragingivally and slightly below the gingival margin for the motivated patient.
  • Toothbrushes penetrate less than 1 mm into the gingival sulcus.[22]

▶ Benefits from removing loosely connected biofilm with the use of an oral irrigator include:
  • Reduction of gingivitis and bleeding.[23,24]
  • Reduction or alteration of subgingival dental biofilm.[25]
  • Subgingival access to pathogenic microorganisms.[26,27]
  • Subgingival delivery of antimicrobial agents.

▶ Supragingival and marginal irrigation are effective for removing loosely attached dental biofilm and reducing gingivitis.

▶ When an antimicrobial agent is used in the irrigator, reduction of the supragingival and subgingival biofilm and of gingivitis is enhanced.[25]

II. Penetration into Pocket: Subgingival Access

▶ The standard jet tip placed supragingivally can penetrate below the gingival margin 44%–71% of the pocket depth.[26]

▶ Specialized tips used for marginal or subgingival delivery have shown penetration between 41% and 90%

depending on tip use, technique, and presence of calculus.[27,28]

III. Power-Driven Device

▶ Generates an intermittent or pulsating jet of fluid with an adjustable dial for regulation of pressure and flow.

▶ Delivers irrigant through a handheld interchangeable tip that rotates 360° for application at or below the gingival margin.

▶ Maintains steady flow or pulsations of irrigant from a reservoir.

DELIVERY METHODS

▶ When a standard delivery tip is directed perpendicular to the long axis of the tooth, two zones of hydrokinetic activity are created.[29]
  • *Zone 1*: impact zone, where the irrigant makes initial contact.
  • *Zone 2*: flushing zone, where the irrigant is deflected from the tooth surface subgingivally.

▶ A pulsating stream has been shown to be superior to a steady stream, a fact to consider when recommending products.

▶ Patient-applied irrigation is divided into three categories based on tip placement and design:
  • Supragingival irrigation
  • Marginal irrigation
  • Subgingival irrigation.

I. Standard Jet Tip

A. Delivery Tips

▶ Monojet (single stream) (Figure 29-14A)
▶ Fractionated microjet (Figure 29-14B)
▶ Pulsating and nonpulsating.

B. Procedure

▶ Described in Box 29-2.
▶ Easy to do for most patients.

C. Special Instructions

▶ Always read and follow manufacturer's instructions regarding use of an irrigator.

▶ Irrigation imparts a clean feeling to the mouth.

▶ It is used as part of a comprehensive oral care regimen.

II. Specialized Tips

A. Delivery Tips

▶ For application at or below the gingival margin for targeted delivery of water or antimicrobial agents.

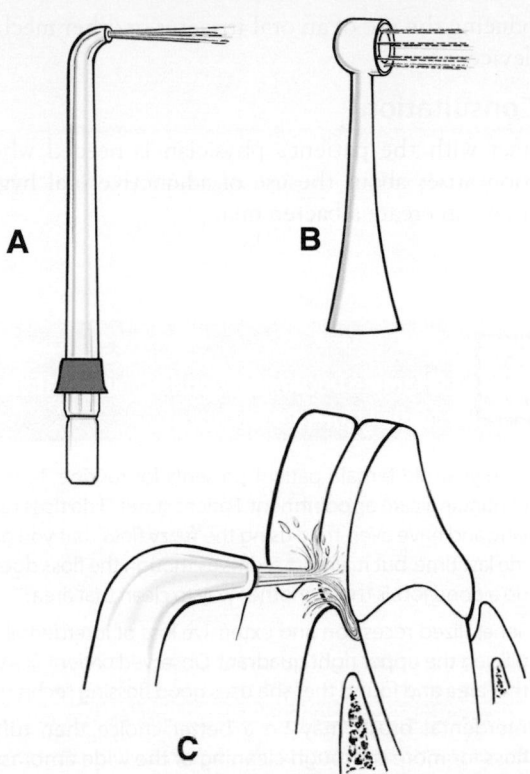

FIGURE 29-14 **Supragingival Irrigation Demonstrating Delivery of Irrigant. A:** Monojet tip (single stream). **B:** Fractionated microjet tip (multiple streams). **C:** Monojet delivery tip showing impact and flushing of subgingival area.

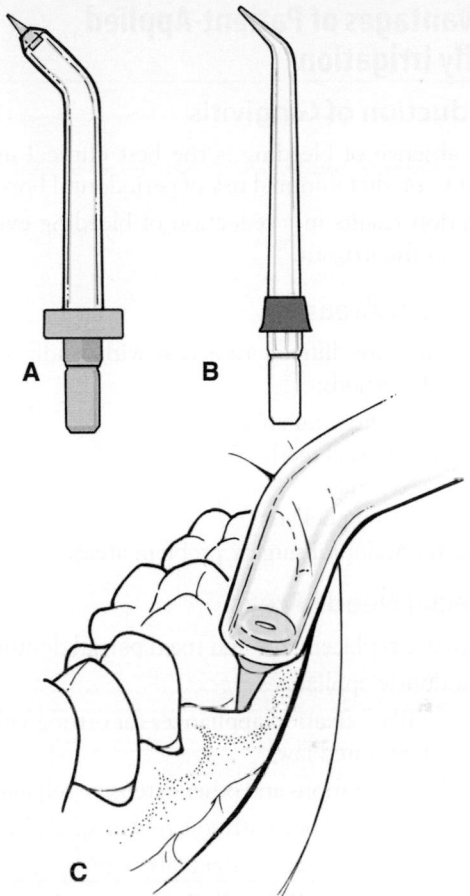

FIGURE 29-15 **Patient-applied Marginal Irrigation. A and B:** Special tips for use by the patient. **C:** Soft rubber tip designed to be placed 2 mm below gingival margin.

BOX 29-2

How to Irrigate

▷ Lean over the sink to allow the irrigant to flow from the oral cavity.

▷ Direct the jet tip toward the interdental area until almost touching the tooth surface.

▷ Hold tip at a right angle (90°) to the long axis of the tooth.

▷ This is generally referred to as supragingival irrigation (Figure 29-14C).

▷ Increase pressure slightly over time depending on gingival inflammation and comfort.

▷ Follow a definite pattern around the teeth: maxillary arch first, then the mandibular, facial, palatal, and lingual.

▶ Types
  • Soft rubber tip designed to be placed 2 mm below the gingival margin (Figure 29-15A).
  • Tapered plastic tip designed to be placed at the gingival margin (Figure 29-15B).

B. Procedure

▶ Identify appropriate areas for use (e.g., specific pocket, furcation, or implant).

▶ Set unit pressure on lowest setting or follow the manufacturer's instructions.

▶ Direct the tip at or below the gingival margin according to the manufacturer's directions. The use of a soft rubber tip or a tapered plastic tip is generally referred to as marginal irrigation (Figure 29-15C).

▶ Activate flow of solution for a few seconds into designated area; stop flow and move to next designated area.

▶ When using a metal or plastic cannula, care must be given to ensure the patient can place the tip subgingivally and deliver the agent accurately and safely. Proper use of a cannula tip is considered subgingival irrigation.

APPLICATIONS FOR PRACTICE

Regular use of daily personal oral irrigation is beneficial.[30] Use a patient-centered approach to evaluate each patient's needs individually to determine which techniques, products, or devices are appropriate.

I. Advantages of Patient-Applied Daily Irrigation

A. Reduction of Gingivitis

▶ The absence of bleeding is the best clinical measurement to predict minimal risk of periodontal breakdown.

▶ Irrigation results in a reduction of bleeding even with water as the irrigant.[30]

B. Problem Areas

▶ Areas that are difficult to access with traditional mechanical methods:
- Open interdental areas
- Malpositioned teeth
- Exposed furcas
- Periodontal pockets
- Postperiodontal surgery problem areas.

C. Special Needs Areas

▶ Prosthetic replacements and fixed partial dentures.

▶ Orthodontic appliances.

▶ Intermaxillary fixation appliances for orthognathic surgery and fractured jaw.

▶ Complex restorations and other extensive rehabilitation.

▶ Implant maintenance with soft rubber specialized tip.

▶ Immunocompromised individuals who have an exaggerated inflammatory response.

▶ Ineffective interdental technique due to physical ability or lack of compliance.

II. Special Considerations

A. Premedication Requirement

A patient who requires antibiotic premedication for dental and dental hygiene treatment is evaluated before introducing the use of an oral irrigator or other mechanical device.

B. Consultation

Contact with the patient's physician is needed when a question arises about the use of adjunctive oral hygiene aids that can create a bacteremia.

BOX 29-3

Example Documentation: Recommendations for Daily Interdental Care

S –A 46-year-old female patient presents for routine 3-month continuing care appointment. Patient states, "I do floss regularly, and have even tried using the 'fuzzy floss' that you gave me last time, but it almost seems as though the floss doesn't do a good job. Is there another way to clean that area?"

O–Generalized recession and extensive loss of interdental papilla on the upper right quadrant. Observed patient flossing that area and found that she uses good flossing technique.

A–Interdental brush may be a better choice than tufted floss for more thorough cleaning of the wide embrasure spaces in that area of her mouth.

P–Showed her examples of several types of interdental brushes and let her choose two she thought she might be most comfortable using. Provided instructions for use of a small interdental brush with a tapered group of filaments as well as an interdental brush handle with replaceable inserts. Provided additional samples of two sizes of interdental inserts (one with medium-sized filaments and one cone- or "Christmas tree"-shaped) to try out and see which works best for her.

Signed _____, RDH
Date _____

EVERYDAY ETHICS

Jane, at the clinic for a routine continuing care appointment, is excited about information she has just read on the Internet about a new device for interdental biofilm removal. She begins to ask Glenna, the dental hygienist, detailed questions about the product such as whether it really works, where it can be purchased, and how much it costs. Glenna is unfamiliar with the aid but doesn't want to be embarrassed in front of the patient so she tells Jane the product doesn't work and spends an extra 5 minutes at the end of the appointment going over manual flossing techniques.

Questions for Consideration

1. Which of the dental hygiene core values (Table II-1, Section II Introduction) have application in this scenario? Also consider the ethical duty for lifelong learning.

2. From the patient's perspective, what is the role of the dental hygienist in this situation? Consider the roles of dental hygiene in Chapter 1.

3. Is it unethical to mislead the patient about a product when the value is unknown or the dental hygienist prefers the benefits of another (perhaps rival) product? Why or why not?

DOCUMENTATION

Documentation for a patient's interdental care progress notes need to include a minimum of the following:

▶ Initially the complete health history including need or not for premedication to prevent bacteremia; extra- and intraoral examination, radiographs; and study casts if used for help in patient instruction.

▶ Information for special needs concerning halitosis (with tests prescribed or given); xerostomia recommendations for oral care.

▶ Notes on all personal oral care demonstrations and products recommended for use.

▶ A sample documentation may be reviewed in Box 29-3.

Factors To Teach The Patient

▷ By demonstration with disclosing agent, how the toothbrush doesn't clean the interdental area thoroughly.

▷ About dental biofilm and how it collects on the proximal tooth surfaces when left undisturbed.

▷ How vulnerable the interdental area is to gingival infection.

▷ How to use each recommended interdental aid to clean the proximal tooth surfaces.

▷ To ask the dental hygienist and the dentist about new products they see advertised and whether the product meets the patient's individual oral self-care needs.

References

1. Smukler H, Nager MC, Tolmie PC. Interproximal tooth morphology and its effect on plaque removal. *Quintessence Int.* 1989;20(4):249–255.

2. Gher ME, Vernino AR. Root morphology—clinical significance in pathogenesis and treatment of periodontal disease. *J Am Dent Assoc.* 1980;101(4):627–633.

3. Fox SC, Bosworth BL. A morphological survey of proximal root concavities: a consideration in periodontal therapy. *J Am Dent Assoc.* 1987;114(6):811–814.

4. Ciancio SG, Shibly O, Farber GA. Clinical evaluation of the effect of two types of dental floss on plaque and gingival health. *Clin Prev Dent.* 1992;14(3):14–18.

5. Abelson DC, Barton JE, Maietti GM, et al. Evaluation of interproximal cleaning by two types of dental floss. *Clin Prev Dent.* 1981;3(4):19–21.

6. Lobene RR, Soparkar PM, Newman MB. Use of dental floss: effect on plaque and gingivitis. *Clin Prev Dent.* 1982;4(1):5–8.

7. Hanes PJ, O'Dell NL, Baker MR, et al. The effect of tensile strength on the clinical effectiveness and patient acceptance of dental floss. *J Clin Periodontol.* 1992;19(1):30–34.

8. Graves RC, Disney JA, Stamm JW. Comparative effectiveness of flossing and brushing in reducing interproximal bleeding. *J Periodontol.* 1989;60(5):243–247.

9. American Academy of Periodontology. *Proceedings of the World Workshop in Clinical Periodontics.* Chicago, IL: American Academy of Periodontology; 1989:II/11–II/15.

10. Hill HC, Levi PA, Glickman I. The effects of waxed and unwaxed dental floss on interdental plaque accumulation and interdental gingival health. *J Periodontol.* 1973;44(7):411–413.

11. Lamberts DM, Wunderlich RC, Caffesse RG. The effect of waxed and unwaxed dental floss on gingival health, Part I: plaque removal and gingival response. *J Periodontol.* 1982;53(6):393–396.

12. Wunderlich RC, Lamberts DM, Caffesse RG. The effect of waxed and unwaxed dental floss on gingival health, Part II: crevicular fluid flow and gingival bleeding. *J Periodontol.* 1982;53(6):397–400.

13. Beaumont RH. Patient preference for waxed or unwaxed dental floss. *J Periodontol.* 1990;61(2):123–125.

14. Dörfer CE, Wündrich D, Staehle HJ, et al. Gliding capacity of different dental flosses. *J Periodontol.* 2001;72(5):672–678.

15. Masters DH. Oral hygiene procedure for the periodontal patient. *Dent Clin North Am.* 1969;13(1):3–17.

16. Hallmon WW, Waldrop TC, Houston GD, et al. Flossing clefts. Clinical and histologic observations. *J Periodontol.* 1986;57(8):501–504.

17. Super Floss®. Oral B Laboratories, Inc., 600 Clipper Drive, Belmont, CA 94002-4199.

18. Yost KG, Mallatt ME, Liebman J. Interproximal gingivitis and plaque reduction by four interdental products. *J Clin Dent.* 2006;17(3):79–83.

19. Poklepovic T, Worthington HV, Johnson TM, et al. Interdental brushing for the prevention and control of periodontal diseases and dental caries in adults. *Cochrane Database Syst Rev.* 2013;12:CD009857.

20. Lewis MW, Holder-Ballard C, Selders RJ Jr, et al. Comparison of the use of a toothpick holder to dental floss in improvement of gingival health in humans. *J Periodontol.* 2004;75(4):551–556.

21. Hoenderdos NL, Slot DE, Paraskevas S, et al. The efficacy of woodsticks on plaque and gingival inflammation: a systematic review. *Int J Dent Hyg.* 2008;6(4):280–289.

22. Waerhaug J. Effect of toothbrushing on subgingival plaque formation. *J Periodontol.* 1981;52(1):30–34.

23. Barnes CM, Russell CM, Reinhardt RA, et al. Comparison of irrigation to floss as an adjunct to tooth brushing: effect on bleeding, gingivitis and supragingival plaque. *J Clin Dent.* 2005;16(3):71–77.

24. Flemmig TF, Newman MG, Doherty FM, et al. Supragingival irrigation with 0.06% chlorhexidine in naturally occurring gingivitis. I. 6 month clinical observations. *J Periodontol.* 1990;61(2):112–117.

25. Newman MG, Flemmig TF, Nachnani S, et al. Irrigation with 0.06% chlorhexidine in naturally occurring gingivitis. II. 6 months microbiological observations. *J Periodontol.* 1990;61(7):427–433.

26. Eakle WS, Ford C, Boyd RL. Depth of penetration in periodontal pockets with oral irrigation. *J Clin Periodontol.* 1986;13(1):39–44.

27. Braun RE, Ciancio SG. Subgingival delivery by an oral irrigation device. *J Periodontol.* 1992;63(5):469–472.

28. Boyd RL, Hollander BN, Eakle WS. Comparison of a sub-gingivally placed cannula oral irrigator tip with a supragingivally placed standard irrigator tip. *J Clin Periodontol.* 1992;19(5):340–344.

29. Lugassy AA, Lautenschlager EP, Katrana D. Characterization of water spray devices. *J Dent Res.* 1971;50(2):466–473.

30. Husseini A, Slot DE, Van der Weijden GA. The efficacy of oral irrigation in addition to a toothbrush on plaque and the clinical parameters of periodontal inflammation: a systematic review. *Int J Dent Hyg.* 2008;6(4):304–314.

ENHANCE YOUR UNDERSTANDING

thePoint® DIGITAL CONNECTIONS
(see the inside front cover for access information)
- **Audio glossary**
- **Quiz bank**

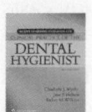

SUPPORT FOR LEARNING
(available separately; visit lww.com)
- *Active Learning Workbook for Clinical Practice of the Dental Hygienist, 12th Edition*

prepU INDIVIDUALIZED REVIEW
(available separately; visit lww.com)
- **Adaptive quizzing with *prepU for Wilkins' Clinical Practice of the Dental Hygienist***

30

Dentifrices and Mouthrinses

Kristeen Perry, RDH, MSDH and Tessie L. Black, RDH, BS

CHAPTER OUTLINE

LEARNING OBJECTIVES

After studying this chapter, the student will be able to:

1. Identify and define the active and inactive components in dentrifices and mouthrinse.

2. Explain the mechanism of action for preventive and therapeutic agents in dentrifices and mouthrinses.

3. Explain the purpose and use of dentifrices and mouthrinses.

4. Discuss the Food and Drug Administration (FDA) and the purpose of FDA.

5. Explain the American Dental Association (ADA) Seal of Acceptance program and purpose.

CHEMOTHERAPEUTICS

Recent advances in understanding the pathogenesis of periodontitis have led to alternative therapies that focus on reduction of inflammation in the oral cavity using both mechanical devices and chemotherapeutics.

▶ Inflammation of periodontal tissues has an impact on the human body beyond the oral cavity, particularly in immunocompromised individuals.

▶ Oral inflammation has been linked to several conditions including stroke and heart disease.[1]

▶ Increased inflammation associated with diabetes can make a patient more susceptible to periodontal disease.[2–4]

▶ Oral pathogens can travel to the lungs to cause healthcare-associated pneumonias[5] as described in Chapter 66.

▶ Either the clinician or the patient can administer chemotherapeutics.

▶ Key words pertaining to chemotherapeutics are defined in Box 30-1.

DENTIFRICES

The benefits of using dentifrices may be preventive, therapeutic, or cosmetic. A dentifrice is a substance applied with a toothbrush or other applicator for:

▶ Removal of biofilm, stain, and other soft deposits from the gingiva and tooth surfaces

▶ Application of therapeutic agents

▶ Superficial cosmetic effects.

PREVENTIVE AND THERAPEUTIC BENEFITS OF DENTIFRICES

I. Prevention of Dental Caries

▶ Although fluoride has long been recognized as an anti-cariogenic agent, the addition of stannous fluoride to a dentifrice was problematic because of lack of compatibility with abrasive agents.[6]

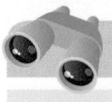

BOX 30-1   KEY WORDS: Dentifrices and Mouthrinses

Acidogenic: acid forming.

Antimicrobial agent: chemical that is bacteriostatic or bactericidal.

Astringent: a substance that causes contraction or shrinkage and arrests discharges.

Chemotherapeutic agent: a chemical that is used for therapeutic reasons.

Chemotherapy: treatment of disease by means of chemical substances or pharmaceutical agents.

CHX: Chlorhexidine.

Copolymer: a substance with a high molecular weight that results from chemically combining two or more monomers.

Efficacy: the benefits of a product or procedure that lead to intended results such as reduction in gingivitis.

Humectant: substance contained in a product (such as in a dentifrice) to retain moisture and prevent hardening upon exposure to air.

Hydrokinetic activity: activity relating to motions of fluids or the forces that produce or affect such motions; opposite of hydrostatic.

Inflammatory mediator: a chemical that impacts the immunoinflammatory process causing either exacerbation (pro-) or reduction (anti-). Proinflammatory mediators include interleukin-1β and (IL-1β), prostaglandin E_2 (PGE_2), and tumor necrosis factor alpha (TNF-α). Interleukin-10 (IL-10) is an anti-inflammatory mediator.

Substantivity: the ability of an agent to bind to the pellicle, tooth surface, and soft tissue and be released over an extended period of time with the retention of its potency.

Synergism: process whereby the joint action of separate agents is greater than the sum of their effects taken separately.

Synergistic effect: coordinated action; acting jointly; for example, one drug might enhance the effect of another drug.

Therapeutic rinse: a chemical with therapeutic properties that is delivered by rinsing or irrigation device.

- The first caries-preventive dentifrice contained stannous fluoride (0.4%). It became available commercially in 1955.[7]
- Additional information about fluoride dentifrices is described in Chapter 36.
- Xylitol, a flavoring agent in some dentifrices, has been shown to provide anticaries benefits.

II. Remineralization of Early Noncavitated Dental Caries

- Fluoride enhances remineralization as described in Chapter 27 and Chapter 36.

III. Reduction of Biofilm Formation

- Agents used:
  - Triclosan
  - Zinc citrate
  - Stannous fluoride.

IV. Reduction of Gingivitis/Inflammation

- An antigingivitis dentifrice can contribute to the improved health of gingival tissue.
- Triclosan is the primary agent that has shown efficacy in reducing gingival inflammation.
- Triclosan combined with a copolymer of polyvinyl methoxyethylene and maleic acid (PVM/MA) increases the substantivity for 12 hours even after eating and drinking.[8]
- Use of a dentifrice-containing triclosan has demonstrated:[9–13]
  - Inhibition of inflammatory mediators in vitro including interleukin-1β and prostaglandin E_2.[11]
  - Reduction in gingival inflammation and gingival bleeding.[10,12,13]
  - Modest reduction in gingivitis using stannous fluoride in a dentifrice.[12,13]
  - There is weak evidence for a reduction in supragingival biofilm formation of about 15%.[13]

V. Reduction of Dentin Hypersensitivity

- The most effective agent in commercial dentifrices for the reduction of dentin hypersensitivity is 5% potassium nitrate.[14,15]
- Patients using a dentifrice for sensitivity are to be instructed to use the dentifrice for no longer than 4 weeks as it is necessary to determine the etiology of the sensitivity in the event it is more serious than exposed dentinal tubules.
- More information on reducing dentin hypersensitivity is discussed in Chapter 44.

VI. Reduction of Supragingival Calculus Formation

- "Tarter control" dentifrices shown to help inhibit supragingival calculus may contain:
  - Pyrophosphate salts[16]
  - Zinc salts (zinc chloride and zinc citrate)[17,18]
  - Sodium hexametaphosphate[19]
  - Triclosan/copolymer.[20]

COSMETIC EFFECTS OF DENTIFRICES

I. Removal of Extrinsic Stain

- The pigments from foods, tobacco use, or chemical agents may become imbedded in the acquired pellicle and dental biofilm.
- Cosmetic results from dentifrice are based on:
  - Mechanical removal of the stained biofilm
  - Delivery of a bleaching agent.
- Each commercially available product needs to be evaluated individually for efficacy and patient acceptance.
- More information on tooth stains is provided in Chapter 22.

II. Reduction of Oral Malodor (Halitosis)

- Certain ingredients added to a dentifrice can reduce oral malodor on a temporary basis by inhibiting the production of volatile sulfur compounds (VSCs).
- Chlorhexidine, cetylpyridinium chloride, and zinc formulations have a beneficial effect on reducing oral malodor via reduction of VSCs.[21]
- Triclosan/copolymer can control the bacteria associated with VSCs, thereby reducing oral malodor.[22]
- Stannous fluoride combined with sodium hexametaphosphate can reduce VSC production.[23]

BASIC COMPONENTS OF DENTIFRICES: INACTIVES

- Most dentifrices share a common composition of ingredients needed for a stable formulation.
- Dentifrices are sold primarily as pastes and gels. The common ingredients and their function are listed in Table 30-1.
- In addition to the inactive ingredients described in Table 30-1, a therapeutic dentifrice will have a drug or chemical agent stated as an active ingredient for a specific preventive or therapeutic action.
- The active ingredient represents approximately 1.5%–2% of the dentifrice's formulation.
- Therapeutic agents are described in Table 30-2.

TABLE 30-1	Ingredients and Function of Commercially Available Dentifrices	
INGREDIENT	**FUNCTION**	**AVERAGE FORMULATION PERCENTAGE (%)**
Surfactant/detergent	Foaming and cleansing	1–2
Abrasive	Cleaning and polishing	20–40
Binder	Thickening agent and stabilizes formula	1–2
Humectant	Prevent water loss/hardening of dentifrice	20–40
Preservative	Prevents microorganisms from destroying the dentifrice in storage	2–3
Flavoring	Sweetener	1–1.5
Water	Maintain the ingredient in formulation	20–40

TABLE 30-2	Therapeutic Active Ingredients in Dentifrices
BENEFIT	**ACTIVE INGREDIENTS**
Antibiofilm/ Antigingivitis	Triclosan/copolymer, stannous fluoride, zinc citrate
Anticalculus	Tetra potassium pyrophosphate, tetra sodium pyrophosphate, sodium hexametaphosphate, triclosan/ copolymer, zinc compounds
Desensitizer	Potassium nitrate, potassium citrate, potassium chloride, stannous fluoride, strontium chloride
Oral malodor	Essential oils, chlorine dioxide, triclosan/ copolymer, stannous fluoride/sodium hexametaphosphate

I. Detergents (Foaming Agents or Surfactants)

▶ *Purposes*
  - Lower surface tension.
  - Penetrate and loosen surface deposits.
  - Suspend debris for easy removal by toothbrush.
  - Emulsify/disperse the flavor oils.
  - Contribute to foaming action.
▶ *Substances used*
  - Sodium lauryl sulfate USP
  - Sodium *N*-lauryl sarcosinate.

II. Cleaning and Polishing Agents (Abrasives)

▶ *Purposes*
  - Cleans well with no damage to tooth surface.

- A polishing agent is used to produce a smooth tooth surface.
- A smooth surface can prevent or delay the reaccumulation of stains and deposits.
▶ *Abrasives used*
  - Calcium carbonate
  - Phosphate salts
  - Hydrated aluminum oxide
  - Silica, silicates, and dehydrated silica gels.

III. Binders (Thickeners)

▶ *Purposes*
  - Stabilize the formulation.
  - Prevent separation of the solid and liquid ingredients during storage.
▶ *Types used*
  - Mineral colloids
  - Natural gums
  - Seaweed colloids
  - Synthetic celluloses.

IV. Humectants (Moisture Stabilizers)

▶ *Purposes*
  - Retain moisture.
  - Prevent hardening on exposure to air.
▶ *Substances used*
  - Xylitol
  - Glycerol
  - Sorbitol.

V. Preservatives

▶ *Purposes*
  - Prevent bacterial growth.
  - Prolong shelf life.

- *Substances used*
  - Alcohol
  - Benzoates
  - Dichlorinated phenols.

VI. Flavoring Agents (Sweeteners)

- *Purposes*
  - Impart a pleasant flavor for patient acceptance.
  - Mask other ingredients that may have a less pleasant flavor.
- *Substances used*
  - Essential oils (peppermint, cinnamon, wintergreen, clove)
  - Artificial noncariogenic sweeteners (xylitol, glycerol, sorbitol).

ACTIVE COMPONENTS OF DENTIFRICES

Today's dentifrice selections offer a variety of active ingredients that may help prevent caries, sensitivity, biofilm, gingivitis, calculus formation, and oral malodor.

- The first active ingredient introduced in a dentifrice was fluoride.
- Since then, there have been major developments in this area. These active ingredients provide benefits in the areas of:
  - Anticaries
  - Antibiofilm/Antigingivitis
  - Anticalculus
  - Antioral malodor (Halitosis)
  - Antisensitivity
  - Specific active ingredients are summarized in Table 30-2.

SELECTION OF DENTIFRICES

I. Prevention or Reduction of Oral Disease

- Dental caries
- Fluoride-containing dentifrice during remineralization program (see Chapter 27 and Chapter 36).
- Dentin hypersensitivity
- Inflammation
- Calculus formation
- Oral malodor/reduction of VSCs.

II. Considerations for the Pediatric Patient

- *Birth to first tooth eruption*
  - Parents can clean the child's gingiva with a soft infant toothbrush or cloth and water.
- *Eruption of first tooth*
  - Parents can begin to start brushing twice daily using fluoridated toothpaste and a soft, age-appropriate sized toothbrush.

- Use a very small "smear" of toothpaste to brush the teeth of a child less than 2 years of age. The small smear of fluoride paste is shown in Figure 50-8, Chapter 50.
- *2–5 year old*
  - The parent can dispense a "pea-sized" amount of toothpaste (Figure 50-8, Chapter 50), and perform or assist child's tooth brushing.
  - Parents need to recognize that young children do not have the ability to brush their teeth effectively without help and supervision.
  - Parents can be role models for their child by brushing their teeth at the same time as the child.
  - Children are supervised until they are able to spit out and not swallow excess toothpaste after brushing.

III. Patient-specific Dentifrice Recommendations

- Dentifrice recommendations are a key part of personal daily care planning and are patient specific.
- Considerations include:
  - Patient's current oral condition
  - Any patient complaint/concern
  - Sensitivities or allergies to a specific ingredient
  - Propensity of staining (stannous fluoride-containing dentifrice)
  - Patient's nontherapeutic/cosmetic choices
  - Expectation of compliance. When a dentifrice does not appeal in either taste or texture, it will not be used no matter what its therapeutic benefits might be.
  - Personal trial is needed before a recommendation is made. Dental hygienists need first-hand experience with each product they recommend.

MOUTHRINSES

- Mechanical aids may not be sufficient to maintain optimum oral health for certain patients and may be supplemented with the use of a chemotherapeutic mouthrinse.
- The benefits of using a mouthrinse may be: preventive, cosmetic, and therapeutic.
- Chemotherapeutic rinses may have active ingredients to reduce inflammation.
- Cosmetic rinses can provide some extrinsic stain removal when it is superficial in unattached biofilm.
- Delivery: rinsing can deliver an agent less than 2 mm into the sulcus or pocket and is not a delivery of choice for patients with moderate or deep pockets.[24]
- Functions: a list of general functions of chemotherapeutic agents is provided in Box 30-2.

PURPOSES AND USES OF MOUTHRINSES

I. Before Professional Treatment

▶ To reduce the numbers of intraoral microorganisms available to aerosols.
▶ To reduce aerosol contamination during use of a handpiece or ultrasonic scaler.

II. Self-Care

▶ As part of personal oral self-care for specific needs
▶ Biofilm control
▶ Dental caries prevention through remineralization of noncavitated early dental caries
▶ Prevention of gingivitis
▶ Contribute to malodor control
▶ Posttreatment therapy following nonsurgical periodontal therapy
  • Periodontal surgery
  • Removal of teeth.

PREVENTIVE AND THERAPEUTIC AGENTS OF MOUTHRINSES

I. Fluoride

A. Mechanism of Action

▶ Stannous:
  • Deposit of fluoride ion on enamel
  • Tin ion from stannous fluoride interferes with cell metabolism for antimicrobial effect.
▶ Sodium:
  • Deposit of fluoride ion on enamel
  • Cariostatic: inhibits demineralization and enhances remineralization.

B. Availability and Use

▶ Available in varying concentrations.

▶ Uses:
  • Prevention of demineralization
  • Reduction of hypersensitivity
  • Reduction of gingivitis.

C. Efficacy

▶ Reduction in biofilm or dental caries when rinse is used topically by the patient.

D. Considerations

▶ Stannous: tooth staining; flavor
▶ Instruct patient to expectorate/not to swallow.

II. Chlorhexidine (CHX)

A. Mechanism of Action[25]

▶ A cationic bisbiguanide with broad antibacterial activity
▶ Binds to oral hard and soft tissues
▶ Attaches to bacterial cell membrane, thereby damaging the cytoplasm causing lysis
▶ Binds to pellicle and salivary mucins to prevent biofilm accumulation
▶ Bactericidal and bacteriostatic depending on concentration
▶ Bactericidal concentrations cause cell lyses
▶ Bacteriostatic concentrations interfere with cell wall transport system
▶ The substantivity of CHX: 8–12 hours
▶ Antimicrobial and antigingivitis agent.

B. Availability and Uses

▶ CHX is the most effective antimicrobial and antigingivitis agent available for clinical use.[25,26]
  • Mouthrinse available by prescription in a 0.12% solution in the United States (higher concentrations are available in other countries); postsurgery for enhanced wound healing (Figure 30-1).

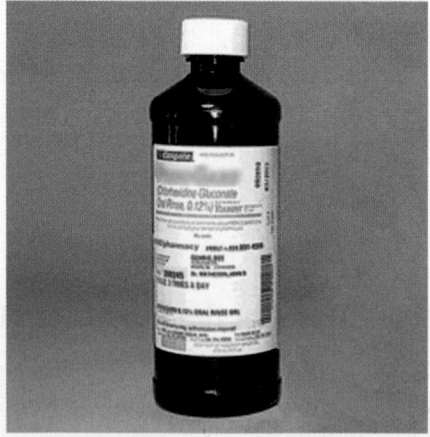

Figure 30-1 Therapeutic Mouthrinse. Chlorhexidine gluconate mouthrinse aids in plaque biofilm control and requires a prescription for purchase. (Reprinted from Nield-Gehrig J, Willmann D. Foundations of Periodontics for the Dental Hygienist. Philadelphia: Wolters Kluwer Health/Lippincott Williams & Wilkins; 2011.)

- Recommend uses:
  - Preprocedural rinse to reduce bacterial load before instrumentation producing aerosols
  - Before, during, and after periodontal debridement
  - Patients who are at a high risk for dental caries
  - Immunocompromised individuals who are more susceptible to infection
  - Postsurgery for enhanced wound healing.

C. Efficacy

- CHX is safe and effective in:
  - Preventing and controlling biofilm formation
  - Reducing viability of existing biofilm
  - Inhibiting and reducing the development of gingivitis[26]
  - Reducing *mutans streptococci*.[26]
- CHX varnish is effective in:
  - Reduction of dental caries for children[27]
  - Reduction of dental caries in people with xerostomia[27]
  - CHX varnish is approved in Canada and Europe.

D. Considerations

- Low level of toxicity due to poor absorption through mucous membranes
- Staining of teeth including smooth surfaces, pits and fissures, restorations, and soft tissues (Figure 30-2)
- Increase in supragingival calculus formation
- Altered taste perception
- Minor irritation to soft tissues, lips, and tongue
- CHX interacts with and is inactivated by sodium lauryl sulfate (a surfactant used in dentifrices) when rinsing is performed immediately after brushing. Wait 30 minutes after brushing before rinsing with CHX.

III. Triclosan

A. Mechanism of Action

- Bisphenol and nonionic antimicrobial agent

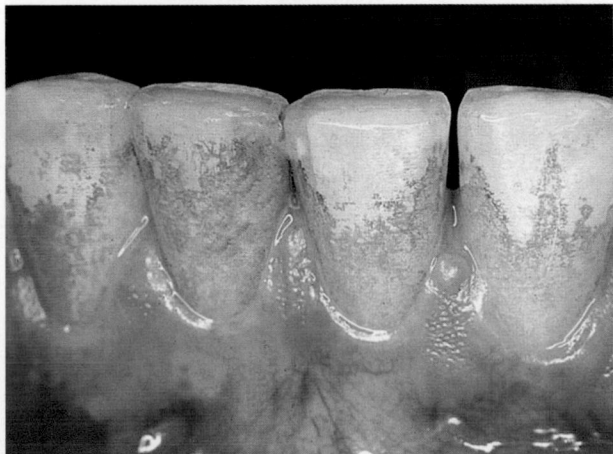

Figure 30-2 Chlorhexidine Stain. (Reprinted from Nield-Gehrig J. Fundamentals of Periodontal Instrumentation and Advanced Root Instrumentation. Philadelphia: Lippincott Williams & Wilkins; 2011.)

- A broad-spectrum agent effective against both gram-negative and gram-positive bacteria
- Acts on the microbial cytoplasmic membrane, causing leakage of the cell contents, or bacteriolysis
- Antimicrobial and antigingivitis agent
- Low toxicity.

B. Availability and Uses

- Triclosan-containing mouthrinse and dentifrice are available.
- Recommended uses:
  - Reduction of biofilm and gingivitis
  - Reduced biofilm accumulation
  - Reduced supragingival calculus formation.

C. Efficacy

- Reduction in biofilm and bleeding on probing (BOP).[28]

D. Considerations

- Easily released from oral tissue binding sites such as tooth surface or soft tissue
- Combining with PVM/MA increases substantivity and efficacy.[28]

IV. Phenolic-related Essential Oils

A. Mechanism of Action

- Phenolics disrupt cell walls and inhibit bacterial enzymes
- Decreases pathogenicity of biofilm
- Antimicrobial and antigingivitis agent.

B. Availability and Uses

- A combination of thymol, eucalyptol, menthol, and methyl salicylate is available as a brand name product and generic product.
- Recommended uses:
  - Individuals unable to perform adequate brushing and flossing.
  - Initially or periodically to help improve oral hygiene.
  - Adjunct for mechanical self-care routines that are not sufficient in reducing biofilm, bleeding, and gingivitis.
  - Preprocedural rinse to reduce bacterial load before instrumentation-producing aerosols.

C. Efficacy

- Significant reduction in the levels of biofilm and gingivitis.[26,29]

D. Considerations

- Burning sensation
- Bitter taste
- Poor substantivity

▶ Efficacy of individual rinses based on following the manufacturer's instructions and not casual use of the rinse

▶ Contraindicated for current or recovering alcoholics due to alcohol content.

V. Quaternary Ammonium Compounds

A. Mechanism of Action[30]

▶ Cationic agents that bind to oral tissues

▶ Rupture the cell wall and alter the cytoplasm

▶ Initial attachment to oral tissue is very strong, but released rapidly

▶ Decreases the ability of bacteria to attach to the pellicle

▶ Low substantivity.

B. Availability and Uses

▶ The most commonly used agent is cetylpyridinium chloride (CPC), at 0.05%–0.07%

▶ Recommended uses:
  • Reduction in biofilm accumulation
  • Adjunct for mechanical self-care routines.

C. Efficacy

▶ Demonstrated reductions in biofilm

▶ Reduction in gingivitis has been demonstrated in limited studies.

D. Considerations

▶ Staining of teeth

▶ Increased supragingival calculus formation

▶ A burning sensation and occasional desquamation.[31]

VI. Oxygenating Agents

▶ *Mechanism of action*
  • Alters bacterial cell membrane increasing permeability
  • Release of oxygen acts to debride area
  • Poor substantivity.

▶ *Availability and uses*
  • The common agents available in commercial rinses are 10% carbamide peroxide and 1.5% hydrogen peroxide.
  • Recommended for short-term use to reduce the symptoms of pericoronitis and necrotizing ulcerative gingivitis.[32]

▶ *Efficacy*
  • Negligible antimicrobial effect
  • Debriding agent.

▶ *Consideration*
  • Does not consistently prevent plaque biofilm accumulation short term, but when used long term some reduction in gingival redness has been noted.[32]

VII. Oxidizing Agents

▶ *Mechanism of action*
  • Neutralization of VSCs that contribute to oral malodor
  • *Availability and uses*
  • The common agents available in commercial rinses are: chlorine dioxide and chlorine dioxide/zinc combination.
  • Recommended short-term use to reduce VSCs in the control of oral malodor.

▶ *Efficacy*
  • Mainly cosmetic.

▶ *Consideration*
  • There is no clinical evidence to support the use of these products for reduction of biofilm or gingivitis.

COMMERCIAL MOUTHRINSE INGREDIENTS

Ingredients and their functions are listed in Table 30-3.

I. Active Ingredients

▶ Commercial mouthrinses generally contain more than one active ingredient and, therefore, may advertise multiple claims for use.

▶ Factors that influence how effective an agent may be:

TABLE 30-3	Typical Commercial Mouthrinse Formulation
INGREDIENT	**FUNCTION**
Alcohol	Enhances flavor impact; contributes to cleansing
Flavor	Adds pleasantness/freshness; makes breath temporarily fresh
Humectant	Adds "body"; inhibits crystallization around closure
Surfactant	Solubilizes the flavor; provides foaming action
Water	Major vehicle to carry other ingredients
Preservative	Preserves aqueous formulation
Dyes	Add color
Sweeteners	Contribute to overall flavor perception
Flavor	Make mouthrinse pleasant to use
Active or functional ingredient	Provide therapeutic and/or benefits

- Dilution by the saliva
- Length of time the agent is in contact with the tissue or bacteria
- Evidence supporting the particular product.

► General characteristics of an effective chemotherapeutic agent are shown in Box 30-3.

II. Inactive Ingredients

A. Water

► Makes up the largest percentage by volume.

B. Alcohol

► Increases the solubility of some active ingredients
► Percentage varies from 0% to 26.9%
► Enhances flavor
► No link to oral cancer.[33]

C. Flavoring

► Essential oils and derivatives (eucalyptus oil, oil of wintergreen)
► Aromatic waters (peppermint, spearmint, wintergreen, or others)
► Artificial noncariogenic sweetener.

III. Patient-specific Mouthrinse Recommendations

Mouthrinses are formulated for a variety of oral benefits including mouth freshening, prevention of caries, biofilm control, control of oral malodor. Several factors are considered when making a mouthrinse recommendation including:

► Is the patient currently able to control biofilm through other methods?
► Does the patient consider rinsing a substitute for other mechanical procedures such as brushing and flossing?

► Does the patient's substance abuse history contraindicate recommending an alcohol-containing mouthrinse?
► Could the patient's xerostomia be worsened by the drying effect of an alcohol-containing mouthrinse?

IV. Contraindications

► The use of a mouthrinse can enhance a patient's personal daily oral care regime. The patient needs to understand why rinsing is not a substitute for brushing or flossing.
► Some agents are contraindicated for children younger than 6 years old who have a tendency to swallow instead of expectorate.
► Review manufacturer's instructions for age limits as they vary by product.
► Contraindicated in patients with physical or cognitive challenges who cannot follow rinsing instructions.

PROCEDURE FOR RINSING

► Many patients, particularly children, must be shown specifically how to rinse. The method can be practiced under supervision.
► Box 30-4 suggests steps for teaching a patient how to rinse.

UNITED STATES FOOD AND DRUG ADMINISTRATION (FDA)[34]

The purpose of the United States FDA is to ensure the safety and efficacy of medical and dental drugs, equipment, and devices that affect living tissue. All drugs require FDA approval. Rinses and dentifrices are classified by the FDA as either cosmetic, therapeutic, or a combination of cosmetic and therapeutic.[34]

I. Brief History of the FDA

▶ Oldest consumer protection agency in the US federal government.

▶ Officially began in 1906 with the passage of the Pure Food and Drug Act.

II. Purposes of the FDA

▶ Regulate drugs, equipment, and devices.

▶ Some devices and equipment are exempt (dental water jets, power and manual toothbrushes, dental floss) if they have existing or reasonably similar characteristics as previously approved devices of the same type.

III. Dental Products Regulated

▶ Infection control products

▶ Dental equipment such as ultrasonic instruments

▶ Diagnostic test kits (i.e., dental caries detection devices)

▶ Prosthetic and restorative materials such as implants

▶ Surgical and periodontal materials such as guided tissue regeneration membranes, bone-filling material, and growth factors

▶ Prescription drugs, controlled and sustained-release devices, and chemotherapeutics

▶ In the case of dentifrice and mouthrinses, FDA has reviewed actives under over-the-counter (OTC) monographs, which are regulations that specify the active ingredients and permissible levels of those ingredients, as well as statements that the product labels must bear. However, the actual formulations of dentifrices excluding triclosan/copolymer have not been subject to any premarket review by FDA.

IV. Research Requirements and Documentation

▶ Table 30-4 outlines the documentation process for a product to receive FDA approval.[34]

AMERICAN DENTAL ASSOCIATION (ADA) SEAL OF ACCEPTANCE PROGRAM[35]

The ADA has promoted safety and effectiveness of dental products for over one hundred years. The ADA Seal of Acceptance Program, which evaluates OTC products offered to consumers, has been in place since 1930, and is internationally recognized. The program is voluntary, and products are awarded the ADA Seal only after the ADA Council on Scientific Affairs has thoroughly evaluated clinical and laboratory studies on a product, and determined that it meets the ADA criteria for safety and effectiveness, when used as directed.

For many years, the Seal Program website has provided a listing of all products that have the ADA Seal. Now there is a new Seal Program feature provides detailed information on each of the accepted products to help

TABLE 30-4	FDA Clearance Documentation Process for Oral Care Products	
PHASE	**STUDY TYPE**	**PURPOSE**
Preclinical	Animal studies	Safety/toxicity
I.	Clinical trial with small sample population (20–80)	Determine: • dosing/safety • how drug is metabolized and excreted • identify side effects.
II.	Clinical trial with a larger sample population (100–200) who have disease or condition that the product is designed to treat. The test drug is compared to a standard treatment or placebo known as a control	Provides further safety data and preliminary evidence of efficacy.
III.	Clinical trial with a large sample population (1,000–3,000) who have a disease or condition to test efficacy, monitor side effects, and identify treatment parameters. The test drug is compared to a standard treatment or placebo known as a control	Identify possible less obvious side effects.
IV.	Clinical trials on products that are already approved and on the market	Continue to measure long-term benefits, risks, and optimal protocol.

consumers and dental professionals select OTC oral care products.

▶ Unlike the FDA, the ADA Seal Program is voluntary and a company must apply to obtain it by making a product submission.

▶ Each product has its ADA-approved Seal Statement that lists the indications for which the product is accepted.

▶ Information is included for each product on the basis for acceptance (i.e., the data on which acceptance is based), indications, directions for use, ingredients, label warnings, and company contact information.

▶ The Seal website also allows comparisons of the attributes of 2–6 products in a given product category.

▶ This information is printable and can be used to help consumers make informed decisions about the oral care products they use.

▶ It can also be useful to dental professionals in recommending OTC oral care products to their patients.

▶ Source of oral health and Seal product information for patients visit http://www.mouthhealthy.org.

▶ Visit http://www.ada.org/seal for more information on the ADA Seal Program and for access to product information on ADA accepted products.

I. Purposes of the Seal Program

The ADA Seal of Acceptance Program is designed to:

▶ Help the public and dental professionals make informed decisions about consumer dental products.

▶ Study and evaluate products for safety and efficacy, when used as directed.

▶ Inform members of the dental team and the public about the safety and efficacy of each product that is accepted.

▶ Maintain liaisons with regulatory agencies and research and professional organizations.

II. Product Submission and Acceptance Process

▶ Information required from the company
  • Complete ingredient listing
  • Objective data from clinical and laboratory studies that support the product's safety, and claimed effectiveness, when used as directed
  • Compliance with specific product category; acceptance guidelines if applicable (http://www.ada.org/3408.aspx)
  • Evidence of good manufacturing processes.

▶ Evaluation.
  • Involves more than 125 expert consultants, members of the ADA Council on Scientific Affairs and Council staff scientists.
  • Acceptance is for a 5-year period, after which the company can reapply for a new 5-year acceptance.
  • When composition, manufacturer, or owner of an accepted product is changed, the company must resubmit for the Seal.

III. Acceptance and Use of the Seal

▶ Claims of product effectiveness on labeling and in advertising and promotional materials must first be approved by the Council on Scientific Affairs.

EVERYDAY ETHICS

Betty, a recent graduate, is just beginning her dental hygiene career in a private practice. Dr Dadaman, the dentist she practices with, has no particular opinions regarding dentifrices and considers one as good as the other. He requests that she simply hand out whatever sample-size products the office receives for free from visiting dental product reps. Betty has read up on the clinical support for many of the currently available products while in school and she is well versed on the differences. However, she is too shy and unsure of herself to challenge her employer and discuss the need to use an evidence-based approach to identifying the correct product for each patient.

When Betty gets home at the end of the day, she reflects that maybe something that she learned in school might help her. She finds her Wilkins textbook and looks up the steps for ethical decision making.

Questions for Consideration

1. By answering some of the questions listed in step three of the decision making steps (in Table 1-1, Chapter 1), identify and develop a rationale to support at least three different choices or alternative actions that Betty could take to resolve this issue.

2. Discuss this scenario in the context of the legal and ethical concepts identified in Table V-1, Section V Introduction. Which of these concepts might help support Betty's choice of actions as she reflects on her own professionalism and determines her responsibilities with regard to making product recommendations for her patients?

3. Whatever course of action Betty takes now will likely set the course for future discussions with her employer regarding patient recommendations or the way Betty practices her profession. Which dental hygienist roles (see Chapter 1) will Betty be filling when she determines the course of action she will take in this situation?

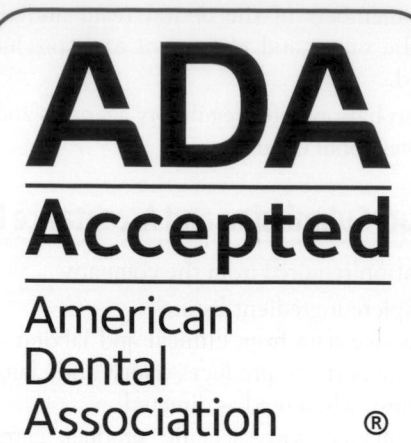

FIGURE 30-3 ADA Seal of Acceptance, The American Dental Association, Council on Scientific Affairs. The Seal is awarded to consumer products that meet ADA guidelines for safety and effectiveness. (Reprinted with permission of the ADA Council on Scientific Affairs.)

▶ The use of the ADA Seal (Figure 30-3) on labeling and in promotional materials must be accompanied by an ADA-approved Seal Statement.

▶ The Seal Statement tells the consumer what specific claims have been reviewed and approved, and indicates why the particular product was accepted.

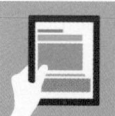

BOX 30-5

Example Documentation: Choosing a Mouthrinse for a Patient with Xerostomia

S –A 76-year-old male presented on time for a routine maintenance appointment. His chief complaint is a dry mouth. He reports no medication and although he has a history of smoking, he quitted 40 years ago. Patient states he eats a lot of apples and other fruits. Patient stated he has been using a "great mouthwash" for the past 25 years. Patient believes it is helping "toughen up his gums" because his mouth is so dry.

O–Extraoral no significant findings. The intraoral exam reveals decreased salivary flow. The peridontal exam reveals generalized 3–4 mm pocket depths with no BOP present.

A–Patient presents with xerostomia and a history of smoking that increases his risk for caries, oral cancer, and periodontal disease.

P–Discussed xerostomia and probable causes and evaluated the amount of alcohol present in mouthwash currently being used. Discussed the effects of alcohol on the oral cavity and recommend mouthwash that does not contain alcohol to reduce the incidence of dry mouth.

Signed _____, RDH
Date _____

DOCUMENTATION

▶ Information to be documented in the patient's permanent record will include a minimum of the following:
  • Recommended dentifrice and mouthrinse for personal oral care daily use: nonalcohol-containing mouthrinse, antibacterial dentifrice.
  • Patient instructed on proper usage including amount and frequency of use.
▶ Summary of current oral findings indicating need for recommendations provided.
▶ Example documentation is provided in Box 30-5.

 Factors To Teach The Patient

▷ Significance of ADA product acceptance seal, especially that it is a voluntary program and lack of a seal on a product does not signify it is unsafe or not effective.

▷ To ask dental hygienist and dentist about new dentifrices and mouthrinses, best way to use, and appropriateness for personal needs.

▷ How to avoid impulse buying with regard to dentifrices, mouthrinses, and other chemical agents. To seek professional advice to avoid contraindications with oral condition and restorations.

▷ To understand that compliance with recommended chemical agent is directly related to expected outcomes (results or improvements).

▷ Why the use of chemotherapeutics is not a substitute for proper and daily mechanical biofilm removal.

▷ To check the ingredients of mouthrinses to prevent the purchase of high-alcohol content if xerostomia is a problem.

References

1. Scannapieco FA, Bush RM, Paju S. Associations between periodontal disease and risk for atherosclerosis, cardiovascular disease, and stroke. A systematic review. *Ann Periodontol.* 2003;8(1):38–53.

2. Löe H. Periodontal disease. The sixth complication of diabetes mellitus. *Diabetes Care.* 1993;16(1):329–334.

3. Nishimura F, Takahshi K, Kurihara M, et al. Periodontal disease as a complication of diabetes mellitus. *Ann Periodontol.* 1998;3(1):20–29.

4. Ryan ME, Carnu O, Kamer A. The influence of diabetes on the periodontal tissues. *J Am Dent Assoc.* 2003;134 (Spec No):34S–40S.

5. Scannapieco FA. Role of oral bacteria in respiratory infection. *J Periodontol.* 1999;70(7):793–802.

6. Mellburg JR. Fluoride dentifrices: current status and prospects. *Int Dent J.* 1991;41(1):9–16.

7. Fischman SL. The history of oral hygiene products: how far have we come in 6000 years? *Periodontol 2000.* 1997;15:7–14.

8. Mariotti AJ, Burrell KH. Mouthrinses and dentifrices. In: American Dental Association. *ADA/PDR Guide to Dental Therapeutics*. 5th ed. Chicago, IL: ADA Publishing Division; 2009:213–223 (Mouthrinses); 223–231 (Dentifrices).

9. Bolden TE, Zambon JJ, Sowinski J, et al. The clinical effect of a dentifrice containing triclosan and a copolymer in a sodium fluoride/silica base on plaque formation and gingivitis: a six-month clinical study. *J Clin Dent*. 1992;3(4):125–131.

10. Lindhe J, Rosling B, Socransky SS, et al. The effect of a triclosan-containing dentifrice on established plaque and gingivitis. *J Clin Periodontol*. 1993;20(5):327–334.

11. Gaffar A, Scherl D, Afflitto J, et al. The effect of triclosan on mediators of gingival inflammation. *J Clin Periodontol*. 1995;22(6):480–484.

12. Mankodi S, Bartizek RD, Winston JL, et al. Anti-gingivitis efficacy of a stabilized 0.454% stannous fluoride/sodium hexametaphosphate dentifrice. *J Clin Periodontol*. 2005;32(1):75–80.

13. Riley P, Lamont T. Triclosan/copolymer containing toothpastes for oral health. *Cochrane Database Syst Rev*. 2013;12:CD010514.

14. Schiff T, Zhang YP, DeVizio W, et al. A randomized clinical trial of the desensitizing efficacy of three dentifrices. *Compend Contin Educ Dent Suppl*. 2000;(27):4–10.

15. Orchardson R, Gillam DG. The efficacy of potassium salts as agents for treating dentin hypersensitivity. *J Orofac Pain*. 2000;14(1):9–19.

16. Sowinski J, Petrone DM, Battista G, et al. The clinical anti-calculus efficacy of a tartar control whitening dentifrice for the prevention of supragingival calculus in a three-month study. *J Clin Dent*. 1999;10(3 Spec No):107–110.

17. Lobene RR, Soparkar PM, Newman MB, et al. Reduced formation of supragingival calculus with use of fluoride-zinc chloride dentifrice. *J Am Dent Assoc*. 1987;114(3):350–352.

18. Segreto VA, Collins EM, D'Agostino R, et al. Anticalculus effect of a dentifrice containing 0.5% zinc citrate trihydrate. *Community Dent Oral Epidemiol*. 1991;19(1):29–31.

19. Schiff T, Saletta L, Baker RA, et al. Anticalculus efficacy and safety of a stabilized stannous fluoride/sodium hexametaphosphate dentifrice. *Compend Contin Educ Dent*. 2005;26(9, Suppl 1):29–34.

20. Volpe AR, Petrone ME, DeVizio W, et al. A review of plaque, gingivitis, calculus and caries clinical efficacy studies with a dentifrice containing triclosan and PVM/MA copolymer. *J Clin Dent*. 1993;4(Spec No):31–41.

21. Seemann R, Conceicao MD, Filippi A, et al. Halitosis management by the general dental practitioner—results of an international consensus workshop. *J Breath Res*. 2014;8(1):017101.

22. Pilch S, Williams MI, Cummins D. In vitro efficacy of Colgate Total advanced fresh. *Compend Contin Educ Dent*. 2003;24(9, Suppl):10–13.

23. Nachnani S. Oral malodor reduction with 3-week use of 0.454% SnF2 dentifrice [640]. *J Dent Res*. 2008;87(Spec Iss B):Abstract 2864.

24. Wunderlich RC, Singelton M, O'Brien WJ, et al. Subgingival penetration of an applied solution. *Int J Periodontics Restorative Dent*. 1984;4(5):64–71.

25. Van Strydonck DA, Slot DE, Van der Velden U, et al. Effect of a chlorhexidine mouthrinse on plaque, gingival inflammation and staining in gingivitis patients: a systematic review. *J Clin Periodontol*. 2012;39(11):1042–1055.

26. Neely AL. Essential oil mouthwash (EOMW) may be equivalent to chlorhexidine (CHX) for long-term control of gingival inflammation but CHX appears to perform better than EOMW in plaque control. *J Evid Based Dent Pract*. 2012;12(3, Suppl):69–72.

27. James P, Parnell C, Whelton H. The caries-preventive effect of chlorhexidine varnish in children and adolescents: a systematic review. *Caries Res*. 2010;44(4):333–340.

28. Ciancio SG. Controlling biofilm with evidence-based dentifrices. *Compend Contin Educ Dent*. 2011;32(1):70–76.

29. Overholser CD, Meiller TF, DePaola LG, et al. Comparative effects of 2 chemotherapeutic mouthrinses on the development of supragingival dental plaque and gingivitis. *J Clin Periodontol*. 1990;17(8):575–579.

30. Sanz M, Serrano J, Iniesta M, et al. Antiplaque and antigingivitis toothpastes. *Monogr Oral Sci*. 2013;23:27–44.

31. Roberts WR, Addy M. Comparison of the *in vivo* and *in vitro* antibacterial properties of antiseptic mouthrinses containing chlorhexidine, alexidine, cetyl pyridinium chloride and hexetidine. Relevance to mode of action. *J Clin Periodontol*. 1981;8(4):295–310.

32. Hossainian N, Slot DE, Afennich F, et al. The effects of hydrogen peroxide mouthwashes on the prevention of plaque and gingival inflammation: a systematic review. *Int J Dent Hyg*. 2011;9(3):171–181.

33. Gandini S, Negri E, Boffetta P, et al. Mouthwash and oral cancer risk quantitative meta-analysis of epidemiologic studies. *Ann Agric Environ Med*. 2012;19(2):173–180.

34. U.S. Food and Drug Administration, Protecting and Promoting Your Health. *Inside Clinical Trials Testing Medical Products in People*. Silver Spring, MD: U.S. Food and Drug Administration. http://www.fda.gov/Drugs/ResourcesForYou/Consumers/ucm143531.htm. Accessed October 15, 2010.

35. American Dental Association, America's Leading Advocate for Health. *ADA Seal and Acceptance Program and Products*. Chicago, IL: American Dental Association. www.ada.org. Accessed February 14, 2014.

ENHANCE YOUR UNDERSTANDING

 DIGITAL CONNECTIONS
(see the inside front cover for access information)

- **Audio glossary**
- **Quiz bank**

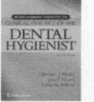 **SUPPORT FOR LEARNING**
(available separately; visit lww.com)

- *Active Learning Workbook for Clinical Practice of the Dental Hygienist, 12th Edition*

prepU **INDIVIDUALIZED REVIEW**
(available separately; visit lww.com)

- **Adaptive quizzing with *prepU for Wilkins' Clinical Practice of the Dental Hygienist***

31

The Patient with Orthodontic Appliances

Jessica August, RDH, BSDH, MSDH and Marylou E. Gutmann, RDH, BS, MA

CHAPTER OUTLINE

CEMENTED BANDS AND BONDED BRACKETS
  I. Advantages of Bonded Brackets
  II. Disadvantages of Bonded Brackets
  III. Fixed Appliance System
  IV. Removable Aligner System

CLINICAL PROCEDURES FOR BONDING
  I. Assessment Examination
  II. Procedural Steps
  III. Characteristics of Bonding Relating to Debonding
  IV. Use of Fluoride-Releasing Bonding System

DENTAL HYGIENE CARE
  I. Complicating Factors: Risk Factors
  II. Disease Control

COMPLETION OF THERAPY

CLINICAL PROCEDURES FOR BAND REMOVAL AND DEBONDING
  I. Band Removal
  II. Clinical Procedures for Debonding

POSTDEBONDING EVALUATION
  I. Enamel Loss
  II. Demineralization (White Spots)
  III. Etched Enamel not Covered by Adhesive

ORTHODONTIC RETENTION

POSTDEBONDING PREVENTIVE CARE
  I. Periodontal Evaluation

  II. Dental Caries
  III. Fluoride Therapy

DOCUMENTATION
EVERYDAY ETHICS
FACTORS TO TEACH THE PATIENT
REFERENCES

LEARNING OBJECTIVES

After studying this chapter, the student will be able to:

1. Recognize key words and terminology used in orthodontic therapy.

2. Explain the advantages and disadvantages of bonded brackets.

3. Summarize the clinical procedures for bonding and debonding.

4. Develop oral self-care recommendations for the orthodontic patient to address effective biofilm removal and reduce risk for dental caries and periodontal disease.

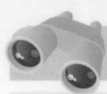

BOX 31-1 | KEY WORDS: Orthodontics

Aligner system: a series of customized transparent and removable aligners utilized in orthodontic therapy to align or straighten teeth.

Appliance: any device designed to influence the shape and/or function of the mouth/jaw system.

Fixed appliance: a bonded or banded appliance affixed to individual teeth or groups of teeth.

Orthodontic appliance: device used to influence growth and/or position of teeth and jaws.

Orthopedic appliance: device used to influence growth and/or position of bones.

Arch wire: curved wire positioned in the brackets around the dental arch and held in place by elastomers or ligatures.

Band: preformed stainless steel ring fitted around a tooth and cemented in place; available in shapes for each tooth form; each band has a bracket attached on the facial side, which is the mode of attachment for the arch wire.

Bonding: process by which orthodontic brackets are affixed to the tooth surface; a fluoride-releasing, light-activated resin is frequently used.

Bracket: attachment that is bonded to the enamel for the purpose of holding the arch wire.

Ceramic: alumina (Al_2O_3) used as a single-crystal material or as a polycrystalline material.

Debonding: removal of brackets and residual adhesive, after which the tooth surface is returned to its normal contour.

Elastomer: elastoplastic ring or latex elastic used to hold an arch wire in a bracket wing.

Fracture toughness: ability of bracket material to resist fracture.

Hawley retainer: a removable plastic and wire appliance used to stabilize teeth; may be modified for special applications during or after orthodontic therapy.

Interceptive/preventive orthodontics: dental services intended to prevent the development of a malocclusion by maintaining the integrity of an otherwise normally developing dentition.

Ligature: cord, thread, elastic, or stainless steel wire used to secure the arch wire to the bracket.

Retainer: an orthodontic appliance, fixed or removable, used to maintain the position of the teeth following corrective treatment.

Space maintainer: prosthetic replacement for prematurely lost primary teeth to prevent closure of the space before eruption of the permanent successors.

Space regainer: appliance used for correction of tooth displacement resulting from premature loss of one or more teeth without timely space maintenance.

Tensile: susceptible to extension; capable of being stretched.

Tensile strength: maximum stress that a material is capable of sustaining; usually expressed in pounds per square inch.

An individualized preventive program that includes a specific plan of instruction, motivation, and supervision is essential for the patient with orthodontic appliances.

▶ The patient needs to understand that much more oral self-care effort is required while in treatment than was required before the appliances were placed.

▶ Terminology used in orthodontic therapy is defined in Box 31-1.

CEMENTED BANDS AND BONDED BRACKETS

▶ Resin-bonded brackets have been used widely in orthodontic treatment.

• Brackets are usually placed on the facial surfaces of the teeth; however, sometimes brackets are bonded to the lingual surfaces.

• Brackets aid in the application and control of applied forces necessary to accomplish tooth movement and bone remodeling for orthodontic therapy.

• Stainless steel or clear ceramic brackets may be used; their function is to retain the arch wire.

• The two types of brackets are illustrated in Figures 31-1 and 31-2.

▶ In some cases, circumferential molar bands are used.

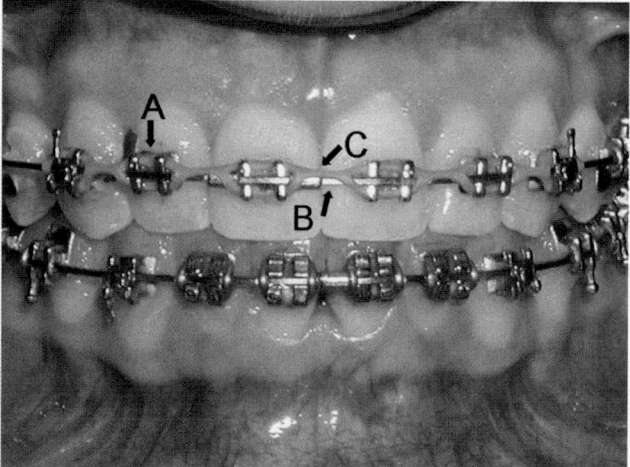

FIGURE 31-1 Fixed Appliance System. A: Bonded brackets **B:** with arch wire **C:** held in place by elastomers.

• For example, for jaw stabilization following orthognathic surgery or when additional strength is needed to hold palatal bars, elastics, or other special devices.

I. Advantages of Bonded Brackets[1]

▶ Improved aesthetics.

▶ Improved gingival condition due to better access for control of dental biofilm at the cervical third of the teeth.

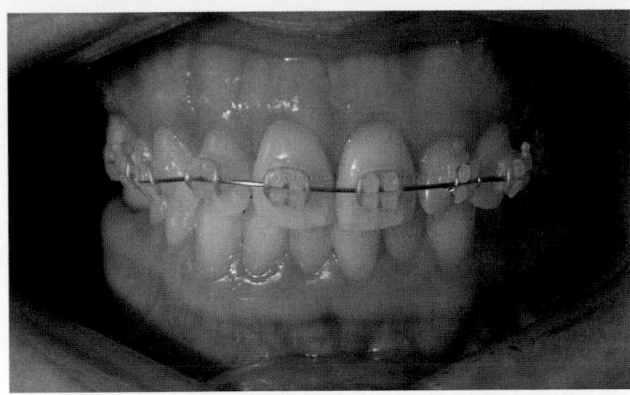

FIGURE 31-2 **Fixed Appliance System.** Bonded clear brackets with arch wire.

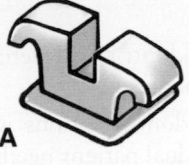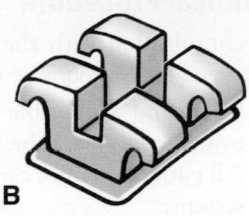

FIGURE 31-3 **Orthodontic Brackets. A:** Single bracket with an incisal and a cervical wing. **B:** Twin, or Siamese, bracket with two wings on each side of the central groove where the arch wire is held. The shape and style of each bracket vary with the tooth on which the bracket will be located.

▶ Proximal surface dental caries can be detected and treated without bracket removal.

▶ Patient can be aware immediately when a bracket loosens, whereas an unsecured band may go undetected.

▶ Placement factors include:
  • No need for tooth separation (as required for band placement); results in less patient discomfort and no band spaces to close at the end of treatment.
  • Lingual brackets ("invisible braces") may be used for specially selected cases.
  • Placement of brackets is faster and easier than placement of bands.

II. Disadvantages of Bonded Brackets[1]

▶ Bond strength of the various materials varies, but self-etching primer results in high bond strength.[2]

▶ Bracket may detach more readily than a band because attachment may be weaker with less surface area is in contact with tooth.

▶ Rebonding a loose bracket is more time consuming and requires more tooth preparation than does recementing a loose band.

▶ Debonding at the end of treatment is more time consuming than debanding, with more potential for damage to the tooth surface because of the higher bond strength.

III. Fixed Appliance System

▶ Figure 31-1 shows bonded metal brackets with arch wire held in place by elastomers.

▶ Figure 31-2 shows bonded clear brackets with arch wire.

A. Brackets

▶ *Materials*
  • Metal (stainless steel).
  • Plastic (polycarbonate).
  • Plastic with metal reinforcements.
  • Ceramic.

▶ *Forms:* Brackets are made in many styles, shapes, and sizes for different teeth, each designed to accomplish a specific objective of treatment. The basic forms are single or twin, as illustrated in Figure 31-3.

▶ *Base:* The base of the bracket is prepared with a mesh backing to assist in retaining the resin bonding agent.
  • The mesh backing, or bonding pad as it is also called, is made to the exact size of the bracket to minimize the gaps between the composite–enamel junction, which can harbor bacteria that cause demineralization.

B. Arch Wire

▶ The arch wire attaches to the bracket to generate and distribute forces that guide orthodontic tooth movement.

▶ Arch wires are made of stainless steel or an alloy of chromium or titanium, and they may be round, rectangular, or multistranded. The arch wire is illustrated in Figures 31-1 and 31-2.

C. Elastomers

▶ Elastomers are available in latex and nonlatex materials and come in a wide variety of colors.

▶ Elastomers are used as chains and on individual teeth for the following purposes:
  • Hold wires in the brackets (Figure 31-1).
  • Apply light continuous force to close spaces between teeth.[3]

IV. Removable Aligner System

Clear aligners systems are an increasingly popular orthodontic technique for aligning teeth and correcting malocclusions.

A. Overview of Removable Aligner System[4]

▶ On the basis of an individual treatment plan, a series of custom, clear thermoplastic aligners are fabricated.

▶ With each set of aligners, the misaligned teeth are progressively moved.

B. Clinical Procedure

▶ A consultation with the orthodontist will determine the need for orthodontic treatment.

- Fixed and removable orthodontic options will be evaluated to meet the individual patient needs.
- All patients are not candidates for removable aligner systems.

▶ Upper and lower impressions are taken and the aligners are fabricated.

▶ The study models are scanned into a computer to make a three-dimensional model of the step-by-step process for movement of the teeth.

▶ Retention attachments are bonded on the teeth so the aligner has a place to clip into place.

▶ A number of aligners are given to the patient to wear per instructions.

- Each tray is worn for approximately 2 weeks.

▶ The patient will visit the orthodontist on a regular basis for adjustments and monitoring of progress.

▶ Impressions will be taken to fabricate retainers to maintain the orthodontic movement.

CLINICAL PROCEDURES FOR BONDING

I. Assessment Examination

Before bonding, documentation of any irregularities of the patient's teeth, such as white spots or cracks, is required to prevent misunderstanding by the patient after debonding.[5]

II. Procedural Steps

▶ The principles for pit and fissure sealants apply for bonding orthodontic brackets.

- Details are not included here, except to point out that calculus must be completely removed.
- Follow procedures described in Chapter 37 for sealant application.
- After bonding, the area around the bracket is carefully cleaned of excess material. Excess material around the bracket serves as a site for biofilm accumulation.[6]

III. Characteristics of Bonding Relating to Debonding

A. Nature of the Bond

▶ The acid etch exposes the prism structure of enamel and creates microclefts (see Figure 37-1 in Chapter 37).

▶ On the bracket side, the resin becomes locked into the mesh base.

B. Effect of Filler Particles

▶ Adding fillers to the resin increases bond strength, hardness, and wear resistance.[7]

- Heavily filled resins (composites) perform better for the posterior teeth because posterior attachments are subject to high forces of mastication.

▶ Ease of debonding can be related to the type of resin and length of etching time.

- Heavily filled composites are thicker and less viscous; they may be more difficult to remove.
- Etching time of 30 seconds significantly improved bond strength for orthodontic brackets.[8]

▶ The bond is stronger when a smaller (thinner) layer of resin is placed between the tooth surface and the bracket.

▶ In summary, anterior brackets may be bonded with a lightly filled resin, whereas posterior teeth may need a heavily filled resin to prevent detachment.

IV. Use of Fluoride-Releasing Bonding System

▶ Demineralization around brackets can result in an increased risk of dental caries for even the most conscientious patient.[9]

▶ Use of fluoride-releasing bonding systems such as glass ionomers have been shown to have positive preventive results.[10]

DENTAL HYGIENE CARE

▶ The patient may be under orthodontic care with regular appointments for a long period, frequently years.

▶ Periodic communication between the orthodontist and the patient's referring dentist and dental hygienist is required to coordinate oral self-care instruction along with other essential dental and dental hygiene care.

▶ Regular dental hygiene preventive care and motivation for oral self-care are essential during orthodontic treatment.[11]

I. Complicating Factors: Risk Factors

A. Age Groups

▶ Many orthodontic patients are in the preteen and teenage years, periods when the incidence of gingivitis is high.

- The incidence of periodontal infection increases from early childhood to late teenage years.

▶ There is a significant increase in the number of adult patients seeking orthodontic treatment.

- As with younger patients, the risk factors for caries and periodontal diseases increase.

- The adult orthodontic patient may be taking medications or have a systemic condition that can complicate therapy.

B. Gingivitis[12]

▶ Dental biofilm retention around orthodontic appliances leads to gingivitis.

▶ The degree can vary from slight to severe with gingival enlargement, particularly of the interdental papillae.

▶ The tissue may greatly enlarge and cover the fixed appliance. The enlarged tissue with pockets provides additional biofilm-retentive areas.

C. Position of Teeth

▶ Teeth that are irregularly positioned are more susceptible to the retention of dental biofilm and are more difficult to clean.

▶ With the severe malocclusions presented by orthodontic patients at the outset, this factor becomes even more significant.

D. Problems with Appliances

▶ Orthodontic appliances retain biofilm and debris.

▶ Accidents may cause a bracket to become detached.

E. Self-care is Difficult

▶ Even the patient who tries to maintain oral cleanliness has difficulty.

- The appliances are in the way and interfere with the application of the toothbrush and other devices used for dental biofilm control.

▶ Instruction needs to be very specific and reviewed at each appointment.

II. Disease Control

A meticulous program for dental caries and periodontal disease control is needed.

▶ The selection of biofilm control procedures for an individual patient is determined by the anatomic features of the gingiva, position of the teeth, and type and position of the orthodontic appliance.

A. General Oral Self-care Instructions[10,11,12]

▶ Give oral self-care instructions before appliances are placed, with the goal of having the oral tissues healthy and the patient motivated to perform thorough daily biofilm removal.

▶ Perform brushing and interdental care in front of a mirror so that technique is accurate and thorough.

- Place emphasis in brushing on sulcular brushing and cleaning the area between the orthodontic bands and brackets and the gingiva.

▶ *Interdental aids*

- A floss threader is needed for biofilm removal from proximal tooth surfaces when the appliance prevents passage of floss from the occlusal aspect.
- Tufted dental floss used in the floss threader can remove the biofilm more efficiently than regular dental floss.
- A single-tuft brush can be particularly beneficial around individual teeth that are hard to access with a regular toothbrush.
- Travel interdental brushes can provide access to areas around and under the arch wires and come in a container that is easy for patients to use away from home.
- Review Chapter 29 for interdental aids, such as tufted floss, interdental brushes, floss threaders, and irrigation options that may be effective for each patient.

▶ Disclosing solution is useful to help the patient self-evaluate biofilm removal.

- A patient wearing an orthodontic appliance may experience difficulty in chewing disclosing wafers without discomfort or pain.
- A disadvantage is that disclosing stains may be difficult to remove from the bonding resin.

▶ Caries prevention is a necessary part of minimizing and preventing white spot lesions.

- Recommend an approved fluoride dentifrice, professionally applied fluoride varnish, and prescribe home fluoride gel or paste to aid in dental caries control (review Chapter 36 for recommendations for fluoride dentifrices, gels, and mouthrinses).[13]
- Sugar-free mints or gum containing xylitol may be used between meals.
- Diet counseling is needed to ensure a patient understands the foods and beverages most likely to impact future dental caries.
- For patients with xerostomia, saliva substitutes and dry mouth products may help reduce caries risk.

▶ Recommend an approved mouthrinse to aid in dental caries control and periodontal inflammation control.

B. Toothbrush Selection

▶ *Power brush*: Used with soft filaments, a light stroke, and at a low speed, power brushes have been shown to be more effective for maintaining gingival health and cleaning around appliances than manual toothbrushes.[14]

▶ Figure 28-9 in Chapter 28 shows various designs of power brushes.

▶ *Manual brush*

- Soft brush: A soft brush with end-rounded filaments is recommended.
- Bilevel: A special bilevel orthodontic brush designed with spaced rows of soft nylon filaments and a shorter middle row that can be applied directly over the appliance is shown in Figure 31-4. It is used with a short horizontal stroke.

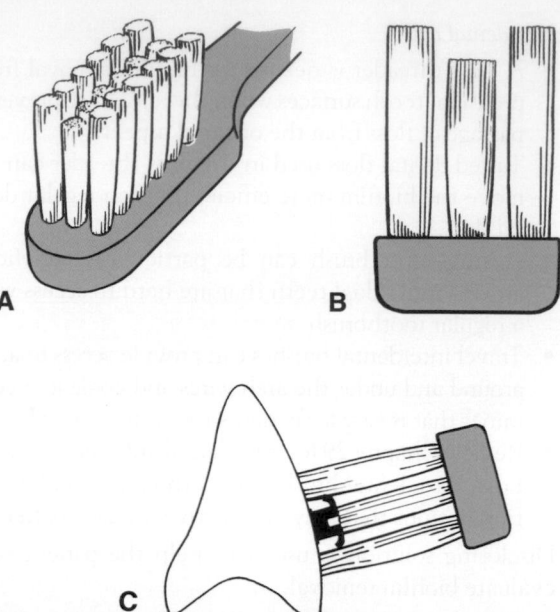

FIGURE 31-4 **Orthodontic Bilevel Toothbrush. A:** Middle row of filaments trimmed shorter to fit over a fixed appliance. **B:** Cross section. **C:** Brush held over a bracket.

C. Toothbrushing Procedure

▶ *Sulcular brushing:* A sulcular method is needed by most patients for cleaning the appliances and maintaining the gingiva.

- Power brushes are adapted for sulcular as well as any other brushing procedures.

▶ *Adapt for appliance:* Special adaptation is required for facial surfaces.

- Place the brush with filament ends directed toward the occlusal surface (Charters' position, Figure 31-5D) to clean under the wire and bracket for mandibular arch, place in Stillman position for the opposite side (Figure 31-5C).

▶ *Clean all surfaces of biofilm and food debris;* To ensure cleanliness, one needs to brush the appliances in any way that the filaments can be manipulated.

- Insert the brush from below, over, and above the arch wire; rotate and vibrate to remove biofilm and debris.

▶ *Lingual and palatal:* Approach to brushing is similar to the basic strokes used on the facial surfaces.

D. Additional Measures

▶ The entire self-care routine is kept as simple as possible; it is a challenge to find the most effective therapeutic aids for the individual needs of the patient.

- When suggesting a new aid, be sure to eliminate one that did not work well for the patient.

▶ Document changes to the oral care plan in the patient's chart.

▶ A rubber tip can be helpful in dislodging biofilm under brackets.

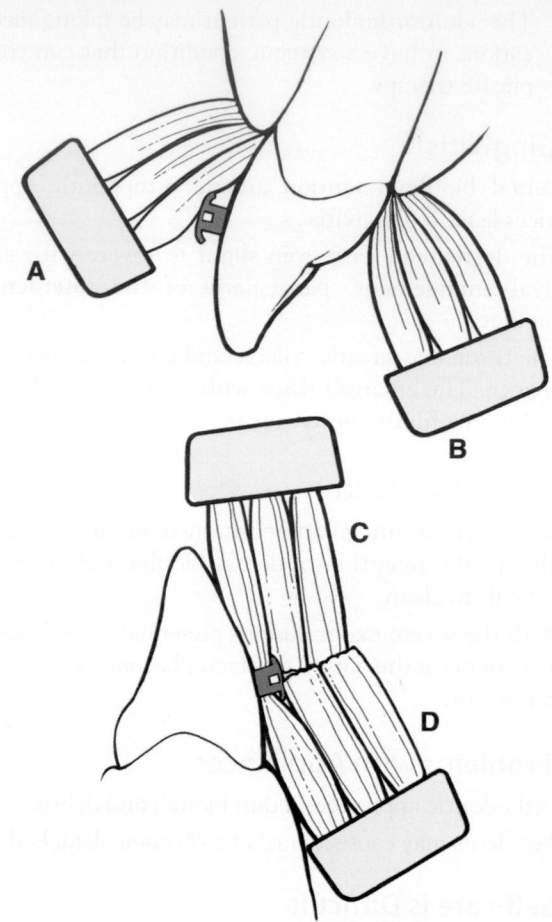

FIGURE 31-5 **Toothbrushing for Orthodontic Appliance. A** and **B:** Sulcular brushing for periodontal tissues. **C:** Brush in Stillman position for occlusal side of bracket and arch wire. **D:** Cleaning the gingival side of bracket using brush in Charters brushing position.

▶ *Oral irrigation:*

- Most patients who wear orthodontic appliances can benefit from the regular use of water irrigation for removal of loose dental biofilm and food debris.
- Oral irrigation, particularly with an orthodontic tip (see Figure 29-14 in Chapter 29), before brushing is recommended so debris is removed to provide access to enamel surfaces for the fluoride dentifrice.

E. Dental Hygiene Instrumentation

▶ It is difficult to instrument manually around orthodontic bands and brackets. The use of an ultrasonic or sonic scaler is helpful.

▶ The use of an air polisher (Chapter 45) may be indicated since the bands and brackets can tear polishing cups and the agent is less abrasive than polishing paste.

COMPLETION OF THERAPY

▶ At the completion of therapy, patients are excited and are looking forward to the removal of the appliances.

▶ Because the patient may forget posttreatment instructions, the dental hygienist provides written as well as verbal instructions on dental biofilm removal, the fluoride regimen, diet, care of the retainer, and follow-up appointments with the orthodontist and general practitioner.

▶ In addition, a description and careful explanation of each step in the procedure for debanding and debonding will alleviate patient apprehension about the process.

▶ Retained excess resin is removed because it retains biofilm, irritating to oral tissues, unsightly, and it must be removed.

CLINICAL PROCEDURES FOR BAND REMOVAL AND DEBONDING

Following active orthodontic therapy, bands and brackets are removed mechanically followed by removal of residual adhesive (cement) and bonding material.

▶ Two types of iatrogenic damage to enamel occur during adhesive and bonding removal include:[15]
  • Loss of enamel from etching, grinding, and polishing.
  • Increased enamel roughness by scratching or creating wear facets.

▶ Objectives for adhesive (cement) and debonding procedure:
  • Remove resin bulk.
  • Minimize damage to pulpal tissue.
  • Avoid damage to enamel surface.
  • Prevent excess enamel loss.

I. Band Removal

▶ Bands are generally removed with orthodontic band-removing pliers.

▶ The dental adhesive (cement) is removed by hand instruments, ultrasonics, or bur.

▶ Complete removal is critical to prevent biofilm retention and support periodontal health.

II. Clinical Procedures for Debonding

A. Method Types

▶ Mechanical, electrothermal, laser, and ultrasonic methods have been studied in an attempt to determine which debonding method is the most efficient and effective, provides the least discomfort for the patient, and causes the least damage to enamel.[15]
  • Tungsten-carbide burs are the fastest and most effective but require a multi-step process to polish the enamel for finishing.
  • The most destructive tools for resin removal included Arkansas stones, green stones, diamond burs, steel burs, and lasers.[15]

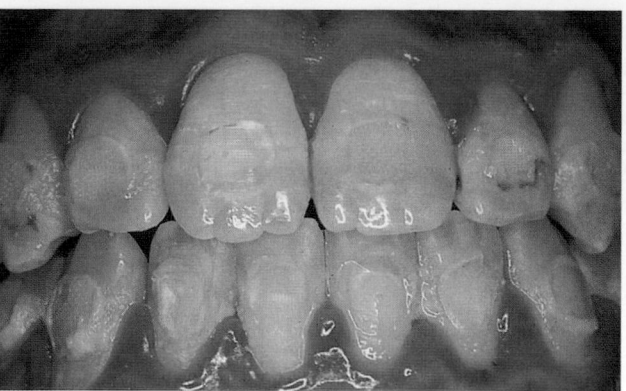

FIGURE 31-6 Facial View of Anterior Teeth with Adhesive Resin Remaining Following Removal of Orthodontic Brackets. (Reprinted with permission from Gutmann ME. Composite adhesive resin removal following orthodontic treatment. *J Pract Hyg.* 1996;5:16.)

BOX 31-2

Steps for Orthodontic Adhesive Resin Removal Using Burs and Polishing Instruments

1. Identify the location and extent of the resin with an explorer, disclosing solution, and patient feedback.
2. Using a tapered, tungsten-carbide finishing bur in a low-speed handpiece, move the bur from the cervical to incisal/occlusal portion of the resin in a light, brushlike stroke.
3. Evaluate progress frequently by rinsing and drying the tooth surfaces.
4. Polish each surface with aluminum oxide polishing points, followed by aluminum oxide polishing cups.
5. Use a rubber cup in a slow-speed handpiece to polish each surface with a fine pumice slurry. Use intermittent strokes.
6. Use a brown polishing cup in a slow-speed handpiece to polish the enamel surfaces.
7. Use a green polishing cup in a slow-speed handpiece to provide the final finish to the enamel surfaces.

B. Removal of Residual Resin bonding

▶ *Examination*
  • Varying amounts of resin remain after the bracket is removed, particularly in normal anatomic grooves, as shown in Figure 31-6.
  • During debonding, frequent examination is necessary using visual and tactile methods.
  • Box 31-2 contains a summary of the steps necessary for complete removal of the orthodontic adhesive resin.

▶ *Identification of residual resin*
  • Patient reports feeling roughness with the tongue.
  • *Visual:* When dry, the resin appears dull and opaque compared with clean, shiny enamel. The use of disclosing solution will also enhance the visibility of the adhesive resin remnant.

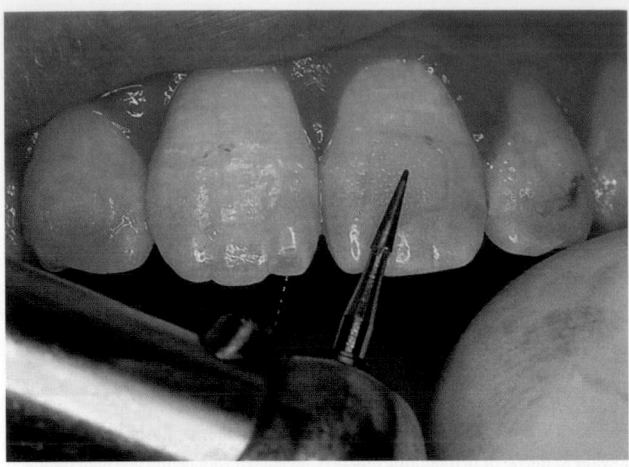

FIGURE 31-7 Use of Tapered, Tungsten-Carbide Finishing Bur on Low-Speed Handpiece to Remove Bulk of Adhesive Resin. (Reprinted with permission from Gutmann ME. Composite adhesive resin removal following orthodontic treatment. *J Pract Hyg*. 1996;5:16.)

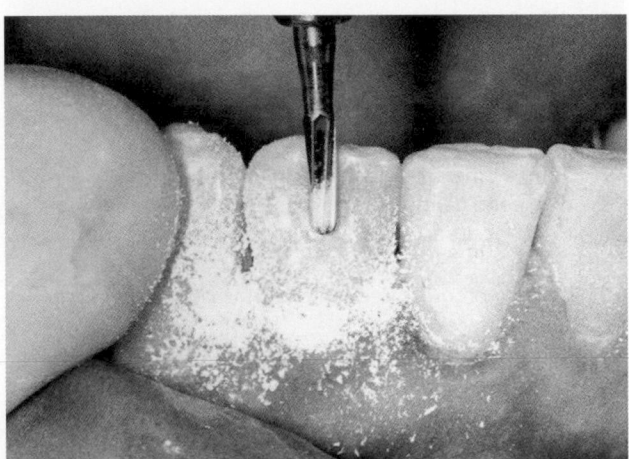

FIGURE 31-8 Adhesive Shavings Following Use of Bur. (Reprinted with permission from Gutmann ME. Debonding orthodontic adhesives. *J Dent Hyg*. 1985;59:369.)

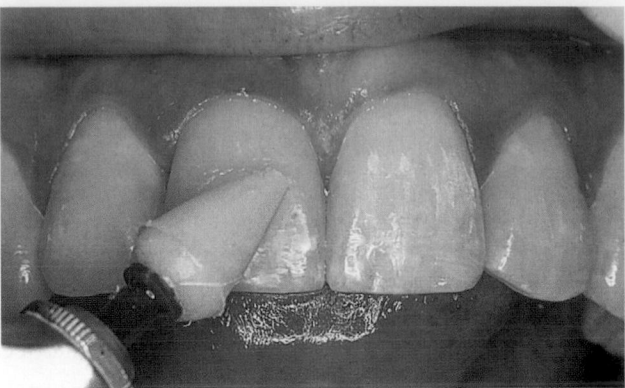

FIGURE 31-9 Aluminum Oxide Finishing Point to Remove Any Enamel Scarring Resulting from Bur. (Reprinted with permission from Gutmann ME. Composite adhesive resin removal following orthodontic treatment. *J Pract Hyg*. 1996;5:16.)

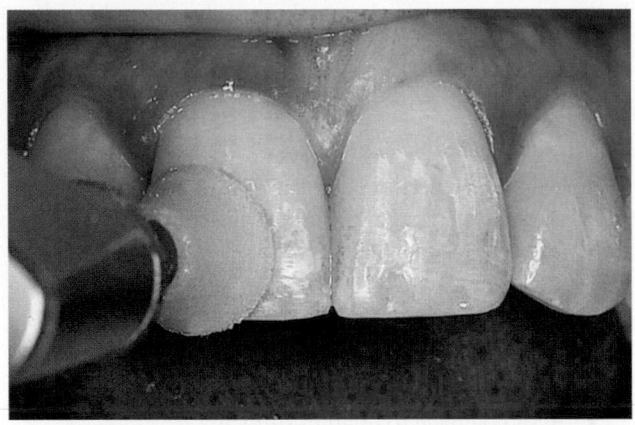

FIGURE 31-10 Aluminum Oxide Finishing Cup to Remove Any Enamel Scarring Resulting from Bur. (Reprinted with permission from Gutmann ME. Composite adhesive resin removal following orthodontic treatment. *J Pract Hyg*. 1996;5:16.)

- *Tactile*: Application of an explorer reveals a rough surface, sometimes with catches along the margin of a resin tag. Filler particles from the resin may abrade the metal explorer tip, leaving a gray line on the resin surface.
- *Use of loupes for magnification of the tooth surface*: A more accurate evaluation of the enamel surface can be made.

▶ *Removal of resin from tooth surface*[15]

- *Bur selection*: Use a tapered, plain-cut, tungsten-carbide finishing bur with a low-speed handpiece, as illustrated in Figure 31-7.
- *Speed*: Use low speed to control heat.
- *Stroke*: Use a smooth, evenly applied, light brush stroke in one direction to prevent faceting.
- *Direction*: Work systematically from cervical portion of the resin; move toward incisal or occlusal third. When removed, the resin resembles fine white shavings, as seen in Figure 31-8.

- *Evaluate frequently* to prevent overinstrumentation, rinse frequently, dry, and evaluate the surface. The resin will appear opaque in contrast to the glossy enamel. Reapply disclosing solution as necessary to visualize small remaining resin particles. Patients may also be helpful in identifying resin remnants with their tongues.

▶ *Final finish*[15]

- *Objective*: Restore pretreatment enamel surface finish.
- *Examination*: Perform visual and tactile examination to distinguish areas of normal enamel from irregularities. Ask patient to feel their teeth by slowly sliding the tongue over the enamel surfaces.
- *Application of aluminum oxide finishing points and cups*
  - Use the finishing points first to remove any fine scarring resulting from the burs (Figure 31-9).
  - Use a low-speed handpiece.
  - Follow with aluminum oxide cups and move from area to area in a cervical to incisal/occlusal direction (Figure 31-10).
- *Application of the rubber cup*

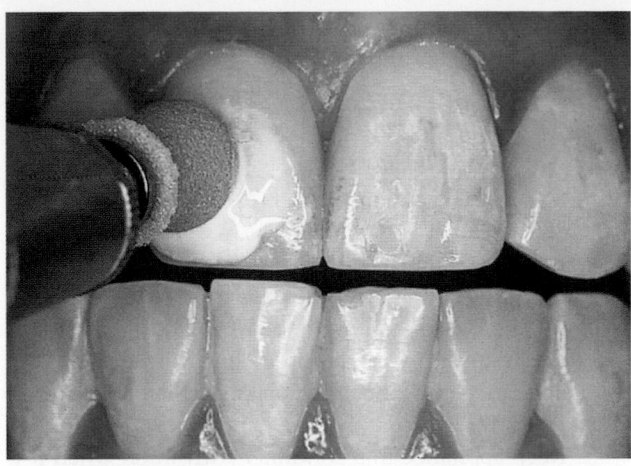

FIGURE 31-11 Polishing with Fine Pumice Slurry and Rubber Cup. (Reprinted with permission from Gutmann ME. Composite adhesive resin removal following orthodontic treatment. *J Pract Hyg*. 1996;5:16.)

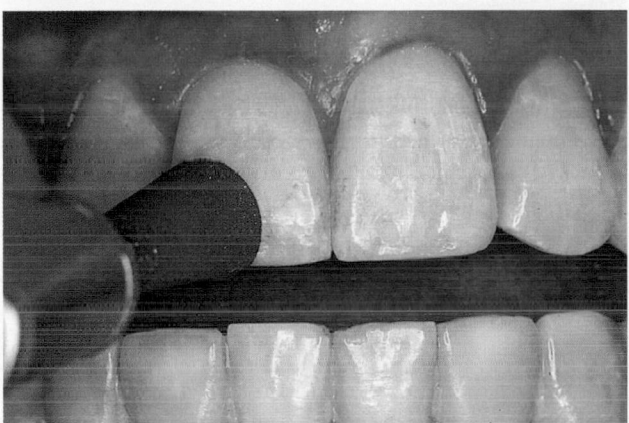

FIGURE 31-12 Brown Polishing Cup Provides Maximum Gloss to Enamel Surface. (Reprinted with permission from Gutmann ME. Composite adhesive resin removal following orthodontic treatment. *J Pract Hyg*. 1996;5:16.)

- Use a fine pumice water slurry, as shown in Figure 31-11.
- Polish in a wet field to prevent overheating.
- Use intermittent strokes to avoid overheating and move from tooth to tooth.
- *Final polish*: Use brown followed by green polishing cups to produce a natural-appearing, glossy enamel surface (Figures 31-12 and 31-13).
- After debonding, topical fluoride varnish application is recommended for caries prevention and to reverse white spot lesions.

POSTDEBONDING EVALUATION

- Each step of bonding and debonding has a deleterious effect on the enamel surface.
- The clinician must avoid unnecessary trauma during the various procedures.

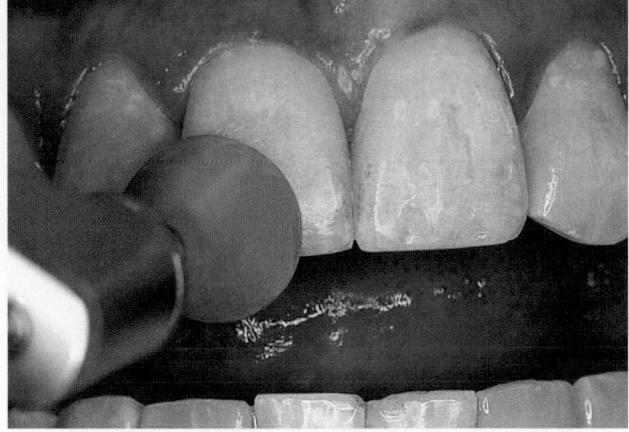

FIGURE 31-13 Final Polishing with Green Polishing Cup. (Reprinted with permission from Gutmann ME. Composite adhesive resin removal following orthodontic treatment. *J Pract Hyg*. 1996;5:16.)

I. Enamel Loss

- Total enamel loss from etching, bracket removal, residual resin removal, surface finishing, and application of pumice averages approximately 55 μm.[15]
  - Use of a tungsten-carbide finishing bur results in enamel loss from 22.7 to 50.5 μm.[15]
- Enamel loss is greater when filled resins (composites) are used for bonding than when unfilled resins are used.
- The loss is also greater when a rotating bristle brush rather than a rubber cup is used with the abrasive for finishing.
- The outer layer of enamel is the most fluoride-rich enamel[14] and is approximately 50 μm deep.
  - Without care during debonding, the entire protective layer can be removed.
- When multiple bonding and debonding procedures are done, such as when a bracket becomes detached, the enamel loss is compounded.
- Careful selection of instruments and abrasives, along with minimal instrumentation, is necessary to minimize enamel loss.

II. Demineralization (White Spots) [9,12]

- White demineralizationed areas or dental caries are relatively common findings after orthodontic treatment.
- Dental biofilm retention on appliances and the resin, along with the difficulty of biofilm removal by the patient, contribute to demineralization and dental caries.

III. Etched Enamel not Covered by Adhesive

- Surface areas etched but not covered with adhesive resin become remineralized when the fluoride contact is increased through personal and professional applications.
- Etched enamel has a high fluoride uptake.

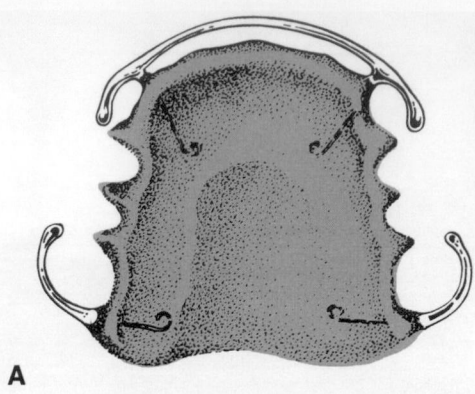

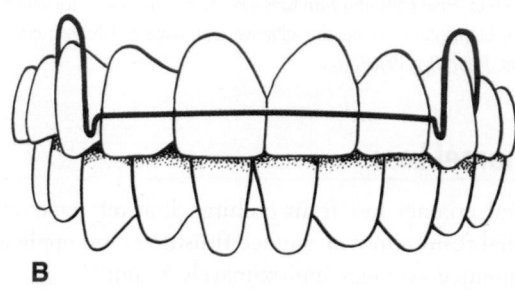

FIGURE 31-14 Hawley Retainer. A: Removable acrylic retainer with facial retaining wire and clasps to be worn after removal of a fixed orthodontic appliance. **B:** Anterior view shows a Hawley appliance in position. The method for cleaning the appliance is similar to that for cleaning a removable denture.

ORTHODONTIC RETENTION

▶ After fixed appliances have been removed, a retainer is worn to give support to the teeth while the bone and other supporting tissues are stabilizing.
  • One type of removable retainer is the Hawley appliance, shown in Figure 31-14.

▶ The use of a retainer provides another source for retention of dental biofilm.
  • Special instruction for care and cleaning of a retainer is needed.
▶ General procedures are suggested here.
  • Clean the appliance after each meal and before bedtime.
  • Instructions for cleaning procedures and agents for removable appliances are described with the care of the removable denture (Chapter 32).
  • Brush and rinse teeth and gingival tissue under the appliance each time the appliance is removed.
  • Brush the mucosa under the appliance.
  • Keep appliance in a container with water when it is out of the mouth.

POSTDEBONDING PREVENTIVE CARE

I. Periodontal Evaluation

▶ A complete examination with a careful periodontal assessment and charting is necessary because many changes take place during treatment.
▶ Calculus removal is completed as needed.
▶ Clinical photographs assist the patient in comparing gingival tissue changes and teeth before and after treatment.
▶ Apply disclosing agent for documentation of biofilm and patient instruction.

II. Dental Caries

▶ Examination for demineralization (white spots) and dental caries is essential.
▶ Dental biofilm retention by orthodontic appliances can be extensive.

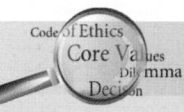

EVERYDAY ETHICS

Dorothy, a patient who had recently completed orthodontic therapy, presents for a maintenance appointment with Caroline, the dental hygienist in her general dentist's practice. The facial surfaces of tooth numbers 4–13 and 20–29 appear to harbor remnants of composite adhesive resin.

Caroline, the dental hygienist, feels an obligation to remove these adhesive remnants but does not want to make any disparaging comments about the orthodontist, whose responsibility it was to remove the adhesive. There is not enough time to remove all of the resin and complete the examination, radiographs, and dental hygiene therapy at the current appointment.

Questions for Consideration

1. Which of the core values (Table II-1, Dental Hygiene Core Values) have particular significance in this setting? How and why?

2. To maintain Dorothy's trust in her orthodontist, how can Caroline inform the patient of the accretions and explain the need for additional appointments?

3. Role play a conversation between Caroline and Dorothy as Caroline explains the problem.

- The configurations of the appliances make biofilm control efforts by the patient extremely difficult.
- Biofilm collects on brackets and some resins even when the patient's oral hygiene is generally good.[6]

▶ Composite resin may be left on the tooth surface around the bracket. The surface of resins is difficult to make smooth; thus, biofilm collects.

III. Fluoride Therapy[13]

▶ A complete program of fluoride treatments, professionally applied at frequent maintenance appointments and used by the patient on a daily basis, is prerequisite both during and following orthodontic therapy.

▶ Application of a fluoride varnish immediately following bonding can help to reduce demineralization by up to 38%–44%.[16,17] Varnish applications need to become a part of every maintenance appointment.

▶ With the loss of fluoride-rich enamel surface during bonding and debonding procedures, the need for remineralization and replenishment of fluoride is clear.

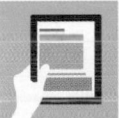

BOX 31-3
Example Documentation: Patient Following Completion of Orthodontic Treatment

S –A 16-year-old female patient presents for 6 month maintenance appointment. Patient has recently completed orthodontic treatment. Patient reports the soreness she had following band removal has subsided.

O–Assessment data collected include marginal redness with bleeding on probing on the mandibular anterior teeth. Hard tissue examination findings include areas of demineralization on the maxillary anterior teeth. Calculus localized to the mandibular anterior teeth.

A –Patient is at a high caries risk level. Caries prevention and remineralization of enamel is essential.

P–Assessment data collected and documented. Health history update, intraoral and extraoral examination, full-mouth periodontal assessment, and biofilm score using disclosing solution. Manually scaled to completion and applied fluoride varnish. Oral self-care instructions reviewed. Demonstrated flossing and positioning of her toothbrush for more effective biofilm removal. Patient observed while brushing and flossing mandibular anterior teeth. Recommended prescription fluoride toothpaste.

Next steps: Schedule continuing care appointment in 3 months to reevaluate demineralized areas.

Signed _____, RDH
Date _____

DOCUMENTATION

Over the long period of treatment, detailed recording of each step, the tissue reactions, and the outcomes are needed.

▶ Patient's personal hygiene, the implements used, and the biofilm observed at individual visits is a significant part of the records.

▶ At dental hygiene appointments, calculus occurrence and removal.

▶ Documentation by the orthodontist includes each step and the summaries of changes noted.

▶ A sample progress note may be found in Box 31-3.

Factors To Teach The Patient

▷ The significance of dental biofilm around orthodontic appliances and the teeth.
▷ How to apply the toothbrush (power or manual) and adjunctive aids to remove dental biofilm from the bracket, the arch wire, and the teeth.
▷ How, when, and why to use fluoride rinses, toothpaste, and brush-on gel.
▷ The frequency for professional follow-up during and after orthodontic therapy.

References

1. Zachrisson BU. Bonding in orthodontics. In: Graber TM, Vanarsdall RL, eds. *Orthodontics: Current Principles and Techniques*. 3rd ed. St. Louis, MO: Mosby; 2000:557–639.

2. Reddy KD, Kishore MSV, Safeena S. Shear bond strength of acidic primer, light-cure glass ionomer, light-cure and self cure composite adhesive systems—an in vitro study. *J Int Oral Health*. 2013;5(3):73–78.

3. Baratieri C, Mattos CT, Alves M Jr, et al. In situ evaluation of orthodontic elastomeric chains. *Braz Dent J*. 2012;23(4):394–398.

4. Rossini G, Parrini S, Castroflorio T, et al. Efficacy of clear aligners in controlling orthodontic tooth movement: a systematic review. *Angle Orthod*. 2014; [Epub ahead of print].

5. Heravi F, Rashed R, Raziee L. The effects of bracket removal on enamel. *Aust Orthod J*. 2008;24(2):110–115.

6. Sukontapatipark W, el-Agroudi MA, Selliseth NJ, et al. Bacterial colonization associated with fixed orthodontic appliances. A scanning electron microscopy study. *Eur J Orthod*. 2001;23(5):475–484.

7. Najafi-Abrandabadi A, Najafi-Abrandabadi S, Ghasemi A, et al. Microshear bond strength of composite resins to enamel and porcelain substrates utilizing unfilled versus filled resins. *Dent Res J*. 2014;11(6):636–644.

8. Firoozmand LM, Brandão JV, Fialho MP. Influence of microhybrid resin and etching times on bleached enamel for the bonding of ceramic brackets. *Braz Oral Res*. 2013;27(2):142–148.

9. Chang HS, Walsh LJ, Freer TJ. Enamel demineralization during orthodontic treatment: aetiology and prevention. *Aust Dent J.* 1997;42(5):322–327.

10. Benson PE, Shah AA, Millett DT, et al. Fluorides, orthodontics and demineralization: a systematic review. *J Orthod.* 2005;32(2):102–114.

11. Migliorati M, Isaia L, Cassaro A, et al. Efficacy of professional hygiene and prophylaxis on preventing plaque increase in orthodontic patients with multibracket appliances: a systematic review. *Eur J Orthod.* 2014. pii:cju044; [Epub ahead of print].

12. Travess H, Roberts-Harry D, Sandy J. Orthodontics, Part 6: risks in orthodontic treatment. *Br Dent J.* 2004;196(2):71–77.

13. Benson PE, Parkin N, Dyer F, et al. Fluorides for the prevention of early tooth decay (demineralised white lesions) during fixed brace treatment. *Cochrane Database Syst Rev.* 2013;12:CD003809.

14. Erbe C, Klukowska M, Tsaknaki I, et al. Efficacy of 3 toothbrush treatments on plaque removal in orthodontic patients assessed with digital plaque imaging: a randomized controlled trial. *Am J Orthod Dentofacial Orthop.* 2013;143(6):760–766.

15. Janiszewska-Olszowska J, Szatkiewicz T, Tomkowski R, et al. Effect of orthodontic debonding and adhesive removal on the enamel—current knowledge and future perspectives—a systematic review. *Med Sci Monit.* 2014;20:1991–2001.

16. Vivaldi-Rodrigues G, Demito CF, Bowman SJ, et al. The effectiveness of a fluoride varnish in preventing the development of white spot lesions. *World J Orthod.* 2006;7(2):138–144.

17. Demito CF, Vivaldi-Rodrigues G, Ramos AL, et al. The efficacy of a fluoride varnish in reducing enamel demineralization adjacent to orthodontic brackets: an in vitro study. *Orthod Craniofac Res.* 2004;7(4):205–210.

ENHANCE YOUR UNDERSTANDING

thePoint° DIGITAL CONNECTIONS
(see the inside front cover for access information)
- **Audio glossary**
- **Quiz bank**

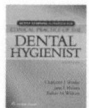

SUPPORT FOR LEARNING
(available separately; visit lww.com)
- *Active Learning Workbook for Clinical Practice of the Dental Hygienist, 12th Edition*

prepU   INDIVIDUALIZED REVIEW
(available separately; visit lww.com)
- **Adaptive quizzing with *prepU for Wilkins' Clinical Practice of the Dental Hygienist***

32

Care of Dental Prostheses

Tammy K. Swecker, BSDH, MED

CHAPTER OUTLINE

After studying this chapter, the student will be able to:

1. Describe the types and components of fixed and removable oral prostheses.

2. List steps to provide professional cleaning of fixed and removable prostheses.

3. Provide a careful evaluation of an oral prosthesis to include clinical examination of the prosthesis, related soft tissue, and patient concerns.

4. Describe the instructions provided for a patient with a new prosthesis.

5. Plan the maintenance program for each patient based on the patient's risk factors and compliance.

Overall health and cleanliness of the oral cavity involves care of all natural teeth, soft tissues, and dental prostheses.

▶ A *prosthesis* is an artificial replacement of a missing part of the body, and a *dental prosthesis* replaces one or more teeth and supporting structures. A *prosthesis* may be fixed or removable.

▶ Awareness of the types and characteristics of *prostheses*, supporting tissues, and the common issues a patient may experience with prostheses is needed to provide information, comprehensive oral hygiene care, and instruction for the patient who has prostheses.

▶ The patient may ask the dental hygienist about options to replace a missing tooth or teeth, how to adjust to a new denture and relearn how to chew, or what to do if a prosthesis feels loose.

▶ Definitions of key words may be studied in Box 32-1.

▶ Daily maintenance by the patient is a vital factor for success and longevity of a prostheses and the health of remaining teeth and oral tissues.

▶ Patients with partial prostheses may be at greater risk for dental caries and periodontal infections because of biofilm adherence to margins of restorations, position of clasps, and tissues under fixed prostheses.

▶ A patient may have more than one prosthesis. A patient with a complete maxillary denture may have both fixed and removable partial dentures (RPDs) in the mandibular arch: an implant-retained RPD or an implant-retained mandibular overdenture.

▶ The regimen for personal care involves the natural teeth as well as the fixed and removable prostheses.

▶ A program of instruction is developed for each patient specific to individual needs.

▶ Examples of types of fixed and removable prostheses and appliances are listed in Box 32-2.

MISSING TEETH

▶ A patient may have one or more missing teeth or may have tooth extractions planned.

▶ A patient is informed of the options to replace missing teeth as well as risk factors associated with not replacing the missing teeth.

▶ Providing objective information on treatment alternatives and acting as a patient advocate allows the patient to make informed, autonomous decisions about personal oral health.

▶ A long history of poor oral hygiene, carious lesions, and periodontal infections may have led to tooth loss; trauma is another common cause of tooth loss.

I. Replacement Options

▶ Replacement options include the following:
  • Fixed prosthesis
  • Removable prosthesis
  • Dental implants (see Chapter 33).

▶ Dental hygienist's role
  • Explain each choice for the patient.
  • Answer questions from the patient.
  • Prepare notes from the patient's medical and dental histories, risk factors, intraoral/extraoral examination, and other pertinent observations to assist the dentist.

II. No Replacement

▶ Replacement for a missing tooth may not be indicated for a patient who has sufficient remaining teeth for function, for example:
  • Third molars are generally not replaced after extraction.
  • Second molars that are extracted and have no opposing teeth.
  • Teeth extracted for orthodontic purposes.

▶ Risks of not replacing missing teeth include:
  • *Migration of adjacent teeth*: Tilting and rotation of teeth may complicate future replacement options or lead to periodontal problems due to difficulty in biofilm control and misdirected occlusal forces when chewing.
  • *Migration of opposing teeth*: An unopposed tooth may supererupt.

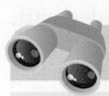 **BOX 32-1** **KEY WORDS:** Dental Prostheses

Abutment: a tooth or an implant used for the support or retention of a fixed or removable prosthesis.

Complete denture: dental prosthesis that replaces the entire dentition and associated structures; may be a complete maxillary denture or a complete mandibular, or both.

Coping: a thin covering or crown.

Denture: artificial substitute for missing natural teeth and adjacent tissues.

Denture adhesive: a soft material used to adhere a denture to the underlying mucosa; also referred to as an adherent.

Denture stomatitis: an inflammation of the oral mucosa that bears a complete or partial removable dental prosthesis, typically a denture.

Fixed partial denture: a replacement for one or more missing teeth that is securely cemented to natural teeth and/or dental implant abutments that furnish the primary support for the prosthesis; also called a fixed prosthesis or bridge.

Immediate denture: any removable dental prosthesis fabricated for placement immediately following the removal of a natural tooth/teeth.

Interim prosthesis: a fixed or removable dental prosthesis designed to enhance esthetics, stabilization, and/or function for a limited period, after which it is to be replaced by a definitive dental or maxillofacial prosthesis. Also referred to as provisional prosthesis, provisional restoration.

Kennedy classification of edentulous areas: a classification system commonly used in dentistry to identify edentulous arches.

Obturator: a prosthesis used to close a congenital or acquired opening, such as for a cleft palate, an area lost because of trauma, or after surgery for removal of a diseased area.

Occlusal vertical dimension: the distance measured between two points when the occluding members are in contact.

Pontic: an artificial tooth on a partial denture that replaces a missing natural tooth, restores its function, and usually occupies the space previously filled by the natural crown.

Precision attachment: a type of connector that consists of a metal receptacle and a close-fitting part; the metal receptacle usually is included within the restoration of an abutment tooth, and the close-fitting part is attached to a pontic or RPD framework.

Prosthesis: artificial replacement of an absent part of the body; may be a therapeutic device to improve or alter function; may be a device employed to aid in accomplishing a desired surgical result.

Removable partial denture: a dental prosthesis that supplies teeth and/or associated structures in a partially edentulous jaw and can be removed and replaced at will.

Residual ridges: the portion of the residual bone and its soft tissue covering that remains after the removal of teeth.

Rest: a rigid, stabilizing extension of a fixed or RPD that contacts a remaining tooth or teeth; prevents movement toward the mucosa and transmits functional forces to the teeth.

Ultrasonic cleaner: a device, in which a denture is placed in water or some type of solvent cleaner, that uses ultrasonic waves to dislodge debris on a denture.

BOX 32-2

Types of Oral Prostheses and Appliances

Fixed

Fixed partial denture
Periodontal splint
Implant-supported complete denture
Orthodontic appliance
Space maintainer

Removable

Removable partial denture (RPD)
Natural tooth supported
Implant supported
Complete denture
Overdenture
Obturator
Removable orthodontic appliance
Removable space maintainer
Hawley appliance

- *Remaining teeth may suffer from the added function and stress:* may lead to fractures and tooth loss.
- *Loss of occlusal vertical dimension:* The bite may become overclosed due to many missing teeth and can lead to temporomandibular joint disorders.
- Loss of vertical dimension may promote angular cheilitis on the corners of the lips from pooling of saliva.

FIXED PARTIAL DENTURE PROSTHESES

I. Description

▶ Fixed partial dentures, commonly called dental *bridges*, are composed of the following, as shown in Figure 32-1:
  - Abutments
  - Connectors
  - Pontics.

▶ Bridges can be fabricated from various materials including:
  - Metals

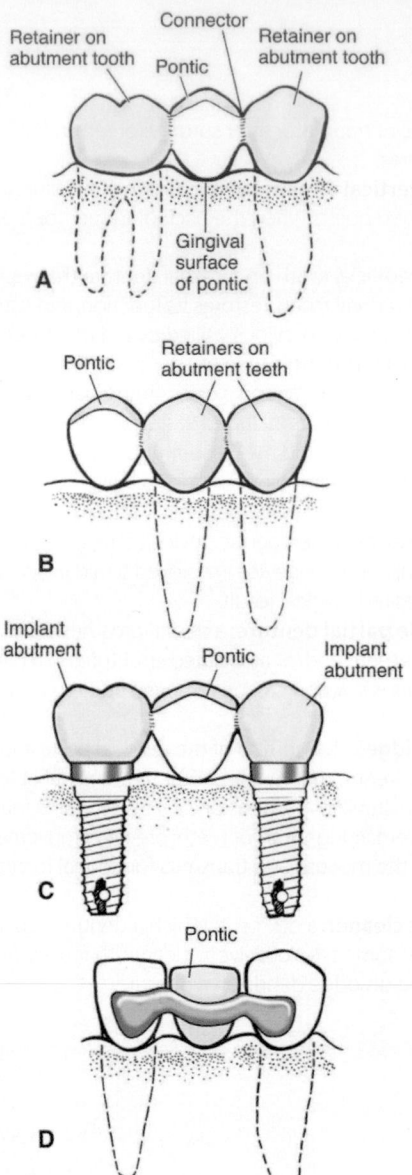

FIGURE 32-1 Fixed Partial Dentures. A: Characteristic parts of a mandibular three-unit fixed partial denture. Cast gold crowns on the abutment teeth serve as the retainers for the bridge. **B:** Cantilever bridge supported by a double abutment. **C:** Fixed partial denture with implant abutments. **D:** Fixed resin–retained partial prosthesis.

- Ceramics
- Combination of both.
▶ A fixed partial denture is affixed to the teeth or implants with a special cement and is not removable.

II. Types of Fixed Partial Dentures

▶ *Natural tooth supported*
- *Traditional/bilateral:* Supported by one or more natural teeth at each end as shown in Figure 32-1A.
- *Cantilever:* Pontic supported by one or more teeth at one end only, as shown in Figure 32-1B.

- *Resin retained:* Wing-like extensions are bonded with a resin cement to etched enamel. Requires minimal or no preparation for tooth structure. Also called a Maryland Bridge and shown in Figure 32-1D.
▶ *Implant supported*
- Shown in Figure 32-1C.
- Blade, cylinder, and crew types of implants used for abutments are shown in Figure 33-4 in Chapter 33.

III. Criteria for Fixed Partial Dentures[1]

▶ Biologically and esthetically harmonious with the teeth and surrounding periodontium.
▶ All parts accessible for cleaning by the patient and the dental professional.
▶ Does not interfere with the cleaning regimen for the remaining natural dentition.
▶ Does not traumatize oral tissues.
▶ Restores functions of the missing tooth or teeth.

CARE PROCEDURES FOR FIXED PROSTHESES

I. Debris Removal

▶ Use an oral irrigator for loose debris removal throughout the dentition for a first step.
▶ Facilitates next step: biofilm removal with a toothbrush and other aids.
▶ Procedure for use of an oral irrigator is described in Chapter 29.

II. Biofilm Removal from Abutment Teeth

▶ Nearly all the methods proposed for dental biofilm control in Chapters 28 and 29 are applicable to abutment teeth.
▶ The proximal surface of an abutment tooth and the gingiva adjacent to a pontic require special attention.
▶ *Toothbrushing*
  Sulcular brushing is generally indicated.
▶ *Dentifrice selection*
- A *nonabrasive* dentifrice is indicated to prevent the abrasion of the prosthesis surfaces and areas of exposed root on abutment teeth.
- A *fluoride-containing* dentifrice is selected for protection of remaining natural tooth surfaces, particularly exposed cementum.
- Acidulated fluoride preparations are contraindicated for implants, porcelain, and composite restorations.[2]
▶ *Additional interdental care*
- Removal of biofilm and food debris from proximal surfaces of teeth, abutment, and pontic is vital.

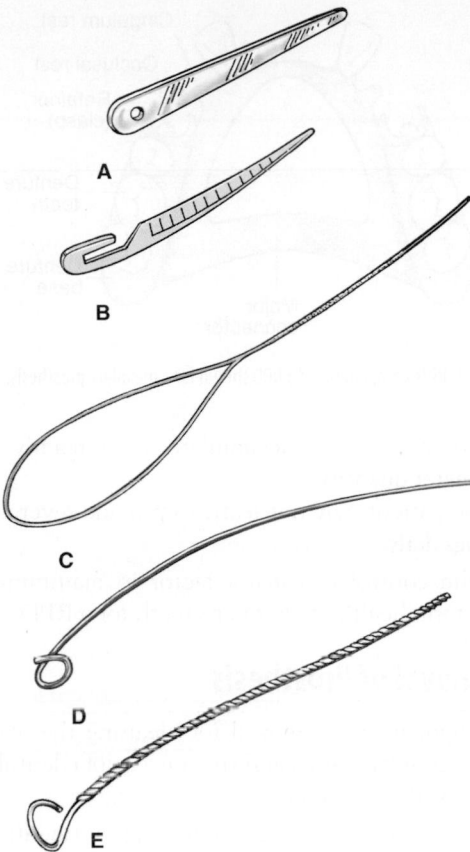

FIGURE 32-2 Floss Threaders. A: Clear plastic with closed eye. **B:** Tinted plastic with open eye. **C:** Soft plastic loop. **D:** Flexible wire. **E:** Twisted wire.

- The method of interdental care is selected based on the manual dexterity of each patient and the type of prosthesis.
- An interdental cleaning device is adapted specifically to the proximal surfaces of the abutments.
- The same interdental cleaning procedures can be applied to the gingival surface of the fixed partial denture.
▶ Interdental cleaning methods and devices are described in Chapter 29.

III. The Prosthesis

▶ *Areas requiring emphasis*
- Restorations may provide areas that retain biofilm and require daily oral hygiene maintenance.
- The gingival surfaces of the pontics and beneath the connectors are particularly prone to biofilm retention.
▶ *Toothbrushing*
- A toothbrush in the Charters position may be helpful for cleaning the gingival surface of the pontic from the facial aspect.
- The filaments can be directed under the pontic to clean the gingival surface.

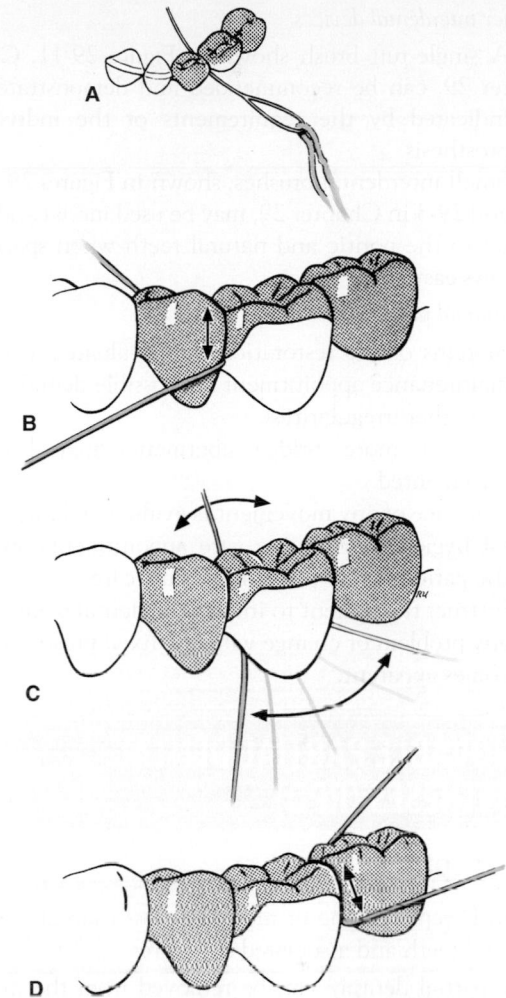

FIGURE 32-3 Use of Floss Threader. A: Use floss threader to draw the floss or tufted floss between abutment and pontic. **B:** Apply floss to the distal surface of the mesial abutment; pull through 1 or 2 inches. **C:** Slide floss under pontic. Move back and forth several times, as shown by the arrows, to remove dental biofilm from the gingival surface of the pontic. **D:** Apply new section of floss to the mesial surface of the distal abutment.

- Charters' brush position is described in Chapter 28.
▶ *Dental floss for threader*
- Tufted dental floss is most efficient for cleaning a fixed partial denture (see Chapter 29).
- Thread a 12- to 15-inch length into a floss threader. Several types are available and are shown in Figure 32-2.
- Apply threader between abutment, pontic, and gingiva.
- Draw the floss through, and using single or double thickness, remove loose debris, as shown in Figure 32-3.
- Apply a new section of the floss with moderate pressure back and forth to the undersurface (gingival surface) of the pontic and then up and down with pressure to the proximal surfaces of each abutment tooth to remove the sticky biofilm.

Other interdental devices

- A single-tuft brush shown in Figure 29-11, Chapter 29, can be recommended and demonstrated as indicated by the requirements of the individual prosthesis.
- Small interdental brushes, shown in Figures 29-10D and 29-3 in Chapter 29, may be used mesial and distal to the pontic and natural teeth when space allows easy entry.

Additional factors

- Margins of the restorations are evaluated at every maintenance appointment for possible dental caries and other irregularities.
- One or more bridge abutments may become uncemented.
- Evidence of any movement is evaluated during dental hygiene continuing care appointments and by the patient while performing daily care.
- Instruct the patient to inform the dental team when any problem or change with the fixed prosthesis becomes apparent.

REMOVABLE PARTIAL DENTAL PROSTHESES (RPD)

I. Description

- A RPD replaces one or more, but less than all, of the natural teeth and associated structures.
- The partial denture can be removed from the mouth and replaced at will.
- The denture base rests on the oral mucosa and carries the artificial teeth.

II. Types

- A typical partial denture consists of a stable metal framework made of chrome cobalt.
- The framework engages abutment teeth or an abutment implant with a wide variety of clasp assemblies and rest seats or precision attachments.
- Depending on the location and number of remaining natural teeth, a partial denture may receive all its support from the teeth or it may be partially tooth borne, partially implant borne, and partially tissue borne.
- The base is made of plastic acrylic resin.
- The teeth are made of porcelain, plastic resin, or metal.
- The basic parts of a RPD are shown in Figure 32-4.

CARE FOR REMOVABLE PARTIAL PROSTHESES

- The health of the underlying tissues can be negatively affected by a RPD because:

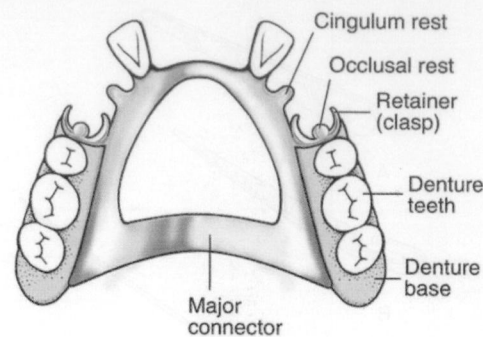

FIGURE 32-4 **RPD.** Components of a RPD shown for a maxillary prosthesis.

- biofilm tends to accumulate more readily and in greater quantities
- the patient may not learn to provide several cleanings daily.
- Biofilm control is a major factor in maintaining the long-term health of abutment teeth for a RPD.

I. Removal of Prosthesis

- The appliance is removed for cleaning the abutment teeth, gingival tissue, and the mucosa of edentulous areas as well as the appliance.
- During professional maintenance appointment:
  - Provide the patient with water and tissue.
  - It is most comfortable to have the patient remove the prosthesis because the patient is familiar with the path of insertion and removal.
- When a patient is unable to remove the appliance, the dental hygienist proceeds as follows:
  - Exert an even pressure on both sides of the denture simultaneously as the clasps slide up over their abutment teeth.
  - The line of insertion and removal of a partial denture is designed and constructed for an even, vertical movement.
  - Avoid grasping the clasp assemblies of the prostheses, which may damage or bend a clasp.

II. Preventing Cross-Contamination

- Prevent cross-contamination when receiving a removable prosthesis from a patient by:
  - Wearing personal protective mask, eyewear, and gloves.
  - Offering a disposable cup in which the patient can place the prosthesis directly.
- Rinse the prosthesis under slowly running water; take care not to splash.
- Place in a cleaning solution in bag in an ultrasonic cleaner as shown in Figure 32-5.
- When the patient has more than one removable prosthesis, place each prosthesis in a separate bag filled with professional prosthesis cleaning solution then place in the ultrasonic cleaner.

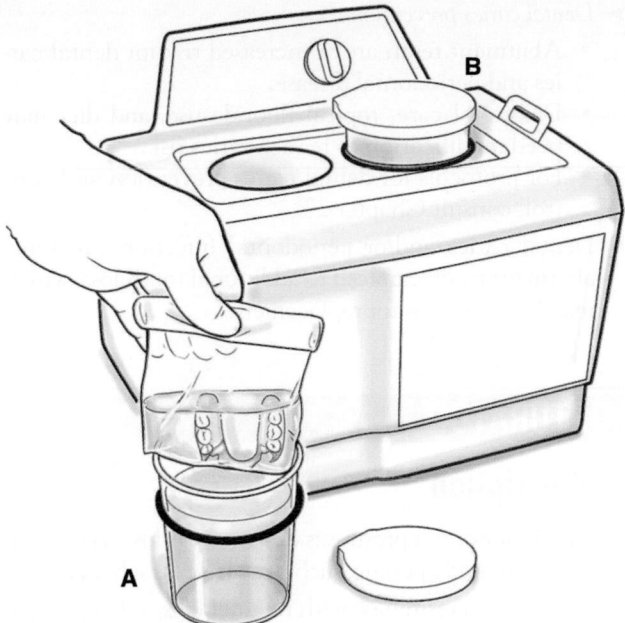

FIGURE 32-5 Ultrasonic Denture Cleaner. A: First, the removable prosthesis is placed in a sealed bag with cleaning solution and placed in a beaker filled with water. **B:** Beaker is then placed in an ultrasonic unit and set according to manufacturer directions.

PATIENT SELF-CARE FOR REMOVABLE PARTIAL PROSTHESES

▶ The significance of the daily care of the RPD is explained to the patient at the initial appointment when the first impression is made.

▶ Instruction is reviewed and continued at every appointment.

▶ The patient needs to learn and appreciate the fact that daily personal debris and biofilm removal is a major step to the comfort and lasting oral tissue health that can result.

▶ The selection of cleansing agents and the procedures for cleaning are complicated by the intricacy of the metallic parts and their relation to the natural teeth, as well as by the dental materials used in construction.

▶ Rinsing, immersing, and brushing methods, as well as the cleansing agents described for the complete denture later in this chapter, may apply to various types of removable prostheses.

▶ At very least after each meal or snack and at bedtime, the appliance is removed and both the appliance and the natural teeth are thoroughly rinsed. Two or three times a day the care needs to be more thorough to remove debris, control halitosis, and appearance especially when the anterior teeth are shown when smiling.

I. Objectives for the Patient

▶ Objective for all patients is to attain and maintain oral health and function.
- The objectives for the natural teeth are to control biofilm for oral sanitation and prevention of dental caries and periodontal infections.
- The care of the natural teeth is described in detail in Chapter 28.
- Interdental care and proximal tooth surfaces of the adjacent teeth are found in Chapter 29.

▶ Cleaning the prosthesis takes on added significance because it is adjacent to natural teeth and rests on soft tissue.

▶ The basic daily oral self-care objective is to:
- Remove all loose debris and attached biofilm.
- Disinfect the appliance to eliminate potential irritants to the teeth and oral tissues that may cause malodor.

▶ A professional care for all removable prostheses is provided at each routine scheduled continuing care appointment.

II. The Prosthesis

A. Rinsing

▶ Partial denture is removed; the mouth is rinsed with fluoridated water; and the water is swished forcefully through the interdental areas. The method for rinsing the mouth is outlined in Box 30-4 in Chapter 30.

▶ The prosthesis is rinsed under running water.

▶ Rinsing does not remove biofilm, which is attached firmly, so it is not a substitute for complete care procedures.

B. Brushing

▶ Precautions are taken during brushing a RPD:
- Too tight a grasp on a partial prosthesis can result in bending or fracture of clasps or bars.
- Filaments of a brush can inadvertently catch the prosthesis and cause it to drop and break.

▶ Partially fill the sink with water and line the sink with a wash cloth or towel to prevent breakage should the prosthesis be dropped.

▶ *Types of brushes: toothbrush*
- The use of a patient's regular toothbrush is not recommended for care of a removable prosthesis because brushing the clasps or other metal parts may deform the toothbrush filaments and make the brush ineffective for use on the natural teeth.
- When a patient insists on using a regular toothbrush, a separate brush is indicated. Demonstrate how difficult it is to fit an adult toothbrush to the partial denture and clasps.

▶ *Power brush*
- A power brush is not used on a removable prosthesis because of the danger of the speeding brush

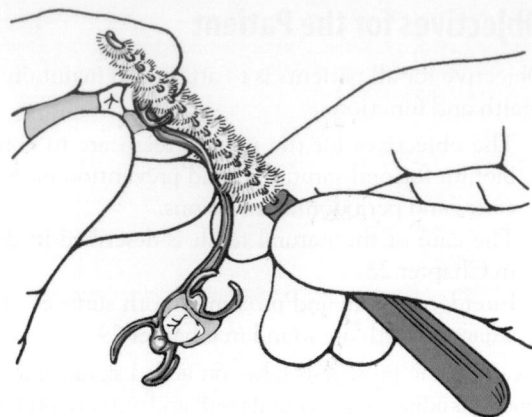

FIGURE 32-6 Clasp Brush. A brush specially designed to remove dental biofilm from the inside surfaces of clasps is available. The denture must be held carefully to avoid accidents.

filaments catching the clasps or other small part and damaging the prosthesis.

▶ *Clasp brush*
  • A specially designed narrow, tapered brush about 2–3 inches long that can be adapted to the inner surfaces of clasps or precision attachments is recommended and shown in Figure 32-6.
  • Difficult-to-clean clasp assemblies have internal surfaces prone to biofilm accumulation that can be removed carefully with a clasp brush.

▶ *Denture brush*
  • A denture brush is shown in Figure 32-9 later in this chapter and is available specifically for brushing complete dentures.
  • Used with careful adaptation it can be useful for cleaning the surfaces and the metal bars of the partial removable denture. Use a clasp brush for the clasps.

C. Immersion

▶ Before immersion, the denture is cleaned by rinsing and brushing to remove all loose surface biofilm and debris.
▶ Avoid agents known to corrode or discolor.
▶ Procedures for immersion cleaning are described later in the chapter.

III. The Natural Teeth

▶ *Biofilm control*
  • The removable prosthesis is taken out of the mouth before biofilm control of implants and remaining natural teeth is performed.
  • Toothbrushing and interdental cleaning methods selected for the particular needs of each patient are followed meticulously.
  • The longevity of the removable appliance depends on the health of the supporting teeth, and the health of the natural teeth depends on the cleanliness of the prosthesis.

▶ *Dental caries prevention*
  • Abutment teeth are at increased risk for dental caries and periodontal disease.
  • Daily oral care, topical fluoride use, and diet may need modification to reduce caries risk.
  • For protocols for dental caries prevention and control, consult Chapter 27.
▶ Dental caries and/or periodontal infection involving abutment tooth can lead to additional tooth loss, which may limit options for replacement.

OBTURATOR

I. Description

▶ An obturator is a prosthesis designed to close a congenital or acquired opening, such as a cleft of the hard palate.
▶ Made with a resin base with retainer clasps that provide stability for the appliance.
▶ Depending on the exact location of the palatal defect, an obturator may extend to include anterior prosthetic teeth.
▶ See Figure 32-7A and B, an example of a palatal defect and corresponding obturator.

II. Purposes and Uses

▶ A variety of medical and physical conditions benefit from use of an obturator including:
  • Cocaine abusers that snort the powder form of the drug develop necrosis of the nasal septum and surrounding tissues.[3]
  • Patient with an area lost due to trauma.
  • Patients with previous cancers involving the maxilla.
  • Patients with cleft palate that fits the dimensions of the palatal defect.[4]
  • More information about obturators for cleft palates can be found in Chapter 51.

III. Clinical Applications

▶ Depending on the size of the palatal defect, the obturator may need to stay in place in the mouth during parts of the intraoral and extraoral examination and treatment procedures to prevent choking or inhalation of materials.
▶ Obturators need to be removed during exposure of radiographic images. An appliance with metal clasps will interfere with the radiolucency of the teeth and surrounding tissues.
▶ Removal of an obturator during dental hygiene therapy may be necessary to ensure access for complete calculus and biofilm removal and treatment of natural tooth surfaces.
▶ Professional care of an obturator follows procedures for a RPD described earlier in this chapter.

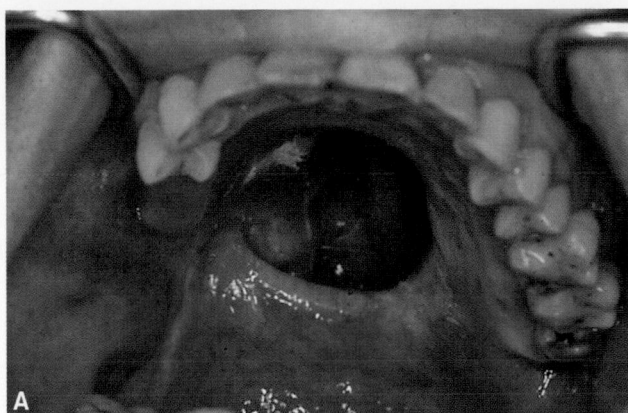

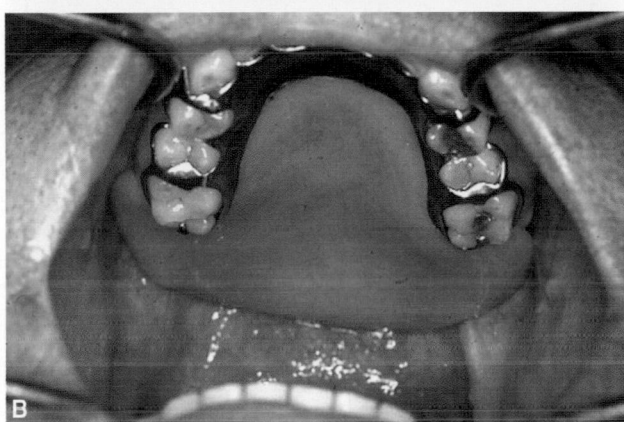

FIGURE 32-7 A: Palatal Defect. B: Corresponding obturator. Picture Courtesy of Altug Kazanoqlu DMD, MS, FAAMP, Virginia Commonwealth University.

▶ Instruction for patient's daily cleaning and care of the obturator is the same as the care given to a RPD.

▶ Patients may need to sleep with the obturator in place when the defect is severe, which may cause the underlying mucosa to become desiccated and the tissue may spontaneously begin to bleed.

▶ Sleeping with an obturator in place increases the risk for demineralization and dental caries in the abutment teeth as well as the incidence of denture stomatitis.

▶ When the patient must sleep with the obturator in place, it is advisable that the obturator be removed for short periods during the day to allow the tissue to rest.

IV. Professional Continuing Care

▶ A minimum of three visits each year to the dentist and dental hygienist is recommended for continuing care depending on patient compliance and risk factors.

▶ The palatal defect will change over time and the dentist will need to adjust the obturator along with routine dental care.

COMPLETE DENTURE PROSTHESIS

▶ The initial adjustment to wearing a prosthesis is challenging for the patient.

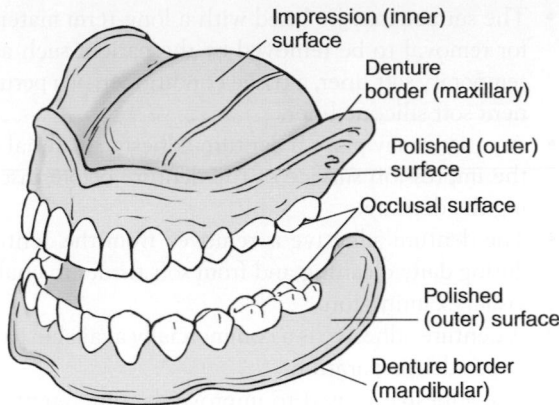

FIGURE 32-8 **Complete Denture.** The surfaces and borders of maxillary and mandibular dentures.

▶ The entire dental team needs to work together to assist the patient through the process of losing teeth and adjusting to a new prosthesis.

▶ A new prosthesis requires several adjustment visits with the dentist.

▶ Components of a complete denture are shown in Figure 32-8.

I. Types of Complete Dentures

▶ *Immediate denture:* Delivered initially at the time the teeth are extracted. Because of the amount of bone remodeling after extraction, the denture is relined or rebased about 6 months later.

▶ *Interim denture:* A temporary denture used for diagnosis and treatment. A conventional denture is made later.

▶ *Conventional denture:* The long-term complete denture prosthesis.

II. Marking Removable Prostheses

▶ All removable appliances are labeled for patient identification purposes.

▶ Methods of identification are described and illustrated in Chapter 54.

III. Components of a Complete Denture

▶ *Denture base*
  • The part of a denture that rests on the oral mucosa and to which the teeth are attached.
  • Most denture bases are made of plastic acrylic resin.
  • Others may be metal such as chrome cobalt or gold, in combination with a plastic resin.

▶ *Impression surface*
  • The tissue or inner surface of the denture.
  • Lies directly on the residual ridges and adjacent tissues.

- The surface may be lined with a long-term material for removal to be removed by the patient such as a temporary soft liner, a tissue conditioner, or a permanent soft silicone liner.
- A patient may place a denture-adhesive material on the impression surface of the denture before inserting the denture.
- The denture adhesive is removed from the denture during daily cleaning and from soft tissues to enable visual examination.
- A denture adhesive is a commercially available paste or powder preparation.
- The adhesive is used to improve denture retention, stabilization, and comfort, as recommended by the dentist.
- A patient may use an adhesive indefinitely in the attempt to cope with ill-fitting dentures that need to be adjusted or remade.

▶ *Polished surface*: The external or outer surface is polished. The impression surfaces are not polished.

▶ *Occlusal surface*: The surface of a denture that makes contact or near contact with the corresponding surface of the opposing denture or natural teeth.

▶ *Teeth*
- The denture teeth may be made of plastic acrylic resin, composite resin, porcelain or polymethyl methacrylate.[5]
- A patient may request to have decorative facings incorporated into certain teeth.
- Metal occlusal surfaces may be present, for example, to maintain a stable vertical dimension of occlusion when opposing teeth may cause excessive wear.

IV. Denture Deposits

▶ Accumulation of stains and deposits on dentures varies between individuals in a manner similar to that on natural teeth. The phases of deposit formation may be divided as follows:

▶ *Mucin and food debris on the denture surfaces*
- Readily removed by rinsing, brushing, and irrigation.

▶ *Denture pellicle and denture biofilm*
- Denture pellicle forms readily after a denture is cleaned.
- Denture biofilm is composed predominantly of gram-positive cocci, rods, and filamentous forms of bacteria in an intermicrobial matrix.
- Biofilm also may include microorganisms related to dental caries and periodontal infections.
- Biofilm serves as a matrix for calculus formation and stain accumulation when the denture is not cleaned.[7]
- Denture biofilm is associated with breath malodor and denture stomatitis.[8]

▶ *Denture calculus*
- Calculus is hard and fixed to the denture surface.
- Calculus can form anywhere on a denture, especially the facial surfaces of the maxillary molars and lingual surfaces of the mandibular anterior.

▶ *Stains*
- Dentures can become stained similarly to natural teeth.
- Frequent causes of stain include tobacco, red wine, coffee, and tea.

V. Removal of Denture

▶ It is most comfortable for the patient to remove the denture.

▶ The clinician may remove dentures for certain patients, particularly those with a physical limitation or in an emergency situation.

▶ Although denture removal may be complicated by anatomic features of an individual mouth, a general procedure is outlined in Box 32-3.

VI. Care of Dentures During Intraoral Procedures

▶ Provide a disposable cup and tissue for the patient's use when requesting the patient to remove or insert the denture.

▶ Rinse in running water to remove any unattached debris without splashing.

▶ Professionally clean the denture in an ultrasonic denture cleaner, following manufacturer's instructions, with appropriate cleaning solution (Figure 32-5).

▶ Follow strict procedures to protect the denture from exposure to unclean areas during transportation and when in the ultrasonic cleaner.

▶ Provide a clean disposable cup or sterile container with a fitted cover to hold the prosthesis after rinsing.

▶ Immerse in antimicrobial solution to disinfect and prevent drying, which can cause distortion of the denture.

▶ Place container in a safe place away from treatment area to prevent spilling or inadvertent discarding.

▶ At the end of the appointment, remember to rinse and return the moist denture before the patient gets out of the dental chair.

VII. Professional Complete Denture Care

▶ At the continuing care appointments, the dental hygienist and the dentist will evaluate the oral mucosa including oral cancer detection, the prosthesis, the patient's compliance with personal care, prosthesis

BOX 32-3

Method for Removal of a Complete Denture

The clinician follows standard procedures for infection control while removing and handling the denture from the patient's mouth.

The Complete Maxillary Denture

1. Clinician is positioned at 11–12 o'clock; left-handed clinician is at 12–1 o'clock.
2. Grasp the anterior portion of the denture firmly with the thumb on the facial surface at the height of the border of the denture under the lip and the index finger on the palatal surface.
3. With the other hand, elevate the lip to expose the border of the denture to break the seal.
4. Remove the denture gently in a downward and forward direction.
5. If the retention of the denture cannot be overcome by elevation of the lip, request the able patient to blow into the mouth with the lips closed to break the suction seal.

The Complete Mandibular Denture

1. Clinician is positioned at 8–9 o'clock; left-handed clinician is at 3–4 o'clock.
2. Grasp the denture firmly on the facial surface with the thumb and on the lingual surface with the index finger.
3. With the other hand, retract the lower lip forward and remove the denture gently.

retention, and any issues the patient has with the appliance.[10]

▶ Commercially available devices include ultrasonic, sonic, and agitating mechanisms that can be combined with an immersion agent.

▶ A professional denture cleaning in a dental office or clinic needs to be completed at least biannually to minimize calculus and biofilm accumulation over time.

▶ The action of the well-functioning ultrasonic cleansing device can be an effective method for cleaning a denture.
  • A cleaning solution is added for additional cleaning and disinfecting benefit.
  • Strict infection control procedures are followed to prevent cross-contamination of the denture and solution inside the cleaning basin.

▶ Avoid scaling the prosthesis with a sharp instrument in the attempt to remove calculus deposits.

▶ An example of dentures placed in sealed bag filled with denture cleaner to be placed in an ultrasonic cleaner is shown in Figure 32-5.

CLEANING THE COMPLETE DENTURE

I. Description

▶ Do not assume the patient who is wearing a denture knows correct methods for caring for the prostheses and intraoral tissue.

▶ During questioning for the patient history, information about the method and frequency of oral care and care of the prostheses is recorded.

▶ When the denture is removed, examine for deposits and stains.

▶ Alternate cleansing agents, devices, or procedures are recommended and demonstrated as needed.

▶ Advise patients, denture cleansing agents are used only to clean the dentures.

▶ Rinse before reinserting the denture into the mouth.[9]

▶ Instruction is individualized for each patient's need, for example:
  • The patient receiving complete dentures for the first time
  • The patient whose dentures have been remade or relined
  • The patient with a single denture that opposes natural teeth.

▶ Record all details of patient instructions and recommendations in the patient's permanent record.

▶ Types of dentures and characteristics of the edentulous mouth are described in Chapter 54.

II. Purposes for Cleaning

Inadequate oral tissue care and denture hygiene practices are major causes of oral lesions under dentures.

▶ Prevent irritation to the soft tissues.

▶ Mechanical irritants: remove rough deposits of biofilm, calculus, *thick stains.*

▶ Chemical irritants: products of putrefaction of food debris and bacterial products

▶ Control infection
  • Reactions to denture biofilm and/or secondary infections of traumatic lesions may occur.

▶ Prevent mouth odors.

▶ Maintain appearance.

III. When to Clean

▶ Several times each day: clean dentures manually after eating and at bedtime.

▶ Each day, clean dentures by chemical immersion, possibly overnight.

IV. Procedure for Cleaning

▶ Rinsing, immersion, followed by brushing, are recommended.

▶ When unable to clean, at least rinsing is advised.

V. Preparation for Cleaning

▶ Rinse the denture thoroughly when it is taken from the mouth to remove saliva and loose debris.

▶ Remove denture-adhesive material with light brushing.

▶ Denture-bearing mucosa: Rinse and clean with a soft toothbrush two or more times daily.

VI. Cleaning by Immersion

The denture is soaked in a solvent or detergent in which chemical action removes or loosens stains and deposits that can then be rinsed or brushed away.

A. Advantages

▶ The solution reaches all areas of the denture for a complete cleaning.

▶ Minimizes the danger of dropping the appliance.

▶ Prevents need for handling, which is required during brushing.

▶ Offers safe storage when dentures are out of the mouth.

▶ Aids patients who have limited ability to manage a brush.

▶ When manual cleaning is not possible, immersion involves the least handling and observation. This advantage is particularly attractive to a caregiver who must clean the denture for a patient.

B. Procedure

▶ The procedure for cleaning a denture by immersion is discussed in Box 32-4.

▶ The solution is changed and the container cleaned daily

▶ Mix fresh solution to prevent contamination and growth of microorganisms.[10]

C. Solutions

1. *Proprietary*: Available in powder or tablet form.
   - *Preparation*: Add measured warm water as directed by the manufacturer.
   - *Length of immersion*:
     - Usually 10–15 minutes or as suggested by the manufacturer.
     - Because the action depends on the mechanical bubbling effect of released oxygen, the solution has little value after the available oxygen has been released.
   - *Effect*: The solutions are only effective against loose debris; denture cleanliness depends on regular daily immersion supplemented by brushing.

BOX 32-4

Procedure for Cleaning a Denture by Immersion

▷ Place denture in a plastic container with a fitted cover that is maintained specifically for this purpose.

▷ Use only warm water, which promotes the action of the cleanser, for rinsing and mixing the solution. Hot water is never used because it can distort plastic resin.

▷ Follow manufacturer's specifications to ensure correct dilution of cleanser and time length for immersion.

▷ Check that the denture is completely submerged in the solution; cover the container.

▷ When the denture is removed, rinse under running water and remove loosened debris and chemicals before proceeding to clean by brushing.

▷ Empty and clean container daily. Mix fresh solution to prevent contamination and growth of microorganisms.[8]

---

2. *Hypochlorite solution*:
   - The use of sodium hypochlorite bleach or products containing sodium hypochlorite is damaging to metal so must not be used for dental prostheses containing metal parts. In addition, soft reline materials can become discolored.
   - Damage to the resin-based materials used to fabricate the denture can compromise the integrity of the appliance.[9,11]

VII. Cleaning by Brushing

▶ Brush with water, soap, or other mild cleansing agent.
   - Abrasive agents cause scratches, which promote biofilm accumulation.

A. Type of Brush

1. *Denture brush*
   - A good-quality denture brush with end-rounded filaments is recommended. The styles of denture brushes vary.
   - One type shown in Figure 32-9 is designed with two arrangements of filaments:
     - Round arrangement to access the inner, curved impression surface
     - Rectangular portion for convenient adaptation to the polished and occlusal denture surfaces.
   - Denture brushes adapted for a patient with one hand or otherwise disabled are shown in Figure 57-6, in Chapter 57.

2. *Other brushes*
   - A few patients prefer not to have a denture brush for personal reasons.
   - A hand scrub brush can be used, provided the filaments are long enough to reach into the deeper portions of the impression surfaces.

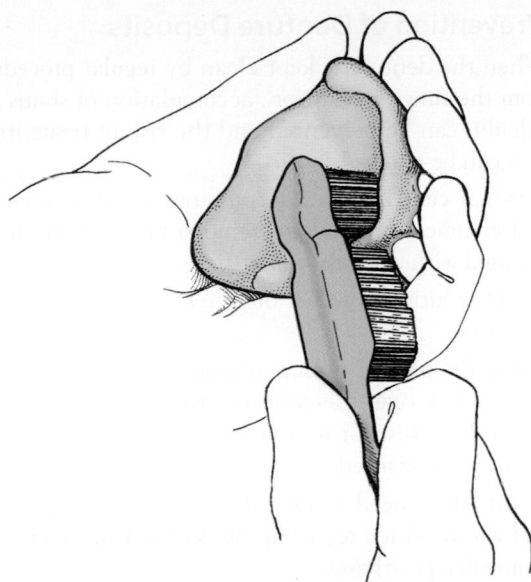

FIGURE 32-9 Denture Brush. The denture is held securely, but without squeezing, in the palm of the nonworking hand. Place a face cloth in the bottom of the sink and partially fill with water. The specially designed brush is preferred because one group of tufts is arranged to provide access to the inner impression surface of the denture, as shown.

BOX 32-5

Procedure for Cleaning Denture by Brushing

1. Spread a towel, wash cloth, or rubber mat over the bottom of the sink to serve as a cushion should the denture be dropped; partially fill the sink with water.
2. Grasp denture in palm of hand securely (Figure 32-9) but without squeezing because dentures can be broken.
3. Apply warm water, nonabrasive cleanser, and brush to all areas of the denture. Pay particular attention to the impression surfaces where configurations of the surface correspond with those of the oral topography. The anterior areas of the inner surfaces of both the maxillary and mandibular dentures require special adaptations of the brush.
4. Rinse denture and brush under running water. Use the brush to remove denture cleanser that may be retained in the grooves.
5. Visually check each area carefully for biofilm.
6. Teach the patient to run a finger over the surfaces to find "slippery" biofilm areas.

- Prerequisite is that each area of each surface of the denture be reached by the brush if denture biofilm formation is to be controlled.
- A multitufted soft nylon regular style brush with end-rounded filaments is acceptable if access to all the inner curvatures is possible without applying undue pressure on certain parts in the attempt to clean others.
- The patient who wears a single denture needs separate brushes for the natural teeth and the denture to maintain the brush for the natural teeth in the best condition possible.
- Adjustments of brush technique may be needed to assist the disabled patient, as described in Chapter 57.

B. Procedure

▶ Procedure for cleaning a denture is listed in Box 32-5.

C. Precautions Related to Brushing

▶ Overzealous brushing and use of an abrasive cleansing agent on the impression surface could damage the fit of the denture.

▶ Plastic resin can be abraded. Scratches make a rough surface; the denture may become more subject to the collection of biofilm, debris, and calculus.

▶ Possibility of incomplete cleaning or cleaning with uneven pressure when the brush is applied more vigorously to accessible areas and misses difficult-to-access areas.

▶ Danger of dropping and breaking the denture is increased when it is wet and slippery.

▶ Advise patients to use their prescription eyewear when brushing to watch the procedure and to observe the cleanliness of the denture after brushing.

VIII. Denture Cleansers

A. Requirements for a Denture Cleanser[12]

▶ Easy for a patient to use.

▶ Bactericidal and fungicidal.

▶ Effective removal of denture deposits (organic and inorganic) without abrasion of the denture surface.[13]

▶ Nontoxic.

▶ Harmless to the dental materials used for RPDs, complete dentures, and obturators.

▶ Reasonably priced.

B. Chemical Solution Cleansers (Immersion)

1. *Alkaline peroxide*
   - Active ingredient: alkaline detergent with an oxygen-liberating agent (sodium perborate or percarbonate).
   - Action: loosens debris and light stains by an oxygen-liberating mechanism. A preventive cleanser is used regularly from the day a denture has been cleaned professionally to prevent accumulation of heavy deposits.
   - Examples: Most proprietary cleansers are in the form of a powder or tablet that is dropped into water to create the alkaline solution of hydrogen peroxide.

2. *Enzymes*
- The enzymes act to break down biofilm proteins and polysaccharides. Enzyme agents have been incorporated into various immersion-type cleansers.

3. *Disinfectants*
- A sanitary denture is necessary for the prevention of inflammation in the oral mucosa under the denture. Types of denture-induced lesions are described in Chapter 54.
- Regular daily maintenance procedures are necessary.
- Patient instruction in disinfection of a denture is needed.
  - The denture needs to be rinsed completely
  - Before disinfection, rinse the denture under running water
  - Take care not to splash and contaminate the area.
- Clinicians need to recommend products to patients that are proven to be safe and effective for denture use.
  - The American Dental Association (ADA) Seal of Acceptance is the clinician's assurance that the product has been evaluated to show the product is effective in accord with the manufacturer's guidelines. See Chapter 30.
  - Following manufacture guidelines is pertinent in protecting the integrity of the denture immersion solutions.[14,15]

C. Abrasive Cleansers (Brushing)

1. *Denture pastes and powders, toothpastes and powders*
- Active ingredient: an abrasive, such as calcium carbonate.
- Action: mechanical removal of biofilm and stains by brushing.
- Disadvantages: can abrade the plastic resin denture base and acrylic teeth.
- Select a product with low abrasiveness.

2. *Household agents*
- Active ingredient: detergent and/or abrasive agent.
- Examples:
  - Salt and bicarbonate of soda are mildly abrasive.
  - Hand soap is cleansing and not particularly abrasive.
  - Avoid scouring powders or other excessively abrasive cleansers.
  - Biofilm will readily attach to scratched, abraded areas on the prosthesis.

IX. Additional Instructions

A. Care of Plastic Resin

▶ Immerse an appliance in cool water or cleansing solution when not in the mouth.

▶ Never place in hot or boiling water as this can cause the denture to warp.[14]

B. Prevention of Denture Deposits

▶ When the denture is kept clean by regular procedures from the time of insertion, accumulation of stains and calculus can be prevented and the risk of tissue irritation can be reduced.

▶ Personal care includes a combination of mechanical and chemical methods to remove microorganisms associated with denture stomatitis.[13]

▶ Avoid scouring powders or other excessively abrasive products.

▶ When the patient notices accumulations or stains not removed by over-the-counter products, a visit to the dental hygienist for a professional cleaning of the appliance is warranted.

▶ Practitioners need to provide education for daily care and the need for regular professional maintenance of removable prostheses.[9]

C. Paste Cleansers

▶ Paste cleansers (dentifrices or denture pastes) may cling and be difficult to rinse from the denture.

▶ Residual chemical agents, such as essential oils, may cause inflammatory or allergic reactions of the oral mucosa, and phenolic agents can have deleterious effects on plastic resin.

D. Soft Lining Materials

▶ Temporary soft lining material may require proprietary cleansers to avoid harm to the material. Washing with cold water and a soft cloth, cotton, or soft brush can be suggested.

▶ Denture biofilm needs to be removed several times each day. Brush outer, polished surfaces in the usual manner.

▶ When the denture is placed in water overnight, the teeth are placed down so that the soft material at the denture border cannot become deformed.

▶ Permanent silicone liners are softer and have a more porous surface to host biofilm accumulation; added diligence is required to remove biofilm and prevent build-up.

E. Denture Adhesives

▶ Some patients prefer the added security of a denture adhesive to ensure stability and retention of a denture.

▶ An adhesive is not a solution for ill-fitting dentures; patient needs evaluation and possible reline, rebase, or new denture.

▶ An adhesive may be necessary for the new denture patient as the immediate, interim denture begins to loosen with healing of the underlying tissues.

▶ Adhesive remaining attached to the tissue is removed to visualize the health status of the tissue underneath.

▶ The practitioner needs to provide education on the use of a denture adhesive. Instruct the patient to follow the manufacturer's guidelines, noting the use of a denture adhesive is temporary.

THE UNDERLYING MUCOSA

▶ The oral mucosa can be negatively affected by contact with a prosthesis, which can result in *denture stomatitis*.

▶ Risk factors include *Candida albicans* and biofilm on the denture, the constant wearing of a denture, amount of tissue covered by the denture, and cigarette smoking.

▶ The residual biofilm may be laden with *Candida albicans* that could lead to regrowth and colonization on a patient's denture.[16,17]

▶ Consistent use of zinc-containing denture adhesives can lead to toxicity with negative systemic side effects including neurological and hematological problems experienced by the patient.

▶ The patient using a denture adhesive needs to read the list of ingredients in the products to avoid zinc toxicity.

▶ Patients need to be trained in applying denture adhesive. If a denture is ill fitting, the patient needs to schedule an appointment with the dentist for evaluation.[9]

▶ Daily cleaning the denture, leaving the denture out for a period of time each day, and proper nutrition are factors in maintaining oral health.

I. Examination

▶ Soft tissue examination and oral cancer screening are recommended at least twice yearly for all patients by a dental professional; more frequently for patients with increased risk factors for oral disease.

▶ Record and refer all changes and concerns to the dentist for evaluation.

▶ Daily examination is performed by patient, taking notice of oral changes and symptoms.

▶ Inform the patient to seek care when experiencing any oral change or when any concerns arise with the prosthesis.

II. Rinsing

▶ Each time the denture is removed, the mouth is rinsed thoroughly with warm fluoridated water or a mild salt solution, unless patient has dietary salt restrictions.

III. Cleaning

▶ At least once daily a soft toothbrush with end-rounded filaments is applied lightly over the ridges and in the vestibules using long, straight strokes from posterior to anterior.

▶ Concurrently, the tongue is cleaned. Use a tongue cleaner as described in Chapter 28.

IV. Massage

▶ For stimulation of circulation and increased resistance to trauma, frequent massage is recommended. Methods for massage that may be suggested and demonstrated are the following:

- *Digital*: Place thumb and index finger over the ridge and apply massage with a press-and-release stroke. The palate may be rubbed with the ball of the thumb.
- *Soft toothbrush*: Apply sides of filaments and vibratory motion to each area. Prevent trauma to the tissue by placing the brush carefully and avoiding scrubbing with undue pressure.

V. Soft Tissue Conditions

▶ Soft tissue changes discussed in Chapter 54 are particularly associated with patients who wear removable prostheses.[18]

▶ Record and call to the dentist's attention suspicious lesions such as the following:
- Traumatic ulcerations
- Denture stomatitis
- Angular cheilitis
- Epulis formation.

VI. Daily Removal of Prostheses

▶ The patient needs to plan a time when the denture will be left out of the mouth for a period of time each day to give the tissue underneath a rest from the constant contact.

▶ The most convenient time to leave denture out of mouth to rest the tissues may be while sleeping.

▶ In certain circumstances, a dentist may advise continual wear.

▶ Dentures are cleaned and immersed in water while out of mouth to avoid warping.

COMPLETE OVERDENTURE PROSTHESES

▶ An overdenture is a complete denture supported by both retained natural teeth and/or implants, and the soft tissue of the residual alveolar ridge.

▶ Overdentures also have been called overlay dentures or coping dentures.

I. Purposes

The advantages of an overdenture compared with a denture in a completely edentulous mouth are that the natural teeth can provide the following:

▶ Help preserve bone, which may improve retention of denture.

▶ Allow the remaining teeth to bear occlusal pressures, thereby reducing the pressures placed on edentulous areas.

▶ Improve stability and retention of the denture.

▶ Improve the patient's tactile and proprioceptive senses by having the periodontal ligament present.

▶ Increase the patient's psychological acceptance of the denture. The patient does not feel that all natural teeth have been lost.

II. Natural Tooth-Retained Overdenture

▶ An overdenture may be possible for any patient whose treatment plan calls for extraction of teeth.
  • Teeth frequently selected for overdenture abutments are the mandibular canines and premolars and the maxillary canines.
▶ *Periodontal condition*
  • Retained teeth must have a healthy periodontium, including healthy gingiva, bone level, and band of attached gingiva.
▶ *Endodontic therapy*
  • Most preserved teeth need endodontic therapy because the crowns will be reduced.
▶ *Restorative*
  • Tooth crowns are reduced to short rounded preparations or to the level and contour of the gingival margin.
  • An amalgam or composite restoration may cover the root canal fillings.

III. Implant-Retained Overdenture

▶ Implants can be placed to help retain dentures and are becoming more widely used than natural teeth for retained overdentures.
▶ Implants are generally placed in an area of each mandibular canine as shown in Figure 32-10.
▶ Implants are not subject to dental caries, which is a factor with retained natural teeth.
▶ Peri-implant hygiene is described in Chapter 33.

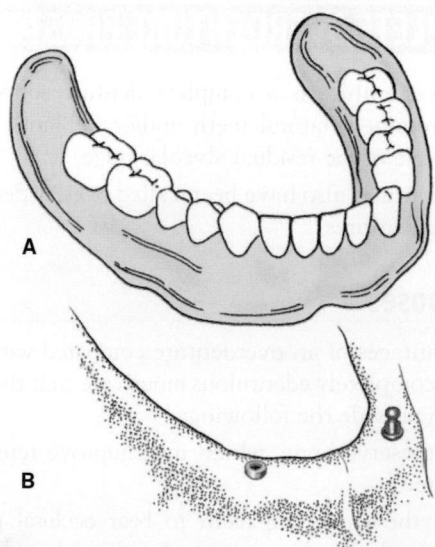

FIGURE 32-10 Overdenture. A: Mandibular complete denture. **B:** Examples of two different types of implant abutments. Generally, the same type of abutments is used in a denture.

DENTAL HYGIENE CARE AND INSTRUCTION

I. General Care

▶ The patient needs to be well informed concerning the care of the retained teeth, implants, the periodontium, and all intraoral and extraoral tissues.
▶ A high degree of motivation to save the remaining teeth is a primary concern.
▶ Patient is provided with the individualized instructions that are appropriate for the type of prosthesis or prostheses present.

II. Instruction for the New Denture Wearer[19]

▶ The dental hygienist plays a valuable role in educating the new prosthesis wearer on its use, limitations, and functions.
▶ The new removable prostheses wearer needs to:
  • Gradually increase the time in which the denture is worn daily.
  • Realize sore areas will arise where the denture rests against the mucosa.
  • Communicate problems with the dentist and schedule appropriate dental appointments for adjustments to the prosthesis.
  • Be aware that hypersalivation will occur during the first 4–6 weeks as the oral cavity gets accustomed to the new appliance.
  • Realize, depending on the size of the prosthesis, alterations in taste may occur as the material used to construct the denture will mask food flavors.
  • Take care to gradually increase seasoning for foods.
  • Start with a soft diet and gradually consume firmer foods cut in small pieces and chewed slowly as chewing effectiveness with a denture is diminished.[20]
  • Understand prostheses may mask the temperature of hot foods leading to burns on the soft tissues of the esophagus.
  • Remember to chew foods on both sides of the mouth to prevent tipping of the prosthesis.
▶ Advise the patient that adapting to a new prosthesis takes time and patience.

III. Fluoride Program for Caries Prevention

▶ A specific fluoride application plan is included for all natural tooth-retained overdentures and any patients with retained natural teeth.
▶ When the teeth have been extracted because of dental caries, caries control measures take on special significance, particularly if dietary habits remain the same.

▶ Current dietary habits are checked by asking the patient to keep a daily food diary for a 3–5 days.
  • Refer to Figure 35-5 in Chapter 35.
  • Discussion on limiting the frequency and consistency of cariogenic food intake is emphasized.
▶ *Fluoride self-application*
  • All patients with any natural teeth need to use a fluoride dentifrice regularly.
  • In addition, a mouthrinse, prescription-strength toothpaste, and/or a gel tray are recommended daily for moderate to high caries risk.
  • The patient's denture, after cleaning, can be used for a custom tray, and the fluoride gel is placed inside at the locations of the natural teeth.
  • Pressure of the denture as it is seated forces the gel around the teeth.
  • Higher concentrations of sodium fluoride (5,000 ppm) have been shown to be more protective for overdenture abutments.[21]
▶ *Professional topical applications*
  • Frequent continuing care appointments are needed to check the health of natural overdenture abutment teeth.
  • Fluoride varnish application is made in accord with patient's caries risk level.
▶ Benefit is derived from fluoride in direct proportion to the frequency of application: the more frequent the application of fluoride, the greater the benefit. Full-time use of fluoridated faucet water is the method of choice.

IV. Sealants

▶ Application of sealants to overdenture abutment teeth has been shown effective in the prevention of dental caries.[22]

V. Continuing Care Appointments

▶ Frequent continuing care appointments are needed to check the health of the gingival tissues along with the prostheses.
▶ Supervision during frequent appointments for scaling, biofilm debridement, topical fluoride applications, motivation, and instruction for biofilm control are essential.
  • Routine extraoral/intraoral examination for potential pathologies, especially early cancerous lesions.
  • Check for periodontal health, integrity of each restoration or sealant, and health of all extraoral and intraoral tissues.
  • Check the condition of the removable prostheses by looking for fractures, cracks, chipped and worn teeth, and broken clasps.
  • More frequent continuing care appointments may be needed for patients at higher risk for periodontitis, dental caries, or other pathology.

DOCUMENTATION

The following items need to be included in the permanent record of a patient with a fixed or removable prosthesis:

▶ Chief complaint will reveal any discomfort the patient is experiencing
▶ Description of the prostheses and stability
▶ Intraoral findings describing soft tissue and any pathologic changes of the attached gingiva, health of abutment teeth to identify mobility, dental caries, or wear facets
▶ Placement of abutment implants
▶ Customized regimen for personal care
▶ Fluoride regimen and recommendations
▶ An example progress note can be found in Box 32-6.

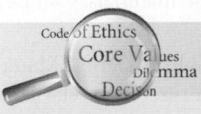

EVERYDAY ETHICS

Mr. Samuel wears an old maxillary complete denture that he has had for almost 30 years. He admits the denture moves around a bit and is sometimes difficult to chew with, but he refuses to have it remade because the removable lower partial denture he finally agreed to have remade last year was so expensive.

Bryce, a very caring dental hygienist who always tries to be sensitive to the financial concerns of his patients, decides to stop bothering Mr. Samuels about getting a new denture. He recommends an over-the-counter temporary soft reline material and the use of denture adhesive every day instead.

Questions for Consideration

1. What legal and ethical concepts (Table V-I, in the Introduction to Section V) are apparent in this scenario?

2. If he was asked, Bryce might say that his recommendations for this patient are supported by the core value of beneficence and that his personal values include helping Mr. Samuels keep the cost of his dental care low in any way he can. Do you agree or disagree? Explain why.

3. Explain how additional core values (Table II-1 in the Introduction to Section II) support a different approach to making recommendations.

BOX 32-6

Example Documentation: Partial Denture

S – A 63-year-old female presents to clinic for an adult prophylaxis appointment with chief complaint "my partial feels loose and lifts off the top of my mouth when I chew meats"

O – Intraoral examination: slight edematous tissue mesial to #6 and #11, with redness noted on palate where RPD rests, probing depths 3 mm or less except the mesial facial #6 and #11; where 4 mm probings are noted, tissue has slight generalized marginal erythema with generalized moderate biofilm. Light generalized stain and calculus on natural dentition, the RPD teeth, and the tissue-supported surface of the RPD.

A – Ill-fitting, unstable RPD with retained calculus is contributing to gingival inflammation and increased risk for oral trauma.

P – RPD placed in sealed bag with cleaning solution and placed in a beaker filled in the ultrasonic unit to remove calculus; upon subsequent visual inspection all calculus was removed and there were no fractures or roughness noted. Advised patient to clean RPD daily, and remove nightly to rest the underlying mucosa. Reminded her to keep the denture soaking in water when it is out of her mouth during the night. Proper technique for denture cleaning was demonstrated and practiced by the patient. Dispensed new denture toothbrush and clasp brush and advised patient to purchase ADA recommended denture cleanser.

Nest steps: schedule with dentist for RPD evaluation to determine possible reline or replacement.

Signed: _____, RDH

Date: _____

Factors To Teach The Patient

▷ How to perform a self-examination of the oral tissues.

▷ How to evaluate the prosthesis.

▷ Why all prostheses need cleaning more than once a day.

▷ How to handle a removable prosthesis while it is cleaned.

▷ The need to adapt toothbrushing, flossing, and use of other aids to the various configurations of abutment teeth whether natural tooth or implant.

▷ How tongue cleaning contributes to complete oral health.

▷ The significance of regular maintenance appointments: intraoral/extraoral screening for pathology, especially oral cancer screening; professional cleaning of remaining teeth and prostheses; and adjustments if needed.

▷ Risks when missing teeth are not replaced.

▷ The importance of seeking professional evaluation if any problems arise with existing prostheses; never attempt to repair or adjust a prosthesis.

Staphylococcus aureus, Streptococcus sobrinus, and *Candia albicans. Quintessence Int.* 2005;36(5):373–381.

7. Paranhos HF, Silva-Lovato CH, de Souza RF, et al. Effect of three methods for cleaning dentures on biofilms formed in vitro on acrylic resin. *J Prosthodont.* 2009;18(5):427–431.

8. Garrett NR. Poor oral hygiene, wearing dentures at night, perceptions of mouth dryness and burning, and lower educational level may be related to oral malodor in denture wearers. *J Evid Based Dent Pract.* 2010;10(1):67–69.

9. Felton D, Cooper L, Duqum I, et al. Evidence-based guidelines for the care and maintenance of complete dentures. *J Am Dent Assoc.* 2011;142(2, Suppl):1S–20S.

10. DePaola LG, Minah GE. Isolation of pathogenic microorganisms from dentures and denture-soaking containers of myelosuppressed cancer patients. *J Prosthet Dent.* 1983;49(1):20–24.

11. Ural C, Sanal FA, Cengiz S. Effect of different denture cleansers on surface roughness of denture base materials. *Clin Dent Res.* 2011;35(2):14–20.

12. American Dental Association, Council on Dental Materials, Instruments, and Equipment. Denture cleansers. *J Am Dent Assoc.* 1983;106(1);77–79.

13. Budtz-Jørgensen E. Materials and methods for cleaning dentures. *J Prosthet Dent.* 1979;42(6):619–623.

14. American Dental Association. ADA accepted denture cleansers. http://www.ada.org/1317.aspx. Accessed June 15, 2015.

15. Davi L, Felipucci D, de Souza RF, et al. Effect of denture cleansers on metal ion release and surface roughness of denture base materials. *Braz Dent J.* 2012; 23(4): 387–393.

16. Jose A, Coco BJ, Milligan S, et al. Reducing the incidence of denture stomatitis: are denture cleansers sufficient? *J Prosthodont.* 2010;19(4):252–257.

References

1. Obreschkow C. Oral hygiene and periodontal considerations in restorative treatment with prefabricated attachments and precision-milled prosthetic devices. *Int J Periodontics Restorative Dent.* 1985;5(4):72–80.

2. American Dental Association, Council on Dental Materials, Instruments and Equipment; and Council on Dental Therapeutics. Status report: effect of acidulated phosphate fluoride on porcelain and composite restorations. *J Am Dent Assoc.* 1988;116(1):115.

3. Brand HS, Gonggrijp S, Blanksma CJ. Cocaine and oral health. *Br Dent J.* 2008;204(7):365–369.

4. Reisberg DJ. Dental and prosthodontic care for patients with cleft or craniofacial conditions. *Cleft Palate Craniofac J.* 2000;37(6):534–537.

5. Lyon C, Yeoh A, Hanson WP. Partial denture care. *Dimens Dent Hyg.* 2010;8(8):16.

6. Yilmaz H, Aydin C, Bal BT, et al. Effects of disinfectants on resilient denture-lining materials contaminated with

17. Ramage G, Tomsett K, Wickes BL, et al. Denture stomatitis: a role for Candida biofilms. *Oral Surg Oral Med Oral Pathol Oral Radiol Endod.* 2004;98(1):53–59.

18. Shulman JD, Rivera-Hidalgo F, Beach MM. Risk factors associated with denture stomatitis in the United States. *J Oral Pathol Med.* 2005;34(6):340–346.

19. Swecker T, Shah A. Eating well for healthy mouth. Educating patients, especially those who require modified diets, about the importance of good nutrition can help them improve their oral and systemic health. *Dimens Dent Hyg.* 2012;10(5):56–59.

20. Berg E. Acceptance of full dentures. *Int Dent J.* 1993; 43:299–306.

21. Ettinger RL, Olson, RJ, Wefel JS, et al. In vitro evaluation of topical fluorides for overdenture abutments. *J Prosthet Dent.* 1997;78(3):309–314.

22. Kurtz KS. Adjunctive caries control in overdenture abutment teeth: a new modality. *J Am Dent Assoc.* 1995;126(2):213–215.

 ENHANCE YOUR UNDERSTANDING

thePoint® **DIGITAL CONNECTIONS**
(see the inside front cover for access information)
- **Audio glossary**
- **Quiz bank**

SUPPORT FOR LEARNING
(available separately; visit lww.com)
- *Active Learning Workbook for Clinical Practice of the Dental Hygienist, 12th Edition*

prepU **INDIVIDUALIZED REVIEW**
(available separately; visit lww.com)
- **Adaptive quizzing with *prepU for Wilkins' Clinical Practice of the Dental Hygienist***

33

The Patient with Dental Implants

Stacy A. Matsuda, RDH, BS, MS

CHAPTER OUTLINE

LEARNING OBJECTIVES

After studying this chapter, the student will be able to:

1. Describe concepts, technology, and terminology relevant to implant dentistry.

2. Develop a knowledge base related to osseointegration and ancillary procedures in oral implantology.

3. Comprehend patient selection factors and education essentials.

4. Understand maintenance of dental implant in the clinical setting.

5. Recognize and manage dental implant problems, complications, and failures.

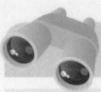

BOX 33-1 | KEY WORDS: Dental Implants

Abutment: segment connecting the submerged implant body to the prosthetic component. The abutment enters the oral cavity providing a platform for attaching crowns or bridges.

Alloplast: an inert foreign body used for implantation within tissue.

Augment: to make greater, more numerous, larger, or more intense.

Augmentation: to increase the size beyond the existing size; in alveolar ridge or maxillary sinus augmentation: to increase the bone to accommodate a dental implant.

Biologic or permucosal seal: functional soft tissue barrier at the base of the peri-implant sulcus; characterized by adhesion of junctional epithelium in the absence of Sharpey's fibers, making it more susceptible to bacterial invasion by periodontal pathogens.

Biocompatible: capable of existing in harmony with the surrounding biologic environment.

Blade form dental implant: tooth root replacement with a wide, thin shape unlike that of a natural tooth.

Endosseous or root form dental implant: tooth root replacement with a cylindrical or conical shape similar to a natural tooth root.

Fibrous encapsulation: layer of fibrous connective tissue between the implant and surrounding bone. Also called fibrous integration; indicative of failed osseointegration.

Guided tissue regeneration: a procedure that attempts to regenerate lost periodontal structures.

Implant thread: endosseous implants with threads resembling a screw.

Occlusal overload: masticatory force applied to an implant exceeding capacity of the bone implant interface or implant component to withstand it. Overload can compromise the integrity of an implant because no periodontal ligament is present to absorb the forces.

Osseointegration: the direct attachment or connection of osseous tissue to an inert alloplastic material without intervening connective tissue.

Peri-implant mucositis: reversible inflammation of the periodontal tissues around an implant with no subsequent bone loss; similar to gingivitis in a natural tooth.

Peri-implantitis: destructive inflammatory process of the periodontal tissues around an implant characterized by progressive bone loss in addition to soft tissue inflammation with hemorrhage and/or exudate; similar to periodontitis in a natural tooth.

Provisional prosthesis or tooth crown: temporary or preliminary appliance or tooth used during healing or osseointegration for purposes of stability or appearance.

Root form dental implant: endosseous implant shaped in the approximate form of a tooth root.

Sinus augmentation (sinus lift): site preparation procedure that elevates the floor of the maxillary sinus to accommodate a dental implant by increasing the vertical height of bone via grafting/augmentation.

Subperiosteal frame dental implant: framework placed under the periosteum that is tacked in place on the bone with a few small screws to support an overdenture; tooth root replacement with a cylindrical or conical shape.

Suppuration: formation or discharge of pus.

Titanium: a uniquely biocompatible metal used for implants either in the commercially pure form or as an alloy.

Titanium alloy: a common titanium alloy (Ti-6A1-4V) used for dental implants that contains 6% aluminum to increase strength and decrease weight and 4% vanadium to prevent corrosion.

Tomography: a 3-dimensional image of the internal structures of a solid object like the mandible.

Dental implants offer a means of tooth replacement to preserve surrounding oral tissues normally compromised by a missing tooth.

▶ Dental implants simulate natural tooth roots. They may be used to replace one tooth or multiple teeth for a partially or completely edentulous patient. The various plates and parts used in the treatment of fractured bones or joint replacements are also implants.

▶ Knowledge of dental implants is essential for all dental hygienists who are responsible for professional maintenance and monitoring of peri-implant health.

▶ Patients often will voice questions and/or concerns to the dental hygienist regarding their treatment options, which presents an opportune time for education to dispel confusion, alleviate fears, or reinforce a decision to proceed with needed treatment.

▶ The success of an implant can depend on many factors, including patient understanding and skills for daily care of the prosthesis and the surrounding soft tissues.

▶ Frequent maintenance appointments for careful supervision and patient motivation are essential components for implant success.

▶ Key words and terminology are defined in Box 33-1.

BONE PHYSIOLOGY

Alveolar bone is of critical importance to the planning and execution of dental implants. A careful assessment of the quantity and quality of bone provides a foundation for proper treatment planning and a more predictable surgical outcome.

▶ Bone is a dynamic tissue that is cellular and vascular.

- Osteocytes: mediate activity.
- Osteoblasts: repair and regeneration.
- Osteoclasts: remodeling and homeostasis.

▶ Key function: to provide structural support to various loads or stresses.

I. Bone Classification[1]

▶ Bone is classified according to its density as follows:

D1 Dense cortical bone

D2 Thick dense to porous cortical bone on crest and coarse trabecular bone within

D3 Thin porous cortical bone on crest and fine trabecular bone within

D4 Fine trabecular bone

D5 Immature, nonmineralized bone.

▶ The density of bone in a potential implant site determines factors such as:
- Time frame for integration of the implant.
- Window of time for prosthetic loading.

II. Biomechanical Force

▶ Wolff's law (1892) states bone is laid down in areas of greatest stress and is resorbed in areas where it is not stressed.[2]

▶ The patient needs to understand the implication of biomechanical force on the alveolar process.
- Bone will resorb when teeth are removed.
- Dental implants *preserve* surrounding bone through function, which supplies the needed load and stress.

III. Grafting and Regeneration[3]

▶ Areas of insufficient bone due to previous resorption or tooth loss can be grafted to create a suitable recipient site for dental implant placement.

▶ Site preparation measures for implant therapy include:
- Atraumatic extraction with ridge and/or socket preservation.
- Ridge augmentation.
- Maxillary sinus augmentation is also called a "sinus lift."

▶ Options for grafting and regeneration of recipient sites include:
- *Autograft*: Bone obtained from the patient, harvested from a donor site.
- *Allograft*: Bone obtained from another human (cadaver bone).
- *Zenograft*: Bone obtained from another species (cow/bovine; horse/equine).
- *Alloplast*: Synthetic derivative of bone (e.g., beta tricalcium phosphate).

OSSEOINTEGRATION

Successful tooth replacement is accomplished by osseointegration, which means direct bone anchorage to an implant body. When viewed at a light microscopic level, osseointegration reveals direct contact between bone and implant with no intervening connective tissue.

▶ Dynamic process

▶ Healing phase takes place between 0 and 12 months.

▶ Remodeling phase takes place between 3 and 18 months.

▶ Steady state takes place 18 months and beyond.

IMPLANT INTERFACES

An implant has an inner interface with the *bone* and a *soft tissue* interface where the abutment, post, or other protruding portion of the implant is surrounded by the mucosal or gingival tissue.

I. Implant/Bone Interface

A. Osseointegration

▶ Refers to direct structural and functional union between the implant and healthy living bone.

▶ Indicates successful placement of the implant.

▶ No mobility evident.

B. Fibrous Encapsulation

▶ Refers to the infusion of connective tissue cells between the implant body and surrounding bone.

▶ Indicates failure of osseointegration.

▶ Mobility of the implant is evident.

II. Implant/Soft Tissue Interface[4,5]

▶ The external environment of an implant is the oral cavity, with saliva, dental biofilm, and debris.

▶ Biologic seal (permucosal seal): between the implant and the soft tissue, a biologic seal exists to prevent microorganisms and inflammation-producing agents from entering the tissues.

▶ Soft tissue connection: sulcular epithelium is in contact with the implant surface.
- Histologically, the tissue appears similar to the epithelial attachment of the junctional epithelium of a natural tooth.
- Hemidesmosomes and basal lamina have been identified.
- The long junctional epithelium of an implant is arranged parallel to the fixture, surrounding it, but with no attachment.
- No connective tissue fibers (Sharpey's fibers) exist to hold the attachment as with a natural tooth.
- Instead, circular connective tissue fibers provide a resilient cuff permitting the overlying epithelial tissue to closely adapt to the implant, much like a rubber band.

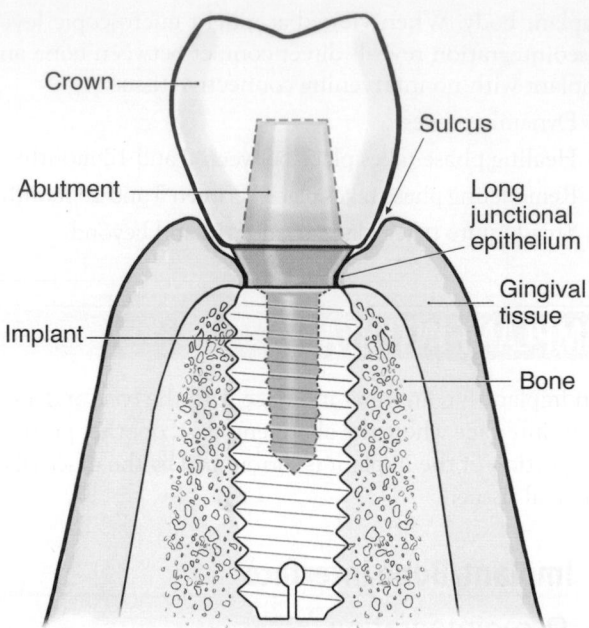

FIGURE 33-1 The Implant/Soft Tissue Interface. At the implant/soft tissue interface, there can be no connective tissue fiber attachment as when bone is present. The attachment resembles a long junctional epithelial attachment.

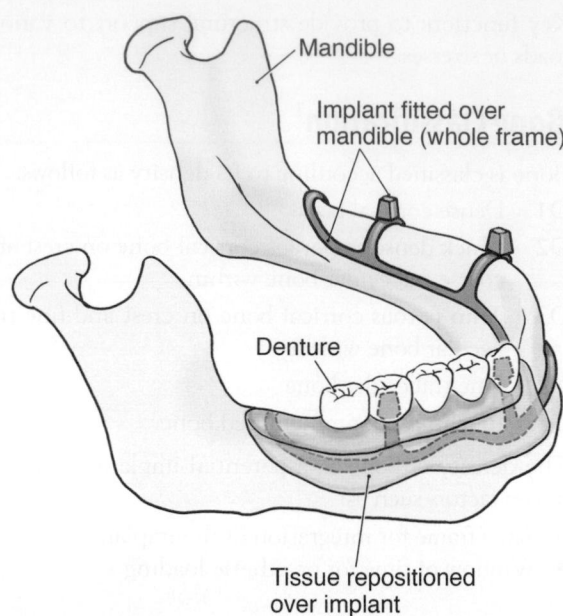

FIGURE 33-2 Subperiosteal Implant. The custom-fabricated framework is shown on the left-hand side of the mandible; on the right-hand side, the framework is shown by dotted lines under the denture.

- The lack of perpendicular fiber attachment leaves the peri-implant space more susceptible to invading periodontal pathogens.
- Figure 33-1 illustrates the implant/soft tissue interface at the junctional epithelium.

TYPES OF DENTAL IMPLANTS

Over the years, a variety of dental implant systems have been tried clinically and studied with research. They are subperiosteal, transosseous, and endosseous. Currently, endosseous or "root form" implants are the most widely used.

I. Subperiosteal

A. Definition

▶ Custom-fabricated framework of metal that rests over the bone of the mandible or maxilla, under the periosteum: complete arch or unilateral.

B. Description[6,7]

▶ Material: Titanium or vitallium (cobalt–chromium–molybdenum).
▶ *Two step*: In the first step, a surgical flap is used to reflect mucosal tissues and to expose the underlying bone. An impression is made of the bony ridge. The metallic unit is cast and then placed in a second surgical step.

Usually, four posts protrude into the oral cavity to hold the complete denture.
▶ *One step*: Computer-assisted tomography design and manufacturing have been applied, using a reformatted computed tomography scan from which approximate casts of the maxilla or mandible can be made. The implant is designed on this replica and is placed in one surgical procedure (Figure 33-2).

II. Transosseous (Transosteal)

A. Definition

▶ A dental implant that penetrates both cortical plates and passes through the full thickness of the alveolar bone.
▶ Also known as a *mandibular staple implant* or *staple bone implant*.

B. Description[8,9]

▶ Materials: stainless steel, ceramic-coated materials, and titanium alloy.
▶ A metal plate, fitted to the inferior border of the mandible, has five to seven pins extending toward the occlusal surface.
▶ Usually, two terminal pins protrude into the oral cavity to hold the overdenture. The pins are connected by a crossbar (Figure 33-3).
▶ The transosteal implant can be used when the patient has an atrophic edentulous mandible or a congenital or traumatic deformity of the mandible.

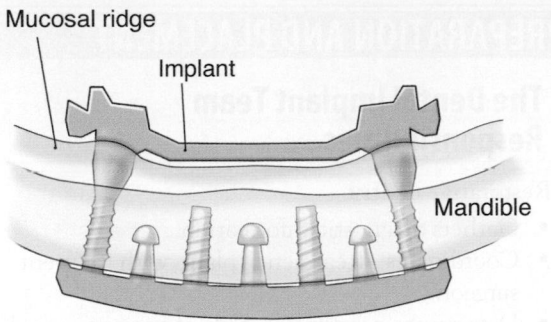

FIGURE 33-3 **Transosteal Implant.** Mandibular staple bone plate in the anterior region shows metal plate at the lower border of the mandible, with pins extending toward the occlusal surface. Terminal pins protrude into the oral cavity to hold the overdenture.

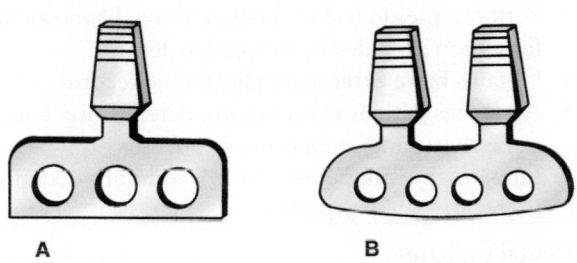

FIGURE 33-4 **Endosseous Blade Implants: A:** Single implant and **B:** implant to replace two teeth.

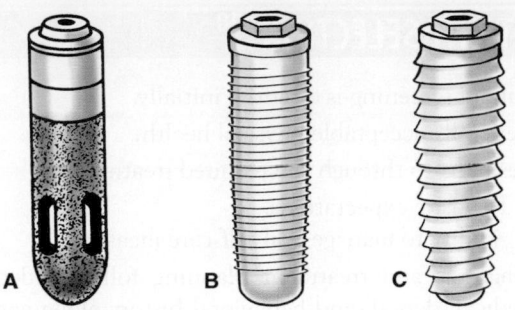

FIGURE 33-5 **Endosseous Root Form Implants. A:** Cylinder type. **B** and **C:** Screw types.

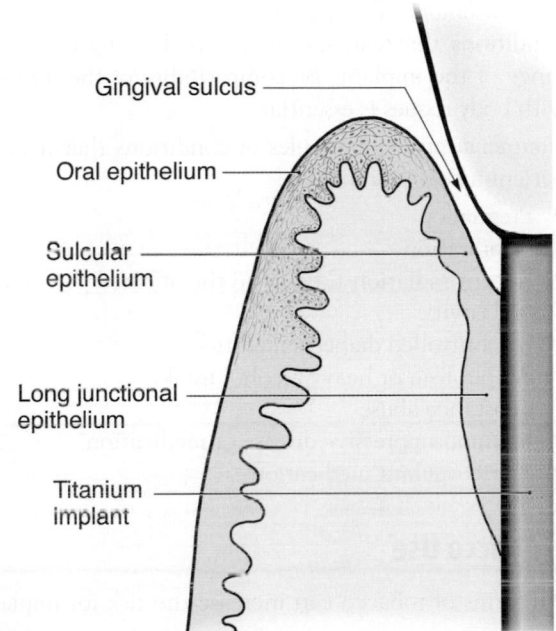

FIGURE 33-6 **Parts of an Endosseous Implant.** The crown, abutment, and implant are shown in relation to the surrounding bone and periodontal tissues.

III. Endosseous (Endosteal) Implant

A. Definition

▶ An implant placed within the bone to replace a single tooth or provide support for the replacement of complete or partial loss of teeth.

▶ Early forms (endosteal): blade or plate form (Figure 33-4).

▶ Current forms (endosseous): "root form" or cylindrical; can be threaded, smooth, perforated, or solid (Figure 33-5).

B. Description

▶ Material: primarily plasma-sprayed titanium.

▶ May be placed in one or two phases.

▶ Immediate: the implant is placed immediately following extraction of the tooth it will replace.

▶ Two phase: the support, body, or fixture is placed in bone during the first surgical step and left covered by a periodontal flap for several months while the implant integrates with the bone. The abutment post is then exposed through the soft tissue at a second-stage surgical procedure. Placement of the crown or prosthesis follows.

▶ Figure 33-6 illustrates the parts of an endosseous implant and the surrounding biologic tissues.

C. Surgical Preparation for Implant Placement

▶ The surgical procedure requires a sterile placement of the implant into the bone.

▶ Whenever microorganisms are introduced during a surgical procedure, healing can be impaired.

▶ Manufacturers prepare implants made of biocompatible material in sterile packages.

▶ Atraumatic surgical technique:
  • Insertion of implant precisely controlled, at less than 2,000 RPM.
  • Adequate irrigation prevents overheating of bone.

D. Prosthodontic Steps

▶ Attention to ideal requirements for acceptable prostheses is necessary.

▶ Margins, embrasure shapes, crown contours, contact areas, and occlusal harmony are designed to prevent dental biofilm collection and permit thorough disease control procedures by the patient.

PATIENT SELECTION[3,10]

▶ Careful screening is essential initially.

▶ Generally acceptable physical health.

▶ Desire to go through the required treatment.
  • Realistic expectations.
  • Ability to manage oral self-care measures.

▶ Diagnosis and treatment planning follow a detailed medical, dental, and behavioral history along with an oral and radiographic examination.

I. Systemic Health

▶ *Medical history*: The patient must be free of systemic conditions that can interfere with healing or acceptance of the implant. Biocompatibility of the implant with body tissues is essential.

▶ *Contraindications*: Examples of conditions that make a patient a poor risk include:
  • Pregnancy
  • Debilitation
  • Recent radiation therapy to the affected part of the oral cavity
  • Uncontrolled diabetes mellitus
  • Alcoholism or heavy alcohol intake
  • Substance abuse
  • Immunosuppressive disease or medication
  • Anticoagulant medication

II. Tobacco Use

▶ All forms of tobacco can increase the risk for implant failure.

▶ During implant placement, it has been recommended that the patient cease at least 1 week before surgery and continue to avoid tobacco at least until healing is completed.

▶ For implant health, a tobacco cessation program is advised (see Chapter 34).

III. Oral Examination

▶ Evidence of adequate depth of alveolar bone
  • Radiographic or other measurements for bone can be made.
  • In the absence of adequate bone, or an intruding maxillary sinus, treatment planning may include bone grafting to augment the proposed treatment site.

▶ Periodontal health
  • The presence of active periodontitis contraindicates implant placement until the disease is treated and under control.
  • The patient must demonstrate consistent and effective personal oral self-care.

PREPARATION AND PLACEMENT[10]

I. The Dental Implant Team Responsibilities

▶ Restorative dentist
  • Gathers diagnostic information.
  • Coordinates treatment plan with patient and surgeon.
  • Determines prosthetic needs of patient, coordinating with dental laboratory technician.
  • Develops surgical guide for occlusal/esthetic optimization.

▶ Implant surgeon
  • Performs presurgical evaluation, using diagnostic information provided by restorative dentist.
  • Obtains more extensive radiographic records.
  • Addresses patient expectations, determining potential esthetic and/or functional concerns.
  • Provides prosthetic insight to restorative dentist from a surgical perspective.

▶ Dental hygienist
  • Information resource for the patient, with thorough understanding of: rationale for implant therapy; site preparation/regenerative procedures; and various protocols and time frames for treatment.
  • Understanding and clinical proficiency in dental implant assessment and maintenance protocol.
  • Providing patient with feedback and tailored instruction for biofilm control is critical to long-term success of dental implants.
  • Reinforcing the value of oral rehabilitation with dental implants, the importance of professional maintenance visits, and motivating patients toward excellent oral self-care.

▶ Implant treatment coordinator (surgical office)
  • Oversees inventory of surgical and prosthetic supplies and ordering from implant manufacturer.
  • Coordinates appointment logistics and communication between restorative dentist, surgeon, laboratory, and implant manufacturer.

▶ Dental laboratory technician
  • Designs/fabricates radiographic/surgical guides, assists with selection of abutments, and fabricates provisional and final prosthesis.

▶ The patient
  • Thorough understanding of the treatment options available for tooth replacement and long-term ramification of each.
  • Understanding and acceptance of their role as a cotherapist in the long-term maintenance requirements for implant therapy to be successful.

II. Information for the Patient

▶ Explanation of procedures to be performed and the time frame for scheduling appointments.

▶ Review of possible complications.

▶ Understand the role of oral self-care and need for daily dental biofilm control.

▶ Understand that a past history of inflammatory periodontal disease may increase the risk of similar problems around dental implants.

▶ Agreement to follow through with the recommendations for personal and professional care.

▶ Sign an informed consent statement and agreement of understanding.

III. Collaborative Treatment Planning

▶ Preliminary dental and dental hygiene treatment is completed to insure a disease-free mouth before commencing the implant therapy.

▶ The treatment sequence is carefully coordinated between the restorative dentist and the periodontist or oral surgeon placing the implant.

▶ A surgical guide is developed to facilitate proper alignment and placement of the implant according to the prosthetic treatment plan.

▶ The surgeon placing the implant uses the surgical guide for precise positioning.

IV. Limiting Factors During Treatment[3]

The success of implant therapy can be compromised by many factors. Problems can occur in any of the following ways:

▶ Tissue damage during surgery because of overheating of the bone.

▶ Infection.

▶ Premature biomechanical loading before osseointegration.

▶ Retained cement[11]

  • Prosthetic crowns attached to implant abutments using cement can and often do leave remnants of cement behind at the crown–abutment interface.

  • Residual cement allows retention of biofilm in the same way as subgingival calculus; however, unlike calculus, resin-based cements cannot be removed nonsurgically.

  • Iatrogenic peri-implantitis can initiate in the sulcular epithelium overlying areas of residual cement on an otherwise stable implant, causing bony destruction.

▶ Bruxism and/or parafunction

  • Excessive lateral forces with inflammation can result in bone loss and breakdown of the implant-to-bone interface.

▶ Insufficient training and/or experience of the dentist performing surgery.

POSTRESTORATIVE EVALUATION

Once the implant is fully integrated in the bone and restorative work is complete, a postrestorative evaluation is made to establish a baseline for maintenance. Using radiographs, clinical examination, and close visual inspection, evaluate and document the following:

▶ *Radiographic*

  • Absence of prosthetic cement

  • Bone level relative to the threads on the implant

  • No space between implant and abutment

  • No space between abutment and prosthesis.

▶ *Peri-implant tissue health*: no inflammation, no calculus or biofilm, no suppuration or bleeding.

  • Use lightweight filament-type floss to check for possible residual cement on cement-retained crowns.

  • Wrap the floss around the abutment 360° subgingivally and gently pull to determine if there is any catching or resistance, which may indicate cement.

▶ *Peri-implant probing*: initial data serve as baseline for comparison during the maintenance phase.

  • Use light pressure and a gentle lateral stroke with an end-rounded plastic probe reserved for implants to evaluate for bleeding and to refrain from introducing periodontopathic bacteria into a peri-implant space.

  • Record six readings, indicating "implant baseline" on the chart. Note that probing depths of 4–5 mm may be common and not indicative of pathology.

▶ *Test for mobility*: no movement.

▶ *Occlusal integrity*: no more than feather contact between implant and opposing tooth.

▶ *Patient function and comfort*: no report of issues related to eating or comfort.

▶ *Sufficiency of patient's oral self-care*: feedback provided and additional instruction as needed with hands-on practice.

PERI-IMPLANT HYGIENE

A key requirement for implant success is the disease control program for the tissue surrounding the implant. Meticulous daily oral self-care is a necessity.

I. Care of the Natural Teeth

▶ Transmission of microorganisms from the natural teeth and periodontal pockets to the peri-implant tissues can occur.

▶ Periodontal pockets around the natural teeth act as natural reservoirs, and periodontal pathogens from the pockets colonize in the tissue around the implants.

▶ Before placement of the implants, it is necessary for the periodontal condition of surrounding natural teeth to be treated and brought to a healthy state.

▶ After the placement of the implants, the maintenance program emphasizes care of the natural teeth and tissues as well as the peri-implant tissues.

II. Implant Biofilm

▶ Biofilm microorganisms around implants with healthy permucosal tissue have been shown to be similar to the flora around natural teeth. Gram-positive, nonmotile, coccoid, and other forms of bacteria predominate.[12,13]

▶ Peri-implant tissues react to toxic byproducts of biofilm in a manner similar to that of the gingiva surrounding natural teeth but inflammation progresses at a more accelerated rate.

▶ Inflammatory infiltrate present in peri-implant tissues can initiate pocket formation with an increase in total number of microorganisms including spirochetes and motile rods.[12]

III. Planning the Disease Control Program

A. Relation to Treatment

Supervision of a patient's oral hygiene begins before the surgical phase for implant placement and carries on throughout the treatment phases.

B. Types of Prostheses

▶ Implant-supported prostheses may be partial, complete, fixed, removable, or single-tooth replacements. Instruction for their care is provided in Chapter 32.

▶ *Examples*
  • Overdenture (Figure 32-10 in Chapter 32)
  • Screw-retained restoration
  • Cemented restoration.

C. Monitoring Prostheses Fit

▶ Instruct and demonstrate to the patient how to monitor the fit of the implant prosthesis on a regular basis by testing the crown, bridge, or superstructure.

▶ Components that have become loose need treatment and are considered true emergencies in the dental practice.

IV. Selection of Biofilm-Removal Methods

▶ Each patient needs an individually planned program so that each type of abutment and prosthesis can be maintained in a biofilm-free environment.

▶ Provide specific directions in a take-home printed form.

▶ Abutments or posts are cleaned daily with meticulous care.

▶ *Precautions*
  • Prevent damage to implant materials. Use implements, dentifrices, or other cleaning agents that will not scratch or abrade the titanium or other material.

  • Each device is checked and selected by the dental hygienist before recommended for use.

▶ *Toothbrushes*
  • Select toothbrush with smooth, soft, and end-rounded filaments to prevent damage to the titanium and the peri-implant tissue.
  • Power toothbrushes with soft, end-rounded filaments can be applied effectively.

▶ *Dental floss*
  • Specialized spongy filament floss is available with a built-in threader (Figure 29-7 in Chapter 29).
  • Commercial floss products include corded varieties.

▶ *Interdental care*
  • Use only smooth plastic coated wires for interdental brushes (Figure 29-10 in Chapter 29).
  • Avoid all metal core brushes.
  • Synthetic yarn or a folded section of gauze bandage can be used to clean abutments under overdentures.
  • A floss threader can be used to position yarn or dental floss around an abutment and under a fixed prosthesis (Figure 32-3 in Chapter 32).
  • The end-tuft brush with soft filaments is particularly useful in lingual and palatal embrasure spaces (Figure 29-11 in Chapter 29).
  • Round, wooden toothpicks used in plastic handles can be effective for cleaning exposed proximal tooth surfaces and "penciling" just under the crest of the gingiva (Figure 29-12 in Chapter 29).

V. Rinsing and Irrigation

A. General Cleaning

▶ Use of an irrigator can remove debris before specific cleaning with toothbrush and auxiliary aids.

B. Chemotherapy

▶ Rinsing or daily irrigation with an approved antimicrobial can be recommended to help minimize bacterial accumulation and inflammation. Specific directions for preparation of the solution and use of the irrigator are demonstrated and practiced with the patient.

▶ Example: Chlorhexidine, 0.12%, has been shown to be effective. A cotton swab, sponge tip, or interdental brush dipped in the solution can be applied directly to the gingival margins to help prevent staining of oral tissues or tooth-color restorations.

VI. Fluoride Measures for Dental Caries Control

▶ For the patient with natural teeth, daily fluoride self-application is incorporated into the regimen.

▶ Avoid acidic fluoride preparations.[14,15]

▶ Neutral sodium fluoride is recommended.

CONTINUING CARE

Periodic care for professional maintenance and monitoring is scheduled according to the complexity of the restoration or prosthetic superstructure and the patient's ability to perform adequate oral self-care.

▶ Continuing supervision of the patient with dental implants is essential.

▶ Episodic nature of periodontal and peri-implant inflammation:
  • A multitude of factors may affect the patient's ability to withstand the critical threshold beyond which pathogenic organisms can overwhelm the host response.
  • Regular in-office periodontal maintenance care is a critical component of implant therapy success.

▶ Patient expectations
  • The well-informed and conscientious patient who devotes time each day on oral self-care procedures expects a continuing care appointment that thoroughly evaluates the health status of the periodontal tissues and adequacy of biofilm control efforts.

I. Probing Dental Implants

▶ Routine probing of dental implants is debated.
  • Because the peri-coronal tissue cuff is positioned around the implant without the benefit of connective tissue fiber insertion, the barrier between oral bacteria and the bone around the implant is weak.
  • Normal probing can easily displace this vulnerable tissue and penetrate to crestal bone while introducing bacteria from the oral cavity.
  • A false-positive indication of bleeding on probing (BOP) can also result from excessive insertion pressure.

▶ The measurement obtained when probing conventionally around an implant represents the length of the abutment and restoration, which can vary widely, rather than being an indication of pathology as with pocket depth on a natural tooth. For this reason, peri-implant probing serves little purpose as a stand-alone diagnostic tool.

▶ In the absence of accompanying clinical signs of infection in the soft tissue or radiographs, routine vertical-insertion probing is not recommended.

▶ If signs indicate a potential problem, light-pressured measurements with a flexible plastic probe can be taken to compare to baseline data collected.
  • Use one-half to one-third the amount of pressure exerted when probing a natural tooth.[16]

▶ Avoid cross-contamination with pathogenic microflora from an adjacent site by confining use of the plastic probe only to implants.
  • The probe can also be dipped in a 0.12% solution of chlorhexidine gluconate as an extra measure of caution.

▶ Technique:
  • For routine implant maintenance with no clinical signs of infection, a gentle lateral sweep just inside the tissue cuff can verify tissue integrity.
  • The technique aims to assess bleeding on provocation rather than conventional vertical insertion to the soft tissue attachment to determine a measurement.

▶ Unlike natural teeth, the most reliable indicator for evaluating peri-implant health is a radiograph depicting threads in sharp focus on mesial and distal surfaces.
  • Since facial and lingual surfaces are not depicted radiographically, it may be prudent to probe these two surfaces gently vertically on an annual basis.

II. Basic Criteria for Implant Success[17]

▶ The long-term success of an implant is assessed during routine, frequent examinations.

▶ Dental hygienists need to recognize the basic criteria by which an ailing/failing implant can be identified.

▶ A healthy implant shows the following:
  • No pain or discomfort reported by the patient.
  • No mobility.
  • Radiograph: no bone loss or peri-implant radiolucency; no space at the implant–abutment interface or at abutment–prosthesis interface with confirmation of a tight fit.
  • No clinical signs of peri-implantitis: close visual inspection shows healthy gingival tissue surrounding the abutment, firm in consistency with no edema.
  • No bleeding or increased depths on gentle probing performed with a rounded, smooth plastic probe.
  • No movement or loose components in the prosthesis; check for cracks, fractures, missing or nonsecured screws by close visual inspection while applying coronally directed force to superstructure using a rigid single-ended instrument such as a mirror handle.
  • No excess occlusal pressure between implant crown and opposing tooth.

III. Frequency of Appointments

▶ The patient's daily oral biofilm removal with regular professional supervision and monitoring directly influence the long-term success of an implant.

▶ When the original teeth were lost because of lack of daily biofilm control by the patient, a more intense program of education and practice may be needed.

▶ Neglect may have been caused by lack of knowledge or appreciation for preventive measures.

▶ An appointment interval based on individual needs is indicated.

▶ The first series of appointments following placement of the implant(s) starts within a week and is scheduled weekly until healing is completed and the patient has demonstrated the ability to control the dental biofilm.

▶ Continuing care appointments during the first year may be at 1- or 2-month intervals.

IV. The Continuing Care Appointment[18,19]

Dental implants represent a sizeable investment for the patient both financially and time devoted. They require close monitoring and continuing care. Responsibility for providing safe professional care that will not pose a threat to the integrity of the restored implant falls to the dental hygienist in the maintenance phase.

A. Health History Review, Vital Signs, and Intraoral/Extraoral Examination

▶ Basic review questions can reveal the present state of health, recent illnesses, changes in medications, and other current information.

▶ Comparisons with previous records permit assessment of vital signs and extraoral/intraoral observations.

B. Selective Radiographs

▶ A standard procedure is used so that comparisons can be made of bone level to implant threads, to determine status of implant stability. Remodeling of bone down to the level of the first thread (1.0–1.5 mm) typically occurs in the first year.

▶ Film placement devices have been developed for consistent positioning of implants.[20,21]

C. Periodontal Assessment

▶ *Peri-implant tissue:* Visual examination shows no signs of inflammation as evidenced by the usual criteria of changes in color, size, shape, and consistency.

▶ *Probing*
  • A smooth plastic probe with rounded end is used.
  • Pressure-sensitive probes are available to guard against excess insertion pressure.
  • Sweep probe gently around the internal surface of the peri-implant gingival cuff (sulcus or pocket wall) to determine bleeding tendency (Figure 33-7).
  • If bleeding occurs, the depth of attachment is carefully measured. Each millimeter of gingival sulcus is lightly probed to detect incipient changes; compare with baseline data collected at postrestorative evaluation.
  • What could seem like a minute area of gingival BOP, whether the pocket is shallow or has started to deepen, can be a warning signal that an area may harbor retained cement, may not be covered adequately by present self-care procedures, or may need additional periodontal treatment.

▶ *Mobility determination*
  • Implant mobility is always present in a failed implant.
  • Careful mobility testing is done with close visual inspection for fluid at the gingival margin; fluid emerging from the peri-implant area around an implant or mobility provocation can be a sign of ailment.

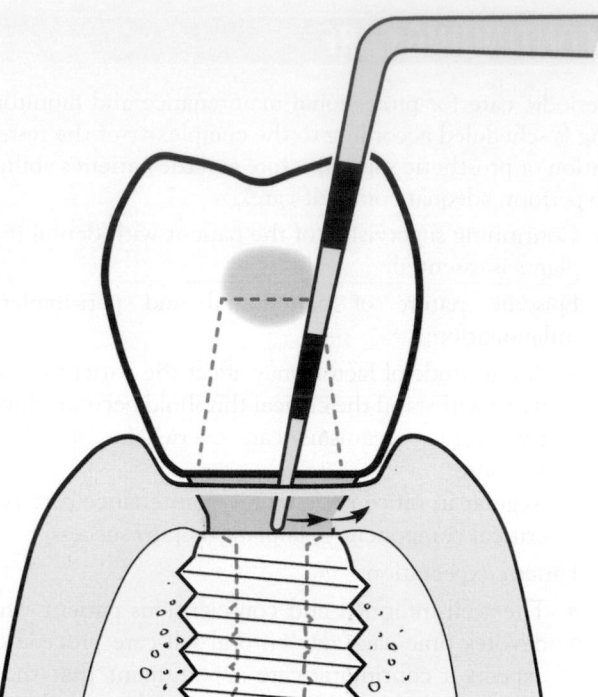

FIGURE 33-7 **Probing an Implant.** Using a plastic probe, sweep gently around the internal surface of the peri-implant gingival cuff (sulcus or pocket wall) to determine bleeding tendency.

  • Inform the dentist and/or implant surgeon immediately of noticeable mobility.

▶ *Dental biofilm*
  • Tested with a disclosing agent.
  • Examined for biofilm accumulation patterns for patient instruction, and documented.

▶ *Calculus*
  • Rarely forms subgingivally on implants when patients adhere to recommendations for professional maintenance and daily oral self-care.
  • Mineralized deposits usually are not extensive, hard, or firmly attached to implant abutments or other protruding parts.
  • Semisoft, partially mineralized deposits can be effectively removed with variations of floss implements.

▶ *Review of personal dental biofilm control procedures*
  • Bleeding points and/or probing depth increases are brought to the attention of the patient along with strategies to address oral self-care problem areas.
  • The patient demonstrates self-care methods, and the clinician provides feedback and recommendations for improvements.

D. Instrumentation

▶ Care is taken not to scratch or alter in any way the surfaces of titanium and other materials making up the implant superstructure.

▶ *Biofilm removal:* Soft deposits are removed from the titanium abutment with gauze strips or sponge-filament dental floss wrapped around the abutment 360°.

- Floss alternatives such as textured cords are often sufficient to remove partially mineralized deposits that are loosely bound to the titanium abutment surface.
- *Calculus removal:* Specialized implant-specific instruments are indicated for hard deposits that remain following soft deposit removal on titanium abutments.
  - Current implant-specific instruments mimic traditional universal curets and sickle scalers in design.
  - Titanium metal instruments safe for use on implants are available in addition to the more traditional nonmetal plastic instruments.
  - Gold-plated instruments are also available but must be monitored for wear to prevent inadvertent scratching of a titanium abutment from the metal beneath the gold.
  - Implant-specific ultrasonic tips and inserts are available for peri-implant debridement. Use *low* power when instrumenting implant abutments with an ultrasonic device.
- *Prevention of damage to the implant surface*
  - Confine manual instrument strokes to the prosthesis and the supragingival area of the abutment.
  - Severe abrasion can result from application of an ultrasonic scaler without a specialized tip designed for implant use.
- *Stain removal:* Unless it is necessary for esthetics, stain removal is not included routinely.
  - When selective stain removal with a rubber cup is indicated, only a nonabrasive agent is used and applied gently.
  - Tin oxide or nonabrasive toothpaste may be suitable for polishing agents.
- *Professional subgingival irrigation:* The use of 0.12% chlorhexidine after professional instrumentation may be a treatment alternative when peri-implantitis has been identified. Irrigation with chlorhexidine gluconate has been shown to be a safe procedure around implants.[22,23]

IMPLANT COMPLICATIONS[9]

I. Factors that Contribute to Implant Failure[24]

A. Systemic Factors

- Not revealed or unknown in initial preparation of medical history
- Undiagnosed or uncontrolled diabetes
- Immunocompromised patient
- Poor vascularity
- Poor bone quality or quantity
- Unanticipated infection
- Cancer, osteoporosis.

B. Surgical Phase of Treatment

- Traumatic insertion
- Break in sterile procedure.

C. Restorative Phase of Treatment

- Premature or excessive loading
- Parafunctional forces
- Prosthetic cement remnants at implant–abutment interface; may not be evident until peri-implantitis develops in the maintenance phase.

D. Maintenance Phase

- Patient neglect; noncompliance with self-care, instruction, and maintenance visits
- Peri-implantitis: soft tissue reactions
- Mechanical/structural complications such as fractured components, broken attachments or mobility.

II. Peri-implant Problems[25]

Prompt intervention when clinical and/or radiographic signs suggest a potential problem is of utmost importance.

- Two prominent factors contributing to breakdown of the peri-implant environment are:
  - Occlusal overload (biomechanical stress).
  - Bacterial infection leading to inflammatory peri-implant disease.
- Patients generally compliant with recommendations who suddenly present with what seems to be idiopathic bone loss on a cement-retained prosthetic crown may be exhibiting the delayed response of residual cement serving as the source of infection.

A. Initial Stage: Peri-implant Mucositis

- Reversible bacterial infection in the soft tissue similar to gingivitis.
- Mild color change with accompanying bleeding may be present.

B. Secondary Stage: Peri-implantitis

- Inflammation has reached the level of the bone resulting in peri-implant bone loss.
- Edema or hemorrhage present in the surrounding tissues.
- Exudate may or may not be present.
- Increase in probing depth.

III. Restorative/Prosthetic Hazards[11]

- When the implant crown is permanently cemented to the abutment, residual cement is a significant risk factor.
- Due to excess cement, iatrogenic peri-implant disease may develop despite optimum patient oral self-care and regular professional care.
- More than three-quarters of peri-implantitis cases in one study were attributed to retained prosthetic cement.[11]

A. Materials

▶ Cement residue goes largely undetected on postrestorative radiographs—particularly buccal and lingual surfaces that cannot be evaluated radiographically.

▶ Glass ionomer-based cements in wide use are difficult to detect even when present in excess on a proximal surface.[26]

▶ Radiopaque cements that are zinc-based *permit* radiographic detection.[26]

▶ Until radiopaque compounds become the standard of care, dental hygienists must be:
  - Aware of this widespread issue.
  - Proactive in immediate referral for reparative treatment.

B. Signs and Symptoms

▶ May occur as early as 4 months in some patients.

▶ Most often a delayed response that may not be apparent for several years.

C. Etiology

▶ Biofilm covering the surface of retained cement can and does form calculus, but the primary etiologic factor appears to be the cement itself; certain prosthetic cements have been shown to be bacteriophilic, hastening the inflammatory process.

▶ Contemporary prosthetic cements are impervious to removal and *cannot be treated nonsurgically* with any degree of assurance.

▶ Until the cement is definitively removed, the problem will remain.

D. Assessment

▶ Document cement-retained implant prosthetics and be vigilant for potential signs of a problem.

▶ Examine postrestorative radiographs carefully for signs of clouds or feathering at proximal implant crown margins.

▶ Be alert to clinical signs of inflammation, especially idiopathic change in an otherwise stable implant, since cement-associated peri-implantitis may not appear for many years following implant restoration.

E. Referral

▶ Residual cement cases are referred back to the implant surgeon for definitive therapy.

▶ The implant is flapped open for surgical debridement using high-speed burs to remove the cement, then grafted with bone and membrane.

CLASSIFICATION OF PERI-IMPLANT DISEASE[27–29]

Peri-implant disease is divided into three stages of severity: ailing implant, failing implant, and failed implant.

I. Ailing Implant (Peri-implant Mucositis)

▶ Inflammation present but no mobility.

▶ Bone may appear normal in the radiograph or incipient bone loss may be evident.

▶ Review/reinforce patient's oral self-care practice.

▶ Perform careful peri-implant debridement, removing all traces of calculus.

▶ Irrigate with an oral antimicrobial rinse (0.12% chlorhexidine gluconate); prescribe for daily home use.

▶ Adjunctive therapy using local delivery antimicrobial placement may also be indicated.

▶ Consultation with the surgeon may be needed if the tissue does not respond favorably to therapy within 2 weeks.

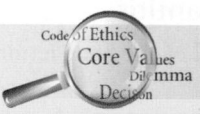 **EVERYDAY ETHICS**

Karen reviewed the permanent record progress notes before receiving Ms. Overly for her routine 4 months' continuing care. Dr. Richards had seen Ms. Overly within the week for an examination and radiograph of tooth #10 where a root canal had been placed 2 years ago and was giving her trouble. The endodontic therapy had failed and Dr. Richards had recorded that the tooth was now indicated for extraction.

While Karen was updating blood pressure and medical history, she noticed that her patient did not seem to be her usual talkative self. "I guess I have to have a bridge put in and *I am not happy* about it," Ms. Overly said.

Karen asked, "Have you discussed this with Dr. Richards?"

Ms. Overly replied, "To tell the truth I'm really confused. My brother asked me why I'm not getting an implant. Dr. Richards just said we need to do a bridge."

Questions for Consideration

1. What obligation does Karen have, and what procedure does Karen need to follow, in terms of assuring that Ms. Overly's treatment options have been fully presented and adequately explained and understood?

2. Is there an issue with societal trust in this incident? Which of the other dental hygiene core values are evident in this scenario? (Refer to Table II-1, Section II Preparation for Dental Hygiene Practice.)

3. With respect to core values and informed consent standards, role-play (1) additional conversation between Karen and Ms. Overly, and (2) a dialogue that could ensue between Karen and Dr. Richards as Karen explains Ms. Overly's concerns about the treatment he has indicated for her.

II. Failing Implant (Peri-implantitis Without Mobility)

▶ Inflammation present; may be accompanied by exudate during mobility testing.

▶ Bone loss has occurred and continues.

▶ Consult the surgeon for prompt intervention treatment when an implant shows signs of failing.

III. Failed Implant (Peri-implantitis with Mobility)

▶ Mobility in a restored implant signifies a serious problem.

▶ Radiographic changes in bone level are apparent when compared with prior films; may show a vertical bony defect.

• Implant mobility coupled with radiographic evidence of bone destruction are conclusive indications of a failed implant.

▶ Patient is referred immediately back to the surgeon for evaluation and removal of the failed implant.

DOCUMENTATION

All members of the implant therapy team are kept informed and up-to-date on the status of the patient from initial consultation through the postrestorative evaluation. Reports and copies of progress notes are sent between surgical and restorative practices.

For documenting appointments concerning a dental implant, the following factors are recorded in the progress note:

▶ Consultation before implant treatment plan:

• Patient advised of all options to replace missing tooth/teeth.

• Patient understands surgical, prosthetic, and maintenance phases of dental implant therapy.

• Expected benefits, principal risks, and potential complications of dental implant therapy have been fully explained.

• Alternatives to suggested dental implant treatment have been outlined.

• Necessary follow-up care and home self-care with ongoing professional maintenance appointments have been fully explained to patient.

▶ Examination: in addition to standard continuing care maintenance procedures, evaluate and document implant-specific assessments as follows:

• Verify dental implant locations with chart and current radiographs.

• Peri-implant tissue tone, color, and texture.

• Presence of inflammation: note erythema, edema, and/or exudate.

• Evidence of pathology: lightly probe peri-implant space if visual signs of inflammation present.

• Radiograph if pathology present, and/or every 12 months to look for changes in bone level.

• Implant mobility.
• Prosthesis integrity and stability.
• Biofilm and calculus accumulation: note quantity and location.

▶ An example of a progress note appears in Box 33-2.

BOX 33-2
Example Documentation: Patient with Implants

S – Patient presents for continuing care 3 months following final seating of implant prosthesis for tooth #3. No chief complaint or concerns.

O – Intraoral/extraoral examination within normal limits. Peri-implant soft tissue appears healthy with no bleeding. Overall biofilm score of <10%. One periapical radiograph within normal limits; no mobility evident of implant fixture or prosthesis; no biofilm or calculus accumulation on tooth #3.

A – Periapical implant appears healthy and well-integrated.

P – Treatment: reinforce implant cleaning procedures with floss threaders, periodontal debridement with manual and ultrasonic scaling. Next: 3-month continuing care. Copy report to surgeon and general dentist.

Signed: _____, RDH
Date: _____.

Factors To Teach The Patient

▷ How tooth loss corresponds to progressive, irreversible bone resorption due to the absence of biomechanical force from masticatory function.

▷ How dental implants preserve and maintain surrounding bone

▷ How to care for implants; special needs related to the titanium surfaces.

▷ How the health of the periodontal tissues and the duration of the implants and prostheses depend on meticulous daily self-care by the patient.

▷ The role of biofilm in periodontitis and peri-implantitis; vulnerability of the implant to infection from periodontal pathogens that may be present on adjacent natural teeth.

▷ How having a history of periodontitis may place a patient at increased risk for peri-implantitis.

▷ How cleaning a mouth with complex restorations takes longer. Time must be allotted in the daily schedule for thorough biofilm removal each day, especially before going to bed.

▷ Why frequent, ongoing professional maintenance care and annual radiographs to document bone height around implants are necessary.

▷ When to call the office to address potential or suspected problems around an implant, for example, peri-implant bleeding, soreness, or pain.

References

1. Misch CE. *Contemporary Implant Dentistry*. 3rd ed. St. Louis, MO: Mosby; 2008:134–135.

2. Wolff J. *The Law of Bone Remodeling*. New York, NY: Springer; 1986. (translation of the German 1892 edition).

3. American Academy of Periodontology. Dental implants in periodontal therapy. *J Periodontol*. 2000;71:1934–1942.

4. Berglundh T, Lindhe J, Ericsson I, et al. The soft tissue barrier at implants and teeth. *Clin Oral Implants Res*. 1991;2(2):81–90.

5. Cochran D. Implant therapy I. *Ann Periodontol*. 1996;1(1):707–791.

6. Harris BW. A new technique for the subperiosteal implant. *J Am Dent Assoc*. 1990;121(9):422–424.

7. Homoly PA. The restorative and surgical technique for the full maxillary subperiosteal implant. *J Am Dent Assoc*. 1990;121(9):404–407.

8. Cranin AN, Sher J, Schilb TP. The transosteal implant: a 17-year review and report. *J Prosthet Dent*. 1986;55(6):709–718.

9. Small IA. The fixed mandibular implant: its use in reconstructive prosthetics. *J Am Dent Assoc*. 1990;121(3):369, 372, 374.

10. American Academy of Periodontology. Parameter on placement and management of the dental implant. *J Periodontol*. 2000;71:870–872.

11. Wilson TG Jr. The positive relationship between excess cement and peri-implant disease: a prospective clinical endoscopic study. *J Periodontol*. 2009;80(9):1388–1392.

12. Mombelli A, Lang NP. Microbial aspects of implant dentistry. *Periodontol 2000*. 1994;4:74–80.

13. Mombelli A, Marxer M, Gaberthüel T, et al. The microbiota of osseointegrated implants in patients with a history of periodontal disease. *J Clin Periodontol*. 1995;22(2):124–130.

14. Siirilä HS, Könönen M. The effect of oral topical fluorides on the surface of commercially pure titanium. *Int J Oral Maxillofac Implants*. 1991;6(1):50–54.

15. Probster L, Lin W, Huttemann H. Effect of fluoride prophylactic agents on titanium surfaces. *Int J Oral Maxillofac Implants*. 1992;7(4):390–394.

16. Gerber JA, Tan WC, Balmer TE, et al. Bleeding on probing and pocket probing depth in relation to probing pressure and mucosal health around oral implants. *Clin Oral Implants Res*. 2009;20(1):75–78.

17. Hultin M, Komiyamma A, Klinge B. Supportive therapy and the longevity of dental implants: a systematic review of the literature. *Clin Oral Implants Res*. 2007;18:50–62.

18. Hempton TJ, Bonacci FJ, Lancaster D, et al. Implant maintenance. *Dimens Dent Hyg*. 2011;9(1):58–61.

19. Christman A, Schrader S, John V, et al. Designing a safety checklist for dental implant placement. *J Am Dent Assoc*. 2014;145(2):131–140.

20. Cox JF, Pharoah M. An alternative holder for radiographic evaluation of tissue-integrated prostheses. *J Prosthet Dent*. 1986;56(9):338–341.

21. Meijer HJ, Steen WH, Bosman F. Standardized radiographs of the alveolar crest around implants in the mandible. *J Prosthet Dent*. 1992;68(2):318–321.

22. Lavigne SE, Krust-Bray KS, Williams KB, et al. Effects of subgingival irrigation with chlorhexidine on the periodontal status of patients with HA-coated integral dental implants. *Int J Oral Maxillofac Implants*. 1994;9(2):156–162.

23. Felo A, Shibly O, Ciancio SG, et al. Effects of subgingival chlorhexidine irrigation on peri-implant maintenance. *Am J Dent*. 1997;10(2):107–110.

24. Chrcanovic BR, Albrektsson T, Wennerberg A. Reasons for failures of oral implants. *J Oral Rehabil*. 2014 Jun;41(6):443-476.

25. American Academy of Periodontology. Peri-implant mucositis and peri-implantitis: a current understanding of their diagnoses and clinical implications. *J Periodontol*. 2013;84(4):436–443.

26. Wadwani C, Hess T, Faber T, et al. A descriptive study of the radiographic density of implant restorative cements. *J Prosthet Dent*. 2010;103:295–302.

27. Lindhe J, Meyle J. Peri-implant diseases: consensus report of the Sixth European Workshop on Periodontology. *J Clin Periodontol*. 2008;35 (Suppl 8):282–285.

28. Sanz M, Chapple IL. Clinical research on peri-implant diseases: consensus report of Working Group 4. *J Clin Periodontol*. 2012;39 (Suppl 12):202–206.

29. Tomasi C, Derks J. Clinical research of peri-implant diseases—quality of reporting, case definitions and methods to study incidence, prevalence and risk factors of peri-implant diseases. *J Clin Periodontol*. 2012;39 (Suppl 12): 207–223.

ENHANCE YOUR UNDERSTANDING

thePoint° DIGITAL CONNECTIONS
(see the inside front cover for access information)
- **Audio glossary**
- **Quiz bank**

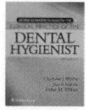

SUPPORT FOR LEARNING
(available separately; visit lww.com)
- *Active Learning Workbook for Clinical Practice of the Dental Hygienist, 12th Edition*

prepU INDIVIDUALIZED REVIEW
(available separately; visit lww.com)
- **Adaptive quizzing with *prepU for Wilkins' Clinical Practice of the Dental Hygienist***

34

The Patient Who Uses Tobacco

Lori Rainchuso, RDH, MS, Elain Benton, RDH, BS, CTTS, and Jane Cotter, RDH, MS

CHAPTER OUTLINE

LEARNING OBJECTIVES

After studying this chapter, the student will be able to:

1. Recognize the health hazards associated with tobacco use.

2. Identify components of tobacco products.

3. Identify various mechanisms for nicotine delivery.

4. Describe the metabolism of nicotine.

5. Recognize the oral manifestations of tobacco use.

6. Recognize the effects of environmental tobacco smoke (ETS).

7. Assess and develop a dental hygiene care plan for the patient who uses tobacco.

8. Recognize protocols for developing a tobacco cessation program.

9. Identify the pharmacotherapies and behavioral therapies used for treatment of nicotine addiction.

▶ There is no safe form of tobacco.

▶ In the 21st century, oral effects from tobacco use are well documented.[1]

▶ Advice from health professionals has been shown to be a powerful influence on patients' decisions to stop or not begin using tobacco.[2]

▶ Dental and dental hygiene professionals are in an ideal position and have a responsibility to provide patients who use tobacco with the opportunity to enter a tobacco cessation program to assist in stopping tobacco use.[2]

▶ Key words related to tobacco use and addiction are defined in Box 34-1. Box 34-2 defines the various forms of tobacco.

HEALTH HAZARDS

▶ Tobacco is toxic to humans. Tobacco use is the single most preventable cause of disease and premature death in the world.[1]

▶ Approximately 25% of adult Americans report using some type of tobacco product: any combustible tobacco product, cigars, cigarillos, regular pipe, water pipe (hookah), electronic cigarettes, and smokeless tobacco.[3]

▶ Offspring of smokers are more likely to become smokers.[1,4,5]

▶ As years of tobacco use accumulate, so do the systemic and oral health effects of all forms of tobacco.[1]

▶ Life expectancy is shortened.[1]

▶ Women who smoke or are exposed to environmental tobacco smoke (ETS) are at risk for the same smoke-related health problems as men.[6]

▶ Approximately 16 million Americans suffer from a disease caused by smoking.[1]

▶ Approximately 90% of men and 80% of women who die from lung cancer is attributed to smoking.[7]

COMPONENTS OF TOBACCO PRODUCTS AND TOBACCO SMOKE

▶ Nicotine is the drug in tobacco products that causes addiction.[8]

▶ Nicotine is considered toxic, and 60 mg can cause fatality.[9]

▶ Once tobacco is ignited, carcinogenic substances become part of mainstream smoke and are emitted in ETS.[10] Figure 34-1 illustrates the smoking process.

▶ Cigarette smoke is a complex mixture containing an estimated 7,357 chemical compounds.[11]

▶ Over 90 of the chemical and chemical compounds in tobacco products and tobacco smoke are identified by the Food and Drug Administration (FDA) as being unsafe or having unsafe potential.[12]

▶ These chemicals or chemical compounds can be categorized as a carcinogen, respiratory toxicant, cardiovascular toxicant, reproductive or developmental intoxicant, an addictive, or a combination of these agents.[12]

▶ The following chemical components in tobacco products have the greatest potential for harmful systemic effects: 1,3-butadiene (cancer), acrolein and acetaldehyde (respiratory), cyanide, arsenic, and cresols (cardiovascular).[1]

▶ Table 34-1 lists differences in the quantity of nicotine delivered by tobacco products: the amount and rate at which a nicotine-containing product delivers nicotine to the bloodstream is a determinant of its addiction potential.[9,12,13]

METABOLISM OF NICOTINE[8,9,11]

▶ Absorption of nicotine occurs through most of the body's membranes: lungs, skin, and oral, buccal, nasal mucosa, and the gastrointestinal tract.

▶ Delivery method affects the way nicotine is absorbed into the body. For example, inhaled tobacco is absorbed via the membranes in the lung.

▶ Another factor affecting absorption is the product's acidity. The more basic the medium the easier absorption. For example, cigar or pipe smoke are less acidic than cigarette smoke.

▶ Several factors influence absorption from smoked tobacco (cigarettes, pipes, and cigars), as identified in Figure 34-1. Regardless of the type of tobacco used, nicotine is primarily metabolized by the liver and excreted through the kidneys as acidic urine.

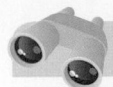

BOX 34-1 KEY WORDS AND ABBREVIATIONS: Tobacco Use

Carcinogen: substance or chemical that has been known to cause cancer.

CDC: Centers for Disease Control and Prevention.

Chemical dependency: generic term relating to psychological or physical dependency, or both, on an exogenous substance.

COPD: chronic obstructive pulmonary disease.

Cotinine: a by-product of nicotine found in body fluids; cotinine levels are used in behavioral research to determine recent use of nicotine-containing products or recent contact with passive smoke and in clinical research to determine correlations between cotinine levels and oral disease.

Drug abuse: any use of a drug that causes physical, psychological, economic, legal, and/or social harm to the person who uses or other persons affected by the user's behavior.

Drug addiction: a chronic disorder leading to negative physical, psychological, or social consequences from compulsive use of substance; characterized by continued use despite negative effects encountered by use.

Dysphoria: generalized feeling of ill being, malaise, restlessness, and discomfort.

FDA: Food and Drug Administration.

Nicotine: a poisonous, addictive stimulant that is the chief psychoactive ingredient in tobacco.

Nicotine gum: polacrilex gum developed to aid in tobacco cessation; available as an over-the-counter (OTC) product.

Nicotine lozenge: lozenge developed to aid in tobacco cessation; available as an OTC product.

Nicotine nasal spray: a prescription nicotine withdrawal product used nasally by the patient to aid in tobacco cessation.

Nicotine patch: a transdermal form of nicotine withdrawal therapy; available as an OTC product.

Nicotine inhaler: a prescription nicotine inhalation system used orally for tobacco cessation.

Nitrosamines: cancer-causing chemicals found in tobacco.

Oral cancer: in this chapter, the term "oral cancer" includes cancer of the lips, tongue, floor of the mouth, palate, gingiva, alveolar mucosa, buccal mucosa, and oropharynx.

OTC: over-the-counter

Placenta abruptio: premature detachment of a normally situated placenta.

Placenta previa: placenta implanted in the lower segment of the uterus extending to the margin of the internal opening of the cervix; may obstruct opening partially or completely.

Psychoactive drug: possessing the ability to alter mood, behavior, cognitive processes, or mental tension.

Pyrolysis: chemical decomposition of a substance by heat.

Smoke: visible vapor and gases given off by a burning substance.

  Environmental tobacco smoke (ETS) or passive smoke: tobacco smoke present in room air resulting from ignited tobacco products burning in an ashtray or exhaled by a smoker (people who are currently smoking are also exposed to other smokers' sidestream smoke).

  Mainstream smoke: smoke inhaled directly into the user's lungs.

  Sidestream smoke: the aerosol emitted directly into the surrounding air from the lit end of a smoldering tobacco product; may be inhaled by the user; is a major component of environmental smoke.

  Third-hand smoke: tobacco smoke residue absorbed by furnishings.

Sudden infant death syndrome (SIDS): Sudden and unexpected death of an apparently healthy infant; typically occurring between the ages of 3 weeks and 5 months.

TSNAs: potent carcinogenic tobacco-specific nitrosamines.

Transdermal: method of drug delivery by patch on skin; a mode for slow release over extended time.

Transmucosal: type of drug delivery by infiltration of mucosal lining.

Use: using the substance of tobacco because of an individual's addiction to nicotine.

User: an individual who either smokes tobacco or places tobacco in the mouth.

I. Nicotine from Smoking[8,13]

A. Absorption: Lungs

Nicotine enters the lungs and quickly passes into arterial circulation by way of blood vessels lining the sacs of the bronchi.

B. Distribution

▸ *To the brain:* Nicotine is delivered efficiently to the brain by the bloodstream in less than 20 seconds.

▸ *Peak plasma concentration:* Figure 34-2 illustrates the peak blood plasma concentrations from various tobacco products and nicotine replacement therapies (NRTs).

  ● Following the onset of smoking, peak plasma concentration of nicotine occurs in approximately 4–5 minutes.

▸ *Dissemination:* Nicotine is spread to all body tissues.

▸ *Changes in the liver:* Nicotine is metabolized in the liver into cotinine.

  ● Cotinine concentrations in the blood, urine, and saliva are used to assess

   ◦ Whether a person uses tobacco.

   ◦ The extent of use.

   ◦ The level of exposure of nonsmokers to passive or environmental smoke.

II. Smokeless Tobacco[13,15]

Smokeless tobacco is the term applied to snuff (moist or dry) and chewing tobacco products (defined in Box 34-2), which are not smoked but are placed in the mouth.

▸ Of the 28 carcinogens found in chewing tobacco and snuff, the most harmful are the tobacco-specific

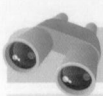

BOX 34-2 KEY WORDS: Forms of Tobacco

Bidis: small, thin hand-rolled cigarettes consisting of tobacco wrapped in a tendu or temburni leaf (plants native to Asia), and may be secured with a colorful string at one or both ends.

Chaw: a golf-ball-sized portion of chewing tobacco held in the user's mouth usually inside the cheek or between the lower lip, gingiva, and mucosa.

Chewing tobacco: tobacco available in loose-leaf, twist, and plug forms manufactured by air-drying tobacco leaves; held inside cheek and/or chewed (chaw).

Cigar: About 1–20 g of air-cured fermented tobacco wrapped in paper that is smoked.

Cigarette: less than 1 g of unfermented tobacco wrapped in a cylindrical paper-enclosed form that is smoked.

Hookah pipe: a water pipe used to smoke specially made flavored tobacco.

Kreteks: referred to as clove cigarettes—are imported from Indonesia and typically contain a mixture of tobacco, cloves, and other additives.

Pipe tobacco: ground leaf tobacco manufactured for smoking through a pipe.

Quid: a pinch of snuff held in the user's mouth for various periods of time.

Sachets: moist snuff in ready to use pouches that look like small tea bags.

Smokeless (spit) tobacco: term used to define all forms of tobacco that are not ignited or inhaled.

Smoking tobacco: any form of tobacco that is ignited and smoked by the user.

Snuff: fire-cured, finely ground, or powdered tobacco sold in both dry and moist forms or baglike pouches; not chewed but a small amount ("pinch" or "quid") is placed and held between cheek and gingiva or lower lip, gingiva, and mucosa. Snuff can also be sniffed or inhaled into the nose.

Snus: moist powder tobacco product that is a smokeless, spitless pouch; originated from a variant of dry snuff used in the 19th century in Sweden.

Tobacco pipe: a tube with a bowl at one end used to smoke tobacco.

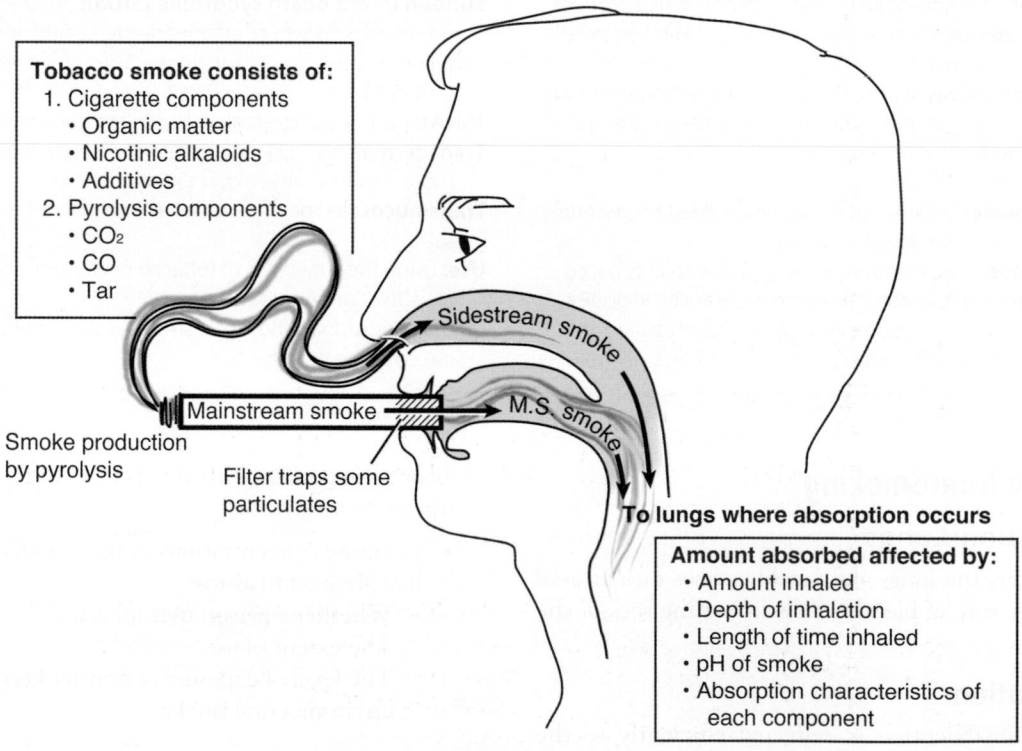

FIGURE 34-1 Components of Mainstream Smoke and Factors Influencing Absorption by the Lungs.

N-nitrosamines (TSNAs). These chemical compounds are usually formed during the growing, curing, fermenting, and aging of tobacco process.

► Other cancer-causing substances found in smokeless tobacco include benzo(a)pyrene, formaldehyde, acetaldehyde, arsenic, nickel, cadmium, and polonium-210.

TABLE 34-1	Nicotine Levels of Various Tobacco Products[13,14]
PRODUCTS	**AMOUNT OF NICOTINE DELIVERY**
Cigarette	0.7–2.0 mg
Bidi	1.5–4.1 mg
Kretek	1.9–2.6 mg
Moist snuff	0.01–7.8 mg/g
Hookah smoking (45 min–1 h)	Equivalent to inhaling 100–200 times the volume of smoke from one cigarette.

A. Absorption: Oral Cavity

▶ Nicotine is directly absorbed through the gingiva and oral mucous membranes.

▶ Once smokeless tobacco is placed in the mouth, the amount of nicotine absorbed is three to four times the amount delivered by a cigarette.[11]

▶ Nicotine concentration declines over 2 hours and is at a negligible level within 24 hours.

▶ Smokeless tobacco users experience nicotine blood plasma levels similar to the nicotine blood levels of smokers.

B. Absorption: Intestinal

▶ Most tobacco juice produced by smokeless tobacco is spit out.

▶ Juice that is intentionally and/or accidentally swallowed by the user is absorbed through the blood vessels lining the small intestine.

III. Electronic Nicotine Delivery Devices[1,16,17]

▶ An electronic cigarette or e-cigarette does not contain tobacco but delivers vaporized nicotine through a device that is made to look similar to a regular cigarette, cigar, or pipe. Additionally, some e-cigarettes are manufactured to look different than a typical cigarette, and more like an everyday item, to conceal its true identity.

▶ To date no clinical trials for e-cigarettes have been submitted for Food and Drug Administration (FDA) approval.

▶ The FDA has not approved e-cigarettes safety or effectiveness.

▶ As a result, there is no way to know how much nicotine is being inhaled, or which chemicals are in an e-cigarette. Long-term use of e-cigarettes may cause health problems.

▶ A serious concern is the different amounts of nicotine found in the cartridges. The nicotine amount in the cartridges varies from the amount advertised leading to unpredictable nicotine dose delivery to the tobacco user.

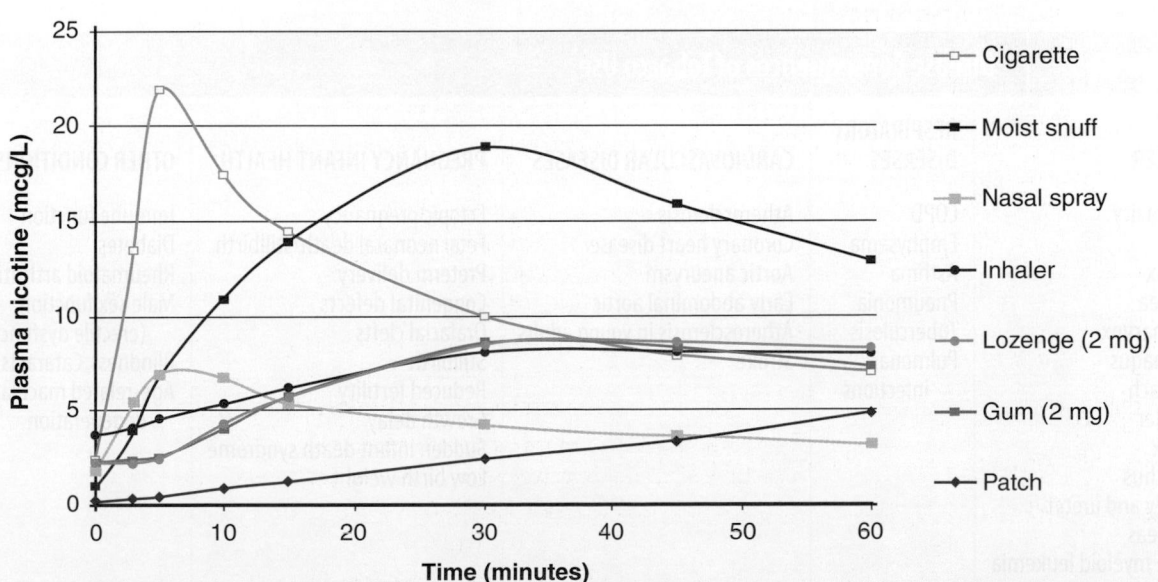

FIGURE 34-2 Plasma Concentrations for Tobacco Products and Nicotine Pharmacotherapies. (*Source*: Choi JH, Dresler CM, Norton MR, et al. Pharmacokinetics of a nicotine polacrilex lozenge. *Nicotine Tob Res.* 2003;5:635–644; Fant RV, Henningfield JE, Nelson RA, et al. Pharmacokinetics and pharmacodynamics of moist snuff in humans. *Tob Control.* 1999;8:387–392; and Schneider NG, Olmstead RE, Franzon MA, et al. The nicotine inhaler: clinical pharmacokinetics and comparison with other nicotine treatments. *Clin Pharmacokinet.* 2001;40:661–684.)

▶ The non-FDA-approved e-cigarette consists of a battery, a heater, and a cartridge containing nicotine, water, propylene glycol, and other chemicals and carcinogens.

▶ Puffing on the device activates the heating element and the solution is then vaporized and inhaled through a mouthpiece.

▶ The device is not FDA approved for nicotine replacement therapy (NRT) or for a method of smoking cessation.

▶ Using e-cigarettes may lead youth/young adults to try conventional tobacco products, which are known to increase morbidity and mortality rates.

SYSTEMIC EFFECTS[1]

▶ The use of tobacco products influences every system of the body. Table 34-2 lists smoking-related conditions.

▶ The diseases that affect each system have consequences ranging from mild to deadly.

I. Cardiovascular Diseases

▶ Smoking aggravates and accelerates the development of atherosclerosis and is a major risk factor for coronary heart disease, the leading cause of death for Americans.

II. Pulmonary Diseases

▶ Smoking is the major cause of chronic obstructive pulmonary disease (COPD), which includes emphysema and chronic bronchitis. More information on COPD is provided in Chapter 66.

▶ Emphysema slowly diminishes a person's ability to breathe.

▶ Chronic bronchitis is a condition in which the airways produce excess mucus, which forces the smoker to cough frequently.

III. Cancer[1,7,10,18,19]

▶ Smoking is responsible for 87% of lung cancers in the United States.

▶ Lung cancer is currently the leading cause of death among cancers, for both men and women.

▶ Smoking can cause many different types of cancers including:

- Lung cancer
- Larynx/throat cancer
- Oropharynx cancer
- Esophagus cancer
- Trachea cancer
- Stomach cancer
- Liver cancer
- Pancreas cancer
- Kidney and ureter cancers
- Bladder cancer
- Cervix cancer
- Colorectal cancer.

▶ Tobacco use causes the most oral cancers. The increase use of tobacco products increases the risk of developing oral cancer.[18]

Table 34-2	Disease Consequences of Tobacco Use[1]			
CANCER	**RESPIRATORY DISEASES**	**CARDIOVASCULAR DISEASES**	**PREGNANCY INFANT HEALTH**	**OTHER CONDITIONS**
Oral cavity	COPD	Atherosclerosis	Ectopic pregnancy	Immune function
Lung	Emphysema	Coronary heart disease	Fetal neonatal death/stillbirth	Diabetes
Larynx	Asthma	Aortic aneurysm	Preterm delivery	Rheumatoid arthritis
Trachea	Pneumonia	Early abdominal aortic	Congenital defects	Male sex function
Orapharynx	Tuberculosis	Atherosclerosis in young adults	Orafacial clefts	(erectile dysfunction)
Esophagus	Pulmonary	Stroke	Stillbirth	Blindness, Cataracts
Stomach	infections		Reduced fertility	Age-related macular
Bladder			Growth delay	degeneration
Cervix			Sudden infant death syndrome	
Bronchus			Low birth weight	
Kidney and ureter				
Pancreas				
Acute myeloid leukemia				
Liver				
Breast				
Colorectal				

IV. Tobacco and Use of Other Drugs[1,7,18]

▶ Smokers are more likely to consume alcohol. The combined use of alcohol and tobacco places the patient at greater risk for neoplasms and other oral problems.

ENVIRONMENTAL TOBACCO SMOKE (ETS)[1,9,10,20]

▶ Also called passive, involuntary, or second-hand smoke when nonsmokers are exposed.

▶ A complex mixture of chemicals are generated during the burning of tobacco products.

▶ The principal contributor is sidestream smoke, the material emitted from burning tobacco products between puffs.

▶ Other components include exhaled mainstream smoke and vaporized compounds diffused through a cigarette wrapper.

▶ In indoor areas, environmental smoke can last for many hours, depending on ventilation. Exposure for certain workers and family members can be extensive.

▶ In the United States, passive smoking is considered the third leading cause of preventable death.

▶ *Third-hand smoke* is defined as tobacco smoke residue absorbed by furnishings.[21,22]

  • Smoke reacts with a common pollutant on indoor surfaces, nitrous acid, which then forms TSNAs.
  • The TSNAs cling to the smoker's body, household dust, and every surface of the home, vehicle, or enclosed area where the smoking takes place. This process represents a health hazard.

I. Toxicity

▶ Many chemicals are contained in passive smoke, including the same carcinogenic compounds as those in mainstream smoke. Some toxic components are actually in higher concentrations in sidestream smoke than in mainstream smoke.

▶ Chemicals present in ETS include irritants and systemic toxicants (hydrogen cyanide and sulfur dioxide), mutagens and carcinogens (benzo[a]pyrene and formaldehyde), and reproductive toxicants (nicotine, cadmium, and carbon monoxide).

▶ Out of the 250 toxic chemicals in ETS, there are at least 50 that are associated with cancer.

II. Lung and Respiratory Effects

▶ Exposure to cigarette smoke, whether active or passive, is the primary cause of lung cancer.[7]

▶ Eye and nasal irritation are the most commonly reported symptoms among adult nonsmokers.[10]

III. Cardiovascular Effects[1,10]

▶ Both active and passive exposure to smoke have similar effects on the cardiovascular system.

▶ ETS is a major preventable cause of cardiovascular disease and death.

▶ A causal relationship exists between second-hand smoke exposure and increased risk of stroke.

PRENATAL AND CHILDREN[1,4,5,10,11,20,23–28]

The fetus, infant, and growing children are exposed to ETS through the following:

▶ Homes and cars where smoking is permitted.

▶ Public environments in which smoking is permitted.

▶ Other enclosed environments that allow smoking, such as restaurants and sporting events.

▶ Nonsmoking mothers who are exposed to ETS, expose their unborn child to tobacco smoke constituents, such as carbon monoxide, nicotine, and continine.

▶ Parental smoking is a strong determinant to smoking uptake among children and adolescents.

I. In Utero

▶ Nicotine and carbon monoxide cross the placenta and concentrate in the fetus at slightly higher levels than the mother.

▶ Adverse pregnancy risks include miscarriage, placenta previa, low birth weight, preterm delivery, and spontaneous abortion.

▶ There is sufficient evidence to conclude a causal relationship between maternal smoking in early pregnancy and orofacial clefts.

▶ There is sufficient evidence to conclude a causal relationship between maternal smoking and ectopic pregnancy.

II. Infancy

▶ Chemicals are passed to the baby in the breast milk of mothers who smoke.

▶ Acute effects include increased incidence of upper respiratory tract illness.

▶ ETS increases risk of an infant developing a lower respiratory illness.

▶ Nicotine can increase the risk of sudden infant death syndrome in infants of smokers.[29]

III. Young Children

▶ ETS affects lung development with symptoms of coughing, phlegm, and wheezing.

▶ Children who are exposed to passive smoking, particularly pre- and postnatal maternal smoking, are at significant risk for onset of wheezing illness and asthma.

▶ Children have an increased incidence of middle ear infections.

ORAL MANIFESTATIONS OF TOBACCO USE[1,19]

▶ The numerous oral conditions attributed to tobacco use vary with the type of tobacco used (smoking or smokeless) and the form in which it is used (cigarettes, pipes, cigars, chewing tobacco, moist and dry snuff).

▶ Pattern and severity of clinical presentation vary with frequency and duration of use.

▶ Table 34-3 lists examples of the wide variety of oral consequences of tobacco use; periodontal diseases and oral cancers provide the most serious destructive effects.

▶ A systematic extraoral/intraoral examination is the most efficient and effective method for detecting tobacco-related conditions in and around the mouth.

▶ The extraoral/intraoral examination gives visual examples for use in encouraging the patient to start a tobacco cessation program.

TOBACCO AND PERIODONTAL INFECTIONS[1,30–39]

Tobacco use is a major risk factor for the development and progression of periodontitis. Users are at a high risk for developing more severe periodontitis at younger ages than nonusers.

I. Effects on the Periodontal Tissues

▶ *Gingivitis*
  • The degree of inflammatory response to dental biofilm accumulation is reduced compared with that in nonsmokers.
  • Smoking may affect treatment and therapeutic outcomes for plaque-induced gingivitis.

▶ *Periodontitis in tobacco users*
  • Increased rate and severity of periodontal destruction.
  • Increased bone loss, attachment loss, and pocket depths.
  • Gingival blood flow and gingival crevicular flow are diminished.
  • Increased tooth loss from periodontal causes.
  • Increased prevalence with increased number of exposures to tobacco.
  • Prevalence and severity lessen with cessation.[40]

II. Mechanisms of Periodontal Destruction

▶ No effect on the rate of dental biofilm accumulation.

▶ Host response: lowered immune response.

▶ Impaired neutrophils: decreased chemotaxis, phagocytosis, and adherence.

▶ Altered antibody production; decreased serum IgG.

▶ Impairment of revascularization; disruption of immune response; impact on healing; increased risk of periodontal disease.

▶ Negative effect on bone metabolism; after menopause, women smokers have a deficit in bone density; smoking can influence osteoporosis.

TABLE 34-3	Oral Consequences of Tobacco Use				
CANCER AND PRECANCER	**PERIODONTAL FACTORS**	**SOFT TISSUE PROBLEMS**	**HARD TISSUE PROBLEMS**	**ESTHETIC FACTORS**	**EXCERBATION— ORAL SIGNS IN SYSTEMIC DISEASES**
Squamous cell leukoplakia (ST)[a] Homogeneous Nonhomogeneous Verrucous	acute necrotizing ulcerative gingivitis (ANUG) and acute necrotizing ulcerative periodontitis (ANUP) Relapse during maintenance Increased risk for peri-implantitis and peri-implant bone loss Localized recession and clinical attachment loss	Nicotine stomatitis (P) Smoker's melanosis Black hairy tongue Median rhomboid glossitis Median rhomboid glossitis Median rhomboid glossitis Leukodema (P) Hyperkeratosis (ST) Dry socket Delayed wound healing	Occlusal or incisal abrasion (P), (ST) Cervical abrasion (ST) Dehiscence of bone (ST) Tooth loss	Halitois Dental stains Prosthesis stains Orthodontic appliance stains Discoloration of restorations Impaired taste and smell	HIV/AIDS Type 1 and Type 2 diabetes

[a]Abbreviations: mainly associated with P = pipe; ST = smokeless tobacco; no notation = smoked tobacco.

III. Response to Treatment[36,41–44]

▶ People who use tobacco products have a weakened response to conventional therapy.

▶ Smoking has a negative impact on bone regeneration after periodontal therapy.

▶ Implants have greater risk for failure due to implantitis.

▶ Delayed healing after surgical and nonsurgical procedures.

NICOTINE ADDICTION[1,9,45,46]

▶ Nicotine is tobacco's psychoactive agent (one that produces feelings of pleasure and well-being), and its use leads to tolerance, dependence, and addiction.

▶ No one starts using tobacco to become addicted to it.

▶ Users seldom can explain why they use tobacco but often say that it helps their physical performance, mood, or ability to think. In fact, physical performance does not improve, mood is not better, and intellectual stimulation is minor.

I. Tolerance

▶ *Physiologic adaptation*
  • Tolerance refers to the user's need for more smoking or chewing the same amount of the same product over time as it becomes less and less effective in creating the desired feeling of well-being.

▶ *Amount of use*
  • To sustain the positive feelings associated with tobacco use, more and more has to be taken as time goes by.

II. Dependence

▶ *Characteristics*
  • As increased amounts are needed over time, the loss of control over the amount and frequency of tobacco use show evidence of dependence.
  • Facts about nicotine dependency are included in Box 34-3, and criteria for nicotine dependency are outlined in Box 34-4.

▶ *Reinforcing effect*
  • Nicotine intensifies the release of dopamine by the brain, thereby increasing a feeling of pleasure and the compulsion to use tobacco.
  • Positive reinforcement is produced with tobacco use, and abrupt stopping produces withdrawal symptoms.

III. Addiction

▶ The US Federal Court has ruled tobacco companies to make the following statements regarding nicotine addiction and nicotine manipulation:

BOX 34-3

Facts About Nicotine Dependency

▷ In 2012, the first federally funded media education Tips from Former Smokers campaign debuted. An estimated 1.6 million quit attempts were attributed to this campaign.

▷ Nicotine addiction is similar to that produced by other substances such as alcohol, cocaine, and heroin.

▷ Those who have a high tolerance to nicotine experience less nausea and dizziness following initial use.

▷ Tobacco abuse: Any use of tobacco products is considered a health hazard. Therefore, the use of any amount is considered abuse.

▷ Nicotine addiction may be the most challenging of all addictions for complete recovery.

▷ On average over half of smokers have attempted to quit for more than 1 day.

▷ Many tobacco users make many unsuccessful quit attempts before stopping use for indefinite or extended periods of time.

▷ Successfully quitting smokeless tobacco use may be equally or more difficult than stopping smoking. Smokeless tobacco is not considered a viable alternative for smokers who can quit.

Source: American Psychiatric Association. *Diagnostic and Statistical Manual of Mental Disorders (DSM-IV)*. 5th ed. Washington, DC: American Psychiatric Association; 2013:571–589; Agaku IT, King BA, Dube SR; and Centers for Disease Control and Prevention (CDC). Current cigarette smoking among adults—United States, 2005–2012. *MMWR Morb Mortal Wkly Rep.* 2014;63(2):29–34.

BOX 34-4

Criteria for Nicotine Dependency

▷ Tolerance:
  ▷ A need for markedly increased amounts of the substance to achieve intoxication or desired effect.
  ▷ Markedly diminished effect with continued use of the same amount.

▷ Withdrawal, as manifested by either:
  ▷ Daily use of nicotine for several weeks.
  ▷ Abrupt stopping or reducing nicotine may result in four or more of the signs of nicotine withdrawal found in Box 34-5 and they will occur within 24 hours.

▷ Used in greater amounts over longer period of time than intended.

▷ A persistent desire or unsuccessful efforts to cut down or quit.

▷ A great deal of time spent using the substance.

▷ Giving up important social, occupational, or recreational activities because of use of the substance.

▷ Continued use despite knowledge of medical problems related to use and/or social and legal problems resulting from use.

Source: American Psychiatric Association. *Diagnostic and Statistical Manual of Mental Disorders (DSM-IV)*. 5th ed. Washington, DC: American Psychiatric Association; 2013:571–589.

Here is the truth: smoking is highly addictive. Nicotine is the addictive drug in tobacco;

Cigarette companies intentionally designed cigarettes with enough nicotine to create and sustain addiction;

It's not easy to quit;

When you smoke, the nicotine actually changes the brain— that is why quitting is so hard;

Defendant tobacco companies intentionally designed cigarettes to make them more addictive;

Cigarette companies control the impact and delivery of nicotine in many ways, including designing filters and selecting cigarette paper to maximize the ingestion of nicotine, adding ammonia to make the cigarette taste less harsh, and controlling the physical and chemical make-up of the tobacco blend.[47]

Addiction is a chronic, progressive, relapsing disease characterized by compulsive use of a substance.

▶ The effects result in physical, psychological, and/or social harm to the user, but use continues despite that harm.

▶ Smoking is more addictive than alcohol and other drugs of abuse in terms of the proportion of those who are exposed and subsequently become dependent.

▶ The pattern of relapse is identical for tobacco, alcohol, and heroin.

▶ Factors affecting the development of addiction include:
  • Properties of psychoactive drug (dose).
  • Family, peer influences, and social acceptance.
  • Existing psychiatric disorders.
  • Cost and availability of the drug.
  • Influence of advertising.

IV. Withdrawal[2,11,45]

▶ Withdrawal refers to the effects of cessation of nicotine use by an individual in whom dependence is established.

▶ When users of nicotine products stop abruptly, within 24 hours they can experience maximal physical and/or psychological withdrawal symptoms.

▶ Box 34-5 identifies typical nicotine withdrawal symptoms.

▶ *Duration*
  • Patients experience withdrawal symptoms almost immediately, and relapse within a week is common.
  • Most symptoms diminish over a few weeks when relapse does not occur.

▶ Cravings for tobacco, increased appetite, and weight gain may persist for months or years.

▶ *Alleviation of symptoms*
  • Table 34-4 lists activities that help to overcome withdrawal symptoms.
  • The goal is to prevent relapse.

TREATMENT[1,2,48]

Tobacco cessation methods or treatment for nicotine addiction fall into two categories: *self-help* and *assisted strategies*.

BOX 34-5
Criteria for Nicotine Withdrawal Syndrome

▷ Dysphoric or depressed mood
▷ Insomnia
▷ Irritability, frustration, and anger
▷ Anxiety
▷ Difficulty concentrating
▷ Restlessness
▷ Decreased heart rate
▷ Increased appetite or weight gain
▷ Cravings for tobacco

Source: American Psychiatric Association. *Diagnostic and Statistical Manual of Mental Disorders (DSM-IV).* 5th ed. Washington, DC: American Psychiatric Association; 2013:571–589.

I. Reasons for Quitting

Success cannot be expected unless the individual makes a concentrated effort and believes in the significance of the effort. Typical reasons include the following:

▶ General health awareness

▶ Specific health problem directly or indirectly related to tobacco use

▶ Effect on family
  • Need to act as a role model
  • Awareness of effects of ETS

▶ Effect of smoking and/or ETS on fetus during pregnancy

▶ Cost

▶ Social pressure and restrictions on smoking in many settings

▶ Personal recognition of the dangers of nicotine addiction and the desire to regain control of one's life.

II. Self-Help Interventions[1,49,50]

About one-third of adult smokers attempt to quit, but only 2%–3% are able to achieve long-term abstinence on their own. The proportion of attempts and successes is similar among high-school students.

▶ Go cold turkey. Consider changing lifestyle, including exercise and diet modifications.

▶ Reduce number of daily tobacco exposures

▶ Select over-the-counter (OTC) nicotine replacement patches, gum, or lozenges.

▶ Join a family member or friend in the tobacco cessation effort.

III. Assisted Strategies[2,51–54]

▶ *Counseling*
  • Provision of practical counseling, including problem solving and skills training.
  • Provision of intratreatment social support: "Our office staff and I are willing to assist you."

TABLE 34-4	Alleviating Nicotine Withdrawal Symptoms
SYMPTOMS	**ACTIVITIES**
Mood changes; anxiety, nervousness, stressed feelings	Breathe deeply; exhale through pursed lips. Take a walk or other relaxation exercise. Know your triggers, get more rest, and take multivitamin. Make a list of things to do instead of smoking. Avoid places where you most commonly used tobacco.
Sleep disturbances	Avoid caffeine, drink a glass of warm milk instead. Avoid alcohol. Take a long walk before bed. Avoid naps, take a warm bath or meditate. Read a book, listen to soothing music.
Appetite increase	Eat only when you are hungry. Eat low-fat, low-calorie snacks. Chew sugarless gum or eat sugarless hard flavorful candy. Drink additional glasses of water. Exercise.
Cravings	*Delay smoking or dipping*: Use tactics such as waiting 1 more minute; often cravings pass in 5 or 10 min. *Distract yourself*: Exercise; take a walk; call a friend. *Drink water*: to fight off cravings. *Deep breaths*: Relax! Close your eyes and take 10 deep breaths; exhale through pursed lips. *Discuss your feelings*: with someone close to you or a support group.[a]

[a]National Advisory Committee on Health and Disability. Guidelines for Smoking Cessation, Revised 2002. Wellington, New Zealand: National Advisory Committee on Health and Disability (National Health Committee); May 2002.

Adapted from Fiore MC, Jaén CR, Baker TB, et al. Treating tobacco use and dependence: 2008 update. In: *Quick Reference Guide for Clinicians*. Rockville, MD: U.S. Department of Health and Human Services. Public Health Service; 2009.

▶ *Pharmacotherapies*

Table 34-5 provides an overview of FDA-approved first-line pharmacotherapies.

▶ *Combination*

Counseling combined with pharmacotherapy has been shown to be effective in helping patients to quit using tobacco.

PHARMACOTHERAPIES USED FOR TREATMENT OF NICOTINE ADDICTION[1,2,51–53]

I. Objectives and Rationale

▶ Make it easier to abstain from tobacco by partial replacement of nicotine or by counteracting nicotine's action.

▶ Reduce withdrawal symptoms.

▶ Fulfill, in part, the craving for tobacco by sustaining tolerance.

▶ Provide some effects (mood, cognitive changes) previously delivered from nicotine.

II. Considerations

▶ Discourage casual use of pharmacotherapies. Failure as a result of improper use can discourage future quit attempts.

▶ Inform patient of signs and symptoms of nicotine overdose: nausea, vomiting, dizziness, weakness, or rapid heartbeat.

▶ Consult primary care provider before use if younger than 18 years or contraindications are present.

III. Contraindications

▶ Self-medication without professional examination and advice.

▶ Pregnancy/breastfeeding: nicotine in the bloodstream, even in small amounts, can reach the fetus.

▶ Nicotine gum or lozenge: hypertension; using medication for asthma, depression, diabetes mellitus, cardiovascular disease, stomach ulcers.

▶ Nicotine patch: same as nicotine gum; in addition, some patients may be allergic to patch adhesives.

▶ Nicotine inhaler: same as nicotine gum; patients need to be cautious if allergy to menthol.

TABLE 34-5	Suggestions for the Clinical Use of Pharmacotherapies for Smoking Cessation				
PHARMACOTHERAPY	**PRECAUTIONS/ CONTRAINDICATIONS**	**SIDE EFFECTS**	**DOSAGE**	**DURATION**	**AVAILABILITY**
Bupropion SR	History of seizure History of eating disorder Using monoamine oxidase inhibitor	Insomnia dry mouth	Day 1–3: 150 mg each morning Day 4—end: twice daily; take evening dose 8 hr before sleep	Start 1–2 wk before quit date Use 2–6 mo	Zyban Wellbutrin SR Generic (prescription only)
Varenicline[b]	Kidney problems or on dialysis Has not been studied In pregnant or nursing women; FDA warning re: potential for agitation, depressed mood, atypical behavior, or suicidal thoughts	Nausea insomnia abnormal, vivid, or strange dreams Constipation, gas, and/or vomiting	Days 1–3: 0–5 mg once in morning Days 4–7: 0.5 mg twice daily Day 8 though end of treatment: 1 mg twice daily	Use 3–6 mo Start 1 wk before quit date	Chantix (prescription only)
Nicotine gum	Temporomandibular disorders disease Caution for denture wearers	Mouth soreness Dyspepsia Headaches	1–24 cigs/day 2 mg gum (up to 24 psc/day) 20+ cigs/day or smokeless tobacco—4 mg gum (up to 24 psc/day)[a]	Up to 12 wk Or as needed	Nicorette ■ Mint (3 kinds) ■ Fruit ■ Cinnamon ■ Original (OTC only) Generic available
Nicotine inhaler	Asthma COPD	Local irritation of mouth and throat	6–16 cartridges/day[a]	Up to 6 mo; taper at end	Nicotrol inhaler (prescription only)
Nicotine nasal spray	Nasal polyps Rhinitis Sinusitis Asthma	Nasal and throat irritation Dependence potential	8–40 doses/day (no more than 48 sprays in 24 hr)	3–6 mo; Taper at end	Nicotrol NS (prescription only)
Nicotine transdermal patch	Allergy to patch adhesive; Do not use if have severe eczema or psoriasis DO NOT CUT PATCHES	Local skin reaction Insomnia Changes in dreams Headache	One patch per day If 10 cigs/day: 21 mg 4 wk 14 mg 2–4 wk 7 mg 2–4 wk If <10/day: 14 mg 4 wk, then 7 mg 4 wk One patch per day	8–12 wk	Nicoderm CQ (OTC only) Generic patches (prescription and OTC) Nicotrol (OTC only)
Nicotine lozenge	One lozenge at a time	Mouth soreness Dyspepsia Nausea Headache Cough Hiccups Heartburn Flatulence	2 mg if smoke/chew after 30 min of waking; 4 mg if smoke/chew within 30 min of waking Maximum 20 lozenges in 24 hr[a]	3–6 mo Wk 1–6: 1 every 1–2 hr Wk 7–9: 1 every 2–4 hr; Wk 10–12: 1 every 4–8 hr	Commit ■ Mint ■ Cherry ■ Original (OTC only) Generic available

TABLE 34-5	Suggestions for the Clinical Use of Pharmacotherapies for Smoking Cessation (*continued*)				
PHARMACOTHERAPY	**PRECAUTIONS/ CONTRAINDICATIONS**	**SIDE EFFECTS**	**DOSAGE**	**DURATION**	**AVAILABILITY**
Nicotine mini lozenge	Same as above	Same as above	2 mg if smoke/chew after 30 min of waking; 4 mg if smoke/chew within 30 min of waking Maximum 24 mini lozenges/day[a]	Same as above	Nicorette mini ▪ Mint (OTC only)

[a]Nothing to eat or drink 15 min prior to or during use.

Adapted from Fiore MC, Jaén CR, Baker TB, et al. Treating tobacco use and dependence: 2008 update. In: *Quick Reference Guide for Clinicians*. Rockville, MD: U.S. Department of Health and Human Services. Public Health Service; 2009.

[b]Varenicline (Chantix) information. 2014 March 17. Available from: https://www.chantix.com/index.aspx

▶ Nicotine gum, lozenge, and inhaler: Avoid eating or drinking acidic beverages for 15 minutes before and during use due to decreased nicotine absorption.

IV. Nicotine Replacement Therapy (NRT)

▶ The objective of NRTs is to help prevent withdrawal symptoms and to promote tobacco cessation.

▶ NRTs are less likely to cause dependence when compared to tobacco products.

▶ Dental hygienists are in an ideal position to discuss the immediate delivery of nicotine to the brain during smoking and to educate patients about the differences in nicotine delivery of various NRTs, particularly those that are available OTC.

▶ *Nicotine gum*
  • *Transmucosal delivery*: Nicotine is released in the mouth during "chewing."
  • *Description*: Nicotine gum is sweetened with xylitol and has either a mild mint, cinnamon, or orange flavor.
  • *Directions*: Chew one piece slowly until tingling or peppery taste is achieved; "park" gum in buccal vestibule; resume chewing when peppery taste or tingle fades; and repeat chew/park activity.

▶ *Nicotine patch*
  • *Transdermal delivery*: Nicotine is released through skin.
  • *Directions*: Place a new patch on a hairless location upon rising; if sleep disruption occurs, remove 24-hour patch before bedtime or use 16-hour patch.

▶ *Nicotine inhaler*
  • *Transmucosal delivery*: Nicotine is released in mouth during inhalation or puffing; hold vapor in oral cavity for absorption, do not inhale.
  • *Requirements*: Store inhaler and cartridges in a warm place when temperatures drop below 40°F to prevent

a decline in delivery of nicotine from the inhaler to the oral cavity.

▶ *Nicotine nasal spray*
  • *Nasal mucous membrane delivery*: Nicotine is released through lining of nose.
  • *Dose delivery*: Avoid sniffing, swallowing, or inhaling while administering doses, as these increase irritating effects.
  • *Directions*: Tilt head slightly back while delivering spray.
  • *Precaution for heavy smoker*: Increased dose.

▶ *Nicotine lozenge*
  • *Transmucosal delivery*: Nicotine is released in mouth as lozenge dissolves.
  • *Description*: The lozenge is sweetened with mannitol and aspartame and flavored with a mild mint or cherry.
  • *Dose delivery*: see Table 34-5.
  • *Directions*: Do not bite or chew lozenge as it dissolves in the mouth; this can cause more nicotine to be swallowed quickly and may result in indigestion and/or heartburn.

NICOTINE-FREE THERAPY

I. Bupropion SR

▶ The first nonnicotine medication shown to be effective for tobacco cessation and approved by the FDA for that use.

▶ Mechanism of action is presumed to be mediated by its capacity to block neural uptake of dopamine and/or norepinephrine.

▶ Additional dosing information is listed in Table 34-5.

▶ Take second dose 8 hours after first and with evening meal to reduce sleep disturbances.

▶ Bupropion SR can be used in combination with NTRs.

II. Varenicline Tartrate

▶ The second nonnicotine medication shown to be effective for smoking cessation and approved by the FDA for that use.

▶ Mechanism of action is: a partial nicotine agonist (blocks nicotine receptors in brain). It also causes reduction in dopamine release.

- Always take after meals with full glass of water, to reduce nausea.
- Take second dose 8 hours after first and with evening meal to reduce sleep disturbances.
- Additional dosing information is listed in Table 34-5.

▶ Not currently recommended for use in combination with NTRs.

III. Combination Therapies

▶ Certain combinations of first-line medications have been shown to be effective smoking cessation treatments.

▶ Effective combination medications are:

- Long-term (>14 weeks) nicotine patch + nicotine gum or spray
- Nicotine patch + nicotine inhaler
- Nicotine patch + bupropion SR.

IV. Second-Line Medications

▶ Second-line medications are pharmacotherapies for which there is evidence of efficacy for treating tobacco dependence, but they have a more limited role because of the following reasons:

- The FDA has not approved them for a tobacco dependence treatment indication.
- There are more concerns about potential side effects than those exist with first-line medications.
- Second-line treatments, clonidine and nortriptyline, can be considered for use on a case-by-case basis after first-line treatments have been used or considered and while under a primary care provider's supervision.

DENTAL HYGIENE CARE FOR THE PATIENT WHO USES TOBACCO[2,55–57]

▶ The majority of people who smoke state they would like to quit, and almost half say that they have tried to quit in the past 12 months.

▶ The tobacco-using patient presents a unique challenge to the oral health team. Specific treatment modifications are indicated.

▶ Helping the patient to quit using tobacco becomes an integral part of the dental hygiene care plan.

ASSESSMENT

I. Patient History

▶ Tobacco use status is assessed at each appointment.

▶ The basic history form in Chapter 10 used by all patients includes one or two questions to determine whether the patient currently uses tobacco and, if so, the types of tobacco (smoking and/or smokeless). A tobacco use assessment form from the National Cancer Institute is shown in Figure 34-3.

▶ Concomitant use of alcohol and other psychoactive drugs, with tobacco may necessitate modifications of clinical procedures.

▶ Some health care providers consider tobacco use status as a vital sign along with temperature, pulse, respiratory rate, and blood pressure.[58]

II. Extraoral Examination[1,22]

▶ *Breath and body odor*
- Halitosis.
- Electropositive smoke: Smoke from cigars and other smoked tobacco products clings to skin, hair, and clothes and results in body odor.

▶ *Fingers*
Smokers of nonfiltered cigarettes have a yellowish-brown discoloration of the fingers and fingernails.

▶ *Skin*
Smokers experience premature and more extensive facial wrinkling.

▶ *Lips*
Pipe and cigar smokers are at risk for development of precancerous and cancerous lip lesions.

III. Intraoral Examination[18,19,59]

An excellent outline for conducting a thorough intraoral examination for the patient who uses tobacco is provided in Table 12-1, Chapter 12. Oral consequences of tobacco use are listed in Table 34-3.

▶ *Detection of an intraoral lesion or problem*
Upon detecting a problem or lesion that may or may not be tobacco related, the clinician will:

- *Show the patient:* Provide a simple but thorough explanation related to the nature of the condition.
- *Explain:* Make certain that the patient understands the consequences of continuing tobacco use as it relates to the progress of the problem or lesion.
- *Record:* Provide a detailed description of the problem or lesion and note the information given to the patient in the dental record for the dentist's review.

TOBACCO USE ASSESSMENT FORM

Name: _____   Date_____

1. Do you use tobacco in any form?   ☐ Yes ☐ No
1A. If no, have you ever used tobacco in the past?   ☐ Yes ☐ No
    How long did you use tobacco?   Years____   Months____
    How long ago did you stop?   Years____   Months____

If you are not currently a tobacco user, no other questions should be answered. Thank you for completing this form.

Question 2-10 are for current tobacco users only.

2. **If you smoke,** what type (check)   How many? (Number)
    ☐ Cigarettes   Cigarettes per day____
    ☐ Cigars   Cigars per day____
    ☐ Pipes   Bowls per day____
3. **If you chew/use snuff,** what type?   How much?
    ☐ Snuff   Days a can lasts____
    ☐ Chewing   Pouches per week____
    ☐ Other (describe)   Amount_____per_____
3A. **How long** do you keep a chew in your mouth? ____minutes
4. **How many days** of the week do you first use tobacco?   7 6 5 4 3 2 1
5. **How soon** after you wake do you first use tobacco?
    Within 30 minutes?____   More than 30 minutes?____
6. Does the person **closest to you** use tobacco?   ☐ Yes   ☐ No
7. **How interested are you** in stopping your use of tobacco?
    ☐ not at all ☐ a little ☐ somewhat ☐ Yes ☐ very much
8. Have you ever **tried to stop** using tobacco before?   ☐ Yes ☐ No
9. Have you **discussed stopping** with your physician?   ☐ Yes ☐ No
10. If you decided to stop using tobacco completely during the next two weeks, **how confident are you** that you would succeed?
    ☐ not at all ☐ a little ☐ somewhat ☐ very confident

FIGURE 34-3 Tobacco Use Assessment Form. (Reprinted from Mecklenburg, RE, Greenspan D, Kleinman DV, et al. *Tobacco Effects in the Mouth: A National Cancer Institute and National Institute of Dental Research Guide for Health Professionals.* Washington, DC: U.S. Department of Health and Human Services, National Institutes of Health; 2007. NIH Publication No. 07-3330.)

▶ *Referral indications*

If a lesion persists for more than 2 weeks, a biopsy is indicated (Chapter 12).
- *Refer* the patient for biopsy.
- *Ascertain:* Check to be certain that the patient undergoes the biopsy and receives results.
- *Consult:* Ensure the pathologist that reviews the biopsy provides the pertinent information.
- *Document:* Ensure that results are entered into the patient's treatment record.

▶ *Oral self-examination*
- It is imperative to teach oral self-examination to all patients who use tobacco. The significance of oral self-examination in this high-risk group cannot be overstated.
- Teach patients to perform an oral self-examination by using the same techniques and components of the professional extraoral and intraoral examinations.

▶ *Detect, relate, motivate*
- Lesions that are a potential direct consequence of tobacco use are pointed out to the patient.
- The presence of tobacco-related problems/lesions can serve as a powerful motivational tool to encourage a quit attempt.
- The demonstration of the arrest or elimination of tobacco-related problems/lesions as the patient continues a nonuse status will aid in achieving permanent cessation.

IV. Consultation

▶ Patients who do not seek routine medical care need referral to a primary care provider for evaluation.
▶ Detection of underlying medical problems is essential so that necessary dental treatment modifications may be utilized.

CLINICAL TREATMENT PROCEDURES[1,57]

▶ Patients who use tobacco may require longer and more frequent appointments due to the presence of increased risk for the following:
- dental stain
- calculus
- dental caries
- periodontal problems.

I. Dental Biofilm Control

▶ Self-care for daily dental biofilm control is the first priority in the care plan.

▶ Immaculate oral hygiene is required by this group of high-risk patients owing to their susceptibility to dental caries, periodontal infections, and other soft-tissue alterations.

II. Nonsurgical Periodontal Therapy[44,60]

▶ Inform the patient that healing will be jeopardized by continued tobacco use and users cannot expect the same treatment results as nonusers.

▶ Inform the patient that tobacco cessation would improve the results of treatment.

▶ When using power-driven instruments:
- Take precautions to protect the patient from aerosols containing bacteria and debris (smokers often have pulmonary and cardiovascular complications).[1]
- Other precautions may be necessary when using power instrumentation (as described in Chapter 41).

III. Other Patient Instruction

▶ *Diet and nutrition*
- Tobacco users may be poorly nourished because tobacco use decreases appetite. Conversely, the desire to control body weight through tobacco use may impede a patient's willingness to quit.
- Suggestions about diet and exercise are included as a part of the cessation program.
- Most smokeless tobacco products are sweetened with sugar or molasses, which increases cariogenic potential. Appropriate instruction is needed.

TOBACCO CESSATION PROGRAM[1,2,53,61,62]

▶ A program for tobacco cessation is an essential component of the dental hygiene care plan for all tobacco using patients.

▶ The treatment of tobacco use and dependence will often require multiple appointments, repeated interventions, and multiple attempts to quit.

▶ The dental setting provides an excellent opportunity to assist tobacco users in tobacco cessation.

▶ The majority of users admit that they would like to quit or "know" that they need to, and about one-third of them are willing to try.

▶ Interventions and their outcomes will vary depending on the motivation and experience of the clinician and the patient's acceptance of, and adherence to, the regimen.

▶ Even a minimal intervention conducted by a clinician may help a patient become tobacco free.

MOTIVATIONAL INTERVIEWING[61]

Motivational interviewing techniques, described in Chapter 26, can be useful in conversing with patients concerning behavior change.

THE "5 A'S"[1,2]

The "5 A's"—ask, advise, assess, assist, arrange—provide the basis for a brief, simple, but effective tobacco dependence intervention for clinicians.[41] A cessation program flowchart is presented in Figure 34-4.

I. Ask

▶ *Health history*
- Ask all patients about tobacco use.
- Include questions about tobacco use on the health history (Health History Form in Chapter 10) and document tobacco use at every appointment.

▶ *Present questions carefully*
- During review of the health history, present questions related to tobacco use nonjudgmentally.
- Address tobacco use as a health issue, not as a moral and/or social issue.
- Obtain facts without placing the patient on the defensive.

▶ *Obtain patient's confidence*
- Express empathy and support patient's decision to choose or reject change.
- Social disapproval of tobacco use is increasing, and patients may hesitate to disclose their habit.

▶ *Children and adolescents*[1,5,63–65]
- The two greatest factors that impact a child or adolescent smoking are parents who smoke and parental nicotine dependence.
- Education and brief counseling needs to be implemented to prevent initiation of tobacco use.
- In the United States 9% of school-aged children reported smoking a whole cigarette before 13 years of age.
- Many minors use tobacco without their parents' knowledge or consent.

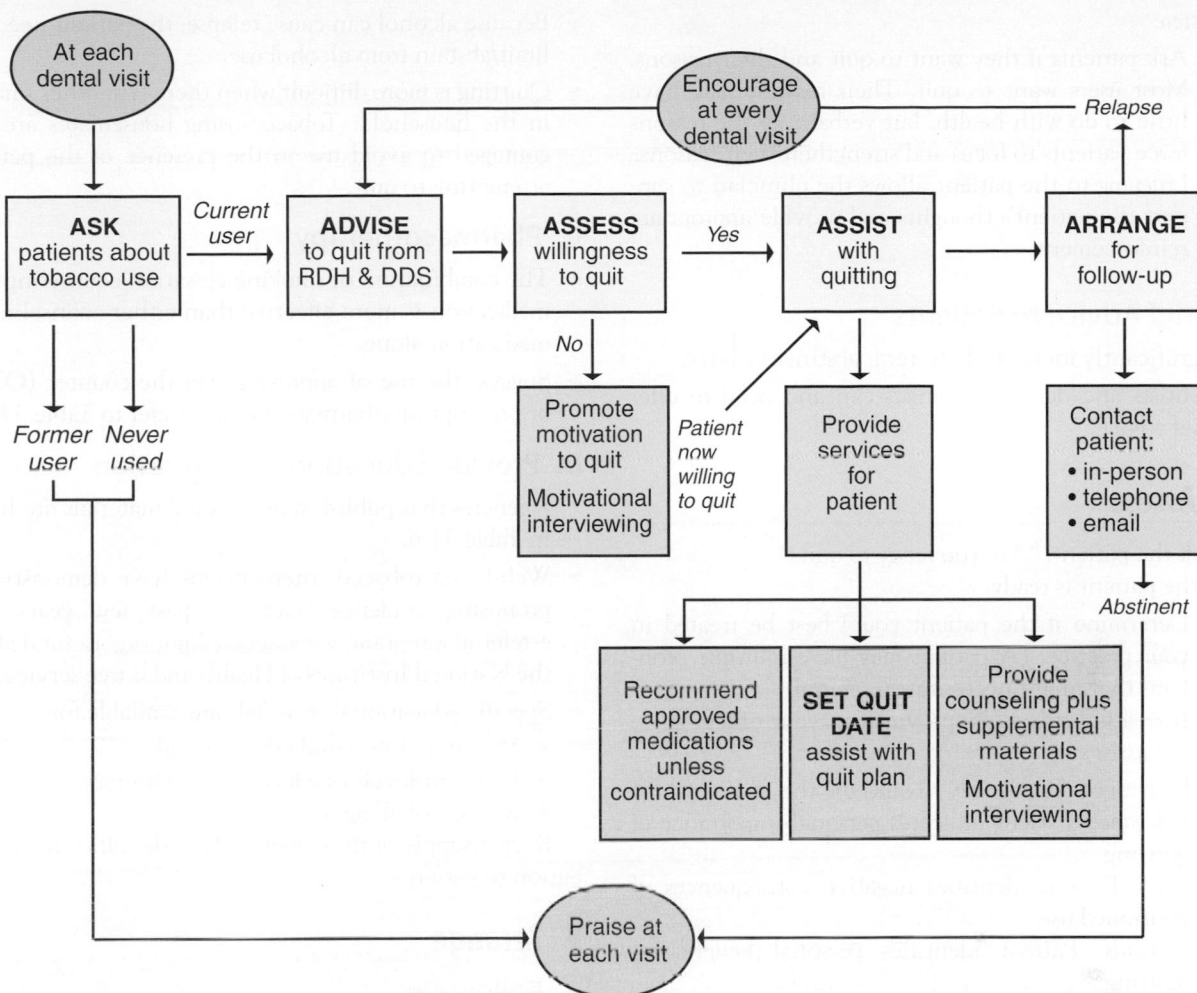

FIGURE 34-4 Tobacco Cessation Flowchart. Flowchart to show how the 5 A's can be incorporated into the clinical setting. (Adapted from Fiore MC, Jaén CR, Baker TB, et al. Treating tobacco use and dependence: 2008 update. In: *Quick Reference Guide for Clinicians*. Rockville, MD: U.S. Department of Health and Human Services. Public Health Service; 2009.)

- Most smokers try their first cigarette at approximately 11 years of age.
- Tobacco companies develop advertisement campaigns to portray tobacco use as cool.
- Children need to hear negative impact messages that counter messages produced by the tobacco industry.
- Ask parents about tobacco use in the home.
- Discuss with the parents, the effects of ETS on health, developmental risks, and how tobacco use sets a bad example for children.

II. Advise

A. Never Users/Former Users

▶ Advise every patient about tobacco use.

▶ Praise "never users" and "former users" for their tobacco-free behavior.

▶ Reinforcement counters the tobacco industry's message and other enticements to begin tobacco use and can help prevent relapse.

B. Current Users: Stop–Look–Listen Approach

1. *Stop now*: Clearly advise the patient about the importance of *stopping* now. Present the advice in a caring, compassionate manner so that patients realize that clinicians are interested in their health and well-being.

2. *Show*: Have patients *look* in their mouths during the initial oral examination to observe the clinical effects of tobacco use.

- Patients may or may not be impressed by a discussion of possible future health problems or of the effect of tobacco use on others.
- Advice needs to be relevant to existing conditions.
- Existing oral conditions that may serve as strong motivators to quit include:
  - Extrinsic stain
  - Supragingival calculus accumulation
  - Halitosis
  - Gingival and/or periodontal infection
  - Soft-tissue lesions

3. *Listen*:
- Ask patients if they want to quit and their reasons. Most users want to quit. Their reasons may have little to do with health, but verbalizing the reasons force patients to focus and strengthen their reasons.
- *Listening* to the patient allows the clinician to support the patient's thoughts and provide appropriate reinforcement.

C. Brief Advice to Patients

▶ Significantly increases long-term abstinence rates.

▶ Dentists and dental hygienists can and need to offer brief advice.

III. Assess

1. Ask the patient: "Are you ready to quit?"
2. If the patient is ready:
- Determine if the patient could best be treated in your practice. (A patient may have multiple problems that might necessitate a referral.)
- If treatment is to be provided in your office, go to the *assist* step.
3. If the patient is not ready to quit, use the "5 R's":
- *Relevance*: Patient indicates personal importance of quitting.
- *Risks*: Patient identifies negative consequences of continued use.
- *Rewards*: Patient identifies personal benefits of quitting.
- *Roadblocks*: Patient identifies barriers to quitting and clinician helps address barriers.
- *Repetition*: Reinforce the motivational message at every visit.

IV. Assist

A. Establish a Quit Plan

▶ Set a quit date, preferably within 2 weeks.

▶ Have the patient tell family, friends, and coworkers about quitting and request their understanding and support.

▶ Warn the patient to anticipate challenges to the planned quit attempt, particularly during the first few weeks. This includes nicotine withdrawal symptoms.

▶ Ask the patient to remove all tobacco-related products from home and work sites.

B. Provide Practical Counseling

▶ Total abstinence is essential: "not even a single puff or dip after the quit date."

▶ Review past quit attempts and identify what helped and what factors contributed to relapse.

▶ Discuss challenges/triggers and how the patient will overcome them successfully.

▶ Because alcohol can cause relapse, the patient needs to limit/abstain from alcohol use.

▶ Quitting is more difficult when there is another smoker in the household. Tobacco-using housemates are encouraged to avoid use in the presence of the patient attempting to quit.

C. Pharmacotherapy

▶ The combination of smoking cessation counseling and medication is more effective than either counseling or medication alone.

▶ Suggest the use of approved over-the-counter (OTC) or prescription pharmacotherapy. Refer to Table 34-5.

D. Provide Educational Information

▶ Agencies that publish motivational materials are listed in Table 34-6.

▶ Web-based tobacco interventions have demonstrated promising evidence over the past few years. An e-referral program www.decide2quit.org is funded by the National Institutes of Health and is free service.[66,67]

▶ Specific educational materials are available for
- Various cultures and ethnic groups.
- Different levels of education and literacy.
- Readers of all ages.

Keep a supply of these materials in the office for distribution to patients.

V. Arrange

A. Follow-up

▶ Essential for successful quit rates.

▶ Provide written documentation as a reminder, listing their quit date.

▶ Suggest posting quit-date reminders in visible locations such as refrigerator door or bathroom mirror or placing index card with the quit date between cellophane and paper of the cigarette package.

B. Contact the Patient Before the Quit Date

▶ Assure patient of care provider's sincere interest in their tobacco cessation attempt via telephone call or e-mail.

▶ Inquire:
- If information provided at initial contact has been helpful.
- If there are any questions regarding the information received.

▶ *Follow-up contact*
- Follow-up, either in person or via telephone or e-mail.
- Timely intervals would be once within the first week after the quit date when the patient's physical withdrawal symptoms are most intense, and again at the end of the first, second, and third months of their tobacco cessation.

TABLE 34-6	Sources for Tobacco Cessation Patient Educational Materials		
NAME OF SOURCE		**QUIT LINES**	**LINKS**
American Cancer Society		1–877—yes quit 1–877—937–7848	www.yesquit.com www.cancer.org
American Lung Association			www.lungusa.org
National Cancer Institute			www.cancer.gov
CDC Tobacco Information and Prevention Tips			www.cdc.gov/tobacco/
Nicotine Anonymous			www.nicotine-anonymous.org
QuitNet			www.quitnet.com
National Alliance for Tobacco Cessation			www.becomeanex.org
You Can Quit Smoking—Agency for Healthcare Research and Quality			www.ahrq.gov/consumer/tobacco
Smokefree.gov		National Quit Line 1–800—Quit-Now (1–800–784–8669)	www.smokefree.gov
American Dental Hygienists' Association (Ask. Advise. Refer)			www.adha.org

- More than four contacts with patient help to increase long-term abstinence.
- Follow-up at regularly scheduled continuing care appointments.

▶ *Actions during follow-up contact*

- Congratulate and praise patients who have remained tobacco free.
- Provide the opportunity for patients to ask questions. If they have none, encourage the patient to contact you if questions arise.
- If relapse has occurred, ask the patient to recall and record the circumstances that led to reuse.
- Encourage the patient to set another quit date, reminding the patient that a lapse can be a learning experience.
- Review the use of pharmacotherapy.
- Provide agencies and local contact numbers for the patient who requests a more intensive cessation program.

THE TEAM APPROACH[2,53]

Evidence concludes that oral health professionals are more effective than other healthcare professionals in providing tobacco cessation interventions.[53]

I. Organize the Clinic Team

▶ *Select a team coordinator*

The coordinator does not do everything, but sees that everything is done.

▶ *Responsibilities*

- Identify tobacco use status at patient's first visit.
- Record appropriate documentation in patient's records.
- Ensure that all tobacco-using patients are offered the opportunity to enter a cessation program.
- Contact patients for follow-up.
- Act as a coach for patients who relapse.
- Maintain a supply of literature for patients.

▶ *Team members*

Tobacco users are interviewed to determine readiness to quit and are encouraged to enter a cessation program.

II. Organize a Tobacco-Free Environment

▶ Remove ashtrays and post "Thank you for not smoking" signs.
▶ Display tobacco use prevention and cessation materials prominently.
▶ Eliminate magazines that contain tobacco advertising from reception area.

III. Organize a Tobacco User Tracking System

▶ *Tobacco use assessment form:* Figure 34-3.
▶ *Patient permanent progress report:* Records include dated case notes for all advice to quit, responses and interest in quitting, and progress.
▶ *Tobacco status on records:* Clearly mark records (paper or electronic) so that status can be immediately seen by any clinic staff.

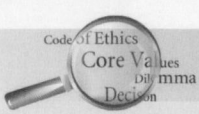

EVERYDAY ETHICS

Fifteen-year-old Jason comes with his mother for a regular maintenance appointment. During the oral examination, Edith, the dental hygienist who has been providing dental hygiene treatment for Jason and his family for many years, notices small red and white patches in the vestibular areas of the mandible adjacent to the molar teeth. She also records moderate brownish staining on the teeth and plans to use the air-powder polisher after scaling. She questions Jason about smoking and the use of smokeless tobacco, but he states that he has tried cigarettes only once or twice.

Questions for Consideration

1. What approach can Edith use to further assess and enhance Jason's understanding of the oral effects of tobacco use if she suspects he is not telling the truth?

2. What alternatives does Edith have in reporting her assessment findings that will maintain Jason's right to confidentiality but still inform his mother of the potentially serious oral tissue changes she has observed?

3. Which legal and ethical concepts, listed in Table VII-1 in the Section VII Introduction, apply to this situation?

BOX 34-6

Example Documentation: Tobacco Use Assessment and Cessation Treatment

S –A 45-year old African American male presents for second quadrant scaling, upper left (UL) with local anesthesia, and postscaling evaluation of first quadrant, upper right (UR). Cigarette smoker for 15 years; 1–2 packs a day. Patient states his oral self-care has improved since the initial quadrant scaling. Patient's chief complaint: Gums still sore from previous scaling appointment.

O –Intraoral assessment reveals slow healing for first quadrant scaling with localized inflammation and erythematous areas, evidence of nicotine stomatitis, other oral cancer finding negative, and no cavitated carious lesions charted. Periodontal exam findings: UL quadrant with generalized 5–6 mm pocket depths, and 7 mm pocket on #15 MB, bleeding on probing #14 and 15 buccal.

A –Patient presents with a high risk for oral and systemic disease due to tobacco dependence. Provided patient with smoking cessation basics, and explanation of oral and systemic effects of tobacco use. Brief discussion indicated patient is motivated to quit because he and his wife are expecting their first baby, but reports previous attempts to quit "Cold Turkey" were unsuccessful due to weight gain, mood swings, and increased stress.

P –Patient congratulated on wanting to quit, and reminded that previous attempts at quitting should not be looked upon as failures. Introduced various options for cessation support. Patient agreed to Internet option www.smokefree.gov, with quitting apps; walked patient through the website. Additionally, patient agreed to 21 mg nicotine transdermal patch, transitioning to 14 mg, then 7 mg patch over 8–10 weeks, combining patch therapy with nicotine gum to help prevent weight gain and provide relief for additional withdrawal symptoms and cravings. Follow-up by telephone in 1 week and re-evaluate at next visit scheduled in 2 weeks.

Next Visit: Scale lower right quadrant with local anesthesia, reassess UL quadrant, and continue tobacco cessation counseling.

Signed: _____, RDH

Date: _____

ADVOCACY[1]

I. Public Health Policy

▶ The Surgeon General's Report on Oral Health was the first report of a Surgeon General that focused on oral health and the report specifically identified tobacco use as a risk factor for oral cavity and pharyngeal cancer.[68]

▶ Healthcare providers can help tobacco users quit and can become partners with one another and with community programs to prevent diseases and promote good health habits.

▶ The Centers for Disease Control and Prevention has been supporting state-based tobacco control coalitions in all 50 states. Many local communities and municipalities are considering or have adopted smoke-free workplace ordinances.

▶ Oral health professionals can be valuable and collaborative partners in these programs.

II. Community Oral Health Educational Programs

No community oral health program can be considered complete without inclusion of tobacco prevention, control, and cessation education. Excellent materials are available from many nonprofit and professional organizations.

DOCUMENTATION

▶ Careful and complete documentation of tobacco use is a component of each patient assessment. It is part of the health history for new patients and part of the clinical (progress) notes for maintenance patients.

▶ Include tobacco history and/or current use, type of tobacco, and amount typically used.

▶ Age, ethnicity, gender, periodontal, and overall dental status as well as oral cancer screening findings.

▶ Patient interest/confidence motivation/readiness to quit and previous quit attempts and techniques used.

▶ Options for cessation presented to patient and referrals to primary care provider for examination/treatment.

▶ Box 34-6 contains an example for tobacco use assessment and cessation treatment.

Factors To Teach The Patient

▷ The most effective method to stop using tobacco is never to start.

▷ How to perform a regular self-examination of the oral cavity.

▷ Pregnant women who use tobacco products can harm the developing fetus and the newborn infant.

▷ Young children may experiment with or use tobacco products. Parents can be educated so they are prepared to provide guidance.

▷ All forms of social tobacco use can lead to addiction.

▷ Nonsmokers who breathe ETS can incur the same serious health problems as smokers; children are especially susceptible.

▷ Smokeless tobacco use is *not* a safe alternative to smoking.

▷ Oral health team members can help patients become tobacco free.

▷ Learn about local or state tobacco legislation and public health policy to make informed choices related to a tobacco smoke-free society.

References

1. U.S. Department of Health and Human Services. *The Health Consequences of Smoking—50 Years of Progress: A Report of the Surgeon General*. Rockville, MD: Office of the Surgeon General; 2014.

2. Fiore MC, Jaen CR, Baker TB, et al. Treating tobacco use and dependence: 2008 update. In: *Quick Reference Guide for Clinicians*. Rockville, MD: U.S. Department of Health and Human Services, Public Health Service; 2009.

3. Agaku IT, King BA, Husten CG, et al. Tobacco product use among adults—United States, 2012–2013. *MMWR Morb Mortal Wkly Rep*. 2014;63:1–6.

4. Agrawal A, Scherrer JF, Grant JD, et al. The effects of maternal smoking during pregnancy on offspring outcomes. *Prev Med*. 2010;50(1/2):13–18.

5. U.S. Department of Health and Human Services. *Preventing Tobacco Use Among Youth and Young Adults: A Report of the Surgeon General*. Rockville, MD: Office of the Surgeon General; 2012.

6. U.S. Department of Health and Human Services. *Women and Smoking: A Report of the Surgeon General*. Atlanta, GA: U.S. Department of Health and Human Services, Office on Smoking, Centers for Disease Control and Prevention, National Center for Chronic Disease Prevention and Health Promotion; 2001.

7. American Cancer Society. Cancer facts and figures. http://www.cancer.org/research/cancerfactsstatistics/cancerfacts-figures2014/. Updated 2014. Accessed June 20, 2014.

8. Benowitz NL, Hukkanen J, Jacob P. Nicotine chemistry, metabolism, kinetics, and biomarkers. *Handb Exp Pharmacol*. 2009;192:29–60.

9. Maisto SA, Galizio M, Connors GJ. *Drug Use and Abuse*. 7th ed. Stamford, CT: Cengage Learning; 2014:144–172.

10. Office on Smoking and Health. Centers for Disease Control and Prevention (CDC). *The Health Consequences of Involuntary Exposure to Tobacco Smoke: A Report of the Surgeon General*. Atlanta, GA: Centers for Disease Control and Prevention; 2006:29.

11. U.S. Department of Health and Human Services. How Tobacco Smoke Causes Disease: The Biology and Behavioral Basis for Smoking-Attributable Disease: A Report of the Surgeon General. Atlanta, GA: U.S. Department of Health and Human Services, Office on Smoking and Health, Centers for Disease Control and Prevention, National Center for Chronic Disease Prevention and Health Promotion; 2010.

12. Food and Drug Administration. Harmful and potentially harmful constituents in tobacco products and tobacco smoke; established list. Federal Register. 2012. FDA-2012-N-0143(77).

13. Djordjevic MV, Doran KA. Nicotine content and delivery across tobacco products. *Handb Exp Pharmacol*. 2009;(192):61–82.

14. World Health Organization (WHO). Waterpipe Tobacco Smoking: Health Effects, Research Needs, and Recommended Actions by Regulators. Geneva: WHO Tobacco Free Initiative; 2005.

15. National Cancer Institute at the National Institutes of Health, ed. *Monograph 2: Smokeless Tobacco or Health: An International Perspective* [Smoking and Tobacco Control Monographs]. Bethesda, MD: US Department of Health and Human Services; 1992.

16. U.S. Food and Drug Administration. Electronic cigarettes (e-cigarettes). http://www.fda.gov/newsevents/publichealth-focus/ucm172906.htm. Updated 2014. Accessed March 20, 2014.

17. U.S. Food and Drug Administration. Summary of results: laboratory analysis of electronic cigarettes conducted by FDA. http://www.fda.gov/NewsEvents/Public Health Focus/ucm173146.htm. Updated 2009. Accessed March 20, 2014.

18. National Institute of Dental and Craniofacial Research. Oral cancer. http://www.nidcr.nih.gov/oralhealth/Topics/OralCancer/. Updated 2013. Accessed April 26, 2014.

19. National Cancer Institute at the National Institutes of Health. What you need to know about oral cancer. U.S. Department of Health and Human Services. NIH Publication No. 09-1574.

20. National Cancer Institute at the National Institutes of Health. *Health Effects of Exposure to Environmental Tobacco Smoke: The Report of the California Environmental Protection Agency*. Smoking and Tobacco Control Monograph No 10. Bethesda, MD: U.S. Department of Health and Human Services, Public Health Service, National Institutes of Health, National Cancer Institute; 1999:ES-3-10.

21. Sleiman M, Gundel LA, Pankow JF, et al. Formation of carcinogens indoors by surface-mediated reactions of nicotine with nitrous acid, leading to potential thirdhand

smoke hazards. *Proc Natl Acad Sci USA.* 2010;107(15): 6576–6581.

22. Schick SF, Farraro KF, Perrino C, et al. Thirdhand cigarette smoke in an experimental chamber: evidence of surface deposition of nicotine, nitrosamines and polycyclic aromatic hydrocarbons and de novo formation of NNK. *Tob Control.* 2014;23(2):152–159.

23. Hackshaw A, Rodeck C, Boniface S. Maternal smoking in pregnancy and birth defects: a systematic review based on 173 687 malformed cases and 11.7 million controls. *Hum Reprod Update.* 2011;17(5):589–604.

24. Cornelius MD, Day NL. The effects of tobacco use during and after pregnancy on exposed children. *Alcohol Res Health.* 2000;24(4):242–249.

25. Centers for Disease Control and Prevention (CDC). Vital signs: nonsmokers' exposure to secondhand smoke—United States, 1999–2008. *MMWR Morb Mortal Wkly Rep.* 2010;59(35):1141–1146.

26. Tong VT, Dietz PM, Morrow B, et al. Trends in smoking before, during, and after pregnancy—pregnancy risk assessment monitoring system, United States, 40 sites, 2000–2010. *MMWR Morb Mortal Wkly Rep.* 2013;62(6):1–19.

27. Burke H, Leonardi-Bee J, Hashim A, et al. Prenatal and passive smoke exposure and incidence of asthma and wheeze: systematic review and meta-analysis. *Pediatrics.* 2012;129(4):735–744.

28. Leonardi-Bee J, Jere ML, Britton J. Exposure to parental and sibling smoking and the risk of smoking uptake in childhood and adolescence: a systematic review and meta-analysis. *Thorax.* 2011;66(10):847–855.

29. American Academy of Pediatrics Task Force on Sudden Infant Death Syndrome. SIDS and other sleep-related infant deaths: expansion of recommendations for a safe infant sleeping environment. *Pediatrics.* 2011;128(5): 1030–1039.

30. Johannsen A, Susin C, Gustafsson A. Smoking and inflammation: evidence for a synergistic role in chronic disease. *Periodontology 2000.* 2014;64:111–1126.

31. Haber J, Wattles J, Crowley M, et al. Evidence for cigarette smoking as a major risk factor for periodontitis. *J Periodontol.* 1993;64(1):16–23.

32. Mavropoulos A, Brodin P, Rosing KC, et al. Gingival blood flow in periodontitis patients before and after periodontal surgery assessed in smokers and non-smokers. *J Periodontol.* 2007;78(9):1774–1782.

33. Bergström J, Eliasson S, Dock J. A 10-year prospective study of tobacco smoking and periodontal health. *J Periodontol.* 2000;71(8):1338–1347.

34. Calsina G, Ramón JM, Echeverría JJ. Effects of smoking on periodontal and tissues. *J Clin Periodontol.* 2002;29: 771–776.

35. Mavropoulos A, Aars H, Brodin P. Hyperaemic response to cigarette smoking in healthy gingiva. *J Clin Periodontol.* 2003;30(3):214–221.

36. Gelskey SC. Cigarette smoking and periodontitis: methodology to assess the strength of evidence in support of a causal association. *Community Dent Oral Epidemiol.* 1999;27(1):16–24.

37. Hanioka T, Ojima M, Tanaka K, et al. Causal assessment of smoking and tooth loss: a systematic review of observational studies. *BMC Public Health.* 2011;11:221.

38. The American Academy of Periodontology. The parameters of care (supplement). *J Periodontol.* 2000;71(5):847–848.

39. Bergström J. Periodontitis and smoking: an evidence-based appraisal. *J Evid Based Dent Pract.* 2006;6(1):33–41.

40. Rosa EF, Corraini P, de Carvalho VF, et al. A prospective 12-month study of the effect of smoking cessation on periodontal clinical parameters. *J Clin Periodontol.* 2011;38(6):562–571.

41. Patel RA, Wilson RF, Palmer RM. The effect of smoking on periodontal bone regeneration: a systematic review and meta-analysis. *J Periodontol.* 2012;83(2):143–155.

42. Carcuac O, Jansson L. Peri-implantitis in a specialist clinic of periodontology. Clinical features and risk indicators. *Swed Dent J.* 2010;34(2):53–61.

43. Strietzel FP, Reichart PA, Kale A, et al. Smoking interferes with the prognosis of dental implant treatment: a systematic review and meta-analysis. *J Clin Periodontol.* 2007;34(6):523–544.

44. Chambrone L, Preshaw PM, Rosa EF, et al. Effects of smoking cessation on the outcomes of non-surgical periodontal therapy: a systematic review and individual patient data meta-analysis. *J Clin Periodontol.* 2013;40(6): 607–615.

45. American Psychiatric Association. Tobacco-related disorders. In: *Diagnostic and Statistical Manual of Mental Disorders (DSM-5).* 5th ed. Arlington, VA: American Psychiatric Association; 2013:571–576.

46. Picciotto MR, Mineur YS. Molecules and circuits involved in nicotine addiction: the many faces of smoking. *Neuropharmacology.* 2014;76:545–553.

47. Tobacco Control Legal Consortium, The Verdict Is In: Findings from United States v. Philip Morris. The Hazards of Smoking (2006).

48. National Center for Chronic Disease Prevention and Health Promotion (US), Office on Smoking and Health. *The Health Consequences of Smoking—50 Years of Progress: A Report of the Surgeon General.* Atlanta, GA: U.S. Department of Health and Human Services, Office on Smoking and Health, Centers for Disease Control and Prevention, National Center for Chronic Disease Prevention and Health Promotion; 2014.

49. Lancaster T, Stead LF. Self-help interventions for smoking cessation. *Cochrane Database Syst Rev.* 2002;(3): CD01118.

50. Hartmann-Boyce J, Lancaster T, Stead LF. Print-based self-help interventions for smoking cessation. *Cochrane Database Syst Rev.* 2014;6:CD001118.

51. Stead LF, Lancaster T. Combined pharmacotherapy and behavioural interventions for smoking cessation. *Cochrane Database Syst Rev.* 2012;10:CD008286.

52. Stead LF, Perera R, Bullen C, et al. Nicotine replacement therapy for smoking cessation. *Cochrane Database Syst Rev.* 2012;11:CD000146.

53. Carr AB, Ebbert J. Interventions for tobacco cessation in the dental setting. *Cochrane Database Syst Rev.* 2012;6:CD005084.

54. Aveyard P, Begh R, Parsons A, et al. Brief opportunistic smoking cessation interventions: a systematic review and meta-analysis to compare advice to quit and offer of assistance. *Addiction.* 2010;107(6):1066–1073.

55. Centers for Disease Control and Prevention (CDC). Vital signs: current cigarette smoking among adults aged ≥18 years—United States, 2005–2010. *MMWR Morb Mortal Wkly Rep.* 2011;60(35):1207–1212.

56. Mecklenburg RE, Greenspan D, Kleinman DV, et al. Tobacco Effects in the Mouth: A National Cancer Institute and National Institute of Dental Research Guide for Health Professionals. Washington, DC: Department of Health and Human Services, National Institutes of Health; 2007.

57. Kumar PS, Matthews CR, Joshi V, et al. Tobacco smoking affects bacterial acquisition and colonization in oral biofilms. *Infect Immun.* 2011;79(11):4730–4738.

58. Fiore MC. The new vital sign: assessing and documenting smoking status. *JAMA.* 1991;266(22):3183–3184.

59. American Dental Association. For the dental patient. Give tobacco the boot. *J Am Dent Assoc.* 2011;142(3):352.

60. Heasman L, Stacey F, Preshaw PM, et al. The effect of smoking on periodontal treatment response: a review of clinical evidence. *J Clin Periodontol.* 2006;33(4):241–253.

61. Lai DT, Cahill K, Qin Y, et al. Motivational interviewing for smoking cessation. *Cochrane Database Syst Rev.* 2010;1:CD006936.

62. Ramseier CA, Warnakulasuriya S, Needleman IG, et al. Consensus report: 2nd European workshop on tobacco use prevention and cessation for oral health professionals. *Int Dent J.* 2010;60(1):3–6.

63. Moyer VA; and US Preventive Services Task Force. Primary care interventions to prevent tobacco use in children and adolescents: U.S. Preventive Services Task Force recommendation statement. *Pediatrics.* 2013;132(3):560–565.

64. Centers for Disease Control and Prevention (CDC). Tobacco use among middle and high school students—United States, 2000–2009. *MMWR Morb Mortal Wkly Rep.* 2010;59(33):1063–1068.

65. Kann L, Kinchen S, Shanklin S, et al. Youth risk behavior surveillance—United States, 2013. *MMWR Surveill Summ.* 2014;63 (Suppl 4):1–168.

66. Ray MN, Funkhouser E, Williams JH, et al. National dental PBRN collaborative group. Smoking-cessation e-referrals: a national dental practice-based research network randomized controlled trial. *Am J Prev Med.* 2014;46(2):158–165.

67. Sadasivam RS, Kinney RL, Delaughter K, et al.; National Dental PBRN Group, and QUIT-PRIMO Collaborative Group. Who participates in web-assisted tobacco interventions? The QUIT-PRIMO and national dental practice-based research network hi-quit studies. *J Med Internet Res.* 2013;15(5):e77.

68. U.S. Department of Health and Human Services. *A National Call to Action to Promote Oral Health.* Rockville, MD: U.S. Department of Health and Human Services, Public Health Service, National Institutes of Health, National Institute of Dental and Craniofacial Research; 2003. NIH Publication No. 03-5303.

ENHANCE YOUR UNDERSTANDING

thePoint® **DIGITAL CONNECTIONS**
(see the inside front cover for access information)
- **Audio glossary**
- **Quiz bank**

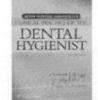

SUPPORT FOR LEARNING
(available separately; visit lww.com)
- *Active Learning Workbook for Clinical Practice of the Dental Hygienist, 12th Edition*

prepU **INDIVIDUALIZED REVIEW**
(available separately; visit lww.com)
- **Adaptive quizzing with *prepU for Wilkins' Clinical Practice of the Dental Hygienist***

35

Diet and Dietary Analysis

Luisa Nappo-Dattoma, RDH, RD, EdD

CHAPTER OUTLINE

LEARNING OBJECTIVES

Upon completion of this chapter, the reader will be able to:

1. Recognize oral manifestations of vitamin and mineral deficiencies.

2. Explain the function of each nutrient in maintaining oral and overall health.

3. Identify good food sources for each macro- and micronutrient.

4. Determine the caries risk potential of a patient's food record.

5. Access and utilize the MyPlate website for diet analysis and as a tool for patient education.

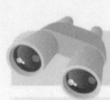

BOX 35-1   KEY WORDS: Diet and Dietary Analysis

Anticariogenic: substance that inhibits or arrests dental caries formation.

Antioxidant: a compound that stops the damaging effects of reactive substances seeking an electron (oxidizing agent).

Ariboflavinosis: a condition resulting from a lack of riboflavin.

Cariogenic: foods and beverages that lower oral pH and are conducive to dental caries; the degree of cariogenicity depends on many factors, including physical form, texture, and consistency of the carbohydrate-containing food; its retention and clearance time from the oral cavity and the frequency of use.

Cariogenic exposure: individual ingestion of a cariogenic food that lowers the pH in the dental biofilm and exposes the tooth surface to demineralization.

Clearance time: the time from the cariogenic exposure until the food is cleared from the oral cavity; influenced by consistency and quantity of saliva; by the action of the tongue, lips, and cheeks; and by the consistency of food.

Diet: customary amount and kind of food and drink taken by an individual from day to day.

Dietary assessment: separation of a dietary food record into individual components of the MyPlate; assessment of quality, of whether the individual is consuming an adequate diet, and of where modifications are needed.

Malnutrition: poor nourishment resulting from improper diet or some defect of metabolism that prevents the body from utilizing the intake of food properly.

Meal plan: a selectively planned or prescribed regimen of food to meet certain needs of the individual.

Noncariogenic food: does not support or promote bacterial growth responsible for caries formation.

Nutrient: a chemical substance in foods needed by the body for growth and repair; the six classes of nutrients are proteins, fats, carbohydrates, minerals, vitamins, and water.

Macronutrients: energy-yielding nutrients needed in larger amounts in the diet: carbohydrate, protein, and fat.

Micronutrients: nutrients needed in small amounts in the diet and are not energy yielding: vitamins and minerals.

Nutrient density: assessment of nutritional quality of a food by comparing the nutrient content with the amount of energy (kilocalories) it provides.

Nutrition: sum of processes involved in taking nutrients into the body, assimilating and utilizing them; includes ingestion, digestion, absorption, transport, utilization of nutrients, and excretion of waste products.

Nutritional deficiency: inadequacy of nutrients in the tissues; the result of inadequate dietary intake or impairment of digestion, absorption, transport, or metabolism.

Registered dietitian: a healthcare professional with a minimum of a bachelor's degree in nutrition or dietetics who has attended an internship program or equivalent and passed the registration examination, all under the approval of the American Dietetic Association. Continuing education is required to keep credentials current.

Synthesis: the process involved in the formation of a complex substance from simpler elements or compounds; the process of building up.

Vegan diet: a diet consisting of only plant foods. Other varieties of the vegan diet are: the fruitarian: fruits, nuts, honey, and vegetable oils; lacto-vegetarian: vegan based with the inclusion of dairy products; lacto-ovo-vegetarian: vegan based with the inclusion of dairy products and eggs.

Nutrition is an integral part of an individual's general health as well as the health status of the oral cavity. The health of oral tissues can be affected by nutrition, diet, and food habits.

▶ Box 35-1 defines relevant terms of standards, diet, nutrition, and oral health. Box 35-2 provides relevant abbreviations.

▶ The interrelationship between nutritional status, systemic diseases, and oral conditions supports the need for timely and effective diet intervention.

▶ Within the scope of practice, the dental hygienist has a responsibility to assess, screen, and deliver nutritional information and instruction as part of comprehensive education in health promotion and disease prevention and intervention.

▶ Dietary and nutritional counseling, as part of a dental caries control program and periodontal maintenance, is an essential part of the dental hygiene care plan.

NUTRIENT STANDARDS FOR DIET ADEQUACY IN HEALTH PROMOTION

▶ Patient education centers on helping patients learn about selection of foods that make up a healthy diet.

I. Government Standards

A. Purposes of Standards

▶ Facilitate education for individuals about dietary needs and goals to achieve and maintain health.

▶ Prevent deficiency diseases and help achieve diet adequacy for the public.

▶ Make recommendations relative to poor food habits such as missed meals, omission of essential foods and nutrients, and fad dieting.

▶ Make specific recommendations for oral health.

▶ Motivate for behavioral modification.

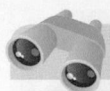

BOX 35-2 KEY WORDS ABBREVIATIONS: Diet and Dietary Analysis

AIs: adequate intakes. The recommended nutrient intake utilized when there is not enough information to establish an EAR.

Body mass index (BMI): a measure of body fat based on height in centimeters (cm) and weight in kilograms (kg).

DRIs: dietary reference intakes. A comprehensive term for categories of reference values that concentrate on maintaining a healthy state for the healthy general population to avoid overeating and prevent chronic disease.

EARs: estimated average requirements. Estimates the nutrient requirements of the average individual.

RDAs: recommended dietary allowances; recommendations for the average amounts of nutrients recommended to be consumed daily by healthy people to achieve adequate nutrient intake to prevent deficiency.

ULs: tolerable upper intake levels, or upper levels; maximum intake by an individual that is unlikely to create risks of adverse health effects in almost all healthy individuals.

USDA: United States Department of Agriculture.

USDHHS: United States Department of Health and Human Services.

B. Guidelines

▶ Provide guidelines through printed and web-based educational materials.

▶ Guidelines reflect public health concerns as they relate to nutrition.

II. Dietary Standards

A. Dietary Reference Intakes (DRIs)[1]

▶ DRIs: a comprehensive term for categories of reference values to meet the general nutrient needs for the healthy population to prevent deficiencies, toxicities, and chronic disease.

▶ Encompasses the current nutrient recommendations made by the Institute of Medicine, National Academy of Sciences, Food and Nutrition Board.

▶ The categories include:
  • RDA (Recommended Dietary Allowance)
  • AL (Adequate Level)
  • EAR (Estimated Average Requirement)
  • UL (Tolerable Upper Level)

▶ Established for vitamins and minerals.

B. Estimated Average Requirements[1]

▶ Estimates the nutritional requirements of the average individual.

▶ Categorized by age and gender.

▶ Provide the foundation for the recommended dietary allowances (RDAs).

C. Recommended Dietary Allowances[2]

▶ Recommendations for the average amounts of nutrients recommended to be consumed daily by healthy people to achieve adequate nutrient intake to prevent deficiency.

▶ Categorized by age and gender; do not include special needs such as illness.

▶ Based on gender and age; do not include special needs such as in illness.

D. Adequate Intakes (AIs)[2,3]

▶ The recommended nutrient intake utilized when there is not enough information to establish an EAR.

▶ AIs have been established for calcium, vitamin D, and fluoride for all age groups.

E. Tolerable Upper Intake Levels, or ULs[2,3]

▶ Maximum intake by an individual that is unlikely to create risks of adverse health effects in almost all healthy individuals.

▶ ULs were established to avoid toxicity due to excess intake of specific nutrients from food, fortified food, water, and nutrient supplements.

III. Dietary Guidelines for Americans

▶ Established by USDA (US Department of Agriculture) and USDHHS (US Department of Health and Human Services) as the basis for a federal nutrition policy based on the most recent scientific evidence review.

▶ Provides information and advice for choosing healthy eating patterns that focus on achieving and maintaining a healthy weight and include food safety principles to avoid foodborne illness.

▶ Used as the basis for developing nutrition-related programs, educational materials, and consumer health messages.

▶ Box 35-3 lists key recommendations in the 2010 Dietary Guidelines for Americans.

IV. MyPlate Food Guidelines[4]

▶ Originally developed as a "Food Pyramid" by the USDA in 1991.

▶ Newest version established June 2011 using the graphic representation of a "dinner plate" icon as illustrated in Figure 35-1.

▶ Colorful graphic provides a visual reminder of the approximate proportions of five food groups necessary for a healthy diet.

BOX 35-3

Key Recommendations: Dietary Guidelines for Americans, 2010

▷ Balance calories to manage weight
  ▷ Prevent overweight and obesity
▷ Increase physical activity
▷ Foods and food components to reduce
  ▷ Sodium
  ▷ Saturated and trans fats
  ▷ Added sugars
  ▷ Refined grains
  ▷ Alcohol
▷ Foods and nutrients to increase
  ▷ Vegetables and fruits
  ▷ Whole grains
  ▷ Fat-free or low-fat milk and milk products
  ▷ Protein foods, including seafood and vegetarian options
  ▷ Oils instead of solid fats
  ▷ Nutrients of concern, particularly potassium, dietary fiber, calcium, and vitamin D
▷ Build healthy eating patterns
  ▷ Meet nutrient needs at appropriate caloric levels
  ▷ Follow food safety to reduce foodborne illnesses

Source: U.S. Department of Agriculture; and U.S. Department of Health and Human Services. *Dietary Guidelines for Americans, 2010.* 7th ed. Washington, DC: U.S. Government Printing Office; 2010. http://health.gov/dietaryguidelines/. Accessed April 25, 2011.

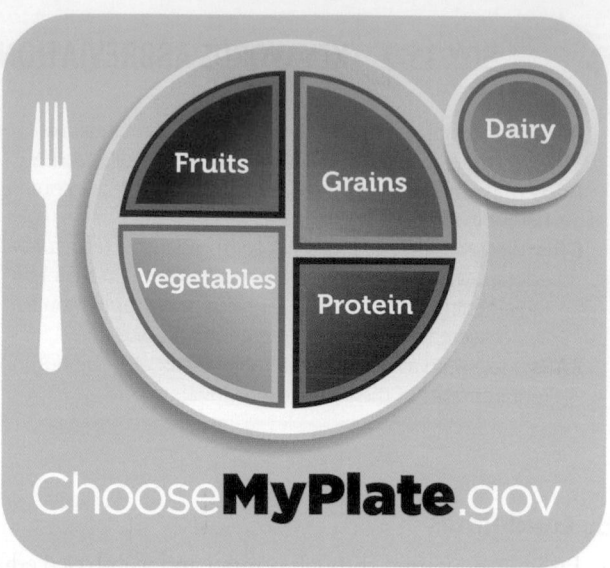

FIGURE 35-1 ChooseMyPlate Guidelines Icon.
Source: U.S. Department of Agriculture, Center for Nutrition Policy and Promotion. ChooseMyPlate guidelines. 2011. http://www.choosemyplate.gov. Accessed February 13, 2014

▶ Twelve caloric patterns ranging from 1,000 to 3,200 kilocalories provide specific amounts of food consumption from the five food groups, oils, and discretionary kilocalories, as illustrated in Table 35-2.

ORAL HEALTH RELATIONSHIPS

▶ Nutrition, diet, and oral health are closely interrelated.
▶ The oral cavity is the gateway to the body.
▶ Healthy masticatory function of the dentition contributes to proper dietary selection for maintenance of the nutritional status of the entire body.
▶ Healthy diet selection provides essential nutrients for optimum health of oral tissues and prevention of nutritional deficiencies.

I. Skin and Mucous Membrane

▶ Relevant vitamins: vitamin A, B complex, and ascorbic acid.
▶ Relevant minerals: zinc and iron.
▶ Table 35-3 outlines the nutrients, their function, and food sources.

II. Periodontal Tissues

Periodontal diseases are not caused by nutritional deficiencies, but malnutrition may contribute to the progression of periodontal disease symptoms and influence healing following treatment.

▶ *Nutritional deficiencies do not cause periodontal diseases.* Without local factors, including the periodontal pathogens in biofilm, biofilm-retentive factors (such as calculus

---

▶ Educational materials accompanying the MyPlate food guidance system encourage consumers to build a healthy plate:

  • Make half the plate vegetables and fruits.
  • Switch to fat-free or low-fat milk.
  • Choose whole grains.
  • Vary protein choices to include seafood and legumes and keep meat portions small.
  • Cut back on foods high in solid fat, added sugars, and salt.
  • Eat the right amount of calories to maintain a healthy weight.
  • Enjoy food, but eat less and keep track of what is consumed.
  • Cook more often at home and choose lower calorie options when eating out.
  • Limit alcoholic beverages.
  • Be physically active.

V. Recommended Food Intake Patterns

▶ Including estimated calorie needs and recommended amounts of food from each food group accompany the MyPlate food guidelines.
▶ Caloric recommendations based on gender, age, and activity level are illustrated in Table 35-1.

TABLE 35-1	Estimated calorie needs per day by age, gender, and physical activity level

Estimated amounts of calories[a] needed to maintain calorie balance for various gender and age groups at three different levels of physical activity. The estimates are rounded to the nearest 200 calories for assignment to a USDA Food Pattern. An individual's calorie needs may be higher or lower than these average estimates.

		MALE	ACTIVITY LEVEL[b]		FEMALE[c]	
AGE (YEARS)	SEDENTARY	MODERATELY ACTIVE	ACTIVE	SEDENTARY	MODERATELY ACTIVE	ACTIVE
2	1,000	1,000	1,000	1,000	1,000	1,000
3	1,200	1,400	1,400	1,000	1,200	1,400
4	1,200	1,400	1,600	1,200	1,400	1,400
5	1,200	1,400	1,600	1,200	1,400	1,600
6	1,400	1,600	1,800	1,200	1,400	1,600
7	1,400	1,600	1,800	1,200	1,600	1,800
8	1,400	1,600	2,000	1,400	1,600	1,800
9	1,600	1,800	2,000	1,400	1,600	1,800
10	1,600	1,800	2,200	1,400	1,800	2,000
11	1,800	2,000	2,200	1,600	1,800	2,000
12	1,800	2,200	2,400	1,600	2,000	2,200
13	2,000	2,200	2,600	1,600	2,000	2,200
14	2,000	2,400	2,800	1,800	2,000	2,400
15	2,200	2,600	3,000	1,800	2,000	2,400
16	2,400	2,800	3,200	1,800	2,000	2,400
17	2,400	2,800	3,200	1,800	2,000	2,400
18	2,400	2,800	3,200	1,800	2,000	2,400
19–20	2,600	2,800	3,000	2,000	2,200	2,400
21–25	2,400	2,800	3,000	2,000	2,200	2,400
26–30	2,400	2,600	3,000	1,800	2,000	2,400
31–35	2,400	2,600	3,000	1,800	2,000	2,200
36–40	2,400	2,600	2,800	1,800	2,000	2,200
41–45	2,200	2,600	2,800	1,800	2,000	2,200
46–50	2,200	2,400	2,800	1,800	2,000	2,200
51–55	2,200	2,400	2,800	1,600	1,800	2,200
56–60	2,200	2,400	2,600	1,600	1,800	2,200
61–65	2,000	2,400	2,600	1,600	1,800	2,000
66–70	2,000	2,200	2,600	1,600	1,800	2,000
71–75	2,000	2,200	2,600	1,600	1,800	2,000
76+	2,000	2,200	2,400	1,600	1,800	2,000

[a]Based on Estimated Energy Requirements (EER) equations, using reference heights (average) and reference weights (healthy) for each age-gender group. For children and adolescents, reference height and weight vary. For adults, the reference man is 5 feet 10 inches tall and weighs 154 pounds. The reference woman is 5 feet 4 inches tall and weighs 126 pounds. EER equations are from the Institute of Medicine. Dietary Reference Intakes for Energy, Carbohydrate, Fiber, Fat, Fatty Acids, Cholesterol, Protein, and Amino Acids. Washington (DC): The National Academies Press; 2002.

[b]Sedentary means a lifestyle that includes only the light physical activity associated with typical day-to-day life. Moderately active means a lifestyle that includes physical activity equivalent to walking about 1.5 to 3 miles per day at 3 to 4 miles per hour, in addition to the light physical activity associated with typical day-to-day life. Active means a lifestyle that includes physical activity equivalent to walking more than 3 miles per day at 3 to 4 miles per hour, in addition to the light physical activity associated with typical day-to-day life.

[c]Estimates for females do not include women who are pregnant or breastfeeding.

Source: U.S. Department of Agriculture, Center for Nutrition Policy and Promotion. 2011.

TABLE 35-2	USDA Food Patterns

The Food Patterns suggest amounts of food to consume from the basic food groups, subgroups, and oils to meet recommended nutrient intakes at 12 different calorie levels. Nutrient and energy contributions from each group are calculated according to the nutrient-dense forms of foods in each group (e.g., lean meats and fat-free milk). The table also shows the number of calories from solid fats and added sugars (SoFAS) that can be accommodated within each calorie level, in addition to the suggested amounts of nutrient-dense forms of foods in each group.

DAILY AMOUNT OF FOOD FROM EACH GROUP

Calorie Level[a]	1,000	1,200	1,400	1,600	1,800	2,000	2,200	2,400	2,600	2,800	3,000	3,200
Fruits[b]	1 cup	1 cup	1½ cups	1½ cups	1½ cups	2 cups	2 cups	2 cups	2 cups	2½ cups	2½ cups	2½ cups
Vegetables[c]	1 cup	1½ cups	1½ cups	2 cups	2½ cups	2½ cups	3 cups	3 cups	3½ cups	3½ cups	4 cups	4 cups
Grains[d]	3 oz-eq	4 oz-eq	5 oz-eq	5 oz-eq	6 oz-eq	6 oz-eq	7 oz-eq	8 oz-eq	9 oz-eq	10 oz-eq	10 oz-eq	10 oz-eq
Protein Foods[e]	2 oz-eq	3 oz-eq	4 oz-eq	5 oz-eq	5 oz-eq	5½ oz-eq	6 oz-eq	6½ oz-eq	6½ oz-eq	7 oz-eq	7 oz-eq	7 oz-eq
Dairy[f]	2 cups	2½ cups	2½ cups	3 cups	3 cups	3 cups	3 cups	3 cups	3 cups	3 cups	3 cups	3 cups
Oils[g]	15 g	17 g	17 g	22 g	24 g	27 g	29 g	31 g	34 g	36 g	44 g	51 g
Limit on calories from SoFAS[h]	137	121	121	121	161	258	266	330	362	395	459	596

VEGETABLE SUBGROUP AMOUNTS PER WEEK

Calorie Level	1,000	1,200	1,400	1,600	1,800	2,000	2,200	2,400	2,600	2,800	3,000	3,200
Dark-green vegetables	½ c/wk	1 c/wk	1 c/wk	1½ c/wk	1½ c/wk	1½ c/wk	2 c/wk	2 c/wk	2½ c/wk	2½ c/wk	2½ c/wk	2½ c/wk
Red and orange vegetables	2½ c/wk	3 c/wk	3 c/wk	4 c/wk	5½ c/wk	5½ c/wk	6 c/wk	6 c/wk	7 c/wk	7 c/wk	7½ c/wk	7½ c/wk
Beans and peas (e.g. pintos, lentils, split peas)	½ c/wk	½ c/wk	½ c/wk	1 c/wk	1½ c/wk	1½ c/wk	2 c/wk	2 c/wk	2½ c/wk	2½ c/wk	3 c/wk	3 c/wk
Starchy vegetables	2 c/wk	3½ c/wk	3½ c/wk	4 c/wk	5 c/wk	5 c/wk	6 c/wk	6 c/wk	7 c/wk	7 c/wk	8 c/wk	8 c/wk
Other vegetables	1½ c/wk	2½ c/wk	2½ c/wk	3½ c/wk	4 c/wk	4 c/wk	5 c/wk	5 c/wk	5½ c/wk	5½ c/wk	7 c/wk	7 c/wk

PROTEIN FOODS SUBGROUP AMOUNTS PER WEEK

Calorie Level	1,000	1,200	1,400	1,600	1,800	2,000	2,200	2,400	2,600	2,800	3,000	3,200
Seafood	3 oz/wk	5 oz/wk	6 oz/wk	8 oz/wk	8 oz/wk	8 oz/wk	9 oz/wk	10 oz/wk	10 oz/wk	11 oz/wk	11 oz/wk	11 oz/wk
Meat, poultry, eggs	10 oz/wk	14 oz/wk	19 oz/wk	24 oz/wk	24 oz/wk	26 oz/wk	29 oz/wk	31 oz/wk	31 oz/wk	34 oz/wk	34 oz/wk	34 oz/wk
Nuts, seeds, soy	1 oz/wk	2 oz/wk	3 oz/wk	4 oz/wk	4 oz/wk	4 oz/wk	4 oz/wk	5 oz/wk	5 oz/wk	5 oz/wk	5 oz/wk	5 oz/wk

[a]**Calorie Levels** are set across a wide range to accommodate the needs of different individuals. The attached table "Estimated Daily Calorie Needs" can be used to help assign individuals to the food pattern at a particular calorie level.
[b]**Fruit Group** includes all fresh, frozen, canned, and dried fruits and fruit juices. In general, 1 cup of fruit or 100% fruit juice, or ½ cup of dried fruit can be considered as 1 cup from the fruit group.
[c]**Vegetable Group** includes all fresh, frozen, canned, and dried vegetables and vegetable juices. In general, 1 cup of raw or cooked vegetables or vegetable juice, or 2 cups of raw leafy greens can be considered as 1 cup from the vegetable group.

TABLE 35-2	USDA Food Patterns *(Continued)*

[d]**Grains Group** includes all foods made from wheat, rice, oats, cornmeal, barley, such as bread, pasta, oatmeal, breakfast cereals, tortillas, and grits. In general, 1 slice of bread, 1 cup of ready-to-eat cereal, or ½ cup of cooked rice, pasta, or cooked cereal can be considered as 1 ounce-equivalent from the grains group. **At least half of all grains consumed should be whole grains.**

[e]**Protein Foods Group** includes meat, poultry, seafood, eggs, processed soy products, and nuts and seeds. In general, 1 ounce of lean meat, poultry, or seafood, 1 egg, 1 Tbsp peanut butter, or ½ ounce of nuts or seeds can be considered as 1 ounce-equivalent from the protein foods group. Also, ¼ cup of beans or peas may be counted as 1 ounce-equivalent in this group.

[f]**Dairy Group** includes all milks, including lactose-free products and fortified soymilk (soy beverage), and foods made from milk that retain their calcium content, such as yogurt and cheese. Foods made from milk that have little to no calcium, such as cream cheese, cream, and butter, are not part of the group. Most dairy group choices should be fat-free or low-fat. In general, 1 cup of milk or yogurt, 1½ ounces of natural cheese, or 2 ounces of processed cheese can be considered as 1 cup from the dairy group.

[g]**Oils** include fats from many different plants and from fish that are liquid at room temperature, such as canola, corn, olive, soybean, and sunflower oil. Some foods are naturally high in oils, like nuts, olives, some fish, and avocados. Foods that are mainly oil include mayonnaise, certain salad dressings, and soft margarine.

[h]**SoFAS** are solid fats and added sugars. The limits for calories from SoFAS are the remaining amount of calories in each food pattern after selecting the specified amounts in each food group in nutrient-dense forms (forms that are fat-free or low-fat and with no added sugars).

ESTIMATED DAILY CALORIE NEEDS

To determine which food intake pattern to use for an individual, the following chart gives an estimate of individual calorie needs. The calorie range for each age/sex group is based on physical activity level, from sedentary to active.

	CALORIE RANGE		
CHILDREN	**SEDENTARY**	→	**ACTIVE**
2–3 years	1,000	→	1,400
FEMALES			
4–8 years	1,200	→	1,800
9–13	1,600	→	2,200
14–18	1,800	→	2,400
19–30	2,000	→	2,400
31–50	1,800	→	2,200
51+	1,600	→	2,200
MALES			
4–8 years	1,400	→	2,000
9–13	1,800	→	2,600
14–18	2,200	→	3,200
19–30	2,400	→	3,000
31–50	2,400	→	3,000
51+	2,200	→	2,800

Sedentary means a lifestyle that includes only the light physical activity associated with typical day-to-day life.

Active means a lifestyle that includes physical activity equivalent to walking more than 3 miles per day at 3 to 4 miles per hour, in addition to light physical activity associated with typical day-to-day life.

Source: U.S. Department of Agriculture, Center for Nutrition Policy and Promotion. 2011. www.cnpp.usda.gov.

TABLE 35-3	Nutrients Relevant to Oral Health		
NUTRIENT	**FUNCTION**	**DEFICIENCY DISEASE**	**FOOD SOURCE**
Vitamin A (retinol, provitamin A carotene)	■ Fat soluble ■ Antioxidant ■ Bone and tooth development ■ Skin and mucous membrane integrity ■ Cell differentiation; essential for reproduction ■ Vision in dim light ■ Immune system integrity	■ Night blindness ■ Xerophthalmia ■ Poor growth ■ Keratinization of epithelium ■ Dry, scaly skin ■ Toxic in large doses: (double vision, hair loss, dry mucous membranes, joint pain, liver damage)	Egg yolk, liver, fish liver oils, fortified milk, cream, cheeses; green leafy vegetables, orange, red, yellow pigmented fruits and vegetables
Vitamin D (calciferol)	■ Fat soluble ■ Aids in the absorption of calcium and phosphorus ■ Mineralization of bone	■ Rickets in children ■ Osteomalacia in adults ■ Osteoporosis ■ Toxic in large doses: (calcification of soft tissues, growth retardation)	Exposure to UV sunlight, fortified milk, fish oils
Vitamin E (tocopherol)	■ Fat soluble ■ Antioxidant	■ Low incidence of deficiency ■ Low toxicity	Whole grains, wheat germ, plant oils, margarines, legumes, seeds, nuts, greens
Vitamin K (quinone)	■ Fat soluble ■ Synthesis of prothrombin in blood clotting and bone proteins	■ Prolonged clotting time ■ Hemorrhage ■ Toxic in large doses; (patients on blood thinners need to limit use in diet)	Synthesized by intestinal bacterial flora; dark green leafy vegetables, liver
Thiamin (B$_1$)	■ Acts as coenzyme in carbohydrate and amino acid metabolism	■ Essential for synthesis of acetylcholine for healthy nerves ■ Beriberi: weight loss, fatigue, edema, depression ■ Toxicity: not seen	Enriched whole grains and cereals, pork, meats, poultry, nuts, seeds, legumes
Riboflavin (vitamin B$_2$)	■ Coenzyme in energy metabolism of fat, carbohydrate, and protein	■ Ariboflavinosis ■ Angular cheilosis ■ Growth failure ■ Eye disorders ■ Toxicity: not seen	Milk, cheese, enriched and whole grains and cereals, rice, mushrooms, liver
Niacin (vitamin B$_3$)	■ Coenzyme in energy metabolism of fat, carbohydrate, and protein	■ Pellagra: diarrhea, dermatitis, dementia, and death ■ Toxicity not seen in food sources ■ Toxicity with large doses of supplements for treatment of hypercholesterolemia: (skin redness and flushing, gastric ulcers)	Enriched whole grains and cereals, rice, meat, poultry, fish, green leafy vegetables
Pyridoxine (vitamin B$_6$)	■ Coenzyme in amino acid and lipid metabolism ■ Hemoglobin synthesis ■ Homocysteine metabolism	■ Dermatitis ■ Depression ■ Convulsions ■ Peripheral neuritis ■ Toxicity not seen in food sources ■ Toxicity from supplements: neuropathy, irreversible nerve damage	Widespread food sources with exception of fat and sugar
Cobalamin (vitamin B$_{12}$)	■ Maturation of RBC ■ Requires intrinsic factor from parietal cells for absorption ■ Cofactor in folate and homocysteine metabolism	■ Pernicious anemia secondary to lack of intrinsic factor and total vegan diet ■ Toxicity: not seen	All animal foods, fortified cereals

TABLE 35-3	Nutrients Relevant to Oral Health (*Continued*)		
NUTRIENT	**FUNCTION**	**DEFICIENCY DISEASE**	**FOOD SOURCE**
Folate (folic acid)	■ Maturation of RBC ■ DNA synthesis ■ Homocysteine metabolism	■ Megaloblastic anemia, ■ Neural tube defects: spina bifida ■ Masks B12 deficiency ■ Toxicity not seen	Green leafy vegetables, fruits, legumes, fortified grains
Ascorbic acid (vitamin C)	■ Antioxidant ■ Collagen synthesis ■ Wound healing ■ Aids in absorption of iron	■ Scurvy ■ Poor wound healing ■ Petechial hemorrhages ■ Increased periodontal symptoms ■ Toxicity: potential for rebound scurvy	Citrus fruits, broccoli, strawberries, peppers, tomatoes, cantaloupe
Calcium	■ Muscle contraction ■ Blood clotting ■ Nerve impulse transmission ■ Calcification of bone and tooth structure	■ Osteoporosis ■ Incomplete calcification of hard tissues ■ Toxicity: not seen	Dairy products, tofu, fortified orange juice, and soy milk, green leafy vegetables, canned salmon, and sardine bones
Phosphorus	■ Required for bone and teeth strength ■ Acid–base balance ■ Muscle contraction	■ Poor bone maintenance ■ Incomplete calcification of teeth ■ Compromised alveolar integrity ■ Toxicity: skeletal porosity	Dairy products, meat, poultry, processed foods, soft drinks, nuts, legumes, whole grain cereals
Magnesium	■ Bone strength and rigidity ■ Hydroxyapatite crystal formation ■ Nerve impulse ■ Muscle contraction	■ Muscle weakness ■ Alveolar bone fragility ■ Toxicity seen in medications containing magnesium	Wheat bran, whole grains, green leafy vegetables, legumes, nuts, chocolate
Fluoride	■ Prevention of dental caries ■ Remineralization	■ Increased incidence of caries ■ Toxicity: tooth mottling, enamel hypoplasia	Fluoridated water, tea, seaweed, toothpaste
Iron	■ Component of hemoglobin ■ Carries oxygen to cells ■ Immune function ■ Cognitive development	■ Anemia: pallor of face, conjunctiva, lips, mucosa, and gingiva ■ Shortness of breath ■ Fatigue ■ Decreased immunity ■ Toxicity: gastrointestinal upset, pigmentation, seen in persons with hemochromatosis	Meat, poultry, fish, whole grains, dried fruit, enriched grains
Zinc	■ Required for over 100 enzymes ■ Normal growth and development ■ Taste and smell sensitivity ■ Sexual development and reproduction ■ Immune integrity ■ Wound healing	■ Altered taste ■ Growth retardation ■ Decreased wound healing ■ Impaired immunity ■ Toxicity: rare (stomach irritation, cramps, diarrhea, vomiting)	Seafood, meats, whole grains, greens
Copper	■ Aids in iron metabolism ■ Collagen formation	■ Anemia ■ Poor growth ■ Low white blood cells ■ Bone demineralization ■ Tissue fragility ■ Decreased trabeculae of alveolar bone ■ Toxicity: vomiting, diarrhea	Whole grains, nuts, dried fruits, meats legumes, shell fish, organ meats

Source: Palmer CA, ed. *Diet and Nutrition in Oral Health*. 2nd ed. Upper Saddle River, NJ: Pearson Prentice Hall; 2007; Chapter 8, Palmer CA, Papas A. The minerals and mineralization; Chapter 9, Palmer CA. Vitamins today: 163, 169–171, 204–205, 222–225.

and defective restorations), and lack of the oral self-care to remove biofilm, periodontal infections cannot occur.

▶ *Severe deficiencies are rare in developed countries.* Symptoms of deficiencies such as those listed in Table 35-4 may be seen in cases of severe deprivation, starvation, and long-term patients with alcoholism or other drug addictions.

▶ *RDAs are essential to the health of the periodontal tissues.* As part of total body health, the daily diet nourishes the oral tissues.

▶ *The physical character of the diet contributes.* A soft sticky diet that stays on the tooth surfaces, especially cervical third and proximal areas, encourages biofilm buildup and proliferation of bacteria, including the periodontal pathogens.

▶ *Malnutrition suppresses the immune system and impairs the host's reaction to infections.* Increased activity of pathogenic microorganisms may result in increased periodontal disease.

▶ *Nutrients contribute to healing and tissue repair.*[5] The elements strongly associated with wound healing include the vitamin B complex, vitamin C (ascorbic acid), and dietary calcium.

- *B complex* refers to all the water-soluble vitamins except vitamin C. They are thiamin (vitamin B_1), riboflavin (vitamin B_2), niacin (vitamin B_3), pyridoxine (vitamin B_6), cobalamin (vitamin B_{12}), biotin, folic acid, and pantothenic acid. Each member of the B complex has individual functions.
- *Vitamin C* is needed for collagen formation and intercellular material, and healing tissues after procedures including scaling and root planing.

- *Dietary calcium.* About 99% of the calcium in the body is in the bones and teeth; 1% is in the body tissues and fluids; essential for cell metabolism, muscle contraction, and nerve impulse transmission. Vitamin D is necessary for the continuous exchange of calcium between the blood, skeletal bones, and other cells.
- *Low dietary intake of calcium can impact alveolar bone integrity in periodontal disease.* Loss of alveolar bone and soft tissue attachment are typical of periodontal disease symptoms.[6]
- *Current and former smokers with low dietary vitamin C intake are at risk for more severe periodontal disease.*[7] No current research has shown whether intake of vitamin C can improve periodontal health.[7]

▶ *Obesity and periodontal disease*
- Obesity and periodontal disease have an association with each other and inflammation is the proposed mechanism for this relationship.[8,9]
- As with all chronic diseases, it is the dental professional's role to promote healthy lifestyle choices including, but not limited to oral self-care, tobacco cessation, healthy nutrition, adequate physical exercise, and weight control to manage and/or prevent progression of disease.

▶ *Dietary assessment for periodontal conditions*
- Following surgical intervention patients may need to alter diet consistency during the healing period.

TABLE 35-4	Oral Manifestations of Nutrient Deficiencies
	NUTRIENT DEFICIENCY
ORAL SYMPTOMS ASSOCIATED WITH THE TONGUE	
Altered taste sensations	Riboflavin, thiamin, zinc, vitamin A, vitamin B_{12}
Glossitis	Folate, niacin, riboflavin, vitamin B_6, vitamin B_{12}
Glossodynia	Niacin, vitamin B_6, vitamin B_{12}
Sore or burning tongue	Iron, niacin, riboflavin, thiamin, vitamin B_6, vitamin B_{12}
ORAL SYMPTOMS ASSOCIATED WITH MUCOSAL TISSUE	
Angular cheilosis	Folate, iron, riboflavin, vitamin B_6, vitamin B_{12}
Candidiasis	Folate, iron, zinc, vitamin A, vitamin C
Delayed wound healing	Riboflavin, zinc, vitamin A, vitamin C
Mucositis/Stomatitis	Folate, niacin, thiamin, vitamin B_{12}

Source: Palmer CA, ed. *Diet and Nutrition in Oral Health.* 2nd ed. Upper Saddle River, NJ: Pearson Prentice Hall; 2007; Chapter 8, Palmer CA, Papas A. The minerals and mineralization; Chapter 9, Palmer CA. Vitamins today:163, 1691–71, 204–205, 222–225.

- A soft diet of high-quality protein is indicated for adequate wound healing. Puddings, scrambled eggs, milkshakes, yogurt, and cottage cheese have high-quality protein to promote healing.
- Chewing firm foods increases salivary flow. Saliva acts as a buffer, and increased saliva aids in oral clearance.

III. Tooth Structure and Integrity

▶ *Nutrients and health of tooth structure*
- Adequate nutrition during tooth development is essential for mineralization.
- Relevant minerals: calcium, phosphorus, magnesium, and fluoride.
- Relevant vitamin: vitamin A.
- Table 35-3 outlines nutrients, their function, and food sources.

▶ *Dietary assessment*
- Diet assessment during early tooth development is essential to assist parents in caries prevention.
- Anticipatory guidance for the parents of infants, children, and adolescents can be found in Chapters 49 and 50.

IV. Dental Caries

▶ *Prevention*[10]
- Fluoride is an essential mineral for dental caries prevention.
- The complexity of dental caries formation is illustrated in Figure 35-2.

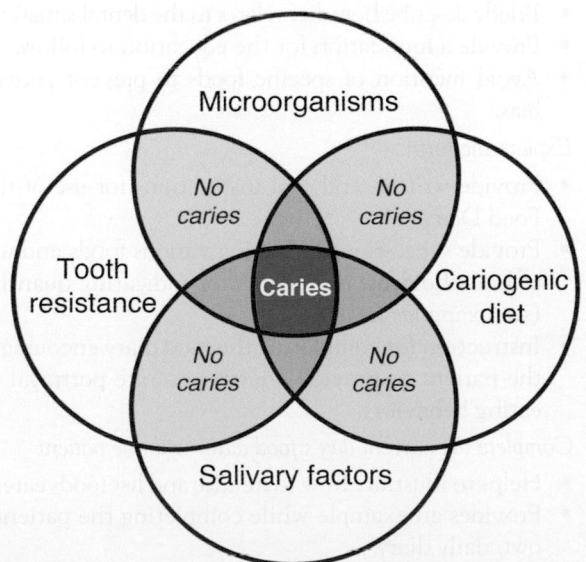

FIGURE 35-2 Dental Caries Process. Four overlapping circles illustrate the factors involved in the development of dental caries. All four act together, and as shown by the center, dental caries results. (Adapted from U.S. Department of Health and Human Services, Public Health Service, National Institute of Dental Research. *Broadening the Scope. Long-range Research Plan for the 1990s.* Washington, DC: United States Government Printing Office; 1990. NIH Publication No. 90-1188.)

▶ *Role of cariogenic foods*[11]
- Dental caries is a result of biofilm and excess cariogenic foods, not a nutrient deficiency.
- *Streptococcus mutans, Lactobacilli,* and other acid-forming organisms use fermentable carbohydrate from the diet to produce acids.

▶ *Consistency of food*[11]
- Soft, sticky foods cling to the teeth and gingiva and encourage biofilm accumulation.
- Microorganisms are protected and nourished in dental biofilm on the tooth leading to increased acid formation.

▶ *Dietary assessment and counseling*
- Use of dietary assessment and patient instruction relative to dental caries control.
- Personal recommendations foster behavioral modification in disease prevention.

COUNSELING FOR DENTAL CARIES CONTROL

▶ *Risk factors (see Chapter 27)*
- Inadequate biofilm removal.
- Inadequately mineralized tooth enamel such as in enamel hypoplasia or demineralization.
- Frequent snacks beverages between meals with fermentable carbohydrates.
- Altered salivary flow such as in drug-induced xerostomia.
- Figure 35-2 illustrates the intricate relationship of all four factors in the development of dental caries.

▶ *Preventive measures that support dietary control*
- Adequate plaque biofilm removal.
- Modification of intake of cariogenic foods and beverages.
- Strengthening the tooth surface to resist caries activity with appropriate office and home fluorides.
- Pit and fissure sealants.
- Restoration of existing carious lesions.

THE DIETARY ASSESSMENT

▶ The dietary assessment is an integral part of disease prevention and health promotion in the scope of dental hygiene care.
▶ The patient and dental hygienist have the opportunity to collaborate in the evaluation of diet adequacy and in diet intervention.

I. Purposes of a Dietary Assessment[12]

▶ Identify the patient who may be at nutritional and oral health risk.

▶ Refer to a registered dietitian nutritionist (RD or RDN) when intervention beyond the scope of dental hygiene practice is indicated.

▶ Provide an opportunity for a patient to study personal dietary habits objectively.

▶ Obtain an overall picture of the types of food in the patient's diet, food preferences, and quantity of food eaten.

▶ Study the food habits and snacking patterns.

▶ Record frequency of use and consumption of cariogenic food.

▶ Determine the overall consistency of the diet.
  • Identify fibrous foods regularly consumed.
  • Identify soft sticky foods regularly consumed.

▶ Identify the nutritional status of an individual with regard to overall requirements, and then collaborate with the patient to make suggestions for modification in nutritional adequacy of the diet in health promotion.

▶ Plan with the patient for necessary changes to improve the health of the oral mucosa and periodontium, and prevent dental caries.

II. Preliminary Preparation for Dietary Assessment

A. Patient History

▶ Information obtained from medical, dental, and social histories is essential in assessing oral health and nutritional status:
  • Disease states
  • Medications
  • Disabilities
  • Learning limitations
  • Significant unintentional change in body weight
  • Factors influencing food use and food intake.

▶ Dietary influences can be identified by intra- and extraoral examination, which may reveal oral tissue changes suggestive of nutritional deficiencies.

B. Clinical Evaluation

▶ Evaluation detects high-risk patients by noting factors suggestive of a dietary problem.

▶ Clinical examination and charting of cavitated carious lesions and demineralizing areas.

▶ Identification of any abnormalities in the patient's overall appearance; weight, skin, nails, and hair.

▶ Table 35-4 lists oral manifestations of severe deficiencies.

III. Forms Used for Assessment

A. Food Diary (Table 35-5)

▶ A diary of the patient's dietary intake over the previous 24 hours.

▶ Obtained by interview with patient.

▶ Assesses nutrients, food groups, diet adequacy, form and frequency of the carbohydrate intake, and snacking patterns.

▶ Results are reviewed and appropriate instruction given at appointment or a follow-up appointment.

▶ It is quick and easy to administer and can be done chairside in one visit.

▶ Is limited to one day's intake; therefore, it is not necessarily representative of a patient's normal diet.

B. Dietary Analysis Recording Form 3–7 Days (Table 35-6)

▶ A more accurate account of a patient's intake.

▶ Patient completes food diary for 3, 5, or 7 days, inclusive of one weekend day.

▶ Affords the patient a more active role in the dietary assessment and a chance to observe areas that require modification.

▶ Provide patient with three to seven copies of the Food Diary (Table 35-5). Request patient return the forms at follow-up visit.

▶ At follow-up visit the patient's diary is evaluated for:
  • Eating patterns
  • Consumption and frequency of fermentable carbohydrates
  • Nutritional adequacy.

IV. Presentation of the Food Diary to the Patient

▶ *Explain the purpose*
  • Briefly describe how diet relates to the dental situation.
  • Provide a foundation for the education to follow.
  • Avoid mention of specific foods to prevent patient bias.

▶ *Explain the form*
  • Provide written and oral instructions for use of the Food Diary.
  • Provide suggestions for listing various foods and use of household measurements for indicating quantity (see examples in Box 35-4).
  • Instruction for completing the food diary encourages the patient to provide a more accurate portrayal of eating behaviors.

▶ *Complete the current day's food diary with the patient*
  • Helps to illustrate how to itemize and list foods eaten.
  • Provides an example while completing the patient's own daily diary.

▶ *General directions*
  • Emphasize importance of completing the diary for each meal as soon after eating as possible to avoid forgetting.
  • Encourage use of typical days, uncomplicated by illness, dieting, holidays, or other unusual events.

TABLE 35-5	Food Diary Form

Sample of a form for patients to use to record the daily intake of foods. Can be used for the 24-hour recall or multiple forms used in the 3-to-7-day food diary.

NAME_____TEL_____

AGE_____SEX_____Height_____Weight_____BMI_____

TYPE OF FOODS/BEVERAGES	QUANTITY EATEN (CUP, OZ, TBSP, TSP, ETC.)	PREPARATION METHOD
BREAKFAST		
7:30 AM Orange juice	½ cup	Bagel shop
Bagel	Whole	
Cream cheese	2 tablespoons	
Coffee	2 cups	
Milk and sugar	½ cup, 2 packets	
SNACK		
10:00 AM Chocolate cookies	2	
Orange soda	12 oz can	
LUNCH		
1:00 PM Mushroom pizza	2 slices	School cafeteria
Orange soda	12 oz can	
Cheese cake	1 slice	
SNACK		
4:00 PM Whole wheat pretzels	1 bag	Vending machine
DINNER		
7:00 PM Turkey	6 oz	Roasted
Potato	1 medium	Baked
Sour cream	2 tablespoons	
Broccoli	1 cup	Sautéed
Oil	2 tablespoons	
Gravy	½ cup	Canned
SNACK		
9:30 PM Popcorn	3 cups	Microwave

- Review details of recording the component parts of a combination dish, such as a sandwich: 2 slices of whole wheat bread, 4 oz of turkey, 1 teaspoon of mayonnaise, 2 slices tomato with lettuce, and 1 slice of cheddar cheese.
- Indicate need for recording nutritional supplements and all fluids consumed, including water and alcoholic beverages.
- The patient needs to indicate where the meal was eaten such as at home, restaurant, or friend's house.
- Instruct patient to select consecutive days and at least one weekend day for a realistic representation of diet pattern.

V. Receiving the Completed Food Diary

► *Obtain supplemental data*

- Receive the Food Diary soon after its completion.
- Question the patient to clarify presented information.
- Does food diary represent a typical day or week?
- Identify influences on appetite such as illness or stress.
- Identify food likes and dislikes; food preferences; intolerances; food allergies.
- Frequency of dining out.
- Identify special diets being followed in the home.
- Average alcohol intake.
- Which family member is doing the cooking and food shopping?

TABLE 35-6	Dietary Analysis Recording Form

From the food diary kept by the patient (Table 35-5), each serving is entered as a check in the space beside the appropriate food group. Each category is totaled, averaged, and compared with the recommendation on the right.

Name_____

Date_____ Age_____

Dietary Analysis

FOOD GROUPS	DAY 1	2	3	4	5	6	7	DAILY AVERAGE	"USDA FOOD PATTERNS FOR SIX MOST USED CALORIC LEVELS (12 TOTAL LEVELS)						
									1000 kcals	1600 kcals	1800 kcals	2200 kcals	2800 kcals	ADEQUATE	
														Yes	No
Grains									3 oz-eq	5 oz-eq	6 oz-eq	7 oz-eq	10 oz-eq[a]		
Vegetables									1 cup	2 cups	2.5 cup	3 cups	3.5 cups		
Fruits									1 cup	1.5 cups	1.5 cups	2 cups	2.5 cups		
Milk									2 cups	3 cups	3 cups	3 cups	3 cups		
Meat & beans									2 oz-eq	5 oz-eq	5 oz-eq	6 oz-eq	7 oz-eq		
Oils									3 tsp	5 tsp	5 tsp	6 tsp	8 tsp		
Discretionary calories									165 kcals	132 kcals	195 kcals	290 kcals	426 kcals[b]		

[a]eq is the abbreviation for the word equivalents. See MyPyramid Food Intake Patterns (Figure 32-3) for more details on equivalents.
[b]kcals = kilocalories.

SWEETS									TOTAL	
Liquid	With meal									Total all liquid exposures and multiply by 20 minutes and divide by total number of days to equal daily acid attack from liquid. **Total Liquid Minutes_____**
	End of meal									
	Between meal									
Soft/ Solid Sticky/ retentive	With meal									Total all soft and hard solid exposures and multiply by 40 minutes and divide by total number of days to equal daily acid attack from solids. **Total Solid Minutes_____**
	End of meal									
	Between meal									
Hard/ Solid Slowly dissolving	With meal									Add Both liquid and solid totals to determine number of minutes per day teeth are under acid attack. **Total Daily Minutes of Acid Attack _____**
	End of meal									
	Between meal									

BOX 35-4
Food Diary Instructions

▷ Write down everything eaten on the food diary form (Table 35-5).

▷ Record each meal as soon after eating as possible to avoid forgetting.

▷ Do not choose days when dieting, fasting, or ill.

▷ Be accurate in determining the amounts eaten, using household measurements (e.g., 1/2 cup cereal, 1 tsp margarine, 3 oz fish). A 3-oz serving size can be compared to the size of a deck of cards.

▷ Use brand names whenever possible.

▷ Record added sauces, gravies, condiments, and all extras (e.g., sugar or cream in coffee, mayonnaise, chewing gum, cough drops).

▷ Record food preparation methods (e.g., baked, fried, boiled, grilled).

▷ Record all fluids; include water and alcoholic beverages.

- Ask about common food habits, such as snacking at night.

▶ *Review patient's Food Diary*

Common omissions include:

- Garnishes: frosting, whipped cream, butter or margarine on vegetables, salad dressings, oil.
- Beverages: quantity, sweetened.
- Snacks: type, brand, quantity.
- Chewing gum or mints: sugarless, nonsucrose sweetener such as xylitol, quantity.
- Canned fruit: packed in water, heavy or light syrup, own juices, or nonsucrose sweetened, quantity.
- Fruit and vegetables: canned, fresh, or frozen.
- Cereal: sugar-treated or low sugar brand, type of milk and/or sugar added, quantity.
- Potato: baked, mashed, fried.
- Seasonings or sauces: quantity, type.

VI. Analysis of Dietary Intake

Three principal parts of the food diary to analyze are the number of servings in each food group, frequency of cariogenic foods, and consistency of the diet.

A. Nutritional Analysis for Adequacy of 24-Hour Recall Intake

▶ When time is a factor, a 24-hour analysis is appropriate.

▶ Compare food groups represented in the patient's 24-hour food diary with that of MyPlate.

▶ Determine nutritional adequacy.

▶ Calculate the patient's "sweet score" as outlined in Table 35-7.

▶ Cariogenic foods are listed and categorized as solid, liquid, or slowly dissolving.

▶ Totals for the one day are multiplied by respective time factors and a score determines patient's caries risk.

B. Nutritional Analysis for Adequacy of Food Intake from the Food Diary

▶ Use the Dietary Analysis Recording Form to summarize adequacy of daily portions of each food group (Table 35-6).

▶ Each food eaten is entered into a food group with number of servings.

▶ Comparison of patient's food diary with the MyPlate Food Guidelines (Figures 35-1; Tables 35-1, 35-2).

▶ Totals for the week are added and the average per day calculated.

▶ The average is compared to the recommended servings for each food group.

▶ Web-based nutrition analysis program available at choosemyplate.gov to analyze a 3-, 5-, or 7-day diary:
  - Charts comparing patient's averages to the RDA.
  - Tables comparing patient to MyPlate recommendations.

▶ Assist patient when inadequacies or deficiencies are identified.

▶ Analysis of cariogenic foods.

▶ Identify physical form of carbohydrate.
  - Liquids: sweetened or unsweetened soft drinks; fruit juice with added sugars.
  - Soft solid/sticky and retentive: retentive cakes, cookies, chips, pretzels, jellybeans, and chewy, sticky candies.
  - Hard solid/slowly dissolving: hard candies, mints, and cough drops.

▶ Identify frequency of meals and snacks.
  - When snacks are consumed.
  - Number of between-meal snacks consumed daily.
  - Circle in red and tally the number of cariogenic foods, both solid and liquids.
  - Frequency more relevant than quantity in caries incidence.
  - High frequency of eating events decrease the ability of calcium and phosphate to remineralize teeth between episodes.

▶ During counseling appointment, show the patient how to:
  - Select and circle in red the cariogenic foods on the Scoring the Sweets form (Table 35-7).
  - Select liquid, soft solid, hard solid, and time of eating.
  - Total the number of sweets for liquid and solids and multiply total by 20 minutes (liquids) and 40 minutes (solids).
  - Divide by number of days (3-, 5-, or 7-day diary).
  - Add the liquid and solid score for total minutes teeth are exposed to sweets and acid attack (Table 35-6).

C. Analysis of Diet Consistency

▶ Help patient to identify the types of firm and fibrous foods from the Food Diary such as:
  - Uncooked fruits and vegetables.
  - Cooked; crisp–tender vegetables.

TABLE 35-7	Scoring the Sweets

Form to be used to determine patient's caries risk when doing a 24-hour recall at chairside. (Adapted with permission from Carole A. Palmer Ed. D., R.D. Division of Nutrition and Oral Health Promotion, Department of General Dentistry, Tufts University School of Dental Medicine.)

SCORING THE SWEETS   (Caries-Promoting Potential)

FOOD ITEMS (from patients 24 hour recall)	REFERENCE FOODS CONSIDERED CARIOGENIC	FREQUENCY (Place a check for each exposure to cariogenic food)	WEIGHTED SCORE	TOTAL POINTS EACH CATEGORY
1.	**Liquid**	—	X 1	
2.	Soft drinks, fruit drinks, cocoa, sugar and honey in beverages, nondairy creamers, ice cream, sherbet, flavored or frozen yogurt, pudding, custard, jello	—		
3.		—		
4.		—		
1.	**Solid & sticky**	—	X 2	
2.	Cakes, cupcakes, doughnuts, sweet rolls, potato chips, pretzels, pastry, canned fruit in syrup, bananas, cookies, chocolate candy, caramel, toffee, jelly beans, other chewy candy, chewing gum, dried fruit, marshmallows, jelly, jam	—		
3.		—		
4.		—		
5.				
6.				
1.	**Slowly dissolving**	—	X 3	
2.	Hard candies, breath mints, antacid tablets, cough drops	—		
3.		—		

TOTAL SCORE _____

Using the 24 hour recall diary:

- Classify each sweet into liquid, solid and sticky, or slowly dissolving. (Use reference food list)
- For each time a sweet was eaten, either at a meal or between meals (at least 20 minutes apart) place a check in the frequency column.
- In each category tally the number of sweets eaten and multiply by the weighted score. Record the category points in the respective column.
- Tally all the category points to determine the total score.

SWEET SCORE: (Risk for dental caries)	HOW TO LOWER YOUR RISK FOR CARIES:
0–1 low risk	1. Cut down on the frequency of between-meal sweets
2–4	2. Don't sip constantly on sweetened beverage
5–7 moderate risk	3. Avoid using slowly dissolving items like hard candy, cough drops etc.
8–9	4. Eat more non-decay promoting foods such as: (low fat cheese, raw
>10 high risk	(vegetables, crunchy fruits, nuts, popcorn, bottled water)

▶ Help patient to identify the frequency of use:
- Daily or occasionally.
- During meal, end of meal, or between meals.

D. Benefits of Food Diary Analysis

▶ Patient can identify appropriate and inappropriate practices for dental caries control.

▶ Corroborate findings with clinical findings and patient's oral health problems in preparation for counseling session.

PREPARATION FOR ADDITIONAL COUNSELING

I. Define Objectives

▶ To help patient understand the individual oral problems and appreciate the need for changing habits.

▶ To explain specific alterations in the diet necessary for improved general and oral health.

▶ For dental caries control.
- To promote the minimal consumption of cariogenic foods, particularly between meals.
- To substitute noncariogenic foods when possible into the diet.

II. Planning Factors

A. Patient Attitude

▶ Consider patient's willingness and ability to cooperate as evidenced by keeping appointments and following personal oral care procedures.

▶ Consider patient's healthcare beliefs and nutrition and dental knowledge.

B. Possible Barriers

▶ Difficulty and resistance to change of normal habits.

▶ Patient dissatisfaction with loss of usual or customary foods.

▶ Patient may not attempt to make modifications if recommendations are numerous or overwhelming.

▶ Lack of appreciation of need for change due to limited knowledge of diet, nutrition, and oral health relationship.

▶ Common misconception about concentrated sugar as an indispensable energy source.

▶ Cultural and religious patterns significant to food selection and preparation.

▶ Financial considerations in food purchasing.

▶ Emotional eating patterns and cravings for sweets.

▶ Parental attitude toward sweets in the diet.
- Elimination of all sugars would deprive a child of normal childhood pleasures.
- All sugars may be viewed as "bad" foods for children. Foods are not "good" and "bad", rather it is the frequency and amount that may be a concern for oral and overall health.

III. Appropriate Teaching Materials

▶ Patient's radiographs, dental charting, and food diary.

▶ Diagrams, food models, food labels, or charts of dietary standards and requirements.

▶ Educational leaflets to illustrate patient's special dietary or oral health needs.

▶ An outline of a realistic diet plan with specific suggestions for food substitutes.

▶ A list of snack suggestions.

COUNSELING PROCEDURES

I. Setting

▶ An environment free from interruptions and distracting background sounds.

▶ Apart from the clinical treatment room.

▶ Patient comfort promotes environment conducive to learning.

▶ Provide limited but pertinent educational information.
- Posters and pamphlets.
- Food labels and food models of portion sizes.
- Avoid overloading with too much new information to minimize confusion.

▶ Persons involved in promoting change:
- For a younger patient, the primary caregiver is present since this individual supervises the child's eating and oral care.
- Person preparing meals and grocery shopping needs to be present to learn about appropriate food choices.

II. Setting the Stage for a Successful Counseling Session

▶ Be prepared and on time.

▶ Plan for only a few simple visual aids.

▶ Concentrate on the factors related to the patient's diet-based dental problem.

▶ Encourage parents to exclude small children (other than the patient) from the conference; they may create distractions.

▶ Develop a friendly atmosphere; establish eye contact with a warm, nonthreatening environment.

▶ Adequately discuss all questions from patient or parent using a conversational tone without lecturing.

▶ Keep session brief, informative, and engaging for the patient without taking notes.

III. Presentation of Findings

A. Review Purpose of the Meeting

▶ Provide explanation of the relevance between diet and patient's oral disease.

▶ Emphasize health promotion and disease prevention.

B. Clarification of "Cariogenic" Foods

▶ Calculate the sugar score from the Scoring the Sweets or Dietary Analysis Recording Form to emphasize caries risk.

▶ Clarify confusion of hidden sugars, added sugars, and natural sugars.

▶ Clarify the moderation of sugar intake and select substitutions.

C. Review of Dental Caries Initiation

▶ The sucrose from cariogenic food on the tooth surface can be changed to acid in minutes.

▶ The pH drops to below 5.5, which is the critical level for demineralization of enamel.

▶ Acid left undisturbed will be cleared from the mouth from 20 minutes to up to 2 hours, depending primarily on salivary flow. For a patient with xerostomia, clearance takes much longer.

▶ Figure 35-3 illustrates how the frequent intake of sucrose lowers the pH for several hours in the course of the day.

D. Frequency and Time of Exposure

▶ Each exposure of the tooth surface to sucrose or other cariogenic food in a meal or snack increases the amount of acid on the tooth.

▶ The quantity of a cariogenic food is not as significant as when and how often the tooth is exposed.

▶ Prolonged intake of a cariogenic liquid or solid, such as continuous sipping of a sucrose-containing beverage while working at a desk, does not allow for a remineralization period to occur in which the pH can rise above the critical level.

E. Retention

▶ Vigorous rinsing with (fluoridated) water immediately after eating a cariogenic food can help remove the sucrose before it is metabolized by the acid-forming bacteria and reaches the tooth surface.

▶ Cariogenic foods consumed after brushing and flossing before bedtime are not cleared readily because salivary flow decreases during sleep.

▶ Cariogenic liquids are removed from the teeth in relatively less time than are solids.

▶ Oral retentiveness of cariogenic foods is related to length of time food debris with fermentable carbohydrate remains on the teeth and exposure to decreased biofilm pH.[13–15]

  • Highly retentive fermentable carbohydrates have a delayed rate of oral clearance increasing exposure of teeth to a decreased pH and higher potential for demineralization.[13,14]

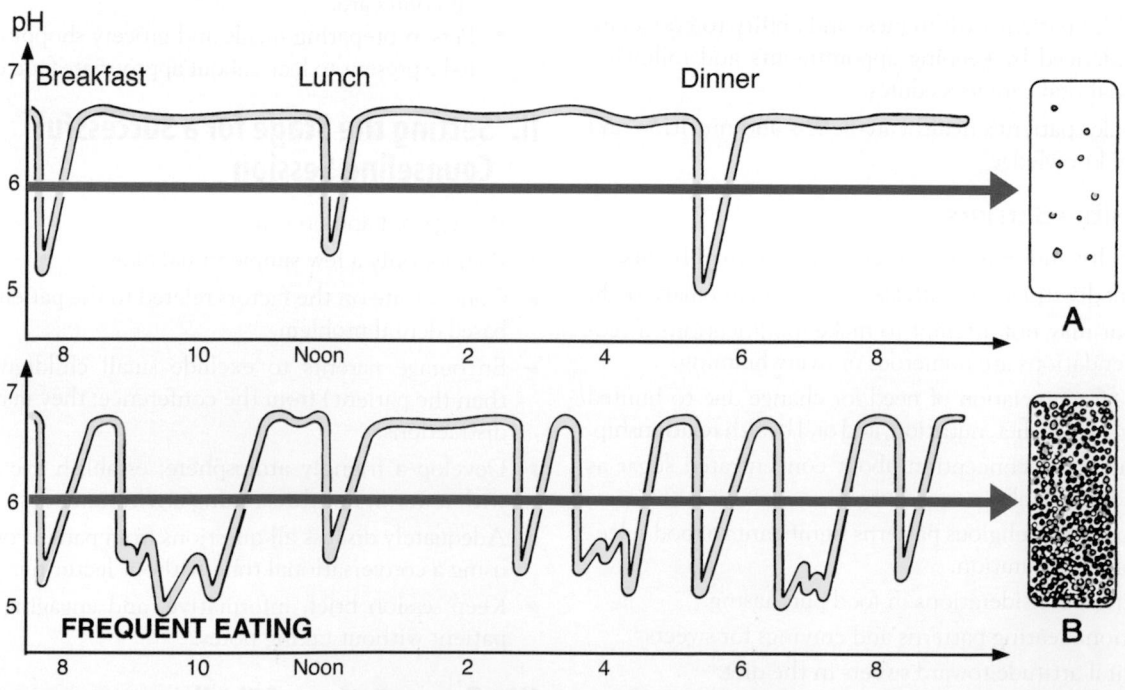

FIGURE 35-3 **Cariogenic Foods and Biofilm pH.** The range of pH in dental biofilm from 5 to 7 is shown on the left. Time intervals are shown across the bottom of each graph. The double-line curve represents the variations in biofilm pH throughout a day. Each time sugar or a cariogenic food is taken in, the pH of the dental biofilm drops to or below the critical pH (5.2–5.5). As shown in the lower graph, frequent eating keeps the pH at the critical level below which enamel demineralization can occur. On the right, **(A)** shows that bacterial counts are lower, whereas in **(B)**, aciduric microorganisms are greatly increased in numbers. The critical pH for the root surfaces is 6.0–6.7. (Adapted with permission from Larmas, M. Simple test for caries susceptibility. *Int Dent J.* 1985;35(2):109–117.)

- Sequence of food consumption within a meal pattern is related to caries incidence.[15–18]
  - Eating fermentable carbohydrates at the beginning of a meal or between other noncariogenic foods (protein and fat) is less cumulative in cariogenic potential.
  - Protein and fat are not metabolized by oral or broken down by salivary amylase bacteria and are recommended to be eaten at the end of a meal.
  - Cheese eaten after sweets or at the end of a meal prevents the decrease in pH and production of acids in the oral cavity.[18]
- Noncariogenic sweeteners contribute to caries prevention.[19]
- Sugar-free gums decrease lactic acid production and increase salivary flow potentially buffering acids.
  - Chewing a gum with xylitol immediately after each meal reduces the levels of *Streptococcus mutans* and promotes remineralization.
  - Xylitol is the sugar substitute of choice because it is not fermentable by caries-promoting bacteria. Sorbitol can be fermented by *Streptococcus mutans* at a very slow rate.[20]

IV. Specific Dietary Recommendations

A. Examination of the Patient's Food Diary

- After analyzing the diet, assist the patient in identifying the deficiencies and excesses in intake.
- Consult Chapter 26 for guidance on working collaboratively with the patient to develop a plan.
- Try to retain as many as possible of the patient's present food habits.
- Make recommendations that can be adapted to the patient's pattern of living.
- Discuss foods from each food group that the patient likes and can be added to the diet.
- Limit the use of cariogenic foods to mealtimes.
  - Evaluate the final food in a meal because it may remain on the teeth if rinsing is not possible.
  - Recommend chewing a gum containing xylitol at the end of each meal especially for a caries-susceptible person.
  - Recommend specific stores in the area where patients can purchase gum containing xylitol.
- Assist patient in finding acceptable substitutions for the cariogenic food choices.
  - Unflavored milk.
  - Cheese.
  - Peanut butter (check the label of the peanut butter to choose one without added sugar) on sliced apples.
  - Sugar-free gelatin or pudding.
- Explore ways to decrease sugar in food preparation and when purchasing ready-made food.
  - Decrease the amount of granulated or brown sugar by half when baking.

- Consider substituting nonsucrose sweeteners such as xylitol.
- Observe care in the purchase of prepared foods and include more foods such as unsweetened fruit juice and canned fruits with no sugar added.
- Natural sugars are just as detrimental as refined sugars (e.g., honey, maple syrup).
- To enhance compliance, help patients create their own meal plans for one day.
  - Incorporate the principles discussed during the counseling.
  - Collaborate on modifications the patient can achieve realistically and is willing to try.
  - Avoid too many changes that may be overwhelming.
  - Determine patient comprehension of information presented and patient's motivational level.
  - Include morning, afternoon, and evening snacks as well as breakfast, lunch, and dinner in a meal plan for a day.
- Encourage daily use of fluoride in water, foods, dentifrices, and rinses.
- When toothbrushing and flossing are not possible, encourage rinsing with water.

EVALUATION OF PROGRESS

I. Immediate Evaluation

- The patient's verbal and nonverbal interest, comprehension, and participation in the dietary analysis and counseling session.

II. Three-Month Follow-up

- Request patient to keep a 3-, 5-, or 7-day food diary for assessment and evaluation.
- Review personal oral care procedures and provide suggestions as needed.
- Scaling as needed; fluoride varnish application.
- Collaborate on ideas for further modifications when indicated. Smaller goals may need to be established for greater compliance.
- Document progress, additional material reviewed, and plan for continued behavior modification.

III. Six-Month Follow-Up

- Perform examination and clinical procedures.
  - Charting of carious lesions and demineralized areas.
  - Disclose and evaluate biofilm score and reteach as needed with new biofilm removal brush, interdental, and tongue-cleaning devices.
  - Scaling as needed; fluoride varnish application.

▶ Compare dental caries incidence with previous chartings and completed restorative dentistry.

▶ Make collaborative dietary recommendations with patient in accord with new assessment.

▶ Document progress, education provided, and plan.

IV. Overall Evaluation

▶ Consistent reduction in dental caries rate in the years following the initial counseling shows sustained change in habits.

▶ Patient's and parents' attitudes toward maintaining adequate oral health habits.

▶ Attempts to maintain a diet containing minimum cariogenic foods.

▶ Compliance with keeping regular appointments for professional dental care.

DOCUMENTATION

The following factors are included when documenting patient care that includes diet analysis and patient counseling:

▶ Rationale for dietary analysis

▶ The type of dietary intake utilized for dietary assessment

▶ The results of the dietary analysis

▶ The results of the sugar score and the level of caries risk

▶ Instructions given on completing the food diary

▶ Box 35-5 contains an example progress note for a patient receiving dietary analysis and counseling.

BOX 35-5

Example Documentation: Patient Receiving a Dietary Analysis and Counseling

S –A 24-year-old, Hispanic female arrived for her annual examination and preventive care appointment. Her medical and dental history were unremarkable.

O –Caries, periodontal, and oral cancer risk assessments were performed. A comprehensive periodontal examination reveals plaque-induced gingivitis with localized bleeding on probing. Dental examination reveals three new carious lesions.

A –Risk assessment indicates the patient is at high risk for dental caries because of the frequency of snacks. A 24-hour recall was performed chair side. Dietary analysis revealed a sweet score of 9, indicating a moderate caries risk. Evaluation of diet for nutritional adequacy revealed an inadequate representation of fruits and vegetables.

P –Preventive education included review of toothbrushing, flossing, and dietary changes to reduce the risk for caries. Reducing the frequency of snacks between meals was discussed. Recommendations including having desserts or sodas during meals. Rinsing with water or chewing xylitol gum were provided as options following desserts or sodas consumed between meals to reduce the caries risk. The patient was also provided with a prescription for a home fluoride for daily application prior to bedtime. A follow-up appointment was made in 2 weeks.

Signed: _____, RDH
Date: _____.

EVERYDAY ETHICS

Ms. Carlson presents with Type I diabetes and several significant changes in her oral cavity since her last dental hygiene appointment including angular cheilosis, glossitis, and several proximal carious lesions. The hygienist, Bettina, believes that Ms. Carlson has advanced dietary needs beyond the scope of practice of a dental hygienist and, therefore, avoids any chairside dietary assessment with the patient. Routine oral self-care instructions are given. On completion of the examination, Bettina mentions her concerns about Ms. Carlson's dietary status to the dentist but does not record any recommendations in the patient's permanent record.

Questions for Consideration

1. What professional protocol for referrals can be followed by the dental hygienist since she believes giving dietary advice to a patient with diabetes is beyond the scope of practice for a dental hygienist?

2. By eliminating the chairside dietary assessment for dental caries prevention did Bettina act nonmaleficently toward the patient? Explain your response.

3. Which ethical principles would be ignored if Bettina does not educate the patient about the preventive measures for her dental caries or document this information in the patient's record?

Factors To Teach The Patient

Medications with Sucrose

▷ The need to avoid liquid or chewable forms containing sucrose.

▷ Reasons to avoid frequent daily use of medications with sucrose.

▷ Reasons for rinsing with water after a medication contained in a sucrose mixture.

Medications with Side Effect of Xerostomia

▷ Drugs the patient is using that cause xerostomia (dry mouth).

▷ How xerostomia increases the risk of dental caries development.

▷ Why it is necessary to use saliva substitutes, chew gum containing xylitol, and avoid slowly dissolving in the mouth candies containing sucrose.

▷ Effect of xerostomia on chewing and swallowing and how it compromises nutrient intake.

Facts About Dental Caries

▷ How dental caries on the tooth surface starts and progresses.

▷ How the interaction of cariogenic foods, tooth surface, saliva, and microorganisms act together contributing as factors in the dental caries process (Figure 35-2).

▷ How repeated, frequent acid production and the pH in the dental biofilm adversely affect the teeth.

▷ Why there is a need to avoid frequent episodes of eating or drinking food or beverages that contain sucrose (Figure 35-3).

References

1. National Research Council. *Dietary Reference Intakes: Applications in Dietary Planning.* Washington, DC: The National Academies Press; 2003.

2. National Research Council. *Dietary Reference Intakes: The Essential Guide to Nutrient Requirements.* Washington, DC: The National Academies Press; 2006.

3. Institute of Medicine. Dietary Reference Intakes for Thiamin, Riboflavin, Niacin, Vitamin B6, Folate, Vitamin B12, Pantothenic Acid, Biotin, and Choline. Washington, DC: The National Academies Press; 1998.

4. Department of Agriculture, Center for Nutrition Policy and Promotion. ChooseMyPlate guidelines. 2011. http://www.choosemyplate.gov. Accessed February 13, 2014.

5. Neiva RF, Steigenga J, Al-Shammari KF, et al. Effects of specific nutrients on periodontal disease onset, progression and treatment. *J Clin Periodontol.* 2003;30(7):579–589.

6. Nishida M, Grossi SG, Dunford RG, et al. Calcium and the risk for periodontal disease. *J Periodontol.* 2000;71(7):1057–1066.

7. Nishida M, Grossi SG, Dunford RG, et al. Dietary vitamin C and the risk for periodontal disease. *J Periodontol.* 2000;71(8):1215–1223.

8. Moura-Grec PG, Marsicano JA, Carvalho CA, et al. Obesity and periodontitis: systematic review and meta-analysis. *Cien Saude Colet.* 2014;19(6):1763–1772.

9. Linden GJ, Lyons A, Scannapieco FA. Periodontal systemic associations: review of the evidence. *J Periodontol.* 2013;84(4, Suppl):S8–S19.

10. Chou R, Cantor A, Zakher B, et al. Preventing dental caries in children <5 years: systematic review updating USPSTF recommendation. *Pediatrics.* 2013;132(2):332–350.

11. Bradshaw DJ, Lynch RJ. Diet and the microbial aetiology of dental caries: new paradigms. *Int Dent J.* 2013;63 (Suppl 2):64–72

12. Marshall TA. Chairside diet assessment of caries risk. *J Am Dent Assoc.* 2009;140(6):670–674.

13. Kashket S, Van Houte J, Lopez LR, et al. Lack of correlation between food retention on the human dentition and consumer perception of food stickiness. *J Dent Res.* 1991;70(10):1314–1319.

14. Kashket S, Zhang J, Van Houte J. Accumulation of fermentable sugars and metabolic acids in food particles that become entrapped on the dentition. *J Dent Res.* 1996;75(11):1885–1891.

15. Lingström P, van Houte J, Kashket S. Food starches and dental caries. *Crit Rev Oral Biol Med.* 2000;11(3):366–380.

16. Linke HA, Birkenfeld LH. Clearance and metabolism of starch foods in the oral cavity. *Ann Nutr Metab.* 1999;43(3):131–139.

17. Rugg-Gunn AJ, Edgar WM, Geddes DA, et al. The effect of different meal patterns upon plaque pH in human subjects. *Br Dent J.* 1975;139(9):351–356.

18. Linke HA, Riba HK. Oral clearance and acid production of dairy products during interaction with sweet foods. *Ann Nutr Metab.* 2001;45(5):202–208.

19. Hayes C. The effect of non-cariogenic sweeteners on the prevention of dental caries: a review of the evidence. *J Dent Educ.* 2001;65(10):1106–1109.

20. Fontana M, Gonzalez-Cabezas C. Are we ready for definitive clinical guidelines on xylitol/polyol use? *Adv Dent Res.* 2012;24(2):123–128.

ENHANCE YOUR UNDERSTANDING

thePoint® DIGITAL CONNECTIONS
(see the inside front cover for access information)
- **Audio glossary**
- **Quiz bank**

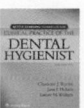

SUPPORT FOR LEARNING
(available separately; visit lww.com)
- *Active Learning Workbook for Clinical Practice of the Dental Hygienist, 12th Edition*

prepU   INDIVIDUALIZED REVIEW
(available separately; visit lww.com)
- Adaptive quizzing with *prepU for Wilkins' Clinical Practice of the Dental Hygienist*

36

Fluorides

Durinda J. Mattana, RDH, BSDH, MS and Erin E. Relich, RDH, BSDH, MSA

CHAPTER OUTLINE

LEARNING OBJECTIVES

After studying this chapter, the student will be able to:

1. Describe the mechanisms of action of fluoride in the prevention of dental caries.

2. Explain the role of community water fluoridation on the decline of dental caries incidence in a community.

3. Recommend appropriate over-the-counter (OTC) and professionally applied fluoride therapies based on each patient's caries risk assessment.

4. Compare use of fluoride home products (OTC and prescription).

5. Incorporate fluoride into individualized prevention plans for patients of various ages and risk levels.

The use of fluorides provides the most effective method for dental caries prevention and control. Fluoride is necessary for optimum oral health at all ages and is made available at the tooth surface by two general means:

▶ *Systemically*, by way of the circulation to developing teeth (preeruptive exposure).

▶ *Topically*, directly to the exposed surfaces of teeth erupted into the oral cavity[1] (posteruptive exposure).

▶ Maximum caries inhibiting effect occurs when there is systemic exposure before tooth eruption and frequent topical fluoride exposure throughout life.[2]

▶ Key words associated with fluoride and fluoride therapy are defined in Box 36-1.

FLUORIDE METABOLISM[1,3]

I. Fluoride Intake

▶ Sources
 • Drinking water that contains fluoride naturally or has been fluoridated
 • Prescribed dietary supplements
 • Foods, in small amounts
 • Foods and beverages prepared at home or processed commercially using water that contains fluoride
 • Varying small amounts ingested from dentifrices, mouthrinses, supplements, and other fluoride products used by the individual.

II. Absorption

A. Gastrointestinal Tract

▶ Fluoride is rapidly absorbed as hydrogen fluoride through passive diffusion in the stomach:
 • Rate and amount of absorption depend on the solubility of the fluoride compound and gastric acidity.
 • Most is absorbed within 60 minutes.

▶ Fluoride that is not absorbed in the stomach will be absorbed by the small intestine.

▶ There is less absorption when the fluoride is taken with milk and other food.

B. Blood Stream

▶ Plasma carries the fluoride for its distribution throughout the body and to the kidneys for elimination.

▶ Maximum blood levels are reached within 30 minutes of intake.

▶ Normal plasma levels are low and rise and fall according to intake.

III. Distribution and Retention

▶ Fluoride is distributed by the plasma to *all* tissues and organs. There is a strong affinity for mineralized tissues.

▶ Approximately 99% of fluoride in the body is located in the mineralized tissues.

▶ Concentrations of fluoride are highest at the surfaces next to the tissue fluid supplying the fluoride.

▶ The fluoride ion (F) is stored as an integral part of the crystal lattice of teeth and bones.
 • Amount stored varies with the intake, the time of exposure, and the age and stage of the development of the individual.
 • The teeth store small amounts, with highest levels on the tooth surface.

▶ Fluoride that accumulates in bone can be mobilized slowly from the skeleton due to the constant resorption and remodeling of bone.

▶ Once tooth enamel is fully matured, the fluoride deposited during development can be altered by cavitated dental caries, erosion, or mechanical abrasion.[1]

IV. Excretion

▶ Most fluoride is excreted through the kidneys in the urine, with a small amount excreted by the sweat glands and the feces.

▶ There is limited transfer from plasma to breast milk for excretion by that route.[1]

FLUORIDE AND TOOTH DEVELOPMENT

▶ Fluoride is a nutrient essential to the formation of sound teeth and bones, as are calcium, phosphorus, and other elements obtained from food and water.

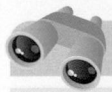

BOX 36-1   KEY WORDS AND ABBREVIATIONS: Fluorides

Abrasive system: cleaning or polishing substances used in dentifrice; best when compatible with fluoride compounds and other ingredients, and does not alter the tooth structure unfavorably.

Acidogenic: producing acid or acidity.

AAPD: American Association of Pediatric Dentistry.

ADA: American Dental Association.

ADACSA: American Dental Association Council on Scientific Affairs.

APF: acidulated phosphate fluoride.

AWWA: American Water Works Association.

Apatite: a group of minerals of the general formula $Ca_{10}(PO_4)X_2$ wherein the X might include hydroxyl (OH), carbonate (CO), fluoride (F), or oxygen (O); crystalline mineral component of hard tissues (bones and teeth).

Cariogenic challenge: exposure of a tooth surface to an acid attack; acid is from the action of dental biofilm and cariogenic food ingested.

Cariostatic: exerting an inhibitory action on the progress of dental caries.

CDC: Centers for Disease Control and Prevention.

Defluoridation: lowering the amount of fluoride in fluoridated water to an optimum level for the prevention of dental caries and dental fluorosis.

Demineralization: breakdown of the tooth structure with a loss of mineral content, primarily calcium and phosphorus.

Dilution: the reduction in the absolute measurable benefits of the effectiveness of an intervention.

DMFT/dmft: decayed, missing, and filled teeth (permanent and primary dentition, respectively).

Efficacy: with reference to a product: an efficacious product produces a statistically and clinically significant benefit under ideal testing conditions in carefully controlled clinical trials.

Enamel hypocalcification: defect of enamel maturation caused by hereditary or systemic irregularities.

FDA: Food and Drug Administration.

Fluorapatite: the form of hydroxyapatite in which fluoride ions have replaced some of the hydroxyl ions; with fluoride, the apatite is less soluble and therefore more resistant to the acids formed from carbohydrate intake.

Fluorhydroxyapatite: apatite formed when low concentrations of fluoride react with tooth mineral; at higher concentrations, calcium fluoride is formed.

Fluoride: a salt of hydrofluoric acid; the ionized form of fluorine that occurs in many tissues and is stored primarily in bones and teeth.

Fluorosis: form of enamel hypomineralization due to excessive ingestion of fluoride during the development and mineralization of the teeth; depending on the length of exposure and the concentration of the fluoride, the fluorosed area may appear as a small white spot or as severe brown staining with pitting.

Gel: semi-solid or solid phase of a colloidal solution.

Glycolysis: process by which sugar is metabolized by bacteria to produce acid.

Hydroxyapatite: $Ca_{10}(PO_4)_6(OH)_2$; the form of apatite that is the principal mineral component of teeth, bones, and calculus.

Hypocalcification: deficient calcification.

Halo or diffusion effect: occurs when foods and beverages processed in a fluoridated community are imported and consumed in a nonfluoridated community.

Maturation: stage or process of becoming mature or attaining maximal development; with respect to tooth development, maturation results from the continuous dynamic exchange of ions into the surface of the enamel from pellicle, dental biofilm, and oral fluids.

NaF: neutral sodium fluoride.

O.T.C.: over the counter.

Prevented fraction: the proportion of disease occurrence in a population that is averted due to an intervention.

ppm: parts per million; measure used to designate the amount of fluoride used for optimum level in fluoridated water, dentifrice, and other fluoride-containing preparations (1 ppm is equivalent to 1 mg/L).

Remineralization: restoration of mineral elements in a tooth surface; enhanced by the presence of fluoride; remineralized lesions are more resistant to initiation of dental caries than is normal tooth structure.

Rx: prescription.

SnF₂: stannous fluoride.

Subsurface lesion: demineralized area below the surface of the enamel created by acid that has passed through micropores between enamel rods; subject to remineralization by action of fluoride.

Thixotropic: type of gel that sets in a gel-like state but becomes fluid under stress; the fluid form permits the solution to flow into interdental areas.

USPHS: United States Public Health Services.

USDHHS: United States Department of Health and Human Services.

"White spot": term used to describe a small area on the surface of enamel that contrasts in appearance with the rest of the surface and may be visible only when the tooth is dried; two types of white spots can be differentiated: an area of demineralization and an area of fluorosis (also referred to as an "enamel opacity").

▶ A comprehensive review of the histology of tooth development and mineralization is recommended to supplement the information included here.[4,5]

I. Preeruptive: Mineralization Stage

▶ Fluoride is deposited during the formation of the enamel, starting at the dentinoenamel junction, after the enamel matrix has been laid down by the ameloblasts.

- Figure 36-1A shows the distribution of fluoride in all parts of the teeth during mineralization.
- The hydroxyapatite crystalline structure becomes *fluorapatite*, which is a less soluble apatite crystal.[2]
- Pre-eruptive fluoride may contribute to shallower occlusal grooves, and reduce the risk of fissure caries.[2]

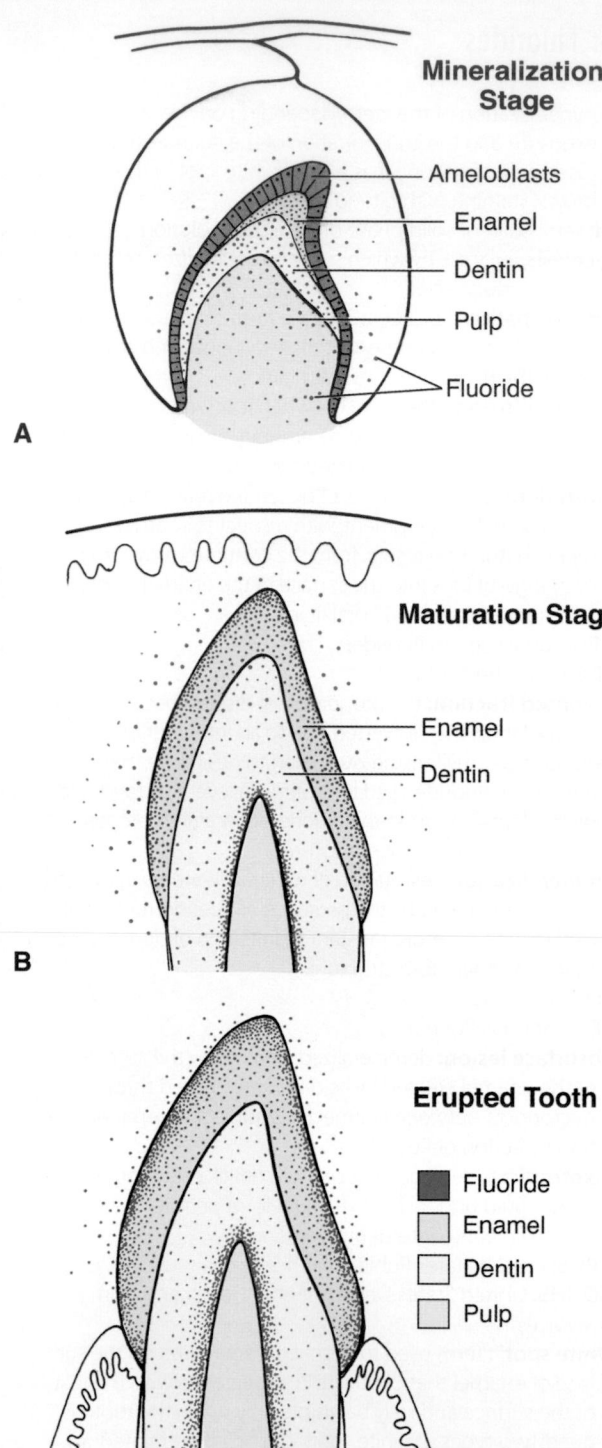

Mineralization Stage

- Ameloblasts
- Enamel
- Dentin
- Pulp
- Fluoride

A

Maturation Stage

- Enamel
- Dentin

B

Erupted Tooth

- ■ Fluoride
- ▨ Enamel
- □ Dentin
- ▢ Pulp

C

FIGURE 36-1 Systemic Fluoride. Green dots represent fluoride ions in the tissues and distributed throughout the tooth. **A:** Developing tooth during mineralization shows fluoride from water and other systemic sources deposited in the enamel and dentin. **B:** Maturation stage before eruption, when fluoride is taken up from tissue fluids around the crown. **C:** Erupted tooth continues to take up fluoride on the surface from external sources. Note concentrated fluoride deposition on the enamel surface and on the pulpal surface of the dentin.

▶ Table 50-4, in Chapter 50, lists the weeks in utero when the hard tissue formation begins for the primary teeth.

▶ The first permanent molars begin to mineralize at birth as listed in Table 16-1, in Chapter 16.

▶ Effect of excess fluoride (fluorosis)[6,7]

- Dental fluorosis is a form of hypomineralization that results from systemic ingestion of an excess amount of fluoride during tooth development.
- During mineralization the enamel is highly receptive to free fluoride ions.
- The normal activity of the ameloblasts may be inhibited, and the defective enamel matrix that can form results in discontinuity of crystal growth.

▶ Dental fluorosis can appear clinically in varying degrees from white flecks or striations to cosmetically objectionable stained pitting as listed in Tables 23-2 and 23-3, in Chapter 23.

II. Preeruptive: Maturation Stage

▶ After mineralization is complete and before eruption, fluoride deposition continues in the surface of the enamel.

- Figure 36-1B shows fluoride around the crown during maturation.
- Fluoride is taken up from the nutrient tissue fluids surrounding the tooth crown.

III. Posteruptive

▶ After eruption and throughout the life span of the teeth, the concentration of fluoride on the outermost surface of the enamel is dependent on:

- Daily topical sources of fluoride to prevent demineralization and encourage remineralization for prevention of dental caries.
- Sources for daily topical fluoride include fluoridated drinking water, dentifrices, mouthrinses, and other fluoride preparations used by the patient.
- The fluoride on the outermost surface is available to inhibit demineralization and enhance remineralization as needed on a daily basis.
- Figure 36-2 depicts the areas on the tooth that acquire fluoride after eruption.
  - The continuous daily presence of fluoride provided for the tooth surfaces can inhibit the initiation and progression of dental caries.
  - Uptake is most rapid on the enamel surface during the first years after eruption.
  - Repeated daily intake of drinking water with fluoride provides a topical source as it washes over the teeth throughout life.

TOOTH SURFACE FLUORIDE

Fluoride concentration is greatest on the surface next to the source of fluoride.

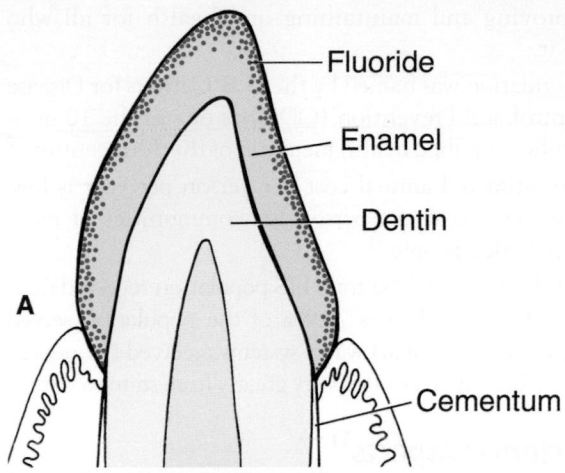

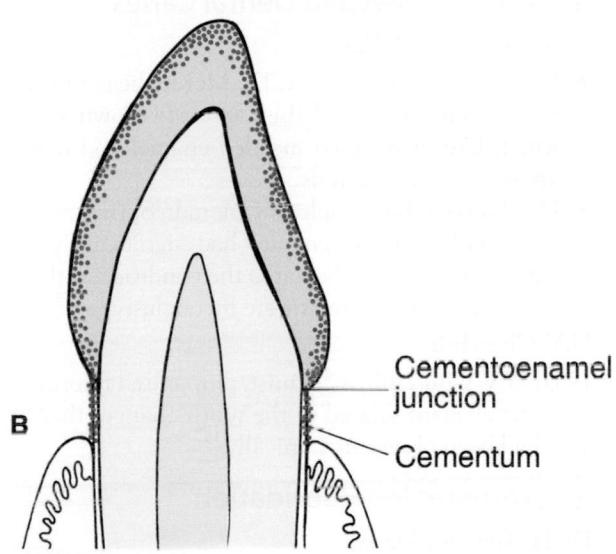

FIGURE 36-2 **Fluoride Acquisition after Eruption. A:** Fluoride represented by green dots on the enamel surface is taken up from external sources, including dentifrice, rinse, topical application, and fluoridated drinking water passing over the teeth. **B:** Gingival recession exposes the cementum to external sources of fluoride for the prevention of root caries and the alleviation of sensitivity.

► For the enamel of the erupted tooth, highest concentration is at the outer surface exposed to the oral cavity.

► For the dentin, the highest concentration is at the pulpal surface.

► Periodontal attachment loss (gingival recession) can often cause the root surface and cementum to become exposed to the oral cavity and external fluoride sources.

I. Fluoride in Enamel

A. Uptake

► Uptake of fluoride depends on the level of fluoride in the oral environment and the length of time of exposure.

► Hypomineralized enamel absorbs fluoride in greater quantities than sound enamel; it incorporates into

the hydroxyapatite crystalline structure to become fluorapatite.[6]

► Demineralized enamel that has been remineralized in the presence of fluoride will have a greater concentration of fluoride than sound enamel.

B. Fluoride in the Enamel Surface

► Fluoride is a natural constituent of enamel.

► The intact outer surface has the highest concentration that falls sharply toward the interior of the tooth.[8]

II. Fluoride in Dentin[9]

► The fluoride level may be greater in dentin than in enamel.

► A higher concentration is at the pulpal or inner surface, where exchanges take place.

► Newly formed dentin absorbs fluoride rapidly.

III. Fluoride in Cementum[9]

► The level of fluoride in cementum is high and increases with exposure.

  • With recession of the clinical attachment level, the root surface is exposed to the fluids of the oral cavity.

  • Figure 36-2B shows fluoride acquisition to exposed cementum.

  • Fluoride is then available to the cementum from the saliva and all the sources used by the patient, including drinking water, dentifrice, and mouthrinse.

DEMINERALIZATION– REMINERALIZATION[8]

Figure 36-3 illustrates the comparative levels of fluoride that may be found in the tooth surface and the sublevel lesion in early dental caries.

I. Fluoride in Biofilm and Saliva

► Saliva and biofilm are reservoirs for fluoride; saliva carries minerals available for remineralization when needed.

► Fluoride helps to inhibit demineralization when it is present at the crystal surface during an acid challenge.

► Fluoride enhances remineralization forming a condensed layer on the crystal surface, which attracts calcium and phosphate ions.

► High concentrations of fluoride can interfere with the growth and metabolism of bacteria.

► Dental biofilm may contain 5–50 ppm fluoride. The content varies greatly and is constantly changing.

► Fluoride may be acquired directly from fluoridated water, dentifrice, and other topical sources and brought by the saliva or by an exchange of fluoride in the biofilm to the demineralizing tooth surface under the biofilm.

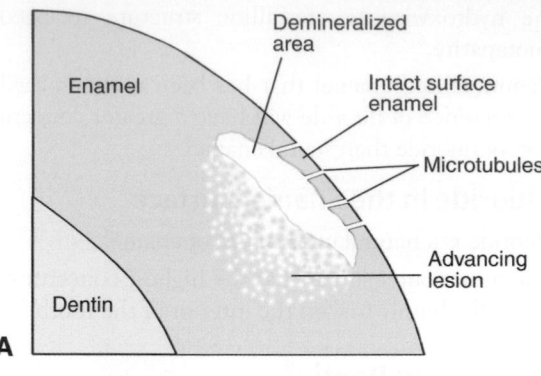

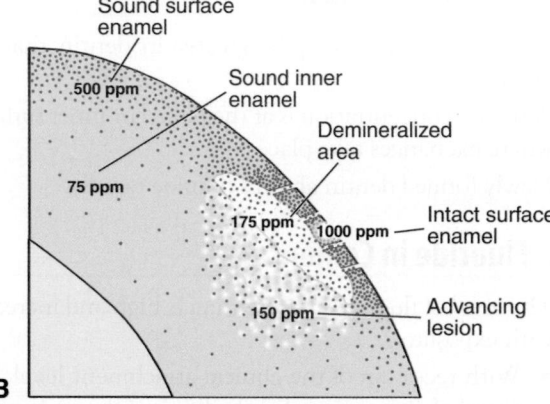

FIGURE 36-3 **Examples of Enamel Fluoride Content. A:** Early stage of dental caries with an intact surface enamel and subsurface demineralized area. **B:** A demineralized area readily takes up available fluoride. As shown, the fluoride content (1,000 ppm) of the relatively intact surface over a subsurface demineralized white spot is higher than that of the sound surface enamel (500 ppm). The body of the advancing lesion has a higher fluoride content (150 ppm) than does the sound inner enamel (75 ppm). (Source: Melberg JR, Ripa LW, Leske GS. *Fluoride in Preventive Dentistry: Theory and Clinical Applications*. Chicago, IL: Quintessence; 1983:31.)

II. Summary of Fluoride Action

Having fluoride available topically to the tooth posteruptively is key to its effectiveness.

▶ Frequent exposure to fluoride, such as from fluoridated water, dentifrice, and mouthrinse, is recommended.

▶ There are three basic topical effects of fluoride to prevent dental caries.[8]

• Inhibit demineralization.

• Enhance remineralization of incipient lesions.

• Inhibit bacterial activity by inhibiting *enolase*, an enzyme needed by bacteria to metabolize carbohydrates.

FLUORIDATION

▶ *Fluoridation* is the adjustment of the natural fluoride ion content in a municipal water supply to the optimum physiologic concentration that will maximize caries prevention and limit enamel fluorosis.[10]

▶ Fluoridation has been established as the most efficient, effective, reliable, and inexpensive means for improving and maintaining oral health for all who use it.

▶ Fluoridation was named by the U.S. Centers for Disease Control and Prevention (CDC) as one of the 10 most significant public health measures of the 20th century.[10]

▶ The estimated annual cost per person per year is low, with lower cost per person for communities of more than 20,000 people.[11]

▶ In 2010, 66.2% of the total US population received fluoridated water, whereas 73.9% of the population served by public (municipal) water systems received fluoridated water. These percentages vary greatly from state to state.[12]

I. Historical Aspects[13]

A. Mottled Enamel and Dental Caries

▶ Dr. Frederick S. McKay

• Early in the 20th century, Dr. McKay began his extensive studies to find the cause of "brown stain," which later was called mottled enamel and now is known as *dental fluorosis*.

• He observed that people in Colorado Springs, Colorado, with mottled enamel had significantly less dental caries.[14] He associated the condition with the drinking water, but tests were inconclusive.

▶ H.V. Churchill

In 1931, H.V. Churchill, a chemist, pinpointed fluorine as the specific element related to the tooth changes that Dr. McKay had been observing clinically.[15]

B. Background for Fluoridation

▶ Dr. H. Trendley Dean

• Epidemiologic studies of the 1930s, sponsored by the US Public Health Service (USPHS) and directed by Dr. Dean, led to the conclusion that the level of fluoride in the water optimum for dental caries prevention averages 1 ppm in moderate climates.

• Clinically objectionable dental fluorosis is associated with levels well over 2 ppm.[16]

• From this knowledge and the fact many healthy people had lived long lives in communities where the fluoride content of the water was much greater than 1 ppm, the concept of adding fluoride to the water developed.

• It was still necessary to show the benefits from controlled fluoridation could parallel those of natural fluoride.

C. Fluoridation—1945

▶ The first communities were fluoridated in 1945.

▶ Research in the communities began before fluoridation was started to obtain baseline information.

D. Control Cities

▶ Aurora, Illinois, where the natural fluoride level is optimum (1.2 ppm), was used to compare the benefits of natural fluoride in the water supply with those of fluoridation, as well as with a fluoride-free city, Rockford, Illinois.

▶ Original cities with fluoridation and their control cities in the research are shown in Box 36-2.

▶ The research conducted in those cities, as well as throughout the world, has documented the influence of fluoride on oral health.

II. Water Supply Adjustment

A. Fluoride Level

▶ Since 1962, the USPHS recommended the optimal fluoride concentration of 0.7 ppm (for warmer climates) to 1.2 ppm (for colder climates) to prevent dental caries and minimize fluorosis.[17]

- The range in fluoride concentration was based on the assumption that people in warmer climates drink more water and therefore receive more fluoride.

▶ In 2015, the US Department of Health and Human Services (USDHHS) updated the recommendation for the optimal concentration of water fluoridation to 0.7 ppm for all communities.

- The decision is based on the fact that Americans have access to many more sources of fluoride today than they did when water fluoridation was introduced in the United States.[18]
- The change still provides an effective level of fluoride to reduce the incidence of dental caries while minimizing the rate of fluorosis.

B. Chemicals Used

▶ All fluoride chemicals must conform to the appropriate American Water Works Association (AWWA) standards to ensure that the drinking water will be safe.[17]

▶ Sources

- Compounds from which the fluoride ion is derived are naturally occurring and are mined in various parts of the world.
- Examples of common sources are fluorspar, cryolite, and apatite.

▶ Criteria for acceptance of a fluoride compound for fluoridation include:

- Solubility to permit regular use in a water plant.
- Relatively inexpensive.
- Readily available to prevent interruptions in maintaining the proper fluoride level.

▶ Compounds used:

- Dry compounds: sodium fluoride (NaF) and sodium silicofluoride.
- Liquid solution: hydrofluorosilicic acid.

EFFECTS AND BENEFITS OF FLUORIDATION

Fluoridated water is a systemic source of fluoride for developing teeth and a topical source of fluoride on the surfaces of erupted teeth throughout life.[19]

I. Appearance of Teeth

▶ Teeth exposed to an optimum or slightly higher level of fluoride appear white, shining, opaque, and without blemishes.

- When the level is slightly more than optimum, teeth may exhibit mild enamel fluorosis seen as white areas in bands or flecks. Without close scrutiny, such spots blend with the overall appearance.

▶ The majority of fluorosis today is mild and not considered an esthetic problem.[10,20]

II. Dental Caries: Permanent Teeth

A. Overall Benefits

▶ Maximum benefit is seen with continuous use of fluoridated water from birth.

▶ Estimates have shown the reduction in caries due to water fluoridation alone (factoring out other sources of topical fluoride) among adults of all ages is 27%.[19]

▶ The effects are similar to communities with optimum levels of natural fluoride in the water.

▶ Many more individuals are completely caries-free when fluoride is in the water.

B. Distribution

▶ Anterior teeth, particularly maxillary, receive more protection from fluoride than do posterior teeth.[16]

- Anterior teeth are contacted by the drinking water as it passes into the mouth.

C. Progression

▶ Not only are the numbers of carious lesions reduced, but the caries rate is slowed.

▶ Caries progression is also reduced in the surfaces that receive fluoride for the first time after eruption.[21]

III. Root Caries

▶ Root caries experience in lifelong residents of a naturally fluoridated community is in direct proportion to the fluoride concentration in the water compared with the experience of residents of a fluoride-free community.[22]

▶ The incidence of root caries is approximately 50% less for lifelong residents of a fluoridated community.[23]

IV. Dental Caries: Primary Teeth

▶ With fluoridation from birth, the caries incidence is reduced up to 40% in the primary teeth.[10]

▶ The introduction of fluoridation into a community significantly increases the proportion of caries-free children and reduces the decayed, missing, and filled teeth (dmft/DMFT) scores when compared to areas that are nonfluoridated over the same time period.[20]

▶ For example, children aged 6–9 years in Newburgh, New York, had five times as many caries-free primary teeth present as did the children of Kingston, where fluoride was not present in the community drinking water.[24]

V. Tooth Loss

▶ Tooth loss due to dental caries is much greater in both primary and permanent teeth without fluoride[24] because of increased dental caries, which progresses more rapidly.

VI. Adults

▶ When a person resides in a community with fluoride in the drinking water throughout life, benefits continue.

▶ In Colorado Springs, adults aged 20–44 years who had used water with natural fluoride showed 60% less caries experience than did adults in fluoride-deficient Boulder, Colorado. In Boulder, adults also had three to four times as many permanent teeth extracted.[25]

▶ In a survey of adults in Rockford, Illinois (no fluoride), there were about seven times as many edentulous persons as there were in a comparable group in Aurora, Illinois (natural fluoride).[26]

VII. Periodontal Health

▶ Indirect favorable effects of fluoride on periodontal health can be shown.
  • Fluoride works to decrease dental caries. The presence of carious lesions favors biofilm retention

which can lead to periodontal infection, particularly adjacent to the gingival margin.

▶ With the use of fluorides, particularly water fluoridation, fewer teeth are lost because of dental caries at younger ages. Periodontal disease prevention and control is to be emphasized in communities with fluoride in the drinking water.

PARTIAL DEFLUORIDATION

▶ Water with an excess of natural fluoride does not meet the requirements of the USPHS.

▶ Several hundred communities in the United States had water supplies that naturally contained more than twice the optimal level of fluoride.

▶ Defluoridation can be accomplished by one of several chemical systems.[27] The efficacy of the methods has been shown.

▶ Examples: The water supply in Britton, South Dakota, has been reduced from almost 7 to 1.5 ppm since 1948, and in Bartlett, Texas, from 8 to 1.8 ppm since 1952. Examinations have shown a significant reduction in the incidence of objectionable fluorosis in children born since defluoridation.[27,28]

SCHOOL FLUORIDATION

▶ To bring the benefits of fluoridation to children living in rural areas without the possibility for community fluoridation, adding fluoride to a school water supply has been an alternative.

▶ Because of the intermittent use of the school water (only 5 days each week during the 9-month school year), the amount of fluoride added was increased over the usual 1 ppm.

▶ Example: 12 years of fluoride at 5 ppm in the school drinking water of Elk Lake, Pennsylvania.
  • Children who had attended that school regularly had 39% fewer decayed, missing, and filled teeth than did those in the control group.
  • The greatest benefits were found on proximal tooth surfaces.[29]

▶ Example: In the schools of Seagrove, North Carolina, after 12 years with the fluoride level at 6.3 ppm, the children experienced a 47.5% decrease in DMF surfaces compared with those in the control group.[29]

▶ Such systems have significance in the long history of efforts for fluoridation for all people in the United States.

▶ School fluoridation has been phased out in several states, and the current extent of this practice is unknown. Operations and maintenance of small fluoridation systems are problematic.[10]

DISCONTINUED FLUORIDATION

▶ When fluoride is removed from a community water supply that had dental caries control by fluoridation, the effects can be clearly shown.

▶ Example: In Antigo, Wisconsin, the action of antifluoridationists in 1960 brought about the discontinuance of fluoridation, which had been installed in 1949.

  • Examinations in the years following 1960 revealed the marked drop in the number of children who were caries-free and the steep increases in caries rates.

  • From 1960 to 1966, the number of caries-free children in the second grade decreased by 67%.[30]

  • Fluoridation was reinstated in 1966 by popular demand.

FLUORIDES IN FOODS

I. Foods[31]

▶ Certain foods contain fluoride, but not enough to constitute a significant part of the day's need for caries prevention.

▶ Examples: meat, eggs, vegetables, cereals, and fruit have small but measurable amounts, whereas tea and fish have larger amounts.

▶ Foods cooked in fluoridated water retain fluoride from the cooking water.

II. Salt[32–34]

▶ Fluoridated salt has not been promoted in the United States, but is widely used in Germany, France, and Switzerland where 30%–80% of the domestic marketed salt is fluoridated.

▶ Another 30 countries or more use fluoridated salt worldwide for its effectiveness as a community health program.

▶ Fluoridated salt results in a reduced incidence of dental caries, but there is insufficient evidence for its overall effectiveness.

▶ Fluoridated salts currently available supply about one-third to one-half of the amount of fluoride ingested daily from 1 ppm fluoridated water.

▶ Fluoridated salt is recommended by the World Health Organization as an alternative to fluoridated water to target underprivileged groups.

III. Halo/Diffusion Effect

▶ Foods and beverages that are commercially processed (cooked or reconstituted) in optimally fluoridated cities can be distributed and consumed in nonfluoridated communities.

▶ The halo or diffusion effect can result in increased fluoride intake by individuals living in nonfluoridated communities, providing them some protection against dental caries.[31]

IV. Bottled Water

▶ Bottled water usually does not contain optimal fluoride unless it has a label indicating that it is fluoridated.

▶ Patients need to be advised to fill their drinking water bottles from a fluoridated water supply.

V. Water Filters[35]

▶ Reverse osmosis and water distillation systems remove fluoride from the water, but water softeners do not.

▶ Carbon filters (for the end of a faucet or in pitchers) vary in their removal of fluoride.

▶ Carbon filters with activated alumina remove fluoride.

▶ Patients need to be warned that water filters may remove fluoride from the drinking water and need to be checked with the manufacturer before purchase.

VI. Infant Formula[36–38]

▶ There has been an increase in breast feeding in the United States, but infant formula remains a major source of nutrition for many infants.

▶ Ready-to-feed formulas do not need to be reconstituted, but water is added to powdered and liquid concentrate formulas.

▶ Breast milk may contain 0.02 ppm fluoride and all types of infant formula themselves contain a low amount of fluoride (0.11–0.57 ppm).[37]

▶ The level of fluoride in the water supply used to reconstitute powdered or liquid concentrate formulas determines the total fluoride intake.

▶ The American Dental Association (ADA) recommends continuing to use optimally fluoridated water to reconstitute infant formula while being aware of the possible risk of mild enamel fluorosis in the primary teeth.[38]

DIETARY FLUORIDE SUPPLEMENTS[10,39,40]

▶ Prescribed dietary supplements were introduced in the late 1940s and are intended to compensate for fluoride-deficient drinking water.

▶ The current supplementation dosage schedule developed by the ADA and the American Association of Pediatric Dentistry (AAPD) and revised in 1994 includes children aged 6 months through 16 years.

  • Table 36-1 contains the daily dosage amounts based on the age of the child and the amount of fluoride in the primary water supply.

TABLE 36-1	Fluoride Supplements Dose Schedule (Mg NaF/d)ᵃ		
	WATER FLUORIDE ION CONCENTRATION (PPM)		
AGE OF CHILD (Y)	**LESS THAN 0.3**	**BETWEEN 0.3 AND 0.6**	**GREATER THAN 0.6**
Birth–6 mo	0	0	0
6 mo–3 y	0.25 mg	0	0
3–6 y	0.50 mg	0.25 mg	0
6–16 y	1.0 mg	0.50 mg	0

ᵃAbout 2.2 mg of sodium fluoride provides 1 mg of fluoride ion.
Source: American Dental Association and the American Academy of Pediatrics.

▶ Clinical recommendations from the American Dental Association Council on Scientific Affairs (ADACSA) include the use of fluoride supplements for children:
- At high risk of developing dental caries
- Those whose primary source of drinking water is deficient in fluoride.[41]

I. Assess Possible Need

▶ Review the patient's history to be certain the child is not receiving other fluoride in such preparations as vitamin–fluoride supplements.

▶ Determine the fluoride level of all sources of drinking water is below 0.6 ppm.

▶ Refer to the list of fluoridated communities available from state or local health departments.

▶ Request water analysis when the fluoride level has not been determined, for example, in private well water.

▶ Determine the child's risk for dental caries is high or moderately high before considering the use of fluoride supplements.[39]

▶ Reassess the caries risk at frequent intervals as the status may be affected by the child's development, personal and family situations, and behavioral factors such as changes in oral hygiene practices.[33,41]

II. Available Forms of Supplements

▶ NaF supplements are available as tablets, lozenges, and drops in 0.25, 0.50, and 1.0 mg dosages.

▶ Prescribed on an individual patient basis for daily use at home.

A. Tablets and Lozenges

▶ Tablets are chewed thoroughly, swished/rinsed around in the oral cavity, and forced between the teeth before swallowing.

▶ Lozenges are dissolved for one to 2 minutes in the mouth to provide both preeruptive and posteruptive benefits.[41]

▶ Best taken at bedtime after teeth are brushed.
- Avoid drinking, eating, or rinsing before going to sleep to gain maximum benefit.

B. Drops

▶ A liquid concentrate with directions that specify the number of drops for the prescription dose daily.

▶ Primary use for child 6 months to 3 years, and patient of any age unable to use other forms that require chewing and swallowing.

III. Prescription Guidelines

▶ No more than 264 mg NaF (120 mg fluoride ion) to be dispensed per household at one time.

▶ Take supplements with juice or water.
- Avoid taking with dairy products because fluoride can combine with calcium and be poorly absorbed.

▶ Storage
- Keep products out of reach of children.
- Keep tablets in the original container, away from heat and direct light, and away from damp places such as a bathroom or kitchen sink area.

▶ Missed dose
- Take as soon as remembered.
- If near next dose time, skip that dose and go to next regular time.

IV. Benefits and Limitations

▶ Prenatal use by pregnant women
- Administration of prenatal dietary fluoride supplements is not recommended.
- Some evidence has shown that fluoride crosses the placenta during the fifth and sixth months of pregnancy and may enter the prenatal deciduous enamel.[42]
- Overall, there is weak evidence to support the use of fluoride supplements to prevent dental caries in primary teeth.

▶ Daily fluoride supplements offer caries preventive benefits in permanent teeth. School-aged children who chewed, swished, and swallowed 1 mg fluoride tablets daily on school days had significantly lower caries experience than children who did not use fluoride supplements.

▶ The use of fluoride supplements in children over 6 years of age shows a 24% decrease in DMF tooth surfaces in permanent teeth compared to no fluoride supplements.[43]

▶ Consider the child's age, caries risk, and all sources of fluoride exposure before recommending the use of fluoride supplements.[33,41]

PROFESSIONAL TOPICAL FLUORIDE APPLICATIONS

Topical fluorides are an essential part of a total preventive program for patients of all ages.

▶ Fluoridated water and fluoride toothpaste are the primary sources of topical fluoride for patients of all ages and levels of caries risk.

▶ Additional topical fluoride sources may be professionally applied and/or self-applied by the patient, primarily for those at an elevated caries risk.

I. Historical Perspectives

▶ Professionally applied fluoride has been instrumental in the reduction of dental caries in the United States and other industrialized countries since the early 1940s.

▶ Dr. Basil G. Bibby conducted the initial topical NaF study using Brockton, Massachusetts schoolchildren.[44]

▶ More than one-third fewer new carious lesions resulted from a 0.1% aqueous solution applied at 4-month intervals for 2 years applied by a dental hygienist.

▶ The research led to extensive studies by Dr. John W. Knutson and others sponsored by the USPHS.

• The aim was to determine the most effective concentration of NaF, the minimum time required for application, and procedural details.[45,46]

• Their results provided the basis for the applications currently used and described in the following sections of this chapter.

• Professionally applied fluorides are available as gels or foams delivered in trays, or varnish that is applied with a soft brush on the teeth.

II. Indications

▶ The professional application of a high-concentration fluoride preventive agent is based on caries risk assessment for the individual patient.

▶ See Table 27-1 in Chapter 27 for the criteria to determine low, moderate, and high caries risk.

▶ Indications for a professional fluoride application are outlined in Box 36-3.[47]

III. Compounds

▶ Table 36-2 provides a summary of the available professional fluoride applications.

• 2.0% NaF as gel or foam delivered in trays.

BOX 36-3

Indications for Professional Topical Fluoride Application[47]

▷ Patients at an elevated (moderate or high) risk of developing caries

See Table 27-1 in Chapter 27 for the criteria to determine low, moderate, and high caries risk.

▷ **5% NaF varnish** at least every 3–6 months (for all ages and adult root caries)

Or

▷ **1.23% APF gel** 4-minute trays at least every 3–6 months (for 6 years and older and adult root caries)

▷ Patients at a low risk of developing caries may not benefit from additional topical fluoride other than OTC-fluoridated toothpaste and fluoridated water daily.

Source: American Dental Association Council on Scientific Affairs. Topical fluoride for caries prevention: executive summary of updated clinical recommendations and supporting systematic review. *J Am Dent Assoc.* 2013;144(11):1279–1291.

• 1.23% acidulated phosphate fluoride (APF) as a gel or foam delivered in trays.

• 5% NaF as a varnish brushed on the teeth.

▶ *2.0% NaF gel*

• NaF, also called "neutral sodium fluoride" due to its neutral pH of 7.0, contains 9,050 ppm fluoride ion.

• Clinical trials demonstrating the efficacy of neutral NaF are based on a series of four or five applications on a weekly basis.[48]

• Quarterly or semiannual applications are most common in clinical practice.

▶ *2.0% NaF foam*

• There is limited clinical evidence to demonstrate foam's effectiveness in caries prevention.

▶ *1.23% APF gel*

• Contains 12,300 ppm fluoride ion.

• A 4-minute tray application is recommended at least every 3–6 months per year for individuals 6 years of age and older at an elevated risk for dental caries.[47]

• Widely used because of its storage stability, acceptable taste, and tissue compatibility.

• Low pH of 3.5 enhances fluoride uptake, which is greatest during the first 4 minutes.[49]

• APF may etch porcelain and composite restorative materials, so it is not indicated for patients with porcelain, composite restorations, and sealants.[50]

• The hydrofluoride component of APF can dissolve the filler particles of the composite resin restorations.

• Macroinorganic filler particles of composite materials demonstrate noticeable etched patterns generated by APF, whereas many of the more recently available microfilled composites/resins are not as sensitive to the APF.[50]

TABE 36-2	Professionally Applied Topical Fluorides			
AGENT	**FORM**	**CONCENTRATION**	**APPLICATION MODE/FREQUENCY**	**NOTES**
NaF neutral or 7 pH	2% Gel or foam[a]	9,050 ppm 0.90% F ion	Tray (4 min)/no currently recommended interval	Do not overfill: see Figure 36-5
Acidulated phosphate 3.5 pH	1.23% Gel or foam[a]	12,300 ppm 1.23% F ion	Tray (4 min)/at least every 3–6 mo[47]	Do not overfill: see Figure 36-5
NaF neutral or 7 pH	5% Varnish	22,600 ppm 2.6% F ion	Apply thin layer with a soft brush (1–2 min)/at least every 3–6 mo[47]	Sets up to a hard film

[a]There is limited published clinical evidence supporting the effectiveness of foam.[47]

- The prevented fraction of dental caries ranged from 18% to 41% with the use of APF or NaF gels.[51]

▶ *1.23% APF foam*
- There is limited clinical evidence to show the effectiveness of foam in caries prevention.

▶ *5% NaF varnish*
- Fluoride varnishes were developed during the late 1960s and early 1970s to prolong contact time of the fluoride with the tooth surface.[52]
- Varnishes are safe and effective, fast and easy to apply, and patient acceptance is good.
- The use of fluoride varnish 2–4 times per year is associated with a 43% decrease in DMFT surfaces in permanent teeth and 37% in primary teeth.[53]
- Varnish has a higher concentration of fluoride than gel or foam (22,600 ppm fluoride ion), but an overall less amount of fluoride is used per application (<7 mg varnish versus 30 mg of gel for a child).
- Varnish sets quickly and remains on the teeth for a number of hours releasing fluoride into the pits and fissures, proximal surfaces, and cervical areas of the tooth where it is needed the most.[54]
- Application is recommended at least every 3–4 months per year for individuals at an elevated risk for dental caries.[47]
- Varnish is effective in reversing active pit and fissure enamel lesions in the primary dentition[55] and remineralizing enamel lesions regardless of whether the varnish is applied over or around the demineralizng lesion.[56]
- Varnish is also effective in reducing demineralization (white areas) around orthodontic brackets.[57]
- Varnish is the fluoride application of choice for those with dentin hypersensitivity; see Chapter 44.

- Varnish is the only professional topical fluoride to be used for children under the age of 6 years.
- Varnish received approval from the United States FDA in 1994 for use as a cavity liner and for treatment of hypersensitive teeth.
- Its use in the United States as a caries preventive agent is considered off-label, but has become a standard of care in practice.[54]

CLINICAL PROCEDURES: PROFESSIONAL TOPICAL FLUORIDE

I. Objectives

▶ *Prevention of dental caries*
- Identify special problems, including areas adjacent to restorations, orthodontic appliances, xerostomia, and other risk factors.
- Box 36-3 contains indications for the application of a professional fluoride.
- Examples: Active or secondary caries, exposed root surfaces, current orthodontic treatment, low or no fluoride exposure, or compromised salivary flow.

▶ *Remineralization of demineralized areas*
- Demineralized white areas on the cervical third, especially under dental biofilm.

▶ *Desensitization*
- Fluoride aids in blocking dentinal tubules, as explained in Chapter 44.

▶ Varnish covers and protects a sensitive area, and fluoride is slowly released for uptake.

II. Preparation of the Teeth for Topical Application

▶ *General preparation for tray and varnish applications*
- Instruct patients about all methods of caries prevention and how they work together.

- Most patients will receive the professional topical application following their routine continuing care appointment with complete dental hygiene procedures of personal oral hygiene care instruction, scaling, and stain removal.
- When the fluoride application is to be applied at a time other than following scaling and debridement, rubber cup polishing is not routinely necessary because fluoride will penetrate biofilm and provide the same benefits with or without prior polishing.[47,58]
- Calculus and stain removal are completed first.
- After calculus removal, apply principles of selective polishing for stain removal.

- Select an appropriate cleaning or polishing agent that will not harm the tooth surface or the restorative material present.
- A fluoride-containing polishing paste is not effective as a fluoride application.[59]
- Preparation and procedure for gel or foam tray application is included in Table 36-3; preparation and procedure for varnish application is described in Table 36-4.

III. Patient and/or Parent Counseling

▶ Help patients understand the purposes and benefits as well as the limitations of topical applications.

TABLE 36-3	Procedure for Topical Gel or Foam Professional Tray
Patient	■ Determine need based on caries risk assessment (not to be used for children under age 6 y) ■ Choose the type of fluoride (APF or NaF and gel or foam); data support use of APF Gel ■ Seat upright ■ Explain procedure including length: 4 min ■ Instruct not to swallow ■ Tilt head forward slightly
Tray coverage	■ Choose appropriate size for full coverage ■ Complete dentition must be covered, including anterior and posterior vertical coverage, distal dam depth, and close fit to teeth ■ Check for coverage of areas of recession (if unable to cover exposed root surfaces use varnish application) ■ Proper and improper tray coverage is shown in Figure 36-4
Place gel or foam	■ Use minimum amount of gel or foam in the trays, as shown in Figure 36-5 ■ Fill tray 1/3 full with gel; completely fill, but do not overfill with foam
Dry the teeth	■ Place a saliva ejector in the mouth during the drying procedure ■ Dry the teeth before insertion of trays starting with the maxillary teeth; facial, occlusal, and palatal surfaces and then the mandibular teeth; lingual, occlusal, and facial surfaces
Insert trays	■ Place both filled trays in mouth ■ A two-step procedure (one tray at a time) may be required; if so, patient may not rinse but must expectorate after the removal of each tray to prevent swallowing
Isolation	■ Use a saliva ejector with maximum efficiency suction
Attention	■ Do not leave patient unattended
Timing	■ Use a timer; do not estimate (4 min) ■ Procedure will take 8 min when a two-step procedure is used
Completion	■ Tilt head forward for removal of tray ■ Request patient to expectorate for several minutes; do not allow swallowing ■ Wipe excess gel or foam from teeth with gauze sponge ■ Use high-power suction to draw out saliva and gel ■ Instruct patient that nothing is to be placed in the mouth for 30 min; do not rinse, eat, drink, or brush teeth

TABLE 36-4	Procedure for Varnish Application (5% NaF)
Patient	■ Determine need based on caries risk assessment (only professional fluoride recommended for children under age 6 y) ■ Explain procedure ■ Seat supine ■ For the infant and toddler the parent and clinician can sit knee to knee with the child held across the knees (Figure 49-4) ■ Instruct not to swallow during the procedure
Prepare product	■ Dispense from a tube or open a single-dose packet ■ Have applicator brush available
Dry teeth	■ Varnish sets up in the presence of saliva, but it is recommended to remove excess saliva by wiping the teeth with a gauze square
Apply varnish	■ Dip applicator brush in varnish and mix well ■ Systematically brush a thin layer over all tooth surfaces ■ For prevention of early childhood caries in the infant, toddler, or very young child, apply to the maxillary anterior teeth first and then proceed to other areas of the dentition if patient is cooperative ■ For all other patients, use a systematic approach. Begin with mandibular teeth; facial, occlusal, and lingual surfaces and then the maxillary teeth; palatal, occlusal, and facial surfaces ■ Provide full coverage to all areas of the teeth including areas of recession and the cervical third of facial, lingual, and palatal surfaces and occlusal surfaces ■ Application time is approximately 1–3 min
Completion	■ Instruct patient that the teeth will feel like they have a coating or film, but this is not visible if clear product has been used ■ Ask the patient to avoid hard foods, drinking hot or alcoholic beverages, brushing, and flossing the teeth until the next day or at least 4–6 hr after application ■ It is advisable to drink through a straw for the first few hours after application

▶ Fluoride is one part of the total prevention program that includes daily biofilm control and limitation of cariogenic foods.

IV. Tray Technique: Gel or Foam

▶ *Tray application appointment preparation*
- Schedule the appointment to end at least 30 minutes before the patient's eating time.
- Prepare the patient for any discomfort, for example, the 4-minute timing when tray application is to be used.
- Explain the need not to swallow but to expectorate immediately after the tray is removed.

▶ *Tray selection and preparation*
- Figure 36-4 shows tray selection for coverage of all exposed root surfaces.
- Design of trays: maxillary and mandibular trays may be hinged together or separated, are of a natural rounded arch shape to hold the gel and prevent ingestion, and are available in various sizes and brands.

- Figure 36-5 shows the amount of gel to be placed in each tray.
- Most gels are thixotropic to offer better physical and handling characteristics for use in trays.
- Procedures for a professional gel or foam tray fluoride application are listed in Table 36-3.

V. Varnish Technique[54]

▶ *Varnish application appointment sequence:*
- Schedule the appointment when the patient can refrain from consuming hard foods and hot liquids.
- Avoid toothbrushing and flossing for 4–6 hours after the application or until the next morning.

▶ Dispense varnish: If dispensed from a tube (rather than a single-dose packet), discard any clear varnish because the ingredients have separated and will contain only a fraction of the intended amount of fluoride.[60]

▶ Unit-dosed 5% NaF varnish is available in premeasured wells or individual packets of different dosages with an applicator brush to mix the varnish and then apply.

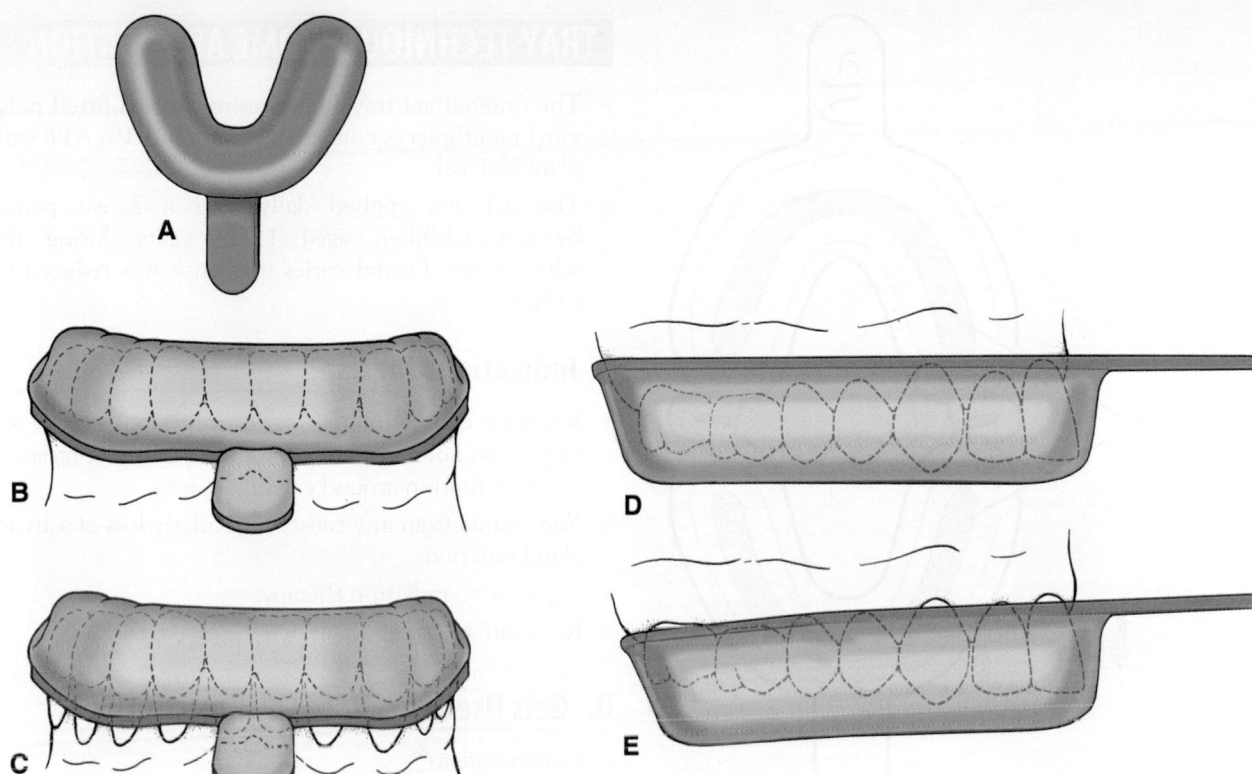

FIGURE 36-4 Tray Selection. A: Mandibular tray held for try-in. **B:** Tray over teeth is deep enough to cover the entire exposed enamel above the gingiva. **C:** In the patient with recession and areas of root surfaces exposed, the tray may not be deep enough to cover the root surfaces where fluoride is needed for prevention of root caries or hypersensitivity. A custom made tray is needed. **D:** Tray adequately covers the distal surface of the most posterior tooth. **E:** If the tray does not cover the distal surface of the most posterior tooth or the cervical third of canine and central incisor adequately, the tray may need to be repositioned to cover the distal surface, or a larger stock or custom tray is needed.

▶ Unit dosages are generally 0.25, 0.4, or 0.5 mL for the primary, mixed, and permanent dentitions, respectively, and are available in different flavors and colors (yellow, white, and clear).

▶ Procedures for a professional varnish fluoride application are listed in Table 36-4.

VI. After Application

▶ *Tray application*
  • Instruct patients not to rinse, eat, drink, brush, or floss until at least 30 minutes after gel or foam applications.
  • Rinsing immediately after a tray application has been shown to significantly lessen the benefits.[61]

▶ *Varnish application*
  • Instruct patients to avoid hot drinks and alcoholic beverages, eating hard foods, and brushing or flossing the teeth until the next morning to allow fluoride uptake to continue undisturbed.
  • Varnish is removed by the patient using toothbrushing and flossing the next day.

SELF-APPLIED FLUORIDES

▶ Self-applied fluorides (prescription (Rx) and OTC products) are available as dentifrices, mouthrinses, and gels.

▶ Concentrations of 1,500 ppm fluoride or less can be sold OTC.[39] Some products containing less than 1,500 ppm of fluoride are available only by Rx.

▶ May be applied by toothbrushing, rinsing, or trays that are custom made or disposable.

I. Indications

▶ Patient needs are determined as part of total care planning.

▶ Indications for use of tray, rinsing, and/or toothbrushing depend on the individual patient prevention needs and caries risk assessment.

▶ Certain patients need multiple procedures combined with professional applications at the regular continuing care appointments. Special indications are suggested as each method is described in the following sections.

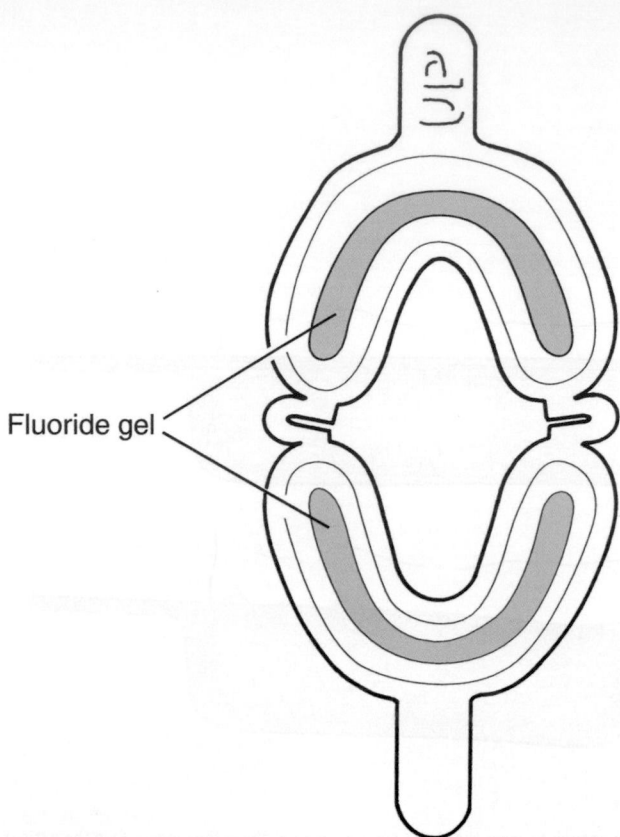

Fluoride gel

FIGURE 36-5 Measured Gel in Tray. No more than 2 mL of gel is placed in each tray for children, and no more than 5 mL is placed in each tray for adults. This amount fills each tray size one-third full.

II. Methods

The three methods for self-application are by tray, rinsing, and toothbrushing.

▶ *Tray*
  • Custom-made or disposable tray: The tray is selected to fit the individual mouth and completely cover the teeth being treated.
  • Figure 36-4 shows adequate and inadequate tray coverage on the teeth.
  • Instruction is provided not to overfill the tray.

▶ *Rinsing*
  • The patient swishes for 1 minute with a measured amount of a fluoride rinse and expectorates.
  • Certain patients will need to learn how to rinse properly to force the solution between the teeth. Box 30-4, in Chapter 30, lists steps for teaching how to rinse.

▶ *Toothbrushing*
  • A fluoride-containing dentifrice is used for regular brushing after breakfast and before going to bed without further eating.
  • Brush-on gel is used after regular brushing to provide additional benefits.
  • Use an interdental brush to apply fluoride to proximal surfaces or open furcations.

TRAY TECHNIQUE: HOME APPLICATION

▶ The original gel tray studies using custom-fitted polyvinyl mouthpieces compared the use of 1.1% APF with plain NaF gel.
▶ The gel was applied daily over a 2-year period by schoolchildren aged 11–14 years during the school years. Dental caries incidence was reduced up to 80%.[62]

I. Indications for Use

▶ Rampant enamel or root caries in persons of any age to prevent additional new carious lesions and promote remineralization around existing lesions.
▶ Xerostomia from any cause, particularly loss of salivary gland function.
▶ Exposure to radiation therapy.
▶ Root surface hypersensitivity.

II. Gels Used (Available by Prescription)

▶ *Concentrations*[39]
  • 1.1% NaF; 5,000 ppm fluoride.
  • 1.1% APF; 5,000 ppm fluoride.
▶ *Precautions*[39]
  • Dispense small quantities.
  • Maximum adult dose is 16 drops per day (4–8 drops on the inner surface of each custom-made tray).
  • Use neutral sodium preparations on porcelain, composites, titanium, or sealants.
  • Patients with mucositis may experience irritation with the APF due to the high acidity.
▶ *Patient instructions*
  • Use the gel tray once each day, preferably just before going to bed without further eating and after tooth brushing and flossing.
  • Box 36-4 outlines the procedures for the patient to follow for a home tray application.
  • A printed copy of the instructions is given to the patient.

FLUORIDE MOUTHRINSES

▶ Mouthrinsing is a practical and effective means for self-application of fluoride for individuals at moderate or high caries risk.
▶ Do not use for patients age 6 or younger, or for patients unable to rinse for a physical or other reason.[63]
▶ Rinsing can be part of an individual care plan or can be included in a group program conducted during school attendance.

BOX 36-4

Instructions for Home Tray Application

1. One daily application just before bedtime; do not eat or drink until morning. If applied at other time of day, do not eat or drink for at least 30 minutes.
2. Brush and floss before applying tray to remove biofilm and food debris.
3. Use prepared custom-made polyvinyl trays. Disposable trays can be used if the appropriate fit can be obtained.
4. Distribute no more than 4–8 drops or a thin ribbon of the gel on the inner surface of each tray. Each drop is equivalent to 0.1 mL.
5. Expectorate to minimize saliva in the mouth.
6. Apply one tray at a time. Hold head upright.
7. Apply the mandibular tray first; close gently to hold the tray in place.
8. Time by a clock for 4 minutes. Do not swallow.
9. Expectorate several times when the tray is removed to prevent swallowing gel, and prepare the mouth for the other tray.
10. Apply the maxillary tray and follow steps 7–9 as for the mandibular tray.
11. After tray removal, do not eat, drink, or brush teeth for at least 30 minutes.
12. After both trays are removed, rinse the trays under running water and brush them clean.
13. Keep in open air for drying.

I. Indications

▶ Mouthrinsing with a fluoride preparation may be an additional benefit for the following:
- Young persons during the high-risk preteen and adolescent years.
- Patients with areas of demineralization.
- Patients with root exposure following recession and periodontal therapy.
- Participants in a school health group program for children older than 6 years.
- Patients with moderate to rampant caries risk who live in a fluoridated or nonfluoridated community.
- Patients whose oral health care is complicated by biofilm-retentive appliances, including orthodontics, partial dentures, or space maintainers.
- Patients with xerostomia from any cause, including head and neck radiation and saliva-depressing drug therapy
- Patients with hypersensitivity of exposed root surfaces.

II. Limitations

▶ Children under 6 years of age and those of any age who cannot rinse because of oral and/or facial musculature problems or other disability.

▶ Alcohol content:
- Use of alcohol-based mouthrinses are not recommended; aqueous solutions are available.
- Alcohol content of commercial preparations is not advisable for children, especially adolescents.
- Alcohol-containing preparations are never to be recommended for a recovering alcoholic person; however, a history of former alcoholism would not necessarily be known to the clinician.

▶ Compliance is greater with a daily rinse than with a weekly rinse when practiced on an individual basis at home.

III. Preparations[39]

▶ Oral rinses are categorized as low-potency/high-frequency rinses or high-potency/low-frequency rinses.

▶ Most low-potency rinses may be purchased directly OTC, whereas most high potency rinses are provided by Rx.

▶ Table 36-5 contains the compounds, concentration, and recommended frequency of use for currently available self-applied fluoride rinses.

▶ *Low potency/high frequency (available OTC)*
- *Preparations*
  - 0.05% NaF; 230 ppm
  - 0.044% NaF or APF; 200 ppm. (available by Rx or OTC depending on the brand)
  - 0.0221% NaF; 100 ppm.
- *Specifications*
  - No more than 264 mg NaF (120 mg of fluoride) can be dispensed at one time.
  - A 500-mL bottle of 0.05% NaF rinse contains 100 mg of fluoride.
  - Bottle is required to have a child-proof cap.

TABLE 36-5	Patient-Applied Fluoride Mouthrinses (age 6 y and older)	
TYPE/ PERCENTAGE (RX OR OTC)	CONCENTRATION IN PPM	FREQUENCY OF USE (10 ML OR 2 TEASPOONS SWISHED FOR 1 MIN)
0.2% NaF (Rx)	905	Once daily or once weekly
0.044% NaF and APF (Rx and OTC)	200	Once daily
0.05% NaF (OTC)	230	Once daily
0.0221% NaF (OTC)	100	Twice daily

- Rinses are not to be used by children under 6 years of age or by children or adults with a disability involving oral and/or facial musculature.
- Young children do not have sufficient control to expectorate and they tend to swallow quickly.
- The rinse is to be fully expectorated without swallowing.
- *Procedure for use*
  - Low-potency rinses are used once or twice daily with 2 teaspoonfuls (10 mL) after brushing and before retiring. Follow manufacturer's ADA-approved specifications.
  - The adult and pediatric maximum dose is 10 mL of solution.
  - Swish between teeth with lips tightly closed for 60 seconds; spit out.
  - See directions for rinsing in Box 30-4, in Chapter 30.
  - Have the patient practice rinsing at the dental chair.
  - Instruct patient: Do not eat or drink for 30 minutes after rinsing.
- *High potency/low frequency (available by Rx)*
  - *Preparation*
    - 0.20% NaF; 905 ppm
    - Originally recommended as a weekly rinse, but can be used up to once per day.[47]
  - *Procedure for use*: the same as for high-frequency/low-potency rinses.

The prevented fraction of dental caries ranges from 30% to 59%, with the use of 0.2% fluoride rinse on various rinsing schedules.[51]

IV. Benefits

- Benefits from fluoride mouthrinsing have been documented many times since the original research using various percentages of various fluoride preparations.[64,65]
- Frequent rinsing with low concentrations of fluoride has the following effects:
  - A 26%–29% average reduction in dental caries incidence.[66]

- Greater benefit for smooth surfaces, but some benefit to pits and fissures.
- Greatest benefit to newly erupted teeth.
- The program needs to be continued through the teenage years to benefit the second and third permanent molars.
- Added benefits for a community with fluoridation.[66]
- Effective in preventing and reversing root caries.[67]
- Primary teeth present in school-aged children benefit by as much as a 42.5% average reduction in dental caries incidence.[68]

BRUSH-ON GEL

- Brush-on gel has been used as an adjunct to the daily application of fluoride in a dentifrice and as a supplement to periodic professional applications.
- Regular use has been shown to help control demineralization about orthodontic appliances.[69]
- Provides protection against postirradiation caries in conjunction with other fluoride applications.[70]

I. Preparations

Table 36-6 contains the type, concentration, and daily usage guidelines for currently available self-applied fluoride gels.

- *1.1% NaF (Neutral pH) or 1.1% APF (3.5 pH); 5,000 ppm*
  - Available as a gel to be used separate from toothbrushing.
- 1.1% neutral NaF is also available as a dentifrice with an abrasive system added.
  - The rationale for the dentifrice product is to increase compliance with one step (brushing only) rather than brushing, followed by application of the high-concentration gel with a toothbrush.
  - Requires a prescription.
- *Stannous fluoride (SnF$_2$) 0.4% in glycerin base (1,000 ppm)*
- Available as a gel to be used separate from toothbrushing.
- Available OTC.

TABLE 36-6	Patient-Applied Fluoride Gels: Brush-on or Use in Custom Trays (age 6 y or older)	
TYPE/PERCENTAGE (RX OR OTC)	**CONCENTRATION IN PPM**	**DAILY USAGE GUIDELINES**
1.1% NaF gel or paste (Rx)	5,000	Brush-on teeth, twice per day or 4–8 drops on inner surface of custom tray or brush-on teeth
1.1% APF (Rx)	5,000	Brush-on teeth, preferably at night or 4–8 drops on inner surface of custom tray
0.4% SnF (OTC)	1,000	Brush-on teeth, preferably at night

II. Procedure

▶ Teeth are cleaned first with thorough brushing and flossing before gel application with a separate toothbrush.

▶ Use once a day or more as recommended, preferably at night after toothbrushing and flossing.

▶ Place about 2 mg of the gel over the brush head and spread over all teeth.

▶ Brush 1 minute, then swish to force the fluid between the teeth several times before expectorating.

▶ Do not rinse.

FLUORIDE DENTIFRICES

I. Development

▶ Historically tried with various compounds, including stannous fluoride, NaF, sodium monofluorophosphate, and amine fluoride.

▶ Early research objectives: to find compatible fluoride, abrasive systems, and formulations containing available fluoride for uptake by the tooth surface.

▶ In 1960 the first fluoride dentifrice gained approval by the ADA, Council on Dental Therapeutics: 0.4% stannous fluoride.[71]

II. Indications

▶ *Dental caries prevention*
  • Fluoride dentifrice approved by the ADA is an integral part of a complete preventive program and is a basic caries prevention intervention for all patients.[71]
  • All patients regardless of their caries risk
  • Toothbrushing that covers all the teeth on all sides at least twice per day with a fluoride toothpaste is the foundation for all patients' fluoride regimen.
  • Patients with moderate to rampant dental caries are advised to brush three or four times each day with a fluoride-containing dentifrice and to chew xylitol gum after a meal when they cannot brush.
  • Expectorate, but do not rinse after toothbrushing, to give the fluoride a longer time to be effective.

III. Preparations

Fluoride dentifrices are available as gels or pastes. Amine fluorides are used in other countries, but not available in the United States.

▶ *Current fluoride constituents*[72]
  • NaF 0.24% (1,100 ppm).
  • Sodium monofluorophosphate (Na_2PO_3 F) 0.76% (1,000 ppm).
  • Stannous fluoride (SnF_2) 0.45% (1,000 ppm).

▶ *Guidelines for acceptance*

The requirements for acceptance of a fluoride-containing toothpaste by the ADA are described in Chapter 30. The Seal of Acceptance is illustrated in Figure 30-1.

IV. Patient Instruction: Recommended Procedures

Advise the patient in the selection of a fluoride dentifrice, the need for frequent use, the method for application to all the tooth surfaces, and the importance of using a fluoride dentifrice to promote oral health.

▶ Select an ADA accepted fluoride-containing dentifrice.

▶ Place recommended amount of dentifrice on the toothbrush.

▶ *Children (age less than 3 years)*: Twice daily brushing (morning and night) with no more than a "smear" or the size of a grain of rice of fluoride dentifrice spread along the brushing plane.[73,74] Figure 50-8, in Chapter 50, illustrates a small smear.
  • Daily oral care begins with the eruption of the first primary tooth.
  • At this time, the oral hygiene of parents and family with attention to daily biofilm removal by toothbrushing can make a significant impact on the small child's oral health.

▶ The paste is then spread over all the teeth before starting to brush so that all teeth benefit and large amounts of paste are not available for swallowing.

▶ *Older child (ages 3–6 years)*: Twice daily brushing (morning and night) with fluoride toothpaste the size of a small pea.
  • Demonstrate spreading this amount over the ends of the filaments, and explain that the child is not to swallow excess amounts of dentifrice.[73,74]

▶ *Adults*: Use 1/2 inch fluoride dentifrice twice daily.

▶ Spread dentifrice over the teeth with a light touch of the brush.

▶ Proceed with correct brushing positions for sulcular removal of dental biofilm (see Chapter 28).

▶ Do not rinse after brushing to keep fluoride in the oral fluids.[73,75]

▶ Keep dentifrice container out of reach of children.

V. Benefits

▶ Twice daily use has greater benefits than once daily use.[63]

▶ Moderate and high caries risk patients and patients who live in a nonfluoridated community benefit from using a dentifrice several times per day to maintain salivary fluoride levels.

▶ The dentifrice is a continuing source of fluoride for the tooth surface in the control of demineralization and the promotion of remineralization.

▶ The use of a dentifrice with a fluoride concentration of 1,000 ppm and above compared to a dentifrice without fluoride can prevent dental caries up to an average of 23%.[76]

COMBINED FLUORIDE PROGRAM

▶ All patients, regardless of caries risk, benefit from at least twice daily use of a fluoridated dentifrice and consumption of fluoridated water multiple times during each day.

▶ Patients at moderate to high caries risk benefit from additional methods of fluoride exposure.

▶ Additional caries reduction can be expected when another topical fluoride such as a mouthrinse or gel tray is combined with a fluoride dentifrice.[77]

▶ When self-administered methods are chosen, patient cooperation is a significant factor.

▶ Age and eruption pattern influence the method selected.

▶ Newly erupted teeth need frequent fluoride exposure as soon after eruption as possible and continued indefinitely to control demineralization.

▶ Continuing care appointments are to be scheduled for frequent professional topical applications for those at moderate and high caries risk and for continuing instruction and motivation regarding daily fluoride use for all patients.

▶ All methods are supplements to the daily use of fluoridated water and a dentifrice with fluoride.

FLUORIDE SAFETY

▶ Fluoride preparations and fluoridated water have wide margins of safety.

▶ Fluoride is beneficial in small amounts, but it can be injurious if used without attention to correct dosage and frequency.

▶ All dental personnel need to be familiar with the following:
  • Recommended approved procedures for use of products containing fluoride.
  • Potential toxic effects of fluoride.
  • How to administer general emergency measures when accidental overdoses occur as listed in Table 8-3 and the section on Internal Poisoning in Table 8-4 in Chapter.

I. Summary of Fluoride Risk Management

▶ Use professionally and recommend only approved fluoride preparations for patient use.
  • Products may have approval from the Food and Drug Administration (FDA) and the ADA in the United States.

• Read about the programs of the ADACSA and the Seal of Approval of Products in Chapter 30.

▶ Use only researched, recommended amounts and methods for delivery.

▶ Know potential toxicity of the various products, and be prepared to administer emergency measures for treating an accidental toxic response.

▶ Instruct patients in proper care of fluoride products.
  • Dentist prescribes no more than 120 mg of fluoride at one time (no more than 480 of the 0.25 mg tablets or 240 of the 0.5 mg tablets).[39] Do not store large quantities in the home.
  • Request parental supervision of a child's brushing or other fluoride administration. Rinses, for example, are not to be used by children under 6 years of age.
  • Fluoride products have child-proof caps and are to be kept out of reach of small children and other persons, such as the mentally challenged, who may not understand limitations.
  • In school health programs, dispensing of the fluoride product is to be supervised by responsible adults. Containers are to be stored under lock and key when not in active use.

II. Toxicity

▶ *Acute toxicity* refers to rapid intake of an excess dose over a short time.
  • Acute fluoride poisoning is extremely rare.[78]

▶ *Chronic toxicity* applies to long-term ingestion of fluoride in amounts that exceed the approved therapeutic levels.

▶ *Accidental ingestion* of a concentrated fluoride preparation can lead to a toxic reaction.

▶ *Certainly lethal dose (CLD)*[79]
  • A lethal dose is the amount of a drug likely to cause death if not intercepted by antidotal therapy.
  • *Adult CLD:* About 5–10 g of NaF taken at one time. The fluoride ion equivalent is 32–64 mg of fluoride per kilogram body weight (mg F/kg; Box 36-5).
  • *Child:* Approximately 0.5–1.0 g, variable with size and weight of the child.

▶ *Safely tolerated dose (STD): one-fourth of the CLD*
  • *Adult STD:* About 1.25–2.5 g of NaF (8–16 mg F/kg).
  • *Child:* Box 36-5B shows STDs and CLDs for children.
    ∘ Weights given for each selected age are minimal, and calculations for the doses are conservative.
    ∘ As can be noted in Box 36-5B, less than 1 g (1,000 mg) may be fatal for children 12 years old and younger, and 0.5 g (500 mg) exceeds the STD for all ages shown.

BOX 36-5
Lethal and Safe Doses of Fluoride

A. Lethal and Safe doses of Fluoride for A 70-Kg Adult CLD

5–10 g NaF
Or
32–64 mg F/kg
STD = 1/4 CLD
1.25–2.5 g NaF
Or
8–16 mg F/kg

B. CLDS AND STDS of Fluoride for Selected Ages

Age (years)	Weight (lbs/kg)	CLD (mg)	STD (mg)
2	22/10	320	80
4	29/13	422	106
6	37/17	538	135
8	45/20	655	164
10	53/24	771	193
12	64/29	931	233
14	83/38	1,206	301
16	92/42	1,338	334
18	95/43	1,382	346

Reprinted with permission from Heifetz SB, Horowitz HS. The amounts of fluoride in current fluoride therapies: safety considerations for children. *ASDC J Dent Child*. 1984;51(4):257–269.

- For children under 6 years of age, however, 500 mg could be lethal.[79]

III. Signs and Symptoms of Acute Toxic Dose

Symptoms begin within 30 minutes of ingestion and may persist for as long as 24 hours.

▶ *Gastrointestinal tract*

Fluoride in the stomach is acted on by the hydrochloric acid to form hydrofluoric acid, an irritant to the stomach lining. Symptoms include:

- Nausea, vomiting, diarrhea.
- Abdominal pain.
- Increased salivation, thirst.

▶ *Systemic involvements*

- *Blood*: Calcium may be bound by the circulating fluoride, thus causing symptoms of hypocalcemia.
- *Central nervous system*: Hyperreflexia, convulsions, paresthesias.

- *Cardiovascular and respiratory depression*: If not treated, may lead to death in a few hours from cardiac failure or respiratory paralysis.

IV. Emergency Treatment

▶ *Induce vomiting*

- *Mechanical*: Digital stimulation at back of tongue or in throat.

▶ *Second person*

- Call emergency service; transport to hospital.

▶ *Administer fluoride-binding liquid when patient is not vomiting*

- Milk.
- Milk of Magnesia.
- Lime water ($CaOH_2$ solution 0.15%).

▶ *Support respiration and circulation*

▶ *Additional therapy indicated at emergency room*

- Calcium gluconate for muscle tremors or tetany.
- Gastric lavage.
- Cardiac monitoring.
- Endotracheal intubation.
- Blood monitoring (calcium, magnesium, potassium, pH).
- Intravenous feeding to restore blood volume, calcium.

V. Chronic Toxicity

▶ *Skeletal fluorosis*[78]

- Isolated instances of osteosclerosis, an elevation in bone density, can result from chronic toxicity after long-term (10 or more years) ingestion of water with 8–10 ppm fluoride or from inhalation of industrial fumes or dust.
- Skeletal fluorosis in its early stages is characterized by stiff and painful joints and becomes crippling in its later stages.
- It has never been a public health concern in the United States, even in communities that have had high levels of fluoride in the water for generations.
- Is endemic in certain countries such as China and India with high levels of natural fluoride in the water.
- Predisposing factors, dietary deficiencies, and population differences with regard to fluoride metabolism may play a role in its development in addition to exposure.
- Methods for defluoridation have been developed, as described in the section on Defluoridation in this chapter.

▶ *Dental fluorosis*

- Ingestion of naturally occurring excess fluoride in the drinking water and/or fluoride dental products can produce visible fluorosis only when used during the years of development of the crowns of the teeth, namely, from birth until age 16 or 18 years or when the crowns of the third permanent molars are completed.

- No systemic symptoms result from the fluoride, and the individual has protection against dental caries.
- Scoring system used to describe dental fluorosis is found in Chapter 23, Tables 23-2 and 23-3.

▶ *Mild fluorosis*

1. *Clinical evaluation*

- Mild and very mild forms, dental fluorosis appears as white opacities in the enamel surface.
- No esthetic or health problem is involved. Many such white spots are not visible except when scrutinized under a dental light and the surface is dried.
- All white spots in the enamel are not related to fluoride intake; distinction can be made by reviewing the patient's dental and fluoride-intake history, by noting the location and distribution of

the white spots, and by considering the sequence of tooth development.

2. *Relation to fluoride sources*

- Mild fluorosis may result from inadvertent ingestion of excess fluoride by young children during topical procedures both self-applied and professional.
- No problem exists when care is taken to follow basic steps, such as those listed in Tables 36-3 and 36-4 for professional applications.
- Mouthrinses are not indicated for children less than 6 years of age.
- Small amounts of dentifrice may be swallowed incidentally at each brushing. A child of 4 years who lives in a nonfluoridated community uses a daily supplement (0.5 mg), and swallows two or three small amounts of dentifrice ingests far less than the STD of 106 mg shown in Box 36-5B.

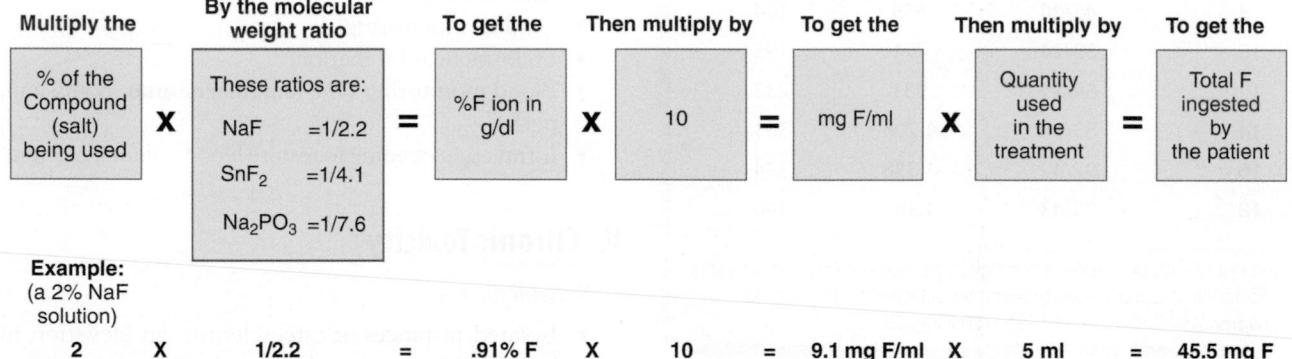

FIGURE 36-6 **Fluoride Calculation.** Flowchart shows steps in the calculation of the amount of fluoride in a compound used in treatment. The example shows that 5 mL of a 2% solution of NaF contains 45.5 mg F, an amount slightly greater than half of the STD for a 2-year-old child (Box 36-5B). (Source: Heifetz SB, Horowitz HS. The amounts of fluoride in current fluoride therapies: safety considerations for children. *ASDC J Dent Child*. 1984;51(4):257–269.)

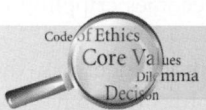

EVERYDAY ETHICS

Daniel was a well-behaved and cooperative 4 1/2-year-old boy at an elevated risk for dental caries due to having one carious lesion and living in a nonfluoridated area. At the time for the fluoride treatment, the dental hygienist, Nina, spent a few extra minutes explaining to Daniel how she will brush a coating on his teeth to make them stronger. Although Daniel's parents did not have insurance coverage, the hygienist decided it would be important for him to receive a fluoride application regardless of the fee. Daniel tolerated the procedure well. After the appointment, Nina explained to Daniel's mother the varnish postoperative instructions. Daniel's mother became upset and said, "why did you give my son a fluoride treatment without my permission? My husband just lost his job and I cannot afford this added cost."

Questions for Consideration

1. Because Daniel's mother brought him to the clinic for a scheduled appointment, Nina assumed *implied consent* for Daniel to receive dental hygiene treatment. Was it appropriate for Nina to assume consent for the fluoride application was also implied? Why or why not?

2. Discuss ways in which the legal/ethical concepts of professional liability, scope of practice, standard of care, and informed consent are related to this scenario.

3. Answer the questions in Box 1-10 for resolving ethical issues or dilemmas found in the Ethical Applications section of Chapter 1. Use the answers to determine at least one course of action Nina can take now to resolve the issue. Make sure to consider all individuals who might be affected by the decision.

VI. How to Calculate Amounts of Fluoride[79,80]

Figure 36-6 is a flowchart that shows the steps necessary to determine the amount of fluoride in a fluoride compound. By doing so, one can then calculate the amount ingested by the patient.

▶ Multiply the percentage of fluoride ion in the compound by the molecular weight conversion ratio, as shown in Figure 36-6.

▶ Obtain the ratio by dividing the molecular weight of the compound by the atomic weight of fluoride.

▶ Example: The molecular weight of NaF is 42 (Na = 23, F = 19). When divided by 19, a 1–2.2 ratio results, as used in the example in Figure 36-6.

DOCUMENTATION

A patient receiving a topical fluoride application and/or counseling regarding fluoride needs the following documented in the permanent record:

▶ Caries risk level (document as low, moderate, high, or extreme).

▶ Current use of fluoride toothpaste and exposure to fluoridated water.

▶ Type, concentration, mode of delivery, and postoperative instructions if a professional fluoride application is provided.

▶ Type, amount, and instructions for the use of any Rx or OTC patient-applied fluoride products recommended.

▶ A sample documentation using the SOAP format is provided in Box 36-6.

BOX 36-6
Example Documentation: Professional Fluoride Application and Prescribing Home Fluoride

S –A 26-year-old male patient presents for a periodic oral examination, radiographs, and dental prophylaxis. Patient states that he drinks high-sucrose beverages on a frequent, daily basis. He also states that he uses toothpaste with fluoride twice daily and consumes fluoridated water.

O –Patient presents with medication induced xerostomia. Two proximal cavitated lesions were discovered on bitewing X-rays.

A –Patient was classified as being high risk for caries after conducting a caries risk assessment analysis.

P –Applied 5% NaF varnish to the entire dentition and provided postoperative instructions. Prescribed 1.1% NaF gel (2 refills) to apply with a separate toothbrush at night. Discussed the need for an additional varnish application in three months to help prevent the future onset of dental caries.

Signed: _____, RDH

Date: _____

Factors To Teach The Patient

I.   Personal Use of Fluorides
▷ Purposes, action, and expected benefits relative to the specific forms of fluoride treatment the patient will receive based upon individual caries risk.
▷ Specific instructions concerning self-applied techniques that will be performed at home.

II. Need for Parental Supervision
▷ Supervise daily care of child's teeth and mouth with the recommended amount of fluoridated toothpaste to prevent excess ingestion of fluoride.
▷ Keep fluoride products out of reach of small children.

III. Determine Need for Fluoride Supplements
▷ Must determine child is at high caries risk and consumes fluoride-deficient drinking water.
▷ Where to send private water source sample for fluoride analysis.

IV. Fluorides Are Part of the Total Preventive Program
▷ Emphasize fluoride toothpaste and fluoridated water as the cornerstone for prevention of dental caries.
▷ Regular professional supervision and care.

V. Fluoridation
▷ How drinking fluoridated water helps people of all ages.
▷ How to access the CDCP Community Water Fluoridation website to obtain reliable information about fluoridation in the United States.

VI. Bottled Drinking Water/Water Filters
▷ When bottled water does not have a label indicating that it is fluoridated, recommend filling a water bottle from a fluoridated water supply.
▷ Check with the water filter manufacturer to be certain the fluoride will not be removed through filtration.
▷ Distillation and reverse osmosis systems remove fluoride from drinking water, but water softeners do not.

VII. Infant Formula
▷ Educate parents that powdered or liquid concentrate infant formula and the water used to reconstitute this formula may contain fluoride.

References

1. Ellwood R, Fejerskov O, Cury JA, et al. Chapter 18: Fluorides in caries control. In: Fejerskov O, Kidd E, eds. *Dental Caries The Disease and its Clinical Management.* 2nd ed. Oxford: Blackwell Munksgaard; 2008:293–294.

2. Newbrun E. Systemic benefits of fluoride and fluoridation. *J Public Health Dent.* 2004;64 (Suppl S1):35–39.

3. Ekstrand J. Chapter 4: Fluoride metabolism. In: Fejerskov O, Ekstrand J, Burt BA, eds. *Fluoride in Dentistry.* 2nd ed. Copenhagen: Munksgaard; 1996:55–67.

4. Bath-Balough M, Fehrenbach M. *Dental Embryology, Histology, and Anatomy.* 2nd ed. St. Louis, MO: Saunders; 2006: 179–189.

5. Melfi RC, Alley KE. *Permar's Oral Embryology and Microscopic Anatomy.* 10th ed. Philadelphia, PA: Lippincott Williams & Wilkins; 2000:43–87.

6. Levy S. An update on fluorides and fluorosis. *J Can Dent Assoc.* 2003;69(5):286–291.

7. Aoba T, Fejerskov O. Dental fluorosis: chemistry and biology. *Crit Rev Oral Bio Med.* 2002;13(2):155–170.

8. Featherstone JD. The science and practice of caries prevention. *J Am Dent Assoc.* 2000;131(7):887–899.

9. Yoon SH, Brudevold F, Gardner DE, et al. Distribution of fluoride in teeth from areas with different levels of fluoride in the water supply. *J Dent Res.* 1960;39:845–856.

10. Centers for Disease Control and Prevention. Recommendations for using fluoride to prevent and control dental caries in the United States. *MMWR Recomm Rep.* 2001;50 (RR-14):1–42.

11. Centers for Disease Control and Prevention. Populations receiving optimally fluoridated public drinking water–United States, 1992–1996. *MWWR Morb Mortal Wkly Rep.* 2008;57(27):737–741.

12. Department of Health and Human Services, Centers for Disease Control and Prevention. *Community Water Fluoridation.* Atlanta, GA: Water Fluoridation Data and Statistics; 2010. [about 4 screens]. http://www.cdc.gov/fluoridation/index.htm. Updated July 13, 2013. Accessed August 25, 2013.

13. Herschfeld JJ. Classics in dental history: Frederick S. McKay and the "Colorado brown stain." *Bull Hist Dent.* 1978;26(2):118–126.

14. McKay FS. The relation of mottled enamel to caries. *J Am Dent Assoc.* 1928;15:1429–1437.

15. Churchill HV. Occurrence of fluorides in some waters of United States. *J Ind Eng Chem.* 1931;23:996–998.

16. Dean HT, Arnold FA Jr, Elvove E. Domestic water and dental caries. V. Additional studies of the relation of fluoride domestic waters to dental caries experience in 4425 white children, aged 12 to 14 years, of 13 cities in 4 states. *Public Health Rep.* 1942;57:1155–1179.

17. Centers for Disease Control and Prevention. Engineering and administrative recommendations for water fluoridation, 1995. *MMWR Recomm Rep.* 1995;44 (RR-13):1–40.

18. Department of Health and Human Services (US). U.S. Public Health Service Recommendation for Fluoride Concentration in Drinking Water for the Prevention of Caries. [Internet] Public Health Reports July/August 2015. [Cited 2015 June 12] 130; 1-14. Available from: http://www.cdc.gov/fluoridation/index.htm

19. Griffin SO, Regnier E, Griffin PM, et al. Effectiveness of fluoride in preventing caries in adults. *J Dent Res.* 2007;86(5):410–415.

20. Yeung CA. A systematic review of the efficacy and safety of fluoridation. *Evid Based Dent.* 2008;9(2):39–43.

21. Dirks OB, Houwink B, Kwant GW. Some special features of the caries preventive effect of water fluoridation. *Arch Oral Biol.* 1961;4:187–192.

22. Burt BA, Ismail AI, Eklund SA. Root caries in an optimally fluoridated and a high-fluoride community. *J Dent Res.* 1986;6(9):1154–1158.

23. Stamm JW, Banting DW, Imrey PB. Adult root caries survey of two similar communities with contrasting natural water fluoride levels. *J Am Dent Assoc.* 1990;120(2):143–149.

24. Ast DB, Fitzgerald B. Effectiveness of water fluoridation. *J Am Dent Assoc.* 1962;65:581–587.

25. Russell AL, Elvove E. Domestic water and dental caries. VII. A study of the fluoride-dental caries relationship in an adult population. *Public Health Rep.* 1951;66(43):1389–1401.

26. Englander HR, Wallace DA. Effects of naturally fluoridated water on dental caries in adults: Aurora-Rockford, Illinois, Study III. *Public Health Rep.* 1962;77(10):887–893.

27. Horowitz HS, Maier FJ, Law FE. Partial defluoridation of a community water supply and dental fluorosis. *Public Health Rep.* 1967;82(11):965–972.

28. Horowitz HS, Heifetz SB. The effect of partial defluoridation of a water supply on dental fluorosis—final results in Bartlett, Texas, after 17 Years. *Am J Public Health.* 1972;62(6):767–769.

29. Horowitz HS. Effectiveness of school water fluoridation and dietary fluoride supplements in school-aged children. *J Public Health Dent.* 1989;49(5 Spec No):290–296.

30. Lemke CW, Doherty JM, Arra MC. Controlled fluoridation: the dental effects of discontinuation in Antigo, Wisconsin. *J Am Dent Assoc.* 1979;80(4):782–786.

31. Jackson RD, Brizendine EJ, Kelly SA, et al. The fluoride content of foods and beverages from negligibly and optimally fluoridated communities. *Community Dent Oral Epidemiol.* 2002;30(5):382–391.

32. Burt BA, Marthaler TM. Chapter 16: Fluoride tablets, salt fluoridation, and milk fluoridation. In: Fejerskov O, Ekstrand J, Burt BA, eds. *Fluoride in Dentistry.* 2nd ed. Copenhagen: Munksgaard; 1996:291–310.

33. Espelid I. Caries preventive effect of fluoride in milk, salt and tablets: a literature review. *Eur Arch Paediatr Dent.* 2009;10(3):149–156.

34. European Academy of Paediatric Dentistry. Guidelines on the use of fluoride in children: an EAPD policy document. *Eur Arch Paediatr Dent.* 2009;10(3):129–135.

35. American Dental Association. *Fluoridation Facts.* Chicago, IL: American Dental Association; 2005.

36. Hujoel PP, Zina LG, Moimaz SA, et al. Infant formula and enamel fluorosis: a systematic review. *J Am Dent Assoc.* 2009;140(7):841–854.

37. Siew C, Strock S, Ristic H, et al. Assessing the potential risk factor for enamel fluorosis: a preliminary evaluation of fluoride content in infant formulas. *J Am Dent Assoc.* 2009;140(10):1228–1236.

38. Berg J, Gerweck C, Hujoel P, et al. Evidence-based clinical recommendations regarding fluoride intake from reconstituted infant formula and enamel fluorosis. *J Am Dent Assoc.* 2011;142(1):79–87.

39. Burrell KH. Chapter 10: Fluorides. In: Mariotti AJ, Burrell KH, eds. *American Dental Association, Council on Scientific Affairs: ADA/PDR Guide to Dental Therapeutics.* 5th ed. Chicago, IL: American Dental Association and Thomson PDR; 2009:323–337.

40. Ismail AI, Hasson H. Fluoride supplements, dental caries, and fluorosis: a systematic review. *J Am Dent Assoc.* 2008;139(11):1457–1468.

41. Rozier RG, Adair S, Graham F, et al. Evidence-based clinical recommendations on the prescription of dietary

fluoride supplements for caries prevention. *J Am Dent Assoc.* 2010;141(12):1480–1489.

42. Toyama Y, Nakagaki H, Kato S, et al. Fluoride concentrations at and near the neonatal line in human deciduous tooth enamel obtained from a naturally fluoridated and a non-fluoridated area. *Arch Oral Biol.* 2001;46(2):147–153.

43. Tubert-Jeannin S, Auclair C, Amsallem E, et al. Fluoride supplements (tablets, drops, lozenges or chewing gums) for preventing dental caries in children. *Cochrane Database Syst Rev.* 2011;(12):CD007592.

44. Bibby BG. Use of fluorine in the prevention of dental caries. II. The effects of sodium fluoride applications. *J Am Dent Assoc.* 1944;31:317.

45. Knutson JW. Sodium fluoride solutions: technique for application to the teeth. *J Am Dent Assoc.* 1948;36(1):37–39.

46. Galagan DJ, Knutson JW. The effect of topically applied fluorides on dental caries experience; experiments with sodium fluoride and calcium chloride; widely spaced applications; use of different solution concentrations. *Public Health Rep.* 1948;63(38):1215–1221.

47. Weyant RJ, Tracy SL, Anselmo T, et al. Topical fluoride for caries prevention: Executive summary of the updated clinical recommendations and supporting systemic review. *J Am Dent Assoc.* 2013;144(11):1279–1291.

48. Warren DP, Chan JT. Topical fluorides: efficacy, administration, and safety. *Gen Dent.* 1997;45(2):134–140, 142.

49. Ripa LW. An evaluation of the use of professionally (operator applied) topical fluorides. *J Dent Res.* 1990;69 (Spec No):786–796.

50. Soeno K, Matsumura H, Atsuta M, et al. Influence of acidulated fluoride agents and effectiveness of subsequent polishing on composite material surfaces. *Oper Dent.* 2002;27(3):305–310.

51. Poulsen S. Fluoride-containing gels, mouth rinses and varnishes: an update of evidence of efficacy. *Eur Arch Paediatr Dent.* 2009;10(3):157–161.

52. Beltrán-Aguilar ED, Goldstein JW, Lockwood SA. Fluoride varnishes: a review of their clinical use, cariostatic mechanism, efficacy and safety. *J Am Dent Assoc.* 2000;131(5):589–596.

53. Marinho VC, Worthington HV, Walsh T, et al. Fluoride varnishes for preventing dental caries in children and adolescents. *Cochrane Database Syst Rev.* 2013;(7):CD002279.

54. Bawden JW. Fluoride varnish: a useful new tool for public health dentistry. *J Public Health Dent.* 1998;58(4):266–269.

55. Autio-Gold JT, Courts F. Assessing the effect of fluoride varnish on early enamel carious lesions in the primary dentition. *J Amer Dent Assoc.* 2001;132(9):1247–1253.

56. Castellano JB, Donly KJ. Potential remineralization of demineralized enamel after application of fluoride varnish. *Am J Dent.* 2004;17(6):462–464.

57. Demito CF, Vivaldi-Rodrigues G, Ramos AL, et al. The efficacy of fluoride varnish in reducing enamel demineralization adjacent to orthodontic brackets: an in vitro study. *Orthod Craniofac Res.* 2004;7(4):205–210.

58. Ripa LW. Need for prior toothcleaning when performing a professional topical fluoride application: review and recommendations for change. *J Am Dent Assoc.* 1984;109(2):281–285.

59. Vrbic V, Brudevold F, McCann HG. Acquisition of fluoride by enamel from fluoride pumice pastes. *Helv Odontol Acta.* 1967;11(1):21–26.

60. Shen C, Autio-Gold J. Assessing fluoride concentration uniformity and fluoride release from three varnishes. *J Am Dent Assoc.* 2002;133(2):176–182.

61. Stookey GK, Schemehorn BR, Drook CA, et al. The effect of rinsing with water immediately after a professional fluoride gel application on fluoride uptake in demineralized enamel: an in vivo study. *Pediatr Dent.* 1986;8(3):153–157.

62. Englander HR, Keyes PH, Gestwicki M, et al. Clinical anti-caries effect of repeated topical sodium fluoride applications by mouthpieces. *J Am Dent Assoc.* 1967;75(3):638–644.

63. Adair SM. Evidence-based use of fluoride in contemporary pediatric dental practice. *Pediatr Dent.* 2006;28(2):133–142.

64. Torell P, Ericsson Y. The potential benefits derived from fluoride mouth rinses. In: Forrester DJ, Schulz EM, eds. *International Workshop on Fluorides and Dental Caries Reductions.* Baltimore, MD: University of Maryland School of Dentistry; 1974:114–176.

65. Birkeland JM, Torell P. Caries-preventive fluoride mouthrinses. *Caries Res.* 1978;12 (Suppl 1):38–51.

66. Driscoll WS, Swango PA, Horowitz AM, et al. Caries-preventive effects of daily and weekly fluoride mouthrinsing in a fluoridated community: final results after 30 months. *J Am Dent Assoc.* 1982;105(6):1010–1013.

67. Heijnsbroek M, Paraskevas S, Vav der Weijden GA. Fluoride interventions for root caries: a review. *Oral Health Prev Dent.* 2007;5(2):145–152.

68. Ripa LW, Leske GS, Varma A. Effect of mouthrinsing with a 0.2 percent neutral NaF solution on the deciduous dentition of first to third grade school children. *Pediatr Dent.* 1984;6(2):93–97.

69. Stratemann MW, Shannon IL. Control of decalcification in orthodontic patients by daily self-administered application of a water-free 0.4 percent stannous fluoride gel. *Am J Orthod.* 1974;66(3):273–279.

70. Wescott WB, Starcke EN, Shannon IL. Chemical protection against postirradiation dental caries. *Oral Surg Oral Med Oral Pathol.* 1975;40(6):709–719.

71. American Dental Association, Council on Dental Therapeutics. Evaluation of Crest toothpaste. *J Am Dent Assoc.* 1960;61:272.

72. Mariotti MJ, Burrell K. Mouthrinses and dentifrices. In: *American Dental Association, Council on Scientific Affairs: ADA/PDR Guide to Dental Therapeutics.* 5th ed. Chicago, IL: American Dental Association and Thomson PDR; 2009:305–321.

73. American Academy of Pediatric Dentistry Liaison with Other Groups Committee; and American Academy on Pediatric Dentistry Council on Scientific Affairs. Guideline on fluoride therapy. *Pediatr Dent.* 2013;36:171–174.

74. American Dental Association Council on Scientific Affairs. Fluoride toothpaste use for young children. *JADA.* 2014;145(2):190–191.

75. Sjogren K, Melin NH. The influence of rinsing routines on fluoride retention after toothbrushing. *Gerodontology.* 2001;18(1):15–20.

76. Walsh T, Worthington HV, Glenny AM, et al. Fluoride toothpastes of different concentrations for preventing

dental caries in children and adolescents. *Cochrane Database Syst Rev.* 2010;(1):CD007868.

77. Marinho VC. Cochrane reviews of randomized trials of fluoride therapies for preventing dental caries. *Eur Arch Paediatr Dent.* 2009;10(3):183–191.

78. Whitford GM. Acute and chronic fluoride toxicity. *J Dent Res.* 1992;71(5):1249–1254.

79. Heifetz SB, Horowitz HS. The amounts of fluoride in current fluoride therapies: safety considerations for children. *ASDC J Dent Child.* 1984;51(4):257–269.

80. Bayless JM, Tinanoff N. Diagnosis and treatment of acute fluoride toxicity. *J Am Dent Assoc.* 1985;110(2):209–211.

ENHANCE YOUR UNDERSTANDING

thePoint **DIGITAL CONNECTIONS**
(see the inside front cover for access information)
- Audio glossary
- Quiz bank

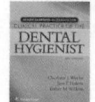

SUPPORT FOR LEARNING
(available separately; visit lww.com)
- *Active Learning Workbook for Clinical Practice of the Dental Hygienist, 12th Edition*

prepU **INDIVIDUALIZED REVIEW**
(available separately; visit lww.com)
- Adaptive quizzing with *prepU for Wilkins' Clinical Practice of the Dental Hygienist*

37

Sealants

Jill C. Moore, RDH, BSDH, MHA

CHAPTER OUTLINE

LEARNING OBJECTIVES

After studying this chapter, the student will be able to:

1. Describe the development and purposes of dental sealant materials.

2. Explain types of sealant material and list criteria of an ideal dental sealant material.

3. List indications and contraindications for placement of dental sealants.

4. Describe clinical procedures for placement and maintenance of a dental sealant.

5. Explain factors that affect sealant penetration.

6. Identify factors to document a dental sealant placement in the patient record.

INTRODUCTION

A pit and fissure sealant is an organic polymer (resin) that flows into the pit or fissure of a posterior tooth and bonds by mechanical retention to the tooth.

▶ Placement of dental sealants is an evidence-based preventive recommendation that can significantly reduce the incidence of dental caries.[1]

▶ As part of a complete preventive program, pit and fissure sealants are indicated for selected patients.

▶ Topically applied fluorides protect smooth tooth surfaces more than occlusal surfaces; dental sealants reduce the incidence of occlusal dental caries.

▶ Incidence of new pit and fissure caries can be lowered by 86% if the sealant is retained at 1 year, 78.6% at 2 years, and 58.6% at 4 years.[2]

▶ Sealant application is a part of a complete prevention program, not an isolated procedure.

▶ As an isolated procedure, patient (and parent) may misunderstand the specific role of sealants in prevention.

▶ Other surfaces and other teeth still need other methods of preventive protection.

▶ Box 37-1 provides definitions and terminology related to sealants and their application.

I. Development of Sealants

Sealants were developed by Dr. Michael Buonocore and the group of dental scientists at the Eastman Dental Center in Rochester, New York.

▶ The focus of the early research was on the need to prepare the enamel surface so a dental material would adhere.

▶ They demonstrated that by using an acid-etch process, the enamel could be altered to increase retention.

▶ The research proved to be a major breakthrough, particularly in esthetic and preventive dentistry.[3,4]

II. Purposes of the Sealant

▶ To provide a physical barrier to "seal off" the pit or fissure.

▶ To prevent oral bacteria and their nutrients from collecting within the pit or fissure to create the acid environment necessary for the initiation of dental caries.

▶ To fill the pit or fissure as deep as possible and provide tight smooth margins at the junction with the enamel surface.

▶ When sealant material is worn or cracked away on the surface around the pit or fissure, the sealant in the depth of the micropore can remain and provide continued protection while sealant material is added for repair and to reseal the enamel/sealant junction.

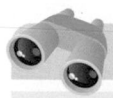

BOX 37-1 **KEY WORDS:** Pit and Fissure Sealants

Acid etchant: in sealant placement, the enamel surface is prepared by the application of phosphoric acid, which etches the surface to provide mechanical retention for the sealant.

Articulating paper: paper treated with dye or wax used to mark points of contact (occlusion) between the maxillary and mandibular teeth.

Bibulous: absorbent; a flat bibulous pad, placed in the cheek over the opening of Stensen's duct, is used to aid in maintaining a dry field while placing sealants.

Biocompatibility: the ability of things to exist together without harm.

Bis-GMA: bisphenol A–glycidyl methylacrylate; plastic material used for dental sealants.

Bonding (mechanical): physical adherence of one substance to another; the adherence of a sealant to the enamel surface is accomplished by an acid-etching technique that leaves microspaces between the enamel rods; the sealant becomes mechanically locked (bonded) in these microspaces.

Bond strength: expression of the degree of adherence between the tooth surface and the sealant.

Conditioner: a substance added to another substance to increase its usability; in sealant placement, the acid etchant is added to the enamel to prepare it for bonding with the sealant.

Curing: the process is used for polymerization of resin-based sealant and composites so the material hardens by which plastic becomes rigid.

Incipient caries: early or beginning caries, caries limited to the enamel.

In vitro: under laboratory conditions.

In vivo: within the living body.

Micropores: tiny openings.

Polymer: a compound of high molecular weight formed by a combination of a chain of simpler molecules (monomers).

Polymerization: a reaction in which a high-molecular-weight product is produced by successive additions of a simpler compound.

  Photopolymerization: polymerization with the use of an external light source.

  Autopolymerization: self-curing; a reaction in which a high-molecular-weight product is produced by successive additions of a simpler compound; hardening process of pit and fissure sealants.

Sealant: organic polymer that bonds to an enamel surface by mechanical retention accommodated by projections of the sealant into micropores created in the enamel by etching; the two types of sealants, filled and unfilled, both are composed of Bis-GMA.

  Filled sealant: contains, in addition to Bis-GMA, microparticles of glass, quartz, silica, and other fillers used in composite restorations; fillers make the sealant more resistant to abrasion.

Viscosity: in general, the resistance to flow or alteration of shape by any substance as a result of molecular cohesion.

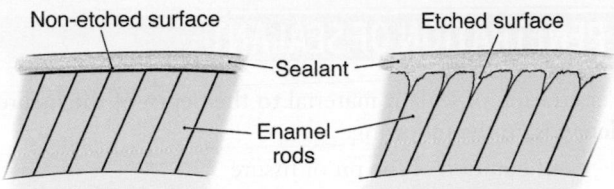

FIGURE 37-1 Enamel–Sealant Interface. Diagram of enamel–sealant interface to compare nonetched with etched surface. Etching produces microscopic porosities in the enamel to increase the area of retention. The unpolymerized resin flows into the porosities and hardens in taglike projections, as shown on the right. (Source: Buonocore MG, Matsui A, Gwinnett AJ. Penetration of resin dental materials into enamel surfaces with reference to bonding. *Arch Oral Biol.* 1968;13(1):61–70.)

III. Purposes of the Acid Etch

▶ To produce irregularities or micropores in the enamel.

▶ To allow the liquid resin to penetrate into the micropores and create a bond or mechanical locking.

▶ Figure 37-1 illustrates the sealant placed on a smooth enamel surface in contrast with placement on an etched surface with retention.

SEALANT MATERIALS

I. Criteria for the Ideal Sealant[3]

▶ Achieve prolonged bonding to enamel.

▶ Be biocompatible with oral tissues.

▶ Offer a simple application procedure.

▶ Be a free-flowing, low-viscosity material capable of entering narrow fissures.

▶ Have low solubility in the oral environment.

II. Classification of Sealant Materials

▶ A majority of sealants in clinical use are made of Bis-GMA (bisphenol A–glycidyl methylacrylate). The techniques of application vary slightly among available products.

A. Classification by Method of Polymerization

▶ *Self-cured or autopolymerized*
  • Preparation: material supplied in two parts. When the two are mixed they quickly polymerize (harden).
  • Advantage: no curing light required.
  • Disadvantages: mixing required; working time limited because polymerization begins when the material is mixed.

▶ *Visible light–cured or photopolymerized*
  • Preparation: material hardens when exposed to a special curing light.

  • Advantages: no mixing required; increased working time due to control over start of polymerization.
  • Disadvantages: extra costs and disinfection time required for curing light, protective shields, and/or glasses.

B. Classification by Filler Content

▶ *Filled*
  • Purpose of filler: To increase bond strength and increase resistance to abrasion and wear.
  • Fillers: Glass and quartz particles give hardness and strength to resist occlusal forces.
  • Effect: Viscosity of the sealant is increased. Flow into the depth of a fissure varies.

▶ *Unfilled*
  • Clear, does not contain particles.
  • Less resistant to abrasion and wear.
  • May not require occlusal adjustment after placement, so provides an advantage for school and community health programs where sealants are placed.

▶ *Fluoride releasing*
  • Purpose: enhance caries resistance.
  • Action: remineralization of incipient caries at base of pit or fissure.

C. Classification by Color

▶ Available: clear, tinted, and opaque.

▶ Purpose: quick identification for evaluation during maintenance assessment.

▶ Effect: clear, tinted, or opaque sealants do not differ in retention.

INDICATIONS FOR SEALANT PLACEMENT

I. Patients with Risk for Dental Caries (Any Age)

▶ Xerostomia: from medications or other reasons.

▶ Patient undergoing orthodontics.

▶ Incipient pit and fissure caries (limited to enamel) with no radiographic evidence of caries on adjacent proximal surface.

▶ Low socioeconomic status.

▶ Diet high in sugars.

▶ Inadequate daily oral health care.

II. Selection of Teeth

▶ Newly erupted: place sealant as soon as tooth is fully erupted.

▶ Occlusal contour: when pit or fissure is deep and irregular as illustrated in Figure 37-2.

▶ Caries history: other teeth restored or have carious lesions.

▶ Figure 37-3 is a flowchart to assist in decision making.

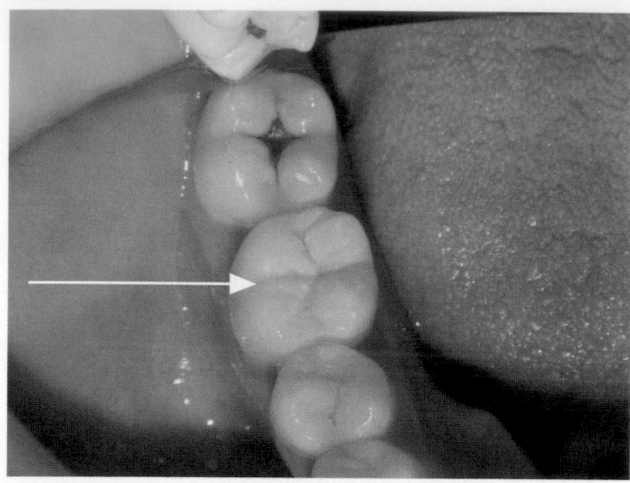

FIGURE 37-2 Molar Tooth with Pits and Fissures. Tooth #30 with deep fissures is selected for placing a dental sealant. Note the amalgam filling on tooth #31, which is evidence of previous dental caries experience. (Photograph courtesy of Jill Moore, RDH, BSDH, MHA, Sealant Coordinator, Michigan Department of Health and Human Services.)

III. Contraindications for Sealant Placement

▸ Radiographic evidence of adjacent proximal dental caries.

▸ Pit and fissures are well coalesced and self-cleansing; low caries risk.

▸ Tooth not completely erupted.

▸ Primary tooth near exfoliation.

PENETRATION OF SEALANT

Penetration of sealant material to the depth of the fissure depends on the following:

▸ Configuration of the pit or fissure

▸ Presence of deposits and debris within the pit or fissure

▸ Properties of the sealant itself.

I. Pit and Fissure Anatomy

The shape and depth of pits and fissures vary considerably even within one tooth. Anatomic differences include:

▸ *Wide V-shaped* (Figure 37-4B) or *narrow V-shaped fissures*.

▸ *Long narrow pits* and grooves reach to, or nearly to, the dentinoenamel junction (Figure 37-4C).

▸ *Long constricted fissures with a bulbous terminal portion* (Figure 37-4D) that may take a wavy course, which may not lead directly from the outer surface to the dentinoenamel junction.

II. Contents of a Pit or Fissure

A pit or fissure may contain the following:

▸ Dental biofilm, pellicle, debris

▸ Rarely but possibly intact remnants of tooth development.

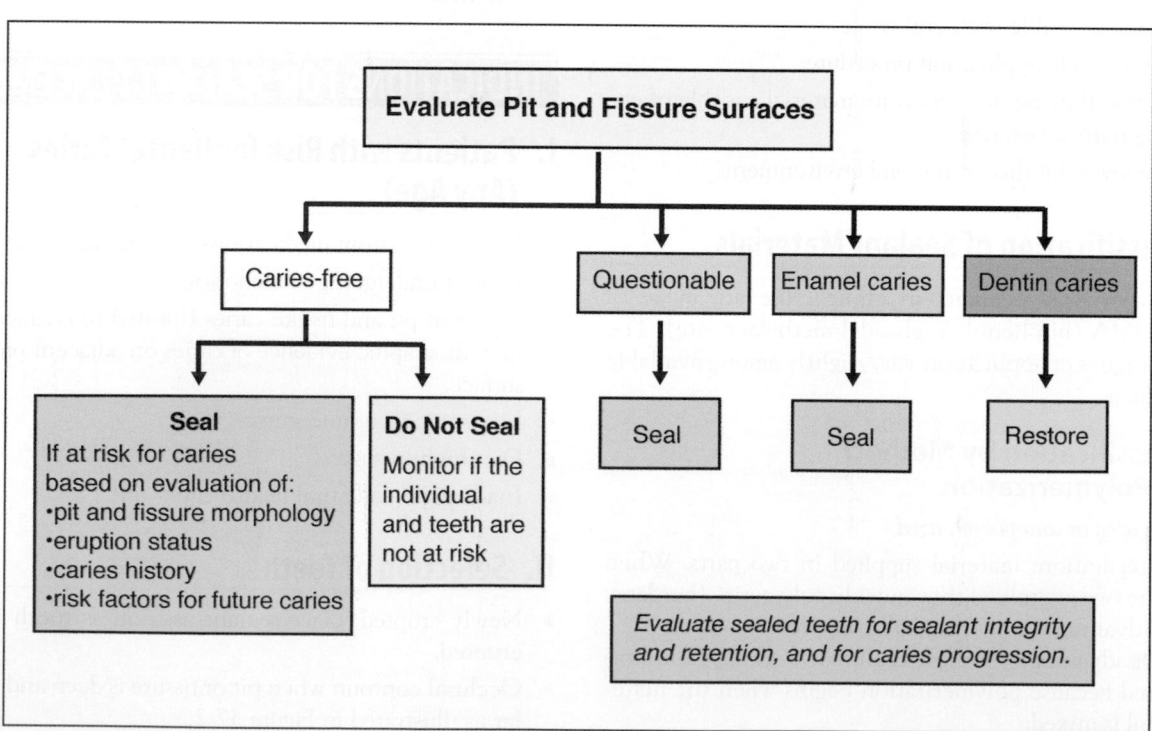

FIGURE 37-3 Tooth Selection for Sealant Placement. Flowchart to assist in decision making for placement of sealants. (Adapted from Workshop on guidelines for sealant use: recommendations. The Association of State and Territorial Dental Directors, the New York State Health Department, the Ohio Department of Health and the School of Public Health, University of Albany, State University of New York. *J Public Health Dent.* 1995;55(5 Spec):263–273.)

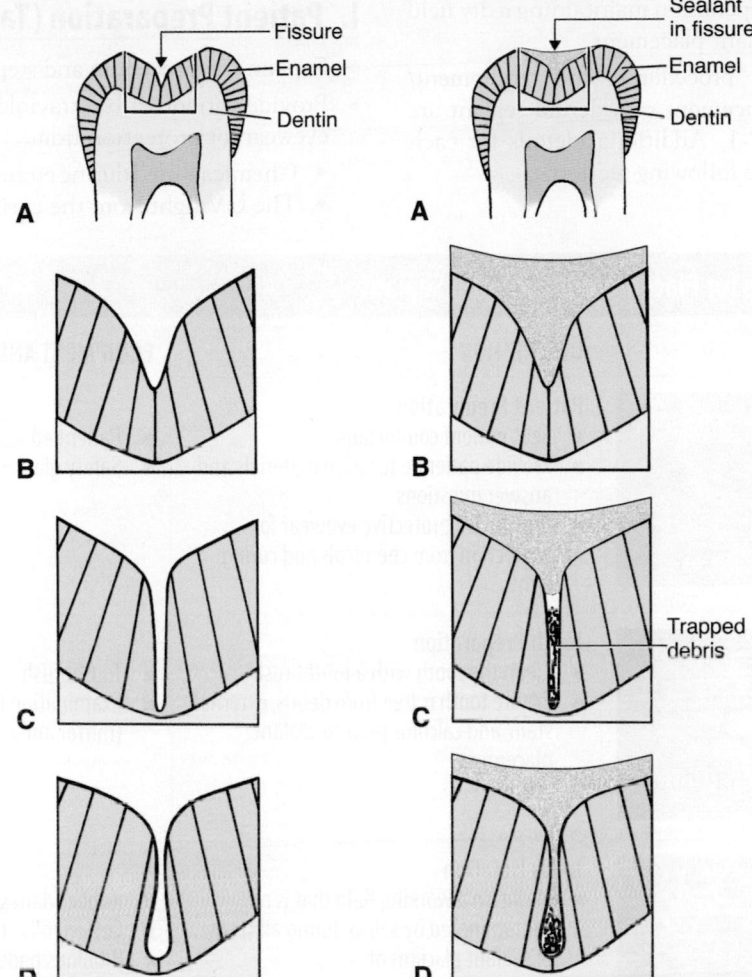

FIGURE 37-4 Occlusal Fissures. Drawings made from microscopic slides show variations in shape and depth of fissures both before and after sealant placement. **A:** Tooth with section enlarged for B, C, and D. **B:** Wide V-shaped fissure shows full sealant penetration. **C:** Long narrow groove that reaches nearly to the dentinoenamel junction. **D:** Long constricted form with a bulbous terminal portion.

III. Effect of Cleaning

▶ The narrow, long fissures are difficult to clean completely.

▶ Cleaning the tooth with pumice prior to dental sealant placement is avoided; if used, complete removal of pumice is necessary.

▶ Retained cleaning material can block the sealant from filling the fissure and can also become mixed with the sealant.

▶ Removal of pumice used for cleaning and thorough washing are necessary for retention of the sealant.

IV. Amount of Penetration

▶ Wide V-shaped and shallow fissures are more apt to be filled by sealant (Figure 37-4B).

▶ Although ideally the sealant penetrates to the bottom of a pit or fissure, such penetration is frequently impossible.

▶ Microscopic examination of pits and fissures after sealant application has shown that the sealant material often does not penetrate to the bottom because residual debris, cleaning agents, and trapped air prevent passage of the material (Figure 37-4C and D).

▶ The bacteria in incipient dental caries at the base of a well-sealed pit or fissure have no access to nutrients required for survival.

CLINICAL PROCEDURES

▶ Treat each quadrant separately while placing sealants on all eligible teeth.

▶ Use four-handed method with an assistant
  • To ensure moisture control.
  • To work efficiently and save time.

▶ Follow manufacturer's directions for each product.

▶ Success of treatment (retention) depends on the precision in each step of the application.

▶ Retention of sealant depends on maintaining a dry field during etching and sealant placement.

▶ Step-by-step clinical procedures and equipment/supplies needed for placement of a dental sealant are illustrated in Table 37-1. Additional details for each step are provided in the following section.

I. Patient Preparation (Table 37-1, Step 1)

▶ Explain the procedure and steps to be performed.

▶ Provide patient with ultraviolet (UV) protective safety eyewear for protection from:
- Chemicals used during etching and sealant placement
- The UV light from the curing lamp.

Table 37-1	Steps for Placement of a Dental Sealant		
STEP	**ILLUSTRATION**	**DESCRIPTION**	**EQUIPMENT AND SUPPLIES**
Step 1		**Patient Preparation** ■ Seat patient comfortably ■ Provide patient education materials and answer questions ■ Provide UV protective eyewear for protection from chemicals and curing light	■ Patient education materials ■ Safety glasses for patient
Step 2		**Tooth Preparation** ■ Clean the tooth with a toothbrush ■ Ensure tooth is free from debris, external stain, and calculus prior to sealant placement	■ Toothbrush ■ Examination instruments (mirror and explorer)

Step 3		**Tooth Isolation**
		■ Maintain a working field that is not contaminated by saliva during all steps of sealant placement
		■ Options include:
		  • rubber dam (not shown)
		  • cotton rolls on the mandibular arch (top left)
		  • triangular bibulous pad to cover the parotid duct for the maxillary arch (lower left)
		■ Note: Take care to moisten all cotton prior to removal to avoid sticking to dry mucosa
			■ Rubber dam setup (optional)
			■ Cotton rolls and holders (Figure 37-3)
			■ Bibulous pads (lower left)

Step 4		**Acid Etch** ■ Dry entire area for 20–30 seconds with air/water syringe ■ Maintain a dry field ■ Use commercial etchant applicator (shown), brush, or cotton pellet to dispense etchant material ■ Place the acid etch only within the grooves and fissures where the sealant will be placed (shown at lower left) ■ Note: Follow product manufacture directions for application time; usually between 15 and 60 seconds	■ Air/water syringe ■ Acid-etch material and applicator, brush, or cotton pellet

STEP	ILLUSTRATION	DESCRIPTION	EQUIPMENT AND SUPPLIES
Step 5		**Rinse and Air Dry Tooth** ■ Place the high-velocity evacuation over the tooth ■ Rinse the tooth with the air/water syringe. ■ Spray water until surface is free of etch (30–60 seconds) ■ Spray air with air/water syringe until dry ■ Reisolate if necessary	■ High-velocity evacuation system ■ Air/water syringe
Step 6		**Evaluate for Complete Etching** ■ A completely etched tooth will have a chalky-white appearance when dry ■ If surface is not chalky appearing, repeat the acid-etch step	■ Air/water syringe ■ Mouth mirror for retraction and indirect vision
Step 7		**Place Sealant Material** ■ Continue to maintain a dry field ■ Use external fulcrum (fingers resting lightly on patient's chin or cheek) ■ Place the wet sealant material in the prepared pits and fissures ■ Adjust flow so sealant material is deposited only within the grooves, pits, and fissures	■ Sealant material and applicator ■ Slow-speed saliva ejector to help maintain dry field

Step 8		**Cure Sealant**
		■ If using light-polymerized sealant material:
		  • Ensure clinician and patient UV protective eye protection
		  • Cover entire tooth with light and cure for 20–30 seconds in accordance with manufacturer instructions
		■ If using self-curing sealant material:
		  • Maintain dry field and allow drying time as indicated in manufacturer's instructions
			■ UV protective goggles/glasses for patient and clinicians.
			■ Curing light
			■ Saliva ejector to help maintain dry field

Step 9		**Final/Cured Sealant** ■ Gently check for voids in sealant material with explorer ■ Additional material can be added if the surface has not been contaminated or wet	■ Mirror and explorer ■ Saliva ejector to help maintain dry field ■ Additional sealant material if needed to fill voids
Step 10		**Check Occlusion** ■ Use articulating paper to locate high spots and adjust as needed ■ Unfilled sealant material will wear down via normal attrition ■ Filled sealant material will require occlusal adjustment	■ Articulating paper ■ Holder

(continues)

Table 37-1	Steps for Placement of a Dental Sealant (*continued*)		
STEP	**ILLUSTRATION**	**DESCRIPTION**	**EQUIPMENT AND SUPPLIES**
Step 11		**Follow-up** ■ Provide patient education materials for the patient to take home. ■ Answer patient's questions ■ Re-evaluate sealants at each subsequent maintenance appointment	■ Excellent patient education materials are available for free from the National Institute of Dental and Craniofacial Research website. Available at: https://www.nidcr.nih.gov/orderpublications/

Photographs in Steps 2, 4a, 7, 8, and 10 courtesy of Susan J. Jenkins, RDH, MS, CAGS, Forsyth School of Dental Hygiene, MCPHS University. Additional photographs courtesy of Jill Moore, RDH, BSDH, MHA, Dental Sealant Coordinator, Michigan Department of Health and Human Services.

II. Tooth Preparation (Table 37-1, Step 2)

A. Purposes

▶ Remove deposits and debris.

▶ Permit maximum contact of the etch and the sealant with the enamel surface.

▶ Encourage sealant penetration into the pit or fissure.

B. Methods

▶ Examine tooth surfaces: remove calculus and stain.

▶ For the patient with no stain or calculus, apply toothbrush filaments straight into occlusal pits and fissures. (see Figure 28-14A in Chapter 28).

▶ Suction the pits and fissures with high-velocity evacuator.

▶ Gently use explorer tip to remove debris and bacteria from the pit or fissure and suction again to remove loosened material.

▶ Evaluate need for additional cleaning; the brushing may be sufficient.

III. Tooth Isolation (Table 37-1, Step 3)

A. Purposes of Isolation

▶ Maintaining a dry tooth is the single most important factor in sealant retention.

▶ Keep the tooth clean and dry for optimal action and bonding of the sealant.

▶ Eliminate possible contamination by saliva and moisture from the breath.

▶ Keep the materials from contacting the oral tissues, being swallowed accidentally, or being unpleasant to the patient because of flavor.

B. Rubber Dam Isolation

▶ Rubber dam application is the method of choice because the most complete isolation is obtained. This method is especially helpful when more than one tooth in the same quadrant is to be sealed.

▶ Rubber dam is essential when profuse saliva flow and overactive tongue and oral muscles make retraction and consistent maintenance of a dry, clean field impossible.

▶ When a quadrant has a rubber dam and anesthesia for restoration of other teeth, teeth indicated for sealant can be treated at the same time.

▶ Use anesthesia when application of the clamp cannot be tolerated by the patient.

▶ Rubber dam may not be possible when a tooth that is essential for holding the clamp is not fully erupted.

C. Cotton-Roll Isolation

▶ Patient position: tilt head to allow saliva to pool on the opposite side of the mouth.

▶ Position cotton-roll holder. Figure 37-5 shows the placement of two types of cotton role holders.

▶ Place saliva ejector.

▶ Apply triangular saliva absorber (bibulous pad) over the opening of the parotid duct in the cheek.

▶ Take care to prevent saliva contamination from entering the area to be etched.

D. Additional Isolation Options

▶ Commercially available isolation systems that can be attached to the dental unit offer intraoral quadrant isolation, illumination, and suction.

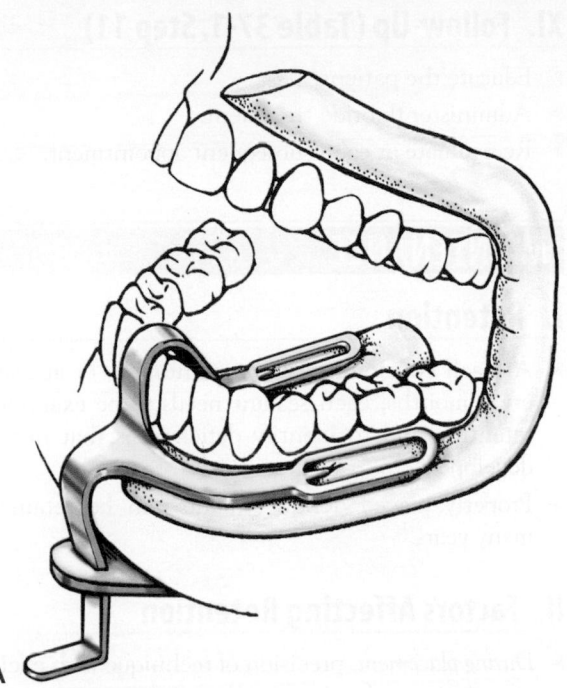

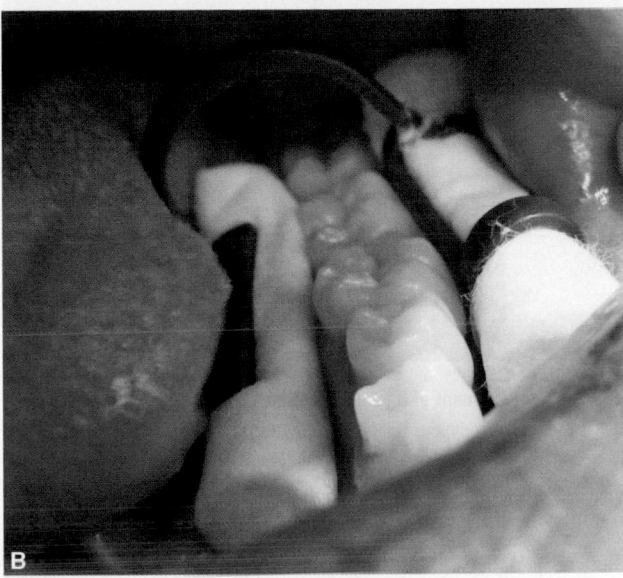

FIGURE 37-5 Tooth Isolation. A: Demonstrates a garmer-type cotton-roll holder, which can be used to treat two quadrants simultaneously. A continuous cotton role extends from the mandibular anterior vestibule to the maxillary anterior vestibule. **B:** Illustrates a disposable plastic cotton-roll holder used to isolate teeth in a mandibular quadrant. (Photograph courtesy of Jill Moore, RDH, BSDH, MHA, Sealant Coordinator, Michigan Department of Health and Human Services.)

IV. Acid Etch (Table 37-1, Step 4)

A. Dry the Tooth

▶ Purposes
  • Prepare the tooth for acid etch.
  • Eliminate moisture and contamination.
▶ Use clean, dry air
  • Clear water from the air/water syringe by releasing the spray into a sink.
  • Test for absence of moisture by blowing on a mouth mirror or other dry surface.
▶ Air dry the tooth for at least 10 seconds.

B. Apply Etchant

▶ Action
  • Creates micropores to increase the surface area and provide retention for the sealant.
  • Removes contamination from enamel surface.
  • Provides antibacterial action.
▶ Etchant solution forms
  • *Phosphoric acid:* 15%–50%, depends on product and manufacturer.
  • *Liquid:* Low viscosity allows good flow into pit or fissure but may be difficult to control.
  • *Gel:* Tinted gel with thick consistency allows increased visibility and control but may be difficult to rinse off the tooth surface.
  • *Semigel:* Tinted, with enough viscosity to allow good visibility, control, and rinsing ease.

▶ Etchant timing varies from 15 to 60 seconds. Follow manufacturer's instructions for each product.
▶ Etchant delivery
  • *Liquid etch:* Use a small brush, sponge, or cotton pellet; continuously pat rather than rub, when applying to keep the surface moist.
  • *Gel and semigel:* Use a syringe, brush, or manufacturer-supplied single-use cannula.

V. Rinse and Air Dry Tooth (Table 37-1, Step 5)

▶ Rinse thoroughly; apply continuous suction to prevent saliva from reaching the etched surface.
▶ Dry for 15–20 seconds; maintain dry isolation ready for sealant application.

VI. Evaluate for Complete Etching (Table 37-1, Step 6)

▶ Dry, and examine the etched surface.
▶ Repeat etching process if the surface does not appear chalky white.

VII. Place Sealant Material (Table 37-1, Step 7)

Follow manufacturer's instructions included in the sealant material package. General instructions include:

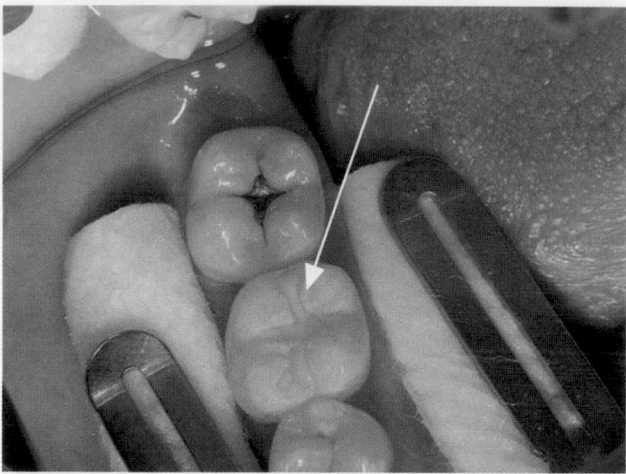

FIGURE 37-6 Placement of Dental Sealant Material. Appropriate placement of a dental sealant will completely fill pits and fissures, but not compromise occlusion by overfilling to a high, flat surface. (Photograph courtesy of Jill Moore, RDH, BSDH, MHA, Sealant Coordinator, Michigan Department of Health and Human Services.)

▶ Avoid overmanipulation of sealant materials to prevent producing air bubbles.

▶ Use disposable implement supplied in the sealant material package for application.

▶ Flow minimal amount into all pits and fissures; do not overfill to a high, flat surface.

▶ Figure 37-6 illustrates a correctly filled dental sealant surface.

VIII. Cure Sealant (Table 37-1, Step 8)

▶ If using a light-cured sealant material:
- Leave liquid sealant material in place for 10 seconds to allow for optimum penetration.
- Use UV blocking eye protection for both clinician and patient.
- Apply the curing light for 20–30 seconds in accordance with manufacturer's instructions. Cover entire tooth surface with the light to ensure complete polymerization.

▶ If using an autopolymerized sealant material, consult manufacturer's instructions for curing time.

IX. Evaluate Cured Sealant (Table 37-1, Step 9)

▶ Check for voids gently with explorer: Additional sealant material can be added if surface has not been contaminated or wet.

X. Check Occlusion (Table 37-1, Step 10)

▶ Use articulating paper to locate high spots; adjust as required.

▶ Occlusal wear: unfilled sealants wear down via normal attrition to correct height; filled sealants require occlusal adjustment.

XI. Follow-Up (Table 37-1, Step 11)

▶ Educate the patient.

▶ Administer fluoride treatment.

▶ Re-evaluate at each subsequent appointment.

MAINTENANCE

I. Retention

▶ At each continuing care appointment, or at least every 6 months, each sealant needs to be examined for retention and to identify deficiencies that may have developed.

▶ Properly placed dental sealants can be retained for many years.[1]

II. Factors Affecting Retention

▶ *During placement*: precision of technique with exclusion of moisture and contamination.

▶ *Patient self-care*: Advise patient to avoid biting or chewing on hard surfaces such as a pencil or ice cubes.

▶ *Dental hygiene care*: Avoid using an air-powder polisher on intact existing sealants during maintenance appointments.[5]

III. Replacement

▶ Consult the manufacturer's instructions.

▶ Tooth preparation: same as for original application.

▶ Removal of firmly attached sections of retained sealant is not usually necessary.

▶ Re-etching of the tooth surface prior to replacement of a dental sealant is always essential.

SCHOOL-BASED DENTAL SEALANT PROGRAMS

▶ Delivery of dental sealants in school-based settings is a proven strategy[6,7] that can:
- Effectively increase the percent of children in communities who receive dental sealants.
- Reduce risk for decay for high-risk children.

▶ Many such school-based programs provide additional preventive services such as screening, prophylaxis, topical fluoride application, and oral health education.[5]

▶ Programs that provide sealants on sound surfaces and noncavitated lesions are an effective adjunct to preventive care provided in traditional dental care settings.[8]

▶ Figure 37-7 shows a portable dental unit set up in a school library.

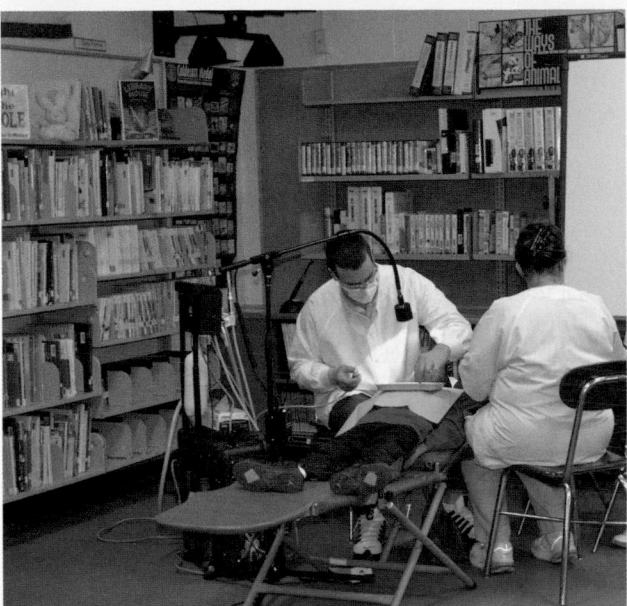

FIGURE 37-7 Delivery of dental sealants in a school-based program using portable dental equipment set up in the school library. (Photograph courtesy of Jill Moore, RDH, BSDH, MHA, Sealant Coordinator, Michigan Department of Health and Human Services.)

DOCUMENTATION

Documentation in the record of a patient receiving a sealant contains a minimum of the following:

► Reason for selection of certain teeth for sealants; informed consent of patient, parent, or other caregiver.

► Type of sealant used, preparation of tooth, manner of isolation, patient cooperation during administration; postinsertion instructions given.

► Sample documentation for placement of dental sealants may be reviewed in Box 37-2.

BOX 37-2
Example Documentation: Placement of Dental Sealants

S –A 12 year-old male patient presents for dental sealant placement.

O –Occlusal contour and previous history of dental caries in primary dentition indicate need for sealant placement for 2nd molars; X-rays indicate no dental caries on proximal surfaces of 2nd molars. Tooth #30 partially erupted with operculum.

A –Need to wait until #30 is completely erupted to place sealant.

P –Reviewed sealant education materials with mother and patient. Mother provided consent for placement of the recommended sealants. Sealants placed on #3-O, 14-O, 14-L, 19-O, 19-B pit using right side, then left side isolation. Autopolymerized opaque sealant material used with 15% acid etch applied with manufacturer's directions. Patient tolerated treatment well, no gagging, minimal saliva, easy isolation.

Next steps: Schedule in 1 month to re-examine for sealant placement on #30 and retention check on 3, 14, and 19.

Signed: _____, RDH

Date: _____

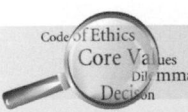

EVERYDAY ETHICS

Lillian had always enjoyed doing sealants when she was in dental hygiene school. They had been required to do quite a few, and as students they got to participate in "Sealant Day," a volunteer program carried out by the local dental hygienists every spring.

Now, when she came back from the state dental hygiene meeting, she was all excited about the new interpretation of the practice act by the Dental Board and greeted her employer, Dr. Fine, with the news first thing Monday morning. The Board had voted that the dental hygienist who had been in practice for 2 years full-time (or part-time equivalent) could make the decision whether a pit or fissure needed a sealant. There was a continuing education course and an examination required.

Lillian added: "Remember Jack—that teenager that was here last week? He had some really deep fissures that I was sure would benefit from sealants. Can I go ahead and schedule him? I told him he needed them. He has an

appointment with you to have a few cavities filled, but that wouldn't fit in your book until nearly the end of the month. They are giving the exam and CE next week."

Dr. Fine continued quietly to tie on his gown for the first patient, and then he smiled and said, "Well, Lil, let's wait until he comes in for his appointment with me and I'll look at them."

Questions for Consideration

1. Professionally, what action(s) can Lillian take to initiate a system of calibration between her and Dr. Fine to pursue the new practice protocols?

2. What ethical issues may be involved here? How can they be resolved?

3. Which of the core values describe the friendly relationship between Lillian and Dr. Fine? And which core values describe Lillian's wishes to extend the services for Jack's (the patient's) benefit?

Factors To Teach The Patient

▷ Sealants are part of a total preventive program. Sealants are not substitutes for other preventive measures. Limitations of dietary sucrose, use of fluorides, and dental biofilm control are major factors with sealants for prevention of dental caries.

▷ What a sealant is and why such a meticulous application procedure is required.

▷ What can be expected from a sealant; how long it lasts, and how it prevents dental caries.

▷ Need for examination of the sealant at frequent, scheduled maintenance appointments, and need for replacement when missing or chipped.

▷ Avoid biting hard items such as a pencil or ice cubes to increase sealant retention.

References

1. Ahovuo-Saloranta A, Forss H, Walsh T, et al. Sealants for preventing dental decay in the permanent teeth. *Cochrane Database Syst Rev*. 2013;(3):CD001830. doi:10.1002/14651858.CD001830.pub4.

2. Beauchap J, Caufiel PW, Crall JJ, et al. Evidence-based clinical recommendations for the use of pit-and-fissure sealants: a report of the American Dental Association Council on Scientific Affairs. *J Am Dent Assoc*. 2008;139(3):257–268.

3. Handleman SL, Shey Z. Michael Buonocore and the Eastman Dental Center. A historic perspective on sealants. *J Dent Res*. 1996;75(1):529–534.

4. Cueto EI, Buonocore MG. Sealing of pits and fissures with an adhesive resin: its use in caries prevention. *J Am Dent Assoc*. 1967;75(1):121–128.

5. Huennekens SC, Daniel SJ, Bayne SC. Effects of air polishing on the abrasion of occlusal sealants. *Quintessence Int*. 1991;22(7):581–585.

6. Children's Dental Health Project. *Dental Sealants: Proven to Prevent Decay*. Washington, DC: Children's Dental Health Project; 2014:21. https://www.cdhp.org/resources/314-dental-sealants-proven-to-prevent-tooth-decay. Accessed May 16, 2014.

7. PEW Center on the States. *Falling Short: Most States Lag on Dental Sealants*. Washington, DC: The PEW Charitable Trusts; 2013. http://www.pewstates.org/research/reports/falling-short-85899434875. Accessed May 16, 2014.

8. Gooch BF, Griffin SO, Gray SK, et al. Preventing dental caries through school-based sealant programs: updated recommendations and reviews of evidence. *J Am Dent Assoc*. 2009;140(11):1356–1365.

ENHANCE YOUR UNDERSTANDING

thePoint® DIGITAL CONNECTIONS
(see the inside front cover for access information)
- Audio glossary
- Quiz bank

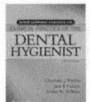

SUPPORT FOR LEARNING
(available separately; visit lww.com)
- *Active Learning Workbook for Clinical Practice of the Dental Hygienist*, 12th Edition

prepU INDIVIDUALIZED REVIEW
(available separately; visit lww.com)
- Adaptive quizzing with *prepU for Wilkins' Clinical Practice of the Dental Hygienist*

SECTION VII

Implementation: Treatment

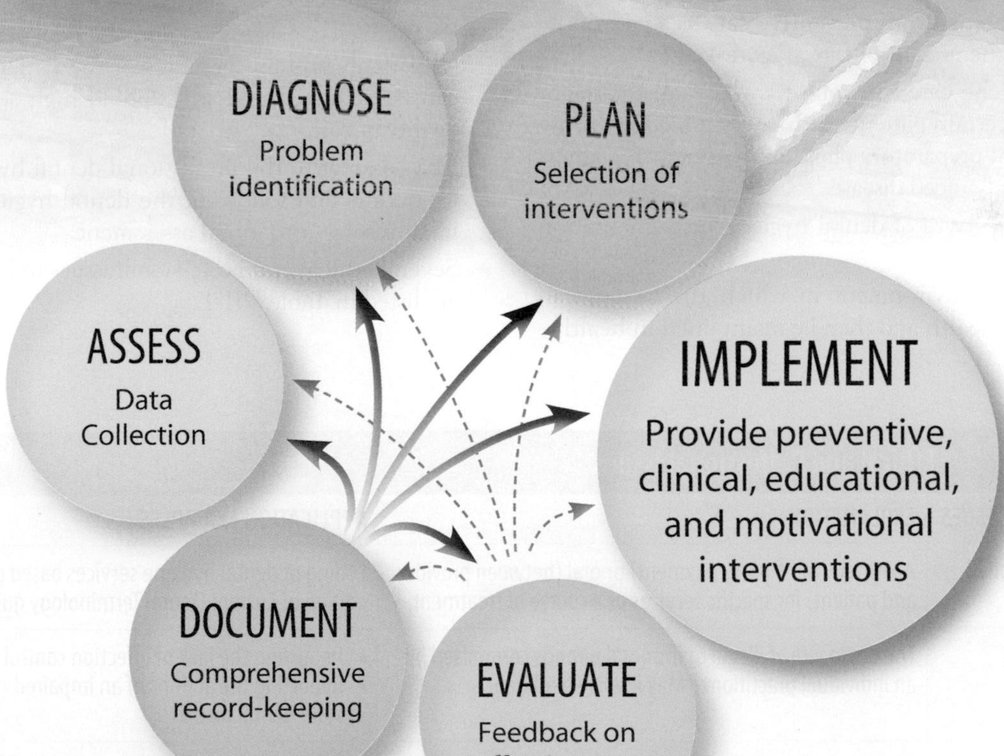

FIGURE VII-1 The Dental Hygiene Process of Care.

INTRODUCTION FOR SECTION VII

The first objective of dental hygiene treatment is to create an environment in which the tissues can return to health.

In the sequence of patient care, introduction to preventive measures occurs first, to help ensure the success of dental hygiene treatment. Professional treatment interventions make a limited contribution to arresting the progression of disease without daily biofilm control measures performed by the patient. Dental hygiene treatment interventions include:

▶ Anxiety and pain control
▶ Instrumentation for scaling and root planing
▶ Extrinsic stain removal
▶ Care of dental restorations
▶ Posttreatment care procedures
▶ Placement and removal of dressings
▶ Removal of sutures
▶ Treatment of hypersensitive teeth
▶ Immediate evaluation, short-term follow-up, and maintenance assessment of treatment outcomes.

THE DENTAL HYGIENE PROCESS OF CARE

▶ Dental hygiene treatment uses nonsurgical periodontal therapy combined with preventive care as a part of the dental hygiene process of care (Figure VII-1).
▶ Dental hygiene care can comprise the total treatment needed for certain patients with uncomplicated disease or the initial preparatory phase of treatment for others with more advanced disease.
▶ General objectives of dental hygiene instrumentation are as follows:
  • Create an environment in which the tissues can return to health and then be maintained in health.

• Aid in the prevention and control of gingival and periodontal infections by removal of periodontal pathogenic microorganisms and factors that predispose to the retention of dental biofilm.
• Provide the patient with smooth tooth surfaces that are easier to clean and keep biofilm free by daily oral self-care procedures.
• Help the patient appreciate the appearance and feeling of a thoroughly clean mouth as a motivation toward development of adequate habits for personal oral care.
• Prepare the teeth and gingiva for dental procedures, including those performed by the restorative dentist, prosthodontist, orthodontist, pedodontist, and oral surgeon.
• Improve oral esthetics and sanitation of the oral cavity.

ETHICAL APPLICATIONS

▶ The professional dental hygienist acknowledges the ethical implications of all aspects of providing patient care.
▶ Many ethical facets of dental hygiene care can:
  • Relate directly to the provider–patient or intraprofessional relationships.
  • Affect the overall delivery of dental services.
▶ Practicing a consistent and professional demeanor with all patients and all members of the patient care team can be achieved and will uphold high standards and quality of care.
▶ The conduct of the professional dental hygienist prior to, during, and following the dental hygiene appointment is subject to moral assessment.
▶ Several ethical and professional issues to be considered are listed in Table VII-1.

TABLE VII-1	Ethical and Professional Issues	
PROFESSIONAL ISSUES	**EXPLANATION**	**APPLICATION EXAMPLES**
Expressed or implied contracts	A written (third-party payment) or oral (between provider and patient) for specific services or a course of treatment.	Coding of dental hygiene services based on current edition of Current Dental Terminology guidelines.
Whistle-blowing	The disclosure of illegal or immoral wrongs committed by an individual practitioner. May involve negligent acts.	• Reporting the lack of infection control procedures. • Reporting the actions of an impaired colleague to a state dental board.
Privacy rights	Involves the handling of health information through protection of privacy, insurance access, preventing fraud and abuse, and standardization within the healthcare industry.	Health Insurance Portability and Accountability the confidentiality of dental records, especially where computers are used to document patient data.
Supervision	The ethical and legal working relationship between the dentist, dental hygienist, and other healthcare providers.	A dental hygienist in a collaborative practice treating patients that reside in a nursing home.

38

Anxiety and Pain Control

Debra November-Rider, RDH, MSDH and Donna J. Stach, BS, RDH, MEd

CHAPTER OUTLINE

LEARNING OBJECTIVES

After studying this chapter, the student will be able to:

1. Describe the components of pain.

2. Summarize the advantages and disadvantages of nitrous oxide–oxygen administration.

3. Define titration and explain application during nitrous oxide–oxygen sedation.

4. List the local anesthetics of short, intermediate, and long duration and indications for use.

5. Give examples of absolute and relative contraindications for local anesthetic administration.

6. Identify items in local anesthesia armamentarium and describe the purpose of each.

7. Summarize the different local and systemic complications from the administration of local anesthesia and how to manage them.

8. List the components of a complete patient record entry following the administration of local anesthesia or nitrous oxide/oxygen sedation.

According to the 2000 United States Surgeon General's Report—Oral Health in America, 50% of Americans are afraid of visiting the dental office, with one-third so frightened that they avoid seeking any type of oral health services.[1,2]

▶ There are many contributing causes, one of which is the association of pain with dental procedures. Ranking of negative dental stimuli is presented in Box 38-1.

▶ Concern for patient anxiety and pain is an integral part of a dental hygiene appointment.

▶ Recognizing and managing a patient's anxiety and pain is an essential part of dental hygiene care planning.

▶ The decision to use a pharmacologic agent for management of anxiety and pain is dependent on a number of factors including the following:

  • Periodontal health status, the treatment being rendered.

  • Patient's pain threshold.

▶ Box 38-2 provides terminology and definitions relative to anxiety and pain and to their management.

BOX 38-1

Ranking of Negative Dental Stimuli

1. Getting an injection (68.1%)
2. Dental radiographs (61.4%)
3. Use of curets and scalers (56%)
4. The sight of the dental needle (54.1%)
5. The sight of curets and scalers (49.4%)
6. The use and sound of power instruments (45.7%)
7. Use of air or water spray (36.4%)
8. Wearing of personal protective equipment (7.5%)

Source: Doebling S, Rowe MM. Negative perceptions of dental stimuli and their effects on dental fear. *J Dent Hyg*. 2000;74(2):110–116.

COMPONENTS OF PAIN

When discussing pain, the three factors to consider are the following:

I. Pain Perception

▶ Relates to the physical process of receiving a painful stimulus and transmitting the information through the nervous system to the brain where it is interpreted as pain.

▶ Little variability in pain perception between individuals with intact nervous systems.

II. Pain Reaction

▶ Pain reaction is a combination of interpretation of and response to the pain message.

▶ It is highly variable between individuals and even in the same individual at different times.

▶ Accounts for much of the variability seen between patients in personal pain management needs.

▶ Many factors influence pain reaction including: age, fatigue, emotional state, both cultural and ethnic learned behaviors.

▶ Anxiety has special significance: the anxious patient is predisposed to feel pain. Current research has shown an association between individuals with red hair and higher levels of dental fear and anxiety.[3]

III. Pain Threshold

▶ Varies between individuals.

▶ Highly reproducible.

▶ May be altered by drugs such as local anesthesia.

▶ Low and high pain threshold are defined in Box 38-2.

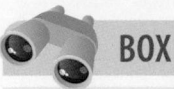

BOX 38-2   KEY WORDS: Anxiety and Pain Control

Absolute contraindication: under no circumstances should the local anesthetic or vasoconstrictor be administered.

Ambient air: surrounding atmosphere.

Analgesia: reduction or elimination of pain in the conscious patient.

Anesthesia: loss of feeling or sensation, especially loss of tactile sensitivity, with or without loss of consciousness.

Anxiety: a negative, emotional response to an anticipated event, the outcome of which is unknown. This is a learned response from personal experience or the stories of others.

ASA classification: developed by the American Society of Anesthesiologists, is a grading system to assess the patient's medical and physical state prior to receiving anesthesia or undergoing surgery.

Aspiration: recommended technique for preventing injection of local anesthetic directly into circulatory system. Negative pressure is created in anesthetic cartridge. If needle tip is in artery or vein, blood will be visible in cartridge.

Block anesthesia: induced by injecting the anesthetic close to a nerve trunk; may be at some distance from the area to be treated; involves multiple teeth and surrounding hard and soft tissues.

Conscious: state in which patient is capable of rational response to commands and protective reflexes are intact, including the ability to maintain a patent airway independently and continuously.

Conscious sedation: the combination of medications to help a patient relax (sedation) and block pain (anesthesia) during a medical or dental procedure.

Epinephrine: a hormone secreted by the adrenal medulla that, among many functions, causes vasodilation of blood vessels of skeletal muscles, vasoconstriction of arterioles of skin and mucous membranes, and stimulation of heart action; used in local anesthetics for its vasoconstrictive action.

General anesthesia: the elimination of all sensations, accompanied by the loss of consciousness.

Hypoxia: diminished availability of oxygen to body tissues.

Diffusion hypoxia: lack of adequate amounts of oxygen that can result from the rapid diffusion of nitrous oxide molecules from the blood stream into the lungs.

Iatrosedation: reduction of anxiety as a result of the clinician's behavior or actions. A psychosomatic method of pain control.

Infiltration anesthesia: induced by injecting the anesthetic directly into or around the area to be anesthetized; anesthetizes the smaller terminal nerve endings of the tooth.

Local anesthesia: loss of sensation, especially pain, in a circumscribed area without loss of consciousness; also called regional anesthesia.

Metered spray: a method for dispensing topical anesthetic that administers a fixed volume of drug and then stops automatically.

Maximum Recommended Dose (MRD): maximum safe dose in milligrams (mg) of a local anesthetic based on patient body weight.

Noninjectable local anesthesia: a thermosetting anesthetic gel extruded into the periodontal pocket results in loss of sensation to the adjacent soft tissue and partial dental/pulpal anesthesia.

Occupational exposure: subject to an action or influence, usually negative, as a result of one's occupation or work environment.

Pain: a sensation in which a person experiences discomfort, distress, or suffering; may vary in intensity from mild discomfort to intolerable agony.

Pain threshold: point at which a sensation starts to be painful and a response results. Varies between individuals based on interpretation of sensation. May be altered by some drugs.

High pain threshold: a greater than average tolerance to a painful stimulus.

Low pain threshold: a strong or rapid reaction to a painful stimulus.

Potency: strength of a drug. Amount of a medication or drug necessary to achieve a desired effect.

Psychosomatic method: any nonpharmacologic technique that reduces anxiety and improves pain control. Effective because the mind influences the body's perception and interpretation of pain.

Relative contraindication: the offending drug (either local anesthetic or vasoconstrictor) can be administered after careful review of the medical history and assessment of risk factors. Use minimal effective amount; stay below the MRD.

Scavenging device: that part of the nitrous oxide equipment that collects exhaled nitrous oxide and removes it. The main component is the scavenging nasal hood. The American Dental Association recommends that effective scavenging devices be installed whenever nitrous oxide is used to reduce occupational exposure.

Sedation: one of the stages of anesthesia in which the patient is still conscious but is under the influence of a central nervous system depressant drug.

Titration: a technique for individualization of drug dose. Administration of small, incremental dose of a drug until the desired clinical action is observed.

Vasoconstrictor: a drug that constricts blood vessels. An additive to most local anesthetic solutions to offset the vasodilating actions of the local anesthetic.

PAIN CONTROL MECHANISMS

▶ Match the pain control method to the patient's treatment needs and medical status.

▶ All pain management techniques are more effective if utilized before the patient experiences pain. The following five pain control mechanisms are often combined for optimum effect:

I. Remove the Painful Stimulus

▶ Affects pain perception.

▶ Examples: clinician repositions fulcrum to avoid pinching the patient's lip during instrumentation.

II. Block the Pathway of the Pain Message

▶ Affects pain perception.

▶ Examples: use of local anesthetic, topical anesthetic.

III. Prevent Pain Reaction by Raising Pain Reaction Threshold

▶ Affects pain reaction.

▶ Examples: use of nitrous oxide–oxygen conscious sedation; nonopioid analgesics such as nonsteroidal anti-inflammatory drugs (NSAIDs).

IV. Depress Central Nervous System

▶ Affects pain reaction.

▶ Example: use of general anesthesia.

V. Use Psychosedation Methods (Also Called Iatrosedation)

▶ Affects both pain perception and pain reaction.

▶ Includes any nonpharmacologic technique to reduce patient anxiety.
  • Builds a trust relationship.
  • Lets the patient feel more in control.

▶ May be used alone or combined with pharmacologic pain management.

▶ Examples: Explain procedures carefully; allow patient to express concerns; use relaxation or distraction techniques.

NONOPIOID ANALGESICS[4,5]

Over-the-counter (OTC) analgesics are an effective adjunct for preventing or reducing the mild-to-moderate discomfort patients experience during dental hygiene therapy or postoperatively.

I. Drugs

▶ NSAIDs.
  • Block prostaglandin synthesis at peripheral nerve endings to inhibit generation of pain message.
  • Suppress onset of pain.
  • Decrease pain severity.
  • The drugs of choice for dental pain.
  • If hemostasis is a consideration during treatment or postoperative bleeding is a concern, use caution when recommending NSAIDs

▶ Acetaminophen.

II. Indications for Use

▶ Mild-to-moderate pain during treatment and postoperative healing.

NITROUS OXIDE–OXYGEN SEDATION[6,7]

▶ Nitrous oxide–oxygen sedation (N_2O-O_2) has been safely used in dental settings for pain control and anxiety management.

▶ A state of conscious sedation is produced with the patient awake, relaxed, responsive to commands, able to cooperate with treatment, and having intact protective reflexes.

▶ The patient has some degree of analgesia and a higher pain reaction threshold.

CHARACTERISTICS OF NITROUS OXIDE

▶ Gaseous agent (nitrous oxide) is absorbed from the lungs into the cardiovascular system.

▶ Onset: rapid, less than 30 seconds; peak effect occurs less than 5 minutes.
  • Duration: terminated as soon as delivery of nitrous is stopped.
  • The clinician has the unique ability to control the amount of sedation based on the patient's psychological needs and level of pain control.
  • Inhalation sedation with nitrous oxide has significant advantages over other techniques of sedation and possesses no significant disadvantages.

I. Anesthetic, Analgesic and Anxiolytic Properties

▶ Produces analgesia.
  • Achieves optimum analgesia and patient cooperation at 20%–40% nitrous oxide for most patients.
  • The need for higher or lower concentrations depends on individual biologic variability.
  • Reduces the intensity of pain but does not block it; only mildly potent as an anesthetic gas.

- Use with local anesthetics when the patient experiences significant discomfort.
- ► Anxiolytic (sedative) effects.
  - Sedation reduces patient's level of fear and anxiety; has a positive effect on pain threshold.
- ► Possesses slight amnestic properties.

II. Chemical and Physical Properties

- ► Gas at room temperature and pressure.
- ► Heavier than air.
- ► Colorless; sweet smelling.
- ► Nonirritating and nonallergenic. No allergic reaction has ever been reported.
- ► Nonflammable but will support the combustion of flammable substances.

III. Blood Solubility

- ► Relatively insoluble in blood; primary saturation of blood occurs in 3–5 minutes.
- ► The gas molecules at the alveoli–blood interface and blood–brain interface pass readily to the tissue with the lowest concentration of nitrous oxide.
- ► Results in rapid onset and recovery.
- ► Results in potential diffusion hypoxia at completion of sedation procedure if 100% oxygen is not administered.

IV. Pharmacology of Nitrous Oxide

- ► Is not metabolized in the body; remains unchanged in blood and tissues.
- ► Enters and exits almost entirely through the lungs.

EQUIPMENT FOR NITROUS OXIDE–OXYGEN

- ► Available as a portable unit or a central storage system with gas piped to individual treatment rooms.
- ► Units have several built-in safety features to ensure a minimal level of oxygen is delivered and the two gases cannot be reversed during delivery.
- ► The equipment can be divided into three basic parts:
  - Gas storage cylinders
  - A gas delivery system
  - A scavenger system with the nasal hood (mask) having components of both the gas delivery and scavenger portions.

I. Compressed Gas Cylinders

- ► *Nitrous oxide*
  - *Color code*: Light blue.
  - *Physical state*: Gas and liquid.

  - *Pressure*: Constant at 750 pounds per square inch (psi) until almost empty.
- ► *Oxygen*
  - *Color code*: Green (International = white).
  - *Physical state*: Gas.
  - *Pressure*: Falls at a uniform rate with use from a full pressure of 2,000 psi or 2,200 psi for size E or H cylinders, respectively.
  - *Use ratio*: About 2.5 cylinders of oxygen are used for each comparably sized cylinder of nitrous oxide.
- ► *Handle carefully*
  - Use no grease, oil, lubricant, or hand cream around the cylinder valves or any fittings that come in contact with the gases.
  - Store vertically on a rack or in another stable and secure manner.
  - Open cylinder valves slowly in a counterclockwise direction.

II. Gas Delivery System

- ► *Regulator or reducing valve*
  - Converts high pressure of gas in the cylinders to a usable, lower level.
  - Subject to extreme high temperature if compressed gas cylinders are opened quickly.
- ► *Flow meter*
  - Visual indicator of liters per minute (L/min) flow of oxygen and nitrous oxide.
  - Gas flow rates of nitrous oxide and oxygen are adjusted independently and the sum of the two is the total gas flow rate.
  - A total combined gas flow rate is established and respective concentrations of the two gases are adjusted concurrently.
- ► *Reservoir bag*
  - Reservoir of gases to accommodate an exceptionally deep breath.
  - Allows for visualization of respirations for monitoring.
  - Degree of inflation can be used to help establish total flow rate of gas needed by the patient for comfortable respirations.
  - May be used to provide oxygen in assisted ventilation if attached to a full-face mask with relief valve.
- ► *Conducting or breathing tubes*

III. Nasal Hood, Nose Piece, Mask

- ► Deliver gas for patient inhalation.
- ► Collect exhaled gas and direct it into scavenger system.
- ► Good fit and seal around patient's nose are essential in size selection.
- ► Ideally, use a disposable item or sterilize before each use.

IV. Scavenger System

▶ Removes exhaled gas to keep nitrous oxide levels low in the ambient air of the treatment room.

▶ Connects to the office central evacuation system.

▶ Vents to outside of building and away from windows and air intakes.

V. Safety Features[6]

▶ *Universal color coding* of cylinders, hoses, flow controls for each gas.

▶ *Pin index* and *diameter index* safety systems physically prevent gas cylinders or hoses from being mistakenly interchanged between the gases due to incompatible placement of pins (projections) and diameter differences in the couplings.

▶ *Minimum oxygen flow,* 30% or 3 L/min.

▶ *Oxygen fail-safe system* automatically shuts off nitrous oxide if the oxygen falls below a minimum level.

▶ *Emergency air inlet* to provide room air if system shuts down.

▶ *Oxygen flush button* to supply 100% oxygen quickly.

VI. Equipment Maintenance

▶ *Function checks*
  • Maintain working order and safe practice by periodic checking of equipment.

▶ *Gas leaks*
  • All equipment connections and rubber goods are subject to leaking. Figure 38-1 shows the places that need to be examined for tight connections, defects, and wear. Apply soapy water to connections; bubbles will form if leaks are present.

PATIENT SELECTION

I. Indications

▶ Patient with mild-to-moderate anxiety.

▶ Medically compromised patient who would benefit from additional oxygen and/or anxiety reduction.
  • Examples: patient with cardiovascular or cerebrovascular disease, or stress-induced bronchial asthma.

▶ Procedures of short duration with low level of pain. The analgesic effect is most pronounced on soft tissues,

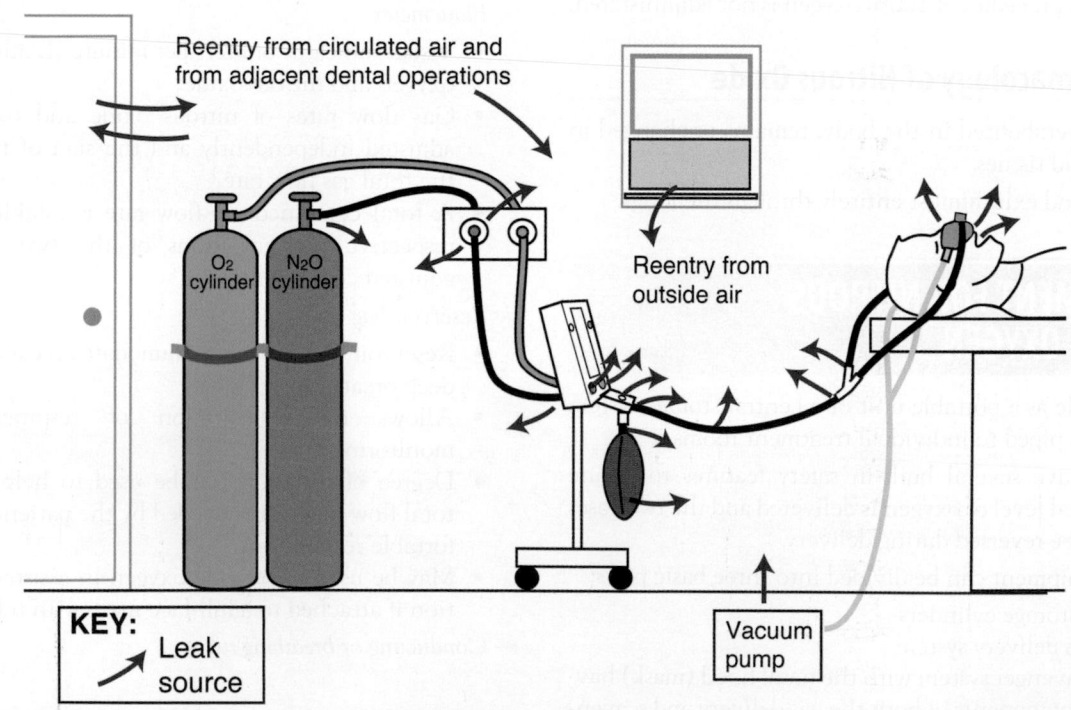

FIGURE 38-1 Potential Sources of Leaks from Nitrous Oxide/Oxygen Delivery Systems. Arrows show locations where regular inspection and testing is necessary. The most common sites of leakage are: *High-pressure connections:* from the gas delivery cylinders, the wall connectors, the hoses connecting to the anesthetic machine, and the anesthesia machine itself (especially the on-demand valve). *Low-pressure connections:* from the anesthetic flow meter and the scavenging mask. Look for loose-fitting connections, loosely assembled or deformed slip joints and threaded connections, defective or worn seals, and gaskets. *Rubber goods:* hoses and reservoir bag. Look for cracks and tears. (Adapted from National Institute for Occupational Strend Health (US). *Alert: Controlling Exposures to Nitrous Oxide During Anesthetic Administration* [Joint Publication of Public Health Service, Centers for Disease Control, National Institute for Occupational Safety and Health]. Cincinnati, OH: U.S. Department of Health, Education, and Welfare; 1994:5. Publication No. 94-100.)

making it especially useful during dental hygiene procedures.

▶ Patient with strong gag reflex.

II. Contraindications

There are no absolute contraindications to the administration of nitrous oxide–oxygen sedation. Individuals with the following conditions needs to be carefully evaluated before nitrous oxide–oxygen sedation:

▶ Patients with a compulsive personality: low success rate, need to be in charge, will fight the effects of the drug.

▶ Claustrophobic patients: cannot tolerate the nasal hood; nasal cannula alternative, but not recommended due to risk to dental professionals.

▶ Children with behavior problems: degree of cooperation required; won't be breathing through nose if crying, screaming, and moving.

▶ Mental illness, autism, Alzheimer's disease: need patient compliance.

▶ Patients with severe personality disorders undergoing psychiatric treatment require medical consultation to ensure there are no contraindications.
  • May want to avoid altering consciousness as the clinician may not be able to assess stage of sedation.

▶ Upper respiratory tract infection or other acute respiratory conditions (cold, sinus problems, mouth breather, allergies, bronchitis, cough): if nose breathing would be difficult or breathing apparatus cannot be sterilized or replaced.

▶ Chronic respiratory conditions: chronic obstructive pulmonary disease, emphysema, cystic fibrosis, chronic bronchitis, tuberculosis.

▶ Recent ophthalmic surgery using intraocular gases: vision damage could result from increased pressure on the eye during healing.[8,9]

▶ Current or recovering drug addiction: may trigger an episode or promote addictive behavior.

▶ Pregnancy: first trimester nitrous oxide crosses the placenta; effects on fetus are inconclusive; not metabolized in the body; safest of all anxiety lowering techniques; consult with physician.[10]
  • Prudent practice would suggest no elective drugs be administered during pregnancy, especially during the first trimester.
  • Second and third trimester: dose and exposure need be kept to a minimum.

▶ Conditions of confined air spaces within the body that would be adversely affected by increased pressure: middle ear or tympanic membrane problems, middle ear or sinus blockage, bowel obstruction.

▶ Latex allergy: concern if equipment (nasal hood, tubing or reservoirs) are made with latex materials.

▶ Patient who does not want nitrous oxide–oxygen: for any of a variety of personal reasons.

CLINICAL PROCEDURES FOR NITROUS OXIDE–OXYGEN ADMINISTRATION[6,7]

Box 38-3 lists the sequence of steps for nitrous oxide–oxygen administration.

I. Patient Preparation

▶ *Inform before appointment*
  • No specific food limitations but generally avoid fasting or heavy meals just before the appointment.
  • Wear comfortable clothing and loosen tight collars.

▶ *Inform at time of appointment*
  • Explain procedure in positive terms.
  • Stress the pleasant sense of relaxation; the patient will be aware and in control at all times.
  • Obtain informed consent.

▶ *Assess and perform*
  • Evaluate patient's medical status; determine the American Society of Anesthesiologists' (ASA) classification (Table 24-1, in Chapter 24).
  • Take and record vital signs.
  • Place patient in a supine position.

II. Equipment Preparation

▶ *Nasal hood*
  • Select the appropriate size for optimum comfort and minimum gas leakage.
  • Attach to tubing.

▶ *Scavenger system*
  • Connect, usually to high-speed volume evacuation, and activate system.
  • Adjust setting of scavenger system.

BOX 38-3

Steps in Nitrous Oxide/Oxygen Administration

1. Assess patient's medical status.
2. Take and record pretreatment vital signs.
3. Educate patient and secure informed consent.
4. Prepare delivery equipment (open tanks, select nasal hood).
5. Activate scavenger system.
6. Turn on oxygen to a flow rate of 5–7 L/min.
7. Place nasal hood and adjust to fit.
8. Adjust gas flow rate.
9. Begin nitrous oxide at about 10%–20%.
10. Titrate to optimum level.
11. Monitor throughout treatment.
12. Return to 100% oxygen.
13. Take and record posttreatment vital signs.
14. Remove nasal hood when patient feels fully recovered.
15. Record progress notes.

▶ *Turn on gas cylinders*
  • Open slowly, first oxygen, then nitrous oxide.
  • Confirm that all equipment is operating correctly.

III. Technique for Gas Delivery[6,7]

A. Establish Volume of Gas Flow

▶ Based on patient's size and medical/psychological condition; determine the total liters flow per minute.
▶ Begin with 6 L 100% oxygen/minute for adults.
▶ Gas flow rate between 6 and 7 L/min for average adults, 4–5 L/min for most children.[6]
▶ Place nasal hood, adjust for comfort; patient may assist in positioning; establish good seal.
▶ Adjust flow using the inflation of the reservoir bag and feedback from the patient.

B. Titration

Individualized drug dose is determined by increasing the percentage of nitrous oxide in small increments until the optimum sedation level is achieved based on clinical signs and symptoms.

▶ *Initial concentration*: Start titration at about 10%–15% concentration of nitrous oxide.
  • Because of the rapid uptake of nitrous oxide in the lungs and distribution through the body, the effect of each dose can be assessed after 1–2 minutes.
▶ *Patient response*: Observe the patient for signs of relaxation or other changes.
  • Ask the patient what is felt. Use the patient's signs and symptoms to determine when the optimum level of sedation has been reached.
  • Table 38-1 lists signs and symptoms for various levels of nitrous oxide–oxygen sedation.
▶ *Adjust dose*: Increase or decrease the nitrous oxide by 5%–10% when the optimum individual dose has not been achieved. Wait 1–2 minutes and reassess. Repeat as needed.
  • Distribution of optimum sedation dose for different individuals follows a bell curve. Generally 20%–40% nitrous oxide results in adequate sedation for dental treatment.

  • At high altitudes, greater nitrous oxide concentrations will be needed because of the change in the partial pressure of the gases.
▶ *Time*: Allow approximately 5 minutes for titration.
▶ *Monitor*: Continue to monitor and adjust the concentration throughout the appointment.
  • As the appointment proceeds or during less anxiety-producing parts of the appointment, a lower dose may be more comfortable.
  • Avoid excessive fluctuations.
▶ *Attend patient*: Never leave a sedated patient unattended; sedation can become deeper without some stimulation or interaction.
▶ *Outcome*: Titration increases clinical success rate of nitrous oxide–oxygen conscious sedation and decreases adverse responses.
▶ *Advantages*: Only the amount of drug required by the patient is given.
  • Allows for individual biovariability.
  • Uncovers idiosyncratic reactions early.
  • Minimizes negative experiences with oversedation.

IV. Completion of Sedation

▶ *Recovery*
  • *Procedure*: At the completion of sedation, return the patient to 100% oxygen for a minimum of 5 minutes; longer if needed for full recovery.
  • *Factors affecting recovery time*: Biologic variation, duration of sedation procedure, and concentration of nitrous oxide administration. Generally, the more nitrous oxide administered, the longer the recovery time.
  • *Signs of recovery*: Patient's report of feeling "back to normal."
  • Comparable presedation and postsedation vital signs are recorded.
  • *Elimination*: Within 5–10 minutes, 99% removed completely from the body.
▶ *Diffusion hypoxia*
If patient is returned directly to room air rather than 100% oxygen, diffusion hypoxia can result.
  • Nitrous oxide diffuses into an area of lower concentration more rapidly than oxygen, causing

TABLE 38-1	Signs and Symptoms of Nitrous Oxide–Oxygen Sedation
LEVEL OF SEDATION	**SIGNS AND SYMPTOMS**
Minimal sedation (ideal)	Comfortable/relaxed; reduced fear and anxiety; tingling of extremities and/or near mouth; body warmth; glazed eyes; responds to directions; intact protective cough and gag reflex; light feeling; vasodilation of neck and face
Oversedation	Disassociation from surroundings; hallucinating; feeling of floating or flying Inability to follow directions and keep mouth open; dizziness; drowsiness
Oversedation (serious)	Delayed responses; slurred words; agitated and/or combative behavior; vomiting; loss of consciousness

inadequate oxygen in the alveoli if the patient is not given supplemental oxygen at the completion of sedation.

- Hypoxia can result in patient discomfort or syncope.
- Inadequate postsedation oxygen may result in a feeling of lethargy, headache, or nausea.
- Prevention: administer 100% oxygen for no less than 5 minutes.

▶ *Dismissal follows full recovery*

- Patients should be fully alert and show no signs of disorientation.
- Usually the patient is able to return to all normal activities, including driving.
- Vital signs can be expected to return to base line readings.
- Important to note that recovery time varies for each patient.

▶ *Record keeping*

As with every dental procedure, complete documentation is essential and good practice. The following items need to be included in the patient's record when administering nitrous oxide–oxygen analgesia (see Box 38-4):

- Medical and psychological history review including determination of the ASA classification.
- Reason for nitrous oxide use.
- Presedation and postsedation vital signs.
- Concentrations of both nitrous oxide and oxygen administered.
- Total gas flow rate (L/min).
- Length of time for sedation procedure.
- Length of time on recovery oxygen.

- Statement of patient's recovery status and any postcare instructions given.
- Any adverse reactions. Summary of patient's response to nitrous oxide can be helpful for subsequent appointments.
- Signature and date.

POTENTIAL HAZARDS OF OCCUPATIONAL EXPOSURE[11–17]

Chronic occupational exposure to nitrous oxide may have deleterious effects on healthcare providers. Overexposure must be prevented.

I. Issues of Occupational Exposure

▶ *Potential health problems*

- Reduced fertility with unscavenged nitrous oxide exposure.
- Spontaneous abortion.
- Increased rate of neurologic, renal, and liver disease.
- Decreased mental performance, audiovisual ability, and manual dexterity.

▶ *Recommended exposure levels*

- Consensus has not been reached on occupational exposure limits; there is currently no exposure standard.
- National Institute of Occupational Safety and Health recommends no more than 25 parts per million (ppm) during administration.

II. Methods for Minimizing Occupational Exposure

▶ Use an effective scavenging system that can move 45 L/min of air.

▶ Maintain equipment and inspect regularly for gas leaks, especially at the locations shown in Figure 38-1. Shut off and secure equipment at the end of each day's use.

▶ Improve general air quality:

- Introduce fresh air
- Use a nonrecycling air-conditioning system, or open a window.
- Vent the scavenger system gases outside the building and away from windows and air intakes.

▶ Use an air sweep fan to direct nitrous oxide away from the clinician's breathing zone; periodically monitor air quality in the clinicians' breathing zone.

▶ Minimize patient conversations and mouth breathing; fit the nasal hood carefully to avoid leaks.

▶ Set conservative limits on the duration and concentration of nitrous oxide use per patient.

BOX 38-4
Example Documentation: Nitrous Oxide/ Oxygen Conscious Sedation

S - Patient presents with gag reflex and anxiety about dental treatment.

O - Medical history non-significant. ASA I.

A - No contraindication for use of nitrous oxide/oxygen.

P - Total gas flow rate: 5 L/min; 35% (2 L/m) nitrous oxide and 65% (4 L/min) oxygen for 40 min. Patient reports tingling in extremities and relaxed feeling. 100% oxygen administered for 5 min. following treatment; patient said he felt fully recovered.

VITAL SIGNS	PRETREATMENT	POSTTREATMENT
Blood pressure	124/84	120/82
Pulse	75	70
Respirations	12	12

Signed: _____, RDH Date: _____.

ADVANTAGES AND DISADVANTAGES OF NITROUS OXIDE/OXYGEN SEDATION ANESTHESIA

I. Advantages

▶ Both a mild analgesic and sedative: reduces patient's reaction to pain by raising pain threshold.

▶ Increases relaxation and cooperation during treatment.

▶ Reduces the gag reflex.

▶ Very safe with few side effects and few medical contra-indications. Excellent for management of many medically compromised patients:
  - Respiratory disease: asthma–nitrous is nonirritating and will not precipitate an attack.
  - Cerebrovascular disease: elevated level of oxygen given, which is beneficial.
  - Hepatic disease: nitrous not metabolized in body like other drugs.
  - Epilepsy: does not increase risk of seizure development.
  - Diabetes: no contraindication.

▶ Allergy: no reported allergy to nitrous oxide.

▶ Provides oxygen enrichment as well as stress reduction.

▶ Helps prevent emergencies because of anxiety and pain management.

▶ Readily absorbed and excreted from the body; rapid onset and recovery from drug effect.

▶ Able to titrate to optimum level.

▶ Recovery complete so patient can be dismissed to return to normal activities.

▶ Appointments less stressful for clinician because of relaxed, conscious, cooperative patient.

II. Disadvantages

▶ A low-potency analgesic drug.
  - Not effective with all patients because of low potency; does not block all perception.
  - Severely distressed or phobic patient may need a more potent drug or combination of drugs.

▶ Patient must be able and willing to breathe through the nose.

▶ Equipment and gases are expensive.

▶ Use of poor techniques such as failure to titrate or use a scavenger system results in undesirable patient experiences and potential staff health risks.

▶ Potential for recreational abuse by health professionals.

▶ May stimulate sexual fantasies in some patients, and any resulting accusations can result in embarrassment, loss of reputation, and/or license.

LOCAL ANESTHESIA

▶ Local anesthesia is the main modality for the management of dental pain.

▶ It blocks sensations, especially of pain, from teeth, soft tissues, and bone in the anesthetized area.

▶ Root instrumentation without discomfort requires a profound pulpal and periodontal tissue anesthesia to increase patient comfort and compliance during the appointment.

PHARMACOLOGY OF LOCAL ANESTHETICS

▶ Local anesthetics are the most frequently used drugs for dental and dental hygiene treatment.

▶ When administered correctly, local anesthesia is a safe and effective method for pain control.

I. Contents of a Local Anesthetic Cartridge

A dental cartridge is prefilled by the manufacturer. Cartridges contain either 1.7 or 1.8 mL of solution. Anesthetic cartridges include the following:

▶ *Amide anesthetic*: Blocks the transfer of ions across the nerve membrane, which stops the transmission of pain messages.

▶ *Vasoconstrictor*: Constricts local blood vessels to offset the vasodilation caused by the amide anesthetic. Provides greater duration, more profound anesthesia and hemostasis to the immediate area.

▶ *Antioxidant*: Preservative added to prevent the oxidation of the vasoconstrictor, usually sodium metabisulfite or sodium bisulfite.

▶ *Sterile water*: Diluting agent.

▶ *Sodium chloride*: Creates a biocompatible solution with the body.

II. Ester and Amide Anesthetic Drugs[18]

Dental local anesthetic drugs can be divided chemically into two major groups: esters and amides. The first dental anesthetic was procaine (Novocain), an ester, which has not been available in dental cartridges in the United States since 1996.

A. General Characteristics of Ester Anesthetics

▶ Widely used in topical anesthetic agents.

▶ Causes vasodilation of local blood vessels.

▶ High incidence of allergic reactions from byproduct, para-aminobenzoic acid (PABA).

▶ Hydrolyzed in plasma by the enzyme pseudo-cholinesterase.

- Elimination via the kidneys.
- Atypical plasma cholinesterase may result in slow removal of the drug from the blood resulting in toxicity (see General Medical Considerations section).

B. General Characteristics of Amide Anesthetics

- Cause vasodilation of local blood vessels.
- Extremely low incidence of allergic reactions.
- Metabolized by the liver (all amides with the exception of articaine are primarily biotransformed in the liver) see General Medical Considerations section.
- Elimination via the kidneys.
- Potential for toxicity or drug overdose make attention to detail in technique of administration and total drug dose critical.

C. Duration of Amide Drugs

- There are three categories of duration for dental local anesthetics:
  - Short acting (~30 minutes of pulpal anesthesia).
  - Intermediate acting (~60 minutes of pulpal anesthesia).
  - Long acting (~90 minutes of pulpal anesthesia).
- Factors influencing the duration include:
  - Individual response to the drug.
  - Type of injection administered (supraperiosteal/infiltration versus nerve block).
  - Accuracy of the injection.
  - Anatomical barriers (ligaments, tendons, fascial planes, density of bone).
  - Vascularity at site of injection.
  - Presence of inflammation and/or infection.
  - Injecting a plain local anesthetic versus a local anesthetic with a vasoconstrictor.

III. Specific Characteristics of Amide Drugs[18,19–23]

A. Lidocaine Hydrochloride (HCL)

- *Properties*
  - Proprietary name: Xylocaine.
  - Duration: intermediate acting.
  - Considered the "gold standard" of all the local anesthetics.
  - Metabolized in the liver and excreted by the kidneys
- *Dosage*
  - Concentration: 2%
  - Vasoconstrictor: Epinephrine 1:50,000 (for hemostasis) or 1:100,000
  - mg/cartridge: 36 mg (1.8 mL), 34 mg (1.7 mL).
- *Safety and precautions*
  - MRD (Maximum Recommended Dose) = 500 mg; 3.2 mg/lb; 7.0 mg/kg.

- Food and Drug Administration (FDA) pregnancy category: B (Box 38-5).
- Calculate the MRD; confirm a negative aspiration prior to depositing, deposit a full cartridge no less than 1 minute.
- *Absolute contraindication*: allergy to the local anesthetic or sodium bisulfite; cocaine or methamphetamine use in the previous 24 hours.
- *Relative contraindication*: cardiovascular disease, angina, CVA, hypertension, hyperthyroidism, significant liver or kidney disease, patients taking beta blockers, cimetidine on a regular basis, steroid-dependent asthmatics, avoid 1:50,000 for ASA 3 cardiac, CVA, hyperthyroidism, and patients sensitive to epinephrine.
- *Recommended for*: pediatric patients, pregnant women, most procedures and treatment requiring intermediate duration; best choice for bleeding control (1:50,000).

BOX 38-5
FDA Pregnancy Categories

Category A

Adequate and well-controlled studies have failed to demonstrate a risk to the fetus in the first trimester of pregnancy (and there is no evidence of risk in later trimesters).

Category B

Animal reproduction studies have failed to demonstrate a risk to the fetus and there are no adequate and well-controlled studies in pregnant women.

Category C

Animal reproduction studies have shown an adverse effect on the fetus and there are no adequate and well-controlled studies in humans, but potential benefits may warrant use of the drug in pregnant women despite potential risks.

Category D

There is positive evidence of human fetal risk based on adverse reaction data from investigational or marketing experience or studies in humans, but potential benefits may warrant use of the drug in pregnant women despite potential risks.

Category X

Studies in animals or humans have demonstrated fetal abnormalities and/or there is positive evidence of human fetal risk based on adverse reaction data from investigational or marketing experience, and the risks involved in use of the drug in pregnant women clearly outweigh potential benefits.

Source: Food and Drug Administration. Content and format of labeling for human prescription drug and biological products; requirements for pregnancy and lactation labeling. *Fed Regist*. 2008;73(104):30831–30868. http://www.gpo.gov/fdsys/pkg/FR-2008-05-29/pdf/E8-11806.pdf.

B. Mepivacaine HCL

▶ *Properties*

- Proprietary name: Carbocaine.
- Duration: short acting (3% plain solution); intermediate acting (2% 1:20,000 levonordefrin).
- Weak vasodilator.
- Metabolized in the liver and excreted by the kidneys.

▶ *Dosage*

- Concentration: 2% (with vasoconstrictor), 3% (plain)
- Vasoconstrictor: levonordefrin 1:20,000
- mg/cartridge: 2% = 36 mg (1.8 mL); 34 mg (1.7 mL)
- mg/cartridge: 3% = 54 mg (1.8 mL), 51 mg (1.7 mL).

▶ *Safety and/or precautions*

- MRD = 400 mg; 3.0 mg/lb; 6.6 mg/kg.
- FDA pregnancy category: C.
- Calculate the MRD; confirm a negative aspiration prior to depositing, deposit a full cartridge in no less than 1 minute.
- *Absolute contraindication*: allergy to the local anesthetic or sodium bisulfite; cocaine or methamphetamine use in the previous 24 hours (2% 1:20,000).
- *Relative contraindication*: patients taking tricyclic antidepressants (TCAs)—interacts with levonordefrin, significant liver or kidney disease.
- *Recommended* for: short duration (3% plain solution), when a vasoconstrictor is contraindicated (3% plain solution), pediatric patients, patients who are epinephrine sensitive.

C. Prilocaine HCL

▶ *Properties*

- Proprietary name: Citanest.
- Duration: short acting administered as an infiltration; intermediate acting when administered as a nerve block.
- Weak vasodilator.
- Metabolized: liver, small percentage by lungs as alternate site and excreted by the kidneys.

▶ *Dosage*

- Concentration: 4%
- Vasoconstrictor: epinephrine 1:200,000
- mg/cartridge: 72 mg (1.8 mL); 68 mg (1.7 mL).

▶ *Safety and precautions*

- MRD = 600 mg; 3.6 mg/lb; 8.0 mg/kg.
- FDA pregnancy category: B.
- Calculate the MRD, confirm a negative aspiration prior to depositing, deposit a full cartridge in no less than 1 minute; may cause increased risk of paresthesia with an inferior alveolar nerve block.[24–26]
- Metabolic by-products may cause acquired methemoglobinemia, a condition that reduces the blood's oxygen-carrying capacity (see Specific Medical Considerations).

- *Absolute contraindication*: allergy to the local anesthetic or sodium bisulfite; cocaine or methamphetamine use in the previous 24 hours.
- *Relative contraindication*: significant liver or kidney disease, methemoglobinemia, sickle cell anemia, anemia, respiratory or cardiac failure, patients on acetaminophen long term.
- *Recommended* for: patients when a vasoconstrictor is contraindicated (4% plain solution); plain solution provides intermediate duration when administered as a nerve block.

D. Articaine HCL

▶ *Properties*

- Duration: intermediate acting.
- Shortest half-life of all the amide anesthetics; reported to diffuse through soft and hard tissues better than other amides.[18]

▶ *Dosage*

- Concentration: 4%
- Vasoconstrictor: epinephrine 1:100,000 and 1:200,000
- mg/cartridge: 72 mg (1.8 mL); 68 mg (1.7 mL)
- MRD = determined by weight; 3.2 mg/lb; 7.0 mg/kg
- Metabolized: blood plasma (approx. 90%–95%) and the liver (approx. 5%–10%)
- Excreted: kidneys
- FDA pregnancy category: C
- Calculate the MRD, confirm a negative aspiration prior to depositing, deposit a full cartridge in no less than 1 minute; may cause increased risk of paresthesia with an inferior alveolar nerve block block.[24–26]
- *Absolute contraindication*: allergy to the local anesthetic or sodium bisulfite; cocaine or methamphetamine use in the previous 24 hours.
- *Relative contraindication*: significant liver or kidney disease.
- *Recommended* for: patients with moderate systemic disease (liver, cardiac); lowest risk of systemic toxicity; shortest half-life allows for safer reinjections.

E. Bupivacaine HCL

▶ *Properties*

- Proprietary name: Marcaine.
- Duration: long acting; longest onset of all the local anesthetics.
- Most potent of the local anesthetics.
- Metabolized by the liver and excreted by the kidneys.

▶ *Dosage*

- Concentration: 0.5%
- Vasoconstrictor: Epinephrine 1:200,000
- mg/cartridge: 9 mg (1.8 mL), 8.5 mg (1.7 mL)

▶ *Safety and precautions*

- MRD = 90 mg per appointment; mg/kg; use smallest effective dose.

- FDA pregnancy category: C.
- Safety and/or precautions: calculate the MRD, confirm a negative aspiration prior to depositing; deposit a full cartridge in no less than 1 minute; highly toxic, stay below the MRD, use caution with reinjection.
- *Absolute contraindication*: allergy to the local anesthetic or sodium bisulfite; cocaine or methamphetamine use in the previous 24 hours.
- *Relative contraindication*: children or adults that are prone to self-mutilation postinjection.
- *Recommended* for: posttreatment pain control; procedures requiring greater than 60 minutes of pulpal anesthesia.

IV. Vasoconstrictors[18,27]

A. Reasons for Use

▶ *Safety*: Potential for toxic reaction (overdose) to the local anesthetic is reduced by slowing the rate at which it enters circulation.

▶ *Longevity*: Duration of anesthetic effect is increased.

▶ *Effectiveness*: Depth and profoundness of anesthetic is increased.

▶ *Hemostasis*: Only if drug is locally injected directly into the area; epinephrine 1:50,000 is most effective.

B. Potential Risks with Use of Vasoconstrictors

▶ Hypersensitivity to the drugs.

▶ Medical problems (see Specific Medical Considerations).

▶ Drug interactions (see Potential Drug Interactions).

▶ Degree of risk to medically compromised patients, including those with heart disease varies. The use of vasoconstrictors in low doses is considered safe.

C. Preservatives

▶ *Sodium bisulfite*
- Preservative added to local anesthetic cartridges that contain a vasoconstrictor.
- Prevents the oxidation of the vasoconstrictor.
- Provides a shelf life of approximately 18 months.
- Most likely offending agent in a dental cartridge when an allergic reaction occurs.
- Avoid administering any local anesthetic with a vasoconstrictor for patients that have a confirmed bisulfite allergy.
- Best alternative choice: 4% prilocaine plain as a nerve block or 3% mepivacaine.

D. Drugs

▶ *Epinephrine (Adrenalin)*
- Potent sympathomimetic amine.
- Rare occurrences to have an allergy since it is produced endogenously.
- Concentrations: 1:50,000, 1:100,000, or 1:200,000.
- MRDs for healthy patients and for medically compromised, especially those with cardiac disease are listed in Table 38-2.
- Absolute contraindication: bisulfite allergy, myocardial infarction (MI; within 6 months), coronary bypass surgery (within 6 months), uncontrolled angina, arrhythmias, hypertension, hyperthyroidism or diabetes, pheochromocytoma (catecholamine producing tumors), cocaine, or methamphetamine use within 24 hours.
- Relative contraindication: cardiac conditions (ASA 3), taking nonselective β-blockers or antidepressants, controlled hypertension, hyperthyroidism, or diabetes.

TABLE 38-2	Vasoconstrictors: Concentrations and Maximum Recommended Dose (MRD)			
VASOCONSTRICTORS AND CONCENTRATIONS	**MRD IN HEALTHY PATIENTS**		**MRD IN MEDICALLY COMPROMISED PATIENTS**	
	MG/APPT	**CARTRIDGES/APPT**	**MG/APPT**	**CARTRIDGES/APPT**
Epinephrine (based on 1.8 mL)				
1:50,000 (0.036 mg/cart.)	0.2	5.5	0.04	1.1
1:100,000 (0.018 mg/cart.)	0.2	11	0.04	2.2
1:200,000 (0.009 mg/cart.)	0.2	22[a]	0.04	4.4
Levonordefrin (based on 1.8 mL)				
1:20,000 (0.09 mg/cart.)	1.0	11.1	0.2	2.2

[a]Local anesthetic is the limiting drug.

▶ *Levonordefrin (Neo-Cobefrin)*
- About 15% as potent as equal doses of epinephrine and with less cardiac and central nervous system stimulation. Used at higher concentration (1:20,000) to accomplish adequate vasoconstriction.
- Not a good choice if hemostasis is required.
- Absolute contraindications: bisulfite allergy, uncontrolled angina, arrhythmias, blood pressure, hyperthyroidism or diabetes; cocaine or methamphetamine within 24 hours.
- Relative contraindication: patients taking tricyclic antidepressants (TCAs).
- MRDs for healthy patients and for medically compromised, especially those with cardiac disease, are given in Table 38-2.

V. Criteria for Local Anesthetic Selection

▶ Length of time needed for pain control is a primary criterion for drug selection. Table 38-3 lists the typical duration of action for common local anesthetics.
▶ Need for hemostasis.
▶ Medical status of the patient.
▶ Potential for prolonged discomfort after treatment.
▶ Potential for self-inflicted injury before anesthetic wears off.

INDICATIONS FOR LOCAL ANESTHESIA

▶ Local anesthesia is indicated for treatment that has the potential to cause discomfort or pain.
▶ Anesthesia prevents both the patient and clinician from the anticipation of discomfort, thus allowing both to relax and make treatment comfortable.

I. Dental Hygiene Procedures

▶ Scaling and root planing in areas with probing depths of 4 mm or greater and subgingival biofilm debridement in all other areas.
▶ Extensive instrumentation with either manual or power-driven instruments.
▶ Treatment in areas of challenging pocket topography, furcations, or other difficult root anatomy.
▶ Instrumentation of sensitive root surfaces.
▶ Instrumentation in areas of painful, inflamed soft tissue.
▶ Treatments that involve soft tissue manipulation.
- Gingival curettage.
- Suture removal.
- Removal of subgingival overhanging restoration.
▶ Treatment in areas of excessive hemorrhage.

TABLE 38-3	Duration of Local Anesthetics (Currently available in the U.S.)		
LOCAL ANESTHETIC DRUGS	**SOFT TISSUE (MINUTES)**	**PULPAL (MINUTES)**	**DURATION CATEGORY**
4% Articaine 1:100,000 Epinephrine	180–360	60–75	Intermediate
4% Articaine 1:200,000 Epinephrine	120–300	45–60	Intermediate
0.5% Bupivacaine 1:200,000 Epinephrine	240–540	90–180	Long
2% Lidocaine 1:50,000 Epinephrine	180–300	60	Intermediate
2% Lidocaine 1:100,000 Epinephrine	180–300	60	Intermediate
3% Mepivacaine plain	120–180	20 (infiltration) 40 (nerve block)	Short Intermediate
2% Mepivacaine 1:20,000 levonordefrin	180–300	60	Intermediate
4% Prilocaine plain	90–120 (infiltration) 120–240 (nerve block)	10–15 (infiltration) 40–60 (nerve block)	Short Intermediate
4% Prilocaine 1:200,000 Epinephrine	180–480	60–90	Intermediate

II. Patient Factors

▶ Extent of patient's oral status and periodontal condition directly influence the extent or rigor of the needed treatment.

▶ Patient's pain reaction or pain threshold.

PATIENT ASSESSMENT

The goal of patient assessment is to ensure an effective and safe local anesthesia experience. Pretreatment evaluation is the first and most important step for avoiding a medical emergency.

I. Sources of Information for Complete Preanesthetic Assessment

▶ Chief complaint.

▶ Vital signs.

▶ Medical history; ASA status (Table 24-1, in Chapter 24).

▶ Current medications.

▶ Emotional status/anxiety level.

▶ Dental history related to local anesthesia.

▶ Presence of infection or inflammation.

II. Treatment Considerations Based on Assessment Findings

Amide local anesthetics and the vasoconstrictor normally incorporated into the dental anesthetic cartridge can be administered safely to almost all patients. Options for treatment include:

▶ Use local anesthetic without special precautions.

▶ Avoid use of local anesthetic or of a specific local anesthetic because of high medical risk.

▶ Select an alternative drug that will minimize or avoid risk.

▶ Limit the dose of drug given at any specific appointment.

▶ Use local anesthesia combined with stress reduction techniques; use in combination with nitrous oxide–oxygen conscious sedation.

▶ Seek medical intervention, consult, or additional testing before proceeding.

▶ Administer block or regional injections rather than infiltration in inflamed tissue which has a low pH that inhibits drug distribution and effectiveness.

III. General Medical Considerations

▶ Regular utilization of safeguards such as medical history questionnaire, dialogue history, physical examination, vital screenings (blood pressure, heart rate, and respiration) can help prevent most medical emergencies in the dental office or clinic.

▶ The ASA Classification System is a tool to help assess medical risk of a patient receiving anesthesia and undergoing surgical procedures. (Table 24-1 in Chapter 24).

• ASA 4 patients and some ASA 3 patients (especially those who are anxious about injections) may not have the functional reserve to tolerate the injection procedure and the subsequent treatment.

• Elective treatment for patients who are too medically compromised for local anesthesia (ASA 4 and some ASA 3) are not performed except in the case of emergency procedures until medical status improves; may not be appropriate for any elective dental therapy.

▶ When performing a risk–benefit analysis for use of local anesthesia, consider the potential for medical distress that can result from inadequate pain control.

▶ Seek a medical consult when there is doubt about the safety of a local anesthetic choice.

▶ Calculate the MRD for all patients especially children or adults weighing less than 150 pounds. Every drug has a MRD in mg/lb and mg/kg that is used for the calculation (see Table 38-2).

• Determine and administer the smallest effective dose for each patient.

• Always use the smallest effective dose.

▶ *Contraindications to local anesthesia administration*

The administration of a local anesthetic drug or vasoconstrictor is generally safe requiring no modifications.

▶ The clinician may need to either limit or completely avoid use of a local anesthetic drug or vasoconstrictor depending on specific medical or psychological considerations of the patient or medications. The two categories to be considered are:

▶ Absolute: under no circumstance should the drug choice be administered to the patient because of the possibility that toxic or lethal reactions will occur.

▶ Relative: the drug in question may be administered after careful determination of the risk factors; only administer the smallest effective dose.

IV. Specific Medical Considerations[18,28]

A. Allergy[29]

▶ *Amide anesthetics*: True allergy is rare. If confirmed, avoid offending drug, choose a different amide, a slight chance of cross-allergenicity may occur; refer to allergist for testing.

▶ *Ester anesthetics*: Allergy is fairly common. If confirmed, avoid all ester anesthetics including topical anesthetics.

▶ *Bisulfites*: Sodium bisulfite and sodium metabisulfite are used as the preservatives for the vasoconstrictor. If allergy is known, avoid anesthetics containing vasoconstrictors.

▶ Best choice: 3% mepivacaine or 4% prilocaine plain if sodium bisulfite is the allergen.

B. Hyperthyroidism

▶ *Uncontrolled*: Avoid vasoconstrictor.

▶ *Controlled*: Can choose local anesthetic with a vasoconstrictor, but stay below the MRD and use the weakest vasoconstrictor concentration.

▶ Best choice: 4% prilocaine plain, 3% mepivacaine plain, 2% mepivacaine 1:20,000 or vasoconstrictor with 1:200,000 (articaine, prilocaine, or bupivacaine).

C. Impaired Liver or Kidney Function

▶ Only severe impairment is clinically relevant (ASA 3 or 4).

▶ Half-life of amide anesthetic could be prolonged, which could result in overdose.

▶ Best choice: 4% articaine (1:100,000 or 1:200,000) since very little is biotransformed through the liver.

D. Malignant Hyperthermia (MH)

▶ Life-threatening complications associated with the administration of general anesthesia.

▶ Syndrome—transmitted genetically; defect in the distribution of myoplasmic calcium.

▶ MH most often occurs after first exposure to general anesthesia.

▶ Clinical signs: tachycardia, high fever, tachypnea, cardiac dysrhythmias, muscle rigidity, cyanosis, and death.

▶ Absolute contraindication for patients to receive general anesthesia (succinylcholine).

▶ Local anesthetics with or without vasoconstrictors can be used. No current evidence to support avoidance of local anesthetics or vasoconstrictors.

▶ Medical consult is recommended prior to treatment.

▶ Best choice: no restrictions, choose most appropriate for procedure.

E. Methemoglobinemia[30]

▶ A congenital or acquired condition; hemoglobin molecule is converted to methemoglobin, which has less oxygen-carrying capacity. A cyanosis-like state may develop if a high percentage of molecules convert.

▶ Prilocaine, articaine, and topical benzocaine can cause a dose-related methemoglobinemia. Avoid their use in patients with a pre-existing condition.

▶ Avoid prilocaine or benzocaine if on long-term acetaminophen use.

▶ Best choice: lidocaine, mepivacaine, or bupivacaine.

F. Heart Failure

▶ Reduced circulation resulting from heart failure slows elimination of amide anesthetic, which increases potential for anesthetic overdose.

▶ Patient is stress intolerant—pain and anxiety must be carefully managed. Consider use of nitrous oxide–oxygen sedation alone or in combination with local anesthesia.

▶ Obtain medical consult and clearance before treating.

▶ Best choice: 2% lidocaine 1:100,000.

G. Coronary Heart Disease, MI, Recent Heart Surgery, and Stroke

▶ Do not treat within the first 6 months; higher risk of a subsequent event or complication. Consult with the cardiologist.

▶ Concern is for the use and amount of vasoconstrictor. Epinephrine cardiac dose = 0.04 mg per appointment; levonordefrin cardiac dose = 0.2 mg per appointment; do not use 1:50,000 epinephrine concentration for these patients.

▶ Decision based on patient ASA category, procedure to be performed, duration needed for pain control, medical consultation recommended.

▶ Best choice: plain anesthetic*; 1:200,000 epinephrine concentrations (if hemostasis is not a consideration); 2% meprivacaine 1:20,000.

H. Angina

▶ Uncontrolled—avoid all dental procedures; controlled—limit amount of vasoconstrictors.

▶ Best choice: plain local anesthetic*; 2% mepivacaine 1:20,000 or 1:200,000 anesthetics.

I. Hypertension

▶ Uncontrolled—avoid all dental procedures; controlled—limit amount of vasoconstrictors.

▶ Best choice: plain anesthetics*; 1:200,000 epinephrine concentrations (if hemostasis is not a consideration); 2% meprivacaine 1:20,000.

J. Hemophilia

▶ Excessive bleeding may result from needle contact with a blood vessel.

▶ Decision based on severity of condition can range from treatment in hospital to avoiding injections into highly vascularized areas [example: the posterior superior alveolar (PSA)].

▶ Best choice: local anesthetic that has a vasoconstrictor; avoid plain anesthetics.

K. Pregnancy and Lactation

▶ Local anesthetics and vasoconstrictors are not teratogens and may be safely administered.

▶ Select a drug in the FDA pregnancy risk category B (lidocaine or prilocaine). The FDA classifies drugs according to their safety for the fetus. Refer to Box 38-5 for FDA pregnancy categories.

- ▶ All local anesthetics are expressed in breast milk; use smallest effective dose.
- ▶ It is prudent practice to limit any elective drug administration, especially during the first trimester.
- ▶ There are no clinical trials showing the safety of local anesthetics and breast feeding.
- ▶ Best choice (pregnancy): 2% lidocaine 1:100,000; 4% Citanest plain or 1:200,000 (FDA drug category B).
- ▶ Best choice (lactation): articaine 1:200,000 due to its half-life compared to the other anesthetics.

L. Diabetes

- ▶ Epinephrine opposes action of insulin (not significant when administering small amount of vasoconstrictor and staying below MRD); do not treat if uncontrolled.
- ▶ Best choice: plain local anesthetic*; 1:200,000 concentrations; 2% mepivacaine 1:20,000.

M. Glaucoma

- ▶ Avoid or limit amount of vasoconstrictor, can increase ocular pressure.
- ▶ Best choice: plain local anesthetic*; 1:200,000 concentrations; 2% mepivacaine 1:20,000.

N. Atypical Plasma Cholinesterase

- ▶ Inability to metabolize ester drugs.
- ▶ Avoid all ester anesthetics including topicals (benzocaine) and articaine.
- ▶ Best choice: any amide anesthetic with the exception of articaine.

*plain local anesthetics (if can achieve adequate depth and duration of pain control).

O. Potential Drug Interactions[18,19,22,27]

All medications reported in a patient's medical history need to be reviewed for potential drug interactions before selecting the local or topical anesthetic.

- ▶ Following are examples of frequently prescribed or OTC drugs that interact with an anesthetic or a vasoconstrictor. Precaution is needed.
  - Histamine (H_2) receptor blockers (e.g. Zantac, Tagamet) and amide anesthetic: reduce liver ability to metabolize amide drugs; limit amount of lidocaine especially if have congested heart failure (ASA 3) and taking a histamine blocker.
  - Nonselective beta blockers (e.g. Inderal, Corgard) and vasoconstrictors: increased risk of serious hypertension, cardiac dysrhythmias, and a potential cardiac event; use plain anesthetic unless hemostasis is needed.
  - Tricyclic antidepressants (TCAs) (e.g. Elavil, Norpramin) and vasoconstrictors: increased risk of hypertension and cardiac dysrhythmias; limit epinephrine and avoid levonordefrin.

- Phenothiazines (e.g. Thorazine) and vasoconstrictors: possible severe hypotension; be aware of potential postural hypotension; use cardiac dose and avoid 1:50,000.
- Cocaine, methamphetamine, and vasoconstrictors: increased risk of hypertensive crisis, MI or stroke; avoid all vasoconstrictors for 24 hours of using offending drug.

ARMAMENTARIUM FOR LOCAL ANESTHESIA

I. Syringe

- ▶ *Nondisposable types*
  - Breech-loading, metallic, aspirating (most frequently used).
  - Breech-loading, metallic, aspirating, petite (smaller thumb ring diameter makes handling easier for clinicians with small hands).
  - Breech-loading, metallic, self-aspirating (easier aspiration for smaller hand clinicians).
  - Breech-loading, plastic, aspirating.
  - Pressure syringe for periodontal ligament (PDL) injection.
  - Jet injector (needleless syringe); used for topical anesthesia of the palate.
- ▶ *Safety syringes* (single use, self sheathing to prevent needle stick injury) (Figure 38-2).
  - Computer-controlled local anesthesia delivery system.
- ▶ *Design features of syringes*
  - Durable metal or plastic can be sterilized and reused with the addition of a new needle and cartridge.
  - Single-use, disposable safety syringes have features to prevent inadvertent needle stick after use.
  - Provide good visibility of the cartridge to determine whether a positive aspiration has occurred.
- ▶ *Promote easy aspiration*
  - Manual aspiration is the traditional design.
  - Self-aspirating syringe works well for small hands.

II. Needle

- ▶ *Disposable*
Intended only for single patient use.
- ▶ *Parts and lengths of the needle* (Figure 38-3)
Needle lengths are not standardized and therefore can vary depending on the manufacturer.
  - *Long needle*: approximately 30–35 mm (1½ inches).
  - *Short needle*: approximately 20–25 mm (1 inch).
  - *Extra-short needle*: approximately 10–12 mm (1/2 inch); used for palatal injections.
- ▶ *Gauge or needle diameter*
  - *Size*: Ranked from largest to smallest, 25-, 27-, and 30-gauge needles are used in dentistry.

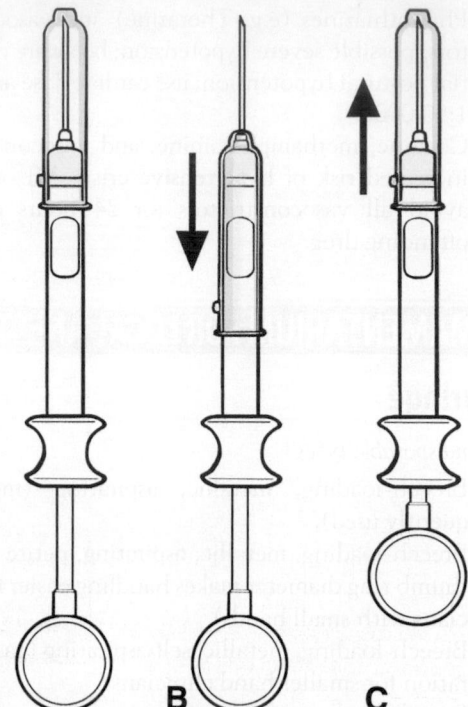

FIGURE 38-2 **Prevention of Percutaneous Injury: Self-sheathing Safety Needle. A:** Syringe with protective sheath over the needle. **B:** As the injection is made, the sheath slides back. **C:** After injection, the sheath returns to cover the needle and protect the clinician during disposal.

- *Rigidity:* 25-gauge needles are stiffer and have less needle deflection as it passes through tissue. Increased accuracy with deep tissue penetration (inferior alveolar (IA) and Gow–Gates (GG) nerve blocks).
- *Aspiration:* Larger-gauge needles provide easier and more accurate aspiration.

III. Cartridge or Carpule

▶ Volume: 1.7 or 1.8 mL of solution.

▶ Storage
  - Store at cool room temperature and away from the light.
  - Do not store in an alcohol or disinfectant solution.

▶ Label on each cartridge: drugs, manufacturer, and expiration date.

▶ Color coding: local anesthetic drug is identified by color on cartridge. Color codes are standardized and shown in Box 38-6.

IV. Additional Armamentarium

▶ Topical antiseptic (e.g., povidone–iodine) to prevent postinjection infections.

▶ Topical anesthetic to increase patient comfort.

▶ Cotton gauze to wipe the injection site to clean, dry, and remove the topical anesthetic. May also be used to improve grasp for lip or cheek retraction.

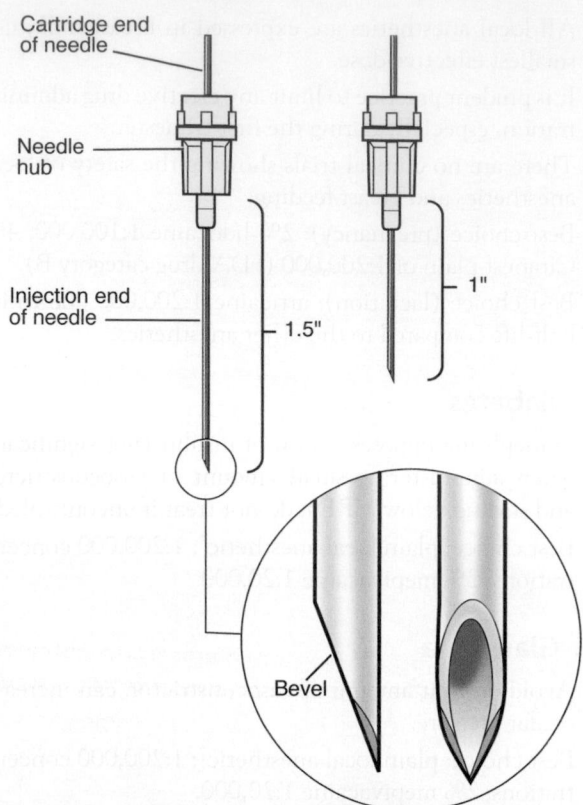

FIGURE 38-3 **The Dental Anesthetic Needle.** Dental needles are available in three lengths, *long, short,* and *extra-short*. Lengths vary slightly between manufacturers. The components of the needle are *cartridge end,* which penetrates the rubber diaphragm of the dental cartridge; *hub,* which attaches the needle to the syringe (made of plastic or metal); *injection end* or shank or shaft, which penetrates the oral tissue so that anesthetic solution is deposited at the desired site. Inset: Shows an enlargement of the tip of the needle with sharp terminus and bevel. When giving an injection, the needle is oriented so that the bevel is parallel to the bone to help prevent the needle from catching the periosteum, the sensitive covering over the bone. Needles should be changed after 3–4 uses to prevent unnecessary discomfort to the patient from a dull or barbed needle.

BOX 38-6

Anesthesia Color Code

Color Codes for Local Anesthetics Currently Available in the United States

A uniform system for easy recognition and safety

Lidocaine 2% with epinephrine 1:100,000	
Lidocaine 2% with epinephrine 1:50,000	
Mepivacaine 2% with levonordefrin 1:20,000	
Mepivacaine 3% plain	
Prilocaine 4% with epinephrine (1:200,000	
Prilocaine 4% plain	
Articaine 4% with epinephrine 1:100,000	
Articaine 4% with epinephrine 1:200,000	
Bupivacaine 0.5% with epinephrine 1:200,000	

▶ Needle recapping device, if self-recapping needle is not used.

▶ Hemostat for broken needle removal from soft tissues if it occurs.

▶ Sharps disposal system to meet safe practice standards for used needle disposal.

V. Sequence of Syringe Assembly

▶ Figure 38-4A illustrates the assembly of the conventional, metallic, breech-loading anesthetic syringe; sequence makes the attachment between the harpoon and rubber stopper easier without applying excess force to the glass cartridge.

▶ Figure 38-4B demonstrates attachment of the dental needle to the needle adapter end of the syringe.

VI. Computer-Controlled Anesthesia Delivery System

▶ Pressure, volume, and rate of deposit of local anesthetic delivery are precisely regulated by a computer.

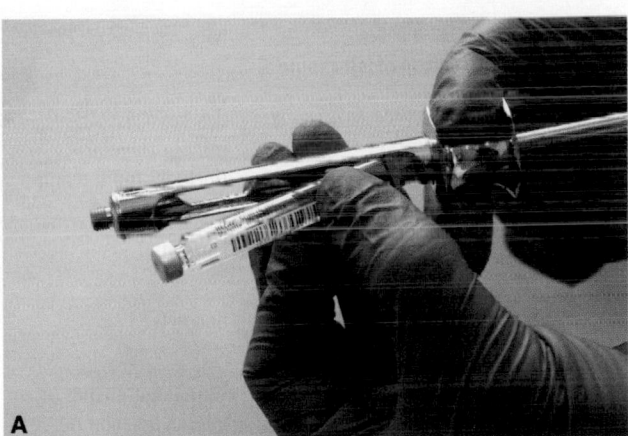

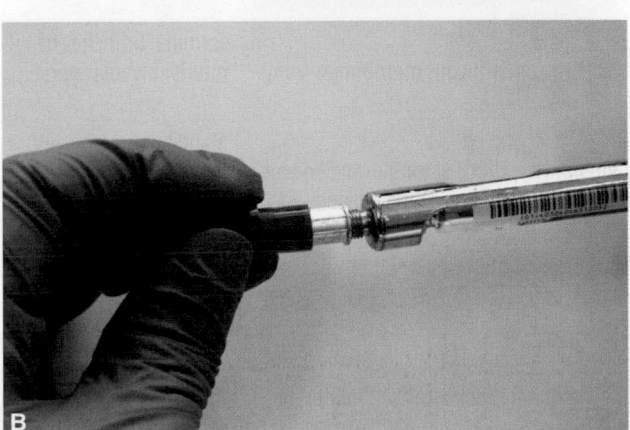

FIGURES 38-4 **Sequence for Assembling a Breech-Loading Aspirating Syringe. A.** 1. Pull back on thumb ring. 2. Insert anesthetic cartridge, rubber stopper end first, toward the thumb ring, then the diaphragm end toward the needle opening. 3. Set harpoon and test for lock into rubber stopper. 4. Remove safety cap from needle. 5. **B.** Screw needle onto the syringe.

▶ Device includes a light, penlike handpiece attached to a computer-controlled motor that is activated by a foot or finger control. Any gauge Luerlock needle and standard anesthetic cartridge may be used.

▶ Slow, controlled delivery of anesthesia solution promotes more comfortable injections, especially palatal and PDL injections; allows unique injections, the anterior middle superior alveolar (AMSA) and the palatal anterior superior alveolar (P-ASA), as well as all traditional dental injections.

▶ Good option for needle phobic and pediatric patients.

CLINICAL PROCEDURES FOR LOCAL ANESTHETIC ADMINISTRATION

Administer the most comfortable injections possible by using gentle tissue manipulation, careful needle penetration, slow deposition of solution, and good patient communication. An example progress note for a patient receiving local anesthesia is found in Box 38-7.

I. Injection(s) Selection

▶ *Basic injections*

Table 38-4 lists injections with hard and soft tissues anesthetized, and the branches of the trigeminal nerve involved.

▶ *Areas anesthetized*

• Figure 38-5 shows the areas to be anesthetized.

▶ *Steps and procedures*

• Box 38-8 outlines the sequence and procedures for the administration of local anesthesia.

BOX 38-7

Example Documentation: Local Anesthesia

S –Patient reported general root sensitivity and gum bleeding when brushing.

O –Reviewed medical history, no contraindications to treatment, ASA I; IOE—negative; BP = 115/75, HR 65.

A –Moderate generalized chronic periodontitis. Plaque score: 50%.

P –NSPT on mandibular left quadrant; 20% benzocaine topical applied; 1:00 pm administered 1 cartridge of 2% Xylocaine 1:100,000 epinephrine; 36 mg lidocaine and 0.018 mg epinephrine given for a left inferior alveolar and buccal nerve blocks. Patient tolerated procedure well, no adverse reactions. Post-BP = 120/76; HR=66; Written post-treatment instructions given to the patient.

Signed: _____, RDH

Date: _____

TABLE 38-4	Common Local Anesthetic Injections for Dental Hygiene Procedures	
INJECTION	**TISSUES ANESTHETIZED**	**BRANCH OF THE TRIGEMINAL NERVE**
Maxillary Arch		Maxillary Division
Supraperiosteal	*Teeth:* individual teeth *Periodontium and soft tissues:* periodontium of teeth anesthetized including facial or buccal tissue overlying individual teeth	Individual terminal branches
PSA	*Teeth:* second and third molars; first molar including mesiobuccal root (72% completely anesthetized) *Periodontium and soft tissues:* periodontium of teeth anesthetized including overlying buccal tissues	PSA
MSA	*Teeth:* first and second premolars, mesiobuccal root of first molar (28%) *Periodontium and soft tissues:* periodontium of teeth anesthetized including overlying buccal tissues	MSA
ASA	*Teeth:* canine and incisors *Periodontium and soft tissues:* periodontium of teeth anesthetized and overlying facial tissues and lip	ASA
Infraorbital (IO)	*Teeth:* incisors, canine, premolars, and MB root of 1st molar if MSA nerve is present (28%) *Periodontium and soft tissues:* periodontium of teeth including overlying facial tissues including the lower eye lid, side of nose cheek, and upper lip	IO (includes both anterior and middle superior alveolar)
Greater palatine (GP)	*Teeth:* none *Periodontium and soft tissues:* lingual gingiva and palatal tissue from distal of third molar to mesial of first premolar medial to midline of palate	GP
Nasopalatine (NP)	*Teeth:* none *Periodontium and soft tissues:* palatal tissues from distal of right canine to distal of left canine	NP
Mandibular Arch		Mandibular Division
IA	*Teeth:* entire quadrant of teeth *Periodontium and soft tissues:* buccal periosteum and soft tissues from premolars to midline	Inferior alveolar (includes mental and incisive nerves)
Lingual (L)	*Teeth:* none *Periodontium and soft tissues:* lingual gingiva, floor of the mouth, anterior two-thirds of tongue	Lingual
Long buccal (LB)	*Teeth:* none *Periodontium and soft tissues:* buccal periosteum and soft tissues of molars	Buccal (LB)
Mental (M)	*Teeth:* none *Periodontium and soft tissues:* buccal gingival tissue and mucous membranes from mental foramen to midline, lower lip, skin of chin	Terminal branches of inferior alveolar nerve
Incisive (I)	*Teeth:* premolars to central incisor in same quadrant *Periodontium and soft tissues:* buccal periosteum, gingival tissue and mucous membranes from premolars to midline, lower lip, skin of chin	Terminal branches of inferior alveolar nerve
GG technique	*Teeth:* entire mandibular quadrant of teeth *Periodontium and soft tissues:* buccal and lingual tissues; anterior two-thirds of tongue and floor of mouth; lower lip; skin over the zygoma; posterior portion of the cheek and temporal regions	Mandibular nerve—V_3 nerve block (includes inferior alveolar, mental, incisive, lingual, mylohyoid, auriculotemporal, and buccal nerves)
Either Arch		
Intraseptal	*Teeth:* unreliable; primarily soft tissue anesthesia; good technique for hemostasis of moderate inflamed tissue (e.g., curettage) *Periodontium and soft tissues:* periosteum and gingiva of anesthetized area	Terminal nerve endings
PDL	*Teeth:* individual tooth *Periodontium and soft tissues:* periosteum, gingiva and mucous membrane associated with anesthetized tooth	Terminal nerve endings

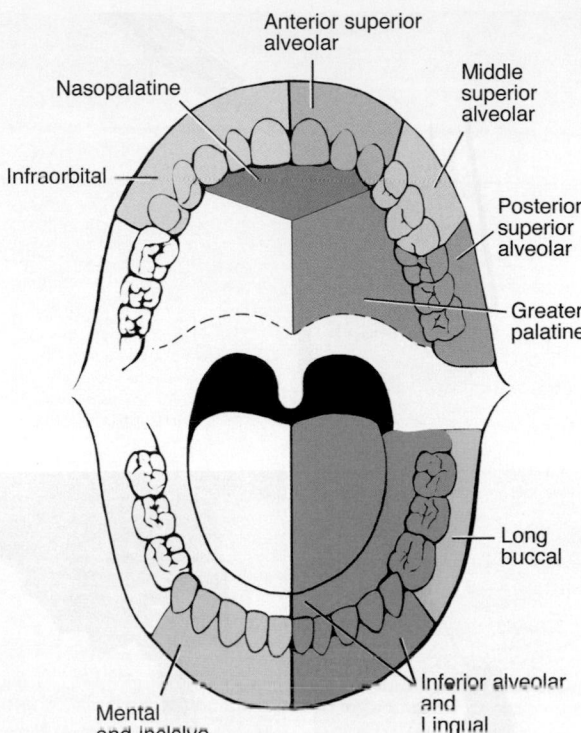

Anterior superior alveolar

Nasopalatine

Middle superior alveolar

Infraorbital

Posterior superior alveolar

Greater palatine

Long buccal

Inferior alveolar and lingual

Mental and incisive

FIGURE 38-5 **Diagrammatic Representation of Teeth and Soft Tissues Anesthetized by Common Dental Injections.**

II. Aspiration

► *Purpose*
- To confirm the tip of the needle is not within a blood vessel prior to depositing the local anesthetic.
- An anesthetic solution must be deposited extravascularly to be effective and to prevent toxicity.

► *When to aspirate*
- Before depositing anesthetic solution.
- Periodically throughout injection to confirm that the needle has not moved and is now in a blood vessel; to slow the rate of deposit.

► *Procedure*
- Hold the needle steady so that the tip does not change position.
- Create negative pressure within the dental cartridge.
  - *Standard harpoon-style syringe*: Pull back gently on the thumb ring. Movement is small, if any (approx. 1–2 mm).
  - *Self-aspirating syringe*: Stop applying positive pressure to the thumb ring.
- Rotate the syringe by a quarter turn and repeat aspiration (prevents a false negative).

► *Interpretation*
- Any fluid at the tip of the needle will be drawn into the cartridge. If the tip of the needle is in an artery

---

BOX 38-8

Steps in the Administration of Local Anesthesia

1. Assess patient medical status, treatment, and pain control needs in order to select injection(s) and anesthetic drug.
2. Assemble and test the syringe setup (**Figure 38-4 A & B**).
   a. Orient the needle so the bevel will be toward the bone during the injection.
   b. Test the assembled syringe.
3. Position patient for good visibility and to prevent syncope with head level with or lower than heart.
4. Use topical anesthetic.
   a. Apply topical to dry tissue at the injection site for the appropriate time. For benzocaine, 1–2 minutes is optimal.
   b. Remove residual topical anesthetic.
5. Wipe injection site with gauze to dry and clean surface bacteria, saliva, and topical anesthetic from the area before injection.
6. Retract the lip or cheek for good visibility; gently stretch the tissue for easier needle penetration.
7. Keep the syringe out of the patient's sight.
8. Pick-up the syringe so that the large window is facing the clinician.
9. Establish a fulcrum or hand rest for stability during the injection.
10. Insert the needle into the tissue and gently advance to desired site for administration of anesthetic.
11. Aspirate before depositing solution; reaspirate as needed throughout procedure.
12. Deposit the anesthetic solution slowly (1–2 minutes for full cartridge) to prevent patient discomfort and to reduce potential for a toxic reaction.
13. Withdraw the needle carefully at the completion of the injection, and recap the needle using a safe technique.
14. Remain with and observe the patient. Adverse drug reactions (ADRs) are most likely to occur during or shortly after the injection.
15. Record injection information in patient chart.
16. Use positive, supportive communication with the patient throughout the procedure.

or vein, blood will become visible; it may only be a small amount at the needle end of the cartridge.

- *Negative aspiration*: No blood in cartridge; proceed with injection.
- *Positive aspiration*: Blood in the cartridge.
  - A small amount of blood with most of the cartridge clear: move to a new location and re-aspirate.
  - Cartridge generally bloody: withdraw needle, replace cartridge, and repeat injection.

III. Sharps Management[31,32]

▶ *Needle recapping*
- Needles are recapped immediately following an injection utilizing a needle cap holder that allows a one-handed recapping technique. Examples of devices are shown in Figure 38-6.
- *Correct and incorrect methods:*
  - One-handed "scoop" technique (Figures 38-7 A-D).
  - Unsafe recapping of a contaminated needle (Figures 38-8A and B).
▶ *No manipulation*
- Do not manipulate needles; do not bend or break.

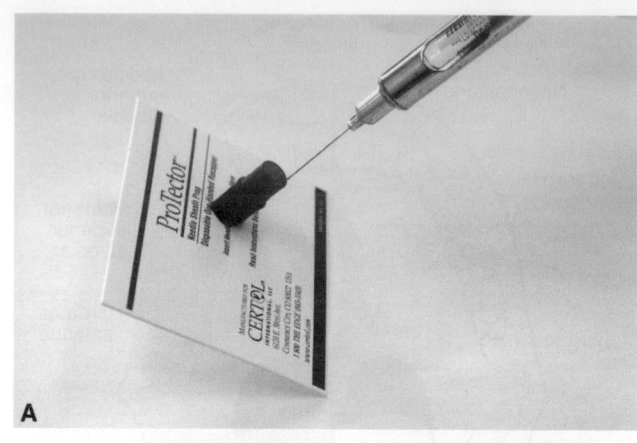

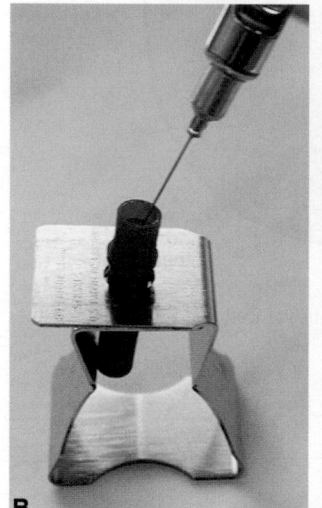
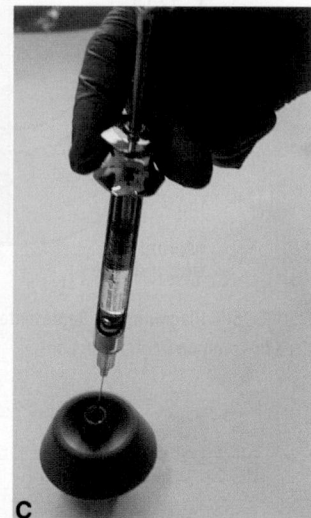

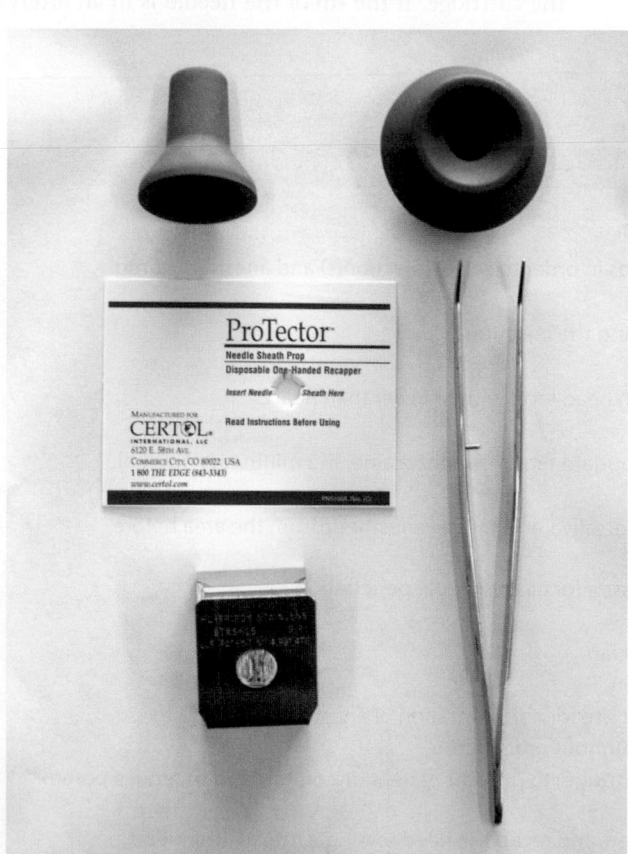

FIGURE 38-6 **Commercially Available Holders for Needle Caps.** One-handed capping or recapping with a safety mechanical device to hold the needle sheath is acceptable.

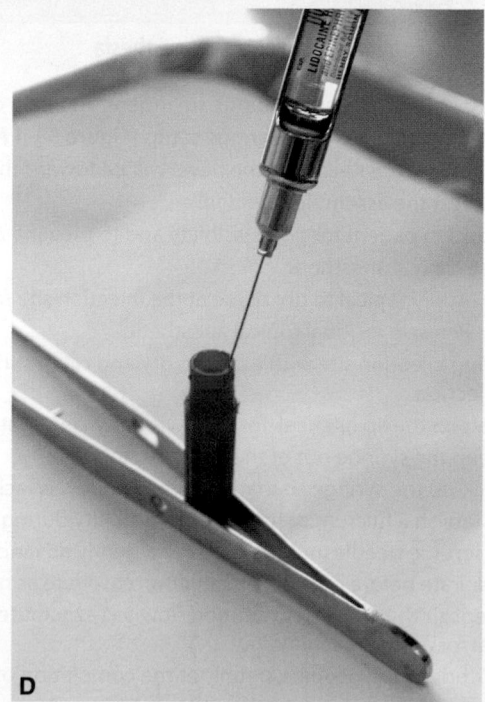

FIGURE 38-7 A-D **Safe Needle Recapping Techniques.** Correct utilization of the various needle cap holders will allow for a safe one-handed needle recapping method.

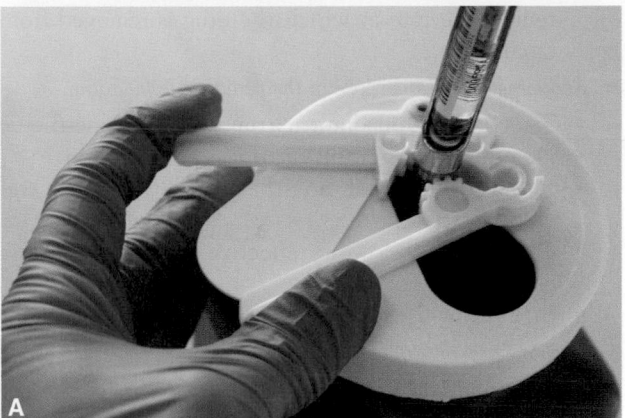

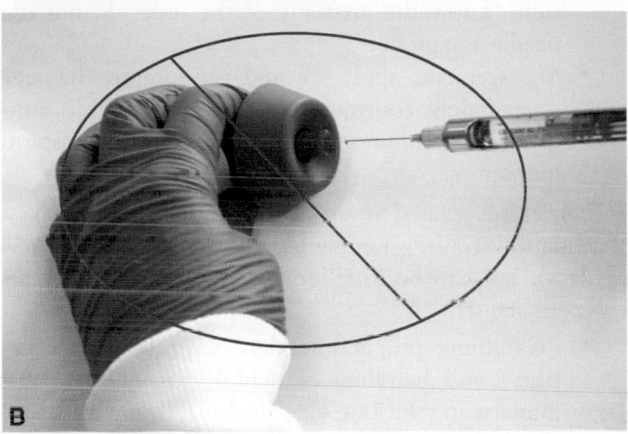

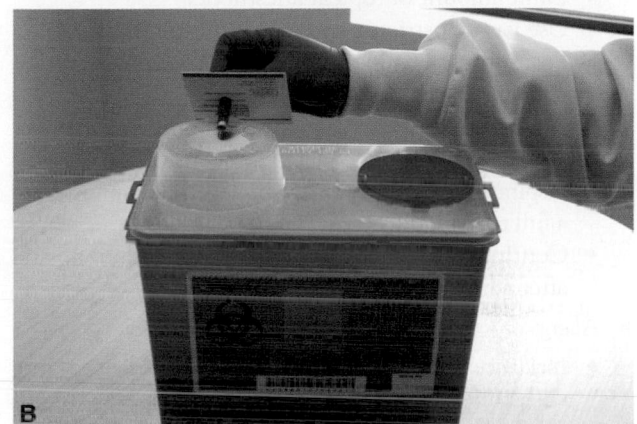

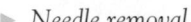

FIGURE 38-8 A & B. **UNSAFE Needle Recapping Techniques.** Increases risk of needle exposure to the clinician.

▶ *Needle removal*
- Disposal containers for contaminated sharps are placed so they are readily accessible and located as close as possible to the area of use (Figures 38-9A-C).
- Discard full sharps containers according to local, state, and federal regulations.

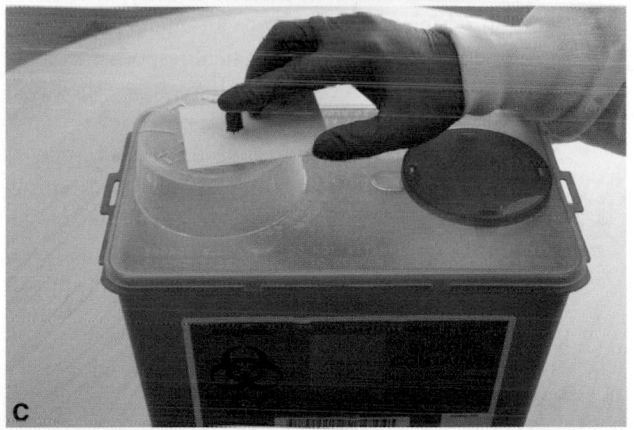

FIGURE 38-9 A-C **Needle Disposal Technique.** Dental needles must be disposed of in the appropriate sharps containers using a one-handed technique.

POTENTIAL ADVERSE REACTIONS TO LOCAL ANESTHESIA

I. Adverse Drug Reactions (ADR) [18,19,22,27]

▶ *Overdose (Toxicity)*
- Overdose is the most common ADR.
- Occurs when the circulating blood level of the drug becomes too high and reaches a toxic level for the individual.
- Reaction continues as long as the local anesthetic plasma level remains above threshold for overdose.

▶ *Typical causes of overdose*
- *Intravascular injection*: prevented by aspiration before deposition of the anesthetic drug.

- *Excessive total drug dose*: affected by drug volumes; drug choice; patient's lean weight, age, physical/medical status.
- *Rapid absorption into the circulatory system*: affected by rate of injection, presence or absence of a vasoconstrictor, or vascularity of injection site.
- *Reduced elimination and/or metabolism of drug*: reduced kidney or liver function or reduced circulation as a result of congestive heart failure may

reduce the rate at which the drug is removed from circulation.

▶ *Reducing risk of overdose in the pediatric population*
  • Treat only one quadrant at a time with local anesthesia.
  • Do not administer full cartridges per injection.
  • Avoid using local anesthetic solutions with no vasoconstrictor.
  • Choose the lowest effective local anesthetic concentration.
  • Stay below the MRD specific for that patient.

▶ *Primary prevention*
  • Thorough review of medical history including any anxiety, fear, or phobias.
  • Limit amount of topical anesthetic.
  • Use vasoconstrictor when not contraindicated.
  • Position patient in a supine or semi-supine position to prevent syncope.
  • Administer lowest concentration and amount necessary to achieve adequate pain control.
  • Aspirate and inject slowly (no less than 1 minute for a full cartridge).
  • Continue to observe patient before, during, and after administration.

▶ *Allergy*[29]
  • *Incidence*: Although often reported, incidence is rare with amide drugs. (Review allergy in Specific Medical Considerations section above.)
  • *Definition*: An allergic reaction is a hypersensitive state in which an exposure to an allergen results in a subsequent exaggerated physical response. In local anesthesia, the most common allergens are the bisulfite antioxidant or ester topical anesthetic.
  • *Symptoms*: Response may range from mild, such as localized erythema or itching, to life threatening, such as generalized anaphylaxis or laryngeal edema.
  • *Onset*: May range from a few seconds to hours.
  • *Management*: Table 8-3 (Chapter 8) presents procedures for managing an allergic reaction.

II. Psychogenic Reactions

▶ *Cause*
  Anxiety response to the injection procedure.

▶ *Symptoms*
  • Vasodepressor syncope (fainting) and hyperventilation are most common.
  • Symptoms can be highly varied and may mimic drug reactions or other medical conditions.
  • Reactions reported by patients as allergies are often psychogenic in nature.

III. Local Complications[18,23–26]

Local and topical anesthetics can cause a variety of local complications ranging from mild to severe; transient to permanent. The clinician is responsible to recognize, prevent, and manage any complications that may arise.

▶ *Trismus*: caused from trauma to muscles resulting in spasm of the jaw muscles that restricts opening or is painful; most often results from IA nerve block.
  • Prevention: use aseptic technique; do not contaminate the needle; avoid repeated insertions into muscle.
  • Management: apply warm, moist cloth to outside of face; warm saline rinses; analgesics for pain; light physiotherapy to exercise jaw.

▶ *Hematoma* (bruise): blood from a nicked artery or vein leaks into the surrounding tissue.
  • Prevention: minimize number of needle penetrations; know the anatomy of the area; do not use needle as a probe.
  • Management: apply ice and pressure to the area immediately, continue over next 6 hours (20 minutes on/20 minutes off) for first day; avoid aspirin for pain.

▶ *Paresthesia*: caused from physical trauma to nerve or chemical insult; generally last for short period (hours–days), but can be long-term lasting months to years (permanent).[24–26]
  • Prevention: proper infection control (needle sterility) and handling of dental cartridge (do not immerse in solutions, e.g., alcohol); thorough assessment whether to administer 4% solution for an inferior alveolar nerve block.
  • Research has shown an increased risk of paresthesia from injecting with a 4% anesthetic (articaine or prilocaine). Must determine the benefit to be gained from your choice of anesthetic outweighs the risk.
  • Management: reassure patient; determine extent of paresthesia and document; re-evaluate 1–2 months for any changes; refer to oral surgeon for consult if no improvement.

▶ *Facial paralysis*: from injecting anesthetic into parotid gland capsule.
  • Prevention: good inferior alveolar injection technique; must touch periosteum prior to depositing; use alternative techniques: PDL, GG nerve block.
  • Management: discontinue treatment; manually close patient's eye (have patient remove contact lenses if wearing them) on affected side, place a gauze patch over eye and tape closed; paralysis lasts as long as the duration of soft tissue anesthesia.

▶ *Broken needle*: caused from bending the needle, sudden movement by patient, using smaller gauge needles for deep insertions (e.g., 30 gauge); inserting needle to the hub.
  • Prevention: use larger gauge needles (25 or 27); do not insert the needle to the hub; do not bend the needle; do not force against resistance.
  • Management: instruct patient to keep mouth open, do not allow the patient to close; if visible, use a

hemostat or locking cotton pliers to remove needle from soft tissue; if unable to retrieve, refer to oral surgeon for consult.

▶ *Epithelial desquamation* (tissue sloughing): may follow prolonged application of topical anesthetic.
  • Prevention: apply topical anesthetic correctly (follow manufacturer's instructions); avoid high concentrations of vasoconstrictor (1:50,000 on palatal injections).
  • Management: topical analgesics for pain.

▶ *Infection*: caused by non-sterile technique; injecting into an area of infection.
  • Prevention: use sterile armamentarium; change needle if injecting into area of infection.
  • Management: evaluate as soon as possible; antibiotics may need to be prescribed.

▶ *Pain on injection*: caused by careless injection technique; fast rate of deposit; using a dull or barbed needle.
  • Prevention: follow proper injection technique; use topical anesthetic prior to injection; use a sharp needle; slow rate of deposit; anesthetic solutions need to be kept at room temperature.

▶ *Burning on injection*: low pH of anesthetic solution containing a vasoconstrictor; contaminated solutions.
  • Prevention: use a higher pH solution; inject small amount of a plain local anesthetic solution prior to injecting local anesthetic with a vasoconstrictor (patient will then not feel burning from the low pH of anesthetic with a vasoconstrictor).
  • Management: reassure patient; will subside by the time the injection is completed.

▶ *Self-inflicted soft tissue injury*: occurs mainly in children.
  • Prevention: use shorter duration local anesthetics; inform parent/caregiver of duration of soft tissue anesthesia; insert cotton roll to prevent biting of lip.
  • Management: analgesics for pain; lukewarm saline rinses; topical analgesics.

ADVANTAGES AND DISADVANTAGES OF LOCAL ANESTHESIA

I. Advantages

▶ Patient experiences no pain or discomfort during treatment procedure.
▶ Clinician has increased confidence to provide complete treatment when the patient is pain free.
▶ Local effect results in loss of sensation in area of treatment without a change in level of consciousness or patient cooperation.
▶ Completely reversible without residual side effects.
▶ Rapid onset of action.

▶ Adequate duration of clinical action that is reasonably predictable and that can be varied by choice of commercially available drugs.
▶ Relatively free of allergic reactions.
▶ Achieves hemostasis if injected directly into area where bleeding is a factor.

II. Disadvantages

▶ Anticipating and receiving dental injections may cause high anxiety for patient. Effects may include:
  • Need for special anxiety reduction technique.
  • Undesirable psychogenic reactions.
  • Avoidance of needed care.
▶ Significant potential exists for toxicity (overdose).
▶ There are systemic side effects from both the local anesthetic drug and vasoconstrictor.
▶ Potential for soft tissue injury post-injection especially for the pediatric population and mentally challenged adolescents and adults.

NONINJECTABLE ANESTHESIA

The anesthetic drugs are applied to the surface of the pocket lining tissue making this a topical application. It provides adjacent soft tissue anesthesia and in varying degrees of dental anesthesia.[32]

▶ Trade name: Oraqix®.
▶ Drugs: 2.5% lidocaine and 2.5% prilocaine; subgingival liquid-to-gel delivery thermo-setting system.
▶ Indications: adults who require localized anesthesia during scaling and/or root planing; initial or maintenance treatment of periodontal pockets where profound pulpal anesthesia is not needed; needle phobic adults.
▶ Steps for application:
  1. Wipe tissue with gauze.
  2. Dispense a thin layer of the anesthetic gel at the gingival margin; wait 30 seconds.
  3. Insert blunt-tipped applicator into the subgingival pocket, dispense product until pocket begins to overflow, then repeat in adjacent area.
▶ Onset: ~1 minute; duration: ~20 minutes with a range of 14–31 minutes.
▶ MRD: 5 cartridges/appointment.
▶ Pregnancy category: B (see Box 38-5).
▶ Contraindicated: allergy to amides; history of methemoglobinemia; children (not approved for use).
▶ Precautions: do not inject.

I. Armamentarium and Pharmacology

A unique dispenser with a blunt-tipped applicator delivers a gel containing both lidocaine and prilocaine into the periodontal pocket. Both the dispenser and the anesthetic gel are contraindicated for injections.

▶ *Dispenser cartridge and blunt-tipped applicator*
- Packaged together; for single-patient use.
- For use only with special dispenser and not for injection.
- Blunt-tipped applicator is individually bent by clinician with either a single or double bend.
- Cartridge contains 42.5mg lidocaine & 42.5mg prilocaine;1.7mL cartridge.
- Store at room temperature.

▶ *Anesthetic gel*
- Gel contents
  - *Anesthetics:* 2.5% lidocaine and 2.5% prilocaine amide anesthetics.
  - *Poloxamers:* thermosetting agents.
  - *pH adjuster:* hydrochloric acid.
  - *Purified water.*

▶ *Gel characteristics*
- Low-viscosity fluid at room temperature.
- Gel at oral temperature.

II. Technique

▶ *Administration*
- Wipe tissue with gauze.
- Dispense a thin layer of the anesthetic gel at the gingival margin; wait 30 seconds.
- Insert blunt-tipped applicator into the subgingival pocket, dispense product until pocket begins to overflow, then repeat in adjacent area.

TOPICAL ANESTHESIA

▶ A topical anesthetic is a drug applied directly to the surface of the mucous membrane to produce a loss of sensation.

▶ A topical anesthetic is used with varying degrees of success for short-duration desensitization of the gingiva, but it does not influence sensations in the teeth.

▶ Topical anesthetic is not a substitute for local anesthetic administered by injection.

I. Indications for Use

A topical anesthetic can be used conservatively for selected dental hygiene and dental services, including the following:

▶ Reduce discomfort of an injection.

▶ Prevention of gagging in radiographic techniques and impression taking.

▶ Temporary relief of pain from localized diseased areas, such as oral ulcers, wounds, or inflammation.

▶ Suture removal.

II. Action of a Topical Anesthetic

▶ *Purpose*
- The purpose of a topical anesthetic is to desensitize the mucous membrane by anesthetizing the terminal nerve endings.

- The superficial anesthesia produced is related to the amount of absorption of the drug by the tissue.

▶ *Factors that affect efficacy*
- Type of drug.
- Duration of application.
- Site of application: thickness of stratified squamous epithelial covering; degree of keratinization.
  - Highly resistant: skin, lips, palatal mucosa.
  - Slow absorption: attached gingiva, palatal gingiva.
  - Fast absorption: tissue without keratinization, such as vestibular mucosa or over the pterygomandibular space.

III. Agents Used in Surface Anesthetic Preparations

Table 38-5 provides onset and duration of topical anesthetics.

▶ *Benzocaine (ester)*
- Types and formulations: Used in 6%–20% (20% most common in dentistry) formulations; available as liquid, gel, ointment, spray, and gel patch; most widely used topical agent.
- Onset: 30 seconds—2 minutes; duration: 5–15 minutes.
- Not readily absorbed into circulation; potential for toxicity is minimal.
- May cause allergic reaction at site of application after prolonged or repeated use.
- Precautions: fast absorption on nonkeratinized tissue—concern for toxicity; can cause methemoglobinemia (dose related); children.
- Pregnancy category: C (see Box 38-5).

▶ *Tetracaine HCL (ester)*
- Types and formulations: Used in 0.25%–0.5% formulations; typically available as part of a combination of drugs in liquid, gel, and controlled-dose spray.
- Most potent; readily absorbed causing deeper penetration, longer effect, and more potential for toxicity. Not to be used over a large area.
- Onset: slow, within 20 minutes; duration: 20–60 minutes.
- Precautions: rapid absorption on mucous membranes, abraded tissues; children.
- Pregnancy category: C (see Box 38-5).

▶ *Lidocaine HCL (amide)*
- Types and formulations: Used in 2% or 5% formulations; available in ointment, metered spray, and in combination with prilocaine.
- The only amide used alone as a topical.
- Toxicity unlikely from topical alone but would be additive with other amide anesthetics. Greatest risk from sprays.
- Onset: 1–2 minutes, peak between 5 and 10 minutes; duration: 15 minutes.
- Precautions: abraded tissues; large areas; children.
- Pregnancy category: B (see Box 38-5).

TABLE 38-5	Topical and Noninjectable Anesthetic Characteristics				
TYPES	**DRUG**	**MRD**	**ONSET**	**DURATION**	
Noninjectable local anesthetic	Amide *2.5% Lidocaine and 2.5% prilocaine*	5 cartridges per appointment	~1 min	14–31 min 20 min average	
Topical anesthetics	Ester *Benzocaine (6%–20%)*	No established MRD; follow manufacturer's recommendations	30 sec–2 min	5–15 min	
	Ester *Tetracaine (0.25%–0.5%); combined with other drugs*	20 mg (1 mL of 2% solution)	Slow–up to 20 min	20–60 min	
	Amide *Lidocaine ointment (2% and 5%)*	2% and 5%—200 mg	1–2 min	15 min	
	Ketone *Dyclonine HCL (0.5%)*ᵃ	200 mg or 40 mL of 0.5% solution	Up to 10 min	30–60 min	

ᵃNot currently available.

▶ *Dyclonine HCL (ketone)*
- Types and formulations: 0.5% or 1% formulation from a compounding pharmacy; available as a liquid, lozenges and spray.
- As a gargle is good for gag reflex suppression.
- Onset: slow, up to 10 minutes; duration: 30 minutes (average), but up to 1 hour.
- Precautions: abraded tissues; reduce dosage in children and medically compromised adults.
- Pregnancy category: C (see Box 38-5).

IV. Topical Drug Mixtures

▶ *Eutectic Mixture of Local Anesthetics (EMLA; amide)*[32]
- EMLA is a combination of two or more drugs; provides more rapid onset on intact skin.
- Types and formulations: 2.5% lidocaine and 2.5% prilocaine; cream; lidocaine and prilocaine periodontal gel (Oraqix®).
- Pregnancy category: B (see Box 38-5).

▶ *Benzocaine, butamben and tetracaine (ester)*
- Types and formulations: 14% benzocaine, 2% butamben, 2% tetracaine; by prescription only as a liquid, spray, and gel.
- Onset: rapid, less than 1 minute; duration: 30–60 minutes.
- Pregnancy category: C (see Box 38-5).
- Precautions: fast absorption into tissues—higher risk for toxicity; not to be injected.

V. Adverse Reactions of Topical Anesthetics

▶ Ester topical anesthetics have a higher incidence of allergic reactions from primary metabolite, para-aminobenzoic acid (PABA).
▶ Redness.
▶ Tissue sloughing.
▶ Edema.
▶ Pain and burning at site.
▶ Greater risk of toxicity compared to local anesthetics (higher drug concentrations).

APPLICATION OF TOPICAL ANESTHETIC

I. Patient Preparation

▶ Consult medical and dental history for pertinent information concerning patient's previous experiences with anesthetics. A patient with an allergy to a local anesthetic may also be allergic to a topical anesthetic.
▶ Determine the most appropriate anesthetic agent and method of application.
▶ Explain purpose and anticipated effect to the patient.

II. Application Techniques

Several application techniques are available. Not all methods are applicable to all products. Select the most appropriate method from the following:

▶ *Surface application*
  - May be used with liquid, gel, or ointment formulations of any of the available topical agents.
  - Topical is applied with a cotton-tipped swab or cotton roll.
  - Time before becoming effective varies with the drug used.
  - After application, excess topical is removed by rinsing or gentle wiping.

▶ *Aerosol spray*
  - Prevent inhalation by avoiding spray preparations when another method would be as effective. A spray must never be directed toward the throat.
  - Use metered- or controlled-dose spray dispensers to prevent inadvertent overdose.

III. Completion of Topical Anesthetic Application

▶ Wait appropriate length of time for anesthetic to take effect before proceeding.

▶ Limit drug exposure.
  - Apply only to the area of need.
  - Use the smallest effective amount.
  - Remove residual drug after application time.

▶ Apply to a limited area when using a drug with a short duration of action for a long procedure such as scaling.

▶ Record topical anesthetic drug information in the patient's record.

I. Anesthesia Reversal Agent[33]

A. Properties

▶ Drug: phentolamine mesylate (OraVerse®); nonselective alpha adrenergic blocking agent.

▶ Formulation: 0.4 mg/1.7 mL.

▶ Indications: reversal of soft tissue anesthesia (~50% reduction time). Recent research has shown that it will impact to a lesser degree reversal of pulpal anesthesia.[33]

▶ Metabolized by the liver and excreted by the kidneys.

▶ Onset: rapid; duration: 30–45 minutes.

▶ Dosage and MRD: 1:1 ratio (cartridge containing a vasoconstrictor).

▶ *Contraindicated*: children under 6 years of age and/or 33 pounds; postsurgical patients; post-PDL or intraosseous injections.

▶ Pregnancy category: C (see Box 38-5).

B. Advantages

▶ Patients can return to normal function faster.

▶ Decrease risk of soft tissue injury from prolonged anesthesia.

C. Technique

▶ Administered by injection in same location and with same technique as the local anesthesia being reversed approximately 20–30 minutes prior to the end of the procedure.

▶ Dosage
  - Adult: 1:1 ratio; 1 cartridge of phentolamine mesylate per cartridge of anesthetic containing a vasoconstrictor, not to exceed 2 cartridges.
  - Children: (1/2 cartridge MRD).

EVERYDAY ETHICS

Mr. Denver, in for a dental hygiene appointment, stated that he has not been to a dental office for the past 5 years because he is fearful of oral treatment owing to past painful experiences. Oral examination revealed bleeding on probing, generalized 5- to 6-mm pockets, and heavy biofilm and calculus deposits. Proposed treatment is four appointments for nonsurgical periodontal therapy (NSPT) with anesthesia and patient instruction, followed by a re-evaluation. Mr. Denver does not want local anesthesia because he is fearful of the needle and wants to try the NSPT without it.

Questions for Consideration

1. What anxiety and pain management methods could be used for this patient? Refer to pain control mechanisms to make your list as complete as possible. Which of these methods are legal for a dental hygienist to utilize in your state or province?

2. In the past, this patient has had painful treatment, you plan to provide comfortable treatment, how do the core values of dental hygiene (Table II-I in Section II Introduction) relate to these two approaches for patient care?

3. Thinking of ethics as expressed by the core values is the patient's expectation for pain management different if a dentist or a dental hygienist provides the NSPT? Explain.

▶ Candidates for use: adult patients with no contraindications to use; pediatric patients; geriatric patients; diabetic patients; special needs patient.

▶ Not candidates: sensitivity to phentolamine mesylate; children less than 6 years of age or weighing less than 33 lbs; postsurgical patients; (increased bleeding); history of MI, angina; coronary artery disease.

II. Buffered Local Anesthetic

A. Properties

▶ Buffered local anesthetic; sodium bicarbonate (8.4% neutralizing additive solution); e.g. Onset.

▶ Increases the pH of the local anesthetic solution to a more physiologic range.

▶ Reduces stinging on injection; current research challenges this claim.[34]

▶ Faster onset; current research challenges this claim.[34]

▶ Increased effectiveness in areas of inflammation.

B. Advantages

▶ Greater patient comfort.

▶ More rapid onset.

▶ Decreased post-injection tissue injury.

III. Intranasal Dental Anesthetic[35]

A. Properties

▶ Not yet FDA approved

▶ Intranasal anesthesia.

▶ 3% Tetracaine and 0.05% oxymetazoline (vasoconstrictor)

▶ Provides maxillary anesthesia.

B. Advantages

▶ Anesthesia of maxillary teeth with no needle.

▶ Good for pediatric and needle phobic patients.

DOCUMENTATION

Documentation in the permanent record for each appointment when a pain control drug or technique is used includes a minimum of the following factors:

▶ Date.

▶ Medical status and vital signs (both pre and post treatment). Document any contraindications to the administration of either the local anesthetic or vasoconstrictor.

▶ Review of dental and psychological history as it pertains to the administration of local anesthesia.

▶ Informed consent was obtained (oral or written).

▶ Rational for pain control use.

▶ Location and type of injection.

▶ Time of administration.

▶ Number of cartridges; type and concentration of the local anesthetic including milligram of drugs administered.

▶ Type and concentration of vasoconstrictor including mg administered if applicable.

▶ Any adverse reactions that occurred.

▶ Post-operative instructions given (specify written or oral).

▶ Full signature.

▶ Example documentation for a patient receiving nitrous oxide–oxygen conscious sedation is found in Box 38-4 and for a patient receiving local anesthesia in Box 38-7.

Factors To Teach The Patient

I. Nitrous Oxide–Oxygen Conscious Sedation

▷ Inform the clinician if the sedation becomes too strong or is too weak so that adjustments can be made. The level of sedation should be adjusted individually for optimum relaxation and comfort.

▷ The gas will not result in unusual or undesirable behavior; the patient will maintain control of all personal actions.

▷ Eat normally before treatment; avoid fasting or heavy meals.

II. Local and Topical Anesthesia

▷ Be careful not to bite lip, cheek, or tongue while tissues are without normal sensations. Warn and watch children to prevent injury. Do not test anesthesia by biting the lip.

▷ Avoid chewing hard foods and avoid hot food and drinks until normal sensation has returned.

References

1. Department of Health and Human Services. *Oral Health in America: A Report of the Surgeon General*. Rockville, MD: U.S. Department of Health and Human Services, National Institute of Dental and Craniofacial Research, National Institutes of Health; 2000.

2. Doebling S, Rowe M. Negative perceptions of dental stimuli and effects on dental fear. *J Dent Hyg*. 2000;74(2): 110–116.

3. Brinkley CJ, Beacham A, Neace W, et al. Genetic variations associated with red hair color and fear of dental pain, anxiety regarding dental care and avoidance of dental care. *J Am Dent Assoc*. 2009;140(7):896–905.

4. Henry MA, Hargreaves KM. Peripheral mechanisms of odontogenic pain. *Dent Clin North Am*. 2007;51:19–44.

5. Jeske A, Zahrowski J. Good evidence supports ibuprofen as an effective and safe analgesic for postoperative pain. *J Am Dent Assoc*. 2010;141(5):567–568.

6. Clark MS, Brunick AL. *Handbook of Nitrous Oxide and Oxygen Sedation.* 3rd ed. St. Louis, MO: Mosby; 2008.

7. Brunick A, Clark MS. Nitrous oxide and oxygen sedation: an update. *Dent Assist.* 2013;82(4):12, 14–16, 18–19.

8. American Dental Association. Nitrous oxide use dangerous after intraocular gas injection: FDA. *J Am Dent Assoc.* 2002;133(11):1476.

9. Lockwood AJ, Yang YF. Nitrous oxide inhalation anaesthesia in the presence of intraocular gas can cause irreversible blindness. *Br Dent J.* 2008;204(5):247–248.

10. Malamed SF. *Sedation: A Guide to Patient Management.* 4th ed. St. Louis, MO: Mosby; 2003.

11. National Institute for Occupational Safety and Health. *Control of Nitrous Oxide in Dental Operatories.* Washington, DC: National Institute for Occupational Safety and Health. http://www.cdc.gov/niosh/nitoxide.html. Updated March 2, 1998. Accessed September 21, 2010.

12. American Academy on Pediatric Dentistry Clinical Affairs Committee; and American Academy on Pediatric Dentistry Council on Clinical Affairs. Policy on minimizing occupational health hazards associated with nitrous oxide. *Pediatr Dent.* 2008–2009;30(7, Suppl):64–65.

13. ADA Council on Scientific Affairs; and ADA Council on Dental Practice. Nitrous oxide in the dental office. *J Am Dent Assoc.* 1997;128(3):364–365.

14. Donaldson M, Donaldson D, Quarnstrom FC. Nitrous oxide-oxygen administration: when safety features no longer are safe. *J Am Dent Assoc.* 2012;143(2):134–143.

15. Rowland AS, Baird, DD, Weinberg CR, et al. Reduced fertility among women employed as dental assistants exposed to high levels of nitrous oxide. *N Engl J Med.* 1992;327(14):993–997.

16. Cohen EN, Gift HC, Brown BW, et al. Occupational disease in dentistry and chronic exposure to trace anesthetic gases. *J Am Dent Assoc.* 1980;101(1):21–31.

17. National Institute for Occupational Safety and Health (US). *Alert: Controlling Exposures to Nitrous Oxide During Anesthetic Administration* [Joint Publication of Public Health Service, Centers for Disease Control, National Institute for Occupational Safety and Health]. Cincinnati, OH: U.S. Department of Health, Education, and Welfare; 1994:1. Publication No. 94-100.

18. Malamed SF. *Handbook of Local Anesthesia.* 6th ed. St. Louis, MO: Mosby; 2013.

19. Moore PA, Hersh EV. Local anesthetics: pharmacology and toxicity. *Dent Clin North Am.* 2010;54:587–599.

20. Haas DA. An update on local anesthetics in dentistry. *J Can Dent Assoc.* 2002;68(9):46–51.

21. Becker DE, Reed KL. Essentials of local anesthetic pharmacology. *Anesth Prog.* 2006;53:98–109.

22. Becker DE, Reed KL. Local anesthetics: review of pharmacological considerations. *Anesth Prog.* 2012;59:90–102.

23. Ogle OE, Mahjoubi G. Local anesthesia: agents, techniques, and complications. *Dent Clin North Am.* 2012;56:133–148.

24. Haas DA, Lennon D. A 21 year retrospective study of reports of paresthesia following local anesthetic administration. *J Can Dent Assoc.* 1995;61(4):319–330.

25. Garisto GA, Gaffen AS, Lawrence HP, et al. Occurrence of paresthesia after dental local anesthetic administration in the United States. *J Am Dent Assoc.* 2010;141(7):836–844.

26. Moore PA, Haas DA. Paresthesias in dentistry. *Dent Clin North Am.* 2010;54:715–730.

27. Hersh EV, Giannakopoulos H. Beta-adrenergic blocking agents and dental vasoconstrictors. *Dent Clin North Am.* 2010;54:687–696.

28. Becker DE. Preoperative medical evaluation, Part 2: pulmonary, endocrine, renal and miscellaneous considerations. *Anesth Prog.* 2009;56:135–145.

29. Speca SJ, Boynes SG., Cuddy MA. Allergic reactions to local anesthetic formulations. *Dent Clin North Am.* 2010;54:655–664.

30. Trapp L, Will J. Acquired methemoglobinemia revisited. *Dent Clin North Am.* 2010;54:665–675.

31. Organization for Safety and Asepsis Procedures. *Infection Control in Practice.* Annapolis, MD: Organization for Safety and Asepsis Procedures; 2002.

32. Dentsply Pharmaceutical. *Oraqix: The Only FDA-Approved Needle-Free Anesthetic.* York, PA: Dentsply Pharmaceutical; 2010. http://www.oraqix.com/. Accessed September 22, 2010.

33. Elmore S, Nusstein J, Drum M, et al. Reversal of pulpal and soft tissue anesthesia by using phentolamine: a prospective randomized, single-blind study. *J Endod.* 2013;39(4):429–434.

34. Hobeich P, Simon S, Schneiderman E, et al. A prospective, randomized, double-blind comparison of the injection pain and anesthetic onset with 2% lidocaine with 1:100,000 epinephrine buffered with 5% and 10% sodium bicarbonate in maxillary infiltrations. *J Endod.* 2013;39(5):597–599.

35. Ciancio SG, Hutcheson MC, Ayoub F, et al. Safety and efficacy of a novel nasal spray for maxillary dental anesthesia. *J Dent Res.* 2013;92(7, Suppl):43S–48S.

36. Occupational Safety and Health Administration (US). Occupational exposure to bloodborne pathogens; needlestick and other sharps injuries. Final Rule. *Fed Regist.* 2001;66(12): 5317–5325.

ENHANCE YOUR UNDERSTANDING

 thePoint **DIGITAL CONNECTIONS**
(see the inside front cover for access information)
- **Audio glossary**
- **Quiz bank**

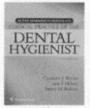 **SUPPORT FOR LEARNING**
(available separately; visit lww.com)
- *Active Learning Workbook for Clinical Practice of the Dental Hygienist, 12th Edition*

prepU **INDIVIDUALIZED REVIEW**
(available separately; visit lww.com)
- **Adaptive quizzing with *prepU for Wilkins' Clinical Practice of the Dental Hygienist***

39

Instruments and Principles for Instrumentation

Esther M. Wilkins, BS, RDH, DMD and Linda D. Boyd, RDH, RD, EdD

CHAPTER OUTLINE

LEARNING OBJECTIVES

After studying this chapter, the student will be able to:

1. Name and describe types, features, and properties of manual instruments used for removal of calculus and biofilm deposits during nonsurgical periodontal therapy.

2. List and describe the five basic principles for use of instruments.

3. Apply clinical factors relating to patient and clinician to provide appropriate lighting and visibility.

4. Relate the choice of each selected instrument to tooth and soft tissue anatomy.

5. Prepare treatment plans for patients of varying ages and disease severity and elect appropriate instruments to meet diagnostic parameters and treatment needs of the patient.

Instrumentation begins with the identification of the specific types of instruments and knowledge of the parts of each instrument during dental hygiene assessment and treatment.

▶ Requirements for putting the instruments into action to accomplish a particular task are:

- *Stabilization* by means of a correct *grasp*, finger *rest*, and fulcrum.
- Instrument *adaptation*, *angulation*, *lateral pressure*, and *stroke*.

▶ Key words related to basic instrumentation are defined in Box 39-1.

▶ A study of oral and dental anatomy and histology needs to accompany learning instrumentation procedures and skills.

▶ Development of a thorough, efficient, and safe procedure for treatment depends on an understanding of the normal, healthy, and diseased characteristics of the dental and periodontal tissues being treated.

▶ A high degree of skill in the care and use of the instruments is required.

▶ Skill depends on knowledge and understanding of the goals of therapy and how the goals can be reached through application of the fundamental principles of instrumentation.

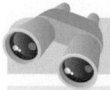

BOX 39-1 KEY WORDS: Principles of Instrumentation

Adaptation: relationship between the working end of an instrument and the tooth surface being treated.

Angulation: the angle formed by the working end of an instrument with the surface to which the instrument is applied for treatment.

Blade: working end of an instrument with special design for a particular clinical treatment.

Curet: a curved, rounded dental instrument utilized for scaling, root planing, and gingival curettage.

  Area-specific curet: a specialized instrument designed with specific angles in the shank for adaptation to a certain group of tooth surfaces.

  Universal curet: a curet designed for use on any tooth surface where the adaptation, angulation, and other principles of instrumentation can be correctly and effectively accomplished.

Curettage: removal of the inflamed soft tissue lining of a pocket wall.

Dominant hand: the hand generally used for performing tasks such as writing and holding instruments for scaling.

Finger rest: for an intraoral rest, the place on a tooth or teeth where the third or ring finger of the hand holding the instrument is placed to provide stabilization and control during activation of the instrument.

Fulcrum: the support upon which a lever rests while force intended to produce motion is exerted.

Indirect vision: use of a dental mouth mirror to view the area of instrumentation. Indirect lighting is provided by the mirror.

Instrumentation zone: section of the tooth where treatment is indicated and instrumentation is performed.

Lateral pressure: the minimal pressure that is required of an instrument against the tooth to accomplish the objective of the assessment or treatment.

Offset blade: the blade of an area-specific Gracey curet in which the lower shank is at a 70° angle to the face of the blade; contrasts with a universal curet blade, which is at a 90° angle with the lower shank.

Scaler: instrument designed for initial removal of calculus, prior to finishing with a curet.

Scaling: instrumentation of a tooth surface to remove calculus and biofilm.

Shank: the part of the instrument between the handle and the working end.

Lower or terminal shank: the part of the shank next to the blade.

Stroke: a single unbroken movement made by an instrument against a tooth surface during an examination or treatment procedure to accomplish a particular objective; the motion made for activation of an instrument.

INSTRUMENT IDENTIFICATION

The instruments needed for assessment and evaluation are described in Chapter 20. The instruments for assessment include the mouth mirror, explorers, and periodontal probe. Instruments for scaling and related procedures are described in this chapter.

I. Recognition of Treatment Instruments

▶ Each instrument is recognized by sight and distinguished at a glance by the design of the instrument.

▶ The clinician is able to designate the names and numbers, and to associate each instrument promptly with the various phases of instrumentation.

▶ The ability to quickly identify instruments contributes to organization of instrument cassettes and efficiency of services rendered.

II. Classification for Treatment Instruments

▶ *Scalers:* sickle, Jacquette, file, hoe, chisel

▶ *Curets:* universal

▶ *Curets:* area specific
- Standard Gracey
- After five Gracey
- Minibladed Gracey
- Micro-minibladed Gracey

III. Description on the Instrument Handle

▶ *Design name:* The university or individual responsible for the design or development.

▶ *Design number:* The traditional number used to identify the specific instrument. The same instrument may be made by various manufacturers using the same number.

INSTRUMENT PARTS AND BALANCE

The three major parts are the *working end* or blade, the *shank*, and the *handle*. The relationship of these parts is illustrated by the curet in Figure 39-1.

I. Working End

▶ The working end refers to the part used to carry out the purpose and function of the instrument. Each working end is unique to the particular instrument.

▶ The working end of a scaler or curet is called a blade.

▶ The parts of a sharp blade are:
- *Cutting edge:* A very fine line where two surfaces meet. For example, the *face* and the *lateral surface* meet to form the sharp cutting edge of a curet (Figure 39-2).
- *Lateral surfaces:* The lateral surfaces meet or are continuous (as in the round back of a curet) to form the *back* of the instrument.

II. Shank

▶ The shank connects the working end with the handle, as shown in Figure 39-1.

▶ The shape, length, and rigidity of the shank govern the access of the working end to accomplish the intended purpose for which the instrument was designed.

▶ The section of the shank adjacent to the blade is called the *lower* or *terminal shank* as labeled in Figure 39-1.

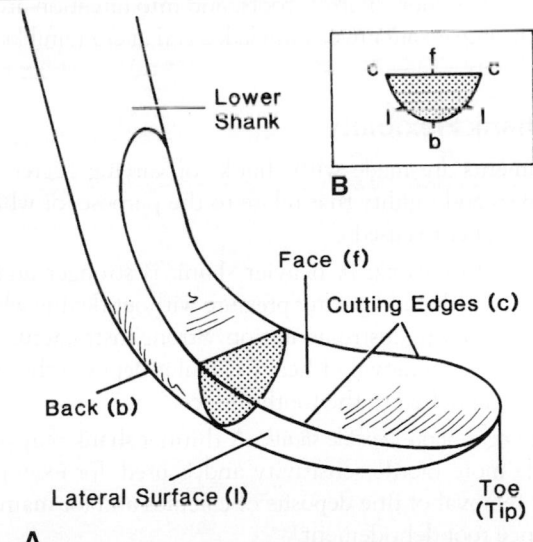

FIGURE 39-2 **Parts of a Curet. (A)** Curet with parts labeled. Lower shank is also called the terminal shank. The curet has a rounded toe, whereas the scaler has a pointed tip. **(B)** Cross section of a curet labeled f (face), c (cutting edges), l (lateral surfaces), and b (back).

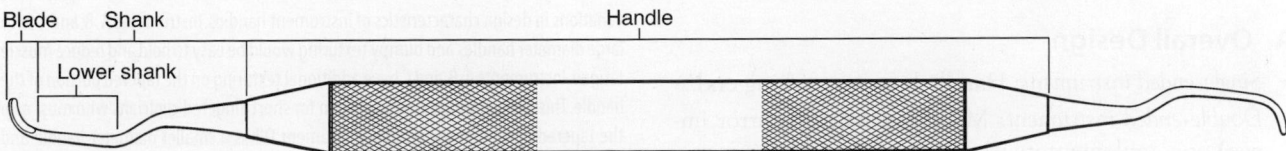

FIGURE 39-1 **Parts of an Instrument.** Curet shows the relationship of the working end (blade), shank, and handle. The section of the shank next to the blade is referred to as the terminal or lower shank.

A. Shape

▸ *Straight (flat)*: For adaptation to tooth surfaces with unrestricted access, such as for anterior teeth. With many instruments, the straight lower shank can provide the line-up for correct positioning for treatment.

▸ *Angled*: For adaptation to tooth surfaces with restricted access, such as proximal surfaces of posterior teeth, deep periodontal pockets on narrow roots, and furcation areas.

- In general, the more restricted the access, the more angulated a shank needs to be and the sharper the bends of the angles.
- Examples: Gracey curets 11/12, 13/14, and 15/16, each of which has three bends.
- Because the *distal* surfaces of molars and premolars are much less accessible than are the mesial surfaces, the angles in the shanks of 13/14 and 17/18 are designed with deeper bends to make access possible.

B. Effect of Shank Length

▸ The distance from the cutting edge (working end) of the blade to the junction of the shank and handle in most instruments is 35–40 mm (1½ inches).

▸ Too short a distance limits action.

▸ Extended lower shank length.

- Adding on 3 mm permits the blade to access deep pockets along narrow roots, and into furcation areas.
- Examples: after five, minibladed and micro-minibladed curets.

C. Shank Flexibility

Instruments are made with shanks of varying degrees of thickness and rigidity that relate to the purpose for which the instrument is used.

▸ *Rigid, thick shank*: A heavier shank is stronger and is able to withstand greater pressure without flexing when applied during instrumentation. Strong instruments are needed for removal of heavy calculus deposits that are firmly attached to the tooth surface.

▸ *Less rigid, more flexible shank*: A thinner shank may provide more tactile sensitivity and is used, for example, for removal of fine deposits of calculus and for maintenance root debridement.

III. Handle

The position and grasp of the handle in conjunction with the finger or hand rest are significant in the tactile sensitivity and the activation of the working end.

A. Overall Design

▸ *Single-ended instrument*: Handle has one working end.

▸ *Double-ended instrument*: May have paired (mirror image) or complementary working ends.

- Paired working ends may be an instrument with its mirror image on the opposite end. One is used for

access to proximal surfaces from the facial and the other for a lingual or palatal approach.

- Complementary working ends may be used during examination with a probe on one end and an explorer at the other end.

▸ *Cone socket handles*: Separable from the shank and working end. They permit screw-in instrument exchanges and replacements.

B. Weight

Handles with lighter weight enhance tactile sensitivity and lessen fatigue related to a tighter grasp. They are sometimes referred to as ergonomic handles.

C. Diameter[1]

▸ Diameters of instrument handles vary widely from the standard handle, which is 6.5 mm to larger more ergonomic handles that are 10 mm in diameter (Figure 39-3 shows a few the types of handles available).

▸ Ergonomically the ideal instrument has a 10 mm diameter handle and weighs less than 15.0 g.

- Instruments with small diameter handles increase muscle activity and pinch force, which over time can lead to musculoskeletal injuries.

D. Surface Texture: Handle

▸ Instrument handles may be smooth, ribbed, or knurled.

- A thinner, smooth handle may require a tighter grasp to prevent slipping, which can lessen tactile sensitivity and increase clinician's fatigue.

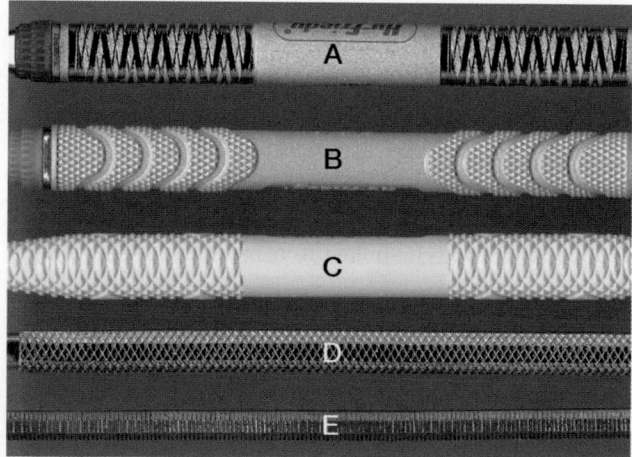

FIGURE 39-3 Handle Diameter and Texturing. The diameter and texturing of a handle varies greatly from manufacturer to manufacturer. Shown here are examples of the variations in design characteristics of instrument handles. Instruments A, B, and C with large diameter handles and bumpy texturing would be easy to hold and reduce muscle fatigue. Instruments A, B, and C have additional texturing on the tapered portion of the handle. This feature reduces muscle strain for short-fingered clinicians who must grip the tapered portion of the handle. Instrument D has a smaller diameter handle and less pronounced texturing. Instrument E has a small diameter handle and very limited texturing. (Reprinted from Nield-Gehrig J, Willmann D. Foundations of Periodontics for the Dental Hygienist, 3rd Ed. Philadelphia: Lippincott Williams & Wilkins; 2011.)

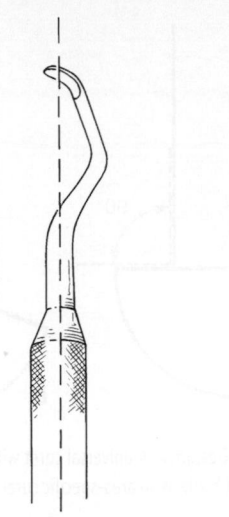

FIGURE 39-4 **Instrument Balance.** The working end of a balanced instrument is centered in line with the long axis of the instrument handle.

- The padded handle with a wider diameter can provide better control with a firm, but lighter grasp without lessening tactile sensitivity.[1]

IV. Instrument Balance

- ▶ The working end of a balanced instrument is centered in line with the long axis of the handle (Figure 39-4).
- ▶ The design of the balance of each instrument provides the ability for adaptation, angulation, and activation to accomplish the objectives of the treatment plan.

THE TREATMENT INSTRUMENTS

- ▶ Each instrument is designed for a specific type of application during treatment procedures.
  - An instrument may be categorized first by whether it is intended primarily for supragingival or for subgingival treatment procedures.
  - Scalers and curets are designed with the blade size and anatomy of the cutting edges to meet the purpose of the treatment.

I. Categories

A. Curets
- ▶ Universal
- ▶ Area Specific
- ▶ After five
- ▶ Minibladed
- ▶ Micro-minibladed

B. Scalers
- ▶ Scaler
  - Curved scaler/sickle scaler
  - Straight scaler/Jacquette
- ▶ File scaler
- ▶ Hoe scaler
- ▶ Chisel scaler

II. Instrument Blade Anatomy

- ▶ Parts of the blade of a scaler or a curet include:
  - *Face* (inner surface)
  - *Lateral surface*
  - *Back*
  - *Tip* (scaler) or *toe* (curet)
  - *Cutting edges*
  A cutting edge is formed by the junction of the face and the lateral surface.
- ▶ Figure 39-2 shows a curet with each part labeled.
- ▶ Parts of the blade of a scaler are named the same way. The differences are the pointed tip and the V-shaped back of the scaler shown in Figure 39-9. Each type of instrument is described in the following sections of the chapter.

UNIVERSAL CURET

A universal curet can be adapted for instrumentation on any tooth surface.[1] The working ends are paired mirror images on a single handle.

I. Description

A. Blade

1. *Face*
   - Perpendicular (at a 90° angle) to the lower shank (Figure 39-6A).
   - Flat in cross section (Figure 39-2B) and curved lengthwise.
2. *Cutting edges*
   - Two parallel cutting edges on a curved blade (Figure 39-2A).
   - Continuous around the face; used and therefore sharpened on both sides and around the toe.
3. *Back or undersurface*: Rounded.
4. *Cross section of the blade*: Shaped like a half circle (Figure 39-2B).
5. *Internal angles*
   - Angles of 70° to 80° are formed where the lateral surfaces meet the face.
   - Figure 39-5 shows the cross section of a curet with the internal angles marked.

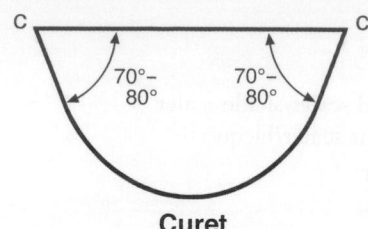

FIGURE 39-5 Internal Angles of a Curet. Cross section of a curet shows the 70° to 80° internal angles at the cutting edges. These angles are restored by sharpening techniques.

B. Shank

▶ Angles or curves in the shank are specific for each of the many different universal curets available.

II. Purposes and Uses

▶ Removal of calculus and root debridement for patients of all ages.

▶ Standard instrument for subgingival scaling to be followed by root planing with Gracey curets.

▶ After ultrasonic or sonic scaling to complete the removal of residual calculus, to be followed by Gracey curets to smooth the tooth surface as needed.

▶ Removal of supragingival calculus: especially the fine supragingival calculus close to the gingival margin.

- The rounded instrument is best adapted to the cervical area of the tooth.
- Round back does not traumatize the gingival margin or base of sulcus or pocket when placed subgingivally.

▶ Useful for obtaining a sample of subgingival biofilm to place on a glass slide for the phase microscope or for microbiologic tests.

AREA-SPECIFIC CURETS

The Gracey curets are area specific, which means that each curet is designed for adaptation to specific surfaces.

I. Description

A. Gracey Curets

▶ *Working ends*: Paired mirror image, usually placed on a single handle. The typical pairs are numbers 1/2, 3/4, 5/6. 7/8, 9/10, 11/12, 13/14, 15/16, and 17/18.

▶ *Face*: "Offset" (at an angle of approximately 70°) in relation to the lower shank (Figure 39-6B).

▶ *Cutting edge*: Each Gracey has one long sharpened cutting edge around the entire blade ending with the curved toe.

- Only the longer, outer cutting edge, which is lower when the handle is held vertically, is sharpened and used during instrumentation.

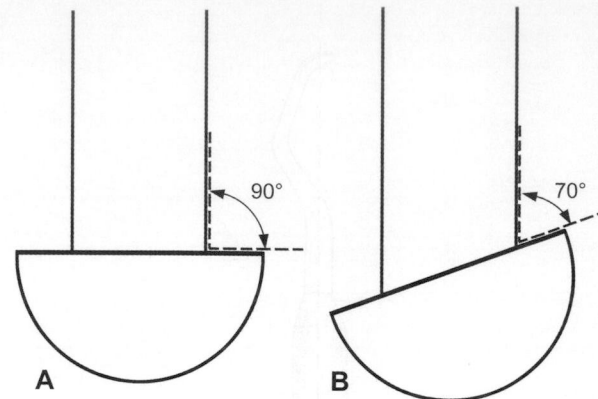

FIGURE 39-6 Curet Design. A: A universal curet with the blade at a 90° angle to the lower shank. **B:** Offset blade of an area-specific curet at a 70° angle to the lower shank.

B. Extended Gracey Curets[2]

Variations of area-specific curets provide clinicians with greater opportunities to complete deep subgingival instrumentation on narrow roots and in furcations.

▶ *Objectives*
- To facilitate access to the base of deep pockets.
- To conform to the curvatures of roots on multirooted teeth and single-rooted teeth with moderate-to-severe loss of attachment.

▶ *Shank*: Terminal (lower) shank elongated by 3 mm to adapt in deep pockets. The total length of the shank from blade to handle not changed.

A. After five (Figure 39-7B)
- Longer terminal shank is 3 mm longer and the blade width is decreased by 10%.
- Allows improved access to pocket depths beyond 5 mm.

B. Minibladed (Figure 39-7C)
- Blade length is 50% shorter than a traditional Gracey curet.
- Reduced length facilitates adaptation to the curved features of root morphology including concavities; longitudinal depressions on proximal surfaces; root surfaces within furcations; and interradicular convexities.

C. Micro minibladed (Figure 39-7D)
- Blade is one-half the length of the minibladed Gracey curet.
- It is narrower and 20% thinner with increase in rigidity of the shank to allow pressure when very deep calculus deposit is firmly attached.

II. Purposes and Uses

▶ Standard instruments for subgingival scaling and root planing.

▶ Necessary after ultrasonic or sonic scaling to complete the procedure as needed.

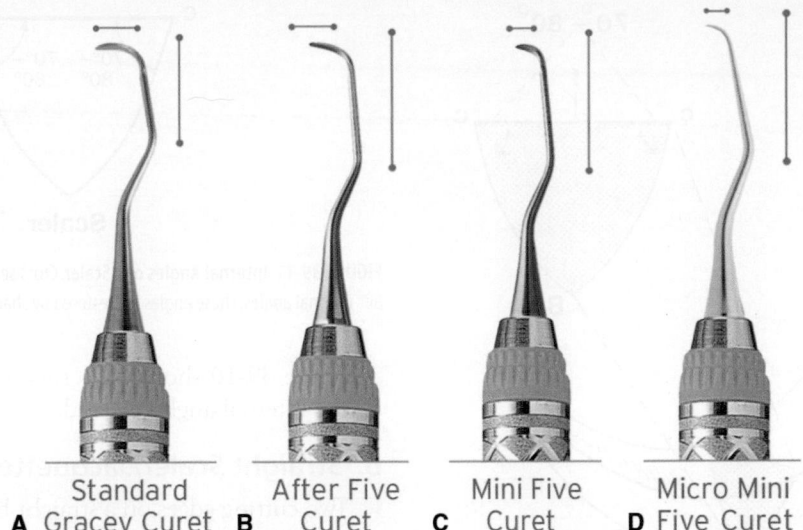

FIGURE 39-7 **Gracey Tip Comparison. (A)** Shows a standard Gracey curet. **(B)** The After Five curet had a 3mm longer shank than (A). **(C)** The Mini-bladed curet has a 50% shorter blade and 3 mm longer shank than (A). **(D)** The Micro-Mini bladed curet has a 50% shorter blade that is narrower and 20% thinner than (A). (Courtesy of Hu-Friedy)

▶ A universal curet or a rigid Gracey curet is used for scaling for removal of as much of the calculus as possible.

▶ Area-specific curets follow for fine scaling and root planing.

▶ Design of the curet with a slender shank allows entrance into the sulcus or pocket with minimal trauma to the gingival margin.

▶ The curved blade with rounded end permits access to the base of the sulcus or pocket.

▶ The rounded back minimizes possible trauma at the base of the sulcus or pocket.

III. Application

A. Angulation

Blade is applied to the tooth so that the face forms a 70° angle with the tooth surface to be treated.

B. Adaptation

Principles of adaptation are described later in this chapter.

▶ Toe third or lower third of the cutting edge is maintained on the tooth surface at all times.

▶ Minimize soft tissue trauma caused by toe extending away from the tooth in the narrow pocket.

▶ Changes in tooth surface contour require constant attention so that safe contact is maintained.

▶ On line angles, only 1 or 2 mm near the toe may be used.

C. Curet Selection

▶ Universal curets are used for scaling for removal of as much of the calculus as possible.

▶ Area-specific curets follow for fine scaling and root planing.

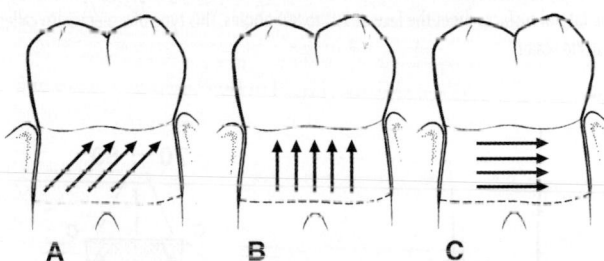

FIGURE 39-8 **Directions of Instrument Strokes.** Arrows on root surface represent **(A)** diagonal or oblique strokes, **(B)** vertical strokes, and **(C)** horizontal strokes.

D. Design

▶ Design of the curet with a slender shank allows entrance into the sulcus or pocket with minimal trauma to the gingival margin.

▶ The curved blade with rounded end permits access to the base of the sulcus or pocket.

▶ The rounded back minimizes possible trauma at the base of the sulcus or pocket.

E. Stroke

▶ *Stroke:* Pull stroke is applied in vertical, horizontal, or oblique directions (Figure 39-8).

▶ Cutting edge is prepared when the instrument is sharpened for use at 70°. When the instrument is applied at a different angle, a bevel will be created, and the instrument will no longer be sharp.

SCALERS

I. Types of Scalers: Sickles and Jacquettes

The "sickle" scaler (Figure 39-9) and the "Jacquette" scaler (Figure 39-10) may be referred to simply as "scalers,"

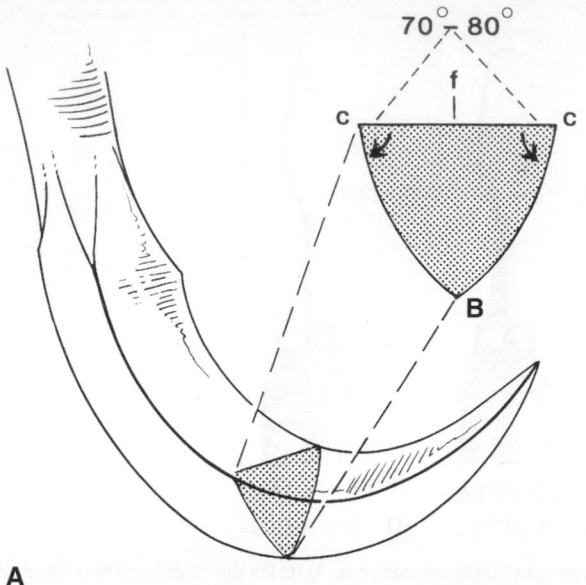

FIGURE 39-9 Curved Scaler (Sickle scaler). (A) The curved blade terminates in a point. **(B)** Cross section shows the face (f) and the two cutting edges (c) formed where the lateral surfaces meet the face at 70° to 80° angles. This type of scaler is also called a sickle scaler.

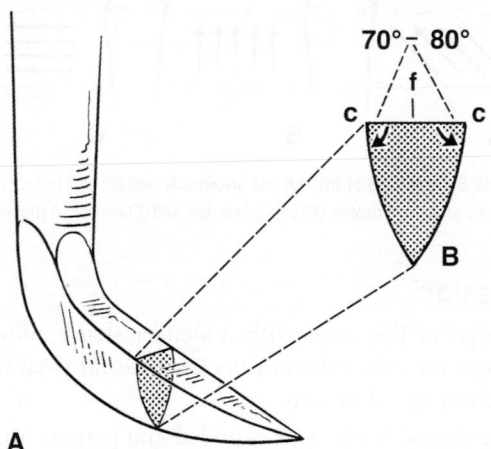

FIGURE 39-10 Straight Scaler (Jacquette). (A) The straight blade converges to a point where the two cutting edges meet at the tip. **(B)** Cross section of the scaler shows the face (f), the two cutting edges (c), and the 70° to 80° internal angles. This type of scaler is also known as the Jacquette scaler.

either curved or straight, respectively. Scalers may have a straight, curved, or contra-angled shank. The blades and cutting edges may be straight or curved.

A. Curved Scaler/Sickle Scaler

▶ Two cutting edges on a curved blade (Figure 39-9).

▶ Face is flat in cross section and curved lengthwise.

▶ The face converges with the two lateral surfaces to form the *tip* of the scaler, which is a sharp point.

▶ In cross section, the blade is triangular (Figure 39-9B).

▶ Internal angles of 70° to 80° are formed where the lateral surfaces meet the face at the cutting edges.

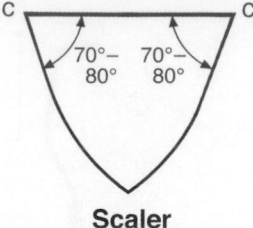

FIGURE 39-11 Internal Angles of a Scaler. Cross section of a scaler shows the 70° to 80° internal angles. These angles are restored by sharpening techniques.

Figure 39-10 shows the cross section of a scaler with the internal angles marked.

B. Straight Scaler/Jacquette

▶ Two cutting edges on a straight blade (Figure 39-10).

▶ Face (between the cutting edges) is flat.

▶ The face converges with the two lateral surfaces to form the tip of the scaler, which is a sharp point.

▶ Cross section of the blade is triangular (Figure 39-10B).

▶ Internal angles of 70° to 80° are formed where the lateral surfaces meet the face at the cutting edges (Figure 39-11).

C. Angulation of the Shank

▶ *Straight*: Single instrument in which the relationships of the shank, blade, and handle are in a flat plane; adaptable primarily for anterior teeth, although may be used for scaling premolars when the lips and cheeks permit retraction for correct angulation.

▶ *Modified or contra-angle*: Paired instruments that are mirror images of each other to provide access to the proximal surfaces of posterior teeth; one adapts from the facial and the other from the lingual and palatal aspects.

D. Purposes and Uses of Scaler

▶ Principally for removal of supragingival calculus.

▶ May be useful for removal of gross calculus that is slightly below the gingival margin when the calculus is continuous with the supragingival calculus, and when the gingival tissue is spongy and flexible to permit easy insertion of the instrument.[3]

  • Extreme caution must be used since the pointed tip of the blade and back of the sickle scaler can traumatize the tissue.

E. Contraindications for Use of Scalers Subgingivally

▶ Cause undue trauma to the gingival tissue because of the large size, thickness, and length of the blade.

▶ Pointed tip and straight cutting edges cannot be adapted to the curved root surfaces. Risk of grooving or scratching the cemental surface is increased.

▶ Tactile sensitivity decreased with larger, heavier blades.

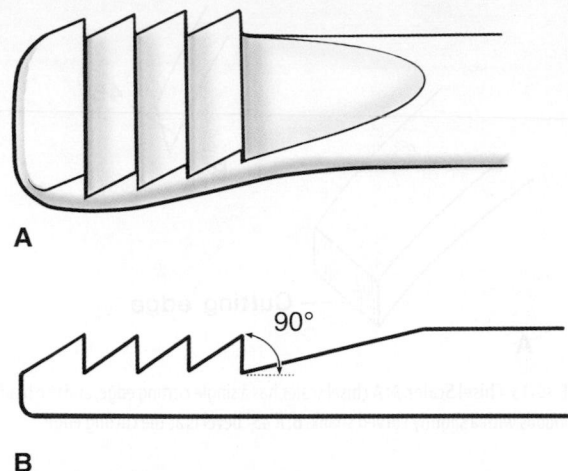

A

B

FIGURE 39-12 File Scaler. A: A file has multiple cutting edges. **B:** Each blade is at a 90° angle with the shank.

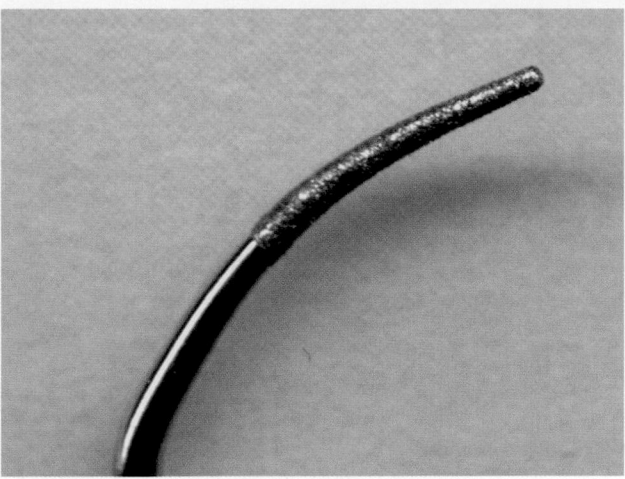

FIGURE 39-13 Diamond-Coated File. A close-up view of a working end on a diamond-coated file. Note the textured coating on the working-end. (Reprinted from Nield-Gehrig J. Fundamentals of Periodontal Instrumentation and Advanced Root Instrumentation. Philadelphia: Lippincott Williams & Wilkins; 2011.)

F. Application

▶ *Angulation.* The face of the blade is adapted to the tooth surface at an angle of approximately 70°.

▶ *Stroke:* Pull stroke only for this type of blade.

▶ Small scalers can be useful for removal of fine supragingival deposits directly under contact areas and between overlapping teeth.

II. File Scaler

A. Characteristics

▶ Stainless steel file scalers include Hirshfeld and Orban files.

- Multiple cutting edges lined up as a series of miniature hoes on a round, oval, or rectangular base (Figure 39-12A).
- The metal multiple blades are at a 90° angle with the shank (Figure 39-12B).
- Shanks are variously angulated: most are paired instruments.
- Reduced tactile sensitivity because of the series of blades.

▶ Diamond-coated file scaler.[4]

- Designs vary by manufacturer.
- There are paired ends (buccal/lingual and mesial/distal) like other file scalers.
- These are not true files, scalers, or curets because there are no blades, the diamond coating is placed 180° to 360° around the tip depending on the manufacturer, and the diamond coating is used to remove the calculus (Figure 39-13).

B. Purposes and Uses of a File Scaler

▶ Traditional file scaler

- Crushes and fractures heavy calculus into fragments prior to use of curets.

- Burnished calculus that is impervious to removal with other bladed instruments can be removed with the file scaler.
- Gross deposits of calculus on patients for whom ultrasonic use is contraindicated.
- Smoothing of overextended or rough amalgam restorations, particularly on proximal surfaces or in cervical areas.

▶ Diamond-coated file scaler

- Use for finishing of root surfaces and accessing furcation areas.
- Early research suggests the use of diamond-coated scalers after conventional curets may provide a tooth surface more compatible with attachment of periodontal ligament fibroblasts.[4]

C. Application

▶ Hirschfeld or Orban file scalers

- *Adaptation:* entire working surface is placed flat against the area to be treated.
- Pressure applied permits the cutting edges to grasp the surface.
- *Stroke:* pull only, using a linear motion.
- *File use:* is always followed with curet(s) to leave a smooth surface on roots.

▶ Diamond-coated file scaler

- Working surface is placed flat against the root surface.
- Very light pressure is used to prevent damage to root surface.
- Strokes are multidirectional (horizontal, vertical, and oblique) in a push–pull motion.[5]

III. Hoe Scaler

A. Characteristics

▶ Single straight cutting edge (Figure 39-14A).

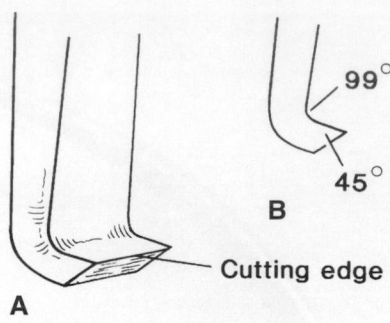

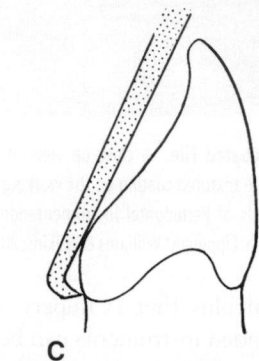

FIGURE 39-14 Hoe Scaler. A: The hoe has a single cutting edge. **B:** The blade is turned at an angle of 99° to the shank, and the cutting edge is beveled at a 45° angle. **C:** Adaptation to a tooth for removal of calculus is with a two-point contact where possible.

▶ *Blade*: Turned at a 99° angle to the shank.

▶ *Cutting edge*: Beveled at a 45° angle to the end of the blade (Figure 39-14B).

▶ *Shank*: Variously angulated for adaptation of cutting edges to accessible tooth surfaces; some are paired.

B. Purposes and Uses of a Hoe Scaler

▶ Removes supragingival calculus, particularly large, accessible, tenacious pieces.

▶ *Contraindications for use subgingivally:*

• Insertion of the thick-bladed instrument into the sulcus can cause unnecessary distention of the pocket wall.

• Lack of adaptability of the wide straight cutting edge to the curved root surface.

• Difficulty of use without gouging the cemental surface. The sharp "corners" are rounded with sharpening (see Chapter 40).

• Lack of sensitivity because of the bulk of the instrument and the marked angulation of the shanks of some hoes.

C. Application

▶ Full width of the cutting edge may be in contact with the calculus.

▶ Two-point contact is maintained with the tooth to stabilize the instrument during the positioning and activation. Two-point contact means contact of the

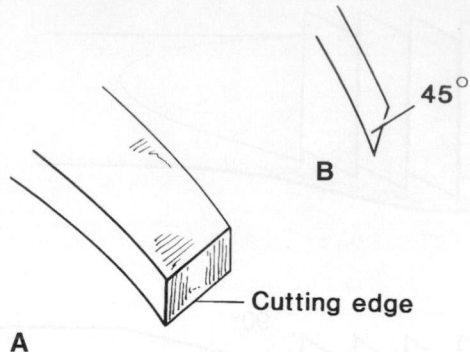

FIGURE 39-15 Chisel Scaler. A: A chisel scaler has a single cutting edge, and the blade is continuous with a slightly curved shank. **B:** A 45° bevel is at the cutting edge.

cutting edge and the side of the shank with the tooth (Figure 39-14C).

▶ Hoes are not generally applied to proximal surfaces except the surface adjacent to an edentulous area.

▶ *Pull stroke* is used in a coronal direction.

IV. Chisel Scaler

A. Characteristics

▶ Single straight cutting edge (Figure 39-15A).

▶ Blade is continuous with a slightly curved shank.

▶ End of blade is flat and beveled at 45° (Figure 39-15B).

B. Purposes and Uses of a Chisel Scaler

▶ Removal of supragingival calculus from exposed proximal surfaces of anterior teeth where interdental gingiva is missing.

▶ Dislodgement of heavy calculus from the proximal areas of mandibular anterior teeth. When the calculus on the lingual surfaces may form a continuous bridge across several teeth, the chisel can be pushed horizontally from the facial aspect to break up the large masses of calculus.

▶ Proximal surfaces of premolars when flexibility of the lips and cheeks permits retraction for proper positioning of the cutting edge.

C. Application

▶ *Apply full width of cutting edge*: Sharp corners can nick and groove the tooth surface. Round the sharp "corners" during sharpening (see Chapter 40).

▶ *Stroke*: Horizontal only, from facial to lingual on proximal surfaces of anterior, particularly mandibular, teeth.

PRINCIPLES FOR INSTRUMENT USE

Understanding the purpose of each instrument and developing dexterity in the effective use of the instruments are fundamental to clinical dental hygiene practice.

▶ *Stability* is essential for effective, controlled action of an instrument.

▶ The correct use depends on maintaining *control* of the movement of the instrument through use of an effective *grasp* and the establishment and maintenance of an appropriate, firm fulcrum (*finger rest*).

INSTRUMENT GRASP

I. Functions of the Instrument Grasp

A. Dominant Hand

▶ The right hand is the dominant hand for the right-handed clinician and vice versa for the left-handed clinician.

▶ A few rare people are completely ambidextrous, and others are partially dexterous with the nondominant hand, a useful capability when carrying out dental and dental hygiene procedures.

▶ Exercises for developing dexterity are provided later in this chapter.

▶ The dominant hand is used to hold and activate the treatment instrument. The manner in which the instrument is held influences the entire procedure.

B. Nondominant Hand

▶ The right-handed clinician uses the left hand and the left-handed clinician uses the right hand for essential supplementary functions to assist the dominant hand.

▶ The mouth mirror is held by the nondominant hand.

▶ With the appropriate grasp and finger rest, the following effects can be provided:
  • Control of the position of the mirror for indirect vision, indirect lighting, and retraction.
  • Assistance in providing the dominant hand with an auxiliary finger rest.

C. Grasp Dynamics

▶ A rigid grasp, in which the instrument is gripped tightly, lessens the tactile sensitivity and, hence, the effectiveness of instrumentation.

▶ The appropriate grasp is controlled, displays the confidence of the clinician in the work being done, and provides the following effects:
  • Increased fingertip tactile sensitivity.
  • Positive control of the instrument with balance and flexibility during motion.
  • Decreased hazard of trauma to the dental and periodontal tissues, which in turn results in less postcare discomfort for the patient.
  • Prevention of fatigue to clinician's fingers, hand, and arm.

▶ Figure 39-15 shows the recommended modified pen grasp for each hand.

II. Types of Grasps

A. Modified Pen Grasp for Internal Finger Rests

▶ *Description*: The modified pen grasp is a three-finger grasp with specific target points of the thumb, index finger, and middle finger all in contact with the instrument.
  • *Thumb*: the center of the upper aspect of the pad.
  • *Index finger*: the center of the upper aspect of the pad.
  • *Middle finger*: the inside upper corner of the pad, behind the upper corner of the nail.

▶ *Location on handle*
  • The instrument is held by the thumb and index finger on the handle.
  • The upper corner of the middle finger is placed on the upper portion of the shank to hold and guide the movement (Figure 39-16).

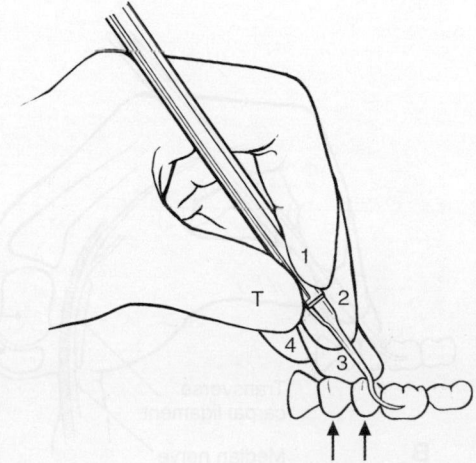 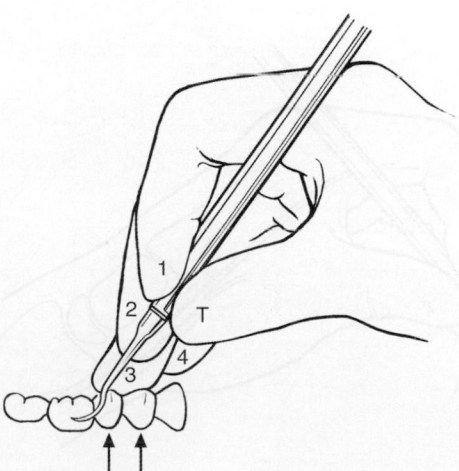

FIGURE 39-16 Modified Pen Grasp for Left and Right Hands. An instrument is held by the thumb (T), index finger (1), and the second, or "middle," finger (2), which also provides support. The third, or "ring," finger (3) serves as the finger rest, and the fourth, or "little," finger (4) is positioned beside the ring finger to supplement the finger rest.

► *Role of middle finger*
  • The shank of the instrument is held against the inside upper corner of the pad of the middle finger.
  • The instrument *is not* held across the fingernail or the side of the middle finger, as in a pen grasp usually used for writing.
  • The specific position of the middle finger is essential to instrument control to prevent the instrument from slipping during adaptation and activation and to optimize application of lateral pressure.

► *Role of ring finger:* The ring finger is used to establish a finger rest/fulcrum.

► *Additional support:* The side-to-side contact of index, middle, and ring fingers allows for greater stability, strength, and control during instrumentation.

B. Palm Grasp

► *Description:* The handle of the instrument is held in the palm by cupped index, middle, ring, and little fingers. The thumb is free to serve as the fulcrum (Figure 39-17).

► *Limitations of use:* Instruments for calculus removal, root planing, and maintenance root debridement are

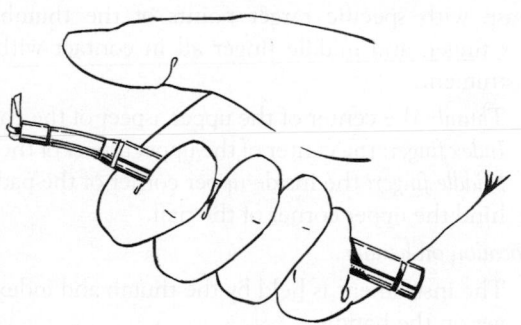

FIGURE 39-17 Palm Grasp of Instrument. The instrument handle is held in the palm by cupped index, middle, ring, and little fingers. Thumb is free and serves as the finger rest.

not used with a palm grasp. The possible exception is a chisel scaler when it is used to remove gross calculus by a push stroke.

► *Examples of uses for palm grasp*
  • Air syringe
  • Rubber dam clamp holder
  • Chisel for restorative work
  • Nondominant hand stabilizing the instrument for sharpening (Figures 40-7 and 40-8 in Chapter 40).

NEUTRAL POSITIONS

Neutral positions for the wrist, forearm, elbow, and shoulder are basic to the following:

► Efficient performance directed at the prevention of occupational pain risks, particularly those risks related to cumulative trauma disorders.

► Clinical activities to prevent cumulative trauma disorders, particularly prevention of carpal tunnel syndrome described in Chapter 7, Figure 7-4 and Table 7-1.

► General clinician and dental chair positioning and neutral body positioning are described in Chapter 7.

I. Wrist

► The wrist is straight, and the forearm and the hand are in the same horizontal plane when in the neutral position.

► Figure 39-18 illustrates the straight wrist and the effect of a bent wrist.

► Carpal tunnel syndrome, brought on by pressure on the median nerve in the carpal tunnel, is one of the nerve entrapment conditions that results from inappropriate work habits, such as working with a bent wrist.

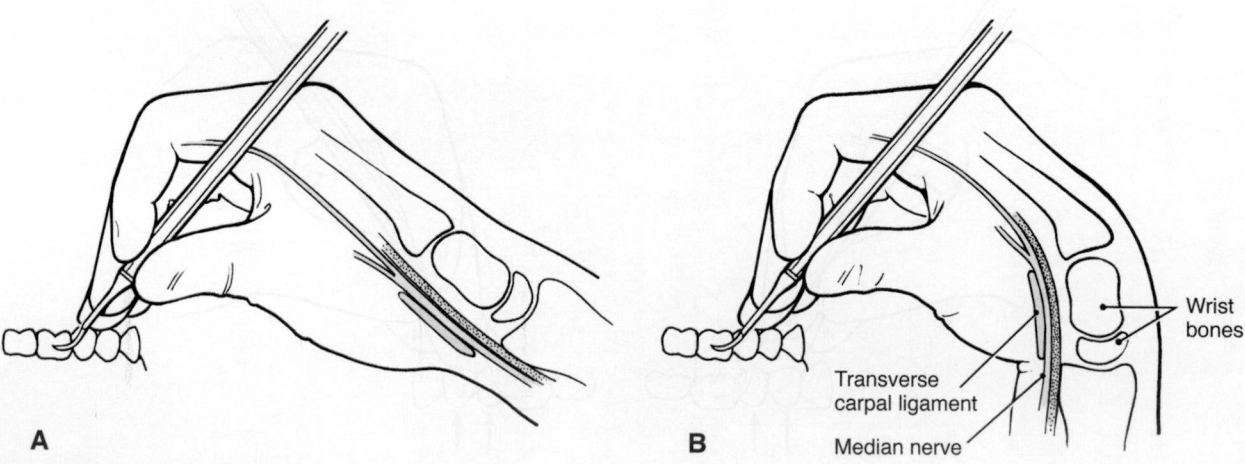

A   **B**

Wrist bones

Transverse carpal ligament

Median nerve

FIGURE 39-18 Effect of Wrist Position. A: Wrist in neutral position in straight line with forearm. **B:** Bent wrist shows cramping of median nerve in the carpal tunnel of the wrist. Repeated pressure on the median nerve can cause carpal tunnel syndrome.

II. Elbow

The neutral elbow is 90° or greater, with the forearm positioned horizontally or slightly oblique. The hand is in straight alignment with the forearm.

III. Shoulder

In neutral, both shoulders are level and relaxed to their lowest position. From a lateral position, each is vertically in line with, and beneath, each ear. The upper arms are straight down to the elbow.

FULCRUM: FINGER REST

A finger rest is always used when instruments are applied to the teeth and gingiva.

I. Definition

A. Fulcrum

The support, or point of rest, on which a lever turns in moving a body.

B. Finger Rest

The support, or point of finger rest on the tooth surface, on which the hand turns in moving an instrument.

II. Objectives

An effective, well-established finger rest is essential to the following:

A. Stability

For controlled action of the instrument.

B. Unit Control

Provides a focal point from which the whole hand can move as a unit.

C. Prevention of Injury

Injury to the patient's oral tissues can result from irregular pressure and uncontrolled movement.

D. Comfort for the Patient

Confidence in the clinician's ability, which results from the feeling of a securely applied instrument.

E. Control of Length of Stroke

With instrument grasp, the finger rest limits the instrumentation to where it is needed.

III. Intraoral Fulcrums

The intraoral fulcrum (finger rest) is essentially a total hand-coordinated effort to provide stabilization.

Figure 39-16 shows the fingers grouped together with the fulcrum where the ring finger (no. 3 in Figure 39-16) maintains its position on a tooth near the tooth being treated.

A. Digits Used for Finger Rest

▶ *Modified Pen Grasp*
- *Ring finger*: Little finger is held close beside ring finger (finger nos. 3 and 4 in Figure 39-16).
- *Supplementary*: Middle finger is held beside ring finger to provide total hand unity; ring finger maintains regular fulcrum position, and middle finger maintains its grasp on the instrument.
- *Palm grasp*: Thumb.

B. Location of Finger Rest

▶ *Purposes*: The location of a finger rest is selected for the following reasons:
- Convenience to area of instrumentation
- Ease in instrument adaptation
- Maintenance of an effective grasp
- Application of the appropriate angulation
- Stability and control of instrument during the activation (strokes)
- Safety of the clinician. A finger rest is not placed in line of the stroke direction to prevent a finger injury if the patient moved suddenly or the instrument slips for any reason.

▶ *Principles*[6]
- The first choice for an intraoral finger rest is the tooth or teeth adjacent to the tooth being treated.
- Maintain the rest on firm stable tooth or teeth. The patient's chin, lips, and cheeks are mobile and flexible and therefore less reliable for stability.
- Where possible, the rest is placed in the same arch, maxillary or mandibular, as the instrumentation; also in addition, where possible, the rest is placed in the same quadrant.

IV. Extraoral Fulcrum

An intraoral fulcrum cannot always be used because of access, especially in maxillary posterior areas and an extraoral fulcrum may be more effective.[6,7]

A. Elements of Extraoral Fulcrum[6,7]

▶ Maximize the contact of the clinician's instrumentation hand with the patient's face.
▶ A secure fulcrum is dependent on pressure against the face and underlying bone.
  - A reinforcing finger from the nondominant hand may also help stabilize the instrument.
▶ The position of the grasp on the instrument will need to be modified so that it is farther from the working end than in a traditional intraoral fulcrum.

B. Location of Extraoral Fulcrum

▶ Cheek and chin are most commonly used.

V. Alternative Fulcrums

▶ When a variation in finger fulcrum is used, basic rules for stability and control are applied, and fulcrums on movable tissues are avoided.

▶ Reasons for Use of an Alternative Fulcrum
  • Limitations of oral anatomic features:
    • Access to posterior teeth.
    • Patient's facial musculature.
    • Mouth opening (microstomia).
    • Size of tongue.
    • Arrangement of the teeth or malocclusions of individual teeth.
    • Physical disability affecting the oral cavity indirectly may interfere with customary positioning for instrumentation.
  • Tenacious calculus in difficult access areas cannot be removed from root surfaces by the usual procedures.
    • Greater support and pressure to the instrument are required.
  • When the problem in instrumentation seems to be related to space and accessibility, the height and position of the dental chair and the patient's head position may need to be adjusted. In addition, a change in the clinician's working position may be necessary.

▶ Three types of variations are suggested here: *substitute*, *supplementary*, and *reinforced* finger rests.

A. Substitute

▶ Missing teeth where finger rest is usually applied.
  • For an edentulous area, a cotton roll or gauze sponge may be packed into the area to provide a dry finger rest.
  • Otherwise, a rest across the dental arch or in the opposite arch may be required to provide stability.

▶ Mobile teeth, or teeth with inadequate bony support.
  • Avoid mobile teeth for finger rests or use only with minimal pressure for brief periods.
  • Not only would the rest on a mobile tooth be unstable, but also pressure, movement, and undue stress on the tooth could traumatize and tear the periodontal ligament fibers.

▶ Index finger of nondominant hand may be placed in the vestibule over a cotton roll or a dry gauze square.
  • The usual finger rest can be placed on the index finger to aid retraction and visibility, particularly in the mouth of a small child.

B. Supplementary

▶ Place the index finger of the nondominant hand on the occlusal surfaces of teeth adjacent to the working area. The finger rest can then be applied to the nondominant index finger.
  • This is known as a "finger-on-finger" rest.
  • Such supplements are helpful for achieving a parallel orientation of the terminal shank to proximal surfaces.
  • Supplemental rests are not useful for certain distal surfaces where the mouth mirror is essential for vision.

C. Reinforced

▶ In this type, a support is placed between the instrument handle and the working end to provide additional strength and force, particularly for hard, tenacious calculus in pockets.
  • Index finger of nondominant hand can be rested on the tooth adjacent to the one being scaled, while the thumb is placed on the instrument shank (or handle) for a reinforcement.
  • Greater control of the instrument can result and, when applied correctly, the danger of instrument breakage is reduced.
  • A definite rest for both hands is needed to distribute the pressure.

VI. Touch or Pressure Applied to Finger Rest

A. Balance

▶ The fulcrum finger rest maintains a secure hold with variable pressure to balance the action of the instrument being applied.

▶ A balance is needed between the pressure exerted against the tooth and on the pressure of the finger rest.

B. Effects of Excess Pressure

▶ Decreased stability

▶ Diminished control

▶ Fatigue of patient caused by use of mandibular fulcrums; heavy pressure on the movable mandible can cause fatigue in the temporomandibular joint and related muscles and discomfort for the patient

▶ Fatigue in clinician's fingers and hand.

ADAPTATION

With an appropriate grasp and finger rest, the instrument is next ready for application. The working end of the instrument is adapted to the surface of the tooth where instrumentation is to take place.

I. Relation to Tooth Surface

▶ Select the correct end of a double-ended paired instrument.

- The side of the tip or toe is maintained in close approximation to the surface being examined or treated.
- The blade of an instrument is divided into thirds referred to as the shank third, the middle third, and the toe (or tip) third.

II. Characteristics of a Well-Adapted Instrument

A. Working End

- The working end of the instrument is positioned correctly for the task to be accomplished.
  - Example: when scaling, the angle formed by the face of the instrument and the tooth surface is crucial for effective calculus removal. ("Angulation" is described in a following section.)
- The instrument is adapted for maximum usefulness of the working end.
  - Example: About 2–3 mm of the toe third of a curet may be adaptable when on a "flat" surface of the tooth, whereas at a line angle or convex surface of a narrow root, less than 2 mm may be adaptable.
- The working end is applied to conform to the contour of the tooth surface.
- As the instrument is activated, it is adjusted to changes required by variations in the tooth surface topography.

B. Soft Tissue

A properly adapted instrument harms neither the tissue being treated nor the surrounding or adjacent tissues.

III. Problem Areas

Areas where instrument adaptation is most difficult and requires more attention, time, and careful application of skill include the following:

A. Line Angles

- All line angles require the instrument be rolled between the fingers to turn the working end as the instrument is activated.
  - At each change of direction around a line angle, the instrument must be rolled to keep the toe third adapted to the tooth surface.
  - Figure 39-19 shows the adaptation of an explorer tip to a line angle.

B. Convex and Rounded Surfaces

Particularly of narrow roots.

C. Cervical Area

Where the root is constricted.

D. Proximal Root Surface

Root surfaces may be concave, have longitudinal grooves, or have narrow furcation openings.

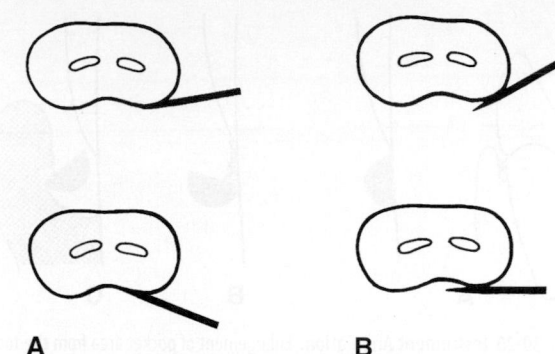

A   **B**

FIGURE 39-19 Instrument Adaptation. Cross section of maxillary first permanent premolar to show adaptation of the tip of an explorer. **A:** Appropriate adaptation in which the tip of the explorer is maintained on the tooth surface in a series of strokes to explore around a line angle. **B:** Incorrect adaptation with the tip of the explorer extended away from the tooth surface.

ANGULATION

A factor closely related to and directly influencing instrument adaptation is angulation.

- Angulation refers to the angle formed at the cutting edge of an instrument between the tooth surface and the face of the instrument.
- Each instrument is applied to a surface in a specific manner for optimum adaptation and angulation.

I. Probe

- The usual adaptation of a probe is to maintain the side of the working tip on the tooth, with the long axis of the working end nearly parallel with the tooth surface.
- As used for a bleeding index, the tip is placed inside the pocket wall and pressed lightly on the wall as the probe is moved horizontally around the tooth (see Figure 23-11 in Chapter 23).

II. Explorer

- The side of the explorer tip is kept on the tooth at all times to feel for changes in the surface such as roughness.
- The angle is 5° or less. Figure 20-3 in Chapter 20 illustrates the use of the subgingival explorer.

III. Scalers and Curets

- Angulation for a scaler or a curet means the angle formed by the face at the cutting edge of the instrument with the surface to which the instrument is applied.
  - Figure 39-20 shows the various angles for curet adaptation.
  - At zero angulation, the curet face is flat against the tooth surface (Figure 39-20A).

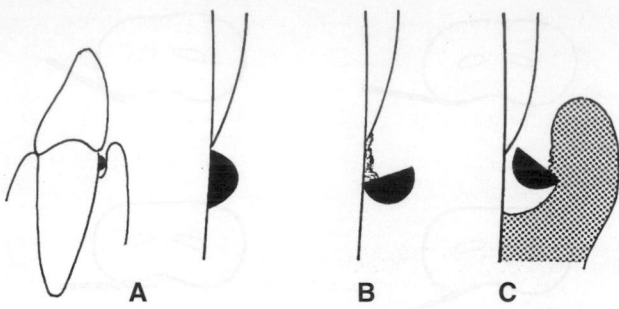

FIGURE 39-20 Instrument Angulation. Enlargement of pocket area from the tooth on the left shows cross section of a curet blade in black. **A:** The curet is angulated at 0° with the tooth surface when used in an exploratory or insertion stroke. At 0° the face of the blade is flat against the tooth surface. **B:** Blade angulated at approximately 70° with the tooth surface for scaling and root planing. **C:** Open blade angulated toward the pocket wall in position for gingival curettage. The face of the blade forms an angle of approximately 70° with the soft tissue pocket wall.

A. Scaling and Root Planing

▶ For curets and scalers, an angle of 70° between the face of the instrument and the tooth surface permits effective calculus removal (Figure 39-20B).

▶ Markedly closed angulation uses only the side of a sharp cutting edge and can result in burnishing.

▶ Burnishing produces a smooth veneer, making the calculus difficult or impossible to detect with an explorer.

B. Gingival Curettage

The face is turned toward the soft tissue wall of the pocket. The angle formed by the face of the curet blade and the soft tissue pocket wall being treated is approximately 70° (Figure 39-20C).

LATERAL PRESSURE

Lateral pressure refers to the pressure of the instrument against the tooth surface during activation. It is described as light, moderate, or heavy pressure.

I. Detection Instruments

Explorers and probes are used with light pressure to maximize the sense of touch in detecting irregularities.

II. Treatment Instruments

A. Assessment Stroke

A light pressure equal to that used by an explorer is applied as the curet blade is moved across the tooth surface. The purpose of the assessment stroke is to do the following:

▶ Assess the surface texture of the root.

▶ Confirm positioning of the back of the curet below the apical margin of the calculus at the soft tissue attachment.

▶ Rehearse the movement of the curet before activating a working stroke to confirm correct adaptation.

B. Scaling Stroke or Working Stroke

A definite, well-controlled, firm stroke of moderate-to-heavy pressure is used for calculus removal.

C. Root Planing Stroke

▶ A varying amount of pressure is applied, dependent upon the surface textures of the root surface.

▶ Lateral pressure begins as moderately firm if deposits are present.

▶ As strokes continue, a lighter pressure is applied progressively as the root surface becomes smooth and all the calculus has been removed.

D. Root Debridement Stroke

Lighter pressure is applied as a curet disrupts and removes dental biofilm from the root surface of a previously root planed tooth.

III. Errors in Technique

A. Effects of Insufficient Pressure

▶ Burnishing of calculus.

▶ Loss of control when both fulcrum and lateral pressure are insufficient.

B. Effects of Excessive Pressure

▶ Excess removal of tooth structure; gouging of root surfaces.

▶ Loss of instrument control.

▶ Potential damage to soft tissue, pocket lining; bleeding.

▶ Patient discomfort; discomfort during healing later.

▶ Clinician fatigue

ACTIVATION: STROKE

▶ A stroke is an unbroken movement made by an instrument; it is the action of an instrument in the performance of the task for which it was designed.

▶ Strokes may be identified by the instrumentation being performed. Examples are the "probing or exploring stroke," "scaling stroke," or "root planing stroke."

　• Technique for each type is described in the chapters covering the specific procedures.

I. Characteristics of Strokes

A. Types of Strokes by Action

▶ *Pull.* Example: scaler removing calculus.

▶ *Placement.* Example: exploratory stroke when a curet is being positioned.

- *Combined push and pull*. Example: explorer in a walking stroke, which is moving the instrument up and down with equal pressure on the surface (see Figure 20-3 in Chapter 20).
- *Walking stroke*. Example: probe is moved up and down, gently touching the coronal border of the periodontal attachment with each down stroke (see Figure 20-11 in Chapter 20).

B. Types of Strokes by Function

- *Assessment stroke*
  - Used to detect irregularities of the tooth surface such as the presence of calculus, a carious lesion, or a rough overhanging margin.
  - The assessment stroke is also called an exploratory stroke. The grasp pressure is light so that tactile sense is magnified. Examples include:
    - Probe is used to locate the attachment at the bottom of the periodontal pocket and to estimate the amount of deposit present on the root surfaces while probing.
    - Explorer is used to evaluate for surface smoothness following treatment.
    - Ultrasonic tip is used prior to activation to confirm the soft tissue attachment to determine adequate access to the base of the pocket.
- *Working stroke*
  The stroke applied to accomplish a task such as calculus removal or reshaping an overhanging margin.

C. Types of Strokes by Direction (Figure 39-8)

- *Diagonal or oblique*: Diagonal to the long axis of the tooth across the surface being treated (Figure 39-8A).
- *Vertical*: Strokes parallel with the long axis of the tooth being treated (Figure 39-8B).
- *Horizontal*: Strokes parallel with the occlusal surface of the tooth being treated (Figure 39-8C).
  - They are sometimes called circumferential, which should not be interpreted to mean that a stroke can be made to go around a tooth or large segment of a tooth.
  - A horizontal stroke will be a short, controlled stroke because of the constant changes in the topography of the tooth surface.
- Curvilinear or circular
  - Stroke used with a handpiece. A small circular stroke is used with varying pressure to:
    - Apply polishing agent with a rubber cup.
    - Polish amalgam restorations using stones, burs, rubber cups, and points.
  - Assessment stroke with an explorer, to check a surface for residual calculus.

II. Factors that Influence Selection of Stroke

- Size, contour, and position of gingiva

- Surface and section of surface where the instrument is used
- Probing depth
- Size and shape of instrument used
- Procedure objective, for example, nature of the deposit to be removed.

III. Nature of Stroke

A. Grasp

- The grasp of a scaler or curet is light while the working end is positioned for the stroke, and then the instrument is held more firmly during the activation stroke.
- An explorer and a probe are held lightly for tactile sensitivity at all times.

B. Hand Stability

- During a stroke, the whole hand pivots or rotates on the fulcrum.

C. Motion

- The motion for a stroke is generated by a unified action of the shoulder, arm, wrist, and hand.

D. Length

- The length of the scaling stroke is limited by the extent of calculus deposit and by the anatomic features of the area where the deposit is located.
- The stroke is short, controlled, decisive, and directed to protect the tissues from trauma.
- Instrumentation is applied to the section of the tooth where treatment is indicated. This section is called the *instrumentation zone*.
- Avoid strokes long enough to pass over the whole crown when the calculus represents only a small area at the cervical third of the tooth.
- The length of a stroke varies with each instrument and purpose. A description of strokes for each instrument is included in the respective sections of this chapter.
- Figure 39-8 shows direction of strokes for various instruments.

IV. Balance of Pressure

For control, a balance or an equalization of pressure is established between the instrument blade against the tooth surface and pressure on the fulcrum. Keeping the two forces equal will facilitate a stable, intentional control of the instrument as it is activated.

A. Assessment

- When exploring the tooth surface, the pressure of the instrument on the tooth is light.
- The grasp pressure of the fingers holding the instrument is also light, in order to achieve tactile sensitivity.

▶ The pressure of the rest, whether a fulcrum finger or hand, is light but secure and stable.

B. Calculus Removal

▶ When moving from assessment to activation of a working stroke, the pressure on the tooth and on the fulcrum increases significantly.

▶ The lateral pressure on the handle of the instrument engages the blade for the working stroke. This is equal to the pressure of the instrument against the tooth.

▶ As the working stroke is initiated to remove calculus on a tooth surface, the pressure of the instrument against the tooth is firm. It may vary from medium heavy to heavy depending on the age of the calculus and the strength of its attachment to the tooth.

▶ The pressure of the finger or hand rest (fulcrum) is equally firm to achieve stability and control of the instrument as it is activated.

C. Maintenance Root Debridement

▶ When removing dental biofilm from a tooth surface with minimal deposit, the pressure of the instrument on the tooth is light to moderate.

▶ The pressure of the specific grasp fingers supplying lateral pressure to the handle of the instrument equals the pressure of the blade on the tooth.

▶ The pressure of the finger/hand rest is similarly moderate.

▶ Pressures vary with the textures encountered.
  • When the texture changes from grainy to rough, the pressure of both finger/hand rest and blade against the tooth surface will increase in order to remove the deposit on the tooth surface.
  • Pressure is, therefore, responsive to the tactile information transmitted as the instrument progresses along the tooth surface.

VISIBILITY AND ACCESSIBILITY

I. Effects of Adequate Vision and Accessibility

▶ Instrumentation is more thorough.
▶ Trauma to the oral tissues is minimized.
▶ Length of time required for treatment may be lessened, thereby decreasing fatigue for patient and clinician.
▶ Patient cooperation can be increased because of shortened treatment time and less discomfort.

II. Contributing Factors

▶ Patient and clinician positions.
▶ Efficient use of direct or reflected illumination by mouth mirror for each tooth surface.

▶ Adequate, yet gentle, retraction of lips, cheeks, and tongue with consideration for the patient's comfort and clinician's convenience.

▶ Magnification: use of loupes.

DEXTERITY DEVELOPMENT

▶ The dental hygiene student or dental hygienist returning to practice after a temporary leave of absence can appreciate the need for exercises to develop dexterity and strength for the efficient and effective use of instruments.

▶ In addition, all students, returning retirees, and dental hygienists continuing in practice need an understanding of preventive measures to preserve the health of their hands, arms, shoulders, and all muscles and joints involved when undertaking patient care.

▶ However generally dexterous a person may be, the use of new or unusual instruments requires different procedures for coordination. Control is essential, and guided strength contributes to control.

▶ Proficiency during procedures comes from repeated correct use of the instruments.
  • Exercises for the fingers, hands, and arms supplement experience.
  • Directed exercises are needed for both hands, separately and together.
  • During the training period, a regular period of time each day can be set aside for exercises.

I. Squeezing Therapy Putty or a Soft Ball

A. Purpose

▶ Develop strength and control.

B. Procedure

▶ Hold putty in palm of hand; grip with thumb and all fingers (Figure 39-21A).
▶ Tighten and release grip at regular intervals.
▶ One hand rests while other is exercising.
▶ Use a ball in each hand to exercise at the same time.

II. Stretching

A. Purposes

▶ To strengthen finger and hand muscles.
▶ To develop control of finger movements.

B. Rubber Band on Finger Joints

▶ Place band at joint between first phalanx and second phalanx.
▶ Stretch band by separating middle and ring fingers (Figure 39-21B).
▶ Place band at joint between second phalanx and third phalanx and proceed as before.
▶ Place bands on both hands and do exercises together.

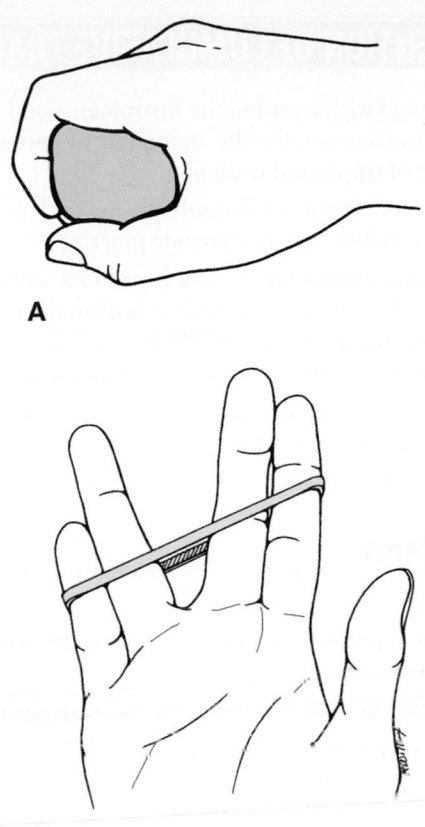

FIGURE 39-21 Exercises for Dexterity Development. A: Squeezing therapy putty can aid in developing strength and control. **B:** A rubber band can be applied at each group of finger and thumb joints and stretched.

C. Rubber Band on Finger Joints with Use of Fulcrum

▶ Place band on joint between first phalanx and second phalanx.

▶ Establish fulcrum (ring finger) on tabletop with little finger closely adjacent to it; elbow and forearm are free, as they are during instrumentation. Keep wrist straight, in same horizontal line as the forearm, and hold elbow at 90°. Stretch band by separating middle and ring fingers.

▶ Touch thumb and index and middle fingers to simulate a modified pen grasp for holding an instrument. Stretch band by separating middle and ring fingers.

▶ Variations
 • Hold instrument in modified pen grasp while doing the exercise.
 • Do writing exercise with rubber band in place.

▶ Rest one hand while other is being exercised.

III. Writing

A. Purposes

▶ To develop correct modified pen grasp.

▶ To propel instrument by activation from wrist and arm, without moving fingers.

▶ To practice use of instruments when mouth mirror is required.

▶ To develop control and precision.

B. Circles and Vertical Lines

▶ Hold long, well-sharpened pencil with modified pen grasp.

▶ Establish fulcrum (ring finger) on a piece of paper on tabletop. Keep wrist straight in line with forearm; elbow is at 90°, and shoulder is in neutral position. Forearm and elbow are free.

▶ Inscribe counterclockwise small circles and vertical lines on paper, rapidly and lightly at first, slowly and with more pressure later.

▶ Accomplish writing by activation of the hand by the upper arm, without flexing or extending the thumb and fingers holding the pencil.

▶ Practice with each hand separately at first; then use a pencil in each hand at the same time, alternating writing action to simulate adaptation of the mirror first and then the explorer or scaler.

C. Using Mouth Mirror

▶ Hold mouth mirror with modified pen grasp in nondominant hand close to pencil while practicing writing exercises (previous section) through the mirror. Reverse hands.

▶ Using engineer's graph paper and modified pen grasp with fulcrum as described earlier, follow the lines of the small squares while looking in mirror held with opposite hand.

D. Everyday Penmanship

▶ Use modified pen grasp whenever possible for writing.

▶ Practice word writing with the left hand (with the right hand for left-handed person) to increase dexterity for handling instruments.

IV. Mouth Mirror, Cotton Pliers, and Explorer

A. Purposes

▶ To develop ability to turn mouth mirror at various angles.

▶ To develop dexterity in holding objects with cotton pliers.

▶ To establish desired grasp of explorer to ensure maximum touch sensitivity.

B. Mouth Mirror

▶ Hold mouth mirror with modified pen grasp, ring finger on tabletop as fulcrum finger with little finger closely adjacent to it; elbow and forearm are free. The mirror is used most frequently in the nondominant hand.

▶ Practice turning mirror with fingers, adjusting as to the several surfaces of the tooth.

▶ Hold a small object in the dominant hand for viewing in mirror held in nondominant hand.

▶ Practice crossing the mirror over fulcrum finger as in position for retracting lower lip while viewing lingual surfaces of mandibular anterior teeth in mouth mirror.

C. Cotton Pliers

▶ Make small, tight cotton pellets with thumb and index and middle fingers of each hand; then make one in each hand simultaneously.

▶ Hold cotton pliers with modified pen grasp and establish fulcrum finger on tabletop; elbow and forearm are free.

▶ Practice picking up cotton pellets using mirror vision (right hand, then left).

• Use in wiping motion on tabletop or other object.

• Move to different area to release pellet as if to a waste-receiving cup.

V. Tactile Sensitivity

A. Explorer

▶ Mount small pieces of various grades of fine-grain sandpaper on a card.

▶ Hold explorer with modified pen grasp, and establish fulcrum finger on tabletop, with upper arm and forearm free. With eyes closed, compare roughness of the various grades of sandpaper. Use a light, exploring stroke.

▶ Use extracted teeth to feel with explorer tip until a light grasp permits maximum security of grasp and maximum sense of touch. Extracted teeth can be used to provide a contrast between exploring enamel, cementum, calculus, or other rough area of tooth surface.

B. Probe

▶ Repeat exercises described for explorer.

▶ Compare with explorer.

PREVENTION OF CUMULATIVE TRAUMA

Hand in hand with learning the instruments and attaining dexterity in their use for the treatment of patients is the well-being of the dental hygienist.

▶ Primary occupational hazards are related to personal everyday habits during chairside practice.

▶ The symptoms of carpal tunnel syndrome are caused by compression of the median nerve within the carpal tunnel as shown in Figure 39-18B. Figure 7-7 in Chapter 7 shows the anatomy of the carpel tunnel wrist area.

Along with the exercises for the development of strength and control in the hands, other types of exercises are needed for maintaining general musculoskeletal health.

I. Problems

▶ Posture.

▶ Extended periods of time spent in the same work position.

▶ Repetitive movements during actual instrumentation.

▶ Study and plan for action in advance, before serious disability can occur.

II. Exercises

▶ Stretching exercises for stress release, improvement of posture, and counteracting repetitive movements used during instrumentation are suggested in Figure 39-22.

▶ Additional exercises are shown in Figure 7-8, Chapter 7.

III. Clinical Application

▶ Exercises performed chairside, between appointments, can contribute greatly to long-range prevention.

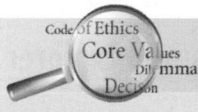 **EVERYDAY ETHICS**

Brittany joins a new private practice office. There is a long time hygienist, Connie, at the practice and all the patients love her. After working with the practice for several months, Brittany notices some of Connie's regular patients have been put into her schedule. When updating the bite-wing radiographs on several of the patients, she sees large ledges of calculus on proximal surfaces. When updating the periodontal examination, Brittany finds many pockets 2–3 mm deeper than noted in previous records. Brittany reviews the findings and radiographs with the dentist and it is determined that quadrant nonsurgical periodontal therapy is required. The patients involved become quite upset when the treatment plan is presented because she has been coming in every 6 months for maintenance care. At a team meeting, Brittany and Connie discuss what

instruments should be ordered and it comes to Brittany's attention that Connie uses only a Barnhart 5/6 and sickle scaler. Connie also states that she doesn't like to do scaling and root planing.

Questions for Consideration

1. Given Brittany's novice status as a clinician, how will she approach Connie—an experienced practitioner—with her concerns? Which core values of dental hygiene (Table II-1 in Section II, Introduction) are involved in this scenario?

2. What harm, if any, is affecting the patients?

3. Utilizing an ethical decision framework (see Chapter 1), describe realistic alternatives for Brittany's course of action in this situation.

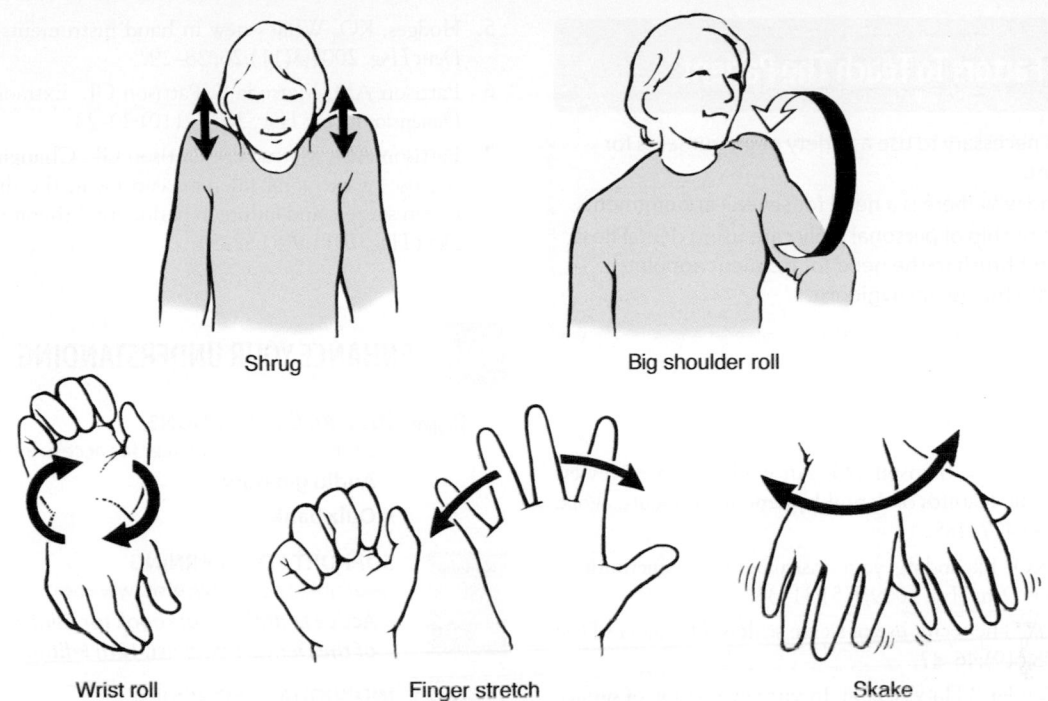

Shrug

Big shoulder roll

Wrist roll

Finger stretch

Shake

FIGURE 39-22 Chairside Stretching Exercises. Stretching exercises to relax the back, shoulders, and neck are shown with the shrug and rolling the head around with the big shoulder roll. Hand and finger rolls, stretches, and shaking can be performed anytime, even while attending a patient.

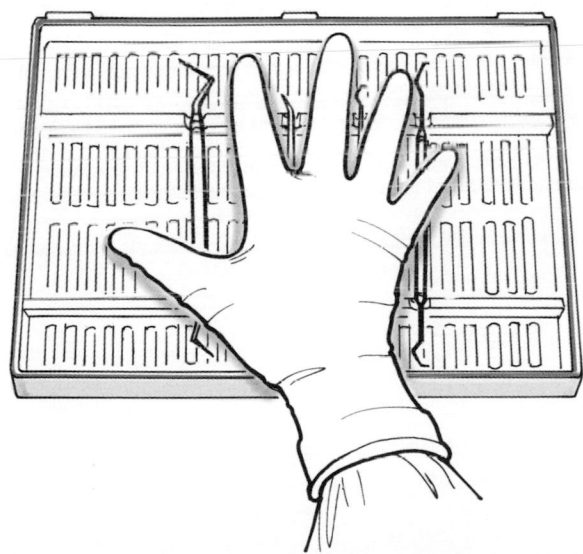

FIGURE 39-23 Stretching Fingers Prior to Instrument Retrieval. One of the exercises that can be used during actual clinical practice.

▶ One idea for an exercise during patient treatment is shown in Figure 39-23. Each time an instrument is returned to the cassette, fingers and wrists can be stretched before picking up the next instrument needed.

DOCUMENTATION

Documentation of instrument selection and instrumentation techniques in a patient record can provide guidance during subsequent dental hygiene care. For example, notes made in the patient record may include the following:

▶ Identification of specific instruments used in specific areas, such as minicurets used to access a particularly deep pocket area.

▶ Areas in the patient's dentition that require more careful attention or careful application of skill.

▶ An example progress note is found in Box 39-2.

BOX 39-2

Example Documentation: Specialized Instruments Used on Select Tooth Surface

S –Female patient, 48 years old and in good health, presents for third in a series of non-surgical periodontal therapy (NSPT) appointments (maxillary left quadrant).

O –Previously documented assessment findings for maxillary left quadrant include: heavy generalized calculus, generalized 4–5 mm probing depths, and 8 mm probing depth on the mesial of #12 and distal of #15 (furcation involvement).

A –In addition to the ultrasonic and standard manual instruments, area-specific after five and minicuret instruments may be needed to assess and scale and debride in deeper pocket areas.

P –Completed quadrant debridement with ultrasonic and manual instruments. Minicurets with a long lower shank were used, with both diagonal and horizontal strokes, to root plane the deep pocket in the mesial concavity of #12 and distal furcation of #15.

Next steps: Scheduled for NSPT on mandibular left quadrant and re-evaluate all areas of previously treated quadrants, particularly deep pocket areas.

Signed: _____, RDH
Date: _____

Factors To Teach The Patient

▷ Why it is necessary to use a variety of instruments for treatment.

▷ When and why there is a need for several appointments.

▷ The relationship of personal daily care using dental floss and a toothbrush to the need for frequent appointments with the dental hygienist.

References

1. Simmer-Beck M, Branson BG. An evidence-based review of ergonomic features of dental hygiene instruments. *Work.* 2010;35(4):477–485.

2. Hodges KO. Expanding your instrument armamentarium. *Dimensions Dent Hyg.* 2009;7(5):31–33.

3. Pattison A. The secret use of sickle scalers. *Dimensions Dent Hyg.* 2008;6(9):46–47.

4. Eick S, Bender P, Flury S, et al. In vitro evaluation of surface roughness, adhesion of periodontal ligament fibroblasts, and Streptococcusgordonii following root instrumentation with Gracey curettes and subsequent polishing with diamond-coated curettes. *Clin Oral Investig.* 2013;17(2):397–404.

5. Hodges, KO. What's new in hand instruments. *Dimensions Dent Hyg.* 2005;3(11):26, 28–29.

6. Pattison AM, Matsuda S, Pattison GL. Extraoral fulcrums. *Dimensions Dent Hyg.* 2004;2(10):20–23.

7. Pattison AM, Matsuda S, Pattison GL. Changing the rules: the use of extraoral fulcrums can mean the difference between success and failure in periodontal therapy. *Dimensions Dent Hyg.* 2011;9(5):52–54.

ENHANCE YOUR UNDERSTANDING

thePoint® DIGITAL CONNECTIONS
(see the inside front cover for access information)

· **Audio glossary**

· **Quiz bank**

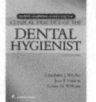

SUPPORT FOR LEARNING
(available separately; visit lww.com)

· *Active Learning Workbook for Clinical Practice of the Dental Hygienist, 12th Edition*

prepU INDIVIDUALIZED REVIEW
(available separately; visit lww.com)

· **Adaptive quizzing with *prepU* for Wilkins' *Clinical Practice of the Dental Hygienist***

40

Instrument Care and Sharpening

Esther M. Wilkins, BS, RDH, DMD and Linda D. Boyd, RDH, RD, EdD

CHAPTER OUTLINE

LEARNING OBJECTIVES

After studying this chapter, the student will be able to:

1. Describe benefits of using sharp instruments.

2. Describe the consequences of using dull instruments.

3. Demonstrate proper technique for sharpening procedures for a variety of periodontal instruments.

4. Explain how to preserve optimal instrument design when sharpening.

INSTRUMENT SHARPENING

*Objectives for techniques of sharpening emphasize the **preservation of the original shape of the blade** while restoring a sharp cutting edge.*

▶ Instruments designed for a particular purpose need to continue to be used in the manner for which they were designed.

- Inaccurate sharpening techniques can distort the blade and render the instrument useless for its intended purpose.

▶ Sharpening is an essential and integral part of instrumentation.

- Sharpening procedures are technique sensitive and require skill and patience to become proficient.
- Instrument sharpness is checked at the beginning and during each appointment.

▶ Successful clinical outcomes with bladed instruments are dependent on correctly contoured and sharpened instruments.

▶ Frequent (daily) sharpening prevents loss of blade structure so recontouring to restore the original shape is not necessary.

▶ Terms related to instrument sharpening are defined in Box 40-1.

I. Benefits from Use of Sharp Manual Instruments

Instruments must be sharp if scaling, root planing, or debridement is to be completed efficiently with minimal trauma to the tissues. When the instrument blade is maintained with its original contour and sharp cutting edges, the following may be expected:

▶ Greater precision of treatment, improved quality of results, and less working time involved.

▶ Increased tactile sensitivity during instrumentation. A sharp instrument does not have to be gripped as firmly as a dull one.

▶ Greater control of the instrument because of the lighter grasp needed; less pressure on the tooth being scaled or planed and decreased pressure on the finger rest are required.

▶ Fewer strokes required.

▶ Less possibility of burnishing rather than removing the calculus.

▶ Prevention of unnecessary trauma to gingival tissues and, therefore, less discomfort experienced by the patient.

▶ Decreased possibility of nicking, grooving, or scratching the tooth surfaces.

▶ Less fatigue for the clinician.

II. Consequences of Using Dull Manual Instruments

▶ Stress and frustration of using ineffective instruments.

▶ Wasted time, effort, and energy.

▶ Loss of control and increased likelihood of slipping with instrument and lacerating the gingival tissue.

▶ Loss of patient confidence in clinician's ability.

▶ Increased likelihood of developing work-related musculoskeletal disorders (WMDs) from excessive muscle strain and increased number of stroke repetitions.

III. Dynamics of Sharpening[1]

Instrument sharpening is accomplished by filing the surface or surfaces that form the cutting edge.

A. Cutting Edge

▶ The cutting edge is a very fine *line* formed where the face and lateral surface meet at an angle (see Figure 40-1).

▶ The edge becomes dull when pressed against a hard surface (the tooth), or it may be nicked when drawn over a rough surface.

▶ A dull edge is rounded and therefore has thickness (Figure 40-2). *The object in sharpening is to reshape the cutting edge to a fine line.*

- Approximately 45 scaling strokes creates a very rounded cutting edge, even 15 strokes results in a slightly rounded cutting edge.[1]

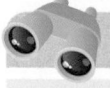

BOX 40-1 | **KEY WORDS: Sharpening**

Arkansas stone: fine-grained sharpening stone quarried from natural mineral deposits.

Burnish: to smooth and polish; an effect that can result when a dull scaler or curet is passed over tenacious calculus in an attempt to remove the deposit.

Cutting edge: the fine line formed where the face and lateral surfaces of a scaler or curet meet when the instrument is sharp; when the instrument is dull, the line has thickness and may even reflect light.

Hone: a sharpening stone (noun).
Honing: sharpening (verb).
Sharpness: when a scaler or curet is sharp, the cutting edge is a fine line that does not reflect light.
Testing stick: plastic 1/4-inch rod, 3 inches long, used to test the sharpness of a scaler or a curet.

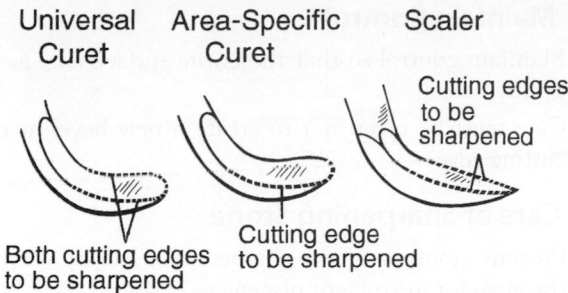

FIGURE 40-1   **Selection of Cutting Edge to Sharpen.** Both cutting edges and the rounded toe are sharpened for a universal curet. An area-specific curet is sharpened on the longer cutting edge and the rounded toe. A scaler is sharpened on the two sides, and the tip is brought to a point.

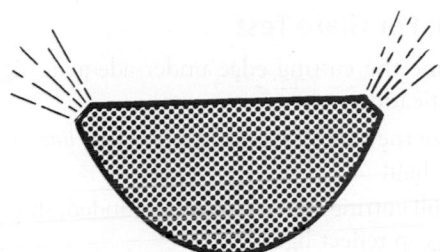

FIGURE 40-2   **Cross Section of a Dull Curet.** A sharp curet has a fine line at the cutting edge that will not reflect light. A dull cutting edge is like a small surface and reflects light as shown.

B. Sharpening Stone Surface

▶ A sharpening stone acts as an abrasive to reshape a dulled blade by grinding the surface until the cutting edge is restored.

▶ The surface of the stone is made up of masses of minute crystals, which are the abrasive particles that accomplish the grinding of the instrument.

▶ A smaller particle size or a finer grit abrades or reduces more slowly and produces a finer cutting edge.

IV. Types of Sharpening Devices

A. Stones

▶ *Natural abrasive stones:* Quarried from mineral deposits.

• Manual sharpening with an Arkansas stone (fine grit) produces a better cutting edge than synthetic stones or power-driven devices (Figure 40-3A).[2,3]

• India stones are also used for manual sharpening and come in a variety of grits (Figure 40-3B).

▶ *Artificial materials*

• Hard, nonmetallic substances impregnated with aluminum oxide, silicon carbide, or diamond particles. Examples: ruby stone, carborundum stones, and the diamond hone.

• Ceramic aluminum oxide (Figure 40-3C).

• Steel alloys are metals that are harder than most dental instrument steel and, therefore, are capable of sharpening the instrument.

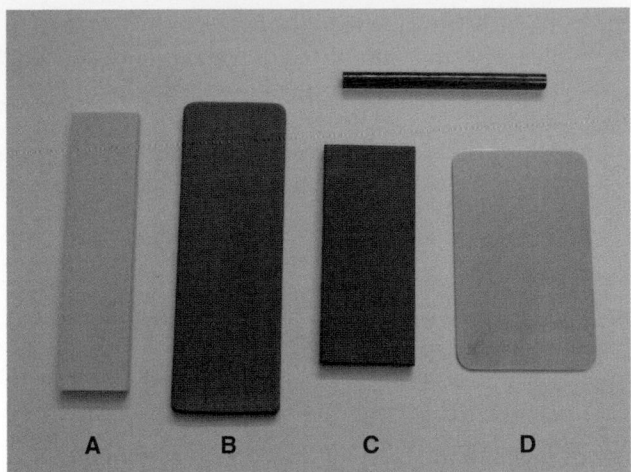

FIGURE 40-3   **Types of Sharpening Stones. A:** Arkansas stone. **B:** India stone. **C:** Ceramic stone. **D:** Diamond-sharpening stone.

• Diamond-coated stainless steel sharpening card is about the size of a credit card and used in the same way as other sharpening stones (Figure 40-3D).

B. Power-Driven or Mechanical Sharpening Devices

▶ A number of manufacturers offer power-driven sharpening devices.

▶ Research suggests a better cutting edge is created with manual sharpening.[2]

BASIC SHARPENING PRINCIPLES

I. Sterilization of the Sharpening Stone

▶ A sterile sharpening stone and testing stick are parts of a basic clinical setup for a scaling appointment.

▶ Sterilization of stones may be accomplished using any of the acceptable sterilization methods described in Chapter 6, in accordance with specific manufacturer's recommendations.

▶ Over time, the steam autoclave may dry out an Arkansas stone and lead to chipping or breakage.

II. Instrument Handling

All instruments must be handled with care to preserve sharpness and prevent accidental damage to the cutting edges.

III. Preparation of Stone for Sharpening

A. Dry Stone

▶ *Advantage:* The problems related to maintaining a sterile stone and preventing contamination when oil, tap water, or a lubricant is applied are eliminated.

▶ A dry stone contributes to the following effects:
- Sharpens the cutting edge without nicks in the blade; nicks can be created from particles of metal suspended in a lubricant.
- Allows the stone to be completely sterilized without the problem of interference by the oil left in and on the stone.

B. Water on Stone

▶ Water can be used for lubrication of ceramic stones, but they may also be used dry.

C. Lubricated Stone

▶ Oil lubrication is recommended with certain quarried stones such as the Arkansas stone to prevent drying out.

▶ Instruments are autoclaved before sharpening, and the stone and instruments are sterilized again after nonsterile lubricant is used.

▶ The lubricant can facilitate the movement of the instrument blade over the stone to prevent scratching of the stone.
- Suspend the metallic particles removed during sharpening.
- Help to prevent clogging of the pores of the stone (glazing).

IV. Sharpening Overview

A. Objectives

The objectives during sharpening are twofold:
▶ To produce a sharp cutting edge.
▶ To preserve the original shape of the instrument.
- Instrument shape is also known as contour.
- The contour of a curet toe is a smooth, continuous curvature with no points or flat edges.

B. When to Sharpen

▶ Sharpen at the first sign of dullness during an appointment.

▶ When instruments become grossly dulled, recontouring wastes the instrument.

▶ Restoring original contour to a grossly dull instrument often leaves a blade that is not functional.

▶ Replace severely dulled instruments.

C. Angulation

▶ Before starting to sharpen, analyze the cutting edge and establish the proper angle between the stone and the blade surface.

▶ Maintain the angle through the firm grasp, secure hand rest, moderate pressure, short stroke, and other features of the technique appropriate to the individual instrument.

D. Maintain Control

▶ Maintain control so that the entire surface is reduced evenly.

▶ Care must be taken not to create a new bevel at the cutting edge.

E. Care of Sharpening Stone

▶ Prevent grooving of the sharpening stone by varying the areas for instrument placement.

▶ Cleaning and stain removal procedures are described in section on Care of Sharpening Equipment in this chapter.

V. Tests for Instrument Sharpness[4]

A. Visual or Glare Test

▶ Examine the cutting edge under adequate light using magnification.

▶ Because the sharp cutting edge is a fine *line*, it does not reflect light.

▶ The dull cutting edge presents a rounded, shiny *surface*, which can reflect light.
- Figure 40-2 shows the cross section of a dull universal curet.
- The dull cutting edges are tiny surfaces that reflect light.
- Compare the cutting edges in Figure 40-2 with Figure 39-2 in Chapter 39, which shows the sharp cutting edges, at the points labeled "c," on a universal curet.

B. Plastic Testing Stick (See Figure 40-4)

▶ Use a sterile plastic or acrylic 1/4-inch rod, 3 inches long.
▶ Place the fulcrum finger on the end of the stick.
▶ Apply the heel (shank end) of the cutting edge to the plastic stick, first at 90°, then closed to the correct angle for scaling (70°).
▶ Press lightly but firmly.

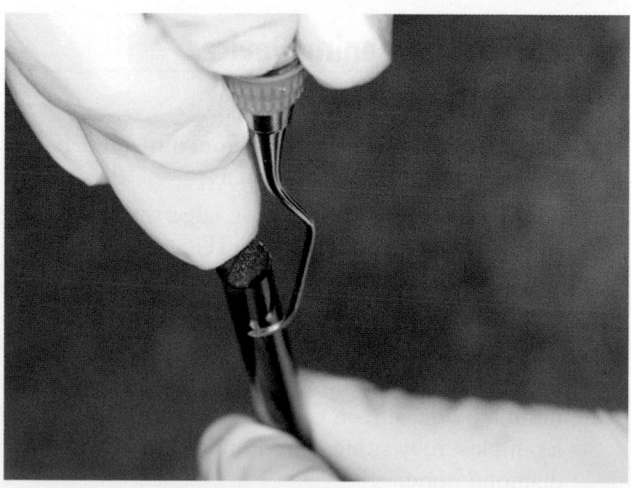

FIGURE 40-4 Plastic Testing Stick. Sharpness can be evaluated using a test stick. A test stick is a cylindrical rod made of plastic or acrylic. (Reprinted from Nield-Gehrig J. Fundamentals of Periodontal Instrumentation and Advanced Root Instrumentation. Philadelphia: Lippincott Williams & Wilkins; 2011.)

► Roll the cutting edge forward from the shank end to the toe by turning or rolling the instrument handle in the fingers to test the entire length of the blade.

C. Confirming Sharpness Using the Plastic Testing Stick

► The *sharp* cutting edge engages or grips the plastic as the length of the blade is tested. Each portion of the cutting edge will engage the plastic uniformly as the blade advances.

► The *dull* cutting edge does not catch without undue pressure and slides easily over the surface of the stick.

► Because the edge is not uniformly dulled during use, there will be portions of a blade that exhibit varying degrees of sharpness or dullness.

► As the instrument blade is rolled along the testing stick, the degree of slipping versus engagement will indicate the degree of sharpness or dullness. If only limited portions of the blade exhibit dullness, attempt to note the segments that slip as the blade is rolled along the testing stick.
  • The entire length of the cutting edge is always sharpened to maintain the original form.
  • Awareness of the portion(s) exhibiting dullness can guide pressure and the number of strokes.
  • This helps to minimize oversharpening.
  • Careful evaluation will increase efficiency and raise the likelihood that dull portions of the blade are restored to sharpness.

VI. Evaluation of Technique

► Observe closely the stabilization of both the instrument and stone, each kept aligned in a single plane, to evaluate sharpening technique.
  • *Self-check:* As the stone is activated for sharpening, observe the top of the instrument to ensure it is secure and not moving.
  • *Self-check:* Observe stone to ensure it remains in a single plane of movement back and forth as it is activated.

► Evaluate by turning the instrument over to examine the back of the lateral surfaces under well-lit magnification.

► A solid, consistent bevel results from:
  • Instrument and stone positioned at the correct angle.
  • Movement occurring in a single plane.

► Irregular bevel is revealed by:
  • Breaks in the fine line of the blade edge.
  • Varying facets indicating the improper stone placement/movement.

VII. After Sharpening

A. Finishing the Instrument

Newly sharpened instruments are finished by carefully inspecting the edges for a clean consistent bevel with no particles or "wire edge" remaining.

B. How the Wire Edge Is Produced

► During sharpening, some of the metal particles removed during grinding remain attached to the edge of the instrument and create the wire edge (Figure 40-5).

► If allowed to remain, the tiny particles may be removed when the instrument is applied to the tooth surface during treatment.

C. Removal of Wire Edge

► Wipe the instrument carefully with a dry gauze square or an alcohol wipe to remove particles.

VIII. Instrument Wear

► As curets are used, the cutting edge wears down, leaving a narrower face and shorter length over a period of time.

► Sharpening also contributes to the size reduction.

► After sufficient reduction, instruments must be retired and discarded.
  • Blades will no longer access or adapt to the tooth surface.
  • Thinner blades are more susceptible to breakage with lateral pressure.

► Used instruments that have become excessively narrow are reserved for patients with minimal deposit and require biofilm debridement only.

► Exert care when using overly thinned curets. If strong lateral pressure is applied, they may break off at the tip, leaving the last few millimeters embedded in the sulcus or pocket.

► Evaluation during sharpening procedures provides the opportunity for proper attention to instrument maintenance.
  • Consider usefulness and suitability of instruments for various procedures as they are sharpened and assigned to tray setups or instrument cassettes.

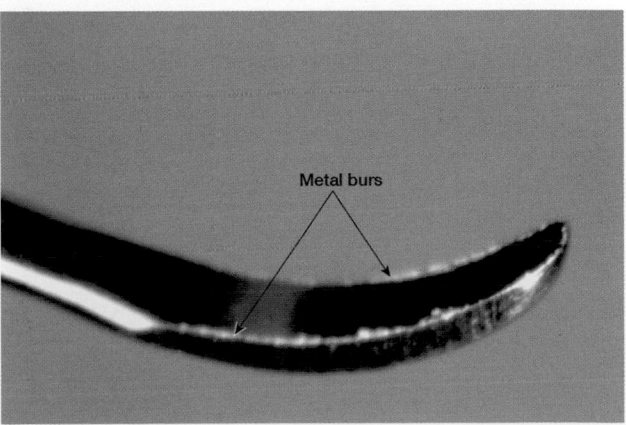

FIGURE 40-5 Wire Edge After Sharpening. Sharpening can produce minute metal burs that project from the cutting edge. (Reprinted from Nield-Gehrig J. Fundamentals of Periodontal Instrumentation and Advanced Root Instrumentation. Philadelphia: Lippincott Williams & Wilkins; 2011.)

- Assign thinner-bladed instruments for use with patients who do not require moderate or heavy calculus removal.
- Discard or recycle instruments that have outlived their usefulness with shortened blades that cannot access proximal surfaces sufficiently.

SHARPENING CURETS AND SCALERS

In the following sections, procedures for a variety of sharpening techniques are outlined.

I. Technique Objectives

▶ Preserve the original contour of the blade.

▶ Sharpen frequently to prevent need for excessive recontouring of the blade.

II. Selection of Cutting Edges to Sharpen

A. Scalers/Sickles

▶ Most scalers are universal instruments.

▶ Cutting edges on both sides of the face are sharpened (Figure 40-1).

▶ A two-step sharpening procedure is used.

B. Curets: Universal

▶ Cutting edges on both sides of the face and the toe are sharpened (Figure 40-1).

▶ A three-step sharpening procedure is used.

C. Curets: Area Specific

▶ Cutting edge on one side of the face and the toe are sharpened.

▶ Sharpen the longer cutting edge; generally it will be the one farthest from the handle. In Figure 40-1, it is indicated by the dotted line.

▶ A two-step sharpening procedure is used: one side of the face and the toe.

MOVING FLAT STONE: STATIONARY INSTRUMENT

▶ The side of the cutting edge formed by the lateral surface is reduced by this method.

▶ The technique described applies to both curets and scalers.

▶ Because the scaler has a pointed tip and the curet has a round toe end, a variation is necessary in the adaptation of the sharpening stone to that portion of the blade.

I. Examine the Cutting Edge to Be Sharpened

Test for sharpness to determine specific areas that are dull, but plan to sharpen the whole cutting edge(s) to maintain original contour.

II. Review the Angulation to Be Restored at the Dull Cutting Edge

▶ Internal angle of the blade at the cutting edge(s) is 70° to 80° (Figures 39-5 and 39-11 in Chapter 39).

▶ Visible angle at which the stone will be placed will be 110°, as shown in Figure 40-6.

III. Stabilize and Position the Instrument[3,4]

▶ Grasp the instrument in the nondominant hand in a palm grasp.

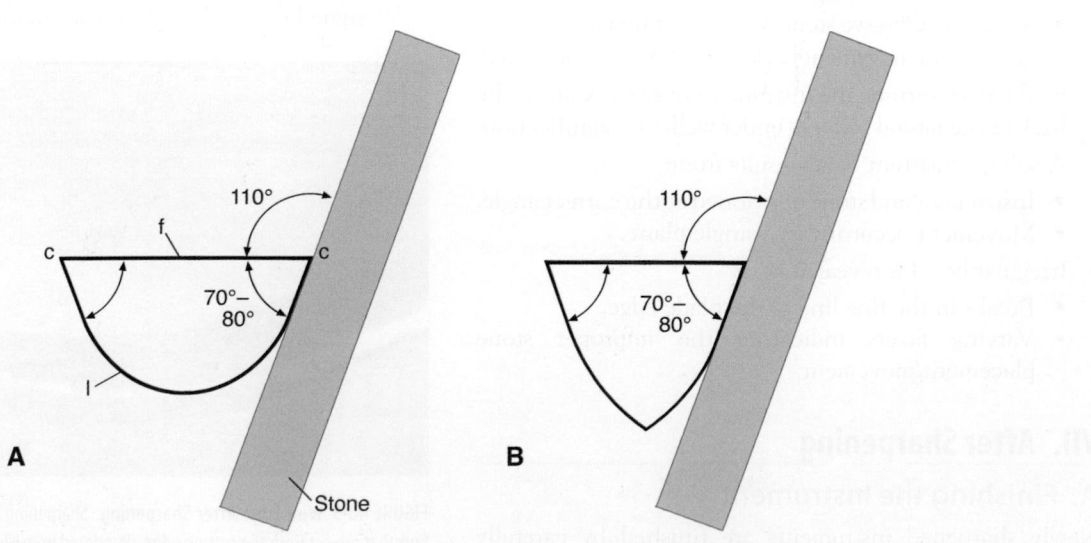

FIGURE 40-6 Angulation for Sharpening. A: Cross sections of a curet and **(B)** a scaler show correct angulation of the face (f) of the blade with the flat sharpening stone to reproduce the internal angle of the instrument at 70°. Note the cutting edges (c) and the lateral surfaces (l).

▶ Lean the hand against the edge of an immovable workbench or table under bright light (Figure 40-7A).

▶ The instrument is positioned low enough to allow the clinician to see the cutting edges clearly.

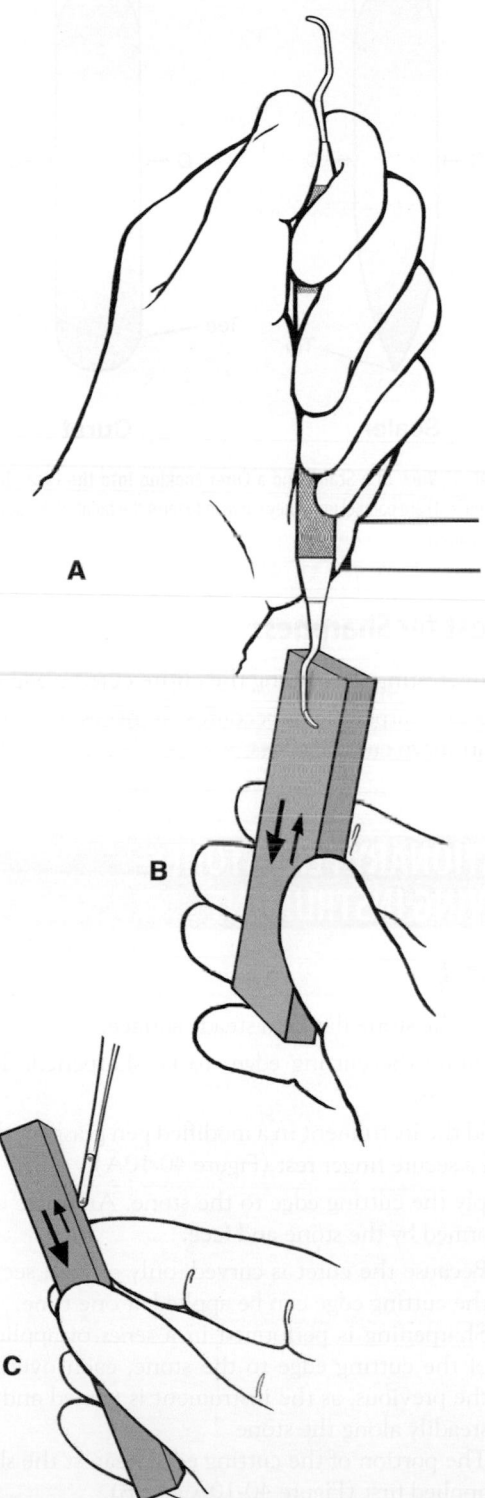

A

B

C

FIGURE 40-7 **Stationary Instrument—Moving Stone Technique. A:** Grasp the instrument with the nondominant hand. Stabilize the hand on the edge of a stationary table or bench and provide good light on the instrument. **B:** The stone is angled with the face of the instrument at 110° to maintain the internal angle of the blade at 70° to 80°. **C:** Stone reversed to sharpen the opposite cutting edge of a universal curet.

▶ Turn the face of the instrument up and parallel with the floor. Point the curet toe (or scaler tip) toward the clinician to provide better access for moving the stone (Figure 40-8B).

▶ Note the shape of the face as shown in Figure 40-9.

▶ The cutting edges begin at the lower shank.

▶ The cutting edges are parallel, until they converge.

▶ For the curet, the cutting edges curve to form the toe.

▶ For the scaler, the cutting edges taper to make the pointed tip.

IV. Apply the Sharpening Stone

▶ Hold the stone perpendicular to the floor, at the shank third of the cutting edge.

▶ From the 90° angle with the face of the instrument, open the stone to make an angle of 110° (Figures 40-7C and 40-8A).

V. Activate the Sharpening Stone

A. Steps One and Two

▶ Maintain the stone in contact with the blade and at the proper angle throughout the procedure.

▶ Tighten the grasp on the instrument (nondominant hand) while applying a smooth even pressure to the cutting edge to keep the instrument stable and motionless.

▶ Move the stone up and down with short rhythmical strokes about ½-inch high. Place more pressure on the down stroke. Maintain the 110° angle precisely. Finish each area with a down stroke.

▶ *For the universal curet*
 • Follow the cutting edge to where the curvature for the toe begins, applying 3 or 4 down strokes overlapping at each millimeter of the cutting edge.
 • Proceed to the opposite side to sharpen, repeating the steps just described (Figure 40-7).
 • Next, proceed to the third step to sharpen the toe.

▶ *For the area-specific curet:* Apply sharpening strokes **only** to the one selected side: proceed to the third step to sharpen all around the toe.

▶ *For the scaler:* Follow the same procedure to where the cutting edge tapers to form the sharp tip and continue in that direction to finish that side of the blade. Proceed to the other side to sharpen the opposite cutting edge.

B. Step Three: The Toe of a Curet[1]

▶ Tip curet down to make the toe parallel with floor.

▶ Apply stone to make a 90° angle with the toe.

▶ Open the stone to make a 110° angle.

▶ Apply strokes for sharpening as described for the sides of the face of the blade.

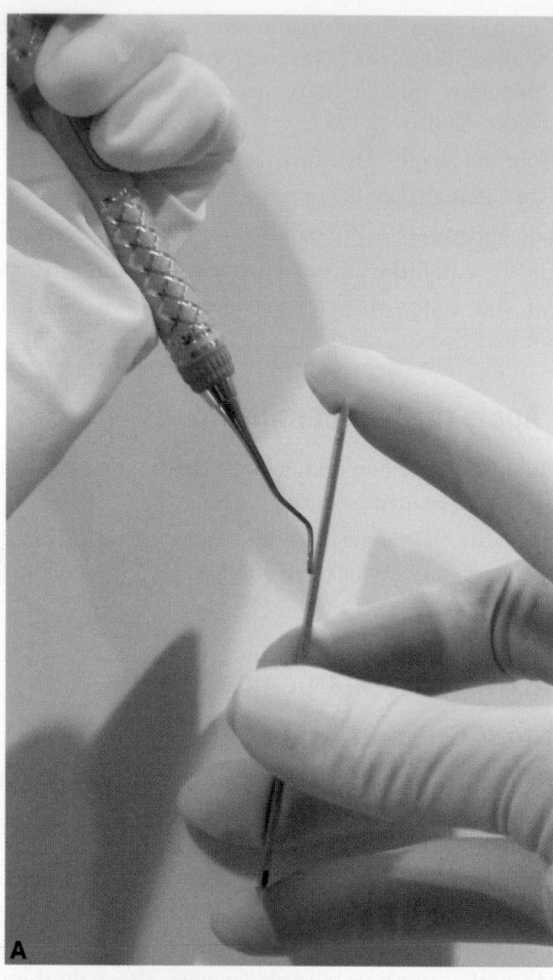

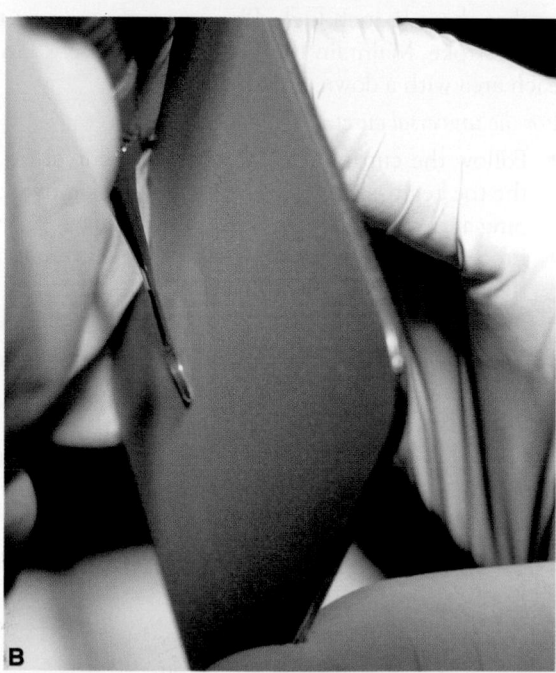

FIGURE 40-8 Stationary Instrument—Moving Diamond-Sharpening Card (A and B) Grasp the instrument with the nondominant hand. Stabilize the hand. The card is angled with the face of the instrument at 110° to maintain the internal angle of the blade at 70° to 80°. **B:** This image shows how the orientation of the diamond-sharpening card to the instrument face and blade look to the clinician during the sharpening process.

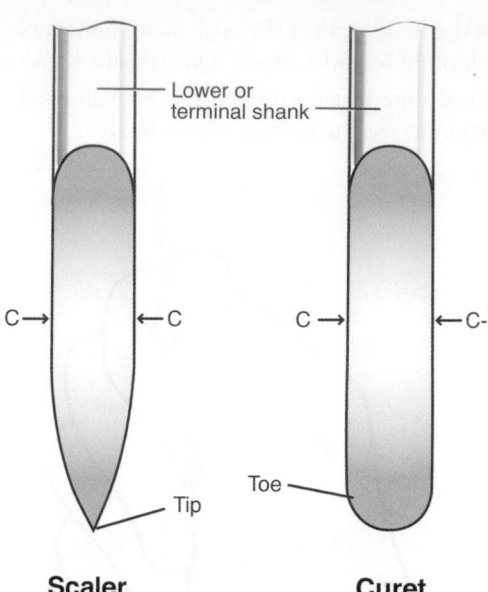

Scaler   **Curet**

FIGURE 40-9 View of a Scaler and a Curet Looking Into the Face. The cutting edges (c and c-1) are parallel until they curve in to form the pointed tip (scaler) or the round toe (curet).

VI. Test for Sharpness

▶ Apply testing stick along the entire cutting edges.

▶ Repeat sharpening procedures as necessary to retain clean sharp cutting edges.

STATIONARY FLAT STONE: MOVING INSTRUMENT

I. Curet

▶ Place the stone flat on a steady surface.

▶ Examine the cutting edges to be sharpened. Test for sharpness.

▶ Hold the instrument in a modified pen grasp, and establish a secure finger rest (Figure 40-10A).

▶ Apply the cutting edge to the stone. An angle of 110° is formed by the stone and face.

   • Because the curet is curved, only a small section of the cutting edge can be applied at one time.

   • Sharpening is performed in a *series* of applications of the cutting edge to the stone, each overlapping the previous, as the instrument is turned and drawn steadily along the stone.

   • The portion of the cutting edge nearest the shank is applied first (Figure 40-10A and B).

▶ Apply moderate to light but firm pressure while the instrument is activated.

▶ Use a slow, steady stroke to maintain control and to ensure that each portion of the cutting edge receives equal treatment.

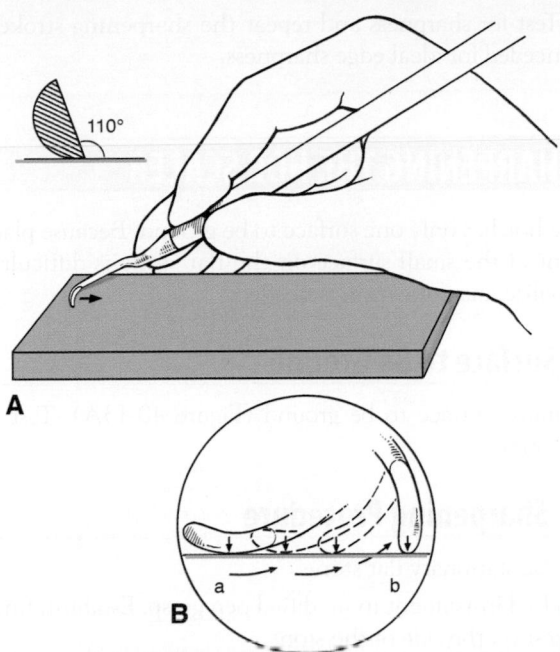

FIGURE 40-10 **Stationary Stone—Moving Instrument Technique for a Curet.** **A:** Stone placed flat with blade in position at the beginning of the sharpening stroke. With the finger rest stabilized on the edge of the stone, the cutting edge is maintained at the proper angulation (110°) as the instrument is drawn along the stone with an even, moderate pressure. **B:** The movement of the blade is shown by the arrows, which indicate each portion of the cutting edge as the blade is turned on the stone from the beginning (a) to the completion (b) of the stroke at the center of the round toe of the curet. For a universal curet, the instrument is turned over and the opposite cutting edge is sharpened.

▶ Move the blade forward into the cutting edge. Turn the instrument continuously until the center of the round end of the blade is reached (Figure 40-10A and B).

▶ Test for sharpness along the entire cutting edge; reapply to stone as necessary for ideal sharpness.

▶ Turn the instrument to sharpen the second cutting edge. Overlap at the center of the round toe. Universal curets are sharpened on both sides and around the toe. Gracey curets are sharpened on one side only and around the toe (see Figure 40-1).

▶ Carefully wipe the instrument with a gauze square or an alcohol wipe to remove the wire edge.

II. Scaler: Sickle or Jacquette

▶ Place the stone flat on a firm table or bench top under adequate light. Do not tilt the stone while sharpening.

▶ Examine cutting edges to be sharpened. Test for sharpness.

▶ Hold the instrument with a firm pen grasp, using thumb, index, and middle (second) fingers to prevent the instrument from rotating or changing angles during sharpening (Figure 40-11A).

▶ Establish finger rest on side of stone using ring and little fingers.

▶ Stabilize stone with fingers of opposite hand.

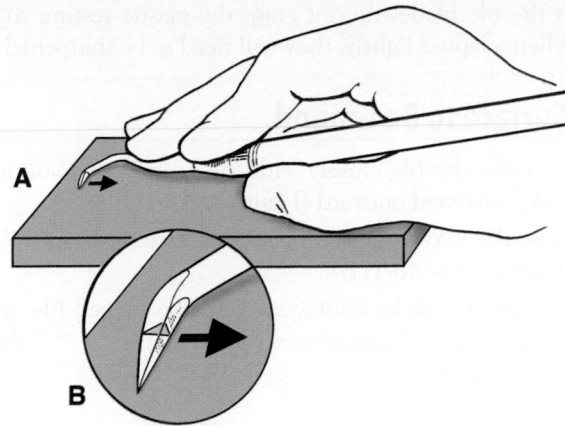

FIGURE 40-11 **Stationary Stone Technique for a Straight Scaler. A:** With a modified pen grasp and a finger rest established on the side of the stone, the scaler is positioned for sharpening. **B:** The portion of the cutting edge nearest the lower shank is applied first with an angle of 110° between the face and the stone. The instrument is turned continuously to follow the arclike shape of the blade. The cutting edges are sharpened to the pointed tip.

▶ Apply cutting edge to be sharpened to the stone. Maintain 70° to 80° internal angle of the instrument (Figure 40-11B). The portion of the cutting edge nearest the shank is applied first.

▶ Apply moderate to light but firm pressure while instrument is in motion. Heavy pressure can reduce control of instrument, cause scratching of the stone, and produce an unfavorable bevel at the cutting edge.

▶ Use a short, slow stroke to maintain the exact relation of the cutting edge to the stone.
- Pull blade forward, toward the cutting edge.
- All fingers move with the arm as a unit.
- Use a slow, steady stroke to maintain control and to ensure that each portion of the cutting edge receives equal treatment.
- Turn the instrument continually to follow the shape of the blade to the pointed tip.

▶ Test for sharpness after one or two strokes. Repeat as needed for ideal sharpness.

▶ Turn instrument and proceed to sharpen other lateral surface. When instrument placement is awkward for a modified contra-angle scaler, use a narrow side of the stone.

SHARPENING THE FILE SCALER

▶ Files are sharpened with a flat sharpening instrument called a *tanged file*.
- Diamond-coated files are *not* sharpened.

▶ Use of magnification and good illumination are necessary when sharpening files to ensure correct placement of the tanged file.

▶ Use a testing stick to check for the degree of sharpness to determine whether the file will need to be sharpened.

▶ If the file blades do not grasp the plastic testing stick when adapted lightly, they will need to be sharpened.

I. Surface to Be Ground

▶ Examine the file closely with the head of the working end positioned outward (Figure 40-12A).

▶ Note the two angular surfaces that meet to form a "V" shape (Figure 40-12B).

▶ The surface to be contacted with the tanged file and ground during sharpening is the surface of the "V" that is farthest away.

II. Sharpening Procedure

▶ Prepare a workplace with good illumination and some means of magnification such as loupes or a magnified light ring.

▶ Place the sterile file on a clean surface. Secure it with the series of teeth facing up.

▶ Position the right end of the tanged file in the channel as shown in the illustration (Figure 40-12A). (Left-handed clinicians reverse the process, positioning the left end of the tanged file in the channel.)

▶ With light-to-moderate steady pressure, pull the tanged file through the channel, moving in a straight line from one end to the other in one direction only.

▶ Release pressure and reposition the tanged file back at the starting point. Repeat the process. Two or three passes with the tanged file are usually sufficient to bring each edge back to sharpness.

▶ Sharpen the remaining blades using the same technique.

▶ Test for sharpness and repeat the sharpening stroke as needed for ideal edge sharpness.

SHARPENING THE HOE SCALER

The hoe has only one surface to be ground. Because placement of the small surface on the flat stone is difficult to visualize, magnification is needed.

I. Surface to Be Ground

Examine surface to be ground (Figure 40-13A). Test for sharpness.

II. Sharpening Procedure

▶ Use stationary flat stone.

▶ Hold instrument in modified pen grasp. Establish finger rest on the side of the stone.

▶ Apply the surface to be ground to the stone in correct relationship to maintain the 45° bevel (Figure 40-13B).

▶ With moderate, steady pressure, pull the instrument toward the cutting edge a short distance. Allow the whole hand to move with the arm as a unit to aid in maintaining the correct angulation.

▶ Release pressure and slide the instrument back. Repeat.

▶ Test for sharpness and reapply as needed for ideal sharpness.

▶ Wipe the instrument carefully with a dry gauze square or an alcohol wipe to remove particles.

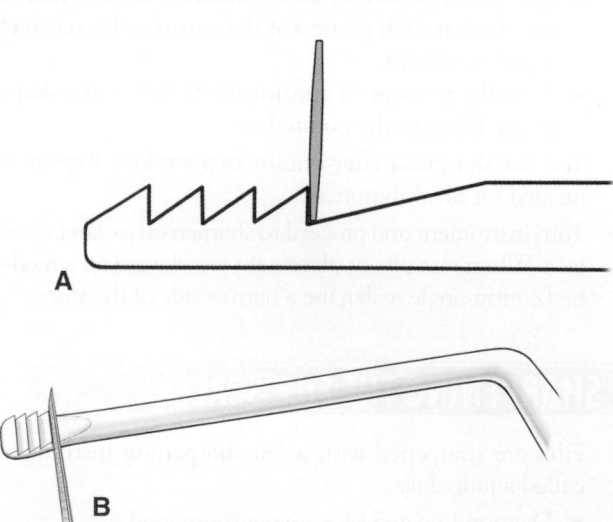

FIGURE 40-12 Sharpening a File Scaler. A: Tanged file in position against one of the several surfaces to be ground. **B:** With the file scaler stabilized to prevent movement, the tanged file is pulled through the channel using a moderate, steady pressure against the surface to be ground.

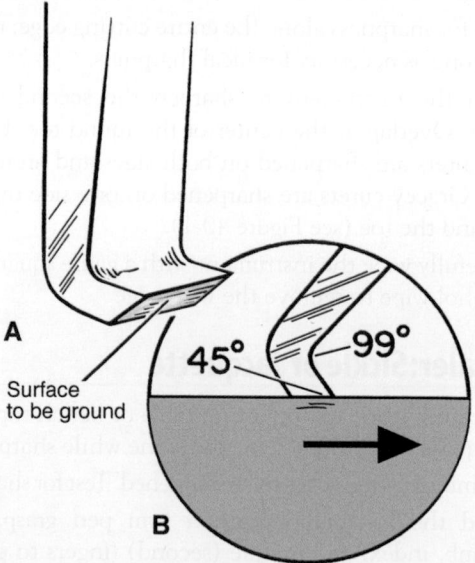

FIGURE 40-13 Sharpening a Hoe Scaler. A: Surface to be ground. **B:** Hoe adapted to the surface of a stationary flat stone at the proper angle to maintain the original bevel of 45°. Arrow indicates direction of the sharpening stroke leading into the cutting edge.

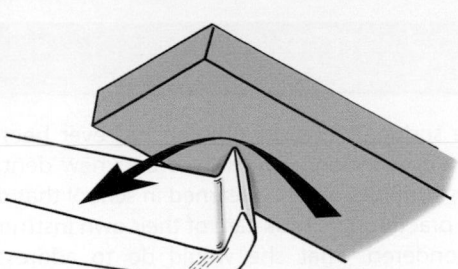

FIGURE 40-14 **Rounding a Hoe Scaler.** To round the sharp corners of the hoe scaler, a flat stone is rubbed over the instrument with a gentle rolling motion. The sharp corners of a chisel are rounded in the same way.

III. Round Corners

Corners need to be rounded at each end of the cutting edge.

▶ Rounded corners help to prevent laceration of soft tissue or grooving of tooth surface.

▶ Hold instrument in nondominant hand with corners of cutting edge directed inward.

▶ Rub the surface of the sharpening stone across each corner with a gentle rolling motion (Figure 40-14). Two or three applications are usually sufficient.

SHARPENING THE CHISEL SCALER

Sharpening procedures for the chisel are similar to those for the hoe. Again, the surface is small, the angulation is difficult to visualize, and the use of magnification is needed.

I. Surface to Be Ground

Examine surface to be ground (Figure 40-15A). Test for sharpness.

II. Sharpening Procedure

▶ Hold instrument with a modified pen grasp, establish finger rest, and apply the surface to be ground to the stone in the correct relationship to maintain the 45° bevel (Figure 40-15B).

▶ With moderate, steady pressure, push the instrument forward, toward the cutting edge, without changing the relationship with the stone.

▶ After two or three applications, test for sharpness and reapply as necessary for an ideal cutting edge.

▶ Wipe the instrument carefully with a dry gauze square or an alcohol wipe to remove particles.

III. Round Corners

Round the corners at each end of the cutting edge. In a manner similar to that shown in Figure 40-14 for the hoe

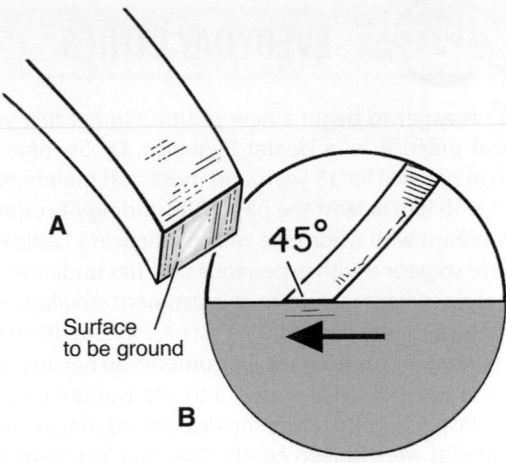

FIGURE 40-15 **Sharpening a Chisel Scaler. A:** Surface to be ground. **B:** Chisel is adapted to the surface of a stationary flat stone at the proper angle to maintain the original bevel of 45°. Arrow indicates direction of the sharpening stroke leading into the cutting edge.

scaler, rub the surface of the flat stone across each corner of the chisel with a gentle, even, rolling motion. Two or three applications are usually sufficient.

SHARPENING EXPLORERS

I. Tests for Sharpness

A. Visual

When examined under concentrated light, a dull explorer tip appears rounded.

B. Plastic Testing Stick

A sharp explorer grips the plastic tester on light pressure and moves with resistance when pulled over the surface. A dull explorer does not catch and will slide.

II. Recontour

Small-nosed pliers can be used to straighten a bent tip.

III. Sharpening Procedure

▶ Use flat stone.

▶ Instrument is held with a modified pen grasp. Finger rest is established on side of stone.

▶ Placement and movement of the tip over the stone resemble somewhat the procedure for the curet on the stone (see Figure 40-10B).

▶ Place side of tip on stone at approximately a 15° to 20° angle of stone with shank of explorer.

▶ As tip is moved over the surface, the handle is rotated so that even pressure can be applied to each part of the tip.

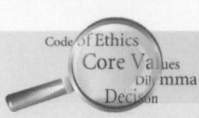

EVERYDAY ETHICS

Leslie is eager to begin a new position in her first year of clinical practice as a dental hygienist. Dr. Shepherd has been in practice for 15 years and most staff members have been with him at least the past 10, including Ann, the dental hygienist with whom she will be practicing. Leslie is glad to have someone with experience take her under her wing. A dental assistant takes care of instrument sterilization and tray setups for the dental hygienists. As she sat down to her first patient, she noticed the instruments on her instrument cassette were all sickle scalers and she wanted curets. On closer inspection, however, she discovered that all but one instrument were indeed curets; they had just been sharpened incorrectly, leaving them with no contour (curvature) at the toe. She excused herself to go into the instrument supply room only to find that all of the curets had sharp, pointed toes. Going back to the clinical area, she peeked in to ask Ann if the assistant did the sharpening for her (as she glanced at Ann's tray she noted the curets were equally sharpened to a distinct point). Ann answered, "No, I do all the sharpening myself because I am very picky."

Leslie suddenly realizes nothing has ever been said in a work description about who orders new dental hygiene instruments. She had learned in school that dental hygiene practitioners took care of their own instruments. Leslie pondered what she would do to address this situation—especially how to approach it without alienating her new coworkers.

Questions for Consideration

1. Given Leslie's novice status as a clinician, how will she approach her new colleague—an experienced practitioner—with her concerns? Which core values of dental hygiene (Table II-1 in Section II, Introduction) are involved in this scenario?

2. What harm, if any, is affecting Dr. Shepherd's patients? Discuss whether or not the dentist needs to be notified about the condition of the instruments.

3. Utilizing an ethical decision framework (see Chapter 1), describe realistic alternatives for Leslie's course of action in this situation.

CARE OF SHARPENING EQUIPMENT

I. Flat Sharpening Stone

A. Prepare for Sterilization

Submerge in ultrasonic cleaner or scrub with soap and water to remove metal particles left from sharpening.

B. Stain Removal

▶ Check manufacturer's recommendation

▶ Alternate cleaning suggestions: Use powdered cleanser when stone becomes discolored. If the stone becomes "glazed" by metal particles ground into the surface, rub sandpaper over the stone placed on a flat, solid surface.

C. Storage

▶ Keep in sealed, sterilized packages for sharpening at instrument preparation area.

▶ A stone and testing stick are stored with each instrument setup in the cassette for use during the treatment appointment.

II. Care of the Tanged File

Because the tanged file corrodes easily when exposed to moisture, it may require special handling.

▶ Wipe the tanged file with a sterile gauze soaked with isopropyl alcohol after use.

▶ Sterilize in a dry heat oven or chemical vapor sterilizer (Chapter 6).

III. Manufacturer's Directions

Follow manufacturer's directions for all artificial stones.

DOCUMENTATION

▶ Example documentation is found in Box 40-2.

BOX 40-2

Example Documentation: Monitoring of Sharpness of Instruments

S –Female patient, 48 years old and in good health, presents for third in a series of scaling and root planing appointments (maxillary left quadrant).

O –Previously documented assessment findings for maxillary left quadrant include: heavy generalized calculus, generalized 4–5 mm probing depths, and 8 mm probing depth on the mesial of #12 and distal of #15 (furcation involvement).

A –Burnished calculus was noted on the quadrants completed.

P –Instrument sharpness carefully monitored. File scaler was used to break up burnished calculus and rigid Gracey curettes used for removal. Completed quadrant debridement with ultrasonic and manual instruments. Extended shank minicurets were used for root debridement in the mesial concavity of #12 and distal furcation of #15.

Next steps: Scheduled for scaling and root planing on mandibular left quadrant and re-evaluate completed quadrants, particularly pocket areas >4mm.

Signed: _____, RDH
Date: _____

Factors To Teach The Patient

▷ Benefits of using a finely sharpened instrument for calculus removal.
▷ Harmful effects of using dull instruments.

References

1. Scaramucci MK. Hone your sharpening technique. *Dimensions Dent Hyg.* 2014;12(2):32–33.
2. Nahass HE, Madkour GG. Evaluation of different resharpening techniques on the working edge of periodontal scalers: a scanning electron microscopic study. *Life Sci J.* 2013;10(1):589–593.
3. Silva MV, Gomes DA, Leite FR, et al. Sharpening of periodontal instruments with different sharpening stones and its influence upon root debridement—scanning electronic microscopy assessment. *J Int Acad Periodontol.* 2006;8(1):17–22.
4. Hu-Friedy. Reference guide: anatomy of a dental instrument. https://www.hu-friedy.com/products/mastercontrol/index/file/id/132. Accessed January 16, 2015.

ENHANCE YOUR UNDERSTANDING

thePoint® DIGITAL CONNECTIONS
(see the inside front cover for access information)
• **Audio glossary**
• **Quiz bank**

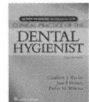

SUPPORT FOR LEARNING
(available separately; visit lww.com)
• *Active Learning Workbook for Clinical Practice of the Dental Hygienist, 12th Edition*

prepU INDIVIDUALIZED REVIEW
(available separately; visit lww.com)
• **Adaptive quizzing with *prepU for Wilkins' Clinical Practice of the Dental Hygienist***

41

Nonsurgical Periodontal Therapy and Adjunctive Therapy

Linda D. Boyd, RDH, RD, EdD and Esther M. Wilkins, BS, RDH, DMD

CHAPTER OUTLINE

LEARNING OBJECTIVES

After studying this chapter, the student will be able to:

1. Explain the goals and desirable clinical endpoints or outcomes for nonsurgical periodontal therapy.

2. Write a care plan for a patient with slight-to-moderate chronic periodontitis.

3. List the steps in manual and ultrasonic instrumentation and the advantages and disadvantages of each.

4. Describe the changes in the subgingival bacteria after periodontal debridement.

5. Describe current evidence related to laser therapy for initial therapy.

6. Develop postoperative instructions for a patient following a nonsurgical periodontal therapy appointment.

7. List the steps in re-evaluation of nonsurgical periodontal therapy and the decisions that must be made based on the clinical outcomes.

8. Compare and contrast the risk and benefits of systemic antibiotics and local delivery antimicrobials.

9. Critically evaluate the benefit of local delivery antimicrobials on changes in pocket depth and clinical attachment level (CAL).

▶ *Periodontal debridement* remains the "gold standard" for initial therapy in inflammatory gingival and periodontal infections and includes the following therapeutic interventions:[1-3]

- Disruption and removal of dental biofilm.
- Scaling and root planing (manual and power-driven) to remove supra- and subgingival calculus.
- Root debridement to eliminate bacterial toxins.

▶ Nonsurgical periodontal therapy consisting of periodontal debridement can provide the definitive or complete treatment for many patients with slight-to-moderate periodontitis. Research shows the following outcomes:[2,3]

- Reduction in infection and inflammation.
- Reductions in pocket depth.
- Increases in CAL.

▶ Adjunctive agents may be utilized for localized active periodontal infection remaining after re-evaluation of nonsurgical periodontal therapy.

▶ Box 41-1 contains key words related to nonsurgical periodontal therapy.

▶ The long-range success of treatment depends on *control* of the dental biofilm by the patient on a daily basis. Therefore, instruction and monitoring biofilm-control procedures precedes, continues simultaneously with, and follows nonsurgical periodontal therapy.

THE SCOPE OF NONSURGICAL PERIODONTAL THERAPY

This chapter is devoted to techniques for the removal of supragingival and subgingival deposits using manual and power-driven scaling procedures. Nonsurgical periodontal therapy may include a combination of the following procedures:

▶ Removal of dental biofilm, endotoxins, other bacterial products, and calculus.

▶ Root planing to remove residual calculus and create a smoother tooth surface.

▶ Adjunctive agents such as sustained-release antibiotic or antimicrobial agent particularly for refractory infections.

▶ Removal of iatrogenic biofilm retainers.
  • Overhanging margins of restorations.
  • Unfinished, poorly contoured, or unpolished restorations.

▶ Concurrent dental therapeutic interventions. Examples include:

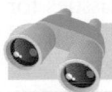

BOX 41-1 KEY WORDS: Nonsurgical Periodontal Therapy

Antibiotic: a form of antimicrobial agent produced by or obtained from microorganisms that can kill other microorganisms or inhibit their growth; may be specific for certain organisms or may cover a broad spectrum

Antimicrobial therapy: use of specific chemical or pharmaceutical agents for the control or destruction of microorganisms, either systemically or at specific sites.

Attachment: with reference to the clinical attachment level, which is the position of the periodontal attached tissue at the base of a sulcus or pocket as measured from a fixed point.
  New attachment: the union of connective tissue or epithelium with a root surface that has been deprived of its original attachment apparatus; the new attachment may be epithelial adhesion and/or connective tissue adaptation or attachment, and it may include new cementum.
  Reattachment: the reunion of epithelial and connective tissues with root surfaces and bone occurs after an incision or injury.

Bacteremia: presence of bacteria in the blood.

Bioabsorbable: available for absorption by the body.

Biodegradable: susceptible of degradation by biological processes, as by bacterial or other enzymatic action.

Cannula: tubular instrument placed in a cavity to introduce or withdraw fluid.

Chemotherapy: treatment by means of chemical or pharmaceutical agents.

Controlled release: local delivery of a chemotherapeutic agent to a site-specific area; may be a patch worn on the skin or a polymeric fiber, such as that used to deliver an agent to a periodontal pocket.

Endoscopy: a minimally invasive diagnostic procedure used in medicine to examine inaccessible tissues by inserting a fiber-optic tube into the body.

Endotoxin: LPS complex found in the cell wall of many gram-negative microorganisms; contained superficially within periodontally involved cementum.

Furcation: anatomic area between the roots of a multirooted tooth.
  Furcation invasion: pathologic resorption of bone within a furcation.

Instrumentation zone: area on tooth where instrumentation is confined; area where calculus and altered cementum are located and treatment is required.

Infection: invasion and multiplication of microorganisms in body tissues.
  Endogenous infection: caused by microorganisms that are part of the normal microbiota of the skin, nose, mouth, and intestinal and urogenital tracts.
  Exogenous infection: caused by organisms acquired from outside the oral cavity or the host.
  Opportunistic infection: occurs in a systemically or locally impaired host; opportunistic pathogens may not be highly virulent, but they can cause disease when the host defense is altered.

Nonsurgical periodontal therapy: dental biofilm removal and control, supragingival and subgingival scaling, root planing, and adjunctive treatments such as the use of chemotherapy; the basic objectives are to restore periodontal health; arrest or slow the progression of early periodontal disease; or, for more advanced disease, to prepare the tissues for more complex periodontal therapy.

PARQ (Procedures, Alternatives, Risks/benefits, and Questions): used to explain therapies planned that address the patient's problem(s), to answer all questions and obtain their consent.

Refractory: not responding to usual treatment.

Root planing: a definitive treatment procedure designed to remove altered cementum or surface dentin that is rough, impregnated with calculus, or contaminated with toxins or microorganisms. Also termed **debridement** or **root preparation.**

Scaling: instrumentation of the crown or root surfaces to remove dental biofilm and calculus.

- Restoration of advanced carious lesions to aid gingival healing by preventing food impaction and making personal biofilm removal possible.
- Analysis of occlusal irregularities.

PREPARATION OF THE CLINICIAN

▶ Knowledge of the anatomic, histopathologic, and physiologic characteristics of the teeth and supporting tissues is foundational for nonsurgical periodontal therapy.

▶ Recognition of the clinical manifestations of the tissues in disease and health is essential to differentiate the two.

TREATMENT GOALS

I. Patient with Uncomplicated Gingivitis

▶ Complete scaling.

▶ Patient compliance in personal daily biofilm removal.

▶ *Therapeutic goal*: Reversal of inflammation to establish gingival health through elimination of etiologic factors.[4]

II. Patient with Early-to-Moderate Periodontitis

▶ Control of infection may be attained through nonsurgical periodontal therapy.

▶ Maintaining the healthy state requires continuing routine appointments for professional scaling and supervision of the patient's biofilm removal methods.

▶ *Therapeutic goals*:[5]
- Reduction in gingival inflammation and bleeding on probing (BOP).
- Reduction in pocket depths.
- Clinical attachment levels (CALs) are stabilized or improved.
- Decrease in detectable dental biofilm to a level consistent with health.

III. Patients with Advanced Periodontal Conditions, or Patients with Poor Response to Routine Therapy

▶ Supplemental therapeutic measures may be needed.

▶ Specialized instruments may be required for deep pockets, furcations, and complex anatomical features of involved diseased root surfaces.

▶ *Therapeutic goals*:[6]
- Same goals as slight-to-moderate periodontal conditions.
- Radiographic improvement in osseous lesions.
- Occlusal stabilization.

IV. Patients Who Require Surgical or Other Advanced Periodontal Therapy

▶ Certain periodontal conditions will require surgical or other advanced therapeutic procedures. Examples include:[6]
- *Mucogingival defects*: periodontal plastic surgery.
- *Exposed root surfaces*: connective tissue grafting; free gingival grafting.
- *Crown lengthening*: functional, restorative, or esthetic.
- *Regenerative procedures*: bone grafting, guided tissue regeneration.
- *Resective therapy*: osseous surgery, root resective therapy, gingivectomy.

▶ For these patients, complete periodontal scaling and root planing (root preparation) prepare the tissues for the added treatment by reducing the bacterial load and reducing inflammation.

COMPONENTS OF NONSURGICAL PERIODONTAL THERAPY

I. Preventive Services

▶ Personal counseling for patients with systemic conditions for which periodontal infection is a risk factor (pregnancy, cardiovascular disease, diabetes).

▶ Fluoride applications and other preventive measures, especially for root caries prevention for the patient with periodontal recession.

▶ At-home rinsing, irrigation, other selective use of antimicrobials, and fluorides (dentifrice, chlorhexidine, water fluoridation).

▶ Smoking cessation assistance.

▶ Desensitization of teeth.

▶ Care for dental implants and prostheses.

▶ Dietary assessment and counseling.

II. Dental Biofilm Removal[2]

▶ Gingival inflammation and periodontal destruction result from the action of pathogenic microorganisms in dental biofilm.

▶ Endotoxin[7–10]
- Lipopolysaccharides (LPSs) or endotoxins, derived from the cell walls of gram-negative pathogenic microorganisms, are toxic to human tissue and lead to inflammation and destruction of the periodontal attachment.
- Endotoxins exist in biofilm and can be removed readily from the parts of the teeth and tissues that the patient can reach with toothbrush, dental floss, interdental brushes, and whatever system works best for the individual patient.

- Cementum
  - The cementum is thin at the cervical third of the root. Some or even complete removal of the cementum during instrumentation for calculus removal is inevitable.
  - Excess removal of the cementum and dentin beyond the point of tactile smoothness is not necessary.[8,9] However, a smooth surface is preferable, since the microorganisms collect and colonize on a rough surface much more rapidly than on a smooth surface.[11]

III. Calculus Removal

- Calculus is not directly a cause of gingival inflammation, but the irregular surface provides a nidus for bacteria of the biofilm to collect and multiply.[2]
- Calculus must be removed to provide a healing environment for the periodontal tissues.

IV. Restorative Biofilm-Retentive Factors

- Overhanging margins and rough surfaces of restorations create a niche for microorganisms to collect, multiply, and mature into gram-negative strains.[11]
- Personal oral self-care efforts by the patient are impeded by overhanging margins, irregular margins that are breaking down, and poorly contoured restorations.
- Removal of overhanging margin or replacement is a critical component of facilitating returning the periodontium to health.

AIMS AND EXPECTED OUTCOMES

The effects and benefits of complete, carefully performed nonsurgical periodontal therapy are summarized here.

I. Interrupt or Stop the Progress of Disease[3]

- Reduce formation of dental biofilm.
- Delay repopulation of pathogenic microorganisms.

II. Create an Environment to Encourage Healing and Resolution of Inflammation[3]

- Convert pocket (disease) to sulcus (health).
- Shrink enlarged spongy tissue.
- Reduce probing depths.
- Eliminate BOP.
- Regenerate the gingival tissues to normal color, size, and contour.
- Change the quality of the tissues from spongy to firm.
- Increase CAL.
- Remove calculus and restorative dentistry irregularities to reduce biofilm retention.

III. Induce Positive Changes in Quality and Quantity of Subgingival Bacterial Flora[2]

- Before instrumentation, the predominant microorganisms are anaerobic, gram-negative, motile forms with many spirochetes and rods, high counts of all types of microorganisms, and many leukocytes.
- After instrumentation, the composition of the bacterial flora shifts to a predominance of aerobic, gram-positive, nonmotile, coccoid forms with lowered total counts and fewer leukocytes (Table 41-1).

IV. Provide Initial Preparation (Tissue Conditioning) for Surgical Periodontal Therapy in Advanced Disease[6]

- Reduce or eliminate etiologic and predisposing factors.
- Permit reevaluation. Surgical procedures may be lessened in extent.

TABLE 41-1	Effect of Instrumentation on Pocket Microflora	
PERIODONTAL INFECTION BEFORE TREATMENT	**PERIODONTAL HEALTH AFTER TREATMENT**	
Predominant flora is Anaerobic Gram negative Motile Spirochetes, motile rods; pathogenic	**Predominant flora is** Aerobic Gram positive Nonmotile Coccoid forms; nonpathogenic	
Total count microorganisms Very high total count of all types of microorganisms	**Total count microorganisms** Much lower total counts of all types of microorganisms	
Leukocyte count Many leukocytes	**Leukocyte count** Lower leukocyte counts	

V. Educate and Motivate the Patient

▶ To appreciate the value of a healthy mouth.

▶ To assume a co-therapist role in maintaining the health established in the treatment phase.

▶ To make a commitment to perform daily personal bio-film control measures.

▶ To continue with periodic maintenance appointments at the recommended interval for ongoing monitoring of periodontal health.

CARE PLAN FOR INSTRUMENTATION[6]

▶ The needs of the individual patient are identified through patient assessment (refer to Chapter 20).

▶ The course of treatment is defined by the dental hygiene diagnosis and care plan (refer to Chapters 24 and 25). Included in the care plan are the following:

• Special considerations required for the individual patient.

• Distribution and severity of the periodontal infection.

• Treatment sequence needed for the individual.

• Length and number of appointments required to complete treatment.

• Plan for re-evaluation and continuing care (described in Chapters 47 and 48).

OVERALL APPOINTMENT SYSTEMS

▶ Whether a single or multiple appointment plan is required, the initial step is patient instruction.

▶ The overall care plan is described and the informed consent of the patient, parent, or guardian obtained.

▶ Treatment begins with the patient taking responsibility for daily removal of biofilm.

▶ In this chapter, the portion of the appointments devoted to instrumentation to remove calculus, subgingival dental biofilm, and overhanging restorations is described.

I. A Single Appointment

▶ The diagnosis may be gingivitis or early periodontitis (Tables 19-1 and 19-2 in Chapter 19) with small areas of deposits readily accessible; local anesthesia may not be needed.

▶ Only a few teeth are present; limited areas of local anesthesia are required.

▶ Patient presents with an acceptable biofilm score, and evidence of reasonable oral self-care without need for time to provide extended follow-up instruction.

▶ Patient acts responsibly in keeping appointments for periodontal maintenance and continued monitoring for disease control.

II. Multiple Appointments

The extent of periodontal involvement as shown by probing measurements, distribution and extent of calculus deposits, and oral cleanliness, which provides evidence of the patient's personal care or lack of it, are major determinants in the number of appointments needed.

A. Quadrant Scaling Appointments

▶ One efficient system for appointment planning is by quadrants or sextants with local anesthesia for more advanced disease at 1-week intervals to permit patient learning and progressive healing.

▶ With less severe periodontitis and a compliant patient, two quadrants on the same side (maxillary and mandibular arches) may be completed at an appointment.

▶ The patient is informed that after the scaling is completed, an appointment for re-evaluation is needed.

▶ The concept of periodic maintenance care is introduced.

B. Tissue Conditioning

▶ At the initial appointment, daily oral self-care for dental biofilm removal is introduced.

• Interdental devices to complement the use of a toothbrush can be added as the patient demonstrates readiness.

▶ At each successive appointment, a biofilm score is shown to the patient, and procedures are reviewed.

▶ With a motivated patient, the tissues will show changes toward a healthy state each week.

▶ The patient is self-treating and at the same time is *conditioning* the tissue for the clinician.

• As a result, there is less debris and less bleeding during instrumentation and fewer bacteria for the aerosol contamination created during instrumentation.

▶ The effect is a cleaner environment in which the clinician can carry out the professional treatment procedures and the patient can appreciate the feeling of a healthy mouth.

C. Evaluation

▶ At each appointment, the quadrants previously treated are examined for evidence of healing.

▶ Calculus left inadvertently can be removed by remedial scaling procedures.

▶ Best done 4–8 weeks following completion of scaling and root planing to allow for connective tissue healing.[12]

III. Full-Mouth Disinfection

A. Definition

▶ System of scaling and root planing of all pockets in two long appointments completed within a 24-hour period with adjunctive chlorhexidine mouthrinse.[13]

▶ The procedures are best accomplished under local anesthesia with a chairside dental assistant.

▶ Systematic review of the research on full-mouth disinfection reveals traditional scaling and root planing in multirooted teeth with deep pockets had greater gains in CAL and less BOP.[13]

- The opposite was true of single-rooted teeth with 5–6 mm pockets, full-mouth disinfection had greater reduction in pocket depths.
- On the basis of inconsistent outcomes across tooth types and pocket depths, the approach for nonsurgical periodontal therapy selected needs to be based on patient preference and scheduling options.

B. Rationale

▶ Periodontal diseases are infections; ridding the mouth of as many of the pathogens as possible at one time can encourage healing.

▶ In the quadrant system, it is possible for a scaled quadrant to become reinfected from pathogens left in untreated quadrants.

C. Limitations

▶ Case selection: Many patients would not be able to withstand such intense treatment.

▶ Patient instruction: Opportunities for review and repeated instruction at the patient's learning pace are not available without a series of appointments with time in between for patient practice of oral self-care.

▶ The ability to re-evaluate healing of each quadrant is lost.

IV. Definitive Nonsurgical Periodontal Therapy

A. Segmental Approach

▶ Quadrant or sextant treatments to completion are recommended to prevent the aforementioned problems associated with incomplete scaling.

▶ Decisions are made according to what can reasonably be completed by the individual clinician within the time frame of a given appointment.

▶ Treatment appointments are scheduled accordingly.

B. Care Planning Factors to Consider

▶ *Access*: the relative ease of insertion to base of the soft tissue pocket.

- Fibrosity and tissue tone of the free gingiva.
- Probing depths: attachment pattern around the full circumference of each tooth.

▶ *Deposit on tooth surfaces*
- Extent and distribution of calculus.
- Age of calculus/degree of mineralization.
- Strength of attachment of calculus to the tooth.

▶ *Root anatomy*
- Multirooted teeth with furcation involvement.
- Deep concavities.

▶ *Patient factors*
- Need for local anesthetic or nitrous oxide/oxygen sedation.
- Limited capacity for opening mouth.
- Behavioral factors such as apprehension.

PREPARATION FOR INSTRUMENTATION

I. Review the Patient's Assessment Record

▶ *Note special needs*: from medical history and previous appointment experiences.

▶ *Identify*: systemic or physical problems with potential for emergency.

II. Review Radiographic Findings

A. Findings Applicable During Instrumentation

▶ Anatomic features of roots, furcations, and bone level, which may need special adaptations of curets.

▶ Overhanging restorations to be removed or scheduled for replacement.

B. Use Radiographs as Guide

▶ Keep radiographs on lighted viewbox or computer screen throughout the treatment for reference to observe bone level and root anatomy for each area.

III. Review Care Plan and Treatment Records

▶ Note flow and sequence of planned appointments.

▶ Note findings that apply to the instrumentation process.
- Examine periodontal probings to review attachment topography and access limitations.
- Assemble procedure tray setup or cassette to include appropriate instruments.

▶ Review previous appointment progress notes.
- Read details of prior treatment, noting segments completed, which will be reassessed for healing.
- Ascertain how previous treatment appointments have been tolerated by the patient.
- Anticipate anesthesia requirements.

▶ Keep periodontal probing chart prominently displayed throughout the treatment for reference.

IV. Patient Preparation

A. Premedication Requirements for High Risk Patient

▶ Transient bacteremia can occur during and immediately after scaling procedures.

- Flossing and a single quadrant of scaling and root planing result in the same incidence and magnitude of bacteremia, so only high-risk patients are in need of antibiotic premedication.[14]

▶ Consult with the primary care provider to determine if premedication is required (see Box 10-2A in Chapter 10 to identify patients who may be at risk for bacterial endocarditis and be in need of prophylactic premedication).

B. Provide Preprocedural Bactericidal Rinse[15]

C. Prepare for Anesthesia as Indicated

V. Supragingival Examination

A. Visual

▶ Gross deposits and tooth surface irregularities can be seen by direct vision. Fine, unstained, white, or yellowish calculus is frequently invisible when wet with saliva.

▶ Observe tooth surfaces closely while a gentle stream of compressed air is applied. Dry calculus is more visible than wet calculus.

B. Tactile

▶ Without deposits or anatomical irregularities, the enamel surface is smooth.

▶ An explorer tip passed over the surface slides freely, smoothly, and quietly.

▶ When rough calculus deposits are present, the explorer tip does not slide freely but meets with resistance over varying textures.

▶ Deposits can produce a scratchy sound or an audible click as the explorer passes over them.

VI. Subgingival Examination

A. Visual

▶ *Gingiva:* The clinical appearance suggestive of underlying calculus may be the following:

- Soft, spongy, bluish-red gingiva, with enlargement of the interdental papillae over proximal surface calculus.
- Dark-colored area beneath relatively translucent marginal gingiva.

▶ *Calculus*

- A loose, resilient pocket wall can be deflected from the tooth surface with a gentle stream of compressed air.
- Dark, subgingival calculus can be seen within the pocket on the root.

B. Tactile

▶ *Periodontal charting*

- Use probing depth recordings as a basic guide for the depth of insertion of the curet.
- Confirm recorded probing depths of segment to be instrumented.
- Study the soft tissue attachment pattern to select effective procedures.

▶ *Identify shallow pockets (sulci)*

- Scaling in shallow pockets of fewer than 3 mm can lead to loss of periodontal attachment due to detachment of periodontal ligament fibers.[1]
- Root surfaces free of calculus may require minimal lateral pressure for comprehensive biofilm removal.

▶ *Determine distribution and extent of deposits*

- Figure 41-1 illustrates probing. As the probe passes over the surface, it may be intercepted by calculus (Figure 41-1B).
- Use an explorer for distinction of fine hard deposits.

▶ *Evaluate tooth topography*

- Detect grooves and furcations using a horizontal stroke (Figure 41-1C).
- Use a Naber's furcation probe to examine furcations (see Chapter 20).
- Note anatomic root and furcation variations (Figure 41-2).

▶ *Evaluate restorative margins*

- Detect overhanging restorations that need to be evaluated and treatment planned for replacement or margination.
- Detect marginal irregularities that retain biofilm.

VII. Formulate Strategy for Instrumentation

▶ Combine clinical findings with information documented in the patient's record.

▶ Review overall treatment objectives for the patient.

▶ Determine a strategy for instrumentation.

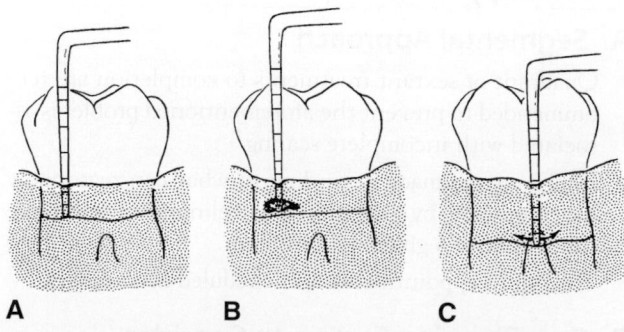

A   **B**   **C**

FIGURE 41-1 Subgingival Examination Using a Probe. A: Probe inserted to the bottom of a pocket for complete examination prior to subgingival scaling. **B:** As the probe passes over the root surface, it may be intercepted by a hard mass of calculus. **C:** Using a horizontal probe stroke to examine the topography of a furcation area. Keep the side of the tip of the probe on the tooth surface and slide over one root, into the furcation, and across to the other root.

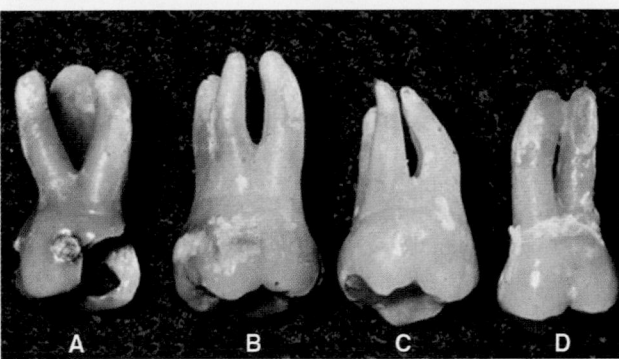

FIGURE 41-2 Anatomic Variations of Furcations. A: Divergent roots with the furcation in the coronal one-third of the root with a short root trunk. **B:** Convergent roots with the furcation in the middle one half of the root with a longer root trunk. **C:** Very convergent roots. **D:** Fused roots with the furcation in the coronal one third of the root. (Reprinted from Scheid R, Weiss G. Woelfel's Dental Anatomy. Philadelphia: Lippincott Williams & Wilkins; 2016.)

CALCULUS REMOVAL

I. Prerequisites

▶ Position of clinician to prevent cumulative tissue trauma.

▶ Good visibility with excellent lighting.

▶ Magnification with loupes and light-emitting diode (LED) light to improve visual acuity.[16]

▶ Sharp instruments with proper contour.

II. Location of Instrumentation

Figure 41-3 illustrates the location of instrumentation. Instrumentation and the selection of the correct instrument depend on the following:

▶ Type of pocket (gingival or periodontal)

▶ Location of calculus (on crown or root surface)

▶ Position of gingival margin (recession or covering cementoenamel junction)

▶ Level of clinical attachment (normal or clinical attachment loss)

III. The Scaling Process

The process is the series of procedures and events that lead to achievement of a specific result.

A. Definitions

▶ *Scaling*: removal of calculus and dental biofilm from supragingival and subgingival exposed tooth surfaces (clinical crown).

▶ *Periodontal debridement*: removal of all residual calculus and toxic materials from the root to produce a clean, smooth tooth surface. Other terms include *root planing*, *root detoxification*, and *root preparation*.

B. Instrumentation Zone

▶ Area of the tooth where instrumentation is performed for scaling and root planing.

▶ *Location*: above the clinical attachment of the periodontal fibers; extends the height and width of the hard and soft deposits of calculus and biofilm to be removed.

▶ Scaling and root planing strokes for deposit removal are limited to the instrumentation zone. Extending the strokes to clean areas where no deposits or biofilm exist can be harmful to the tooth, increase risk for the clinician to lose control, dull the instrument, and waste time.

C. Systematic Deposit Removal

▶ Tooth to tooth

▶ Section to section of deposit on each tooth surface

▶ Strokes overlap in channels

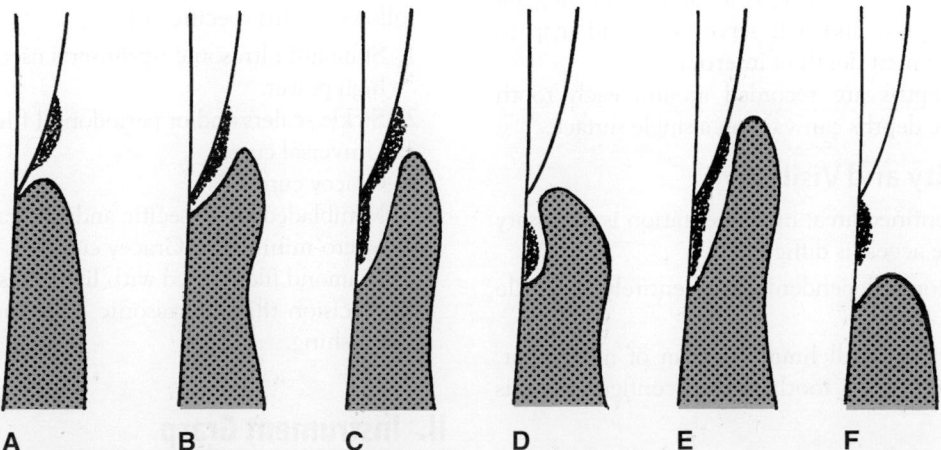

FIGURE 41-3 Location of Instrumentation. The location of calculus deposits, level of periodontal attachment, depth of pocket, and position of the gingival margin determine the site of instrumentation. **A:** Supragingival calculus on the enamel. **B:** Gingival pocket with both supragingival and subgingival calculus on enamel. **C:** Periodontal pocket with both supragingival and subgingival calculus. **D:** Periodontal pocket with subgingival calculus only on root surface. **E:** Periodontal pocket with subgingival calculus on both enamel and root surface. **F:** Calculus on root surface exposed by gingival recession.

▶ The instrument is positioned progressively along the area of the deposit, within the *instrumentation zone*.

▶ *Nature of the deposit* (see Chapter 21).

  • The oldest calculus, located next to the tooth surface, is more calcified and likely to be more difficult to remove.

  • The outermost calculus is covered with a layer of dental biofilm that has not yet started to mineralize.

IV. Special Subgingival Considerations

Although the basic steps described for calculus removal apply to both supragingival and subgingival deposits, subgingival techniques are unique and complicated by several significant factors. Some of the variables are included here.

A. Subgingival Anatomy

▶ *Tooth surface pocket wall*

  • As shown in Figure 41-3C and E, some subgingival instrumentation is on the crown (enamel), and some on the root (cementum or dentin).

  • In the cervical third of the root, the cementum is thin (0.03–0.06 mm) and may have been removed during previous instrumentation.

▶ *Soft tissue pocket wall*

  • The pocket wall hugs closely to the tooth surface covered with rough calculus, which in turn is covered with bacterial biofilm.

  • Only a narrow area is available for manipulation of instruments.

  • The pocket narrows in the deeper area next to the clinical attachment.

  • Bleeding during instrumentation is inevitable because of the inflammation in the wall of the pocket.

▶ *Variations in probing depths*

  • The periodontal charting is a guide to subgingival instrumentation and will serve as a road map to guide instrument depth of insertion.

  • Probing depths are recorded around each tooth because the depths can vary on a single surface.

B. Accessibility and Visibility

▶ Pocket is a confined area; instrumentation is necessary in areas where access is difficult.

▶ Instrumentation is dependent almost entirely on tactile sensitivity.

▶ Soft tissue pocket wall limits freedom of movement. Careful adaptation to tooth surface configurations is essential.

C. Subgingival Calculus

▶ *Location*: Subgingival calculus may be located on the enamel, the root, or both (Figure 41-3B–E).

▶ *Attachment*

  • Calculus attaches to the cementum in minute irregularities and in areas of cemental resorption.

  • It is more tenacious than on the enamel and requires a different technique for removal.

  • On the enamel it is attached primarily by means of an acquired pellicle, which makes calculus removal much easier.

▶ *Morphology of calculus*

  • Subgingival calculus is irregularly deposited. It occurs in nodular, ledge, smooth veneer, and other forms (Table 21-1 in Chapter 21).

  • Previously scaled or burnished calculus: Subgingival calculus that has been partially scaled and left after incomplete instrumentation may be smooth and may not be detected when an explorer is used to check the area.

MANUAL SUBGINGIVAL SCALING STEPS

Types of instruments and the basic principles for their use are included in Chapter 39. This chapter continues from Chapter 39 to describe the use of the instruments for deposit removal. Box 41-2 summarizes the steps.

I. Selection and Sequence of Instruments

▶ The order in which instruments are selected and used can have an effect on the efficiency and quality of final product, similar to the woodworking process. Heavy coarse grit sanders are always used prior to finer grain tools in order to achieve a uniformly smooth surface.

▶ Instrument selection sequence is recommended as follows, in this specific order:

  1. Standard ultrasonic tips/inserts used on moderate to high power.
  2. Sickle scalers and/or periodontal files.
  3. Universal curets.
  4. Gracey curets.
  5. Minibladed area-specific and/or Gracey curets.
  6. Micro-minibladed Gracey curets.
  7. Diamond files—used with light pressure only.
  8. Precision-thin ultrasonic tips/inserts for final finishing.

II. Instrument Grasp

▶ *Apply a modified pen grasp* (Figure 39-13 in Chapter 39).

  • Thumb and index and middle fingers make up the grasp points.

BOX 41-2

Steps for Calculus Removal Using Manual Instruments

Assessment

▷ Probe to determine pocket/sulcus characteristics and confirm soft tissue attachment topography.

▷ Explore to determine location and extent of deposits and tooth surface irregularities.

▷ Select correct instruments that will adapt and conform to concavities and other root morphology characteristics for areas being treated.

Preparation: Instrument Control

▷ Hold instrument with a modified pen grasp.

▷ Identify correct cutting edge of blade for surface being scaled.
  ▷ For area-specific curets: terminal shank parallel with surface being scaled.
  ▷ For universal curets: terminal shank *less* than parallel with surface being scaled (approximately 20°).

▷ Establish a light hand rest for instrument placement to allow for adjustment and repositioning.

▷ Insert: use placement or exploratory stroke to locate apical edge of deposit.

▷ Adjust working angulation (average at 70°).

Action: Strokes

▷ Secure a stable, functional extraoral hand rest or intraoral finger rest that can support instrument placement and activation at correct working stroke angulation.
  ▷ Pressure into the fulcrum equals the pressure against the tooth.
  ▷ Balance fulcrum pressure with lateral pressure of the strokes.

▷ Activate for working stroke.
  ▷ Apply firm lateral pressure for calculus removal.
  ▷ Apply moderate lateral pressure to smooth the surface.
  ▷ Apply light lateral pressure for biofilm debridement.
  ▷ Control length and direction of stroke: respect the instrumentation zone.
  ▷ Maintain continuous adaptation throughout the stroke.

Channels: Overlap to Completion

▷ Continue channel scaling with overlapping multidirectional strokes.
  ▷ Apply placement stroke to reposition blade for next stroke.
  ▷ Activate instrument circumferentially around tooth.
  ▷ Keep toe adapted around line angles by rolling handle.
  ▷ Cover all surfaces comprehensively to remove all traces of calculus and biofilm.

Evaluation

▷ Use explorer to determine end point of treatment.

▶ *Use a light grasp for*:
  • Instrument insertion and positioning.
  • Assessment strokes.
  • Root debridement strokes to remove biofilm.

▶ *Keep the grasp firm and secure* during calculus removal.

▶ *Apply a light grasp with light lateral pressure after calculus removal*.
  • To remove small irregularities.
  • To leave the treated area smooth.

III. Stabilization: Establish the Fulcrum (Finger Rest)

A. Primary Rest Fingers

▶ Ring and little fingers (numbers 3 and 4 in Figure 39-16 in Chapter 39).

▶ Rest fingers are kept close to the middle finger (number 2) and join the total hand motion during activation.

B. Location

▶ *Intraoral rests*
  • Placed on the tooth adjacent to the one being scaled, or as near as convenient.
  • Avoid position in the path of the strokes to protect from accidental instrument puncture of finger.

▶ *Distance rests*: A long span between the rest and the point of instrument application.
  • Requires an extended grasp.
  • Requires a secure finger rest.

▶ *Variations*: Substitute, supplementary, and reinforced rests are described in Chapter 39.

▶ *Dry the rest position*
  • Biofilm and saliva make tooth surfaces slippery.
  • Use compressed air or dry with gauze sponge.

IV. Select Correct Cutting Edge

A. Universal Curets

▶ Curets are paired and usually mounted on double-ended handles. Single-ended handles may be selected for certain patients or procedures.

▶ Correct cutting edge for scaling: when positioned on the tooth surface, only the back of the blade can be seen.

▶ Incorrect blade adaptation: the open face of the blade will be seen.
  • It would be impossible to angulate at 70° for scaling.
  • The *open* blade is in the correct position for gingival curettage to remove the inner soft tissue lining of the pocket wall.

B. Gracey Curets

▶ Hold instrument with the terminal shank perpendicular to the floor.

▶ Look into face.

▶ Select longer, lower cutting edge.

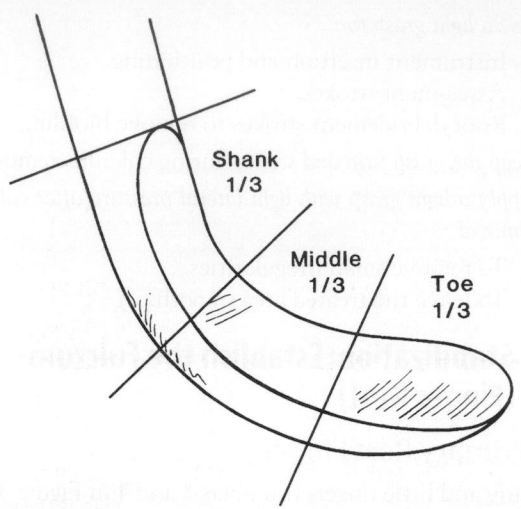

FIGURE 41-4 **Curet Divided into Thirds.** The toe third is kept in contact with the tooth surface during instrumentation. Because of tooth contours, most strokes for scaling and root planing are accomplished using the toe third. Adaptation of the toe third is shown in Figure 41-5.

V. Adaptation of Cutting Edge

A. Apply Blade to Conform to Tooth Surface Being Treated

▶ Because of tooth contours, only a portion of a blade can be adapted.

▶ The toe and middle thirds of a curet blade are used most frequently (Figure 41-4).

B. Maintain Adaptation

▶ Roll the handle around line angles and other tooth convexities.

▶ Maintain close adaptation of the cutting edge to prevent trauma of the adjacent soft tissue (Figure 41-5B).

▶ At the same time maintain the 70° angulation.

VI. Angulation

A. Insertion

Close the angle to nearly flat against the tooth surface (0°) as the instrument is inserted to the base of a pocket (Figure 41-6A and B).

B. Establish Optimal Angle for Scaling

A 70° angle is effective for deposit removal using a scaler or a curet.

VII. Lateral Pressure

A. Degree of Pressure of Blade against Tooth

Whether a light, moderate, or heavy pressure is needed will depend on the nature of the deposit and the type of therapy being performed.

▶ *Light pressure*
  • Assessment.
  • Instrument insertion.
  • Exploration to get below the calculus deposit.
  • Confirmation of the soft tissue attachment.

▶ *Moderate-to-heavy lateral pressure*
  • Calculus removal.
  • Working strokes require heavy-to-moderate lateral pressure depending on the degree of mineralization of the calculus.

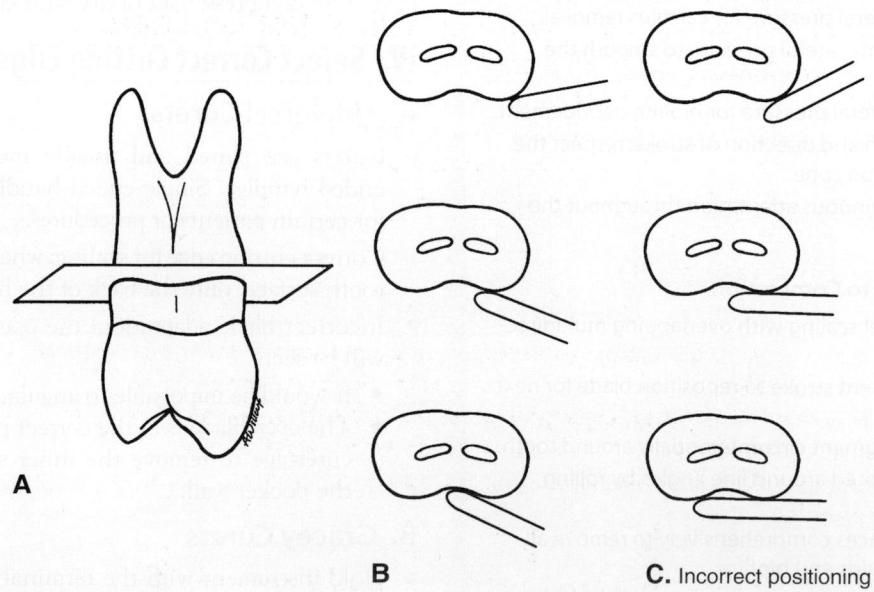

A   **B**   **C.** Incorrect positioning

FIGURE 41-5 **Instrument Adaptation. A:** Maxillary first premolar shows cross section of root drawn for (B) and (C). **B:** Diagram of three positions of a curet shows correct adaptation at a line angle and on the concave mesial surface with toe third of the instrument maintained on the tooth as the instrument is adapted. **C:** Diagram shows **incorrect** adaptation with toe of curet extended away from the tooth surface.

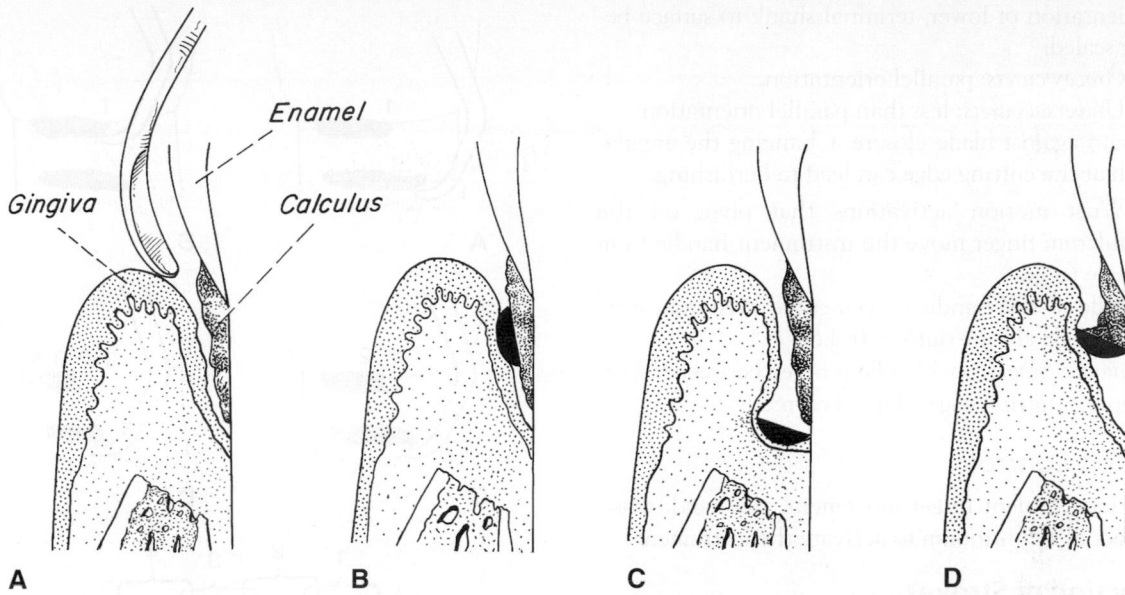

FIGURE 41-6 Subgingival Scaling and Root Planing. A: The curet is inserted gently under the gingival margin. **B:** With a placement stroke, the blade is passed over the surface of the tooth or calculus. Note 0° angle of the face of the curet with the calculus. **C:** The curet is lowered to the base of the pocket until the tension of the soft tissue is felt with the rounded back of the curet. The curet then is positioned at an angle of 70° to 80° with the tooth surface beneath the calculus deposit. **D:** The blade is moved along the root surface in a scaling stroke to remove the calculus.

- Recently formed calculus can be removed more readily than established calculus.
▶ *Biofilm debridement*
  - When the root surface is free of calculus, confine instrumentation to light-pressured debridement over the entire subgingival surface.
  - The tactile sense transmits vibrations felt from any irregularities present.
  - Unnecessary and unwarranted tooth structure removal can be minimized.

B. Balance of Pressure During Stroke

Careful control is accomplished by a balance of pressure between:
▶ Grasp of the instrument,
▶ Pressure on the finger rest,
▶ Lateral pressure against the tooth.

C. Factors Affecting Lateral Pressure

▶ *Sharp instrument*
  - A minimum degree of pressure allows the cutting edge to "grab" the calculus.
  - Engaging the deposit provides strong leverage for effective, clean removal.
  - Less time, with fewer strokes, is required.
  - Fatigue is kept to a minimum.
▶ *Dull instrument*
  - When dull, the blade cannot engage the deposit and will slide over it, burnishing it on the surface.
  - The more the deposit is burnished with repeated strokes, the more difficult it becomes to remove.

- More strokes are taken, causing increased fatigue.
- Inefficiency increases treatment time.
- Grasp and lateral pressure increase to compensate for the sliding effect.
- Stroke control is reduced with the heavier pressure needed to activate a dull blade; this can lead to instrument slippage and trauma to the patient's gingival tissues.
- Loss of confidence by the clinician.
- Loss of patient confidence in the clinician.

VIII. Activation: Stroke

A. Tighten the Grasp

▶ Renew the stability of the rest position.
  - Whether an intraoral finger rest or an extraoral hand rest, the pressure of the rest will equal the pressure against the tooth.
▶ Move the instrument firmly and deliberately, making each stroke intentional.
▶ Wrist and arm bear the weight during the stroke, rather than flexing the fingers in the grasp.

B. Maintain Cutting Edge Evenly During the Stroke

▶ *Adaptation:* Keep blade closely aligned with the surface of the tooth.
▶ *Angulation:* Maintain blade position by observing lower shank from beginning to end of each stroke.
  - Relationship of the angle of the lower shank to the tooth surface stays consistent for the full length of the stroke.

- Orientation of lower, terminal shank to surface being scaled:
  - *Gracey curets*: parallel orientation.
  - *Universal curets*: less than parallel orientation.
- Guard against blade closure. Changing the angulation at the cutting edge can lead to burnishing.
  - Wrist motion activations that pivot on the fulcrum finger move the instrument handle from side to side.
  - Side-to-side handle movement is often indicative of blade closure during stroke.
- ▶ *Maintain the adaptation*: Handle is rolled between fingers to keep the cutting edge adapted correctly.

C. Motion Control

Without independent finger movement, the hand, wrist, and arm act as a continuum to activate the instrument.

D. Direction of Strokes

- ▶ Select overlapping vertical, oblique (diagonal), or horizontal strokes to accommodate the anatomical features of the tooth surfaces (Figure 39-8 in Chapter 39).
- ▶ Strokes are applied systematically, not haphazardly.
- ▶ Avoid horizontal strokes at the bottom of a pocket to avoid damage to the clinical attachment.

E. Length of Stroke: Within Instrumentation Zone

- ▶ Short, smooth, decisive strokes permit accommodation of the cutting edges to changes in the topography of the tooth surface.
- ▶ Confine the strokes to the pocket to prevent the need for repeated removal and reinsertion of the curet; prevent trauma to the gingival margin.

IX. Channels of Strokes: Coverage

A. Make Strokes in Channels (Figure 41-7)

- ▶ At the completion of each stroke, move the instrument laterally a very short distance to assure overlap.
- ▶ Maintain the same finger rest.

B. Overlap Strokes in Channels

- ▶ Ensure complete coverage of every square millimeter of subgingival surface for thorough removal of deposits.

C. Repeat Strokes

- ▶ Continue until surface has been completely debrided.

X. Plane the Root Surface

A. Finishing Techniques

- ▶ *Purpose*: smoothing the tooth surfaces to lessen immediate recolonization of bacteria.

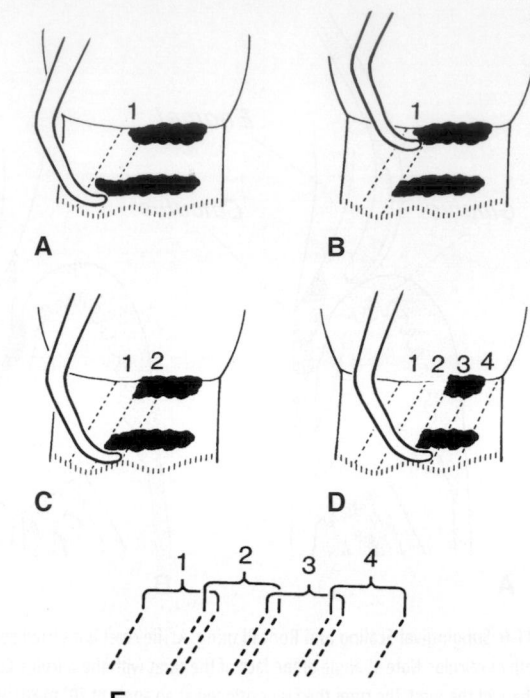

FIGURE 41-7 Channel Scaling. A: Curet adapted in position for channel 1 stroke from the base of the pocket under the calculus deposit. **B:** Completion of stroke for channel 1. **C:** Using an exploratory stroke, the curet is lowered into the pocket and is positioned for calculus removal in channel 2. **D:** Curet positioned for channel 3. Several strokes in each channel may be needed to ensure complete calculus removal. **E:** Strokes of each channel overlap strokes of the previous channel. (Adapted from Parr RW, Green E, Madsen L, et al. *Subgingival Scaling and Root Planing.* Berkeley, CA: Praxis; 1976.)

- ▶ *Procedure*: instrumentation is basically the same as for scaling.
- ▶ *Application*: only where deemed necessary after exploration with an explorer, such as an extended ODU 11/12 explorer, capable of accessing the farthest reaches of pocket depths.

B. Touch and Pressure

- ▶ Specific differences in technique are related to touch and pressure.
  - A lighter grasp will increase tactile sensitivity.
  - Light lateral pressure is applied for maximum sensitivity to minute irregularities of the surface.
  - A lighter stroke can be used for final smoothing of the root surface; increased pressure is not needed.
- ▶ Sharp instruments are essential for tactile transmission.

C. Strokes

- ▶ Use smooth strokes that overlap systematically.
- ▶ As the surface becomes smoother, longer strokes with reduced pressure help to remove small lines, scratches, or grooves without gouging the surface.
- ▶ *Stroke direction*

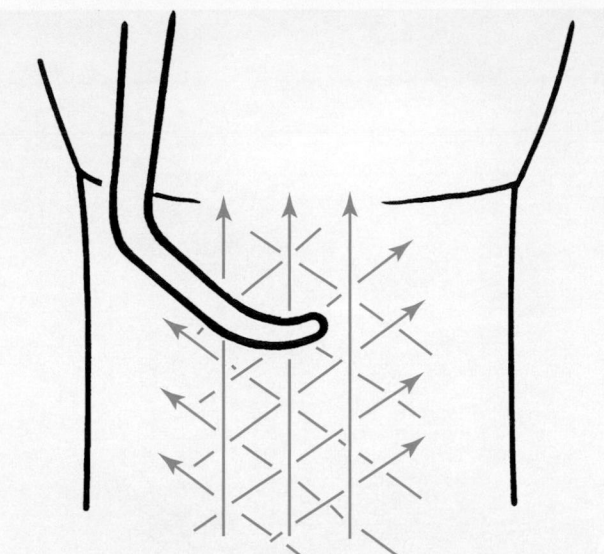

FIGURE 41-8 Root Surface Strokes. The use of strokes in vertical and oblique directions with light lateral pressure can help to eliminate grooves left after scaling. A smooth surface results. (Adapted from: Parr RW, Green E, Madsen L, et al. *Subgingival Scaling and Root Planing.* Berkeley, CA: Praxis; 1976:42.)

- Multidirectional stroke patterns create the ideal finished surface.
- Vertical and then oblique strokes may be used (Figure 41-8).
- Keep horizontal strokes away from the attachment epithelium.
▶ *Adaptation*
- Careful adaptation of the curet to the unique anatomic features of the roots is needed.
- Convex surfaces, constricted cervical areas, concavities and grooves of the proximal surfaces, and the variations in furcations all require precise adaptation.
- Mini- and micro-minibladed Gracey curets are designed specifically to access and adapt to concavities and convexities where standard-length blades either can span across or protrude beyond (Figure 41-5C).
- As a surface area becomes smooth, a gradual change in the sound of the instrument stroke may occur. At completion, the instrument may be as quiet as when used on polished enamel.

XI. Evaluation

▶ Use a subgingival periodontal explorer to examine for completion of calculus removal and smoothness of the treated surfaces.
▶ Apply explorer in both vertical and diagonal strokes to detect irregularities (Figure 41-8).
▶ Refine spots of roughness with a sharp curet.
▶ Adapt curet with light lateral pressure for maximum sensitivity to minute irregularities of the surface. Avoid grooving the treated surface.

▶ Postcare patient instructions (see section on Instruction after Scaling and Root Planing in this chapter).

ADVANCED INSTRUMENTATION

I. Specialized Debridement Instruments

▶ Clinical attachment loss of ≥4–6 mm exposes contours of the root that complicate nonsurgical instrumentation.
▶ Longitudinal grooves, proximal depressions, and concavities and convexities of root morphology make comprehensive debridement covering every square millimeter of tooth surface difficult to accomplish.
▶ Examples of instruments for problem areas:
- Minibladed area-specific curets.
- Periodontal files.
- Diamond-coated files.
- Precision-thin ultrasonic tips/inserts.

II. Definitive Debridement of Furcations

The complex morphology of a furcation necessitates meticulous care during root preparation. Skillful use of specialized instruments designed for use in furcations can enhance treatment outcomes.

A. Components of Furcation Debridement

▶ Optimum blade sharpness and contour.
▶ Instrumentation sequence observed.
▶ Instrumentation fundamentals observed:
- Close adaptation of blade and/or tip/insert to the root surfaces.
- Confined, precision movement of blade and/or tip/insert.
▶ Use of specialized instruments:
- Minibladed hoes and furcation curets: specialized semilunar blades—use with light pressure.
- Minibladed Gracey numbers 5–6, 11–12, 13–14.
- Micro-minibladed Gracey numbers 1–2, 11–12, 13–14.
- Diamond files: *use only with light pressure.*
▶ Precision-thin ultrasonic tips/inserts: *use at low power for final finishing.*
▶ Definitive assessment following instrumentation:
- Use specific periodontal explorer with lightest pressure to assess root texture for uniform smoothness.
- Examples include: TU-17 explorer shown in Figure 20-1 and extended 3A explorer shown in Figure 20-2 in Chapter 20. The regular or extended ODU 11/12 is another option.

III. Endoscope-Assisted Periodontal Debridement

The dental endoscope is a device developed to visualize below the gingival margin for use during diagnosis and instrumentation for treatment of periodontally diseased root surfaces.

A. Objectives

▶ Visualization of the root surface during instrumentation.

▶ Explore, instrument, and evaluate the root surface using indirect visual observation on the device monitor.

▶ Increase the effectiveness and thoroughness of root debridement.[17,18]

▶ Augment subjective data collection with objective confirmation.

B. Description (See Figure 41-9)

▶ *Subgingival probe*: adapted to provide fiber-optic imaging with magnification.

▶ *Sheath* to provide a sterile barrier between the patient and the endoscope.

▶ *Peristaltic pump* to provide irrigation to the working field.

▶ *LED lamp* to provide illumination to the working field.

▶ *Video camera* to capture images of the working field for display.

▶ *Video monitor* for live viewing of the working field.

▶ *Specialized probes, curets,* and *retracting instruments* to maximize tissue visualization.

C. Indications for Use

▶ During maintenance to detect and remove remaining deep burnished calculus deposits, which are the cause of continued BOP (Figure 41-10A and B).

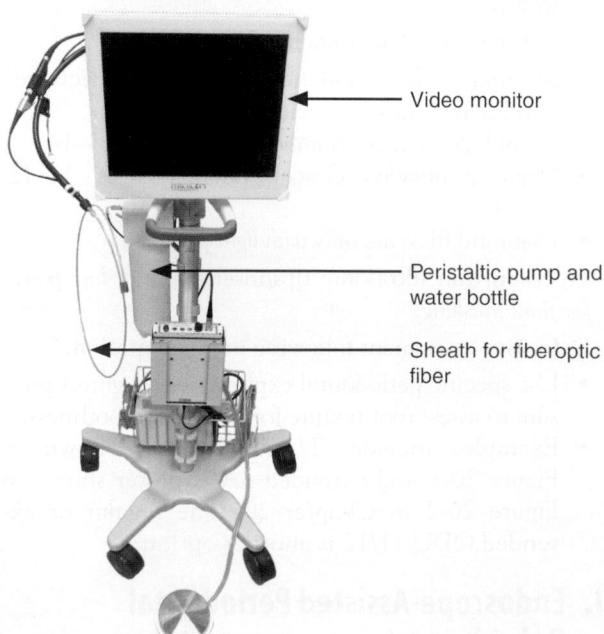

FIGURE 41-9 Dental Endoscope. A device used in subgingival pockets to visualize residual calculus and assist with removal. (Courtesy: John Y. Kwan, DDS)

Video monitor

Peristaltic pump and water bottle

Sheath for fiberoptic fiber

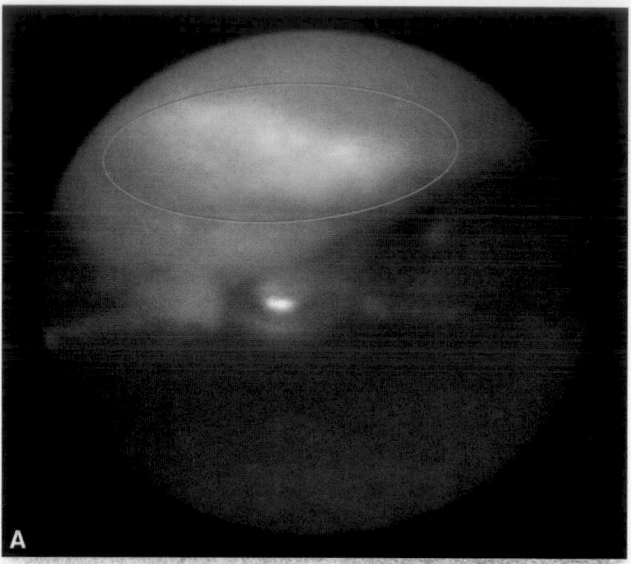

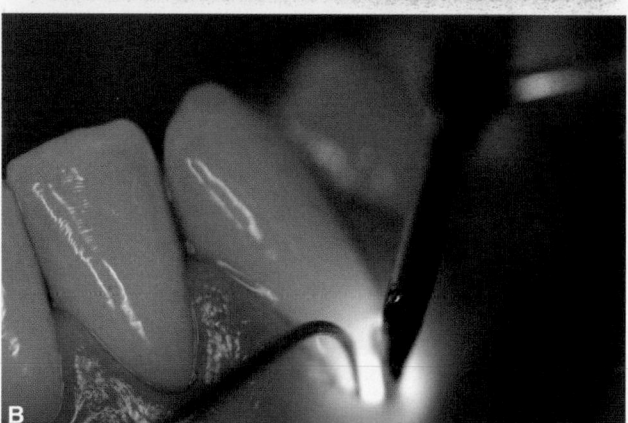

FIGURE 41-10 Endoscope-Assisted Calculus Detection and Removal. A: The calculus is a cream white color due to the mineralization. The explorer for the endoscope is to at the bottom of the picture. **B:** In this image, the precision or slimline ultrasonic tip (left) is being used with the endoscope to the right. (Courtesy: Judy Carroll, RDH.)

▶ Advanced root therapy for patients unable or unwilling to have recommended surgical procedures.

D. Advantages

▶ *Quality of end product*: Enhance the quality of instrumentation by providing an objective means of evaluating root surface.

▶ *Tactile sensitivity*: Over a period of time, instill a greater tactile sense in the clinician, improving subjective evaluation skill.

▶ *Patient education*: Create a new means of engaging, motivating, and educating the patient in the treatment.

▶ Provide opportunity for noninvasive, definitive root therapy:
  • When access is limited during routine instrumentation.
  • For sites unresponsive to traditional nonsurgical therapy.

- In anterior regions where preservation of soft tissue is necessary for optimum esthetics.
- When surgical therapy may be contraindicated for the patient.
▶ Provide confirmation of clinical findings that might otherwise go undiagnosed or require surgical intervention.
  - Root fractures.
  - Restorative post perforations.
  - Open margins.
  - Subgingival caries.
  - Residual cement.
  - Anatomical anomalies.

E. Disadvantage

▶ *Learning curve*: Using the endoscope to visualize root accretions is of significant benefit, but learning to utilize the endoscope is challenging and takes regular use to become proficient. Some of the challenges include:
  - The clinician must work two-handed and hold the endoscope in the left hand while adapting instruments and ultrasonic to the root surface with the right hand.
  - The clinician has to watch the monitor in order to assess the presence of calculus and adaptation for removal.

ULTRASONIC AND SONIC SCALING

Ultrasonic and manual nonsurgical instrumentation can produce equivalent results in calculus and dental biofilm removal when the instruments are applied correctly and sensitive posttreatment evaluation is made.[1]

▶ Long-term goals of therapy are accomplished through a blended approach utilizing both methods of instrumentation.

▶ The patient benefits from therapy incorporating the strengths of each approach.
▶ Manual instrumentation was the only method available for the safe removal of supragingival and subgingival calculus until the ultrasonic scaling device was introduced in the 1950s.[19]
▶ The power-driven scaling device converted high-frequency electrical energy into mechanical energy in the form of rapid vibrations.
▶ Technologic advances in ultrasonics improved and allowed for rapid calculus removal that resulted in much less hand fatigue for the clinician.
▶ Later, sonic scalers were developed that worked on the same principle but utilized an air turbine as an energy source.
▶ Terminology related to power-driven instrumentation is defined in Box 41-3.

MODE OF ACTION[19]

Although the main action of the ultrasonic and sonic scalers is mechanical, cavitation and irrigation also play a role in debridement.

I. Mechanical Vibration

▶ Power-driven scaling devices convert electrical energy (ultrasonic) or air pressure (sonic) into high-frequency sound waves.
▶ Sound waves produce rapid vibrations in the specially designed scaling tips.
▶ Calculus is incrementally shattered from the tooth surface when the vibrations are applied to the deposit.

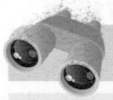

BOX 41-3　KEY WORDS: Ultrasonic and Sonic Instrumentation

Acoustic turbulence: agitation in the fluids surrounding a rapidly vibrating ultrasonic tip; has potential to disrupt the bacterial matrix.

Cavitation: action created by the formation and collapse of bubbles in the water by high-frequency sound waves surrounding an ultrasonic tip.

Ferromagnetic: type of rod with unusually high magnetic permeability used in magnetostrictive ultrasonic unit inserts.

Kilohertz (kHz): a unit of energy equal to 1,000 cps.

Lavage: the therapeutic washing of the pocket and root surface to remove endotoxins and loose debris.

Magnetic field: space occupied by magnetic lines of force.

Magnetostrictive: ultrasonic scaling device that generates a magnetic field and produces tip vibrations by the expansion and contraction of a metal stack or rod.

Piezoelectric: ultrasonic scaling device activated by dimensional changes in crystals housed in the handpiece.

Sonic scaler: type of mechanical power-driven scaler that functions from energy delivered by a vibrating working tip in the frequency of 2,500–7,000 cps; driven by compressed air, the handpiece connects directly to a conventional rotary handpiece tubing.

Stack: magnetostrictive inserts made of flat metal strips stacked, or sandwiched, together; metal in stack acts like an antenna to pick up magnetic field and cause vibration.

Transducer: a device that converts energy or power from one form to another.

Ultrasonic scaler: power-driven scaling instrument that operates in a frequency range between 25,000 and 50,000 cps to convert a high-frequency electrical current into mechanical vibrations.

II. Cavitation

▶ Water is required to dissipate the heat produced at the vibrating tip.

▶ Cavitation occurs when the water meets the vibrating tip. Minute bubbles are created that collapse and release energy.

▶ *Effect of cavitation*: Cavitation is capable of destroying surface bacteria and removing endotoxin from the root surface.[20,21]

III. Irrigation[21]

▶ The water spray penetrates to the base of the pocket to provide a continuous flushing of debris, microorganisms, and endotoxin.

▶ Oscillation of the ultrasonic tip causes hydrodynamic waves to surround the tip. This acoustic turbulence is believed to have a disruptive effect on surface bacteria.

▶ Ultrasonic debridement following manual instrumentation provides cleansing and rinsing of scaled and root planed surfaces, which can promote healing of soft tissues.

IV. Variable Elements

Power-driven scaling devices feature varying elements but are mainly distinguished by their frequency output and the direction and pattern of tip motion, as shown in Figure 41-11.

▶ *Amplitude*: distance of tip movement measured in micrometers.

　• Distance of tip movement determines power output of the instrument, which is an adjustable component on all ultrasonic devices.

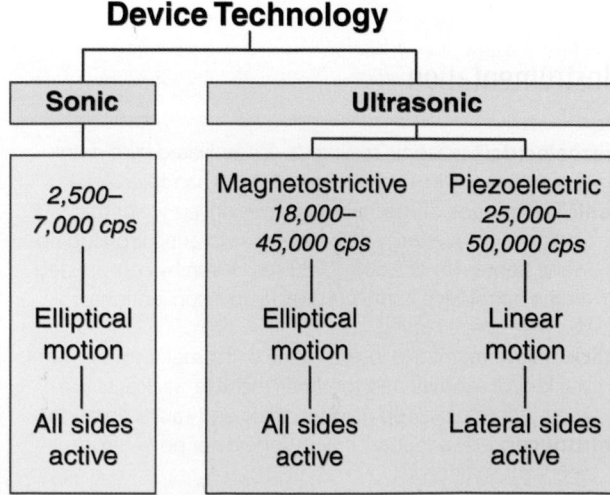

Device Technology

FIGURE 41-11 Power-Driven Scaling Devices Technology. For sonic and both magnetostrictive and piezoelectric ultrasonic scalers, the speed (cps), the motion (linear or elliptical), and the active part of the tip (lateral sides only or all sides) identified.

▶ *Frequency*: speed of movement.

　• Number of cycles per second (cps) the tip moves.

　• Adjustable component available only on manually tuned ultrasonic devices.

　• Majority of available devices have tuning preset or "automatic."

ULTRASONIC SCALING DEVICES

I. Two Types

▶ Magnetostrictive ultrasonic scalers.

▶ Piezoelectric ultrasonic scalers.

II. Equipment

Ultrasonic scaling devices share certain attributes and are differentiated by others.

A. Unit Parts

▶ Electric generator

▶ Handpiece assembly

▶ Set of interchangeable scaling tip inserts

▶ Foot control to activate the handpiece.

B. Tip Activation

▶ Vibrations in the tip occur when electric current is applied to the handpiece.

C. Water Source

▶ Necessary for delivery of water to the handpiece.

▶ Water is carried through or around the instrument tip.

▶ Cools tip. Rapid tip movement creates friction and/or temperature increase in the tooth.

▶ Flushes subgingival debris.

III. Magnetostrictive Ultrasonic Scalers[21]

A. Composition

▶ *Conventional magnetostrictive units*: Utilize a longitudinal stack of metal strips in the handpiece.

▶ *Ferromagnetic units*: Utilize a fragile ferric rod that generates less heat than the conventional metal stack.

B. Activation

▶ Vibrations in the tip occur when electric current is applied to the handpiece.

▶ A magnetic field is created by expansion and contraction of metal strips in the handpiece.

C. Tip Motion

▶ Conventional tip moves in an elliptical pattern; all surfaces of the tip are active.

▶ Ferromagnetic tip rotates 360° in three different planes; equal effectiveness on all sides of the tip.

D. Tip Shape

Cross section of tip is round.

E. Frequency

▶ Conventional units range from 18,000 to 45,000 cps.
  • Older units are designed to operate at 25,000 cps and are called 25-kilohertz (kHz) machines.
  • Newer units are designed to operate at 30,000 cps and are called 30-kHz machines.
▶ Ferromagnetic units operate at 42,000 cps.

IV. Piezoelectric Ultrasonic Scalers

▶ *Composition*: Scaler devices feature a ceramic rod in the handpiece.
▶ *Activation*: As a result of dimensional changes in crystal transducers housed in the handpiece.
▶ *Tip motion*: Moves in a linear pattern, forward and backward.
  • Only the lateral surfaces of the tip are active.
  • Handpiece position will adjust at each line angle to maintain adaptation of the lateral surface of the tip to the tooth; accomplished by pivoting the wrist to approximate a 90° turn of the instrument to move from facial or lingual surfaces to proximal surfaces and back again.
▶ *Technique*: Placement and movement of the tip is specific.
  • Position the lateral surface of the tip in contact with the tooth.
  • Use only the terminal 2–3 mm of the tip's lateral surface.
  • Keep terminal lateral surface adapted at all times around curvatures and line angles using wrist pivot.
▶ *Tip shape*: Cross section of tip varies from trapezoidal with angular edges to round to bladed.
▶ *Frequency*
  • Varies according to manufacturer
  • Ranges from 25,000 to 50,000 cps.

SONIC SCALING DEVICES[21]

I. Equipment: Unit Parts

▶ Handpiece.
▶ Interchangeable scaling tips.
▶ Handpiece attaches directly to the dental unit and is activated with the conventional handpiece foot control.

II. Tip Activation

A. Tip Motion

▶ Driven by compressed air from the dental unit rather than electrical energy.

▶ Moves in an orbital pattern, but varies depending on tip and type of sonic scaler.
▶ All surfaces of the tip are active.

B. Amplitude

▶ Less powerful than ultrasonic scalers.

C. Frequency

▶ Producing vibrations at the tip; range between 3,000 and 8,000 cps.
▶ Because of fewer vibrations produced, calculus removal is more difficult.

D. Water Source

▶ Water is required to cool the friction between the instrument tip and the tooth surface.
▶ Heat is not generated by the scaling tip.

PURPOSES AND USES FOR POWER-DRIVEN SCALERS[21]

I. Indications for Use

▶ Removal of dental biofilm, extrinsic stain, and supra- and subgingival calculus.
▶ *Subgingival periodontal debridement, including:*
  • Removal of calculus, attached biofilm, and endotoxins from the root surface
  • Reduction of bacterial load in the periodontal pocket.
▶ *Initial debridement*
  • For a patient with necrotizing ulcerative gingivitis or other conditions that can be relieved by removal of deposits.
  • Loose debris and microorganisms are first removed by preprocedural rinse,[15] brushing, and flossing during patient instruction to prevent or reduce contaminated aerosol production.
▶ Debridement of furcation areas following manual instrumentation.
▶ Debridement of deposits before oral surgery.
▶ Removal of orthodontic cement; debonding.
▶ Removal of overhanging margins of restorations.

II. Contraindications

A. Systemic Health Conditions

▶ *Communicable disease*: Patient with a communicable disease that can be transmitted by aerosols, such as tuberculosis.
▶ *Susceptibility to infection*
  • Compromised patient with marked susceptibility to infection.
  • Examples: immunosuppression from disease or chemotherapy, uncontrolled diabetes, or kidney or other organ transplant.

▶ *Respiratory risk*: patient with a respiratory risk. Septic material and microorganisms from biofilm and periodontal pockets can be aspirated into the lungs.[22]

- History of chronic obstructive pulmonary disease, including asthma, emphysema, or cystic fibrosis.

▶ *Swallowing difficulty*

- Patient with a swallowing problem (dysphagia) or prone to gagging.
- Dysphagia results in liquids being aspirated into the lungs along with oral bacteria and increases the risk of aspiration pneumonia.[23] Consultation with the primary care provider is needed prior to dental treatment.
- Examples: amyotrophic lateral sclerosis, muscular dystrophy, Parkinson's disease, paralysis, multiple sclerosis, and after stroke.

▶ *Cardiac pacemaker*

- Newer pacemaker devices are shielded. Consultation with the patient's cardiologist is necessary.

B. Oral Conditions

▶ *Avoid demineralized areas*

- Ultrasonic vibrations can remove the delicate remineralizing cover of a demineralized area.[24]

▶ *Exposed dentinal surfaces*

- Tooth structure can be removed in excess and create sensitivity with too much lateral force and high power settings.[24]
- The smear layer can be removed and dentinal tubules uncovered, which can increase sensitivity or aggravate existing sensitivity.

▶ *Thermal injury*

- Thermal damage to the pulp can occur if the ultrasonic tip overheats because of inadequate water cooling or excess pressure.[19,24]
- Gingival tissues can be experience thermal injury if water cooling is inadequate.

▶ *Children*

- Young, growing, developing tissues are sensitive to ultrasonic vibrations.
- Primary and newly erupted permanent teeth have large pulp chambers. Vibrations and heat from the ultrasonic scaler may damage pulp tissue.

III. Precautions

A. Damage to the Integrity of Restorations[25]

▶ Improper tip application may increase roughness such as scratches chips, or notches in restorative materials.

- *Porcelain*: may remove the glaze of the porcelain and create pores on the surface where the tip was in contact with the porcelain.

- *Amalgam*: may cause scratches, loss of material, and create pores in the restorative material.
- *Composites*: roughened surfaces.

B. Titanium Implant Abutments

Ultrasonic instrumentation will damage titanium surfaces unless the insert is designed for use with implants and covered with a specially designed plastic tip.[26]

IV. Risk Considerations

A. Clinician

▶ *Cumulative trauma*

- Many dental hygienists suffer from musculoskeletal injuries related to cumulative trauma.
- Powered scaling reduces the pinch force and finger–hand muscle activity needed to remove deposits, which is hypothesized to reduce nerve compression disorders like carpal tunnel syndrome and other musculoskeletal disorders.[27]
- However, work with instruments that vibrate, such as the ultrasonic scaler, are associated with sensorineural dysfunction that include loss of tactile sense in the fingertips.[20] In one study, dental hygienists using vibrating tools had higher rates of carpel tunnel syndrome suggesting more research is needed in this area.[28]

▶ *Magnetic fields*

- Ultrasonic scalers produce weak, time-varying magnetic fields similar to those produced by common household appliances.
- There is no scientific evidence that cumulative exposure to weak, time-varying magnetic fields has caused any biological harm to any dental personnel.[29]

B. Patient

▶ *Hearing shifts*

- Extended exposure to noises above a certain level, such as the noise of a high-speed handpiece or an ultrasonic scaler, may be damaging.
- Temporary hearing shifts have been demonstrated for a group of patients.[19]

ULTRASONIC AND SONIC TIP DESIGN

I. Parts

The parts are illustrated in Figure 41-12. The design of the instrument tip will vary according to the intended use. Figure 41-13 shows examples of various tip designs.

II. Size and Type

A. Conventional or Standard Tip

▶ Traditional ultrasonic and sonic tips, bulkier than most curet tips. Also called *universal* tips.

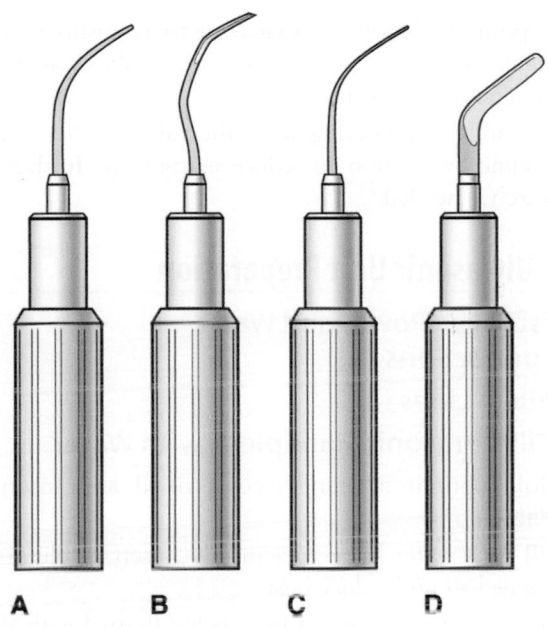

Point   Tip   Grip   O-Ring   Magnetostrictive stack

FIGURE 41-12 Ultrasonic Handpiece Insert. With parts labeled.

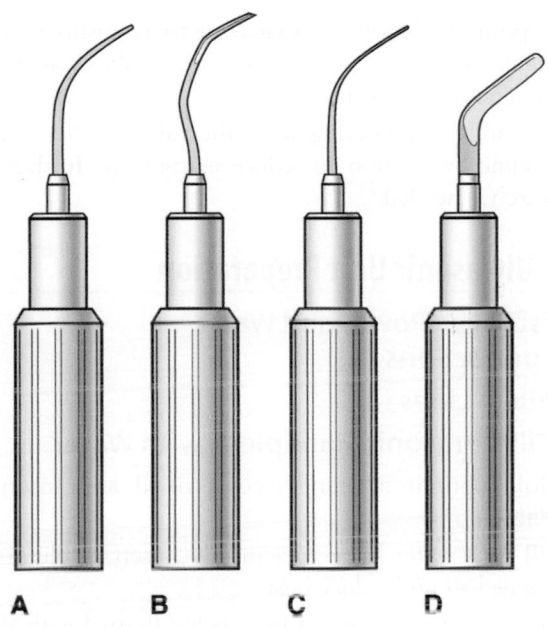

FIGURE 41-13 Ultrasonic Tip Designs. A: Straight tip with internal flow water delivery. **B:** Triple bend tip for moderate-to-heavy calculus. **C:** Thinner tip. **D:** Beavertail for supragingival surfaces needing removal of heavy calculus or cement.

- Generally used for moderate-to-heavy deposit removal from supragingival or relatively shallow subgingival surfaces.
- Standard tips for both magnetostrictive and piezoelectric devices may be used on any power setting.

B. Periodontal or Narrow-Profile Tip

- Thinner and longer tips provide better access to subgingival surfaces.
- Allow superior coverage of deep pockets and furcations.
- Most magnetostrictive thin tips are used on low-to-medium power to prevent breakage.
- Piezoelectric thin tips may be used on high power, which will not burnish calculus.
- Tip design innovations continue to emerge in answer to the demands of advanced nonsurgical therapy.
- Bladed and beveled tips are capable of removing calculus rapidly.

- Diamond-coated tips used on low power are effective for fine scaling and root planing.[30]

C. Plastic, Silicone, or Carbon Composite Tip[26]

- An insert with a plastic, silicone, or carbon composite tip may be used to protect vulnerable restorative surfaces such as titanium abutments of implants or esthetic materials surfaces.
- Dentin and titanium surfaces can be safely instrumented with the plastic tip. A low power, light pressure is all that is needed to remove biofilm and mineralizing deposits.

III. Shape

- *Universal:* Tip slightly curved in one direction; to be used throughout the dentition (Figure 41-14 shows a piezoelectric handpiece and universal tip).
- *Triple bend:* A design with beveled edges for removal of heavy stain and calculus.
- *Contra-angled:* Instrument tips have curvatures to left and right designed to adapt to posterior surfaces of the teeth.

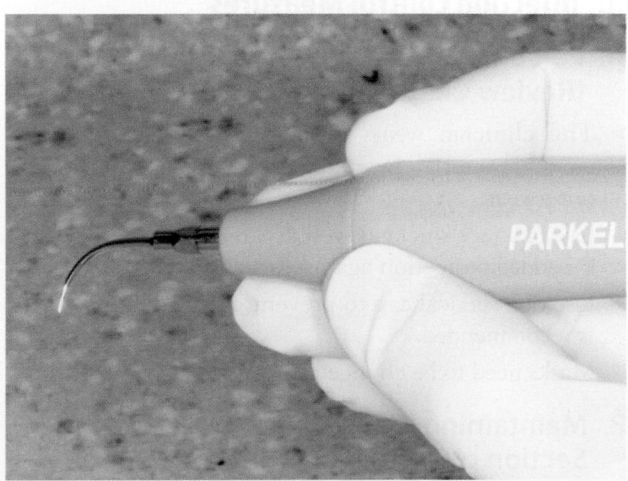

FIGURE 41-14 Piezoelectric Handpiece and Universal Tip. An example of a piezoelectric ultrasonic handpiece and powered tip. (Reprinted from Nield-Gehrig J. Fundamentals of Periodontal Instrumentation and Advanced Root Instrumentation. Philadelphia: Lippincott Williams & Wilkins; 2011.)

▶ *Beavertail*: Designed to be used on supragingival surfaces for the removal of heavy calculus, stain, and orthodontic cement.

▶ *Thin periodontal*: Straight or contra-angled tip designed for light subgingival instrumentation used on low-power setting.

IV. Water Delivery

▶ *External tube*: An external tube delivers the water to the tip of the instrument.

▶ *Internal tube*: Water is delivered from the unit to cool the tip through the internal structure of the insert.

CLINICAL PREPARATION

I. Dental Hygiene Care Plan

A. Review Patient's Medical History and Treatment Records

B. Oral Examination

▶ Review the risk assessment, examination data (review Chapter 20), radiographs, and care plan to determine the following:
  • Location of deposits.
  • Depth of pockets and soft tissue attachment topography.
  • Location and grade of furcation involvement.

C. Instrumentation Plan

▶ Plan a systematic sequence.

▶ Complete one quadrant before starting another, instrumenting each tooth to completion.

II. Infection Control Measures

A. Personal Protective Equipment (Review Chapter 5)

▶ The clinician wears protective eyewear, high-efficiency bacterial face mask, gloves, and protective outerwear.

▶ Use of a face shield as well as a regular mask is needed for added protection against aerosols.

▶ Use of a surgical cap to prevent contamination of hair is recommended.

▶ Masks need to be changed at the first sign of moisture.

B. Maintaining Water Lines[31,32] (Review the Section on Unit Water Lines in Chapter 6)

▶ Biofilm forms on the internal surfaces of dental tubing, as found in the dental unit and ultrasonic unit.

▶ Risk of exposure to dental personnel through the aerosol emerging in the vicinity of the treatment area up to 20 feet.

▶ Risk of exposure to the patient through aspiration and/or bacteremia.

▶ To reduce bacterial contamination, water lines maintained as follows:
  • Chemical treatment of water lines and frequent testing of water quality is required.
  • Flush for 20–30 seconds between patients.
  • Flush for 30 seconds before sterile insert is placed in the handpiece.

C. High-Volume Evacuation

▶ Deposition of tooth-associated microorganisms into the pulmonary system during ultrasonic scaling can result in pulmonary infection.[22]

▶ Research is conflicting about the value of use of high-volume evacuation to reduce aerosols, so further research is needed.[25]

III. Ultrasonic Unit Preparation

A. Establish Power and Water Connections

B. Flush Lines

C. Fill Ultrasonic Handpiece with Water

▶ Hold upright as handpiece is filled and insert is placed.

▶ Fill with water before placing the insert to eliminate trapped air and reduce heat.

▶ To prevent sterile insert from being flushed with stagnant water in pipes.

D. Select Insert

▶ Insert needs to be compatible with ultrasonic unit available.

▶ The metal stacks in the 30-kHz inserts are much shorter than the 25-kHz inserts.

▶ The tip is selected according to the intended use.
  • Standard tip for calculus removal.
  • Slender profile elongated thin tips for biofilm debridement during maintenance phase.

E. Set Power Level

▶ Select the power setting according to the task at hand.
  • *Calculus*: medium-high to high power is needed.
  • *Soft deposit*: low-to-medium power is sufficient for removal of attached and unattached biofilm.

▶ Consistent use of the unit on the lowest power setting for all case types will burnish the calculus present.

F. Adjust Water

▶ Water provides cooling and irrigation.

▶ Proper water setting will create a fine mist at the tip of the instrument.

▶ Increase water if heat is produced.

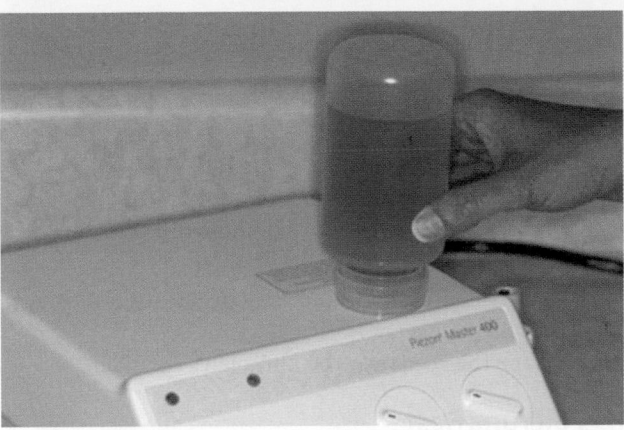

FIGURE 41-15 Reservoir for Ultrasonic Unit. This ultrasonic device has an optional reservoir system for dispensing irrigant solutions—such as chlorhexidine gluconate—to an ultrasonic tip. (Reprinted from Nield-Gehrig J, Willmann D. Foundations of Periodontics for the Dental Hygienist. Philadelphia: Wolters Kluwer Health/Lippincott Williams & Wilkins; 2011.)

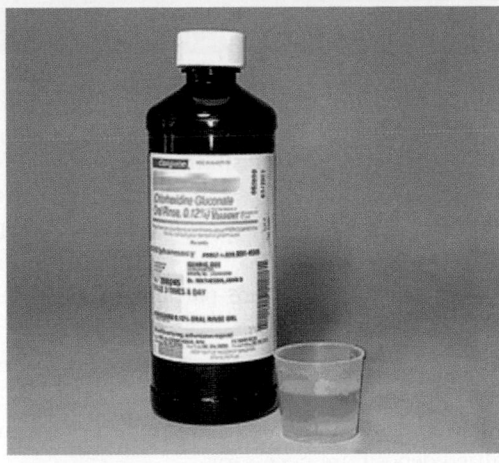

FIGURE 41-16 Preprocedure Rinse. Administering a preprocedural rinse is recommended to reduce the numbers of bacteria and other oral pathogens in aerosols. (Reprinted from Nield-Gehrig J, Willmann D. Foundations of Periodontics for the Dental Hygienist. Philadelphia: Wolters Kluwer Health/Lippincott Williams & Wilkins; 2011.)

G. Use of an Antimicrobial Solution

▶ Some ultrasonic units have reservoirs (see Figure 41-15) so an antimicrobial solution can be used as the coolant since the lavage of ultrasonics can penetrate to the base of the pocket.[19]

▶ Antimicrobial solutions will reduce the number of pathogens present in the contaminated aerosol.[15]

IV. Sonic Unit Preparation

▶ Flush water lines in slow-speed-handpiece line for 2 minutes.

▶ Attach sonic handpiece to slow-speed-handpiece line.

▶ Select and screw sonic tip into handpiece.

V. Patient Preparation

A. Review Health History

▶ Check to ensure that any patient requiring preprocedural antibiotic has taken the prescribed medication. Bacteremia is produced in a high percentage of patients treated by powered instrumentation, as well as manual instrumentation.[28]

▶ Identify contraindications to ultrasonic instrumentation.

B. Explain Procedure

▶ Describe and demonstrate sound and spray, vibration, and the purpose for use.

▶ Request hearing-impaired patient turn off hearing aid; ultrasonic use creates interference and feedback in hearing aids.

C. Provide Protection for Patient

▶ Safety glasses to prevent eye infections or injury.

▶ Fluid-resistant drape over patient to keep moisture from skin and clothing.

D. Preprocedural Rinse[15]

▶ Ultrasonic and sonic instrumentation generates aerosols that are heavily contaminated by microorganisms.

▶ Prior to treatment, patients are directed to rinse with an antimicrobial mouthrinse for 30 seconds.

▶ The use of 0.12% chlorhexidine is preferred for the preprocedural rinse because of its substantivity (Figure 41-16).

E. Patient Position

Place the patient in a supine position for maximum visibility.

F. Patient Breathing

▶ Explain to the patient, and request breathing/air exchange only through the nose.

▶ Reduces potential for aspiration of oral pathogens into lung tissue.

▶ Allows water to pool for evacuation with saliva ejector.

▶ Less fogging of mouth mirror.

▶ More comfort for patient.

G. Pain Control

Use local anesthesia for pain management.

H. Water Control

▶ Prepare to use evacuation with saliva ejector or high-volume evacuator with a dental assistant as indicated by the severity and degree of sepsis and communicability of infection from the patient.[32]

▶ Shape and position saliva ejector so the patient can hold it in place to collect water pooling in the mouth.

ULTRASONIC INSTRUMENTATION

As with manual instrumentation, power instrumentation depends on skill and technique.

▶ Tactile sensitivity and visibility are reduced when power instrumentation is used, so knowledge of tooth morphology is essential for debriding periodontal pockets efficiently and safely.

▶ Ultrasonic instrumentation, particularly piezoelectric, is technique dependent.

• Care in adapting the terminal 3-mm portion of the working end to the tooth surface and methodical activation using sufficient power to disrupt the mineralized deposit are necessary.

I. Principles for Technique

A. Power Setting

▶ *Low power*

• While more comfortable for the patient, low power is not capable of removing moderate-to-heavy calculus effectively.

• Deposit can become burnished on the root surface and leave a polished exterior surface that is difficult to detect and remove.

• Remnants of burnished calculus can harbor pathogenic contaminants.

▶ *High-to-medium power*

• Moderate-to-heavy calculus can be removed using higher power settings, provided the proper technique is employed.

• Use of local anesthesia permits maximum thoroughness while keeping the patient comfortable.

B. Transfer of Energy

▶ The full length of the tip is vibrating, but only the terminal few millimeters will transfer maximum energy capable of disrupting calculus.

C. Adaptation

▶ Position side of tip against tooth, with the few millimeters nearest the end of the tip closely adapted on the surface at all times (Figure 41-17).

▶ May be difficult to accomplish, since the end segment of the tip is generally straight in contrast to anatomical curvatures of the tooth anatomy.

D. Activation

▶ Adequate time is needed for energy to transfer from the active tip to the deposit to break up the mineralized component effectively.

▶ Speed of movement is critical to this transfer.

▶ The tip is moved constantly at a slow-to-moderate pace.

II. Ultrasonic Scaling

A. Grasp

▶ Use a modified pen grasp.

▶ A light grasp will increase tactile sensitivity.

▶ The weight of the cord tends to pull on the handpiece and place additional strain on the wrist. Manage cord drag by the following:

• Loop the cord and hold it between the ring finger and little finger.

• Drape the cord over the clinician's shoulder.

B. Fulcrum/Rest

▶ A hard tissue fulcrum is not required because force and pressure against the tooth surface are not indicated.

▶ A gentle finger rest is used to stabilize and guide the instrument tip in anterior segments.

▶ Extraoral and soft tissue rests allow for proper access and adaptation to deeper posterior segments.

C. Adaptation

▶ Keep the side of the instrument tip closely adapted to the tooth surface (Figure 41-17).

▶ Do not hold the tip perpendicular to the tooth surface at any time because damage to the tooth surface can result.

▶ *Narrow periodontal pockets*

• Narrow subgingival pockets interfere with proper adaptation and impede visibility.

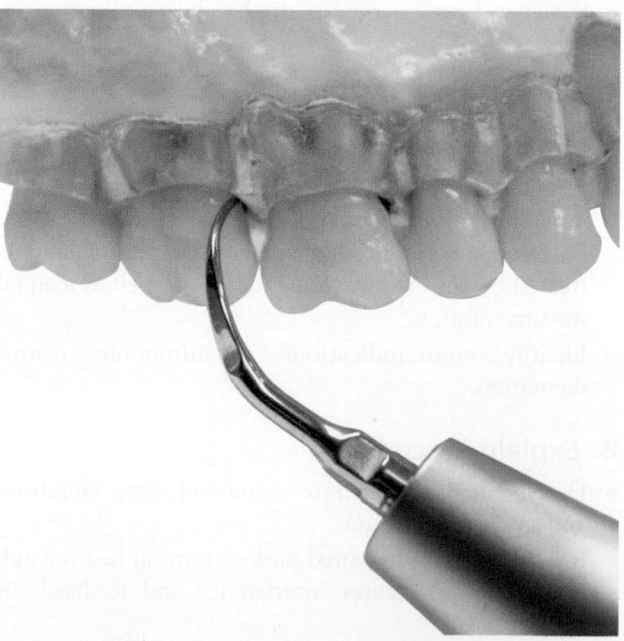

FIGURE 41-17 **Adaptation of Ultrasonic Tip.** The side of the point of a tip is placed parallel to the tooth surface to prevent damage to the tooth structure. Damage occurs when the point is held perpendicular to the surface. (Courtesy of Hu-Friedy).

- When instrumenting narrow pockets use an insert with appropriate length and limited width.
- Direct the tip apically and confirm access to the attachment prior to activating the tip.

D. Stroke

▶ Keep the instrument tip moving at a moderate-to-slow pace with a feather-light touch at all times to prevent the following:
- Scratches or gouging on the tooth surface.
- Excessive heat build-up.
- A galvanic shock-like effect to the patient.

▶ Use featherlike pressure to prevent tooth damage. Excessive lateral pressure can result in the following:
- Damage to the tooth surface.
- Dampening and deactivation of the tip vibrations.
- Burnishing of calculus.

▶ *Overlap strokes*
- For comprehensive coverage of all surfaces.
- Strokes may be horizontal, vertical, oblique, or a combination.

▶ Procedure when the tip binds in an embrasure.
- Deactivate the power; remove the instrument tip from the embrasure.
- Reposition the instrument and reactivate the power.

E. Microultrasonics[33,34]

▶ Microultrasonics is a term used to describe the use of slimmer ultrasonic tips in concert with a dental endoscope to visualize subgingival calculus for debridement (Figure 41-18).

▶ Advantages of microultrasonics include:
- Reduce overinstrumentation.
- Minimize excessive removal of cementum.
- Improves outcomes and minimizes the need for periodontal surgery.

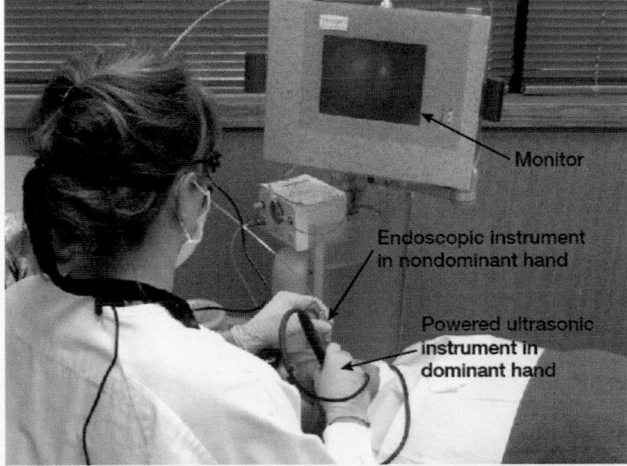

FIGURE 41-18 **Dental Endoscopic System.** The clinician holds the endoscopic instrument in her nondominant hand. In this photo to visualize calculus and the root surface. The clinician uses microultrasonics in her dominant hand. (Courtesy of John Y. Kwan, DDS.) Reprinted from Nield-Gehrig J. Fundamentals of Periodontal Instrumentation and Advanced Root Instrumentation. Philadelphia: Lippincott Williams & Wilkins; 2011.)

III. Water Control

A. Foot Pedal

▶ Release the foot pedal at regular intervals to aid in water control.

▶ Stop periodically to evaluate tooth surfaces.

B. Mirror Use

▶ Water is continuously sprayed onto the mirror surface, making indirect vision difficult.

▶ Wipe the wet surface of the mirror with a gloved finger to coalesce the drops into a clear wet surface. When water is allowed to pool on the surface in this manner, a clearer image of the working area can be seen through the water.

IV. Manual Scaling

▶ Complete the procedure with manual instruments directly following ultrasonic instrumentation.

▶ Check subgingival areas with a subgingival explorer.

▶ Remove remaining subgingival irregularities and smooth the surface with curets.

V. Evaluation

A. Use a Periodontal Subgingival Explorer

▶ To evaluate the effectiveness of instrumentation periodically during treatment.

▶ There may be areas of root contour where it is not possible to adapt the ultrasonic insert tip, thus leaving portions of the root surface untreated.

▶ Portions of the root that cannot be accessed by the ultrasonic tip must be instrumented using curets that will adapt to the root surface; after five, mini- or micro-mini-bladed Gracey curets are well suited for this purpose.

B. Ultrasonic Tip Without Power Can Be Used as Explorer

▶ To confirm access to the soft tissue attachment.

▶ There is insufficient tactile sensitivity to accomplish a careful assessment of the root surface smoothness with the insert.

VI. Troubleshooting

There may be a number of reasons for the ultrasonic instrument to produce unacceptable instrumentation. The causative factor is analyzed to remedy the problem.

A. Tip Wear

▶ As an ultrasonic tip is used over a period of time, the length of the tip is reduced. With each millimeter of tip length lost, there is a corresponding loss of power.

▶ Tips need to be checked periodically for wear and replaced when length has reached a point beyond which the tip is incapable of producing sufficient vibration.

▶ *To monitor tip wear*:

- Use a tip wear indicator template provided by the manufacturer (see Figure 41-19A and B).
- Reserve one of each tip in use as a prototype to compare length reduction.
- Check for loss in length; a 2 mm or more loss in length renders the tip ineffective for calculus removal.

B. Improper Adaptation

▶ Failure to adapt the terminal few millimeters of the tip to the tooth surface.

▶ Root morphology has many curvatures featuring convex and concave surfaces.

▶ Straight instruments do not adapt well to curved surfaces.

▶ Curets, specifically minibladed Gracey curets, are designed to conform to root contours.

▶ Supplement ultrasonic instrumentation with manual instrumentation to access the highly curved portions of the root.

C. Stroke Too Rapid

▶ Moving the tip too quickly across the tooth surface.

▶ Keep tip moving slowly and methodically.

▶ Brisk tip movement is ineffective for deposit removal.

D. Inadequate Coverage

▶ Failure to keep strokes confined to close, overlapping channels.

- Move the tip in overlapping segments or channels that cover each square millimeter of root surface.

▶ Moving the tip in a random, scribbling pattern can treat effectively only those limited portions of the root surface that were contacted by the moving tip.

E. Tip Pressure

▶ Exerting lateral pressure with the tip against the tooth surface rendering the vibrations ineffective due to a dampening effect.

- The tip is held with only a light but secure contact and close adaptation against the tooth surface.

LASER THERAPY

▶ Use of lasers in periodontal treatment is controversial, but continues to increase despite conflicting research findings.[32]

- The American Academy of Periodontology suggests there is inadequate evidence to support use of lasers for treatment of chronic periodontitis. Research has not shown it to be superior to traditional scaling and root planing.[32–37]

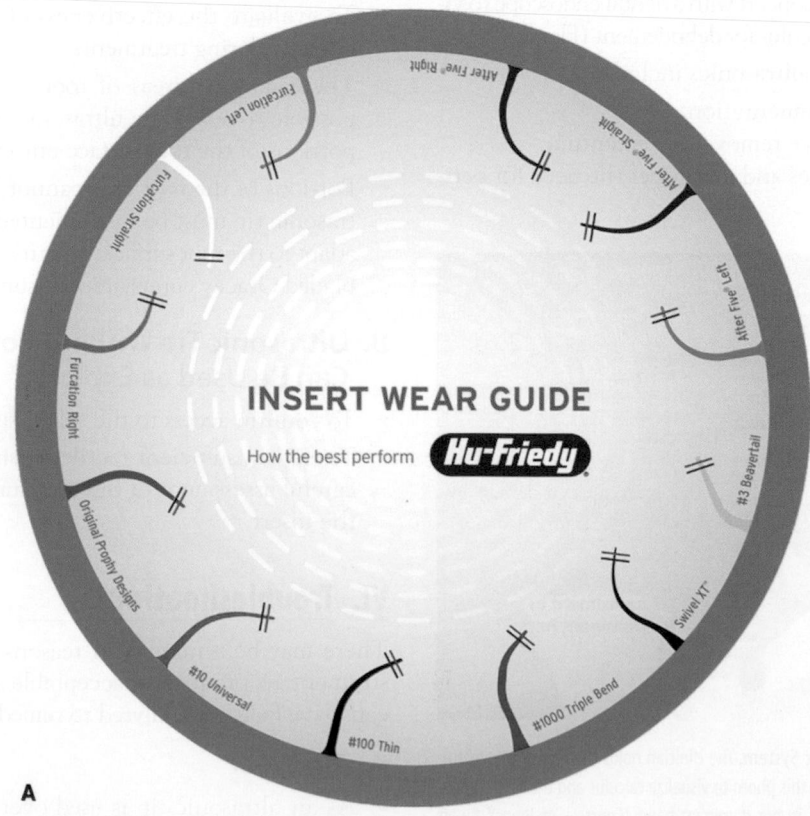

A

FIGURE 41-19 A and B: Ultrasonic Tip Wear. Scaling efficiency is diminished with worn insert tips and should be assessed regularly with a wear guide. About 1 mm loss results in 25% loss of efficiency and 2 mm loss results in 50% loss of efficiency in calculus removal. (Courtesy Hu-Friedy.)

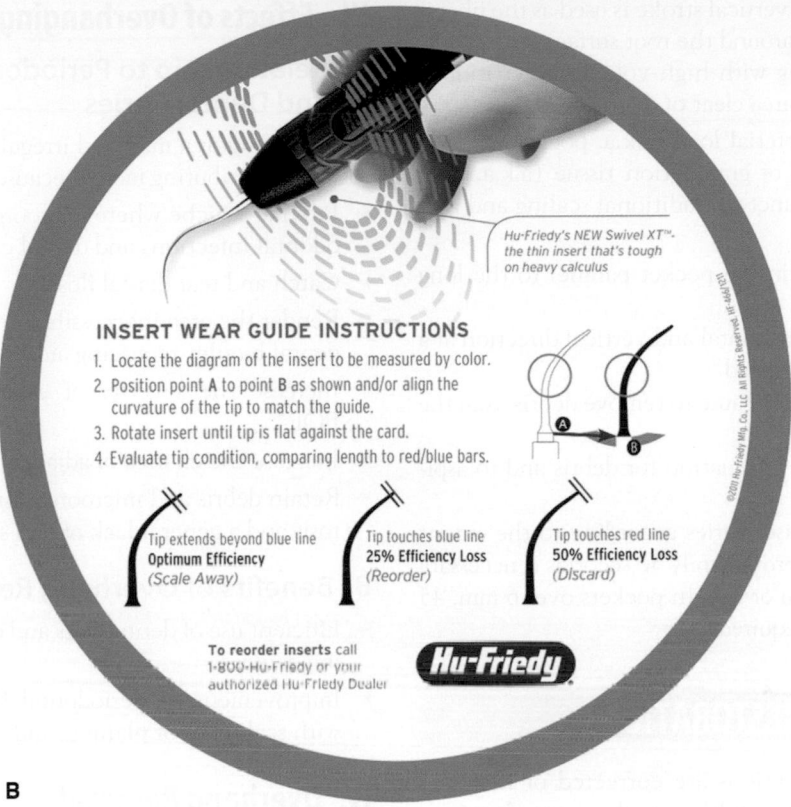

FIGURE 41-19 (*continued*)

I. Types of Lasers

▶ Lasers emit light through a process called stimulated emission.
  • When the light reaches the tissue, it is reflected, scattered, absorbed, or transmitted to surrounding tissues.
  • The wavelength of the light influences how the light interacts with the tissue.
▶ The wavelength of lasers most often used in periodontal treatment is 635–10,600 nm and includes:[36]
  • Semiconductor diode lasers
  • Solid-state lasers: neodymium-doped; yttrium, aluminum, and garnet (Nd:YAG); neodymium-doped yttrium, aluminum, and perovskite (Nd:YAP); erbium-doped: yttrium, aluminum and garnet (Er:YAG); and erbium, chromium-doped yttrium scandium, gallium and garnet (Er,Cr:YSGG).
  • Gas lasers (CO_2)
▶ A thorough knowledge of the effect of the various emission wavelengths of the laser on biologic tissues to choose the most appropriate device for treatment.
▶ The equipment for laser therapy is expensive and cost–benefit over traditional scaling and root planing has not been evaluated in current literature.
  • Each manufacturer requires the purchaser contract with them for training to use the equipment, which further impacts the cost.

II. Purported Benefits of Lasers in Nonsurgical Periodontal Therapy[38–40]

▶ Pocket debridement
  • There is little evidence of benefit of laser therapy beyond traditional scaling and root planing.
▶ Reduction of subgingival bacterial load
  • Results of research have been inconsistent in demonstrating that lasers reduce the subgingival bacterial load beyond traditional SRP.
▶ Scaling and root planing
  • Erbium lasers (Er:YAG) show the most potential for effective root debridement.
  • There is potential for damage to the root surface because the Er:YAG is a hard tissue laser.
  • Research is inconsistent regarding increases in clinical attachment with the Er:Yag versus scaling and root planing.[38]

III. Technique

▶ For calculus removal:[40]
  • Insert laser fiber in the pocket parallel to the long axis of the tooth.
  • Angulation is 45°.

- A horizontal and vertical stroke is used as the fiber is slowly advanced around the root surface.
- Water spray along with high-volume evacuation is used to keep the area clear of debris.

▶ For reduction of bacterial load (a.k.a. pocket sterilization) and curettage of granulation tissue (a.k.a. laser curettage) as an adjunct to traditional scaling and root planing:[41]

- Insert laser fiber in the pocket parallel to the long axis of the tooth.
- Move fiber in a horizontal and vertical direction at a slow-to-moderate speed.
- Use moistened 2 × 2 gauze to remove debris from the fiber periodically.
- Use high-volume evacuation for debris and to aspirate fumes.
- Time for use of laser varies according to the extent of disease, but approximately 30 seconds is necessary in pocket of 6 mm or less. In pockets over 6 mm, 45 seconds may be required.[41]

OVERHANGING RESTORATIONS

All overhanging restorations are corrected or removed and replaced for the health of the periodontium. Whether an overhang can be recontoured or needs to be replaced with a new restoration requires a professional decision.

I. Overhanging Margins

Overhangs may occur on any tooth surface, supragingivally or subgingivally. Proximal surface overhangs result primarily from

▶ Improper placement of the matrix band and/or wedge.
▶ Incorrect manipulation of the dental material.
▶ Finishing errors.

II. Identification

A. Clinical

An overhang is identified by the:

▶ Detection of excess amalgam or composite material beyond the level of the tooth surface with an explorer.
▶ Information from the patient relative to floss breakage and food impaction.

B. Radiographic

▶ Limited to proximal surfaces viewed in the radiograph.
▶ Visibility changed by angulation of the X-ray.
▶ Supplement radiographic examination with a clinical examination using an explorer.
▶ Use of magnification to detect dental caries adjacent to an overhang.

III. Effects of Overhanging Restorations

A. Relationship to Periodontal Disease and Dental Caries

An overhang or a marginal irregularity is a significant iatrogenic contributing factor because it can do the following:

▶ Provide a niche where microorganisms that cause periodontal infections and dental caries can proliferate.
▶ Catch and tear dental floss.
▶ Render the area inaccessible to a toothbrush and other dental biofilm-removing aids.
▶ Increase the severity of existing inflammation and BOP.[42]
▶ Increase the chance of adjacent bone loss.
▶ Retain debris and microorganisms contributing to halitosis and a general lack of oral sanitation.

B. Benefits of Overhang Removal

▶ Efficient use of dental floss and other interdental cleaning devices.
▶ Improvement in periodontal health when combined with scaling, root planing, and dental biofilm control.[43]

IV. Overhang Removal

A. Procedural Overview

▶ Remove excess amalgam.
▶ Finish margins to ensure they are continuous and smooth.
▶ Smooth all surfaces of the restoration.

B. Manual Instruments

General suggestions for use:

▶ Select on basis of accessibility of the filling, amount of reduction required, and surface finish indicated.
▶ Instruments: chisel, file, scalers, curets, finishing strips, and unwaxed extra-fine floss.
▶ *Technique*
  1. Maintain sharp instruments.
  2. Hold the instrument with a modified pen grasp.
  3. Use short, well-controlled, overlapping shaving strokes; remove amalgam in small increments to prevent fracture risk.
  4. Work deliberately to prevent damage to gingival tissue and surrounding tooth surfaces, especially cementum.
  5. Use the tooth surface as a guide to contour the restoration.
  6. Move a bladed instrument parallel to, or slightly toward, the margin of the prepared tooth.
     - For a curet, use oblique strokes over the junction of the material and the tooth.
     - For a chisel, position the blade across the tooth structure and amalgam; activate chisel horizontally across the junction.

- For files, position perpendicular to the long axis of the tooth on the proximal surface and activate horizontal stroke.
7. Keep instruments in contact with the tooth surface to reduce risk of ditching.
8. For proximal adaptation, move chisel away from gingiva to prevent pushing bits of amalgam into the tissue; evacuate continuously.
9. Follow removal of overhang with a chisel or file use a curet for final finishing.
10. Unwaxed extra-fine floss is used to assess complete removal of the overhang.

C. Power-Driven Instruments

▶ Some state practice acts include removal of overhangs with high- or slow-speed handpiece.
  - For high-speed handpieces, a flame-shaped finishing bur is often used.
  - Care is taken not to cause tissue trauma or gouge the restoration or tooth surface.
  - Slow-speed handpieces can also be used.
▶ Ultrasonic instrumentation can be used to remove overhanging margins in concert with manual instruments.
  - Use medium-to-high power for bulk of removal; then switch to manual instruments to finish.
  - *Standard tip*: vertical strokes on proximal surface.
  - *Beavertail design*: horizontal strokes on proximal surface.

COMPLETION OF INITIAL THERAPY

▶ After each nonsurgical instrumentation appointment, an immediate evaluation is made and special instructions are given to the patient for the initial tissue healing period.
▶ A follow-up telephone call, e-mail, or text to the patient during the evening after the appointment can be a welcome gesture that conveys professional responsibility and concern.
▶ A short-term follow-up appointment is scheduled in a minimum of 2 weeks when initial healing will be in progress.
▶ After health has been attained, it must be maintained. Planning for a long-term maintenance program is described in Chapter 48.

I. Ongoing Evaluation

A. Teeth

▶ Observation and exploration reveal the immediate effects of instrumentation on the teeth.
▶ The goal of nonsurgical periodontal therapy is thorough mechanical removal of biofilm and calculus from root surfaces.[1]

▶ The effect of specific instrumentation is to facilitate the patient's self-care by removing local factors, particularly calculus and overhanging fillings, that encourage dental biofilm retention.

B. Gingiva

▶ The gingival changes are not apparent immediately after instrumentation.
▶ Tissue regeneration and initial healing begin in a few days, and by 2 weeks, the area can be gently probed.
▶ Maturation of connective tissue and keratinization of epithelium continues up to 8 weeks after completion of initial therapy and may continue for 9 months.[12]
▶ The objective of treatment is to *create an environment in which the gingival tissue can heal and be maintained in health by the patient.*

II. Examination

When scaling is accomplished over a series of appointments, each previously scaled quadrant or area is examined and rescaled as needed. Visual and tactile methods are applied carefully to each tooth surface.

A. Visual

▶ Compressed air is used with a mouth mirror and adequate lighting to examine the supragingival areas and just below the gingival margins.
▶ Transillumination methods are applied.

B. Tactile

▶ Evaluation with an explorer immediately after completion of instrumentation is made to ascertain the tooth surfaces are smooth and all detectable calculus has been removed.

III. Instruction After Scaling and Root Planing Appointment

Personalized instructions are provided for each patient during each dental hygiene and periodontal appointment. Instruction pertaining to periodontal dressings and sutures is outlined in Table 43-2 in Chapter 43. Many of the same principles can be applied for postcare instruction when a dressing has not been applied.

IV. Printed Take-Home Instructions

▶ Personalized printed instructions give the patient a handy reference.
  - Verbal instructions alone can easily be forgotten or misinterpreted by even the most conscientious patient.
▶ An added personal note or underlining of significant parts of the printed materials can let a patient sense the caring attitude of the professional team.

A. Information to Include

▶ Possible discomfort to expect

▶ Rinsing

▶ Oral self-care

▶ Eating

▶ Where to call in case of a problem or question.

B. Rinsing

A warm solution is soothing to the tissues and improves the circulation, thereby helping healing.

▶ *Solutions suggested for use*

• *Hypertonic salt solution:* 1/2 teaspoonful of table salt in 1/2 cup (4 ounces) of warm water; provides 3 or 4 mouthfuls for holding and swishing thoroughly before expectorating.

• *Sodium bicarbonate solution:* 1/2 teaspoonful of baking soda in 1 cup (8 ounces) of warm water.

• *Directions for salt or bicarbonate solutions:* Every 2 hours; after eating; after toothbrushing; before retiring.

▶ *Chlorhexidine 0.12%:* Chlorhexidine rinsing is advised following instrumentation for necrotizing ulcerative gingivitis, necrotizing ulcerative periodontitis, and advanced periodontitis.

• *Directions:* twice daily, after breakfast and before going to bed, without eating after rinsing to take advantage of the substantivity property of chlorhexidine.[36]

• Rinsing is not a substitute for personal biofilm removal with toothbrush and interdental aids.

C. Toothbrushing

The use of a soft brush may be recommended for a few days after scaling and root planing. The patient needs to understand the significance of daily biofilm disruption/removal.

D. Diet

Dietary and nutritional factors to consider include:

▶ Patients who have received local anesthesia are instructed to avoid chewing solid food until the anesthetic has worn off to avoid trauma to the tongue, cheek, and lips.

▶ If the tissues are tender during healing, use bland foods without strong, spicy seasonings, as well as continuing use of nutrient-dense, high-protein foods to promote healing.

▶ Foods for a liquid or a soft diet are suggested in Chapter 55.

EFFECTS OF NONSURGICAL PERIODONTAL THERAPY

▶ The essential components of successful nonsurgical instrumentation are thorough supra- and subgingival debridement by the clinician and effective dental biofilm control by the patient.

▶ The focus of treatment and the aims and expected outcomes are described earlier in this chapter.

▶ Tissue response is the most significant measure of success in periodontal debridement.

▶ Tissue response is manifested by clinical features commonly referred to as the endpoints of therapy.

I. Clinical Endpoints

▶ *BOP (bleeding on probing):* eliminated.

▶ *Probing depths:* reduced.

▶ *Attachment levels:* same or improved.

▶ *Inflammation:* resolved.

▶ *Gingival appearance:* size reduced, color normal.

▶ *Subgingival microflora:* lowered in numbers, delay in repopulation.

▶ *Dental biofilm control record:* improvement in scores approaching 100% biofilm free.

▶ *Tooth surfaces:* smooth; no biofilm-retentive irregularities.

▶ *Quality of life factors:* oral comfort with freedom from pain.

II. Healing

A. Factors Affecting Healing

▶ Severity of the infection and clinical features at the start of treatment.

▶ Noncompliance of the patient with:

• Control of dental biofilm.

• Completion of the recommended treatment plan.

▶ *Tobacco use:* see Chapter 34.

▶ Systemic influences

• Glycemic control of diabetes (refer to Chapter 69).

• *Lowered defense:* compromised immunity due to conditions such as HIV/AIDs, medications such as prednisone, or therapy such as chemotherapy in cancer.

▶ Root surface irregularities from incomplete debridement: retained calculus, endotoxins, and microorganisms.

B. Healing Process

▶ *Resolution of inflammation:* Edema recedes, necrotic cells are cleared away, and tissue regenerates.

▶ *Clinical attachment:* A long epithelial attachment can be expected.

III. Effect on Microorganisms[2]

A. Changes in Pocket Flora

▶ The subgingival bacterial flora is changed after debridement, as listed in Table 41-1.

▶ Before instrumentation for treatment of periodontitis, the subgingival microorganisms are primarily anaerobic, gram-negative, motile forms.

▶ After scaling and root planing, the total number of subgingival organisms decreases substantially. A shift to aerobic, gram-positive, nonmotile forms occurs.

B. Effect of Conversion of Microorganisms

▶ The disease-producing gram-negative pocket microorganisms are changed to a health-producing gram-positive flora.

▶ The gingiva reflects the changes. Gingival BOP is lessened, and the color, size, shape, and other characteristics assume a normal appearance.

C. Repopulation

▶ Without personal daily biofilm control, the microorganisms can return to pretreatment levels within an average of 42 days.[42]

▶ With biofilm control, the repopulation of the pocket takes longer, even in susceptible patients.

▶ In many patients, nonsurgical periodontal therapy results in a gingival condition that can be maintained free from reinfection.

D. Endotoxins[8,9]

▶ Endotoxins are LPSs (lipopolysaccharides) released from gram-negative bacterial cell walls.

▶ They occur in the bacteria covering the cementum and superficially in the cementum itself. Endotoxins have been shown to be toxic to human cells. Endotoxins do not penetrate deeply into cemental surfaces.

▶ Retained endotoxins are held by calculus not removed during instrumentation as well as by new microorganisms recolonizing on the surfaces.

RE-EVALUATION

▶ Recommendations are for the initial therapy re-evaluation to occur 4–8 weeks after nonsurgical periodontal therapy.[12]

I. Re-evaluation Procedure[41]

A. Periodontal Examination

▶ Complete periodontal examination is performed and documented.

▶ Bleeding points are noted as probings are made and documented in the periodontal record.

▶ Patient biofilm control efforts are evaluated.
  • Obtain biofilm score after the soft tissue visual examination has been completed.

• Provide feedback for the patient's efforts and the degree of improvement noted, as well as areas needing further attention.

B. Tactile Evaluation

▶ Areas demonstrating bleeding points are carefully assessed with a periodontal explorer and compressed air for residual calculus deposits.

▶ Special checks for difficult-to-access areas.
  • Concavities and depressions of the root anatomy.
  • Subgingival margins of crowns, fixed partial denture, or overhanging restoration.
  • Furcation invasions.

II. Reinstrumentation

▶ *Remove remaining calculus*
  • Use only optimally sharpened instruments.

▶ *Anticipate effects*
  • Smooth root surfaces that are free of calculus create a biologically compatible root surface that can support healing in the overlying tissues.

III. Response to Treatment

▶ Once treatment has been completed and the re-evaluation is complete, a decision is made as to the relative success of the therapy.
  • The patient may have reached the point of being able to be managed under the care of the dental hygienist.
  • There may be localized activity and adjunctive therapy may be considered.
  • In case of advanced disease that has not responded adequately to nonsurgical periodontal therapy, a referral to a periodontist is necessary as described in Chapter 48.

IV. Maintenance Interval Determined

▶ Assessment findings indicate the relative success of therapy delivered.

▶ On the basis of the findings, a determination is made about recommended intervals for subsequent maintenance appointments.

▶ Factors taken into account include the following:
  • Soft tissue response to instrumentation and degree of healing.
  • Changes and/or stabilization in probing depth.
  • *Patient factors*: use of tobacco; systemic influences such as diabetes.
  • Currently demonstrated biofilm control efforts; level of skill.
  • Motivation and responsibility assumed for daily personal oral self-care.
  • Psychosocial factors; stress.

ADJUNCTIVE THERAPY

▶ Pharmacologic agents are used as a adjuncts to mechanical therapy.

ANTIMICROBIAL TREATMENT

I. Objectives of Antimicrobial Therapy

▶ By arresting the infection using antimicrobial drugs, further loss of periodontal attachment and other periodontal tissue destruction caused by microorganisms can be prevented.

▶ Treatment using antimicrobials aims to suppress and eliminate pathogenic microorganisms to allow the recolonization of the microbiota compatible with health.

II. Types of Delivery of Antimicrobials

▶ *Systemic administration*
  - Systemic administration of antibiotics is well known and highly successful in the world of medical care. Antibiotics have saved the lives of many people with generalized infectious diseases.
  - A significant disadvantage to use of systemic antibiotics over the past 50 years is an increase in antibiotic resistance, so they need to be used with caution with careful cost–benefit analysis.

▶ *Local delivery*
  - The knowledge that periodontal diseases are site-specific infections has led to the development of methods for placing antimicrobials directly at the site of the infection—the pocket (see Table 41-2 for examples).

SYSTEMIC DELIVERY OF ANTIBIOTICS

I. Action of Systemically Administered Antibiotic

▶ In contrast to locally applied agents placed directly into a pocket, antibiotics administered systemically reach the pathogenic organisms in the pocket through the circulation.

▶ The antibiotic is absorbed into the circulation from the intestine. From the bloodstream, the drug is passed into the body tissues.

▶ The antibiotic enters the periodontal tissues and passes into the pocket by way of the gingival sulcus fluid.

II. Selection of Antibiotic[44]

▶ Ideally, the specific microorganism causing a certain periodontal disease needs to be determined, and the antibiotic selected needs to be specific for the organism.[7]
  - Microbiological testing is available and can be used to guide clinical decisions.
  - Periodontal diseases are caused by mixed infections of microorganisms. The pathogens tend to work in clusters, that is, in combination with other organisms so microbiological testing has limitations in mixed infections.

▶ Antibiotics regimens used with scaling and root planing include the following:
  - Metronidazole is effective against *Porphyromonas gingivalis* and *Prevotella intermedia*.

TABLE 41-2	Local Delivery Antimicrobials	
	ARESTIN	**ATRIDOX**
Active ingredient	Minocycline HCl (1 mg)	Doxycycline hyclate (10%)
Method of delivery	Unit-dose cartridge inserts into cartridge handle.	Doxycycline hyclate (10%); single use syringe suspended in 450 mg of ATRIGEL [poly(DL-Lactide): NMP].
Mechanism of action	Exerts antimicrobial activity by inhibiting protein synthesis in the bacterial cell wall that causes leakage and destroys the cell.	Subgingival controlled release; upon contact with crevicular fluid, the liquid product solidifies and then permits controlled release for a period of 7 days.
Indications	As an adjunctive therapy to scaling and root planing for reduction of pocket depth and BOP in patients with adult periodontitis.	For use in the treatment of chronic adult periodontitis for reduction in probing depth, reduction in BOP, and a gain in clinical attachment.
Contraindications	Sensitivity to minocycline and/or tetracycline; children; pregnant or nursing women.	Sensitivity to doxycycline or any of the tetracycline class.

- Tetracycline, specifically doxycycline or minocycline, to treat *Aggregatibacter actinomycetemcomitans* in aggressive periodontitis.
- Clindamycin, ciprofloxacin, and azithromycin have also been used to stop progression of disease, but are used less often.
▶ Antibiotics used for acute periodontal abscesses along with debridement:
  - Amoxicillin
  - Azithromycin or Clindamycin for patients with penicillin allergy.

III. Limitations[44]

▶ The precautions and adverse effects, as well as the acquisition of antibiotic resistance by the organisms, preclude the widespread use of systemic antibiotics for periodontal problems.
▶ Limitations include the following:
  - Side effects of certain antibiotics.
  - Potential for the development of resistant strains.
  - Local concentration diluted by the time the drug reaches the pathogens; drug is "wasted" in that it covers a large area not needing the treatment.
  - Superimposed infection can develop, such as candidiasis.
  - Low compliance of the patient in following the prescription for the required number of days.

IV. Use of Systemic Therapy

▶ Most periodontal infection responds well to nonsurgical periodontal therapy, meticulous biofilm control, and antimicrobial mouthrinses/dentifrices. However, there are groups of people who do not respond to initial therapy who would benefit from systemic antibiotics including:[44]
  - Continued loss of attachment despite initial therapy and thorough biofilm control.
  - Recurrent or refractory periodontitis.
  - Acute periodontal infection such as necrotizing ulcerative gingivitis or periodontitis, periodontal abscess.
  - Aggressive types of periodontitis
  - Medical conditions predisposing to periodontal disease such a poorly controlled diabetes.

LOCAL DELIVERY OF ANTIMICROBIALS

▶ The concept of a controlled local delivery system for treatment of periodontal pathogens in a pocket infection was developed over many years by Goodson and coworkers with the introduction of a subgingival tetracycline fiber.[45]
  - Improvements in probing depth, CAL, BOP, and reduction of sites with periodontal pathogenic

microorganisms laid the groundwork for continuing research and development in local delivery agents.[45,46]
▶ Local delivery means the medication used to treat the periodontal infection is concentrated at the site of the infection.
▶ Local drug agents can be divided into two classes:[47]
  - Sustained-release formulations release a drug for a period less than 24 hours and are used in a variety of ways. The nicotine patch, used to assist a person trying to break a smoking addiction, is an example.
  - Controlled delivery refers to providing the medication over an extended period of time that exceeds 1 day.

I. Requirements

A local delivery method can place high concentrations of the antimicrobial in an infected pocket. To be successful, the medication must:[48]

▶ Provide adequate bactericidal drug concentration.
▶ Reach site of disease activity such as the bottom of the pocket and furcation.
▶ Stay in contact long enough in the effective concentration for the antimicrobial action to take place.
  - *Comparison with systemic*: When systemic treatment is used, much less of the antimicrobial medication reaches the actual site of the infection where pathogens are concentrated because the agent becomes diluted as it passes through the body.
▶ Ease of application.
▶ Biodegradability.
▶ Cost and the benefit for the patient must be carefully evaluated given the average reduction in pocket depth ranges from 0.25 to 0.50 mm and the gains in CAL range from 0.10 to 0.50 mm.[46]

II. Uses for Slow-Release Local Delivery[46]

▶ Local delivery agents have the potential to enhance therapy at sites unresponsive to conventional treatment.
▶ Antimicrobials used in individual sites may be considered by the clinician according to patient needs and professional judgment.

A. Initial Therapy

▶ Periodontal diseases result from local infection with a pathogenic microflora.
  - The periodontal pocket contains microorganisms and may also contain subgingival calculus, which further acts to harbor bacteria.
▶ Scaling and root planing are highly effective procedures for controlling periodontal infections, reducing

inflammation, reducing probing depths an average of 1.5 mm, and resulting clinical attachment gains of 1.5 mm or more.[46]

▶ The adjunctive use of local antimicrobials may enhance the effect of the mechanical instrumentation, particularly in areas of compromised access such as furcations and deep root concavities.

- Use of a controlled-release antimicrobial in addition to scaling and root planing may result in an additional 0.30–0.50 mm pocket depth reduction and 0.25–0.50 mm gain in clinical attachment.[46]

B. Adjunctive Treatment: At Re-evaluation

▶ At the completion of initial periodontal therapy, a re-evaluation is completed 4–6 weeks later.

- Residual calculus is removed.
- Control of dental biofilm is assessed and reinforcement is provided for the patient.
- For areas of residual pocket depth and/or BOP, adjunctive therapy may be considered such as systemic antibiotics or a local delivery antimicrobial agent.

C. Recurrent Disease

▶ Periodontal disease tends to be cyclical with periods of stability and progression.

▶ Recurrence or progression of periodontal disease may be due to:[49]

- Noncompliance with periodontal maintenance schedule.
- Inadequate daily control of dental biofilm.
- Inadequate periodontal debridement.
- Continued tobacco use.
- Unknown.

▶ Recurrence of periodontal infection may be localized, particularly in pockets associated with root concavities, furcations, and areas of complex root morphology, where definitive debridement is most challenging.

- Burnished calculus is difficult to detect with an explorer and becomes recolonized with pathogenic microbes soon after debridement, which interferes with healing.
- Bleeding may indicate residual burnished calculus from insufficient instrumentation.

▶ Localized areas of recurrence of disease are candidates for application of an antimicrobial agent.

D. Peri-implantitis

The ailing or failing implant may respond to a localized slow-release antimicrobial.[50]

III. Types of Local Delivery Agents

▶ Available for treatment of periodontal infections are bioabsorbable polymers, minocycline and doxycycline.

▶ For all products, the manufacturer's advice and directions are followed.

▶ Benefits include:[46]

- Pocket depth reductions range from 0.7 to 1 mm, with a mean effect size of 0.49 mm.
- Clinical attachment gains range from 0.43 to 0.80 mm, with a mean effect size of 0.46 mm.

MINOCYCLINE HYDROCHLORIDE (HCL)

▶ Bioresorbable minocycline HCl is a sustained-release agent delivered in powdered microsphere form to be placed in periodontal pockets in conjunction with scaling and root planing.[46] Research indicates the following benefits to use of the minocycline HCl microspheres with SRP:[46]

- Overall pocket depth reduction was an additional 0.49 mm over SRP alone.
- Gain in clinical attachment was an average of 0.46 mm.

I. Description

▶ Unit dose cartridge contains 1 mg minocycline.

▶ Once the minocycline microspheres come in contact with gingival crevicular fluid, they hydrolyze allowing them to adhere to the surrounding surfaces.

▶ Sustained release 14 days.

▶ Does not block the flow of subgingival fluid.

▶ Contraindications:[51]

- Patients sensitive to tetracycline.
- Women who are pregnant or breastfeeding.
- Acute periodontal abscess.

II. Administration

A. Site Selection

▶ Use as an adjunct to scaling and root planing.

▶ Probing depth of at least 5 mm.

B. Cartridge Loading

▶ Insert unit cartridge into dispenser handle.

▶ Exert slight pressure.

▶ Twist cartridge until it snaps securely into place.

C. Tip Preparation

1. Cartridge tip can be manipulated to reposition the angle for difficult-to-reach areas.
2. Leave cap covering the cartridge in place prior to manipulating the angle to prevent agent from being inadvertently expelled.
3. Tip opening can be narrowed for ease of subgingival insertion if needed.

- Remove cap.
- Using the end of a mirror handle, gently compress the last millimeter of the tip.

D. Delivery of Agent

1. Place cartridge tip into the site selected for treatment.
2. Keep tip parallel to the long axis of the tooth as it enters the periodontal pocket (Figure 41-20).
3. Do not force the tip to the base of the pocket.
4. Gently press thumb ring of handle to express the agent while withdrawing cartridge tip coronally from the base of the pocket.
5. With delivery complete, retract thumb ring and remove cartridge with free hand.
   - Discard contaminated cartridge.
   - Sterilize handle prior to reuse.
6. The bioadhesive microspheres activate and adhere on contact with moisture.
7. Caution patient to avoid disruption of activated material within pocket.

III. Posttreatment Instructions

Instruct patient on proper care of treated areas. Give written guidelines to prevent misunderstanding.

▸ Avoid touching treated area(s).

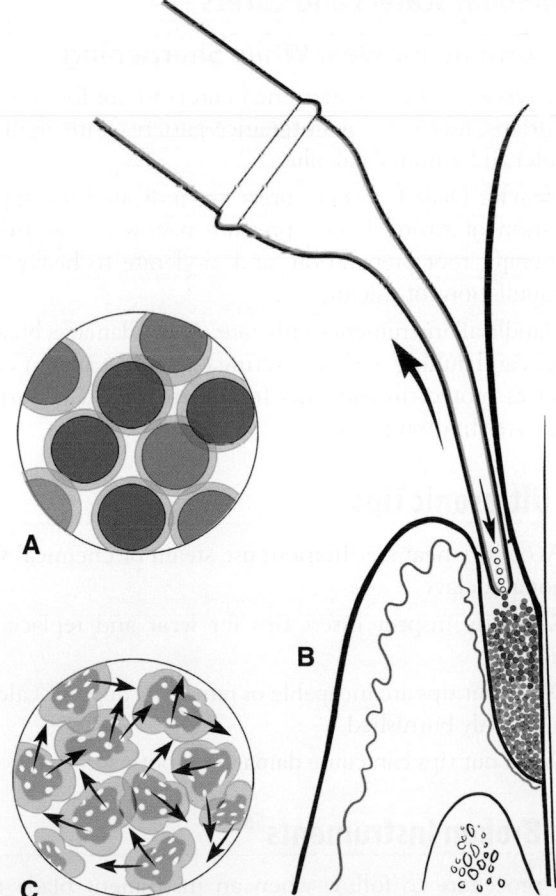

FIGURE 41-20 Minocycline HCl. A: Minocycline microspheres intact within cannula, prior to application. **B:** Deposition: cannula is withdrawn from periodontal pocket as plunger is depressed. **C:** Once deposited, microspheres dissipate, releasing activated minocycline HCl into the subgingival space.

▸ Do not use interdental cleaners or floss between teeth that have been treated for at least 10 days.
▸ Avoid eating hard, crunchy, or sticky foods that could disturb retention of the product for 1 week.
▸ Some mild-to-moderate sensitivity may be present the first week after scaling and root planing and placement of minocycline HCl, but the patient needs to contact the dentist if pain or swelling occurs.
▸ Schedule a follow-up appointment for continuing maintenance care.

IV. Maintenance Appointments

▸ Probe carefully to evaluate treated area(s).
▸ Reinforce home oral self-care measures and adherence to continuing care.
▸ Re-evaluate at the periodontal maintenance appointment.
   - Referral to a periodontist needs to be considered if the disease activity is still not controlled.[52]

DOXYCYCLINE HYCLATE

Biodegradable doxycycline polymer in liquid form is controlled-release agent delivered by cannula into a pocket and solidifies on contact with the dampness of the sulcus fluid.

▸ Research indicates the following benefits to use of the minocycline doxycycline hyclate with SRP:[46]
   - Overall pocket depth reduction was an additional 0.47 mm over SRP alone.
   - Gain in clinical attachment was an average of 0.24 mm.

Beneficial effects include reduction of probing depths, gain of attachment, and destruction of periodontal pathogenic microorganisms in comparison to scaling and root planing alone.[53]

I. Description

A. Equipment

▸ *Syringe*: Two syringe mixing system consisting of the following:[54,55]
   - Syringe A contains 450 mg of the bioabsorbable polymeric formulation.
   - Syringe B contains 50 mg of doxycycline hyclate.
   - Once combined the solution contains 10% doxycycline hyclate.
▸ *Cannula*: Blunt ended, 23-gauge, narrow diameter.
▸ Controlled release of drug for 7 days.
▸ Contraindications:
   - Patients sensitive to tetracycline.
   - Women who are pregnant or breastfeeding.

II. Administration[55]

A. Site Selection

▶ Use as an adjunct to scaling and root planing.

▶ Probing depth of at least 5 mm.

B. Preparation of Agent

▶ If refrigerated, take pouches with product out of refrigerator at least 15 minutes before mixing.

▶ *Mixing:* Two syringes are coupled and the substances are passed back and forth, which is one mixing cycle. Mixing continues for 100 mixing cycles (Figure 41-21A). Follow the manufacturer's instructions.

▶ *Adapt cannula:* Attach 23-gauge blunt cannula to syringe. As the cap is removed, the cannula is held part way and bent against the wall of the cover to provide an angle appropriate for insertion into the periodontal pocket (Figure 41-21B).

C. Delivery of agent

1. Place cartridge tip into the site selected for treatment.
2. Keep tip parallel to the long axis of the tooth as it enters the periodontal pocket.
3. Do not force the tip to the base of the pocket.
4. Express the agent as the cannula is withdrawn to just over the gingival margin (Figure 41-21C).
5. Use a blunt instrument to pack the agent down. Wet the instrument to prevent sticking to the agent.

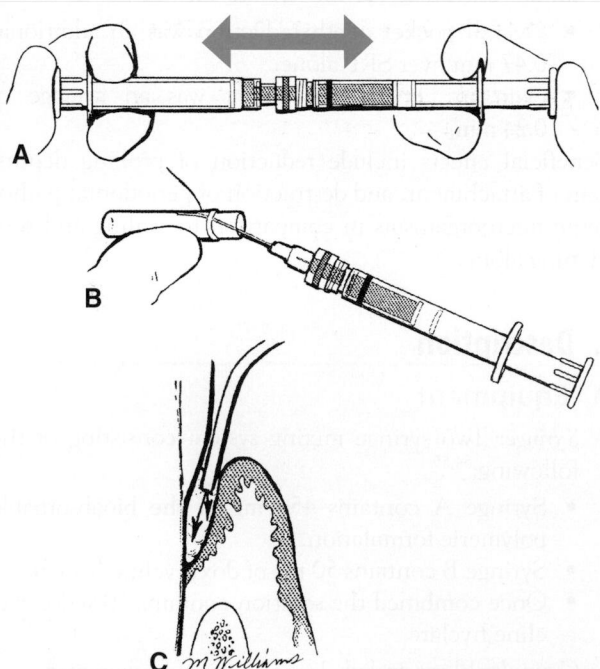

FIGURE 41-21 Doxycycline Polymer Gel. A: Syringes are coupled and the contents passed back and forth until mixed. **B:** The cannula is attached to the syringe with the agent; as the cap is removed, the cannula is pressed against the side to bend it to an angle appropriate for accessing the pocket to be treated. **C:** The cannula is inserted to the base of the pocket, and the agent is released to fill the pocket.

• Add more if necessary to fill the pocket.

• On contact with the moisture of the pocket, the agent will solidify.

6. Placing a periodontal dressing over the area aids retention.

III. Posttreatment Instructions

Instruct patient on proper care of treated areas. Give written guidelines to prevent misunderstanding.

▶ Prevent accidental removal.

▶ Routine brushing and other oral self-care on all other areas, but avoid tooth brushing or flossing the treated areas for 7 days.[55]

▶ Schedule a follow-up appointment to remove periodontal dressing.

• Evaluate tissue; evaluate biofilm removal.

▶ Plan routine maintenance.

INSTRUMENT MAINTENANCE

I. Manual Scalers and Curets

A. Examine for Wear While Sharpening

▶ Reserve thinned or shortened curets to use for conscientious, motivated maintenance patients with shallow sulci and minimal calculus.

▶ Heavier bladed, newer curets are indicated for application of strong lateral pressure necessary for initial therapy, root preparation, and moderate to heavy accumulations of calculus.

▶ Handle all instruments with care. Avoid damage, breakage, and dulling of sharp cutting edges; instrument cassettes protect instruments from wear and tear during the sterilization process.

II. Ultrasonic Tips

▶ Avoid dry heat sterilization; use steam or chemical vapor autoclave.

▶ Regularly inspect insert tips for wear and replace as needed.

▶ Worn out tips are incapable of removing deposit; calculus is only burnished.

▶ Worn out tips can cause damage to tooth surfaces.

III. Broken Instruments[56]

The procedure to follow when an instrument blade tip breaks in a patient's mouth during treatment will be in accord with policy developed in each individual practice. *The principal objective in the location of a broken instrument tip is to know positively that the tip has been recovered.* A general procedure is suggested in Box 41-4.

EVERYDAY ETHICS

Lorna and Caroline practice as dental hygienists in the same office approximately 2½ days per week. Lorna graduated from dental hygiene school about 15 years ago, while Caroline was licensed just 3 years ago. The front desk tries to schedule patients with the same hygienist. One day Mrs. Border, a patient routinely scheduled with Lorna, showed up in Caroline's appointment book because she wanted to fit in her regular maintenance appointment before going to live with her daughter for several months. The receptionist scheduled her with the first available hygienist. Caroline reviewed the patient's medical history and recorded the blood pressure. During the periodontal examination, she found many areas of pocket depth increases with BOP in molar areas. Upon review of the radiograph taken that day, subgingival calculus was noted in many areas. Caroline raised Lorna's chair to an upright position to discuss the findings. She showed Mrs. Border the radiographs with the calculus and then reviewed the periodontal charting comparing today's numbers with her last examination. Caroline then went to get Dr. Bennett to discuss the need for nonsurgical periodontal therapy with Ms. Border. The patient was outraged at the recommendation for quadrant scaling and root planing with local anesthesia and complained that Caroline "should have used the sprayer-machine like Lorna usually does."

Questions for Consideration

1. Is this an ethical dilemma or an issue for Caroline? For Lorna? For Dr. Bennett? Why?

2. Caroline realizes the deep calculus could not all have formed since the previous appointment. How should Caroline have addressed this problem with the patient? With Lorna? With Dr. Bennett?

3. Using the questions in Table VI, in Section VI Introduction, outline three or four possible avenues for Caroline to consider in resolving this difficult situation.

BOX 41-4

Care of a Broken Instrument

Preparatory Planning

▷ Discuss with dentist during early practice days.
▷ Determine practice policy.

Objective

Know positively that the broken segment (i.e., tip of scaler) has been completely recovered.

Immediate Action

▷ Cease procedure, retain retraction.
▷ Do not move patient's head.
▷ Isolate with gauze sponge.
▷ Do not use air/water syringe.
▷ Adjust saliva ejector to opposite side.
▷ Do not alarm the patient by describing what happened.

Examination of Area

▷ Do not dry with air.
▷ Use careful, gentle retraction to examine the immediate area including the floor of the mouth and mucobuccal fold.

▷ Blot the gingival tissue dry with a cotton roll to examine around the tooth.
▷ Use transilluminating light or mouth light.
▷ Examine gingival sulcus
  1. Use a curet applied gently with a spoonlike stroke
  2. Take great care not to push the tip into the base of the pocket (in case the broken segment is there).

Treatment

▷ Consult with the supervising dentist for assistance in accord with previously discussed policy.
▷ Prepare a radiograph of the area.
▷ If the broken tip is not retrieved during any of above procedures:
  ▷ Arrange for a periodontal surgical procedure.

Source: Schwartz M. The prevention and management of the broken curet. *Compend Contin Educ Dent.* 1998;19:418.

DOCUMENTATION

Documentation for the second in a series of appointments for a quadrant of scaling and root debridement with local anesthesia.

▶ Complete health history and assessment examination findings.

▶ Record new blood pressure

▶ Oral preliminary examination for (1) healing and progress of the treatment of the previously treated quadrant, with comments from the patient and (2) specific reexamination of quadrant to be treated that day.

▶ Note patient's biofilm successes: provide instructions for care of newly treated area.

▶ A sample progress note may be reviewed in Box 41-5.

BOX 41-5

Example Documentation: Special Attention to Instrument Adaptation on a Compromised Tooth Surface

S—Female patient, 26 years old, presents for routine continuing care after being away for 2 years in the Peace Corps in Africa. Patient states she had tried hard to care for her teeth daily, but safe water was never assured, and she ran out of floss without a place to shop for more. She pointed to the upper left quadrant and said it was sore and bleeding up there. No basic changes in health history

O—Vital signs normal (BP 121/70). Generalized moderate calculus, with generalized 4 mm probing depths. Tooth #12 mesial has 6 mm pocket, BOP, and calculus (visible on the BW radiograph).

A—Tooth #13 may have a mesial concavity that requires careful adaptation of both hand and ultrasonic instrument tips.

P—Careful adaptation of the ultrasonic tip and a mini curet on the mesial surface of #13 to assure the base of a mesial concavity has been reached to remove calculus and root plane the root surface, followed by careful evaluation with an explorer.

Next Steps: Appointment made in 2 weeks for re-evaluation of #13 mesial.

Signed: _____, RDH

Date: _____

Factors To Teach The Patient

▷ The significance of dental biofilm to periodontal infection.
▷ The nature, occurrence, and etiology of calculus; its role as a biofilm reservoir.
▷ The importance of and necessity for complete removal of calculus to the health of the oral tissues in the prevention of periodontal infections.
▷ Reasons for multiple appointments to complete the scaling and root planing.
▷ The rationale for re-evaluation following the completion of scaling and root planing.
▷ Relationship of personal oral self-care measures to accumulation/maturation of dental biofilm.
▷ The importance of the patient's role in maintenance of therapeutic gains.
▷ The limits of what can be accomplished nonsurgically and the rationale for referral to a specialist.
▷ The rationale for combining manual instrumentation with ultrasonic instrumentation.
▷ The rationale for adjunctive therapy to control disease.
▷ The harmful effects of overhanging margins: producing a niche for biofilm that cannot be cleansed, contributing to gingival disease and caries, and the necessity of overhang removal.

References

1. Drisko CL. Periodontal debridement: still the treatment of choice. *J Evid Based Dent Pract.* 2014;14 Suppl:33–41.
2. Cobb CM. Microbes, inflammation, scaling and root planing, and the periodontal condition. *J Dent Hyg.* 2008;82 (Suppl 3):4–9.
3. Suvan JE. Effectiveness of mechanical nonsurgical pocket therapy. *Periodontol 2000.* 2005;37:48–71.
4. American Academy of Periodontology. Parameter on plaque-induced Gingivitis. *J Periodontol.* 2000;71:851–852.
5. American Academy of Periodontology. Parameter on chronic periodontitis with slight to moderate loss of periodontal support. *J Periodontol.* 2000;71(5, Suppl):853–855.
6. American Academy of Periodontology. Parameter on chronic periodontitis with advanced loss of periodontal support. *J Periodontol.* 2000;71(5, Suppl):856–858.
7. Nyman S, Westfelt E, Sarhed G, et al. Role of "diseased" root cementum in healing following treatment of periodontal disease: a clinical study. *J Clin Periodontol.* 1988;15(7):464–468.
8. Moore J, Wilson M, Kieser JB. The distribution of bacterial lipopolysaccharide (endotoxin) in relation to periodontally involved root surfaces. *J Clin Periodontol.* 1986;13(8):748–751.
9. Cadosch J, Zimmermann U, Ruppert M, et al. Root surface debridement and endotoxin removal. *J Periodontal Res.* 2003;38(3):229–236.
10. Drisko CH. Root instrumentation. Power-driven versus manual scalers, which one? *Dent Clin North Am.* 1998;42(2):229–244.
11. Teughels W, Van Assche N, Sliepen I, et al. Effect of material characteristics and/or surface topography on biofilm development. *Clin Oral Implants Res.* 2006;17 (Suppl 2):68–81.
12. Sweeting LA, Davis K, Cobb CM. Periodontal treatment protocol (PTP) for the general dental practice. *J Dent Hyg.* 2008; 82 (Suppl 3):16–26.
13. Segelnick SL, Weinberg MA. Reevaluation of initial therapy: when is the appropriate time? *J Periodontol.* 2006;77(9):1598–1601.
14. Eberhard J, Jepsen S, Jervøe-Storm PM, et al. Full-mouth disinfection for the treatment of adult chronic periodontitis. *Cochrane Database Syst Rev.* 2008;(1):CD004622.
15. Zhang W, Daly CG, Mitchell D, et al. Incidence and magnitude of bacteraemia caused by flossing and by scaling and root planing. *J Clin Periodontol.* 2013;40(1):41–52.
16. Shetty SK, Sharath K, Shenoy S, et al. Compare the efficacy of two commercially available mouthrinses in reducing viable bacterial count in dental aerosol produced during ultrasonic scaling when used as a preprocedural rinse. *J Contemp Dent Pract.* 2013;14(5):848–851.
17. Eichenberger M, Perrin P, Neuhaus KW, et al. Influence of loupes and age on the near visual acuity of practicing dentists. *J Biomed Opt.* 2011;16(3):035003.
18. Geisinger ML, Mealey BL, Schoolfield J, et al. The effectiveness of subgingival scaling and root planing: an evaluation of therapy with and without the use of the periodontal endoscope. *J Periodontol.* 2007;78(1):22–28.

19. Wilson TG Jr, Carnio J, Schenk R, et al. Absence of histologic signs of chronic inflammation following closed subgingival scaling and root planing using the dental endoscope: human biopsies—a pilot study. *J Periodontol.* 2008;79(11):2036–2041.

20. Arabaci T, Ciçek Y, Canakçi CF. Sonic and ultrasonic scalers in periodontal treatment: a review. *Int J Dent Hyg.* 2007;5(1):2–12.

21. Baehni P, Thilo B, Chapuis B, et al. Effects of ultrasonic and sonic scalers on dental plaque microflora in vitro and in vivo. *J Clin Periodontol.* 1992;19(7):455–459.

22. Khosravi M, Bahrami ZS, Atabaki MS, et al. Comparative effectiveness of hand and ultrasonic instrumentations in root surface planing in vitro. *J Clin Periodontol.* 2004;31(3):160–165.

23. Scannapieco FA, Bush RB, Paju S. Associations between periodontal disease and risk for nosocomial bacterial pneumonia and chronic obstructive pulmonary disease. A systematic review. *Ann Periodontol.* 2003;8(1):54–69.

24. Garcia JM, Chambers E IV. Managing dysphagia through diet modifications. *Am J Nurs.* 2010;110(11):26–33.

25. Paramashivaiah R, Prabhuji ML. Mechanized scaling with ultrasonics: perils and proactive measures. *J Indian Soc Periodontol.* 2013;17(4):423–428.

26. Arabaci T, Ciçek Y, Ozgöz M, et al. The comparison of the effects of three types of piezoelectric ultrasonic tips and air polishing system on the filling materials: an in vitro study. *Int J Dent Hyg.* 2007;5(4):205–210.

27. Mann M, Parmar D, Walmsley AD, et al. Effect of plastic-covered ultrasonic scalers on titanium implant surfaces. *Clin Oral Implants Res.* 2012;23(1):76–82.

28. Dong H, Barr A, Loomer P, et al. The effects of finger rest positions on hand muscle load and pinch force in simulated dental hygiene work. *J Dent Educ.* 2005;69(4):453–460.

29. Cherniack M, Brammer AJ, Nilsson T, et al. Nerve conduction and sensorineural function in dental hygienists using high frequency ultrasound handpieces. *Am J Ind Med.* 2006;49(5):313–326.

30. Kim DW, Choi JL, Kwon MK, et al. Assessment of daily exposure of endodontic personnel to extremely low frequency magnetic fields. *Int Endod J.* 2012;45(8):744–748.

31. Ribeiro FV, Casarin RC, Nociti Júnior FH, et al. Comparative in vitro study of root roughness after instrumentation with ultrasonic and diamond tip sonic scaler. *J Appl Oral Sci.* 2006;14(2):124–129.

32. Garg SK, Mittal S, Kaur P. Dental unit waterline management: historical perspectives and current trends. *J Investig Clin Dent.* 2012;3(4):247–252.

33. Kohn WG, Collins AS, Cleveland JL, et al; and Centers for Disease Control and Prevention (CDC). Guidelines for infection control in dental health-care settings—2003. *MMWR Recomm Rep.* 2003;52 (RR-17):1–61.

34. Desarda H, Gurav A, Dharmadhikari C, et al. Efficacy of high-volume evacuator in aerosol reduction: truth or myth? A clinical and microbiological study. *J Dent Res Dent Clin Dent Prospects.* 2014;8(3):176–179.

35. Kwan JY. Enhanced periodontal debridement with the use of micro ultrasonic, periodontal endoscopy. *J Calif Dent Assoc.* 2005;33(3):241–248.

36. Bains VK, Mohan R, Bains R. Application of ultrasound in periodontitis, Part II. *J Indian Soc Periodontol.* 2008;12(3):55–61.

37. American Academy of Periodontology. Statement on efficacy of lasers in the non-surgical treatment of inflammatory periodontal disease. *J Periodontol.* 2011;82(4):513–514.

38. Schwarz F, Aoki A, Sculean A, et al. The impact of laser application on periodontal and peri-implant wound healing. *Periodontol 2000.* 2009;51:79–108.

39. Cobb CM. Lasers in periodontics: a review of the literature. *J Periodontol.* 2006;77:545–564.

40. García-Caballero L, Quintas V, Prada-López I, et al. Chlorhexidine substantivity on salivary flora and plaque-like biofilm: an in situ model. *PLoS One.* 2013;8(12):e83522.

41. Sgolastra F, Petrucci A, Gatto R, et al. Efficacy of Er:YAG laser in the treatment of chronic periodontitis: systematic review and meta-analysis. *Lasers Med Sci.* 2012;27(3):661–673.

42. Andreana S. The use of diode lasers in periodontal therapy: literature review and suggested technique. *Dent Today.* 2005. http://www.dentistrytoday.com/technology/lasers/1361. Accessed December 30, 2014.

43. Pack AR, Coxhead LJ, McDonald BW. The prevalence of overhanging margins in posterior amalgam restorations and periodontal consequences. *J Clin Periodontol.* 1990;17(3):145–152.

44. Slots J; Research, Science and Therapy Committee. Systemic antibiotics in periodontics. *J Periodontol.* 2004;75(11):1553–1565.

45. Goodson JM, Haffajee A, Socransky SS. Periodontal therapy by local delivery of tetracycline. *J Clin Periodontol.* 1979;6(2):83–92.

46. Bonito AJ, Lux L, Lohr KN. Impact of local adjuncts to scaling and root planing in periodontal disease therapy: a systematic review. *J Periodontol.* 2005;76(8):1227–1236.

47. Singh M, Shreehari AK, Garg PK, et al. Clinical efficacy of chlorhexidine chips and tetracycline fibers as an adjunct to non surgical periodontal therapy. *Eur J Gen Dent.* 2014;3(20);134–139.

48. Greenstein G, Polson A. The role of local drug delivery in the management of periodontal diseases: a comprehensive review. *J Periodontol.* 1998;69:507–520.

49. American Academy of Periodontology. Parameter on periodontal maintenance. *J Periodontol.* 2000;71(5, Suppl):849–850.

50. Esposito M, Grusovin MG, Worthington HV. Treatment of peri-implantitis: what interventions are effective? A Cochrane systematic review. *Eur J Oral Implantol.* 2012;5 Suppl:S21–S41.

51. Lexicomp for Dentistry. *Minocycline Hydrochloride (Periodontal) (Dental Lexi-Drugs).* Hudson, OH: Lexi-Comp. Accessed January 1, 2015.

52. American Academy of Periodontology. Statement on local delivery of sustained or controlled release antimicrobials as adjunctive therapy in the treatment of periodontitis. *J Periodontol.* 2006;77(8):1457–1458.

53. Garrett S, Johnson L, Drisko CH, et al. Two multi-center studies evaluating locally delivered doxycycline hyclate, placebo control, oral hygiene, and scaling and root planing in the treatment of periodontitis. *J Periodontol.* 1999;70(5):490–503.

54. Lexicomp for Dentistry. *Doxycycline Hyclate Periodontal Extended-release Liquid (Dental Lexi-Drugs)*. Hudson, OH: Lexi-Comp. Accessed January 1, 2015.

55. Food and Drug Administration. Package insert: Atridox. http://www.accessdata.fda.gov/drugsatfda_docs/label/2003/50751scs011_atridox_lbl.pdf. Accessed January 2, 2015.

56. Schwartz M. The prevention and management of the broken curet. *Compend Contin Educ Dent.* 1998;19(4):418–420, 422, 424–425.

ENHANCE YOUR UNDERSTANDING

thePoint® DIGITAL CONNECTIONS
(see the inside front cover for access information)
- **Audio glossary**
- **Quiz bank**

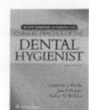

SUPPORT FOR LEARNING
(available separately; visit lww.com)
- *Active Learning Workbook for Clinical Practice of the Dental Hygienist, 12th Edition*

prepU INDIVIDUALIZED REVIEW
(available separately; visit lww.com)
- **Adaptive quizzing with *prepU for Wilkins' Clinical Practice of the Dental Hygienist***

42

Acute Periodontal Conditions

Susan J. Jenkins, RDH, MS, CAGS

LEARNING OBJECTIVES

After studying this chapter, the student will be able to:

1. Identify the oral/clinical characteristic signs and symptoms of necrotizing periodontal diseases (NPDs), primary herpetic gingivostomatitis (HG), and periodontal abscess.

2. Differentiate NPD from primary gingivostomatitis and the periodontal abscess from the endodontic abscess.

3. Identify risk factors associated with NPDs, primary HG, and periodontal abscess.

4. Recognize the systemic conditions that can contribute to the inception of NPDs, primary HG, and the periodontal abscess.

5. Explain the care plan/treatment options for NPDs, primary HG, and periodontal abscess.

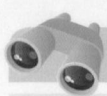

BOX 42-1 KEY WORDS AND ABBREVIATIONS: Acute Periodontal Conditions

Abscess: localized collection of pus in a circumscribed or walled-off area formed by the disintegration of tissues.

Acute: sudden onset, runs a relatively short course; produces pain and local inflammation.

Chronic: long term, slow development with little evidence of inflammation; usually an intermittent pus discharge; may follow an acute abscess.

Fetor oris: foul, offensive odor from the mouth; halitosis.

Fistula: a pathologic sinus or abnormal passage/track that leads from an abscess to the surface of the gingiva or mucosa.

Gingival: localized in the gingiva or interdental papilla but not involving bone.

Gum boil: a lay term for a circumscribed swelling (abscess) in the tissue over the alveolar process, usually at the level of the root apices; may break and drain periodically, thus preventing pain.

Herpetic gingivostomatitis or primary herpetic gingivostomatitis: a viral infection (herpes simplex) of the oral mucosa.

Linear gingival erythema (LGE): a well-demarcated band of intense erythema at the gingival margin, not associated with dental biofilm, and which does not respond to conventional biofilm removal procedures; common with HIV-positive patients.

Malaise: feeling of general indisposition, uneasiness, discomfort; may be early indication of illness.

Necrosis: death of tissue; morphologic changes indicative of cell death caused by enzymatic degradation.

Necrotizing periodontal diseases (NPD): a collective term that includes both NUG and NUP since they may be different stages of the same disease.

Periapical: at or around the apex of a tooth root.

Pericoronitis: gingival inflammation around the crown of an incompletely/partially erupted tooth; most frequently occurs about a mandibular third molar.

Periodontal: localized in the periodontal tissues.

Pseudomembrane: false membrane; false layer of tissue covering a surface.

Purulent: accompanied by or containing pus.

Sequestra: small bone spicules working to the surface after surgery; singular, sequestrum.[1]

Sinus tract: a channel connecting with an abscess or suppurating area.

Ulceration: formation or development of an ulcer with loss of epithelial surface and sloughing of necrotic inflammatory tissue.

Vesiculation: formation or presence of vesicles, small fluid filled blisterlike elevations on the skin or mucosa.

This chapter will describe common acute periodontal conditions the dental hygienist may encounter. Key words for acute conditions are defined in Box 42-1.

Acute periodontal diseases are clinical conditions. The patient may present with some or all of the following:

▶ Rapid onset

▶ Involve the periodontium and associated structures

▶ May be characterized by pain and discomfort

▶ Infection will be present.

▶ May be related to gingivitis, periodontitis, or both.

▶ May be localized or generalized, in the periodontium with possible systemic manifestations.[2]

NECROTIZING PERIODONTAL DISEASES

▶ Necrotizing ulcerative gingivitis (NUG) and necrotizing ulcerative periodontitis (NUP) are acute inflammatory, destructive diseases related to diminished systemic resistance to bacterial infection of the periodontal tissues.[2,3]

▶ Other names used include necrotizing gingivitis, acute NUG, trench mouth, Vincent's infection, Vincent's disease, and ulceromembranous gingivitis.

I. Necrotizing Ulcerative Gingivitis

▶ Although NUG may occur at any age, it is usually seen among young people between ages 15 and 30 years.

▶ It is rare in children under 10 years of age in the United States, but not uncommon in young children from low socioeconomic groups studied in sub-Saharan Africa and other developing countries.[4]

II. Necrotizing Ulcerative Periodontitis

▶ Destructive infection of periodontal tissues with ulceration of interdental papillae (punched-out papilla), cratering of interdental bone and soft tissue, and clinical attachment loss (Figures 42-1 and 42-2).

▶ An increased incidence of NUG/NUP has been strongly associated with HIV-infected patients (Figure 42-1D).[5]

  • A more severe, rapidly progressive breakdown of the periodontium occurs.

  • Because of the rapid breakdown and tissue necrosis with severe attachment loss, the condition usually is not associated with deep pockets.[5]

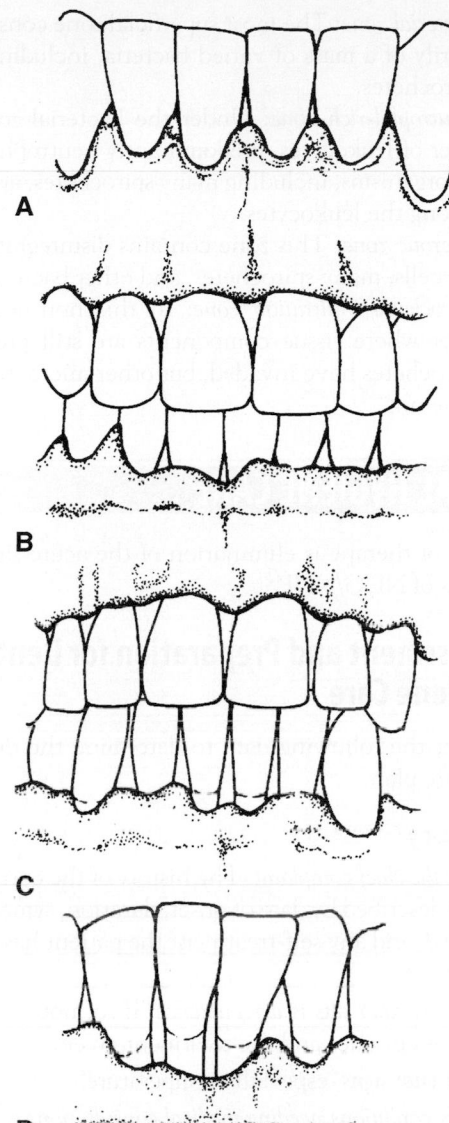

A

B

C

D

FIGURE 42-1 **NUG/Periodontitis. A:** Early lesion with blunted papillae and interdental necrosis. **B:** Increased destruction with loss of interdental tissue; rolled margins of the gingiva. **C:** More advanced destruction with recession and interdental cratering. **D:** Very advanced lesions, with loss of attached gingiva, recession, and tooth mobility. (Reprinted from Nield-Gehrig J, Willmann D. Foundations of Periodontics for the Dental Hygienist. Philadelphia: Wolters Kluwer Health/Lippincott Williams & Wilkins; 2011.)

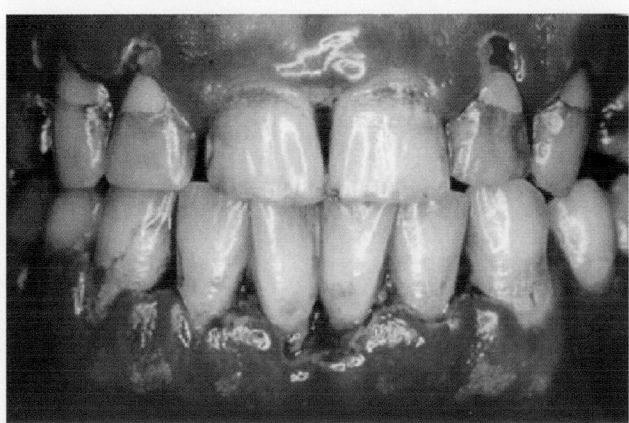

FIGURE 42-2 **NUP.**

RISK FACTORS

I. Local Factors

► NUG is rarely found in a clean, healthy, and professionally supervised mouth.
► Many of the factors predisposing to NUG are the same as those that predispose to chronic marginal gingivitis.
► Predisposing factors include:
  • Pre-existing gingivitis and/or periodontitis.
  • Inadequate personal oral care with general neglect of personal hygiene.
  • Factors related to retention of microorganisms and deposits.
  • Smoking.

II. Stress Factors

► Acute anxiety related to life situations is common.
► Occurs and reoccurs during periods of stress.
► Examples include:
  • Students during examination periods
  • Military men in combat.
► Emotional stress is frequently accompanied by poor oral care, improper diet, excessive smoking, overexertion, interrupted sleep, and other deviations in health habits.

III. Systemic: Disease-Resistance Factors

► Dietary and nutritional inadequacies including malnutrition and vitamin deficiencies.
► Compromised immune system or recent illnesses; frequent upper respiratory infections, infectious mononucleosis, pernicious anemia, hepatitis, leukemia, and HIV infection.
► Side effects of chemotherapy and radiation.
► Fatigue; insufficient sleep.

IV. Microbiology

► NUG and NUP are acute inflammatory conditions with characteristic microflora.
  • Of the many types of organisms found in NUG lesions, fusiform bacilli, and medium-sized spirochetes predominate.
  • The constant flora has been shown to include *Prevotella intermedia*[3], *Treponema* and *Selenomonas* species, *Bacteroides melinogenicus, intermedius, and Fusobacterium species*.[3,6]

CLINICAL RECOGNITION

I. Initial Signs and Symptoms

▶ Sudden onset.

▶ Pain and soreness caused by slight pressure, such as during chewing and tooth brushing; may be intensified by hot or highly seasoned foods. Gentle probing may produce an exaggerated pain response and bleeding.

▶ Poor appetite.

▶ Metallic or other unpleasant taste.

II. Characteristic Clinical Findings

▶ *Interdental necrosis*

• Ulceration of the papillae produces crater-like defects in the col areas.

• In early disease, only the tips of papillae are involved, followed by progressive destruction of entire papillae and extension to the marginal gingiva facially and lingually (Figures 42-1 and 42-2).

▶ *Pseudomembrane*

• Forms over the necrotic area.

• Gray, loose, necrotic slough; when wiped off, exposes a red and shiny hemorrhagic gingiva.

• Consists primarily of fibrin, necrotic tissue, leukocytes, and masses of microorganisms.

• Localized or generalized membranous ulceration

▶ *Other clinical findings*

• Debris and biofilm collect profusely because the patient avoids brushing the sensitive teeth and gingiva.

• Fetor oris (bad breath) is often severe; caused by necrotic tissue, stagnant saliva, and breakdown products of blood and debris.

• Increased salivation.

▶ *Signs of systemic involvement*

Examination is made to detect the presence of the following:

• Elevation of body temperature.

• Malaise.

• Lymphadenopathy of submandibular and cervical nodes.

III. Course of Development

▶ *Clinical characteristics of the lesion*

• NPD is superimposed on gingivitis and/or periodontitis.

• Ulceration and necrosis begin in the interdental papilla.

• Both epithelial tissue and connective tissue are involved.

• The disease process progresses to involve the entire papilla and, eventually, the marginal gingiva on the facial and lingual surfaces.

▶ *Microscopic examination*

Four zones in the lesion have been described from observations made by electron microscopy.[7] All layers contain spirochetes.

• *Bacterial zone*: The most superficial zone consists primarily of a mass of varied bacteria, including a few spirochetes.

• *Neutrophil-rich zone*: Under the bacterial zone is a layer of leukocytes, predominantly neutrophils. Microorganisms, including many spirochetes, are found among the leukocytes.

• *Necrotic zone*: This zone contains disintegrating tissue cells, many spirochetes, and other bacteria.

• *Spirochetal infiltration zone*: In this non-necrotized layer where tissue components are still preserved, spirochetes have invaded, but other microorganisms have not.

DENTAL HYGIENE CARE

The goal of therapy is elimination of the acute signs and symptoms of NUG/NUP.[2]

I. Assessment and Preparation for Dental Hygiene Care

▶ Collect the following data to determine the diagnosis and care plan.

A. History

▶ *Record the chief complaint*: The history of the current disease is described by date of onset, duration, symptoms as reported, and any self-treatment the patient has already performed.

▶ *Record whether this is a recurrence*: If so, note details of previous episodes and the treatment given.

▶ *Record vital signs*, especially temperature.

▶ *Identify conditions needing medical consultation.*

• Need for premedication for pre-existing condition. (Refer to Chapter 10 for information on conditions that require antibiotic premedication).

• Allergies

▶ *Use knowledge of predisposing factors for NPD to record pertinent information*

• Tobacco habits.

• Recent illnesses or types of therapy may explain a lowered resistance.

• Record previous 24-hour food intake. When the mouth has been sore and eating has been painful, a patient's usual intake will be negatively impacted.

• Variations of normal sleeping hours and routine; stress.

B. Clinical Examination

▶ *Extraoral/intraoral examination* (refer to Chapter 12).

• Observe face and skin to determine whether flushed, damp.

• Observe signs of malaise.

▶ Preliminary clinical examination can be made.

• Overall appearance of the gingival tissue recorded.

- The dentist may prefer to see the gingiva as it appears initially, before instrumentation or rinsing, to make the diagnosis and prepare the treatment plan.

II. Care Plan

The dental hygiene care plan is formulated within the total treatment plan. Only a partial treatment plan is made until after the acute phase of the disease has passed.

III. Acute Phase: First Appointment

A. Patient Oral-Self Care Instruction

Instructions for home use: Instructions for home procedures are carefully explained. Written directions are needed.

- ▶ *Toothbrushing*
  - Use a soft nylon brush gently, but thoroughly.
  - Clean all surfaces of teeth as much as possible especially before going to bed.
- ▶ *Rinsing directions*
  - Vigorous rinsing with warm water or weak saline solution is necessary every hour during the period of acute symptoms.
  - Using 3% hydrogen peroxide with equal parts of water is preferred by some clinicians. If used, it needs to be recommended for only a few days and then discontinued.
  - Rinse with chlorhexidine (0.12%) twice daily:
    - After breakfast, brush and use 0.5 ounce to swish.
    - After brushing and flossing before retiring; swish each side of the mouth between the teeth for 1 minute.

Instructions for continuing care: Inform the patient that treatment will not be complete when the pain is eliminated. Explain the underlying gingival or periodontal infection and how NPD recurs if the periodontal condition is not treated.

B. General Debridement

- ▶ Clean away loose debris: Apply hydrogen peroxide (3% solution mixed with equal parts of water) with cotton pellets at proximal areas; request patient to swish and rinse.
- ▶ Avoid use of compressed air or water spray to prevent reaction from sensitivity and dispersion of contaminated aerosols.
- ▶ Use topical anesthetic, local anesthesia, or nitrous oxide–oxygen sedation as needed to manage pain.
- ▶ Use manual or ultrasonic instruments for scaling; use high-speed evacuation to manage aerosols. Ultrasonic instrumentation may be preferred as it applies less pressure to the gingiva and the lavage (flushing) of the pockets may help healing.

C. Subgingival Instrumentation

The gingiva responds sooner with definitive scaling if the patient can tolerate it at the first appointment.

- ▶ Perform instrumentation with ultrasonic or well-honed instruments carefully but thoroughly.
- ▶ Have assistant evacuate continuously to minimize contaminated aerosols and to protect the patient from inhaling microorganisms.

- ▶ Irrigate and evacuate frequently to clear all debris and calculus removed during instrumentation.

D. Adjunctive Treatment

- ▶ Recommend a multivitamin/mineral supplement with at least 100% of the RDAs.
- ▶ Systemic antibiotic therapy
  - Prescribed conservatively; only to prevent infective endocarditis or for joint replacement (see Chapter 10).
- ▶ Tobacco cessation
  - *Inform patient*: Describe the effect of smoked or smokeless tobacco on the oral cavity, with special emphasis on facts about the gingival tissues.
  - *Avoid tobacco products*: The heavy smoker who is not ready for cessation can be requested to limit use while treatment for NPD is under way.
- ▶ *Diet*
  - Recommend frequent, small, high-protein meals incorporating daily requirements from the *MyPlate* guidelines (Chapter 35).
  - Drink plenty of water to stay hydrated.
  - No carbonated beverages.
  - A liquid or soft bland diet is advised for the first day, particularly for the patient with systemic symptoms or pronounced sensitivity when chewing.
  - Avoid highly seasoned foods, between meal snacks, high-sugar-containing foods/drinks, and alcoholic beverages.

IV. Acute Phase: Second Appointment

Ideally the second appointment is the next day or very soon after the initial appointment.

A. Patient Examination

- ▶ Improvement can be seen within 24 hours.
- ▶ Pseudomembrane gone, and tissue enlargement reduced.
- ▶ Evaluate oral self-care by applying disclosing solution and showing the patient areas missed.

B. Scaling and Root Debridement

- ▶ Objective: be as thorough as possible; biofilm retained over residual calculus and altered cementum can keep the tissues from healing completely.
- ▶ Begin individual quadrant nonsurgical periodontal therapy with subgingival scaling.
- ▶ Use local anesthesia or other pain management as needed.

C. Oral Self-care Instruction: Second Day

- ▶ *Rinsing*: When healing is progressing favorably, change rinsing schedule to every 2 hours.
- ▶ *Proximal surfaces*:
  - Use of floss or a small interdental brush is advised at this or the third appointment, depending on the readiness of the patient and the tissue.

- Other proximal cleaning devices may be useful. When the interdental embrasures are open as a result of papillary necrosis (Figure 42-1C and D), an interdental brush or other proximal device is indicated to clean the surface. The importance of complete biofilm removal is explained.
- ▶ *Diet*: A high-protein liquid diet may still be indicated after the first day, but patient can add begin to add soft, bland foods once chewing is comfortable.

V. Re-evaluation

- ▶ Once the acute condition is resolved, a comprehensive periodontal evaluation is scheduled.
- ▶ Repeated scaling and debridement is performed as needed.
- ▶ The complete plan for dental care is prepared and oral self-care instructions are reviewed.

VI. Maintenance

- ▶ Periodontal health will be carefully monitored with regular periodontal maintenance appointments for the following reasons:
  - Gingival and bony craters remaining after the initial healing phase are vulnerable to continuing disease and episodic recurrence of NPD.
  - Biofilm and debris can collect readily in the misshapen proximal areas and are difficult to clean with routine biofilm control techniques.
  - When bony craters exist, treatment may involve periodontal surgery.

HERPETIC GINGIVOSTOMATITIS

A viral infection of the oral mucosa caused by *Herpes simplex*. It may be mistaken for NPD. Characteristics for differential diagnosis are listed in Table 42-1. Additional information on herpes simplex virus can be found in Table 4-1 (Chapter 4).

I. Etiology

HSV1 is spread by infected saliva or active perioral lesions.

- ▶ Causative agent: HSV; usually HSV1 but HSV2 possible and clinically the same.
- ▶ Saliva can contain and transmit the virus when infected individuals are asymptomatic. Two patterns of clinically evident infections:
  - Primary infection
    - When an individual without antibodies is initially exposed.
    - Typically at a young age.
    - May be symptomatic but often is asymptomatic.
    - Virus usually enters a latent state in the trigeminal ganglion.
  - Secondary or recurrent infection
    - Occurs when latent virus is reactivated.
    - Most frequent location is at the vermilion border and adjacent skin of the lips where it is known as herpes labialis, cold sore, or fever blister.
- ▶ HSV has a short period of viability in the external environment.

TABLE 42-1	Comparison Between Necrotizing Periodontal Disease (NPD) and Herpetic Gingivostomatitis (HG)	
	NPD	**HG**
Cause	Bacteria and lower immunity	*Herpes simplex* virus
Who	Young adult	Child
Where	Interdental papilla. Rarely beyond periodontium	Entire oral mucosa including gingiva
Signs and symptoms	Ulcerations, necrotic tissue, and gray pseudomembrane Fetor oris Sometimes fever	Multiple vesicles followed by small round fibrin-covered ulcerations Fetor oris Fever
How long	1–2 days if treated	1–2 weeks
Contagious	No	Yes
Treatment focus	Behavior modification to support immune system Biofilm control Complete debridement	No specific treatment Counseling for nutrition, fluid intake, biofilm control Avoid contact (contagious)
Immunity to recurrence	No	Partial
Long-term effect	Permanent damage to periodontal tissue	No permanent tissue change

II. Pathogenesis

▶ HG is a primary infection of HSV in an individual without antibodies.

▶ Occurs most often in children from 6 months to 6 years, usually between ages 1 and 3; can occur at any age.

▶ Typical incubation period is 3–9 days.

▶ HG is self-limiting and resolves in 7–14 days with or without treatment.

▶ Primary infection is usually asymptomatic (subclinical) or may manifest as pharyngitis that mimics a common cold or may be mistaken as a difficult teeth episode.

▶ Transmission is by physical contact with contaminated saliva or an active lesion often by kissing, shared utensils, or contaminated hands.

III. Clinical Recognition and Diagnosis

A. Initial Signs and Symptoms

▶ Onset is abrupt.

▶ Initial symptoms may include any combination of the following:
  • Anterior cervical lymphadenopathy
  • Fever (103°–105°F) sore throat, and/or headache
  • Malaise, nausea, and irritability
  • Sore mouth, drooling, and/or refusal of food (anorexia).

B. Oral Presentation

▶ Oral lesions may be simultaneous with lymphadenopathy and fever or may follow after 1–2 days.

▶ A generalized sore mouth develops (Figure 42-3).
  • Diffuse, erythematous, shiny involvement of the gingiva and the adjacent oral mucosa, with varying degrees of edema and gingival bleeding.[8]
  • Gingiva is painful, erythematous, enlarged and may have spontaneous bleeding from the gingival sulcus.

▶ Any oral mucosal tissue can be involved both keratinized and nonkeratinized mucosa.
  • Mucosa develops numerous discrete, spherical gray, pinhead-sized vesicles.

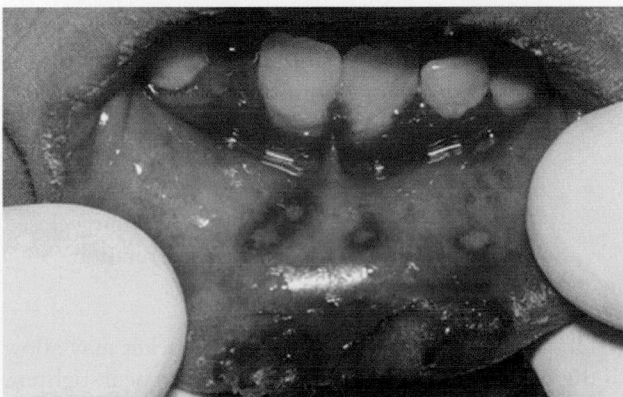

FIGURE 42-3 Herpetic Gingivostomatits. (Reprinted from Lippincott Williams & Wilkins' Comprehensive Dental Assisting. Philadelphia: Wolters Kluwer Health/Lippincott Williams & Wilkins; 2011.)

• May occur on the gingiva, labial and buccal mucosae, soft palate, pharynx, sublingual mucosa, and tongue.[8]
• May be missed because they collapse or rupture quickly, after 24 hour to form small superficial red ulcers.[8]
• Initial ulcers enlarge slightly or may coalesce to from a larger, shallow irregular ulceration.
• Central area of the ulcer is covered by yellow fibrin and is surrounded by a red ring of inflammation.
• Number of lesions is variable.

▶ Affected gingiva often has punched-out erosions at the midfacial of the free gingival margin.

▶ Lips and perioral skin are often involved.

IV. Management and Treatment

▶ Primary goal is pain relief and maintenance of nutrition and hydration.

▶ Antiviral medication may be considered[8,9]; antiviral medication is most effective during the earliest phase of viral infection but is rarely identified soon enough in Primary Herpetic Gingivostomatitis (PHG).

▶ Medical consult or referral may be indicated if secondary infection or dehydration is suspected.

▶ Reassure that condition is self-limiting; usually of 1–2 weeks duration.

▶ Advise that *Herpes simplex* virus is contagious during the acute stages of the disease especially when vesicles or ulcerated lesions are present.

▶ Treatment recommendation:
  • Avoid dental and dental hygiene treatment including debridement of the teeth due to the infective nature of the virus both to the clinician and to other areas of the patient's mucosa.

▶ Patient counseling includes:
  • Instruction in adequate nutrition and fluid intake.
  • Dehydration is the most common cause of hospitalization of small children with PHG.
  • Normal oral hygiene is discontinued during the few days of the acute painful stage; gentle oral hygiene can begin again during healing.

V. Palliative Treatment

A. Diet

▶ Soft high-protein diet of bland warm or cold foods.

▶ Cold foods such as ice cream or sherbet may be soothing.

▶ Avoid acidic or carbonated drinks.

B. Mouthrinses

Palliative mouthrinses to relieve pain and inflammation may include:

▶ Rinse, but do not swallow, warm saline and bicarbonate rinses (½ teaspoon table salt, ½ teaspoon baking soda, 8 ounces warm water) swished, held in the mouth for a few minutes then expectorated.

▶ Acyclovir oral suspension as prescribed[10]
  • Can be used after meals and at bedtime in place of toothbrushing during the most painful phase.
▶ Diphenhydramine elixir and an antacid such as Kaopectate or Maalox mixed in equal parts.
▶ Viscous lidocaine, Diphenhydramine elixir, and an antacid such as Kaopectate or Maalox mixed in equal parts (can be mixed at compounding pharmacy).
  • Instruct patient to swish between their teeth a teaspoonful for 30–60 seconds and expectorate.
  • Especially helpful before meals.
  • Caution about swallowing: difficulties due to numb mouth.

VI. Resolution

▶ Fever typically subsides after 2 days.
▶ Oral lesions begin to heal 3 days after appearance.
▶ Mild cases resolve in 5–7 days with more severe cases lasting 2 weeks.
▶ Lesions heal completely and without scaring.

PERIODONTAL ABSCESS

▶ An abscess is a localized purulent inflammatory lesion.
▶ Gingival and periodontal abscesses occur within the periodontal tissues.
  • An abscess is called *gingival* when it is limited to the marginal area or interdental papilla.
  • An abscess is called *periodontal* when it is in the deeper periodontal tissues.
  • The lesion may be acute or chronic.
  • May also be known as *lateral abscesses* because they occur along the lateral surfaces of teeth.

I. Development of a Periodontal Abscess

▶ Pus or exudate collects in the tissue as a result of bacterial infection.
▶ The infection may be:
  • A complication of an existing periodontal infection.
  • An immediate result of microorganisms from biofilm forced into the tissue by some form of trauma.
▶ The body's reaction is to send large numbers of defense cells to the area, particularly polymorphonuclear leukocytes (PMNs), which are major constituents of the purulent exudate (pus) that collects.
▶ Pus is a thick fluid product of inflammation.
  • Contains many living and dead PMNs mixed with debris from cells and tissues destroyed by the enzymes released by the PMNs.
  • Without a means for drainage, the pus collects and forms an abscess.

▶ A sinus tract or fistula may form.
  • Drainage may occur through the sinus port and release the pressure within the abscess, thereby relieving the patient's pain.

II. Clinical Signs and Symptoms

Clinical manifestations may vary. The classic signs and symptoms are:
▶ *Area of abscess*
  • Area of the abscess is enlarged, with a red, shiny, smooth surface.
  • The abscess may appear domelike or pointed, and on slight digital pressure, pus may appear.
▶ *The tooth*
  • *Sensitivity*: The tooth may be slightly mobile and sensitive to percussion. When extruded, it may be sensitive to touching the tooth in the opposing jaw.
  • *Pulp vitality test*: Pulp testing usually reveals a vital tooth, responding within the normal range.
▶ *Radiographs*
  • A radiolucency may be noted along the lateral wall beside the tooth, but such a finding is variable.
  • Early lesions do not present with bone loss.
  • The amount of bone destruction and the location of the abscess influence the possible radiographic findings.
▶ *General physical condition*
  Patient shows evidence of systemic involvement:
  • A slight elevation in body temperature.
  • Malaise.
  • Lymphadenopathy.
▶ *Chronic abscess*
  • In the chronic state, a sinus tract usually opens on the gingival surface and drains periodically.
  • Before drainage, the patient may have a dull pain from the pressure of the fluid within the abscess area.
  • Acute symptoms may be expected from time to time unless definitive periodontal therapy is completed.

III. Etiologic Factors

A. Periodontal Pockets

▶ Deep pockets of chronic inflammatory periodontal infection provide an environment for abscess formation.
  • Intrabony pockets those extending into bifurcation or trifurcation areas.
  • Complex pockets that develop in winding or irregular shapes are particularly susceptible to becoming closed and, therefore, susceptible to abscess formation.

B. Instrumentation

▶ Incomplete scaling in the depth of a pocket may allow the tissue at the opening of the pocket to heal, tighten, and prevent drainage of the infectious material deep in the pocket.

▶ Biofilm and calculus remaining in the sealed off part of the pocket attract the collection of more bacteria and PMNs, and an abscess develops.

C. Trauma

▶ Foreign objects may enter by way of the sulcus or pocket and become embedded along with microorganisms. The infection leads to abscess formation.[11]

▶ Implanted or impacted material:
- A popcorn hull
- Small fish bone or shellfish fragment, seeds, seed coverings, or other material from food
- Oral hygiene devices such as a toothbrush bristle or filament.

D. Oral and Systemic Relationship

▶ Risk for abscess formation within the gingival tissue is increased by any of the etiologic factors that have been mentioned when the patient's resistance to infection is lowered.

▶ Patients with uncontrolled diabetes or who are receiving immunosuppressive medication are examples of those at greater risk.

IV. Comparison of Periapical (Endodontic) and Periodontal Abscesses

The dentist often needs to make a differential diagnosis between a periodontal abscess and a periapical abscess of pulpal origin. Certain signs and symptoms are similar for both.

▶ Under certain circumstances, left untreated, the following may occur:
- The periapical abscess can lead to the destruction of bone.
- The spread of infection to soft tissue and muscle spaces, resulting in a severe, life-threatening infection.[12]
- Hospitalization may be necessary for patients with advanced infections requiring more invasive treatment, such as intravenous antibiotic medications and surgical incisions with intraoral or extraoral drainage under general anesthesia and supportive care.[12]
- The economic burden associated with a periapical abscess is increased.[12]

A few of the potentially distinguishing findings are noted here.

▶ *Pulpal abscess*
- Nonvital response to pulp test; sensitivity to percussion.
- May have no periodontal pocket.
- Swelling related to apex of tooth with or without fistulous tract.
- Pain often severe; may be difficult to locate specifically.

▶ *Radiographic examination*
- Early stages of either a periapical or a periodontal abscess are not evident in a radiograph.
- A widening of the periodontal ligament space may appear.

▶ *Combined periodontal/periapical (endodontic) lesion*
- *Etiology:* the lesion may originate primarily from pulpal infection expressing itself through the periodontal tissues or bacteria from a deep periodontal pocket may invade the pulp. It may be the result of a fractured tooth.
- Communication may exist between a deep periodontal pocket and the pulp by way of a lateral or accessory canal through the dentin, often in the area of a furcation.

V. Care Plan

Two phases of treatment are used for the patient with a periodontal abscess.
- The first: for immediate relief of acute symptoms.
- The second: the definitive diagnosis and treatment followed by preventive maintenance.
- The entire plan is explained to the patient at the outset.

▶ *Objectives of emergency treatment*
- Relieve pain.
- Establish drainage.
- Determine need for systemic antibiotic therapy.
- Manage patient comfort.

▶ *Review medical history*
- Determine necessary preappointment precautions, such as the need for antibiotic premedication.

▶ *Examination for systemic involvement*
- Antibiotic medication may be prescribed by the dentist when systemic involvement is definite.
- Determine and record the patient's body temperature.
- Examine submandibular and neck nodes for lymphadenopathy.

▶ *Provide anesthesia*
- When the abscess is confined to the gingival area, and the drainage may be expected to cause little if any discomfort, a topical anesthetic may suffice.
- Usually, block anesthesia is indicated.

▶ *Methods for drainage: Via pocket or sulcus opening*
- Local anesthetic injection for pain management.
- Isolate the area, swab with a topical antiseptic, and use a probe to gain admission into the sulcus or pocket.
- Gently probe circumferentially until an opening into the abscess is found.
- Drainage usually begins immediately.

▶ *Methods for drainage: Curet area*
- Use a curet to open the area, and locate and remove a foreign body irritant when it is known to be present from the history obtained from the patient.
- Scaling and subgingival debridement are performed as needed.

▶ *Posttreatment instructions and follow-up*
- Rinsing with warm saline solution every 2 hours is advised; over-the-counter analgesics as needed.

- The patient returns for observation in 24–48 hours. Relief from pain and discomfort can be expected and appointments for definitive treatment planned.
- Oral self-care instruction is initiated or continued to control biofilm, and scaling and debridement are completed.

▶ *Anticipated results*

- Acute symptoms are resolved.
- Pain relief occurs within a short time following the initiation of drainage because the pressure is released from within the abscessed area.
- Extruded tooth returns to its normal position.
- Swelling is reduced.
- Temporary comfort is obtained for the patient; the lesion is reduced to a standard chronic lesion that requires additional treatment.
- If drainage is not complete, an acute lesion may develop into a lesion with a chronic sinus or pocket drainage.

VI. Definitive Therapy

▶ When a pocket elimination procedure is indicated, it needs to be completed within a reasonable time to prevent further complications.

▶ Careful and regular dental biofilm control with scaling and subgingival debridement are essential on a maintenance basis.

GINGIVAL ABSCESS

I. Development of a Gingival Abscess

▶ An acute, localized purulent infection that involves the marginal gingiva or interdental papilla with no history of previous disease.[13,14]

II. Etiologic Factors[14]

▶ Microbial biofilm infection
▶ Trauma
▶ Foreign body impaction.

III. Clinical Signs and Symptoms[14]

▶ Clinical features may include:
- A red, smooth swelling
- Sometimes painful
- Fluctuant and pointed swelling
- Purulent exudate may be present.

IV. Definitive Therapy

▶ Removal of foreign body.

PERICORONAL ABCESS/ PERICORONITIS[13–15]

▶ Inflammation of the gingiva surrounding the crown of a partially erupted tooth.
▶ May be acute, subacute, or chronic.

I. Development of a Pericoronal Abscess

▶ An operculum, a flap of gingival tissues that covers the partially erupted tooth
- Creates an opportunity for food debris and microorganisms to be trapped beneath the flap of the partially erupted tooth.
▶ Infection ensues.

EVERYDAY ETHICS

Mr. Rufus, who has been a patient in the office for many years, shows up this afternoon without an appointment because he is suddenly having mouth pain and a "horrible metallic taste." Susan, the dental hygienist, is overtaken by a strong mouth odor when he speaks. Dr. Janus is on vacation this week, but according to the laws of her state, Susan practices under *general supervision* and may provide dental hygiene care for a patient of record even when the dentist is not in the office. Susan seats Mr. Rufus in the dental chair to assess the situation.

Susan determines that there have been no changes in Mr. Rufus' health history, but he describes the heart-breaking details of his divorce proceedings. He confides in Susan that he has hardly eaten or brushed his teeth for weeks.

Susan begins an extraoral and intraoral examination, but Mr. Rufus says it is too painful for her to retract his cheeks and lips. During the brief examination, she noticed punched out papillae and pseudomembrane formation over much of his gingiva. She immediately suspects NUG, or perhaps NUP.

Questions for Consideration

1. Which of the core values (Table II-1, in Introduction to Section II) apply to this scenario? Discuss their meaning in this situation. Are "informed consent" or "implied consent" a concern if all Susan has done to help Mr. Rufus is assess and examine his oral cavity?

2. Would it be legal for Susan to provide acute phase (first appointment) care for Mr. Rufus today, even though Dr. Janus is not in the office? Why or why not?

3. Mrs. Rufus, who comes in for her appointment later in the month, does not share any information about the divorce. However, she asks Susan why Mr. Rufus was billed for several appointments for quadrant scaling and debridement when he was just to "clean his teeth." What ethical principles guide how Susan responds to any questions Mrs. Rufus might ask?

BOX 42-2
Example Documentation: Patient with NUG

S –A 23-year-old male presents with chief complaint of painful bleeding gingiva of 4 days duration. Patient has a clear medical history taking no medications. Patient states he smokes 1 pack/day. Patient also reports recent high-stress levels.

O–Intraoral assessment reveals slightly enlarged, glossy, bright red, marginal gingiva throughout, BOP with slight contact. The papilla between 3–4, 4–5, and 28–29 have yellowish gray coating. Patient has pronounced oral malodor. Tissue is so painful to touch that full-mouth probing was deferred to a future appointment. Bone levels look normal on radiographs.

A–Acute pain and discomfort due to NUG.

P–Patient education—Discussed etiology of NUG and probable causes including stress and smoking, lack of sleep, poor nutrition, and long-standing gingivitis due to poor biofilm control and lack of professional care.

Oral Self-care: Oral self-care instructions given using a soft TB, recommend twice daily using Bass technique. Discussed smoking cessation, he is currently not interested but willing to talk about it again in future.

Treatment plan: Initial visit—gentle full-mouth debridement of supragingival biofilm/calculus and patient education. Patient committed to try the following behavior modifications: Get at least 6 hours of sleep a night, eat 3 meals a day and add one fruit and vegetable a day, and take a multivitamin daily. He did not think he could reduce stress at this time.

Treatment Provided: Pre-tx rinse with CHX; debridement with hydrogen peroxide: water mix (50:50) applied generously to the gingival with a cotton swab; full-mouth supragingival ultrasonic instrumentation. Patient was somewhat uncomfortable but said to continue and generally tolerated procedure well. High-speed evacuation was used to manage aerosol.

Next visit: following day, assess healing, and evaluate biofilm removal and behavior modification. Modify as needed; add flossing. Begin definitive debridement, by quadrant, under local anesthesia. Patient gave consent.

Signed _____, RDH
Date _____

- As inflammation increases the operculum can:
  - Increase in size.
  - When biting, become trapped between the mandibular and maxillary dentitions.
  - Trismus, a limited ability to open the mouth, may occur.
- Most common location mandibular 3rd molars.

II. Systemic Implications[13]

- Possible elevated temperature
- Possible lymphadenopathy.

III. Treatment[13]

- Administer local anesthesia, as needed.
- If pus is present, drain; irrigate under the operculum.
- Dentist may prescribe an antibiotic to decrease the infection.
- Definitive treatment—extraction of impacted tooth.

DOCUMENTATION

Documentation is the permanent record for each appointment when a patient presents with complaint of pain. It includes a minimum of the following factors:

- Description of signs, symptoms, location, and duration of condition.
- Diagnosis or differential diagnosis.
- Treatment plan.
- Description of treatment.
- Description of patient education and postoperative instructions.
- Future plan.
- An example progress note documenting an appointment for a patient with NUG is given in Box 42-2.

Factors To Teach The Patient

- Premature discontinuation of treatment for NUG because acute signs have subsided can lead to recurrence of the infection.
- The role of diet, rest, and dental biofilm control in the prevention of NUG.
- The avoidance of an oral irrigating device in the presence of acute inflammatory conditions. Microorganisms may be forced into the tissues beneath a pocket, and bacteremia can be produced.

References

1. Dofka C. *Dental Terminology*. 2nd ed. 2007. http://www.r2library.com.ezproxy.mcphs.edu/resource/detail/1428015229/pr0002. Accessed August 25, 2013.
2. American Academy of Periodontology. Parameter on acute periodontal diseases. *J Periodontol*. 2000;71(5, Suppl):863–866.
3. Lang N, Soskolne WA, Greenstein G, et al. Consensus report: necrotizing periodontal diseases. *Ann Periodontol*. 1999;4(1):78.
4. Enwonwu CO, Phillips RS, Savage KO. Inflammatory cytokine profile and circulating cortisol levels in malnourished children with necrotizing ulcerative gingivitis. *Eur Cytokine Netw*. 2005;16(3):240–248.
5. Mataftsi M, Skoura L, Sakellari D. HIV infection and periodontal diseases: an overview of the post-HAART era. *Oral Dis*. 2011;17:13–25.

6. Loesche WJ, Syed SA, Laughon BE, et al. The bacteriology of acute necrotizing ulcerative gingivitis. *J Periodontol.* 1982;53(4):223–230.

7. Listgarten MA. Electron microscopic observations on the bacterial flora of acute necrotizing ulcerative gingivitis. *J Periodontol.* 1965;36:328–339.

8. Klokkevold PR, Carranza FA. Chapter 10: Acute gingival infections. In: Newman MG, Takai H, Klukkevold PR, et al., eds. *Carranza's Clinical Periodontology.* 11th ed. St. Louis, MO: Saunders; 2012:97–103.

9. Nasser M, Fedorowicz Z, Khoshnevisan MH, et al. Acyclovir for treating primary herpetic gingivostomatitis. *Cochrane Database Syst Rev.* 2008;(4):CD006700.

10. Stoopler ET, Balasubramanian R. Topical and systemic therapies for oral and perioral herpes simplex virus infections. *J Calif Dent Assoc.* 2013;41(4):259–262.

11. Gillette WB, Van House RL. Ill effects of improper oral hygiene procedure. *J Am Dent Assoc.* 1980;101(3):476–480.

12. Shah AC, Leong KK, Lee KM, et al. Outcomes of hospitalizations attributed to periapical abscess from 2000 to 2008: a longitudinal trend analysis. *J Endod.* 2013;39(9):1104–1110.

13. Lang N, Soskolne WA, Greenstein G, et al. Consensus report: abscesses of the periodontium. *Ann Periodontol.* 1999;4(1):83.

14. Meng, HX. Periodontal abscess. *Ann Periodontol.* 1999; 4(1):79–82.

15. Melnick P, Takei HH. Chapter 42: Treatment of periodontal abscess. In: Newman MG, Takei HH, Klokkevold PR, et al., eds. *Carranza's Clinical Periodontology.* 11th ed. St. Louis, MO: Saunders; 2012:443–447.

ENHANCE YOUR UNDERSTANDING

thePoint° DIGITAL CONNECTIONS
(see the inside front cover for access information)
- **Audio glossary**
- **Quiz bank**

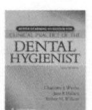

SUPPORT FOR LEARNING
(available separately; visit lww.com)
- *Active Learning Workbook for Clinical Practice of the Dental Hygienist, 12th Edition*

prepU INDIVIDUALIZED REVIEW
(available separately; visit lww.com)
- **Adaptive quizzing with *prepU for Wilkins' Clinical Practice of the Dental Hygienist***

43

Sutures and Dressings

Susan J. Jenkins, RDH, MS, CAGS and Marilyn Cortell, RDH, MS

CHAPTER OUTLINE

LEARNING OBJECTIVES

After studying this chapter, the student will be able to:

1. State the functions and purposes of sutures and periodontal dressings.

2. Describe the differences between absorbable and nonabsorbable sutures.

3. Describe the procedure for suture removal.

4. Describe the procedure for periodontal dressing placement and periodontal dressing removal.

5. Explain approaches for managing biofilm with the periodontal dressing in place and upon removal.

Many periodontal surgical procedures require sutures and dressings. The dental hygienist will often participate in the patient's oral self-care instruction at initial placement and postcare. Knowledge of the surgical and posttreatment procedures will support continuity of treatment. Key words related to sutures and dressings are defined in Box 43-1.

SUTURES

A suture is a strand of material used to ligate blood vessels and approximate tissue. Sutures are necessary in many oral surgical procedures when a surgical wound must be closed, a flap positioned, or tissue grafted.

Through the centuries, a wide range of suture materials has been used, including silk, cotton, linen, and animal tendons and intestines. Today's suture materials are designed for specific procedures, thus decreasing potential for postsurgical infections while providing patient comfort and convenience.

I. Functions of Sutures

▶ Close periodontal wounds and secure grafts in position

▶ Assist in maintaining hemostasis

▶ Reduce posttreatment discomfort

▶ Promote primary intention healing

▶ Prevent underlying bone exposure

▶ Protect a healing surgical wound from foreign debris and trauma.

II. Characteristics of Suture Materials

▶ Sterile

▶ Handle comfortably and easily

▶ Pass through tissue with minimal trauma

▶ Cause little or no tissue reaction throughout healing

▶ Possess a high tensile strength.

III. Classification of Suture Materials

▶ By *number of strands*
   • *Monofilament suture*: single strand of material
   • *Multifilament suture*: several strands twisted or braided together.

▶ By *material used*
   • *Natural*: capable of causing adverse tissue reaction
   • *Synthetic*: developed to reduce tissue reactions and unpredictable rates of absorption commonly found in natural sutures.

▶ By *absorption properties*
   • *Natural absorbable sutures*: digested by body enzymes
      ◦ *Plain gut*: Most common, monofilamentous, derived from purified collagen of sheep or cattle.[1]
      ◦ *Chromatic gut*: Chromatic salts to delay enzyme resorption.[1]
   • *Synthetic resorbable sutures*: Broken down by hydrolysis, a process in which water slowly penetrates the suture filaments to cause a breakdown of the suture's polymer chain.

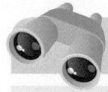

BOX 43-1   KEY WORDS: Sutures and Dressing

Alveolectomy: surgical removal of a portion of the alveolar bone to allow for fitting of a prosthesis.

Border mold: the shaping of the edges of a dressing by manual manipulation of the tissue adjacent to the borders (e.g., lips, cheeks) to duplicate the contour and size of the vestibule.

Chemical cure: mode of self-cure or setting of a dressing in which the ingredients unite in a chemical process that starts as soon as the blending is complete; the setting time is influenced by warm temperature and the addition of an accelerator.

Coapt: to approximate, as the edges of a wound; bring edge to edge with no overlap.

Eugenol: constituent of clove oil; used in early periodontal dressings with zinc oxide for its alleged antiseptic and anodyne properties; more recently found to be toxic, to elicit allergic reactions, and to hinder, more than promote, healing.

Hemostasis: the termination of bleeding by mechanical or chemical means or by the complex coagulation process of the body that consists of vasoconstriction, platelet aggregation, and thrombin and fibrin synthesis.

Hydrolysis: a process in which water slowly penetrates the suture filaments, causing breakdown of the suture's polymer chain. Hydrolyzation yields a lesser degree of tissue reaction.

Ligation: application of a wire or thread (suture) to hold or constrict tissue.

Septic: presence of potentially pathogenic microorganisms; opposite of **Asepsis:** absence of infectious material.

Suture: a stitch or series of stitches made to secure apposition of the edges of a surgical or traumatic wound.

   Suture apposition: a suture that holds the margins of an incision close together.

Swage: the fusion of a suture material to the needle, which allows for a smooth eyeless attachment. The suture will then pass through the tissue as smoothly as possible.

Tensile strength: amount of strength the suture material will retain throughout the healing period. As the wound gains strength, the suture loses strength.

Visible light–cure: light activation using a photocure system; shorter curing time than self-cure (chemical cure); does not start setting until the light is activated, thereby allowing longer working time for adapting the dressing material.

- Example: Polyglactin (Vicryl), Poliglecaprone (Monocryl) and polydioxanone (PDS II).
- *Nonabsorbable sutures*: not digested by body enzymes or hydrolyzation; patient returns for removal usually after 1 week
  - *Natural nonabsorbable*
    - Braided silk
  - *Synthetic nonabsorbable*
    - Nylon (Ethilon)
    - Polyester (Ethibond)
    - Polypropylene (Prolene)
    - Polytetrafluoroethylene (Gore-Tex).
▶ By *diameter of suture material*
- Diameters range from 1–0 to 11–0.
- More zeros, smaller the diameter.
- Fewer zeros, larger the diameter.
- Example: 3–0 is larger than 5–0.

IV. Selection of Suture Materials

Choosing the appropriate suture material for a specific procedure is critical both for patient comfort and tissue health. Suture selection is based on
▶ Preference of surgeon
▶ Delicacy of tissue
▶ Cosmetic implications
- Examples of suture types surgeons may use for specific procedures are listed in Table 43-1.

NEEDLES

Many types of suturing needles are available. Their use and selection are primarily based on specific procedures, location for use, and clinician's preference.

I. Needle Components

▶ *Swaged end (eyeless)*
- Swaged allows suture material and needle to act as one unit (Figure 43-1).

▶ *Body*
- *Shape/curvature*
  - Straight
  - Half-curved
  - Curved 1/4, 3/8, 1/2, 5/8 (Figure 43-2).

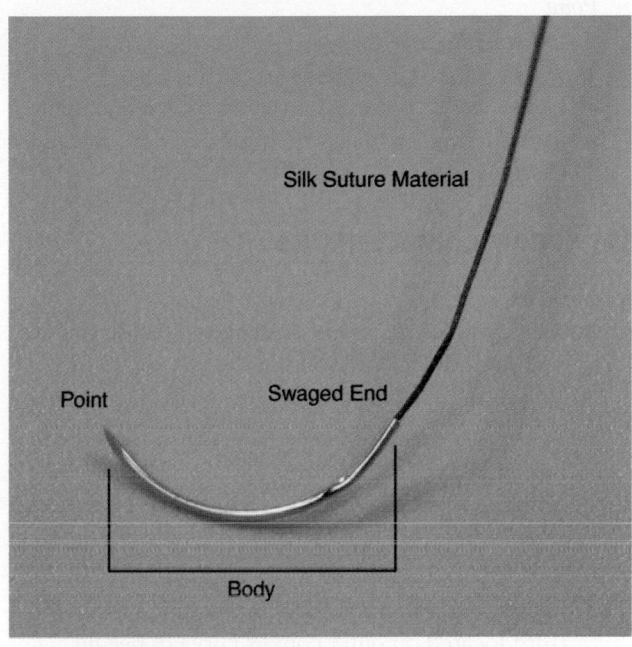

FIGURE 43-1 Suture Needle Components. (Courtesy of Susan Jenkins, MCPHS University Forsyth School of Dental Hygiene.)

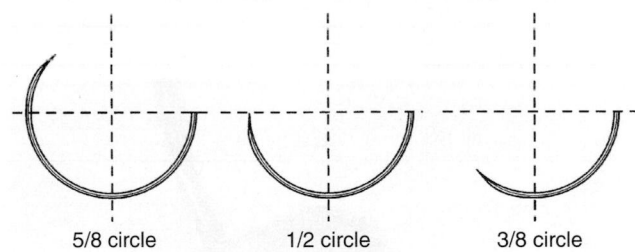

FIGURE 43-2 Suture Needles. A curved needle is manipulated with a needleholder. The 3/8 curve is most effective for closure of skin and mucous membranes and is a needle of choice in many dental and periodontal surgeries.

TABLE 43-1	Selection of Suture Material
SUTURE TYPES	**SPECIFIC DENTAL PROCEDURES**
Silk, nonresorbable, braided	Periodontal flaps and closure
Nylon, monofilament	Periodontal flaps and closure
Polyester, braided	Periodontal flaps and closure
Gut, resorbable	Extraction socket, bone grafting, free-gingival grafting
Resorbable preferred: Nonresorbable used when pain and swelling may be anticipated	Implant flap closure

- *Diameter*
  - Gauge or size; finer for delicate surgeries.
  - Body is the strongest part of the needle that is grasped with the needleholder during the surgical procedure.
  - Swaged end is the weakest part of the body.
- *Point*
  - Point of the needle extends from the extreme tip of the needle to the widest part of the body.
  - Each needle point is designed and manufactured to penetrate tissue with the highest degree of sharpness.

II. Needle Characteristics

- *Material*
  - Most needles are made of stainless steel formulated and sterilized for surgical use.
- *Attachment*
  - Majority of needles are permanently attached to suture material.
  - Eliminates need for threading and unnecessary handling.
- *Cutting edge* (Figure 43-3)
  - *Reverse cut*: Has two opposing cutting edges, with a third located on outer convex curve of needle.
  - *Conventional cut*: Consists of two opposing cutting edges and a third within the concave curvature of the needle.

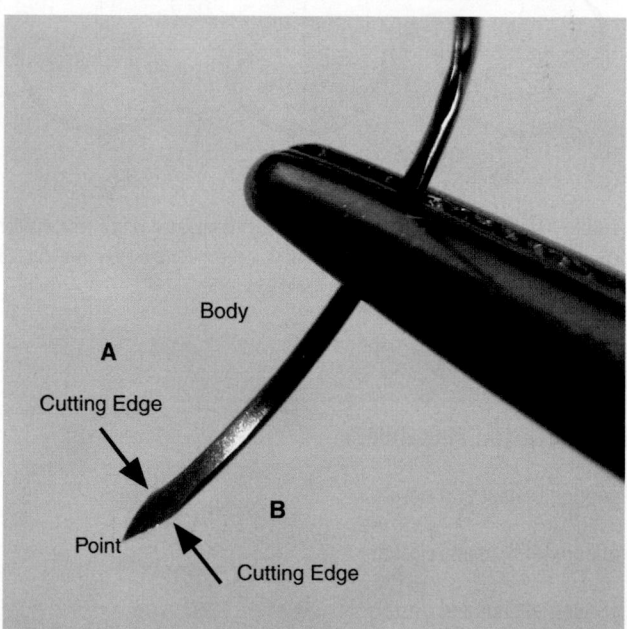

FIGURE 43-3 Suture Needles. Shapes of Points. Triangle shows cross section of needle point. **A:** Conventional cutting with third cutting edge on the inside of the needle curvature. **B:** Reverse cutting with third cutting edge on the outer curvature of the needle, used for difficult-to-penetrate tissue, such as skin. (Courtesy of Susan Jenkins, MCPHS University Forsyth School of Dental Hygiene.)

- *Requirements*
  - *Needle point*: Designed to meet the needs of specific surgical procedures.
  - *Surgical needles*: Intended to carry suture material through tissues with minimal trauma.
  - Needle points:
    - Sharp enough to penetrate tissues with minimal resistance.
    - Rigid enough to resist bending, yet are flexible.
    - Sterile and corrosion resistant.

KNOTS

The book *Surgical Knots and Suturing Techniques*[2] describes a variety of surgical knots. Only a few are used in dentistry.
- Type of knot used will depend on the specific procedure.
- Location of the incision.
- Amount of stress the wound will endure.
- Square knots are most frequently used in dentistry because they are the easiest and most reliable.

I. Knot Characteristics

- A knot is tied as small as possible.
- Completed knot needs to be firm to reduce slipping.
- Excessive tension is avoided to prevent breakage or trauma to the tissue.

II. Knot Management

- Tie knots on facial aspect for easier access for removal.
- Leave 2- to 3-mm suture "tail" to assist in locating at the time of removal.

SUTURING PROCEDURES

- Many different patterns of suturing are used. Assisting and observing during the surgical procedure can be an educational experience for the dental hygienist.
- General types of sutures frequently used in the oral cavity are described here (Figure 43-4).

I. Blanket (Continuous Lock)

- Each stitch is brought over a loop of the preceding one, thus forming a series of loops on one side of the incision and a series of stitches over the incision (Figure 43-4A).
- Uses: To approximate the gingival margins after alveolectomy.

II. Interrupted

- Figure 43-4B shows a series of interrupted sutures.

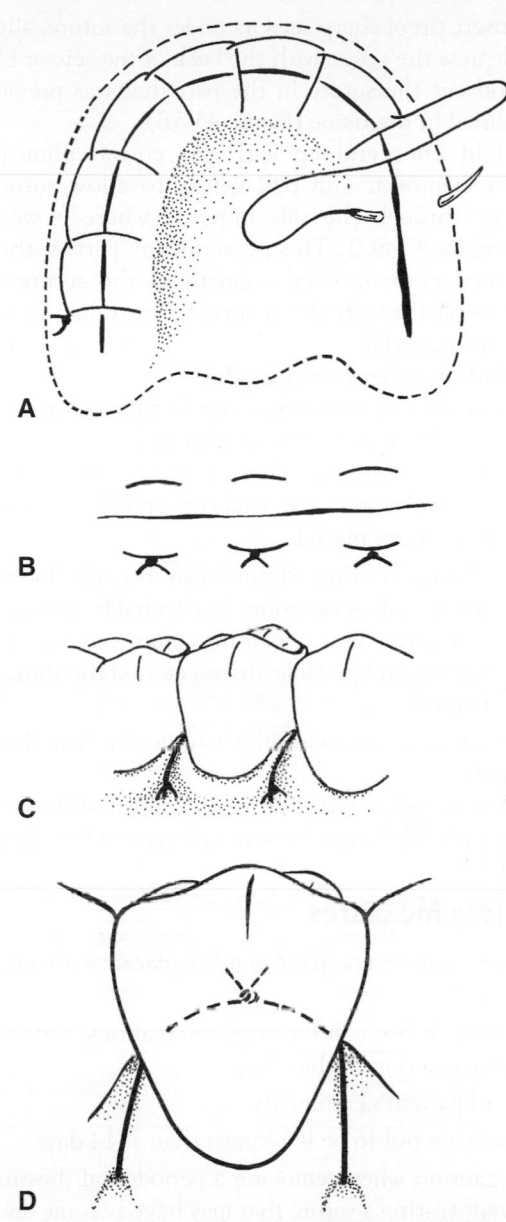

III. Continuous Uninterrupted

▶ A series of stitches tied at one or both ends.

▶ Examples of sutures that may be applied in a series are the sling or suspension and the blanket.

IV. Circumferential

▶ Suture that encircles a tooth for suspension and retention of a flap.

V. Interdental

▶ Flaps are on both the lingual and facial sides, interdental ligation joins the two by passing the suture through each interdental area (Figure 43-4C). Coverage for the interdental area can be accomplished by coapting the edges of the papillae.

VI. Sling or Suspension

▶ When a flap is only on one side, facial or lingual, the sutures are passed through the interdental papilla, around the tooth, and into the adjacent papilla (Figure 43-4D).

▶ The suture is adjusted so that the flap can be positioned for correct healing.

PROCEDURE FOR SUTURE REMOVAL

Removal schedule: 7 days after the surgery or no longer than 14 days to prevent tissue infection and promote healing. When chlorhexidine rinse was initiated after surgery, it is continued to support healing.

I. Review Previous Documentation

▶ Medical history
▶ Surgical procedures
▶ Patient reactions to healing
▶ Current surgery: number and type of sutures placed.

II. Sterile Clinic Tray Setup

▶ Sterile mouth mirror
▶ Sterile cotton pliers
▶ Sterile curved sharp scissors with pointed tip (suture scissors)
▶ Gauze sponges
▶ Topical anesthetic: type that can be applied safely on an abraded or incompletely healed area to be used
▶ Cotton pellets
▶ Saliva ejector tip.

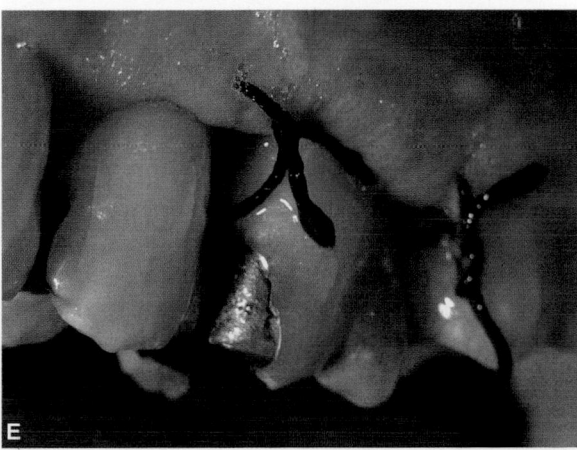

FIGURE 43-4 Types of Sutures. A: Blanket stitch. **B:** Interrupted, individual sutures. **C:** Interdental individual sutures. **D:** Sling or suspension suture tied on the lingual (*dotted line*) **E:** Interrupted silk sutures in place one-week post surgery. (Courtesy of Dr. Robert Lewando, Boston, MA.)

III. Preparation of Patient

▶ *Patient history check*

- Suture removal can cause bacteremia.[2,3]
- High-risk patients may need antibiotic premedication for suture removal. Consultation with patient's physician is indicated.

▶ *Patient examination*

- Observe healing tissue around the suture(s) (Figure 43-4E).
- Record any deviations in color, size, shape of the tissue, adaptation of a flap, or coaptation of an incision healing by first intention.

▶ *Preparation of the sutured area*

- Sutures placed without a dressing may have a crust over them at the time of removal.
- Apply a water-based gel with a cotton swab or pellet.
- In a short time, the crust will soften and can be wiped away.
- If the suture is removed with the crust, it can cause unnecessary patient discomfort and bleeding.
- Debride and rinse the area to remove debris particles.
- Use a cotton-tipped applicator or a cotton pellet dipped in 3% peroxide.
- Follow with another rinse, or wipe gently with a gauze sponge.
- Place and adjust saliva ejector.
- Retract and pat area with gauze sponge to remove surface moisture.
- Swab area with topical antiseptic. Maintain retraction to prevent dilution.
- Apply topical anesthetic.

▶ *Retraction*

- Three hands are really needed for efficient clinical procedure: one for retraction, one for cotton pliers to hold and remove the suture, and one for cutting the suture.
- When an assistant is not available, place a cotton roll in the vestibule to provide enough retraction along with the finger rest and little finger of the nondominant hand holding the cotton pliers.

IV. Steps for Removal

▶ The suture removal procedure described here and illustrated in Figure 43-5 is for a single interrupted suture.

▶ The same principles apply for the ends and each segment of a continuous suture, wherever septic suture material can pass through the soft tissue.

▶ *Steps*

1. Grasp the suture knot with the cotton plier held in the nondominant hand. Gently draw the suture up about 2 mm and hold with slight tension (Figure 43-5A). A finger rest is needed for control.

2. Insert tip of sharp scissors under the suture, slightly depress the tissue with the back of the scissor blade, and cut the suture in the part that was previously buried in the tissue (Figure 43-5B).

3. Hold knot end up with the cotton plier locking hemostat and pull gently to allow suture to exit through the side opposite where it was cut (Figure 43-5C). This prevents any part of the exposed contaminated segment of the suture from passing through the tissue and introducing infectious material.

4. Withdraw gently and steadily.

5. Place each suture on a sponge for final counting, and proceed to remove the next suture.

6. Count the total number of sutures removed. The number of sutures removed corresponds to the number of sutures placed.

   - During healing, sutures can become loosened, misplaced, or occasionally covered by tissue.
   - The effect of a remaining suture can lead to infection and possible abscess around the suture left behind.

7. Apply gauze sponge with slight pressure on bleeding spots.

8. Request patient to close on the sponge while dressing is readied (when a dressing replacement is indicated).

V. Safety Measures

▶ Count sutures; compare number placed with number removed.

▶ Observe all tissue and record observations, noting any adverse reactions or bleeding.

▶ Record patient's comments.

▶ Sutures are not to be left longer than 7–14 days.

▶ Use caution when removing a periodontal dressing to prevent tearing a suture that may have become embedded in the dressing.

▶ Provide proper postappointment instructions both verbally and in writing.

PERIODONTAL DRESSINGS

A dressing may be placed over the surgical wound following periodontal surgery. Dressings are not used to cure the wound but serve to protect the tissue. Some clinicians use dressings for all surgical procedures, some occasionally, and some others rarely.

I. Purposes and Uses

▶ Provide protection for a surgical wound against external irritation or trauma.

▶ Help prevent posttreatment bleeding by securing initial clot formation.

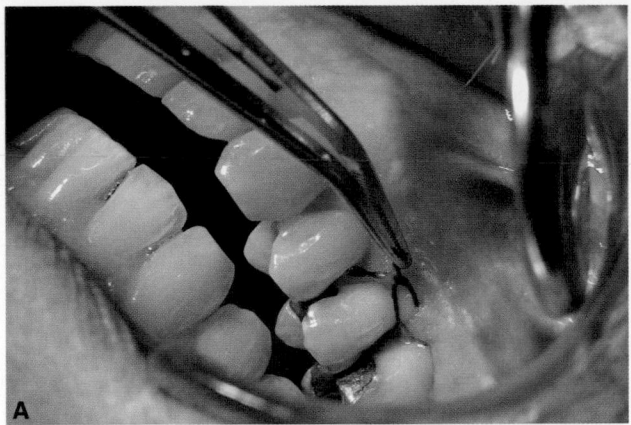
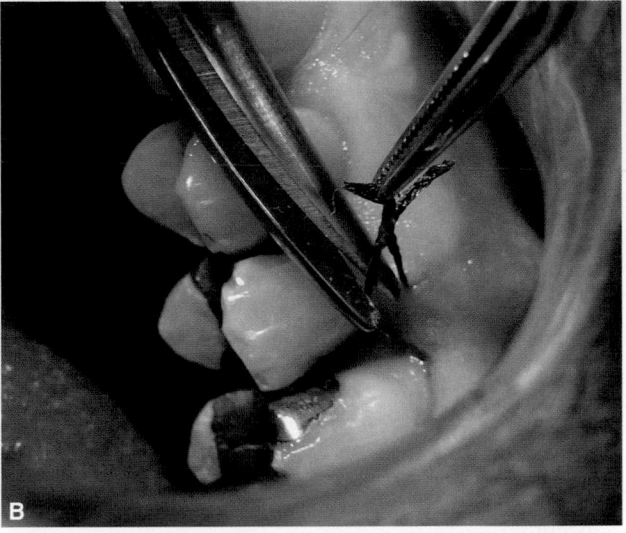
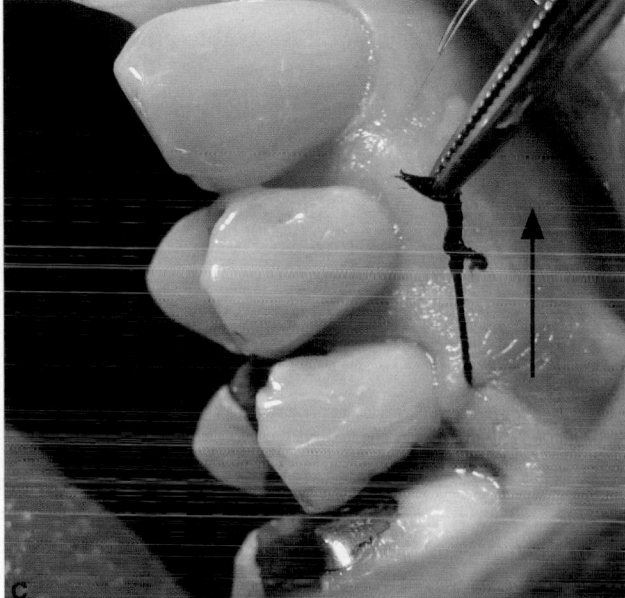
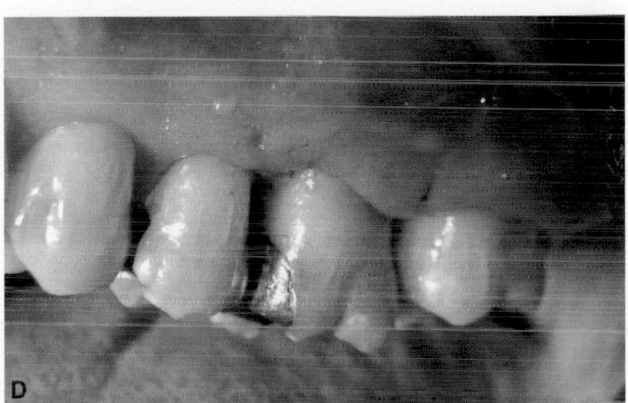

FIGURE 43-5 Suture Removal. A: Suture grasped by pliers near the entrance into tissue. **B:** Suture pulled gently up while scissor is inserted close to the tissue. Suture is cut in the part previously buried in the tissue. **C:** Suture is held up for vertical removal. **D:** Suture is pulled gently to bring it out on the side opposite from where it was cut. The object is to prevent the external part of the suture from passing through the tissue and introducing infectious material. (Courtesy of Dr. Robert Lewando, Boston, MA.)

▶ Support mobile teeth during healing.

▶ Assist in shaping or molding newly formed tissue, in securing a flap, or in immobilizing a graft.

II. Characteristics of Acceptable Dressing Material

An acceptable dressing material has the following characteristics:

▶ Preparation, placement, and removal will take place with minimal discomfort to the patient.

▶ Material adheres to itself, teeth, and adjacent tissues, and maintains retention within interdental areas.

▶ Provides stability and flexibility to withstand distortion and displacement without fracturing.

▶ Is nontoxic and nonirritating to oral tissues.

▶ Possesses a smooth surface that will resist accumulation of dental biofilm.

▶ Will not traumatize tissue or stain teeth and restorative materials.

▶ Possesses an aesthetically acceptable appearance.

TYPES OF DRESSINGS

Traditionally, dressings were classified into two groups: those that contained eugenol and those that did not. With the development of new products, "noneugenol-containing" dressings have been reclassified into *chemical-cure* and *visible light–cure (VIC) materials*. They are available as ready-mix, paste–paste, or paste–gel preparations.

I. Zinc Oxide with Eugenol Dressing

A. Basic Ingredients

▶ *Powder*: zinc oxide, powdered rosin, and tannic acid.

- *Liquid*: eugenol, with oil (such as peanut or cotton-seed) and thymol. Check patient's medical history for allergies.
  - Example: Kirkland Periodontal Pack.

B. Advantages

- *Consistency*: firm and heavy—provides support for tissues and flaps.
- *Slow setting*: extended working time.
- *Preparation and storage*: can be prepared in quantity and stored (frozen) in work-size pieces.

C. Disadvantages

- *Taste*: sharp, unpleasant taste.
- *Tissue reaction*: irritating; hypersensitivity reactions can occur.
- *Consistency*: the dressing is rough, hard, brittle, breaks easily, and encourages dental biofilm retention.

II. Chemical-Cured Dressing

The ingredients of commercial products are trade secrets, but general information about available dressings can be found. Two examples of chemical-cured dressings are PerioCare® and Coe-Pak™.

A. Basic Ingredients

- *PerioCare®*: Paste–gel mix
  - Paste: zinc oxide, magnesium oxide, calcium hydroxide, and vegetable oils.
  - Gel: resins, fatty acids, ethyl cellulose, lanolin, calcium hydroxide.
- *Coe-Pak™*: Paste–paste mix.
  - Base: rosin, cellulose, natural gums and waxes, fatty acid, chlorothymol, zinc acetate, and alcohol.
  - Accelerator: zinc oxide, vegetable oil, chlorothymol, magnesium oxide, silica, synthetic resin, and coumarin.
  - Coe-Pak™ is available in a hard and fast set.

B. Advantages

- *Consistency*: pliable, easy to place with light pressure.
- *Smooth surface*: comfortable to patient; resists biofilm and debris deposits.
- *Taste*: acceptable.
- *Removal*: easy, often comes off in one piece.

III. Visible Light–Cured Dressing

- VIC dressing (*Barricaid®*) is available in a syringe for direct application or from a mixing pad for indirect application.
- The same light-curing unit used for composite restorations and sealants is used.

A. Basic Ingredients

- *Gel ingredients*: polyester urethane dimethacrylate resin, silanated silica, VIC photoinitiator, accelerator, stabilizer, and colorant.

B. Advantages

- *Color*: more like gingiva than other dressings.
- *Setting*: begins when activated by the light-curing unit. (Exposure before placement is limited: daylight may begin the activation process.)
- *Removal*: easy, often comes off in one piece.

IV. Collagen Dressing

- Absorbable collagen dressings used to promote wound healing.
- Special use in periodontal surgery for a collagen patch dressing: for protection of graft sites of the palate during healing.
- One form prepared in a bullet shape to use for deep biopsy sites.
- Available in individual unit sterile packages.
- Collagen dressing may be placed on clean moist or bleeding wounds.

CLINICAL APPLICATION

I. Dressing Placement

- *General procedure*
  - For all types of dressing, follow the manufacturer's instructions. Each product has unique properties that require special handling.
- *Retention*
  - Mold the dressing by pressing at each interproximal site to cover interdental tissue (Figure 43-6A). Do not extend over the height of contour of each tooth.
  - Border mold to prevent displacement by the tongue, cheeks, lips, or frena (Figure 43-6 B and C).
  - Check the occlusion and remove areas of contact.

II. Characteristics of a Well-Placed Dressing (Figure 43-6)

- Dressings placed in keeping with biologic principles contribute to healing and are tolerated more comfortably by the patient.
- A satisfactory dressing (Figure 43.6D) has the following characteristics:
  - Is secure and rigid. A movable dressing is an irritant and can promote bleeding.
  - Has as little bulk as possible, yet is bulky enough to give strength.

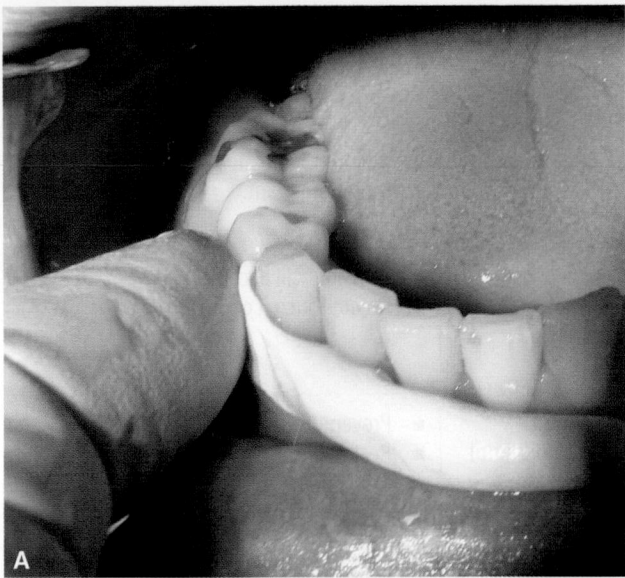
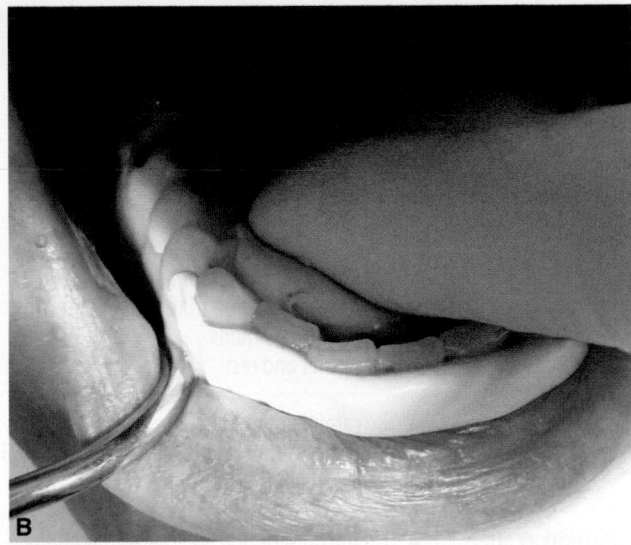
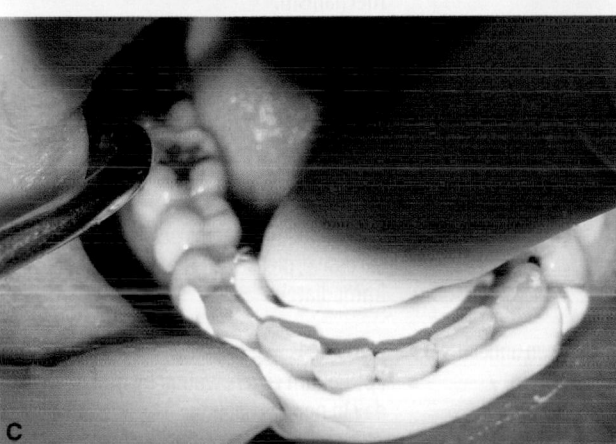
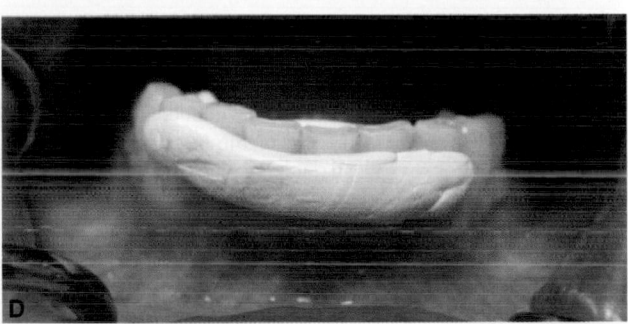

FIGURE 43-6 Periodontal Dressing. A: Gently pressing the facial periodontal dressing into the interproximal space. **B:** Gently pushing the lingual periodontal dressing into the interproximal space. **C:** Gently pressing the dressing from the buccal and lingual to help "lock" the dressing in place. **D:** Correct Placement of the Periodontal Dressing. A dressing must cover the surgical wound without unnecessary overextension and fill interdental areas to lock the dressing between the teeth. It is molded in the vestibule and around frena to allow movement of the lips, cheeks, and tongue with no displacement of the dressing. (Courtesy of Susan Jenkins, MCPHS University Forsyth School of Dental Hygiene.)

- Locks mechanically interdentally and cannot be displaced by action of tongue, cheek, or lips.
- Covers the entire surgical wound without unnecessary overextension.
- Fills interdental area and adequately covers the treated area to discourage retention of debris and dental biofilm.
- Possesses a smooth surface to prevent irritation to cheeks and lips while resisting debris and biofilm retention.

III. Patient Dismissal and Instructions

▶ Patient is not dismissed until bleeding or oozing from under a dressing has ceased.

▶ Written instructions are necessary to reinforce those that are provided verbally. Table 43-2 lists items to discuss with the patient before discharge.

DRESSING REMOVAL AND REPLACEMENT

During healing, epithelium begins to cover a wound in 5–6 days, and complete restoration of epithelium and connective tissue can be expected by 21 days. The dressing may be left in place from 7 to 10 days, as determined by the surgeon.

Keep the following factors relative to dressings in mind:

▶ If the dressing becomes dislodged before the removal appointment, the healing tissue needs to be evaluated.

▶ When the dressing remains intact for 4 or 5 days, replacement may not be necessary.

▶ When replacement is indicated, the dressing is replaced in its entirety rather than patched.

▶ Instruct the patient to proceed with daily frequent biofilm removal and rinsing using an antimicrobial agent.

▶ Schedule patient's follow-up appointment.

TABLE 43-2	Instructions for Posttreatment Care	
FACTOR	**INSTRUCTIONS TO PATIENT**	**PURPOSE OF INSTRUCTION**
Information for the patient about the dressing	■ Dressing will protect the surgical wound. ■ Do not disturb the dressing. ■ Allow it to remain until the next appointment.	■ An informed patient is more likely to be more compliant.
Care during the first few hours	■ Dressing will not set for a few hours. ■ Do not eat anything that requires chewing. ■ Use only cool liquids. ■ Stay quiet and rest.	■ Dressing will become hard. ■ Do not touch it or disturb it.
Anesthesia	■ Be careful not to bite lip or cheek. ■ Avoid foods that require chewing, hot liquids, and spicy foods until anesthesia has worn off.	■ Prevent trauma to lips and cheeks. ■ Rest and be quiet.
Discomfort after anesthesia wears off	■ Fill the prescription and follow directions. ■ Do not take more than directed. ■ Avoid aspirin. ■ Call the dental office if pain persists.	■ Pain control. ■ Aspirin can interfere with blood-clotting mechanism. ■ The patient will be more prepared to manage any postoperative discomfort when appropriately informed.
Ice pack or cold compress	■ Apply every 30 min for 15 min; or 15 min on, then 15 min off. ■ Use as directed only.	■ Prevent swelling from edema.
Bleeding	■ Slight bleeding within the first few hours is not unusual. ■ Do not suck on the area or use straws. ■ Blood clot is left alone.	■ When bleeding seems persistent or excessive, please call the dental office immediately.
Dressing care and retention	■ Avoid disturbing the dressing with the tongue or trying to clean under it. ■ Small particles may chip off, which is no problem unless sharp edges irritate the tongue or the dressing becomes loose. ■ Call the dentist if the entire dressing or a large portion falls off before the fifth day. ■ Rinse with a saline solution; rinse with chlorhexidine 0.12% morning and evening after brushing teeth.	■ Dressing is needed for wound protection. ■ Epithelium covers wound by fifth or sixth day in normal healing.
Use of tobacco and tobacco products	■ Do not smoke; avoid all tobacco products. ■ A heavy smoker must make every effort to decrease quantity of tobacco used.	■ Heat and smoke irritate the gingiva and delay healing.
Rinsing	■ Do not rinse on the day of the treatment. ■ Second day: Use saline solution made with 1/2 teaspoon (measured) in 1/2 cup of warm water every 2–3 hr. ■ Begin chlorhexidine 0.12% b.i.d. (twice a day)	■ Might disturb blood clot. ■ Saline cleanses and aids healing.
Toothbrushing and flossing	■ Continue to maintain optimal personal oral care in untreated areas. ■ Lightly brush occlusal surface over dressing material. ■ Use soft brush with water, and carefully clean film from dressing. ■ Clean the tongue.	■ Dental biofilm control essential to reduce the number of oral microorganisms. ■ Odor and taste control. ■ Oral sanitation.
Diet	■ Use highly nutritious foods for healing. ■ Follow the MyPlate guide (Chapter 35) ■ Use soft-textured diet. ■ Avoid highly seasoned, spicy, hot, sticky, crunchy, and coarse foods.	■ Healing tissue requires a healthy diet and specific comfort foods. ■ Use soft foods to protect the dressing from breakage or displacement.
Mastication	■ Avoid foods that require excessive chewing. ■ Chew only on the untreated side. ■ Use ground meat or cut meat into small, bite-sized pieces.	■ To protect the dressing while it protects the surgical site.

I. Patient Examination

▶ Question patient about and record posttreatment effects or discomfort. Record length of time the dressing remained in place.

▶ Examine the mucosa around the dressing and record its appearance.

II. Procedure for Removal

▶ Insert a smooth instrument under the border of the dressing and gently apply lateral pressure.

▶ Watch for sutures lodged in the dressing. They may need to be cut.

▶ Remove fragments of dressing gently with cotton pliers to avoid scratching the thin epithelial covering of the healing tissue.

▶ Observe tissue and record its appearance. Note any deviations from normal healing that is expected within the number of days.

▶ Use a scaler for removal of fragments adhering to tooth surfaces; use a curet for particles near the gingival margin. All calculus and roughness is eliminated to prevent new dental biofilm retention.

▶ Use an air–water syringe with a gentle stream of *warm* water. *W*arm diluted mouthrinse may soothe the traumatized area.

III. Dressing Replacement Procedure

1. Topical anesthetic to prevent patient discomfort.
2. Use a soft dressing with minimal pressure during application.

IV. Patient Oral Self-care Instruction

Biofilm control follow-up is essential after final dressing removal.

1. Use a soft brush on the treated area, paying careful attention to biofilm removal at the gingival margin.
2. Increase intensity of care on the treated area each day, with a return to uncompromised oral hygiene procedures by 3 or 4 days.
3. Rinse: 0.12% chlorhexidine gluconate twice daily during the healing period. Gently force liquid between the teeth when swishing.
4. Recommend a dentifrice with sodium fluoride for root caries prevention to be used regularly and indefinitely.
5. If the patient experiences postsurgical sensitivity, recommend a dentifrice containing a desensitizing agent. Suggestions for coping with sensitivity are found in Chapter 44.

V. Follow-up

The return for observation of the surgical areas can be scheduled in 1–2 weeks, depending on the patient's progress and treatment planning.

DOCUMENTATION

Detailed documentation is required at each patient visit. The appointment is dated and signed by the attending clinician.

▶ At the time of surgical treatment include in the patient's permanent record at least the following:
- Vital signs
- Anesthesia: type, location, number and size of carpules, and patient response to anesthesia
- Sutures: type, location, number placed
- Dressing: specific type and area placed
- Instructions to patient at dismissal
- Date and signature by attending dentist or periodontist and surgical assistant.

▶ Dressing and suture removal
- Tissue examination: tissue response
- Patient comments of posttreatment effects, discomfort
- Number of sutures removed: compare with number placed
- Patient instruction for continued care
- Date and signature by attending dental hygienist.

Sample documentation may be reviewed in Box 43-2.

BOX 43-2

Example Documentation: Sutures and Dressings

S –Patient presents for postsurgical dressing removal between teeth 11 and 15. Patient states no postsurgical problems.

O –Tissue bled slightly during dressing removal. Removed four sutures; confirmed four sutures placed (see documentation of previous appointment). Patient responded well.

A –Dr. examined area; no additional dressing needed; patient discharged with postremoval instructions.

P –Patient instructed to call if any problems; Patient to return for 3-month maintenance appointment.

Signed:_____, RDH

Date: _____

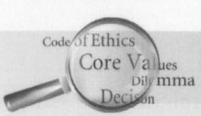

EVERYDAY ETHICS

Ms. Jean arrived for a suture removal appointment with Susan, the dental hygienist, and immediately explains the discomfort she is feeling. When asked why she didn't come in sooner to have the area observed, she said it was so close to the removal appointment she might as well wait. Susan notes from the record that no dressing was placed. The area appeared inflamed, with a slight cyanotic appearance circumscribing the suture area. The patient prerinsed with a 0.12% chlorhexidine, and Susan began removing the sutures. Moderate bleeding and discomfort were present.

Upon removal, Susan noted that only three sutures could be found, but four had been placed. When she conferred with Dr. Wynn, the periodontist, Susan was told to dismiss the patient and "prepare a prescription for an antibiotic to prevent an infection. Eventually the suture will be absorbed by body tissues."

Questions for Consideration

1. Given the sequence of events, what issues of ethical principles may be applied?

2. Does it seem clear that the patient understood the postoperative instructions? What suggestions do you have to improve communication?

3. Was the treatment provided within an acceptable standard of care for this patient? Which of the core values have application here? (See Section II Introduction, Table II-1).

4. Prepare examples of progress notes that you suggest Susan could write in the permanent record for Ms. Jean's appointment. Which example would you prefer and why?

Factors To Teach The Patient

▷ Explanations for the items in Table 43-2.

▷ Care of the mouth during the period after treatment while wearing a periodontal dressing.

▷ Reasons for not using aspirin for pain relief.

▷ Inform and explain why tobacco use is detrimental and delays healing. Encourage cessation of use of all forms of tobacco.

▷ Discuss the importance of regular maintenance after treatment is formally over.

References

1. Takei, H, Carranza, FA. Caranzza's clinical periodontology. 11th ed. St. Louis, MO: Saunders; 2012.

2. Giddings FD. *Book of Surgical Knots and Suturing Techniques*. 3rd ed. Fort Collins, CO: Giddings Studio Publishing; 2009.

3. King RC, Crawford JJ, Small EW. Bacteremia following intraoral suture removal. *Oral Surg Oral Med Oral Pathol*. 1988;65(1):23–27.

4. Giglio JA, Rowland RW, Dalton HP, et al. Suture removal-induced bacteremia: a possible endocarditis risk. *J Am Dent Assoc*. 1992;123(1):65–70.

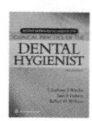

ENHANCE YOUR UNDERSTANDING

thePoint® [THEPOINT LOGO] **DIGITAL CONNECTIONS**
(see the inside front cover for access information)
• Audio glossary
• Quiz bank

[WORKBOOK COVER IMAGE] **SUPPORT FOR LEARNING**
(available separately; visit lww.com)
• *Active Learning Workbook for Clinical Practice of the Dental Hygienist, 12th Edition*

prepU [PREPU LOGO] **INDIVIDUALIZED REVIEW**
(available separately; visit lww.com)
• *Adaptive quizzing with prepU for Wilkins' Clinical Practice of the Dental Hygienist*

44

Dentin Hypersensitivity

Terri S.I. Tilliss, RDH, PhD and Janis G. Keating, RDH, MA

CHAPTER OUTLINE

HYPERSENSITIVITY DEFINED
I. Stimuli that Elicit Pain Reaction
II. Characteristics of Pain from Hypersensitivity

ETIOLOGY OF DENTIN HYPERSENSITIVITY
I. Anatomy of Tooth Structures
II. Mechanisms of Dentin Exposure
III. Hydrodynamic Theory

NATURAL DESENSITIZATION
I. Sclerosis of Dentin
II. Secondary Dentin
III. Smear Layer
IV. Calculus

THE PAIN OF DENTIN HYPERSENSITIVITY
I. Patient Profile
II. Pain Experience

DIFFERENTIAL DIAGNOSIS
I. Differentiation of Pain
II. Data Collection by Interview
III. Diagnostic Techniques and Tests

HYPERSENSITIVITY MANAGEMENT
I. Assessment Components
II. Educational Considerations
III. Treatment Hierarchy
IV. Reassessment

ORAL HYGIENE CARE AND TREATMENT INTERVENTIONS
I. Mechanisms of Desensitization
II. Behavioral Changes
III. Desensitizing Agents
IV. Self-Applied Measures
V. Professionally Applied Measures
VI. Additional Considerations

DOCUMENTATION

EVERYDAY ETHICS

FACTORS TO TEACH THE PATIENT

REFERENCES

LEARNING OBJECTIVES

After studying this chapter, the student will be able to:

1. Describe stimuli and pain characteristics specific to hypersensitivity, and explain how this relates to differential diagnosis.

2. Describe factors that contribute to dentin exposure and behavioral changes that could decrease hypersensitivity.

3. Explain the steps in the hydrodynamic theory.

4. Describe two mechanisms of desensitization and their associated treatment interventions for managing dentin hypersensitivity.

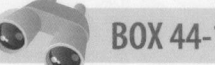

BOX 44-1 KEY WORDS AND ABBREVIATIONS: Dentin Hypersensitivity

Abfraction: wedge- or V-shaped cervical lesion created by the stresses of lateral or eccentric tooth movements during occlusal function, bruxing, or parafunctional activity resulting in enamel microfractures.

ADA: American Dental Association.

Burnishing: repeated rubbing of a tooth surface with a toothpick or wooden stick.

Dentin hypersensitivity: transient pain arising from exposed dentin, typically in response to a stimulus, which cannot be explained as arising from any other form of dental defect or pathology and subsides quickly when stimulus is removed.

FDA: Food and Drug Administration.

Hydrodynamic theory: currently accepted mechanism for pain impulse transmission to the pulp as a result of fluid movement within the dentinal tubule, which stimulates the nerve endings at the dentinopulpal interface.

Intertubular dentin: dentin located between dentinal tubules.

Intratubular or peritubular dentin: increased deposition of minerals into tubules that become more mineralized with increasing age, resulting in thicker, sclerotic dentin.

Neural depolarization mechanism (sodium/potassium pump): reduction of the resting potential of the nerve membrane so that a nerve impulse is fired. At rest, the inner surface of the nerve fiber is negatively charged and impermeable to sodium ions. A stimulus temporarily alters the membrane, making it permeable so that potassium

leaks out and sodium rushes into the nerve fiber. This mechanism is known as the sodium–potassium pump. The reversal of electrical charge, or **depolarization**, creates the nerve impulse. The process then reverses, and the membrane potential is restored, or **repolarized**.

Osmosis: the passage of fluids and solutions of lesser concentration through a selective membrane to one of greater solute concentration.

OTC: over the counter.

Patent: open, unobstructed; a patent dentinal tubule allows fluid flow to signal pain; many desensitizing agents work by decreasing the patency of the tubule.

Randomized Clinical Trials (RCT): a specific type of scientific experiment that is the gold standard for a clinical trial. RCTs are often used to test the efficacy and/or effectiveness of various types of interventions within a patient population.

Secondary dentin: dentin that is secreted slowly over time after root formation to "wall off" the pulp from fluid flow within dentinal tubules following a stimulus; results in narrower pulp chamber and root canals.

Smear layer: has been referred to as "grinding debris" from instrumentation or other devices applied to the tooth; consists of microcrystalline particles of cementum, dentin, tissue, and cellular debris; serves to plug tubule orifices.

Tertiary/reparative dentin: a type of dentin formed along the pulpal wall or root canal as a protective mechanism in response to trauma or irritation, such as caries or a traumatic cavity preparation.

The dental hygienist is often the first oral health professional to become aware of the presence of hypersensitive teeth when a patient presents for care. Individuals who suffer from hypersensitivity may be uncomfortable during dental hygiene treatment, since exposure to stimuli such as a cold water spray or contact with metal instruments can elicit the pain of hypersensitive teeth.

▶ Patients often report that activities of daily living such as eating or drinking cold foods or beverages cause pain and request information about causes and treatment for their discomfort.

▶ Hypersensitivity is often difficult to diagnose because the presenting symptoms can be confused with other types of dental pain with a different etiology.

▶ Management of hypersensitivity can be a challenge because there are numerous treatment approaches with varying degrees of efficacy.

▶ Knowledge of the predisposing factors that lead to gingival recession and loss of enamel or cementum and dentin can assist patients in preventing conditions that cause or exacerbate dentin hypersensitivity.

▶ Box 44-1 provides definitions for terms related to hypersensitivity.

HYPERSENSITIVITY DEFINED

A definitive characteristic associated with dentin hypersensitivity is pain elicited by a stimulus and alleviated upon its removal. Numerous types of stimuli can lead to pain response in individuals with exposed dentin surfaces.

I. Stimuli That Elicit Pain Reaction

▶ *Tactile:* contact with toothbrush and other oral hygiene devices, eating utensils, dental instruments, and friction from prosthetic devices such as denture clasps.

▶ *Thermal:* temperature change caused by hot and cold foods and beverages, and cold air as it contacts the teeth. Cold is the most common stimulus for pain.

▶ *Evaporative:* dehydration of oral fluids as from high-volume evacuation or application of air to dry teeth during intraoral procedures.

▶ *Osmotic:* alteration of pressure in dentinal tubules through a selective membrane.

▶ *Chemical:* acids in foods and beverages such as citrus fruits, condiments, spices, wine, and carbonated beverages;

acids produced by acidogenic bacteria following carbohydrate exposure; acids from gastric regurgitation.

II. Characteristics of Pain from Hypersensitivity

▶ Sharp, short, or transient pain with rapid onset.

▶ Cessation of pain upon removal of stimulus.

▶ Presents as a chronic condition with acute episodes.

▶ Pain in response to a non-noxious stimulus, one that would not normally cause pain or discomfort.

▶ Discomfort that cannot be ascribed to any other dental defect or pathology.[1]

ETIOLOGY OF DENTIN HYPERSENSITIVITY

A review of tooth anatomy facilitates an understanding of the mechanism of hypersensitivity.

I. Anatomy of Tooth Structures

A. Dentin

▶ The portion of the tooth covered by enamel on the crown and cementum on the root.

▶ Composed of fluid-filled dentinal tubules that narrow and branch as they extend from the pulp to the dentinoenamel junction (Figure 44-1).

▶ Only the portions of the dentinal tubules closest to the pulp are innervated with nerve fiber endings from the pulp chamber.

▶ Tubules are wider and more numerous in sensitive areas.[2]

B. Pulp

▶ Highly innervated with nerve cell fiber endings that extend just beyond the dentinopulpal interface of the dentinal tubules.[3]

▶ Body portions of odontoblasts (dentin-producing cells) located adjacent to the pulp extend their processes from the dentinopulpal junction a short way into each dentinal tubule (Figure 44-1).

C. Nerves

▶ Nerve fiber endings extend just beyond the dentinopulpal junction[4] and wind around the odontoblastic processes as shown in Figure 44-1.

▶ Nerves react via the same neural depolarization mechanism (sodium potassium pump, defined in Box 44-1), which characterizes the response of any nerve to a stimulus.

II. Mechanisms of Dentin Exposure

▶ The sequential events of gingival recession, loss of cementum or enamel, and subsequent dentin exposure, as seen in Figure 44-2, can result in hypersensitivity.

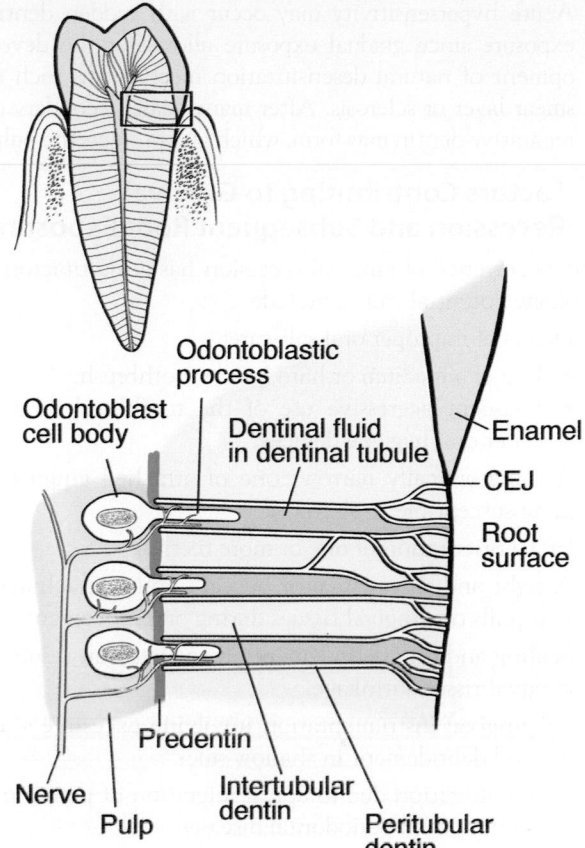

FIGURE 44-1 Relationship of Dentin Tubules and Pulpal Nerve Endings. Nerve endings from the pulp wrap themselves around the odontoblasts that extend only a short distance into the tubule. Fluid-filled dentin tubules transmit fluid disturbances through the mechanism known as hydraulic conductance.

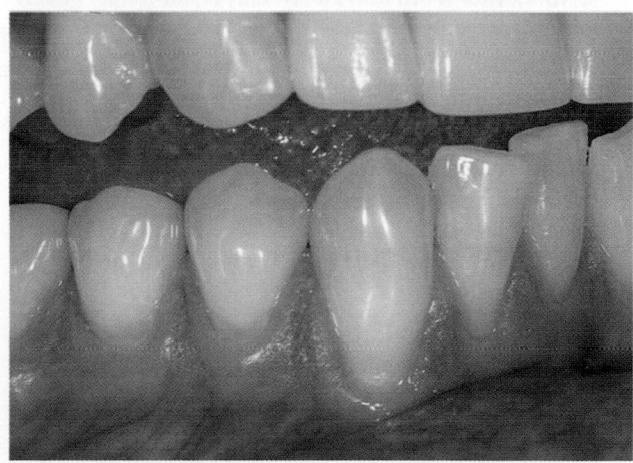

FIGURE 44-2 Gingival Recession. Note recession from the mandibular right central incisor to the 2nd premolar. If the thin cemental layer of the exposed root surface is lost, dentin hypersensitivity can develop.

▶ Loss of enamel or cementum can expose dentin gradually or suddenly as in tooth fracture.

▶ As a result of the lower mineral content of cementum and dentin compared with enamel, demineralization occurs more rapidly and at a lower critical pH.

▶ Acute hypersensitivity may occur with sudden dentin exposure since gradual exposure allows for the development of natural desensitization mechanisms such as smear layer or sclerosis. After many years, secondary or reparative dentin may form, which also protects the pulp.

A. Factors Contributing to Gingival Recession and Subsequent Root Exposure

The occurrence of gingival recession has a multifactorial etiology. Potential causes include:

▶ Effects of improper oral self-care:
  • Use of a medium or hard bristle toothbrush.
  • Frequent aggressive use of the toothbrush and/or other oral hygiene devices.
▶ An anatomically narrow zone of attached gingiva is more susceptible to abrasion.
▶ Facial orientation of one or more teeth.
▶ A tight and short labial or buccal frenum attachment that pulls on gingival tissues during oral movement.
▶ Scaling and root debridement procedures that result in gingival tissue shrinkage.
▶ Subgingival instrumentation involving excessive scaling and debridement in shallow sulci.[5]
▶ Tissue alteration due to apical migration of junctional epithelium from periodontal diseases.
▶ Periodontal surgical procedures can alter the architecture of gingival tissues resulting in recession.
▶ Periodontal surgery procedures such as crown lengthening, repositioning of gingival tissues, or tooth extractions can affect gingival coverage of adjacent teeth.
▶ Orthodontic tooth movement may result in loss of periodontal attachment.
▶ Restorative procedures, such as crown preparation, that abrade marginal gingival tissues.
▶ Metal jewelry used in an oral piercing of the lip or tongue that repeatedly traumatizes the adjacent facial or lingual gingival tissue.

B. Factors Contributing to Loss of Enamel and Cementum

▶ Loss of tooth structure rarely develops from a single cause but rather from a combination of contributing factors.
▶ Cementum at the cervical area is thin and easily abrades when exposed.
▶ Enamel and cementum do not meet at the cementoenamel junction (CEJ) in about 10% of teeth, leaving an area of exposed dentin, as shown in Figure 18-10 (Chapter 18).

C. Attrition, Abrasion, and Erosion

▶ Effects of attrition and abrasion are exacerbated when acid erodes the tooth surface or when the tooth is brushed immediately after consumption of acidic foods and beverages.
▶ Hypersensitivity may be a clinical outcome of erosion.[6]

▶ Erosion can occur from dietary acids, such as citrus fruits/juices, wine, and carbonated drinks.[7]
▶ Dietary acid intake results in an immediate drop in oral pH; after normal salivary neutralization, a physiologic pH of 7 re-establishes within minutes.
▶ Frequent acid consumption is a critical factor; holding or "swilling" of acidic agents, holding low pH foods such as citrus fruits against teeth, or continual snacking increases erosion risk.
▶ Gastric acids from conditions such as gastric reflux, morning sickness, or self-induced vomiting (bulimia) repeatedly expose teeth to a highly acidic environment.

D. Abfraction

▶ Abfraction, a wedge-shaped cervical lesion, has a questionable etiology.[8–11]
▶ A cervical lesion caused by lateral/occlusal stresses or tooth flexure from bruxing.
▶ Microscopic portions of the enamel rods chip away from the cervical area of the tooth resulting in loss of tooth structure (Figure 44-3).
▶ Lesion appears as a wedge- or V-shaped cervical notch.
▶ Is a co-factor with abrasion for loss of tooth structure and potential sensitivity.

E. Other Factors

▶ Crown preparation procedures that remove enamel or cementum can expose dentin at the cervical area.
▶ Instrumentation during scaling or root debridement procedures on thinning cementum.
▶ Frequent or improper stain-removal techniques, in which abrasive particles wear away the cementum and dentin.
▶ Root surface carious lesions.
▶ Removal of proximal enamel using a sandpaper disk or strip to create additional space for orthodontic movement of crowded teeth, also known as "enamel stripping."

III. Hydrodynamic Theory

Hydrodynamic theory is a currently accepted explanation for transmission of stimuli from the outer surface of the dentin to the pulp.

▶ Described by Brannstrom in the 1960s,[12] who theorized that a stimulus at the outer aspect of dentin will cause fluid movement within the dentinal tubules.
▶ Fluid movement creates pressure on the nerve endings within the dentinal tubule, which transmits the pain impulse by stimulating the nerves in the pulp.
▶ Credibility for this theory is supported by the greater number of widened dentin tubules seen in hypersensitive teeth compared with nonsensitive teeth.[2] Figure 44-4 depicts open dentinal tubules at the microscopic level. Figure 44-5 depicts partially occluded dentinal tubules.

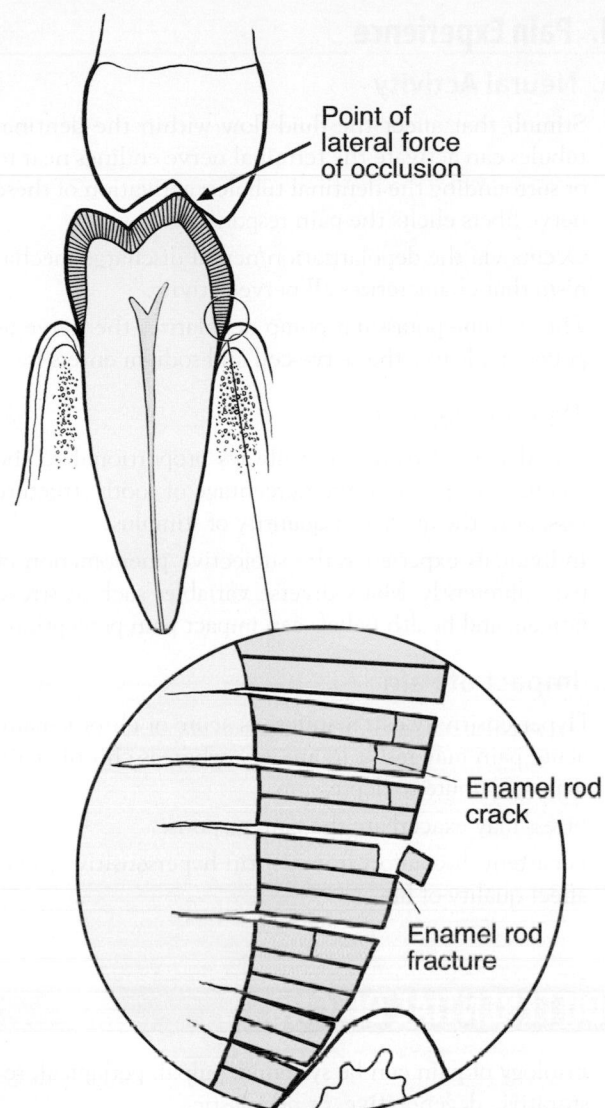

FIGURE 44-3 **Process of Abfraction.** Lateral occlusal forces stress the enamel rods at the cervical area, resulting in enamel rod fracture over time. In an advanced stage, a wedge- or V-shaped cervical lesion is visible. Although minute cracks in the enamel rods may not be clinically evident, the tooth can exhibit hypersensitivity.

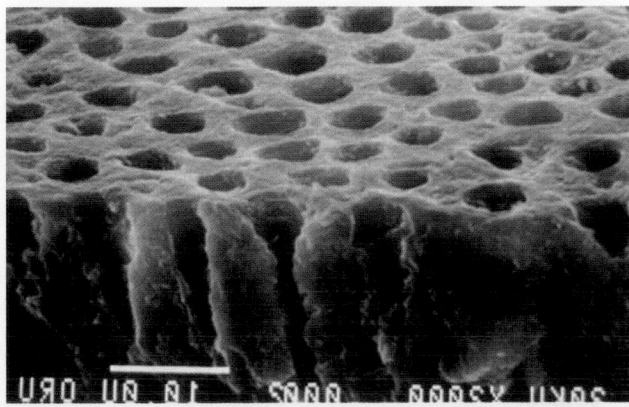

FIGURE 44-4 **Open Dentin Tubules.** Note cross-section and transverse views of tubules. Courtesy of Dr. Sheldon Newman.

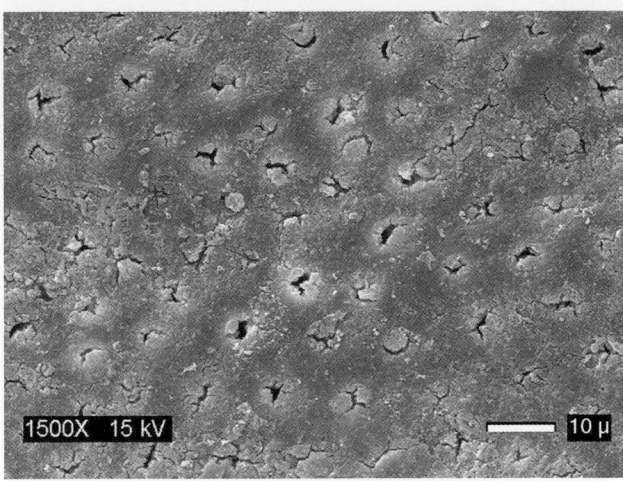

Figure 44-5 **Partially Occluded Dentin Tubules.** These dentin tubules are nearly filled. Courtesy of Anthony Giuseppetti.

NATURAL DESENSITIZATION

▶ Hypersensitivity can decrease naturally over time, even without treatment interventions.

▶ There are several mechanisms by which desensitization can occur naturally over time, including the following:

I. Sclerosis of Dentin

▶ Occurs by mineral deposition within tubules as a result of traumatic stimuli, such as attrition or dental caries.

▶ Creates a thicker, highly mineralized layer of peritubular dentin (deposited within the periphery of the tubules).

▶ Results in a smaller-diameter tubule that is less able to transmit stimuli through the dentinal fluid to the nerve fibers at the dentinopulpal interface.

II. Secondary Dentin

▶ Deposited gradually on the floor and roof of the pulp chamber after teeth are fully developed.

▶ Secreted more slowly than primary dentin formed before tooth eruption; both types of dentin are created by odontoblasts.

▶ Creates a "walling off" effect between the dentinal tubules and the pulp to insulate the pulp from dentin fluid disturbances caused by a stimulus such as dental caries.

▶ With aging, secondary dentin accumulates, resulting in a smaller pulp chamber with fewer nerve endings and less sensitivity.

III. Smear Layer

▶ Consists of organic and inorganic debris that covers the dentinal surface and the tubules.[13]

▶ Accumulates following scaling and root instrumentation, use of toothpaste (abrasive particles), cutting with a bur, attrition, or abrasion (burnishing with a toothbrush or toothpick, or other device).

▶ Occludes the dentinal tubule orifices, forming a "smear plug" or a natural "bandage" that blocks stimuli.

▶ The nature of the smear layer changes constantly since it is subject to effects such as mechanical disruption from ultrasonic debridement, or dissolution from acid exposure.

IV. Calculus

▶ Provides a protective coating to shield exposed dentin from stimuli.

▶ Postdebridement sensitivity can occur after removal of heavy calculus deposits; dentinal tubules may become exposed as calculus is removed.

THE PAIN OF DENTIN HYPERSENSITIVITY

Individuals react differently to pain based on factors such as age, gender, situation and context, previous experiences, pain expectations, and other psychological and physiological parameters.

I. Patient Profile

The prevalence of reported hypersensitivity varies due to differences in the stimulus, and whether data are gathered by patient report or standardized clinical examination. Patient accounts may not represent true hypersensitivity since the pain can be confused with other conditions.

A. Prevalence of Hypersensitivity

▶ A large multipractice cross-sectional survey found a prevalence of dentin hypersensitivity of 12.3%, with an average of 3.5 hypersensitive teeth; the highest prevalence occurred in those 18–44 years of age.[14]

▶ Higher prevalence has been reported in periodontally involved populations.[15]

▶ Incidence and severity declines with advancing age, due to the effects of sclerosis and secondary dentin.[16]

▶ Gingival recession is more prevalent with aging.[17] Dentin hypersensitivity is not more prevalent with aging.

▶ Hypersensitivity, when measured objectively, occurs more often in women.[14]

B. Teeth Affected

▶ Hypersensitivity has been reported to occur primarily at the cervical one-third of the facial surfaces of premolars and mandibular anterior teeth,[18] or on premolars and molars.[14]

▶ Can occur on any tooth exhibiting predisposing factors.

II. Pain Experience

A. Neural Activity

▶ Stimuli that affect the fluid flow within the dentinal tubules can activate the terminal nerve endings near to or surrounding the dentinal tubules; activation of these nerve fibers elicits the pain response.

▶ Occurs via the depolarization/neural discharge mechanism that characterizes all nerve activity.

▶ The sodium–potassium pump depolarizes the nerve as potassium leaves the nerve cell and sodium enters it.

B. Pain Perception

▶ The degree of pain is not always proportional to the amount of recession, the percentage of tooth structure loss, or to the quality or quantity of stimulus.

▶ Individuals experience the subjective phenomenon of pain differently. Many diverse variables such as stress, fatigue, and health beliefs can impact pain perception.

C. Impact of Pain

▶ Hypersensitivity can manifest as acute or chronic pain; acute pain may result in anxiety, whereas chronic pain may contribute to depression.

▶ Stress may exacerbate the pain response.

▶ Persistent discomfort from dentin hypersensitivity may affect quality of life.

DIFFERENTIAL DIAGNOSIS

▶ Etiology of pain can be systemic, pulpal, periapical, restorative, degenerative, or neoplastic.

▶ A differential diagnosis can rule out other causes of pain before treating for hypersensitivity.

▶ Skilled interviewing and diagnostics contribute to the differential diagnosis.

▶ Components to consider in the differential diagnosis of tooth pain are detailed in Table 44-1.

I. Differentiation of Pain

▶ Hypersensitivity pain elicited by a non-noxious stimulus, such as cold water, can mimic pain elicited by a noxious agent, such as cavitated dental caries.

▶ The pain of hypersensitivity subsides when the stimulus is removed.

▶ It is difficult to distinguish between the pain of hypersensitivity and other causes of dental pain when both are in the mild-to-moderate range. Many types of dental pain can be intensified by thermal, sweet, and sour stimuli.

▶ Chewing pain (occlusal pressure) can be indicative of pulpal pathology.

TABLE 44-1	Differential Diagnosis of Tooth Pain	
CONDITION	SIGNS AND SYMPTOMS	CLINICAL ASSESSMENT
Dentinal hypersensitivity	Thermal, mechanical, evaporative, osmotic, chemical sensitivity Sharp, sudden, transient pain	Clinical examination: gingival recession and loss of tooth structure
Caries extending into dentin	Thermal sensitivity Pain on pressure Pain with sweets	Clinical examination Radiographic examination
Pulpal caries	Thermal sensitivity Severe, intermittent or throbbing pain Pain on chewing	Clinical examination Radiographic examination
Fractured restoration	Thermal sensitivity Pain on pressure	Clinical examination
Fractured tooth	Thermal sensitivity Pain on pressure	Occlusal examination Transillumination
Recently placed restoration	Thermal sensitivity Pain on pressure	Dental history Clinical examination Occlusal examination
Occlusal trauma	Chemical sensitivity Thermal sensitivity Pain on pressure Mobility	Occlusal examination
Pulpitis	Severe, intermittent throbbing pain	Thermal and electric pulp tests Percussion
Sinus infection	"Nondescript" tooth pain Nasal congestion (drainage) Sinus pressure Headache	Clinical examination, including extraoral sinus palpation Radiographic examination
Galvanic pain	Sudden, sharp stabbing pain on tooth to tooth contact	Examination for contact between restoration of dissimilar nonprecious metals
Periodontal ligament inflammation	Pain on chewing Clinical examination, including palpation for apical tenderness	Percussion
Abfraction	"Cratered" areas of enamel or dentin at CEJ in the shape of a wedge- or V-shaped notch	Clinical examination Occlusal examination

▶ Pulpal pain is severe, intermittent, and throbbing. The pain results from deep dental caries, pulpal inflammation, vertical tooth fracture, or infection, and may occur without provocation and persist after stimulus is removed.

II. Data Collection by Interview

▶ Utilize direct, open-ended and non-leading questions.
- Establish the location, degree of pain, onset/duration, source of stimulus, intensity, and alleviating factors

related to the painful response; patients may have difficulty characterizing the pain.
- Ask trigger questions as suggested in Box 44-2 to elicit detailed information to characterize the pain and assist in the dental hygiene diagnosis.

▶ Establish rapport, combined with effective listening and counseling skills to develop collaborative treatment/management strategies.

▶ Record a thorough dental history, including pain chronology, nature, location, aggravating and alleviating factors, and history of dental treatment/restorations.

BOX 44-2

BOX 44-2

Trigger Questions for Data Collection

▷ Which tooth or teeth surfaces is/are sensitive?
▷ On a scale from 1 to 10, with 10 being the most painful, what is your pain intensity?
▷ How long does the pain last?
▷ Which words best describe the pain: sharp, dull, shooting, throbbing, persistent, constant, pressure, burning, intermittent?
▷ Does it hurt when you bite down (pressure)?
▷ On a scale from 1 to 10, with 10 being a major impact, how much does the pain impact your daily life?
▷ Is the pain stimulated by certain foods? Sweet? Sour? Acidic?
▷ Does sensitivity occur with hot or cold food or beverages?
▷ Does discomfort stop immediately upon removal of the painful stimulus, such as cold food or beverage, or does it linger?
▷ Have you whitened your teeth lately?

III. Diagnostic Techniques and Tests

When patients have difficulty describing and localizing their pain, the following diagnostic techniques and tests can aid in differentiating among the numerous causes of tooth pain.

▶ Visual assessment of tooth integrity and surrounding tissues.
▶ Palpation of extra- and intraoral soft tissues.
▶ Evaluation of nasal congestion, drainage, or sinus expressed as tooth pain.
▶ Occlusal examination with use of marking paper to detect a premature contact or hyperfunction following placement of a new restoration.

▶ Radiographic assessment to determine signs of pulpal pathology, vertical tooth fracture, or other irregularities of the teeth or surrounding structures.
▶ Percussion with use of an instrument handle to lightly tap on each tooth. A pain response may indicate pulpitis.
▶ Mobility testing may detect trauma or periodontal pathology.
▶ Pain from biting pressure with use of a bite stick to assess pain indicative of tooth fracture.
▶ Transillumination with a high-intensity focused light to enhance visualization of a cracked tooth; dye may also indicate a fracture line.
▶ Pulpal pathology assessment with thermal or electric pulp tests.

HYPERSENSITIVITY MANAGEMENT

When the differential diagnosis indicates dentinal hypersensitivity, the dental hygiene care plan includes further assessment and patient counseling combined with treatment interventions.

I. Assessment Components

▶ Determine extent and severity of pain.
  • Solicit a self-report of symptoms, including the eliciting stimuli.
  • Quantify and record the baseline pain intensity using objective measures such as the visual analog scale (VAS) and/or the verbal rating scale (VRS), as described in Box 44-3.
▶ Determine if oral self-care procedures contribute to loss of gingiva or tooth structure.
▶ Use a diet analysis to assess the frequency of acidic food and beverage intake; correlate intake with timing of toothbrushing.

BOX 44-3

Subjective Pain Assessment Form

Name: _____
Date: _____
Teeth: _____

VAS—Visual Analog Scale

Please place an "X" on the line at a position between the two extremes to represent the level of pain that you experience.

No Discomfort |————————————| Severe Discomfort

VRS—Verbal Rating Scale

Please describe the pain you experience on a scale from 0 to 3:

0 = No discomfort/pain, but aware of stimulus
1 = Slight discomfort/pain
2 = Significant discomfort/pain
3 = Significant discomfort/pain that lasted more than 10 seconds

► Explore parafunctional habits, such as bruxing, that may contribute to abfraction.

II. Educational Considerations

► Provide education regarding etiology and contributing factors. Explain the natural mechanisms for resolution of hypersensitivity over time.

► Discuss realistic oral self-care measures that the patient is likely to maintain and include technique demonstrations.

► Utilize effective communication and motivational interviewing skills to promote compliance and to decrease patient anxiety (see Chapter 26).

III. Treatment Hierarchy

► There are two basic treatment goals:
  • Pain relief.
  • Modification or elimination of contributing factors.

► Address mild-to-moderate pain with conservative approaches or agents; more severe pain may require an aggressive approach.

► Sequence treatment approaches from the most conservative and least invasive measures to more aggressive modalities.

► Prognosis of pain resolution is difficult to predict due to variable success with different treatment options among individuals.

  • Historically, a vast array of treatment approaches have been utilized with varying degrees of success; no one best method has been identified due to lack of quality randomized clinical trial (RCT) data, difficulties inherent in dentin hypersensitivity research design, and a significant placebo effect.
  • A trial-and-error approach may be necessary to determine the most effective treatment option.
  • Characteristics of an ideal desensitizing agent are listed in Box 44-4 and can be useful evaluation criteria when selecting a desensitizing agent.

► Treatment options that include both oral self-care measures and professional interventions with the same objective of reducing hypersensitivity have a synergistic effect.

IV. Reassessment

► Evaluate treatment interventions.
  • Allow sufficient time to elapse (2–4 weeks) to evaluate effectiveness of treatment recommendations; assess and reinforce behavioral changes.
  • Repeat the VAS and/or the VRS to compare changes in pain perceptions from baseline.

► If pain persists, a different option may provide relief.

ORAL HYGIENE CARE AND TREATMENT INTERVENTIONS

I. Mechanisms of Desensitization

Desensitization agents and oral self-care measures disrupt the pain transmission as described by the hydrodynamic theory in one of two ways:[19]

► Prevent nerve depolarization that interrupts the neural transmission to the pulp. This physiologic process is the mechanism of action for potassium-based products.[20]

► Prevent a stimulus from moving the tubule fluid by occlusion of dentin tubule orifices or reduction in tubule lumen diameter.

II. Behavioral Changes

Encourage habits that allow tubules to remain occluded or that occlude patent tubules.

► Use a motivational interviewing approach (Chapter 26) to help the patient commit to appropriate oral hygiene self-care and dietary habits before or in conjunction with self-applied or professionally applied desensitizing agents.

► Educate the patient that some products may take 2–4 weeks to decrease sensitivity.

A. Dietary Modifications

► Have patient analyze acidic food and beverage habits that incite pain from dissolution of the smear layer which covered open dentinal tubules.[21] Examples include citrus fruits and juices, acidic soda/cola beverages, sharp flavors and spices, pickled foods, wines, and ciders.

► Counsel patient regarding change in dietary habits.

► Help patient determine if brushing is sequenced immediately after consuming acidic foods and beverages. Advise altering sequence to eliminate combined effects of erosion and abrasion, which can accelerate tooth structure loss.[22]

► Guide patient toward mouthrinses with a non-acidic formulation.

BOX 44-4

The Ideal Desensitizing Agent

▷ Minimal application time
▷ Easy application procedure
▷ Does not endanger the soft tissues
▷ Inexpensive
▷ Requires few dental appointments
▷ Does not cause pulpal irritation or pain
▷ Rapid and lasting effect
▷ Causes no staining
▷ Consistently effective
▷ Acceptable taste

▶ Provide professional treatment referrals for patients with eating disorders such as bulimia or systemic conditions such as acid reflux that repeatedly create an acidic oral environment.

▶ The acidic environment created by bulimia and acid reflux can be neutralized by rinsing with water (particularly fluoridated water) or an alkaline rinse such as bicarbonate of soda in water.

▶ Counsel patient to eliminate extremes of hot and cold foods and beverages to avoid discomfort.

B. Dental Biofilm Control

▶ In the presence of dental biofilm, the dentinal tubule orifices increase to three times the original size; with re-establishment of biofilm control measures, there is a 20% decrease in size.[23]

▶ The presence/amount of dental biofilm on exposed root surfaces does not directly correlate with the degree of dentin sensitivity,[17] suggesting biofilm composition maybe a factor.

C. Toothbrush Type and Technique

▶ Brush one or two teeth at a time with a soft or ultra-soft toothbrush, rather than using long horizontal strokes over several teeth to prevent further recession and loss of tooth structure.

▶ Identify brushing sequence and adjust by beginning in least sensitive areas and ending with more sensitive areas. In the initial phases of brushing, toothbrush filaments are stiffer and brushing is more aggressive.

▶ Explore option of brushing with the nondominant hand, if dexterity permits; nondominant hand exerts less pressure than the dominant hand.

▶ Help patient investigate current toothbrush grip. Adjust to a modified pen grasp rather than a traditional palm grasp to reduce the amount of pressure applied.

▶ Explore receptivity to use of a power toothbrush because it removes dental biofilm effectively with less than half the pressure of a manual toothbrush; an individual using a manual toothbrush typically exerts 200–400 g of pressure; 70–150 g of pressure is usually exerted with a power toothbrush.[24] Some power toothbrushes have a self-limiting mechanism to reduce filament action if too much pressure is applied.

▶ Recommend and demonstrate dental biofilm control measures that are meticulous, yet gentle, and do not contribute to abrasion of hard or soft tissues.

D. Burnishing

A wooden toothpick is repeatedly rubbed over the root surface with moderate pressure. Figure 44-6 shows placement of a toothpick.

▶ The toothpick may be dipped into fluoride dentifrice or other desensitization agents, although it is the burnishing process that forms a smear layer over dentin, occluding the dentinal tubule orifices.[25]

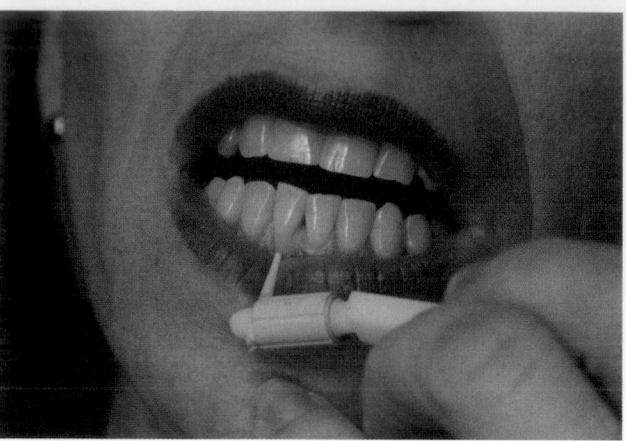

FIGURE 44-6 Burnishing Sensitive Root Surface. A small amount of a fluoride dentifrice or other fluoride agent can be burnished into the sensitive area with a toothpick or wooden point. Moderate pressure with a "rubbing" or circular stroke is applied. A toothpick holder facilitates effective use of a toothpick to burnish an exposed root surface.

▶ May stimulate the production of secondary or reparative dentin; a very slow process.

E. Eliminate Parafunctional Habits

▶ Help patient assess bruxing and clenching behaviors and whether additional treatment is indicated.

▶ Determine need for occlusal adjustments to eliminate abfractive forces.

▶ Coach patient to monitor occurrence of subconscious parafunctional behaviors and levels of stress. Identify whether stress reduction protocols are needed.

III. Desensitizing Agents

▶ There are study design challenges when researching desensitization due to subjectivity of the pain response, the strong placebo effect, and the process of natural desensitization.

▶ Despite widespread professional recommendation and use, there is little in vivo scientific evidence validating the efficacy and mechanisms of action of desensitizing agents.

▶ Randomized controlled trials (RCTs) are needed to support professional recommendation and treatment. The exception is fluoride, with a substantial body of knowledge validating its usefulness as a desensitizing agent.

▶ Desensitizing agents can be categorized according to their mechanisms of action, either depolarization of the nerve or occlusion of the dentinal tubule. Potassium salts are the only agents that are theorized to work by depolarization.

A. Potassium Salts

▶ Formulations containing potassium chloride, potassium nitrate, potassium citrate, or potassium oxalate reduce depolarization of the nerve cell membrane and transmission of the nerve impulse.[22]

▶ Potassium nitrate dentifrices containing fluoride are widely used[20] and readily available OTC.

B. Fluorides

▸ Precipitate calcium fluoride (CaF_2) crystals within the dentinal tubule to decrease the lumen diameter.[22]

▸ Create a barrier by precipitating CaF_2 at the exposed dentin surface, to block open dental tubules.[26]

   • Fluoride varnishes are FDA approved for tooth desensitization and a cavity liner; although they are frequently used "off-label" for dental caries prevention.

   • Fluoride gels and varnishes are most commonly used and are a successful treatment modalilty.[27,28]

C. Oxalates

▸ Block open dental tubules.[29]

▸ Oxalate salts such as potassium oxalate and ferric oxalate precipitate calcium oxalate crystals to decrease the lumen diameter.[29]

D. Gluteraldehyde

▸ Coagulates proteins and amino acids within the dentinal tubule to decrease the dentinal tubule lumen diameter.[29]

▸ Can be combined with HEMA, a hydrophilic resin, which seals tubules.[29]

▸ Creates calcium crystals within the dentinal tubule to decrease the lumen diameter.[30]

E. Calcium Phosphate Technology

▸ Advocated for use as a caries control agent to reduce demineralization and increase remineralization by releasing calcium and phosphate ions into saliva for deposition of new tooth mineral (hydroxyapatite).[31]

   • Calcium phosphates can compromise the bioavailability of fluorides since calcium and fluoride react to form calcium fluoride.[32]

   • May be effective for patients with poor salivary flow and consequent deficient calcium phosphate levels.[33]

▸ Agents that support remineralization may lessen dentinal hypersensitivity by occluding dentinal tubule openings.

▸ Most studies in support of calcium phosphate technology are animal, in vitro, or *in situ* models designed to analyze remineralization rather than hypersensitivity.

   • One *in vivo* study found a reduction in bleaching-induced sensitivity at days 5 and 14 when amorphous calcium phosphate (ACP) was added to a bleaching gel.[34]

   • Additional research related to calcium phosphate technologies is needed.[35]

▸ ACP

   • Theorized to plug dentinal tubules with calcium and phosphate *precipitate*; promotes an ACP reservoir within the saliva.

   • Enhances fluoride delivery in calcium and phosphate-deficient saliva.[33]

   • May remineralize areas of acid erosion and abrasion, and reduce hypersensitivity.[33]

▸ Calcium sodium phosphosilicate (CSP)

   • Contains sodium and silica in addition to calcium and phosphorous.

   • Delivered in solid bioactive glass particles that react in the presence of saliva and water to release calcium and phosphate ions and create a calcium phosphate layer that crystallizes to hydroxyapatite.

   • Reacts with saliva; sodium buffers the acid, and calcium and phosphate saturate saliva to fill demineralized areas with new hydroxyapatite.

   • Claims include remineralizing enamel and dentin, positive impact on acid erosion and abrasion, a bactericidal effect, and reduction in hypersensitivity.

   • RCT comparing a CSP and a potassium nitrate toothpaste found, using a VAS, that CSP paste was significantly better at reducing dentin hypersensitivity.[36]

▸ Casein phosphopeptide–amorphous calcium phosphate (CPP-ACP)

   • CPP is a milk-derived protein that stabilizes ACP and allows it to be released during acidic challenges.

   • Researchers are exploring benefits such as remineralization of acid erosion, caries inhibition and reduction of dentinal hypersensitivity.

▸ Tricalcium phosphate (TCP)

   • Developed in an effort to create a calcium material that can coexist with fluoride to provide greater efficacy than fluoride alone.[33] Additional components are added to β-TCP to "functionalize" it. Increased remineralization has been demonstrated in vitro[37]; in vivo evidence is needed.

F. Arginine and Calcium Carbonate Technology

▸ Desensitization approach that occludes the dentinal tubules utilizing arginine, a naturally occurring amino acid, bicarbonate (pH buffer), and calcium carbonate.

▸ Marketed as a prophylaxis paste to be applied before instrumentation, using a slow-speed handpiece with a rubber cup and moderate pressure.

▸ Randomized controlled trials that adhere to clinical research standards are still necessary.

IV. Self-Applied Measures

A. Dentifrices

▸ In many OTC sensitivity-reducing dentifrices, 5% potassium nitrate, sodium fluoride, or stannous fluoride separately or in combination are the active desensitizing agents. Studies have suggested that some of the desensitizing effects of dentifrices may be due to the blocking action of the abrasive particles.[22]

▸ Tartar control dentifrices may contribute to increased tooth sensitivity for some individuals, although the mechanism is unclear.

▸ Dentifrices containing highly concentrated fluoride (5,000 ppm fluoride) combined with an abrasive to facilitate extrinsic stain control are available by prescription. This formulation is also available with the addition of potassium nitrate.

B. Gels

▶ Gels containing 5,000 ppm fluoride are a prescription product brushed on for generalized hypersensitivity or burnished into localized areas of sensitivity.

▶ Contain no abrasive agents for biofilm and stain control.

▶ Can be self-applied with custom or commercially available fluoride or whitening trays.

C. Mouthrinses

▶ Mouthrinse containing 0.63% stannous fluoride mouthrinse can be prescribed for daily use to treat hypersensitivity.

▶ Short-term use (2–4 weeks) will limit staining concerns.

V. Professionally Applied Measures

A. Tray Delivered Fluoride Agents

▶ A tray delivery system can be used to apply a 2% neutral sodium fluoride solution.

▶ Select trays of adequate height and fill with sufficient fluoride agent to cover the cervical areas of each tooth.

B. Fluoride Varnish

▶ A 5% sodium fluoride varnish maintains prolonged contact with the tooth surface by serving as a reservoir to release fluoride ions in response to pH changes in saliva and biofilm.[38]

▶ Does not require a dry tooth surface, which is advantageous since drying the tooth can be a painful procedure for a patient with dentin hypersensitivity.

▶ Use a microbrush to apply the varnish to the exposed dentin surface.

▶ Instruct the patient to avoid oral hygiene self-care for several hours to allow the fluoride to stay in contact with the tooth surface for as long as possible, preferably overnight.

C. 5% Gluteraldehyde

▶ Use a microbrush to apply to the affected tooth surface.

▶ Prevent excess flow into soft tissues with cotton roll isolation since contact with soft tissues may cause gingival irritation.

D. Oxalates

▶ Oxalate preparations are applied (burnished) to a dried tooth surface.

▶ May provide immediate and short- rather than long-term relief.

E. Unfilled or Partially Filled Resins

▶ Used to cover patent dentinal tubules.

▶ Resins are applied following an acid etch step that may remove the smear layer, and cause discomfort.

▶ The tooth surface must be dehydrated before resin application, which can create discomfort.

▶ Use of local anesthetic may facilitate patient comfort during this procedure.

F. Dentin-Bonding Agents

▶ Obturates the tubule opening and does not require use of acid etch or dehydration; a single application may protect against further erosion for 3–6 months.

▶ Methylmethacrylate polymer is a common dentin sealer.

G. Composite/Glass Ionomer

▶ Glass ionomer may be placed in the presence of moisture, which eliminates the need for drying the tooth.

▶ In addition to the glass ionomer restoration physically blocking the dentinal tubule, there is an added benefit of slow fluoride release.

H. Soft Tissue Grafts

▶ Surgical placement of soft tissue grafts to cover a sensitive dentinal surface.

I. Lasers

▶ Nd:YAG laser treatment can obliterate dentinal tubules through a process called "melting and resolidification." When used with an appropriate protocol, there is no resulting damage to the pulp or dentin surface cracking.[39,40]

▶ Long-term, in vivo studies are needed to establish safety and efficacy of laser treatment for dentin hypersensitivity. The Food and Drug Administration (FDA) has not approved these devices for this therapeutic modality.

VI. Additional Considerations

A. Periodontal Debridement Considerations

▶ *Preprocedure*

- Explain potential for sensitivity resulting from calculus removal and/or instrumentation of teeth with areas of exposed cementum or dentin.
- Patients are likely to respond more favorably to treatment when prepared for what might occur.
- When multiple teeth in the same treatment area are hypersensitive during scaling and root planing procedures, local anesthetics and/or nitrous oxide analgesia can be utilized.
- Desensitizing agents that are marketed for immediate relief from severe hypersensitivity can be used.

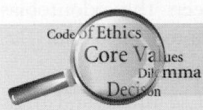

EVERYDAY ETHICS

Marcy, the dental hygienist, practices with Dr. Goldman, who only schedules time to examine a patient at alternate dental hygiene visits unless requested for special needs. Mrs. Stuart arrives for her dental hygiene appointment but is not scheduled to see Dr. Goldman until her next visit. She is complaining of discomfort "on the lower back teeth" when she chews and when she eats or drinks something cold. The pain may last up to an hour.

When she completes the scaling and debridement, Marcy determines that Dr. Goldman is running behind schedule. She knows it will be difficult to get him to come to her treatment room to examine her patient in a timely manner. Marcy gives Mrs. Stuart a sample of desensitizing toothpaste and suggests they will see how it is at the next appointment. Marcy then advises Mrs. Stuart to "Call if it gives you more trouble." The patient is not classified

as having a periodontal condition, is considered low-to-medium risk for dental caries. Her next visit will be in 4 months.

Questions for Consideration

1. How do each of the core values (Table II-1, Section II Introduction) apply in this event? Does the issue of informed consent enter this discussion? Explain why or why not.

2. What ethical issues can arise if Marcy and Dr. Goldman do not take time during this appointment to thoroughly assess Mrs. Stuart's situation to establish a differential diagnosis?

3. Answer the questions provided in the "Questions to Ask" column of Table VI-1 (Section VI Introduction) to determine at least two ethical alternative actions Marcy could have taken.

▶ *Postprocedure*
- Professionally applied desensitization agents can be used.
- Patient is instructed in daily oral health behavior changes and use of self-applied desensitizing agents.

B. Research Developments

▶ The search for the ideal desensitizing agent is ongoing.

▶ Evidence-based scientific research is indicated as new products are developed; *in vivo* research protocols are needed to support clinical application.

C. Tooth Whitening–Induced Sensitivity

Tooth whitening agents, such as hydrogen peroxide and carbamide peroxide, may contribute to increased dentinal hypersensitivity.

▶ Thought to result from by-products of 10% carbamide peroxide (3% hydrogen peroxide and 7% urea) readily passing through the enamel and dentin into the pulp; the reversible pulpitis is caused from the dentin fluid flow and pulpal contact of the hydrogen peroxide without apparent harm to the pulp.[41]

▶ Hypersensitivity may dissipate over time, lasting from a few days to several months.

▶ Exposed dentin and pre-existing dentin hypersensitivity increase hypersensitivity risk secondary to whitening.

▶ Some whitening products contain fluoride or potassium nitrate to eliminate or minimize the effects of sensitivity.

▶ Recommendations outlined in Table 46-3, Chapter 46 to prevent or reduce tooth whitening–induced sensitivity include:

- Use of a potassium nitrate, fluoride, or other desensitization product before, or concurrently with whitening.
- Some take home whitening gels incorporate, 5% potassium nitrate, fluoride and amorphous calcium phosphate.
- Home-use whitening products are usually less concentrated than professionally applied in-office treatment options, with less hypersensitivity risk.
- Allow for a "recovery period" between whitening sessions during which desensitizing agents are used. Decrease frequency of use by whitening every second or third day.

DOCUMENTATION

The permanent record for a patient with a history of tooth sensitivity needs to include at least the following information:

▶ Medical and dental history, vital signs, extra- and intraoral examinations, consultations, and individual progress notes for each appointment and maintenance appointments.

▶ For dentin hypersensitivity: identify teeth involved, differential diagnosis, and all treatments, along with patient instruction for ideal oral self-care, diet, and other for preventive recommendations.

▶ Outcomes and posttreatment directions.

▶ A progress note example for the patient with hypersensitive dentin may be reviewed in Box 44-5.

BOX 44-5
Example Documentation: Patient with Dentin Hypersensitivity

S–Patient complains of pain when eating/drinking cold foods/beverages that disappears immediately after.

O–Generalized facial gingival recession of 1–2 mm on all teeth in the mandibular arch.

A–Based on patient symptoms, exposed roots, and no other evidence of dental disease, the working diagnosis is dentin hypersensitivity.

P–Applied fluoride varnish and gave post-op instructions; advised patient to avoid acidic beverages: or not to brush immediately after ingestion of citrus fruits or beverages; also advised rinse with fluoridated water to buffer acidic conditions (to raise pH). Recommended purchase and use of an OTC potassium nitrate-containing dentifrice. Explained that relief from the dentifrice can take between 2 and 4 weeks. Advised to recontact the office if pain persists or worsens.

Next Steps: Follow-up at next visit.

Signed _____, RDH

Date _____

Factors To Teach The Patient

▷ Etiology and prevention of gingival recession.

▷ Factors contributing to dentin hypersensitivity.

▷ Mechanisms of dentin tubule exposure, which can allow various stimuli to trigger pain response.

▷ Natural desensitization mechanisms that may lessen sensitivity over time.

▷ Appropriate oral hygiene self-care techniques, such as using a soft toothbrush and avoiding a vigorous brushing technique that may contribute to gingival recession and subsequent abrasion of root surfaces.

▷ Connection between an acidic diet and dentin sensitivity; need to eliminate specific foods and beverages that can trigger sensitivity.

▷ Toothbrushing is not recommended immediately after consumption of acidic foods or beverages.

▷ The challenges of managing hypersensitivity, hierarchy of treatment measures, and variable effect of treatment options.

References

1. Addy M. Etiology and clinical implications of dentine hypersensitivity. *Dent Clin North Am.* 1990;34(3):503–514.

2. Absi EG, Addy M, Adams D. Dentine hypersensitivity: the development and evaluation of a replica technique to study sensitive and non-sensitive cervical dentine. *J Clin Periodontol.* 1989;16(3):190–195.

3. Frank RM. Attachment sites between the odontoblast process and the intradental nerve fibre. *Arch Oral Biol.* 1968;13(7):833–834.

4. Thomas HF, Carella P. Correlation of scanning and transmission electron microscopy of human dentinal tubules. *Arch Oral Biol.* 1984;29(8):641–646.

5. Dufour LA, Bissell HS. Periodontal attachment loss induced by mechanical subgingival instrumentation in shallow sulci. *J Dent Hyg.* 2002;76(3):207–212.

6. Absi EG, Addy M, Adams D. Dentine hypersensitivity: the effect of toothbrushing and dietary compounds on dentine in vitro. *J Oral Rehabil.* 1992;19(2):101–110.

7. Prati C, Montebugnoli L, Supp P, et al. Permeability and morphology of dentin after erosion induced by acidic drinks. *J Periodontol.* 2002;74(4):428–436.

8. Staninec M, Nalla RK, Hilton JF, et al. Dentin erosion simulation by cantilever beam fatigue and pH change. *J Dent Res.* 2005;84(4):371–375.

9. Litonjua LA, Andreana S, Bush OJ, et al. Wedged cervical lesions produced by toothbrushing. *Am J Dent.* 2004;17(4):237–240.

10. Estafan A, Furnari PC, Goldstein G, et al. In vivo correlation of noncarious cervical lesions and occlusal wear. *J Prosthet Dent.* 2005;93(3):221–226.

11. Sarode GS, Sarode CS. Abfraction: a review. *J Oral Maxillofac Pathol.* 2013;17(2):222–227.

12. Brannstrom M, Linden LA, Astrom A. The hydrodynamics of the dental tubule and of pulp fluid: a discussion of its significance in relation to dentinal sensitivity. *Caries Res.* 1967;1(4):310–317.

13. Eldarrat AH, High AS, Kale GM. In vitro analysis of "smear layer" on human dentine using ac-impedance spectroscopy. *J Dent.* 2004;32(7):547–554.

14. Cunha-Cruz J, Wataha JC, Heaton LJ, et al. The prevalence of dentin hypersensitivity in general dental practices in the northwest United States. *J Am Dent Assoc.* 2013;144(3):288–296.

15. Taani Q, Awartani F. Clinical evaluation of cervical dentin sensitivity (CDS) in patients attending general dental clinics and periodontal specialty clinics (PSC). *J Clin Periodontol.* 2002;29(2):118–122.

16. Addy M, Pearce N. Aetological, predisposing and environmental factors in dentine hypersensitivity. *Arch Oral Biol.* 1994;39 (Suppl):33S–38S.

17. Kassaba MM, Cohen RE. The etiology and prevalence of gingival recession. *J Am Dent Assoc.* 2003;134(2):220–225.

18. Gillam DG, Aris A, Bulman JS, et al. Dentine hypersensitivity in subjects recruited for clinical trials: clinical evaluation, prevalence and intraoral distribution. *J Oral Rehabil.* 2002;29(3):226–231.

19. Addy M. Dentine hypersensitivity: new perspectives on an old problem. *Int Dent J.* 2002;52 (Suppl 1):367–375.

20. Orchardson R, Gillam DG. The efficacy of potassium salts as agents for treating dentin hypersensitivity. *J Orofac Pain.* 2000;14(1):9–19.

21. Correa FO, Sampaio JE, Rossa C, et al. Influence of natural fruit juices in removing the smear layer from root surfaces—an in vitro study. *J Can Dent Assoc.* 2004;70(10):697–702.

22. Orchardson R, Gilla DC. Managing dentin hypersensitivity. *J Am Dent Assoc.* 2006;137(7):990–998.

23. Kawasaki A, Ishikawa K, Sug T, et al. Effects of plaque control on the patency and occlusion of dentine tubules in situ. *J Oral Rehabil.* 2001;28(5):439–449.

24. Van Der Weijden GA, Timmerman MF, Reijerse E, et al. Toothbrushing force in relation to plaque removal. *J Clin Periodontol.* 1996;23(8):724–729.

25. Pashley DH, Leibach JG, Horner JA. The effects of burnishing NaF/kaolin/glycerin paste on dentin permeability. *J Periodontol.* 1987;58(1):19–23.

26. Suge T, Ishikowa K, Kawasaki A, et al. Effects of fluoride on the calcium phosphate precipitation method for dentinal tubule occlusion. *J Dent Res.* 1995;74(4):1079–1085.

27. Ritter AV, de L Dias W, Miguez P, et al. Treating cervical dentin hypersensitivity with fluoride varnish: a randomized clinical study. *J Am Dent Assoc.* 2006;137(7):1013–1020.

28. Cunha-Cruz J, Wataha, JC, Zhou, L, et al. Treating dentin hypersensitivity, therapeutic choices made by dentists of the Northwest PRECEDENT network. *J Am Dent Assoc.* 2010;141(9):1097–1105.

29. Haywood VB. Dentine hypersensitivity: bleaching and restorative considerations for successful management. *Int Dent J.* 2002;52 (Suppl 1):376.

30. Pashley DH, Kalathoor S, Burnham D. The effects of calcium hydroxide on dentin permeability. *J Dent Res.* 1986;65(3):417–420.

31. Featherstone JD. The continuum of dental caries-evidence for a dynamic disease process. *J Dent Res.* 2004;83 (Spec No C):C39–C42.

32. Karlinsey RL, Mackey AC, Walker ER, et al. Surfactant-modified B-TCP: structure, properties, and in vitro remineralization of subsurface enamel lesions. *J Mater Sci Mater Med.* 2010;21(4):2009–2020.

33. Chow L, Wefel JS. The dynamics of de-and remineralization. *Dimensions Dent Hyg.* 2009;7(2):42–46.

34. Giniger M, MacDonald J, Ziemba S, et al. The clinical performance of professionally dispensed bleaching gel with added amorphous calcium phosphate. *J Am Dent Assoc.* 2005;136(3):383–392.

35. Yengopal V, Mickenautsch S. Caries-preventive effect of casein phosphopeptide-amorphous calcium phosphate (CPP-ACP): a meta-analysis. *Acta Odontol Scand.* 2009;21:1–12.

36. Pradeep AR, Sharma A. Comparison of clinical efficacy of a dentifrice containing calcium sodium phosphosilicate to a dentifrice containing potassium nitrate and to a placebo on dentinal hypersensitivity: a randomized clinical trial. *J Periodontol.* 2010;81(8):1167–1173.

37. Karlinsey RL, Mackey AC, Walker ER, et al. Preparation, characterization and in vitro efficacy of an acid-modified β-TCP material for dental hard-tissue remineralization. *Acta Biomater.* 2010;6(3):969–978.

38. Shen C, Autio-Gold J. Assessing fluoride concentration uniformity and fluoride release from 3 varnishes. *J Am Dent Assoc.* 2002;133(2):176–182.

39. Kara C, Orbak R. Comparative evaluation of Nd:YAG laser and fluoride varnish for the treatment of dentinal hypersensitivity. *J Endod.* 2009;35(7):971–974.

40. Lopes AO, Aranha ACC. Comparative evaluation of the effects of Nd:YAG laser and a densensitizer agent on the treatment of dentin hypersensitivity: a clinical study. *Photomed Laser Surg.* 2013;31(3):132–138.

41. Li Y, Greenwall L. Safety issues of tooth whitening using peroxide-based materials. *Br Dent J.* 2013;215(1):29–34.

 ENHANCE YOUR UNDERSTANDING

thePoint° **DIGITAL CONNECTIONS**
(see the inside front cover for access information)
- **Audio glossary**
- **Quiz bank**

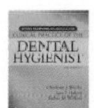 **SUPPORT FOR LEARNING**
(available separately; visit lww.com)
- ***Active Learning Workbook for Clinical Practice of the Dental Hygienist, 12th Edition***

prepU **INDIVIDUALIZED REVIEW**
(available separately; visit lww.com)
- **Adaptive quizzing with *prepU for Wilkins' Clinical Practice of the Dental Hygienist***

45

Extrinsic Stain Removal

Caren M. Barnes, RDH, BS, MS

LEARNING OBJECTIVES

After studying this chapter, the student will be able to:

1. Describe the difference between a cleaning agent and a polishing agent.

2. Explain the basis for selection of the grit of polishing paste for each individual patient.

3. Discuss the rationale for avoiding polishing procedures on areas of demineralization.

4. Explain the effect abrasive particle shape, size, and hardness have on the abrasive qualities of a polishing paste.

5. Explain the types of powdered polishing agents available and their use to remove tooth stains.

6. Explain patient conditions that contraindicate the use of air-powder polishing.

INTRODUCTION

After treatment by scaling, root planing, and other dental hygiene care, the teeth are assessed for the presence of remaining dental stains.

▶ The cleaning or polishing agents used must be *selected* based on the patient's individual needs such as the type and amount of stain present and whether or not restorations are present.

▶ Preliminary examination of each tooth will reveal that the surfaces to be treated may be tooth structure (enamel, or with recession cementum or dentin) or when restored, a variety of dental materials (metal or esthetic, tooth-color restorations).

▶ *Preservation of the surfaces of both the teeth and the restorations is of primary importance during all cleaning and polishing procedures.*

▶ Stain removal will require the use of prophylaxis polishing agents that contain various abrasive grits. The smallest, least abrasive grit is used.

▶ Some patients will not consider their teeth "cleaned" unless they have been polished. This situation is ideal for a *cleaning agent* that will not abrade the dental hard tissues, but will remove dental biofilm and the patient's teeth will have the same clean feeling as they would if an abrasive prophylaxis paste were used.

▶ *One size grit prophylaxis paste is not appropriate for every patient and is unethical and clinically the wrong choice. To use such a practice is to ignore a patient's individual needs, can worsen hypersensitivity, and cause significant damage to esthetic restorations.*

▶ The longevity, esthetic appearance, and smooth surfaces of dental restorations depend on appropriate care by the dental hygienist and the daily personal care by the patient.

▶ It is a responsibility of the dental hygienist to be current in knowledge of the procedures to prevent damage to the restorations during professional healthcare appointments.

▶ The dental hygienist is responsible for educating the patient about proper daily oral self-care that will contribute to the maintenance of the restorations, such as recommending the least abrasive dentifrices.[1,2]

▶ Terms related to extrinsic stain removal are defined in Box 45-1.

PURPOSES FOR STAIN REMOVAL

Stains on the teeth are not etiologic factors for oral disease or destructive process.

▶ The removal of stains is for esthetic, not for therapeutic or health, reasons.

  • Stain removal procedures have been an integral part of the oral prophylaxis since the inception of tooth cleaning procedures and patients have come to expect to have their teeth polished as a part of the oral prophylaxis.

▶ The American Dental Hygienists' Association and the Academy of Periodontology include tooth polishing in their definitions of the term "oral prophylaxis."[3,4]

▶ Key words related to stain removal, polishing, instruments, coronal polishing, air-powder polishing, cleaning agent, prophylaxis polishing agent, tribiology, two-body abrasion and three-body abrasion are defined in Box 45-1.

SCIENCE OF POLISHING

▶ Polishing is intended to produce intentional, selective and controlled wear. Within the science of tribology, polishing is considered to be two-body or three-body abrasive polishing.

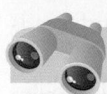

BOX 45-1   KEY WORDS AND ABBREVIATIONS: Extrinsic Stain Removal

Abrasion: wearing away of surface material by friction.

Abrasive: a material composed of particles of sufficient hardness and sharpness to cut or scratch a softer material when drawn across its surface; available in various particle sizes.

Air-powder polisher: air-powered device using air and water pressure to deliver a controlled stream of specially processed sodium bicarbonate slurry through the handpiece nozzle; also called air abrasive, airpolishing, air-powered abrasive, or airbrasive.

Binder: substance used to hold abrasive particles together; examples are ceramic bonding used for mounted abrasive points, electroplating for binding diamond chips for rotary instruments, and rubber or shellac for soft discs.

Coronal polishing: polishing of the anatomic crowns of the teeth to remove dental biofilm and extrinsic stains; does not involve calculus removal.

Glycerin: clear, colorless, syrupy fluid used as a vehicle and sweetening agent for drugs and as a solvent and vehicle for abrasive agents.

Grit: with reference to abrasive agents, grit is the particle size.

Polishing: the production, especially by friction, of a smooth, glossy, mirrorlike surface that reflects light; a very fine agent is used for polishing after a coarser agent is used for cleaning.

psi: pounds per square inch.

rpm: revolutions per minute.

Slurry: thin, semi-fluid suspension of a solid in a liquid.

Three-body abrasion: involves loose abrasive particles that move in the interface space between the surface being polished and the polishing application device.

Two-body abrasion: involves abrasive particles attached to a medium (polishing application device) that move directly against the surface being polished.

Tribiology: tribiology incorporates the study and application of the principles of friction, lubrication, and wear as they apply to polishing.

- Two-body abrasive polishing involves the abrasive particles attached to a medium, such as a rubber cup impregnated with abrasive particles that would not require a prophylaxis polishing paste.
- Three-body abrasive polishing is the type most commonly used by dental hygienists, in which loose abrasive particles (the abrasive particles in prophylaxis polishing paste) move in the interface space between the surface being polished and the polishing application device (rubber cup or brush).[6–8]

EFFECTS OF CLEANING AND POLISHING

Attention is given to the positive and negative effects of polishing so that evidence-based decisions can be made for the treatment of each patient. *Professional judgment based on a patient's needs and requests determines when a service is to be included in a dental hygiene care plan, and if services are warranted, they should be selected carefully.*

I. Precautions

▶ As with all gingival manipulation with instruments, including a toothbrush,[9,10] bacteremia can be created during the use of power-driven stain removal instruments. Rotation of the rubber cup can force microorganisms into the tissues.

▶ An inflammatory response can be expected, and bacteria may gain access to the bloodstream to create a bacteremia.

▶ The response is a normal expectation and not of concern in healthy patients.

▶ It is a concern for a patient who requires prophylactic antibiotic coverage before dental treatment; another reason why the medical history is such an essential part of patient assessment and is recorded before all treatments.

▶ The medical history is reviewed and updated at each succeeding appointment.

▶ For patients at risk, particularly those with damaged or abnormal heart valves, prosthetic valves, and other conditions listed in Chapter 10 (Box 10-2) may require antibiotic prophylaxis as specified by the patient's cardiologist.

II. Environmental Factors

A. Aerosol Production

▶ Aerosols are created during the use of all rotary instruments, including a prophylaxis handpiece with a rubber cup to hold polishing paste, the air and water sprays used during rinsing, and air-polishing.[11]

- The biologic contaminants of aerosols stay suspended for long periods and provide a means for disease transmission to dental personnel, as well as to other patients.

- Use of power-driven instruments is limited when a patient is known to have a communicable disease, a serious or chronic respiratory disease, or is immunocompromised.

- Standard personal protective procedures are used.

B. Spatter

- Protective eyewear is needed for all dental team members and for the patient.

- Serious eye damage has occurred because of spatter from polishing paste or from instruments.[12]

III. Effect on Teeth

A. Removal of Tooth Structure

- Polishing with coarse abrasive prophylaxis pastes may remove a few micrometer of the outer enamel. This is justification for using the least abrasive prophylaxis paste necessary to meet the patient's needs for polishing procedures.

- The fluoride-rich outer surface of the enamel is necessary for protection against dental caries[13] and care is taken for it to be preserved. The use of a cleaning agent in place of an abrasive prophylaxis polishing agent will prevent any removal of the outermost layer of enamel.

B. Areas of Demineralization

- *Demineralization*: Polishing demineralized white spots of enamel is contraindicated. More surface enamel is lost from abrasive polishing over demineralized white spots than over intact enamel.[14]

- *Remineralization*: Demineralized areas of enamel can remineralize as these areas are exposed to fluoride from saliva, water, dentifrices, and professional fluoride applications.

  • Since remineralization cannot be detected visually, it is necessary to remember that polishing procedures can interrupt enamel surface remineralization.

C. Areas of Thin Enamel, Cementum, or Dentin

- Areas of thin enamel are contraindicated for polishing.

  • Amelogenesis imperfecta is an example of thin enamel resulting from imperfect tooth development in Chapter 22.

- *Exposure of dentinal tubules*: cementum and dentin are softer and more porous than enamel, so greater amounts of their surfaces can be removed during polishing than from enamel. When cementum is exposed because of

gingival recession, polishing of the exposed surfaces is avoided.

- Smear layer could be removed and dentinal tubules exposed.[15]

- When surface structure is removed, unnecessary tooth sensitivity can result.[16]

D. Care of Restorations and Implants

- Use of coarse abrasives may create deep, irregular scratches in restorative materials. Figure 45-1 shows a scanning electron photomicrograph of the damaged surface of a composite restoration polished with a rubber cup and coarse prophylaxis paste.

- Microorganisms collect and colonize on a rough surface much more rapidly than on a smooth surface.[17]

- It is imperative that prophylaxis polishing agents are not used on restorative materials. Polishing pastes not intended for use on restorative materials can destroy the surface integrity of the dental material.[18]

  • Select a cleaning agent or a polishing agent recommended by the manufacturer of the restorative materials.[18,19]

E. Heat Production

- Steady pressure with a rapidly revolving rubber cup or bristle brush and a minimum of wet abrasive agent can create sufficient heat to cause pain and discomfort for the patient.

- The pulps of children are large and may be more susceptible to heat.

- The rules for the use of cleaning or polishing agents are:
  • Use light pressure, slow speed of the rubber cup.
  • Use a moist agent.
  • Cleaning or polishing agents are never to be used as dry powders applied directly on teeth.

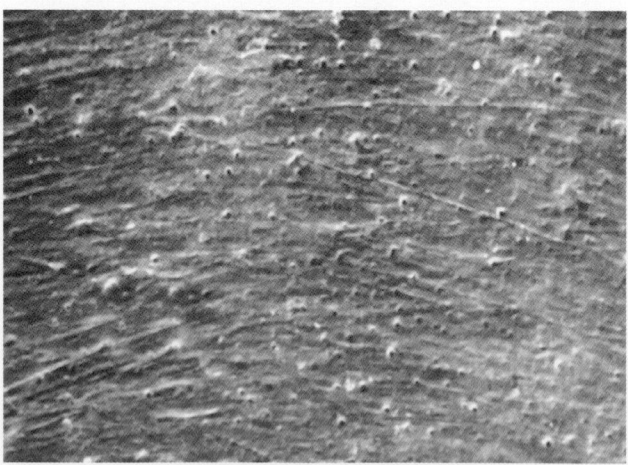

FIGURE 45-1 Scanning Electron Photomicrograph of A Composite Restoration Polished with Coarse Prophylaxis Paste.

IV. Effect on Gingiva

▶ Trauma to the gingival tissue can result, especially when the prophylaxis angle is run at a high speed with heavy pressure and the rubber cup is applied for an extended period adjacent to gingival tissues.

▶ Stain removal after gingival and periodontal treatments, including scaling and root planing, is not recommended on the same day. The diseased lining of the pocket usually has been removed during scaling and incidental curettage, leaving the pocket wall wide open ready to receive abrasive particles and microorganisms that can become embedded out of reach of the most careful irrigation and rinsing.

INDICATIONS FOR STAIN REMOVAL

I. Removal of Extrinsic Stains

A. Patient Instruction

▶ Discuss source of stain and how it can be prevented.

▶ Encourage patient to make necessary habit changes, especially to seek counseling for smoking cessation if that is the cause of the patient's stain. Tobacco cessation is described in Chapter 34.

▶ Practice toothbrushing to remove stains incorporated in dental biofilm.

• For example: The patient can be taught that chlorhexidine stain can be prevented and/or lessened with dental biofilm removal during personal oral care procedures. The less dental biofilm the patient has, the less chlorhexidine may stain the teeth.

B. Scaling and Root Planing

▶ In addition to the use of cleaning or polishing agents during polishing procedures, stains can also be removed during scaling and root planing instrumentation.

• Example: Black line stain has been compared to calculus because it may be elevated from the tooth surface and may need to be removed by instrumentation. It is described in Chapter 22.[20]

II. To Prepare the Teeth for Caries-Preventive Procedures

A. Placement of Pit and Fissure Sealant

▶ Follow manufacturer's directions. Sealants vary in their requirements.

▶ Avoid commercial oral prophylaxis pastes that contain glycerin, oils, flavoring substances, or other agents. Glycerin and oils can prevent an optimum acid-etch and interfere with the adherence of the sealant to the tooth surface, causing the sealant to fail.

▶ Air-powder polishing is one method of choice for preparing tooth surfaces for sealants (see Chapter 37).[21,22]

▶ An alternative is the use of a plain, fine pumice mixed with water when precleaning is determined to be necessary.

• After the use of pumice, the tooth surface(s) needs to be rinse thoroughly to remove the particles.

B. Professional Application of Fluoride Varnishes, Solutions, or Gels

▶ Tooth polishing is not necessary before fluoride application.[23]

• Biofilm and debris removal can be accomplished adequately by the patient using a toothbrush and dental floss, after complete calculus removal.

▶ The pellicle on the tooth surface does not act as a barrier to fluoride, and fluoride uptake in the enamel from a fluoride application is similar whether the teeth are brushed by the patient or polished with a cleaning or polishing agent.[23]

III. To Contribute to Patient Motivation

Removal of biofilm is a *daily* procedure to be carried out *by the patient*. When accomplished thoroughly at least twice daily and for some patients three times daily, infection can be controlled, the sanitation of the mouth maintained, and staining can be minimized or prevented.

A. Development of Biofilm

▶ It is known that pellicle returns to cover the teeth within minutes after complete polishing.

▶ Biofilm begins to collect on the pellicle within 1 or 2 hours, increasing in thickness until, by 12–24 hours, biofilm is thick enough to show clearly when a disclosing agent is applied.

▶ Undisturbed, biofilm may begin to calcify within a few days in a calculus-susceptible patient.

B. Motivation

Smooth polished tooth surfaces may contribute in part to the following effects:

▶ Help the patient to obtain more satisfactory results from oral self-care procedures. A smooth surface can be easier to achieve once the patient understands what a biofilm and debris-free mouth feels like after having the teeth professionally polished with a cleaning or polishing agent.

▶ Show the patient the appearance and feeling of a clean mouth for motivational purposes. The change in behavior, or the true learning, can be obtained through patient participation in the use of a disclosing agent and personal visualization of the biofilm followed by removal of the biofilm with floss and toothbrush.

CLINICAL APPLICATION OF SELECTIVE STAIN REMOVAL

The decision to polish teeth is based on the individual patient's needs.

I. Summary of Contraindications for Polishing

The following list suggests some of the specific instances in which polishing either can be performed with a cleaning agent or is contraindicated.

A. No Unsightly Stain

▶ Polishing is a procedure based on the patient's individual needs. If no stain is present, polishing with an abrasive polishing agent is not necessary; however, this is an ideal situation for using a cleaning agent.

▶ If cleaning agents will not remove the stain that is present, the choice is the least abrasive polishing agent that will remove the stain.

▶ Appearance is important to patients, but maintaining the integrity of the tooth surface for disease prevention is more important.

▶ When the abrasive paste is a medium, coarse, or extra coarse paste, those pastes need to be followed by the use of the next least abrasive paste in succession until the final paste used is fine paste.

B. Characteristics of Patients at Risk for Dental Caries

▶ Patients at risk for dental caries need extra fluoride to protect their tooth surfaces and fluoride-rich enamel surfaces need to be preserved. Examples include:
- Rampant caries, nursing caries, root caries, all ages
- Noncavitated dental caries in early stages of demineralization
- Xerostomia, from any reason.

C. Patients with Respiratory Problems

Polishing procedures typically require rinsing of the patient's mouth several times throughout the procedure.

▶ Care is taken to minimize the spray from the air–water syringe as much as possible as the aerosols are contraindicated for such conditions as asthma, emphysema, cystic fibrosis, lung cancer, patients requiring oxygen, or when breathing is a problem.

▶ This caution also applies to the use of air-powder polishers and spatter from prophylaxis polishing pastes.

D. Tooth Sensitivity

▶ Abrasive agents can uncover ends of dentinal tubules in areas of thin cementum or dentin.

▶ The polishing of dentin and cementum is contraindicated and needs to be avoided to every extent possible.

E. Restorations

▶ Restorations and titanium implants may be scratched by abrasive prophylaxis polishing pastes.
- However, a cleaning agent will not scratch restorative materials or titanium implants.[19]

▶ Tooth-colored restorations need to be polished with a cleaning agent, a polishing paste specifically formulated for use on esthetic restorations, or the paste recommended by the manufacturer of the restorative material.[18]

F. Conditions that Require Postponement for Later Evaluation

▶ When instruction for personal biofilm removal (daily care) has not yet been given or when the patient has not demonstrated adequate biofilm control.

▶ Soft spongy tissue that bleeds on brushing or gentle instrumentation.

▶ Communicable disease potentially disseminated by aerosol.

II. Suggestions for Clinic Procedure

A. Give Instruction First

▶ Daily dental biofilm removal to assist in dental stain control.

▶ Explain to the patient that drinking coffee, tea, and color-added soft drinks and/or use of tobacco is responsible for most dental stains.

▶ Patients need information about the types of dentifrices that are safe for stain control and those that are contraindicated due to excessive abrasiveness or chemical harshness.

▶ Tobacco cessation introduction when stain is primarily from tobacco use (Chapter 34).

B. Remove Stain by Scaling

▶ Whenever possible, stains can be removed during scaling, root planing, and debridement.

▶ Assist in planning a preventive plan for stain control.

C. Stain Removal Techniques

▶ Cleaning agent or low-abrasion oral prophylaxis paste.
▶ Use the lightest pressure necessary for stain removal.
▶ Low-speed handpiece.
▶ Minimal heat production.
▶ Soft rubber cup at 90° to tooth surface with intermittent light applications.

CLEANING AND POLISHING AGENTS

There are two distinct types of agents used for "polishing" teeth: one is a cleaning agent, and the other is a polishing agent.[1]

I. Polishing Agents

▶ Traditionally, abrasive agents have been applied with polishing instruments to remove extrinsic dental stains and leave the enamel surface smooth and shiny.

▶ Polishing agents act by producing scratches in the surface of the tooth or restoration created by the friction between the abrasive particle and the softer tooth or restorative surface.

▶ The cleaning and polishing process progresses from coarse abrasion to fine abrasion until the scratches are smaller than the wavelength of visible light, which is 0.05 μm.[1]

▶ When scratches this size are created, the surface appears smooth and shiny—the smaller the scratches, the shinier the surface.

▶ Unless the abrasive agent has been specially formulated for esthetic restorative surfaces, the use of prophylaxis polishing pastes is contraindicated for application to any esthetic restorative surfaces.[19,24]

II. Cleaning Agents

▶ Unlike polishing agents, cleaning agents are round, flat, nonabrasive particles, and do not scratch surface material but produce a higher luster than polishing agents.

▶ The most readily available cleaning agent (ProCare, Young Dental Mfg. Earth City, MO) is made of a combination of feldspar, alkali (sodium and potassium) and aluminum silicates. This feldspar, sodium–aluminum silicate cleaning agent is formulated into a powder and can be mixed with water or sodium fluoride to make a paste for cleaning.[25,26]

▶ Because of the extremely low level of abrasion, cleaning agents can be used on any tooth surface, restorative surface, or implant surface without fear of creating deep scratches.

▶ Cleaning agents will not harm restorative surfaces and any other polishing agent selected for restorative surfaces is selected based on the formulation and appropriateness for the restorative material.[27]

▶ Dental hygienists must be mindful that many esthetic restorations are virtually undetectable due to color and surface match; therefore, it is imperative that the patient's dental chart and radiographs be examined to locate the esthetic restorations before applying polishing agents.

III. Factors Affecting Abrasive Action with Polishing Agents

During polishing, sharp edges of abrasive particles are moved along the surface of a material, abrading it by producing microscopic scratches or grooves. The rate of abrasion, or speed with which structural material is removed from the surface being polished, is governed by hardness and shape of the abrasive particles, as well as by the manner in which they are applied.

A. Characteristics of Abrasive Particles

▶ *Shape*: Irregularly shaped particles with sharp edges produce deeper grooves and thus abrade faster than do rounded particles with dull edges.

▶ *Hardness*: Particles must be harder than the surface to be abraded; harder particles abrade faster.

• Many of the abrasives used in prophylaxis polishing pastes are 10 times harder than the tooth structure to which they are applied.[27]

• Table 45-1 provides a comparison of the Mohs hardness value of dental tissues compared to agents commonly used in prophylaxis polishing pastes and substances used in cleaning agents.

▶ *Body strength*: Particles that fracture into smaller sharp-edged particles during use are more abrasive than those that wear down during use and become dull.

TABLE 45-1	Mohs Hardness Value of Dental Tissues Compared to Commonly Used Polishing Abrasive Particles
	MOHS HARDNESS VALUE
DENTAL TISSUES	
Enamel	5
Dentin	3.0–4.0
Cementum	2.5–3.0
ABRASIVE AGENTS IN POLISHING PASTES	
Zirconium silicate	7.5–8.0
Pumice	6.0–7.0
Silicone carbine	9.5
Boron	9.3
Aluminum oxide	9
Garnet	8.0–9.0
Emery	7.0–9.0
Zirconium oxide	7
Perlite	5.5
Calcium carbonate	3
Aluminum silicates	2
Sodium	0.5
Potassium	0.4

The Mohs hardness value of enamel, cementum, and dentin compared to the Mohs hardness value of abrasive materials commonly used in prophylaxis polishing pastes. The Mohs hardness value is indicative of a material's resistance to scratching. Diamonds have a maximum Mohs value of 10; talc has a minimum of Mohs hardness of 1.

▶ *Particle size (grit)*

- The larger the particles, the more abrasive they are and the less polishing ability they have.
- Finer abrasive particles achieve a glossier finish.
- Abrasive and polishing agents are graded from coarse to fine based on the size of the holes in a standard sieve through which the particles will pass.
- The finer abrasives are called powders or flours and are graded in order of increasing fineness as F, FF, FFF, and so on.
- Particles embedded in papers are graded 0, 00, 000, and so on.

B. Principles for Application of Abrasives

▶ *Quantity applied*: The more particles applied per unit of time, the faster the rate of abrasion.

- Particles are suspended in water or other vehicles for frictional heat reduction.
- Dry powders or flours represent the greatest quantity that can be applied per unit of time.
- Frictional heat produced is proportional to the rate of abrasion; therefore, the use of *dry agents* is *contraindicated* for polishing natural teeth because of the potential danger of thermal injury to the dental pulp.

▶ *Speed of application*: The greater the speed of application, the faster the rate of abrasion.

- With increased speed of application, pressure must be reduced.
- *Rapid abrasion* is *contraindicated* because it increases frictional heat.

▶ *Pressure of application*: The heavier the pressure applied, the faster the rate of abrasion.

- *Heavy pressure* is *contraindicated* because it increases frictional heat.

▶ *Summary*: When cleaning and polishing are indicated after patient evaluation, the following are observed:

- Use wet agents.
- Apply a rubber polishing cup, using low speed.
- Use a light, intermittent touch.

IV. Abrasive Agents

The abrasives listed here are examples of commonly used agents. Some are available in several grades, and the specific use varies with the grade.

- For example, while a superfine grade might be used for polishing enamel surfaces and metallic restorations, a coarser grade would be used only for laboratory purposes.

Abrasives for use daily in a dentifrice necessarily are of a finer grade than those used for professional polishing accomplished a few times each year.

A. Silex (Silicon Dioxide)

▶ *XXX Silex*: Fairly abrasive.

▶ *Superfine Silex*: Can be used for heavy stain removal from enamel.

B. Pumice

▶ Powdered pumice is of volcanic origin and consists chiefly of complex silicates of aluminum, potassium, and sodium.

▶ Pumice is the primary ingredient in commercially prepared prophylaxis pastes. The specifications for particle size are listed in the *National Formulary*[28] as follows:

- *Pumice flour or superfine pumice*: Least abrasive, and may be used to remove heavy stains from enamel.
- *Fine pumice*: Mildly abrasive.
- *Coarse pumice*: Not for use on natural teeth.

C. Calcium Carbonate (Whiting, Calcite, Chalk)

▶ Various grades are used for different polishing techniques.

D. Tin Oxide (Putty Powder, Stannic Oxide)

▶ Polishing agent for teeth and metallic restorations.

E. Emery (Corundum)

Not used directly on the enamel.

▶ *Aluminum oxide (alumina)*: The pure form of emery. Used for composite restorations and margins of porcelain restorations.

▶ *Levigated alumina*: Consists of extremely fine particles of aluminum oxide, which may be used for polishing metals but are destructive to tooth surfaces.

F. Rouge (Jeweler's Rouge)

▶ Iron oxide is a fine red powder sometimes impregnated on paper discs.

▶ It is useful for polishing gold and precious metal alloys in the laboratory.

G. Diamond Particles

▶ Constituent of diamond polishing paste for porcelain surfaces.

V. Cleaning Ingredients

▶ Particles for cleaning agents differ from abrasive agents in shape and hardness.

▶ Particles used for cleaning agents include feldspar, alkali, and aluminum silicate.

A. Clinical Applications

Numerous commercial preparations for dental prophylactic cleaning and polishing preparations are available. Clinicians need more than one type available to meet the requirements of individual restorative materials.

B. Packaging

▶ Commercial preparations are in the forms of pastes or powders.

▶ Some are available in measured amounts contained in small plastic or other individual packets that contribute to the cleanliness and sterility of the procedure.

▶ Selection of a preparation is based on qualities of abrasiveness, consistency for convenient use, or flavor for patient pleasure.

C. Enhanced Prophylaxis Polishing Pastes

Additives are included in prophylaxis polishing pastes to provide a specific function, such as enhancing the mineral surface of enamel, diminishing dentin hypersensitivity, or tooth whitening.

▶ *Fluoride prophylaxis pastes*

- Application of fluoride by use of fluoride-containing prophylaxis polishing pastes **cannot** be considered a substitute for or the equivalent of a conventional topical fluoride treatment.

- There is no scientific evidence that the amount of fluoride in prophylaxis paste is sufficient to have a preventive effect for dental caries. The fluoride ions in the prophylaxis paste mix with the saliva; fluoride is not burnished into enamel with prophylaxis paste.

- *Enamel surface*: The greatest benefit of fluoride as a prophylaxis polishing paste additive occurs when the fluoride ions in the prophylaxis paste are released into the saliva.
  - The fluoride ions that become mixed in the saliva may become incorporated into the hydroxyapatite structure of the tooth, thus aiding in the remineralizing of the tooth and improving enamel hardness.

- *Clinical application*: Use only an amount sufficient to accomplish stain removal to prevent a child patient from swallowing unnecessary fluoride. The paste may contain 4,000–20,000 ppm fluoride ion.[29]

▶ *Amorphous calcium phosphate and other forms of calcium and phosphate*

- Amorphous calcium phosphate and other formulations of calcium and phosphate, as an additive to prophylaxis polishing pastes, have been shown to hydrolyze the tooth mineral to form apatite.

- When these additives are included in oral prophylaxis paste, the benefit is not solely from burnishing them into the tooth surface.

- When prophylaxis polishing pastes containing calcium and phosphate become mixed with saliva, the mineral ions may become incorporated into the hydroxyapatite structure of the tooth, thus aiding in remineralizing the tooth and improving enamel hardness.

- Polishing agents containing amorphous calcium phosphate have the potential to enhance tooth smoothness and the luster of the enamel surface.[30,31]

▶ *Fluoride, calcium, and phosphate*

- Fluoride, calcium, and phosphate prophylaxis pastes have an edge over those pastes that contain only calcium and phosphate, in that there are three minerals that can be incorporated into the tooth surface. Just as with the pastes that contain amorphous calcium and phosphate, the mineral ions, including the fluoride ions, may become incorporated into the hydroxyapatite structure of the tooth, thus aiding in remineralization to improve enamel hardness.

▶ *Tooth whitening*

- In addition to removing extrinsic stains, there are commercially available prophylaxis polishing pastes that contain 35% hydrogen peroxide to provide a whitening benefit.

- A hydrogen peroxide gel is applied to the tooth and then "polished" into the tooth surface with a rubber cup and prophylaxis polishing paste.[32]

- Prophylaxis polishing pastes with the hydrogen peroxide additive are not intended to be a primary delivery system for professional tooth whitening but can be used as an aid to maintain whitening results.

▶ *Dentin hypersensitivity*

- Topical desensitizing products work either by occluding dentinal tubules thereby blocking fluid flow or by interfering with nerve transmission.

- Topical products that occlude dentinal tubules do so by physically occluding the tubules.

- The desensitizing products that block nerve transmission utilize the active ingredient 5% potassium nitrate (KNO_3). Nerve transmission is blocked by KNO_3 by penetration of dentinal tubules and depolarization the nerve.[33–35]

- Dentifrices for patients that have dentinal hypersensitivity have long been available and some prophylaxis polishing pastes have been formulated for this purpose.

- Prophylaxis polishing pastes that contain arginine, calcium, and bicarbonate/carbonate have the purpose of minimizing dentin hypersensitivity. Mixing these ingredients produces arginine bicarbonate and calcium carbonate. When applied with a rubber cup these adjunctive ingredients can aid in sealing the dentinal tubules.[36] However, the sealing of the dentinal tubules is not permanent.

PROCEDURES FOR STAIN REMOVAL (CORONAL POLISHING)

I. Patient Preparation for Stain Removal

A. Instruction and Clinical Procedures

▶ Review medical history to determine premedication requirements.

▶ Review intraoral charting and radiographs. The intraoral chart and radiographs need review before any polishing procedures to locate all restorations. Some tooth-colored restorations are so artfully created and color matched that they are almost impossible to detect.

▶ After review, a plan for polishing can be made that includes the appropriate polishing agents for the restorations that are present.

▶ Practice biofilm control.

▶ Complete scaling, root planing, and overhang removal.

▶ Inform the patient that polishing is a cosmetic procedure, not a therapeutic one.

▶ After scaling and other periodontal treatment, an evaluation is made to determine the need for stain removal of teeth, polishing restorations, and dental prostheses.

▶ Check all restorations to ensure that the correct polishing agent has been selected.

▶ Explain the difference between cleaning and polishing agents.

B. Explain the Procedure

▶ Describe the noise, vibration, and grit of the polishing paste.

▶ Explain the frequent use of rinsing and evacuation with the saliva ejector.

C. Provide Protection for Patient

▶ Safety glasses worn for scaling are kept in place to prevent eye injury or infection.

▶ Fluid-resistant drape over patient to keep moisture from skin and clothing.

D. Patient Position

▶ The patient is positioned for maximum visibility.

E. Patient Breathing

▶ Encourage the patient to breath only through the nose.

▶ Reduce potential for aspiration of oral pathogens into the lungs.

▶ Allow water to pool for evacuation with saliva ejector.

▶ Less fogging of mouth mirror.

▶ Enhanced patient comfort.

II. Environmental Preparation

Environmental factors are described in Chapter 6.

A. Procedures to Lessen the Extent of Contaminated Aerosols

▶ Flush water through the tubing for 2 minutes at the beginning of each work period and for 30 seconds after each appointment.

▶ Request the patient rinse with an antimicrobial mouthrinse to reduce the numbers of oral microorganisms before starting instrumentation.

▶ Use high-velocity evacuation.

B. Protective Barriers

▶ Protective eyewear and bib are necessary for the patient.

▶ The clinician wears the standard barrier protection, namely, eyewear, mask, gloves, and clinic gown to cover clothing.

HISTORICAL PERSPECTIVE: THE PORTE POLISHER

▶ *Design*

● The porte polisher is a manual instrument designed especially for extrinsic stain removal or application of treatment agents such as for hypersensitive areas.

● It is constructed to hold a wood point at a contra-angle. The wood points may be cone or wedge shaped and made of various kinds of wood, preferably orangewood. Figure 45-2 illustrates a typical porte polisher.

▶ *Grasp:* The instrument is held in a modified pen grasp, Figure 39-16, or palm grasp, as shown in Figure 39-17 in Chapter 39.

▶ *Application:* The wood point is applied to the tooth surface using firm, carefully directed, massaging, circular or linear strokes to accommodate the anatomy of each tooth.

● A firm finger rest and a moderate amount of pressure of the wood point provide protection for the gingival margin and efficiency in technique.

▶ *Features*

● The porte polisher is useful for instrumentation of difficult-to-access surfaces of the teeth, especially malpositioned teeth.

● No heat generation, no noise compared with powered handpieces, and minimal production of aerosols.

● The porte polisher is readily portable and therefore is useful in any location, for example, for a bed bound patient.

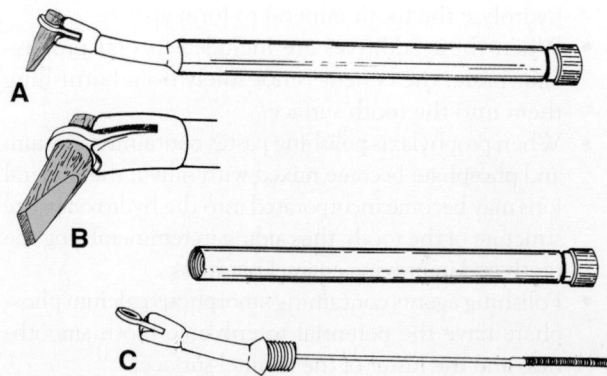

FIGURE 45-2 **Porte Polisher. A:** Assembled instrument shows position of wood point ready for instrumentation. **B:** Working end shows wedge-shaped wood point inserted. **C:** Disassembled, ready for autoclave.

THE POWER-DRIVEN INSTRUMENTS

I. Handpiece

▶ A handpiece is used to hold rotary instruments.

▶ The three basic designs are straight, contra-angle, and right angle.

▶ Instruments have been classified according to their rotational speeds, designated by revolutions per minute (rpm) as high speed and low (or slow) speed.

▶ Handpiece must be maintained and sterilized according to manufacturer's directions.

A. Ultra or High Speed

▶ *Speed*: 100,000–800,000 rpm; air driven.

▶ *Uses*: For cavity preparation and other restorative preparations.

▶ *Fiberoptic light*: Better visibility is provided when a fiberoptic light is built into the head of the handpiece. The beam of light is projected onto the field of operation when the handpiece is activated.

▶ Ultra and high-speed handpieces operate at very high speeds and therefore are *not* used for cleaning or polishing teeth with a prophylaxis angle and rubber cup.

B. Low Speed

▶ *Speed*: Typical range is up to 5,000 rpm for low-speed handpieces manufactured for dental hygienists. Other low-speed handpieces may have a higher range of rpms; air driven.

▶ Low speed handpieces are used for cleaning or polishing the teeth with a prophylaxis angle and rubber cup.

II. Types of Prophylaxis Angles

▶ Types of prophylaxis angles are described in Table 45-2.

▶ Contra- or right-angle attachments to the handpiece for which polishing devices (rubber cup, bristle brush) are available.

▶ Contra-angle prophylaxis angles may have a longer shank and a wider angle between the rubber cup and shank to allow for greater reach when polishing posterior teeth and surfaces.

▶ Disposable with rubber cup impregnated with polishing agent abrasive particles embedded in the rubber cup.[1]

▶ Stainless steel with hard chrome, carbon, steel, or brass bearings.

▶ Figure 45-3 shows examples of disposable for one-time use[37] contra-angle and right-angle prophylaxis angles and a stainless steel prophylaxis angle.

▶ Stainless steel prophylaxis angles that are sealed will not allow saliva and debris into the head of the angle nor will they allow grease and debris to leak out of the head of the angle.[38,39]

▶ Unless they are disposable, only instruments that can be sterilized are selected.

TABLE 45-2	Types of Prophylaxis Polishing Angles		
Comparison of disposable prophylaxis angles and stainless steel prophylaxis angles[a]			
TYPE OF ANGLE	**DISPOSABLE PROPHYLAXIS ANGLE**	**DISPOSABLE ANGLE WITH ABRASIVE IMPREGNATED RUBBER CUP**	**STAINLESS STEEL PROPHYLAXIS ANGLE**
Maintenance and care	One-time use, discard	One-time use, discard	Requires maintenance, sterilization
Attachments	Supplied with rubber cup from the manufacturer	Supplied with rubber cup from the manufacturer that is impregnated with one type of abrasive	Accepts variety of attachments: cups, brushes, and cone-shaped rubber points
Screw-in or snap-on rubber cups	Usually screw-in type cup		Will accept screw-in or snap-on cups and brushes
Advantages	Requires no maintenance or sterilization	Requires no additional prophylaxis paste	Can be used hundreds of times if maintained properly
Disadvantages	Not package with other attachments Creates refuse that is not biodegradable	Must have water and/or saliva as lubricant Creates refuse that is not biodegradable	Does require time to clean and maintain

[a]A comparison of the features of a disposable prophylaxis angle to a disposable prophylaxis angle with abrasive-impregnated rubber cup and a sterilizable stainless steel prophylaxis angle.

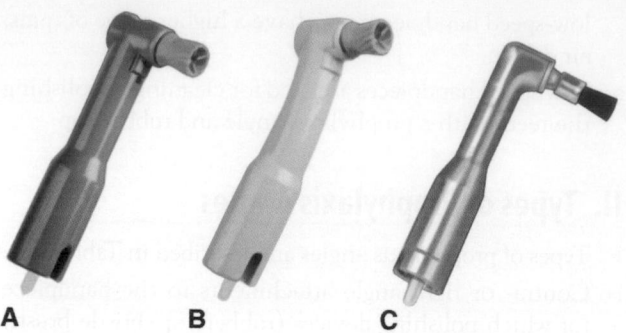

FIGURE 45-3 Prophylaxis Angles. A: Disposable right-angled prophylaxis angle with rubber cup attached. **B:** Disposable contra-angled prophylaxis angle with an attached rubber cup impregnated with a polishing agent (abrasive particles). **C:** Sterilizable stainless steel prophylaxis angle holding a cleaning or polishing brush on a mandrel.

- Stainless steel or any other type of metal autoclavable prophylaxis angle must be sterilized after every use and the manufacturer's instructions followed for the proper maintenance and care as well as the correct sterilization procedures.

III. Prophylaxis Angle Attachments

A. Rubber Polishing Cups

▶ *Types:* Figure 45-4 shows several types of rubber polishing cups from which to choose. The internal designs and sizes have the same purpose, which is to aid in holding the prophylaxis polishing paste in the rubber cup while polishing. The ideal rubber cup design retains the prophylaxis polishing paste in the cup and will release the paste at a steady rate.
  - *Slip-on (snap-on):* with ribbed cup to aid in holding polishing agent.

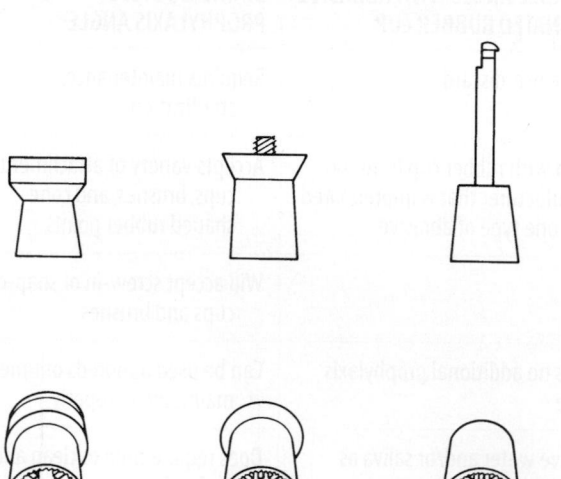

FIGURE 45-4 Rubber Cup Attachments. A: Slip-on or snap-on for button-ended prophylaxis angle. **B:** Threaded for direct insertion in right angle. **C:** Mandrel stem for latch-type prophylaxis angle.

- *Threaded (screw type):* with plain ribbed cup or flange (webbed) type.
- Mandrel mounted.
▶ *Materials*
  - *Natural rubber:* more resilient; adapts readily to fit the contours of the teeth.
  - *Synthetic:* stiffer than natural rubber.

B. Bristle Brushes

▶ *Types*
  - *For prophylaxis angle:* slip-on or screw type.
  - *For handpiece:* Mandrel mounted.
▶ *Materials:* synthetic.

C. Rubber Polishing Points

▶ Figure 45-5 shows an example of a rubber point that screws into a prophylaxis angle.
▶ *Material*
  - *Natural rubber:* Flexible so that tip adapts to proximal surfaces, embrasures, and around orthodontic bands and brackets.
▶ *Use:* Because the ribs for holding the prophylaxis polishing paste onto the rubber polishing point are on the external surface, the polishing paste will have to be reapplied frequently.

IV. Uses for Attachments

A. Handpiece with Straight Mandrel

▶ Dixon bristle brush (type C, soft) for polishing removable dentures.
▶ Rubber cup on mandrel for polishing facial surfaces of anterior teeth.

B. Prophylaxis Angle with Rubber Cup, Brush, or Rubber Point

▶ *Rubber cup:* for removal of stains from the tooth surfaces and polishing restorations.
▶ *Brush:* for removing stains from deep pits and fissures and enamel surfaces away from the gingival margin. A brush is contraindicated for use on exposed cementum or dentin.
▶ *Rubber polishing point:* for removing stains and biofilm from proximal surfaces, embrasures, and around orthodontic bands and brackets.

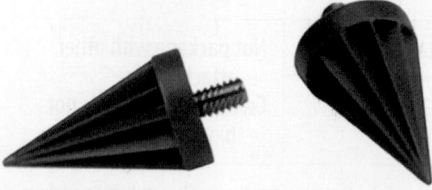

FIGURE 45-5 Flexible Rubber Point has Screw Connection for a Prophylaxis Angle. Made with ribs or grooves to carry cleaning or polishing agent to difficult-to-reach areas.

USE OF THE PROPHYLAXIS ANGLE

I. Effects on Tissues: Clinical Considerations

▶ Can cause discomfort for the patient if care and consideration for the oral tissues are not exercised to prevent unnecessary trauma.

▶ Tactile sensitivity of the clinician while using a thick, bulky handpiece is diminished and unnecessary pressure may be applied inadvertently.

▶ The greater the speed of application of a polishing agent, the faster the rate of abrasion. Therefore, the handpiece is applied at a low rpm.

▶ Trauma to the gingival tissue can result from too high a speed, extended application of the rubber cup, or use of an abrasive polishing agent.

▶ Tissue damage and the need for antibiotic premedication for risk patients are described in Chapter 10.

II. Prophylaxis Angle Procedure

▶ Apply the polishing agent only where it is needed, that is, where there is unsightly stain. See section Contraindications.

▶ As with all oral procedures, a systematic order is followed.

A. Instrument Grasp

▶ Modified pen grasp (Figure 39-16).

B. Finger Rest

▶ Establish a fulcrum firmly on tooth structure or use an exterior rest.

▶ Use a wide rest area when practical to aid in the balance of the large instrument. For example, place cushion of rest finger across occlusal surfaces of premolars while polishing the molars.

▶ Avoid use of mobile teeth as finger rests.

C. Speed of Handpiece

▶ Use lowest available speed to minimize frictional heat.

▶ Adjust rpm as necessary.

D. Use of Rheostat

▶ Apply steady pressure with foot to produce an even, low speed.

E. Rubber Cup: Stroke and Procedure

▶ Observe where stain removal is needed to prevent unnecessary rubber cup application.

▶ Fill rubber cup with polishing agent, and distribute agent over tooth surfaces to be polished before activating the power.

▶ Establish finger rest and bring rubber cup almost in contact with tooth surface before activating power source.

▶ Using slowest rpm, apply revolving cup at a 90° angle lightly to tooth surfaces for 1 or 2 seconds. Use a light pressure so that the edges of the rubber cup flare slightly. The rubber cup needs to flare slightly underneath the gingival margin and onto the proximal surfaces.

▶ Move cup to adjacent area on tooth surface; use a patting or brushing motion.

▶ Replenish supply of polishing agent frequently.

▶ Turn handpiece to adapt rubber cup to fit each surface of the tooth, including proximal surfaces and gingival surfaces of fixed partial dentures.

▶ Start with the distal surface of the most posterior tooth of a quadrant and move forward toward the anterior; polish only the teeth that require stain removal. For each tooth, work from the gingival third toward the incisal third of the tooth.

▶ When two polishing agents of different abrasiveness are to be applied, use a separate rubber cup for each.

▶ Rubber cups, polishing points, and polishing brushes cannot be sterilized and are used only for one patient and then discarded.

F. Rubber Polishing Points (Figure 45-5)

▶ Rubber polishing points can be used around orthodontic bands and brackets, on fixed bridges and in wide interproximal spaces or embrasures.

▶ Rubber points are loaded with the cleaning or polishing agent in the grooves around the sides. The rubber points will need to be replenished frequently with paste after use on every 1–2 teeth.

G. Bristle Brush

▶ Bristle brushes are used selectively and limited to occlusal surfaces.

▶ Lacerations of the gingiva and grooves and scratches in the tooth surface, particularly the roots and restorations can result when the brush is not used with caution.

▶ Soak stiff brush in hot water to soften bristles.

▶ Distribute mild abrasive polishing agent over occlusal surfaces of teeth to be polished.

▶ Place fingers of nondominant hand in a position that both retracts and protects cheek and tongue from the revolving brush.

▶ Establish a firm finger rest and bring brush almost in contact with the tooth before activating power source.

▶ Use slowest rpm as the revolving brush is applied lightly to the occlusal surfaces only. Avoid contact of the bristles with the soft tissues.

▶ Use a short stroke in a brushing motion; follow the inclined planes of the cusps.

▶ Move from tooth to tooth to prevent generation of excessive frictional heat. Avoid overuse of the brush. Replenish supply of polishing agent frequently.

H. Irrigation

▶ Irrigate teeth and interdental areas thoroughly several times with water from the syringe to remove abrasive particles. Avoid heavy water pressure to prevent forcing particles into the tissue.

▶ The rotary movement of the rubber cup or bristle brush tends to force the abrasive into the gingival sulci, thereby creating a potential source of irritation to the soft tissues.

POLISHING PROXIMAL SURFACES

▶ Care must be exercised in the use of floss, tape, and finishing strips.

▶ Understanding the anatomy of the interdental papillae and their relationship to the contact areas and proximal surfaces of the teeth is prerequisite to the prevention of tissue damage.

▶ As much polishing as possible of accessible proximal surfaces is accomplished during the use of the rubber cup in the prophylaxis angle.

▶ This can be followed by the use of dental tape with polishing agent when indicated.

▶ Finishing strips are used only in selected instances, when all other techniques fail to remove a stain.

I. Dental Tape and Floss

A. Features

▶ Floss and tape are described in Chapter 29.

▶ The wax covering affords some protection for the tissues, facilitates the movement of the floss or tape, prevents excessive absorption of moisture, and helps prevent shredding.

▶ Dental tape is flat and has relatively sharp edges, whereas floss is round. Either floss or tape may injure the tissue when used incorrectly or carelessly.

▶ The use of dental floss or tape for dental biofilm control on proximal tooth surfaces is an essential part of self-care by the patient.

B. Uses During Cleaning and Polishing

▶ Techniques for tape and floss application are described in Chapter 29 and illustrated in Figures 29-4, 29-5, and 29-6.

▶ The same principles apply whether the patient or the clinician is using the floss.

▶ Finger rests are used to prevent snapping through contact areas.

▶ *Stain removal with dental tape:* Polishing agent is applied to the tooth, and the tape is moved gently back and forth and up and down curved over the area where stain was observed.

▶ *Cleaning gingival surface of a fixed partial denture:* A floss threader is used to position the floss or tape over the gingival surface. Floss threaders are described and illustrated in Chapter 32 in Figure 32-3. The agent is applied under the pontic, and the floss or tape is moved back and forth with contact on the bridge surface.

▶ *Flossing:* Particles of abrasive agent can be removed by rinsing and by using a clean length of floss applied in the usual manner.

▶ *Rinsing and irrigation:* Irrigate with water-spray syringe to clean out all abrasive agent.

II. Finishing Strips

A. Description

▶ Finishing strips are thin, flexible, and tape shaped.

▶ Available in four widths: extra narrow, narrow, medium, and wide.

▶ Available in extra fine, fine, medium, and coarse grit. *Only extra narrow or narrow strips with extrafine or fine grit are suggested for stain removal, and then only with discretion.*

▶ Most finishing strips are now made of plastic; however, linen abrasive strips are available. Finishing strips have one side that is smooth and the other side serves as a carrier for abrasive agents bonded to that side.

▶ "Gapped" strips are available with an abrasive-free portion to permit sliding the strip through a contact area without abrading the enamel.

▶ Finishing strips are available with two different grits on one strip. One-half of the strip may have fine abrasives and the other one-half will have medium grit abrasives. These strips are available in several different combinations.

B. Use

▶ *For stain removal on proximal surfaces of anterior teeth; when other techniques are unsuccessful.*

▶ *Precautions for use*

• Edge of strip is sharp and may cut gingival tissue or the lip.

• Use of a finishing strip is limited to enamel surfaces and some restorative materials, such as composite. It is of upmost importance to ensure the finishing strip selected has an appropriate grit abrasive for the surface to be polished. Manufacturers make finishing strips intended for use solely on composites or porcelain; other types of finishing strips are available for use on enamel.

C. Technique for Finishing Strip

▶ *Grasp and finger rest*

• A strip no longer than 6 inches is most conveniently applied.

• Grasp and finger rest must be well controlled.

• Protection of the lip by retraction with the thumb and index finger holding the strip is a helpful safety measure.

▶ *Positioning*
- Direct the abrasive side of the strip toward the proximal surface to be treated as the strip is worked slowly and gently between the teeth with a slight sawing motion.
- Bring strip just through the contact area. If the strip breaks, immediately use floss to remove abrasive particles that may have separated from the finishing strip.
- When a space is clearly visible through an embrasure and the interdental papilla is missing, a narrow finishing strip may be threaded through. Prepare strip by cutting the end on a diagonal to facilitate threading.

▶ *Stain removal*
- Press abrasive side of strip against tooth. Draw back and forth in a 1/8-inch arc two or three times, rocking on the established fulcrum.
- Remove strip. Do not attempt to turn the strip while it is in the interdental area.

▶ *Dental floss:* Follow each application of a finishing strip with dental floss to remove abrasive particles.

AIR-POWDER POLISHING

▶ Principles of selective stain removal are applied to the use of the air-powder polishing system. After biofilm control instruction, instrumentation, and periodontal debridement are completed, follow with an evaluation of need for stain removal.

I. Principles of Application

▶ Air-powder systems manufactured by several companies are efficient and effective methods for mechanical removal of stain and biofilm.[40,41]
▶ Air-powder polishing systems use air, water, and specially formulated powders to deliver a controlled spray that propels the particles to the tooth surface.
- Only powders approved by each air-powder polishing manufacturer are used in each brand of air-powder polishing unit. The use of an unapproved powder in an air-powder polishing unit could void the warranty on the unit.[42]
▶ The equipment is operated using inlet air pressure between 40 and 100 psi and inlet water pressure between 20 and 60 psi. Internal air polishing unit air and water pressures will vary according to manufacturer and are not to be adjusted from their original settings.
▶ The handpiece nozzle is moved in a constant circular motion, with the nozzle tip 4–5 mm away from the enamel surface.
▶ The spray is angled away from the gingival margin.
▶ The periphery of the spray may be near the gingival margin, but the center is directed at an angle less than 90° away from the margin.

▶ Complete directions for care of equipment and preparation for use of the device are provided by the individual manufacturer.

II. Specially Formulated Powders for Use in Air-Powder Polishing

Several manufacturers make and sell air-powder polishing powders.
▶ The abrasiveness of one brand of powder may differ from another brand, even though it is the same type of powder.[43]

A. Sodium Bicarbonate[42]

▶ Sodium bicarbonate is the original powder used in air-powder polishing.
▶ It is specially formulated with scant amounts of calcium phosphate and silica to keep it free flowing.
▶ The Mohs hardness number for sodium bicarbonate is 2.5 and the particles average 74 μm in size.
▶ Warning: over-the-counter sodium bicarbonate cannot be used in airpolishing equipment as it will clog the unit.
▶ The *only* type of sodium bicarbonate that can be used in air-powder polishing units is the type specially formulated for air-powder polishing.
▶ Sodium bicarbonate air-powder is available with flavorings. However, the patient will taste the salt and smell the flavor.

B. Aluminum Trihydroxide

▶ Aluminum trihydroxide was the first air-powder developed as an alternative to sodium bicarbonate for patients who are sodium bicarbonate intolerant.[44]
▶ Aluminum trihydroxide has a Mohs hardness value of 4 and the particles range in size from 80 to 325 μm.

C. Glycine

▶ Glycine is an amino acid. For use in powders, glycine crystals are grown using a solvent of water and sodium salt.
▶ Glycine particles for use in airpolishing have a Mohs hardness number of 2 and are 20 μm in size.

D. Calcium Carbonate

▶ Calcium carbonate is a naturally occurring substance that can be found in rocks.
▶ It is a main ingredient in antacids, and is also used as filler for pharmaceutical drugs.
▶ Calcium carbonate has a Mohs number of 3.[42]

E. Calcium Sodium Phosphosilicate (Novamin)

▶ Calcium sodium phosphosilicate (Novamin) is a bioactive glass and has a Mohs hardness number of 6, making it the hardest air polishing particle used in air-powder polishing powders.[42] The particles vary from 25 to 120 μm in size.

▶ Since calcium sodium phosphosilicate was first introduced, research on the effects of this air polishing powder has determined that it is highly abrasive and destructive to enamel, hybrid composites, and glass ionomers. The investigators concluded this powder should not be used on any tooth structure or restorative material.[44]

III. Uses and Advantages of Air-Powder Polishing

▶ Requires less time, is ergonomically favorable to the clinician, and generates no heat.[40–42,45]

▶ Sodium bicarbonate is less abrasive than traditional prophylaxis pastes, which makes the air-powder polisher ideal for stain and biofilm removal. However, some air-polishing powders are much more abrasive than sodium bicarbonate and should only be used on surfaces that they will not damage.[42]

▶ Removal of heavy, tenacious tobacco stain and chlorhexidine-induced staining.[40–42,45]

▶ Stain and biofilm removal from orthodontically banded and bracketed teeth[45,46,47] and dental implants.[48,49]

▶ Before sealant placement or other bonding procedures.[21,22]

▶ Root detoxification for periodontally diseased roots by the periodontist during open periodontal surgery.[50,51]

IV. Technique

Proper angulation of the air-powder polishing handpiece is essential to reduce the amount of inherent aerosols created[52–54] and to remove stain and biofilm without iatrogenic soft tissue trauma.

A. For Anterior Teeth

▶ Place the handpiece nozzle at a 60° angle to the facial and lingual surfaces of anterior teeth (Figure 45-6A).

B. For Posterior Teeth

▶ Place the handpiece nozzle at an 80° angle to the facial and lingual surfaces (Figure 45-6B).

C. For Occlusal Surfaces

▶ Place the handpiece nozzle at a 90° angle to the occlusal plane (Figure 45-6C).

D. Incorrect Angulation

▶ Incorrect angulation of the handpiece is probably the single most common cause of excess aerosol production.

▶ The handpiece nozzle is never directed into the gingival sulcus or into a periodontal pocket with little bony support remaining, as this could result in facial emphysema[42] (also known as a subcutaneous emphysema).

▶ Facial emphysemas occur due to the abnormal introduction of air into subcutaneous tissues or interstitial spaces.[42]

▶ Facial emphysemas can be prevented by avoiding the use of high-speed handpieces during third molar extractions,[55] air/water syringes near extraction or surgical sites or lacerations,[56–59] and airpolishing[60,61] spray in these areas.

▶ Facial emphysemas exhibit symptoms such as facial swelling, a "crackling" sensation of the face and neck area when touched, tenderness, and pain. If detected early, patients with facial emphysemas usually require observation, antibiotics, and analgesia.[42]

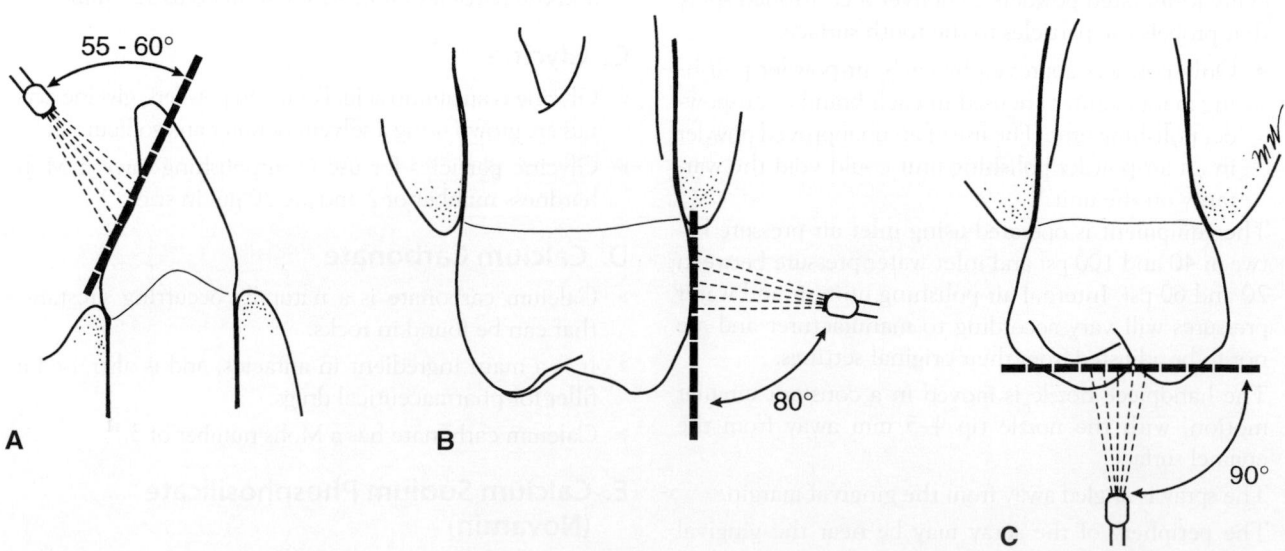

FIGURE 45-6 Air-Powder Polishing. Direct the aerosolized spray for **A:** the anterior teeth at a 60° angle. **B:** The posterior teeth facial and lingual or palatal at an 80° angle. **C:** The occlusal surfaces at a 90° angle to the occlusal plane.

Sequelae that Can Develop as a Result of Compressed Air Forced into Soft Tissues of the Head and Neck

Bilateral pneumothorax
Cerebral air embolism
Cervicofacial emphysema
Facial emphysema
Mediastinal emphysema
Pneumediastinum
Pneumothorax
Retropharyngeal emphysema

Sequelae that Can Develop as a Result of Facial Emphysema

Bilateral pneumothorax
Cerebral air embolism
Embolism
Pneumediastinum
Pneumothorax
Thrombosis

- Box 45-2 Contains a list of the sequelae that can develop as a result of compressed air forced into soft tissues of the head and neck.
- Box 45-3 contains a list of sequelae that can develop as a result of a facial emphysema.
▶ The closer the nozzle is held to the enamel, the more spray will deflect back into the direction of the clinician.
▶ When a clinician directs the handpiece at a 90° angle toward a facial, buccal, and some lingual surfaces, the result is an immediate reflux of the aerosolized spray back onto the clinician.
▶ Changing the angle of incidence to the proper angulations of 60° and 80° will result in a change in the angle of the reflection, thus reducing the amount of reflux of aerosolized spray.

V. Recommendations and Precautions

A. Aerosol Production

A copious spray containing oral debris and microorganisms is produced. As with all contaminated aerosols, a health hazard can exist. Suggestions for minimizing contamination and the effects of the aerosols include the following:
▶ Patient uses a preprocedural antibacterial mouthrinse.[62]
▶ High-volume evacuation is needed, using a wide tip held near the tooth where the spray is released from the nozzle or using a high-volume scavenger attachment for a high-volume evacuation suction tip or saliva ejector.[52–54]

B. Protective Patient and Clinician Procedures

▶ Use protective eyewear, protective gown, and hair cover.
▶ Lubricate patient's lips to prevent drying effect of the sodium bicarbonate using a nonpetroleum lip lubricant.
▶ Do not direct the spray on the gingiva, directly into the gingival sulcus or other soft tissues, which can create patient discomfort, undue tissue trauma, or more seriously, a facial emphysema.
▶ Avoid directing the spray into periodontal pockets with bone loss or into extraction sites as a facial emphysema can be induced.

VI. Risk Patients: Air-Powder Polishing Contraindicated

The information from the patient's medical history is used and appropriate applications made. Antibiotic premedication is indicated for all the same patients who are at risk for any dental hygiene procedure (Chapter 10).

A. Contraindications[42]

▶ Physician-directed sodium-restricted diet (only for sodium bicarbonate powder).
▶ Respiratory disease or other condition that limits swallowing or breathing, such as chronic obstructive pulmonary disease.
▶ Patients with end-stage renal disease, Addison's disease or Cushing's disease.
▶ Communicable infection that can contaminate the aerosols produced.
▶ Immunocompromised patients.
▶ Patients taking potassium, antidiuretics, or steroid therapy.
▶ Patients who have open oral wounds, such as tooth sockets, from oral surgery procedures.

B. Other Contraindications

▶ *Root surfaces:* Avoid routine polishing of cementum and dentin.
  - There is some evidence they can be removed readily during air-powder polishing.[63]
  - However, much more research on the effect of air polishing and the removal of cementum and dentin needs to be conducted.
▶ *Soft, spongy gingiva:* The air-powder can irritate the free gingival tissue, especially if not used with the recommended technique.
  - When heavy stain calls for the use of an air-powder polisher, instruct the patient in daily bacterial biofilm removal.
  - Following scaling and periodontal debridement, postpone the stain removal until soft tissue has healed.

TABLE 45-3	Recommendations for Use of Air Polishing on Restorative Materials	
	POLISHING POWDER CONTAINING	
RESTORATIVE MATERIAL	SODIUM BICARBONATE	ALUMINUM TRIHYDROXIDE
Amalgam	Yes	No
Gold	Yes[a]	No
Porcelain	Yes[a]	No
Hybrid composite	No	No
Microfilled composite	No	No
Glass ionomer	No	No
Compomer	No	No
Luting agents	No	No

[a]Only if margin is avoided.

▶ *Restorative materials:* The use of air-powder polishing on composite resins, cements, and other nonmetallic materials can cause removal or pitting.[18,19,25,63]

- Table 45-3 provides a guide as to which restorative materials can be safely treated with air-powder polishing agents, the sodium bicarbonate powder, and the aluminum trihydroxide powder.[37]
- Significant damage to margins of dental castings has been shown.[50]

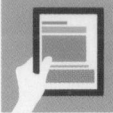

BOX 45-4

Example Documentation: Selection of Polishing Agent for a Patient with Esthetic Restorations

S–A 36-year-old male patient presents for regular maintenance appointment, grinning to show that his new implant crown and other esthetic restorations are not distinguishable from the color of his teeth. Updated medical history, medications, no changes.

O–Blood pressure (115/75); extra-intraoral exams no findings periodontal examination with complete probing localized 3–4 mm, with BOP in 4 mm pockets in molar areas with supragingival calculus mand ant.; minimal biofilm with sparse and isolated areas of yellowish staining.

A–Checked his dental records for the material used for the various restorations and found that the patient has porcelain crowns on teeth numbers #2, 14, and anterior microhybrid composite restorations in teeth numbers #6, 7, 8, 10, and 11. Patient has an implant and porcelain crown on #9. Note: Microhybrid composite restorations and implant crown match the patient's natural teeth to the extent that it is difficult to identify the restorations.

P–Gave patient new toothbrush with tongue cleaner on back, and demonstrated the tongue cleaner. Went over places he had been missing on his teeth and gingiva. Calculus removal. Avoided use of airpolishing with sodium bicarbonate (the only powder I have available) and also avoided prophy paste. Selected a cleaning agent to remove biofilm and isolated areas of yellowish staining.

Next regular appointment 4 months made at front desk.

Signed _____, RDH

Date _____

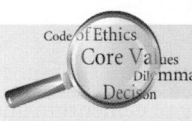

EVERYDAY ETHICS

Mr. Jackson, the 62-year-old chief executive officer of a major oil company, presents for his routine 3-month maintenance with Carol, his dental hygienist of several years. Mr. Jackson is meticulous about his appearance and is always handsomely dressed. He is well-known internationally and frequently seen in the news media being interviewed and having pictures taken for news articles.

Mr. Jackson had a complete cosmetic restoration of his teeth a year ago. Previously his teeth had been stained by the numerous cups of tea he drank every day. He has had porcelain veneers placed on his maxillary anterior teeth, and all restorations are now tooth colored. The color match of the restorations to his teeth is perfect. Unfortunately, Mr. Jackson has not cut back on drinking tea and during her assessment, Carol notes that generalized stain is starting to

discolor most of the new restorations. Before the cosmetic restorations were placed, Carol used a coarse prophy paste to eliminate the tea stains and now Mr. Jackson asks her to "just use that gritty stuff again." He states that he absolutely does not want his teeth to appear stained.

Questions for Consideration

1. What role does each of the dental hygiene core values play as Carol contemplates a course of action to take in this situation?

2. What alternative actions are available that would respect Mr. Jackson's rights as well as allow Carol to provide treatment that meets standards of care?

3. What financial or legal considerations will Carol need to consider as she determines her course of action?

DOCUMENTATION

Documentation for a patient receiving tooth stain removal as part of the dental hygiene care plan for a maintenance appointment would include a minimum of the following:

▶ Review patient medical history with questions to determine health problems, recent medical examinations and treatments, and changes in medications.

▶ *Current clinical examination findings*: intraoral, extraoral, periodontal, and dental.

▶ *With dental charting*: identification of dental materials used in restorations that can influence choice of polishing agents. Identification would require use of radiographs and the intraoral dental charting.

▶ Dental hygiene examination for state of patient's personal daily self-care, calculus and biofilm deposits, sources for dental stains, products used for oral care, and dietary factors influencing the dentition and all oral tissues: questions answered about best choices for various products.

▶ A sample progress note may be reviewed in Box 45-4.

Factors to Teach the Patient

▷ How dental biofilm and stains form on the natural teeth and their replacements.

▷ The meaning of selective polishing and why it is not necessary to polish all teeth at every appointment when daily care is effective.

▷ Stains and biofilm removed by polishing can return promptly if biofilm is not removed faithfully on a schedule of two or three times each day.

▷ Polishing agents used during professional coronal polishing are too abrasive for daily home use.

References

1. Barnes CM. The science of polishing. *Dimensions Dent Hyg.* 2009;7(11):18–20, 22.

2. Liljeborg A, Tellefsen G, Johannsen G. The use of a profilometer for both quantitative and qualitative measurements of toothpaste abrasivity. *Int J Dent Hyg.* 2010;8(3):237–243.

3. American Academy of Periodontology. *Glossary of Periodontal Terms.* 3rd ed. Chicago, IL: American Academy of Periodontology; 1992:40.

4. American Dental Hygienists' Association. *Position Paper on the Oral Prophylaxis.* Chicago, IL: ADHA; 1998. www.adha.org/profissues/prophylaxis.htm.

5. Jeffries SR. Abrasive finishing and polishing in restorative dentistry: a state-of-the-art review. *Dent Clin North Am.* 2007;51(2):379–397.

6. Hutchings IM. Abrasion process in wear and manufacturing. *Proc Inst Mech Eng Part J: J Eng Tribol.* 2002;216(2):55–62.

7. Rémond G, Nockolds C, Phillips M, et al. Implications of polishing techniques in quantitative x-ray microanalysis. *J Res Natl Inst Stand Technol.* 2002;107(6):639–662.

8. Williams JA. Wear and wear particles: some fundamentals. *Tribiol Int.* 2005;38(10):863–870.

9. Fine DH, Furgang D, McKiernan M, et al. An investigation of the effect of an essential oil mouthrinse on induced bacteraemia: a pilot study. *J Clin Periodontol.* 2010;37(9):840–847.

10. Lucas V, Roberts GJ. Odontogenic bacteremia following tooth cleaning procedures in children. *Pediatr Dent.* 2000;22(2):96–100.

11. Cristina ML, Spagnolo AM, Sartini M, et al. Investigation of organizational and hygiene features in dentistry: a pilot study. *J Prev Med Hyg.* 2009;50(3):175–180.

12. Farrier SL, Farrier JN, Gilmour AS. Eye safety in operative dentistry: a study in dental practice. *Br Dent J.* 006;200(4):218–223.

13. Featherstone JD. Prevention and reversal of dental caries: role of low level fluoride. *Community Dent Oral Epidemiol.* 1999;27(1):31–40.

14. Honório HM, Rios D, Abdo RC, et al. Effect of different prophylaxis methods on sound and demineralized enamel. *J Appl Oral Sci.* 2006;14(2):117–123.

15. Kubinek R, Zapletalova Z, Vujtek M, et al. Examination of dentin surface using AFM and SEM. In: Méndez-Vilas A, Díaz J, eds. *Modern Research and Educational Topics in Microscopy,* Vol. 2. Zurbarán, Spain: Formatex; 2007:593–598.

16. Miglani S, Aggarwal V, Ahuja B. Dentin hypersensitivity: recent trends in management. *J Conserv Dent.* 2010;13(4):218–224.

17. Anusavice KJ. Finishing and polishing materials. In: Anusavice KJ, ed. *Phillips' Science of Dental Materials.* 11th ed. St Louis, IL: Saunders; 2003:352.

18. Barnes CM. Polishing esthetic restorative materials. *Dimensions Dent Hyg.* 2010;8(1):24, 26–28.

19. Barnes CM. Care and maintenance of esthetic restorations. *J Prac Hyg.* 2004;14:19–22.

20. Essex GA. Predilection for polishing. *Dimensions Dent Hyg.* 2005;3(3):36, 38.

21. Scott L, Greer D. The effect of an air polishing device on sealant bond strength. *J Prosthet Dent.* 1987;58(3):384–387.

22. Ahovuo-Saloranta A, Hiiri A, Nordblad A, et al. Pit and fissure sealants for preventing dental decay in the permanent teeth of children and adolescents. *Cochrane Database Syst Rev.* 2008;4:CD001830. Review.

23. Azarpazhooh A, Main PA. Efficacy of dental prophylaxis (rubber cup) for the prevention of caries and gingivitis: a systematic review of literature. *Br Dent J.* 2009;207(7):E14.

24. Barnes CM, Covey DA, Walker MP, et al. Essential selective polishing: the maintenance of aesthetic restorations. *J Prac Hyg.* 2003;12(5):18–24.

25. Putt MS, Kleber CJ, Davis JA, et al. Physical characteristics of a new cleaning and polishing agent for use in a prophylaxis paste. *J Dent Res.* 1975;54(3):527–534.

26. Putt MS, Kleber CJ, Muhler JC. Enamel polish and abrasion by prophylaxis pastes. *J Dent Hyg.* 1982;56(9):38, 40–43.

27. Barnes CM. Adapting polishing procedures to maintain aesthetic restorations. *J Prac Hyg.* 2005;15:22.

28. United States Pharmacopeia. *The National Formulary.* Rockville, MD: United States Pharmacopeia Convention; 1995:1342.

29. Burrell KH, Chan JT. Fluorides. In: *American Dental Association, Council on Scientific Affairs: ADA Guide to Dental Therapeutics.* 3rd ed. Chicago, IL: ADA; 2003:238.

30. Tung MS, Eichmiller FC. Amorphous calcium phosphates for tooth mineralization. *Compend Contin Educ Dent.* 2004;25 (9, Suppl 1):9–13.

31. Tung M, Malerman R, Huang S, et al. Reactivity of prophylaxis paste containing calcium phosphate and fluoride salts. *J Dent Res.* 2005;84 (Special Issue A). Abstract #2156, IADR Abstracts, 2005.

32. Daniels A. Professionally applied enhanced polishing agents. *J Prac Hyg.* 2006;15:26.

33. Wolff MS, Kleinberg I. Duration of reduction of dentinal hypersensitivity after prophylaxis with a calcium/arginine bicarbonate carbonate paste. *J Dent Res.* 2003;82 (Special Issue A). Abstract 180.

34. Canadian Advisory Board on Dentin Hypersensitivity. Consensus-based recommendations for the diagnosis and management of dentin hypersensitivity. *J Can Dent Assoc.* 2003;69(4):221–226.

35. Addy M. Dentine hypersensitivity: new perspectives on an old problem. *Int Dent J* 2002;52 (5, Suppl 1):367–375.

36. Mattana D. Reducing dentin Hypersensitivity. *J Prac Hyg.* 2006;15:24.

37. Barnes CM, Fleming LS. An in vitro evaluation of commercially available disposable prophylaxis angles. *J Dent Hyg.* 1991;65(9):438–441.

38. Barnes CM, Anderson NA, Li Y, et al. Effectiveness of steam sterilization in killing spores of *Bacillus stearothermophilus* in prophylaxis angles. *Gen Dent.* 1994;42(5):456–458.

39. Barnes CM, Anderson NA, Michalek SM, et al. Effectiveness of sealed dental prophylaxis angles inoculated with *Bacillus stearothermophilus* in preventing leakage. *J Clin Dent.* 1994;5(2):35–37.

40. Gutmann ME. Air polishing: a comprehensive review of the literature. *J Dent Hyg.* 1998;72(3):47–56.

41. Weaks LM, Lescher NB, Barnes CM, et al. Clinical evaluation of the Prophy-Jet as an instrument for routine removal of tooth stain and plaque. *J Periodontol.* 1984;55(8):486–488.

42. Barnes CM. An in-depth look at air polishing. *Dimensions Dent Hyg.* 2010;8(3):32, 34–36.

43. Barnes CM, Covey DA, Walker MP, et al. An in vitro evaluation of the effects of aluminum trihydroxide delivered via the Prophy Jet on dental restorative materials. *J Prosthet Dent.* 2004;13(3):166–172.

44. Barnes CM, Covey DA, Watanabe H, et al. An in vitro comparison of the effects of various airpolishing powders on enamel and selected esthetic restorative materials. *J Clin Dent.* 2014;25(4):76-87.

45. Orton GS. Clinical use of an air-powder abrasive system. *Dent Hyg.* 1987;61(11):513–518.

46. Barnes CM, Russell CM, Gerbo LR, et al. Effects of an air-powder polishing system on orthodontically bracketed and banded teeth. *Am J Orthod Dentofac Orthop.* 1990;97(1):74–81.

47. Shultz PH, Brockmann-Bell SL, Eick JD, et al. Effects of air-powder polishing on the bond strength of orthodontic bracket adhesive systems. *J Dent Hyg.* 1993;67(2):74–80.

48. Barnes CM, Fleming LS, Mueninghoff LA. An SEM evaluation of the in-vitro effects of an air-abrasive system on various implant surfaces. *Int J Oral Maxillofac Implants.* 1991;6(4):463–469.

49. Barnes CM, Toothaker RW, Ross J. Polishing dental implants and dental implant restorations. *J Prac Hyg.* 2005;14(8):6–8.

50. Berkstein S, Reiff RL, McKinney JF, et al. Supragingival root surface removal during maintenance procedures utilizing an air-powder abrasive system or hand scaling: an in vitro study. *J Periodontol.* 1987;58(5):327–330.

51. Agger MS, Hörsted-Bindslev P, Hovgaard O. Abrasiveness of an air-powder polishing system on root surfaces in vitro. *Quintessence Int.* 2001;32(5):407–411.

52. Barnes CM. The management of aerosols with airpolishing delivery systems. *J Dent Hyg.* 1991;65(6):280–282.

53. Harrel SK, Barnes JB, Rivera-Hidalgo F. Aerosol reduction during air polishing. *Quintessence Int.* 1999;30(9):623–628.

54. Worrall SF, Knibbs PJ, Glenwright HD. Methods of reducing bacterial contamination of the atmosphere arising from use of an air-polisher. *Br Dent J.* 1987;163(4):118, 119.

55. Davies DE. Pneumomediastinum after dental surgery. *Anaesth Intensive Care.* 2001;29(6):638–641.

56. Tan WK. Sudden facial swelling: subcutaneous facial emphysema secondary to use of air/water syringe during dental extraction. *Singapore Dent J.* 2000;23 (1, Suppl):42–44.

57. Josephson GD, Wambach BA, Noordzji JP. Subcutaneous cervicofacial and mediastinal emphysema after dental instrumentation. *Otolaryngol Head Neck Surg.* 2001;124(2):170, 171.

58. Yang SC, Chiu TH, Lin TJ, et al. Subcutaneous emphysema and pneumomediastinum secondary to dental extraction: a case report and literature review. *Kaohsiung J Med Sci.* 2006;22(12):641–645.

59. Heyman SN, Babayof I. Emphysematous complications in dentistry, 1960–1993: an illustrative case and review of the literature. *Quintessence Int.* 1995;26(8):535–543.

60. Arai I, Aoki T, Yamazaki H, et al. Pneumomediastinum and subcutaneous emphysema after dental extraction detected incidentally by regular medical checkup: a case report. *Oral Surg Oral Med Oral Pathol Oral Radiol Endod.* 2009;107(4):e33–e38.

61. Finlayson RS, Stevens FD. Subcutaneous facial emphysema secondary to use of the Cavi-Jet. *J Periodontol.* 1988;59(5):315–317.

62. Fine DH, Mendieta C, Barnett ML, et al. Efficacy of preprocedural rinsing with an antiseptic in reducing viable bacteria in dental aerosols. *J Periodontol.* 1992;63(10):821–824.

63. Atkinson DR, Cobb CM, Killoy WJ. The Effect of an air-powder abrasive system on in vitro root surfaces. *J Periodontol.* 1984;55(1):13–18.

ENHANCE YOUR UNDERSTANDING

thePoint® **DIGITAL CONNECTIONS**
(see the inside front cover for access information)
- **Audio glossary**
- **Quiz bank**

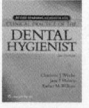

SUPPORT FOR LEARNING
(available separately; visit lww.com)
- *Active Learning Workbook for Clinical Practice of the Dental Hygienist, 12th Edition*

prepU **INDIVIDUALIZED REVIEW**
(available separately; visit lww.com)
- **Adaptive quizzing with *prepU for Wilkins' Clinical Practice of the Dental Hygienist***

46

Tooth Bleaching

Pamela S. Kennard, BSN, CRDH, MA

CHAPTER OUTLINE

LEARNING OBJECTIVES

After studying this chapter, the student will be able to:

1. Discuss the mechanism, safety, and efficacy of tooth bleaching agents.

2. Identify specific tooth conditions and staining responses to tooth bleaching.

3. Discuss reversible and irreversible side effects associated with the tooth bleaching process.

4. List appropriate interventions for tooth bleaching side effects.

INTRODUCTION

Patients of all ages have concerns about the appearance of their teeth and expect their dental hygienists to provide information to guide them in their esthetic choices. Because there are many causes of tooth discoloration, a review of Chapter 22 is recommended.

▶ Tooth bleaching may improve a patient's appearance and contribute to a patient's self-confidence.

▶ A whiter smile may motivate the patient to maintain improved oral health, which is a significant benefit.

I. Bleaching Versus Whitening

The terms bleaching and whitening have been used interchangeably, but two separate descriptions can define them more accurately.[1]

▶ Tooth whitening refers to use of abrasive agents contained in a dentifrice to remove extrinsic stain.

▶ Bleaching involves free radicals and the breakdown of pigment, which occurs in the tooth bleaching procedures.

▶ Key words and abbreviations are defined in Box 46-1.

II. Vital Tooth Bleaching Versus Nonvital Tooth Bleaching

▶ External tooth bleaching is used for both vital and nonvital teeth.

▶ Vital teeth can be stained intrinsically and extrinsically.

▶ Agents for bleaching are applied to the external surfaces of the teeth.

▶ Color change can extend into the dentin to produce a whitened tooth.

▶ Nonvital teeth become intrinsically stained by blood breakdown products, or agents from root canal therapy.[1]

▶ Nonvital tooth bleaching is a procedure performed by a dentist after root canal therapy using rubber dam or other type of isolation.

 • The bleaching agents are introduced into the pulp chamber.

 • The color of a single tooth is lightened to help it blend with the adjacent teeth.

III. History

A. Nonvital Tooth Bleaching History

▶ Bleaching of discolored, nonvital teeth was first described as early as 1864.[2,3]

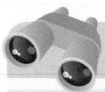

BOX 46-1   KEY WORDS: Tooth Bleaching

Bleaching: a cosmetic dental procedure that uses free radicals and breakdown of pigments to whiten teeth.

Block-out resins: light-cured resin materials that can be used as a rubber dam substitute during bleaching procedure or on study models to create space to hold bleaching material on custom trays.

Color: a phenomenon of light or visual perception that enables the differentiation of otherwise identical objects. Usually determined visually by measurement of hue, saturation, and luminous reflectance of light.

Esthetic: pertaining to the study of beauty and the sense of beautiful; objectifies beauty and attractiveness, elicits pleasure.

Extrinsic: external, extraneous, as originating from or on the outside.

Iatrogenic: resulting from the activity of a clinician; disorders induced in a patient by the clinician.

Intrinsic: from within, incorporation of a colorant within a material.

Laser bleaching and ultraviolet light system: dental office procedure that uses light in combination with hydrogen peroxide to activate bleaching materials and reduce the time necessary to produce a lighter color of teeth; use of

rubber dam or protective light-cured resin on soft tissue required during use, as well as eye protection.

Microabrasion: a proven method for treating tooth discolorations by microreduction of superficial enamel through various methods of mechanical and/or chemical actions.

NGVB: acronym for night guard vital bleaching, which requires development of a custom tray that allows for administration and containment of tooth bleaching material such as carbamide peroxide or hydrogen peroxide.

Potassium nitrate: active ingredient in many antisensitivity dentifrices.

Psoralen: a compound that absorbs ultraviolet radiation, and is used to treat skin problems such as psoriasis, eczema, or alopecia.

Synergism: when the combined effect of the interaction of elements produces a greater total effect than the sum of the individual elements.

Surfactant: a wetting agent.

Translucency: having the appearance between complete opacity and complete transparency; partially opaque.

Whitening: use of abrasive agents in the dentifrice that results in whitening of teeth. Has also been used to describe the process of bleaching.

► In 1961, the "walking bleach" method was introduced. The "walking bleach" method sealed a mixture of sodium perborate and water into the pulp chamber and retained it there between the patient's visits.[4]

► By 1963 the "walking bleach" was modified using water and 30%–35% hydrogen peroxide instead of the sodium perborate and water. Result: improved lighter color of nonvital teeth.[2]

B. Vital Tooth Bleaching History

► In the 1960s, tooth lightening was observed after orthodontic patients used an antiseptic that contained carbamide peroxide to promote tissue healing due to gingivitis.[2,5]

► In the 1980s lighter tooth color was noted after advising patients to use carbamide peroxide in customized trays for antiseptic purposes following periodontal surgery.[5]

► In 1989 the use of carbamide peroxide for the primary purpose of tooth bleaching was introduced.[6]

• A custom tray was used to maintain the bleaching gel on the tooth surface for an extended time.

• The procedure was known as nightguard vital bleaching (NGVB).

► No significant, long-term oral or systemic health risks have been associated with professional at-home tooth bleaching materials containing 10% carbamide peroxide or 3.5% hydrogen peroxide when professionally supervised.[7]

VITAL TOOTH BLEACHING

The bleaching process is being studied and still is not fully understood. The color of the teeth is influenced by thickness of enamel and underlying color of dentin.

I. Mechanism of Bleaching Vital Teeth

► Bleaching products penetrate enamel and dentin reaching the pulp within 5–15 minutes.[7,8]

► Bleaching products break down larger pigmented organic molecules into smaller, less pigmented constituents that are locked in the enamel matrix and dentinal tubules.

► Oxygen released from bleaching products changes the optical qualities of the tooth color.[9]

II. Tooth Color Change with Vital Tooth Bleaching

► Color of both dentin and enamel are changed; primarily the dentin color is changed.[10]

► Dentin color is either yellow or gray and transilluminates through the enamel.

► Darker teeth take more time to lighten.

► Each tooth reaches a maximum color change. Additional bleaching product or contact time will not necessarily result in a lighter color.[10]

► Bleaching products cause teeth to become dehydrated immediately during and after product administration. A lighter shade can result temporarily.

► Color will stabilize approximately 2 weeks after bleaching.[9,10]

III. Materials Used for Vital Tooth Bleaching

► Both hydrogen peroxide and carbamide peroxide are used to lighten vital teeth.

► Hydrogen peroxide is approximately three times stronger than carbamide peroxide.[5]

► Hydrogen peroxide has a short working time; carbamide peroxide has an extended working time.[8] Figure 46-1 compares the release or duration time of carbamide peroxide with that of hydrogen peroxide.

► The chemicals are used alone or in combination with each other.

► Bleaching materials need an appropriate viscosity to flow over the tooth surface but not so excessive as to spread onto gingival and other oral tissues.

A. Hydrogen Peroxide

► Active agent in most bleaching systems in a 15%–35% concentration.

► Used directly or produced through a chemical reaction when carbamide peroxide breaks down.[10] See Figure 46-2.

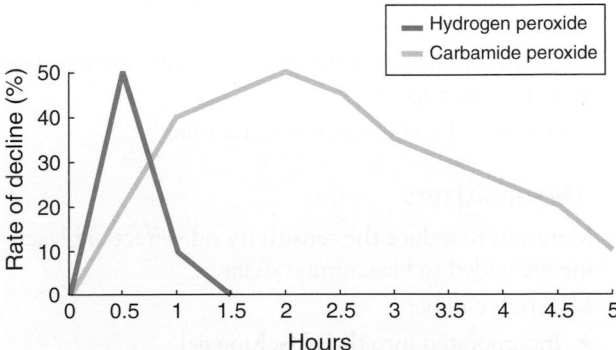

FIGURE 46-1 Release Time of Carbamide Peroxide Compared to Hydrogen Peroxide. Hydrogen peroxide has a much shorter working time than carbamide peroxide and causes more sensitivity. Hydrogen peroxide releases all of the peroxide within 1.5 hours. Carbamide peroxide releases the peroxide over a much longer time. Hydrogen peroxide is approximately three times stronger than carbamide peroxide. (Figures courtesy of Dr. Van Haywood. Reprinted from Haywood VB. Treating sensitivity during tooth whitening. *Compend Contin Educ Dent.* 2005;28(9, Suppl 3):11–20. © 2005, AEGIS Publications, LLC. Used with permission.)

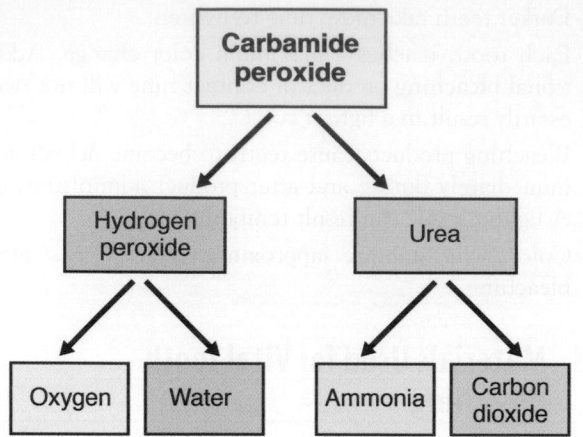

FIGURE 46-2 Hydrogen Peroxide and Carbamide Peroxide Product Breakdown. Flowchart to show breakdown of bleaching products. Hydrogen peroxide breaks down into oxygen and water; carbamide peroxide breaks down into hydrogen peroxide and urea, which further break down as shown.

▶ Has a lower pH than carbamide peroxide, which may result in demineralization when used for longer treatment times than recommended.

▶ Takes less time per day, but more days to change tooth color effectively.[7]

▶ Has high acidic nature; may result in dentin changes which never recover.[11]

B. Carbamide Peroxide

▶ Breaks down into hydrogen peroxide and urea. As shown in the flowchart (Figure 46-2), urea may further break down into ammonia with high pH to facilitate bleaching.

▶ Has slow release: 50% of peroxide released in 2–4 hours and remainder of peroxide in 2–6 hours resulting in less sensitivity.[8] In Figure 46-1 the release time is shown for carbamide peroxide compared with hydrogen peroxide.

▶ At neutral pH, 10% solution is both safe and effective as a bleaching agent.[12]

▶ Takes fewer days but more contact time.[1]

C. Desensitizers

▶ Materials to reduce the sensitivity side effect of bleaching are added to bleaching systems.

▶ Materials can be:
- incorporated into the bleaching gel
- applied to teeth before bleaching
- given for use in trays before, during, and after treatment.

▶ Material used:
- Potassium nitrate creates a calming effect on pulp by affecting the transmission of nerve impulses.[8]
- Sodium fluoride.

- Calcium phosphate and amorphous calcium phosphate aid in remineralization.[8]

D. Other Ingredients

▶ Carbopol: A water-soluble resin used as a thickening agent, which:
- prolongs the release of hydrogen peroxide from carbamide peroxide
- promotes quicker results.

▶ Glycerin: A gel to thicken and control the flow of bleaching agent to prevent overextending onto gingival tissues.

▶ Sodium hydroxide: A chemical base.

▶ Surfactants help to lift and remove extrinsic stains.

▶ Flavoring.

E. Interactions with Bleaching Agents[1]

▶ Coffee and tea may compromise treatment. Advise patient to avoid.

▶ Tobacco may compromise treatment; may have additive carcinogenic effect when combined with hydrogen peroxide. Advise patient to avoid.

IV. Vital Tooth Bleaching Safety

A. Tooth Structure

▶ Both hydrogen peroxide 3.5% and carbamide peroxide 10% are considered safe to lighten the color of teeth when professionally monitored.[7]

▶ Up to two-thirds of patients will experience transitory mild-to-moderate tooth sensitivity.[7]

▶ Higher concentrations of hydrogen peroxide may result in:
- greater sensitivity
- greater color relapses after termination of bleaching.[11]

▶ Hydrogen peroxide at concentrations of 30% or higher may:
- remove the enamel matrix
- create microscopic voids that scatter light
- Result: increase in whiteness until remineralization occurs and color partly relapses.[1]

▶ Carbamide peroxide 10% will cause fewer changes in the enamel matrix.[1]

▶ Pulpal necrosis was noted when material combined with excessive heat or trauma.[12]

B. Soft Tissue

▶ Hydrogen peroxide is caustic and may cause burning and bleaching of the gingiva and any exposed oral tissue.[2]

▶ Hydrogen peroxide 10% concentration or higher has greater incidence of gingival irritation.[7]

▶ Ill-fitting or overfilled tray may cause product spillage onto soft tissues resulting in tissue burning.

C. Restorative Materials

▶ Restorative material color such as porcelain or composite materials will not be changed by bleaching.

▶ After bleaching, new restorative procedures need to be delayed for 2 weeks to allow for color stabilization.[12]

▶ Bonding needs to be delayed for 2 weeks due to significantly reduced bonding strength associated with recently bleached tooth surface.[11]

▶ Bleaching chemicals containing hydrogen peroxide may:

- Have a negative effect on restorations and restorative materials due to lower pH, although impact does not require the renewal of the restoration.[9]
- Increase mercury release from amalgam restorations giving off a green hue.[9]
- Increase solubility of some dental cements.[13]

D. Systemic Factors

▶ The use of tooth-bleaching products containing hydrogen peroxide or carbamide peroxide has not been proven to increase the risk of oral cancer in the general population, including those persons who are alcohol abusers and/or heavy cigarette smokers.[7]

▶ Accidental ingestion of small amounts of the product may cause sore throat, nausea, vomiting, abdominal distention, and ulcerations of the oral mucosa, esophagus, and stomach.[2]

▶ Drugs that may be associated with photosensitivity and hyperpigmentation when light-activated whitening agents are used are listed in Box 46-2.

E. Cautions and Contraindications Associated with Vital Tooth Bleaching

1. *Personal factors that affect acceptance for treatment*
   - Teeth at an acceptable shade, which is subjective.
   - Patients with unrealistic personal expectations.
   - Patients who are unable to be compliant with treatment will not achieve optimal results.
   - Patients with tooth conditions that do not respond favorably to vital tooth bleaching.

2. *Children and adolescents*
   - The American Academy of Pediatric Dentistry[14] discourages full-arch cosmetic bleaching for patients with a mixed dentition, but encourages judicious use of vital and nonvital bleaching due to the negative self-image that may arise from a discolored tooth or teeth.
   - Current American Dental Association recommendations for children and adolescent use include:
     - Delaying treatment until after permanent teeth have erupted.
     - Use of a custom-fabricated tray to limit amount of bleaching gel.
     - Close supervision.[7]

3. *Contraindications*
   - Bleaching products are contraindicated for pregnant and lactating women.
   - Patients taking photosensitive medications. See Box 46-2.
   - Laser light/power bleaching contraindicated for some patients as described in Box 46-3.

V. Factors Associated with Efficacy[1,9]

▶ Some tooth conditions will not respond to tooth bleaching; other tooth conditions will respond slowly (Table 46-1).

▶ The initial color of the teeth and type of stain present will affect the final color change.

▶ Specific indications for bleaching and methods of treatments are listed in Table 46-2.

▶ Patient age: Attrition, incisal, and occlusal wear through enamel exposes the darker underlying dentin.

▶ Concentration of bleaching agent.

▶ Ability of agent to reach the stain molecules.

▶ Duration of contact of the active bleaching agent: longer duration, the greater the degree of bleaching.

▶ Number of types the agent is applied to obtain desired results: darker teeth tend to require more treatment applications.

BOX 46-2

Drugs Associated with Potential Photosensitivity and Hyperpigmentation

▷ Acne medications
▷ Anticancer drugs
▷ Antidepressants
▷ Antiparasitics
▷ Antipsychotics
▷ Diuretics
▷ Hypoglycemics
▷ Nonsteroidal anti-inflammatory drugs

BOX 46-3

Issues Associated with Light-Activated Bleaching

Light-activated bleaching is contraindicated for patients who are:
▷ Light sensitive
▷ Taking a photosensitive medication
▷ Receiving photochemotherapeutic drugs or treatments such as psoralen and ultraviolet radiation.

Exposure to ultraviolet radiation produced by some lights is avoided by those at increased risk for or have a history of skin cancer, including melanoma.

TABLE 46-1	Decision Making for Tooth Bleaching	
TOOTH CONDITION	**RESPONSE TO TOOTH WHITENING**	**SPECIAL CONSIDERATIONS**
Yellow color	Normally excellent.	Resistant yellow may be tetracycline stain.
Enamel white spots	Do not bleach well or may get lighter during whitening.	■ Eventually background color lightens resulting in less noticeable white spots. ■ Goes through splotchy stage before background color whitens. ■ Microabrasion may lessen white spots if less than one-third through enamel.
Brown fluorosis stains	Respond 80% of the time.	Microabrasion techniques done after whitening and color stabilization may improve final result.
Nicotine stains	Require longer treatment.	May take 2–3 mo of nightly application.
Tetracycline stains	Multicolored band may not respond well. ■ Gray most difficult. ■ Dark grays only get lighter. ■ Dark cervical has poorest prognosis.	Requires 2–12 mo of daily whitening.
Minocycline stains	Will respond; will take longer than yellow stain.	■ Type of tetracycline stain. ■ Gives gray hue.
Root exposure	Does not respond to whitening.	Better treated with periodontal coverage.
Dentinogenesis imperfecta and amelogenesis imperfecta	No significant improvement with bleaching.	Inherited condition resulting in defective dentin and enamel, respectively.
Microcracks	Become whiter than rest of tooth.	Bright light or magnification required during assessment to view; may appear streaky during whitening process.
Anterior lingual amalgams	Become more visible after bleaching.	Replacement with very light composite restoration before bleaching.
Dental caries	Not to be bleached.	Decay removal; temporary restoration followed by bleaching and final restoration after color stabilization; carbamide peroxide will increase sensitivity and is bactericidal.
Dark canines	Require longer bleaching.	Isolated canine treatment until color match.
Attrition	Incisal edges do not respond.	Composite restorations added to incisal edges after bleaching.
Aging	Excellent.	More youthful appearance; root surfaces exposure likely.
Translucent teeth	Bleaching will increase translucency at incisal.	Translucent areas will appear darker after whitening due to contrast.

TABLE 46-2	Indications for Tooth Bleaching and Methods of Treatment
INDICATION	**METHOD TO TREAT**
Discolored, endodontically treated tooth	Internal bleaching; in-office or walking.
Single or multiple discolored teeth	External bleaching: in-office 1–3 visits or custom trays worn 2–6 wk.
Surface staining	Brushing with whitening dentifrice.
Isolated brown or white discoloration, shallow depth in enamel	Microabrasion followed by neutral sodium fluoride applications.
White discoloration on yellowish teeth	Microabrasion followed by custom tray whitening.

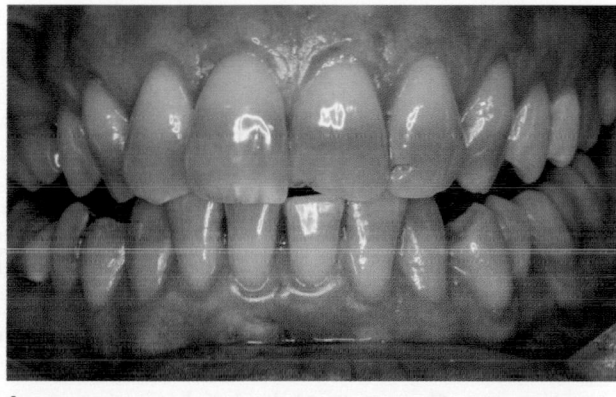 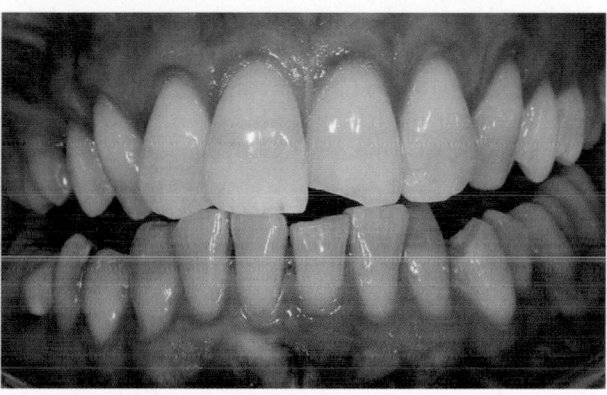

FIGURE 46-3 Before and after Bleaching of Brown Tetracycline-Stained Teeth. A: Patient before treating. **B:** Patient treated with 10% carbamide peroxide for 2 months. Some tetracycline-stained teeth will require up to 12 months to achieve improved results. Those with severe gray stain or banded staining may require porcelain veneers to achieve an acceptable cosmetic result. (Images courtesy of Dr. Van Haywood. Reprinted from Haywood VB. The "bottom line" on bleaching 2008. *Inside Dent.* 2008;4(2):2–5. © 2008, AEGIS Publications, LLC. Used with permission.)

▶ Temperature of agent: heat will result in faster oxygen release, but speed of color change may not be altered.

A. Intrinsic

1. Tetracycline and minocycline staining

- Tetracycline particles incorporate into dentin calcium during mineralization of unerupted teeth. Result: discolored dentin resistant to bleaching.[15]
- Minocycline, a derivative of tetracycline, can discolor erupted teeth.[13]
- Tetracycline and minocycline staining severity varies. A comparison of before and after bleaching of brown tetracycline staining is shown in Figure 46-3.
  - *First category staining*: Light-yellow to light-gray responds to bleaching.
  - *Second category staining*: darker, more extensive yellow-gray responds to extended bleaching time.
  - *Third category staining*: intense dark gray-blue banding stains. Severe third category staining may require porcelain veneers for satisfactory esthetic result.

- Some tetracycline stains will require 1–12 months to achieve a satisfactory result.

2. Fluorosis

- Fluorosis results from ingesting excessive fluoride during tooth development resulting in white or brown spots on teeth.
- Bleaching does not change white spots, but lightens the background color, making the contrast less noticeable.
- White spots go through a splotchy stage during bleaching but will return to baseline.[12]
- Amorphous calcium phosphate may be effective in lessening the white spots if lesion is less than one-third through enamel.[12]
- Brown discoloration responsive to bleach 80% of the time.[12]

3. Nicotine

- Nicotine stains: require 1–3 months of nightly treatment due to the tenacity of the stain.

B. Longevity of Results

▶ Relapse of shade occurs almost immediately as newly bleached, dehydrated teeth rehydrate.

▶ As months and years pass, teeth may discolor and darken again, especially if stain-inducing activities continue.

▶ To maintain shade, periodic bleaching procedures are performed or repeated.

C. Additional Benefits of Bleaching

▶ Hydrogen peroxide used in bleaching has temporary additional effects, which include an antimicrobial action that may lead to a reduction in biofilm and improved gingival health.[16]

▶ Improved motivation to have higher standards of personal daily oral hygiene while participating in bleaching procedures.

▶ Carbamide peroxide may assist with caries control due to raising pH levels to 8 during application.[17]

▶ Carbamide peroxide has been shown to be bacteriocidal to cariogenic bacteria, which benefits elderly xerostomic patients, and orthodontic patients.

VI. Reversible Side Effects of Vital Bleaching: Sensitivity

The most common side effects of bleaching are tooth tingling and sensitivity. Aching sensation can occur because of insult of peroxide on nerves: a reversible pulpitis.[8]

▶ Primarily occur in the first 2 weeks of treatment and may last days to months after cessation of bleaching.

▶ Side effects resolve completely as teeth become accustomed to bleaching.

▶ Not correlated with increased wear time.[8]

▶ Lower concentrations have been used for up to 12 months and do not exhibit greater sensitivity.[8]

▶ Patients with prior history of tooth sensitivity may be more at risk to develop sensitivity during bleaching.

▶ Vulnerable tooth surfaces include:

• Exposed root surfaces and dentin appear to increase risk of developing sensitivity and need to be protected from bleaching material.

• Teeth with unrestored abfraction lesions (see Figure 44-3, Chapter 44) tend to have more sensitivity.

▶ Addition of desensitizing materials decreases sensitivity.

▶ Treatments to reduce tooth sensitivity are listed in Table 46-3.

VII. Irreversible Tooth Damage[1]

A. Root Resorption

▶ Can occur after bleaching, particularly after intracoronal, nonvital tooth bleaching when heat is applied during the technique.

▶ Internal and external resorption may become apparent several years after bleaching.

▶ Occurs usually in cervical third of the tooth.

▶ Cause may be related to a history of trauma.

TABLE 46-3	Desensitization Procedures for Bleaching
Pretreatment	▪ Brush on or use with tray a desensitizing toothpaste containing potassium nitrate, without sodium lauryl sulfate, which removes smear layer from dentin, beginning 2 wk before whitening. ▪ Use toothpaste with prescription strength sodium fluoride. ▪ Use toothpaste that includes calcium carbonate.
During treatment	▪ Continue to use desensitizing toothpaste, which includes sodium fluoride or potassium nitrate, daily between treatments. ▪ Increase time intervals between treatments. ▪ Reduce exposure time of bleaching materials. ▪ Limit the amount in tray to prevent tissue contact.
Postbleaching	▪ Sensitivity diminishes with time. ▪ Continue daily use of desensitizing dentifrice. ▪ Have professional fluoride varnish application. ▪ Avoid foods and beverages with temperature extremes or that contain acidic elements.

▶ May lead to tooth loss.

▶ Bleaching agents are not placed on exposed cementum to avoid complications.

B. Tooth Fracture

▶ May be related to removal of tooth structure or reduction of the microhardness of dentin and enamel.

▶ May lead to tooth loss.

C. Demineralization

▶ Patient with over-the-counter product may not seek or follow professional advice and attempt to get the teeth whiter by using the product more than recommended.

▶ Demineralization with slight surface pitting can result.

▶ Remineralization may be possible if started early enough.

▶ Remineralization protocols are described in Chapter 27.

VIII. Modes of Vital Tooth Bleaching

▶ A comparison of the advantages and disadvantages of professionally applied and professionally dispensed/professionally monitored systems and the over-the-counter systems is listed in Table 46-4.

▶ The different methods of tooth bleaching can achieve similar, effective results, although the mode of delivery, length of treatment, and ease of treatment vary.

A. Professionally Applied

▶ Professionally applied bleaching is performed with high concentrations of 30%–40% hydrogen peroxide or 35%–44% carbamide peroxide.

▶ Some systems use activation or enhancement with a light or heat source.

▶ Teeth are not anesthetized in order to monitor heat-provoked sensitivity.

▶ Heat applied or produced by the use of light may cause an adverse effect such as necrosis of the pulp of the tooth.

▶ The additional issues associated with the use of a light-activated whitening are listed in Box 46-3.

▶ Treatment may take one to six applications for preferred results.

▶ Time for each application varies between different products; ranges from 30- to 60-minute treatment.

▶ Bleaching gels are administered in a professional treatment room. They are not for at-home use.

▶ Rubber dam or an equivalent technique, such as a liquid light-cured resin dam, is applied to isolate the caustic agents from contact with soft tissues.

▶ Care is taken to assure the liquid light-cured resin dam is in the interproximal spaces to protect gingival tissue.

▶ Improvements in paint-on rubber dams, cheek, lip retractors, and lower concentrations of peroxide have made in-office bleaching safer for patient and dentist.

▶ Laser-safe/ultraviolet light protection of eyes for all in treatment room is required.

▶ Gingival sensitivity or irritation may occur.

▶ Laser/power bleaching treatment plan may also involve use of trays for home use.

B. Professionally Dispensed/Professionally Monitored

▶ Also called NGVB, external bleaching, at-home bleaching.

▶ Tray preparation:
  • An impression of the teeth is taken to prepare the cast for fabrication of the tray.
  • Thin, vacuum-formed custom trays are made for each dental arch to be bleached.
  • Trays are fitted to the patient and adjusted to ensure bleaching material will not come into contact with soft tissues.
  • As shown in Figure 46-4, trays are either scalloped at gingival margin or unscalloped and trimmed at mucogingival line.
  • Nonscalloped trays seal better, use less material, and are more comfortable.

▶ Patient instruction:
  • Patient is given instructions and bleaching materials for use in the trays at home.
  • Once or twice daily application for 1–2 weeks is usually recommended if lack of sensitivity and other side effects permit. Maximum color change obtained with consistent compliance. See Figure 46-5.

▶ Patient retains the trays after completion of bleaching to reuse for touch-ups as needed.

▶ Professionally dispensed bleaching products are commonly recommended after professionally applied bleaching procedures to maintain and promote results.

C. Over-the-Counter Products

▶ Also called "at-home" or "self-directed" products.

▶ When asked about use of the self-directed product, a dental hygienist may stress the need for professional examination and supervision; the products can cause harm if misused, may irritate tissues, or cause systemic illness if ingested.

▶ May be recommended to help maintain results of professionally applied and professionally dispensed methods of bleaching.

▶ Patient informs dental professional of proposed use to discuss risks and possible interaction with any proposed dental treatment.

▶ Patient is advised to have thorough oral evaluation before use of the products, as well as appropriate dental

TABLE 46-4	Comparisons of Modes of Tooth Bleaching Systems	
METHODS	**ADVANTAGES**	**DISADVANTAGES**
Professionally applied utilizing laser/ ultraviolet light system procedure	<ul><li>Comprehensive</li><li>Treatment may be combined with trays and professional grade home bleaching materials</li><li>Product selection</li><li>Patient education</li><li>Follow-up, evaluation of effectiveness</li><li>Sensitivity treatment</li><li>Compliance guaranteed</li><li>Quickest result</li></ul>	<ul><li>Higher cost</li></ul>
Professionally dispensed includes professional grade product and trays	<ul><li>Comprehensive</li><li>Dental examination</li><li>Appropriate patient</li><li>Selection</li><li>Product selection</li><li>Patient education</li><li>Follow-up, evaluation of effectiveness</li><li>Sensitivity treatment</li><li>Choice of comfortable time and place for application</li><li>Quicker result</li></ul>	<ul><li>Cost</li><li>Longer time to whiten than professionally applied</li></ul>
Over the counter	<ul><li>Lowest cost</li><li>Immediate start</li><li>Easier access to purchase</li></ul>	<ul><li>No comprehensive exam</li><li>Slowest whitening</li><li>Noncustomized delivery</li><li>Results and tissue response not monitored</li><li>Over-the-counter products have short exposure times, which limit effects</li><li>Unsupervised</li><li>Compliance issues</li></ul>

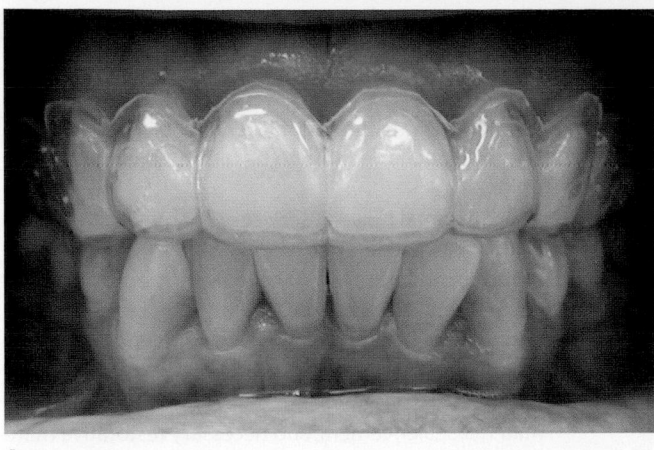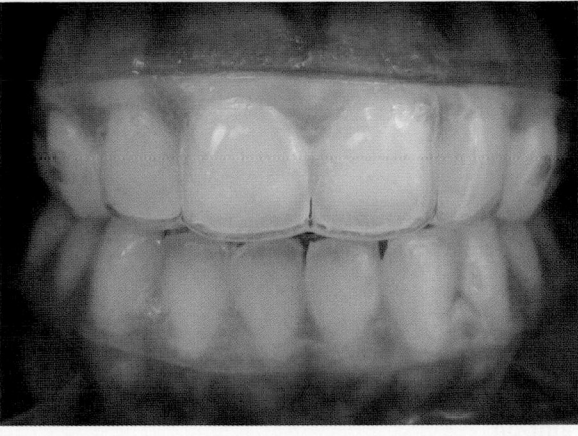

FIGURE 46-4 Scalloped and Unscalloped NGVB Tray Designs. Either scalloped or unscalloped trays may be used. **A:** Scalloped trays aim to protect the gingiva and exposed root surfaces. **B:** Unscalloped trays are more comfortable and take less preparation time. Patients need to be warned to avoid overfilling trays.

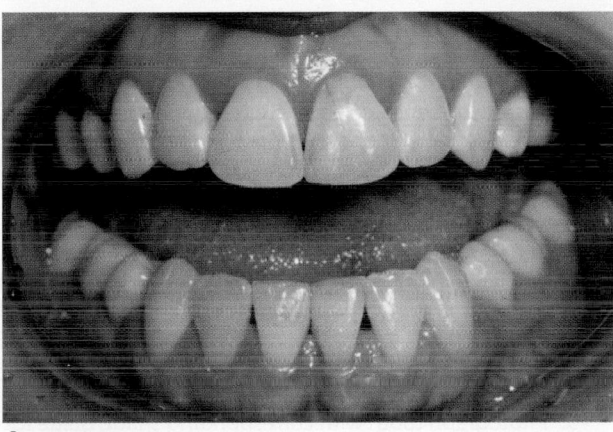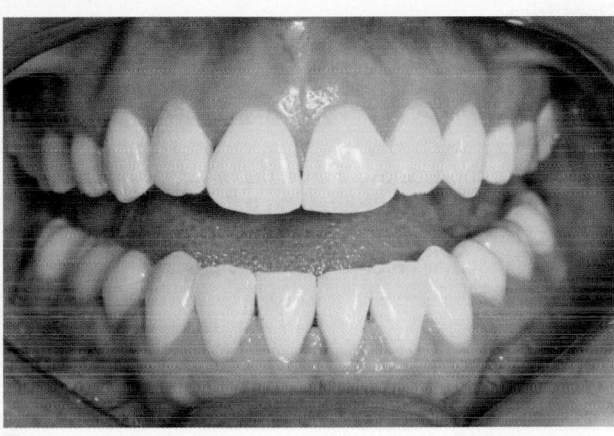

FIGURE 46-5 (A) Before and (B) After Home Tray Bleaching Treatment. (Photo courtesy of Gordon J. Christensen DDS MSD PhD. Used with permission.)

and periodontal treatment including calculus, stain, and biofilm removal.

▶ Delivered through various packaging, viscosities, and flavors (Box 46-4).

NONVITAL TOOTH BLEACHING

▶ Also called "walking bleach" procedure, internal bleaching.

▶ Bleaching of a single, endodontically treated tooth that is discolored can be accomplished by nonvital tooth bleaching procedures.

▶ Alternative to more invasive correction, such as a post and core with crown, or single, discolored, endodontically treated tooth.

▶ Performed by a dentist.

▶ Requirements for procedure:
  • Healthy periodontium.
  • Successfully obturated root canal filling.

• Root canal filling is sealed off with a restorative material before treatment to prevent bleaching agent from reaching periapical tissue.

▶ Hydrogen peroxide and/or sodium perborate is placed in the pulp chamber, sealed, and left for 3–7 days, as outlined in Box 46-5.

▶ Hydrogen peroxide and sodium perborate may be synergistic and very effective in bleaching the tooth.

▶ The process is repeated until a satisfactory result is obtained.

▶ Once satisfactory result is obtained, the pulp chamber is sealed with glass ionomer cement.

▶ Appoint patient 2 weeks later to place permanent, bonded, composite-resin restoration in access cavity to allow dissipation of residual oxygen that would interfere with efficacy of bonding agent.

▶ If unsuccessful after repeated attempts, techniques for vital tooth bleaching can be tried or an alternative restorative procedure, such as a post and core, with crown.

BOX 46-4

Over-the-Counter Bleaching Preparations

Strips

▷ Hydrogen peroxide is delivered on polyethylene film strips.

▷ Strips are placed on the teeth up to two times per day for 30 minutes for about 2 weeks.

Prefabricated Trays

▷ Thin membrane tray loaded with bleaching agent is adapted to maxillary or mandibular arch.

▷ Usually worn 30–60 minutes daily for 5–10 days.

Paint-on

▷ Carbamide peroxide is incorporated into a thick gel that is painted on the teeth selected to be bleached.

▷ An advantage to this method is that individual teeth may be bleached.

Dentifrice

▷ Used to help keep teeth cleaner, and therefore look whiter.

▷ Some have more abrasive materials to remove extrinsic stains.

▷ Owing to short exposure time, the bleaching agent in the dentifrice has little effect on staining.

▷ Some contain hydrogen peroxide; others contain agents that may deter further attachment of stains to the teeth.

Mouthrinse

▷ Content of alcohol is avoided in selection of mouthrinse.

BOX 46-5

Procedure for Nonvital Tooth Bleaching

Periodontally healthy, endodontically treated tooth:

1. Photograph of the tooth to be bleached with shade guide.
2. Provide dental hygiene services to remove extrinsic stain and calculus.
3. Probe circumferentially to determine the outline of the cementoenamel junction.
4. Rubber dam isolation is applied to prevent contamination of root canal therapy.
5. Prepare access cavity. Remove all endodontic obturation material, sealer, cement, and necessary restorative material without removing more dentin than necessary.
6. Remove 2–3 mm of obturation material from the root canal to level below the crest of the gingival margin.
7. Irrigate access cavity with copious amount of water and dry well without desiccating.
8. Root canal therapy is sealed off, commonly with glass ionomer cement or other filling material.
9. Medicament is placed in pulp chamber.
10. Pulp chamber is sealed with a temporary restoration.
11. Patient returns in 3–7 days for evaluation.
    Aforementioned procedure is repeated several times until desired result is obtained.

To finalize procedure:

1. Rubber dam isolation.
2. Temporary restoration on medicament is removed.
3. Pulp chamber is irrigated thoroughly with water.
4. Coronal restoration is placed; generally a composite material.
5. Photograph tooth with corresponding shade guide for records.

▶ Results usually last longer than external tooth bleaching.

▶ There is no universal standard for what is considered acceptable esthetics.

▶ Personal background, culture, and society's and patient's image of esthetics are factors.

▶ The dentist initially may not identify a patient's esthetic issues in the same way that the patient identifies them.

▶ Care is taken to communicate and agree about the course of treatment and the expected result of treatment before the start of bleaching.

DENTAL HYGIENE PROCESS OF CARE

I. Patient Assessment

▶ Review of medical history; identify any contraindications for bleaching.

▶ Complete dental assessment including the following:

• Complete extraoral and intraoral examination including oral cancer screening.

• Updated radiographs.

• The presence of cavitated dental caries is a contraindication for bleaching.

• A lesion is prepared and restored with a temporary restoration to be replaced with permanent matching restoration upon completion of bleaching.

• Updated radiographs to identify abscesses or nonvital teeth, which would require endodontic therapy before bleaching.

• Periodontal examination including areas of recession. Cementum needs to be protected from bleaching material to avoid potential internal and/or external resorption.

• Obtain photographic record of tooth shade without lipstick or strong clothing colors that may interfere with accurate assessment. Use canine for base color. Color will be gray or yellow. Confirm with patient. Figure 46-6 illustrates using a shade guide.

▶ Identify those factors that would lead to a guarded prognosis for bleaching such as:

• History or presence of sensitive teeth.

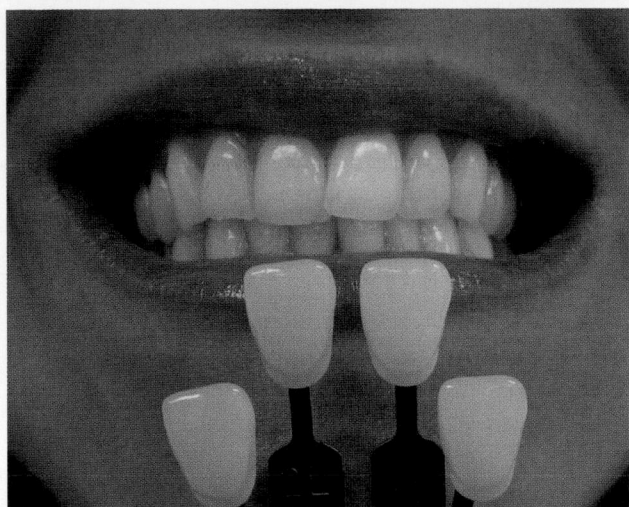

FIGURE 46-6 Digital Photographic Record of Tooth Shade. Patient's shade taken, recorded, and photographed in natural light or color-corrected lighting after extrinsic stain removal before bleaching. Several manufacturers provide color ranges with as many as 29 shades. Electronic digital shade guides provide objective records. Patient's shade and photograph are recorded at each visit while in bleaching treatment. (Photo courtesy of author.)

- Extremely dark gingival third of tooth visible during a smile.
- Extensive white spots that are very visible.
- Temporomandibular joint dysfunction or bruxism that would make wearing NGVB uncomfortable and potential for aggravating condition.
- Very translucent teeth that would become less es thetic due to increased translucency.

▶ Identify contraindications for at-home whitening including the following:
  - Unrealistic expectations of the patient.
  - Unwillingness or inability to comply with at-home treatment routines.
  - Excessive existing restorations not requiring replacement.
  - Inability to tolerate the taste of the product.
  - Pregnancy or lactation.

II. Dental Hygiene Diagnosis

Deficit in wholesome body image as evidenced by patient statement related to dissatisfaction of tooth color.

III. Dental Hygiene Care Plan

▶ *Dental hygiene therapy* with complete removal of all supra- and subgingival calculus and stain along with personal care instruction.

▶ *Patient education*
  - Procedure, product chosen based on patient need.
  - Tooth sensitivity treatment and sensitivity prevention.
  - Emphasis on the following:

- Effective daily biofilm removal before bleaching material use to prevent additional extrinsic stain accumulation.
- Use of nonabrasive whitening dentifrice.
- Removal of excess bleaching material after use.
- Avoidance of over-filling tray to protect soft tissue and exposed cementum.
- Avoidance of foods that stain teeth, coffee, alcohol, and use of tobacco to maximize results.
- Avoidance of swallowing bleaching material due to irritation of materials to mucosa.

▶ Choose appropriate bleaching method.
  - Discussion of procedure, risks, and realistic results.
  - Plan with patient for anticipated needs after bleaching, such as replacement of existing tooth-colored restorations that will not match after bleaching.
  - Obtain informed consent listing procedure and risks with patient's signature (see Chapter 25).

IV. Implementation

▶ Review instructions for use and patient education items previously listed.

▶ *Dental hygiene therapy*: removal of all calculus deposits, and extrinsic stains.

▶ Pretreatment desensitization when indicated. Recommended procedures for pretreatment, during treatment, and postbleaching are listed in Table 46-3.

▶ Premedication with anti-inflammatory pain medication when indicated for sensitivity.

▶ Preparation of trays; impression and construction.
  - Wet teeth before taking impression to ensure teeth are not dehydrated.
  - Monitoring appointments as needed to assess patient compliance, results, sensitivity.

V. Evaluation, Planning for Maintenance

▶ At routine appointments, compare tooth color with tooth color guide. Take follow-up photos as appropriate for records.

▶ Tooth color from bleaching relapses with time.

▶ Plan for repeat of bleaching process at appropriate intervals.

DOCUMENTATION

Documentation in the patient's permanent record when planning tooth bleaching includes a minimum of the following:

▶ Current oral conditions.

▶ Consent to treat related to tooth whitening.

▶ Services provided including necessary records for tooth shade.

▶ Impressions and preparation of the trays.

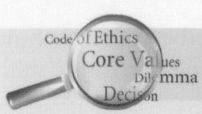

EVERYDAY ETHICS

Julia is a 12-year-old dental hygiene patient who is quite verbal about the appearance of her "dark front tooth." As part of the oral care instructions, Theresa, the dental hygienist, begins to discuss possible options of nonvital bleaching to lighten the tooth. Julia becomes visibly excited and wants to whiten the tooth right away. Following Dr. Leonard's examination, Theresa brings Julia's mother in to discuss the possibility of whitening. The mother quickly tells Julia "You don't want to do that, it's probably too expensive."

Questions for Consideration

1. Is it ethical to discuss treatment options with a child patient before informing the parent or guardian who will make the decision for treatment? Explain.

2. Consider the steps in resolving an issue or a dilemma (Box 1-10 in Chapter 1). What are the rights of each of the individuals involved in this situation? Are there any conflicts of interest that Theresa must identify as she works through the steps in resolving this issue?

3. What financial, legal, or cultural factors need consideration if Theresa is to identify an alternative approach that will lead to a positive outcome? Describe her possible approaches.

▶ Demonstration of tray filling, positioning, timing, and cleaning.

▶ Instructions given to patient.

▶ Planned follow-up care and appointments.

▶ Patient problems or complaints expressed.

▶ An example documentation is shown in Box 46-6.

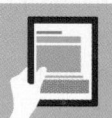

BOX 46-6

Example Documentation: Patient Receiving Vital Tooth Bleaching

S –Patient states she is unhappy with the color of teeth. Patient states she has sensitive teeth.

O –Tooth shade: C-1; appears to have only yellow stain. Patient's medical and dental histories present no contraindications for tooth bleaching. Radiographs and dental examination reveal absence of cavitated caries.

A –Patient presents with a deficit in wholesome body image as evidenced by her statement she is self-conscious of tooth color.

P –Consent for treatment signed and copy given to patient. Completed prophy with all extrinsic stain removed. Intraoral photographs obtained to document tooth color. Impressions and preparation of NGVB trays. Dispensed three syringes of carbamide peroxide 10%. Patient instructed to brush with potassium nitrate product for 2 weeks before beginning bleaching process; after beginning bleaching use of carbamide peroxide 10% every other day.

Patient demonstrated dispensing correct amount of bleaching gel into tray. Patient states: tray provides comfortable fit; understanding of sensitivity treatment; and willingness to return for follow-up appointment.

Next steps: Patient scheduled for follow-up appointment 2 weeks after bleaching process initiated.

Signed _____, RDH

Date _____

Factors To Teach The Patient

▷ Why a complete oral cancer screening and dental examination, including radiographs and periodontal evaluation, are performed before any form of whitening is initiated.

▷ During bleaching, teeth and gingival tissues may become sensitive for a period of time.

▷ If sensitivity is experienced, use a desensitizing product, discontinue bleaching, or delay next treatment.

▷ Regardless of method, color relapse occurs in a relatively short period of time.

▷ Excessive use of bleaching products may be harmful. Follow manufacturer's directions.

▷ Existing tooth-colored restorations will not change color, and therefore may not match and may need to be replaced after bleaching.

References

1. Byrne BE, McIntyre F. Chapter 12: Bleaching agents. In: *ADA/PDR Guide to Dental Therapeutics.* 5th ed. Chicago, IL: American Dental Association; 2009:351.

2. Dahl JE, Pallesen U. Tooth bleaching—a critical review of the biological aspects. *Crit Rev Oral Biol Med.* 2003; 14(4):292–304.

3. Truman J. Bleaching of non-vital discolored anterior teeth. *Dent Times.* 1864;1:69–72.

4. Spasser HF. A simple bleaching technique using sodium perborate. *NY State Dent J.* 1961;27:332.

5. Mokhlis GR, Matis BA, Cochran MA, et al. A clinical evaluation of carbamide peroxide and hydrogen peroxide whitening agents during daytime use. *J Am Dent Assoc.* 2000;131(9):1269–1277.

6. Haywood VB, Heymann HO. Nightguard vital bleaching. *Quintessence Int.* 1989;20(3):173–176.

7. ADA Council on Scientific Affairs. *Tooth Whitening/Bleaching Treatment Considerations for Dentists and Their Patients.* Chicago, IL: American Dental Association; 2009:12.

8. Haywood VB. Treating sensitivity during tooth whitening. *Compend Contin Educ Dent.* 2005;26(9, Suppl 3):11–20.

9. Sweeney MR. Tooth whitening. In: Gladwin M, Bagby M, eds. *Clinical Aspects of Dental Materials.* Philadelphia, PA: Lippincott, Williams & Wilkins; 2009:212–222.

10. Haywood VB. Chapter 1: Diagnosis and treatment planning for bleaching. In: *Tooth Whitening Indications and Outcomes of Nightguard Vital Bleaching.* Chicago, IL: Quintessence; 2007:1–26.

11. Haywood VB. The "bottom line" on bleaching 2008. *Inside Dent.* 2008;4(2):2–5.

12. Matis BA, Wang Y, Eckert GJ, et al. Extended bleaching of tetracycline stained teeth: a 5-year study. *Oper Dent.* 2006;31(6):643–651.

13. Basting RT, Rodrigues AL Jr, Serra MC. The effect of 10% carbamide peroxide, carbopol and/or glycerin on enamel and dentin microhardness. *Oper Dent.* 2005;30(5):608–616.

14. American Academy of Pediatric Dentistry Council on Clinical Affairs. Policy on dental bleaching for child and adolescent patients. *Pediatric Dent.* 2005–2006; 27(7, Suppl):46–48.

15. Mello HS. The mechanism of tetracycline staining in primary and permanent teeth. *J Dent Child.* 1967; 34(6):478–487.

16. Marshall K, Berry TG, Woolum J. Tooth whitening: current status. *Compend Contin Educ Dent.* 2010;31(7):486–492, 494–495.

17. Haywood VB. Bleaching and caries control in elderly patients. *Aesthet Dent Today.* 2007;1(4):42–44.

ENHANCE YOUR UNDERSTANDING

thePoint® **DIGITAL CONNECTIONS**
(see the inside front cover for access information)
- **Audio glossary**
- **Quiz bank**

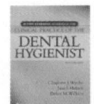

SUPPORT FOR LEARNING
(available separately; visit lww.com)
- *Active Learning Workbook for Clinical Practice of the Dental Hygienist, 12th Edition*

prepU **INDIVIDUALIZED REVIEW**
(available separately; visit lww.com)
- **Adaptive quizzing with *prepU for Wilkins' Clinical Practice of the Dental Hygienist***

Evaluation

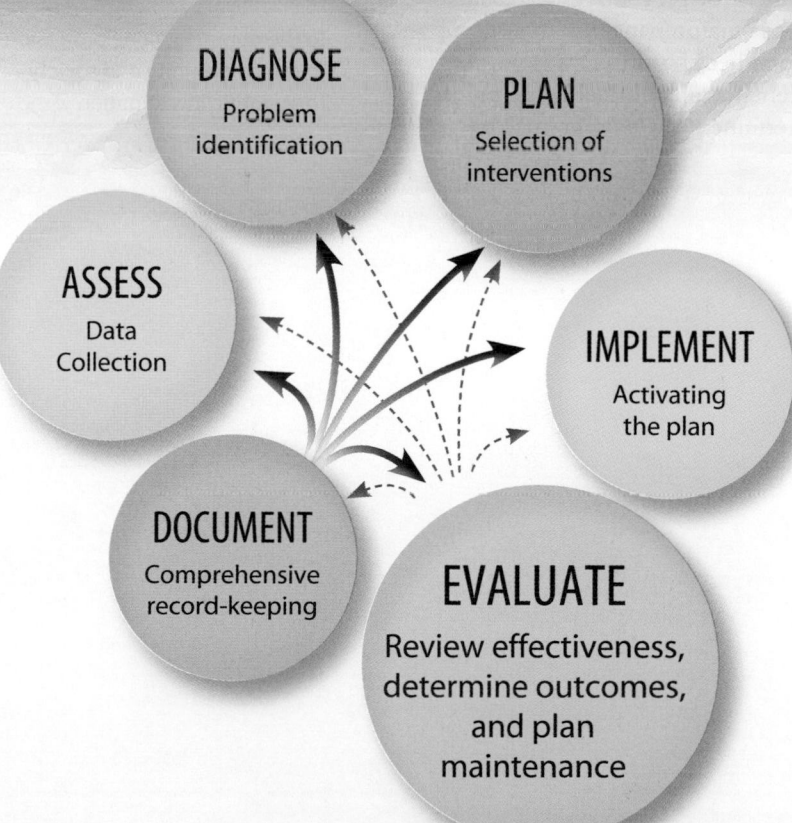

FIGURE VIII-1 The Dental Hygiene Process of Care.

INTRODUCTION FOR SECTION VIII

Evaluation of dental hygiene care is a determination of whether the oral health goals identified in the patient's care plan have been met. The systematic evaluation of dental hygiene prevention and treatment interventions:

▶ Relies on the careful collection of data and comparison of posttreatment information with baseline data.

▶ Determines further treatment needs and appropriate periodontal maintenance interval.

▶ Allows comparison with both previous and future observations to determine changes in the patient's oral health status over time.

THE DENTAL HYGIENE PROCESS OF CARE

▶ Evaluation is an essential component of every step in the dental hygiene process of care, as illustrated by the arrows in *Figure VIII-1*.

▶ The dental hygienist who evaluates each step in the process during each patient appointment will assure that attention is paid to any changing circumstance that affects patient care or treatment outcomes.

▶ As the process of patient care continues:

• A new care plan, based on evaluation data, will address further treatment or preventive needs and/or determine the proper maintenance interval to support the patient's oral health status.

• During the maintenance appointment, the process will be used to determine if the patient's needs have changed and to plan and implement interventions that meet those needs.

ETHICAL APPLICATIONS

▶ It is beneficial to evaluate an ethical situation involving treatment outcomes or self-evaluation of professional skills and abilities based on the *Standards of Professional Responsibility* outlined in the ADHA Code of Ethics and listed in *Box VIII-1*.

▶ The ethical dental hygienist will:

• Assess how a particular decision could potentially affect each of the professional roles of a dental hygienist.

• Evaluate a choice of action that acknowledges each area of professional responsibility.

BOX VIII-1

Standards of Professional Responsibility

Professional dental hygienists acknowledge the following responsibilities:

▷ To ourselves as individuals and professionals
▷ To family and friends
▷ To patients
▷ To employers and employees
▷ To the dental hygiene profession
▷ To the community and society
▷ To scientific investigation

47

Principles of Evaluation

Charlotte J. Wyche, RDH, MS

LEARNING OBJECTIVES

After studying this chapter, the student will be able to:

1. Identify and define key terms and concepts related to evaluation of dental hygiene interventions.

2. Discuss standards for dental hygiene practice.

3. Identify skills related to self-assessment and reflective dental hygiene practice.

PRINCIPLES OF EVALUATION

▶ Evaluation is a systematic determination of worth, value, or significance.[1]

▶ Evaluation of dental hygiene treatment and oral health education outcomes has long been considered the final step in providing evidence-based dental hygiene care.[2,3]

▶ As illustrated in the dental hygiene process of care Figure VIII-1, ongoing evaluation at each step provides feedback that determines success or indicates need to modify procedures throughout the process.

▶ Key terms related to evaluation are defined in Box 47-1.

I. Purposes of Evaluation

▶ Evaluation of dental hygiene care includes assessment of outcomes for both treatment and preventive interventions.

▶ *Formative evaluation*, information collected during any dental hygiene appointment, provides ongoing feedback that will allow the dental hygienist to monitor patient needs (e.g., need for pain control) and adapt to changes in the patient's general health or oral health status during care.

▶ *Immediate evaluation*, for example, use of an explorer to check for residual calculus or evaluating to make sure there has been no undue tissue trauma will help make sure patient care goals have been met at each appointment.

▶ *Ongoing evaluation* of tissue changes and patient self-care abilities during a multiappointment treatment sequence can provide information regarding need for modifications in the original patient care plan.

▶ *Summative evaluation* at the end of a sequence of planned dental hygiene interventions determines whether the oral health goals stated in the patient's care plan have been met.

▶ Assessing the outcome of both clinical and preventive interventions at the completion of a treatment cycle identifies need for further treatment and adapted self-care protocols.

▶ The evaluation process also helps to determine the appropriate continuing care interval to maintain an achieved increase in oral health status.

II. Evaluation Design

▶ A plan for evaluation of patient care outcomes includes informal monitoring, feedback, and modifications in patient care provided during each patient appointment.

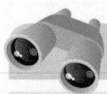

BOX 47-1 · KEY WORDS: Evaluation

Data: information collected during the evaluation procedure that is analyzed to determine oral health outcomes related to dental hygiene interventions.

Evaluation design: a description of the purpose, plans, and strategies that will be needed to gather, process, and interpret the data used to determine treatment outcomes.

Evaluation methods: data collection procedures and strategies that are selected to determine whether or not expected outcomes related to patient specific oral health goals identified in the dental hygiene care plan have been met. (See Figure 25-1.)

Expert witness: a person licensed to perform treatment in a specific health profession or with specialized knowledge, beyond that of the average person, in an area of treatment; a source for determining legal professional standard of care in a court case.

Feedback: communication that occurs among all individuals participating in the patient's care, including the dentist, the dental hygienist, the patient and the patient's physician or caregiver, if necessary. Giving and receiving feedback creates trust and ensures that those involved in all aspects of patient care stay informed at every step.

Formative evaluation: ongoing evaluation to monitor each step in the dental hygiene process of care; ongoing feedback that determines any needed changes in the dental hygiene care plan prior to the completion of a treatment sequence.

Indicators: benchmarks used to measure or test changes. In evaluating dental hygiene interventions, indicators can be quantitative (measurement of probing depth or plaque scores) or qualitative (patient expressions of satisfaction or ability to perform self-care routines).

Objectives: measurable goals; the expected outcomes of clinical treatment, patient education, counseling, or oral hygiene instruction/home care interventions identified in the patient care plan.

Outcomes assessment: a measure of the effectiveness of dental hygiene clinical and educational interventions in meeting oral health goals identified in the patient care plan.

Standard of care: criteria or protocols that define the minimal quality of care required to defend against a legal dispute against the practice of one's profession; usually established by federal laws, state and local statutes and codes and/or testimony from an "expert witness," and is supported by guidelines or recommendations documents published by professional associations.

Summative evaluation: formal, standardized evaluation procedures conducted at the end of a treatment series; includes determination of periodontal maintenance interval and/or identification of further treatment needs.

- Methods for evaluating the success of dental hygiene treatment have traditionally included collecting new clinical data, such as probing depths and areas of bleeding to compare with the patient's health status at the beginning of treatment.
- The evaluation process includes measures that assess the extent to which disease prevention and health promotion interventions have been effective.
- A comparison of pre- and posttreatment values indicates areas of success or areas of need for further intervention.

III. Evaluation Process

- When writing the dental hygiene care plan, indicators (evaluation measures) that will evaluate each oral health goal and objective set in the plan can be determined.
- Following treatment, new complete assessment data are documented.
- An evidence-based decision-making approach is used to determine any necessary modifications to the ongoing treatment sequence or to plan maintenance care.
- All assessment findings and any planned modifications for treatment or oral health education are documented in an evaluation summary.

EVALUATION BASED ON GOALS AND OUTCOMES

- The dental hygiene care plan establishes individualized immediate and long-range patient goals for each dental hygiene intervention.
- The treatment, education, and self-care instruction goals listed in the patient's care plan provide the basis for evaluating whether expected outcomes have been achieved at each level.
- Outcomes that can be evaluated following the completion of dental hygiene treatment and patient education in each area of a three part plan for care are listed in Box 47-2.
- Selected outcomes are used to develop goals for patient care when writing a new dental hygiene care plan.

EVALUATION OF CLINICAL (TREATMENT) OUTCOMES

- Final evaluation of dental hygiene treatment outcomes is made after initial therapy has been completed, when the response of the gingival tissue to therapy is apparent.
- When a treatment sequence consists of multiple appointments, evaluation of the previously treated areas at each subsequent appointment allows immediate

> **BOX 47-2**
> **Expected Outcomes Following Dental Hygiene Interventions**
>
> **Gingival/Periodontal Health Outcomes**
> - Reduced dental biofilm
> - Smooth tooth surfaces with calculus removed
> - Reduced probing depths
> - No bleeding on probing
> - Resolution of erythematous tissue
> - Reduced swelling and edema
> - No further loss in attachment level
> - Decrease or no change in mobility
>
> **Dental Caries Risk Outcomes**
> - No new cavitated lesions
> - Demineralized/noncavitated areas resolved
> - Reduced intake of cariogenic foods/beverages
> - Dental sealants placed
> - Increased fluoride use
>
> **Prevention Outcomes**
> - Elimination of iatrogenic factors (calculus, restoration overhangs)
> - Increased percentage of biofilm-free areas
> - Patient demonstration of recommended oral care procedures
> - Patient report of compliance with daily care recommendations
> - Compliance with recommended continuing care interval
> - Tobacco-free status achieved
> - Modification/stabilization of systemic risk factors

intervention in an area that shows poor response to the previous treatment.
- The clinical examination instruments and procedures used for initial assessment as well as evaluation assessment are described more completely in Chapter 20.

I. Visual Examination

- Obtain biofilm score after the soft tissue visual inspection has been completed so the use of disclosing solution does not interfere with soft tissue examination.
- Gingival examination looks for changes in tissue color, size, shape (contour), and consistency and compares them to examination findings documented prior to treatment.
- Visual examination can also determine whether a goal related to caries risk, such as restorative treatment or sealants, has been completed.

II. Periodontal Probing

- A complete probing is performed and documented using a form that allows comparison with pretreatment assessment data.

- Current pocket depths and bleeding points noted during probing are documented in the periodontal record.
- See Chapter 33 for information about probing around dental implants.

III. Tactile Evaluation

- All tooth surfaces, particularly in areas demonstrating bleeding points, are assessed with a periodontal explorer for residual calculus deposits and other iatrogenic factors.
- Use of an explorer with a long straight terminal shank is needed for areas with pockets of 5 mm or deeper (as shown in Figure 20-3, Chapter 20).
- Residual calculus can be expected on any subgingival surface that demonstrates bleeding on gentle probing.
- Smooth root surfaces free of calculus create a biologically compatible root surface that can support healing in the overlying tissues.
- Special checks for difficult-to-access areas include:
  - Concavities and depressions of the root anatomy
  - Subgingival margins of crowns, fixed partial denture, or overhanging restoration
  - Furcation invasions.

EVALUATION OF HEALTH BEHAVIOR OUTCOMES

- Evaluation of health behavior outcomes provides evidence of:
  - The patient's response to the clinician's counseling and education interventions.
  - Development of oral self-care skills.
- The dental hygiene care plan establishes self-care and health behavior goals determined in collaboration with the patient.
- If the evaluation process indicates that goals have not been met, the data collected during evaluation can provide a baseline from which the dental hygienist can again collaborate with the patient to develop new or next step goals.
- Methods for evaluating self-care and health behavior outcomes are as follows.

I. Visual Examination

- Patient biofilm control is evaluated using the same dental indices used to determine original biofilm levels.
- Self-care skills are evaluated by observing a demonstration of each skill by the patient.

II. Interview Evaluation

- Patient interviewing techniques can be used to determine whether each goal established by the patient for health behavior change and daily self-care has been met.
- Patient interview and discussion can be used to evaluate:
  - Success of factors associated with patient comfort during treatment
  - The patient's understanding of recommendations and self-care instructions
  - Effectiveness of the clinician's communication approaches.

COMPARISON OF ASSESSMENT FINDINGS

- Analysis and comparison of pretreatment and evaluation data determines the relative success of the therapy and can help determine whether the patient:
  - Is able to be managed for the present under the care of the dental hygienist, requiring development of a new dental hygiene care plan.
  - Has not responded adequately to nonsurgical therapy and referral for specialized periodontal care may be necessary.
- On the basis of the findings, a recommended interval for continuing care appointments is determined.
- Additional factors taken into account when determining next steps for patient care are listed in Box 47-3.

STANDARD OF CARE

- In addition to evaluating individual patient outcomes at all points in the dental hygiene process of care, the dental hygienist is responsible for evaluating personal adherence to a professional standard of practice.

BOX 47-3

Factors Considered When Determining Need for Retreatment, Referral, or Maintenance Interval

- ▷ Soft tissue response to instrumentation and degree of healing
- ▷ Changes and/or stabilization in probing depth and attachment loss
- ▷ Patient health behaviors, such as use of tobacco
- ▷ Systemic influences on oral health status, such as diabetes
- ▷ Level of skill and effectiveness in biofilm control
- ▷ Motivation and responsibility assumed for daily personal oral self-care
- ▷ Psychosocial factors that can affect oral status, such as stress

▶ Standards of care in dentistry evolved from early court cases that established a ruling of negligence when healthcare providers failed to possess a minimum standard of special knowledge and ability, or adhere to reasonable and recognized standards while providing patient care.[4]

▶ Standards for delivery of dental hygiene care are defined by the *ADHA Standards for Clinical Dental Hygiene Practice*, based on the dental hygiene process of care and summarized in Table 47-1.[5]

▶ *The Guidelines for Infection Control in Dental Health-Care Settings* (Appendix V) as well as a number of other documents published by both dental and dental hygiene professional associations are additional sources used for establishing a professional standard of care.

▶ Three sources for determining standard of care in a legal dispute are listed in Box 47-4.

▶ Failure to provide a minimally acceptable level of patient care is considered to be professional negligence.

▶ The professional dental hygienist recognizes that standards of care change over time as new knowledge is introduced and becomes commonly accepted by the profession and the public.

▶ Knowledge of and adherence to a professional dental hygiene standard of care is enhanced through continuous evidence-based inquiry and pursuit of life-long learning.

BOX 47-4

Three Sources for Determining Standard of Care in a Legal Dispute

▷ Opinion of expert witnesses
▷ Journals, guidelines, or other published documents from recognized professional associations or other authoritative sources
▷ Federal, state, or local statutes and/or regulations

Source: Curley AW. The legal standard of care. *J Am Coll Dent.* 2005;72(4):20–22.

TABLE 47-1	Standards for Clinical Dental Hygiene Practice	
STANDARD	**DESCRIPTION**	**CRITERIA FOR EVALUATING ADHERENCE TO STANDARD**
Standard 1 ASSESSMENT	Ongoing collection and interpretation of patient data	▪ Collect personal, dental, and health history. ▪ Provide comprehensive clinical examination. ▪ Assess risks to general and oral health.
Standard 2 DENTAL HYGIENE DIAGNOSIS	Analysis and critical decision making	▪ Analyze and interpret all data. ▪ Determine patient needs. ▪ Incorporate dental hygiene diagnosis into overall dental treatment plan.
Standard 3 PLANNING	Making clinical decisions within the context of ethical and legal principles	▪ Identify, prioritize, and sequence interventions. ▪ Coordinate resources and collaborate with other healthcare providers. ▪ Present plan and explain rationale, risks benefits, expected outcomes, alternatives, and prognosis to patient. ▪ Obtain informed consent or refusal.
Standard 4 IMPLEMENTATION	Delivery of dental hygiene interventions	▪ Review, implement, and modify care plan and plan for continuing care. ▪ Communicate with patient.
Standard 5 EVALUATION	Reviewing and documenting outcomes throughout the process of care	▪ Use measurable criteria. ▪ Communicate with patient. ▪ Collaborate with other healthcare providers.
Standard 6 DOCUMENTATION	Complete and accurate recording of information	▪ Document all components of care objectively, legibly, concisely, and accurately. ▪ Recognize ethical and legal aspects of recordkeeping. ▪ Respect and protect patient information.

Source: American Dental Hygienists' Association. *Standards for Clinical Dental Hygiene Practice*. Chicago, IL: American Dental Hygienists' Association; 2008:6–9. http://www.adha.org/resources-docs/7261_Standards_Clinical_Practice.pdf. Accessed September 17, 2014.

SELF-ASSESSMENT AND REFLECTIVE PRACTICE

▶ Ongoing self-assessment of skills and current knowledge is an essential component of evaluating clinical practice.

▶ Although self-assessment and reflection in healthcare practice have been studied mainly in educational settings, there is evidence to suggest that development of these skills can:

- Be taught and developed, mainly through reflective writing[6]
- Be enhanced with practice[6,7]
- Help assure quality and positive outcomes in the delivery of patient care.[8]

I. Purpose

▶ Self-assessment of personal clinical and communication skills and knowledge can guide the dental hygiene practitioner toward an evidence-based approach to finding new information to support best-practice interventions for patient care.

▶ Reflecting on clinical experiences contributes to development of critical thinking skills that can help the practitioner determine and implement new and more successful approaches for patient care.[9]

▶ Self-assessment can assist the dental hygienist to determine a need to enhance specific clinical skills and abilities, or develop a plan for continuing education that supports personal professional goals.

II. Skills and Methods

▶ Key skills for reflective practice include:
- Perceptive self-awareness
- Judgment and self-assessment
- Critical analysis and synthesis
- Access to and application of new knowledge
- Feedback and evaluation (continued reflection).

▶ Methods for informal assessment of professional practice include individual reflection (thinking about one's own practice habits) or discussing clinical issues with colleagues.

▶ Reflective practice can also take on a more formal aspect, as in maintaining a written "critical incident" journal.

III. A "Critical Incident" Approach

A formal approach used to evaluate dental hygiene practice takes the form of answering questions about a specific situation, often called a critical incident, that prompts the practitioner to look for answers.

▶ Three steps, sometimes referred to as the "What? So What? Now What?" approach, can be used to structure

written reflective journal entries or can also be used to guide a less formal means of thoughtful personal self-assessment.

▶ The approach to reflective self-assessment includes a basic progression of reflective actions with questions for each step that can help guide thinking about the situation from a variety of perspectives.

▶ The steps and a brief clinical practice example are provided in Table 47-2. The same steps and similar questions can be used to guide self-assessment reflection about situations involving communication skills, patient education approach, or adherence to ethical and legal standards of practice.

DOCUMENTATION

I. Patient Care Outcomes

▶ Evaluation of such factors as patient comfort, communication efforts, and treatment safety and efficacy is ongoing and occurs at each patient appointment. Documentation in the patient record provides guidance for future patient interactions.

▶ Documentation of outcomes evaluation following clinical dental hygiene treatment is similar to the documentation of clinical data during initial assessment.

▶ Evaluation data following treatment are recorded in an identical format to the pretreatment assessment data, which facilitates comparison and analysis of outcomes.

▶ Box 47-5 has an example progress note that documents evaluation of a patient care situation.

II. Self-assessment and Reflection

Self-assessment and reflective evaluation of personal professionalism and learning can be documented in several ways. Two suggestions are as follows:

▶ Regular written entries in a professional practice reflection journal that describe and critically analyze a variety of clinical, ethical, and professional situations the dental hygienist has found meaningful. Over time, this ongoing record will reflect how the practitioner's professional skills, actions, and knowledge have been enhanced through the process of reflective practice.

▶ A clinical practice portfolio can be developed to document a variety of factors related to professional development and self-evaluation of dental hygiene practice. A portfolio may contain artifacts such as:
- Case presentations describing care provided for patients with special needs.
- A personal practice philosophy describing ethical parameters that impact how the dental hygienist provides care.
- Goals for future continuing education and courses taken or planned for reaching those goals.

TABLE 47-2	Components of a "Critical Incident" Approach to Reflection and Self-assessment		
STEP	SUMMARY/DEFINITION	SOME EXAMPLE QUESTIONS FOR GUIDING REFLECTION	CLINICAL PRACTICE EXAMPLE
DESCRIPTION "What?"	Brief description of what happened and what effect the situation had on those involved in the incident.	What about the situation triggered a need to evaluate what happened? Who was involved? How did those involved feel about or react to the incident? What about this situation is interesting to explore further?	Patient presents for evaluation following scaling and root planing. Residual calculus, resulting in areas of bleeding and need for patient to return for retreatment of those areas. Patient is not happy about need for retreatment. Dental hygienist is concerned about her personal skill in calculus removal.
ANALYSIS "So What?"	Reflective phase that involves analysis and critical thinking to identify: ■ Potential causes and factors that influenced outcome of the situation ■ Gaps related to standards of good practice ■ Changes that need to be made in current practice ■ New knowledge required	Why did this happen? What gaps in knowledge or skill influenced the outcome? Does the knowledge base need to be updated? Were patient and/or clinician's goals met during this situation? How were values or ethical standards related to or applied during this situation?	The dental hygienist analyzes the situation using some of the questions in the previous column, and realizes that this is not the first time the personal patient care goal for complete calculus removal at each appointment has not been met. Recently, while participating in an advanced instrumentation continuing education course, it became clear that the problem is not deficient scaling and root planing skills. Instrument sharpening skills have not been updated (or applied) recently.
APPLICATION "Now What?"	Summary of insights or learning from the situation and a plan for addressing need for new knowledge or alternative action.	What was learned? What next steps can be taken to produce a different outcome in a future situation?	The dental hygienist learned that instrumentation skill alone might not be all that is necessary to meet the goal of complete calculus removal. Next steps: find an instrument-sharpening "how-to" booklet to begin practicing sharpening and attend a continuing education workshop related to instrument sharpening at the first opportunity.

 **EVERYDAY ETHICS**

Mrs. Midoun called in this morning and scheduled during a cancelled appointment time in the afternoon. She states she is in a hurry and just wants her teeth "shined up" as her daughter is graduating this weekend. Salima, one of three dental hygienists in the practice, has not provided care previously for Mrs. Midoun. She quickly scans the patient record, noticing that three months ago Mrs. Midoun received scaling and root planing treatments in all four quadrants. Although she had signed a consent form outlining the entire sequence of appointments, including evaluation, Mrs. Midoun had cancelled the evaluation appointment at the last minute and never rescheduled it.

Salima explains that, before providing any further dental hygiene care, it would be necessary to complete the posttreatment evaluation. Mrs. Midoun objects strenuously to "wasting time" with evaluation of her previous treatment. She states that her oral health is much better now and she notices very little bleeding. Mrs. Midoun states emphatically that, unless Salima cleans her teeth today, she will "just leave now and find another office" where they will clean her teeth. Dr. Kim is out of the office and Salima hesitates, not knowing quite how to handle the situation without consulting him.

Questions for Consideration

1. Is this an ethical issue or a dilemma? Explain.

2. What are Mrs. Midoun's rights in this situation? What core values need to be considered during Salima's decision-making process?

3. What alternative decisions can Salima make about interventions she will provide at Mrs. Midoun's appointment today that will meet the standards of care for dental hygiene practice?

Box 47-5

Example Documentation: Evaluation of Patient Comfort During a Sequence of Treatment Appointments

S –A 79-year-old male patient presents for third in a series of appointments scheduled for scaling and root planing. Patient states: "Following both of the previous appointments, my back has significantly bothered me because of laying back so far in the dental chair for such a long time. Do we need to have such long appointments?"

O –Patient medical history form indicates history of osteoarthritis, but no previous problem with back pain.

A –Analyzed the problem through discussion with patient about how to balance his needs with the time necessary to complete planned care at each appointment. Decided together that placing a small cushion (or his jacket) beneath his knees as well as briefly bringing the chair to an upright position every 15 minutes could help to alleviate his discomfort.

P –Completed third quadrant scaling and provided flossing instruction as indicated in the patient's care plan for this appointment while using the new "comfort protocol." He indicated that he felt much better during this treatment session.

Next steps: Re-evaluate at the next appointment, scheduled in 2 weeks.

Signed: _____, RDH

Date: _____.

References

1. Centers for Disease Control and Prevention. Program Performance and Evaluation Office (PPEO)—program evaluation. http://www.cdc.gov/eval/framework/index.htm. Accessed September 17, 2014.

2. Forrest JL, Miller SA. Evidence-based decision making—a new term for a new concept. *Dimensions Dent Hyg.* 2005;3:12.

3. Niederman R, Richards D. Evidence-based dentistry: concepts and implementation. *J Am Coll Dent.* 2005;72(4):37–41.

4. Graskemper JP. The standard of care in dentistry: where did it come from: how has it evolved? *J Am Dent Assoc.* 2004;135(10):1449–1455.

5. American Dental Hygienists' Association. *Standards for Clinical Dental Hygiene Practice.* Chicago, IL: American Dental Hygienists' Association; 2008. http://www.adha.org/resources-docs/7261_Standards_Clinical_Practice.pdf. Accessed September 17, 2014.

6. Tsang AK. Oral health students as reflective practitioners: changing patterns of student clinical reflections over a period of 12 months. *J Dent Hyg.* 2012;86(2):120–129.

7. Asadoorian J, Schönwetter DJ, Lavigne SE. Developing reflective health care practitioners: learning from experience in dental hygiene education. *J Dent Educ.* 2011;75(4):472–484.

8. Jackson SC, Murff EJ. Effectively teaching self-assessment: preparing the dental hygiene student to provide quality care. *J Dent Educ.* 2011;75(2):169–179.

9. Mould MR, Bray KK, Gadbury-Amyot CC. Student self-assessment in dental hygiene education: a cornerstone of critical thinking and problem-solving. *J Dent Educ.* 2011;75(8):1061–1072.

Factors To Teach The Patient

▷ The need for evaluation to establish the basis for "next step" treatment and maintenance decisions.

▷ Types of evaluation measures and indicators that measure outcomes for each goal.

▷ How outcomes from dental hygiene interventions are used to determine further treatment needs and maintenance interval.

ENHANCE YOUR UNDERSTANDING

thePoint® DIGITAL CONNECTIONS
(see the inside front cover for access information)

• **Audio glossary**
• **Quiz bank**

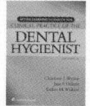

SUPPORT FOR LEARNING
(available separately; visit lww.com)

• *Active Learning Workbook for Clinical Practice of the Dental Hygienist, 12th Edition*

prepU INDIVIDUALIZED REVIEW
(available separately; visit lww.com)

• **Adaptive quizzing with *prepU* for Wilkins' *Clinical Practice of the Dental Hygienist***

48

Continuing Care

Linda D. Boyd, RDH, RD, EdD and Esther M. Wilkins, BS, RDH, DMD

CHAPTER OUTLINE

LEARNING OBJECTIVES

After studying this chapter, the student will be able to:

1. Describe the goals of a continuing care program in dental hygiene practice.

2. Determine appointment intervals based on an individual patient's risk factors, compliance, and oral health history.

3. Name and discuss the contributing factors in recurrence of periodontal disease.

4. List steps in a continuing care appointment including assessment, care plan, and therapy.

5. Outline methods for continuing care systems in the dental office or clinic.

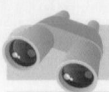

BOX 48-1 | KEY WORDS: Continuing Care

Compliance: action in accordance with request; extent to which a person's health behaviors coincide with dental/medical health advice. Also called *adherence*.

Consultation: the joint deliberation, usually for diagnostic purposes, between two or more practitioners or between a patient and a practitioner.

Continuing care: system of appointments for the long-term maintenance phase of patient care; the system is carried out by computer, telephone, and/or mail. Also called recare or maintenance.

Disease activity: ongoing dynamic process that results in loss of clinical attachment and alveolar supporting bone; an area is quiescent when a diseased site becomes inactive or stable without treatment.

End points: criteria for completion of a particular procedure; therapeutic end points generally have been reached when the clinical signs of the treated pathologic condition have been eliminated or reduced.

PM: periodontal maintenance; also called preventive maintenance, supportive periodontal therapy (SPT); procedures performed at selected intervals as an extension of periodontal therapy to assist the patient in maintaining oral health; includes complete assessment, review of and/or additional instruction in dental biofilm control, and such clinical procedures as scaling and root planing.

Refractory: resistant, not responding to routine therapy.

Risk factor: a characteristic, habit, or predisposing condition that makes an individual susceptible to, or in danger of acquiring, a certain disease or disability.

The overall therapeutic goals of treatment are to arrest disease and provide oral health, function, and comfort for the patient. After active treatment, when evaluation shows the soft tissue is in optimum health and the dentition has been restored in function, the patient enters a new phase of treatment for continuing care.

▶ Terms associated with continuing care are defined in Box 48-1.

GOALS OF THE CONTINUING CARE PROGRAM

▶ Continue the healthy state attained during active therapy.

▶ Prevent recurrence of infection. The patient needs to understand that oral diseases recur, but *control* is possible through combined personal and professional effort.

▶ Prevent initiation of new disease.

▶ Monitor educational and behavioral changes.

▶ Monitor risk and clinical signs of health and disease including:
  • periodontal infection
  • oral mucosal lesions
  • dental caries from demineralization to noncavitated to cavitated lesions.

▶ Provide specialized instruction for new implants, prostheses, orthodontic appliances, and various restorations.

▶ Offer motivational encouragement for oral self-care. The success of the program depends on compliance by the patient with the daily oral self-care and regular professional maintenance.

BOX 48-2

Purposes and Outcomes of Periodontal Maintenance

▷ Resolve inflammation
▷ Eliminate BOP
▷ Restore tissues to normal contour and texture
▷ Create environment for healing
▷ Arrest disease progression
▷ Provide patient comfort
▷ Encourage patient oral self-care
▷ Create environment that deters recurrence of infection
▷ Motivate patient to participate in continuing care

I. Periodontal Maintenance[1]

▶ Patients who comply with regular periodontal maintenance (PM) intervals have less attachment and tooth loss.[1,2]

▶ Evidence suggests patients with a history of periodontal disease need to be seen four times a year to decrease the risk for progression of the disease.[1]

▶ Therapeutic goals of PM are listed in Box 48-2 and include the following[1,3]:
  • Prevent the recurrence of disease and maintain the state of periodontal health attained during periodontal therapy. Such therapy may have been nonsurgical or surgical.
  • Prevent or reduce the incidence of tooth or implant loss with careful monitoring.
  • Increase timely identification of the need for treatment of other conditions or disease manifested in the oral cavity such as poorly controlled diabetes mellitus.

CONTINUING CARE APPOINTMENT PROCEDURES

The dental hygiene process of care is described in Chapter 1. As with preparation of the initial dental hygiene care plan, discussed in Chapters 24 and 25, the steps in the process of care apply for the *dental hygiene continuing care plan*.

I. Assessment

▶ Preparation of assessment data follows the same procedure as that for a new patient.

▶ At every maintenance appointment, whether at 3 or 4 months, or any other interval, a patient of any age needs a complete reassessment, diagnosis, and care plan.

A. Review of Patient History

▶ Supplementary questions are asked to determine the present state of health with emphasis on changes since the previous appointment.

▶ Recent illnesses, hospitalizations, current medications, and other pertinent new data.

▶ Date of last physical examination with primary care provider.

B. Vital Signs

▶ Blood pressure and other vital signs are documented (Chapter 11).

C. Extraoral and Intraoral Examination

▶ A thorough extraoral and intraoral examination is documented as described in Chapter 12.

D. Radiographs

▶ The frequency of radiographic surveys is in accord with the determination of an individual patient's need and recommendations for dental radiographs from the American Dental Association and Federal and Drug Administration (see Table 13-4, in Chapter 13).

E. Periodontal Examination

▶ Observe and record: gingival color, size, shape; mucogingival changes.

▶ Complete periodontal examination: pocket depths, bleeding on probing (BOP), exudate or suppuration, attachment levels, furcation involvement, and gingival recession.[3] Compare findings with previous periodontal examinations and check for changes since treatment was completed.

▶ Occlusion, fremitus, mobility.

▶ Calculus: distribution, amount.

▶ Biofilm and soft deposits.

F. Examination of the Teeth

▶ Integrity of restorations and sealants.

▶ Dental caries: demineralization, early dental caries, and cavitated lesions.

▶ Sensitivity: location.

G. Evaluation of Oral Cleanliness and Adequacy of Self-care Measures

▶ Evaluate biofilm on teeth after applying a disclosing agent to areas of gingival redness, enlargement, and other signs of inflammation.

H. Examination of Specific Areas

▶ Areas of special problems include endodontically treated teeth, postsurgical areas, implants, occlusal factors, and prosthetic appliances.

II. Continuing Care Plan

A care plan is outlined on the basis of new dental hygiene diagnosis and evaluation of the patient's oral condition. Supplemental procedures may be needed.

A. Oral Hygiene Instruction/Motivation

▶ During continuing care, the patient is considered a cotherapist.

▶ To keep etiologic factors under control, compliance with daily oral self-care is a major feature in the total program.

B. Periodontal Scaling and Debridement

▶ The periodontal examination findings may indicate need for subgingival scaling and root planing.

▶ Plan appropriate pain control such as local anesthesia.

▶ Plan for number of appointments.

▶ Local delivery of antimicrobials for isolated periodontal pockets with active disease that is not responding to nonsurgical therapy (see Chapter 41).

▶ For areas of BOP, endoscopic examination or evaluation for surgical therapy may be indicated.

C. Dental Caries Control

▶ Prevention needs to address modifiable caries risk factors with attention to root caries; appropriate use of office and home fluorides, and diet modifications.

▶ Implement or monitor previously introduced remineralization protocol (see Chapter 27).

D. Supplemental Care Procedures

▶ Smoking cessation assistance (see Chapter 34).

▶ Desensitization of sensitive areas (see Chapter 44).

▶ Special care for implants and fixed prostheses (see Chapters 32 and 33).

▶ Referral for retreatment evaluation.

III. Criteria for Referral to a Periodontist

A. Referral from General Practice

General practice dentists may include periodontal surgical therapy in their practice, but referral to a periodontist is recommended for care outside the scope of practice for a general dentist.

▶ Others refer all the severe or complicated periodontal cases to the specialist periodontist.

▶ During patient care in a general practice, the dental hygienist may confer with the dentist to determine the need for referral to a periodontist in the following situations:

• *Initially* when a patient new to the practice is examined and severe advanced periodontitis is evident, or the patient has an uncommon periodontal disease such as an aggressive periodontitis (formerly called "juvenile periodontitis"), necrotizing ulcerative gingivitis or periodontitis, or a drug-induced gingival enlargement (such as phenytoin for seizures).

• *Later during the reevaluation* after nonsurgical periodontal therapy is complete for a nonresponsive or refractory type of moderate or advanced periodontal condition (or any of the conditions mentioned earlier).

• *During periodontal maintenance*: If there are signs of recurrence of periodontal disease including, but not limited to bleeding or suppuration on probing, increasing pocket depths, increasing mobility or migration of teeth, or recurrent periodontal abscesses.

B. Recurrence of Periodontal Disease

▶ Recurrence of signs and symptoms of periodontal infection indicates recolonization of periodontal pathogens.

▶ Recolonization of a pocket can occur in an average of 42 days.[4]

• Without daily personal dental biofilm control and regular professional supervision and maintenance procedures, infection can recur.

• Colonization depends on the number, frequency of exposure, and virulence of the organisms.

• Transmission of periodontal microorganisms has been shown between family members.[5,6]

• How soon after the completion of treatment colonization may reappear will vary with each patient depending on a number of contributing factors.

▶ *Contributing factors for recurrence*: recurrence will vary with each patient depending on a number of factors including the following:

• Inadequate biofilm control.

• Lack of compliance with PM appointments.

• Inadequate professional treatment.

  • *Inadequate scaling and debridement*, especially in areas of difficult access such as furcations and deep proximal pockets.

• *Biofilm retention*: Failure to remove or replace overhanging restorations and other areas that trap biofilm and foster bacterial growth.

• Failure of tobacco cessation including smoking tobacco, smokeless tobacco, or waterpipe tobacco smoking.[1,3,7,8]

• Systemic diseases such as diabetes mellitus,[9] HIV/AIDS,[10] and certain other systemic diseases influence healing and may control factors related to bone loss and severity of infections.

• Genetic factors: future testing for genetic factors may be used as a component of risk assessment.[11,12]

C. Criteria for Referral During PM

During maintenance therapy, any of the types of patients aforementioned may still need referral. Other cases may include:

▶ Pocket depth that prohibits access for complete debridement during nonsurgical periodontal therapy.

▶ Furcation involvements and other deep or complex anatomical areas that cannot be instrumented successfully by nonsurgical methods.

▶ Mucogingival problems; lack of attached gingiva.

▶ Periodontal disease that is refractory, or not responsive to usual treatment.[13]

APPOINTMENT INTERVALS (FREQUENCY)

▶ *Frequency planning*

• The frequency of continuing care or maintenance depends on the needs of each patient.

• Appointment intervals may vary from 2 to 6 months.

• The time interval is re-evaluated periodically and changed in accordance with changing needs.

▶ *Factors to consider in determining continuing care or maintenance frequency*

• Risk for periodontal disease activity.

• Risk for dental carious lesions.

• Risk for oral cancer: tobacco and alcohol users.

• Predisposing diseases, conditions, and behaviors for periodontal diseases including diabetes, HIV/AIDS, host genetic factors, smoking, and stress.

• Compliance: keeping appointments, personal daily biofilm control.

• Previous treatment: patient who has a history of disease, either dental caries or periodontal infection, is at a greater risk for recurrence.

• Local factors: rate of calculus formation.

• Restorative complications: implants, prosthetic replacements.

▶ *Special appointment requirements*

• Intervals of 2 or 3 months are required for many patients. A few are mentioned here.

• *Periodontitis*: Patients who have completed initial nonsurgical or surgical periodontal therapy. The first preventive maintenance appointment is scheduled based on the completion date of the initial scaling and root planing (or nonsurgical therapy).

- *Cognitive or physical disability*: Managing the toothbrush and other oral care devices may be difficult; when the disability involves the mouth area, opening the mouth may be a problem.
- *Diabetes*: Diabetes or other disease can predispose patients to lowered resistance to infection.
- *Cardiovascular disease or other condition*: Those who have been recently hospitalized may find oral self-care tiring and require some modifications to oral self-care routines. Appointments need to be short because of fatigue.
- *Patient undergoing extensive dental care*: When extensive restorative, prosthetic, or other treatment is in progress, frequent tissue maintenance during long-term therapy is essential.
- *Rampant dental caries*: Appointment for continuation of a caries control effort includes fluoride varnish applications, dietary supervision, and personal care factors for biofilm control.
- *Sealants*: Need for regular examination for defects such as chipped or loss of a *sealant to repair*, *replace*, or *extend*.
- *Orthodontic therapy*: Appliances make cleaning and biofilm control difficult; frequent topical fluoride applications may be indicated; response of gingival tissue to irritants can be marked.

METHODS FOR CONTINUING CARE SYSTEMS

▶ The continuing care system is essential for managing the oral health of patients.

▶ Methods for administration of continuing care include prebooking or prescheduling an appointment or a reminder card to schedule an appointment.

I. Prebook or Preschedule Method

▶ Make each patient's appointment before the patient leaves the current appointment in a computer-based electronic or traditional appointment book.

▶ An appointment card is given to the patient with a reminder to enter it on their calendar.

- If the patient uses a calendar application in their cell phone, encourage entering the new appointment before leaving the office or clinic.

▶ Reminders for the appointment can be done by:

- Preparing a postcard for mailing before the scheduled appointment. The card can be prepared by the patient before leaving the office or postcards or labels for postcards can be printed from the patient management system.
- Sending a reminder via e-mail, text, or other electronic media.

EVERYDAY ETHICS

There were two full-time dental hygienists in the practice. Susan had been there more than 15 years, and Jessica less than a year. Jessica had previously practiced with a periodontist in another city for 6 years, and she joined this practice shortly after she moved here. Each hygienist had instruments of their own preference and cared for them relative to sharpening and preparation for the sterilizer. Patients usually had appointments with the same dental hygienist. Susan scheduled a maintenance for 45 minutes, whereas Jessica never felt she had time enough even with an hour.

Occasionally, certain long-standing patients who had been with Susan for many years would be scheduled with Jessica when Susan could not be in the office.

As Jessica saw more of Susan's regular patients, she began to see a pattern of subgingival calculus that could not have formed since the previous 3 or 4 months' maintenance appointment. She had decided to ask the secretary to have Susan's patients wait for her return for their appointments.

Ms. Doubleday, a patient of Susan's, had already been scheduled and came for her appointment the next day. After the usual history review, periodontal charting, and treatment started, Jessica had to tell the patient that she needed two appointments and wanted to complete her scaling with local anesthesia. The patient was confused after having only short appointments faithfully and wanted to know whether to reschedule with Susan to finish since Susan would be back from her vacation soon.

Questions for Consideration

1. Is this an ethical issue or a dilemma? Explain. How do the core values (Table II-1, in Section II Introduction) apply in this scenario?

2. Using the step procedure for solving an issue or a dilemma (Box 1-10 in Chapter 1), suggest various possible actions for Jessica.

3. Prepare possible answers Jessica could use for her reply to Ms. Doubleday's immediate question.

▶ The reminder requests the patient call to confirm the appointment. For unconfirmed appointments, a call to the patient the day before is made.

II. Monthly Reminder Method

▶ If a patient is not prescheduled, a monthly list of patients due for maintenance can be generated.

- For a manual system, postcards can be filed alphabetically by the last name of the patient under the month when the patient is due.
- Practice management systems can easily create patient-specific postcards or letters to be mailed to the patient. Many systems can be set up to automate the process.

DOCUMENTATION

For the permanent patient's record the following needs to be recorded for a patient who is scheduled for routine continuing care:

BOX 48-3
Example Documentation: Continuing Care Appointment

S– A patient presents for 3-month PM appointment and apologized for not being able to clean her teeth after lunch. She described her daily self-care regimen; a remarkable behavior change since her initial periodontal therapy and patient education 4 years ago. She asked which toothpaste she needed to use saying "…one of those new kind for removing calculus?"

O– Medical, dental, and medication reviews, no changes. BP 135/60, Extra- and intraoral nothing remarkable. Vertical bitewings for molar areas were exposed based on patient risk factors. Periodontal examination with probing revealed numerous proximal areas of molars had 3–4 mm areas with BOP, subgingival calculus, and moderate-to-heavy biofilm suggesting lack of flossing.

A– Generalized moderate chronic periodontitis. Interdental biofilm accumulation with need for more specific instruction to include interdental brushes.

P– Asked patient to demonstrate current brushing method and provided additional instruction to modify her technique with emphasis on Bass brushing for interdental cleaning. Advised brushing more than once a day with a focus on every tooth. Demonstrated use of interdental brush. Gave her sample interdental brushes and explained where to purchase them. Recommended anticalculus toothpaste. Completed calculus removal for maxillary and mandibular right quadrant.

Next visit: two weeks to check success of today's instruction and scaling. Complete treatment for both left quadrants with local anesthesia due to extreme sensitivity in maxillary molars.

Signed _____, RDH
Date _____

▶ Medical, dental, medications, histories updated with each continuing care appointment.

▶ Complaints and questions patients may express of significance to the treatment given and the personal self-care expected by the patient.

▶ Findings during routine examinations including vital signs, extraoral and intraoral, periodontal, dental, temporomandibular joint, occlusion, and all special examinations following individual treatments for other reasons.

▶ A sample progress note may be reviewed in Box 48-3.

Factors To Teach The Patient

▷ Purposes of follow-up and continuing care or maintenance appointments.
▷ Relationship of personal oral care habits to the maintenance of cleanliness provided through professional scaling and debridement.
▷ Importance of keeping all maintenance appointments.

References

1. Chambrone L, Chambrone D, Lima LA, et al. Predictors of tooth loss during long-term periodontal maintenance: a systematic review of observational studies. *J Clin Periodontol.* 2010;37(7):675–684.

2. Cohen RE; Research, Science and Therapy Committee, American Academy of Periodontology. Position paper: periodontal maintenance. *J Periodontol.* 2003;74(9):1395–1401.

3. American Academy of Periodontology. Parameter on periodontal maintenance. *J Periodontol.* 2000;71(5, Suppl):849–850.

4. Mousqués T, Listgarten MA, Phillips RW. Effects of scaling and root planing on the composition of the human subgingival microbial flora. *J Periodontal Res.* 1980;15:144–151.

5. Asano H, Ishihara K, Nakagawa T, et al. Relationship between transmission of Porphyromonas gingivalis and fimA type in spouses. *J Periodontol.* 2003;74(9):1355–1360.

6. Doğan B, Kipalev AS, Okte E, et al. Consistent intrafamilial transmission of Actinobacillus actinomycetemcomitans despite clonal diversity. *J Periodontol.* 2008;79(2):307–315.

7. Research, Science and Therapy Committee of the American Academy of Periodontology. Position paper: tobacco use and the periodontal patient. *J Periodontol.* 1999;70(11):1419–1427.

8. Akl EA, Gaddam S, Gunukula SK, et al. The effects of waterpipe tobacco smoking on health outcomes: a systematic review. *Int J Epidemiol.* 2010;39(3):834–857.

9. Salvi GE, Carollo-Bittel B, Lang NP. Effects of diabetes mellitus on periodontal and peri-implant conditions: update on associations and risks. *J Clin Periodontol.* 2008;35(8, Suppl):398–409.

10. John CN, Stephen LX, Joyce Africa CW. Is human immunodeficiency virus (HIV) stage an independent risk factor for altering the periodontal status of HIV-positive patients? A South African study. *BMC Oral Health*. 2013; 13:69.

11. Research, Science and Therapy Committee of American Academy of Periodontology. Informational paper: implications of genetic technology for the management of periodontal diseases. *J Periodontol*. 2005;76(5):850–857.

12. Schaefer AS, Bochenek G, Manke T, et al. Validation of reported genetic risk factors for periodontitis in a large-scale replication study. *J Clin Periodontol*. 2013;40(6): 563–572.

13. American Academy of Periodontology. Parameter on "refractory" periodontitis. *J Periodontol*. 2000;71(5, Suppl):859–860.

ENHANCE YOUR UNDERSTANDING

thePoint® **DIGITAL CONNECTIONS**
(see the inside front cover for access information)
- **Audio glossary**
- **Quiz bank**

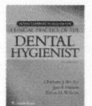

SUPPORT FOR LEARNING
(available separately; visit lww.com)
- *Active Learning Workbook for Clinical Practice of the Dental Hygienist, 12th Edition*

prepU **INDIVIDUALIZED REVTIEW**
(available separately; visit lww.com)
- **Adaptive quizzing with** *prepU for Wilkins' Clinical Practice of the Dental Hygienist*

Patients with Special Needs

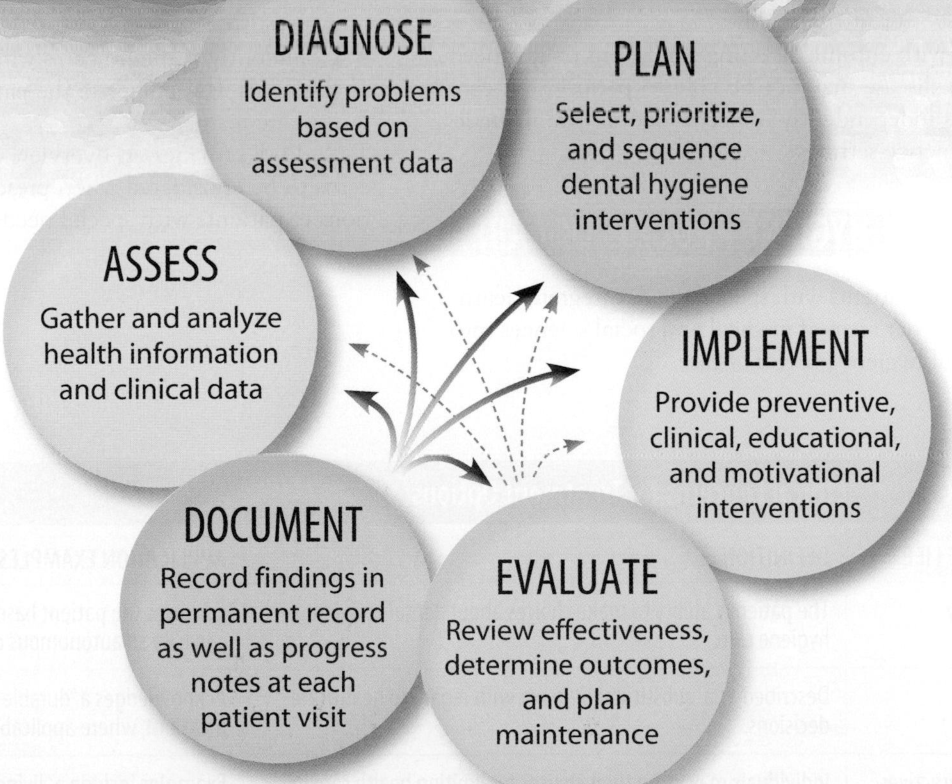

DIAGNOSE
Identify problems based on assessment data

PLAN
Select, prioritize, and sequence dental hygiene interventions

ASSESS
Gather and analyze health information and clinical data

IMPLEMENT
Provide preventive, clinical, educational, and motivational interventions

DOCUMENT
Record findings in permanent record as well as progress notes at each patient visit

EVALUATE
Review effectiveness, determine outcomes, and plan maintenance

FIGURE IX-1 **The Dental Hygiene Process of Care.**

INTRODUCTION FOR SECTION IX

The dental hygienist's obligation is to see that no patient needs special rehabilitative dental or periodontal services because of any condition that could have been prevented by dental hygiene care.

▶ For every patient, dental hygiene interventions are selected and patient management strategies are considered according to individualized needs.

▶ Patients with special needs that may complicate the plan for dental hygiene care are those with significant concerns related to:
  • Their age group.
  • Specific oral and general systemic conditions.
  • Degree of physical or cognitive disability.

▶ Dental hygiene care for patients with special needs may require:
  • A more skillful application of dental hygiene knowledge and ability to accomplish a comparably favorable outcome.
  • Pursuit of current evidence-based information about individuals with specific health concerns and successful patient management strategies.
  • Collaboration with an interprofessional team of both healthcare and home care providers to assure the patient's needs are met.

▶ Optimum oral health is frequently a contributing factor in maintaining or restoring optimum systemic health and enhancing quality of life.

▶ Patients with chronic disabling conditions or advanced stages of disease may not be able to perform self-care regimens independently or access dental care in traditional practice settings.

THE DENTAL HYGIENE PROCESS OF CARE

▶ The care of patients with special needs integrates learning from other areas of medical and social sciences into the dental hygiene process of care.

▶ The importance of each step in the process (Figure IX-1) is enhanced when providing care for a patient with health concerns that affect patient management or increase risk for poor treatment outcomes.

ETHICAL APPLICATIONS

▶ The complex medical and dental conditions of certain patients may translate into a need to identify unique treatment approaches that consider:
  • The quality of care provided.
  • The patient's quality of life.

▶ Increasingly, medically compromised patients are ambulatory and appear in a dental practice or clinic for maintenance and preventive procedures.

▶ A dental hygienist may also provide care in alternative settings such as a long-term care facility or the patient's home.

▶ The ethical dental hygienist:
  • Selects dental hygiene interventions that are consistent with the patient's physical, mental, and personal capabilities.
  • Instructs patients and/or caregivers about oral hygiene problems and needs related to their systemic disorders and medications.
  • Ensures that all appropriate persons are included in all chairside discussions, if someone other than the patient is responsible for making treatment decisions.
  • Confidently communicates with all healthcare professionals who comprise the patient's interdisciplinary care team.

▶ Table IX-1 provides an overview of some ethical concerns to be considered when presenting treatment options to patients with special needs.

TABLE IX-1	Ethical Concerns for Treatment Options	
QUALITY OF LIFE	**DEFINITION**	**APPLICATION EXAMPLES**
Competency	The patient's ability to make choices about dental and dental hygiene care.	Educates the patient based on intellectual capacity so autonomous consent can be given.
Surrogate	Described as a "substitute" or proxy with regard to healthcare decisions.	Acknowledges a "durable power of attorney" for a patient, where applicable.
Advanced directives	Individuals may write their choices for limiting health care in the event that they are unable to make choices in the future.	Examples include a "living will," "do not resuscitate" order, and "patient values" history.

49

The Pregnant Patient and Infant

Lori Rainchuso, RDH, MS, Esther M. Wilkins, BS, RDH, DMD, and Nancy S. Lepeau, RDH, MS, MA

LEARNING OBJECTIVES

After studying this chapter, the student will be able to:

1. Describe the oral implications of fetal development in all stages of pregnancy.

2. Identify common oral findings during pregnancy.

3. Recognize the association between periodontal infection and pregnancy.

4. Assess and develop an appropriate preventive plan for dental hygiene treatment during pregnancy.

5. Recognize special problems that may occur during pregnancy and need for referral.

6. Recognize the importance of infant oral health.

7. Describe anticipatory guidance for the infant to include dietary education for the caretakers.

8. Describe components of and techniques for conducting an infant oral examination.

Pregnancy is a unique time during a woman's life. Attention is focused on healthy lifestyle practices for both the mother and fetus.[1]

▶ *Prenatal care* refers to supervised preparation for childbirth to help the mother enjoy optimum health during and after pregnancy and maximize chances for the baby to be born healthy.[2]

  • Prenatal care involves the combined efforts of the obstetrician and/or midwife, nurse practitioner, dentist, dental hygienist, dietitian, and expectant parents.

▶ There is no indication that dental and dental hygiene treatment during any trimester of pregnancy can cause harm to the mother or developing fetus. However, most research indicates the second trimester as most ideal for dental treatment.[3]

INTRODUCTION

▶ Medical providers (prenatal care specialists) in private and public health settings need to recommend dental and periodontal examinations early in pregnancy.

▶ Referrals from medical providers may bring many women to the private dental practice or dental clinic who would not have regular access to dental care.

  • Many of these women may not have had education about the value of daily oral self-care and diet related to the health of the oral tissues.

  • Numerous misconceptions can be addressed when providing information about the relationship of pregnancy and oral health.

▶ Women who do not receive routine oral health care may appear for emergency dental services and once the emergency situation is resolved, they may be receptive to a preventive program of care and instruction.

▶ The dental hygienist in public health, especially maternal and child health clinics, participates in community educational programs with public health nurses. In these programs, women not well informed about oral health may learn of the need for professional dental and dental hygiene care and education during pregnancy.

Key words for study with this chapter are defined in Box 49-1.

FETAL DEVELOPMENT

▶ Pregnancy is arbitrarily divided into three periods of 3 months each called the first, second, and third trimesters.[4]

▶ Physiologic changes in the mother occur to nearly every body system.

▶ Early development of the embryo is greatly influenced by heredity and the general health of the mother.[5]

▶ Normal pregnancy, or period of gestation, is approximately 40 weeks.[4] Premature birth refers to a birth before 37 weeks' gestation.[6]

I. First Trimester

▶ During the early stages of pregnancy, the embryo is highly susceptible to injuries, malformations, and mortality.[7]

▶ Teratogenic effects can be produced by many sources, including maternal poor nutrition, infections, and drug intake.

▶ All organ systems are formed (organogenesis) during the first trimester. By 12 weeks, the fetus moves and swallows.[6]

A. Oral Cavity Development Includes the Teeth, Lips, and Palate

▶ Tooth buds develop between the 5th and 6th week. Initial mineralization occurs from the 4th to 5th month (Table 50-4 in Chapter 50).[8]

▶ Lips form during the 4th–7th week and the palate forms between the 8th and the 12th week.[8]

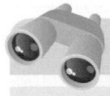 **BOX 49-1   KEY WORDS AND ABBREVIATIONS**

Anticipatory guidance: anticipatory guidance is the process of providing practical, developmentally appropriate information about children's health to prepare parents for the significant physical, emotional, and psychological milestones.

Dental home: An ongoing relationship between the dentist and the patient, including all aspects of oral health care delivered in a comprehensive, continuously accessible, coordinated, and family-centered way.

Early childhood caries (ECC): the presence of 1 or more decayed (noncavitated or cavitated lesions), missing (due to caries), or filled tooth surfaces in any primary tooth in a child younger than 6 years of age.

Fetus: An unborn offspring, from the embryo stage until birth.

Gestational diabetes: diabetes with initial onset or recognition during pregnancy

Gestation: gestation is the period of time between conception and birth.

Severe early childhood caries (S-ECC): the presence of any area of smooth surface decay in a child younger than 3 years of age.

Xylitol: a natural sugar-alcohol that is approved for use in food by the US Food and Drug Administration.

▶ Cleft lip is apparent by the 8th week; cleft palate, by the 12th week (see Chapter 51).

II. Second and Third Trimesters

▶ The organs are completed, and growth and maturation continue.

▶ Rapid fetal growth and weight changes occur during the second and third trimester.

▶ The second trimester is the ideal time for dental treatment.[3]

III. Factors that Can Harm the Fetus

A. Infections

▶ Although numerous epidemiological studies have suggested a statistically significant association between periodontal infection and increase risk for adverse pregnancy outcomes, other studies have not confirmed this relationship.[9,10]

▶ As a result of the numerous studies supporting an association with preterm delivery and low birth weight babies, the American Academy of Periodontology recommends women who are planning to become pregnant or currently are pregnant to have a periodontal examination and receive preventive or therapeutic treatment, when needed.[11]

▶ Protection from infectious diseases is necessary because damage to and infection of the fetus can result.[12]

▶ Women of childbearing age need to take advantage of all available vaccines prior to conception.[12]

▶ Defects, deformities, and life-threatening infections in the fetus can result from infection acquired during pregnancy or during delivery and after birth.[12]

▶ Rubella (German measles), rubeola, varicella, herpes viruses, hepatitis B, human immunodeficiency virus (HIV) infection, syphilis (congenital syphilis), and gonorrhea all can have serious effects on the fetus (see Chapter 4).

B. Pharmacokinetics[13]

▶ During pregnancy normal physiological changes occur; as a result drug movement within biologic systems is unique.

▶ Nearly all drugs pass across the placenta to enter the circulation of the developing fetus, and may have teratogenic effects based on factors such as gestational age, route of administration, absorption, dose, and maternal serum levels.

▶ However, the majority of medications/drugs prescribed by an oral health professional and dispensed during pregnancy are not associated with teratogenic effects or adverse effects of fetal development.

▶ Table 49-1 lists selected drugs with indications, contraindications, and special considerations for pregnant women.

▶ *Effect of tetracycline*
  • Tetracycline is well known for intrinsic staining of tooth structure.
  • The effect occurs during mineralization of the primary teeth beginning at about 4 months of gestation and of the permanent teeth near and after birth (see Table 50-4, in Chapter 50).
  • When an antibiotic is required during pregnancy, the prescribing of tetracycline must be avoided.[13]

▶ *Therapy for HIV infection*
  • Prevention of perinatal HIV transmission and health for the fetus and neonate are considered with the plan for optimal health care for the mother with HIV/AIDS infection.[14]
  • There is a high mortality rate among pregnant and postpartum women with HIV infection who have suspended their antiretroviral therapy (ART).[15]
  • Among HIV-infected pregnant women who are eligible, ART is considered a safe and effective treatment in maternal viral suppression, and in decreasing mother to child transmission and infant mortality.[16]

C. Drugs of Abuse and Dependence

▶ Use of tobacco, alcohol, and substances of abuse during pregnancy can have severe influences on the developing fetus, as well as on the child after birth.[17,18]

▶ Pregnancy is an ideal time to motivate a patient to quit smoking and avoid the use of other harmful substances.[7]

▶ Explain increased risks for reduced birth weight, spontaneous abortions, perinatal deaths, and sudden infant death syndrome.[3,18]

▶ The effects of tobacco use on pregnancy and assistance for smoking cessation are discussed in Chapter 34.

▶ Explain the effects of second-hand and third-hand smoke on the fetus and child after birth.[17,19]

▶ Present the steps in a cessation program, as described in Chapter 34.

▶ Information on the effects of alcohol use during pregnancy and fetal alcohol syndrome is included in Chapter 65.

D. Herbal Dietary Supplements[20]

▶ Herbal dietary supplements are not regulated by the Federal Drug Administration. The public is free to purchase them over the counter to self-medicate.

▶ Questions about the use of herbal dietary supplements, their amount, and duration of use are documented when taking a routine medical history. Information about possible problems when taking the supplements can be presented to the patient.

▶ Common uses are for colds, burns, headaches, allergies, rashes, depression, and insomnia.

TABLE 49-1	Pharmacological Chart

PHARMACOLOGICAL CONSIDERATIONS FOR PREGNANT WOMEN

The pharmacological agents listed below are to be used only for indicated medical conditions and with appropriate supervision.

PHARMACEUTICAL AGENT	INDICATION, CONTRAINDICATIONS, AND SPECIAL CONSIDERATIONS
Analgesics	
Acetaminophen	May be used during pregnancy.
Acetaminophen with Codeine, Hydrocodone, or Oxycodone	
Codeine	
Meperidine	
Morphine	
Aspirin	May be used in short duration pregnancy; 48–72 hr. Avoid in 1st and 3rd trimesters.
Ibuprofen	
Naproxen	
Antibiotics	
Amoxicillin	May be used during pregnancy.
Cephalosporins	
Clindamycin	
Metronidazole	
Penicillin	
Ciprofloxacin	Avoid during pregnancy.
Clarithromycin	
Levofloxacin	
Moxifloxacin	
Tetracycline	Never use during pregnancy.
Anesthetics	Consult with a prenatal care health professional prior to using intravenous sedation or general anesthesia.
Local anesthetics with epinephrine (e.g., Bupivacine, Lidocaine, Mepivacaine)	May be used during pregnancy.
Nitrous oxide (30%)	May be used during pregnancy when topical or local anesthetics are inadequate. Pregnant women require lower levels of nitrous oxide to achieve sedation; consult with prenatal care health professional.
Antimicrobials	Use alcohol-free products during pregnancy.
Cetylpyridinium chloride mouth rinse	May be used during pregnancy.
Chlorhexidine mouth rinse	
Xylitol	

Source: Reproduced with permission from Oral Health Care During Pregnancy Expert Workgroup. *Oral Health Care During Pregnancy: A National Consensus Statement.* Washington, DC: National Maternal and Child Oral Health Resource Center; 2012.

► Several remedies have implications for dental/dental hygiene treatment, such as:
  • Echinacea used for upper respiratory infections (colds) activates cell-mediated immunity: may cause allergic reactions, decreased effectiveness of immunosuppressants, and immunosuppression with long-term use.[21]
  • Valerian used for insomnia and stress has a sedative effect and may increase the sedative effect of

anesthetics and, with long-term use, may increase anesthetic requirements.[22]

ORAL FINDINGS DURING PREGNANCY

I. Gingival Conditions[3,10,23]

▶ Increased gingival inflammation is a well-documented phenomenon occurring during pregnancy and may occur because of the following:
  - Increased circulating levels of estrogen and progesterone hormones in pregnancy.
  - Immunological alterations that are pregnancy induced cause a weakening of the mother's cell-mediated immune response.
  - Exaggerated response of the tissues to dental biofilm and local irritants.
  - Trauma, poor oral self-care, and local irritation from calculus or prostheses may be contributory factors.

▶ Gingival changes in pregnancy usually appear in the first trimester, and can continue throughout the pregnancy unless instruction is given and daily oral self-care is improved.

▶ When the periodontal tissues are in good health and the patient uses adequate oral self-care measures for biofilm control, major adverse gingival changes are not expected.

▶ When left untreated, gingival inflammation continues as the hormones rise to a maximum level by the 8th month.

▶ Symptoms abate after the birth of the child, but a completely healthy condition does not necessarily result. A patient with a gingival disturbance during pregnancy may continue to have the disturbance, to a somewhat lessened degree, after the birth especially if she is breastfeeding.

II. Gingivitis[3]

▶ Most common oral condition associated with pregnancy.
▶ Commonly referred to as pregnancy gingivitis.

A. Clinical Appearance

▶ Shows characteristics of inflamed tissues, including enlargement, redness, smooth and shiny surface.
▶ Bleeding on probing (BOP).

B. Predisposing Factors[10,24]

▶ Maternal immunological changes.
▶ Local irritation and infection because of poor oral self-care leaving dental biofilm on the teeth and gingiva.
▶ Hormonal (estrogen and progesterone) changes during pregnancy that may alter the tissue reaction.[10]

▶ Increased proportions of *Bacteroides melaninogenius* and *Prevotella intermedia* have been found in gingivitis.[24]

III. Gingival Enlargement

A. Oral "Pyogenic" Granuloma[10,24–26]

▶ Also referred to as pregnancy epulis, granuloma gravidarum, pregnancy granuloma, or a pregnancy tumor.
▶ The use of the word *tumor* is misleading; the lesion is not a tumor but a hyperplasia and may also occur in men and nonpregnant women.
▶ Benign, inflammatory lesion; rapid growing gingival mass.
▶ When the lesion is removed during pregnancy, there is some tendency for recurrence.

B. Clinical Appearance

▶ The lesion appears as an isolated, discrete, soft, round enlargement near the gingival margin usually associated with an interdental area, as shown in Figure 49-1.
▶ It forms in a mushroomlike shape with a smooth, glistening surface.
▶ The pressure of the lip or cheek tends to flatten it.
▶ The color depends on the vascularity and may be purplish-red, magenta, or deep blue, sometimes dotted with red.

C. Symptoms

▶ Bleeds readily with slight trauma.
▶ Painless unless it becomes large enough to interfere with occlusion and mastication.

D. Significance

▶ Interference during mastication: can contribute to inadequate nutritive intake for mother and baby because of discomfort when chewing.
▶ Provides a site for bacterial growth; potential development of periodontal attachment loss and eventual bone destruction.

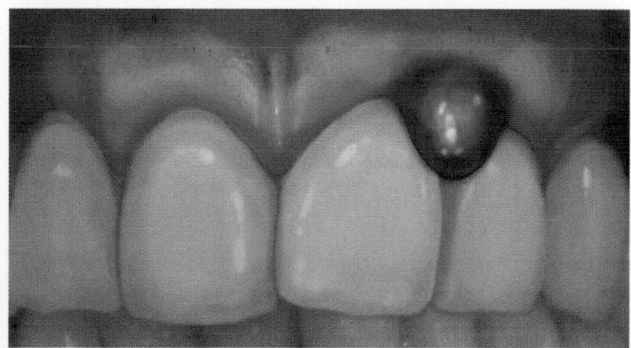

FIGURE 49-1 "Pyogenic" Granuloma or "Pregnancy Tumor. " Isolated, discrete, round, soft enlargement near the gingival margin; smooth, glistening surface, purplish-red in color.

▶ Results in bleeding and pain: may interfere with routine dental biofilm removal using toothbrush and interdental aids.

▶ Creates undesirable esthetic effects.

▶ Lesion must be ruled out for similar appearing malignancies and underlying systemic conditions. Referral for excision and biopsy may be indicated.

IV. Periodontal Infections[3,10,24]

▶ Pregnancy-associated immunologic changes cause a suppression of the mother's cell-mediated immune response, particularly the neutrophil function.

▶ Many epidemiological studies suggest a causal relationship between periodontal infections and several adverse pregnancy outcomes, such as pre-eclampsia, preterm delivery, and low birth weight.

▶ Evidence shows periodontal treatment is safe during pregnancy. The American Academy of Periodontology recommends that a pregnant woman undergo a routine periodontal examination.[11]

▶ Preventive services such as periodontal maintenance care can be rendered during pregnancy.[11]

▶ Periodontal therapeutic services can be rendered during pregnancy.[11]

V. Enamel Erosion[3,27]

A. Development

▶ Morning sickness with vomiting over an extended period can lead to demineralization and acid erosion primarily on the maxillary palatal surfaces.

B. Recommendations for the Patient

▶ Eat small amounts of nutritious yet noncariogenic foods throughout the day.

▶ Use a sodium bicarbonate rinse after vomiting to neutralize acid on teeth; one cup of water to one teaspoon of sodium bicarbonate.

▶ Chew gum containing xylitol after eating.

▶ Use a soft toothbrush and low abrasive fluoride toothpaste to prevent damage to demineralized tooth surfaces.

ASPECTS OF PATIENT CARE[3,23,28]

I. Assessment

▶ Preventive oral health care needs to begin early and continue throughout the pregnancy, to keep the gingival tissues in optimum health and prevent oral infections.

A. Medical History: Health Problems Need Identification During Examination

▶ Gestational diabetes: First recognition during pregnancy; needs insulin adjustment and careful

supervision.[29] More information is included with Chapter 69.

▶ Women with hypertension are considered to be at high risk for having complications during pregnancy. A consultation with the patient's physician and/or obstetrician is necessary.

▶ Adolescent health: When the expectant mother is an adolescent, her own special needs differ from those of a mature woman. Aspects of adolescent development are described in Chapter 50 and Chapter 52.

B. Consultations

▶ Treatment approval is not required when providing routine dental care. Consultation with the patient's physician and/or obstetrician may be indicated, when underlying health conditions are present.[3]

▶ When a patient seeks dental and dental hygiene care and is not under the care of a physician, she is urged and assisted to obtain medical supervision for her health and the health of her baby.

II. Radiography[30,31]

A. Universal Safety Factors

▶ Guidelines for dental radiographs during pregnancy have been established.

▶ ALARA (as low as reasonably achievable) principles to minimize the patient's exposure to radiation needs to be followed (see Chapter 13).

▶ Recommendations advise that dental radiographs are safe throughout pregnancy, and that X-ray exposure for a diagnostic procedure does not cause harmful effects to the developing embryo or fetus.

▶ With contemporary safety factors of modern radiography, the patient can be assured that essential radiographs can be made without question during pregnancy.

▶ When radiographs are required during pregnancy, the patient is covered with a lead apron and a thyroid collar.

III. Overall Treatment Considerations

A. Dental Hygiene Care Goal

▶ The dental hygienist who is well informed about dental care can motivate the patient during her pregnancy and alleviate fears related to certain services.

▶ When treating a pregnant patient, the dental hygienist's goal is to optimize the oral health of both the mother and child.

B. Dental Care[3,32]

▶ *Restorative*: Complete restorative needs with permanent restorative materials. Recommended at any time during pregnancy; however, the second trimester is considered most ideal.

▶ *Elective* esthetic *treatment*: Postpone until postdelivery.

C. Appointment Planning[3,27,28]

▶ Appointment adaptations for the pre-natal patient are listed in Table 49-2.
▶ Frequency depends on patient care plan.
  • Monthly appointments or appointments three times during the 9-month period may be required.
  • Appointment frequency depends on the patient's needs as well as ability and motivation to maintain a healthy oral environment.
▶ Individual appointments
  • Patients are more comfortable with short appointments.

• A series of appointments is indicated when calculus deposits are heavy, and/or periodontal infection is present.
▶ Postpartum continuing care appointments
  • Emphasis is placed on motivating the patient to continue regular appointments for dental hygiene and dental care after the baby is born.

D. Patient Positioning[3,28]

▶ *Effect of supine position*
  • The weight of the developing fetus in the uterus bears down directly on the major vessels, the aorta, and the inferior vena cava.

TABLE 49-2	Appointment Adaptations for the Prenatal Patient
CHARACTERISTIC	**DENTAL HYGIENE IMPLICATION**
Fatigues easily, may even fall asleep	Short appointments; several in series, as needed. Work with an assistant to accomplish more at each appointment
General awkwardness because of new shape and weight gain	Attend to details, such as gently lowering and straightening chair for patient. Make sure rinsing facilities are convenient; or preferably, an assistant attends to evacuation
Frequent urination	Allow sufficient appointment time for interruptions. Suggest at beginning of appointment that patient indicate if a restroom break is needed
Discomfort of remaining in one position too long	Position the patient on her left side and not in supine or trendelenburg position (Figure 49-2)
Backache	Encourage position changes throughout the appointment. Assistance with evacuation during intraoral instrumentation can shorten appointment time
Faintness and dizziness	Be prepared for emergency (Table 8-3, Chapter 8)
Adverse reaction to strong smells and flavors	Recommend less strong-flavored dentifrice
Exaggerated reactions to odors and flavors of medicaments and other office materials	Determine particularly obnoxious odors for an individual patient and remove them; check office ventilation
Unpleasant taste in mouth	Advise: nonalcoholic mouth rinse; use a neutral sodium fluoride rinse. Demonstrate tongue cleaning as in Chapter 28
Nausea and vomiting	To avoid tooth abrasion, do not brush immediately after vomiting. Rinse generously with fluoridated water or water and a teaspoon of sodium bicarbonate (baking soda) mixture after vomiting to neutralize the acid from the teeth
Gagging	Recommend a small toothbrush. Turn head down over sink while brushing; helps to relax throat and allow saliva to flow out. Take care in instrument and radiographic film placement
Physician's recommendation for alleviation of nausea symptoms: frequent eating of small amounts of foods	Encourage use of noncariogenic foods
Unusual food cravings	If cravings are for sweets, clearly define relationship of frequent snacking of cariogenic foods to dental caries. Conduct a dietary analysis. Provide list of nutritious noncariogenic snacks

- The vessels are pressed between the spinal column and the uterus.
- During the third trimester, symptoms of circulatory insufficiency can appear when venous return is decreased.

▶ *Supine hypotensive syndrome: emergency*[33]
- Patient is lying in supine position.
- Abrupt fall in blood pressure.
- Bradycardia, sweating, nausea, weakness, air hunger.
- Symptoms caused by impaired venous return resulting from pressure of the uterus with developing baby on the inferior vena cava.
- Leads to decrease in blood pressure, reduced cardiac output, and loss of consciousness.

▶ *Emergency treatment*
- Roll the patient over to her left side to relieve pressure of uterus on vena cava.
- Blood pressure will return to normal promptly.

▶ *Alternate positions* (Figure 49-2).
- Elevate the right hip to displace the uterus to the left. Use a pillow or rolled-up blanket (Figure 49-2A).
- Patient lies on left side (Figure 49-2B).

IV. Dental Hygiene Care[1,3,23]

A. Preventive Care and Measures

▶ Preventive oral health care needs priority attention, beginning with information and motivation.

- Areas of food impaction are corrected, and all overhanging restorations are reshaped or replaced.
- All nonsurgical periodontal therapy procedures are carefully and thoroughly completed.
- When a patient has gingival enlargement and inflammation, instruction in biofilm control and other preventive measures including diet and eating patterns are needed.
- At the follow-up appointments, evaluation with disclosing agent is made and instruction is continued.

B. Instrumentation

▶ Careful instrumentation for complete calculus removal is indicated.
▶ The use of ultrasonic scalers is not contraindicated for reasons related to pregnancy.
▶ Nonsurgical periodontal therapy may be performed during pregnancy.

C. Anesthesia[3,34]

▶ Local anesthetics containing epinephrine are allowed during pregnancy.
▶ After consultation with the patient's physician, nitrous oxide/oxygen may be used in moderation.
▶ If used in the second or third trimester, precaution is required, including the length minimized to 30 minutes with oxygen percentage at 50%.

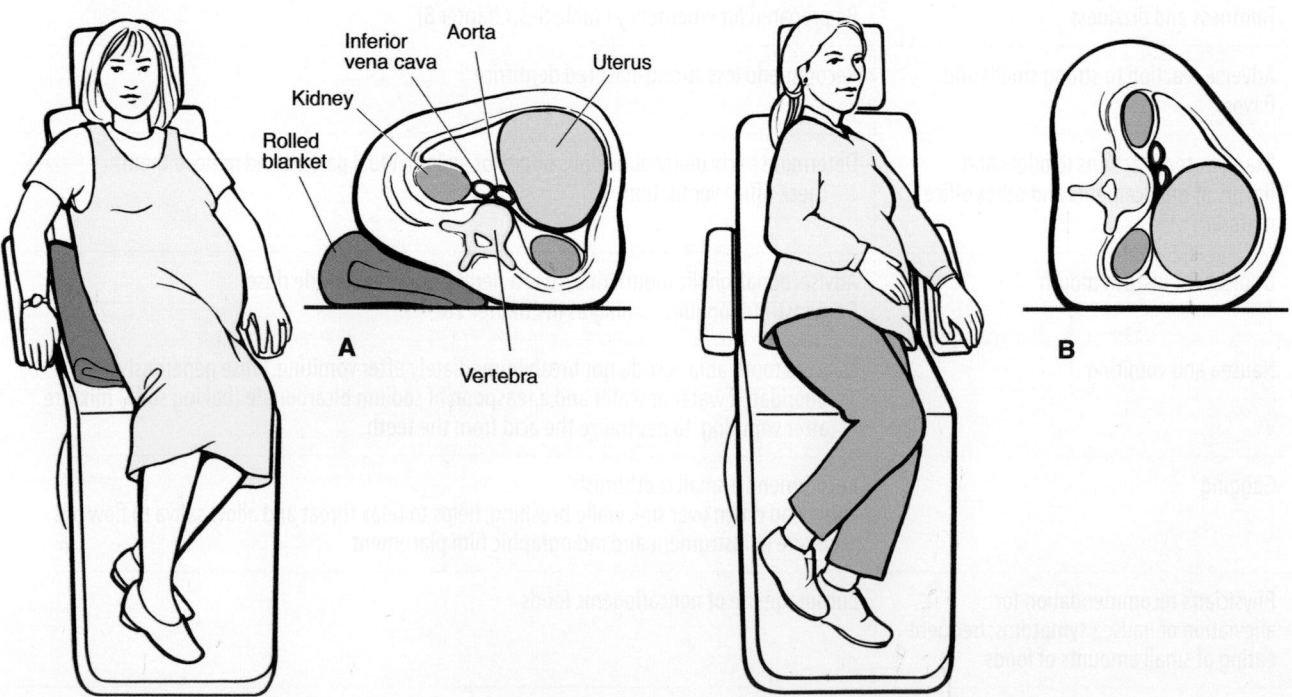

FIGURE 49-2 Positions During Pregnancy. The supine position allows the weight of the developing fetus to bear down directly on the major vessels. **A:** Patient lies on left side with a pillow or blanket roll to elevate right hip. **B:** Patient turned farther to left. Note position of uterus in cross sections of the abdomen.

PATIENT INSTRUCTION

▶ The emphasis on general health during pregnancy provides the ideal setting for instructions relative to many aspects of oral health for the mother, her expected child, and other family members.

▶ New developments in disease prevention and control need to be explained.

▶ Helping the mother learn what to expect before infant arrival is essential.

I. Dental Biofilm Control[3,12,24]

▶ A schedule for oral self-care is established and specific methods are outlined and demonstrated. A series of instructional sessions is better for patient learning.

▶ Increased gingival inflammation is a common phenomenon during pregnancy.

▶ Gingival changes during pregnancy require daily self-care by the patient and periodic professional dental hygiene appointments.

II. Diet[35-37]

▶ Instruction is provided in prevention of dental caries and maintenance of the health of the supporting structures of the teeth.

▶ The use of a varied diet containing the essential protective food groups, with a minimum of cariogenic foods, is necessary. The www.choosemyplate.gov is a valuable resource with specifics for maternal nutrition. The ChooseMyPlate Food Guide is shown in Figure 35-1, Chapter 35.

A. Purposes of Adequate Diet During Pregnancy

▶ Maintain daily strength and feeling of well-being.

▶ Provide the essential building materials for the developing fetus.

▶ Protect and promote the health of the oral tissues of the mother.

▶ Minimize postpartum problems.

B. Dietary Needs During Pregnancy

The mother's diet needs to maintain her own nutritional status and to meet the needs of the growing baby. These particular needs are:

▶ Proteins for general tissue construction.

▶ Minerals, especially calcium and phosphorus, for bone and tooth mineralization; iron for blood corpuscles.

▶ Vitamins, especially vitamin D, for calcium metabolism, folate to prevent neural tube defects and low birth weight.

▶ A prenatal vitamin supplement is commonly recommended during pregnancy.

C. Dietary Assessment and Recommendations for Oral and General Health Include[35]

▶ Intake from food groups.
- Consume a healthy diet from the fruit, vegetable, grain, meat/meat alternatives, and dairy food groups.
- About 800 mg of calcium per day or 3–4 servings of low-fat/fat-free calcium-rich foods.
- About 1,000 mg of calcium per day is recommended for a pregnant adolescent.
- Iron and folic acid supplements and iron and folate-rich foods.

▶ Frequency and types of snacks per day.
- Limit cariogenic food occurrence.
- Healthy snacks, such as carrots, fresh fruits, or almonds.

▶ Intake of sweetened and caffeinated beverages, such as ice tea or soda.
- Limit or avoid drinking beverages that are sweetened with sugar and contain caffeine.
- Substitute with fluoridated water.

▶ Avoiding sugar-containing chewing gum.
- Instead use a sugarless chewing gum containing xylitol.[38,39]

III. Dental Caries Control[3,27]

A. Incidence During Pregnancy

▶ Complete a caries risk assessment survey to indicate patient's caries risk (see Chapter 27).

▶ Some patients believe that they have more dental caries during and because of pregnancy.

▶ Research has shown that this is not true and that any relationship is indirect.[3]

▶ Factors that result in dental caries formation are the same during pregnancy as at other times (Figure 35-2, Chapter 35).

▶ Mothers with poor oral health and high levels of cariogenic bacteria are at a greater risk for infecting their children with the bacteria and increasing their children's caries risk at infancy.[40]

B. Factors that May Contribute to an Increase in Dental Caries Rate

▶ *Previous neglect*: A patient may not have kept a regular dental appointment plan. The existing dental caries during pregnancy may represent years of accumulation.

▶ *Diet during pregnancy*: Increase in intake of cariogenic foods:[35]
- Unusual cravings may be for sweet foods.
- Frequency of eating: patient may be eating every few hours for prevention of nausea, and those foods may be cariogenic.

► *Neglect of personal oral care procedures:* Patient may lack interest in daily dental biofilm removal or be lax about rinsing (with water) immediately following intake of a cariogenic food.

► Vomiting associated with morning sickness may lead to tooth decalcification and erosion.

► The smell of toothpaste or the act of brushing may precipitate nausea and cause reduction in oral care.

C. Relationship of Fluoride[39]

No direct evidence shows prenatal fluoride intake by the mother influences the rate of dental caries in the child.

IV. Fluoride Program[41]

A. Professional Topical Application

► Professional fluoride varnish application for caries prevention has been endorsed by the American Dental Association.

► Applications can be indicated, especially for patients with a tendency toward demineralization and those with numerous restorations. CAMBRA (Caries Risk Management by Risk Assessment) is described in Table 27-1, Chapter 27.

B. Self-applications

► A fluoride dentifrice.

► Drinking fluoridated water is recommended for all patients.[42]

► Other fluoride recommendations are individualized according to patient need.

► A daily fluoride mouth rinse, gel tray, or other mode of application is essential for some patients; review how to rinse thoroughly (Box 30-4, Chapter 30).

SPECIAL PROBLEMS REQUIRING REFERRAL

I. Depression During Pregnancy

Childbearing years place women at greatest risk for depression.[43] Oral healthcare professionals can learn to identify signs and symptoms of depression in pregnant patients. Treatment for depression and dental hygiene care for individuals with depression are described in Chapter 64.

A. Signs of Depression

► Depressed mood; loss of interest or pleasure in ordinary activities

► Fatigue and disturbed sleep

► Loss of appetite

► Difficulty making decisions

► Feelings of worthlessness and suicidal thoughts.[44]

B. Impact on Health of the Fetus

► Higher tendencies for preeclampsia

► Longer labor

► Low birth weight

► Preterm delivery.

C. What to Do

► Explain that depression is a biologically based illness caused by a chemical imbalance in the brain.

► Indicate that depression is treatable, and when treated, can improve the quality of life.

► Refer patient to the physician of record or a community mental health resource center.

II. Domestic Violence[45]

A. Identification

Identification, assessment, and intervention with victims of domestic violence can be a significant part of a dental visit (see Chapter 62).

B. Most Common Sites of Injury

► Head

► Face

► Neck.

C. Obstetrical and Other Manifestations

► Obstetrical: miscarriages and spontaneous or multiple abortions

► Substance abuse

► Depression

► Suicide attempts.

D. What to Do[43]

1. Address the issue with the patient.
2. Refer to a Domestic Violence Intervention Program in the community when domestic violence is suspected.

TRANSITIONING FROM PREGNANCY TO INFANCY

Once the baby is born, the focus shifts to the oral health needs of both mother and child. The next section will address infant oral health and parental guidance through the first year of life.

INFANT ORAL HEALTH[3,28,40,46]

To optimize infant oral health, oral health counseling begins during prenatal dental visits.[3,40]

I. Anticipatory Guidance[47]

▶ Dental care during pregnancy includes educating the mother about the importance of infant oral health, so she can be prepared (Table 49-3).

▶ Anticipatory guidance helps a parent learn what to expect during the infant's early and future developmental stages.

▶ Eruption patterns vary and are familial in nature; the primary maxillary and mandibular central and lateral incisors generally erupt prior to age one.[8] This process is known as teething. See Table 50-4 in Chapter 50 for tooth eruption patterns.

▶ Teething often causes the infant to experience mild irritability, increased salivation, and experience a low-grade fever.

▶ To ease teething discomfort a chilled teething ring or washcloth are recommended.

▶ Over-the-counter teething products containing benzocaine are not recommended for children under 2 years of age.[48]

▶ Over-the-counter teething products containing benzocaine can cause a rare but potentially fatal condition, methomoglobinemia.[48]

TABLE 49-3	Anticipatory Guidance: Birth to 12 Months	
AREA OF CONCERN	**BIRTH TO 6 MO**	**6–12 MO**
Developmental milestone	■ Eruption of first tooth ■ Pattern of eruption	■ Pattern of eruption ■ Expected new teeth
Nutrition and feeding	■ Relation of improper bottle/breast feeding to initiation of dental caries ■ No propping of bottles in bed ■ Avoid use of bottle as pacifier ■ Breastfeeding passage of alcohol and drugs to infant ■ Discuss weaning	■ Begin weaning ■ Discontinue bottle feeding by age 1 y ■ Use small regular cup ■ Avoid at-will access to bottle or sippy cup ■ Discuss sugar use, sugar retention, and caries initiation ■ Discuss consumption of sugar-sweetened beverages ■ Snacking safety (aspiration) ■ Avoid use of food for behavior modification
Oral hygiene and caries prevention	■ Oral health of parents; Streptococcus mutans transmission ■ Clean ridges after each feeding (soft, wet cloth or gauze) ■ Use of brush (water only) ■ Position of infant for brushing	■ Use of brush ■ Review position of infant for brushing ■ Parents look for signs of disease ■ Importance of maintaining primary dentition
Fluoride information	■ Explain the relation of fluoride to teeth ■ Anticipate need to supplement ■ Check water supply for fluoride content at home and daycare	■ When water supply is deficient, prescribe supplement (see Table 36-1) ■ Discuss compliance ■ Review manner of storage: cool, dry, out of reach ■ Possible fluoride varnish application
Trauma prevention	■ Car seat safety	■ Discuss highest accident rate is 1–2 y ■ Car seat safety ■ Trauma proofing ■ Confirm emergency access to dental provider
Habits/function behaviors	■ Discuss teething ■ Discuss nonnutritive sucking	■ Discuss oral/head and neck signs of child abuse
Environmental (passive) smoke	■ Detrimental at all ages; smoking parents encouraged to start tobacco cessation program	■ Provide smoke-free environment
Dental/dental hygienist visit	■ Provide rationale for timing of baby's first dental visit ■ Explain what happens at first dental visit ■ Encourage parents to make appointments for their own dental care to eliminate Streptococcus mutans and maintain oral health	■ Schedule first dental visit within 6 mo of eruption of first tooth ■ Provide information about how to make the first dental/dental hygiene visit a happy experience ■ Review need for parents to complete their own dental care

▶ It is recommended that an infant receive a dental examination at 12 months, or by the eruption of the first primary tooth.

▶ Establishment of a dental home for infants by 12 months of age is recommended. Early establishment of a dental home is crucial in early childhood caries (ECC) prevention and intervention.[47]

▶ When discussing anticipatory guidance include the following: infant daily oral hygiene; fluoride exposure; nutrition and diet; first dental visit; nonnutritive oral habits such as pacifier use, and thumb sucking; and dental trauma and injury avoidance (see Table 49-3).

▶ Developmental milestones to consider when providing patient education are outlined in Table 49-4.

II. Infant Daily Oral Hygiene Care

▶ Advise caregiver to brush the infant's teeth twice daily, with a child size toothbrush.

▶ A smear layer of fluoridated toothpaste is advised for an infant, and up to the age of 3.[49]

▶ Brushing technique involves lifting of the lip to expose the cervical 1/3 portion of the erupted anterior teeth.

▶ Advise caregiver to look frequently at the infant's teeth for demineralization (white chalky appearance) and early carious lesions (Figures 50-2, 50-3, 50-6, and 50-7 in Chapter 50).

A. Inquire of Fluoride Exposure[42]

▶ History of exposure to fluoride.

▶ Fluoride level of current water supply, including childcare environments (check public health department records).

▶ Well water (have water tested for fluoride level).

▶ Use of fluoridated or unspecified bottled water.

▶ Use of fluoride supplementation can begin at 6 months of age.[50] (See Table 36-1 in Chapter 36).

III. Feeding Patterns (Birth to 1 Year)

A. Frequency and Method of Feeding

▶ Explain the cariogenicity of certain foods and beverages, the consequence from frequent consumption of sugary beverages and foods, and the demineralization process. See Chapter 35.

▶ Problems with feeding and sleeping.
  • When the infant falls asleep after sucking, milk collects around teeth and causes demineralization.[28,33]

B. BreastFed

▶ The US Surgeon General and all professional pediatric organizations endorse exclusive breastfeeding for the first 6 months of life, and up to 12 months of age with additional nutritional supplementation after the first 6 months of life.[43]

▶ Discourage prolonged, at-will breastfeeding after tooth eruption.

▶ If the infant sleeps with the mother, discourage at-will breastfeeding, after the eruption of the first tooth.

C. Bottle Fed

▶ The American Dental Association supports the use of fluoridated water with liquid or powdered concentrated infant formula.[51]

▶ Hold the child during feeding.

▶ Discourage putting the infant to bed with a bottle containing anything other than fluoridated water, after the first tooth eruption.

▶ Do not put sweetened milk, juice, or other sweet liquids in a bottle or sippy cup.

▶ Do not use the bottle as a pacifier.

▶ Inquire of the age other children in family were weaned.

▶ Encourage parents to have infant drink from a cup by age one. The American Academy of Pediatrics recommends children be weaned from the bottle before 18 months of age.[52]

TABLE 49-4	Milestones in Child Development: Birth to Age 12 Months	
AREAS	**BIRTH TO 6 MO**	**6–12 MO**
Language	■ 0–2 mo: quiets to sound ■ Reflects displeasure at noises ■ Coos and babbles	■ Says dada or mama ■ Understands name ■ Pays attention to verbalization
Motor	■ 2 mo: head control ■ 6 mo: transfer hand to hand ■ Grasps with forearm (ulnar grasp)	■ 7–9 mo: sits ■ 9–10 mo: plays pat-a-cake ■ Waves bye, bye
Social/emotional	■ 2 mo: gazes at human face ■ Alert to voices	■ Inhibited by word "no" ■ Separation anxiety ■ Stranger awareness

IV. Nonnutritive Sucking

▶ Suggestions for pacifier selection and use:
- The use of pacifiers has been shown to decrease the incidence of sudden infant death syndrome (SIDS).[18]
- The American Academy of Pediatrics Task Force on SIDS recommends the use of a pacifier throughout the first year of life.[18]
- For breastfed infants, delay introduction of pacifier until 1 month old.[44]
- Choose a pacifier with solid construction so it cannot be pulled apart. Figure 49-3 shows two types of pacifiers: one has an orthodontic nipple and the other a nonorthodontic. The orthodontic nipple is designed to be more like a mother's breast nipple during nursing.
- Ventilated shield larger than the child's mouth, at least 1–1/2 inches wide, to prevent swallowing.[53]
- Not tied to the crib, child's clothing, or around the neck or hand, which could lead to strangulation.[53]

▶ Not cleaned in the parent's/caregiver's mouth since caries-producing bacteria could be transferred to the infant.[40]

▶ Clean in warm, soapy water. Replace with a new pacifier regularly.[53]

V. Components of the First Dental Visit[3,47]

A first dental visit is recommended at the eruption of the first tooth, and no later than age one.

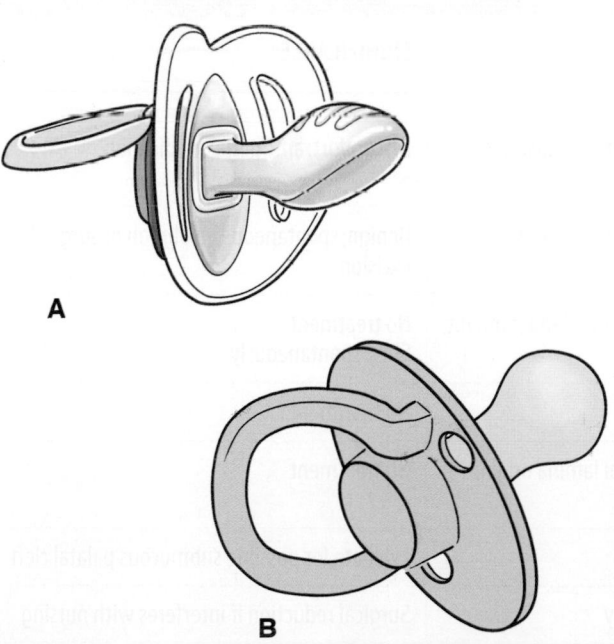

A

B

FIGURE 49-3 **Criteria for Selecting Pacifiers.** Two styles of pacifiers nipples: **(A)** orthodontic and **(B)** conventional. True orthodontic pacifiers expand to support the palate and maintain natural tongue posture. It is important to select the appropriate bulb size for each stage of development (0–2, 3–6, 6–18 months). Criteria for selection of a safe pacifier; size of shield is wider than child's mouth (at least 1¼ inches) in diameter; shield has air vents; plastic portion is of sturdy construction to prevent separation and possible choking; nipple is checked frequently for cracking and stickiness, at which time pacifier is replaced.

▶ One of the major reasons for this first visit is to establish a dental home (see Chapter 50).

A. Components of Dental Hygiene Visit

▶ To ensure patient cooperation, schedule the first visit at a time that is best for baby.

▶ A thorough medical history is necessary prior to beginning the infant oral examination.

▶ Explain to caregiver that crying is a normal reaction during the oral examination.

▶ Complete a caries risk assessment and discuss potential risk factors for Early Childhood Caries (ECC).[54] Some of the risk factors include:
- Diet and feeding patterns.
- Lack of daily oral hygiene care.
- Poor maternal dental health. Research shows a strong association between maternal caries producing bacterial loads, and Early Childhood Caries (ECC) development.[46]
- Limited/No water fluoridation exposure.
- The process known as vertical transmission occurs when mothers/primary caregivers exchange saliva with their infant. This can occur during kissing, sharing of food, drink, eating utensils, and the cleaning of pacifiers via the mother's mouth.[3,55]

B. Oral Examination: Positioning to Access

▶ Seat parent and clinician knee to knee.

▶ Place child's head on the lap of the examiner, as seen in Figure 49-4.

▶ Have caregiver crisscross arms gently across the infant's body, stabilizing the infant's hands and feet.

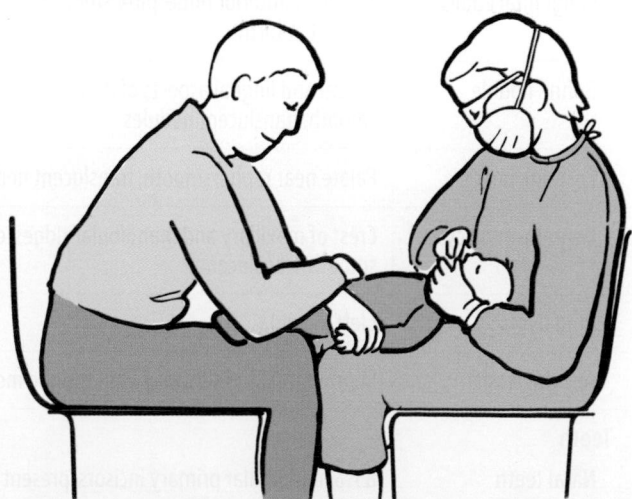

FIGURE 49-4 **Knee-to-Knee Infant Examination.** The clinician makes the oral examination, discusses oral findings, and demonstrates proper oral care for the parent. The position of the infant then is reversed so that the parent has the opportunity to position the child and demonstrate proper oral care.

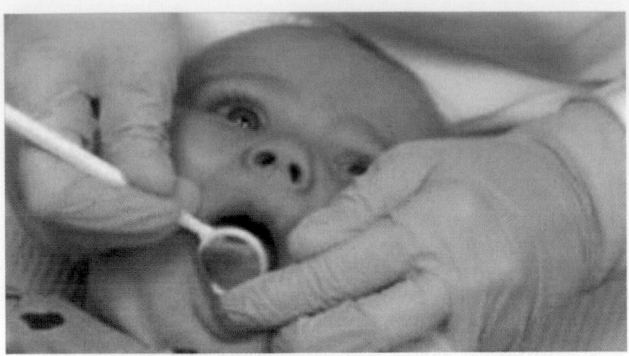

FIGURE 49-5 Infant Oral Examination. Using a plastic mirror. Looking for presence of carious lesions on deciduous teeth.

C. Examination Sequence

▸ Examine the child's head and neck, legs, and arms for evidence of abuse. Signs of abuse are described in Chapter 62.

▸ When teeth are present, lift the lips away from the gingival margin to observe the condition of the anterior teeth (Figure 49-5).

▸ Examine all teeth for evidence of biofilm, discoloration.

▸ Look for malformations (Figure 50-1), dental caries (Figures 50-2), and white spot lesions (Figure 50-6).

▸ Show parents the findings and inform them of the significance.

▸ Make referrals to the dentist if evidence of pathology is noted (Tables 49-5 and 50-1).

D. Treatment[40]

▸ Biofilm removal: use dampened soft infant-size toothbrush.

▸ Fluoride varnish application is recommended for children, beginning at age one, who are moderate-to-high risk for ECC.[47]

DOCUMENTATION

Documentation for the pregnant patient includes a minimum of the following:

▸ Thorough medical history, medications taken, use of tobacco, alcohol, or illicit drugs, history of gestational diabetes, miscarriage, hypertension, and morning sickness.

▸ Consultations with general physician and obstetrician along with their response.

▸ Oral examination findings with areas of concern that need treatment and follow-up.

TABLE 49-5	Oral Soft and Hard Tissue Conditions/Pathology in Infants (1–6 Months)	
CONDITIONS	**FINDINGS**	**SIGNIFICANCE**
Soft Tissue		
Pseudomembranous candidiasis (thrush)	Mucosa or tongue; white, curdlike plaques; wipe-off leaving red and raw area	Discomfort; antifungal medication
Congenital epulis	Maxillary anterior ridge; pink, smooth, pedunculated mass; present at birth	Benign; spontaneous involution or surgical excision
Bohn's nodule	Buccal and lingual aspects of dental ridge; mucous gland remnant; smooth, translucent nodules	No treatment Shed spontaneously
Epstein's pearls	Palate near raphe; smooth, translucent nodules	No treatment
Dental lamina cysts	Crest of maxillary and mandibular ridges; dental lamina origin; smooth, translucent	No treatment
Bifid uvula	Cleft in uvula	Evaluate for possible submucous palatal cleft
Ankyloglossia	Short lingual frenum; may limit tongue mobility	Surgical reduction if interferes with nursing
Teeth		
Natal teeth	85% mandibular primary incisors; present at birth; commonly occur in pairs	Familial tendency; remove if mobile or have sharp edges causing injury
Neonatal teeth	Erupt within 30 days after birth	Same as above

Source: McDonald RE, Avery DR, Dean JA. *Dentistry for the Child and Adolescent.* 8th ed. St. Louis, MO: Mosby; 2004:137–138, 154–155, 183–185, 423.

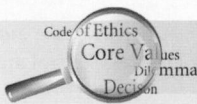

EVERYDAY ETHICS

Anna, the dental hygienist, welcomed her patient Julie, a 20-year-old single woman. She is in the first trimester of pregnancy and was referred by a nurse from the Maternal and Child Health Clinic. Anna notices the way Julie holds a hand over her mouth when she talks. Julie's medical history appears negative except for smoking about a half pack of cigarettes daily. Examination reveals multiple carious lesions, heavy calculus, and 4–5 mm proximal probing depths in several molar areas. After making the radiographic survey and presenting initial patient instruction, there was time for one quadrant of scaling. Follow-up appointments were scheduled to complete treatment. Julie does not show up for any of the appointments.

Questions for Consideration

1. Which of the dental hygiene core values (Section II) apply to this situation? Explain.

2. What is the role of the dental hygienist, if any, to make further contact with this patient, and why? How will she go about it?

3. Describe two or three courses of action and the possible outcomes of the situation through a dental hygiene care plan.

BOX 49-2
Example Documentation: Pregnant Patient

S –A 32-year-old female presents for a 3-month recare appointment. Patient is in her second trimester, 15th week of pregnancy. Patient is currently taking folic acid (vitamin B9) supplement 600 mcg and prenatal vitamin daily. Patient reports mild nausea "morning sickness" during the morning hours. Patient's chief complaint: mild bleeding when brushing. States she tires easily, as her 1-year-old requires a lot of attention, and hasn't been compliant with daily oral self-care.

O –Intraoral assessment reveals generalized gingival inflammation, edematous and erythematous, with generalized light biofilm/plaque, new localized subgingival calculus deposits on mandibular posterior molars. Hard tissue examination: Cavitated carious lesion on #3. Periodontal examination findings: localized BOP #2, 3, 14, 18, 30, 31; localized 4 mm periodontal pocket depths on #2, 3, 14, 18, 31 were noted in periodontal chart.

A –Patient presents at a high caries risk. Periodontal condition: Gingivitis combination of plaque induced and pregnancy.

P –Patient congratulated on keeping the 3-month recall, as last appointment was previously cancelled. Frequent bathroom breaks were given. Dietary analysis completed and reviewed. Patient given resources for improved nutritional intake. Relationship of nutritional intake for patient and baby was discussed, as well as dental caries relationship to carbohydrate foods. Patient demonstrated toothbrushing method, and better angulation was suggested. A powered electric toothbrush was advised for improved oral health. Discussed anticipatory guidance for new baby and 1-year-old son.

Next visit: Restorative #3. Additionally, patient scheduled son for 1-year oral health assessment.

Signed _____, RDH

Date _____

▶ Changes from previous examinations with respect to oral self-care by the patient and record types of instruction provided.

▶ A sample progress note may be found in Box 49-2.

Factors To Teach The Patient

▷ The relationship of oral health of the mother to the general health of the fetus and newborn.

▷ The serious effects of tobacco and other drugs on the health of the fetus, the infant, and the child.

▷ Reasons for dental hygiene appointments early during pregnancy, at regular intervals throughout pregnancy, and after birth of the baby.

▷ Reasons for receiving routine dental care appointments during pregnancy, and most ideal time for scheduling, during second trimester.

▷ The rationale for maintaining good personal oral hygiene care to control dental biofilm throughout the pregnancy and after the baby's birth.

▷ Self-examination of the oral cavity to evaluate the effectiveness of daily dental biofilm removal and the health of the soft tissues.

▷ Reasons for limiting fermentable carbohydrate intake and maintaining a healthy diet from the fruit, vegetable, grain, meat, and meat alternatives, and dairy food groups.

References

1. Oral Health Care During Pregnancy Expert Workgroup. *Oral Health Care During Pregnancy: A National Consensus Statement—Summary of an Expert Workgroup Meeting.* Washington, DC: National Maternal and Child Oral Health Resource Center; 2012.

2. U.S. Department of Health and Human Services, Office on Women's Health. Prenatal care fact sheet. http://www.womenshealth.gov/publications/our-publications/fact-sheet/

prenatal-care.html. Updated July 16, 2012. Accessed September 12, 2014.

3. California Dental Association Foundation. *Oral Health: During Pregnancy & Early Childhood: Evidence-Based Guidelines for Health Professionals.* 2010. www.cdafoundation.org/portals/0/pdfs/poh_guidelines.pdf. Accessed August 2014.

4. Barlow Pugh M, et al. *Stedman's Medical Dictionary.* Vol 2011. 28th ed. Baltimore, MD: Lippincott Williams & Wilkins; 2006.

5. *Stedman's Medical Dictionary.* 28th ed. Baltimore, MD: Lippincott Williams & Wilkins; 2006.

6. Cunningham FG, Leveno KJ, Bloom SL, et al. Chapter 4: Fetal growth and development. In: Cunningham FG, Leveno KJ, Bloom SL, et al., eds. *Williams Obstetrics.* 23rd ed. New York, NY: McGraw-Hill; 2010. http://www.accessmedicine.com.ezproxy.mcphs.edu/content.aspx?aID=6037835. Accessed August 19, 2014.

7. Simpson JL. Incidence and timing of pregnancy losses: relevance to evaluating safety of early prenatal diagnosis. *Am J Med Genet.* 1990;35(2):165–173.

8. Lunt RC, Law DB. A review of the chronology of calcification of deciduous teeth. *J Am Dent Assoc.* 1974;89:599–606.

9. Gibbs RS, Romero R, Hillier SL, et al. A review of premature birth and subclinical infections. *Am J Obstet Gynecol.* 1992;166(5):1515–1528.

10. Armitage GC. Bi-directional relationship between pregnancy and periodontal disease. *Periodontology 2000.* 2013;61: 160–176.

11. American Academy of Periodontology. American Academy of Periodontology statement regarding periodontal management of the pregnant patient. *J Periodontol.* 2004;75(3):495.

12. Advisory Committee on Immunization Practices Centers for Disease Control and Prevention (CDC). Guiding principles for development of ACIP recommendations for vaccination during pregnancy and breastfeeding. 2008;57(21):580.

13. Chisholm CA, Ferguson JE II. Physiologic and pharmacologic factors related to the provision of dental care during pregnancy. *J Calif Dent Assoc.* 2010;38(9):663–671.

14. Watts DH. Management of human immunodeficiency virus infection in pregnancy. *N Engl J Med.* 2002;346(24): 1879–1891.

15. Calvert C, Ronsmans C. The contribution of HIV to pregnancy-related mortality: a systematic review and meta-analysis. *AIDS.* 2013;27:1631–1639.

16. Sturt AS, Dokubo EK, Sint TT. Antiretroviral therapy (ART) for treating HIV infection in ART-eligible pregnant women. *Cochrane Database Syst Rev.* 2010;(3):CD008440.

17. U.S. Department of Health and Human Services. *The Health Consequences of Smoking—50 Years of Progress: A Report of the Surgeon General.* Rockville, MD: Office of the Surgeon General; 2014.

18. American Academy of Pediatrics Task Force on Sudden Infant Death Syndrome. SIDS and other sleep-related infant deaths: expansion of recommendations for a safe infant sleeping environment. *Pediatrics.* 2011;128(5):1030–1039.

19. Office on Smoking and Health. Centers for Disease Control and Prevention (CDC). *The Health Consequences of Involuntary Exposure to Tobacco Smoke: A Report of the Surgeon General.* Atlanta, GA: Centers for Disease Control and Prevention; 2006:29.

20. Ang-Lee MK, Moss J, Yuan C. Herbal medicines and perioperative care. *JAMA.* 2001;286(2):208–216.

21. Barrett BP, Brown RL, Locken K, et al. Treatment of the common cold with unrefined echinacea: a randomized, double-blind, placebo-controlled trial. *Ann Intern Med.* 2002;137(12):939–946.

22. Awang D, Leung A. Valerian. In: Coates P, Blackman M, Cragg G, et al., eds. *Encyclopedia of Dietary Supplements.* New York, NY: Marcel Dekker; 2005:687–700.

23. Giglio JA, Lanni SM, Laskin DM, et al. Oral health care for the pregnant patient. *J Can Dent Assoc.* 2009;75(1): 43–48.

24. Otomo-Corgel J. Periodontal therapy in the female patient. In: Newman MG, Takei HH, Klokkevold PR, et al., eds. *Carranza's Clinical Periodontology.* 11th ed. Philadelphia, PA: Saunders; 2012:412–421.

25. Kornman KS, Loesche WJ. The subgingival microbial flora during pregnancy. *J Periodontal Res.* 1980;15(2):111–122.

26. Fehrenbach MJ, Lemborn UE, Phelan JA. Inflammation and repair. In: Ibsen OA, Phelan JA, eds. *Oral Pathology for the Dental Hygienist.* 6th ed. Philadelphia, PA: Saunders; 2013.

27. Amini H, Casimassimo PS. Prenatal dental care: a review. *Gen Dent.* 2010;58(3):176–180.

28. Kumar J, Samelson R. Oral health care during pregnancy and early childhood practice guidelines. New York, NY: New York State Department of Health; 2006.

29. Lamster IB, Lalla E, Borgnakke WS, et al. The relationship between oral health and diabetes mellitus. *J Am Dent Assoc.* 2008;139 (Suppl 5):19S–24S.

30. American College of Obstetricians and Gynecologists Committee. ACOG committee opinion number 299: Guidelines for diagnostic imaging during pregnancy. *Obstet Gynecol.* 2004;104(3):647–651.

31. American Dental Association, U.S. Department of Health and Human Services. Guidelines for the selection of patients for dental radiographic examinations. http://www.fda.gov/downloads/Radiation-EmittingProducts/RadiationEmittingProductsandProcedures/MedicalImaging/MedicalX-Rays/ucm116505.pdf. Updated 2004. Accessed August 9, 2011.

32. American Dental Association Council of Scientific Affairs. Dental amalgam: update on safety concerns. *J Am Dent Assoc.* 1998;129(4):494–503.

33. Little JW, Falace DA, Miller CS, et al. Pregnancy and breast feeding. In: *Dental Management of the Medically Compromised Patient.* 8th ed. St. Louis, MO: Mosby; 2013:271–282.

34. Santos AC, Braveman FR, Finster M. Obstetric anesthesia. In: Barash PG, Cullen BF, Stoelting RK, eds. *Clinical Anesthesia.* 5th ed. Philadelphia, PA: Lippincott-Raven; 2006.

35. U.S. Department of Agriculture. Center for nutrition policy and promotion. http://www.choosemyplate.gov/2014. Accessed September 12, 2014.

36. Harper LF, Faine MP. Nutrition in pregnancy, infancy, and childhood. In: Palmer CA, ed. *Diet and Nutrition in Oral Health.* 2nd ed. Upper Saddle River, NJ: Prentice Hall; 2007:344–365.

37. Institute of Medicine (US) Committee to Review Dietary Reference Intakes for Vitamin D and Calcium; Ross AC, Taylor CL, Yaktine AL, et al., editors. *Dietary Reference Intakes for Calcium and Vitamin D.* Washington, DC: National Academies Press (US); 2011. http://www.ncbi.nlm.nih.gov/books/NBK56070/.

38. Soderling E. Xylitol, mutans streptococci, and dental plaque. *Adv Dent Res.* 2009;21(1):74–78.

39. Nakai Y, Shinga-Ishihara C, Kaji M, et al. Xylitol gum and maternal transmission of mutans streptococci. *J Dent Res.* 2010;89(1):56–60.

40. American Academy of Pediatric Dentistry, Clinical Affairs Committee-Infant Oral Health Subcommittee. Guideline on infant oral health care. Revised 2011. http://www.aapd.org/media/Policies_Guidelines/G_infantOralHealthCare.pdf. Accessed September 12, 2014.

41. American Dental Association Council on Scientific Affairs. Professionally applied topical fluoride: evidence-based clinical recommendations. *J Am Dent Assoc.* 2006;137(8):1151–1159.

42. Centers for Disease Control and Prevention, National Center for Chronic Disease Prevention and Health Promotion. Community water fluoridation. http://www.cdc.gov/fluoridation/basics/index.htm. Updated 2013. Accessed September 11, 2014.

43. Gwinn C, McClane GE, Shanel-Hogan KA, et al. Domestic violence: no place for a smile. *J Calif Dent Assoc.* 2004;32(5):399–407.

44. American Psychiatric Association. Tobacco-related disorders. In: *Diagnostic and Statistical Manual of Mental Disorders (DSM-5).* 5th ed. Arlington, VA: American Psychiatric Association; 2013:571–576.

45. Jasinksi JL. Pregnancy and domestic violence: a review of the literature. *Trauma Violence Abuse.* 2004;5(1):47–64.

46. American Academy of Pediatrics. Policy statement: oral health risk assessment timing and establishment of the dental home. *Pediatrics.* 2003;111(5):1113.

47. American Academy of Pediatric Dentistry, Council on Clinical Affairs. Guideline on periodicity of examination, preventive dental services, anticipatory guidance/counseling, and oral treatments for infant, children, and adolescents. *Pediatr Dent.* 2013;35(6):114–121.

48. U.S. Food and Drug Administration. FDA drug safety communication: reports of a rare, but serious and potentially fatal adverse effect with the use of over-the-counter (OTC) benzocaine gels and liquids applied to the gums or mouth. http://www.fda.gov/drugs/drugsafety/ucm250024.htm. Updated 2011. Accessed July 25, 2014.

49. American Academy of Pediatric Dentistry; and American Academy of Pediatrics. Policy on early childhood caries (ECC): classifications, consequences, and preventive strategies. *Reference Manual Oral Health Policies.* Revised 2014;36(6). http://www.aapd.org/media/Policies_Guidelines/P_ECC_Classifications.pdf. Accessed July 4, 2015.

50. Rozier RG, Adair S, Graham F, et al. Evidence-based clinical recommendations on the prescription of dietary fluoride supplements for caries prevention: a report of the American Dental Association Council on scientific affairs. *J Am Dent Assoc.* 2010;141:1480–1489.

51. Berg J, Gerweck C, Hujoel PP, et al. Evidence-based clinical recommendations regarding fluoride intake from reconstituted infant formula and enamel fluorosis: a report of the American Dental Association Council on scientific affairs. *J Am Dent Assoc.* 2011;142(1):79–87.

52. American Academy of Pediatrics. Weaning from the bottle. http://www.aap.org/en-us/about-the-aap/aap-press-room/aap-press-room-media-center/Pages/Weaning-from-the-Bottle.aspx. Accessed September 12, 2014.

53. American Academy of Pediatrics. Caring for your baby and young child: birth to age 5. American Academy of Pediatrics Website. http://www.healthychildren.org/English/safety-prevention/at-home/Pages/Pacifier-Safety.aspx. Updated August, 2013. Accessed August 29, 2014.

54. American Academy of Pediatric Dentistry. Guideline on caries-risk assessment and management for infants, children, and adolescents. *Clinical Guidelines.* http://www.aapd.org/media/Policies_Guidelines/G_CariesRiskAssessment.pdf. Accessed July 4, 2015.

55. Chaffee BW, Gansky SA, Weintraub JA, et al. Maternal oral bacterial levels predict early childhood caries development. *J Dent Res.* 2014;93(3):238–244.

 ENHANCE YOUR UNDERSTANDING

thePoint° DIGITAL CONNECTIONS
(see the inside front cover for access information)
- **Audio glossary**
- **Quiz bank**

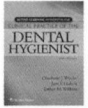 **SUPPORT FOR LEARNING**
(available separately; visit lww.com)
- *Active Learning Workbook for Clinical Practice of the Dental Hygienist, 12th Edition*

prepU INDIVIDUALIZED REVIEW
(available separately; visit lww.com)
- **Adaptive quizzing with *prepU for Wilkins' Clinical Practice of the Dental Hygienist***

50

The Pediatric Patient

Carolynn A. Zeitz, RDH, BS, RDA, MA and Teresa B. Duncan, RDH, BS

CHAPTER OUTLINE

LEARNING OBJECTIVES

After studying this chapter, the reader will be able to:

1. Describe the specialty of pediatric dentistry.

2. Discuss the use of a caries risk assessment tool to identify an individual patient's risk and preventive factors.

3. Identify age-appropriate anticipatory guidance/counseling factors to educate parents/caregivers of toddlers, school-aged children, and adolescents.

4. Identify preventive and therapeutic oral healthcare interventions based on age and caries risk assessment.

5. Discuss oral health home care needs, adjunct aids, and continuing care recommendations for children.

Oral health for toddlers, preschoolers, school-aged children, and adolescents depends primarily on parental intervention for the young child, and gradually transitioning the child through parent involvement to independent management of daily oral self-care. Parents are:

► Provided with education through anticipatory guidance before a child's birth and at regular intervals thereafter.

► Given the information needed to assess their child's oral health status.

► Taught how to intervene and to anticipate the child's oral health needs at various ages and stages of growth and development.

► Box 50-1 defines key words associated with dental hygiene care of pediatric patients.

PEDIATRIC DENTISTRY

I. The Specialty of Pediatric Dentistry

► An age-defined specialty that provides both primary and comprehensive preventive and therapeutic oral health care for infants and children through adolescence, including those with special healthcare needs.[1]

► Requires 2–3 years of additional specialized training (after the required 4 years of dental school) to prepare for treating a wide variety of children's dental problems and children with medical, physical, and mental disabilities.[2]

II. The American Academy of Pediatric Dentistry (AAPD)[2]

► The membership organization representing the specialty of pediatric dentistry.

► The American Academy of Pediatric Dentistry's mission is to advocate policies, guidelines, and programs that promote optimal oral health and oral health care for children.

► Professional and parental information is available at the AAPD website.[3]

THE CHILD AS A PATIENT

The age categories of pediatric patients are:[4]

► Infants: 0–1 year of age (see Chapter 49).

► Toddlers: 1–2 years of age.

► Preschoolers: 3–5 years of age.

► School-aged children (middle childhood): 6–10 years of age.

► Adolescents (teens and young adults): 11–21 years of age.

I. The Dental Home

► *First dental hygiene visit*: The AAPD, American Dental Association (ADA), and the American Academy of Pediatrics have similar policies recommending a first dental examination for children be after the eruption of the first tooth, but no later than 12 months of age.

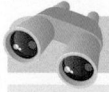

BOX 50-1   KEY WORDS AND ABBREVIATIONS: Pediatric Oral Health Care

Adolescent: child from 11 years of age to 21 years of age; considered teen or young adult.

Anticipatory guidance: provide information to parents and caregivers on what to expect in a child's current and next developmental stage so that the child's needs can be anticipated and properly managed.

CAMBRA: acronym that refers to the phrase "caries management by risk assessment."

Dental home: a dentist of record in the community established early in childhood for continuous and comprehensive preventive interventions, dental hygiene, and dental care.

Grazing: eating or drinking at-will throughout the day or evening.

Infant: child younger than 1 year of age.

Interim therapeutic restoration (ITR): a provisional placement of a fluoride-releasing glass ionomer restoration without using local anesthesia and utilizing a spoon excavator to remove most—all caries; purpose is to prevent the progression of dental caries in young patients, uncooperative patients, patients with special healthcare needs, and situations in which traditional cavity preparation and/

or placement of traditional dental restorations are not feasible. It is necessary to "recharge" the glass ionomer material using fluoridated toothpaste daily and regular –3–6 month professional fluoride applications.

Main caregiver: the person who has primary daily care of the child.

Nonnutritive sucking: sucking fingers, thumb, pacifiers, or other objects for comfort.

Preschooler: child 3–5 years of age; may or may not be attending a preschool program.

PSR (periodontal screening and recording): used as a screening procedure to determine the need for comprehensive periodontal evaluation; described in Chapter 23.

School-age: child from 6 years of age to 10 years of age, considered middle childhood.

Sippy cup: a special cup with a lid that may have a straw or a drinking projection to teach a young child to drink.

Tooth germination: two teeth appear to have developed from one tooth.

Toddler: child from age 1 year to 2 years of age.

Wean: to discontinue breast- or bottle feeding; to nourish the infant with other food.

- However, often a child's first dental home visit isn't scheduled until they are 3–5 years old.
- Early visits include referral to dental specialists when appropriate.
- The ongoing relationship between the dentist and the patient addresses all aspects of oral health care delivered in a comprehensive, continuously accessible, coordinated, and family-centered way.
- Emphasis is placed on early intervention before serious oral health problems can develop.[5]

II. Barriers to Dental Care

- Lack of parental knowledge about prevention of oral disease
- Language
- Cost
- Fear
- No dental home established
- General dentist may not want to provide care for children under the age of 3 years
- Dentist's hours do not fit into parents'/caregivers' schedules
- Dentist does not accept child's insurance
- Transportation.

III. Child Dental Visits

A. Purposes

- The purposes of the dental hygiene visit are to:
  - Establish rapport, teach appropriate behaviors, and prevent management problems.
  - Develop and continue relationship with the child and the family.
  - Initiate and/or strengthen positive age-appropriate preventive measures, such as fluoride usage, appropriate nutritional practices, and daily dental biofilm removal.
  - Discover, intercept, and recommend changes in any parental practices that may be detrimental to the child's oral health.
- Appointments are planned for clinical oral examination, caries-risk assessment, biofilm and calculus removal, professional fluoride application, radiographic assessment, treatment planning of dental disease, evaluation of developing dentition/malocclusion, anticipatory guidance/counseling, and introduction to dental hygiene.

B. Frequency of Continuing Care

- Visits to the dental hygienist and the dentist are scheduled according to the child's specific needs. A common appointment plan for children with little or no oral disease is every 4 or 6 months.

- Some patients may require more or less frequent intervals based upon the child's risk factors, historical, clinical, and radiographic findings.[6]
- Re-evaluation and reinforcement of preventive activities contribute to improved instruction for the parent, child, and adolescent.[6]

C. Scheduling

The best time to schedule dental visits for toddlers, and young school aged children is:

- Early in the morning when the child is well rested and more cooperative
- After naps when the child is not tired and is more apt to listen and cooperate.

PATIENT MANAGEMENT CONSIDERATIONS

Cooperation is usually gained with nonverbal communication such as smiling and talking with the child and the parent.

I. Toddlers (1–2 Years of Age)

- Primary teeth are vulnerable to tooth decay from their very first appearance, on average between the ages of 6 and 12 months.
- Children who wait to have their first dental visit until age two or three are more likely to require restorative and emergency visits.
- Use of child-friendly terms instead of the dental term. See Box 50-2 for examples of child-friendly terms.

BOX 50-2

Child-Friendly Substitution Words for Dental Terminology

Dental Term	Child-Friendly Term
Air/water syringe	Water squirter, wind
Amalgam restoration	Silver star
Dental light	Sunshine light
Explorer, scaler	Tooth counter
Fluoride varnish	Fluoride tooth vitamins
High-speed handpiece	Mr. Whistle
Low-speed handpiece	Tooth tickler, Mr. Bumpy
Mouth mirror	Tooth mirror
Prophy paste	Special toothpaste
Dental hygiene treatment	Teeth cleaning
Saliva ejector	Mrs. Thirsty/special straw
Suction (high-speed)	Vacuum

A. Oral Examination: Positioning for Access

▶ Utilize the knee-to-knee positioning for the oral examination and teach the parent to do at home to provide thorough biofilm removal with toothbrush and floss. Refer to Figures 49-4 and 49-5, Chapter 49.

▶ Prior to performing the examination, explain to the parent proper positioning; child's legs around parent waist, parent's elbows restrain child's legs, and parent holds child's hands on his/her stomach.

▶ It is the clinician's responsibility to control the head during the examination.

▶ Crying during the examination is normal behavior and can provide better visibility of the child's mouth and throat.

B. Examination Sequence

▶ Examine the child's head and neck, legs, and arms for evidence of abuse. Abuse is described in Chapter 62.

▶ Oral soft tissues are assessed (see Table 50-1).[7]

▶ Lift the upper lip to observe the condition of the anterior teeth.

TABLE 50-1	Oral Soft and Hard Tissue Conditions/Pathology in Children Approximately 6 Months to 5 Years	
CONDITIONS	**FINDINGS**	**SIGNIFICANCE**
Soft Tissue		
Eruption cysts	Translucent, smooth; may appear blue to blue-black if bleeding in cystic space	Usually no treatment
Mucocele	Lower lip, floor of mouth, buccal mucosa most common in order of occurrence; fluid-filled vesicle or blister; trauma, tearing of minor salivary duct	May resolve or require surgical excision
Traumatic ulcer	Reaction to puncture wound	Clean wound; possible suture
Alveolar abscess	Smooth, red or yellowish nodule; tender; primary teeth—more diffuse infections; may be acute or chronic	Radiographic evaluation, drainage and antibiotic may be required
Primary herpetic gingivostomatitis	High fever, 102°–104°F; regional lymphadenopathy; diffuse, swollen erythematous gingiva; vesicles form painful ulcers	Urgent care (see Chapter 42) Resolves in 7–10 days
Geographic tongue	Red, smooth areas devoid of filliform papillae on dorsum of tongue; margins well developed, slightly raised; pattern changes	No treatment; brush tongue to reduce bacteria
Verruca vulgaris	Multiple white sessile lesions; fingerlike projections, rough surface; human papilloma virus in origin	May resolve spontaneously or require excision
Teeth		
Enamel hypoplasia	Disturbance of enamel matrix during tooth development; irregular to round pits of varying size on enamel, usually in a row; multiple causes	Esthetics
Fluorosis	Infrequent in primary dentition; may be seen in cervical region of second primary molars	Daily biofilm removal
White-spot lesions	Opaque enamel, usually cervical and proximal areas of teeth at contacts; earliest clinical sign of the carious process; indicates that the surface and underlying enamel are demineralized	Need fluoride for remineralization; daily biofilm removal
Fused teeth	Usually limited to anterior teeth; union of two independently forming primary tooth buds; familial tendency	Possible caries at point of fusion; may be absence of one of corresponding permanent teeth
Gemination	More common in primary teeth; invagination of single tooth germ; bifid crown on single root; crown appears wide	None

Source: McDonald RE, Avery DR, Dean JA. *Dentistry for the Child and Adolescent.* 9th ed. Maryland Heights, MO: Mosby Elsevier; 2011:10–12, 86–90, 95–100, 116–117, 127–128, 132, 136, 156, 250, 369.

II. Preschoolers (3–5 Years of Age)

A. Prepare the Child for the Dental Visit

▶ Make the dental visit as pleasant as possible for the child.

▶ Children are told that the dental hygienist and dentist help them take good care of their teeth.

▶ Parents are instructed to avoid using negative words, such as "hurt, pain, and don't be scared."

▶ When the child is not present, parents are asked if the child has any fears or has had any prior negative experiences.

B. Positioning

▶ For young preschoolers (3-year-old) utilization of the knee-to-knee positioning may still be needed.

▶ May sit in the dental chair without any problems and can be encouraged with "being a big girl or boy."

▶ The dental chair possibly may be modified by removing the head rest or a portion of the backrest to better fit the child.

C. Parental Involvement

▶ Determine the expected developmental milestones of the child according to the chronological age, as outlined in Table 50-2.[8,9]

▶ Ask parents to identify actual developmental milestones so appropriate management can be initiated during the appointment.

▶ Ask parents to provide a general statement regarding the child's temperament and ability to cooperate.

▶ Evaluate whether the parent needs to accompany the child into the treatment room.

TABLE 50-2	Milestones in Child Development: 12 Months to 5 Years				
AREAS	**12–18 MONTHS**	**18 MO TO 2 YEARS**	**2–3 YEARS**	**3–4 YEARS**	**5 YEARS**
Language	■ Repeats a few words ■ Says two or more words ■ Uses expression, "uh, oh" ■ Points to few body parts ■ Follows one-step directions	■ Has up to 50 words and two-word sentences ■ Talks to self ■ Hums or sings simple songs ■ Says names of familiar objects ■ Listens to short rhymes	■ Up to 500 words ■ Converses using simple 2- to 3-word phrases and sentences ■ Responds to simple directions	■ 75%–80% of speech understandable ■ Knows location words ■ Likes familiar stories repeated over and over ■ Knows what, who, why questions	■ Five-word sentences ■ Conversations more mature ■ Links past and present events
Motor	■ Pincer grasp ■ Gives toys on request ■ 15–18 mo: good use of cup and spoon	■ Feeds self ■ Uses straw ■ Walks well ■ Helps wash hands ■ Seats self in chair	■ Dresses with supervision ■ Holds crayon in fist	■ Feeds self well ■ Takes off jacket ■ Holds crayon with fingers	■ Fine motor coordination maturing ■ Buttons clothing ■ May be able to tie shoelaces
Social/emotional	■ Separation anxiety and stranger awareness continue	■ Likes to imitate ■ Independent ■ Difficulty waiting ■ Shy with strangers ■ Likes adult attention ■ May exhibit anger and temper tantrums	■ Likes to see and touch ■ Attached to parent ■ Rarely shares ■ Self-help skills of interest	■ Likes to please ■ Responds to commands	■ Distinguishes fantasy from reality ■ Likes pretend play ■ Longer attention span ■ Tolerates parent separation

Source: Goldson E, Reynolds A. Child development and behavior. In: Hay WW, Levin MJ, Sondheimer JM, et al., eds. *Current Pediatric Diagnosis and Treatment*. 19th ed. New York, NY: McGraw Hill; 2008:66–83.

III. School Age Children (6–10 Years of Age)

▶ Can be an active participant in the dental care visit.

▶ May still display signs of anxiety or uncooperativeness.

▶ Typically once a child is in school full time having a parent present during their appointments is no longer necessary.

▶ Child's dentition may be all primary or mixed dentition, or by 11 or 12 years of age all permanent dentition depending on personal development.

▶ Examine the need for pit and fissure sealants.

▶ A periodontal assessment needs to be completed even if there is no bone loss. Child may have pockets, bleeding, and subgingival calculus.

▶ Child is starting to develop independent skills and ability to perform their own oral care.

▶ Continue to avoid the use of negative words.

▶ Avoid lecturing or reprimanding with a negative tone. Suggest, advise, and highlight the positive.

▶ Use of pictures for explaining proper oral hygiene, calculus, and biofilm may help the child understand.

IV. Adolescents (11–21 Years of Age)

▶ Dental hygiene services provided during adolescence can impact oral health throughout the patient's lifetime.

▶ Adolescent's dentition is all permanent dentition.

▶ Need to assess for periodontal issues and diseases at each hygiene visit.

▶ May respond and wish to be treated as adults or as children at different times.

▶ Are learning to adapt to body changes, sexual impulses, secondary sex characteristics, and independence.

▶ May exhibit the different characteristics to one degree or another. Table 50-3 lists factors related to the psychological development of adolescents.

▶ May have anxiety due to: family issues (i.e., divorce), school performance, sexual issues, peer pressures, violence, or substance abuse.

▶ Concern over physical characteristics and personal appearance. Want to dress/be like their peers.

▶ Teachers, coaches, and health professionals can have a powerful impact at this time.

▶ Additional communication strategies for motivating adolescent patients are discussed in Chapter 3.

COMPONENTS OF THE DENTAL HYGIENE VISIT

Components of the dental visit are essentially the same for all pediatric patients. A clinical examination and diagnostic tools are utilized during a dental hygiene appointment to assess the child's overall oral health based on age and developmental milestones.

I. Initial Interview/New Patient Visit

▶ Parents are seated in a quiet, private place so they are able to concentrate and feel comfortable while supplying the information requested.

▶ As rapport is established with the parent(s), an explanation is given as to why the information is needed.

▶ The initial medical and family history information is collected and reviewed.

II. Child and Family Medical/Dental History

A. Family Configuration

▶ Number of people in the household and their relationship to the child.

▶ Other caregivers, the time periods, and location.

▶ Socioeconomic status and educational level of parents/guardians.

B. Medical History of the Child

▶ An accurate, comprehensive, and up-to-date medical history is necessary for correct diagnosis and effective treatment planning.[8]

▶ Refer to Chapter 10 regarding the medical health history process and an example of a child-specific health history form (Figure 10-2 in Chapter 10).

▶ Other health problems: The child patient with diabetes; cardiovascular disease; a mental, physical, or sensory disability; or other systemic involvement requires special adaptations of procedures as described in the various chapters of Section IX of this book.

▶ Dental caries and periodontal disease infections of parents and children.

III. Intra- and Extra-Oral Examination

▶ Table 50-1 lists child age-specific soft and hard tissue conditions/pathology and identifies significance to dental hygiene care.[7]

▶ Evaluate head and extremities for any abnormalities or signs of child abuse.

▶ Refer to Chapter 12 for performing the intra- and extra-oral examination.

IV. Developing Dentition, Occlusion, and TMJ

A. Evaluation

▶ Retract the lips to expose facial aspect to evaluate cervical areas for demineralization.

▶ Assess and document amount of biofilm present and any discolorations.

TABLE 50-3	Psychosocial Development of Adolescents		
	EARLY ADOLESCENCE APPROXIMATELY 11–13 YEARS OF AGE	**MIDDLE ADOLESCENT APPROXIMATELY 14–17 YEARS OF AGE**	**LATE ADOLESCENT APPROXIMATELY 18–21 YEARS OF AGE**
Environment	■ Home ■ Middle School ■ Extracurricular activities	■ Home ■ High School ■ Extracurricular activities/employment	■ Home/dorm ■ Secondary education ■ Employment
Identity/independence	■ Struggles with identity ■ Increased need for privacy ■ Desire for independence	■ Self-involvement increases; continual change between high expectations and poor self-concept ■ Tendency to distance selves from parents/parent conflicts peak ■ Continual drive for independence	■ Firmer sense of identity ■ Increased independence or completely independent ■ Self-reliant
Physical	■ Puberty is beginning ■ Physical growth : height and weight ■ Uncertain about changing appearance	■ Puberty is complete ■ Physical growth continues for males, decreases for females as puberty progresses ■ Continued uncertainty regarding physical changes/appearance	■ Females typically fully developed ■ Males continue to physically change (hair, muscle mass, height, weight) ■ Acceptance of pubertal changes
Cognitive	■ Growing abstract thinking ■ Deeper moral thinking ■ Intellectual interests become more important and expand	■ Continued growth of abstract thinking ■ Ability to set goals ■ Interest in moral reasoning	■ Ability to think ideas through ■ Think or be interested about the future ■ Continued interest in moral reasoning
Peers	■ Intense relationships with same sex friends ■ Increased influences of peer groups ■ Worried about being "normal"	■ Need for friends, reliance of friends, and need to fit in/popularity ■ Increased sexual activity and experimentation ■ Risk-taking behaviors	■ Peer relationships important ■ Development of intimate/serious relationships

Source: AACAP. *Facts for Families*. Washington, DC: American Academy of Child & Adolescent Psychiatry; 1952–2013. AACAP Facts for Families: Normal Adolescent Development Part 1, No. 57; 2011 December. http://www.aacap.org/aacap/Families_and_Youth/Facts_for_Families/Facts_for_Families_Pages/Normal_Adolescent_Development_Part_I_57.aspx and AACAP. *Facts for Families*. Washington, DC: American Academy of Child & Adolescent Psychiatry; 1952–2013. AACAP Facts for Families: Normal Adolescent Development Part II, No. 58; 2011 December. http://www.aacap.org/aacap/Families_and_Youth/Facts_for_Families/Facts_for_Families_Pages/Normal_Adolescent_Development_Part_II_58.aspx.

▶ Document tooth eruption delays compared with normal averages (in Table 50-4).

▶ Table 16-2 in Chapter 16 lists general features to observe when examining the child's teeth.

▶ Adequate spacing for developing dentition.

▶ Classification of occlusion.

▶ Look for malformations (Figure 50-1) and dental caries (Figure 50-2).

▶ Loss of teeth and condition of present restorations.

▶ Evaluation of pits and fissures for indication for sealants or repair of previously placed sealants.

▶ Temporomandibular joint (TMJ) disorder for clicking, popping, grinding, or discomfort upon opening, closing, or mastication.

B. Indications for Referral

▶ Severely crowded, malposed, or congenitally missing teeth.

▶ Overbite, overjet, crossbites, or other malocclusions requiring intervention.

▶ Early loss of primary molars: this condition, if untreated, usually disrupts the eruption and alignment of permanent molars and premolars, as depicted in Figure 50-3.

TABLE 50-4	Tooth Development and Eruption: Primary Teeth			
TOOTH	**HARD TISSUE FORMATION BEGINS (WEEKS IN UTERO)**	**ENAMEL COMPLETED (MONTHS AFTER BIRTH)**	**ERUPTION (MONTHS)**	**ROOT COMPLETED (YEAR)**
Maxillary				
Central incisor	14	1½	10 (8–12)	1½
Lateral incisor	16	2½	11 (9–13)	2
Canine	17	9	19 (16–22)	3¼
First molar	15½	6	16 (13–19 boys) (14–18 girls)	2½
Second molar	19	11	29 (25–33)	3
Mandibular				
Central incisor	14	2½	8 (6–10)	1½
Lateral incisor	16	3	13 (10–16)	1½
Canine	17	9	20 (17–23)	3¼
First molar	15½	5½	16 (14–18)	2¼
Second molar	18	10	27 (23–31 boys) (24–30 girls)	3

Source: Reprinted with permission from Lunt RC, Law DB. A review of the chronology of deciduous teeth. *J Am Dent Assoc.* 1974;89:372.

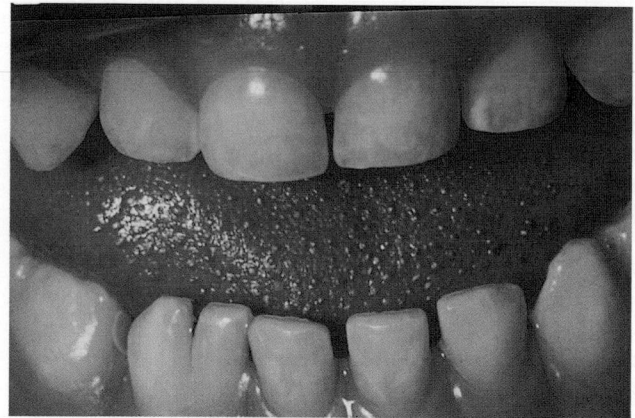

FIGURE 50-1 **Developmental Disturbance of Primary Teeth.** Germination of mandibular right lateral incisor caused by invagination of a single tooth germ and resulting in a notched and grooved crown.

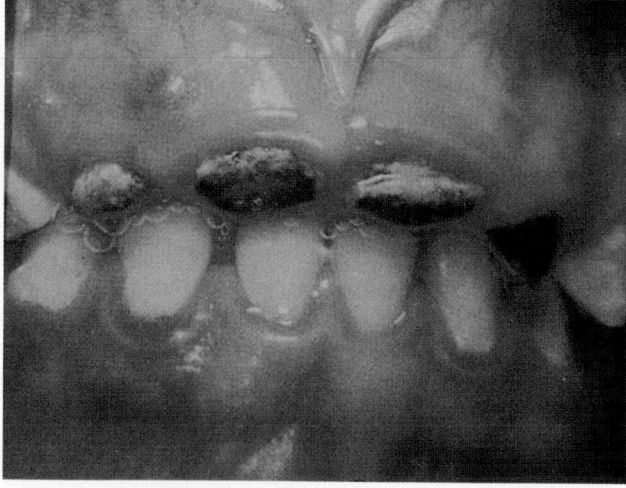

FIGURE 50-2 **S-ECC.** Nearly complete loss of tooth structure of maxillary incisors. Note the abscess on the gingival tissues between the maxillary right central and lateral incisor, and the cervical biofilm on the mandibular incisors.

V. Radiographic Assessment

Radiographs are a valuable diagnostic tool to aid in the overall oral health and developing an individualized treatment plan of the infant, child, or adolescent dental needs.

A. Radiographic Needs

▶ The dentist's professional judgment and ADA/Food and Drug Administration guidelines to prescribing needed dental radiographs for the child. See Table 13-4, Chapter 13.

▶ A patient's age is not the indicator for initial radiographic needs.

▶ Each child is unique and the need can only be determined by the dentist after reviewing the patient's medical and dental histories, completing a clinical examination, and assessing the patient's vulnerability to environmental factors that affect oral health.

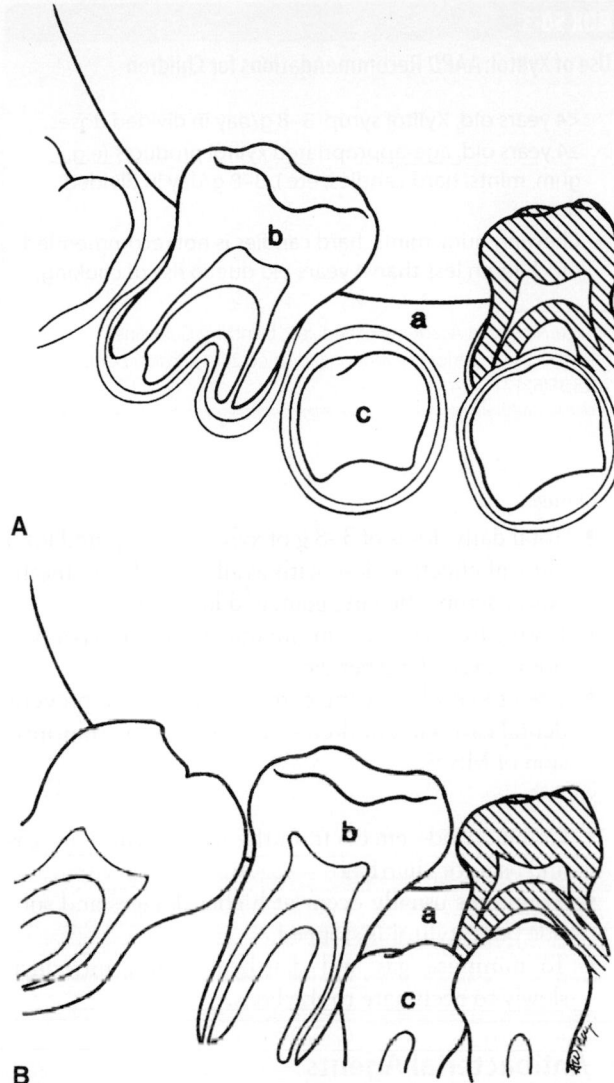

FIGURE 50-3 Premature Loss of Second Primary Molar. A: Developing first permanent molar (b) inclines and drifts mesially into the space (a) from which the second primary molar was removed. Developing second permanent premolar (c) is crowded. **B:** Space from which molar was removed (a) is nearly closed by the mesial drift and eruption of the first permanent molar (b). Developing second premolar (c) is closed in and prevented from eruption. Note that the second permanent molar has impacted against the first molar.

B. Cooperation

▸ Each child is different. Cooperation may depend on age and previous dental experiences.

▸ Use of tell–show–do, assistance of a parent, dental assistant or dentist, and/or using holding devices (see Chapter 13) will aid in taking radiographs.

VI. Dietary Assessment

▸ A study of the child's diet and counseling relative to general nutrition and dental caries control can provide important learning experiences for the parent, parent/ child, or adolescent.

▸ When discussing diet with adolescent patients, responsibility is placed on them and their ability to make choices.

A. Diet Instruction Suggestions

▸ Advice on food choices from the most recent My Plate Food Guide is illustrated in Figure 35-1 in Chapter 35.

▸ The use of the terms "healthy versus unhealthy" snacks instead of "good versus bad" snacks. The young child may not be able to distinguish the difference between "good" snacks that are "bad" for teeth, such as cookies are "good" tasting, but are "bad" for teeth.

VII. Dental Hygiene Treatment

A. Purpose

▸ Removal of biofilm, stain, and calculus for gingival health.

▸ Educate parents and children regarding proper, daily biofilm control procedures, and other preventive measures.

B. Type of Dental Hygiene Treatment

▸ The type of dental hygiene treatment provided for the child depends on the age and oral findings.

▸ The use of a disclosing agent is essential for assessment and education for school-aged children and adolescents.

▸ Perform at beginning of appointment to provide a visual tool for children to understand the presence of biofilm and removal with toothbrushing technique.

▸ Frequency of dental hygiene treatment is based on assessment of caries risk and periodontal health.

C. Instrumentation

▸ Presence of calculus is evaluated at each hygiene appointment for all ages.

▸ Removal of all local irregularities, including inadequate margins of restorations.

▸ When ultrasonic scaling is utilized for a pediatric patient with mixed dentition, it is only used on permanent teeth, never primary teeth.

▸ Ultrasonic scaling is effective for localized moderate-to-heavy calculus and orthodontic patients.

VIII. Prevention

A. Fluoride

Fluoride contributes to the prevention, inhibition, and reversal of caries.[10] Refer to Chapter 36 for additional fluoride information.

▸ *Professional application*
  • Well water—have tested for fluoride level.
  • Use of nonfluoridated bottle water or water systems using reverse osmosis.

- Application of professional fluoride treatment is based on the child's caries risk.
- Children with moderate caries risk need to receive a professional fluoride application every 6 months; high caries risk receive at a greater frequency of 3–6 months.[6]

▶ *Supplementation*

- Fluoride supplementation may be considered if fluoride exposure is not optimal. The ADA and the AAPD guidelines are used for supplementation recommendations (see Table 36-1 in Chapter 36).
- For children with moderate caries risk, over-the-counter fluoride rinses can be recommended as a supplement to daily brushing.

▶ Prescription fluoridated toothpaste is recommended for children with high risk or who have numerous carious lesions on proximal surfaces.

▶ A daily application of a fluoride gel in a custom-made tray may be necessary in selected cases.

▶ *Fluorosis*

- Dental fluorosis occurs as a result of excess fluoride ingestion during tooth formation.[11]
- Enamel fluorosis and primary teeth fluorosis can only occur when teeth are forming.[12]

B. Dental Sealants[13,14]

▶ As many as 90% of dental caries in school-aged children occurs in pits and fissures.

▶ Dentition is evaluated periodically for development defects and deep pits and fissures that may contribute to caries risk.

▶ Dental sealant is evaluated for repair or replacement as part of a periodic dental examination.

▶ Complete information about dental sealants can be found in Chapter 37.

C. Xylitol Use in Caries Prevention[15,16]

▶ *Background*

- A naturally occurring five-carbon sugar polyol (found in various trees, fruits, and vegetables) currently approved for use in foods, pharmaceuticals, and oral health products in more than 35 countries.
- Clinically effective levels of xylitol show mutans streptococci (MS) strains with reduced adhesion to the teeth and other reduced virulence properties such as less acid production.

▶ *Recommendations*

- For moderate or high caries-risk patients.
- Routinely re-evaluate every 6 months for changes in patient's caries-risk status and adjust recommendations accordingly.
- AAPD xylitol recommendations for children are listed in Box 50-3.

BOX 50-3

Use of Xylitol: AAPD Recommendations for Children

▷ <4 years old, Xylitol syrup, 3–8 g/day in divided doses.

▷ ≥4 years old, age-appropriated xylitol products (e.g., gum, mints, hard candies, etc.), 3–8 g/day in divided doses.

▷ Chewing gum, mints, hard candies is not recommended for children less than 4 years old due to risk of choking.

Source: American Academy of Pediatric Dentistry. Guideline on xylitol use in caries prevention [adopted 2011]. *Pediatr Dent.* 2013;35(6):171–174.

▶ *Dosage*

- Total daily doses of 3–8 g of xylitol are required for a clinical effective dose with available delivery methods or syrup, chewing gum, and lozenges.
- Dosing frequency is a minimum of two times per day, not to exceed 8 g per day.
- Use of xylitol chewing gum by mothers can prevent dental caries in children by preventing the transmission of MS.[15]

▶ *Side effects*

- Common side effects from the use of xylitol are gas and osmotic diarrhea.
- Symptoms usually occur at higher dosages and subside once xylitol is stopped.
- To minimize gas and diarrhea xylitol, introduce slowly to acclimate to the body.

D. Antibacterial Agents

▶ Antibacterial mouth rinses are not recommended for children under 12 years of age due to the potential of ingestion.

▶ Main caregiver of the child may rinse once daily rinsing with a 0.12% chlorhexidine gluconate for 1–2 weeks per month to decrease risk of transferring cariogenic bacteria.[17]

PERIODONTAL RISK ASSESSMENT

I. Gingival and Periodontal Evaluation

The AAPD's recommendations for children and adolescents includes placing greater emphasis on prevention, early diagnosis, and treatment of gingival and periodontal disease in children.[18] The risk of periodontal disease is lowered by establishing excellent oral hygiene habits in children, which will carry over to adulthood.

▶ *Periodontal evaluation*

- Periodontal probing, periodontal charting, and radiographic periodontal diagnosis is necessary when providing dental hygiene care for the adolescent.[19]

- The extent and nature of the periodontal evaluation is determined professionally on an individual basis.[19]
- Routine periodontal screening and probing is indicated following the eruption of permanent incisors and first molars.[20]
- The use of the periodontal screening and recording (PSR) method can facilitate the early detection of periodontal diseases in children and the need for a comprehensive periodontal examination.[21] See Chapter 23 for more information about the PSR.

II. Periodontal Infections

▶ Adolescents are at risk for periodontal infections and gingival problems.

▶ Careful probing and study of radiographs are indicated for each patient.

▶ Emphasis is placed on preventive measures, early assessment, early treatment, and regular maintenance appointments.

A. Biofilm-Induced Gingivitis

▶ Incidence and severity may increase during puberty.

▶ Clinical changes and hormonal changes related to increased dental biofilm.

▶ Exaggerated response to dental biofilm.

B. Risk Factors for Periodontitis[22]

▶ Local factors: supragingival and subgingival calculus; dental biofilm accumulations.

▶ Pathogenic microorganisms, viruses.

▶ Untreated dental caries and defective restorations.

▶ Orthodontic appliances.

▶ Oral hygiene: personal habits of care.

▶ Infrequent, inadequate dental and dental hygiene care.

▶ Socioeconomic influences.

▶ Use of tobacco.

▶ Systemic diseases such as diabetes and hematological diseases.

▶ Host immune factors.

▶ Genetic factors.

CARIES-RISK ASSESSMENT

A caries management by risk assessment (CAMBRA) process uses a questionnaire to interview the parent and/or child in combination with other assessment data to determine caries risk level. See Table 50-5.

I. Purpose

▶ To identify and decrease contributing factors (biological and clinical findings).

▶ Identify current protective factors.

▶ Classifies the child's risk level (low, moderate, or high) of developing caries. See Box 50-4.

▶ A communication tool with the parent and/or age-appropriate child in discussing and eliminating risks.

▶ A balance of risk factors and protective factors is needed to prevent the progression of caries as visualized in Figure 50-4.

II. Principles

▶ Provide parent and/or patient education.

▶ Promote remineralization of noncavitated lesions by use of topical fluorides.

▶ Modify oral flora to favor oral health by use of topical antibacterial agents.

▶ Minimal restoration of cavitated lesions and defective restorations.

III. Steps

▶ Complete a caries-risk assessment based on the child's specific age-related risk and preventive factors (Table 50-5).

▶ Determine level of caries risk (Box 50-4).

▶ Implement caries management by risk assessment (CAMBRA) treatment guidelines for ages 0–5 years old as listed in Table 50-6.

▶ CAMBRA treatment guidelines for individuals 6 years and older can be found in Table 27-1, Chapter 27.

IV. Classification of Caries Risk

▶ Low: no or little history of carious lesions, restorations, or extractions due to caries; no risk factors indicated; adequate protective factors.

▶ Moderate: history of carious lesions, restorations, or extractions due to caries but none the last 2 years; some risk factors but show no signs of continuing caries; could easily move to high risk; some protective factors.

▶ Moderate, non-compliant: same classification as moderate but child is noncompliant with recommended protective factors; no reduction in risk factors; balance is unstable.

▶ High: one or more observable and/or radiographic carious lesions present; history of carious lesions, restorations, or extractions due to caries within last year; more than two risk factors; inadequate protective factors; special needs or medically compromised with parent intervention; continuous carious lesions; medications with diminished salivary function.

▶ High, noncompliant: same classification as high; child and/or caregiver is noncompliant with recommended protective factors and risk factor reduction; could easily progress to extreme risk.

Table 50-5	Caries Risk and Protective Factors to Assess at Each Dental Visit

Assessment is based on provider's judgment of balance between risk factors/disease indicators and protective factors

CATEGORY	PATIENT AGE: 1–5	PATIENT AGE: 6 AND OVER
Biological predisposing risk factors Any one of these indicators signifies "high" overall caries risk	■ Mother/primary caregiver has active dental decay ■ Bottle with fluid other than water, plain milk, and/or plain formula ■ Continual bottle or sippy cup use ■ Child sleeps with a bottle or nurses on demand during night ■ Frequent (>3×/day) intake of sugars, cooked starch, or sugared beverages ■ Saliva-reducing factors present, including: ■ Medications ■ Medical (cancer treatment or genetic factors) ■ Developmental delay or special healthcare needs ■ Low caregiver health literacy, WIC participant, and/or child participates in free lunch program and/or early head start	■ Visible, heavy dental biofilm ■ Frequent snacking (>3× daily between meals) ■ Deep pits and fissures ■ Recreational drug use ■ Inadequate saliva flow by observation or measurement ■ Saliva reducing factors: • Medications • Radiation • Systemic/medical condition • Exposed root surfaces • Orthodontic appliances
Disease indicator/risk factors	■ Obvious white spots, decalcification, enamel defects, or decay present ■ New remineralization since last examination ■ Past caries experience (restorations present) ■ Obvious biofilm or easily bleeding gingiva ■ Visually inadequate saliva flow	■ Visible caries or radiographic penetration of the dentin ■ Radiographic proximal enamel lesions (not in dentin) ■ White spots on smooth surfaces ■ Caries experience (restorations) within last three years
Test results/Saliva tests indicated for high risk	■ Child: bacteria/saliva test ■ Caregiver: bacteria/saliva test	■ MS and lactobacillus both medium or high (by culture) ■ Saliva flow rate
Protective factors Necessary protective factor(s) to be utilized to lower overall risk	■ Lives in fluoridated community or takes fluoride supplements ■ Drinks fluoridated water (use of tap water instead of bottled water) ■ Use of fluoridated toothpaste at least once or twice daily ■ Fluoride varnish applied within last 6 mo ■ Xylitol chewing gum or application 2–4 times daily	■ Lives in fluoridated community or takes fluoride supplements ■ Drinks fluoridated water (use of tap water instead of bottled water) ■ Use of fluoridated toothpaste at least once or twice daily ■ Use of 5,000 ppm fluoride toothpaste ■ Use of 0.05% NaF mouth rinse daily ■ Fluoride varnish or office topical fluoride treatment within last 6 mo ■ Chlorhexidine use at least 1 wk of last 6 mo ■ Xylitol chewing gum/lozenges 4 times daily during last 6 mo ■ Saliva flow >1 mL/min stimulated

Child's overall risk (circle): High Moderate Low

Assessed by: _____ Date: _____ Next assessment date: _____

Source: Ramos-Gomez FJ, Ng MW. CAMBRA—caries risk assessment form for age 0 to 5 years. *J Calif Dent Assoc.* 2011;3(10):723–733.

▶ Extreme: rampant decay; chronic medical condition or special needs; hyposalivary function; numerous risk factors, none or minimal protective factors.

V. Early Childhood Caries (ECC)

▶ The disease of ECC is the presence of one or more decayed (noncavitated or cavitated lesions), missing (due to caries), or filled tooth surfaces in any primary tooth in a child under the age of six.

▶ A child under the age of three with any smooth-surface caries (white-spot lesion or cavitated lesion) is indicative of severe early childhood caries (S-ECC).[23]

▶ This form of caries is usually seen in children who routinely have been given a bottle when going to sleep containing a cariogenic liquid (formula, milk, or juice) or have experienced prolong at-will breastfeeding.

▶ Nursing bottle caries, baby bottle tooth decay, and rampant caries are older terms. The AAPD adopted the term ECC to reflect the multifactorial etiology (frequency, tooth-adherent specific bacteria, primarily mutans streptococci (MS), that metabolize sugars to produce acid that, over time, demineralizes tooth structure).[23]

▶ Children experiencing caries as infants or toddlers are at higher risk for developing caries in primary and permanent teeth in the future.[24,25]

▶ ECC and S-ECC case definition criteria are found in Table 23-1, Chapter 23.

A. Prevalence

▶ Tooth decay (dental caries) affects children in the United States more than any other chronic infectious disease.[26]

▶ Tooth decay affects more than one-fourth of US children aged 2–5 years and half of children aged 12–15 years.[27]

B. Microbiology

▶ Dental caries is a common chronic infectious transmissible disease resulting from tooth-adherent specific bacteria, primarily MS.[26] *Lactobacilli* in large numbers are also in the dental biofilm.

▶ Transfer of MS from parent, caregiver, sibling, or other child by saliva sharing behaviors to the infant or young child.[28]

▶ Colonization of MS has been shown to occur before tooth eruption and as early as birth.[29]

▶ High levels of MS in saliva and dental biofilm are a strong risk indicator for ECC.[30]

▶ Avoid saliva sharing behaviors such as kissing on the mouth, tasting food before feeding, cleaning a dropped pacifier by mouth, and sharing of cups, toys, or utensils.[31]

C. Risk Factors

The areas of concern related to disease indicators/risk factors are listed in Table 50-5. Teaching parents about the cause and effects of ECC is a significant part of anticipatory guidance (Table 50-7).

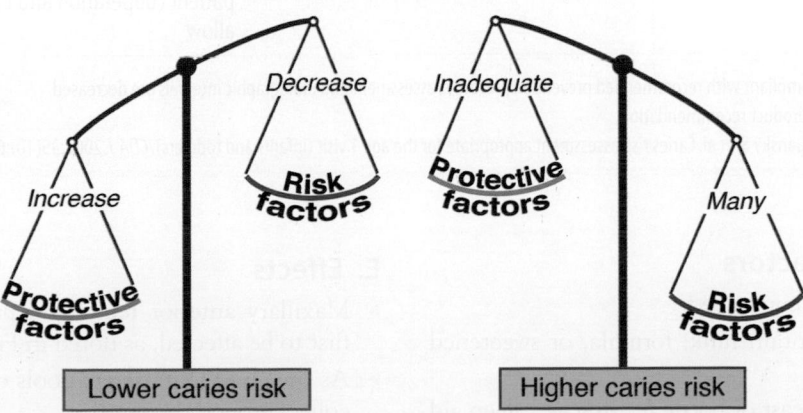

FIGURE 50-4 Visualize the Caries Balance. Individualized assessment of risk factors can help determine the caries-risk level of each patient. Providing interventions that increase protective factors such as adequate biofilm removal and fluoride exposure can change the balance and reduce caries risk.

Table 50-6	Caries Management Based on Risk Level for Patients Up to Age 5 Years Old

RECOMMENDATIONS/ INTERVENTIONS	CARIES-RISK LEVEL			
	LOW	MODERATE[A]	HIGH[A]	EXTREME[A]
Assessment				
Periodic oral examination	Annual	Every 6 mo	Every 3 mo	Every 1–3 mo
Radiographs—unless proximal surfaces can be visually examined	Posterior bitewings 12–24 mo interval	Posterior bitewings 12–24 mo interval	Anterior occlusal film and posterior bitewings 6–12 mo interval	
Saliva test	Optional for Baseline	Suggested	Recommended	
Preventive interventions				
Fluoride: home:	Fluoride toothpaste 2× daily Recommended: Caregiver OTC sodium fluoride rinses			
Fluoride: Office:	Not required	Varnish application at all preventive visits		
Xylitol[b] (wipes, syrup, lollipop, hard candy, mints, or chewing gum)	Not required	Recommended for both child and caregiver		
Sealants	n/a	In deep pits and fissures of fully erupted molars		
Antibacterials	n/a	n/a	Consider chlorhexidine rinse for caregiver	
Anticipatory guidance	Preventive oral health counseling and anticipatory guidance based on age-appropriate and caries risk–specific factors is recommended at all preventive visits			
Self-management goals (for parent)	Not required	Recommended		
White-spot lesions (noncavitated)	n/a	Fluoride application as indicated to promote remineralization		
Restorative interventions				
Existing lesions	n/a		ITR or conventional restorative treatment as patient cooperation and family circumstances allow	

[a]If the parent/guardian is noncompliant with recommended prevention protocols, assessment and radiographic intervals are decreased.
[b]Age-appropriate use of Xylitol product recommendation.
Source: Ramos-Gomez F, Crall J, Gansky S, et al. Caries risk assessment appropriate for the age 1 visit (infants and toddlers). *CDA J.* 2007;35(10):687–702.

D. Predisposing Factors

▶ Placing bottle/sippy cup in bed.
▶ Bottle/sippy cup contain milk, formula, or sweetened fluid with sucrose.
▶ Prolonged at-will breast or bottle feeding as a sleep aid or behavioral control.
▶ Ineffective or no daily biofilm removal from the teeth.

E. Effects

▶ Maxillary anterior teeth and primary molars are the first to be affected, as noted in Figures 50-2 and 50-5.
▶ As the child falls asleep, pools of the sweet liquid can collect around the teeth.
▶ While the sucking is active, the liquid passes beyond the teeth.

TABLE 50-7	Anticipatory Guidance: 12 Months to 6 Years of Age		
AREA OF CONCERN	**12–24 MONTHS**	**2–3 YEARS**	**4–6 YEARS**
Developmental milestone	■ Check tooth contacts ■ Close contacts: teach parents to floss ■ Normal/abnormal eruption pattern	■ Primary dentition complete ■ Evaluate occlusion for crowding, overbite, overjet ■ Bruxing and occlusal wear ■ Evaluate for sealants on primary teeth based on caries risk	■ Discuss exfoliation of primary teeth ■ Eruption patterns and expected new permanent teeth ■ Evaluate for sealants on 1st permanent molars
Nutrition and feeding	■ Nutrition, snacking based on child's diet ■ Reduce snacking frequency ■ Review snacking safety ■ Avoid food as reward for behavior modification ■ Avoid dependence on sippy cup	■ Suggest snacks from fruit, vegetable, dairy, and meat groups ■ Limit juice intake to 4 ounces	■ Snacking: suggest healthy snacks ■ Limit juice and soda
Oral hygiene and caries prevention	■ Complete caries-risk assessment ■ OHI with parent and daily oral hygiene completed by parent ■ Disclose for dental biofilm ■ Review brushing; continue with a "smear" of fluoridated toothpaste ■ Lift upper lip when brushing ■ Parents are the role models ■ Parents look for signs of disease ■ Review position of child for OH—knee-to-knee	■ Complete caries-risk assessment ■ OHI with parents and child. Parent continues with daily oral hygiene and child may "have a turn" ■ Ask about problems ■ Lift upper lip when brushing ■ Brush morning and night ■ Use a "pea" sized amount of fluoridated toothpaste ■ Review signs of disease ■ Review position of child for OH—standing behind child	■ Complete caries-risk assessment ■ OHI including flossing with parents and child; parent continues with daily oral hygiene; child also performs brushing after parent ■ Review signs of disease
Fluoride information	■ Update fluoride status ■ Store fluoride products out of reach of children ■ Use of small, thin smear of fluoride dentifrice on brush ■ Fluoride varnish application	■ Parents control toothpaste ■ Evaluate changes in diet and water ■ Make appropriate fluoride recommendations ■ Fluoride varnish application	■ Parents continue toothpaste control ■ Check fluoride status ■ Varnish applications
Trauma/injury prevention	■ Car seat safety ■ Discuss oral electrical burns and child-proofing home ■ Care of avulsed tooth	■ Provide trauma management plan at daycare or preschool ■ Discuss head and neck, oral signs of child abuse ■ Review other safety measures (i.e., bike helmet, car seats, etc.)	■ Trauma management plan at school ■ Review need for mouth guard ■ Discuss bike safety ■ Monitor for signs of child abuse ■ Review other safety measures
Habits/function behaviors	■ Effects of continued thumb, finger, or pacifier sucking	■ Nonnutritive sucking may still be present ■ Discuss elimination of thumb/finger sucking; possible early orthodontic referral	■ Eliminate thumb/finger sucking; possible orthodontic referral needed
Environmental (passive) smoke	■ Smoke-free environment required	■ Smoke-free environment required	■ Smoke-free environment required
Dental/dental hygiene visit	■ Home preparation for dental visit ■ Frequency depends on caries risk and parent compliance with home preventive measures ■ Parents emphasize helping–caring nature of dentist/dental hygienist ■ Toothbrush dental biofilm removal ■ Discuss findings and recommendations with parents ■ Radiographic evaluation if indicated ■ Discuss findings and recommendations with parents	■ Frequency of preventive care based on caries risk ■ Use disclosing solution to identify dental biofilm ■ Toothbrush or rubber cup dental biofilm removal ■ Radiographic evaluation if indicated ■ Discuss findings and recommendations with parents	■ Frequency of preventive visits and radiographic evaluation based on risk factors ■ Emphasize helping/caring nature of providers ■ Use disclosing solution to identify dental biofilm ■ Assess for calculus requiring scaling ■ Rubber cup polishing ■ Discuss findings and recommendations with parents

Source: American Academy of Pediatric Dentistry. Guideline on Periodicity of Examination, Preventive Dental Services, Anticipatory Guidance/Counseling, and Oral Treatment for Infants, Children, and Adolescents. [Revised 2013];35(6):114–121. http://www.aapd.org/media/Policies_Guidelines/G_Periodicity.pdf. Accessed March 9, 2014.

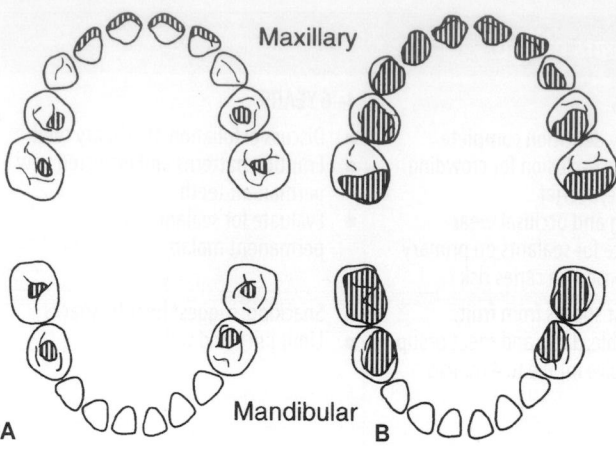

FIGURE 50-5 Progression of ECC. A: Earliest caries affect the maxillary anterior teeth, followed by the molars as they erupt. **B:** Severe extensive lesions develop in all except the mandibular anterior teeth. Protection for the mandibular incisors and canines is provided by the tongue during the sucking process.

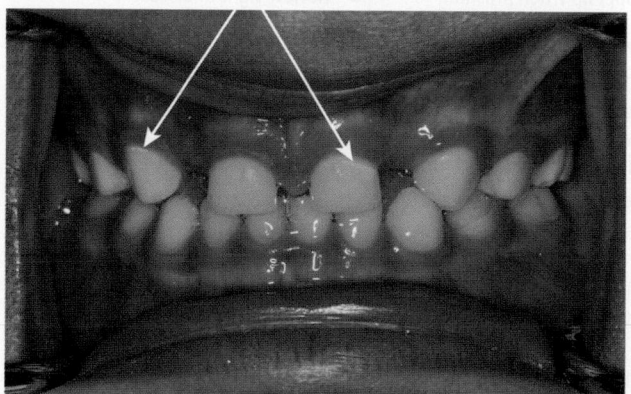

FIGURE 50-6 White-Spot Lesions. Opaque, chalky enamel areas, usually on cervical or proximal areas of teeth at contacts, indicate that the surface and underlying enamel are demineralized. Subtle white lesions (indicated by the arrows) at the cervical margin of the maxillary canine and incisor provide the earliest clinical sign of the carious process. Note that the maxillary lateral incisors are missing. (Photograph courtesy of Dr. Samuel Blanchard, DDS, MS.)

▶ The nipple covers the mandibular anterior teeth; hence, they are rarely affected.

F. Recognition

▶ Demineralization or white-spot lesions may be noted along the cervical third of the maxillary anterior teeth and proximal surfaces when the upper lip is lifted (Figure 50-6).

▶ At a later stage, cavitation occurs and the lesions appear brown or dark brown (Figure 50-7). Eventually, the crowns may be destroyed to the gum line, abscesses may develop, and the child may suffer severe pain and discomfort. An advanced stage of dental caries is shown in Figure 50-2.

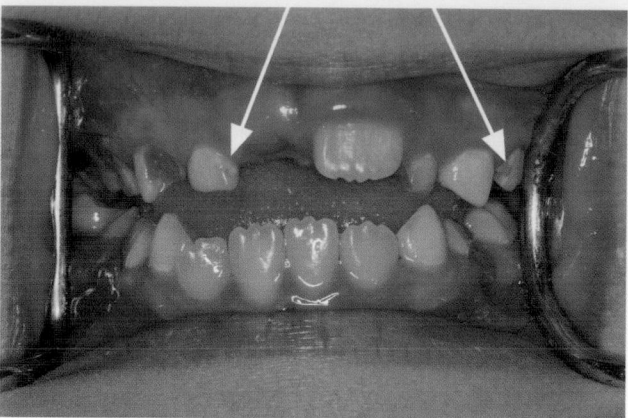

FIGURE 50-7 Cavitation of White Lesion Areas. Small brownish-looking cavitated areas can be seen adjacent to white-spot lesions on the mesial–facial surface of the lateral incisor and the mesial–facial surface of the first primary molar. A large cavitated carious lesion can be seen on the maxillary right canine. Note additional white-spot lesions at the cervical margins of the maxillary left canine, the mandibular canines, and the left mandibular molar. (Photograph courtesy of Dr. Samuel Blanchard, DDS, MS.)

ANTICIPATORY GUIDANCE

▶ Anticipatory guidance is the process of providing practical, developmentally appropriate information about children's health to prepare parents for the significant physical, emotional, and psychological milestones.[6]

▶ Involves both the parent and the child patient (when age appropriate).

▶ Customized patient-centered recommendations presented orally, demonstration provided, and written documentation to be taken home for reference.

▶ Developmental milestones, nutrition and feeding, oral hygiene measures, dental caries prevention, health and safety precautions, and treatment measures are outlined in Tables 50-7 and 50-8.

I. Dietary and Feeding Pattern Recommendations

A. Toddlers and Preschoolers

▶ Children need a series of small, healthy meals during the day.

▶ Healthy snacks include non-cariogenic foods from the grain, vegetable, fruit, meat/meat alternatives, and dairy groups.

▶ Sweetened foods and drinks are limited to 3 or less per day and provided at mealtimes rather than between meals.

▶ Do not allow the child to sip or graze at will on a bottle or sippy cup containing milk or sweet liquids, which promotes demineralization and ECC.

▶ Limit juice to no more than 4–6 ounces per day.

TABLE 50-8	Anticipatory Guidance: Age 6 to Adolescent	
AREA OF CONCERN	**6–12 YEARS**	**12 YEARS AND OLDER**
Developmental milestone	■ Eruption patterns; mixed dentition; missing teeth ■ Evaluate orthodontic needs ■ Evaluate for sealants on permanent molars	■ Eruption patterns; permanent dentition; missing teeth ■ Evaluate orthodontic needs ■ Evaluate for sealants on 2nd permanent molars
Nutrition and feeding	■ Snacking: continue with healthy snack choices ■ Limit juice, soda, and sports drinks ■ Discussion with parent and child on hidden sugars, carbohydrate snacks and frequency	■ Snacking: continue with healthy snack choices ■ Limit juice, soda, and sports drinks ■ Discussion with parent and child on hidden sugars, carbohydrate snacks, and frequency
Oral hygiene and caries prevention	■ Complete caries-risk assessment form ■ OHI with child; parent supervises daily oral hygiene; child performs daily oral hygiene ■ Reinforce daily brushing for 2 min, 2 times daily ■ Teach flossing and use of floss holders if needed; flossing daily ■ Review need for adjunct hygiene care products (disclosing tablets, fluoride rinses, floss threaders) ■ Review signs of disease	■ Complete caries-risk assessment form ■ OHI with child; consult with parent as necessary ■ Reinforce daily brushing for 2 min, 2 times daily ■ Teach flossing and use of floss holders if needed; flossing daily ■ Review need for adjunct hygiene care products (disclosing tablets, fluoride rinses, floss threaders) ■ Review signs of disease
Fluoride information	■ Check fluoride status ■ Varnish applications	■ Check fluoride status ■ Varnish applications
Trauma/injury prevention	■ Trauma management plan at school ■ Review need for mouth guard ■ Discuss bike safety ■ Monitor for signs of child abuse ■ Review other safety measures	■ Trauma management plan at school ■ Review need for mouth guard ■ Discuss bike safety ■ Monitor for signs of child abuse ■ Review other safety measures
Habits/function behaviors	■ Evaluation for need for orthodontic referral	■ Evaluation for need for orthodontic referral
Environmental (passive) smoke	■ Smoke-free environment required ■ Educate regarding tobacco use	■ Smoke-free environment required ■ Educate regarding tobacco use
Dental/dental hygiene visit	■ Frequency of preventive visits and radiographic evaluation based on risk factors ■ Emphasize helping/caring nature of providers ■ Use disclosing solution to identify dental biofilm ■ Evaluate periodontal status as permanent teeth erupt ■ Assess for calculus requiring scaling ■ Rubber cup polishing ■ Discuss findings and recommendations with parents ■ Age-appropriate counseling for substance abuse and/or smoking	■ Frequency of preventive visits and radiographic evaluation based on risk factors ■ Emphasize helping/caring nature of providers ■ Use disclosing solution to identify dental biofilm ■ Evaluate periodontal status as permanent teeth erupt ■ Assess for calculus requiring scaling ■ Rubber cup polishing ■ Discuss findings and recommendations with parents ■ Assessment for removal of 3rd molars ■ Age-appropriate counseling for: substance abuse, intraoral/perioral piercing, and/or smoking

Source: American Academy of Pediatric Dentistry. Guideline on Periodicity of Examination, Preventive Dental Services, Anticipatory Guidance/Counseling, and Oral Treatment for Infants, Children, and Adolescents. [Revised 2013];35(6):114–121. http://www.aapd.org/media/Policies_Guidelines/G_Periodicity.pdf. Accessed March 9, 2014.

B. School Aged

▶ Educate about healthy snacks and drinks; encourage tooth-healthy choices.

▶ School-aged children continue to have problems with likes and dislikes.

▶ Family, friends, and the media (especially TV) influence their food choices.[32]

C. Adolescent

▶ Adolescents' frequency of eating increases due to growth periods, emotional issues, or peer pressures.

▶ Cariogenic foods and drinks are often selected. Incidence of dental caries may increase during adolescence.

▶ Highest caries risk of any time in life for males; exceeded only during pregnancy for females.

▶ Inadequate nutrition is common.
  • Boys: due to over activity and poor food selection.
  • Girls: due to voluntary diet restrictions, with poor food selection and fad diets in the attempt to be trim.
  • Teens with a distorted body image may take concern to extremes.

▶ Eating disorders
  • Anorexia nervosa and/or bulimia can lead to severe health complications and even death.
  • Successful treatment usually requires an interdisciplinary team approach involving medical care, psychotherapy, and nutrition and family counseling (as described in Chapter 64).

▶ Iron-deficiency anemia
  • Common among teenage girls, particularly after the onset of menstruation.
  • Treated with iron supplements, changes in diet, or both.

II. Oral Health Considerations for Toddlers/Preschoolers[33]

A. Gaining Cooperation

▶ At these ages, the child is becoming more independent.

▶ Parents can provide a fun activity by making up and singing a brushing song.

▶ For a 2- to 3-year-old, teach the child to take turns with the parent when brushing by using the phrase, "It's your turn to brush," followed by, "It's my turn to brush."

▶ To gain better cooperation, connect brushing with a fun activity such as first, we brush teeth and then, we read a story.

▶ Provide or recommend 2- or 3-minute timers to be used for motivation during brushing.

B. Brushing and Flossing

▶ Establish a routine: make suggestions as to how to establish and maintain a brushing routine.

▶ Recommend brushing in the morning after breakfast and before bedtime.

▶ Specify that the most critical time for dental biofilm removal is before bedtime.

C. Parental Involvement and Supervision

▶ Parents keep fluoride toothpaste out of reach of the child and are in charge of placing the correct amount of toothpaste on the toothbrush.

▶ Until the child develops fine motor coordination, and is able to effectively remove biofilm, the parents/caregivers assist the child in cleaning the teeth by doing the brushing and flossing. The time to cease assistance depends on parental/caregiver assessment and varies markedly from child to child.

▶ Parents teach the child to brush and then evaluate to ensure effective and complete biofilm removal.

▶ Parents floss closely approximated primary teeth to remove biofilm from proximal surfaces.

D. Toothpaste

▶ Children's toothpastes manufactured in the United States contain the same amount of fluoride as adult toothpastes, whereas manufacturers in several countries around the world reduce the amount of fluoride in children's toothpastes.

▶ Parents/caregivers are informed that they need to prevent problems by controlling the amount of toothpaste used and placing it out of the child's reach.

▶ For children younger than 6 years, regularly ingesting pea-sized amounts or more can lead to mild fluorosis.[34]

▶ Appropriate amount of fluoridated toothpaste is to be used for children of all ages.[35]

▶ Children like the taste of toothpaste and may eat a large amount at one time resulting in acute fluoride toxicity.

E. Instructions for parents:

▶ An adult can brush the child's teeth with a tiny amount of fluoridated toothpaste as soon as the first tooth comes in.

▶ Younger than 3 years old use a small "smear" of fluoride toothpaste (an amount about the size of a grain of rice) as illustrated in Figure 50-8.[34]

▶ Children 3–6 years of age use a "pea-size" amount of fluoride toothpaste.[34] See an illustration in Figure 50-8.

▶ Teach children to spit out toothpaste as soon as they are old enough to do so.[34]

▶ Continue to control the toothpaste and keep it out of reach.

▶ Teach parents how to examine the mouth for signs of gingival inflammation, dental caries, and injury.

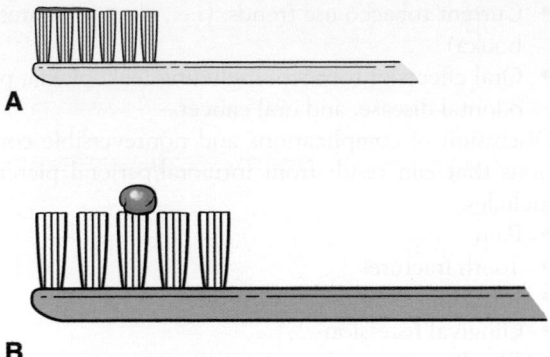

A

B

FIGURE 50–8 **Dentifrice for a Child.** For children under 3 years of age, a parent is instructed to place a small smear of fluoridated toothpaste on a child-sized brush (A). For all children ages 3–6 years of age, the appropriate size is that of a small pea (B). The paste is spread in a thin layer over the brush surface and then spread over all of the teeth before brushing.

▸ Evaluation of pits and fissure for caries-susceptible primary and permanent teeth (molars, premolars, and anterior teeth).

III. Speech and Language Development

▸ Premature loss of primary teeth, digit habits, and malocclusions can have direct implications on a child's development of speech and language.

▸ Early detection and referral can help correct speech or language development.

IV. Digit Habits

▸ Prolong thumb- and finger-sucking habits have been associated with narrow maxillary arch width, anterior open bite, posterior crossbite, increased overjet, and decreased overbite[35] (see Figure 50-9).

V. Accident and Injury Prevention

▸ Age-appropriate accident and injury prevention counseling for oro-facial trauma is provided and/or evaluated at every hygiene visit.

▸ Written information regarding what to do in the event of a traumatic oral injury makes parents feel more prepared.

▸ Table 8-4 in Chapter 8 provides information on a dislocated jaw, facial fracture, and tooth forcibly displaced or avulsed.

A. Toddlers

▸ The greatest incidence of injury to the primary dentition occurs at 2–3 years of age. Toddlers have increased mobility and developing coordination and as a result are subject to injuries.

▸ Provide counseling regarding play objects, pacifiers, car seats, and electrical cords.

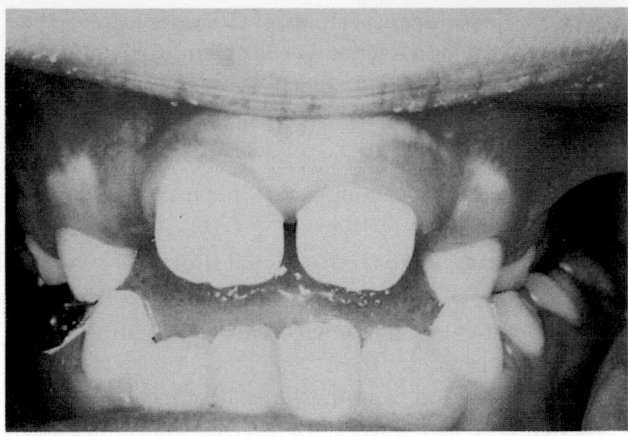

FIGURE 50-9 **Effects of Prolonged Thumb Sucking on Teeth.** Anterior open bite with posterior cross bite.

B. School-Aged Children

▸ House structures/furniture such as floors, steps, tables, and beds are most commonly associated with dental injuries in children under age 7 years.

▸ Parents can be taught to protect the child by close supervision, anticipating problems, and making the environment safe by removing dangers.

C. Adolescents

▸ Common injuries to permanent teeth are related to car accidents, violence, and sports-related trauma.

▸ Counseling and providing athletic mouth guards for all contact sports and activities can enhance trauma prevention.

VI. Oral Malodor

A. Causes

▸ Bacteria at the base of the tongue.
▸ Bacteria between the teeth.
▸ Postnasal drip.

B. What to Teach Parents

▸ Explain bacterial causes.
▸ Emphasize thorough dental biofilm removal through daily brushing of the teeth.
▸ Teach how to floss their child's teeth.
▸ Show how to brush gently the dorsum of the tongue (refer to Chapter 28).

VII. Oral Health Considerations for Adolescents[19]

Increased risk for dental caries and periodontal infections during adolescence has already been described in this chapter. Some additional examples of oral problems related to adolescent development and behavior characteristics, including risky health behaviors, are listed here.

- Assess the presence, position, and development of third molars. Provide a referral if need of removal is indicated.
- Oral manifestations of sexually transmitted infections.
- Potential effects of hormonal fluctuations and use of oral contraceptives on periodontal tissues (Chapter 52).
- Oral findings of anorexia nervosa or bulimia (Chapter 65).
- Traumatic injury to teeth and oral structures.
  - Contact sports and skateboarding are risky behaviors.
  - Automobile and motorcycle accidents can also cause dental injuries.
- If pregnancy and parenting are issues for the adolescent patient, the dental hygienist has the opportunity to use anticipatory guidance to educate about important oral health issues for the mother and infant (Chapter 50).

VIII. Tobacco/Piercings/Substance Abuse

- As the child approaches adolescence, the prevention discussion can be expanded to include the serious health consequences of tobacco use, intraoral/perioral piercings, and substance abuse.
- These topics may require the dental hygienist to obtain additional information from the child and to be comfortable talking with the child/adolescent.
- Discussion of tobacco use (see Chapter 34) includes:
  - Smoking, smokeless tobacco, and exposure to second-hand smoke.

- Current tobacco use trends. (i.e., electric cigarettes, hooka)
- Oral effects of tobacco, including leukoplakia, periodontal disease, and oral cancer.
- Discussion of complications and nonreversible conditions that can result from intraoral/perioral piercings includes:
  - Pain
  - Tooth fractures
  - Infections
  - Gingival recession
  - Bleeding
  - Obstruction of the airway
- The patient who has or is considering an oral piercing is:
  - Educated regarding daily hygiene of the piercing site to avoid infection.
  - Counseled at every dental hygiene visit regarding possible complications
  - Encouraged to remove the piercings.
- A complete discussion about oral complications related to the use of cocaine and other street drugs is found in Chapter 65.

IX. Referral

- Appropriate referrals are made when problems that require intervention by other health providers are identified.
- Conditions requiring referral include:
  - Evidence of systemic illness and pathology

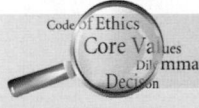

EVERYDAY ETHICS

Maria has practiced as a dental hygienist in the office of Dr. Reynolds for 3 years. Maria recently attended a continuing education course on dental caries-risk assessment and prevention. At the course, recommendations from professionally applied topical fluoride: evidence-based clinical recommendations published by the ADA were reviewed. Maria heard the results of systematic reviews on fluoride varnish, reviewed the ADA's recommendations of fluoride varnish as the only topical fluoride recommended for children under age 6, and learned fluoride varnish can even be used on infants to prevent ECC.

Maria is convinced that she needs to be using fluoride varnish on patients of all ages based upon caries risk. Dental hygienists at Dr. Reynolds' office are currently applying 2.0% sodium fluoride foam to patients under age 18. At the weekly staff meeting, Maria presented an overview of fluoride varnish products, key research findings, a cost comparison of varnish versus fluoride tray and foam, and distributed copies of the ADA fluoride recommendations. The following week, Dr. Reynolds told Maria that she had reviewed the fluoride varnish information and decided to continue using the fluoride foam and trays. When Maria asked why, Dr. Reynolds stated, "the

increased costs of using fluoride varnish would really add up over a year and increasing patient fees is not an option. Anyway, patients expect to have smooth shiny teeth after dental hygiene treatment" Dr. Reynolds concluded.

Questions for Consideration

1. Because fluoride varnish is the safest professional fluoride application and recommended by the ADA for children under age 6, how do the ethical principles of beneficence and nonmaleficence apply in this situation?

2. Do clinical recommendations or guidelines from professional associations, such as the ADA, constitute standards of care? Why or why not?

3. Maria has an ethical responsibility to her employer, who has expressed concerns about cost and patient acceptance of this "new" type of fluoride treatment, as well as to her patients. Which questions in the steps for resolving an ethical situation (Box 1-10, Chapter 1) might help Maria to balance those responsibilities as she makes a decision about an action to take in continuing this discussion with Dr. Reynolds?

- Child abuse or neglect and evidence of poor parenting skills[36]
- Failure to provide safety measures
- Substance abuse in the family.[36]

▶ Understand the reporting and licensing requirements for child abuse and neglect specific to the state.

TREATMENT PLANNING AND CONSENT

▶ The dental hygiene diagnosis is used to develop the dental hygiene care plan (Chapter 24 and Chapter 25).

▶ Before treatment, the care plan is discussed with the dentist in order to integrate the dental hygiene plan into the comprehensive dental treatment plan.

▶ Inform parent/guardian of findings from the assessment and present the care plan both orally and in writing.

▶ Have parent/guardian sign an informed consent before treatment (Chapter 25).

▶ *Medical clearance:* The parent/guardian will need to consent to medical clearance for conditions requiring

antibiotic coverage, local anesthesia, or other medication for a patient under legal age.

▶ *Parental approval:* The dental hygienist care plan requires approval by the parent/guardian.

DOCUMENTATION

The following items are documented in the progress notes of pediatric patients.

▶ Overall appraisal of physical status and key health history findings.

▶ Existing pathology: soft tissue, gingiva, caries, occlusal status.

▶ Oral hygiene status and caries-risk assessment.

▶ Anticipatory guidance provided, parent/patient recommendation, and any adjunct hygiene aids provided (disclosing tablets, prescriptions, proxy brush, floss threader).

▶ Procedures completed: initial examination, recall examination, scaling and polishing, radiographs taken, type of fluoride provided.

▶ Child's behavior throughout the appointment and level of cooperation (e.g., patient's behavior quiet during appointment but cooperative with all aspects of the appointment).

▶ Treatment planned for next visit.

▶ Box 50-5 provides an example of documentation for a child's dental visit.

Box 50-5

Example Documentation: Preventive Dental Hygiene Visit by Child Patient

S –A 8-year-old male presents for continuing care visit. Medical history reviewed w/mother. No health concerns, no medications, no chief complaint. Home care: brushing 1×/day in the morning only and does not floss.

O –I/E oral examination: within normal limits, buccal mucosa: bilateral linea alba, tongue: coated. Class II occlusion, 50% overbite, 3 mm overjet, lower anterior crowding. Clinical findings: sealants on #3, 14, 19, and 30 sound. Radiographic findings: no caries. Oral hygiene: generalized moderate biofilm, localized light calculus: supragingival mandibular anteriors—all surfaces, subgingival mandibular posterior linguals, and supra/subgingival facial of maxillary 1st molars. Perio evaluation of permanent teeth: 1–2 mm w/bleeding on probing.

A –Generalized gingivitis due to moderate biofilm, localized calculus, and generalized slight/moderate bleeding. OH is poor, "plaque-free score" = 20%, no improvement same as last visit, Caries risk = low.

P –Scaled, polished, and flossed. Applied 5% sodium fluoride varnish. OHI and recommendations: using mod bass technique, 2×/day brushing for 2 min w/fluoridated toothpaste, daily flossing using a floss holder, use of disclosing tablets every other day. Goal for next appointment: "plaque-free score" improvement, and reduced areas of calculus present. Patient was well behaved and genuine interest in improving his oral health care. Parent advised to supervise care at home.

Signed _____, RDH

Date _____

Factors To Teach The Parents

▷ How the parents' own oral health affects their child's oral health.

▷ How the bacteria that cause dental caries can be transferred to the baby's mouth from parents or other family members.

▷ How fluoride makes enamel stronger and more resistant to the bacteria that cause dental caries.

▷ Methods to prevent dental caries from developing in a young child's mouth.

▷ How feeding methods and snacking patterns can contribute to dental caries.

▷ How the parent can examine the infant's/child's mouth and what to look for during the examination.

▷ Reasons why the baby's mouth needs to be examined by an oral health professional at 6 months of age or as soon as the first tooth erupts.

▷ Reasons why maintenance of primary teeth is necessary for oral health, growth, and development.

▷ Ways parents can prepare their young children for visits to the dentist and dental hygienist.

▷ How parents can prevent accidents and injury in their infants and children.

References

1. American Dental Association. Specialty definitions. In: ADA: *America's Leading Advocate for Oral Health*. Chicago, IL: American Dental Association; 1995–2013. http://www.ada.org/495.aspx. Accessed October 15, 2013.

2. American Academy of Pediatric Dentistry. About the AAPD: mission and vision. In: *America's Pediatric Dentists the Big Authority on Little Teeth*. Chicago, IL: American Academy of Pediatric Dentistry; 2002–2013. www.aapd.org/about/mission/. Accessed October 15, 2013.

3. American Academy of Pediatric Dentistry. *America's Pediatric Dentists the Big Authority, on Little Teeth*. Chicago, IL: American Academy of Pediatric Dentistry; 2002–2013. www.aapd.org. Accessed October 15, 2013.

4. National Center on Birth Defects and Developmental Disabilities. *Child Development*. Atlanta, GA: Infant Health and Child Development. http://www.cdc.gov/ncbddd/childdevelopment/positiveparenting/index.html. Updated March 11, 2014. Accessed April 23, 2014.

5. Green M, Palfrey JS, eds. Chapter 1: Getting started. In: *Bright Futures: Guidelines for Health Supervision of Infants, Children, and Adolescents*. 2nd ed. Arlington, VA: National Center for Education in Maternal and Child Health; 2002:1–15.

6. American Academy of Pediatric Dentistry. Guideline on periodicity of examination, preventive dental services, anticipatory guidance/counseling, and oral treatments for infant, children, and adolescents. *Pediatr Dent*. 2013;35(6):114–121.

7. McDonald RE, Avery DR, Dean JA. *Dentistry for the Child and Adolescent*. 9th ed. Maryland Heights, MO: Mosby Elsevier; 2011:10–12, 86–90, 95–100, 116–117, 127–128, 132,136,156, 250, 369.

8. Overby KJ. Pediatric health supervision. In: Rudolph AM, Kamei RK, Overby KJ, eds. *Rudolph's Fundamentals of Pediatrics*. 3rd ed. New York, NY: McGraw-Hill; 2002:1–69.

9. Goldson E, Reynolds A. Child development and behavior. In: Hay WW, Hayward AR, Levin MJ, et al., eds. *Current Pediatric Diagnosis and Treatment*. 19th ed. New York, NY: McGraw-Hill; 2008:66–83.

10. American Academy of Pediatric Dentistry. Guideline on fluoride therapy. *Pediatr Dent*. 2013;35(6):167–170.

11. Wong M, Glenny AM, Tsang BLE, et al. Cochrane review: topical fluoride as a cause of dental fluorosis in children. *Evid Based Child Health: A Cochrane Rev J*. 2011;6(2):388–439.

12. DenBesten P, Li W. Chronic fluoride toxicity: dental fluorosis. Fluoride and the oral environment. *Monogr Oral Sci*. 2011;22:81–96.

13. American Academy of Pediatric Dentistry. Policy on third-party reimbursement of fees related to dental sealants. *Pediatr Dent*. 2013;35(6);95–96.

14. Beauchamp J, Caufield PW, Crall JJ, et al. Evidence-based clinical recommendations for the use of pit-and-fissure sealants. *JADA*. 2008;139(3);257–268.

15. American Academy of Pediatric Dentistry. Policy on the use of xylitol in caries prevention. *Pediatr Dent*. 2013;35(6);45–47.

16. American Academy of Pediatric Dentistry. Guideline on xylitol use in caries prevention. *Pediatr Dent*. 2013;35(6):171–174.

17. Ramos-Gomez FJ, Crall J, Gansky SA, et al. Caries risk assessment appropriate for the age 1 visit (infants and toddlers). *J Calif Dent Assoc*. 2007;35(10):687–702.

18. Green M, Palfrey JS, ed. *Bright Futures: Guidelines for Health Supervision of Infants, Children, and Adolescents*. 2nd ed. Arlington, VA: National Center for Education in Maternal and Child Health; 2002:1–15.

19. American Academy of Pediatric Dentistry. Guideline on adolescent oral health care. *Pediatr Dent*. 2013;35(6):142–149.

20. McDonald RE, Avery DR, Dean JA. *Dentistry for the Child and Adolescent*. 9th ed. Maryland Heights, MO: Mosby Elsevier; 2011:10.

21. McDonald RE, Avery DR, Dean JA. *Dentistry for the Child and Adolescent*. 9th ed. Maryland Heights, MO: Mosby Elsevier; 2011:397.

22. Albandar JM, Rams TE. Risk factors for periodontitis in children and young persons. *Periodontology 2000*. 2002;29(1):207–222.

23. American Academy of Pediatric Dentistry. Policy on early childhood caries (ECC): classifications, consequences, and preventive strategies. *Pediatr Dent*. 2013;35(6):50–52.

24. Peretz B, Ram D, Azo E, et al. Preschool caries as an indicator of future caries: a longitudinal study. *Pediatr Dent*. 2003;25(2):114–118.

25. Foster T, Perinpanayagam H, Pfaffenbach A, et al. Recurrence of early childhood caries after comprehensive treatment with general anesthesia and follow-up. *J Dent Child*. 2006;73(1):25–30.

26. National Center for Chronic Disease Prevention and Health Promotion. *Children & Adults; Children's Oral Health*. Atlanta, GA: Centers for Disease Control and Prevention; Division of Oral Health.

27. National Center for Chronic Disease Prevention and Health Promotion. *Children & Adults; Oral Health Strategic Plan for 2011–2014; IV. Goals: Focusing Efforts of the Oral Health Program*. Atlanta, GA: Centers for Disease Control and Prevention; Division of Oral Health. http://www.cdc.gov/OralHealth/strategic_planning/plan4.htm. Accessed April 26, 2014.

28. Berkowitz RJ. Mutans streptococci: acquisition and transmission. *Pediatr Dent*. 2006;28(2):106–109.

29. Wan AK, Seow WK, Purdie DM, et al. Oral colonization of Streptococcus mutans in six-month-old predentate infants. *J Dent Res*. 2001;90(12):2060–2065.

30. Parisotto TM, Steiner-Oliveira C, Silva CM, et al. Early childhood caries and mutans streptococci: a systematic review. *Oral Health Prev Dent*. 2010;8(1):59–70.

31. California Dental Association Foundation. Oral health during pregnancy and early childhood: evidence-based guideline for health professional. *J Calif Dent Assoc*. 2010;38(6):391–426.

32. John Hopkins Medicine Health Library. *School-Aged Child Nutrition*. Baltimore, MD: John Hopkins Medicine Health

Library. http://www.hopkinsmedicine.org/healthlibrary/conditions/pediatrics/school-aged_child_nutrition_90,P02280/. Accessed April 26, 2014.

33. Get it done in year one. mychildrensteeth.org Website. Chicago, IL: American Academy of Pediatric Dentists; Oral Health Campaigns. 2012–2014. http://www.aapd.org/assets/2/7/GetItDoneInYearOne.pdf. Accessed October 17, 2013.

34. Wright JT, Hanson N, Ristic H, et al. Fluoride toothpaste efficacy and safety in children younger than 6 years. *JADA*. 2014;145(2):182–189.

35. American Academy of Pediatric Dentistry. Management of the developing dentition and occlusion in pediatric dentistry. *Pediatr Dent*. 2013;35(6):243–255.

36. American Academy of Pediatric Dentistry. Guidelines on oral and dental aspects of child abuse and neglect. *Pediatr Dent*. 2013;35(6):163–166.

ENHANCE YOUR UNDERSTANDING

thePoint® DIGITAL CONNECTIONS
(see the inside front cover for access information)
- **Audio glossary**
- **Quiz bank**

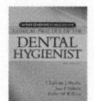

SUPPORT FOR LEARNING
(available separately; visit lww.com)
- *Active Learning Workbook for Clinical Practice of the Dental Hygienist, 12th Edition*

prepU INDIVIDUALIZED REVIEW
(available separately; visit lww.com)
- **Adaptive quizzing with *prepU for Wilkins' Clinical Practice of the Dental Hygienist***

51

The Patient with a Cleft Lip and/or Palate

Sara L. Beres, RDH, MSDH

CHAPTER OUTLINE

LEARNING OBJECTIVES

After studying this chapter, the student will be able to:

1. Describe the types of cleft lip and palate that result from developmental disturbances.

2. Identify and describe the role of the professionals on the interdisciplinary team for the treatment of a patient with cleft lip and/or palate.

3. Identify the oral characteristics of a patient with cleft lip and/or palate may experience.

4. Explain how to adapt the dental hygiene appointment sequence for a patient with cleft lip and/or palate.

Cleft lip and/or palate are the most common of the many types of congenital craniofacial anomalies.[1] Cleft lip and/or palate may occur as isolated conditions, but frequently occur as part of a syndrome with other birth defects.

▶ The prevalence varies between 1 and 2 per 1,000 births, but this ratio varies based on geographic and ethnic distribution.[1]

▶ Cleft lip occurs more frequently in males, while cleft palate occurs more frequently in females.[1]

▶ The person with a cleft lip and/or palate can be dentally dysfunctional unless extensive habilitative care and supervision from birth is available.

▶ An interdisciplinary team of medical and dental specialists is required to provide adequate treatment and family counseling as needed.[1]

▶ The dental hygienist can be a member of the team with responsibilities to coordinate dental and periodontal care.

▶ Speaking ability and appearance are among the first factors considered when the long-range treatment program is planned because the objective is to help the patient lead a normal life.

▶ Dental personnel need to maintain a current list of the health agencies, clinics, and other community resources where the patient and family can obtain assistance for the various phases of treatment and habilitation.

▶ Key words relating to cleft lip and/or palate are defined in Box 51-1.

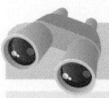

BOX 51-1   KEY WORDS: Cleft Lip and/or Palate

Autograft: graft transferred from one part of the patient's body to another part.

Bifid uvula: cleft of the uvula of the soft palate that divides the uvula into two parts (Figure 51-1, Class 2).

Cheiloplasty: surgical repair of a lip defect.

Cheilorhinoplasty: plastic surgery of nose and lip.

Cleft lip: a unilateral or bilateral congenital fissure of the upper lip, usually lateral to the midline; can extend into one nostril or both and may involve the alveolar process; caused by defect in the fusion of the maxillary and globular processes.

Cleft palate: a congenital fissure of the palate caused by failure of the palatal shelves to fuse; may extend to connect with unilateral or bilateral cleft lip.

Congenital: present at and existing from the time of birth.

Craniofacial: pertaining to the cranium, the part of the skull that encloses the brain, and the face.

Dentally dysfunctional: abnormal functioning of dental structures.

Graft: tissue that is transplanted and expected to become a part of the host tissue.

Haberman feeder: specialty bottle used for infants with cleft palate.

Heredity: genetic transmission of traits from parents to offspring; the hereditary material, chromosomes, is contained within the ovum and the sperm (23 chromosomes each), which unite when the sperm penetrates the ovum.

Mandibular distraction: method used to increase the length of a micrognathic mandible.

Multifactorial: pertaining to, or arising through the action of, many factors.

Nasoalveolar molding technique (NAM): treatment used for unilateral and bilateral cleft palate to reduce the severity of the cleft in the maxillary gingiva or alveolar ridges and to reduce the deformity of the nose.

Obturator: a prosthesis designed to close a congenital or an acquired opening, such as a cleft of the hard palate.

Orthognathic surgery: surgical repositioning of all or parts of the maxilla or mandible.

Orthopedics: branch of surgery dealing with the preservation and restoration of function of the skeletal system, its articulations, and associated structures.

Palatoplasty: plastic reconstruction of the palate.

Premaxilla: anterior part of maxilla that contains the incisor teeth; bilateral cleft lips separate the premaxilla from its normal fusion with the entire maxilla.

Prosthesis: an artificial replacement of an absent part of the human body; a therapeutic device to improve or alter function.

Rehabilitation: the process of restoring a person's ability to live and work as normally as possible after a disabling injury or illness; aims to help the individual to achieve maximum possible physical and psychologic fitness and to regain ability to carry out personal care.

  Habilitation: the same goals and objectives as rehabilitation, but for a person with acquired disability for whom the ability to achieve maximum physical and psychologic fitness is acquired for the first time.

Rhinoplasty: plastic surgery of nose.

Speech aid prosthesis: a prosthetic device with a posterior section to assist with palatopharyngeal closure; also called bulb, speech bulb, or prosthetic speech appliance.

  Pediatric speech aid prosthesis: a temporary or interim prosthesis used to close a defect in the hard and/or soft palate; may replace tissue lost as a result of developmental or surgical alterations; necessary for intelligible speech.

  Adult speech aid prosthesis: a definitive prosthesis to improve speech by obturating (sealing off) a palatal cleft or occasionally assisting an incompetent soft palate.

Syndrome: a combination of symptoms either resulting from a single cause or occurring so commonly together as to constitute a distinct clinical picture.

Tracheostomy: creation of an opening into the trachea through the neck, with insertion of an indwelling tube to facilitate passage of air or evacuation of secretions.

Velopharyngeal insufficiency: anatomic or functional deficiency in the soft palate or the muscle affecting closure of the opening between mouth and nose in speech; results in a nasal speech quality.

Velum: covering structure or veil.

  Velum palatinum: soft palate.

CLASSIFICATION OF CLEFTS

▶ Classification is based on disturbances in the embryologic formation of the lip and palate as they develop from the premaxillary region toward the uvula in a definite pattern.

▶ Interference with normal development of the palate may occur at one stage level of the embryo and the normal pattern may be re-established at a later stage.

▶ The seven classes are illustrated in Figure 51-1. All degrees are found, from an insignificant notch in the mucous membrane of the lip or uvula, which produces no functional disability, to the complete cleft defined by Class 6 of this classification.

ETIOLOGY

I. Embryology[2]

▶ Cleft lip and palate represent a failure of normal fusion of embryonic processes during development in the first trimester of pregnancy.

▶ Figure 51-2 shows the locations of the globular process and the right and left maxillary processes.

▶ With normal fusion, no cleft of the lip results.

▶ Fusion begins in the premaxillary region and continues backward toward the uvula.

▶ Formation of the lip:
  • Occurs between the 4th and 8th week in utero.
  • A cleft lip becomes apparent by the end of the second month in utero.

▶ Development of the palate
  • Takes place during the 6th–12th week.
  • A cleft palate is evident by the end of the third month.

II. Risk Factors

▶ Multifactorial genetic and environmental factors can be significant. Rarely, a single factor can be found as the specific cause.[3]

▶ Highest rates in Asians and Native Americans (1 in 500 births).

▶ Early in the first trimester is the significant time for influences due to the environmental factors including:
  • Use of tobacco.[4–6]
  • Alcohol consumption.[3,7]
  • Teratogenic agents: phenytoin, vitamin A (isotretinoin), corticosteroids, drugs of abuse (Table 49-1, Chapter 49).
  • Maternal age >40 years.[2]
  • Inadequate diet: vitamins, especially folic acid deficiency.
  • Lack of adequate prenatal care and instruction is a risk factor that has influence on all the environmental factors.

GENERAL PHYSICAL CHARACTERISTICS

I. Other Congenital Anomalies

▶ Incidence of multiple congenital anomalies is high with cleft lip and/or palate.

▶ In more than 300 disorders, cleft lip, cleft palate, or both represent one feature of a syndrome.[8]

II. Facial Deformities

Facial deformities may include (see Figure 51-3A and B):

▶ Depression of the nostril on the side with the cleft lip.

▶ Deficiency of upper lip, which may be short or retroposed.

▶ Overprominent lower lip.

III. Infections

▶ Predisposition to upper respiratory and middle ear infections is common.

IV. Airway and Breathing

▶ Craniofacial anomalies of the nose and throat area predispose the child with a cleft palate to airway obstruction and breathing problems.[9]

▶ Early treatment intervention is necessary for the infant to cope with feeding problems.

▶ Speech involves breathing and swallowing.

V. Speech[1]

▶ Patients with cleft lip and/or cleft palate have difficulty making certain sounds and may produce nasal tones.

▶ Anatomic structure, airway and breathing problems, and hearing difficulties all contribute to speech problems.

VI. Hearing Loss

▶ The incidence of hearing loss is significantly higher in individuals with cleft palate than in the noncleft population.

ORAL CHARACTERISTICS

I. Tooth Development

▶ Disturbances in the normal development of the tooth buds occur more frequently in patients with clefts than in the general population.

▶ There is a higher incidence of missing and supernumerary teeth, as well as of abnormalities of tooth form.[10]

▶ Common missing teeth include:
  • Maxillary lateral incisors
  • Maxillary premolars

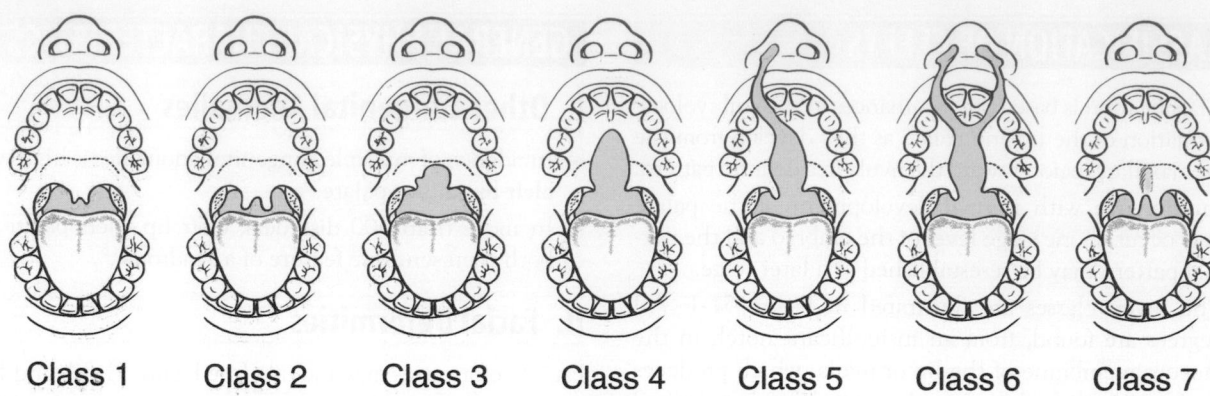

Class 1   Class 2   Class 3   Class 4   Class 5   Class 6   Class 7

FIGURE 51-1 Classification of Cleft Lip and Cleft Palate. Class 1: Cleft of the tip of the uvula; Class 2: cleft of the uvula (bifid uvula); Class 3: cleft of the soft palate; Class 4: cleft of the soft and hard palates; Class 5: cleft of the soft and hard palates that continues through the alveolar ridge on one side of the premaxilla; usually associated with cleft lip of the same side; Class 6: cleft of the soft and hard palates that continues through the alveolar ridge on both sides, leaving a free premaxilla; usually associated with bilateral cleft lip; Class 7: submucous cleft in which the muscle union is imperfect across the soft palate. The palate is short, the uvula is often bifid, a groove is situated at the midline of the soft palate, and the closure to the pharynx is incompetent.

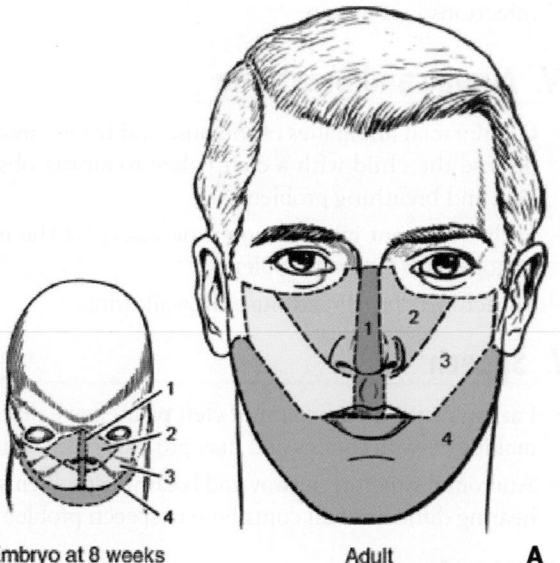

B Embryo at 8 weeks   Adult   **A**

FIGURE 51-2 Developmental Processes of the Face. A: The nose, eyes, and mouth form between the 4th and 6th weeks of development. **B:** Development of the face illustrating derivatives of embryologic development. (1) Median nasal process; (2) lateral nasal process; (3) maxillary process; (4) mandibular process. Clefts can occur at the midline of the maxillary and/or the mandibular process if fusion fails during development. (Reprinted from Lippincott Williams & Wilkins' Comprehensive Dental Assisting. Philadelphia: Wolters Kluwer Health/Lippincott Williams & Wilkins; 2011.)

- Mandibular second premolars
- Usually correspond to the side of the mouth that has the cleft.[10,11]

II. Malocclusion

▶ A high percentage of patients with cleft lip and palate require orthodontic care.[1]

▶ Orthodontic treatment may be required after each stage of surgical treatment for cleft palate.

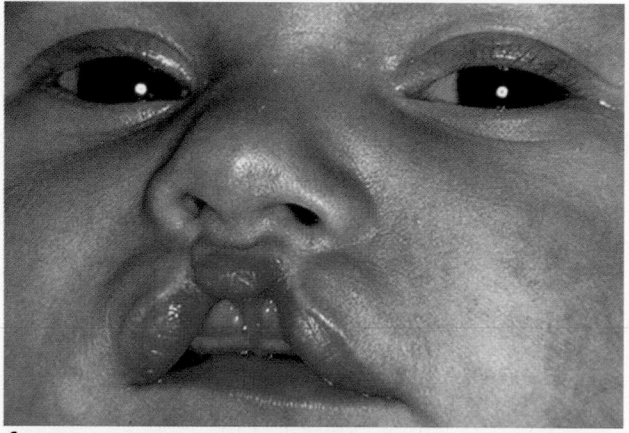

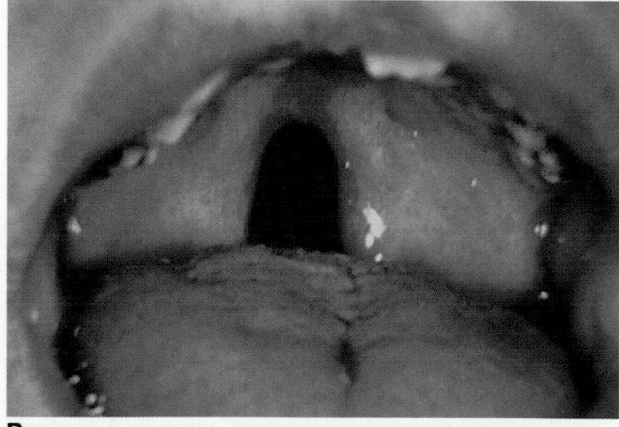

B

FIGURE 51-3 A: Cleft Lip. **B:** Cleft Palate. (Reprinted from Lippincott Williams & Wilkins' Comprehensive Dental Assisting. Philadelphia: Wolters Kluwer Health/Lippincott Williams & Wilkins; 2011.)

III. Open Palate

▶ Before surgical correction, an open palate provides direct communication with the nasal cavity.

- A cleft lip makes it more difficult for a child to suck on a nipple. Special nipples and bottles have been designed to make feeding easier.
- A cleft palate may cause formula or breast milk to pass into the nasal cavity. A prosthetic palatal obturator may be constructed to aid during drinking and eating.

IV. Muscle Coordination

- A lack of coordinated movements of lips, tongue, cheeks, floor of mouth, and throat may exist.
- Compensatory habits may be formed by the patient in the attempt to produce normal sounds while speaking.

V. Periodontal Tissues

- Dental biofilm accumulation is influenced by the irregularly positioned teeth, inability to keep lips closed, mouth breathing, and the difficulties in accomplishing adequate personal oral care, especially around the cleft areas.
- Patients with unilateral and bilateral cleft lip, palate, and alveolus show extensive periodontal lesions in the maxillary anterior region, in comparison to the general population.[12]
- Periodontal tissue loss in later years is greatest at the cleft sites.[13]

VI. Dental Caries

- Children with a cleft lip and/or palate are at higher risk for dental caries.[14,15]
- Risk factors relating to malpositioned teeth, problems of mastication, diet selection, and dental biofilm retention are intensified for the person with a cleft lip and/or palate.
- Feeding difficulties of infants and toddlers have contributed to early childhood caries also known as ECC (see Chapter 50 and Table 23-1 in Chapter 23).

TREATMENT

- Treatment is coordinated by a team of specialists and is based on the patient's progress at each age period.[1]
- Members of the interprofessional patient care team are listed in Box 51-2.
  - The team is responsible for providing integrated case management. Quality and continuity of care are essential.[17]
- Need for attention to gingival health throughout the years of treatment cannot be overemphasized.

I. Cleft Lip

- Surgical union of the cleft lip is made at 2–3 months of age. A general well-known rule for scheduling surgery: when the child is approximately 10 weeks of age,

weighs 10 pounds, and has achieved a serum hemoglobin of 10 mg/mL.[1]
- The infant's general health is a determining factor.

A. Purposes for Early Treatment

- Aid in feeding.
- Encourage development of the premaxilla.
- Help partial closure of the palatal cleft.
- Assist families in adjusting to the birth of a child with cleft lip and/or palate.

B. Orthodontics and Dentofacial Orthopedics

- In preparation for cleft closure, orthodontic and orthopedic treatment may be needed to reduce the protrusion and stabilize the premaxilla.[10]

II. Cleft Palate

- Primary surgery to close the palate is usually undertaken by age 18 months or earlier when possible.[17]
- The combined efforts of many specialists are required as listed in Box 51-2.

A. Goals for Treatment

- Produce anatomic closure.
- Maximize maxillary growth and development.
- Achieve normal function, particularly normal speech.
- Relieve problems of airway and breathing.
- Establish good dental esthetics and functional occlusion.

B. Types of Secondary Surgical Procedures (Box 51-3)

- Secondary surgical care refers to additional surgical procedures after primary closure of the clefts.
- Secondary surgery may involve the lips, nose, palate, and jaws.
- Objectives are to improve function for coherent communication, improve appearance, or both.
- Treatment plans are individualized to fit the needs of the patient.
- Team evaluations on a periodic basis determine the effects of treatment to date and outline the next phase.

C. Use of Bone Grafting[16]

- Bone grafting is used to repair residual alveolar and hard palate clefts.
  1. *Alveolar graft*
     - Placed before eruption of maxillary teeth at the cleft site.
     - Creates a normal architecture through which the teeth can erupt. A need for future prosthetic replacement of missing teeth is reduced.

- Support is provided for teeth adjacent to the cleft areas.
2. *Hard palate graft*
- Provides closure of oronasal fistulae.
- Helps to relieve a compromised airway.
3. *Sources for autogenous bone for graft*
- Rib, iliac crest, skull, mandible, or bone morphogenic proteins.

D. Use of Osseointegrated Implant

After bone grafting, implants can be used to replace individual teeth.

▶ Implants also provide support for a complete prosthesis.

III. Prosthodontics

A. Types of Appliances[18]

▶ *Obturator*: A removable prosthesis may be designed to provide closure of the palatal opening (Figure 51-4).
▶ *Speech aid prosthesis*: A removable appliance to complete the palatopharyngeal valving required for speech.

B. Purposes and Functions of a Prosthesis[18]

The prosthesis may be designed to accomplish one or all of the following:

▶ Closure of the palate.
▶ Replacement of missing teeth.
▶ Scaffolding to fill out the upper lip.
▶ Masticatory function.
▶ Restoration of vertical dimension.
▶ Postorthodontic retainer.

IV. Orthodontics

▶ Treatment may be initiated as early as 3 years of age, depending on dentofacial development.
▶ Each stage of surgery and treatment may require orthodontic intervention and follow-up.[1]
▶ Final formal orthodontic treatment for realigning the teeth and gaining a functional occlusion may start during the mixed dentition years or later.[1]
▶ During the orthodontic treatment period, an intensive program for dental caries prevention and gingival health is maintained.

V. Speech Therapy[1]

▶ Training is started with very young children.
▶ Therapy is essential following surgical or prosthodontic treatment.

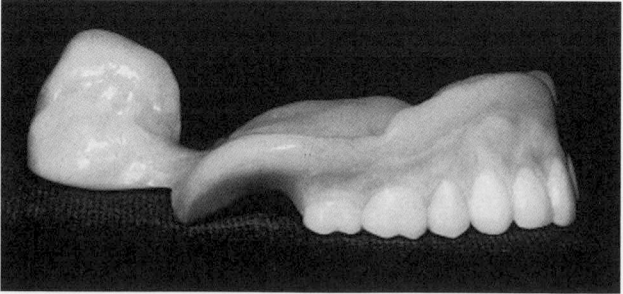

FIGURE 51-4 Maxillary Obturator Prosthesis with Denture. (Reprinted from Thorne C, Bartlett S, Beasley R, Aston S, Gurtner G, Spear S. Grabb and Smith's Plastic Surgery. Philadelphia: Wolters Kluwer Health/Lippincott Williams & Wilkins; 2006.)

VI. Restorative Dentistry

▶ Dental hygienists practicing with a pediatric dentist or general dentist are involved in direct patient care.

▶ A major problem can be dental caries, leading to tooth loss. With missing teeth, major difficulties arise related to all phases of treatment.

▶ Preservation of primary teeth has special significance.

DENTAL HYGIENE CARE

▶ Preventive measures for the preservation of the teeth and their supporting structures are essential to the success of the special care needed for the habilitation of the patient with a cleft lip and/or palate.

▶ Each phase of dental hygiene care and instruction takes on even greater significance in light of the magnified problems of the patient with a cleft lip and/or palate.

▶ Every attempt is made to avoid the need to remove teeth, especially around the cleft area. In an area already weakened by lack of bone, removal of teeth creates further complications.

▶ The presence of teeth encourages optimum arch growth.

I. Parental Counseling: Anticipatory Guidance

▶ Understanding the value of preventive procedures by the patient and the parents is accomplished through explanation and instruction.

▶ When the patient has not had specialized care, the dental team has a responsibility to arrange referral to an available agency, clinic, or private practice specialist.

▶ *Anticipatory guidance:* Items from Table 49-3 in Chapter 49 and Table 50-7 in Chapter 50 pertain to the parents and infant with a cleft lip and/or palate.

▶ Primary concerns are daily dental biofilm removal and prevention of early childhood dental caries.

II. Objectives for Appointment Planning

▶ Frequent appointments, scheduled every 3 or 4 months, are usually needed during the maintenance phase of the patient's care.

▶ *Objectives include* the following:
- To review dental biofilm control measures.
- To provide encouragement for the patient to maintain the health of the supporting structures and cleanliness of the removable prostheses (Chapter 32).
- To remove all calculus and biofilm as a supplement to the patient's personal daily care procedures.
- To supervise a dental caries prevention program for both primary and permanent dentitions with fluorides (Chapter 36) and sealants (Chapter 37).

III. Appointment Considerations

A. Patient Apprehension and Self-esteem

▶ A patient who has been seen often in hospital clinics may become very apprehensive about dental and dental hygiene care.

▶ Lower self-esteem and difficulties in social interaction have also been noted with a patient with cleft lip and/or palate.[19]

B. Communication

▶ *Speech:* Speech may be difficult to understand. With repeated contact, understanding can be developed. Referral for speech assessment, if not already done, is recommended.

▶ *Hearing:* Depending on the severity of hearing loss, the approach is similar to that for speech difficulties. Suggestions for care of patients with hearing problems are described in Chapter 60.

C. Provide Motivation

▶ Use of a motivational interviewing approach can help patients gain an positive attitude toward oral health (see Chapter 26).

IV. Patient Instruction

A. Personal Oral Care Procedures

▶ For a small child, the caretakers may be afraid of damaging the deformed areas or hurting the child if cleaning methods are employed.

▶ An empathetic approach and plan for continued instruction over a long period is needed.
- *Personal daily care:* Select toothbrush, brushing method, and auxiliary aids according to the individual needs.
- *Fluoride:* Instigate daily self-application of fluoride by way of fluoride dentifrice, and diet supplements for a young child in a nonfluoridated community (Table 36-1, Chapter 36).
- *Rinsing instruction:* Only older children (at least age 6 years, and evaluated for ability to rinse without swallowing) are given mouthrinsing for therapy. Instruction in how to rinse is needed when this procedure is new to the patient (Box 30-4, Chapter 30).
- *Prosthesis or speech aid:* Halitosis may be a problem because mucus secreted in the nasal cavity, as well as biofilm, accumulates on the prosthesis and must be thoroughly cleaned on a regular basis (see Chapter 32).

B. Diet

▶ *Need for a varied diet:* Include adequate proportions of all essential food groups (Figure 35-1 MyPlate, Chapter 35).

▶ *Need for prevention of dental caries:* Limit cariogenic foods, particularly for between-meal snacks.

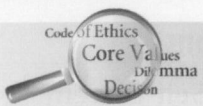

EVERYDAY ETHICS

Leona, a dental hygienist, has been delivering dental hygiene care and providing oral health education for Brian's family since they moved to her town right after he was born. Brian, now 8 years old, was born with a bilateral clefting of the lip with partial involvement of the palate. He recently had another surgical procedure completed on his upper lip. Brian's mother Joyce has been very impressed by the extra time that Leona has taken to research and learn about oral clefting. Joyce has depended on the guidance Leona has provided to help the family anticipate and meet Brian's oral health needs before, during, and after each of his multiple surgeries.

Joyce asks Leona to sign up as a hospital volunteer and share her expertise with parents of children who are receiving surgical care for orofacial clefts. Leona hesitates to agree because she really is not sure she has the time to prepare an educational presentation right now. In addition, she is concerned about how much of her limited free time this volunteer position will take.

Questions for Consideration

1. Consider the Basic Beliefs and Fundamental Principles identified in the ADHA Code of Ethics (Appendix I). Does Leona have an ethical responsibility to share her professional expertise as a volunteer in her community? Why or why not?

2. Are there elements in the ADHA Code of Ethics that help support Lorna's decision if she decides *not* to volunteer? Explain.

3. What elements in the Canadian (CDHA), National (NDHA), or International (IFDH) Codes of Ethics (Appendices II, III, and IV) encourage community volunteerism?

C. Smoking Cessation

▶ The patient or family member who smokes or uses any form of smokeless tobacco is informed about the effects of tobacco on all the oral tissues.

▶ Emphasis on the potential damage to the periodontal tissues can have special significance for the patient with a cleft palate.

▶ Offer assistance with a smoking cessation program.

V. Dental Hygiene Care Related to Oral Surgery

A. Presurgery (Chapter 55)

▶ Objectives have particular significance because the patient with a cleft palate is unusually susceptible to infections of the upper respiratory area and middle ear.

▶ Every precaution is taken to prevent complications.

B. Postsurgery Personal Oral Care

▶ After each feeding (liquid diet for several days, soft diet for the next week), the mouth is rinsed carefully.

▶ Oral care is needed and accomplished with great care, usually by the parent or caregiver, to avoid damage to the healing suture lines.

▶ In selected cases, a toothbrush with suction attachment may be useful (Figure 58-4 in Chapter 58).

DOCUMENTATION

The documentation of care that the patient with cleft lip or palate receives over the individual's lifetime is imperative. Documentation includes the following:

▶ Description of location, classification, and extent of cleft.

▶ History and status of surgical interventions.

▶ Missing teeth and related recommendations for self-care regimens.

▶ Description of prosthetic appliances and recommendations for daily care regimens.

▶ A documentation example for a patient appointment is found in Box 51-4.

BOX 51-4
Example Documentation: Patient with Cleft Lip and/or Palate

S –A 6-year-old patient presented for routine maintenance appointment. Reviewed medical history: patient had a rhinoplasty completed 6 months ago. All vital signs are normal.

O –Extraoral examination: scar on right maxillary lip from cleft lip surgery at age 3 months. Intraoral examination: Missing #D and wears obturator, which was removed during examination. Plaque free score: 50% primarily interproximally.

A –Unilateral right Class 5 cleft lip and palate.

P –Disclosed teeth with disclosing solution to show biofilm, demonstrated modified bass toothbrushing technique and "C" flossing. Showed patient and his mother how to use an interdental brush to clean between # E and #C. A denture brush was provided and instructions for care of the obturator were reviewed. Hand scaled all four quads and applied 5% sodium fluoride varnish. Gave postoperative instructions. Patient tolerated appointment well. Three-month continuing care appointment scheduled.

Signed _____, RDH

Date _____

Factors To Teach The Patient

▷ Parental anticipatory guidance (Tables 49-3 and 50-7).
▷ Biofilm removal methods for cleft areas.
▷ Prevention of mouth odors by proper cleaning of tongue and removable appliances.
▷ Necessity for regular dental hygiene appointments to maintain freedom from infection.
▷ Resources with addresses for team treatment clinics specializing in craniofacial developmental defects.

REFERENCES

1. Robin NH, Baty H, Franklin J, et al. The multidisciplinary evaluation and management of cleft lip and palate. *South Med J.* 2006;99(10):1111–1120.
2. Shkoukani MA, Chen M, Vong A. Cleft lip—a comprehensive review. *Front Pediatr.* 2013;1:53.
3. Slavkin HC. Meeting the challenges of craniofacial-oral-dental birth defects. *J Am Dent Assoc.* 1996;127(5):681–682.
4. Shaw GM, Wasserman CR, Lammer EJ, et al. Orofacial clefts, parental cigarette smoking, and transforming growth factor-alpha gene variants. *Am J Hum Genet.* 1996;58(3):551–561.
5. Little J, Cardy A, Arslan MT, et al. Smoking and orofacial clefts: a United Kingdom-based case-control study. *Cleft Palate Craniofac J.* 2004;41(4):381–386.
6. Källén K. Maternal smoking and orofacial clefts. *Cleft Palate Craniofac J.* 1997;34(1):11–16.
7. Lorente C, Cordier S, Goujard J, et al. Tobacco and alcohol use during pregnancy and risk of oral clefts. Occupational Exposure and Congenital Malformation Working Group. *Am J Public Health.* 2000;90(3):415–419.
8. Wyszynski DF, Sárközi A, Czeizel AE. Oral clefts with associated anomalies: methodological issues. *Cleft Palate Craniofac J.* 2006;43(1):1–6.
9. Perkins JA, Sie KC, Milczuk H, et al. Airway management in children with craniofacial anomalies. *Cleft Palate Craniofac J.* 1997;34(2):135–140.
10. Menezes R, Vieira AR. Dental anomalies as part of the cleft spectrum. *Cleft Palate Craniofac J.* 2008;45(4):414–419.
11. Bartzela TN, Carels CE, Bronkhorst EM, et al. Tooth agenesis patterns in bilateral cleft lip and palate. *Eur J Oral Sci.* 2010;118(1):47–52.
12. Gaggl A, Schultes G, Kärcher H, et al. Periodontal disease in patients with cleft palate and patients with unilateral and bilateral clefts of lip, palate, and alveolus. *J Periodontol.* 1999;70(2):171–178.
13. Brägger U, Schürch E Jr, Salvi G, et al. Periodontal conditions in adult patients with cleft lip, alveolus, and palate. *Cleft Palate Craniofac J.* 1992;29(2):179–185.
14. Bokhout B, Hofman FX, van Limbeek J, et al. Incidence of dental caries in the primary dentition in children with a cleft lip and/or palate. *Caries Res.* 1997;31(1):8–12.
15. Stec-Slonicz M, Szczeparínska J, Hirschfelder U. Comparison of caries prevalence in two populations of cleft patients. *Cleft Palate Craniofac J.* 2007;44(5):532–537.
16. Guo, J, Zhang Q, Zou S, et al. Secondary bone grafting for alveolar cleft in children with cleft lip or cleft lip and palate. *Cochrane Collab.* 2008; 2(4): 1–8.
17. American Cleft Palate-Craniofacial Association. *Parameters for Evaluation and Treatment of Patients with Cleft Lip/Palate or Other Craniofacial Anomalies.* Rev. ed. Chapel Hill, NC: American Cleft Palate-Craniofacial Association; 2009:1–34. http://www.acpa-cpf.org/teamcare/Parameters Rev.2009.pdf. Accessed December 20, 2010.
18. Reisberg DJ. Dental and prosthodontic care for patients with cleft or craniofacial conditions. *Cleft Palate Craniofac J.* 2000;37(6):534–537.
19. Sousa AD, Devare S, Ghanshani J. Psychological issues in cleft lip and cleft palate. *J Indian Assoc Pediatr Surg.* 2009; 14(2):55–58.

ENHANCE YOUR UNDERSTANDING

thePoint® DIGITAL CONNECTIONS
(see the inside front cover for access information)
• **Audio glossary**
• **Quiz bank**

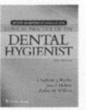

SUPPORT FOR LEARNING
(available separately; visit lww.com)
• *Active Learning Workbook for Clinical Practice of the Dental Hygienist, 12th Edition*

prepU INDIVIDUALIZED REVIEW
(available separately; visit lww.com)
• **Adaptive quizzing with *prepU for Wilkins' Clinical Practice of the Dental Hygienist***

52

The Patient with an Endocrine Disorder or Hormonal Change

Katherine Yee, RDH, MPH
Patricia A. Cohen, RDH, BS, MS

CHAPTER OUTLINE

LEARNING OBJECTIVES

After studying this chapter, the student will be able to:

1. Identify the major endocrine glands and describe the functions of each.

2. Explain signs, symptoms, and potential oral manifestations of each endocrine gland disorder.

3. Describe hormonal effects and oral health risk factors commonly associated with puberty, menses, contraceptives, and menopause.

OVERVIEW OF THE ENDOCRINE SYSTEM

The endocrine glands secrete substances directly into the blood or lymph system. They secrete highly specialized substances (hormones) that, with the nervous system, maintain body homeostasis. Influences of the endocrine system on oral health and patient care are discussed in this chapter. Key words are defined in Box 52-1.

I. Glands of the Endocrine System

▶ The major endocrine glands, shown in Figure 52-1, are the pineal, hypothalamus, pituitary, thyroid, parathyroids, thymus, pancreas, adrenals, and gonads (ovaries and testes).

▶ The anterior pituitary is called the master gland because it regulates the output of hormones by other glands.

▶ In turn, the pituitary itself is regulated by the hormones produced by the other endocrine glands.

▶ The endocrine glands and the hormones produced by each are listed in Table 52-1.

II. Hormones and Their Functions[1]

▶ Hormones affect a number of major functions and are transported by the blood or lymph.

▶ Hormones may act directly on body cells or indirectly to control the hormones of other glands.

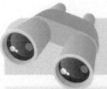

BOX 52-1   KEY WORDS: Endocrine Disorders and Hormonal Change

Acne vulgaris: a chronic skin disorder with increased production of oil from the sebaceous glands; may be inflammatory or noninflammatory; appears on the face, back, and chest.

Adolescence: the period extending from the time the secondary sex characteristics appear to the end of somatic growth, when the individual is mature.

Amenorrhea: absence of spontaneous menstrual periods in a female.

Circumpubertal: on or around the age of puberty.

Dysmenorrhea: difficult and painful menstruation.

Dysphoria: feeling unwell or unhappy, depressed feeling.

Endocrine: pertaining to secretion of a substance directly into blood or lymph rather than into a duct; the opposite of exocrine.

Endometrium: the lining of the uterus.

Endometriosis: a condition of the endometrium that causes pelvic pain.

Epinephrine: a catecholamine hormone that causes the "fight-or-flight" response to physical or emotional stress; increased secretion produces marked dilation of bronchioles and increased blood pressure, blood glucose level, and heart rate.

Gland: organ or structure that secretes or execrates substances.

Gonad: sex gland in which reproductive cells form.

Goiter: enlargement of the thyroid gland, may indicate Graves' disease or Hashimoto's thyroiditis.

Gynecologist: physician who specializes in conditions specific to women, particularly of the genital tract, female endocrinology, and reproductive physiology.

Homeostasis: the tendency of biologic systems to maintain constant internal stability while continually adjusting to external changes.

Hormone: a chemical product of an organ or of certain cells within the organ that has a specific regulatory effect upon cells elsewhere in the body.

Hormone replacement therapy: prescription of a purified or synthetic hormone to correct or prevent undesirable symptoms of menopause.

Hyperkalemia: a higher than normal level of potassium in the bloodstream.

Hypernatremia: elevated sodium level in the bloodstream.

Hypokalemia: a lower than normal level of potassium in the bloodstream.

Libido: sexual urge or desire.

Macrocephaly: head circumference which is greater than 2 standard deviations larger than the average for a given age and sex.

Macrognatia: enlargement or elongation of the jaw.

Mastalgia: fullness, soreness, or pain in the breast.

Maturity: state of complete growth.

Menarche: onset of menstruation; may occur from ages 9 to 17 years.

Menopause: the time of life when a woman ceases menstruation; defined as a period of 12 months of amenorrhea in a woman over 45 years of age.

Menses: menstruation.

Myxedema: a disease caused by decreased activity of the thyroid gland characterized by dry skin, swellings around the lips and nose.

> **Myxedema coma:** blunting of the senses and intellect, labored speech, swelling all over the body associated with hypothyroidism. Condition is life threatening.

Norepinephrine: a catecholamine that functions as a neurotransmitter, sending signals from one neuron to another neuron or to a muscle cell.

Oligomenorrhea: menstrual intervals of greater than 45 days.

Premenstrual syndrome: a cluster of behavioral, somatic, affective, and cognitive disorders that appear in the premenstrual (luteal) phase of the menstrual cycle and that resolve rapidly with the onset of menses.

Puberty: period in which the gonads mature and begin to function.

Pubescence: arriving or having arrived at the age of puberty.

Spermatogenesis: the process of male sperm production.

Thyroiditis: inflammation of the thyroid.

Thyrotoxic crisis (thyroid storm): potentially life-threatening condition for people with hyperthyroidism. The thyroid suddenly releases large amounts of thyroid hormone.

Xerostomia: dry mouth.

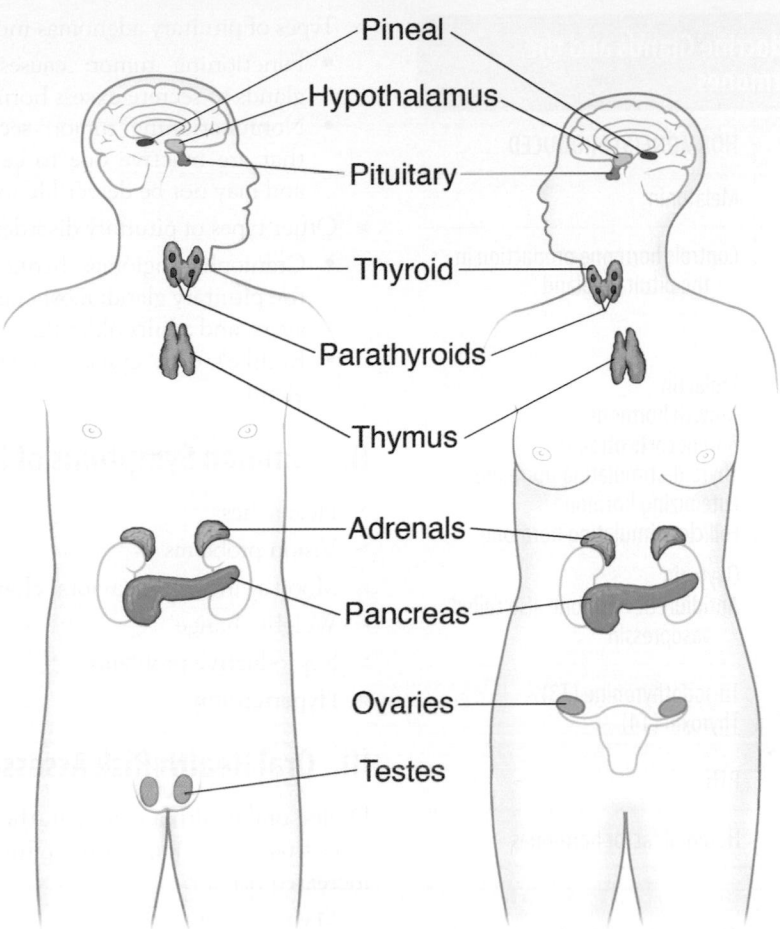

Pineal
Hypothalamus
Pituitary
Thyroid
Parathyroids
Thymus
Adrenals
Pancreas
Ovaries
Testes

FIGURE 52-1 The Major Endocrine Glands. Illustrated here for both male and female, these glands produce hormones that regulate body systems.

▶ Complex and unified actions of hormones produced by endocrine glands augment and regulate many vital functions, including:
- Growth and development
- Energy production
- Food metabolism
- Reproductive processes
- Responses of the body to stress and temperature.

III. Regulation of Hormones

▶ Regulation of hormonal secretion is complex, and the mechanisms are not fully understood. Normally, hormones are secreted when needed.

▶ The stimulus for hormone secretion is often a chemical signal in the blood.
- When the hormone is released the signal disappears.
- As more hormone is required, the signal reappears.

▶ This system of "negative feedback" works to provide hormones in optimal amounts and only in response to a need.

▶ Both hyposecretion and hypersecretion of a hormone can cause physical and mental disturbances.

ENDOCRINE GLAND DISORDERS

▶ When diseases affect the glands, hormones may be underproduced or overproduced, causing physical and biochemical changes that may have profound effects on the body, including the oral cavity.

▶ Presence or absence of a particular hormone may affect oral structures and may cause the host response to infection, healing, or stress to vary.[2]

▶ Many systemic diseases and disorders are risk indicators or risk factors for periodontal disease.

▶ Hormonal fluctuations associated with puberty, pregnancy, and menopause can affect the periodontium and directly modify the tissue's response to local factors.

PITUITARY GLAND

▶ The pituitary gland is composed of two functionally distinct portions:
- Anterior pituitary
- Posterior pituitary.

TABLE 52-1	Endocrine Glands and the Hormones
ENDOCRINE GLAND	**HORMONE(S) PRODUCED**
Pineal	Melatonin
Hypothalamus	Controls hormone production in the pituitary gland
Pituitary	
Anterior	Prolactin Growth hormone Adrenocorticotropin Thyroid-stimulating hormone Luteinizing hormone Follicle-stimulating hormone
Posterior	Oxytocin Antidiuretic hormone also called vasopressin
Thyroid	Tri-iodothyronine (T3) Thyroxin (T4)
Parathyroid	PTH
Thymus	Humoral factor hormones
Adrenals	
Adrenal cortex (outer portion)	Glucocorticoids (such as Cortisol) Mineral corticoids (such as aldosterone)
Adrenal medulla (inner portion)	Epinephrine (adrenaline) Norepinephrine
Pancreas	Insulin
Gonads	
Testes (males)	Testosterone
Ovaries (females)	Estrogen Progesterone Inhibin

▶ Each portion of the pituitary secretes different hormones.
▶ Excess or inadequate secretion of any of these hormones can cause severe problems for bodily functions.
▶ The anterior pituitary is called the "master gland" because of great influence on body organs, other endocrine glands, and overall well-being.

I. Pituitary Tumors

▶ Adenomas are the most common pituitary tumors.
▶ These benign tumors:
  • Usually secrete too much of one hormone
  • Can develop at any age.

▶ Types of pituitary adenomas include: [3]
  • Functioning tumor: causes the other endocrine glands to secrete excess hormones.
  • Nonfunctioning tumor: secretes excess hormones that are inactive due to cell development process and may not be detectible in blood tests.
▶ Other types of pituitary disorders include:
  • Craniopharyngiomas: benign tumors that grow near the pituitary gland; most common in children, teenagers, and adults older than 50.
  • Rathke's cleft cysts: benign cysts in the pituitary gland.

II. Common Symptoms of Pituitary Disorders

▶ Headaches
▶ Vision problems
▶ Mood swings or behavioral changes
▶ Weight change
▶ Reproductive problems
▶ Hypertension

III. Oral Health Risk Assessment

During oral health assessment, the dental hygienist recognizes that the patient with a pituitary gland disorder is at increased risk for:
▶ Macrocephaly
▶ Macrognathia
▶ Disproportionate mandibular growth: mandibular prognathism
▶ Open anterior bite
▶ Large pulp chambers
▶ Delayed eruption of primary and secondary teeth[2]
▶ Increased risk for periodontal disease due to growth factors and hormone imbalances.[4]

IV. Patient Management Considerations

▶ Orthodontic evaluation
▶ Increased risk of hypertension
▶ Increased risk of developing insulin resistance or type 2 diabetes
▶ General anesthesia may be contraindicated due to electrolyte imbalance.

THYROID GLAND

▶ Thyroid hormone receptors are present in almost every tissue in the body.
▶ This hormone plays a big role in normal physiologic function in the body including growth and development and energy metabolism.[5]

▶ Levothyroxine (Synthroid), used to treat thyroid gland disorders, is the third most common drug prescribed in the United States.[6]

I. Hypothyroidism[7]

▶ Hypothyroidism, the most common thyroid disorder, occurs when the thyroid does not produce enough thyroid hormone.

▶ It is more common in women than in men. Hypothyroidism develops slowly and is more common in people over the age of 60.

▶ Untreated or inadequately controlled hypothyroidism may cause an increased susceptibility to infections.

▶ The most common cause is an autoimmune disorder called Hashimoto's disease.

▶ Characteristics and oral manifestations of hypothyroidism[8] are listed in Table 52-2.

▶ Oral health risk assessment: because of the autoimmune response, patients with hypothyroidism are at an increased risk for:
  • Periodontitis[8]
  • Oral candidiasis
  • Easily bleeding gingiva
  • Poor wound healing

▶ Medical management: treatment is levothyroxine, lifelong monitoring.

▶ Patient management considerations
  • Monitor vitals: blood pressure and pulse
  • Avoid aspirin due to increased gingival bleeding and poor wound healing
  • Increased risk for myxedema coma due to longstanding low levels of thyroid hormone in the blood.
  • Myxedema coma is a life-threatening emergency. Triggers for myxedema coma are listed in Box 52-2

II. Hyperthyroidism[7,8]

▶ When the thyroid gland produces too much thyroid hormone, also referred to as overactive thyroid, it is called hyperthyroidism.

▶ This can occur over a short or long period of time.

▶ Causes include:
  • Excess of iodine in the diet
  • Graves' disease (autoimmune disorder that affects the thyroid)
  • Viral infection
  • Taking too much thyroid hormone medication.

▶ Characteristics and oral manifestations of hyperthyroidism are listed in Table 52-2.

▶ Oral health risk assessment
  • Accelerated tooth development, potential for malocclusion

Table 52-2	Characteristics of Thyroid Disorders
Hypothyroidism	
Hashimto's thyroiditis	
Congenital hypothyroidism	
GENERAL CHARACTERISTICS	**ORAL MANIFESTATIONS**
• Fatigue • Intolerant to cold • Weight gain—decreased metabolic rate • Constipation • Decreased concentration • Bradycardia • Muscle cramps and pain • Myxedema	• Macroglossia • Salivary gland enlargement • Facial myxedema • Increased dental caries • Compromised periodontal health • Delayed tooth eruption • Delayed wound healing • Hoarse voice • Burning mouth syndrome • Xerostomia • Lichen planus
Hyperthyroidism	
Graves' disease—autoimmune	
Thyroid storm	
GENERAL CHARACTERISTICS	**ORAL MANIFESTATIONS**
• Fatigue • Intolerant to heat • Increased appetite • Weight loss • Tremor • Protrusion of the eyes • Excess sweating • Enlargement of thyroid gland	• Difficulty swallowing • Increased dental caries • Increased periodontal disease • Macroglossia • Accelerated development of teeth and jaws

BOX 52-2

Triggers for Myxedema Coma in a Patient with Hypothyroidism

▷ Drugs (especially sedatives, narcotics, anesthesia)
▷ Infections
▷ Stroke
▷ Trauma
▷ Heart failure
▷ Gastrointestinal bleeding
▷ Hypothermia
▷ Failure to take thyroid medications

• Analgesics can increase the amount of thyroid hormones, making it more difficult to control hyperthyroidism

- Vasoconstrictors are used with caution in patients with uncontrolled hyperthyroidism, as these may increase symptoms of tachycardia.[7]
▶ Patient management considerations
  - Check vitals: blood pressure and pulse
  - Thyroid crisis (thyroid storm) is a sudden worsening of hyperthyroidism symptoms, which can be caused by an infection or stress. Immediate hospitalization is necessary.

PARATHYROID GLANDS[9,10]

As the parathyroid glands develop, they become embedded in the thyroid gland. Secretion of the parathyroid hormone (PTH) is in response to the serum-ionized calcium.

▶ The hormone controls calcium, phosphorus, and vitamin D levels in the blood and bone.
▶ All parathyroid gland disorders are rare. The most common cause of hypoparathyroidism is when the glands are accidently removed during a thyroidectomy.

I. Hyperparathyroidism

▶ Occurs when the parathyroid glands produce too much PTH.
▶ Can cause long-standing hypercalcemia, which may result in osteoporosis.
▶ Symptoms of hyperparathyroidism
  - Bone pain
  - Depression
  - Fatigue
  - Frequent broken bones
  - Kidney stones
  - Nausea
  - Loss of appetite.
▶ Oral health risk assessment
  - Loss of alveolar bone evident on dental images
  - Spontaneous mandibular fracture
  - Widened pulp chambers
  - Demineralized teeth.
▶ Patient management considerations
  - Home fluoride therapy
  - Increased risk of osteoporosis.

II. Hypoparathyroidism

▶ Hypoparathyroidism occurs when the glands produce insufficient PTH.
  - Causes the blood calcium levels to decrease and phosphorus levels increase.
  - Most common cause is injury to the parathyroid glands during thyroid and neck surgery.
▶ Symptoms[11]
  - Abdominal pain

- Brittle nails
- Dry hair
- Muscle cramps
- Muscle spasms (tetany)
- Increased muscular and peripheral nerve irritability.
▶ Oral care risk assessment[8]
  - Delayed teeth eruption
  - Congenitally missing teeth
  - Shortened roots
  - Delay or cessation of dental development
  - Enamel hypoplasia
  - Poorly calcified dentin
  - Widened pulp chambers
  - Mandibular tori
  - Chronic candidiasis
  - Paresthesia of the tongue or lips
  - Twitching or spasm of the facial muscles.
▶ Medical management: calcium supplements needed.
▶ Patient management considerations
  - Home fluoride therapy
  - Antifungal medication to treat chronic candidiasis.

ADRENAL GLANDS

▶ The adrenal glands consist of a pair of glands that sit at the top of each kidney.
▶ The glands are composed of an outer cortex and an inner medulla.
▶ The adrenal glands work with the hypothalamus and the pituitary gland to produce adrenaline, noradrenaline, dopamine, progesterone, and glucocorticoids.
▶ Treatment for adrenal gland disorders is corticosteroids.

I. Hyperadrenalism/Cushing's Syndrome

Cushing's syndrome is caused by too much cortisol production. Increased production of cortisol can be caused by a tumor in the anterior pituitary, a tumor in the adrenal gland or exogenous administration of steroids.

▶ Symptoms[11]
  - Weight gain
  - Broad, round face
  - "Buffalo hump"
  - Hypertension
  - Impaired healing
  - Hypokalemia
  - Hyperglycemia, glycosuria, polydipsia (mimics diabetes mellitus)
  - Increased bone fractures
  - Mood swings and depression.
▶ Oral health risk assessment
  - Increased melanic pigmentation may develop black-bluish areas affecting the buccal mucosa, palate, tongue, and lips

- Delayed wound healing
- Loss of collagen
- Skin and oral tissues are fragile
- Oral candidiasis.
▶ Medical management: surgery or radiation.
▶ Patient management considerations
  - Antifungal treatment
  - Antiviral medication.

II. Hypoadrenalism/Addison's Disease/ Adrenal Insufficiency

▶ Hypoadrenalism is divided into three categories:
  - Primary acute (adrenal crisis) failure of the gland to produce cortisol and aldosterone
  - Primary chronic adrenocortical insufficiency: Addison's disease (an autoimmune disease)
  - Secondary adrenocortical insufficiency: Rapid withdrawal of steroids or insufficient steroid supplements combined with acute stress (infections, trauma, or surgical procedures) may precipitate an adrenal crisis.
▶ Symptoms of adrenal crisis, a life-threatening emergency, are listed in Box 52-3.
▶ Symptoms of hypoadrenalism include:
  - Progressive weakness, fatigue
  - Gastrointestinal disturbances (anorexia, nausea, vomiting, diarrhea)
  - Hyperkalemia
  - Hypnatremia
  - Hypotension
  - Profuse sweating
  - Weight loss
  - Hypoglycemia.
▶ Oral health risk assessment[11,12]
  - Hyperpigmentation of the skin and mucosal surfaces

Box 52-3

Symptoms of Adrenal Crisis

▷ Abdominal pain
▷ High fever
▷ Loss of appetite
▷ Nausea
▷ Excessive sweating on face or palms
▷ Rapid respiratory rate
▷ Darkening of the skin
▷ Confusion
▷ Dizziness
▷ Low blood pressure
▷ Rapid heart rate
▷ Vomiting
▷ Joint pain
▷ Dehydration

- Long-term immune suppression may lead to Kaposi's sarcoma, lymphoma, or lip cancer[6]
- Oral candidiasis.
▶ Medical management: Treatment is long-term steroid use, which is important to patient management due to increased risk for infection, increased bleeding, and poor healing.
▶ Patient management considerations
  - Monitor vital signs: blood pressure and pulse
  - Provide antifungal medications to treat candidiasis
  - Provide pain control to avoid stress and invoking an adrenal crisis
  - Consider antianxiety medications prior to dental treatment
  - Delay nonemergency dental treatment until condition is stable or well controlled by medication.

PANCREAS

▶ Produces insulin to regulate blood glucose by way of the Islets of Langerhans.
▶ Improper function leads to diabetes.
▶ Diabetes is a disease of metabolism with inadequate production of the hormone insulin.
▶ Diabetes, the most common disorder of the pancreas, is covered in Chapter 69.

PUBERTY

I. Stages of Adolescence

▶ The period of life considered adolescence is represented by the years between ages 11 and 21.
▶ The adolescent years, which include puberty, are marked by hormonal fluctuations as well as many physical and psychosocial changes (Table 50-3, Chapter 50).
▶ From a psychosocial aspect, this period can be divided into three overlapping phases:
  - Early adolescence, approximately ages 11–13.
  - Middle adolescence, approximately ages 14–17.
  - Late adolescence, approximately ages 18–21.

II. Pubertal Changes[13]

▶ Puberty is a dynamic period of development marked by rapid changes in body size, shape, and composition.
▶ Some individuals go through changes earlier and faster than others.
▶ Physiologic changes occur due to hormones production and secretion by the endocrine glands especially the gonads.
▶ In males the testes produce testosterone hormones and in females the ovaries produce estrogen, progesterone, and inhibin hormones.

A. Hormonal Influences

▶ Pituitary hormones control the hormones produced by the ovaries and the testes.

▶ The several hormones produced by the ovaries are known collectively as estrogens, and those produced by the testes are called androgens.

▶ Responsible for the development of the sex organs, the accessory sex organs, and the secondary sex characteristics.

▶ As the levels of these hormones fluctuate during adolescence, they have strong physical, mental, and emotional influences throughout the body.

B. Oral Health Risk Assessment[14]

▶ Gingival inflammation due to the release of increased sex hormones.

▶ Diet analysis recommended to explore dietary-related dental disease patterns.

▶ Hyperplastic gingiva related to orthodontic appliances.

▶ Acute intraoral infections involving the periodontium require immediate treatment (Chapter 42).

▶ Periodontal infection may be localized or generalized (Chapter 19).

III. Patient Management Considerations

Additional information about oral health risk factors and patient management considerations for the adolescent patient are found in Chapter 50.

WOMEN'S HEALTH

I. Menstrual Cycle[15]

▶ The cycle, illustrated in Figure 52-2, is the period from the beginning of one menstrual flow to the beginning of the next menstrual flow.

▶ Each cycle takes approximately 28 days.

▶ Menstruation occurs in cyclical manner (lasting 4–6 days) from puberty to menopause.

▶ The rise and fall of hormone levels during the month control the menstrual cycle.

A. Characteristics

▶ Estrogen levels rise during the first half of the cycle to prepare the endometrium for pregnancy.

▶ If conception does not occur, estrogen levels decrease and menstruation begins.

▶ Variations in the cycle are common.

▶ Factors affecting the cycle: changes in climate, changes in work schedule, emotional trauma, acute or chronic illnesses, weight loss, or excessive exercise.

▶ Premenstrual syndrome may occur 7–10 days before menstruation. Symptoms may include fatigue, headache, bloating, mastalgia, skin breakouts, cramps, food cravings, depression, anxiety, irritability, hostility, tearfulness, mood changes, reduced ability to concentrate.[16]

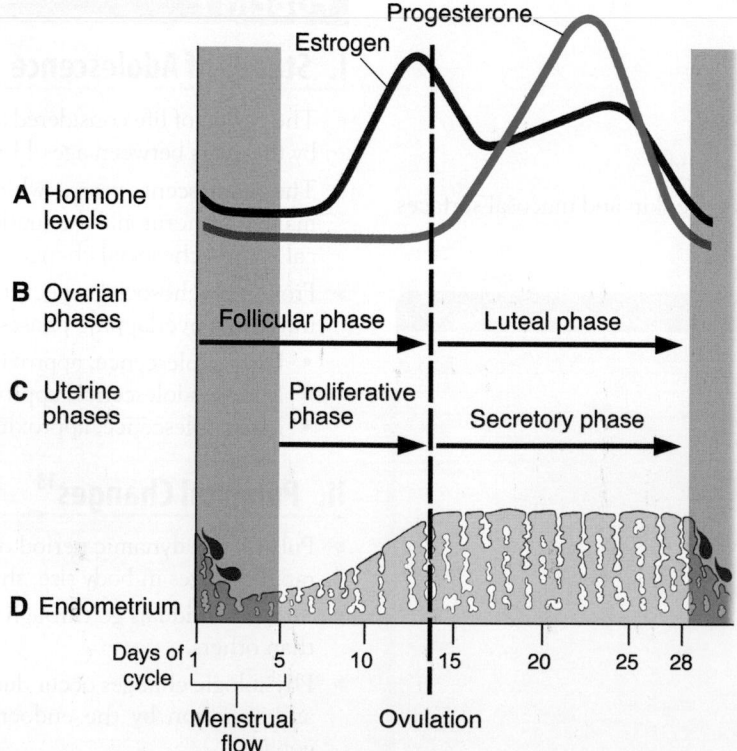

FIGURE 52-2 Changes During the Menstrual Cycle. The 28 days of a normal cycle are shown, with ovulation between days 12 and 15 and the menstrual flow between days 1–5 and again at day 28. Hormonal levels (**A**) show the estrogen peak shortly before ovulation during the follicular phase (**B**) of the ovary and the proliferative phase (**C**) of the uterus. The endometrium (**D**) builds up at the end of each menstrual flow. This prepares the area for possible implantation of a fertilized ovum.

B. Oral Health Risk Assessment[17]

▶ Exaggerated response to local irritants or unusual gingival bleeding may be noted.

▶ Patient may experience no specific gingival changes.

C. Patient Management Considerations

▶ Menstruation is normal and shows the body is healthy and functioning normally.

▶ Question women on regularity of menstrual cycle. Irregularity may reflect general health problems.

▶ Prevention through dental biofilm control, oral self-care measures, and removal of calculus at regular maintenance appointments can reduce oral effects of hormone imbalance during menstruation.

II. Hormonal Contraceptives

A variety of effective forms of hormonal contraceptives containing estrogen and progestin are available by prescription.[18] Delivery methods include:

▶ Oral contraceptives (birth control pills).

▶ Intramuscular injection: contains hormones to prevent pregnancy one shot lasts for 12 weeks.

▶ Patch: a transdermal patch applied to the skin releases hormones to prevent pregnancy.

▶ Ring: a small, flexible ring that releases hormones to prevent pregnancy inserted into the vagina once a month.

▶ Sponge: a round piece of plastic foam inserted into the vagina to block sperm from entering the uterus. Also contains a spermicide.

A. Estrogen and Progestin

▶ Combination of synthetic hormones estrogen and progestin is nearly 100% effective in preventing pregnancy when taken appropriately.

▶ Oral contraceptives inhibit the release of gonadotropin-releasing hormones, without which the ovum cannot be released from the ovary.

B. Oral Health Risk Assessment[18]

▶ An exaggerated response to dental biofilm and other local irritants has been noted in patients who use any type of contraceptives. The gingival response is similar to that described for pregnancy (see Chapter 49).

▶ Record the use of oral contraceptives each time the medical history is updated.

III. Menopause

▶ Menopause is the complete and permanent cessation of menstrual flow.

▶ Menopause generally occurs between the ages of 47 and 55 years.

▶ Signals the end of fertility due to decreased production of estrogen and progesterone by the ovaries.

▶ Menopause is usually confirmed when a woman has no menstrual period for 12 consecutive months and there is no other cause for this change.

A. Characteristics

▶ Before menopause, menstruation changes in frequency, duration, and amount of flow over a period of about 12–24 months.

▶ Menopause is accompanied by a number of characteristic physiologic hormonal-based changes.

▶ Many women experience only minor symptoms; a small percent have increased symptoms during menopause.

B. General Symptoms[19]

As ovarian function declines with diminishing estrogen, physiologic changes in body function include:

▶ Vasomotor reactions
  • Hot flashes, defined as periodic surges of heat involving the whole body; may be accompanied by drenching sweats.
  • Hot flash may begin with a headache; proceed to a flushing of the face, with heart palpitations, and dizziness, followed by a chill.
  • Episodes may last a few minutes or more than 30 minutes.
  • Night sweats and sleeping problems may lead to feeling tired, stressed, or tense.

▶ Mucosal changes
  • Associated with fluctuating and decreasing estrogen levels.
  • Dryness, irritation, and thinning of tissue may occur.
  • Frequent vaginal infections may occur.

▶ Emotional disturbances
  • Alterations in estrogen level may result in mood swings, depression, irritability, and difficulty with concentration or memory.
  • Decreased libido and changes in sexual response.
  • Some women experience anxiety, tension, and irritability and feel useless.
  • Weight gain or increase of body fat around waist.

C. Postmenopausal Effects

▶ Reproductive organs atrophy.

▶ Osteopenia and osteoporosis have been associated with the menopause.

▶ Skin and mucous membranes decrease in thickness and keratinization, becoming fragile and easily injured.

▶ Predisposition to conditions including atherosclerosis, diabetes, and hypothyroidism.

D. Burning Mouth Syndrome[20]

▶ Burning sensation in the mouth with the absence of identifiable oral lesion.

▶ Described as burning, tingling, hot, scalding, numbness.

▶ Cause is unknown. Very common in menopausal women.

▶ Treatment includes benzodiazapam, antidepressants, or analgesics.

E. Oral Health Risk Assessment

▶ Oral changes can be related to menopause, but they are not a common feature.

▶ Gingival changes:

• Gingival changes associated with menopause usually represent an exaggerated response to dental biofilm.

• Hormonal changes influence oral tissue response.

• Menopausal gingivostomatitis may develop. It may also occur after removal of, or radiation therapy to, the ovaries.

▶ Changes to mucous membranes and tongue[21]

• Tissue may appear shiny and may vary in color from abnormal paleness to redness. Dryness with burning sensations may be present.

• Burning mouth syndrome may occur.

• Altered salivary composition in some menopausal women may be due to psychological stress.

• Epithelium may become thin and atrophic with decreased keratinization; tolerance for removable prostheses may lessen, especially with xerostomia.

• Taste perception may be altered, described as salty, peppery, or sour.

• Inadequate diet and eating habits may contribute to the adverse changes of the mucosal tissues. The appearance and symptoms frequently resemble those associated with vitamin deficiencies, particularly B vitamins.

▶ Alveolar bone loss

• As a result of systemic osteoporosis, ridge resorption and loss of teeth can occur.[22]

• Osteoporotic jaws may be unsuitable for conventional prosthetic devices or dental implants.

IV. Patient Management Considerations

▶ During patient education, the relationship of oral conditions to endocrine disorders or hormonal fluctuation is considered.

▶ Emphasize the need for oral self-care measures due to hormonal fluctuations or imbalances.

▶ Consider oral effects of medications used to treat endocrine disorders and conditions.

▶ Control of local factors through preventive dental hygiene appointments will supplement daily personal oral care.

▶ Create an environment that decreases the stress level for the patient.

A. Patient Approach

▶ Review and update the patient's health history.

▶ Rapport begins with the clinician's courtesy, personal attention, and friendly, unhurried manner.

▶ Give particular attention to details, such as seating the patient promptly, handling materials and instruments efficiently and with calm assurance.

B. Instruction of Patient

▶ Saliva substitute may be needed to provide relief from xerostomia and aid in the prevention of dental caries.

▶ Measures for the prevention of periodontal infections can be carefully explained.

EVERYDAY ETHICS

Amy, an 18-year-old female, returns home from her first semester of college and presents with swollen gingiva, weight gain, and stories about considerable amounts of alcoholic beverages being consumed at parties. She also tells Sally, the dental hygienist who has provided care for her since she was a child, that she has just started taking birth control pills and mentions that her mother would be furious if she knew. Sally not only acknowledges Amy's desire to exercise her independence while away at school but also educates her extensively on the health consequences of these new behaviors. When she writes her progress notes for the appointment, Sally indicates the term "risky behaviors" in the patient's chart.

Questions for Consideration

1. What ethical issues come into play when Sally considers her responsibility for discussing this situation with Amy's parents, who are financially responsible for her oral health care?

2. Consider what has been entered into the patient's chart—"risky behaviors." What personal values might Sally be bringing into play when she uses this subjective, judgmental statement in writing her progress notes? Has Sally violated Amy's rights by using this kind of terminology to document her assessment findings?

3. Using the decision-making steps from Box 1-10 in Chapter 1, prioritize the factors Sally must address as she determines actions to take in resolving this ethical dilemma.

▶ Emphasize reasons for frequent calculus removal as a supplement to meticulous daily self-care.

▶ Explain the relationship between good general health and oral health.

C. Diet

▶ Dietary assessment may help the patient identify and correct inadequately balanced food selection (refer to Chapter 35).

▶ Recommend whole grain products, vegetables, and fruits. Choose foods low in fat and cholesterol. Recommend calcium to keep bones strong. Limit alcohol intake.

▶ Caries prevention through selection of nutritious and noncariogenic foods is especially important for the patient who snacks frequently.

D. Fluoride Therapy

Fluoride recommendations are based on assessment of the patient's dental caries risk status (refer to Chapter 27).

DOCUMENTATION

When documenting care for a patient with oral manifestations related to hormonal fluctuations, factors to document include:

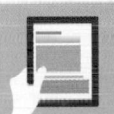

BOX 52-4

Example Documentation: Female Patient with Gingivitis Due to Hormonal Fluctuation

S –A 13-year-old female patient reports for routine dental hygiene care. Patient stated she has stopped flossing because her gums have been bleeding every time she does.

O –Health history review with patient and parent indicates recent on-set of menarche. Examination findings include increased biofilm levels compared to previous findings, extreme maxillary anterior gingivitis, moderate bleeding, and increased sensitivity to instrumentation.

A –Gingival health appears to be exacerbated by hormonal fluctuations related to patient's irregular menstrual cycle as well as her recent reluctance to provide adequate self-care.

P –Motivational interviewing approach to patient education discovers that patient values her beautiful smile. Patient agreed to concentrate on careful, complete daily biofilm removal in order to reduce what she called "disgusting and ugly" gingival redness, swelling, and bleeding. Flossing instruction provided.

Next steps: Patient scheduled for 3-month follow-up maintenance appointment.

Signed _____, RDH

Date _____

▶ Patient's age and gender.

▶ Description of the patient's health status related to any endocrine disorder or hormone fluctuations.

▶ Symptoms and oral manifestations related to hormonal fluctuations.

▶ Box 52-4 provides an example documentation for a patient with an oral manifestation related to reproductive hormone fluctuation.

Factors To Teach The Patient

▷ Self-care procedures that are necessary to maintain good oral health.

▷ The long-term impact of health behaviors, including lifestyle choices and risk reduction.

▷ The benefits of fluoride throughout life.

▷ The importance of nutrition, exercise, and sleep for good health.

▷ The value of seeking professional help when problems arise.

References

1. American Medical Association. *The Endocrine System.* Chicago, IL: American Medical Association; 1995–2013. http://www.ama-assn.org/ama/pub/physician-resources/patient-education-materials/atlas-of-human-body/endocrine-system. Accessed August 24, 2013.

2. Scaramucci T, Guglielmi CAB, Fonoff RD, et al. Oral manifestations associated with multiple pituitary hormone deficiency and ectopic neurohypophysis. *J Clin Pediatr Dent.* 2011;35(4):409–414.

3. Johns Hopkins Medicine. *Types of Pituitary Tumors.* Boston, MA: Johns Hopkins. http://www.hopkinsmedicine.org/neurology_neurosurgery/specialty_areas/pituitary_center/pituitary-tumor/types/. Accessed August 25, 2013.

4. Britto IMPA, Aguiar-Oliveira MH, Oliveira-Neto LA, et al. Periodontal disease in adults with untreated congenital growth hormone deficiency: a case control study. *J Clin Periodontol.* 2011;38:525–531.

5. Little JW. Thyroid disorders, Part II: hypothyroidism and thyroiditis. *Oral Surg Oral Med Oral Pathol Oral Radiol Endod.* 2006;102(2):148–153.

6. Baskin HJ, Cobin RH, Duick DS, et al. American Association of Clinical Endocrinologists medical guidelines for clinical practice for the evaluation and treatment of hyperthyroidism and hypothyroidism. *Endocr Pract.* 2002;8(6):457–469.

7. Rodgers GP. Hypothroidism: symptoms, diagnosis & treatment. *NIH Medline Plus.* 2012;7(1):24–25.

8. Zahid TM, Want BY, Cohen RE. The effects of thyroid hormone abnormalities on periodontal disease status. *J Int Acad Periodontol.* 2011;13(3):80–85.

9. National Institutes of Health. *Hypoparathyroidism.* Bethesda, MD: U.S. Department of Health and Human Services;

1997–2013. http://www.nlm.nih.gov/medlineplus/ency/article/000385.htm. Updated March 22, 2013. Accessed August 25, 2013.

10. Rees TD. Endocrine and metabolic disorders. In: Patton LL, ed. *The ADA Practical Guide to Patients with Medical Conditions* (Practical Guide Series). Chicago, IL: Wiley-Blackwell; 2013:69–94.

11. Fabue LC, Soriano YJ, Perex MGS. Dental management of patients with endocrine disorders. *J Clin Exp Dent.* 2010;2(4):e196–e203.

12. Bornstein, SR. Predisposing factors for adrenal insufficiency. *N Engl J Med.* 2009;360:2328–2339.

13. Medline Plus. *Puberty.* Bethesda, MD: National Institute of Health; 2013. www.nlm.nih.gov/medlineplus/puberty.html. Updated August 7, 2013. Accessed August 24, 2013.

14. American Academy of Pediatric Dentistry. Guideline on adolescent oral health care. *Clin Guide.* 2010;34(6):137–144.

15. WebMD. Normal Menstrual Cycle Guide - Normal Menstrual Cycle. WebMD Web site. http://www.webmd.com/women/tc/normal-menstrual-cycle-normal-menstrual-cycle. Accessed July 21, 2015.

16. Yonkers KA, Casper RF. *Clinical Manifestations and Diagnosis of Premenstrual Syndrome and Premenstrual Dysphoric Disorder.* Waltham, MA: UpToDate; 2013. http://www.uptodate.com/contents/clinical-manifestations-and-diagnosis-of-premenstrual-syndrome-and-premenstrual-dysphoric-disorder. Accessed August 21, 2013.

17. American Academy of Periodontology. *Gum Disease and Women.* Chicago, IL: American Academy of Periodontology. http://www.perio.org/consumer/women.htm. Accessed August 22, 2013.

18. Saini R, Saini S, Sharma S. Oral contraceptives alter oral health. *Ann Saudi Med.* 2010;30(3):243.

19. U.S. Department of Health and Human Services. *Menopause.* Washington, DC: Office on Women's Health. http://womenshealth.gov/menopause/menopause-basics/index.html. Updated September 22, 2010. Accessed August 24, 2013.

20. Dahiya P, Kamal R, Kumar M, et al. Burning mouth syndrome and menopause. *Int J Prev Med.* 2013;4(1):15–20.

21. Meurman JH, Tarkkila L, Tiitinen A. The menopause and oral health. *Maturitas.* 2009;63:56–62.

22. Vishwanath SB, Kumar V, Kumar S, et al. Correlation of periodontal status and one mineral density in postmenopausal women: a digital radiographic and quantitative ultrasound study. *Indian J Dent Res.* 2011;22(2):270–276.

ENHANCE YOUR UNDERSTANDING

thePoint° DIGITAL CONNECTIONS
(see the inside front cover for access information)

- **Audio glossary**
- **Quiz bank**

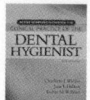

SUPPORT FOR LEARNING
(available separately; visit lww.com)

- *Active Learning Workbook for Clinical Practice of the Dental Hygienist, 12th Edition*

prepU INDIVIDUALIZED REVIEW
(available separately; visit lww.com)

- **Adaptive quizzing with *prepU for Wilkins' Clinical Practice of the Dental Hygienist***

53

The Older Adult Patient

Lisa M. LaSpina, RDH, MS and Janet H. Towle, RN, RDH, BS, MED

CHAPTER OUTLINE

LEARNING OBJECTIVES

After studying the chapter, the student will be able to:

1. Describe physiological and cognitive changes associated with aging.

2. Explain common chronic conditions associated with aging.

3. Identify common oral changes associated with aging.

4. Demonstrate best practices for communicating with the older adult patient.

5. Explain and document the dental hygiene process of care for the older adult patient.

The number of adults over 65 years of age continues to increase. The first of the "baby boom" generation turned 65 in 2011. They are the first generation to benefit from systemic fluoride in community water supplies and topically in toothpastes.

► The older adult population is:
  • Retaining more natural teeth; many with full dentitions.
  • Motivated to maintain and improve oral health.
  • Seeking more preventive procedures for oral health than in previous years.[1]

► Dental hygienists will be challenged by the complex needs of the aging population.

► As the life span of individuals increases, so does the incidence of chronic diseases.

► Dental hygienists need to be competent in providing safe, preventive, and therapeutic services for the older adult patients in all types of dental practices.

► An increasing number of dental hygienists will specialize in the care of the older adults and be employed in long-term care, home health care, and residential facilities for the aging.

► Tooth loss increases with age, but not because of the aging process.

► Dental caries and periodontal diseases are the major causes of tooth loss.

► Periodontal diseases in the older adult population represent the cumulative effects of long-standing, undiagnosed, untreated, or neglected chronic infection.

► Dental caries in the older adult population is associated with:
  • Gingival recession
  • Salivary hypofunction
  • Use of xerostomic medications
  • Diet in fermentable carbohydrates
  • Poor oral hygiene.

► The use of fluoride can provide a valuable protection to teeth and exposed root surfaces for all ages. It is unfortunate that some older adults believe fluoride is only for children.

► Key words relating to older adult patients are defined in Box 53-1.

AGING

I. Biological and Chronological Age

► From a chronological viewpoint, 65 years of age is the entry point for "old age." The period of 65 and older is divided into subgroups:
  • Young-old, adults between the ages of 65 and 74
  • Old-old, adults between the ages of 75 and 84
  • Oldest-old, adults 85 and older
  • Centenarians, adults over the age of 100
  • Supercentenarians, adults over the age of 110.

► Biological age is not synonymous with chronological age:
  • Signs of aging appear at different chronological ages in different individuals.
  • Aging is a process with many physiological changes.
  • A person can be biologically old at age 65; others can be physically fit at age 75.

II. Classification by Function

► The degree of general health and physical activity provides a classification system, functional age, not based on chronological age but on how older adults actually perform.

► Relative to the degree of impairment, older persons may be *functionally independent*, *frail*, or *functionally dependent*.

► Classification by function is more useful and is defined by activities of daily living and instrumental activities of daily living as described in Table 24-3 in Chapter 24.

III. Primary, Secondary, and Optimal Aging[2]

► *Primary aging* (also referred to as normal aging): age-related changes that occur in the body's systems advancing at an individual rate. These age-related changes are universal, intrinsic, and progressive. Example: skin wrinkling.

► *Secondary aging* (also referred to as impaired aging): age-related changes due to disease that leads to impairment. These age-related changes are associated to trauma and chronic diseases. Example: heart disease.

► *Optimal aging* (also referred to as successful aging): aging is slowed or altered due to promoting preventive measures to avoid negative changes. Example: eating a healthy diet.

NORMAL PHYSIOLOGICAL AGING

► Primary normal changes with aging are physiological.

► Secondary pathologic aging influences and accelerates the aging process.
  • Each age level brings changes in body metabolism, activity of the cells, endocrine balance, and mental processes.
  • In a healthy person, free of chronic diseases and medications with their potential side effects, the tissue changes of aging may be more subtle, appear at a later age, and be influenced by the person's lifestyle.

► Skin: thin, wrinkled, and dry, with pigmented spots, and loss of tone.

► Reduced tolerance to temperature extremes and solar exposure.

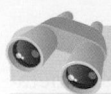

BOX 53-1 | KEY WORDS: The Older Adult Patient

Ageism: discrimination toward/against the older adult population.

Aging: the continuous process (biological, psychological, social) beginning with conception and ending with death, in which the organ systems age.

Alzheimer's disease: a form of irreversible dementia, usually occurring in older adulthood, characterized by gradual deterioration of memory, disorientation, and other features of dementia.

Biological age: the anatomic or physiologic age of a person as determined by changes in organismic structure and function; takes into account features such as posture, skin texture, strength, speed, and sensory acuity.

Chronological age: the actual measure of time elapsed since a person's birth.

Dementia: severe mental deterioration involving impairment of mental ability; organic loss of intellectual function.

Dysphagia: difficulty in swallowing.

Emphysema: pathologic accumulation of air in tissues or organs; general use refers to chronic pulmonary emphysema, in which terminal bronchioles become plugged with mucus, the lung and tissue lose elasticity, and breathing difficulties ensue.

Functional age: how well an older adult performs.

Geriatric dentistry: the branch of dentistry that deals with the special knowledge, attitudes, and technical skills required in the provision of oral health care for older adults.

Geriatrics: the branch of medicine that deals with the problems and illnesses of aging and their treatment.

Gerontology: study of the aging process; includes the biological, psychological, and sociological sciences.

Hemostasis: arrest of the escape of blood by either natural (clot formation or vessel spasm) or artificial (compression or ligation) means, or by the interruption of blood flow to a part.

Isolated systolic hypertension: condition in which only the systolic blood pressure is elevated; once thought to be part of the normal aging process; medical intervention is recommended.

Life expectancy: average number of years that a person can be expected to live; expectancy from birth in 1900 averaged 47 years; in 2010, average life expectancy for white females was 85.3 years; black females, 84.3 years; white males, 82.8 years; and black males 80.9 years.[a]

Lifestyle: relatively permanent organization of activities, including work, leisure, and associated social activities, characterizing an individual.

Osteoid: young bone that has not undergone calcification.

Osteopenia: decreased calcification or density of bone; inadequate osteoid synthesis.

Osteoporosis: low bone mass resulting from an excess of bone resorption over bone formation, with resultant bone fragility and increased risk of fracture.

Polypharmacy: concurrent use of a large number of drugs.

Presbycusis: progressive loss of hearing due to the normal aging process.

Presbyopia: a condition of farsightedness (hyperopia) resulting from a loss of elasticity of the lens of the eye due to the normal aging process.

Psychological age: the age of a person as determined by his or her feelings, attitudes, and life perspective.

Senescence: the process of growing old.

Senility: old age; loss of mental, physical, or emotional control; caused by physical and/or mental deterioration.

Sjögren's syndrome: an immunological disorder characterized by insufficient production of the lacrimal gland to produce tears and the salivary glands to produce saliva that results in abnormally dry eyes and mouth.

Tinnitus: ringing, buzzing, tinkling, or hissing sounds in the ear.

---

[a]Centers for Disease Control and Prevention. Life expectancy by age, race and sex, 2000–2009, U.S. Life Tables. 2009, table 21. http://www.cdc.gov/nchs/data/nvsr/nvsr63/nvsr63_07.pdf. Accessed July 24, 2015.

▶ Normal physiological changes that occur as the individual ages are universal, progressive, intrinsic, and unavoidable. These changes vary between each individual, and the body's systems.

▶ During aging, an overall gradual reduction in functional capacities occurs in most organs, with a decrease in cell metabolism and numbers of active cells.

▶ The following provides a summary of physiological changes that occur due to the normal aging process.

I. Musculoskeletal System

▶ Bone volume (mass) decreases gradually after the age of 40.

▶ Loss of muscle function: diminished muscular strength, and diminished speed of response.

▶ Curvature of cervical vertebrae due to a decrease in bone density and atrophic changes to cartilage and muscle.

▶ Joints may stiffen because of loss of elasticity in the ligaments.

II. Cardiovascular System[3]

▶ Decline in cardiac output; minimal increase in the size of left ventricular wall.

▶ Blood vessels become less elastic and flexible.

- Lumen of vessels decrease in size with resultant reduction of blood supply to organs, especially the liver and kidneys.
- Increased peripheral resistance.

▶ Atherosclerosis (fatty deposits on inner walls of arteries) is associated with aging; diet, smoking, and lack of exercise can be an influence.

▶ Changes in cardiovasculature do not affect function under normal, nonstressful conditions.

III. Respiratory System[4]

▶ Vital capacity is progressively diminished, leading to decreased efficiency of oxygen–carbon dioxide exchange.

▶ Skeletal changes weaken respiratory muscles, which limit chest expansion and reduce effective ventilation.

▶ Less effective cough reflex; increased risk for respiratory infections.

IV. Gastrointestinal System

▶ Production of hydrochloric acid and other secretions gradually decrease.

▶ Peristalsis is slowed.

▶ Decreased absorptive functions can affect nutrition and medications.

V. Central Nervous System

▶ Intellectual or cognitive function is slowed, not lost.

▶ Complex tasks may be more difficult.

▶ Short-term memory declines; long-term memory remains constant.

VI. Peripheral Nervous System

▶ Decrease in tactile sensitivity.

▶ Decreased proprioception (sense of one's position in space); risk for falls.

VII. Sensory Systems

▶ Age-related vision changes include[5]:
- Presbyopia
- Decreases in visual acuity (more light needed), peripheral vision, color clarity (problems with blues and greens)
- Decreased dilation and constriction of pupils results in difficulty adjusting to changes in light and problems with glare.

▶ Age-related hearing changes include[6]:
- Presbycusis
- Thicker and dryer cerumen (wax) contributes to hearing loss
- Decrease in ability to hear high-frequency tones
- Tinnitus.

▶ Management of a dental hygiene patient with vision and hearing impairment is discussed more in Chapter 60.

VIII. Endocrine System

▶ Decrease in thyroid efficiency; decreased basal metabolic rate.

▶ Altered thermoregulatory system; sensitive to cold; may not respond to infection with increased temperature.

IX. Immune System[7]

▶ The immune system declines with age. Among individuals the degree of decline varies greatly.

▶ Age-related changes in the skin and mucous membranes decrease effectiveness of the first line of defense against invading substances.

▶ Thymus gland decreases in size: decline in T cell function.

▶ With age there may be an increase in autoimmune disorders.

▶ Changes in the immune system result in increased incidence of infections. Older adults need to seek immunizations for influenza, varicella–zoster virus, and pneumococcal pneumonia. Vaccinations for hepatitis A, hepatitis B, hepatitis C, varicella, and meningococcal are recommended.

X. Cognitive Change[8]

▶ Cognitive change can distract the individual's attention away from their daily activities.

▶ The older adult patient struggles with numerous demands, which can affect the ability to function, especially the ability to concentrate.

▶ Factors such as excess light and noise can distract the older adult from perceiving relevant information.

▶ Supportive interventions that can aid an older adult with cognitive changes to maintain normal life activities are listed in Table 53-1.

▶ Tooth loss and gingival inflammation are associated with lower cognitive performance.[9]

PATHOLOGY AND DISEASE

I. Factors that Influence Disease

▶ An older person's health status is influenced by many factors. Biologic, environmental, psychosocial, psychologic, and a lifestyle of factors influence longevity.

▶ Genetically, a person may belong to a family that has exhibited resistance to disease factors.

▶ Healthy dietary habits and regular exercise can prevent or minimize disease.

▶ The following risk factors influence disease states:
- Tobacco use: all forms
- Use of alcohol
- Obesity and overweight.

Table 53-1	Supportive Interventions to Aid an Older Adult with Cognitive Changes
SITUATION	**SUPPORTIVE INTERVENTION**
Physical surroundings—environmental	▪ Reduce clutter.
Informational	▪ Use 14-point font for paper and online reading materials. ▪ Avoid unnecessary medical and legal jargon in patient reading materials. ▪ Facilitate use of reminder devices and lists.
Behavioral	▪ When possible, alter situations that restrict behaviors, including transportation and mobility problems. ▪ Provide assistive devices to promote independence and control.
Affective	▪ Assess for personal concerns and worries. ▪ Manage to decrease anxiety.

▶ Decreased immunologic functioning of aging is a factor in increased susceptibility of both men and women to HIV infection, AIDS, and other sexually transmitted diseases (STDs).

▶ Associations between periodontitis and specific systemic diseases include:[10–13]

- Atherosclerotic diseases[10,12,13]
- Diabetes mellitus[10,11,13]
- Respiratory infections[10,13]
- Rheumatoid arthritis.[10,13]

▶ The incidence of disease is higher in individuals from lower educational and socioeconomic backgrounds.[11]

II. Response to Disease

▶ The diseases that affect the older adult age group also occur in younger people, however:

- There are differences such as a lessened reserve capacity.
- An older adult may not view the classic symptoms of disease as a younger person.

▶ Characteristics of the altered response of the older adult to disease are listed in Box 53-2.

BOX 53-2

Characteristics of Altered Response to Disease in the Older Adult

▷ *Course and severity*: disease may occur with greater severity and have a longer course, with slower recovery.

▷ *Pain sensitivity*: may be lessened.

▷ *Body temperature response*: may be altered so that a patient may be very ill without the expected increase in body temperature.

▷ *Healing response*:
  ▷ Decreased healing capacity.
  ▷ More prone to secondary infection.

CHRONIC CONDITIONS ASSOCIATED WITH AGING

▶ Although many older adults function well and live independently in the community, the incidence of chronic diseases increases with advancing age.

▶ Individuals may have more than one chronic illness.

▶ The most common chronic conditions are osteoarthritis, visual and hearing impairments, cardiovascular diseases, and diabetes.

▶ Because of the number of chronic conditions, patients may be taking a large number of medications (polypharmacy), which can exacerbate xerostomia and increase the possibility of drug interactions.

I. Alzheimer's Disease

▶ Dementia is severe impairment of cognitive abilities, notably thinking, memory, and judgment. Alzheimer's disease is a nonreversible type of dementia and the most common of all dementias.

A. Etiology

▶ *Two types*:
  - Early onset: rare, reported in individuals in their 30s and 40s.
  - Late onset: most common, people over 65.

▶ *Etiology unknown*: theories include genetics, environment, nutrition, free radicals, and infectious agents.

▶ Average duration is 8–10 years from onset of symptoms to death.

B. Symptoms and Stages

▶ The common impairments of Alzheimer's disease may be divided into overlapping stages and may extend up to 20 years.

▶ Box 53-3 illustrates the progression of Alzheimer's disease symptoms using a common stage classification system that describes how a person's abilities change from normal function through advanced disability.

▶ Keep in mind that stages are general guides; symptoms vary greatly. Not every individual with Alzheimer's disease will experience the same symptoms or progress at the same rate.

C. Treatment

▶ There is no proven treatment to prevent or cure the disease.

▶ Treatment is designed to support the family as well as the patient.

▶ Requires a prolonged multidisciplinary effort.

▶ Medications are prescribed for patients with mild-to-moderate symptoms.

▶ Medications prescribed to address behavioral problems include:
  - Antidepressants
  - Antianxiety medications
  - Antipsychotics
  - Anticonvulsants may be prescribed for the small percentage of individuals who have seizures.

D. Dental Hygiene Management Considerations

▶ Box 53-4 illustrates guidelines for caregivers of Alzheimer's disease.

▶ Specific dental hygiene care considerations for the patient with early and later stages of Alzheimer's disease are listed in Box 53-5.

▶ Link between periodontal disease and Alzheimer's disease; brain inflammation can result from periodontal bacteria and the entry of pathogen products into the brain.[15]

▶ Goals of dental hygiene care:
  - Preserve oral health and function
  - Prevent future oral and systemic disease
  - Provide comfort.

▶ The dental hygiene care plan:
  - Considers the current stage of the patient's disease.
  - Provides a plan for comprehensive care in anticipation of future decline in oral health.

▶ Undiagnosed patients: when patient's behavior is suspect, a referral to the patient's physician is made.

II. Osteoarthritis

Osteoarthritis is the most common form of arthritis and involves a progressive loss of articular cartilage. Management of the patient with arthritis is discussed in more detail in Chapter 59.

BOX 53-3

Stages of Alzheimer's Disease

Stage 1: Normal Function
▷ No memory problems

Stage 2: Very Mild
▷ Memory lapses; personal awareness of forgetting familiar words or the location of everyday objects
▷ No medical diagnosis of dementia

Stage 3: Mild
▷ Memory lapses; family members/friends begin to notice problems in memory or concentration
▷ Observable difficulties include:
  ▷ Trouble remembering names or the right words
  ▷ Performing tasks
  ▷ Losing objects
  ▷ Trouble organizing

Stage 4: Moderate
▷ Able to clearly detect that there are problems
▷ Observable difficulties include:
  ▷ Forgetting events and personal history
  ▷ Increasing difficulty with complex tasks
  ▷ Withdrawn

Stage 5: Moderately Severe
▷ Noticeable lapses in memory and thinking
▷ Does not remember own address/phone number
▷ *Confused;* does not know what day it is
▷ Still self-sufficient with eating or using the toilet

Stage 6: Severe
▷ Memory worsens/personality changes
▷ Observable difficulties include:
  ▷ Cannot recall recent experience
  ▷ Trouble remembering the name of family members
  ▷ Changes in sleep patterns
  ▷ Needs assistance with toileting/unable to control bladder or bowels
  ▷ Becomes suspicious
  ▷ Compulsive/repetitive behavior: example shredding tissue
  ▷ Wanders easily/can become lost

Stage 7: Very Severe
▷ Loss of ability to respond to environment
▷ Cannot carry on a conversation or easily control movement
▷ Observable difficulties include:
  ▷ Eating
  ▷ Using the toilet
  ▷ Smiling
  ▷ Holding head upright
  ▷ Swallowing

Source: *Seven Stages of Alzheimer's Disease.* Chicago, IL: Alzheimer's Association. http://www.alz.org/alzheimers_disease_stages_of_alzheimers.asp. Accessed October 13, 2013.

Box 53-4

Alzheimer's Disease: Guidelines for Caregivers

▷ Keep the same daily routine. Keep the environment calm.

▷ Promote the use of clocks, calendars, and newspapers to maintain the patient's orientation.

▷ Watch the patient's medical and oral health. Encourage exercise and regular dental visits.

▷ Keep communication open. Use laughter as a tool.

▷ Use positive reinforcement.

Source: Saxon S, Etten MJ, Perkins EA. *A Guide for the Helping Professions Physical Change & Aging*. 5th ed. New York, NY:Springer; 2010:98–99.

BOX 53-5

Dental Hygiene Care Considerations for the Patient with Alzheimer's Disease

Early Stages

▷ Review of the patient's medical and dental history at each maintenance appointment may reveal lapses in memory and other signs of early disease.

▷ An early sign may be a slow decline of interest in oral hygiene and personal care.

▷ Provide routine care with initiation of aggressive preventive regimens.

▷ Three-month intervals for maintenance appointments are recommended.

▷ Topical fluoride applications; fluoride varnish.

▷ Oral hygiene instruction; involve caregivers early in disease process.

Later Stages

▷ Routine intraoral examination to assess lesions due to cancer, medications, or injury.
  ▷ Sedation may be required.
  ▷ Possible need for mouth prop and physical restraint.

▷ Caregivers assume daily oral care. Power toothbrushes may improve dental biofilm removal for caregivers to use.

▷ Patient may reside in a long-term care facility. Dental hygienists who specialize in the treatment of this population may oversee care.

A. Symptoms

▶ Intermittent joint pain

▶ Stiffness upon arising

▶ Crepitation (creaking joints)

B. Treatment

▶ Physical therapy

▶ Exercise

▶ Rest

▶ Reduced stress on joints

▶ Dietary modifications

▶ Drug therapy

C. Dental Hygiene Management Considerations

▶ Keep appointments short

▶ Schedule afternoon appointments

▶ Allow breaks to relax the jaw

III. Alcoholism[16]

A. Effects of Alcohol Use

▶ Owing to age-related primary physiological changes, older drinkers may experience more detrimental health-related effects compared with younger drinkers.

▶ Older adults require less alcohol for adverse effects to occur.

▶ Excessive use of alcohol by older adults may:
  • Have more severe health-related consequences.
  • Exacerbate medical and emotional problems associated with aging.
  • Predispose to adverse drug reactions with prescription and over-the-counter medications.
  • Be associated with major depressive disorder.

B. Dental Hygiene Management Considerations

Management of a dental hygiene patient with a substance-abuse disorder is discussed more completely in Chapter 65.

IV. Osteoporosis

▶ Osteoporosis is a bone disease involving loss of mineral content and bone mass.

▶ Osteoporosis is common in individuals older than age 60, and the incidence increases with age.

▶ Although most prominent in postmenopausal women, the condition may also occur at other ages and in men.

A. Causes

▶ Endocrine: hormonal disturbances; depletion of estrogen after menopause.

▶ Inadequate intake of calcium and/or vitamin D or defective absorption of calcium or vitamin D metabolism.

B. Prevention

Prevention is the first line of defense against osteoporosis.

▶ Adequate calcium and vitamin D intake during adolescence and early adulthood is critical to forming peak bone mass.

▶ The minimum requirements for both calcium and vitamin D increase with age.

▶ Load-bearing exercise is necessary to maintain bone mass.

C. Risk Factors

A number of risk factors have been identified; some of which work together. From the risk factors, a list of methods for long-term prevention can be derived:

▶ Female gender; positive family history.

▶ Caucasian or Asian ethnicity (worldwide, Blacks are least affected).

▶ Low calcium and vitamin D intake (lifelong).

▶ Early menopause or early surgical removal of ovaries; use of corticosteroids; eating disorders.

▶ Sedentary lifestyle; lack of exercise.

▶ Alcohol abuse; tobacco use; high caffeine intake.

▶ High sodium intake.

▶ Low body–mass index.

D. Relationship to Periodontal Disease[17,18]

▶ Relationship exists between the reduced bone mineral density of osteoporosis and oral bone loss in skeletal and mandibular bone; oral bone loss in the edentulous person pertains to:
  • Periodontal bone destruction
  • Residual ridge loss.

▶ Mutual risk factors of osteoporosis and periodontal disease are:
  • Smoking
  • Nutritional deficiencies
  • Alcohol use
  • Hormonal status.

▶ Osteoporotic bone is:
  • Less dense
  • More readily absorbed.

E. Symptoms

Osteoporosis develops over many years; a long asymptomatic period of bone change can occur with no clinical symptoms.

▶ Clinical symptoms may include:
  • Backache: stooping of the posture. Figure 53-1 illustrates the posture of an older adult with osteoporosis.
  • Vertebral fractures or compression fractures cause the spine to curve.
  • Fractures: hip, compression fractures of spine, ends of long bones.
  • Evidence of bone changes in the mandible: residual ridge resorption.

F. Treatment/Medications

▶ A number of medications, with various mechanisms of action, decrease bone resorption, increase bone formation, or both.

▶ Whichever regimen of medications is prescribed, successful treatment and prevention requires simultaneous intake of calcium and vitamin D.

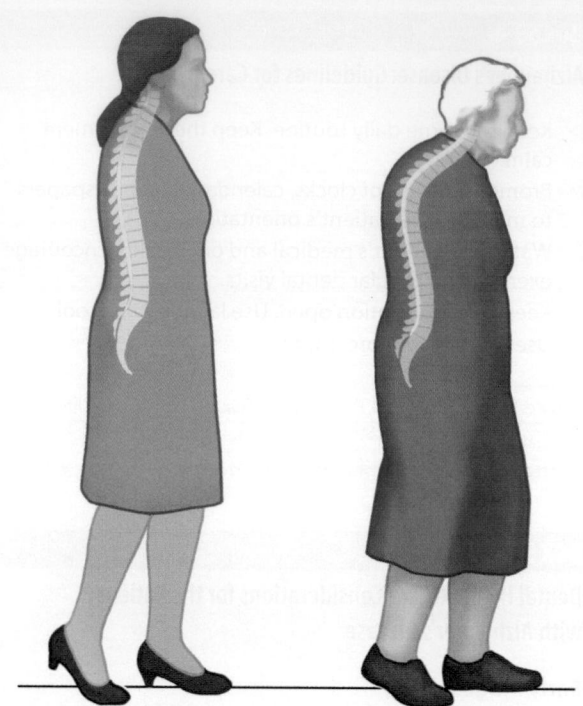

FIGURE 53-1 Example of an older adult's posture with osteoporosis. Vertebral fractures or compression fractures cause the spine to curve.

▶ *Bisphosphonates*: slows bone metabolism/increasing bone density.

▶ *Selective estrogen receptor modulators*: inhibits bone resorption.

▶ *Calcitonin*: inhibits bone resorption.

▶ *Parathyroid hormone*: stimulates bone formation.

G. Treatment and Prevention

▶ Weight bearing physical activity, such as walking, has a beneficial effect on bone mass.

▶ Activities of daily living and physical activity require caution and preventive measures to avoid accidental falls.

▶ Avoid smoking and excessive alcoholic intake.

▶ Severe involvement of the spine may require orthopedic support and medication for pain.

▶ Dental hygiene management considerations:
  • Do not rush; try to prevent falls.
  • Provide extra time for positioning; provide cushioning.
  • Taking bisphosphonates is a contraindication for dental surgery due to increased risk for osteonecrosis (bone destruction) of the jaw.
  • Health promotion opportunities exist for long-term prevention. Encourage:
    ○ Smoking cessation.
    ○ Limiting alcohol consumption.
    ○ Healthy lifestyles involving adequate calcium and vitamin D intake and regular physical activity.

V. Sexually Transmitted Diseases

▶ The most common STDs include:
  • Chlamydia
  • Syphilis
  • HIV/AIDS
  • Genital herpes
  • Gonorrhea
  • Human papilloma virus.
▶ STDs are on the rise in the older adult populations.

A. Incidence in Older Populations

The most common STD in this demographic is HIV/AIDS, with an increase of new HIV/AIDS cases in the over 50 years age group.[19]

▶ Factors that influence the increase in numbers include:
  • Increased use of medications to treat erectile dysfunction.
  • Increased divorce rate.
  • People living longer and generally in better health.
▶ Sexually active senior women more prone to acquiring STDs due to:
  • Thinning of the epithelium of the vaginal area.
  • Diminished immune system.
▶ Increased number of older adults living in assisted living centers or senior housing communities.
▶ Cultural and generational differences may explain why older adults are not as knowledgeable about the need for safe-sex practices.
▶ Older adults might not practice safe sex since the risk of pregnancy is eliminated.

B. Dental Hygiene Management Considerations

▶ Medical referral or consultation
▶ An appointment with the patient's physician is necessary to determine what medication is needed to treat the STD.
▶ Goals of dental hygiene care include:
  • Open, nonjudgmental communication.[20]
  • Increased patient awareness of the transmission of STDs.
  • Importance of communication with the patient's physician.

VI. Respiratory Disease[21]

▶ Older adults are at higher risk for respiratory disease.
▶ Good oral hygiene practices can reduce the progression or occurrence of respiratory diseases among older adult patients.
▶ Chapter 66 provides more information regarding dental hygiene care for patients with respiratory disease

A. Age-Related Disorders of the Respiratory System

▶ Pneumonia
▶ Chronic obstructive pulmonary disease
▶ Asthma

B. Dental Hygiene Management Considerations

▶ Monitor vital signs.
▶ Adjust seating position as needed for comfortable breathing. Refer to Chapter 7 for information related to patient positioning.

VII. Cardiovascular Disease

▶ Heart disease is a common cause of death for the older adult patient over age 65.
▶ Health promotion and healthy behaviors initiated early can prevent heart disease.
▶ Chapter 67 provides more information regarding dental hygiene care for patients with cardiovascular disease.
▶ Age-related disorders of the cardiovascular system include:
  • Arteriosclerosis and atherosclerosis
  • Hypertension postural hypotension
  • Angina pectoris
  • Myocardial infarction
  • Congestive heart failure
  • Heart valve disease
  • Transient ischemic attack (ministroke)
  • Cerebrovascular accident (stroke)
▶ Dental hygiene management considerations:
  • Monitor blood pressure
  • Use of relaxation techniques
  • Lifestyle changes.

ORAL CHANGES ASSOCIATED WITH AGING

▶ Healthy tissue features of primary aging need to be separated from the long-term effects of secondary aging due to chronic disease and medications.

I. Soft Tissues

A. Lips

▶ Tissue changes: dry, purse-string opening results from dehydration and loss of elasticity within the tissues.
▶ Angular cheilitis is not specifically an age-related lesion, but it is seen frequently among older adults.[22]
▶ Etiologic factors may be candidiasis and vitamin B deficiency.

▶ Appears as skin folds with fissuring at the angles of the mouth and can be related to reduced vertical dimension or inadequate support of the lips.

▶ Cheilitis in conjunction with dentures is described in Chapter 54.

B. Oral Mucosa

▶ Atrophic changes: The tissue may become thinner and less vascular, with a loss of elasticity; a smooth shiny appearance is related to thinning of the epithelium.

▶ Hyperkeratosis: White, patchy appearance of tissue may develop because of irritation from sharp edges of broken teeth, restorations, or dentures, and from use of tobacco.

▶ Capillary fragility: Facial bruises and petechiae of the mucosa are common.

C. Tongue

▶ Atrophic glossitis (burning tongue).
  • The tongue appears smooth, shiny, bald, and with atrophied papillae.
  • The condition is usually related to anemia that results from a deficiency of iron or combinations of deficiencies.
  • Deficiency anemia results from nutritional factors.

▶ Taste sensations[23]
  • Taste buds are slower.
  • The acuity of the perception for salt declines with age.
  • The perception of sweet and sour does not decline with age.
  • Olfactory acuity, which significantly affects taste, declines more than taste.
  • Flavoring agents and spices can be added to foods instead of salt and sugar to enhance taste.
  • Tongue cleaning increases taste perception.

▶ Sublingual varicosities
  • Clinical appearance: deep, red or bluish nodular dilated vessels on either side of the midline on the ventral surface of the tongue.
  • Significance: varicosities do not have a direct relation to systemic conditions.

D. Xerostomia[24]

▶ Xerostomia, dryness of the mouth, is:
  • Characterized by the absence or diminished quantity of saliva.
  • Prevalent in the older adult.[25]
  • A symptom, not a disease entity.

▶ Lack of saliva and the effect of a dry mouth are significant contributing factors to oral discomfort and disease, particularly dental caries.

▶ Causes of xerostomia include:
  • Systemic medications, which provide the most common influence. Many drugs that are common prescription items produce dry mouth as a side effect.

  • Autoimmune diseases such as Sjogren's syndrome, rheumatoid arthritis, systemic lupus erythematosus.
  • Diabetes.
  • Radiation to head and neck for cancer therapy: permanent damage to the salivary glands can result.

▶ Clinical symptoms include:
  • Feeling of oral dryness; tongue sticks to palate
  • Difficulty with mastication, swallowing, and speech
  • Impaired taste
  • Burning, and soreness of mucosa and tongue.

▶ Oral effects of xerostomia
  • Heavy dental biofilm, material alba, and debris accumulation can lead to increased:
    ‣ Severity of periodontal infection and demineralization of tooth surface.
    ‣ Predisposition to dental caries, particularly root caries.
    ‣ Problems of denture wearing.
    ‣ Dietary changes during eating; may use increased quantities of liquid to soften food for swallowing.

▶ See Box 53-6 for a partial list of some of the drug groups that may decrease salivary function.

E. Oral Candidiasis

▶ Oral candidiasis is an infection of the oral mucosal tissues.

▶ Denture stomatitis and angular cheilitis represent the two common forms, as described in Chapter 54.

▶ Candidiasis is associated with the use of antibiotics, head and neck radiation therapy, chemotherapy, steroids, and other immunosuppressive drugs.

▶ Medical conditions that alter the immune system, including diabetes and HIV infection, permit an overgrowth of the Candida organisms.

▶ Patients with xerostomia have an increased incidence of candidiasis.

II. Teeth

A. Color

▶ Darkening or yellowing is the result of changes in the underlying dentin.

BOX 53-6

Partial List of Classes of Drugs That Decrease Salivary Function

Anticholinergics

Antihistamines

Antihypertensives

Antianxiety

Anticonvulsants

Diuretics

Antidepressants (tricyclic)

Nonsteroidal anti-inflammatory

► Color changes result from long use of tobacco and beverages such as tea and coffee.

► Dark intrinsic stains from dental restorations.

B. Dental Pulp[26]

► Pulpal changes develop as reactions to wear, dental caries, restorations, bruxism, and other assaults during the elderly person's long life.

► Narrowing of pulp chambers and root canals; increased deposition of secondary and tertiary dentin. Figure 53-2 provides examples of radiographs showing the narrowing of pulp canals with age.

► Progressive deposition of calcified masses (pulp stones or denticles).

C. Attrition

► Signs of wear, which may be the long-term effects of diet, occupational factors, or bruxism.

► Attrition may be accompanied by chipping and teeth may seem more brittle.

D. Abrasion

► Abrasion at the cervical third of a tooth may result from extended use of a hard toothbrush in a horizontal direction with an abrasive dentifrice.

► With current preventive measures, use of soft-textured brushes, and attention to abrasiveness of dentifrices, future generations will be less likely to exhibit such tooth alterations.

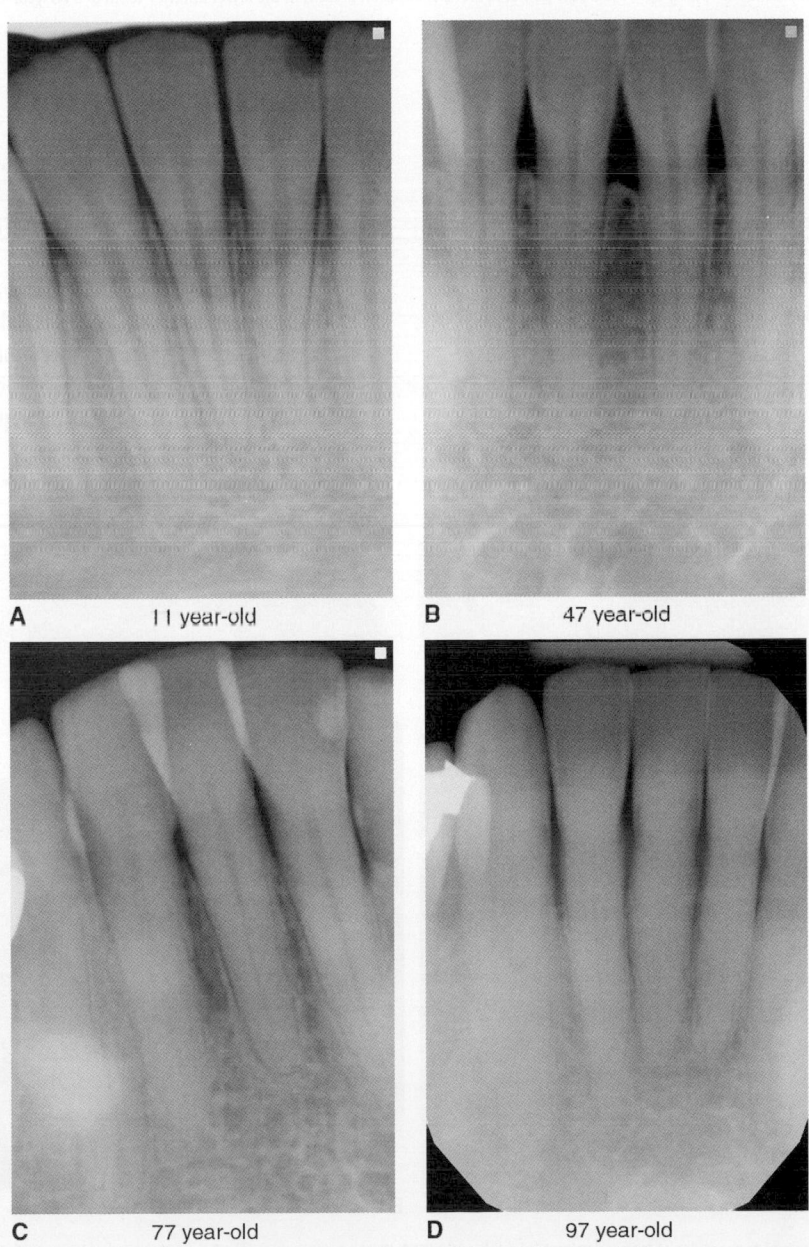

FIGURE 53-2 Radiographs provide an example of narrowing pulp canals with age. The radiograph of the 11-year-old boy (**A**) illustrates pulp canals common in youth, radiographs (**B**) and (**C**) illustrate narrowing with advancing age, and the radiograph of the 97-year-old woman (**D**) shows pulp canals, which are significantly diminished.

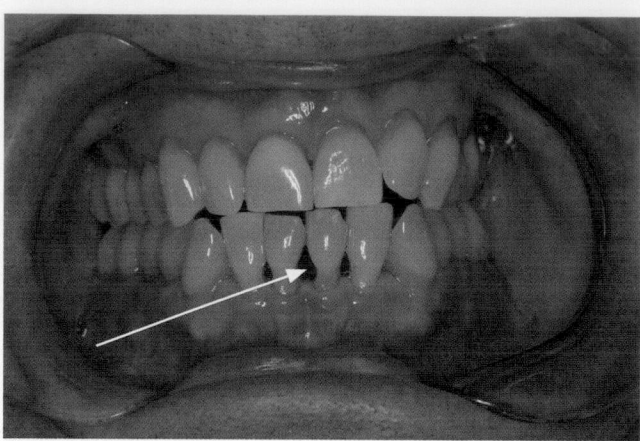
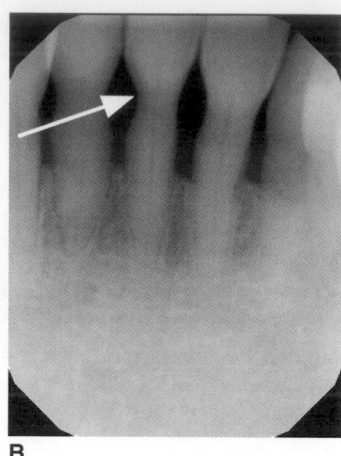

A   **B**

FIGURE 53-3 In both the photograph and the radiograph, the arrow points to areas of abrasion present in the lower anterior teeth of a 66-year-old man. (Photograph courtesy of Dr. Paul Epstein, DMD.)

▶ Figure 53-3 provides a photograph and radiographic image of abrasion.

E. Root Caries[27]

▶ Prevalence: Older adults have more root caries than any other age group, except in communities with natural fluoride or community water fluoridation.

  • A photograph in Figure 53-4 provides examples of root caries.

▶ Risk factors for root caries include:

  • Exposed root surfaces due to:
    ◦ Periodontal infections that cause loss of attachment.

  ◦ Horizontal toothbrushing technique results in abrasion.
  • Biofilm retention due to inadequate oral hygiene. Reasons include:
    ◦ Cognitive and physical disabilities that hinder biofilm removal.
    ◦ Inadequate oral care received.
  • Faulty restorations and partial dentures retain cariogenic food substances and biofilm.
  • Xerostomia and medications.
  • High carbohydrate diet; frequency of snacking on fermentable carbohydrates.
  • Combinations of these factors increase the risk.

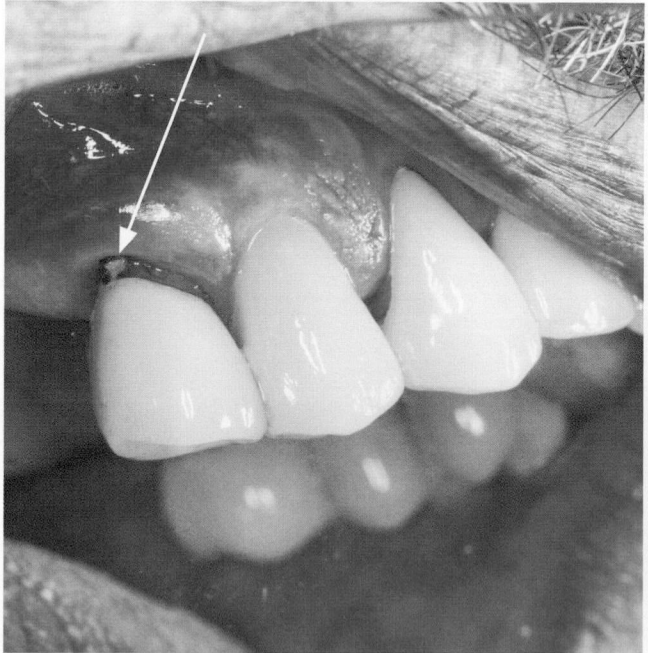
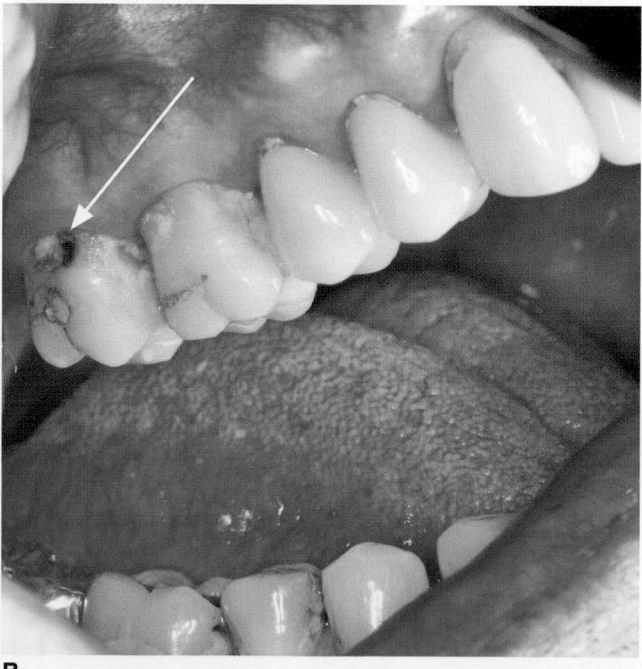

A   **B**

FIGURE 53-4 The two photographs provide examples of root caries in older adult patients. A: Illustrates a cavitated lesion on the exposed root surface apical to the margin of a crown on tooth number 4. The arrow in photograph (B) points to dental caries apical to the cementoenamel junction on tooth #3. Notice the previously restored areas on adjacent teeth. (Photographs courtesy of Dr. Paul Epstein, DMD.)

▶ *Effect of fluoride:*
- Adults with longtime residence in a fluoridated community have substantially fewer root carious lesions than those in a nonfluoridated community.
- The protective factor is especially true for lifelong residents of areas where there is natural fluoride in the water.[28]

▶ *Prevention:*
- Control of risk factors for dental caries is essential for older adults as it is for all age groups.
- Emphasis is placed on periodontal health because attachment loss with resultant root exposure needs to be prevented.
- Caries preventive agents need to be strongly recommended, including the professional application of fluoride varnish.

III. The Periodontium

▶ Bone
- Osteoporosis may be present.
- Depressed vascularity, a reduction in metabolism, and reduced healing ability affect bone.

▶ Cementum
- The average overall thickness of the cementum at 20 years of age was 0.095 mm; cementum from 60-year-old persons measured 0.215 mm.[29]

▶ Gingiva
- Gingival changes can be traced to the effects of infection or to anatomic factors.
- Gingival recession is common in older individuals.
- Predisposing factors: a lack of sufficient attached gingiva: malposition of the teeth.

▶ *Risk factors for periodontal disease*
- Similar to younger individuals.
- May be modified by chronic diseases and medications.

▶ *Clinical findings*
- The periodontal tissues reflect the health and disease of the patient over the years.
- Moderate periodontal disease may be more prevalent than advanced disease.

▶ *The healthy periodontium*
- Healthy tissues that have been maintained over the years may have had a minimum of disease.
- The radiographs show little if any attachment loss, the gingiva are firm, and the appearance is normal.
- Probing reveals minimal sulcus depth with no bleeding.
- The teeth are not mobile.

▶ *The patient with periodontal infection*
- Neglect or omission of preventive measures and therapy over the years may have resulted in a chronic periodontal infection with extension of tissue destruction into the bone, periodontal ligament, and cementum.
- Loss of attachment, deep periodontal pockets, tooth mobility, and radiographic signs of periodontitis may be present.

▶ *The treated patient*
- Although the patient was subject to periodontal infection, treatment was completed, and the tissues were maintained in health through personal oral self-care and professional supervision.
- The tissues may show the effects of the treated disease, such as open interproximal embrasures.
- Areas of recession with exposed cementum may also be evident.
- The teeth are not mobile, especially when occlusal analysis and adjustment has been featured.

DENTAL HYGIENE CARE FOR THE OLDER ADULT PATIENT

▶ The dental hygiene process of care for the older adult is based on individual need as with all patients.
- Many older adults value oral health as a component of overall health and wellness.
- Care for the older adult patient needs to be planned in terms of comprehensive, not palliative treatment.
- Increasing numbers of the older adult population avail themselves of esthetic dental services.
- Adaptations need to be made to the process of care when cognitive, sensory, or physical conditions/limitations are present.
- Long-term maintenance for the prevention of oral disease is the basic objective.

I. Barriers to Care

▶ Lack of perceived need is one of the most common reasons why the older adults do not seek dental care.

▶ Older generations believed a decline in oral health was the result of the aging process.

▶ Economic and access barriers:
- Fixed income after retirement.
- Lack of dental insurance.

▶ Transportation problems:
- Functional disabilities affecting mobility limit access without assistance.

▶ Physical/architectural barriers:
- Accessibility to the dental office or clinic.
- Restrictions to access to care for institutional residents.
- Wheelchair access.
- Hazards, such as small rugs, which can slide on polished floors; loose corners of rugs, which can be

tripped over; and irregularities in floor levels, need to be eliminated.

- Sitting for extended periods, keeping mouth open, and such might be difficult; provide frequent opportunities to change positions.
- Consider several short appointments as opposed to extended appointments.
- Raise the chair to a sitting position slowly due to the possibility of postural hypotension.

II. Assessment

▶ Patient history

Preparation of a careful and detailed medical and dental history takes on particular significance. Suggestions for good communication include the following:

- Allow sufficient time for reviewing complex histories.
- Eliminate distracting background music or sounds.
- Sit facing the patient and speak clearly with a low tone of voice.
- Speak directly to the patient even when a caregiver is present.
- Do not call the patient by his/her first name unless the patient suggests doing so.

▶ Medications

- Because of the prevalence of chronic diseases, older patients are the largest consumers of both prescription and over-the-counter medications.
- Drug usage and the incidence of adverse drug reactions increases with age.
- Obtain a complete list. Include herbal and dietary supplements.
- Ask the patient to bring in either the bottles that contain the various medications (over-the-counter as well as prescription items) or a written copy of the labels so that a list may be kept in the patient's record.

▶ References for checking drugs: Each practice center or clinic needs access to current references, such as the *Physician's Desk Reference*®, *Merck Manual*, or pharmacology reference websites (Lexi-Comp®) specifically directed to the dental practice.

▶ Review the list of medications at each continuing care appointment.

▶ Review each medication to determine:

- Potential adverse side effects. Effects on the oral cavity such as xerostomia and gingival hyperplasia.
- Possible drug interactions with products recommended or used during the appointment.
- Certain medications may require frequent bathroom breaks.

▶ Vital signs

- Blood pressure is determined and recorded at each visit.

▶ Intraoral and extraoral examination

- The need for careful, periodic examination of the oral mucosa from lips to the throat is especially crucial for the older adult patient because oral cancer occurs with increasing frequency with advancing years.
- Many oral lesions exist without the patient being aware of them.
- Document lesions with accurate descriptions and comparisons over time (see Chapter 12).
- When indicated, patient referral for biopsy is planned with the patient.

III. Preventive Care Plan

▶ Older adult patients may need frequent appointments to maintain a high level of oral health.

▶ The content of a care plan will emphasize the control of dental biofilm and recommend fluoride use.

▶ Follow-up to determine complete care, healed gingival tissues, and meticulous daily biofilm removal.

▶ Give printed oral health instructions to partner or caregiver to be posted in bathroom or where the patient will be performing self-care.

IV. Dental Biofilm Control

▶ Implement the basic objectives of dental biofilm control.

▶ Infection needs to be eliminated and controlled.

▶ *Factors affecting adequate biofilm control*

- Patients with cognitive, mental, and physical deficits can provide a challenge to the dental hygienist.
- Gingival recession with wide embrasures resulting from periodontal destruction provides a larger surface area for biofilm retention.
- Exposed cementum with areas of abrasion or dental caries at the cervical third of a tooth can create undercut areas where special adaptation of biofilm removal devices is needed.
- Decreased saliva production reduces or eliminates the cleansing and lubricating effects of saliva.
- Exposed untreated cementum may hold biofilm more readily than enamel. A smooth root surface is less likely to hold biofilm therefore biofilm removal efforts can be more successful.
- Restorations and prostheses provide a more complex dentition and biofilm removal may require more time, patience, and motivation.
- Deficient restorations may have overhanging margins that provide areas for biofilm retention.
- Lack of dexterity related to disabling conditions resulting from chronic diseases, such as arthritis and Parkinson's disease, makes biofilm removal more difficult.

Table 53-2	Strategies for Enhancing Communication with the Older Adult Patient
Before the appointment	■ Schedule extra time for appointment ■ Ask patient to bring a list of medications
During the appointment	■ Provide a friendly greeting ■ Eye contact ■ Be an active listener ■ Speak slowly ■ Present information one topic at a time ■ Use visual aids ■ Have the patient repeat instructions
After the appointment	■ Provide written instructions

Source: Stein P, Aalboe J, Savage M, et al. Strategies for communicating with older dental patients. *J Am Dental Assoc*. 2014;145(2):159–164.

▶ *Approach to instruction*
- Strategies to enhance communication with the older adult patient are listed in Table 53-2.
- Suggestions for providing oral health instruction for the older adult with specific characteristics are listed in Table 53-3.
- Motivation through expression of sincere interest on the part of dental personnel can be an influencing factor in helping the patient to better health.
- Allow sufficient time; do not leave instructions until the end of the appointment. Keep session short and present small amounts of information at any one time.
- When appropriate, include the caregiver in instructions.
- Carefully assess the patient's ability to perform each technique. Avoid sudden changes or surprises.
- Base instruction on the patient's functional status.
- Determine what the patient already knows. Assist the older adult learner to relate new knowledge to past experiences.
- Make changes gradual over time.
- Repeated reinforcement and evaluation are critical.

TABLE 53-3	Strategies for Providing Oral Health Instruction for Older Adult Patient
CHARACTERISTIC OF THE OLDER ADULT PATIENT	**SUGGESTIONS FOR PATIENT INSTRUCTION**
Vision impaired	■ Provide adequate lighting. ■ Provide instructional materials in large print on nonglare paper. ■ Avoid instructional materials in blue and green colors. ■ For the patient who wears prescription eyeglasses, make sure the glasses are worn while instruction is being given. ■ Recommend that eyeglasses be worn at home while performing biofilm control procedures.
Hearing impaired loss of sensitivity to higher tones	■ Speak distinctly in a normal voice. ■ Look directly at patient while speaking; many are lip readers.
Hearing aid	■ Reduce background noise; turn off music. ■ Ask patient if they prefer to turn down or turn off the when the handpiece or ultrasonic is used.
Slowing of voluntary responses Slowing of speed of thought associations Rate of learning slowed, ability to learn not changed Changes in speed of vocalization	■ Make suggestions gradually, over a series of appointments. ■ Be realistic and practical with expectations; go slowly, anticipate difficulties, give cues and clues. ■ Distinguish between slowness of learning and inability to learn. ■ Lower the pitch of your voice
Memory difficulties	■ Provide written instruction; spoken instructions may be forgotten or misunderstood. ■ Provide repeated reinforcement. ■ Give instructions to caregivers.
Apparent frustration with diminished functional abilities	■ Acknowledge frustration; retain positive attitude; provide repeated reinforcement.
Symptoms of depression	■ Acknowledge feelings; positive attitude but avoid overly cheerful demeanor; repeated reinforcement. ■ Appropriate use of affective ("caring") touch.

► *Selection of dental biofilm removal devices*
  • Use of a power toothbrush may help patients with impaired hand function.
  • Power toothbrushes are often easier for caregivers to manage.
  • Adaptations to alter the handle of a manual brush are described in Chapter 57.
  • Interproximal brushes are recommended for open gingival embrasures. Methods for using interproximal brushes are described in Chapter 29.

► Dentifrice selection
  • Fluoride ingredient mandatory for all surfaces including prevention for root caries.
  • Mild abrasive agent to prevent abrasion of root surfaces.
  • Desensitizing ingredient for exposed dentinal tubules.

V. Relief for Xerostomia

► Provide specific instructions for use of a saliva substitute.

► Instruction and motivation techniques are applied gradually and regularly at frequent intervals for best results.

VI. Periodontal Care

The incidence and severity of periodontal diseases tend to increase with age as an effect of disease accumulation. The extent of periodontal destruction reflects the length of time the tissues have been exposed to disease-producing factors, primarily biofilm microorganisms.

► Implementation of periodontal care includes complete debridement of calculus and biofilm.

► Follow-up evaluation to assess the need for additional therapy is essential.

► The patient's cognitive, mental, or physical condition may necessitate shorter appointments.

► Quadrant non-surgical periodontal therapy with anesthesia may be appropriate.

VII. Dental Caries Control

► Assess diet; diet record covering several days.

► Diet adjustment to eliminate cariogenic foods and make appropriate substitutions.

► Emphasis on prevention of root caries.

► Professionally applied topical fluoride treatments: fluoride varnish.

► Daily self-applied fluoride therapy:
  • Fluoride dentifrice.
  • Fluoride rinses and gels; custom trays as applicable for a particular patient.

► Chlorhexidine rinses periodically for individuals with high bacterial counts; effective against *Mutans streptococcus* (Chapter 27).

► Xylitol chewing gum after meals and snacks for patients without chewing and swallowing difficulties.

VIII. Diet and Nutrition

► Dietary and resulting nutritional deficiencies are common in older people.

► Characteristic changes, such as burning tongue, angular cheilitis, and atrophic glossitis, may be related to vitamin B deficiencies.

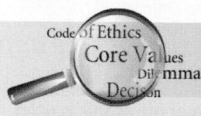

EVERYDAY ETHICS

Mr. and Mrs. Bracken were among Dr. Roberts' first patients when he began his practice almost 30 years ago. They keep a strict 4-month continuing care plan with the dental hygienist. Rosemary, the new hygienist, is looking forward to meeting and treating the Brackens for the first time as she has heard many wonderful things about this lovely older couple.

On completion of the oral examination with Mrs. Bracken, Rosemary recorded significant dental biofilm retention and evidence of xerostomia. She immediately begins to give the patient detailed homecare instructions and asks for a complete listing of medications Mrs. Bracken is taking for her arthritis, angina, and diabetes. Mrs. Bracken left the appointment confused and upset.

Questions for Consideration

1. Which of the ethical core values (Table II-1 in the Section II Introduction) apply in this scenario? Considering that Mrs. Bracken seemed overwhelmed at the end of her appointment, how may Rosemary have erred in her judgment of the patient and the instruction she gave? Suggest alternative approaches.

2. To ensure the autonomy of Mr. and Mrs. Bracken while acknowledging their longevity in the practice, how can the medical status of these patients be clarified?

3. Using the questions in Table VI-1 in Section VI Introduction outline at least three alternative care plans that Rosemary could have used for her appointment with Mrs. Bracken.

▶ Factors contributing to dietary and nutritional deficiencies include:
  • Limited budget.
  • Not eating regular meals; frequently using nonnutritious snacks.
  • Lack of interest in shopping for or preparing food.
  • Acuteness of senses (taste, smell) lowered; may seek highly seasoned or sweetened foods.
  • Inadequate masticatory efficiency because of tooth loss or dentures that no longer fit properly.
  • Adverse food selection may result from social embarrassment over inability to chew.
  • Following dietary fads that provide only a limited and unbalanced diet.
  • Difficulty in swallowing.
  • Alcoholism.

▶ Dietary/nutritional considerations for older adults include:
  • Reduced need for calorie intake as a result of decreased energy needs; to avoid overweight or obesity.
  • Protein, vitamins, minerals, and water are particularly important for body function, repair, and resistance to disease.
  • Increased need for calcium, vitamin D, and folate.

▶ A necessary objective in geriatric nutrition is to slow or prevent the progression of diet-induced chronic diseases. Examples are:
  • Atherosclerosis related to high dietary fat diets
  • Anemias related to iron and folic acid deficiencies
  • Osteoporosis resulting from inadequate intake of calcium and vitamin D.

▶ Fluoride intake over the years is beneficial in the prevention of osteoporosis and bone fractures, and water fluoridation is beneficial for direct application to the teeth.

▶ *Instruction in diet and oral health*
  • Dietary analysis by means of a 4- or 5-day record of the patient's diet can provide information to guide recommended changes.
  • Patients with cognitive and/or memory deficits may be unable to provide an accurate food diary. When possible, enlist the help of family members or caretakers.
  • Minimally, an accurate 24-hour food diary needs to be obtained.
  • Recommendations for older adult patients are based on establishing a well-balanced diet with limited amounts of cariogenic foods for dental caries prevention.
  • Provide patient with dietary educational materials.
  • Refer older adults with complex medical conditions to a registered dietitian nutritionist (RD/RDN).

▶ Patient motivation may be enhanced by discussing the relationship of dietary deficiencies to:
  • Lowered resistance to disease
  • Appearance (weight control)
  • Premature aging.

DOCUMENTATION

The permanent record for an older adult needs complete personal health history followed from initial appointment to include a minimum of the following:

▶ Detailed medical history
▶ Current vital signs
▶ History of medications
▶ Current radiographs with exposure records
▶ Extraoral and intraoral examination with particular emphasis on oral cancer and all pathology
▶ Dental history
▶ Detailed dental charting and periodontal clinical examination including record of probing depths, clinical attachment level, furcations, mobility, occlusion, calculus classification, and biofilm control record.
▶ For each professional visit, a summary of current findings and planned treatment as well as outcomes from previous appointment treatments
▶ A sample of documentation for an older adult dental visit may be reviewed in Box 53-7.

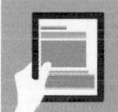

BOX 53-7

Example Documentation: Older Adult Patient with Xerostomia

S–A 78-year-old female presents for a 6 months continuing care appointment. Patient stated "I wake up in the middle of the night with my tongue sticking to the roof of my mouth. My tongue becomes sore."

O–Updating the medical health history, it is noted that the patient is taking a new antihypertensive medication called hydrochlorothiazide. During the intraoral examination, an observation is made of a decrease in the flow of saliva from the patient's three major salivary glands: the parotid, submandibular, and sublingual.

A–Significant decrease in salivary flow is most likely due to the new antihypertensive medication. No previous clinical notes have documentation of complaints of xerostomia from the patient or noted findings of xerostomia from the intraoral examination. Patient is at high risk for caries based on the ADA caries risk assessment tool.

P–Patient is given instructions for the management of xerostomia such as the use of saliva substitute and to drink plenty of water. Additional instructions provided specifically for biofilm control and 5% sodium fluoride gel was prescribed with instructions for use to manage increased risk of dental caries. Fluoride varnish was applied due to high caries risk.

Next step: Re-evaluate at the 3 month continuing care appointment.

Signed _____, RDH

Date _____

Factors To Teach The Patient

▷ To remember to tell the dentist and dental hygienist all changes in personal health, medical care received since the last appointment, and all changes in prescriptions.

▷ The interrelationship of the systemic and oral health.

▷ The dentition can last a lifetime. Daily preventive measures and a healthy lifestyle are essential.

▷ The value of a well-balanced diet with reduced calories and regular exercise to successful aging.

▷ Importance of drinking fluoridated water when it is available.

▷ Dental caries is a transmissible disease; therefore, it is urgent to have all cavitated lesions restored and dental biofilm cleaned from the teeth daily.

References

1. Manski RJ, Cohen LA, Brown E, et al. Dental service mix among older adults aged 65 and over, United States, 1999 and 2009. *J Public Health Dent.* 2014;74(3):219–226.

2. Whitbourne SK, Whitbourne SB. *Adult Development and Aging Biopsychosocial Perspectives.* 5th ed. Hoboken, NJ: John Wiley; 2014:6–7.

3. Govindaraju DR, Pencina KM, Raj DS, et al. A systems analysis of age-related changes in some cardiac aging traits. *Biogerontology.* 2014;15(2):139–152.

4. Lowery EM, Brubaker AL, Kuhlmann E, et al. The aging lung. *Clin Interv Aging.* 2013;8:1489–1496.

5. Chader GJ, Tayloe A. Preface: the aging eye: normal changes, age-related diseases, and sight-saving approaches. *Invest Opthalmol Vis Sci.* 2013;54(14):ORSF1–ORSF4.

6. Bainbridge KE, Wallhagen MI. Hearing loss in an aging American population: extent, impact, and management. *Annu Rev Public Health.* 2014;35:139–152.

7. Castelo-Branco C, Soveral I. The immune system and aging: a review. *Gynecol Endocrinol.* 2014;30(1):16–22.

8. Yam A, Marsiske M. Cognitive longitudinal predictors of older adults' self-reported IADL function. *J Aging Health.* 2013;25 (Suppl 8):163S–185S.

9. Naorungroi S, Schoenbach VJ, Beck J, et al. Cross-sectional associations of oral health measures with cognitive function in late middle-aged adults: a community-based study. *J Am Dent Assoc.* 2013;144(112):1362–1371.

10. Linden GJ, Lyons A, Scannapieco FA. Periodontal systemic associations review of the evidence. *J Periodontol.* 2013;84 (Suppl 4):S8–S19.

11. Patel MH, Kumar JV, Moss ME. Diabetes and tooth loss: an analysis of data from the National Health and Nutrition Examination Survey, 2003–2004. *J Am Dent Assoc.* 2013;144(5):478–485.

12. Kelly JT, Avila-Ortiz G, Allareddy V, et al. The association between periodontitis and coronary heart disease: a quality assessment of systematic reviews. *J Am Dent Assoc.* 2013;144(4):371–379.

13. Berkey D, Scannapieco F. Medical considerations relating to the oral health of older adults. *Spec Care Dentist.* 2013;33(4):164–178.

14. Griffin, SO, Jones JA, Brunson D, et al. Burden of oral disease among older adults and implications for public health priorities. *Am J Public Health.* 2012;102(3):411–418.

15. Uppoor AS, Lhi HS, Nayak D. Periodontitis and Alzheimer's disease: oral systemic link still on the rise? *Gerodontology* 2013;30:239–242.

16. Wang YP, Andrade LH. Epidemiology of alcohol and drug use in the elderly. *Curr Opin Psychiatry.* 2013;26(4):343–348.

17. Passos J, Gomes-Filho I, Vianna M, et al. Outcome measurements in studies on the association between osteoporosis and periodontal disease. *J Periodontol.* 2010;81(12):1773–1780.

18. Anil S, Preethanath RS, Almoharib HS, et al. Impact of osteoporosis and its treatment on oral health. *Am J Med Sci.* 2013;346(5):396–401.

19. Centers for Disease Control and Prevention. HIV among Older Americans. www.cdc.gov/hiv/risk/age/olderamericans/index.html. Accessed July 26, 2015.

20. Guneri P, Epstein J, Botto RW. Breaking bad medical news in a dental care setting. *J Am Dent Assoc.* 2013;144(4):381–386.

21. Vadiraj S, Nayak R, Choudhary GK, et al. Periodontal pathogens and respiratory diseases—evaluating their potential association: a clinical and microbiological study. *J Contemp Dent Pract.* 2013;14(4):610–615.

22. Stoopler ET, Nadeau S, Sollecito TP. How do I manage a patient with angular cheilitis? *J Can Dent Assoc.* 2013;79:d68.

23. Toffanello ED, Inelmen EM, Imoscopi A, et al. Taste loss in hospitalized multimorbid elderly subjects. *Clin Interv Aging.* 2013;8:167–174.

24. Wiener C, Wu B, Crout R, et al. Hyposalivation and xerostomia in dentate older adults. *J Am Dent Assoc.* 2010;141(3):279–284.

25. Villa A, Polimeni A, Strohmenger L, et al. Dental patient's self-reports of xerostomia and associated risk factors. *J Am Dent Assoc.* 2011;142(7):811–816.

26. Tranasi M, Sberna MT, Zizzari V, et al. Microarray evaluation of age-related changes in human dental pulp. *J Endod.* 2009;35(9):1211–1217.

27. Sequeira-Byron P, Lussi A. Prevention of root caries. *Evid Based Dent.* 2011;12(3):70–71.

28. Ghezzi EM. Developing pathways for oral care in elders: evidence-based interventions for dental caries prevention in dentate elders. *Gerodontology.* 2014;31 (Suppl 1):31–36.

29. Zander HA, Hurzeler B. Continuous cementum apposition. *J Dent Res.* 1958;37(6):1035–1044.

 ENHANCE YOUR UNDERSTANDING

thePoint® **DIGITAL CONNECTIONS**
(see the inside front cover for access information)
- **Audio glossary**
- **Quiz bank**

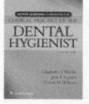 **SUPPORT FOR LEARNING**
(available separately; visit lww.com)
- *Active Learning Workbook for Clinical Practice of the Dental Hygienist, 12th Edition*

prepU **INDIVIDUALIZED REVIEW**
(available separately; visit lww.com)
- **Adaptive quizzing with *prepU for Wilkins' Clinical Practice of the Dental Hygienist***

54

The Edentulous Patient

Esther M. Wilkins, BS, RDH, DMD

CHAPTER OUTLINE

PURPOSES FOR WEARING DENTURES

TYPES OF REMOVABLE COMPLETE DENTURES

THE EDENTULOUS MOUTH
I. Bone
II. Mucous Membrane

THE PATIENT WITH NEW DENTURES
I. Patient Counseling
II. Postinsertion Care

DENTURE-RELATED ORAL CHANGES
I. Bone Changes
II. Oral Mucosal Changes

III. Effect of Xerostomia
IV. Sensory Changes

DENTURE-INDUCED ORAL LESIONS
I. Principal Causes of Lesions Under Dentures
II. Inflammatory Lesions
III. Ulcerative Lesions
IV. Papillary Hyperplasia
V. Denture Irritation Hyperplasia (Epulis Fissuratum)
VI. Angular Cheilitis

PREVENTION
I. Oral Hygiene and Denture Cleaning
II. Oral Mucosa
III. Rest for the Tissues

IV. Diet and Nutrition
V. Relief from Xerostomia

CONTINUING CARE

DENTURE MARKING FOR IDENTIFICATION
I. Criteria for an Adequate Marking System
II. Inclusion Methods for Marking
III. Surface Markers
VI. Information to Include on a Marker

DOCUMENTATION

EVERYDAY ETHICS

FACTORS TO TEACH THE PATIENT

REFERENCES

LEARNING OBJECTIVES

After studying this chapter, the student will be able to:

1. Identify causes and prevention of tooth loss.

2. Describe the anatomical features of an edentulous oral cavity.

3. Explain causes and prevention of denture-induced oral lesions.

4. Describe methods for marking a denture for permanent identification.

5. Outline a plan for continuing care for the patient with a complete denture.

► A fully edentulous patient has no teeth.

- Absence of teeth may be congenital or due to loss from a variety of causes such as a traumatic accident or lack of knowledge about disease prevention.
- Inadequate oral hygiene practices without professional dental and dental hygiene care may have resulted in progression of dental carious lesions and periodontal infections which result in removal of teeth.
- An edentulous patient may have dental implants to improve the function and stability of an overdenture dental prosthesis.

► A partially edentulous patient may have a complete denture opposing an arch with all natural teeth or various fixed or removable partial prostheses.

► Terminology related to the edentulous patient is defined in Box 54-1.

PURPOSES FOR WEARING DENTURES

► Replace missing teeth and adjacent structures.

► Presence of teeth has an esthetic role.

► Restore facial contour including lip support and temporomandibular joint position.

► Provide function.

► Enhance ability to eat a wider variety of healthy foods.

► Promote proper speech and enunciation.

TYPES OF REMOVABLE COMPLETE DENTURES[1]

► *Tissue-supported complete denture*: A removable dental prosthesis that replaces the entire dentition and associated structures of the maxilla or the mandible and rests on the denture foundation area, the mucosal-covered alveolar ridge.

► *Implant denture*: A complete dental prosthesis that is supported in part or whole by one or more dental implants. The denture itself is not an implantable device.

► *Overdenture*: A removable prosthesis that rests on one or more remaining natural teeth and/or dental implants (Figure 33-4 in Chapter 33). Also called an overlay prosthesis.

► *Interim denture prosthesis*: A removable dental prosthesis designed to enhance esthetics, stabilization, and/or function for a limited period, after which it is to be replaced by a definitive prosthesis.

- Often such prostheses are used to assist in determining the therapeutic effectiveness of a specific treatment plan or the form and function of the planned definitive prosthesis.
- Also called a provisional prosthesis.

► *Immediate denture*: A denture fabricated for placement immediately following the removal of a natural tooth or teeth.

- An immediate or interim denture tends to loosen after the significant remodeling of bone and soft tissue that follows surgery.

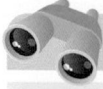

BOX 54-1   KEY WORDS: Edentulous Patient

Anodontia: a rare condition characterized by congenital absence of all teeth, primary and permanent.

Complete denture prosthodontics: that body of knowledge and skills pertaining to the restoration of the edentulous arch with a removable prosthesis.

Denture: an artificial substitute for missing natural teeth and adjacent tissues.

Complete denture: a complete removable dental prosthesis that replaces the entire dentition and associated structures of the maxilla or mandible.

Immediate denture: a complete denture fabricated for placement immediately following the removal of a natural tooth/teeth and/or other surgical preparation of the dental arches.

Overdenture: a removable denture that covers and is partially supported by one or more remaining natural teeth, roots, and/or dental implants and the soft tissue of the residual alveolar ridge; also called overlay denture.

Denture adhesive: a material used to adhere a denture to the oral mucosa.

Denture foundation area: the surfaces of the oral structures available to support a denture.

Denture placement: the process of directing a prosthesis to a desired oral location; introduction of a prosthesis into a patient's mouth; other terms used are denture delivery or denture insertion.

Exostosis: bony projection extending beyond the normal contour of a bony surface.

Implant prosthesis: any prosthesis supported and retained in part or whole by dental implants.

Prosthesis: an artificial replacement of an absent part of the human body. A therapeutic device to improve or alter function.

Dental prosthesis: artificial replacement of one or more teeth and/or associated dental/alveolar structures.

Resection: excision of a segment of any part.

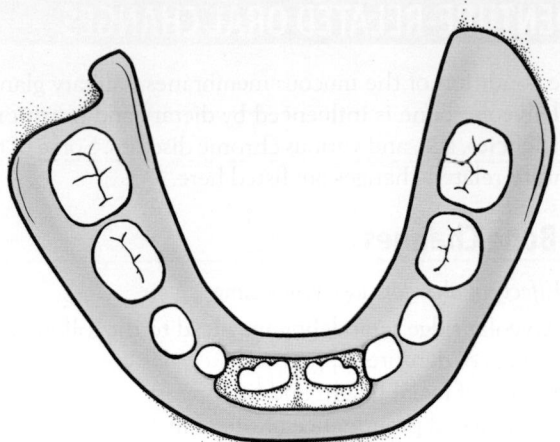

FIGURE 54-1 **Denture for a Young Child.** As permanent teeth erupt, parts of the denture are cut away. Shown is the denture alteration for the erupting permanent mandibular incisors.

- Temporarily, the denture may be relined with a soft liner or a tissue conditioning material.
- The patient may use a denture adhesive until the majority of healing occurs.
- After approximately 6 months, dentures are remade, relined, or rebased.
- *Denture for primary teeth*
  - Dentures occasionally must be constructed to replace primary teeth.
  - The teeth may be congenitally missing (anodontia) or may have been extracted due to rampant caries or trauma.
  - Early childhood dental caries can break down the teeth severely soon after eruption (Figures 50-2 and 50-5, Chapter 50).
  - To provide esthetics and function, dentures can be constructed for the accepting child who is able to cooperate.
  - As the permanent teeth begin to erupt, parts of the denture are cut away as in Figure 54-1.
  - A supervised dental caries prevention program is initiated for protection of the permanent dentition.

THE EDENTULOUS MOUTH

I. Bone

- *Residual ridges*
  - After the teeth are removed, the residual ridges enter into a continuing process of remodeling.
  - The alveolar bone, which had supported the teeth, undergoes resorption. The rate and amount of bony resorption vary with each individual.
  - Major bony changes occur during the first year after the teeth are removed, but changes continue throughout life.
  - Mandibular bone loss is generally as much as four times greater than maxillary bone loss.[2]

- Bone remodeling and soft tissue healing may make it necessary to have dentures rebased, relined, or remade at intervals.
- *Tori and exostoses*
  - Benign bony outgrowths may interfere with the fabrication and wearing of dentures.
  - Because of the size, shape, or location, excess bone often needs to be removed surgically before a denture can be constructed.
  - *Torus palatinus:* Bony enlargement located over the midline of the palate.
  - *Torus mandibularis:* Bony mass generally located on the lingual in the region of the premolars.
  - *Exostosis:* A bony protuberance generally located on the buccal aspects of maxilla and/or mandible.

II. Mucous Membrane

- *Composition: Mucosa*
  - Oral mucosa is composed of masticatory, lining, and specialized mucosa.
  - *Masticatory* mucosa covers the edentulous ridges and the hard palate. The mucous membrane covering the bony ridges is made up of two layers, the lamina propria and the surface-stratified squamous epithelium, which is keratinized in the healthy mouth.
  - *Lining* mucosa covers the floor of the mouth, vestibules, and cheeks.
  - *Specialized* mucosa covers the dorsal surface of the tongue and contains filiform, fungiform, and circumvallate papillae, as shown in Figure 12-5, Chapter 12.
- *Composition: Submucosa*
  - Underneath the mucous membrane is the submucosa, which is attached to the underlying bone.
  - Composed of connective tissue with vessels, nerves, adipose tissue, and glands.
  - The support or cushioning effect for the denture depends on the makeup of the submucosa, which varies in different parts of the mouth.
- *Tension test*
  - Examine the edentulous mouth by retracting the lips and cheeks using a tension test technique described in Chapter 18.
  - A line of demarcation similar to the mucogingival junction is apparent, separating the attached tissue over the bony ridge and the loose lining mucosa of the vestibule.
  - Frenal attachments can be observed.

THE PATIENT WITH NEW DENTURES

I. Patient Counseling

- *Preparation*
  - The preparation for denture insertion has to begin well in advance of the day the dentures are delivered.

- Becoming edentulous may be very emotional for a patient and requires effort to learn to adapt and function with the new prosthesis.
- Anticipatory guidance will help the patient gain a clear idea of what to expect and what procedures to follow.
- Successful after-care and denture satisfaction depend to a large extent on conditioning the patient to the adjustments to be made and to the period of practice and learning with the new dentures that can be expected.

▶ *Adjuncts*

Many dental teams prepare their own printed educational materials, whereas others use those available from outside sources.

II. Postinsertion Care

The preliminary counseling is followed through the initial postinsertion appointments to adjust the prosthesis, teach denture hygiene, and arrange for continuing care appointments.

▶ *Immediate denture*

- The patient is instructed to leave the immediate denture in place for 24–48 hours after tooth removal and surgery to aid in the control of bleeding and swelling.
- When the patient returns and the denture is removed, the mouth is rinsed and appropriate instructions are given.
- After initial healing, the denture care and other instructions are similar to those presented in Table 54-1.

▶ *New dentures over healed ridges*

- Following insertion, appointments are scheduled routinely because adjustments can be expected.
- The first appointment is made within 24–48 hours of the time of insertion.
- Additional appointments are made in as needed for each individual patient.

▶ *Instructions*[3]

- Many verbal instructions given on the day of insertion may confuse the patient; limit instruction to basic denture care and other procedures of immediate concern. Slow repetition over several sessions helps the patient to develop adequate denture management and hygiene habits.
- Written instruction can be helpful for the patient.
- Basic information for the new denture wearer is provided in Table 54-1.
- Denture cleaning methods are described with other biofilm control procedures for the care of dental prostheses in Chapter 32.

DENTURE-RELATED ORAL CHANGES

The condition of the mucous membranes, salivary glands, and alveolar bone is influenced by dietary and nutritional deficiencies, age, and various chronic diseases. Some of the denture-related changes are listed here.

I. Bone Changes

▶ *Effects of alveolar ridge remodeling*

Alveolar ridge remodeling may lead to the following:
- Loss of denture support
- Loss of facial height and lip support
- Increased prominence of the chin
- Temporomandibular joint manifestations
- Occlusal disharmony

▶ *Compensations by the patient*

- Patients may adapt to the bone changes by compensating in the way they wear and manage the dentures.
- Other patients may resort to drug store remedies, such as pads, adhesives, or self-reline materials, which can be detrimental if used improperly.
- Denture adhesives cannot be used to compensate for a poorly designed, poorly constructed, or ill-fitting denture.

▶ *Treatment by the dentist*

- Dentures need adjusting, repairing, relining, rebasing, or remaking periodically.
- Patients are instructed to seek professional care if any issues relating to denture or oral health arise between scheduled continuing care appointments.

II. Oral Mucosal Changes

▶ *Tissue reaction*

- Tissue reaction under a denture varies considerably among individuals.
- One mouth may have thinning of the mucosa, submucosa, and, particularly, the epithelium with an absence of keratinization, and another may have normal keratinization or hyperkeratinization.

▶ *Factors that influence the mucosa*

- Systemic conditions that alter host response
- Aging mucosa tends to become thinner
- Denture and tissue hygiene
- Wearing the denture constantly
- Xerostomia
- Fit and occlusion of the denture itself.

III. Effect of Xerostomia[4]

▶ The causes of xerostomia include:
- Sjogren's syndrome
- Drugs or medications
- Radiation therapy to the oral area.

TABLE 54-1	Patient Instruction for Complete Dentures

ITEM	FACTORS TO TEACH

Food selection	■ Use foods from the MyPlate Food Guide (Figure 35-1). Check each day's diet to fulfill needs for a balanced diet appropriate for each individual patient.
	■ Select foods to prevent nutrient deficiencies and diet-induced chronic diseases.
	■ New denture wearer:
	  • Avoid foods, such as an apple, which need to be incised (bitten through using anterior teeth).
	  • Avoid raw vegetables, fibrous meats, and sticky foods until experience has been gained.
	  • Cut food into small pieces.
	■ Practiced denture wearer:
	  • Select a variety of foods, but do not expect the same chewing efficiency as with the previous denture.

Incision or biting	■ Use the canine and premolar area. Insert for biting at the angle of the mouth. ■ Push back as the food is incised; do not pull or tear the food in a forward direction.
Chewing	■ Take small portions. ■ Try to chew with some food on each side at the same time to stabilize the denture. ■ Be patient, chew slowly, and practice.
Salivary flow	■ Anticipate an increased flow of saliva when a new denture is worn.
Speaking	■ Speak slowly and quietly. ■ Practice by reading aloud at home, preferably in front of a mirror. ■ Repeat and practice words that seem the most difficult.
Sneezing, coughing, yawning	■ Anticipate loss of denture retention. ■ Cover mouth with hand and handkerchief.
Denture hygiene	■ Thoroughly clean dentures at least twice each day. ■ Immerse dentures in chemical solution and brush for biofilm removal; rinse thoroughly. ■ Complete denture care is described in Chapter 32. ■ Devices to aid a person with a disability to clean the denture are shown in Chapter 57.
Mucosa	■ Tissues need to rest each day; consult dentist regarding whether it is best to leave the denture out while sleeping or during an alternative time period. ■ Brush and massage the mucosa to clean away biofilm and debris and stimulate circulation.
Storage of dentures	■ After careful cleaning to remove all bacterial biofilm, store the denture in water (or cleaning solution) in a covered container. ■ Place in a safe place inaccessible to children or house pets. ■ Change water or cleaning solution daily and wash the container.
Over-the-counter products	■ Never attempt to alter the denture for relief of discomfort. ■ Do not buy and use self-reline materials, adhesives, or other additives without consulting the dentist. They may be harmful to the dentures and/or the oral tissues. ■ Consult the dentist for advice about all denture problems.
Continuing care	■ Understand the importance of the dentist's examination of the denture fit, occlusion, wear, and the condition of the oral mucosa, routinely. ■ First year: expect reline, rebase, or remake of dentures because bone remodeling is greatest during the first year after extraction. ■ Subsequent appointments: an examination each year for most patients, provided the denture hygiene is ideal; patients with increased risk for oral cancer need an examination every 3 mo.
Seek care	■ Report any concerns, changes, or problems immediately. ■ Dentures may need adjustments to correct occlusion or traumatic sore spots.

▶ Diminished salivary flow can influence denture retention and tissue lubrication, as well as reduce the resistance of the oral mucosa to trauma and infection.

▶ *Lubrication*: The oral mucosa needs saliva for protection against frictional irritation by the denture.

▶ *Retention*: The film of saliva between the denture and the mucosa contributes to retention and suction of the denture.

IV. Sensory Changes

▶ *Tactile sense*
  • With the dentures in place, sensitivity to small objects in the mouth, such as small bones or bits of nuts may be diminished.
  • Proprioception, which signals how hard to chew and when to stop biting, is lost due to the absence of periodontal ligaments.

▶ *Taste*
  • Patients may indicate that food has a different taste since they have been wearing dentures.
  • Taste buds that are located in the tongue papillae are not affected by the dentures.
  • Taste buds of the palate are covered by a maxillary denture and therefore are ineffective for taste and temperature perception.
  • Dentures may develop thick odoriferous biofilm, which can alter food flavors, if not kept meticulously clean.

DENTURE-INDUCED ORAL LESIONS

When the mouth is examined extraorally and intraorally, the dentures are removed and the mucosa is examined carefully and thoroughly.

▶ A patient may report an area that has been sensitive to help call attention to a lesion.

▶ A patient may be unaware of chronic mucosal lesions, which are often asymptomatic.

▶ Because tissue changes can be important indicators of serious disease, such as oral cancer, the intraoral examination must be conducted thoroughly with good illumination.

I. Principal Causes of Lesions Under Dentures

The factors that singly or in combination cause most oral lesions under dentures are:

▶ *Ill-fitting dentures*
  • Because tissue changes under dentures can occur gradually over a long period, the patient may not be aware of developing disease.
  • The patient may not have been informed of the significance of having regular professional examinations of the dentures and the oral mucosa.

▶ *Inadequate oral hygiene*
  • Dentures and the oral mucosa need daily care.
  • Neglected dentures can accumulate heavy biofilm and calculus that may irritate the mucosa and cause infection and inflammation.

▶ *Continuous wearing of dentures*
  • Dentures need to be removed for a period each day so that the mucosa can have a rest from the pressure of the hard acrylic during occlusion, bruxism, and clenching.
  • A rest period allows the tissue to recover in its natural environment, where the tongue and saliva provide a cleansing effect.

II. Inflammatory Lesions

▶ *Contributing factors*

The following may occur alone or in combination:
  • Denture trauma from the fit, occlusion, or parafunctional habits
  • Inadequate denture hygiene and care of the mucosa
  • Chemotoxic effect from residual cleansing paste or solution not thoroughly rinsed from the denture
  • Allergy to the denture base (rare)
  • Continuous denture wearing without relief for the tissues
  • Patient self-treatment with over-the-counter products for relining
  • Tolerance of the tissues to trauma and resistance to infection can be reduced, for example, with nutritional deficiencies, immunosuppression such as chemotherapy, and systemic diseases such as diabetes.

▶ *Localized inflammation (sore spots)*
  • *Appearance*: isolated, red, inflamed area, sometimes ulcerated.
  • *Contributing factors*: trauma from an ill-fitting denture, a rough spot on a denture surface, a tongue bite, or a foreign object caught under the denture.

▶ *Generalized inflammation, Candida albicans infection*[5]

Oral candidiasis in the form of *denture stomatitis* is a reoccurring disease common to denture wearers and may be characterized by the following:
  • Generalized redness, inflamed mucosa of the tissues that support the denture
  • Burning sensation
  • Discomfort
  • Unpleasant taste
  • Denture wearer may be unaware the condition is present.

▶ Etiologic factors include the following:
  • Trauma from ill-fitting, usually maxillary, denture
  • Continuous denture wearing
  • Reduced salivary flow
  • Lack of denture cleanliness
  • Aging dentures have surface texture favorable to attachment of biofilm.

- Treatment may include:
  - Denture adjustments or fabrication of new denture
  - Antifungal medication
  - Massaging the tissues.
- Patients with the following are more prone to oral candidiasis:
  - Depressed immune system
  - History of head and neck radiation therapy
  - Antibiotic use.

III. Ulcerative Lesions

- Localized ulcerated lesions can be related to an overextended denture border.
- The ulcer may resemble a cancerous lesion and need to be biopsied when it persists longer than expected of a healing traumatic ulcer (7–14 days) after the denture is adjusted.

IV. Papillary Hyperplasia[4,6]

- *Appearance*
  - Inflammatory papillary hyperplasia is located on the palate, rarely outside the confines of the bony ridges (Figure 54-2A).
  - The overall lesion appears as a group of closely arranged, pebble-shaped, red, edematous projections (Figure 54-2B).
- *Contributing factors*
  - The cause is unknown.
  - Associated with poor denture hygiene, ill-fitting dentures, and possible *C. albicans* infection.

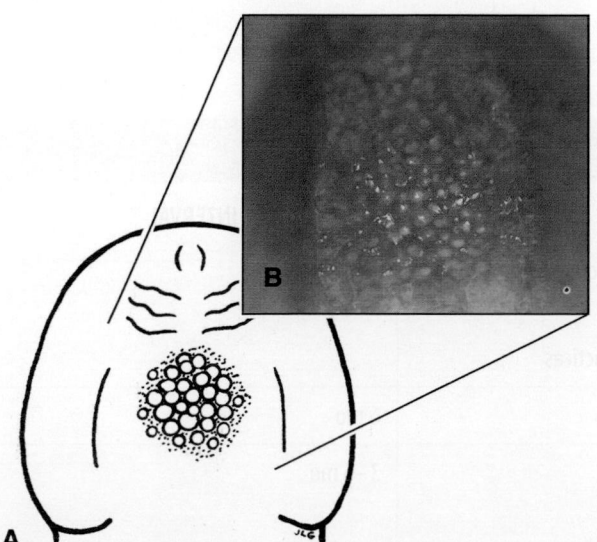

FIGURE 54-2 Papillary Hyperplasia. A: Outline of an edentulous palate shows the characteristic location of papillary hyperplasia within the bony ridges. **B:** Photograph of inflammatory papillary hyperplasia on hard palate. Courtesy of Michael Kahn, DDS, Chairperson, Oral Pathology, Tufts University, School of Dental Medicine.

V. Denture Irritation Hyperplasia (Epulis Fissuratum)[6]

- Long-standing chronic inflammatory tissue appears as tissue growth over the alveolar ridges.
- The etiology is often multifactorial and may include poor oral self-care, smoking, and ill-fitting dentures.
- It may be treated by surgical removal by scalpel or laser.

VI. Angular Cheilitis

- *Appearance*
  - Fissuring at the angles of the mouth, with cracks, ulcerations, and erythema.
  - Moist with saliva or sometimes dry with a crust.
- *Contributing factors[7]*
  - Local factors including contact dermatitis, allergy, and infection by *C. albicans* or other organisms are most common.
  - Irritation from saliva is associated with anatomical changes that make the folds at the corners of the mouth deeper and more pronounced.
  - Overclosure from loss of vertical dimension of occlusion is a common cause of angular cheilitis.
  - Malnutrition with deficiencies in B vitamins and iron can further complicate angular cheilitis, particularly in debilitated and dependent elder patients.[8]
- Prescription antifungal medication may be indicated.

PREVENTION[9]

I. Oral Hygiene and Denture Cleaning

- Dentures are cleaned after each meal, as described in Chapter 32.
- Cleansing solutions are changed daily.

II. Oral Mucosa

- Brush to clean and massage.
- Perform digital massage.

III. Rest for the Tissues

- Recommend the patient remove the dentures overnight to reduce the incidence of oral lesions.[9]
  - The temporomandibular joint will need to be carefully monitored because it could become symptomatic from lack of support from the denture overnight.
  - The patient may prefer not to remove the denture overnight and may prefer a time during the day, such as while bathing.
  - Place dentures in a container with cleaning solution when out of the mouth.
  - Clean and massage the underlying mucosa.

IV. Diet and Nutrition

▶ Patients who wear dentures need dietary counseling to assist them in maintaining a healthy diet.
  • Emphasize foods from the basic food groups as shown in MyPlate, Figure 35-1, Chapter 35.
  • Recommendations need to focus on maintaining a healthy weight and avoidance of cariogenic beverages and snacks between meals.
  • A dietary analysis can provide a foundation for making specific recommendations.

▶ Diet concerns for the older adult patient are described in Chapter 53.

▶ Factors that contribute to dietary deficiencies in patients of any age are magnified when dentures are ill fitting or painful, and masticatory efficiency is decreased.

▶ The patient tends to overlook nutrient dense food choices and select soft foods that are easier to chew or can be swallowed without chewing.

▶ Learning to adapt to an initial denture may affect nutrition. Patient can be instructed to attempt small amounts of a soft diet to relearn to chew.

V. Relief from Xerostomia[4]

▶ Use of saliva substitutes may be recommended.

▶ Hydration can be improved by increasing water intake; especially during meals if swallowing is a problem.

▶ To relieve xerostomia symptoms, recommend use of gels, mouthrinses, and toothpastes specifically formulated to moisturize, lubricate, buffer acids, and provide salivary enzymes like lactoperoxidase.[10]

▶ Use xylitol or sugarless mints, and other sugar-free snacks.

CONTINUING CARE

▶ *Continuing care*
  • The edentulous patient requires regular continuing care appointments for evaluation of the oral tissues and potentially pathology screening.
  • Regular continuing care appointments include evaluation of the fit and function of the prostheses, supervision of daily biofilm control for dentures, as well as care of the soft tissues.
  • After the initial adjustments, the patient may need reline, rebase, or remake of dentures in 6 months to 1 year.
  • Frequency of continuing care appointments is determined by individual needs and risk factors, as listed in Table 54-2.
  • Patients are encouraged to seek care at any time if discomfort or concerns arise with the denture or any tissue area.

▶ *Procedures*
  • Review patient history; make necessary additions to the record.
  • Determine vital signs.
  • Perform an extraoral and intraoral examination.
  • Examine dentures for cleanliness and evidence of patient care.
  • Ask patient to demonstrate the personal hygiene care procedures used routinely.
  • Supplement with additional demonstration and instruction when the care is less than adequate.
  • Clean the dentures to remove calculus and stain.

▶ *Procedures for the dentist*
  • Review the complete assessment.
  • Examine the oral tissues and the fit and occlusion of the dentures.

TABLE 54-2	Continuing Care Recommendations	
RISK LEVEL	**DESCRIPTION OF PATIENT**	**APPOINTMENT INTERVAL**
Low risk	▪ Healthy individual, healthy life-style and diet, no systemic disease ▪ No tobacco or alcohol use ▪ Impeccable denture care and hygiene practices	6–12 mo
Moderate risk	▪ All patients in between low and high risk	6 mo
High risk	▪ Daily tobacco and alcohol use ▪ Previous history of cancer ▪ Systemic diseases such as diabetes ▪ Medication use such as immunosupressants or those that cause xerostomia ▪ Continuously wears denture ▪ Any remaining natural teeth and/or implants	3–6 mo

- *Subsequent appointment*
  - Make necessary appointments for continuing current treatment.
  - All tissues must be examined at least annually for oral cancer screening and other changes indicative of oral or systemic disease.

DENTURE MARKING FOR IDENTIFICATION[11]

The need for denture marking is apparent in a variety of situations. A universal system for marking would be ideal. Marking is required by law in some countries and in most states of the United States.

- In forensic dentistry, or for identification of victims of war, such disasters as flood or fire, or transportation catastrophes, the dentition has been used increasingly as a means of identification.
- Dentures provide a method for immediate identification. Prompt identification can be urgent when an individual is found unconscious from illness or injury or is suffering from amnesia as a result of psychiatric or traumatic causes, as well as from Alzheimer's disease.
- The dentures of people in long-term residence or care facilities must be marked. Mislaid dentures can be returned, and mix-ups by the direct care staff can be prevented. An important contribution to an oral health program is to introduce a plan for denture marking.

I. Criteria for an Adequate Marking System

Information on the denture must be specific so that rapid identification is possible.

- *Relative to the denture*
  - Must have no adverse effects on denture material.
  - Must not change the strength, surface texture, or fit of the denture.
  - Must be cosmetically acceptable; the label must be placed in an unobtrusive position.
- *Relative to the procedure*
  - Readily learned and simple to carry out
  - Inexpensive
  - Durable result. When the information is incorporated during denture processing, indefinite durability can be expected. A surface marker for a denture already in use needs to be able to withstand denture-cleaning methods for a reasonable period of time.
- *Characteristics of the material used*
  - *Fire and humidity resistant*: When the label is placed inside the posterior section of a denture, the surrounding tongue and maxillofacial parts offer protection except in the most severe conflagration.
  - *Radiopaque*: A metal marker can be of use as a means of identification by radiographic examination in the

event the radiolucent acrylic denture is accidentally swallowed.

II. Inclusion Methods for Marking[11]

Inclusion methods are more permanent, but tend to be more expensive, require special equipment, and require trained personnel.

- *ID-Band*
  - A shallow indentation is made on the denture for a stainless steel metal band containing the patient identification and covered with clear acrylic resin.
  - The Swedish ID-Band is the international standard.
- *ID-Strip*
  - Identification information can be placed on the surface of the impression to be incorporated when the denture is fabricated (Figure 54-3).
- *Electronic microchip*
  - A microchip can be incorporated in the denture because of the small size and esthetic acceptability.
  - They have a higher cost than other methods and can only be inscribed by the manufacturer.
- *Laser etching*
  - Copper vapor laser has been used to mark dentures with metal frameworks, removable partial dentures, and other metallic restorations.
  - This method is expensive and requires specialized equipment and personnel.
- *Radio-frequency identification (RFID) tags*
  - RFID tags are small and can be incorporated into the denture resin.
  - They permit rapid identification and can store large amounts of data.
  - Not widely used due to the high cost.

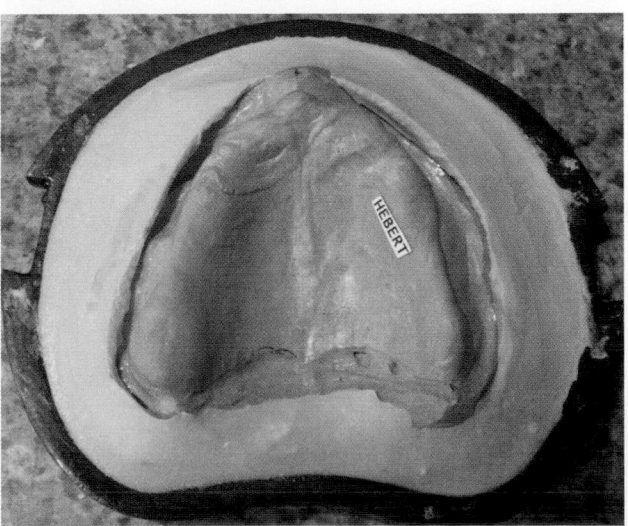

FIGURE 54-3 Inclusion Marker for New Denture. The label is inserted on the impression surface as the denture is being processed.

▶ *Bar codes*
  • Bar codes can be printed on silk and incorporated into a denture with clear acrylic resin.
  • A disadvantage is that it requires expensive special equipment.

III. Surface Markers

Surface markers are not as durable, but instruction can be provided for persons not trained in dental laboratory methods. In a skilled nursing facility or other long-term institution that has no resident dentist or dental hygienist, it may be possible to teach a nurse or other staff member to mark dentures of residents as they are admitted. The methods described as follows have been used for this purpose.

▶ *Indelible pen or ballpoint*
  • After cleaning and drying the denture, a small area near the posterior of the outer or polished denture surface is rubbed with an emery board until it is rough (Figure 54-4).
  • Name, initials, or other identification is printed on the roughened area with an indelible pen and dried.
  • Two or three coats of a fingernail acrylic (heavy nail protector) are painted over the area; each layer is dried before applying the next.
  • Surface markings have been found to last up to 6 months.
  • Light-cured materials may also be used.

▶ *Engraving tool or dental bur*
  • An engraving tool or round dental bur may be used to enter the name on the denture.
  • The engraving should be covered with a denture acrylic and processed to provide a smooth surface that will not retain food debris.

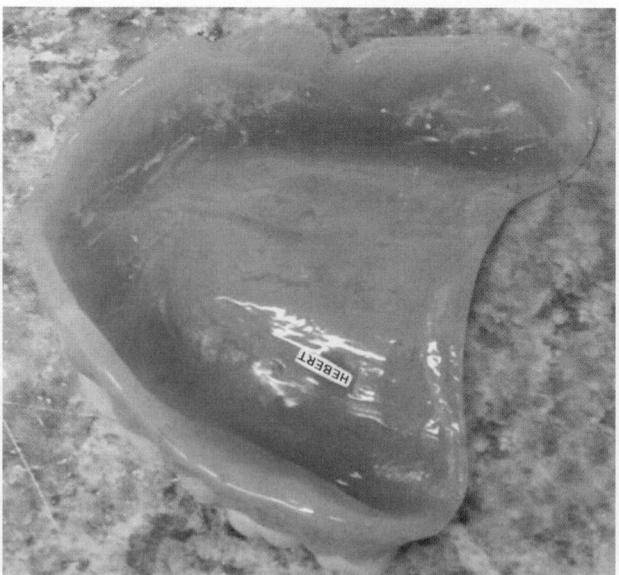

FIGURE 54-4 Surface Markers for Dentures. The labels are placed on the denture surfaces for existing dentures.

IV. Information to Include on a Marker

▶ For residents of a home or institution, using only the person's name and initials can suffice for temporary surface marking.

▶ In a community, country, or international situation, the name alone would not provide enough identification, and the social security number, armed services serial number, or the equivalent in other countries have been included.

▶ Other identification, such as blood type and vital drug or disease condition, has been suggested.

▶ In certain countries, the dentist's registration or hospital number has been used. In Sweden, the patient's date of birth and national registration number have been marked on the dentures.

▶ Markings that can provide *immediate* identification are the most significant.

DOCUMENTATION

Every appointment for a patient wearing a denture or having one made or repaired needs a carefully prepared progress note in the patient's permanent record to include a minimum of the following:

BOX 54-2

Example Documentation: Denture-Related Lesion

S –Female patient presents for routine continuing care; has worn complete maxillary and mandibular dentures for several years now. Chief complaint: soreness under left mandibular denture area for past week.

O –Patient history review no changes; BP 130/65; no MD visits or other health problems. Oral examination showed red lesion (2 mm × 3 mm) on lingual side of maxillary ridge in area of 1st molar. Internal surfaces of both dentures were clean. Calculus was noted on buccal surfaces of maxillary molars and lingual surfaces of mandibular anterior teeth.

A –Dr Frye examined and recommended referral to Dr. Snow the pathologist for an examination and possibly a biopsy. Completed the necessary forms; called and made the appointment before she left.

P –Cleaned the dentures, including calculus removal. Discussed home-cleaning agents used for dentures and frequency. Advised to be careful while rinsing of dentures after using cleaning agents as well as after soaking agents when dentures are out all night. Will call her when biopsy report is available—probably within a week.

Signed _____ , RDH

Date _____

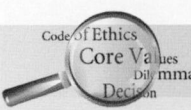

EVERYDAY ETHICS

Mr. Ryan presents for his yearly denture examination and oral cancer screening. He faithfully keeps his appointment every year because the cigarette stains build up on his full upper and lower dentures and he likes the way his dental hygienist, Kaitlin, gets them very clean.

During this visit, Kaitlin notices a small area on the alveolar ridge under the denture near the area of tooth #29. Mr. Ryan is aware of the lesion and sometimes doesn't wear his lower denture, but he indicates that it doesn't really bother him. Kaitlin informs Mr. Ryan that she will ask the dentist to check the area. Mr. Ryan becomes annoyed at her concern. He clearly states he is in a hurry and he just wants to have his denture cleaned and to leave.

Questions for Consideration

1. Since Mr. Ryan has been a heavy smoker for over 40 years, what actions are indicated to document and evaluate the lesion? Which of the core values (Table II-1, in Section II) are evident in this scenario?

2. Is Kaitlin facing an ethical issue or a dilemma? What are Kaitlin's ethical obligations to the patient in communicating the possible serious nature of her findings?

3. Study the questions in Table VI-1 in Section VI to determine possible avenues Kaitlin may take if Mr. Ryan leaves the office without having the lesion evaluated.

▶ Changes in the health history, vital signs, and findings from a careful extra- and intraoral examinations.

▶ Patient reports of tissue changes or difficulty with a denture.

▶ Observation of the denture, fixed or removable, to make necessary changes in the patient's daily care of the denture; new instruction with additional devices or cleaning materials when necessary.

▶ A sample progress note may be reviewed in Box 54-2.

Factors To Teach The Patient

▷ Dentures are not permanent prostheses.

▷ Dentures and tissues must be examined at least once a year for care of the tissue-supported removable prosthesis; for the implant-supported prosthesis and those at higher risk for disease, more frequently.

▷ Why the frequency of maintenance appointments depends, in part, on the individual's ability to clean the dentures and maintain them free of biofilm, stain, and calculus.

▷ Dentures may need replacement periodically. Tissues under the denture change.

▷ Why use of drugstore remedies, reliners, and other home-applied materials is avoided unless the dentist has provided specific instruction.

▷ Specific methods of care for dentures.

▷ Why dentures need to be left out of the mouth overnight in accord with the dentist's directions.

▷ Where to obtain and how to use a saliva substitute.

References

1. Academy of Prosthodontics Foundation. The glossary of prosthodontic terms. *J Prosthet Dent.* 2005;94(1):10–92.

2. Tallgren A. The continuing reduction of the residual alveolar ridges in complete denture wearers: a mixed-longitudinal study covering 25 years. *J Prosthet Dent.* 2003;89(5):427–435.

3. Gallagher JB. Insertion and postinsertion care. In: Clark JW, ed. *Clinical Dentistry.* Vol 5. 5th rev ed. Philadelphia, PA: Lippincott; 1984:1–27.

4. Turner M, Jahangiri L, Ship JA. Hyposalivation, xerostomia and the complete denture: a systematic review. *J Am Dent Assoc.* 2008;139(2):146–150.

5. Ramage G, Tomsett K, Wickes BL, et al. Denture stomatitis: a role for Candida biofilms. *Oral Surg Oral Med Oral Pathol Oral Radiol Endod.* 2004;98(1):53–59.

6. de Arruda Paes-Junior TJ, Cavalcanti SC, Nascimento DF, et al. CO(2) Laser surgery and prosthetic management for the treatment of epulis fissuratum. *ISRN Dent.* 2011;2011:282361.

7. Park KK, Brodell RT, Helms SE. Angular cheilitis, part 1: local etiologies. *Cutis.* 2011;87(6):289–295.

8. Park KK, Brodell RT, Helms SE. Angular cheilitis, part 2: nutritional, systemic, and drug-related causes and treatment. *Cutis.* 2011;88(1):27–32.

9. Felton D, Cooper L, Duqum I, et al. Evidence-based guidelines for the care and maintenance of complete dentures: a publication of the American College of Prosthodontists. *J Am Dent Assoc.* 2011;142 (Suppl 1):1S–20S.

10. Aliko A, Alushi A, Tafaj A, et al. Evaluation of the clinical efficacy of Biotène Oral Balance in patients with secondary Sjögren's syndrome: a pilot study. *Rheumatol Int.* 2012;32(9):2877–2881.

11. Datta P, Sood S. The various methods and benefits of denture labeling. *J Forensic Dent Sci.* 2010;2(2):53–58.

ENHANCE YOUR UNDERSTANDING

thePoint® DIGITAL CONNECTIONS
(see the inside front cover for access information)
- Audio glossary
- Quiz bank

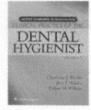

SUPPORT FOR LEARNING
(available separately; visit lww.com)
- *Active Learning Workbook for Clinical Practice of the Dental Hygienist, 12th Edition*

prepU INDIVIDUALIZED REVIEW
(available separately; visit lww.com)
- Adaptive quizzing with *prepU for Wilkins' Clinical Practice of the Dental Hygienist*

55

The Oral and Maxillofacial Surgery Patient

Esther M. Wilkins, BS, RDH, DMD and Deborah Manne, RDH, RN, MSN, OCN

CHAPTER OUTLINE

LEARNING OBJECTIVES

After studying the chapter, the reader will be able to:

1. Discuss the role of the dental hygienist in the pre- and postsurgery care of the oral and maxillofacial surgery patient.

2. Discuss pre- and postsurgical care planning for the maxillofacial surgery patient.

3. Identify types of maxillary and mandibular fractures and discuss treatment options.

4. Describe modifications for dental hygiene treatment, diet, and personal oral care procedures needed after maxillofacial surgery.

5. Explain dental hygiene care needed before and after general surgery.

Oral and maxillofacial surgery is the specialty of dentistry that includes diagnostic, surgical, and adjunctive treatment of diseases, injuries, and defects involving both functional and aesthetic aspects of the hard and soft tissues in the oral and maxillofacial regions.[1] Box 55-1 lists types of treatment included in this specialty.

▶ The oral surgeon may be based in a group clinical setting, in a hospital, or in a private practice with outpatient hospital facilities available.

▶ The oral surgeon is part of a team of specially trained individuals that includes surgical assistants, anesthetists, registered nurses, and dental hygienists.

▶ Terminology relating to maxillofacial surgery is defined in Box 55-2.

▶ The oral surgeon may coordinate the surgical procedures with various dental practitioners, including general dentists, prosthodontists, orthodontists, dental implant specialists, and other specialists caring for the patient.

▶ Surgery for treatment of diseases and correction of defects of the periodontal tissues is categorized specifically as *periodontal surgery*.

　• Within the scope of periodontal surgery are procedures for pocket elimination, gingivoplasty, treatment of furcation involvements, correction of mucogingival defects, treatment for bony defects about the teeth, and placing implants.

　• Preparation for periodontal surgery is not specifically described in this chapter.

BOX 55-1

Categories of Oral and Maxillofacial Treatments

DENTOALVEOLAR SURGERY

Exodontics

Impacted tooth removal

Alveolar bone surgery: alveoloplasty

INFECTION

Abscesses

Osteomyelitis

TRAUMATIC INJURY

Fractures of jaws, zygoma

Fracture of teeth, alveolar bone

NEOPLASM

Cysts

Tumors

DENTAL IMPLANT PLACEMENT

PREPROSTHETIC RECONSTRUCTION

Maxillofacial prosthetics

Immediate denture

ORTHOGNATHIC SURGERY

Prognathism correction

Facial aesthetics

CLEFT LIP/PALATE

TEMPOROMANDIBULAR DISORDERS

SALIVARY GLAND OBSTRUCTION

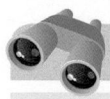

BOX 55-2　　KEY WORDS: Oral and Maxillofacial Surgery

Comminution: act of breaking or condition of being broken into small fragments.

Ecchymosis: a hemorrhagic spot, larger than a petechia, in the skin or mucous membrane caused by extravasation of blood; forms a nonelevated, rounded, or irregular purplish patch.

Exodontics: branch of dentistry dealing with the surgical removal of teeth.

Exostosis: benign new growth projecting from the surface of bone.

Intermaxillary fixation: fixation of the maxilla in occlusion with the mandible held in place by means of wires and elastic bands; the healing parts are stabilized following fracture or surgery.

Maxillofacial: pertaining to the jaws and the face.

Maxillofacial prosthetics: the branch of prosthodontics concerned with the restoration of the mouth and jaws and associated facial structures that have been affected by disease, injury, surgery, or a congenital defect.

Orthognathic surgery: surgery to alter relationships of the dental arches and/or supporting bone; usually coordinated with orthodontic therapy.

Orthognathics: science dealing with the causes and treatment of malposition of the bones of the jaws.

Osteosynthesis: internal fixation of a fracture by mechanical means, such as metal plates, pins, or screws.

　Miniplate osteosynthesis: a method of internal fixation of mandibular fractures utilizing miniaturized metal plates and screws formerly made of titanium or stainless steel and currently made primarily of biodegradable or resorbable synthetic materials.

Trismus: motor disturbance of the trigeminal nerve with spasm of masticatory muscles and difficulty in opening the mouth (lockjaw).

PATIENT PREPARATION

I. Objectives

Dental hygiene care and instruction before oral and maxillofacial surgery may improve a patient's health and well-being by one or more of the following:

A. Reduce Oral Bacterial Count

▶ Aid in the preparation of an aseptic field for the surgery.

▶ Make postsurgical infection less likely or less severe.

B. Reduce Inflammation of the Gingiva and Improve Tissue Tone

▶ Lessen local bleeding at the time of the surgery.

▶ Promote postsurgical healing.

C. Remove Calculus Deposits

▶ Remove a source of dental biofilm retention and thus improve gingival tissue tone.

▶ Prevent interference with placement of surgical instruments.

▶ Prevent pieces of calculus from breaking away.

- Danger of inhalation, particularly when a general anesthetic is used.
- Possibility of calculus falling into a tooth socket or other surgical area and acting as a foreign body to inhibit healing.

D. Instruct in Presurgical Personal Oral Care Procedures

▶ Reduce inflammation and thus improve tissue tone.

▶ Help to prepare the patient for postsurgical care.

E. Instruct in the Use of Foods

▶ Foods that provide the elements essential to tissue building and repair during pre- and postsurgical periods.

▶ For the patient who will have teeth removed and immediate complete or partial dentures inserted, the importance of a diet containing all essential food groups is emphasized.

F. Interpret the Dentist's Directions

▶ Explanation is needed for the immediate presurgical preparation with respect to rest and dietary limitations, particularly when a general anesthetic is to be administered.

G. Motivate the Patient Who Will Have Teeth Remaining

▶ Motivation to prevent further tooth loss through routine dental and dental hygiene professional care and personal oral care procedures.

II. Personal Factors

▶ The extent of the surgery to be performed and previous experiences affect the patient's attitude.

▶ Many patients who are in the greatest need of presurgical dental hygiene care and instruction may be people who have neglected their mouths for many years. They may have been indifferent to or unaware of the importance of obtaining adequate oral care.

▶ Visits to a dentist may have been to have a toothache relieved. Their knowledge of preventive measures may be limited.

▶ A few possible characteristics are suggested here.

A. Apprehensive and Fearful

▶ Apprehensive and indifferent toward need for personal care of teeth.

▶ Fearful of all dental procedures, particularly oral surgery and anesthesia.

▶ Fearful of personal appearance after surgery.

B. Resigned

▶ Feeling of inevitableness of the situation.

▶ Lack of appreciation for preserving natural teeth.

C. Discouraged

▶ Over tooth loss or development of soft tissue lesions.

▶ Toward time lost from work.

▶ By the financial aspects of dental care.

▶ About inconvenience and discomfort.

DENTAL HYGIENE CARE

I. Presurgery Treatment Planning

A. Initial Oral Preparation

▶ The pending date for the surgery and the patient's attitude may limit the time to be spent.

▶ Complete medical and dental history, extra- and intraoral examination, vital signs, photographs, and radiographs are essential; determine need for prophylactic premedication (see Chapter 10).

▶ Develop rapport; explain purposes of presurgical appointments.

▶ Explain and demonstrate dental biofilm control principles. Demonstrate appropriate technique using new soft toothbrush.

▶ Perform scaling to prepare for tissue healing; local anesthesia is used as needed.

▶ Provide postappointment instruction for rinsing with basic saline or with chlorhexidine 0.12% for tissue conditioning.

B. Follow-up Evaluation

▶ Complete or continue the scaling.

▶ More appointments may be needed for patients who will have surgery for oral cancer or who have a cardiovascular or other condition for which all periodontal and dental treatment is completed before surgery.

▶ When radiation or chemotherapy will be used following surgery for oral cancer, or when a prosthetic heart valve or total joint replacement will be involved, complete oral care is needed before surgery.

▶ Scaling and root planing is planned for a few weeks after oral surgery. Emphasis is placed on review and redemonstration of personal daily care.

II. Patient Instruction: Diet Selection

▶ The nutritional status can influence the resistance to infection and wound healing, as well as general recovery powers.

▶ Nutritional deficiencies can occur because of the inability to ingest adequate nutrients orally.

▶ Specific recommendations of what to include and not to include in the diet are provided.

▶ Postsurgical suggestions may differ from presurgical; for example, when difficulty in chewing is a postsurgical problem, a liquid or soft diet may be required.

▶ When major oral surgery requires hospitalization, nasogastric tube feeding may be used during the initial healing period.

A. Nutritional and Dietary Needs

Diets outlined are designed to include the essential foods from the MyPlate Guide (Figure 35-1, Chapter 35).

▶ *Essential for promotion of healing*: Protein and vitamins, particularly vitamin A, vitamin C, and riboflavin.

▶ *Essential for building gingival tissue resistance*: A varied diet that includes adequate portions of all essential food groups.

▶ *Essential for dental caries prevention*: Noncariogenic foods. When a patient has not been able to masticate properly, the diet employed frequently may have included intake of:

• Soft and cariogenic foods.
• Frequent sugary snacks.
• Intake of high sucrose "energy beverages."

B. Suggestions for Instruction

▶ Provide instruction sheets that show specific pre- and postsurgery meal plans. Foods for liquid and soft diets are listed in the Dental Hygiene Care section of this chapter.

▶ Express nutritional needs in terms of quantity or servings of foods so that the patient clearly understands.

▶ For the patient who will receive dentures, careful instruction is provided over a period of time. Information

for the patient with new dentures is described in Table 54-1, Chapter 54.

▶ When the patient loses the teeth because of dental caries, the diet has likely been highly cariogenic. Emphasis needs to be placed on helping the patient include nutritious foods for the general health of the body and, more specifically, the health of the alveolar processes, which will support the dentures.

III. Presurgical Instructions[2]

▶ The objective of presurgical instruction is to educate the patient on what to expect during the oral surgery appointment and immediately afterward.

▶ The patient may have concerns about the anesthesia, the surgical procedure, and the outcome.

▶ For surgery in a hospital setting, the presurgical instructions are often mailed to the patient.

▶ When surgery is done in the dental office, the dental hygienist may be responsible to deliver the instructions.

▶ Verbal instructions are supplemented with printed information.

▶ Instructions may include explanation of:

• *Food and liquid restrictions before surgery*: Specify the number of hours before the time of the surgery when the patient stops further intake of food and fluids.

• *Alcohol and medication restrictions*: The patient may be instructed to discontinue use of certain medications, supplements, and alcohol, which are not compatible with the anesthetic and drugs to be used during and following the surgical procedure.

• *Transport to and from the appointment*: When general anesthetic or light sedation is used, the patient is instructed not to drive. Plans for someone to accompany and assist the patient are made.

IV. Postsurgical Care

A. Immediate Instructions

Printed postsurgical instructions are provided following all oral surgery procedures. The prepared material is reviewed with the patient after surgery. Specific details vary, but basic information for postsurgical instruction sheets includes the following:

▶ *Control bleeding*:

• Keep the gauze square in the mouth over the surgical area for half an hour; then discard it.

• When bleeding persists at home, place a gauze square or cold wet teabag over the area and bite firmly for 30 minutes.

▶ *Rinsing*:

• Do not rinse for 24 hours after the surgical appointment.

• Then use warm salt water [1/2 teaspoonful salt in 1/2 cup (4 ounces) of warm water] after tooth brushing and every 2 hours.

▶ *Dental biofilm control*: Brush the teeth and use interdental aids more carefully than usual. Avoid the surgery site.

▶ *Rest*: Get plenty of rest; at least 8–10 hours of sleep each night. Avoid strenuous exercise during the first 24 hours, and keep the mouth from excessive movement.

▶ *Diet*: Use a liquid or soft diet high in protein. Drink water and fruit juices freely. Avoid spicy, hard or chewy foods.

▶ *Pain*: If needed, use a pain-relieving preparation prescribed by the oral surgeon or general dentist. Adhere to directions.

▶ *Icepack*:
   • When swelling is possible, apply icepack (ice cubes in a plastic bag) for 15 minutes, followed by 15 minutes off, or as directed by the oral surgeon.
   • Heat is not used for swelling.

▶ *Complications*: Include the telephone number to call after office hours, should complications arise. Complications may include:
   • Uncontrolled pain, uncontrolled bleeding
   • Temperature of 101°F or higher
   • Difficulty in opening the mouth
   • Unusual or excessive swelling after the surgery.

B. Follow-up Care

▶ The dental hygienist may participate in suture removal, irrigation of sockets, and other postsurgical procedures when the patient returns.

▶ Instruction concerning biofilm control, rinsing, oral irrigation, and other personal care, as well as diet supervision, can be continued as appropriate.

PATIENT WITH INTERMAXILLARY FIXATION

▶ Limited access for personal oral care procedures and the effect of the liquid diet required for most cases define the need for special dental hygiene care for the patient with intermaxillary fixation (IMF).

▶ Attention to rehabilitation of oral tissues during the period following removal of fixation appliances takes on particular significance to prevent permanent tissue damage and inadequate oral care habits from being continued indefinitely.

▶ Descriptions in this section are related to a fractured jaw, but IMF may be required for a variety of corrective surgeries and other conditions, including temporomandibular joint treatment and reconstructive and orthognathic surgeries.

▶ Regardless of the reason for IMF, instructions for dental hygiene care are similar, and the patient's problems are much the same.

FRACTURED JAW

▶ The patient with a fractured jaw may be hospitalized.

▶ A dental hygienist employed in a hospital would be called upon to assume part of the responsibility for patient care or to give oral hygiene instruction to direct-care personnel.

▶ After dismissal from the hospital, the patient may require special attention in the private dental office for a long period.

▶ Treatment of a fractured jaw can be complex, and the patient may suffer considerably, both physically and mentally.

▶ Basic knowledge of the nature of fractures and treatment is helpful in understanding the patient's needs.

I. Causes of Fractured Jaws

A. Traumatic

Domestic violence, gunshots, sporting injuries, falls, road traffic accidents (including motorcycles and bicycles), and industrial accidents.

B. Predisposing

Pathologic conditions, such as tumors, cysts, osteoporosis, or osteomyelitis, weaken the bone; thus, slight trauma or even tooth removal can cause fracture.

II. Emergency Care

▶ Immediate attention is paid to measures for care of the patient's general condition.

▶ Monitor breathing, airway, and circulation, and prepare for possible basic life support measures (Chapter 8).

▶ Hemorrhage, shock, and skull or internal head injuries are next in the sequence of concern.

▶ Almost any category of emergency care may be required (Tables 8-3 and 8-4 in Chapter 8).

▶ Although treatment for the fractured jaw cannot be postponed for any great length of time, its immediate care takes second place to the vital aspects of patient care.

III. Recognition

A. History

Except for a pathologic fracture, a history of trauma is usually described by the patient.

B. Clinical Signs

▶ Pain, especially on movement, and tenderness on slight pressure over the area of the fracture.

▶ Teeth may be displaced, fractured, or mobile. Because of muscle pull or contraction, segments of the bones may be displaced and the occlusion of the teeth may be irregular.

► Muscle spasm is a common finding, particularly when the fracture is at the angle or ramus of the mandible.

► Crepitation can be heard if the parts of bone are moved.

► Soft tissue in the area of the fracture may show laceration and bleeding, discoloration (ecchymosis), and enlargement.

IV. Types of Fractures

A fracture is classified by using a combination of descriptive words for its *location*, *direction*, *nature*, and *severity*. Fractures may be single or multiple, bilateral or unilateral, complete or incomplete.

A. Classification by Nature of the Fracture (Figure 55-1)

► *Simple*: has no communication with outside.

► *Compound*: has communication with outside.

► *Comminuted*: shattered.

► *Incomplete*: "Greenstick" fracture has one side of a bone broken and the other side bent.
  • It occurs in incompletely calcified bones (young children, usually).
  • The fibers tend to bend rather than break.

B. Mandibular (Described by Location)

► Alveolar process
► Condyle
► Angle
► Body
► Symphysis

C. Midfacial

► *Alveolar process*: The alveolar process fracture does not extend to the midline of the palate.

► *Le Fort*[3]: The Le Fort classification is used widely to identify the three general levels of maxillary fractures, as shown in Figure 55-2.
  • *Le Fort I*: A horizontal fracture line that extends above the roots of the teeth, above the palate, across the maxillary sinus, below the zygomatic process, and across the pterygoid plates.
  • *Le Fort II*: The midface fracture extends over the middle of the nose, down the medial wall of the orbits, across the infraorbital rims, and posteriorly, across the pterygoid plates.
  • *Le Fort III*: The high-level craniofacial fracture extends transversely across the bridge of the nose, across the orbits and the zygomatic arches, and across the pterygoid plates.
  • *Le Fort combination*: A combination of two levels is also possible such as a right Le Fort 1 and a left Le Fort II.

V. Treatment of Fractures[4,5]

Each fracture differs from the next, and the methods used in treatment vary with the individual case.

A. Treatment Planning

► Many factors are involved when the oral surgeon selects the methods to be used, particularly the location of the fracture or fractures, the presence or absence of teeth, existing injuries to the teeth, other head injuries, and the general health and condition of the patient.

► All fractures do not require active intervention. Examples are fractures of the condylar and coronoid processes, nondisplaced fractures of an edentulous mandible, and greenstick fractures of children.

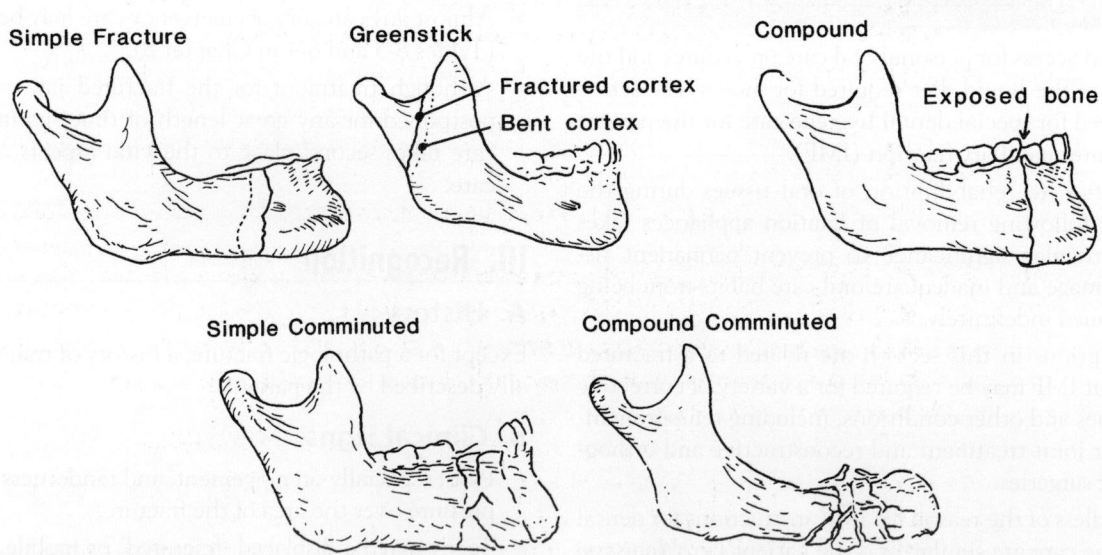

FIGURE 55-1 **Types of Fractures.** (Reprinted with permission from Kruger GO. *Textbook of Oral and Maxillofacial Surgery*. 6th ed. St. Louis, MO: Mosby; 1984.)

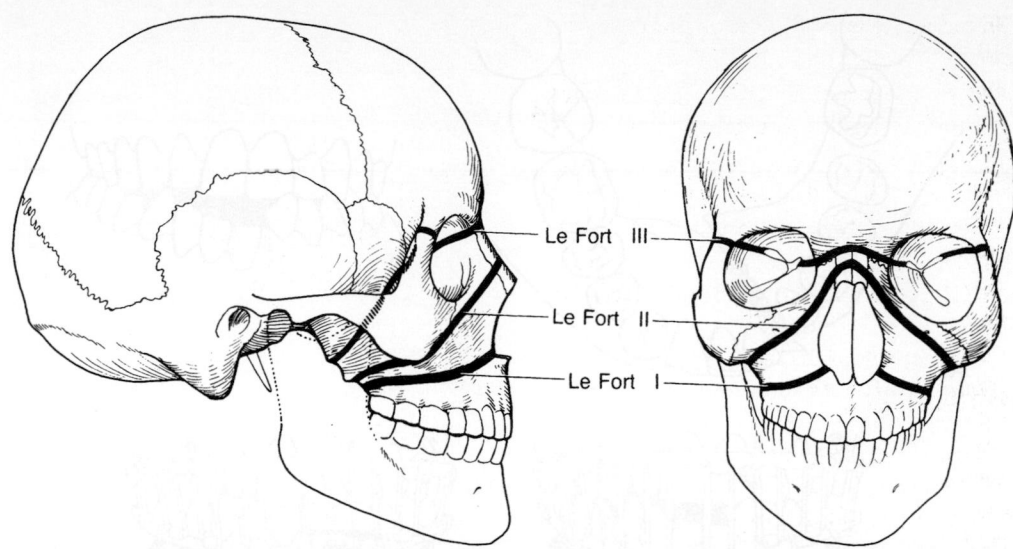

FIGURE 55-2 Le Fort Classification of Facial Fractures. Le Fort I, horizontal fracture above the roots of the teeth, below the zygomatic process, and across the pterygoid plates. Le Fort II, midface fracture over the middle of the nose and across the intraorbital rims. Le Fort III, transversely across the bridge of the nose, across the orbits and the zygomatic bone. (Adapted with permission from Archer WH. *Oral and Maxillofacial Surgery.* 5th ed. Philadelphia, PA: Saunders; 1975. From American College of Surgeons, Committee on Trauma. *Early Care of the Injured Patient.* Philadelphia, PA: Saunders; 1972.)

B. Basic Treatment

▶ *Reduction* (open or closed) restores normal position of the bones.

▶ *Fixation* of the fragments.

▶ *Immobilization* for healing.

▶ Control of treatment complications centers around prevention of infections, misalignment of the parts, and malocclusion of the dentition.

C. Healing

▶ Union is affected by the location and character of the fracture.

▶ Depends on the patient's general health and resistance, as well as on cooperation.

▶ Six weeks is considered the average for the uncomplicated mandibular fracture, and 4–6 weeks for the maxillary.

▶ Major cause of complication is infection.

MANDIBULAR FRACTURES

Reduction means the positioning of the parts on either side of the fracture so they are in apposition for healing and restoration of function.

▶ *Open reduction* refers to the use of a surgical flap procedure to expose the fracture ends and bring them together for healing.

▶ *Closed reduction* is accomplished by manipulation of the parts without surgery.

I. Closed Reduction

▶ The closure of the teeth in normal occlusion for the individual is the usual guide for position of the fracture parts in the dentulous patient.

▶ To identify the customary relation of the teeth can be difficult, especially in the partially edentulous mouth.

II. Intermaxillary Fixation (IMF)

After reduction, a method of fixation and then immobilization that has been used for many years is *IMF.* It still is indicated under certain circumstances and in certain parts of the world.

A. Description

▶ IMF is accomplished by applying wires and/or elastic bands between the maxillary and mandibular arches (Figure 55-3).

▶ *Arch bars:* ready made, contoured arch bars are adapted to fit accurately to each tooth and provide hooks for connecting the arches (Figure 55-3C). A small horizontal elastic may be positioned across the fracture to reduce the lateral displacement (Figure 55-3D).

B. Evaluation: Advantages

▶ Relative simplicity without surgical requirement: noninvasive.

▶ Lower cost; shorter hospital stay (depending on other injuries).

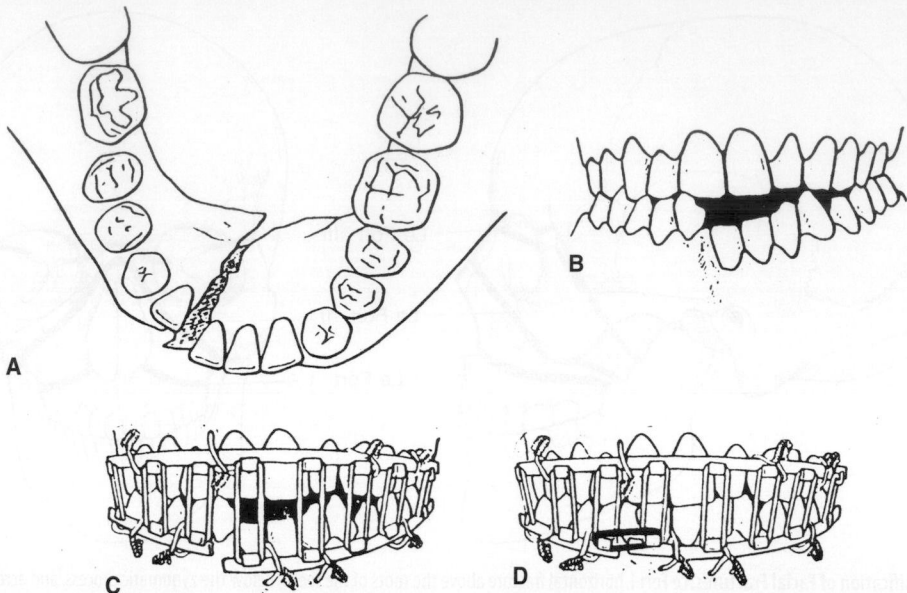

FIGURE 55-3 Intermaxillary Fracture. A: Location of fracture of the mandible. **B:** Segments of bone on either side of the fracture are displaced by muscle pull or contraction. **C:** Arch bars with hooks for metal wires or rubber bands positioned to provide a steady pull for fracture reduction. **D:** Note small horizontal rubber band extending from the hook at the mandibular right central incisor to the mandibular right canine to reduce the lateral displacement. (Adapted with permission from Archer WH. *Oral and Maxillofacial Surgery.* 5th ed. Philadelphia, PA: Saunders; 1975.)

▶ Resources and trained surgeons may be limited in less developed countries.

▶ Patient can return to activity and work sooner; can use outpatient facility for follow-up.

C. Evaluation: Contraindications and Disadvantages

▶ Patients with chronic airway diseases who cough and expectorate: asthma, chronic obstructive pulmonary diseases.

▶ Patients who vomit regularly; notably, during pregnancy.

▶ Patients with a mental illness.

▶ Dietary problems: patients lose weight with liquid, monotonous diet, often with cariogenic content.

▶ Oral hygiene and dietary limitations lead to increased dental caries and periodontal infection.

III. External Skeletal Fixation (External Pin Fixation)

A. Description

Two special bone screws are placed via skin incisions on either side of the fracture (Figure 55-4A). An acrylic bar is molded and, while still pliable, is pressed over the threads of the bone screws and locked into position with the screw nuts (Figure 55-4B).

B. Indications

Management of a fracture cannot always be accomplished satisfactorily by intermaxillary wiring alone. The following are indications for external fixation:

▶ Insufficient number of teeth in good condition for IMF.

▶ As a supplement to IMF when no teeth are present in the fractured portion of the mandible.

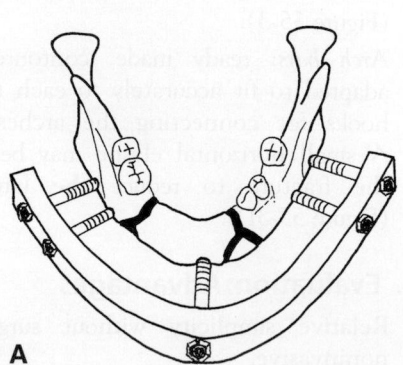
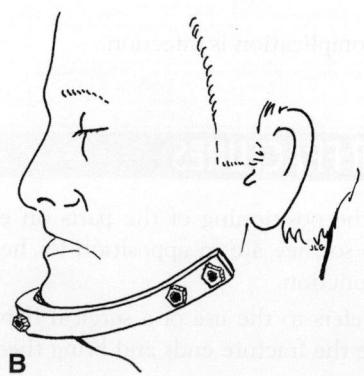

FIGURE 55-4 External Skeletal Fixation. A: Precision bone screws placed on either side of the fractures shown by heavy black lines. **B:** Molded acrylic bar positioned over the bone screws and locked into position with nuts.

- Loss of bone substance.
  - When bone substance is lost because of an accident, a gunshot wound, or a pathologic condition, a bone graft may be indicated.[6]
  - The extraoral fixation is used first to hold the fractured parts in a normal relationship, and then to immobilize the area during healing following the bone graft surgery.
- Some patients may be unable to have the jaws closed for a long period. Examples of these are:
  - Patient with a vomiting problem, such as during pregnancy.
  - Patient with a mental or physical disability, such as cerebral palsy, epilepsy, or mental retardation.
- Edentulous mandible when the fracture fragments are greatly displaced, when the fracture is at the angle of the mandible, or when the mandible is atrophic or thinned.

IV. Open Reduction

A. Principles for Treating Skeletal Fractures

- Anatomic reduction
- Functionally stable fixation
- Atraumatic surgical technique
- Active function
- Prevention of infection

B. Description

- Surgical approach to bring the fracture parts together.
- *Anesthesia:* anesthesia selected in accord with patient history.
- Types of systems used for immobilization include:
  - Transosseous wiring (osteosynthesis)
  - Plates of various sizes
  - Titanium mesh
  - Bone clamps, staples, screws
  - *Materials:* miniplates, screws, and other parts made of biodegradable or resorbable synthetic materials.

C. Clinical Example

- Figure 55-5 illustrates various positions for miniplates to provide stability for the reduced fracture parts.
- Care is needed so that the screws are not placed over a fracture line or over the roots of teeth and so that they do not infringe on the mandibular canal.

MIDFACIAL FRACTURES

I. Principles

- Maxillary fractures are more difficult to manage because of the number of bones, the associated anatomy, and the complications of basal skull fractures.

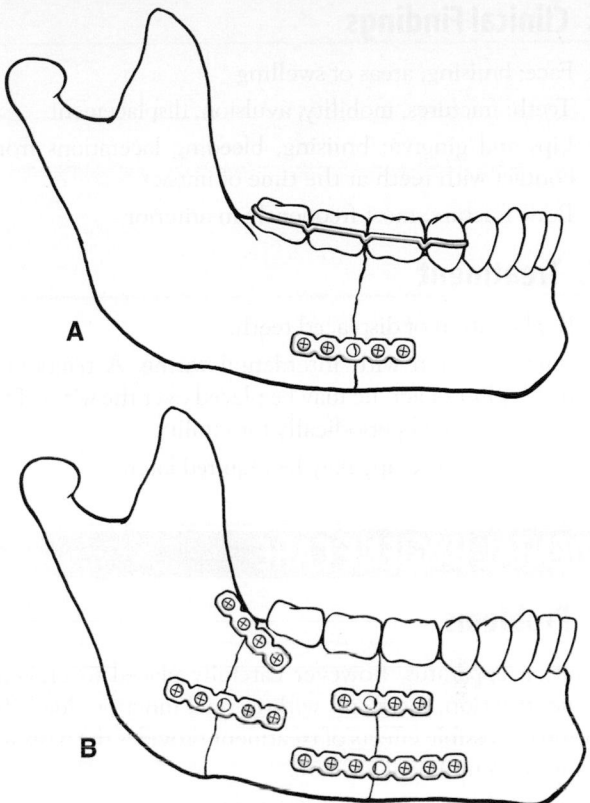

FIGURE 55-5 **Miniplates for Immobilization of Fracture. A:** Tension band on the teeth to aid in maintaining correct occlusion while miniplate holds fracture ends in apposition. **B:** Examples of possible positions for miniplates.

- Not all mid-face fractures need fixation following reduction.
- Function and cosmetics are both involved.

II. Description

A. Older Methods

- Internal wire suspension
- External cranial suspension to a stable bone, such as uninvolved zygoma
- Headcaps

B. Current Therapeutic Interventions

- Open reduction with internal fixation
- Use of bone plates of various sizes
- Grafts for reconstruction of mid-face defects
- Early reconstruction before scarring and soft tissue contracture deform the surrounding area

ALVEOLAR PROCESS FRACTURE

The most common fracture is of the alveolar process, maxillary or mandibular.

I. Clinical Findings

▶ Face: bruising, areas of swelling

▶ Teeth: fractures, mobility, avulsion, displacement

▶ Lips and gingiva: bruising, bleeding lacerations from contact with teeth at the time of impact

▶ Bone fracture: most frequently in anterior

II. Treatment

▶ Replantation of displaced teeth.

▶ Immobilization with interdental wiring. A temporary fixed splint of acrylic may be placed over the wires. The teeth are tested periodically for vitality.

▶ Endodontic therapy may be required later.

DENTAL HYGIENE CARE

I. Problems

Fixation apparatus, however carefully placed to prevent tissue irritation, interferes with normal function. Identification of possible effects of treatment provides the basis for planning dental hygiene care.

A. Development of Gingivitis or Periodontal Complications

▶ Thick biofilm formation and food debris accumulation provide sources of irritation to the gingiva.

▶ Gingivitis can develop in 9–19 days.[7]

▶ Lack of normal stimulation of the periodontium and of cleansing effects usually provided by the action of the tongue, lips, and facial muscles contributes to stagnation of saliva and accumulation of debris and bacteria.

▶ Tender, sensitive gingiva make biofilm control more difficult, even on available surfaces.

B. Initiation of Demineralization

▶ An appetizing soft or liquid diet is difficult to plan using limited cariogenic foods for dental caries prevention.

C. Loss of Appetite

▶ Loss of appetite related to monotonous liquid or soft diet may lead to weight loss and lowered physical resistance.

▶ Secondary infections, including those of the oral tissues, may result.

D. Difficulty in Opening the Mouth

▶ When the temporomandibular joint has been injured, the patient wearing fixation appliances that involve only the mandible has difficulty in applying a toothbrush to the lingual surfaces of teeth.

▶ After removal of appliances, all patients have a degree of muscular trismus that limits personal oral self-care and mastication.

II. Instrumentation

A. Presurgical

Gross calculus is removed, as much possible, before open reduction procedures. Trauma to surrounding soft tissues of lip, tongue, and cheeks limits accessibility.

B. During Treatment

Periodic scaling contributes to oral health. Although access is only from the facial aspect for a patient with intermaxillary wiring, some benefit can be obtained. An assistant provides continual suction during treatment.

C. After Removal of Appliances

A few weeks after removal of appliances, when the patient can open the mouth normally and personal daily oral care has been initiated, complete scaling and root planing can be provided.

III. Diet

Many patients with fractured jaws tend to lose weight, which is generally related to an inadequate nutrient and caloric intake. Objectives in planning the diet are to:

▶ Prevent new carious lesions.

▶ Help the patient maintain an adequate nutritional state.

▶ Promote healing.

▶ Increase resistance to infection.

Attention is given to the patient's willingness and ability to follow the recommendations made. The patient may be in the hospital for a few days to a few weeks, depending on the severity of other injuries. A greater length of time is spent as an outpatient, when the diet is much more difficult to supervise. The patient's understanding of dietary instructions and what is expected may appear more significant than the specific components of the diet recommended.

A. Nutritional Needs

After a surgical fixation procedure, the diet is planned to promote tissue building and repair.

▶ All essential food elements.

▶ Emphasis on protein, vitamins, particularly A, C and D, and minerals particularly calcium and phosphorus.

▶ Usual caloric requirements for patient's age, taking into consideration lack of physical exercise and loss of appetite when ill.

B. Methods of Feeding

▶ *Plastic straw*: Liquid is sucked through the teeth or through an edentulous area. Straw can be bent to accommodate a patient who cannot sit up.

▶ *Spoon feeding*: When a patient's arms are not functional, direct assistance is needed. The mouth may have injuries that prevent sucking food through a straw.

▶ *Tube feeding*: Tube feeding may be indicated following various types of extensive oral surgery, facial trauma, burns, immobilized fractured jaw, and other conditions that prevent ingesting sufficient calories and nutritional foods by way of the mouth.

- A nasogastric tube is used. Blenderized food can be prepared, or special tube formulas are available commercially.
- When commercial preparations are used, contents can be selected to meet the specific nutritional and caloric requirements of an individual patient.

C. Liquid Diet

A *clear liquid* diet to help prevent dehydration may be prescribed initially, but it can be nutritionally inadequate. A *full liquid* diet to provide high protein and other healing elements is of a consistency to be taken by a cup. A *blenderized liquid* diet can be passed through a straw.

▶ Indications
- All patients with jaws wired together.
- Patients with no appliance or single-jaw appliance who have difficulty opening the mouth because of a condition, such as temporomandibular joint involvement or tongue or lip injury, that hinders insertion of food or manipulation of food in the mouth.

▶ *Examples of foods*: fruit juices, milk, eggnog, meat juices and soups, cooked thin cereals, and canned baby foods. Strained vegetables and meats (baby foods) may be added to meat juices and soups.

▶ *Use of a blender*: regular table foods can be mixed in a food blender. With liquid, such as clear soup or milk, added, a fluid consistency can be obtained that will pass through a straw (Figure 55-6).

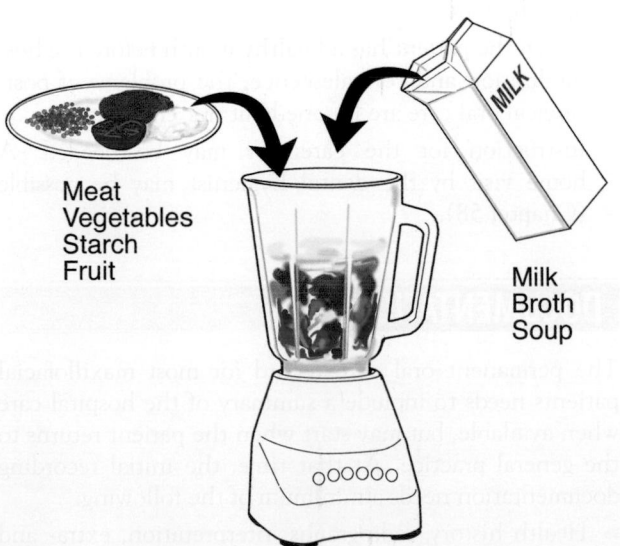

FIGURE 55-6 Preparation of a Liquid or Soft Diet. Regular table foods can be blended with milk or other nutritious liquid.

D. Soft Diet

▶ *Indications*
- Patient with no appliance or with single-jaw appliance without complications in opening the mouth or in movement of the lips and tongue.
- Patient who has been maintained on liquid diet throughout treatment period.
  - After appliances are removed, the soft diet is recommended for several days to 1 week to provide the stomach with foods that are readily digestible rather than making a drastic change to a regular diet.
  - A soft diet can also aid by protecting tender oral tissues from the rough textures of a regular diet until the tissues have had a chance to respond to softer foods.

▶ *Examples of foods*
- Soft-poached, scrambled, or boiled eggs; cooked cereals; mashed soft-cooked vegetables, including potato; mashed fresh or canned fruits; soft, finely divided meats; custards; plain ice cream.

E. Hints for Diet Planning with the Nonhospitalized Patient

▶ Provide instruction sheets that show specific meal plans.
▶ Express nutritional needs in quantities or servings of foods.
▶ Show methods of varying the diet. A liquid or soft diet is at best monotonous because of the sameness of texture.
▶ Encourage limitation of cariogenic foods as an aid to prevention of dental caries.

IV. Personal Oral Care Procedures

▶ Every attempt is made to keep the patient's mouth as clean as possible for comfort and sanitation, and as free of dental biofilm as possible for disease prevention.
▶ The extent of possible care depends on the appliances; the condition of the lips, tongue, and other oral tissues; and the cooperation of the patient.
▶ The patient is encouraged to begin tooth brushing as soon as possible after the surgical procedure, but until the patient is able, a plan for care is outlined for a caregiver.

A. Irrigation

▶ *Indications*: During the first few days after the surgical procedure, while the mouth may be too tender for brushing, frequent irrigations are required; irrigation also serves as an adjunct to tooth brushing.
▶ *Method*: In a hospital, irrigations with suction are possible. At home, the patient irrigates with the head lowered over a sink (Box 29-2, in Chapter 29).
▶ *Mouth rinse selection*: The oral surgeon is consulted for specific instructions. Suggestions include:

- Physiologic saline (1 tsp (5 g) of salt to 1 cup (250 mL) of warm water)
- Chlorhexidine gluconate
- Fluoride rinse.

B. Early Mouth Cleansing

While the patient is in the hospital, a soft toothbrush with suction can be used. The toothbrush with suction is described in Figure 58-4 in Chapter 58.

C. Personal Care by the Patient

- As soon as possible, the patient is instructed in personal care.
- A tooth brushing method and other aids, such as those used for orthodontic appliances, are recommended and demonstrated, as discussed in Chapter 31.
- Interdental and proximal tooth surface care is restricted to access only from the facial approach, making the choice of oral care devices limited.[8] Some spaces permit insertion of an interdental brush. With instruction, most patients can use a toothpick in a holder (Perio Aid®) to disturb biofilm around just under the free gingival margin, as shown in Figure 29-12 in Chapter 29.
- When the tongue is not injured, the patient can be instructed to use the tongue as an aid in cleaning the lingual surfaces of the teeth and massaging the gingiva.
- The ambulatory patient can use a water irrigator. A low-pressure setting is used, and the spray is directed carefully to prevent tissue injury, as illustrated in Figure 29-14 and described in Chapter 29.

D. After Appliances are Removed

- Demineralization and dental caries can result from biofilm retention about the appliances.
- Except for the patient who had practiced good personal oral care before the accident, a step-by-step series of lessons is necessary.
- A method for daily self-applied fluoride, such as a mouth rinse or brush-on gel, can be introduced along with the use of a fluoride dentifrice.

DENTAL HYGIENE CARE BEFORE GENERAL SURGERY

- Completing dental and dental hygiene treatment and bringing the oral cavity to a state of health before surgery have special significance for certain patients who will have surgical procedures other than oral.
- When emergency surgery is performed, preparation of the mouth is not possible, and postsurgical examination and care may be complicated by various limitations.

- When surgery is elective, or planned in advance, the patient can be encouraged to have complete dental and periodontal treatment.
- Types of patients are described briefly here. Other examples are found in the various special patient chapters throughout this section of the book.

I. Patients in Whom Surgical Procedures Affect Their Risk Status

- Patients who receive chemotherapeutic agents following surgery for various types of cancer, and others who use immunosuppressant drugs, require special management to prevent complications during dental and dental hygiene appointments.
- Antibiotic premedication to prevent infective endocarditis and other infections is mandatory for certain patients is described in Chapter 10.
- Before surgery for prostheses, transplants, cancer, and other serious conditions, patients are informed of the need for completing oral care treatments and practicing preventive daily personal care.

II. Preparation of the Mouth Before General Inhalation Anesthesia

- Because the mouth is an entryway to the respiratory system, the possibility always exists that bacteria, debris, and fluids from the mouth may be inhaled.
- Inhalation could occur during the administration of an anesthetic or when the patient coughs.

III. Patient with a Long Convalescence

- Patients whose surgery requires a long convalescence may be unable to keep a regular continuing care appointment.
- When the patient has a healthy mouth before the hospitalization and convalescence, the problems of postsurgical oral care are lessened but not eliminated.
- Instruction for the caregiver may be needed. A home visit by the dental hygienist may be possible (Chapter 58).

DOCUMENTATION

The permanent oral care record for most maxillofacial patients needs to include a summary of the hospital care when available, but may start when the patient returns to the general practice. At that time, the initial recording documentation needs a minimum of the following:

- Health history, radiographs interpretation, extra- and intraoral findings, vital signs.

EVERYDAY ETHICS

Ms. Squires (age 79) was involved in a serious automobile accident that fractured her mandible and required fixation with intermaxillary wiring, which was recently removed. Apparently she is here because of pressure from her adult children who have been taking turns tending to her needs. The daughter who accompanied her to this appointment said her bad breath was bothering them even more than her complaining all the time.

This is her first appointment with William, the dental hygienist, since the accident 10 months ago. He documented the moderate amounts of calculus and heavy dental biofilm throughout the mouth. Mrs. Squires demonstrates difficulty opening her mouth and seems fussy and apprehensive when William attempts to go over a

toothbrushing procedure and continually asks her to "open wider, please."

Questions for Consideration

1. Which of the dental hygiene core values (Table II-1 in Section II) become involved with a patient with such complications? Explain each one.

2. Review the steps for decision making, Box 1-10 in in Chapter 1 to help plan and present optimal oral health services to benefit this patient.

3. Describe the role of the dental hygienist in coordinating preventive care with the posttreatment examinations Mrs. Squires has with the oral maxillofacial surgeon.

▶ Comprehensive periodontal examination and summary of current needs.

▶ Risk factors and dental caries review; complete examination for demineralization.

▶ Care planning for maintenance.

▶ A sample progress note is available for review in Box 55-3.

Factors To Teach The Patient

Accident Prevention

▷ Always use seat belts in automobiles and other vehicles.

▷ Use mouthguards and all safety devices during contact sports.

▷ Wear motorcycle and bicycle helmets.

For the Patient Who Will Have General Surgery

▷ Significance of a clean mouth during general anesthesia.

▷ Postsurgery oral problems related to specific diseases.

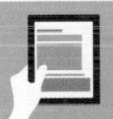

BOX 55-3

Example Documentation: Postsurgical Dental Hygiene Appointment

S –A 20-year-old college student presents for first dental hygiene appointment following a mandibular fracture due to a motorcycle accident. Stabilizing interdental wiring and fixed splint were removed yesterday. Patient complains of "mouth feeling dirty and it smells bad." Past medical history: Patient admits to smoking a pack of cigarettes a day and an occasional beer on the weekends; otherwise unremarkable.

O–Healthy looking young male in no obvious distress. Oral cavity is remarkable for heavy dental biofilm and calculus buildup; tissues are inflamed, bleeding, and edematous. No pocket depths greater than 4 mm were charted. Mandibular fracture appeared completely healed.

A–A 20-year-old male status postwire removal from motorcycle accident with poor oral hygiene.

P–Complete periodontal debridement × 4 quadrants, and polishing; detailed oral hygiene instructions; tobacco cessation education; 4-week follow-up to assess healing and patient compliance to oral care instructions and success with tobacco cessation.

Signed _____, RDH

Date _____

References

1. American Dental Association. Specialty definitions. http://www.ada.org/en/education-careers/careers-in-dentistry/dental-specialties/specialty-definitions Accessed July 20, 2015.

2. Chuong R. Perioperative management of the surgical patient. In: Peterson LJ, ed. *Oral and Maxillofacial Surgery.* Philadelphia, PA: Lippincott; 1992:63–85.

3. Haskell R. Applied surgical anatomy. In: Rowe NL, Williams JL, eds. *Maxillofacial Injuries.* London: Churchill Livingstone; 1985:21–24.

4. Luyk NH. Principles of management of fractures of the mandible. In: Peterson LJ, ed. *Oral and Maxillofacial Surgery.* Philadelphia, PA: Lippincott; 1992:407–434.

5. Banks P, Brown A. Treatment of fractures of the mandible. In: *Fractures of the Facial Skeleton.* Oxford: Wright; 2001:81–106.

6. Boyne PJ. Bone grafts. In: *Osseous Reconstruction of the Maxilla and the Mandible.* Chicago, IL: Quintessence; 1997:64–74.

7. Löe H, Theilade E, Jensen SB. Experimental gingivitis in man. *J Periodontol.* 1965;36:177–187.

8. Phelps-Sandall BA, Oxford SJ. Effectiveness of oral hygiene techniques on plaque and gingivitis in patients placed in intermaxillary fixation. *Oral Surg Oral Med Oral Pathol.* 1983;56(5):487–490.

ENHANCE YOUR UNDERSTANDING

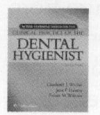

the Point® DIGITAL CONNECTIONS
(see the inside front cover for access information)
- **Audio glossary**
- **Quiz bank**

SUPPORT FOR LEARNING
(available separately; visit lww.com)
- *Active Learning Workbook for Clinical Practice of the Dental Hygienist, 12th Edition*

prepU INDIVIDUALIZED REVIEW
(available separately; visit lww.com)
- **Adaptive quizzing with *prepU for Wilkins' Clinical Practice of the Dental Hygienist***

56

The Patient with Cancer

Dianna S. Weikel, RDH, MS and Deborah S. Manne, RDH, RN, MSN, OCN

CHAPTER OUTLINE

LEARNING OBJECTIVES

After studying this chapter, the student will be able to:

1. Identify healthcare professionals involved in the multidisciplinary oncology team.

2. Explain several systemic medical treatment options utilized in cancer management.

3. Describe common oral complications secondary to cancer treatment.

4. Provide examples of evidenced-based dental hygiene care strategies for mucositis management.

Dental hygiene care of the patient with cancer before, during, and after therapy strives to not only attain but also maintain a patient's oral health at the highest possible level. This contributes to the patient's general health and overall quality of life. Terminology relating to cancer is defined in Box 56-1.

▶ Cancer treatment modalities (radiation therapy, chemotherapy, surgery, and hematopoietic cell transplantation) have the potential to affect the oral cavity significantly.

▶ The patient will be under the care of a team of multidisciplinary specialists. Box 56-2 lists the members of the multidisciplinary team.

DESCRIPTION

▶ Cancer refers to:
  • A group of neoplastic diseases in which there is transformation of normal cells into malignant ones.
  • As cancer cells proliferate, the mass of abnormal tissue that is formed enlarges until it takes over the host site. It then sheds cells that spread to distant sites (metastasis).

▶ Characteristics of benign and malignant neoplasms are compared in Table 56-1.

▶ Cancers are classified on the basis of:
  • Origin of the tissue involved: carcinomas from epithelial tissue, sarcomas from connective tissue
  • Type of cell from which they arise, namely, an epithelial or connective tissue cell.[1]

▶ Staging is:
  • A succinct, standardized description of a tumor based on origin and extent
  • Made up of three components: T (tumor size), N (presence or absence of lymph nodes), and M (presence or absence of distant metastases).

▶ Common signs and symptoms of cancer are listed in Box 56-3.

I. Incidence and Survival

Cancer is the second leading cause of death in the United States for adults under the age of 85.[2] Survival depends on the following:

▶ Type of cancer
▶ Location and size of the tumor
▶ Presence of distant metastases
▶ Tumor sensitivity to treatment
▶ Physical condition: comorbidities, age.

II. Risk Factors[3]

Numerous factors increase a person's risk for developing cancer, including:

▶ *Tobacco*: both cigarette smoking and use of smokeless tobacco products are implicated in head and neck cancer, lung cancer, and bladder cancer.

▶ *Alcohol*: chronic, long-term use especially in combination with tobacco use implicated in head and neck cancer, bladder cancer, and liver cancer.

▶ *Sunlight*: especially occupations requiring work in the sun such as construction workers, farmers, as well as sunbathers.

▶ *Environmental/occupational*: exposure to asbestos, radon, coal dust, and chemicals, to name a few.

▶ *Viruses*:
  • Epstein–Barr virus implicated in Burkett's lymphoma
  • Hepatitis C implicated in liver cancer
  • Human Papillomavirus (16 and 18) implicated in cervical cancer and cancer of the oropharynx (tonsil, base of tongue).

▶ *Socioeconomic*: late diagnosis with poorer prognosis seen in lower socioeconomic populations (inner city, rural, working poor).

III. Types of Cancer[2]

The most common types of cancer are as follows:

▶ Men:
  • Prostate
  • Lung and bronchus
  • Colon and rectum
▶ Women:
  • Breast
  • Lung and bronchus
  • Colon and rectum

IV. How Cancer Is Treated[3,4]

Cancer is treated using a variety of different approaches based on the following:

▶ The location and size of the tumor
▶ Treatment objectives (cure, control, or palliation)
▶ The different approaches include
▶ Surgery
▶ Chemotherapy
▶ Radiation therapy
▶ Hematopoietic cell transplantation
▶ Hormone therapy
▶ Vaccine therapy
▶ Biotherapy
▶ Targeted therapies
▶ A combination of two or more of the above.

SURGERY

Surgery is the most common form of treatment for solid tumors, both malignant and nonmalignant.

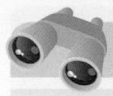

BOX 56-1 | KEY WORDS: Oncology

Alimentation: providing nutrition.

Alopecia: a loss of hair.

Anaplasia: an irreversible alteration in adult cells toward more primitive (embryonic) cell types; characteristic of tumor cells.

Benign: not malignant (Table 56-1).

Biotherapy: use of biological agents to treat cancer.

Carcinogen: an agent that may cause cancer; may be chemical, physical (ionizing radiation), or biologic; biologic carcinogens may be external (e.g., viruses) or internal (genetic defects).

Carcinoma: a malignant tumor of epithelial origin.

Chemotherapy: treatment of illness by chemical means, that is, by medication or drugs.

Dysgeusia: distortion of the sense of taste.

Dysplasia: an abnormality of development; in pathology, alteration in size, shape, and organization of adult cells.

Hematologic profile: an analysis of the blood and blood-forming tissues.

Hematopoiesis: formation and development of blood cells.

Hyperbaric oxygen: the patient is placed in a sealed chamber and given pure oxygen through a face mask. At the same time, compressed air is introduced into the chamber to raise the atmospheric pressure to several times normal. This equalizes the pressure inside and outside of the body, thereby flooding the tissues with oxygen. An increase in oxygen to the irradiated tissues can temporarily compensate for the reduction in circulation.

Imaging: the production of diagnostic images, including radiography, ultrasonography, or scintigraphy.

Infiltration: the diffusion or accumulation in a tissue of cells or substances not normal to it or in amounts in excess of normal; in leukemia, for example, white blood cells infiltrate body tissues.

In situ: in its normal place; confined to the site of origin.

Interstitial: pertaining to, or situated in, the interstices (small spaces) of a tissue.

Intrathecal: within a sheath; through the theca of the spinal cord into the subarachnoid space; in leukemia, for example, the location for the delivery of various chemotherapeutic drugs.

Isogenic (syngenic): having the same genetic constitution.

Leukemia: an acute or chronic progressive malignant neoplasm of the blood-forming organs, marked by diffuse proliferation of immature white blood cells (leukocytes); subsequent reduction in erythrocytes and platelets results.

Lymphadenectomy: excision of one or more lymph nodes.

Malignant: tending to become progressively worse and to result in death; having the properties of anaplasia, invasiveness, and metastasis; said of tumors (Table 56-1).

Metastasis: transfer of disease from one organ or part to another not directly connected with it; for example, regional or distant spread of cancer cells from the site primarily involved.

Nadir: the point at which a patient's blood counts reach their lowest level after chemotherapy administration; dental or dental hygiene care is contraindicated during this time.

Neoplasm: any new and abnormal growth, specifically one in which cell multiplication is controlled and progressive; may be benign or malignant.

Oncology: the study of tumors; the sum of knowledge regarding tumors.

Oral mucositis/stomatitis: inflammation and ulceration of the oral mucous membranes; can increase the risk for pain, oral and systemic infection, and nutritional compromise.

Osteonecrosis of the jaw (ONJ): exposed bone in the maxilla or mandible, of more than 8 weeks duration, in a patient treated with a bisphosphonate or other antiresorptive drug.

Osteoradionecrosis: blood vessel compromise and necrosis of bone exposed to high-dose radiation therapy, resulting in decreased ability to heal if traumatized and in extreme susceptibility to infection.

Palliative/palliation: affording relief, but does not cure.

Pancytopenia: abnormal depression of all cellular elements of the blood.

Pleomorphism: occurrence in more than one form; the assumption of various distinct morphologic types by a single organism or cell.

Radiation therapy: the treatment of disease by ionizing radiation; may be external megavoltage or internal by use of interstitial implantation of an isotope (radium).

Radium: a highly radioactive chemical element found in uranium minerals; used in the treatment of malignant tumors in the form of needles or pellets for interstitial implantation.

Relapse: the return of a disease weeks or months after its apparent cessation.

Remission: diminution or abatement of the symptoms of a disease; the period during which such diminution occurs.

Salivary gland hypofunction: objective reduction in the production of saliva, often a long-term complication of head/neck radiation.

Sarcoma: a tumor, often highly malignant, composed of cells derived from connective tissue such as bone and cartilage, muscle, blood vessel, or lymphoid tissue.

Staging: the succinct, standardized description of a tumor with regard to origin and spread. This clinical classification is based on physical assessments, biopsy, imaging, and endoscopy. Each stage (I–IV) consists of three components: T (size of tumor); N (lymph node involvement); and M (presence or absence of distant metastasis).

Stomatoxic: potential for causing oral ulceration/inflammation of the gastrointestinal tract.

Trismus: limitations of opening because of spasm and/or fibrosis of the muscles of mastication and/or temporomandibular joint located in the field of radiation.

Xerostomia: subjective report of oral dryness—saliva may appear thick or reduced, or increases the risk for infection and compromised chewing, speaking, and swallowing. Persistent dry mouth increases the risk for dental caries.

I. Indications for Surgery[5]

▶ Tumors that are small in size, localized, and easy to remove.

▶ Debulk or remove portions of large tumors before treatment (chemotherapy or radiation therapy).

▶ Provide pain relief or prolong life when no chance of cure is possible (palliation).

CHEMOTHERAPY

Chemotherapy involves the use of drugs that affect the rapidly dividing cancer cells at different points in the cell cycle. The drugs are used as a single agent or in

TABLE 56-1	Characteristics of Benign and Malignant Neoplasms	
CHARACTERISTIC	**BENIGN**	**MALIGNANT**
Cell characteristics	Well-differentiated cells of the tissue from which the tumor originated	Cells are undifferentiated. Anaplastic features (lack of differentiation)
Mode of growth	Tumor grows by expansion and does not infiltrate the surrounding tissues; encapsulated	Tumor grows at the periphery and sends out processes that infiltrate and destroy the surrounding tissues
Rate of growth	Rate of growth is usually slow	Rate of growth is usually relatively rapid and is dependent on level of differentiation; the more anaplastic the tumor, the more rapid the rate of growth
Metastasis	Does not spread by metastasis	Gains access to the blood and lymph systems to metastasize to other organs
Destruction of tissue	Does not usually cause tissue damage unless location interferes with blood flow	Often causes extensive tissue damage as the tumor outgrows its blood supply or encroaches on blood flow to the area; may also produce substances that cause cell damage

Adapted from Porth C. *Pathophysiology: Concepts of Altered Health States.* 7th ed. Philadelphia, PA: J. B. Lippincott; 2005.

combination. Side effects can be severe and frequently involve the oral cavity.

I. Objectives

▶ To destroy cancer cells and keep them from metastasizing.
▶ To prevent cancer from recurring.
▶ To provide an improved quality of life.

II. Indications

▶ Eliminate a localized tumor too large for surgical removal.
▶ Treat cancer that has metastasized to other parts of the body.
▶ Prevent cancer recurrence with maintenance therapy.
▶ Use before surgery to make a tumor easier to remove completely.
▶ Palliative.
▶ Treatment of "liquid tumors" such as leukemia.

III. Types of Chemotherapy

Box 56-4 lists the types of agents used for chemotherapy.

IV. Systemic Side Effects of Chemotherapy

Chemotherapy affects both rapidly dividing cancer cells and rapidly dividing normal cells (hair, oral/gastrointestinal mucosa, and bone marrow). Halting cell division of normal cells may cause side effects that range from mild to life threatening. The most common include the following:

▶ Alopecia (hair loss)
▶ Myelosuppression (bone marrow suppression causing a reduction in blood counts leading to anemia, leukopenia, and thrombocytopenia)
▶ Immunosuppression (inhibition of antibody responses resulting from leukopenia)
▶ Nausea, vomiting, and diarrhea
▶ Loss of appetite
▶ Gastrointestinal mucositis

BOX 56-4

Types of Agents Used for Chemotherapy

Alkylating agents
Antibiotics
Antimetabolites
Plant alkaloids
Steroids/hormones
Proteasome inhibitors, mammalian target of rapamycin inhibitors
Targeted therapies

V. Oral Complications of Chemotherapy

The following are oral complications resulting from chemotherapy:[4,6]

▶ *Oral mucositis/stomatitis*: an inflammation of the oral mucosa characterized by erythema, ulceration, and pain.
▶ *Xerostomia*: subjective report of oral dryness.
▶ *Salivary gland hypofunction*: objective reduction in saliva production.
▶ *Infections*:
  • Bacterial
  • *Viral*: herpes simplex, varicella zoster, cytomegalovirus
  • *Fungal*: *Candida albicans*.
▶ *Bleeding*: anywhere in the mouth; spontaneous or induced.
▶ *Neurotoxicity*: mimics toothache; usually bilateral.
▶ *Osteonecrosis of the jaw*: exposed bone of at least 8 weeks duration in either the maxilla or mandible secondary to use of systemic bisphosphonates and/or other antiresorptive therapies.[7]

RADIATION THERAPY

Radiation therapy uses ionizing radiation to treat cancer.

▶ Radiation impacts the cancer cell's ability to replicate and survive.
▶ Not all tumors are radiosensitive (ability of the radiation therapy to kill the tumor).
▶ Head and neck radiation therapy produces acute short-term and chronic long-term effects in the oral cavity.

I. Indications

▶ Treat a small localized tumor that is radiosensitive.
▶ Shrink a large tumor before surgery.
▶ Increase effectiveness of chemotherapy when used concurrently.
▶ Prevent the spread of cancer or control residual tumor.
▶ Prevent a recurrence of the cancer.
▶ Provide symptom/pain relief for bone metastases or palliative therapy.

II. Types

A. External Beam

▶ Conventional use of ionizing radiation applied outside the body.
▶ Intensity-modulated radiation therapy (IMRT)
  • Developed in the late 1990s.
  • Considered a high precision delivery of radiation.
  • Accomplished via computer-guided images of target anatomy with radiation produced by a linear accelerator.

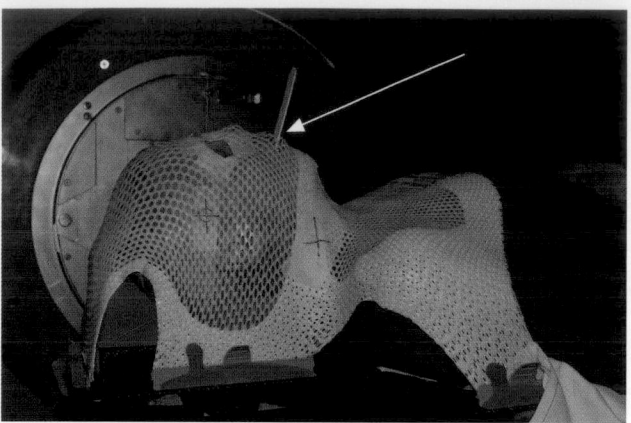

FIGURE 56-1 Custom Patient Mask. This is worn by the patient at each radiation appointment. The mask, made out of firm mesh, snaps into the treatment table to assist immobilizing the patient for precise radiation delivery throughout the course of radiation therapy. A bite block is placed intraorally (arrow) to maintain the mouth in a static position. The linear accelerator (source of radiation) is seen in the background. (Used with permission from Dianna S. Wiekel)

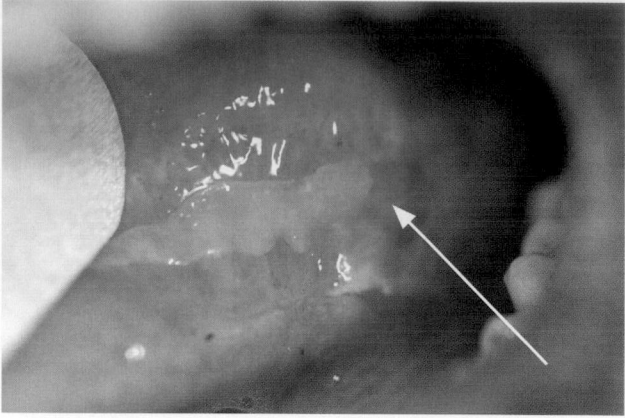

FIGURE 56-2 Mucositis left lateral border of tongue, secondary to radiation to the head and neck tissue. Note erythema distal to the ulcerated area (arrow). This lesion is characterized by pain, complicating the patient's ability to eat, speak, or swallow. (Used with permission from Dianna S. Wiekel)

- Used in treatment of head and neck cancer.
- Radiation dose is elevated at site of the gross tumor while simultaneously sparing surrounding normal tissue.
- Results in decreased side effects, better tumor targeting.
- Figure 56-1 illustrates patient preparation prior to IMRT.

B. Internal Source

▶ Radiation source (such as implants or seeds) is placed within the body.

▶ Less radiation is delivered to surrounding tissues than when an external source is utilized.

III. Doses

▶ Total dose given depends on the type of tumor, treatment goals, and patient's ability to tolerate treatment.

▶ Total radiation dose is approximately 30–70 Gy.

▶ It is divided into equal doses (conventional) or modulated fractions (IMRT) per day.

▶ It is given once a day, 5 days a week, for 5–8 weeks.

IV. Systemic Effects

▶ *Skin reactions*: looks like a bad sunburn

▶ Fatigue

▶ Nausea, vomiting, diarrhea, constipation.

V. Oral Complications[4,6,8]

▶ Oral mucositis (see Figure 56-2)

▶ Xerostomia/salivary gland hypofunction

▶ Radiation caries

▶ Taste loss

▶ *Infection*:
 - Bacterial
 - *Viral*: herpes simplex, varicella zoster
 - Fungal: *Candida albicans*

▶ Trismus

▶ Osteoradionecrosis.

HEMATOPOIETIC STEM CELL TRANSPLANTATION[9,10]

Hematopoietic stem cell transplantation is used to treat cancers involving the bone marrow, including leukemia. The purpose is to substitute peripheral blood stem cells from the patient or a healthy, compatible donor.

I. Types

▶ Autologous: self

▶ Allogeneic: human leukocyte antigen–matched donor, either related or unrelated

▶ Syngeneic: identical twin.

II. Stages of Transplantation Process

A. Patient Selection

▶ *Indications*: patient not responsive to chemotherapy alone; relapse occurs after one or more remissions.

▶ *Evaluation*: medical and dental assessments completed to ensure patient is free of infection and physically able to undergo the preparative regimen.

B. Donor Regimen

▶ Histocompatibility matching

▶ Bone marrow aspirated from iliac crest, ribs, or sternum.

C. Conditioning of Patient to Receive Bone Marrow Graft

▶ Preparative high-dose immunosuppressive regimen: chemotherapy alone or with total body irradiation.
▶ Purposes:
  • Kill malignant cells
  • Suppress immune system so new stem cells/marrow will engraft.

D. Transplantation

▶ Intravenous infusion of donor's marrow/stem cells.

E. Pancytopenia

▶ All cellular elements of the blood are depressed, that is, white blood cells, red blood cells, platelets.
▶ Protective isolation for the patient is required; patient is highly susceptible to infection.
▶ Function of new marrow (to produce peripheral blood elements) begins after 10–20 days.

F. Recovery

▶ Immune recovery 3–12 months; long-term recovery 1–3 years.

III. Acute Complications[6,11]

▶ Acute Graft-Versus-Host Disease (Acute GVHD)
  • Description: The donor's T-lymphocytes see the host cell antigens as foreign and react against the host tissue.
▶ Symptoms:
  • Present during the first 100 days posttransplant.
  • Painful red skin rash starting on the palms of hands and soles of feet and progressing to the upper trunk.
  • Severe, persistent diarrhea.
  • Jaundice, elevated liver enzymes, liver tenderness.
▶ *Infection:*
  • Bacterial
  • *Viral:* herpes simplex, varicella zoster, cytomegalovirus
  • *Fungal: Candida albicans.*
▶ Gastrointestinal, hepatic, cardiac, pulmonary, hematologic, neurologic complications.
▶ *Oral complications:*
  • *Oral mucositis:* appears 10–14 days posttransplant
  • Xerostomia
  • *Viral and fungal infections:* herpes simplex virus and *Candida albicans.*

IV. Chronic Complications[11]

▶ Chronic GVHD
  • May affect all organs of the body.
  • Can appear up to 2 years posttransplant.

▶ *Oral complications:*
  • Oral mucositis
  • Oral infection/periodontal infection
  • Xerostomia/dental caries
  • Poor oral hygiene
  • Difficulty eating/chewing.

MUCOSITIS MANAGEMENT[12–16]

I. Prevention/Oral Health Maintenance

▶ Basic oral care using a soft toothbrush.
▶ As dental flossing is technique sensitive, use may be precluded during cytotoxic treatment.
▶ Use of a bland mouthrinse such as normal saline, 3–4 times/day.
▶ Cryotherapy (ice chips)
  • Recommended for selected patient populations such as multiple myeloma receiving high-dose Melphalan and head and neck patients receiving bolus dosing of 5-fluorouracil.
  • Instruct patient to hold ice chips in mouth immediately prior to and during administration of chemotherapy agent.
▶ Palifermin (a human recombinant keratinocyte growth factor, KGF-1)
  • Intravenous infusion in selected populations prior to peripheral blood stem cell transplant
  • Given for three consecutive days before and after myelotoxic therapy for a total of six doses.
▶ Benzydamine mouthrinse (nonsteroidal anti-inflammatory agent) in patients receiving moderate dose radiation therapy (up to 50 Gy). Note: This drug not available in the United States.

II. Treatment of Established Mucositis

▶ Mouthrinse containing diphenhydramine HCL in combination with other agents (usually coating agent and topical anesthetic).
  • Evidence does not support a direct effect of this antihistaminic on the prevention or treatment of mucositis lesions.
  • This type of rinse is often used to palliate pain topically.
▶ *Systemic pain medication:* Patient controlled analgesia with morphine for the management of pain due to oral mucositis in patients undergoing hematopoietic stem cell transplant.
▶ Transdermal fentanyl patch may be effective in the management of mucositis pain due to conventional and high-dose chemotherapy with or without total body irradiation.
▶ Morphine mouthrinse may reduce the severity and duration of mucositis pain in patients undergoing head and neck area radiation therapy.

▶ Doxepin mouth rinse (0.5%) may be effective for the management of pain due to oral mucositis.

DENTAL HYGIENE CARE PLAN⁶

I. Objectives

It is recommended that patients be in optimal oral health before starting any type of cancer therapy. Overall objectives include the following:

▶ Assess the oral cavity for any signs of hard or soft tissue infection.

▶ Eliminate or minimize sources of dental/periodontal or soft tissue infection.

▶ Eliminate or minimize any areas of chronic trauma or tissue irritation.

▶ Provide preventive oral care education to patient and/ or caregiver.

II. Personal Factors

The very word *cancer* brings fear and anxiety to the patient, and many times is viewed by the patient as *cancer equals death*. This will impact anything taught to the patient. Suggestions include the following:

▶ Encourage the patient to bring a friend or family member along to take notes during teaching visits.

▶ Provide written instructions appropriate to the reading level of the patient. Make sure they are written in the patient's native language.

▶ Provide positive reinforcement and be creative in helping the patient maintain optimal oral health.

▶ Show acceptance and empathy. Acknowledge the appropriateness of the patient's concerns.

▶ Practice active listening skills.

III. Oral Care Protocol

The following sections are adapted from the *Oral Complications of Cancer Treatment: What the Oral Health Team Can Do* from the National Institute for Dental and Craniofacial Research (NIH publication no. 02-4372).

▶ Similarities exist between the three forms of treatment (radiation therapy, chemotherapy, and hematopoietic stem cell transplantation).

▶ There are differences that dental hygienists need to know to provide appropriate oral care.

▶ Numerous grading scales have been developed to assess the severity of oral mucositis, but none for the other oral complications.

▶ Table 56-2 lists an example of one mucositis scale. Scales are useful to:

TABLE 56-2	World Health Organization Oral Mucositis Scale
GRADE	**CLINICAL FEATURES**
0	No oral mucositis
1	Soreness, erythema
2	Oral ulcers, solid foods tolerated
3	Oral ulcers, liquid diet only (due to mucositis)
4	Oral ulcers, alimentation impossible (due to mucositis)

Source: Lalla R, Sonis S, Peterson D. Management of oral mucositis in patients with cancer. *Dent Clin North Am*. 2008;52(1):61–68.

• Measure mucositis in the nursing/medical setting
• Document treatment toxicity in the clinical and/or research setting
• Communicate intraprofessionally.

A. Pretreatment Therapy

▶ It is well recognized that patients who do intensive personal oral care in preparation for and during their cancer therapy have a reduced risk for the development of oral complications.

▶ Box 56-5 provides examples of dental hygiene/dental treatment options that may be beneficial before the start of cancer therapy.

B. Head and Neck Radiation Therapy¹⁷⁻¹⁹

▶ Patients receiving radiation therapy to the head and neck are at high risk for developing severe oral complications that will affect the patient in the short and long term.

▶ Box 56-6 lists an example oral care protocol to be followed during treatment.

▶ *During radiation therapy:*

• Encourage daily oral care including biofilm removal at least twice daily.

• Encourage daily fluoride use (in any form, i.e., tray, brush on, rinse).

• Monitor the patient for trismus; check for pain or weakness in masticating muscles in the radiation field.

• Instruct the patient to exercise three times a day, opening and closing the mouth as far as possible without pain; repeat 20 times.

▶ *After radiation therapy:*

• For the first 6 months after cancer treatment, recall the patient every 4–8 weeks as needed for nonsurgical periodontal therapy.

BOX 56-5

Dental Hygiene/Dental Pretreatment Guidelines for Patients Planning to Undergo Cancer Therapy

DENTAL

▷ Conduct a pretreatment oral health examination.

▷ Schedule dental treatment in consultation with the oncologist (medical or radiation).

▷ Extract teeth with a poor or questionable prognosis at least 2 weeks before the start of cancer therapy.

▷ Restore or repair indicated teeth before the start of cancer therapy.

▷ Perform other necessary oral surgery procedures at least 2 weeks before the start of cancer therapy.

DENTAL HYGIENE

▷ Conduct a pretreatment oral health assessment.

▷ Schedule dental hygiene treatment in consultation with the oncologist (medical or radiation).

▷ Perform dental hygiene treatment (periodontal scaling and root planing, polishing, fluoride applications) before the start of cancer treatment.

▷ Evaluate the patient's oral health knowledge and provide an appropriate oral hygiene regimen based on the cancer management.

▷ Prevent tooth demineralization and dental caries:

  ▷ Instruct the patient in the daily application of fluoride gel at home.

  ▷ If receiving head–neck radiation therapy, fabricate custom gel-applicator trays for the patient.

  ▷ Demonstrate application of a 1.1% neutral pH sodium fluoride gel or a 0.4% stannous, unflavored gel for use in the trays or brush on when tray insertion may not be tolerated.

  ▷ Use only a neutral pH sodium fluoride gel for porcelain crowns or glass or resin ionomer restorations.

  ▷ The trays cover all tooth surfaces and are left in the mouth for 5 minutes. Instruct the patient to have nothing to eat or drink for 30 minutes after using the fluoride. Specific technique is located in Chapter 36.

BOX 56-6

Oral Care Protocol During Treatment

Daily Biofilm Removal

▷ Gently brush teeth with a soft toothbrush and fluoride toothpaste after every meal and at bedtime. The tongue may be brushed with a soft toothbrush and water.

▷ Use interdental aids gently but thoroughly clean between teeth before brushing at least once each day.

Mouthrinsing

▷ Every 2–3 hours while awake, rinse the mouth with a baking soda, salt and water solution, followed by a plain water rinse. (Use 1/4 teaspoon of baking soda and 1/8 teaspoon salt in 1 cup of lukewarm water.)

▷ Use of fluoridated water when available.

Xerostomia

▷ Sip water frequently.

▷ Suck on ice chips or use sugar-free gum or candy.

▷ Use saliva substitute spray or gel or a prescribed saliva stimulant.

▷ Avoid lemon glycerin swabs.

▷ Avoid hot, spicy, salty, sharp, or high-sucrose foods.

▷ Moisten foods with gravy or liquids before eating.

Dental Caries Prevention

▷ Use fluoride toothpaste every day.

▷ If prescribed, brush teeth with 1.1% neutral NaF gel for 60 seconds after usual tooth cleaning, just before going to bed. Do not eat, drink, or rinse for a minimum of 30 minutes afterward.

▷ If using custom-made polyvinyl trays, place gel in trays, apply to teeth, close mouth, and hold in place for 4 minutes. Set timer. Remove trays, expectorate several times, and do not eat or drink for at least 30 minutes afterward.

Oral Pain Management

▷ Swish, and spit a prescribed mouthrinse containing topical anesthetic solution 30 minutes before eating.

- Review instructions for daily oral self-care.
- Reinforce the importance of daily oral self-care.
- After mucositis subsides, consult with the radiation/medical oncologist regarding timing of denture/appliance fabrication.
- Observe for trismus, demineralization, and caries.
- Lifelong, daily applications of prescription fluoride (in any form) are recommended for patients with chronic salivary gland hypofunction.
- Advise against oral surgery on irradiated bone, because of the risk of osteoradionecrosis.
- Tooth extraction, if unavoidable, is conservative.
- Prophylaxis against possible osteoradionecrosis is accomplished with Pentoxifylline 400 mg pre- and postextraction.

C. Chemotherapy[6,20,21]

▶ The extent of oral complications of chemotherapy depends on:

- The degree of preexistent dental and oral disease,
- The chemotherapy drugs used and their dosages,
- The use of concurrent or adjuvant radiation therapy to the head/neck,
- The patient's personal daily oral hygiene.

▶ Before any dental or dental hygiene clinical procedures during chemotherapy:

- Consult the medical oncologist before any dental or dental hygiene clinical procedures.
- Ask the medical oncologist to order blood work 24 hours before oral surgery or other invasive

procedures (such as periodontal scaling/root planing). Postpone when the platelet count is less than 50,000/mm³ or abnormal clotting factors are present, and/or neutrophil count is less than 1,000/mm³.

- In patients with fever of unknown origin as determined by the medical oncologist, check for oral source of viral, bacterial, or fungal infection.
- Encourage thorough oral self-care.
- Review indications for use of antibiotic premedication for patients with central venous catheters or peripherally inserted catheters (also known as central lines). There is no evidence suggesting this is beneficial and as such varies from practitioner to practitioner.
- Consult the medical oncologist for preference on using the American Heart Association prophylactic antibiotic regimen or another antibiotic regimen.

▶ Refer to Box 56-6 for a suggested oral care protocol during treatment.

▶ *After chemotherapy:* Place the patient on a dental hygiene continuing care schedule when chemotherapy is completed and all side effects, including immunosuppression, have resolved.

D. Hematopoietic Stem Cell Transplantation[22,23]

Some hematopoietic cell transplant patients develop acute oral complications, especially patients who had an allogeneic stem cell transplant and develop GVHD.

▶ *After transplantation*

- Monitor for oral infections of the soft tissues. Herpes simplex and Candida albicans are common oral infections.

- Delay elective dental procedures (such as implants) for 1 year.
- Follow patients for long-term oral complications (changes in taste, xerostomia, dental caries). Such problems are strong indicators of chronic GVHD.
- Continue to monitor the patient's oral health for biofilm control, tooth demineralization, dental caries, and oral infection.
- Follow transplant patients carefully for second malignancies in the oral region.

E. Special Care for Children[24,25]

Children receiving chemotherapy and/or radiation therapy are at risk for the same oral complications as adults. Other actions to consider in managing pediatric patients include the following:

▶ Extract loose primary teeth and teeth expected to exfoliate during cancer treatment.

▶ Remove orthodontic bands and brackets if myelosuppressive chemotherapy is planned or if the appliances will be in the radiation field.

▶ Continually monitor craniofacial and dental structures for abnormal growth and development.

▶ Encourage routine daily personal oral care including biofilm removal and fluoride application.

▶ Avoid cariogenic foods and drinks. If these are necessary to improve a child's weight, then have the child rinse with fluoridated water after eating or drinking.

EVERYDAY ETHICS

It's the end of the day and all of the patients, staff, and the dentist had left the office. Ashley, the dental hygienist, was reviewing the next day's patient records at the front desk.

The telephone rang and Ashley answered it. It was Gina, the daughter of a longtime patient, Mr. Prisby. Gina, a pediatric registered nurse, lives out of state, but is visiting her 70-year-old father who is undergoing head and neck radiation therapy and chemotherapy treatments for tongue cancer. When she arrived, she was shocked to find her father having difficulty opening his mouth completely and a white coating on the inside of his cheeks. Gina also noticed multiple sores in his mouth. Her father has been unable to eat anything but the softest of foods due to the severe discomfort and dryness. Gina is concerned that her father cannot maintain a healthy weight during treatment. She asks Ashley what the white coating and the sores are in her father's mouth and what can be done for him.

Ashley puts Gina on hold and pulls Mr. Prisby's record. She sees that he had a complete examination and all treatment performed that left him in good dental health 3 months ago, just before he started his cancer treatment. The white coating that Ashley described may be candidiasis and require medication. But she's not sure how to treat the sores Gina sees. Ashley considers whether to refer Gina back to the oncologists treating her father or phoning in the prescription in the dentist's name to save time.

Questions for Consideration

1. What advice can Ashley give to Gina, considering the stipulations of patient confidentiality?

2. Describe the ethical and legal consequences of Ashley phoning in a prescription for Mr. Prisby.

3. What decisions and/or actions are appropriate for Ashley to pursue within the scope of her legal duties at this time?

DOCUMENTATION

Each patient appointment is carefully documented to include at least the following:

▶ Cancer diagnosis; type of treatment; treatment start and completion dates.

▶ Oncologists' names and contact information; note any consults done with the oncologists.

▶ Oral assessment, clinical care provided, patient teaching on each visit.

▶ Any oral complications present; grading scaling number of oral mucositis; and what symptom management was prescribed.

▶ Planned follow-up visit and plan of care with proposed symptom management treatment outcomes.

▶ Box 56-7 shows an example of a documentation for a patient with oral lesions related to cancer therapy.

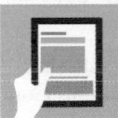

BOX 56-7
Example Documentation: Patient with Oral Lesions Related to Cancer Treatment

S –Patient presents for 3-month perio maintenance appointment; medical history changes include diagnosis of stage IV floor of mouth (FOM) cancer; lesion found at previous perio maintenance visit and patient evaluated by Otolaryngology 3 months ago, surgery completed 10 weeks ago followed by 6 weeks of radiation therapy (total of 62 Gy) ending last week.

O–Complete oral examination performed; unable to perform perio maintenance due to severe oral ulcerations and inflammation involving the tongue bilaterally as well as the mandibular labial mucosa and vestibule; saliva appears thick and ropey; reviewed oral hygiene; patient is not currently using fluoride.

A–Oral mucositis grade 4 and severe xerostomia following radiation to the oral cavity for squamous cell carcinoma of the FOM. Current health status precludes dental hygiene instrumentation today.

P–Recommend:
1. Discuss the above findings and today's recommendations with oncology team (primary oncologist, oncology nurse).
2. Extra soft toothbrush after meals and at bedtime.
3. Interproximal cleansing with appropriate aid.
4. Neutral sodium fluoride gel applied with brush 1 × day following dental biofilm removal.
5. Baking soda mouthrinse—mix 1/4 tsp baking soda and 1/8 tsp salt in 8 oz of warm water; rinse with 20 cc's 3 × day.
6. Avoid mouthrinses containing alcohol.

Will follow 1× week until oral mucositis resolves; next visit assess xerostomia and make treatment recommendations as needed.

Signed _____, RDH

Date _____

Factors To Teach The Patient

▷ How to exercise the jaw muscles three times a day to prevent and treat jaw stiffness from head and neck radiation therapy.
▷ Why to avoid candy, gum, and soda unless they are sugar free.
▷ Why to avoid spicy or acidic foods, and the use of toothpicks.
▷ Why to avoid use of tobacco products and alcohol.
▷ Why the dental hygienist needs to conduct an oral soft tissue screening and complete oral examination at regular frequent intervals.
▷ How and when to use dental biofilm control methods, gel-tray application, use of saliva substitute, and all other details of personal oral care to reduce oral side effects caused by the disease and/or cancer treatment.
▷ Ideas for remembering to follow the instructions to keep the mouth healthier and more comfortable during cancer treatment.
▷ The reasons why a routine schedule of preventive periodontal scaling, fluoride application, and oral hygiene assessment by a dental hygienist contributes to the success of the cancer treatment.

Factors To Teach The Caregiver

▷ How maintaining optimal oral health throughout treatment will contribute to the successful outcome of cancer therapy.
▷ The need to report any changes in the oral cavity to the oncologist and/or dentist/dental hygienist.
▷ Why it is necessary for the patient to receive preventive periodontal scaling, polishing if indicated, fluoride application, and oral hygiene assessment by a dental hygienist on a regular frequent basis.
▷ Why it is important to support the patient in stopping tobacco and alcohol use.

References

1. Hanahan D, Weinberg RA. Hallmarks of cancer. *Cell.* 2011;144(5):646–674.
2. Siegel R, Naishadham D, Jemal A. Cancer statistics, 2013. *CA Cancer J Clin.* 2013;63(1):11–30.
3. American Cancer Society. *CA Facts and Figures.* Atlanta, GA: American Cancer Society; 2013.
4. American Cancer Society. Find support and treatment. http://www.cancer.org/treatment/index. Accessed May 27, 2014.
5. Scarpa R. Surgical management of head and neck Carcinoma. *Semin Oncol Nurs.* 2009;25(3):172–182.
6. National Institutes of Health Consensus Development Conference on Oral Complications of Cancer Therapies:

Diagnosis, Prevention, and Treatment. *NCI Monogr.* 1990;9:1–184.

7. Badros A, Weikel D, Salama A, et al. Osteonecrosis of the jaw in multiple myeloma patients: clinical features and risk factors. *J Clin Oncol.* 2006;24(6):945–952.

8. Elting L, Keefe D, Sonis S, et al. Patient-reported measurements of oral mucositis in head and neck cancer patients treated with radiotherapy with or without chemotherapy. *Cancer.* 2008;113(10):2704–2713.

9. Gooley TA, Chien JW, Pergam SA, et al. Reduced mortality after allogeneic hematopoietic-cell transplantation. *N Engl J Med.* 2010;363(22):2091–2101.

10. Sheppard D, Bredeson C, Allan D, et al. Systematic review of randomized controlled trials of hematopoietic stem cell mobilization strategies for autologous transplantation for hematologic malignancies. *Biol Blood Marrow Transplant.* 2012;18(8):1191–1203.

11. Ferrara JL, Levine JE, Reddy P, et al. Graft-versus-host disease. *Lancet.* 2009;373(9674):1550–1561.

12. McGuire DB, Fulton JS, Park J, et al; and Study Group of the Multinational Association of Supportive Care in Cancer/International Society of Oral Oncology (MASCC/ISOO). Systematic review of basic oral care for the management of oral mucositis in cancer patients. *Support Care Cancer* 2013;21(11):3165–3177.

13. Peterson DE, Ohrn K, Bowen J, et al.; and Mucositis Study Group of the Multinational Association of Supportive Care in Cancer/International Society of Oral Oncology (MASCC/ISOO). Systematic review of oral cryotherapy for management of oral mucositis caused by cancer therapy. *Support Care Cancer.* 2013;21(1):327–332.

14. Raber-Durlacher JE, von Bultzingslowen I, Logan RM, et al.; and Mucositis Study Group of the Multinational Association of Supportive Care in Cancer/International Society of Oral Oncology (MASCC/ISOO). Systematic review of cytokines and growth factors for the management of oral mucositis in cancer patients. *Support Care Cancer.* 2013;21(1):343–355.

15. Nicolatou-Galitis O, Sarri T, Bowen J, et al; and Mucositis Study Group of the Multinational Association of Supportive Care in Cancer/International Society of Oral Oncology (MASCC/ISOO). Systematic review of anti-inflammatory agents for the management of oral mucositis in cancer patients. *Support Care Cancer.* 2013;21(11):3179–3189.

16. Saunders DP, Epstein JB, Elad S, et al.; and Mucositis Study Group of the Multinational Association of Supportive Care in Cancer/International Society of Oral Oncology (MASCC/ISOO). Systematic Review of antimicrobials, mucosal coating agents, anesthetics and analgesics for the management of oral mucositis in cancer patients. *Support Care Cancer.* 2013;21(11):3191–3207.

17. Schuurhuis J, Stokman M, Roodenburg J, et al. Efficacy of routine pre-radiation dental screening and dental follow-up in head and neck oncology patients on intermediate and late radiation effects. A retrospective evaluation. *Radiother Oncol.* 2011;101(3):403–409.

18. Hong CHL, Napenas JL, Hodgson BD, et al. A systematic review of dental disease in patients undergoing cancer therapy. *Support Care Cancer.* 2010;18(8):1007–1021.

19. Bueno A, Ferreira R, Barbosa F, et al. Periodontal care in patients undergoing radiotherapy for head and neck cancer. *Support Care Cancer.* 2013;21(11):969–975.

20. Rubenstein E, Peterson D, Schubert M, et al.; the Mucositis Study Section of the Multinational Association of Supportive Care in Cancer; and the International Society for Oral Oncology. Clinical practice guidelines for the prevention and treatment of cancer therapy-induced oral and gastrointestinal mucositis. *Cancer.* 2004;100(9, Suppl): 2026–2046.

21. Jensen S, Pedersen A, Vissink A, et al. A systematic review of salivary gland hypofunction and xerostomia induced by cancer therapies: prevalence, severity and impact on quality of life. *Support Care Cancer.* 2010;18(8):1039–1060.

22. Morimoto Y, Niwa H, Imai Y, et al. Dental management prior to hematopoietic stem cell transplantation. *Spec Care Dentist.* 2004;24(6):287–292.

23. Meier J, Wolff D, Pavletic S, et al. Oral chronic graft-versus-host disease: report from the International Consensus Conference on clinical practice in cGVHD. *Clin Oral Investig.* 2011;15(2):127–139.

24. da Fonseca MA. Dental care of the pediatric cancer patient. *Pediatr Dent.* 2004;26(1):53–57.

25. Cheng K, Lee V, Li C, et al. Impact of oral mucositis on short-term clinical outcomes in paediatric and adolescent patients undergoing chemotherapy. *Support Care Cancer.* 2013;21(8):2145–2152.

ENHANCE YOUR UNDERSTANDING

 thePoint® DIGITAL CONNECTIONS
(see the inside front cover for access information)
- Audio glossary
- Quiz bank

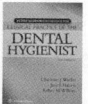 **SUPPORT FOR LEARNING**
(available separately; visit lww.com)
- *Active Learning Workbook for Clinical Practice of the Dental Hygienist, 12th Edition*

prepU INDIVIDUALIZED REVIEW
(available separately; visit lww.com)
- Adaptive quizzing with *prepU for Wilkins' Clinical Practice of the Dental Hygienist*

57

The Patient with a Disability

Charlotte J. Wyche, RDH, MS

LEARNING OBJECTIVES

After studying this chapter, the student will be able to:

1. Identify and define key terms and concepts relating to individuals with disabilities.

2. Identify risk factors for oral disease associated with disabling conditions.

3. Describe factors that enhance the prevention of oral disease for individuals with disabilities and their caregivers.

4. Explain procedures and factors that contribute to safe and successful management of individuals with disabilities during dental hygiene care.

Disabilities can impact the daily activities and function of an individual. People with disabilities may require a modified approach to oral health care in order to achieve and maintain oral health and prevent rampant dental disease.[1] This chapter provides general guidelines for modifying dental hygiene care for the patient with a disability.

▶ Further information about patients with specific disabling conditions is found throughout the chapters in Section IX of this book.

▶ Box 57-1 supplies key words and definitions pertaining to impairments and disabilities.

DISABILITIES OVERVIEW

▶ Obtaining access to oral health services can present challenges for both the patient and dental personnel.

▶ The patient may need to overcome numerous obstacles in daily living before the additional issues of oral self-care and access to dental care are addressed.

▶ Imagination, ingenuity, flexibility, and persistence are necessary in order to individualize and modify dental hygiene interventions when caring for people with disabilities.

▶ Patience, calmness, kindness, and empathy are keys to approaching any special needs patient.

I. Definitions and Classifications

▶ The United States Americans with Disabilities Act (ADA) defines an individual with a disability as a person who:
  • Has a physical or mental impairment that substantially limits one or more major life activities
  • Has a record of such impairment
  • Or is regarded as having such impairment.[2]

▶ Impairment refers to a loss of structure or function that leads to restriction of function.

▶ Use of the term handicap, which implies that an individual with impairment is disadvantaged in some way, is not usually appreciated by a person with a disability.

▶ Table 57-1 outlines a classification system for disability and health that provides a standard language and framework for the description of health and health-related states.[3]

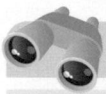

BOX 57-1 KEY WORDS: Impairment and Disability

Americans with Disabilities Act (ADA): prohibits discrimination on the basis of a disability and requires public and commercial facilities to meet standards of accessibility by removing architectural, transportation, and communication barriers.

AwDA: Americans with Disabilities Act; abbreviation sometimes used to prevent confusion with the ADA (American Dental Association).

Barrier free: area freely accessible to all without discrimination on the basis of a disability; obstacles to passage or communication have been removed.

Behavior modification: an approach to correction of undesirable conduct accomplished through systematic manipulation of the environmental and behavioral variables related to the specific behavior to be changed.

Behavior therapy: an approach in which the focus is on the patient's observable behavior rather than on conflicts and unconscious processes presumed to underlie the maladaptive behavior.

Deinstitutionalization: returning patients to home and community rather than housing them permanently or for long periods in custodial institutions; elimination of mental health institutions, for example, made possible by (1) use of new medications to control the symptoms of illness and (2) community health centers to provide support.

Desensitization: the treatment of phobias and related disorders by intentionally exposing the patient, in imagination

or real life, to emotionally distressing stimuli; desensitization to accept dental treatment might consist, for example, of short exposures to the dental chair, instruments, air syringe, and sound of a handpiece along with building trust in the dental team members.

Developmental disability: a substantial handicap of indefinite duration with onset before the age of 18 years. Examples include autism and cerebral palsy.

Disability: (individual dimension) restriction or lack of ability (resulting from an impairment) to perform an activity in the manner or within the range considered normal for a human being of the same age, sex, and background.

Handicap: (social dimension) a disadvantage for an individual, resulting from an impairment or a disability, that limits or prevents fulfillment of a role that is within the normal range for a human of the same age, sex, and social and cultural factors as the affected individual.

Impairment: (organ or body dimension) any loss or abnormality of psychologic, physiologic, or anatomic structure or function.

Mainstreaming: integration of people with disabilities into their community through programs of rehabilitation; process by which persons with special needs (educational, physical, psychologic) are included within the mainstream of society rather than segregated.

Normalization: establishing patterns and conditions of everyday life as close as possible to the norms and patterns of the mainstream of society.

TABLE 57-1	International Classification of Functioning, Disability, and Health

PART 1: FUNCTIONING AND DISABILITY	
BODY FUNCTIONS	
Mental functions	The brain: both global mental functions, such as consciousness, energy and drive, and specific mental functions, such as memory, language, and calculation mental functions.
Sensory functions	Seeing, hearing, tasting, and touch, as well as the sensation of pain.
Voice and speech functions	Producing sounds and speech.
Functions of the cardiovascular, hematological, immunological, and respiratory systems	The heart and blood vessels, blood production, immunity, respiration, and exercise tolerance.
Functions of the digestive, metabolic, and endocrine systems	Ingestion, digestion, and elimination, as well as metabolism and the endocrine glands.
Genitourinary and reproductive functions	Urination and the reproduction, including sexual and procreative functions.
Neuromusculoskeletal and movement-related functions	Movement and mobility, including functions of joints, bones, reflexes, and muscles.
Functions of the skin and related structures	Skin, skin glands, nails, hair, and related structures.
BODY STRUCTURES	
Structures of the nervous system	Brain, spinal cord, meninges, and nervous system, including sympathetic and parasympathetic nervous systems.
The eye, ear, and related structures	Eye socket, eyeball, external ear, middle ear, inner ear, and related structures.
Structures involved in voice and speech	Nose, mouth, pharynx, larynx, and related structures.
Structures of the cardiovascular, immunological, and respiratory systems	Heart, arteries, veins, and capillaries; central lymphoid tissue (bone marrow, thymus) and peripheral lymphoid tissue (lymph nodes, spleen, mucosa-associated lymphoid tissue); and pharynx, trachea, bronchi, and lungs.
Structures related to the digestive, metabolic, and endocrine systems	Salivary glands, esophagus, stomach, intestines, pancreas, liver, gall bladder and ducts, endocrine glands, and related structures.
Structures related to the genitourinary and reproductive systems	Kidneys, ureter, bladder, pelvic floor, and male and female reproductive structures.
Structures related to movement	Head, neck, shoulder, upper and lower extremities, pelvic regions, trunk, musculoskeletal system, and other structures related to movement.
Skin and related structures	Skin, skin glands, nails, hair, and related structures.
PART 2: CONTEXTUAL FACTORS	
ACTIVITIES AND PARTICIPATION	
Learning and applying knowledge	Learning, applying the knowledge that is learned, thinking, solving problems, and making decisions.
General tasks and demands	Carrying out specific single or multiple tasks, organizing routines and handling stress; identifying the underlying features of the execution of tasks under different circumstances.

(continues)

TABLE 57-1	International Classification of Functioning, Disability, and Health (*continued*)
PART 2: CONTEXTUAL FACTORS	
Communication	General and specific features of communicating by language, signs and symbols, including receiving and producing messages, carrying on conversations, and using communication devices and techniques.
Mobility	Moving by changing body position or location or by transferring from one place to another by carrying, moving, or manipulating objects; by walking, running, or climbing; and by using various forms of transportation.
Self-care	Caring for oneself, washing and drying oneself; caring for one's body and body parts; dressing, eating and drinking; and looking after one's health.
Domestic life	Carrying out domestic and everyday actions and tasks; acquiring a place to live, food, clothing, and other necessities; household cleaning and repairing; caring for personal and other household objects; and assisting others.
Interpersonal interactions and relationships	Carrying out the actions and tasks required for basic and complex interactions with people (strangers, friends, relatives, family members, and lovers) in a contextually and socially appropriate manner.
Major life areas	Carrying out the tasks and actions required to engage in education, work, and employment and to conduct economic transactions.
Community, social, and civic life	Actions and tasks required to engage in organized social life outside the family in community, social, and civic areas of life.

ENVIRONMENTAL FACTORS THAT INFLUENCE FUNCTIONING

Products and technology	Natural or human-made products or systems of products, equipment, and technology in an individual's immediate environment that are gathered, created, produced, or manufactured.
Natural and human-made changes to environment	Animate and inanimate elements of the natural or physical environment, and components of that environment that have been modified by people, as well as characteristics of human populations within that environment.
Support and relationships	People or animals that provide practical physical or emotional support, nurturing, protection, assistance, and relationships to other persons in their home, place of work, school, at play, or in other aspects of their daily activities.
Attitudes	The observable consequences of customs, practices, ideologies, values, norms, factual beliefs, and religious beliefs that influence individual behavior and social life; individual or societal attitudes about a person's value as a human being that may motivate positive, honorific practices, or negative and discriminatory practices.
Services, systems, and policies	Governmental and private programs, infrastructure, regulations, and standards designed to meet the needs of individuals.

II. Types of Conditions

▶ Types of disabilities include:
- Developmental: hereditary conditions that manifest symptoms before age 21.
- Acquired: caused by chronic disease (such as multiple sclerosis), acute medical conditions (such as stroke), or trauma (such as spinal cord injury).
- Age associated: usually after age 65 and related to a chronic health condition (such as arthritis or Parkinson's disease).

▶ Some types of impairment can manifest as a stable condition; others may cause progressive disability.

▶ A temporary disability can result from a physical impairment such as a broken leg or because of a physiologic condition such as the limitations that occur during pregnancy.

- A variety of impairments are found among persons with disabilities, and an individual may have more than one type of disability.
- Many diseases and syndromes with associated symptoms of disability or impairment are described in various chapters throughout Section IX of this book.

III. Occurrence

- An estimated 8% of individuals 16–64 and almost 6% of children 5–15 are affected by a disability and the number is increasing.[4]
- Progress in medical care has increased initial survival of those born with a disability and increased the survival rate of those experiencing a disabling condition.
- As life expectancy increases, so does the likelihood of acquiring a disability.[4]

IV. Access to Oral Health Services

- People with disabilities experience a diminished oral health status and reduced access to dental services compared to the general population.[5-8]

- Progress is being made to ensure adequate access to dental care, but barriers that exist can involve the patient, family, caregivers, guardians, and dental professionals, as described in Table 57-2.
- Having adequate access to dental and dental hygiene services can make a significant contribution to the oral health, well-being, independence, and sense of personal esteem of a patient with a disability.
- Although providing care for patients with disabilities is challenging, training, experience, empathy, patience, and a desire to be successful can help.[7]

V. Trends in Community-Based Delivery of Services

A. Overview

- Most individuals with physical and intellectual impairments have community-based living, educational, and work arrangements.
- Barrier-free or assisted-living housing for individuals and staffed community-based residential facilities for group living are available for those who need daily assistance.

TABLE 57-2	Examples of Barriers to Access for Dental Care		
	PATIENT	**FAMILY, CAREGIVER, GUARDIAN**	**DENTAL PROFESSIONAL**
Attitude barriers	■ May not comprehend importance of dental health. ■ May not be aware of needing dental care. ■ May not want to or be able to cooperate.	■ May not care for own dental health. ■ May be overstressed with other patient health issues that seem more important than dental need.	■ May not feel adequately trained to or want to or be able to treat safely a physically, cognitively, or medically compromised patient.
Health literacy barriers	■ May not understand the relationship of oral health to systemic health. ■ May have difficulty understanding insurance coverage, locating a provider, making appointments, or completing paperwork.	■ May not understand the relationship of oral health to systemic health. ■ May have difficulty understanding insurance coverage, locating a provider, making appointments, or completing paperwork.	■ May not understand that the patient has many barriers to accessing dental care. ■ May not have adequately assessed the patient's health literacy when providing previous care.
Physical barriers	■ Fear of not being able to cope with architectural barriers. ■ Fear of falling. ■ Fear of attracting attention in an embarrassing way.	■ May not be able to transport patient with wheelchair. ■ May not be able to lift or support patient in car or dental chair.	■ Office facility or treatment rooms may not provide a barrier-free environment.
Financial barriers	■ May have limited income. ■ May not have adequate dental insurance coverage or cannot find a provider who accepts specific insurance.	■ May not be able to take time from employment to accompany patient to appointments.	■ Cost of building accessible features or buying specialized equipment. ■ Lack of reimbursement for the additional cost of longer appointment times needed for care.

- Many home-care and community-based services are available for individuals with disabilities; however, access to dental services is often limited by traditional office-based dental care delivery systems.

- New healthcare delivery system models are being proposed to provide access to dental services where people live, work, play, go to school, or receive other social services.[9–11]

B. New Models

- Development of delivery system focused on screening, triage, prevention, and education, with only complex treatment, needs being referred to a private dental practice or hospital clinic.

- Integration of oral health into general health and social services systems.

- Integration of licensed "health facilities" in public and private residential facilities and training of staff and other caregivers to play a more major role in oral health.

- Delivery of services in residence homes using mobile equipment.

- Expansion of "direct access" regulations that increase the ability of dental hygienists to provide preventive services in alternative settings and function as members of interprofessional patient care teams.[12–15]

- The development of new midlevel oral health providers trained to provide less complex dental care.[16,17]

- Use of technology to facilitate consultation between oral health professionals as well as communication between patient and providers.

- Reform of the oral health insurance/Medicaid reimbursement systems to increase payment for extra time needed when providing care for special needs populations.

BARRIER-FREE ENVIRONMENT

- Healthcare facilities are required to follow guidelines and specifications for a barrier-free physical environment based on governmental regulations for accessibility standards.[18]

- In general, a facility that is barrier free for a patient in a wheelchair is accessible to all other individuals. The patient in a wheelchair requires more space for turning and positioning.

- Additional features are needed for other specific disabilities, for example, braille floor indicators can be installed beside the numbers on elevators; doorways, steps, and stairways can be outlined with bright colors to contrast with the background for people with limited vision.

I. External Features

A. Parking

- A reserved area, clearly marked, near the building entrance and 13-feet wide (8-foot car space with 5-foot access aisle permits opening car doors for exiting and reboarding).

- Curb ramps (cuts) from the street and from the parking area.

B. Walkways

- A 3-foot-wide walkway is needed for wheelchair accommodation.

- The surface is solid and nonslip, without irregularities.

C. Entrance

- At least one entrance to the building on ground level accessible by a gently sloping ramp (rise of 1 inch for every 12 inches).

- An easily grasped handrail (height 30–34 inches) is needed on both sides, to accommodate left- and right-handed cane and one-crutch users.

D. Door

The lightweight door with a lever type of handle opens at least 32 inches for a person using a tall crutch and for a wheelchair as shown in Figure 57-1.

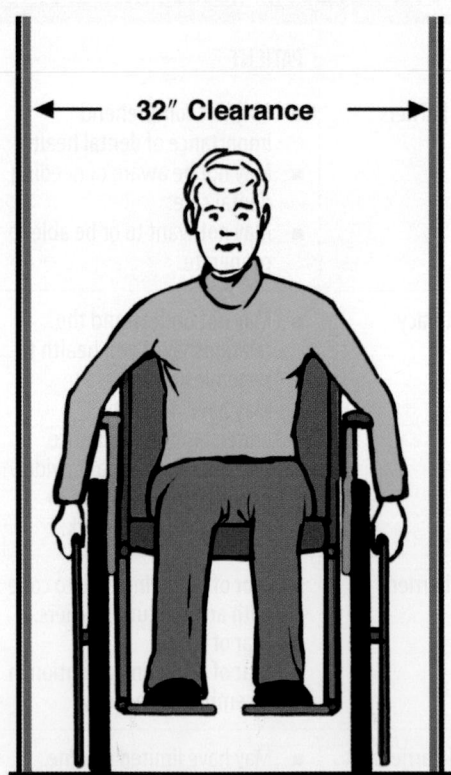

FIGURE 57-1 Wheelchair Accessibility. Wheelchairs designed for adults vary in width from 2 feet 3 inches to 2 feet 8 inches. A clear door width of 32 inches to accommodate these wheelchairs has been accepted as the official regulation.

II. Internal Features

Official regulations specify dimensions for accessibility of all aspects, including passageways, floors, drinking fountains, and restrooms. A few are described here.

A. Passageways

▶ The passageways are at least 3 feet wide, with handrails along the sides.

▶ Passageways are free from obstructions, such as hanging signs that a tall blind person could collide.

B. Floors

▶ Level floors with nonslip surfaces.

▶ Thick or small, unattached movable rugs or carpets present obstacles for wheelchairs or walkers and hazards for a patient with crutches, cane, or leg brace.

C. Reception Area

▶ At least part of the furniture will permit easy access during seating and rising.

▶ Preferred are chairs with 18-inch-high, flat, firm seats, and arms for support when pushing oneself up by the arms.

▶ Select chairs that do not slide or tip as the person rises.

III. The Treatment Room

▶ Space is needed for the dental chair, related dental equipment, and the wheelchair.

▶ The doorways are at least 32 inches wide.

▶ The wheelchair is placed beside and parallel to the dental chair for patient transfer. In a small facility, the dental chair can be rotated to allow for turning the wheelchair.

▶ The dental chair selected is able to lower to 19 inches from the floor and accessible from both sides for wheelchair transfer.

▶ An X-ray machine in the same treatment room can simplify the problems of moving the patient into a separate radiography room.

RISK ASSESSMENT

▶ Patients with disabilities may be at higher risk for oral disease due to characteristics related to the specific disability or disease.

▶ Risk factors associated with specific disabilities and medical conditions are described more completely in the chapters devoted to the particular condition.

▶ Assessment of oral disease risk factors for a patient with a disability includes assessment of oral conditions, functional ability, and medical status.

I. Oral Manifestations[19]

People with disabilities have an increased risk for oral problems.

▶ Dental caries is common, often associated with diet and poor oral hygiene.

▶ Periodontal disease can occur more often and develop at an earlier age.

▶ Malocclusion is associated with muscular abnormalities, developmental delays, delayed tooth eruption, and oral habits such as bruxism or tongue thrusting.

▶ Oral and craniofacial anomalies may be present, particularly in individuals with developmental disabilities.[19] Examples include:
   • Enamel defects
   • High lip lines and dry gingiva due to air exposure
   • Variations in number, size, or shape of teeth
   • Facial asymmetry and hypoplasia of the midfacial region
   • Cleft lip or palate (see Chapter 51).

▶ Damaging oral habits can affect both soft and hard oral tissues. Examples include:
   • Bruxism
   • Mouth breathing
   • Tongue thrusting
   • Self-injurious behavior
   • Rumination (regurgitation of chewed food)
   • Pica (eating unusual objects and substances such as cigarette butts or clay).

▶ Evidence of trauma or injury may be present, especially in individuals with a seizure disorder or physical disability.

▶ Weakness or paralysis of facial muscles can compromise mastication and self-cleaning motion of the tongue. Food pouching is common.

▶ Drooling or impaired swallowing of saliva is a common feature of some disabling conditions involving head and neck musculature.[20]

▶ Potential oral side effects of medications include:
   • Increased dental caries risk due to sweetened elixirs or medication induced xerostomia.
   • Drug-induced gingival enlargement, a potential side-effect of treatment with phenytoin or other antiepileptic medication (see Chapter 63).
   • Oral ulcerations, mucositis, and susceptibility to infection, frequent manifestations following chemotherapy cancer treatment or radiation to head and neck area are discussed in Chapter 56.

II. Functional Ability

▶ Functional ability refers to the ability of an individual to accomplish daily living skills (bathing, toothbrushing, dressing, etc.).

▶ Assessment of functional ability determines what oral self-care tasks an individual can do alone, what range or degree of assistance is needed, or whether the person depends on others for complete care.

▶ An individual patient's functional level may be affected by:
- Decrease in cognitive capability
- Behavioral problems
- Mobility problems
- Uncontrolled body movements.

▶ Functioning levels and implications for oral self-care are described in Box 57-2 and in Table 24-3 in Chapter 24.

III. Medical Status

▶ Assessment and monitoring of the patient's medical status during treatment can reduce the risk of a medical emergency.

▶ Individuals with a disability may also experience additional medical comorbidities and health challenges such as[19]:
- Cardiac disorders
- Gastroesophageal reflux
- Seizures
- Visual and hearing impairments
- Latex allergies (due to spina bifida or frequent surgeries).

BOX 57-2

Level of Function and Implications for Oral Self-care

HIGH FUNCTION LEVEL: *ADL/IADL[a] LEVEL 0*

▷ The high-functioning, self-care group includes those capable of flossing and brushing their own teeth.

▷ Many patients, particularly children and those of all ages who are disabled mentally, need varying degrees of encouragement, motivation, and supervision.

MODERATE FUNCTIONING LEVEL: *ADL/IADL LEVELS 1 & 2*

▷ The moderate-functioning, partial-care group includes those capable of carrying out at least part of their oral hygiene needs but who require considerable training, assistance, and direct supervision.

▷ The assistance may be verbal, gestural, or hand over hand.

LOW FUNCTIONING LEVEL: *ADL/IADL LEVEL 3*

▷ The low-functioning, total-care group includes those who are unable to attend to their own care and are therefore dependent.

▷ Patients in this group may be bedridden and nonambulatory, although others may be confined to wheelchairs. With training, some may be able to attempt a part of their own care.

---

[a]Based on: ADL/IADL Measures of Patient Functioning in Table 24-3 in Chapter 24.

▶ Medications the patient takes may enhance risk for oral disease.
- Medications with a side effect of xerostomia contribute to dental caries.
- Medications that diminish appetite as a side effect influence diet habits.
- Sucrose-based liquid medications contribute to dental caries incidence.[21]

ORAL DISEASE PREVENTION AND CONTROL

I. Objectives

Whether care is being delivered in a traditional private practice, residential or educational facility, or community-based clinical setting the dental team has as its objectives to:

▶ Provide regular professional examinations and treatment at intervals established by the patient's level of risk for oral disease.

▶ Motivate the patient and caregiver to establish and maintain healthy oral tissue with freedom from infection.

▶ Contribute to the patient's general health through preventing tooth loss and maintaining ability to masticate food, which prevents malnutrition and increases resistance to infection.

▶ Prevent the need for extensive dental and periodontal treatment the patient may not be able to tolerate because of lowered physical stamina or the inability to cooperate.

▶ Prevent the need for dentures or other removable prostheses, which can be hazardous, difficult, or impossible for certain patients to tolerate.

▶ Aid in personal appearance, the perception of healthy oral status, and social acceptance without halitosis.

II. Preventive Care Introduction

▶ Preventive interventions are selected based on individualized risk factors and level of assistance needed for daily oral care.

▶ Depending on the disability and level of function, the patient may need:
- Complete assistance.
- Partial assistance.
- No assistance with daily biofilm removal.

▶ If assistance is needed, caregiver cooperation and motivation are essential for success.

▶ Daily personal oral hygiene care can be compromised due to:
- Lack of patient or caregiver knowledge and understanding about oral disease prevention and how it is accomplished.

- Lack of patient or caregiver motivation to carry out the necessary daily routines.
- Lack of the necessary cognitive and/or physical coordination to carry out oral hygiene measures.
- Lack of assistance from a caregiver.

III. Dental Biofilm Removal

A. Provide Basic Information

▶ Individualized instruction is provided for each patient according to the patient's unique needs and functional ability.

▶ Determine the current daily care routine to identify what modifications are needed.

▶ Biofilm formation and disease development are described on a level at which the patient and caregiver can learn and be motivated.

▶ Approaches for motivating the patient or caregiver's health behavior change are described in Chapter 26.

B. Toothbrushing

▶ Basic information about toothbrushes and methods is found in Chapter 28.

▶ Biofilm removal is more important than the specific technique used, as long as damage is not done to the gingiva or teeth.

▶ Use of a soft toothbrush and a scrub-brush or circular Fones method may be appropriate and within the capability of certain patients.

▶ Alternative positions for a parent or caregiver providing toothbrushing assistance are discussed more completely later in this chapter.

▶ Adaptations for brush handles and other self-care aids can promote or make possible a patient's independent biofilm removal.

C. Dentifrice

▶ A dentifrice containing fluoride is recommended for patients who can use a dentifrice.
  - When a patient cannot control saliva, rinse, or expectorate, use of a dentifrice may be contraindicated.
  - A dentifrice may increase a gag reflex for certain patients.
  - Dentifrice is not essential to biofilm removal, and another method of daily fluoride application may be more appropriate.
  - When a parent or other caregiver is assisting, the paste may limit visibility for thorough biofilm removal.
  - When a paste is used, only a small amount is placed on the brush (pea size, Figure 50-8, in Chapter 50).

▶ The person who is severely disabled may be treated with a suction brush, as described in Chapter 58 to help prevent aspiration.

D. Dental Floss

▶ If standard use of dental floss is not possible, due to limited dexterity or use of only one hand, the use of a floss holder described below can make flossing possible.

▶ The holder may also be useful for the caregiver.

▶ Methods for increasing the size of a toothbrush handle may be adapted for the handle of a floss holder.

▶ Some patients will need to use other interdental aids, described in Chapter 29.

IV. Adaptive Aids

▶ Although a caregiver may be willing to brush the patient's teeth, as much as possible is carried out by the patient.

▶ Benefits to the patient may include feelings of self-esteem and accomplishment when able to manage the important task of brushing, particularly for patients who have physical but no cognitive disability.

▶ For patients whose main deterrent to oral self-care is related to grasp, manipulation, or control of a toothbrush, adaptations and self-care aids can help accommodate specific needs.

A. General Prerequisites for a Self-care Aid

▶ Disinfectable

▶ Durable; can withstand exposure to water and saliva

▶ Resistant to absorption of oral fluids

▶ Replaceable

▶ Inexpensive

B. Manual Toothbrush

▶ Figure 57-2 illustrates attachments to insert and hold the brush handle against the patient's hand. This attachment is useful for a patient
  - With fingers permanently fixed in a fist
  - Who cannot grasp and hold.

▶ Aids to enlarge the diameter of the toothbrush handle, useful for a patient with limited hand closure, are illustrated in Figure 57-3.

▶ For patient with limited shoulder or elbow movement, lengthen handle of the brush using a material strong or rigid enough to provide sufficient lateral pressure to remove biofilm from the tooth surfaces. Examples include:
  - Cylinder of wood with brush handle cemented inside.
  - Two brushes. Cut the head from an old brush and fasten the handle to the end of the new brush handle with glue or tape.
  - Tongue depressors taped to the brush handle, then one or two other tongue depressors taped to overlap and provide an extension.
  - Bicycle spoke, coat hanger, or other means for elongation fixed with a handle of acrylic resin. The metal tip may be heated and pushed into the toothbrush handle. Use double or triple thickness to avoid flexibility.

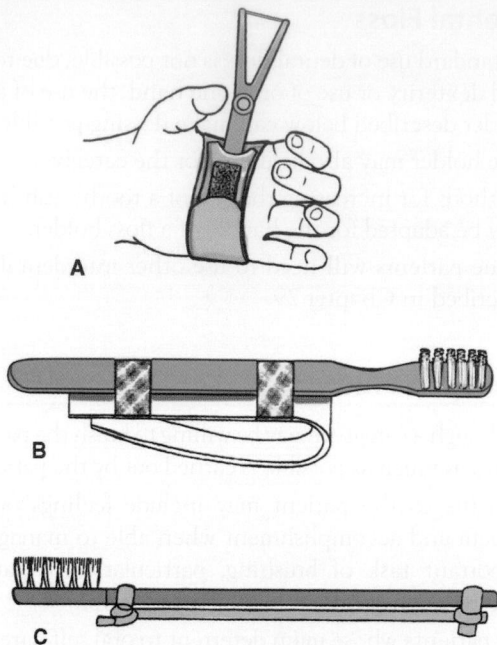

FIGURE 57-2 Aids for Patient Who Cannot Grasp and Hold. A: Adjustable Velcro strap around hand has a pocket designed to hold the toothbrush handle or floss aid. **B:** Handle of a fingernail brush attached to toothbrush by adhesive tape. **C:** Rubber tubing attached firmly to toothbrush handle enables patient to hold brush across the palm of the hand. A floss holder also may be held by these methods.

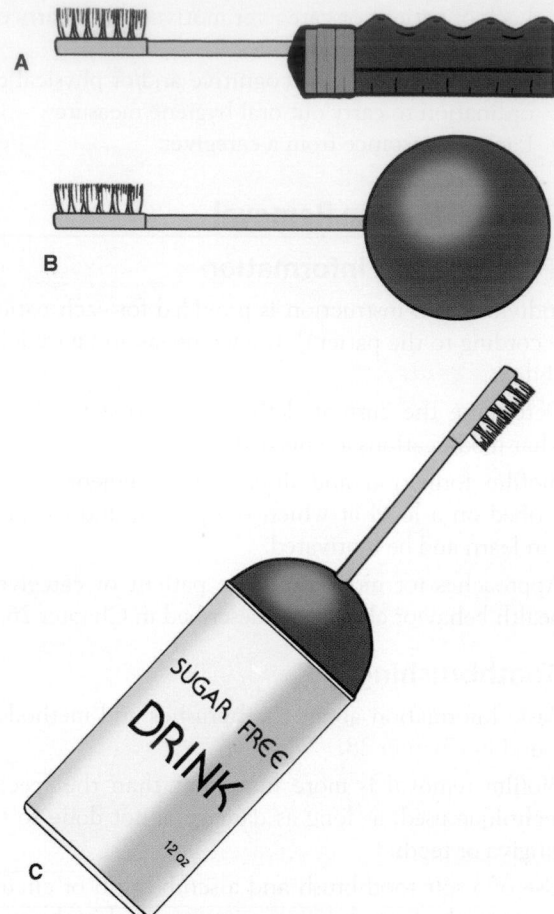

FIGURE 57-3 Aids for Patient with Limited Grasp. A: Toothbrush inserted into a bicycle handle grip. **B:** Toothbrush inserted into a soft rubber ball. **C:** Toothbrush in soft rubber ball inserted into a juice or soda pop can provide a handle of appropriate diameter for patients with limited hand closure.

▶ A specially designed toothbrush curved outer filaments and a short stiff center row of filaments that brush exposed tooth surfaces simultaneously is shown in Figure 57-4.

- For patient who can hold and position the toothbrush, but cannot make strokes for biofilm removal.
- For patient with hand tremors, such as with Parkinson's disease.
- Can be used with patient moving the head side to side and up and down instead of moving hand.
- Can be used by caregiver who provides toothbrushing assistance.
- Provides similar reduction in biofilm compared with use of a conventional brush.[22]

C. Power Aided Devices

▶ Use of a power toothbrush can provide independence and more effective biofilm removal for many patients and can motivate patients who have difficulty with a manual toothbrush.

- Can cause trauma if used incorrectly by, for example, a patient unable to hold the heavier weight of the power toothbrush or one lacking the comprehension for proper use.
- The extra size and weight of the handle may be advantageous for some patients or difficult for others with limited strength.

- The on/off mechanism may be difficult to use for those lacking finger strength and coordination.
- The larger handle can aid those who have difficulty grasping objects.
- The vibrations created during use cannot be tolerated by certain patients.
- Additional cost of the brush may be a consideration for some patients.

▶ Additional power aided devices, such as flossers, are available and are recommended based on assessment of an individual patient's need and abilities.

▶ Patients are instructed to follow manufacturers' instructions for proper use as indicated on each package.

▶ A patient with limited grasp can adapt a cuff around the handle to aid in holding the power-aided brush, similar to those shown in Figure 57-2.

▶ Cross contamination can be a problem, particularly in group living situations. Ensure each patient has a separate marked toothbrush and is kept apart from others.

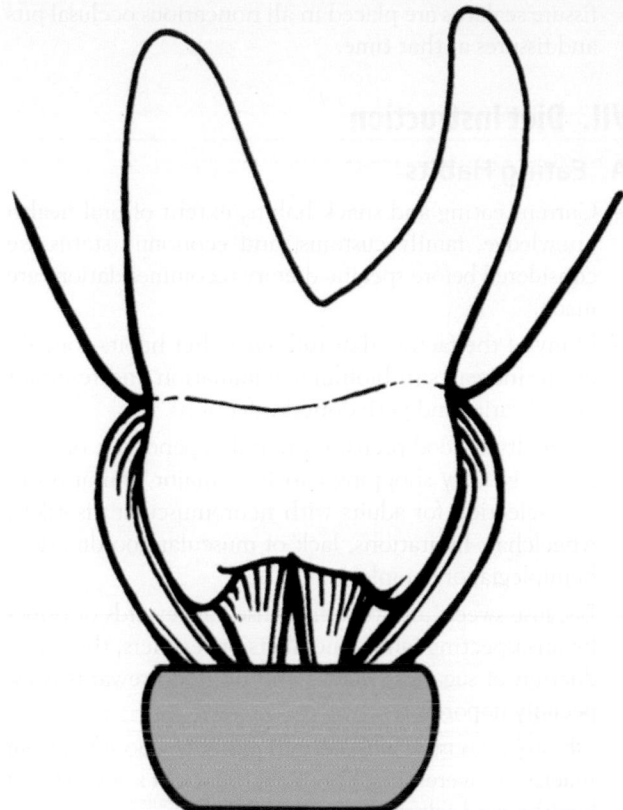

FIGURE 57-4 **Aid for Patient with a Brushing Problem.** A specially designed toothbrush is shown on the mesial of a maxillary second primary molar. Used with a back-and-forth motion, the filaments remove debris and dental biofilm simultaneously from the facial, lingual (palatal), and occlusal tooth surfaces.

D. The Floss Holder

▸ Careful instruction for use, as illustrated in Figure 57-5, and supervision is provided to avoid cutting the papilla and prevent tissue damage.

- Use a rest or fulcrum to prevent snapping through the contact.
- Pull the floss mesially while moving up and down (to clean the distal surface of a tooth) or push distally (to clean the mesial surface) to allow floss to be positioned on the side of the papilla.

E. Cleaning Removable Dental Prostheses

▸ The details for cleaning removable prostheses are described in Chapter 32.

▸ For the patient with difficulty grasping or holding the brush, a denture brush handle may be adapted by any of the methods described for the regular toothbrush.

▸ A fingernail brush may be used instead of a standard denture brush provided all denture surfaces can be reached for biofilm removal.

▸ For the patient with use of only one hand or who needs to grasp the denture with two hands to prevent accidents, the following are recommended:

- Fingernail brush with suction cups.

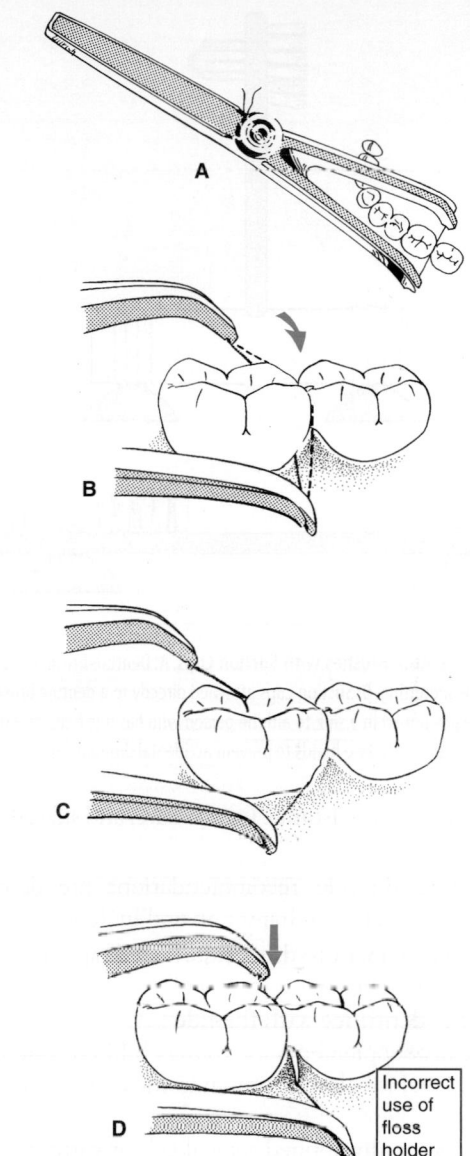

FIGURE 57-5 **Use of a Floss Holder. A:** The floss is held over the proximal contact for insertion. A hand rest is maintained on the chin to prevent excess pressure. **B:** As the floss is lowered gently and drawn through the contact area, the holder is pulled mesially when the floss is applied to the distal surface and pushed distally when the floss is applied to the mesial surface. **C:** Floss is lowered slightly below the gingival margin. **D:** Floss cut in the papilla when used incorrectly.

- Denture brush in mounting that has suction cups, as shown in Figure 57-6A.
- Denture brush with suction cups, as shown in Figure 57-6B, can attach low inside the sink bowl.

V. Fluorides

▸ Selection of a fluoride program for any patient depends on assessment of the individual's caries risk status (see Chapter 27).

▸ The patient with a disability may be at increased risk for caries due to barriers that limit access to preventive services, decreased ability to provide or

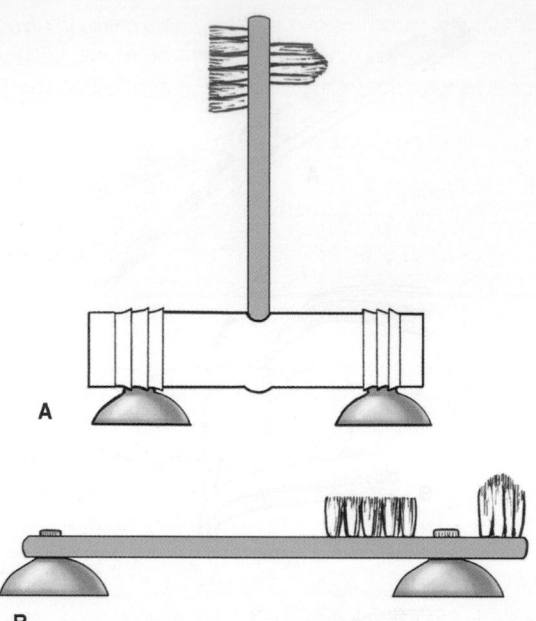

FIGURE 57-6 Denture Brushes with Suction Cups. A: Denture brush in a commercially available mounting. **B:** Suction cups attached directly to a denture brush. Either brush may be positioned in a sink to aid the person who has one hand or who needs to grasp the denture with two hands to prevent accidental dropping and breakage.

cooperate with assistance for self-care, and side effects of medications.

► Risk-based fluoride recommendations are described more completely in Chapter 36 and include:

- Encouragement to drink fluoridated tap water where available
- Use of dentifrice with fluoride
- Dietary supplements for young children, when fluoride level is below optimum in the community water supply
- Professionally applied topical gels or varnish
- Self-applied home fluoride

► For a dependent, low-functioning person, brushing with a fluoride gel rather than a toothpaste can be recommended.

VI. Pit and Fissure Sealants

► Pit and fissure sealants can be provided for cooperative patients with developmental disabilities with satisfactory results.

► The principles for application are the same as those for all patients, as described in Chapter 37.

► Use of a dental assistant is imperative to help with patient management and enhance ability to maintain a dry field to assure sealant retention.

► The use of a rubber dam is particularly helpful for patients with excess saliva, hyperactivity of the tongue, or other management difficulties.

► When a severely disabled patient will be administered general anesthesia for restorative procedures, pit and

fissure sealants are placed in all noncarious occlusal pits and fissures at that time.

VII. Diet Instruction

A. Eating Habits

► Current eating and snack habits, extent of oral health knowledge, family customs, and economic status are considered before specific dietary recommendations are made.

► Many of the factors that influence diet habits contribute to increases in biofilm accumulation and resultant dental caries and periodontal infections.

► Difficulty of food preparation and dependence on others for grocery shopping can be a major limitation to diet selection for adults with neuromuscular disorders, wheelchair limitations, lack of muscular coordination, hemiplegia, or paraplegia.

► Because sweets are sometimes used as rewards or bribes by unsuspecting family members or teachers, the introduction of sugarless snacks and nonfood rewards is especially important.

► Obesity is an issue with certain patients who suffer from inactivity, overeating, boredom, or lack of knowledge of healthy food selection.

B. Oral Factors

► Problems with mastication and swallowing can lead to use of a soft diet, often composed mainly of carbohydrates.

► Conditions that affect the integrity of facial musculature can compromise self-cleansing of oral structures and contribute to food pouching in the buccal vestibule.

C. Food Record

► A high-functioning patient may be able to keep a food diary, and participation is encouraged.

► The parent, advocate, or caregiver can assist or, in the case of a low- or moderate-functioning person, may complete the entire diary.

► With the aid of the daily food record and the information from the medical and dental histories, items for counseling can be selected.

D. Recommendations

► General procedures for dietary assessment and counseling are described in Chapter 35.

► Adaptations involve long-range planning for gradual modification of the patient's diet.

► The person who selects and prepares the food for the patient is involved in the planning.

► In an institutional setting, the dental hygienist can work as a member of the interprofessional patient care team with the administrative and medical personnel, teachers, dietitians, and aides to introduce dietary modifications.

PATIENT MANAGEMENT

▶ With a few modifications and attention to managing specific factors related to each individual's situation, most patients with disabilities can be treated in a clinical setting.

▶ Only a relatively small number need hospitalization due to difficulties in management or a systemic condition that requires special medical supervision.

I. Objectives

▶ Increase the efficacy, efficiency, and safety of dental and dental hygiene treatment.

▶ Make patient appointments pleasant and comfortable.

II. Communication

▶ Basic behavioral support strategies, such as tell–show–do, modeling, positive reinforcement, and desensitization, can be adapted to address the unique needs of the patient with a disability.[23]

▶ Unless the patient has an extreme cognitive impairment, the patient is always addressed first and the caregiver secondarily.

▶ The patient's ability to understand what is said is not underestimated; assessment of the patient's cognitive ability is essential and respect is indicated by addressing and making eye contact with the patient.

▶ Kindness, patience, and empathy will help the clinician build trust; each patient is unique, and members of the dental team can watch, listen, and learn procedures that will develop the patient's cooperation.

▶ Parents and other caregivers can explain how best to communicate with the patient, help interpret the changing moods of the patient, identify problems, and note changes in behavior that may indicate a dental problem.

▶ Nonverbal communication using facial expressions, pointing, body language, and demonstration helps certain patients to respond.

▶ A patient may prefer to write messages on a pad of paper or use sign language, a language board, or other devices the dental personnel can learn to use.

III. Pretreatment Planning

A. Preliminary Contact

▶ Information may be obtained from the patient, or with legal authority from the guardian, parent, relative, advocate, or other person responsible for the patient.

▶ The essential information can be obtained in advance by telephone interview, or medical forms can be mailed to the home for completion.

▶ Advanced information permits the dental team to be prepared to make the appointment a successful and positive experience for the patient and clinician.

B. Legal Guardianship

▶ When a person is declared incapacitated by a legal process, a guardian is appointed.

▶ The guardian then provides consent for any treatment, including signatures on consent forms.

▶ Written proof of legal guardianship is obtained and kept in the patient record.

C. Information to Obtain

▶ In addition to the usual topics covered by the medical, personal, and dental histories, additional information is requested, using questions listed in Box 57-3.

▶ To avoid unpleasant situations and misunderstanding, ask direct questions about a patient's disability rather than making assumptions.

D. Consultation with Interprofessional Care Team

▶ Management of a patient with disabilities can be very complex because the patient is medically compromised.

▶ Consultation with physicians, other medical providers, and the social worker who form the team of professionals involved in the patient's care may be required to help determine a plan to meet the patient's oral health needs.

▶ Extra time may be required to access information about the conditions and medications before an appointment.

E. Interaction with Caregiver

▶ A patient with a disability may depend on a caregiver for daily life activities.

▶ Caregivers may or may not be the legal guardian of patient or contact person to plan appointments.

▶ If the caregiver is not the legal guardian, the adult patient is consulted to determine the limits of the caregiver's role.

▶ Caregivers can be an excellent source of information, help prepare the patient for the appointment, and offer suggestions for gaining cooperation from the patient.

▶ Invite the caregiver to the office before the appointment to see the facility and become familiar with the surroundings and staff.

IV. Appointment Scheduling

A. Special Requirements

▶ Allow time in the schedule for preparation needed before appointment, for example, to move furniture, retrieve and set up special equipment, or premedicate the patient.

BOX 57-3

Patient with a Disability: Additional Information to Obtain Before the Appointment

Basic Information

▷ Has a guardian been legally appointed? Obtain written documentation.

▷ Is there a caregiver, case worker, or counselor who works with the patient?

▷ Will someone accompany the patient to appointments?

▷ Does the patient give consent to discuss care with other individuals?

▷ Degree of independence, self-care, and communication preferences of the patient.

Medical History

▷ Specific list of disabilities or disabling conditions.

▷ When diagnosed.

▷ History of treatments, hospitalizations, or institutionalization.

▷ Current medications and other therapy.

▷ Names and addresses of specialists.

▷ Any restrictions, such as dietary or for safety (leg braces, helmet).

Dental History

▷ Previous dental experiences and patient's attitude.

▷ Difficulties in obtaining appointments, barriers to dental care experienced.

▷ Most recent care: procedures, setting, success.

▷ History of oral infections and oral habits.

▷ Fluoride history, including fluoridation levels in drinking water and self- or professionally applied topical methods.

▷ Current home-care methods: aids and special devices, frequency, degree of self-care.

▷ Concepts of perceived needs, attitudes, and apparent emphasis on dental care.

▷ Modifications and successful techniques used before and during appointments.

Supplemental Information

Are any of the following affected by disability?

▷ Muscular coordination, mobility, walking

▷ Sitting tolerance

▷ Sitting position

▷ Ability to cooperate/involuntary movements

▷ Communication: speech, hearing, vision

▷ Breathing, including when reclined

▷ Swallowing, control of saliva

▷ Bowel or bladder control

▷ Mental capacities

▷ Dexterity, ability to brush and floss teeth

▷ Ability to chew or eat.

Open-Ended Other Information

▷ Does patient require any additional assistance or have any other issues of concern?

▶ Identify special aids the patient is asked to bring to the appointment, such as a transfer board for transfer into the dental chair, hearing aid, dental prostheses, and biofilm control devices currently in use.

▶ Some individuals with disabilities are accompanied by service dogs, such as guide dogs for the blind and hearing and signal dogs, which are allowed by law into all public buildings and on public transportation. Additional information about guide dogs for the blind is found in Chapter 60.

B. Transportation

▶ A patient may rely on the caregiver or another source for transport to an appointment.

▶ A wheelchair patient may need to reserve a wheelchair transport vehicle and be limited by the time schedule.

▶ Patient may arrange a ride transportation service that is contacted when the patient has completed the appointment; forms may need to be completed.

C. Time Considerations

▶ Determine how the patient's daily schedule influences time selection for scheduling appointments.

▶ Inquire about the schedule of the caregiver who accompanies the patient.

▶ The cooperation of the patient may be decreased if basic routines are disturbed; for example:

• Appointment for the patient with diabetes does not interfere with medication, meal, or between-meal eating schedules.

• The elderly person who rises early may feel better during a morning appointment.

• Patients with arthritis may have greater mobility late in the morning or in the afternoon.

• Child's nap schedule may preclude afternoon appointments.

• Early morning appointment may be difficult for a patient who requires a long time for morning preparation, such as a patient with a spinal cord injury or colostomy.

▶ Arrange a time when the patient will not have to wait a long time after arrival.

▶ Allow sufficient time so the patient is not rushed; many persons with disabilities cannot hurry.

▶ Consider incontinence issues, including time needed for rest room visits; encourage emptying bladder before entering treatment room.

D. Patient Reception: The Initial Appointment

▶ The orientation of a patient with a disability paves the way for long-term success of dental and dental hygiene supervision and care.

▶ The first appointment includes and, when necessary, may be devoted entirely to a basic orientation to the facilities, the dental chair, and the personnel.

▶ Several orientation visits may be necessary to acclimate the patient to surroundings and to desensitize.

▶ Desensitization techniques and a "show–tell–do" approach can help reduce anxiety, particularly for a patient with cognitive impairment or one who is fearful.

▶ Assessment procedures and preventive personal care instructions are initiated, and participation of the caregiver is solicited as indicated.

E. Follow-up

The frequency of continuing care appointments for all patients is individualized, but frequent appointments are encouraged for persons with a disability for the following reasons:

▶ To decrease length of single appointment by keeping the oral tissues at an optimum level of health.

▶ To assist the patient whose disability limits the ability to perform personal oral self-care adequately.

▶ To provide motivation through monitoring biofilm and review of procedures for the patient and the caregiver involved.

V. Assistance for the Ambulatory Patient

▶ A patient may walk with one or more assistive aids such as braces, a cane, crutches, or a walker.

▶ Certain patients do better without assistance because they have developed their own method of balancing; many patients gain balance by holding both hands on the partially flexed forearm of a person walking beside them.

A. Seating the Patient

▶ Ask patient how much and what kind of assistance is needed.

▶ Raise chair slightly above the patient's knee level and adjust chair arm out of the way.

▶ Stand aside or assist while patient moves until back of legs touch chair and then bends knees to lower into dental chair.

▶ If assistance is needed grasp ankles, lift legs, and turn patient into dental chair.

▶ Remove assistive aides and store out of the way; service dogs that accompany a patient are allowed to lie quietly nearby during the dental appointment.

B. The Seated Patient

▶ After telling the patient, tilt chair back slowly. Balance can be precarious while sitting as well as standing; patient may fall forward.

▶ If necessary, position supportive padding to maintain patient comfort.

C. Rising from the Chair

▶ After telling patient, slowly raise the chair to upright position, with the seat slightly higher than the patient's knee level to minimize need to bend knees when rising.

▶ Allow time for adjustment to upright position in order to avoid the effects of postural hypertension.

▶ Ask or assist patient to move feet down to the floor.

▶ Retrieve assistive aids and hold them for patient to grasp with the dominant hand.

▶ Ask patient and, if assistance is needed to rise from the chair, offer support by placing arm under the patient's arm on the nondominant side until balance is obtained for walking.

VI. Patient Positioning

▶ The objectives for patient positioning during treatment are to let the patient feel comfortable while the clinician provides care in a position that provides adequate illumination, visibility, and accessibility.

▶ Extreme care is given to slightly raising the head of any patient with a swallowing defect or respiratory compromise; the patient may be unable to prevent aspiration of fluids or object placed in the mouth during treatment.

A. Adapt Chair Position

▶ Adapt chair position slowly, in steps to allow the patient to adjust.
  • Bring the feet up first to provide balance so that the patient cannot fall.
  • While tipping the chair back, place one hand on the patient's shoulder to offer assurance and support.

▶ A patient with a respiratory or cardiac complication is positioned with the chair back raised to a level that is comfortable for the patient. The patient can be asked, "How many pillows do you use at night?" and the chair can be adjusted accordingly.

B. Body Adjustments

▶ Patients with a spinal cord injury do a "push up" and patients with quadriplegia shift their weight every 20 minutes for 10–15 seconds to maintain good circulation in the tissues that do not have sensation, such as the buttocks.

▶ The procedure is a preventive measure for decubitus ulcers and is a particular consideration during long dental procedures.

VII. Supportive and Protective Stabilization

▶ The objectives for patient stabilization are to enhance patient comfort and safety while intraoral treatment is provided.

▶ Patients who are hyperactive, lack muscular control, or have a mental impairment can provide many challenges for keeping the head and mouth positioned.

▶ In addition, control of profuse saliva and an oversized or hyperactive tongue can be difficult.

▶ With basic knowledge of methods for maintaining patient stability, adequate visibility of working area, secure instrument grasps and finger rests, and well-controlled strokes, instrumentation can be effectively accomplished.

▶ Supportive stabilization, such as padding under flexed knees or bite block positioned to rest jaw muscles, can be used to facilitate patient comfort.

▶ Protective stabilization or medical immobilization techniques described below can help prevent injury to the patient and the dental practitioner; however, the use of restraint is controversial and has the risk of causing injury or resulting in a lawsuit.[24]

▶ Protective stabilization is never used as a form of punishment.

▶ When protective support of any type is to be used, it is explained completely to the patient and/or the legal guardian and a signed informed consent is obtained.

▶ The least restrictive method of stabilization is selected for each patient and communication-based or desensitizing techniques are tried first.

A. Body Enclosure

▶ Although a small patient may be held by a parent, such positioning can be tiring for the parent, insecure, and may not provide good body mechanics for the clinician.

▶ *Pediwrap or papoose board*: Adjustable arm or leg immobilizer wraps with velcro closures or a padded board with wide fabric wraps around upper body, middle body and legs are available in adult and pediatric sizes, but not recommended unless the clinician has specialized training and informed consent has been obtained.

B. Head Stabilization

▶ *Arm of clinician*: From a working position at 12 o'clock (top of the patient's head), the nondominant arm is placed around the patient's head to stabilize it in position.

C. Oral Stabilization

A mouth prop can be used to assist the patient who has difficulty maintaining an open mouth. Patience, a gentle but firm touch, and continuing experience are essential. Training on technique for safe use of mouth props is required. Verbal encouragement of the patient continues throughout the appointment.

▶ The most stable mouth prop is a sterilized ratchet type (Molt's mouth prop) that can be nearly closed for insertion between the teeth.
  • It can be opened gradually to hold the jaws to the necessary position.
  • The tips are covered with rubber tubing and are positioned over the maxillary and mandibular teeth

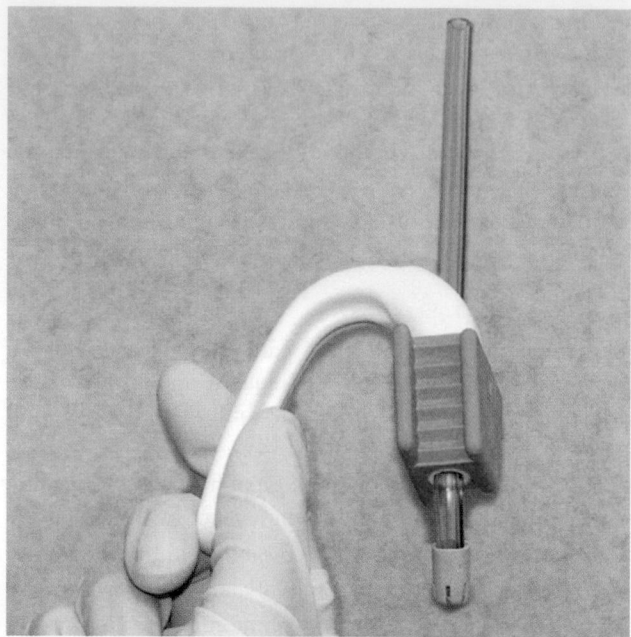

FIGURE 57-7 Rubber Bite Block Mouth Prop with Saliva Ejector.

on one side while the clinician treats the opposite side.

▶ Different types of rubber bite blocks are available; for example, Figure 57-7 shows one that allows for placement of a suction tip.

▶ A long piece of dental floss is tied through the holes in a commercially available rubber mouth prop so that, in case of a sudden respiratory change, the prop can be quickly pulled out and breathing normalized.

D. Precautions for the Use of a Mouth Prop

▶ Patient and caregivers are informed of the risks and reassured that all stabilization devices are for comfort and to make the work easier and that they are in no way meant to hurt or punish.

▶ Mobile teeth could be knocked out and aspirated.
  • Loose primary teeth in young patient.
  • Mobile teeth in advanced periodontal infection.

▶ Fatigue of the patient's facial and masticatory muscles and temporomandibular joint.

VIII. Four-Handed Dental Hygiene

▶ The use of a dental hygiene assistant during the appointment can enhance:
  • Efficiency
  • Patient management
  • Patient safety and comfort
  • Safety and comfort for clinician
  • Visibility during intraoral procedures

▶ Excess drooling, common with some disabilities, requires continuous suction to maintain a clear visual field for instrumentation and to decrease the risk of aspiration.

▶ A patient with impaired respiratory function, swallowing, or gag reflex is at risk for aspiration; attention to patient position and continuous suction to keep passageways clear are vital.

▶ When the patient's disorder involves orofacial muscles and nerves, the risk for splashing of aerosols into the eye is increased during dental hygiene care.

IX. Instrumentation

▶ Biofilm control instruction precedes scaling to provide a clean mouth for professional instrumentation.

▶ Unbreakable mirrors are recommended for use with a patient subject to spasm or sudden closure.

▶ Use single-end sharp instruments to prevent accidents. When an unrestrained patient moves involuntarily, the nonworking end of an instrument can be a hazard.

▶ Use of an ultrasonic scaler is contraindicated for a patient at risk for aspiration and for patients who overreact to sensory stimuli, such as a patient with autism.

▶ Introduce each procedure and sound to prevent startling a patient: Follow the basic instruction rule to "show, tell, then do."

▶ Finger rests: Firm, dependable finger rests are needed. Supplemental or reinforced rests can contribute to instrument stability. External finger and hand rests may be safer for the clinician.

▶ The occurrence of generalized heavy calculus deposits in disabled patients is not unusual due to factors related to the disabling condition.

X. Pain and Anxiety Control

▶ For many patients with a disability, treatment can be easily accomplished in a dental clinic.

▶ Some patients with behavioral or cognitive disabilities may need intervention beyond standard communication techniques and local anesthesia in order to receive dental care.

▶ Alternative methods of pain and anxiety control for patients who are unable to cooperate during dental treatment include[25]:

- Pharmacologically induced sedation: minimal, moderate, or deep sedation; provided by trained dentist or anesthesiologist.
- General anesthesia: delivered in hospital, surgery centers, or dental offices; provided by trained anesthesiologists.

WHEELCHAIR TRANSFER[26]

▶ Selection of a transfer technique is influenced by the size, weight, and mobility of the patient, along with any special physical conditions and patient preferences.

▶ The patient may prefer to transfer from the left or the right side of the dental chair, depending on which side of the body is stronger.

▶ Transfer from the wheelchair can be a frightening experience to the patient owing to fear of falling and injury.

▶ Always inform the patient of intended actions before starting.

I. Preparation for Wheelchair Transfer

A. Clear the Area

▶ Before starting a transfer, clear the area: move the clinician's stool, bracket tray, portable unit, and dental light.

▶ After the transfer, release the wheelchair brake to move it aside.

▶ In a small treatment room, the wheelchair may be folded and set aside.

B. Special Needs of Patient

▶ *Chair padding*: Special padding is used in a wheelchair as protection from pressure sores. Depending on the length of the appointment, the patient will decide whether the padding is moved to the dental chair. Pressure sores (decubitus ulcers) are described in Chapter 59.

▶ *Bags and catheters*: Patients who do not have control of urine discharge, such as those with paraplegia or quadriplegia, have a bag with tubing for collection. The bag may be attached to the leg of the patient or to the wheelchair. After transfer, the tubing is checked to be sure it is not bent or twisted.

▶ *Spasms*: Ask the patient about susceptibility to spasms and about procedures to follow for prevention.

▶ *Advice concerning transfer*: Ask the patient, family member, or caregiver how best the clinician can help during the transfer. The patient is allowed to do as much as possible.

II. Mobile Patient Transfer

When a patient can support his or her own weight, the "stand and pivot" technique can be used, as shown in Figure 57-8.

A. Position the Wheelchair

Face the wheelchair in the same direction as the dental chair at approximately an angle of 30°; set brakes; remove footrests and wheelchair armrests. The patient will adjust a power-driven chair and set the brakes before turning it off.

B. Prepare Dental Chair

Adjust the dental chair to the same height as or lower than the wheelchair; clear a path for transfer by uplifting the dental chair arm.

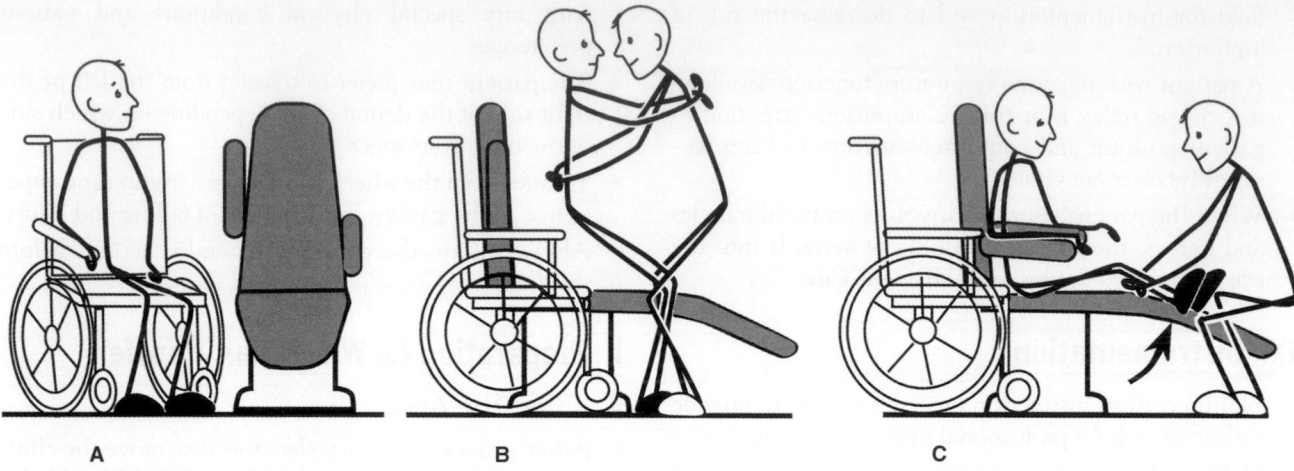

FIGURE 57-8 **Wheelchair Transfer for a Mobile Patient. A:** Position the wheelchair at level of or lower than the dental chair; set wheel locks, remove footrests and armrests, and raise the dental chair arm. **B:** Clinician places feet outside of the patient's feet, grasps the patient around the waist under the arms, locks hands, or grasps belt in back; patient holds clinician around shoulders or neck; patient is lifted up and pivoted to dental chair side. **C:** Patient is gently lowered to sitting position; dental chair arm is lowered; clinician grasps legs together to lift onto dental chair.

C. Approach to Patient

▶ Detach patient's safety belt.

▶ Face the patient and place feet outside the patient's feet for pivoting. Clinician's knees are placed close to or against the patient's knees to prevent buckling.

▶ Place hands under the patient's arms and grasp the waist belt in back. Patient places arms around clinician's neck or places hands on wheelchair to push up.

▶ Clinician lifts patient to standing position, as in Figure 57-8B.

D. Pivot to Dental Chair

▶ Pivot together slowly until the patient is backed up to the side of the dental chair, with the backs of the legs touching. The patient is gently lowered to a sitting position. Reposition the arm of the dental chair.

▶ Grasp the patient's legs together between the ankles and knees, and lift them onto the dental chair, as shown in Figure 57-8C.

E. Repeat in Reverse

After the appointment, return the patient to the wheelchair in the reverse order of procedure.

III. Immobile Patient Transfer

When the patient is unable to support his or her own weight, two aides are required. The parent or other caregiver may serve as the second person.

A. Position the Wheelchair

▶ Position the wheelchair in the same direction and parallel with the dental chair; set brakes; remove footrests.

▶ Adjust the dental chair to the same height as or lower than the seat of the wheelchair.

▶ Move the arm of the dental chair out of the transfer area, and remove the arm of the wheelchair.

B. Assistant I

▶ Assistant I is positioned behind the wheelchair.

▶ Place feet, one on either side of the rear wheel nearest the dental chair; place hands under the patient's arms below the elbows, pressing forearms against the patient's lower thorax area.

▶ Clasp hands or wrists under the patient's rib cage.

C. Assistant II

Assistant II may do either of the following, depending on the size and weight of the patient.

▶ Face patient and grasp hands under the patient's knees.

▶ Face dental chair; place one arm under the thighs and the other under the calves of the lower legs.

D. Transfer

On a prearranged signal and a steady motion, lift and gently transfer the patient to the dental chair.

E. Repeat in Reverse

After the appointment, the patient is returned to the wheelchair in the reverse order of procedure.

IV. Sliding Board Transfer

A patient may bring a sliding board or one may be kept in the office or clinic. A transfer board is shown in Figure 57-9.

A. Position the Wheelchair

▶ Position the wheelchair in the same direction as and parallel with the dental chair; set the brakes; remove the footrests.

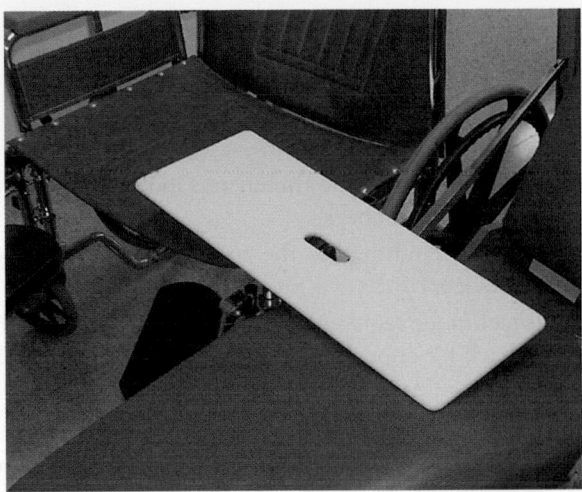

FIGURE 57-9 **Transfer Board.** Transfer board placement between wheelchair and dental chair.

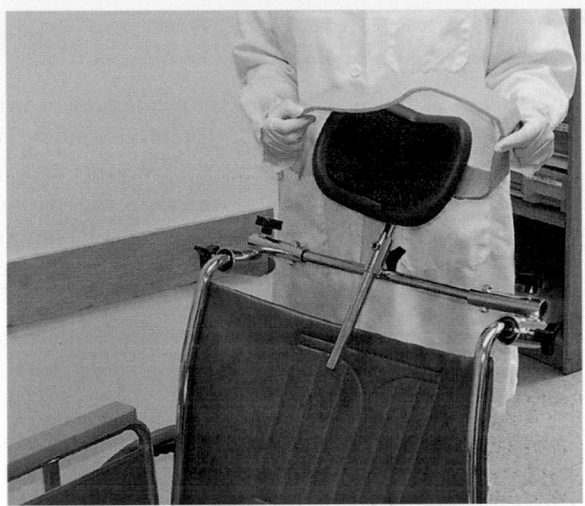

FIGURE 57-10 **Portable Headrest Attached to Wheelchair.**

▶ Adjust the seat of the dental chair to slightly lower than the wheelchair seat.

▶ Move the arm of the dental chair out of the transfer area, and remove the arm of the wheelchair.

B. Adjust the Sliding Board

▶ Patient or clinician places the sliding board well under the hip of the patient.

▶ The board is extended across the dental chair.

C. Transfer

▶ Patient shifts weight, balances on hands, and walks the buttocks across the board. The clinician can assist or do the transfer by holding the patient under the axillae. Two persons are needed when the patient is heavy or less mobile.

▶ Board is removed and replaced after the appointment.

D. Repeat in Reverse

Dental chair is positioned slightly higher than the wheelchair seat for the return transfer.

V. Wheelchair Used During Treatment

When the patient is in a total support wheelchair, transfer to the dental chair may not be advisable. The wheelchair can be positioned for direct utilization.

▶ Some wheelchairs are self-reclining and have headrests (Figure 58-2, Chapter 58).

▶ A portable headrest may be attached to the wheelchair handles, as shown in Figure 57-10.

▶ The dental chair can be swiveled to permit the wheelchair to be placed so the dental light can be directed into the patient's oral cavity.

▶ An automatic wheelchair lift that tilts the chair back can be obtained for a clinical facility where wheelchair patients are treated frequently.

▶ When a teaching area is planned for patient instruction, attention is given to ensure accessibility for a patient in a wheelchair, as shown in Figure 57-11.

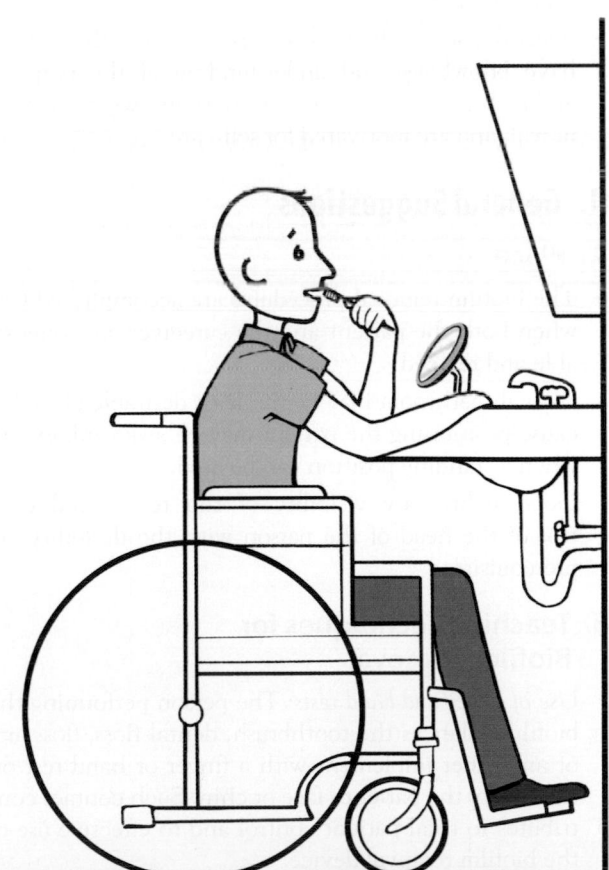

FIGURE 57-11 **Biofilm Control Station.** The tabletop and washbasin in a patient instruction area or lavatory are built at a height of 32–34 inches to provide clearance underneath for knees of the patient and arms of the wheelchair. A magnifying mirror, preferably on a pedestal that tilts, can provide an excellent aid for viewing the disclosed biofilm and the devices for biofilm removal. Hot pipes under a sink are covered or insulated because patients with no sensation could be burned.

INSTRUCTION FOR CAREGIVERS

▶ Individuals who need partial or total care present with varying degrees of ability to cooperate, depending on the type of disability.

▶ The size of the patient and whether the patient is ambulatory, bedridden, or in a wheelchair are among the factors that influence the technique for management.

▶ The instructions for the caregiver are given where the specific techniques can actually be demonstrated as they will be done at home.

▶ When the patient lies down with the head in the parent's lap, for example, a suitable couch is used, or chairs can be placed together.

▶ Time and repeated practice sessions may be needed for successful biofilm removal.

I. Self-care and Attitude

▶ Whenever possible, instruction for the parents, family members, or other caregivers begins with their own personal oral care.

▶ Success comes when those who care for the patient have knowledge and understanding of the purposes and techniques, can demonstrate their own biofilm removal, and are motivated for self-care.

II. General Suggestions

A. Place

▶ The biofilm removal procedures are accomplished best when both the patient and the caregiver are comfortable and relaxed.

▶ A small bathroom may be the least desirable place because positioning the patient may be awkward, except when a standing position can be used.

▶ Good light, easy visibility of the teeth, and control of the head of the person with the disability are prerequisites.

B. Teaching Techniques for Biofilm Removal

▶ *Use of finger and hand rests*: The person performing the biofilm balances the toothbrush, dental floss, floss aid, or any other implement with a finger or hand rest on the side of the patient's face or chin. Such contact contributes to total patient control and to effective use of the biofilm removal device.

▶ *Use of a mouth prop*: For certain patients, biofilm removal is impossible without a mouth prop, and demonstration for insertion on both sides is needed. For home use, a rolled and moist washcloth may be appropriate.

III. Positions

A. Caregiver Standing

▶ With the caregiver standing from behind, the arm is brought around the patient's head and the chin is cupped while using the thumb and index finger to retract the lips and cheeks.

▶ The other hand applies the toothbrush, floss aid, or other device.

▶ This technique requires the patient be able to bend the head back far enough for the parent to see the maxillary teeth.

▶ The procedure may be applicable for the following:
  • Short patient standing in front of and backed up to the caregiver.
  • Tall patient seated in a chair with the head tipped back to lean against the caregiver, or seated in a large chair or sofa with the head stabilized against the top of chair back.
  • Patient in a wheelchair leaning back against the caregiver. Wheelchair brakes are set.

B. Caregiver Seated

▶ Patient seated on pillow on floor in front of parent, with back close to the chair and head turned back into parent's lap, as shown in Figure 56-12A. The caregiver may place his/her legs over the shoulders of the patient to restrain arms and body movements, as shown in Figure 56-12B.

▶ Caregiver is seated at the end of a sofa or couch, and patient is lying down with the head in parent's lap, as shown in Figure 56-12C.

▶ For a bedridden patient, the caregiver may sit at the patient's head and place the head in the lap. When body and arm movements need to be controlled, the caregiver can sit beside the patient, lean across the patient's chest, and hold the patient's arm against the body with the elbow. The hand of the restraining arm can hold the mouth prop, retract, or do whatever is necessary.

C. Two People

▶ In any of the positions previously mentioned, the parent may need the assistance of a second person to hold the hands and arms or otherwise restrain the patient.

▶ A small child may be placed across the laps of two persons seated facing each other. One stabilizes the head and brushes and flosses while the other person holds hands, arms, and legs as needed, as shown in Figure 56-12D.

GROUP IN-SERVICE EDUCATION

▶ In-service programs are provided for teachers, registered nurses, other health professionals, parents, and

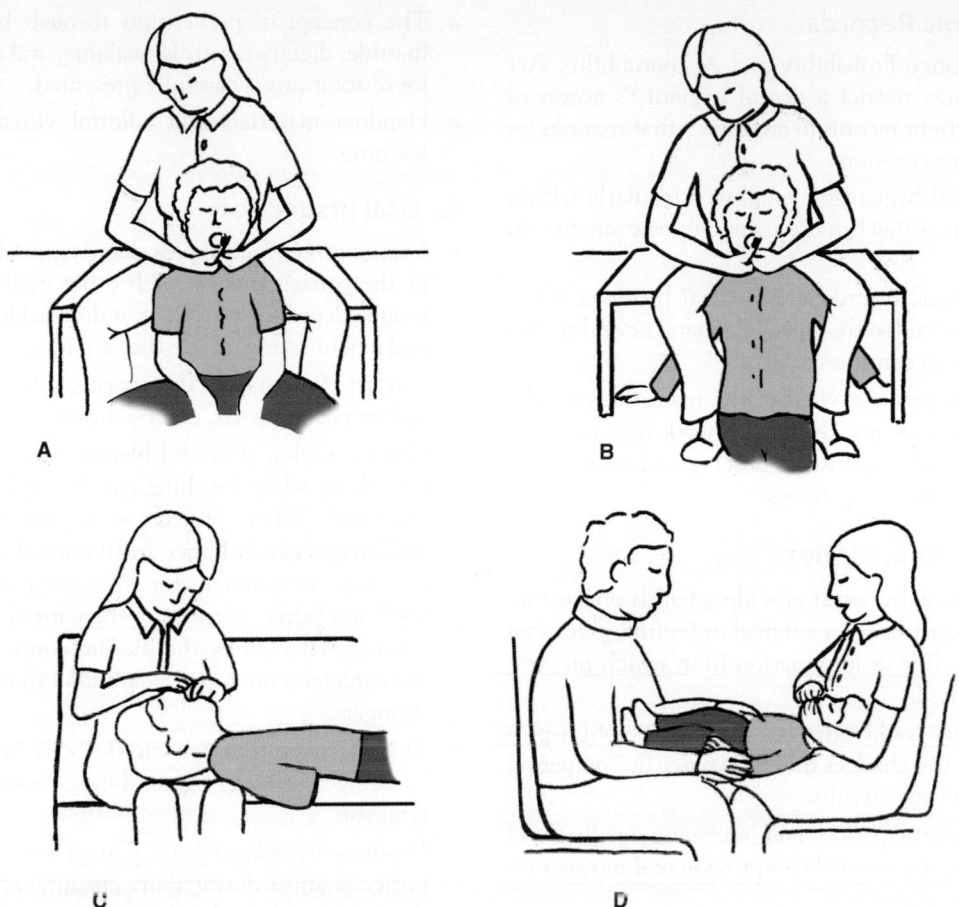

FIGURE 57-12 Positions for Child or Disabled Patient During Biofilm Removal. A: Patient seated on floor with head turned back into the lap of the caregiver. **B:** Patient's arms restrained by legs of caregiver. **C:** Patient reclining on couch with head in lap of caregiver. **D:** Two people participating with small child between. One holds patient for stabilization while the other holds the head for toothbrushing and flossing.

volunteers in school and community preventive programs. For example, all persons mentioned could be involved in the preparation of a program about classroom weekly rinsing with a fluoride mouthrinse. When a program is citywide and many dental hygienists are involved, in-service preparation for the dental hygienists themselves is necessary to provide coordination for the event.

▶ A special need exists for in-service instruction in oral health measures for caregivers in extended care institutions. Many patients in such facilities are unable to care for their own needs and may require total care, partial assistance, supervision, or regular reminders.

▶ The dental hygienist is able to work with the caregivers to teach them appropriate techniques and to motivate them to incorporate oral care into the daily routine for each resident or patient.

▶ The general suggestions outlined in the following sections pertain to preparation and content for in-service workshops for the oral care of long-term patients.

I. Preparation for an In-Service Program

A. Planning

▶ An in-service program needs careful planning. A leading factor contributing to the success of a program is the genuine concern and enthusiasm of the program leader in motivating the participants.

▶ Effective learning materials are clear and to the point, interestingly presented with appropriate visual aids, and stimulating for learning. Objectives are defined in writing and serve as a guide to preparation and evaluation.

▶ Problems of the staff are recognized and addressed during the program. Some members may have negative oral health attitudes, minimal educational background, and poor personal oral health.

▶ Initially, basic preparation includes learning about the functioning levels of the patient and assessing the procedures used for oral care. A survey of the biofilm control materials and devices available and in current use, methods for labeling or storing individual brushes, and the frequency of use is important.

B. Use of Clinic Records

▶ Health Insurance Probability and Accountability Act regulations may restrict a dental hygienist's access to individual patient records in an agency that requests an oral health presentation.

▶ When a dental hygienist is employed regularly within an institution, a much more complete assessment can be made.

▶ If possible, clinic records and medical histories of patients are reviewed so that special general or oral health problems can be considered.

▶ The dental hygienist invited to the institution for the specific purpose of presenting the workshop needs to arrange a preworkshop visit to observe and get to know the caregivers and the patients.

C. Gingival/Biofilm Index

▶ When the dental hygienist providing hands-on instruction for oral care, use of a gingival or biofilm index can provide a baseline of information from which progress can be evaluated.

▶ The caregivers could carry out the daily biofilm program and see the changes that take place by comparing the before and after results.

▶ Continuing participation and receiving feedback of successful biofilm removal can provide real motivation to caregivers.

II. Program Content

An oral health in-service program will be more successful if the content presented is based on an assessment of specific needs identified by the institution, patients, and caregivers. Some topics that can be considered are as listed.

A. The Caregivers' Own Biofilm Control

▶ Caregivers who are motivated to care for their own mouths may have a clearer understanding of the effects and importance of oral care and give a higher priority to the time spent providing oral health care for their patients.

▶ A biofilm-free score or another evaluation index can be used, as described in Chapter 23.

▶ A group may be willing to work in pairs and learn to evaluate and score each other, thereby learning the techniques to be applied to their patients.

B. Facts About Cause and Prevention of Oral Disease

▶ Basic information about biofilm, its formation, and how gingivitis and dental caries develop are important to most groups.

▶ The progress of disease from reversible gingivitis to severe periodontitis can be explained, as can the process of dental caries.

▶ The concept of prevention through biofilm control, fluoride, dietary controls, sealants, and early treatment for restorations is carefully presented.

▶ Handout materials and colorful visual aids promote learning.

C. Oral Inspection

▶ *Oral mucosa*: Techniques demonstrated and practiced by the participants on each other include the use of a tongue depressor to retract, a disposable mouth mirror, and a light source to see the oral mucosa.

▶ *Tongue*: How to hold the tongue, using a sponge to lift and inspect all parts, can be shown.

▶ *Gingiva*: Color, size, and bleeding that occurs spontaneously or while brushing can be explained and demonstrated. When projection is possible, illustrations and images can enhance instructional material. When a camera is available for intraoral photography, "before" and "after" pictures of the patients can be shown. Changes effected by the biofilm control supervised by the caregivers are more meaningful than are pictures of strangers.

▶ *Biofilm*: Inspection for biofilm can be demonstrated by using disclosing agent during biofilm scoring and removal.

▶ *Denture-supporting mucosa*: Caregivers can be trained to notice changes during daily cleaning and massaging of the mucosa while the denture is out of the mouth for cleaning and call them to the dentists' attention at the next visit.

▶ *Dentures*: Sample dentures may be used to help the participants learn to examine each denture for cracks or sharp edges. Examination for deposits can be made by the patient and the caregivers and compared with the denture after it has been cleaned.

D. Techniques of Mouth Care and Disease Control

▶ Staff members working in pairs can be more efficient, particularly in the care of challenging patients.

▶ A plan for each patient can be worked out with the caregivers so individual problems relative to dental caries prevention, gingival disease control, or complete or partial denture care can be solved.

▶ *Biofilm control*: Instruction includes: positioning of the patient, application of disclosing agent, examination for biofilm on the teeth, toothbrush selection and technique, use of a mouth prop, and flossing with or without a floss aid. The use of a portable or bedside suction unit for removing debris from a patient's mouth can be practiced by a paired team.

▶ *Fluoride application*: The objectives and techniques for brushing with a gel, swabbing with a mouthrinse, assisting the patient with a chewable tablet, or applying a gel tray can be included.

▶ *Denture care*: Procedures for care of dentures and of the mucosa under the denture are shown.

▶ *Saliva substitute*: Use of saliva substitute for dry mouth is demonstrated; instruction includes how to use a swab with saliva substitute to provide relief for certain patients.

E. Denture Marking Procedure

▶ All dentures are marked for patient identification.

▶ Most dentures are marked during processing.

▶ The techniques for denture marking are outlined in Chapter 32.

III. Records

▶ An oral care documentation form completed for each patient is essential to evaluate the success of the in-service presentation.

▶ During the instruction periods, the staff can learn how to complete the record and where to file the copies.

▶ The form can be designed with spaces to record information obtained during the oral examination, the functioning level and degree of cooperation, the procedures needed for dental caries control, periodontal health, and/or denture care.

▶ In addition, the instruction provided, the implements and materials used, the planned future instruction, the prognosis, and any other notes can be included. Successful techniques are described, and suggestions for future appointments can be made.

IV. Follow-up

▶ After caregivers have tried their newly learned procedures, an opportunity to have questions answered is provided.

▶ Direct observation by the dental hygienist of techniques performed with and for the patients, advice concerning oral problems of particular patients, and corrections when necessary can motivate and encourage both patient and caregiver.

▶ Disclosing and recording the biofilm for comparison of scores before and after the program can show the progress being made.

V. Continuing Education

▶ Individual instruction is provided for each new employee during the orientation period for that employee.

▶ Periodic updating for all employees can be accomplished at regular intervals. Questions and problems can be discussed, and plans can be introduced for changing a certain procedure based on new research evidence.

▶ A specific plan for scheduled oral health programs may be a requirement for licensure of a healthcare facility.

▶ Advanced education programs are available for extensive training in care of the disabled patient.

THE DENTAL HYGIENIST WITH A DISABILITY

▶ Disability is not necessarily an obstacle to dental hygiene licensure and provision of clinical care.[27]

▶ Adaptive technology, tax incentives for accessibility construction, and creative thinking can facilitate any necessary workplace modifications.

▶ Additional dental hygiene roles, such as manager, advocate, or educator may provide employment opportunities for the dental hygienist with a disability.

DOCUMENTATION

In addition to the standard information recorded for a patient visit, documentation of care provided for a patient who has a disability includes:

▶ Individualized information about the patient's condition or level of functioning that will affect modifications needed during dental hygiene care. Some suggestions for information needed are listed in Box 57-4.

▶ Specific details related to patient management or communication strategies used during the dental hygiene appointment, and an indication of whether or not those strategies were successful.

▶ Identification of self-care aids, modifications to standard oral hygiene instructions, and details of any recommendations or instructions provided for caregivers.

▶ Box 57-5 provides an example of documentation for an appointment with a patient with a disability.

BOX 57-4

Basic Planning Questions for a Patient with Disability

▷ What is the patient's functioning level?

▷ Is the patient capable to do all or part of the daily biofilm removal independently or will the patient require partial or total care?

▷ Is the patient involved in any community dental health programs (home, school, or day activity), and can the dentist and/or dental hygienist in such a program be contacted to coordinate the instruction given?

▷ Which disabilities have the greatest influence on the extent of self-care possible and the anticipated success of the overall preventive program? Mental? Physical? Sensory? Learning? Oral?

▷ Which techniques and procedures will best fit the situation of the particular patient and the caregiver?

▷ How can the patient be helped to be as independent as possible?

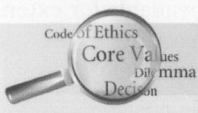

EVERYDAY ETHICS

When Mrs. Becker has her dental appointment, Lauren, the dental hygienist, needs to rush to finish the previous patient so she can have time to go to the storage closet in the basement and get the transfer board so Mrs. Becker can slide over to the dental chair from her wheelchair. Mrs. Becker has numerous medical and dental problems that she tends to complain about. She has been very difficult to motivate to perform daily biofilm control. Her current dental status indicates that she needs to be placed on more frequent 2- to 3-month maintenance appointments. Lauren feels overstressed to prepare for and treat Mrs. Becker in the time she is allowed for appointments. Lauren is considering ignoring the plan for more frequent maintenance visits and scheduling Mrs. Becker in 6 months to avoid another unpleasant experience for both of them.

Questions for Consideration

1. Which core values of dental hygiene ethics apply in this situation?

2. In terms of every patient's right to expect the best of care, how can Lauren fulfill her professional obligations of beneficence and fairness if Ms. Becker is not appointed at intervals appropriate for her oral health needs?

3. What are the legal implications related to standard of care if Lauren follows through with her plan to reduce the frequency of Mrs. Becker's maintenance visits?

BOX 57-5

Example Documentation: Self-care Management for Patient with a Disability

S –A 25-year-old male patient with Down's syndrome, who lives in an assisted-living group home, presents for routine 3-month periodontal maintenance appointment. Patient and his caregiver both state that the curved bristle toothbrush, introduced at the last appointment, is working quite well for him and that his caregiver has affixed a rubber band to the handle in order to help stabilize the toothbrush in his hand.

O–No changes in medical history. His biofilm index is now below 20%.

A–Next step in patient's care plan is to help develop a system that will help patient take more personal responsibility for his own oral self-care with less need for caregiver assistance.

P–Congratulated patient and caregiver on their successful reduction in biofilm. Worked with caregiver to develop a personal "Daily Oral Care" list to identify all the steps and materials necessary for his daily oral care regimen. Caregiver will make up a large poster of the steps using pictures and will laminate and hang the poster by the bathroom sink in order to help the patient be more independent with his daily oral care regimen. Maintenance scaling and root planing completed. Used a "tell–show–do" approach to provide basic instructions for using a floss holder. First time efforts were clumsy, but patient is motivated to practice.

Next steps: Evaluate success at next visit scheduled in 3 months.

Signed _____, RDH

Date _____

Factors To Teach The Patient and Caregiver

▷ Seek regular dental and medical examinations.

▷ Learn about disability; know status, disease, names, and doses of medications including over-the-counter medications, and other changes in medical history.

▷ Recognize the early warnings of complications of disease.

▷ Recognize the side effects of treatments and medications.

▷ Seek immediate medical attention for any complications.

▷ Practice a healthy lifestyle, including healthy diet, daily exercise, no tobacco products, alcohol avoidance, attainment of ideal weight, and stress reduction. Accept assistance for smoking cessation.

▷ Practice meticulous oral hygiene to prevent dental and periodontal diseases and adapt techniques as needed.

▷ Ways to overcome barriers to dental care.

References

1. National Institute of Dental and Craniofacial Research. Developmental disabilities and oral health. http://www.nidcr.nih.gov/OralHealth/Topics/DevelopmentalDisabilities/. Accessed July 31, 2014.

2. United States Department of Justice. Americans with Disabilities Act of 1990 as Amended. http://www.ada.gov/pubs/adastatute08.htm. Accessed July 2, 2014.

3. World Health Organization. International Classification of Functioning, Disability and Health (ICF). http://www.who.int/classifications/icf/en/. Accessed July 21, 2014.

4. Cornell University. Online Resource for U.S. Disability Statistics.http://www.disabilitystatistics.org/reports/census.cfm?statistic=1. Accessed July 22, 2014.

5. Hall JP, Chapman SL, Kurth NK. Poor oral health as an obstacle to employment for Medicaid beneficiaries with disabilities. *J Public Health Dent.* 2013;73(1):79–82.

6. Rouleau T, Harrington A, Brennan M, et al. Receipt of dental care and barriers encountered by persons with disabilities. *Spec Care Dentist.* 2011;31(2):63–67.

7. Glassman P, Subar P. Improving and maintaining oral health for people with special needs. *Dent Clin North Am.* 2008;52(2):447–461.

8. Douglass CW, Glassman P. The oral health of vulnerable older adults and persons with disabilities. *Spec Care Dentist.* 2013;33(4):156–163.

9. Garcia RI, Inge RE, Niessen L, et al. Envisioning success: the future of the oral health care delivery system in the United States. *J Public Health Dent.* 2010;70 (Suppl 1):S58–S65.

10. Glassman P, Harrington M, Namakian M, et al. The virtual dental home: bringing oral health to vulnerable and underserved populations. *J Calif Dent Assoc.* 2012;40(7):569–577.

11. Glassman P, Subar P. Creating and maintaining oral health for dependent people in institutional settings. *J Public Health Dent.* 2010;70 (Suppl 1):S40–S48.

12. Naughton DK. Expanding oral care opportunities: direct access care provided by dental hygienists in the United States. *J Evid Based Dent Pract.* 2014;14 (Suppl):171–182.

13. Nash DA. Expanding dental hygiene to include dental therapy: improving access to care for children. *J Dent Hyg.* 2009;83(1):36–44.

14. American Dental Hygienist's Association. Advocacy: direct access. http://www.adha.org/directaccess. Accessed July 22, 2014.

15. National Governors Report. *The Role of Dental Hygienists in Providing Access to Oral Health Care.* Washington, DC: National Governors Association; 2014:18.

16. Friedman JW, Mathu-Muju KR. Dental therapists: improving access to oral health care for underserved children. *Am J Public Health.* 2014;104(6):1005–1009.

17. Self K, Born D, Nagy A. Dental therapy: evolving in Minnesota's safety net. *Am J Public Health.* 2014;104(6):e63–e68.

18. United States Department of Justice. ADA standards for accessible design. http://www.ada.gov/2010ADA standards index.htm. Accessed July 15, 2014.

19. National Institute of Dental and Craniofacial Research. Practical care for people with developmental disabilities. http://www.nidcr.nih.gov/OralHealth/Topics/Developmental-Disabilities/ContinuingEducation.htm. Accessed July 22, 2014.

20. Meningaud JP, Pitak-Arnnop P, Chikhani L, et al. Drooling of saliva: a review of the etiology and management options. *Oral Surg Oral Med Oral Pathol Oral Radiol Endod.* 2006;101(1):48–57.

21. Neves BG, Farah A, Lucas E, et al. Are paediatric medicines risk factors for dental caries and dental erosion? *Community Dent Health.* 2010;27(1):46–51.

22. Chava VK. An evaluation of the efficacy of a curved bristle and conventional toothbrush. A comparative clinical study. *J Periodontol.* 2000;71(5):785–789.

23. Lyons RA. Understanding basic behavioral support techniques as an alternative to sedation and anesthesia. *Spec Care Dentist.* 2009;29(1):39–50.

24. Romer M. Consent, restraint, and people with special needs: a review. *Spec Care Dentist.* 2009;29(1):58–66.

25. Glassman P, Caputo A, Dougherty N, et al; and Special Care Dentistry Association. Special Care Dentistry Association consensus statement on sedation, anesthesia, and alternative techniques for people with special needs. *Spec Care Dentist.* 2009;29(1):2–8.

26. National Institute of Dental and Craniofacial Research. Wheelchair transfer: a health care provider's guide. http://www.nidcr.nih.gov/OralHealth/Topics/DevelopmentalDisabilities/WheelchairTransfer.htm. Accessed July 23, 2014.

27. Smith DS. Challenges in dental hygiene employment for dental hygienists with disabilities. *Access.* 2010;24(8):35–37.

 ENHANCE YOUR UNDERSTANDING

thePoint® DIGITAL CONNECTIONS
(see the inside front cover for access information)

- **Audio glossary**
- **Quiz bank**

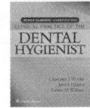 **SUPPORT FOR LEARNING**
(available separately; visit lww.com)

- *Active Learning Workbook for Clinical Practice of the Dental Hygienist, 12th Edition*

prepU INDIVIDUALIZED REVIEW
(available separately; visit lww.com)

- **Adaptive quizzing with *prepU for Wilkins' Clinical Practice of the Dental Hygienist***

Dental Hygiene Care in Alternative Settings

Charlotte J. Wyche, RDH, MS

LEARNING OBJECTIVES

After studying this chapter, the student will be able to:

1. Identify and define key terms and concepts related to oral health care in alternative settings.
2. Identify materials necessary for providing dental hygiene care in alternative settings.
3. Plan and document adaptations to dental hygiene care plans and oral hygiene instructions for the patient who is homebound, bedridden, unconscious, or terminally ill.

▶ In recent years, increased attention has been paid to the oral health needs of individuals who are not able to access oral health services in a traditional dental practice setting.[1]

▶ Individuals confined to hospitals, hospices, institutions, nursing homes, skilled nursing facilities, or private homes:

- Experience barriers accessing routine dental services
- Are likely to have poor oral health status and diminished quality of life
- May need special adaptations for oral care.

▶ Many states now have laws that allow direct access for dental hygiene services through collaborative practice or relaxed supervision requirements in certain public health settings.[2]

▶ An important role for the dental hygienist is to provide triage to insure optimum use of available dental care resources.

▶ Key words and definitions related to caring for patients in alternative settings are found in Box 58-1.

ALTERNATIVE PRACTICE SETTINGS

Providing dental hygiene care in alternative settings can address the needs of individuals who otherwise experience barriers to accessing traditional private practice-based oral care.

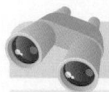

BOX 58-1   KEY WORDS: Dental Hygiene Care in Alternative Settings

Advanced dental hygiene practitioner or advanced dental therapist: a dental hygienist with advanced education and certification in specialty areas who is licensed to provide a wide range of services including, but not limited to, diagnostic, preventive, restorative, and therapeutic services directly to the public; the model for this midlevel practitioner is similar to that of a nurse practitioner.

ADL/IADL (activities of daily living/instrumental activities of daily living): a measure of ability to carry out the basic tasks needed for self-care.

Ambulate: to walk or move about.

   Nonambulatory: inability to walk or move about freely.

Collaborative practice: an alternative oral care delivery model in which dental hygienists collaborate autonomously with members of interprofessional teams to provide dental hygiene services in a variety of nontraditional settings.

Coma: state of unconsciousness from which the patient cannot be aroused.

   Irreversible coma: brain death.

   Comatose: pertaining to or affected with a coma.

Depression: temporary mental state or chronic disorder characterized by feelings of sadness and low self-esteem.

Direct Access: ability to maintain a direct patient provider relationship; allows dental hygienist to deliver care without the specific or previous authorization of a dentist and provide treatment without the presence of a dentist.

Disability: physical, mental, or functional impairment that restricts a major activity; may be partial or complete.

Frail elderly: medically and/or physically fragile, delicate, or weak older person; usually refers to those older than 80 years.

Functional dependence: inability to perform one or more ADL without help; the level of functional dependence is based on the level of assistance needed to perform ADL or the number of activities for which assistance is needed.

Hospice: an interprofessional practice program providing a continuum of home and inpatient palliative and supportive care to meet the physical, emotional, spiritual, social, and economic needs experienced by terminally ill individuals and their families during the final stages of illness and during dying and bereavement.

Interprofessional collaborative practice (ICP): patient care team consists of specialists from many fields; combines expertise and resources to provide insight into all aspects of the patient's needs.

Nurse practitioner (NP): a licensed registered nurse who has had advanced preparation for practice that includes clinical experience in diagnosis and treatment of illness; NPs may work in collaborative practice with physicians or independently in private practice or nursing clinics; in some states NPs can prescribe medications.

Nursing home: a residential facility for persons with chronic illness or disability; often care for the frail elderly. Also called skilled-care or long-term care facility.

Palliative: affording relief but not cure.

Polypharmacy: regular use of three or more drugs or medications; often a concern with elderly or medically compromised patients.

Residence-bound (homebound): inability to leave home because of illness or injury; leaving requires considerable and taxing effort. Can be temporary or permanent situation.

Sordes: foul matter that collects on the lips, teeth, and oral mucosa in patients with low fevers or dehydration; consists of debris, microorganisms, epithelial elements, and food particles; forms a crust.

Teledentistry: a model of healthcare delivery that uses web-based technology to send electronic information such as patient history and digital radiographs, between on-site and off-site practitioners; this model can be used to support collaborative practice between dentists and dental hygienists who are caring for patients in nontraditional settings.

Terminally ill patient: a person who is experiencing the end stages of a life-threatening disease and for whom there is no longer hope of a cure.

Triage: screening and classification of individuals in order to make optimal use of treatment resources; sorting and allocating relative priority for patient treatment needs.

I. Barriers to Access[3,4]

- ▶ Few on-site dental clinics in nursing homes or residential facilities
- ▶ Limited availability of general and specialty practitioners who provide home-based services
- ▶ Ageism or other negative attitudes of practitioners
- ▶ Cost
- ▶ Limited Medicaid coverage for adult dental services
- ▶ Nonpayment of Medicare for dental services
- ▶ Limited mobility
- ▶ Nonavailability of transportation
- ▶ Fear
- ▶ Patient's health attitudes and beliefs
- ▶ Patient's daily pain or discomfort levels.

II. Eliminating Barriers

- ▶ Many services, including visiting nurses and personal/household assistance, are being delivered to homebound individuals by home health agencies.
- ▶ Midlevel allied health professionals, such as nurse practitioners, oversee programs that provide direct medical services for patients.
- ▶ New models for healthcare delivery use web-based communication tools to enhance potential for collaboration between onsite and supervising health team members.
- ▶ Current public health programs in numerous states allow dental hygienists to provide direct access care for certain underserved populations.
- ▶ Midlevel, direct access care providers can address access issues related to shortage of dentists, limited availability of safety net options for low-income populations, and need for care in nontraditional settings.[5,6]
- ▶ Several midlevel oral health provider models are currently being explored; some models are based on increased scope of practice for dental hygienists who have received additional education and certification.

III. Portable Delivery of Care

- ▶ For patients who cannot be transported to a dental treatment room, dental and dental hygiene services can be provided in a variety of surroundings using mobile equipment.
- ▶ Dental hygiene assessment and care:
  - Can be provided in any setting within the limits of state practice acts,
  - Particularly lend themselves to care for residence-bound individuals because most dental hygiene treatment can be completed with manual instruments.

RESIDENCE-BOUND PATIENTS

- ▶ The individual who is residence bound may be:
  - Limited in one or more activities of daily living (Table 24-3 in Chapter 24).
  - An American Society of Anesthesiologists' classification of III or higher (Table 24-1 in Chapter 24).
  - Functionally dependent on caregivers.
- ▶ Potential homebound patients are listed in Box 58-2.
- ▶ Instruction in personal oral preventive procedures has particular significance for comfort and quality of life, as well as the systemic health of these individuals.

I. Private Homes

- ▶ A private, traditional neighborhood residence.
- ▶ Individuals who are homebound can live alone or with partner, spouse, friend, family members, or other caregivers.
- ▶ Often a variety of home-based healthcare and personal care services are utilized.

II. Residential Facilities

- ▶ Residential facilities can include:
  - Nursing homes that provide skilled nursing care
  - Rehabilitation centers that provide temporary support for patients
  - Independent and assisted living facilities for seniors or disabled individuals.
- ▶ United States federal regulations on dental services require residential facilities that receive Medicaid or Medicare funding to contract with qualified dental personnel.
- ▶ Medicare coverage does not include payment for dental services.[7]
- ▶ Medicaid-eligible residents are covered only for dental services included in the state plan; most state plans have limited coverage for adults.[8]

BOX 58-2

Potential Homebound Patients

- ▷ Frail elderly
- ▷ Severely medically compromised
- ▷ Critically ill
- ▷ Physically disabled
- ▷ Developmentally disabled
- ▷ Chronically mentally ill
- ▷ Terminally ill

▶ Under US federal guidelines, nursing homes are not required to cover the costs of dental care, but are required to help individuals residing in the facility obtain the following:

- Comprehensive assessment of dental status
- Routine as well as emergency dental services
- Transportation to dental appointments
- Prompt referral to a dentist for lost or damaged dentures
- Supplies related to oral health (e.g., toothbrush and dental floss) at no cost to the individual.

▶ Regulations in each state regarding the provision of dental services for both Medicaid-eligible and -noneligible individuals vary greatly.[8]

▶ A few states provide guidelines in terms of frequency of examinations or spell out elements included in routine or emergency care.

▶ Some states require facilities contract with a dentist to advise on policies and education.

▶ However, studies[3,9] indicate that generally individuals residing in nursing homes:

- Have poor oral health status
- Do not receive adequate daily oral care
- Cannot adequately access routine dental services.

III. Community-Based Settings

Community-based settings for alternative dental hygiene practice may include:

▶ Senior centers and aggregate meal sites
▶ Work/activity centers for disabled individuals
▶ Medical practices
▶ Homeless shelters
▶ Churches
▶ Elementary and secondary schools (some already provide school-based medical care)
▶ Head Start and day care centers.

DENTAL HYGIENE CARE

I. Common Oral Problems[9,10]

▶ Periodontal infections
▶ Lack of daily personal oral care
▶ Need for routine dental check-up
▶ Difficulty biting and chewing
▶ Losing weight/not eating because of oral problems
▶ Toothache/pain and abscess/swelling
▶ Trauma/fractured teeth
▶ Loose teeth
▶ Lost fillings/crowns

▶ Dental caries
▶ Loose, uncomfortable, or lost dentures

II. Significance of Oral Health to Overall Health

▶ Although more research is indicated, a growing body of evidence supports the idea that oral health can affect systemic conditions.[11]

▶ Oral pain/discomfort can compromise nutritional status.

▶ Physical limitations can compromise daily personal oral care abilities.

▶ Oral health status and oral cleanliness can affect patient self-esteem, quality of life, and ability to communicate with family and caregivers.

III. Objectives of Care

The objectives of dental hygiene care of homebound individuals will vary according to the patient's situation and needs. A dental hygienist providing care in a home-based setting may:

▶ Provide intraoral/extraoral screening to triage patients who need treatment by a dentist.

▶ Assist in preventing further complication of the patient's health status by identifying oral infections and other problems.

▶ Provide routine screening to detect lesions that may be pathologic, particularly those that may be early cancer.

▶ Provide dental hygiene treatment and education interventions to prevent dental caries and periodontal infections that require extensive treatment.

▶ Encourage adequate daily personal oral care, whether performed by the patient or a caregiver.

▶ Provide palliative care for the individual with a shortened life span.

▶ Contribute to the patient's general well-being and quality of life.

IV. Preparation for the Home Visit

A. Understanding the Patient

▶ When providing patient care in any situation, the rule is "know before you go."

▶ The following steps will help prepare for a homebound patient visit.

▶ Review patient's medical history.

- Provide the medical history form in advance for patient to complete and return.
- Monitor medication lists carefully, especially when the patient takes multiple prescription or over-the-counter preparations.
- Telephone before visit to clarify responses or ask questions.

- Consider specific characteristics and special problems associated with the patient's age, chronic medical condition, medications, disability, or physical limitations.
- Chapters 49–69 review considerations for a variety of individuals with special needs.
- Determine precautions necessary for the individual patient's care and safety.
- Arrange with dentist or attending physician when premedication or other prescription is required.
- Include arrangements for local anesthesia if indicated.
- Arrange with patient or caregiver for items, such as extra towels or pillows, needed to support patient comfort during dental hygiene care.

B. Instruments and Equipment

- Routine dental hygiene care can often be provided using manual instruments and without the need for powered equipment.
- Several dental equipment companies, listed in Box 58-3, manufacture portable dental delivery units, suctions, X-ray units, and autoclaves.
- Self-contained power-driven scalers can be transported and set up in the patient's home, but require the use of suction.
- Additional equipment and supplies that can be transported by the clinician to the patient's residence are listed in Box 58-4.
- Covered plastic tubs or boxes, labeled for "clean" or "contaminated," are useful for carrying materials.
- The Organization for Safety, Asepsis, and Prevention provides infection control guidelines for safe delivery of oral care outside the dental office.[12]

C. Appointment Time

- Arrange the dental hygiene visit during a time when the patient is usually awake.
- Consult with patient or caregivers to schedule as convenient a time as possible in relation to nursing care and mealtime schedule.

V. Approach to Patient

A. Communication

- The dental hygienist may find approaching a relatively helpless, disabled, or ill person to be difficult.
- Clinician empathy and understanding, as well as good interpersonal and communication skills, can help project a caring attitude toward the patient.
- An oversolicitous attitude may not contribute to development of a cooperative patient relationship; a gently firm approach is most successful.
- Direct communication with the patient is most appropriate; however, communication with a caregiver may be necessary.

BOX 58-3

Commercial Sources for Portable Equipment

DENTAL DELIVERY SYSTEMS

A-Dec, Inc.
Website: www.a-dec.com
Toll free phone: (800) 547-1883

Aseptico
Website: www.aseptico.com
Toll free phone: (866) 244-2954

ASI Medical, Inc.
Website: www.asimedical.net
Toll free phone: (800) 566-9953

Bell Dental
Website: www.belldental.com
Toll free phone: (800) 920-4478

DNTLworks Equipment Corporation
Website: www.dntlworks.com
Toll free phone: (800) 847-0694

Mobile Dental Systems
Website: www.mobiledentalsystems.com
Toll free phone: (800) 321-6332

Safari Dental, Inc.
Website: www.safaridental.com
Toll free phone: (800) 567-0013

HAND-HELD X-RAY SYSTEM

Aribex, Inc.
Website: www.aribex.com
Toll free phone: (866) 340-5522

AUTOCLAVE

Alfa Medical
Website: www.statimsales.com
Toll free phone: USA: (800) 839-0722

HEADLAMPS

Orascoptic
Website: www.orascoptic.com
Toll free phone: (800) 369-3698

PeriOptix, Inc.
Website: www.perioptix.com
Toll free phone: (800) 445-0345

SUCTION TOOTHBRUSHES

Sage Products, Inc.
Website: www.sageproducts.com
Toll free phone: (800) 323-2220

Trademark Medical
Website: www.trademarkmedical.com
Toll free phone: (800) 325-9044

BOX 58-4

Instruments and Equipment to Provide Dental Hygiene Care for Homebound Patients

PERSONAL PROTECTIVE EQUIPMENT

▷ Mask, protective eyewear, gloves, and gown

Patient Education/Oral Hygiene Instruction Materials

▷ Toothbrushes, floss, tongue cleaner
▷ Denture brush if needed
▷ A variety of interdental aids
▷ Hand mirror
▷ Examples of adaptive aids
▷ Written or printed patient education materials

STERILE INSTRUMENTS

▷ The clinician's selection of instruments and other items required for patient care
▷ Transported before treatment in the sealed packages in which they were sterilized
▷ Transported after use in special plastic containers labeled for contaminated instruments

DISPOSABLE ITEMS—PREPARED IN "SINGLE TREATMENT" PACKAGES THAT ARE CONVENIENT TO OPEN AND USE AT BEDSIDE

▷ Napkins
▷ Gauze sponges
▷ Cotton rolls and pellets
▷ Fluoride application trays
▷ Additional essential disposable items

COVERALL

▷ A large plastic drape (helpful if patient's coordination is limited during rinsing)

ADDITIONAL EQUIPMENT

▷ Emesis basin (kidney-shaped basin facilitates the rinsing process)
▷ Portable headrest (attached to wheelchair or straight back chair to provide head support during treatment)

PHARMACEUTICALS

▷ Pretreatment mouthrinse
▷ Disclosing agent
▷ Topical fluoride preparation (varnish)

LIGHTING

▷ Adequate wattage to facilitate visibility
▷ Headlamp or reflector
▷ Photography spotlight or gooseneck lamp with narrow, concentrated beam

MISCELLANEOUS ITEMS—USUALLY AVAILABLE AT THE PATIENT'S HOME

▷ Large towels (for covering pillows)
▷ Pillows (firm enough to assist in maintaining patients head in stationary position)
▷ Hospital bed (can be adjusted to position patient most effectively)
▷ Wheelchair or chair with high back for head support
▷ Container for prostheses
▷ Power toothbrush

B. Personal Factors

▶ A patient who is comfortable with home-delivered care and aware of the difficulties under which the clinician is working may show significant appreciation.

▶ Establishment of rapport with the patient may depend on whether:
- The patient has requested and anticipated the appointment.
- Caregivers have insisted on and arranged the appointment.

▶ Cooperation may depend on the patient's attitude toward the illness or disability.

▶ Prolonged illness, suffering, the effects of inactivity, and monotonous confinement can contribute to depression.

▶ A patient who is depressed requires extra attention to communication because that individual may:
- Have difficulty maintaining a cooperative attitude.
- Appear indifferent to personal appearance and general rules of personal hygiene.
- Be noncompliant with the clinician's recommendations.
- Have increased risk for dental disease because of effects of medications, poor oral hygiene, and high carbohydrate diet.

▶ Caring for the patient with depression is described in Chapter 64.

C. Suggestions for General Procedure

▶ Request the caregiver to be present to assist as needed and to demonstrate current method of personal daily oral care.

▶ Prevent distraction by asking that other visitors remain out of the room during treatment.

▶ Introduce each step slowly to be sure patient knows what is being done. Do not make the patient feel rushed.

▶ Listen attentively; socializing is one of the best ways to establish rapport.

▶ Plan multiple appointments when extensive scaling is required to:
- Avoid tiring the patient.
- Observe tissue response.
- Provide encouragement in biofilm control procedures.

VI. Treatment Location

▶ Because many residence-bound individuals can sit in a chair or wheelchair at least part of the day, only rarely is dental hygiene care provided while the patient is in bed.

▶ A kitchen or large bathroom may be the most satisfactory treatment location to provide access to water and counter space.

▶ Dental hygiene treatment is complicated by instability of the patient's head. Ingenuity is needed to arrange

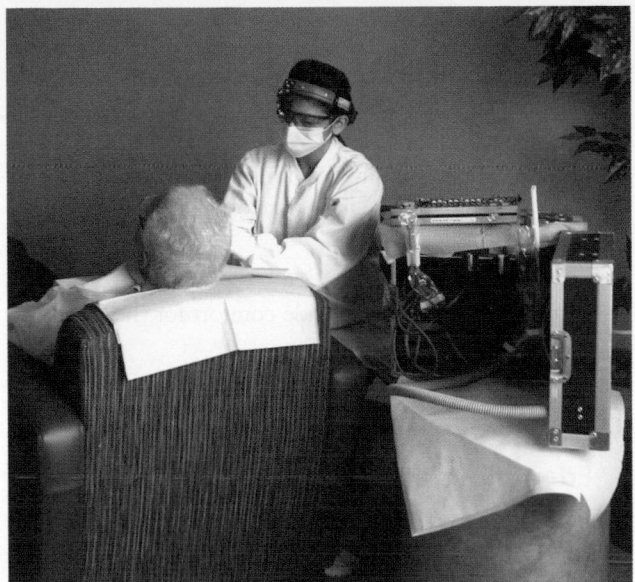

FIGURE 58-1 A dental hygiene student provides patient care using a headlamp and a portable dental unit that folds into a small suitcase-like container.

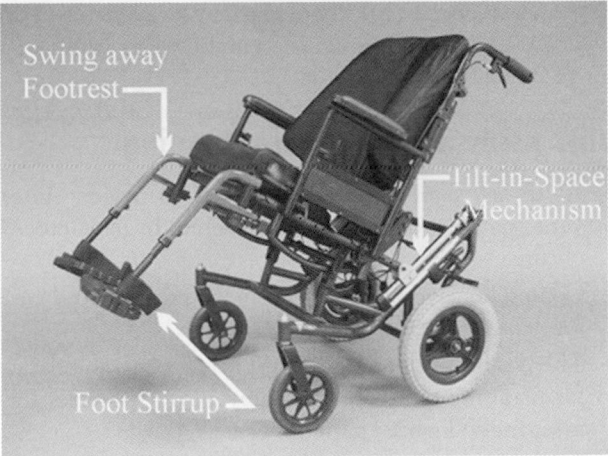

FIGURE 58-2 A wheelchair that is designed to tilt back, providing comfort and easy access for dental care. (From Frontera WR, DeLisa's Physical Medicine and Rehabilitation, 5th Edition. Philadelphia: Wolters Kluwer Health, 2010.)

patient position to provide access for treatment as well as maintain comfort for both the patient and the clinician (Figure 58-1).

A. Patient in Bed

▶ *Hospital bed*: Adjust to lift patient's head to desirable height.

▶ *Ordinary bed, sofa, or cushioned chair*: Use firm pillows to support and stabilize patient's head.

▶ *Small patient*: Positions for biofilm control described in Chapter 57 and shown in Figure 57-12 may be applicable during treatment.

B. Patient in Wheelchair

▶ A portable headrest can be attached to back of a straight chair or wheelchair (Figure 57-10, in Chapter 57).

▶ A straight chair or wheelchair can be backed against a wall to provide a stable headrest.

▶ Some wheelchairs tilt or slightly recline to facilitate patient positioning for care (Figure 58-2).

▶ A firm pillow can be inserted between the chair back and the patient's head to provide a cushioned resting surface.

VII. Additional Considerations

▶ Use instruments directly from a sterile package or cassette.

▶ Place instrument packets and other supplies in a small tray on a bed or chair side table or on the bathroom/kitchen counter.

▶ Provide adequate lighting.

  • Turn off overhead lighting to reduce shadows in the mouth.

  • A headlamp is usually the most convenient, efficient, concentrated form of light (Figure 58-3).

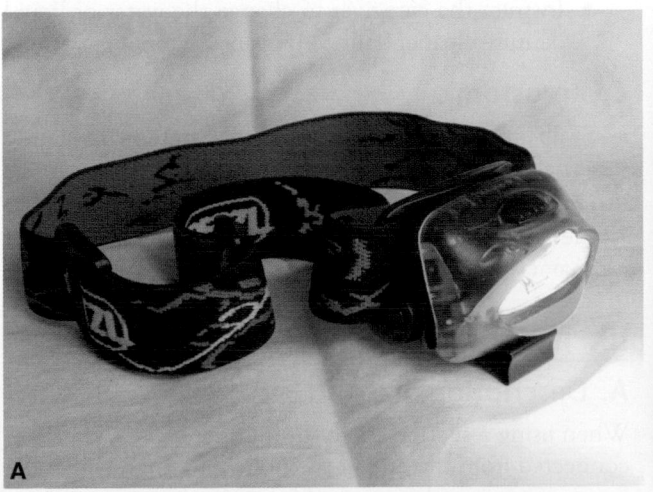

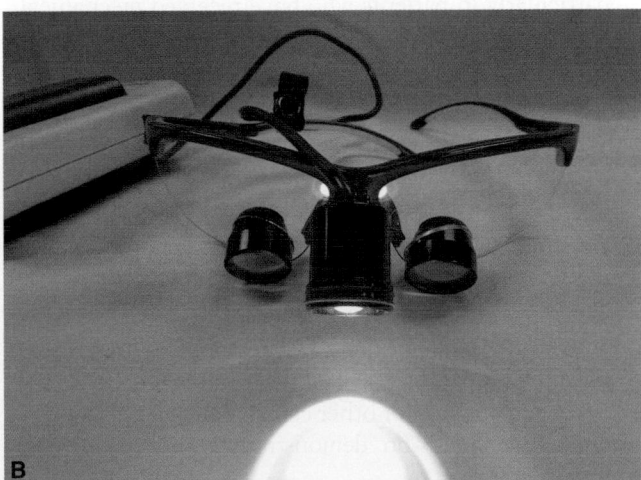

FIGURE 58-3 **A:** A small light-emitting diode (LED) light with an attached headband, sometimes called a "camping" headlamp. **B:** Safety glasses with loupes and an attached LED headlamp. With either lighting system, the beam can be adjusted so that it is focused directly into the patient's oral cavity.

- A gooseneck-type floor lamp may be available in the patient's home or can be purchased as part of the clinician's mobile setup.

VIII. Assessment and Care Planning

▶ As in any patient care setting, dental hygiene interventions are provided using the dental hygiene process of care.

▶ Comprehensive patient assessment provides the basis for dental hygiene diagnoses.

▶ The dental hygiene diagnosis provides the foundation for planning treatment and prevention strategies that meet individualized patient needs.

▶ Follow-up appointments for maintenance and ongoing evaluation of the patient's oral condition determine whether treatment goals are met.

IX. Protocols for Prevention

▶ Table 58-1 identifies special considerations for developing a personalized prevention plan for residence-bound individuals.

▶ Additional strategies for preventing poor oral status can include:
  - Training caregivers
  - Consulting with members of interprofessional healthcare teams.

THE CRITICALLY ILL OR UNCONSCIOUS PATIENT

▶ Maintenance of oral cleanliness for the acutely ill or unconscious patient requires special procedures because of the complete helplessness of a patient who is not able to cooperate.

▶ Effective oral care can reduce the odds of pneumonia, particularly in patients who have received mechanical breathing assistance.[11,13,14]

▶ Methods need adaptation when the patient's head cannot be elevated.

▶ When the patient's illness or injury involves the oral cavity, the advice and recommendations of the attending physician and/or oral surgeon are followed.

▶ Personal oral care procedures for the unconscious patient are accomplished by the caregiver.

▶ The role of the dental hygienist is to:
  - Evaluate patient's oral care needs
  - Plan and conduct an oral health in-service program for nursing staff or other caregivers
  - Include hands-on demonstration and practice in training
  - Motivate the caregiver to provide daily care.

I. Objectives of Care

▶ Observe the overall health of the oral tissues and provide routine screening to detect lesions that may be pathologic.

▶ Prevent debris and microorganisms in the mouth from being aspirated and reduce risk for aspiration pneumonia (see Chapter 66).

▶ Minimize the possibility of oral infection.

▶ Clean the mouth and provide comfort for the patient.

▶ Relieve mouth dryness.

II. Instructions for Caregivers

A. Edentulous and Dentulous

▶ Clean the mouth at least twice a day to prevent dryness and sordes.

▶ A soft toothbrush or gauze wrapped finger can be used to wipe the oral mucosa.

▶ A power toothbrush used with a very light touch or a suction toothbrush may be more efficient and thorough.

▶ Gently brush or wipe all surfaces of the lips, teeth, gingiva, tongue, and oral mucosa to remove biofilm.

▶ A mouth prop can be placed in one side of the mouth while the other side is being retracted and cleaned.

B. Removable Prosthesis

▶ If dentures or other removable prostheses are present, remove before providing oral care; often hospital policy requires removal of dentures when a patient is unconscious.

▶ Procedure for removing dentures is described in Box 32-3 in Chapter 32.

▶ When the dentures are removed:
  - Clean and mark them as described in Chapter 54.
  - Store in water in a covered container.
  - Instruct the caregiver to change the water or liquid denture cleaner daily to prevent bacterial growth.

C. Xerostomia

▶ Swab oral mucosa using a saliva substitute as frequently as needed throughout the day and night.

▶ Lemon and glycerin swabs are contraindicated due to the acidic effect of lemon on the demineralization of enamel[15] and the drying effect of glycerin.

III. Toothbrush with Suction Attachment

A. Description of Brush

When using a suction toothbrush (Figure 58-4), tubing is connected from the end of the hollow toothbrush handle to an aspirator outlet or portable suction unit.

TABLE 58-1	Protocols for Prevention: Homebound, Unconscious, or Hospice Patients

COMMON PROBLEMS	STRATEGIES FOR PLANNING DENTAL HYGIENE CARE (Based on Assessment of Individualized Patient Needs)
Need for professional oral care	■ Provide complete intraoral examination ■ Provide dental hygiene care ■ Triage patient needs and refer/facilitate access for dental treatment ■ Recognize and facilitate treatment for oral pain ■ Facilitate treatment for oral lesions ■ Facilitate reline/replacement of lost, broken, or poor-fitting dentures/prostheses
Inadequate biofilm removal	■ Educate regarding the role of biofilm in oral and systemic disease ■ Assess patient ADL levels, emotional status, and knowledge levels related to ability to perform self-care regimens ■ Provide oral hygiene aids or develop adaptive measures that facilitate self-care ■ Train caregivers, as necessary, to provide adequate daily oral cleaning
Increased risk for dental caries	■ Identify/treat/prevent xerostomia ■ Provide for professional and/or home fluoride application ■ Provide dietary analysis ■ Educate about reducing intake of fermentable carbohydrates ■ Demonstrate daily oral self-care technique
Increased risk for periodontal infections	■ Provide periodontal therapy ■ Provide regularly scheduled maintenance care ■ Educate regarding the effect of oral disease on systemic health ■ Provide oral hygiene aids or develop adaptive measures that facilitate self-care ■ Train caregivers, as necessary, to provide daily oral care
Oral pain	■ Document and follow-up on patient complaints of oral pain ■ Provide oral examination to identify oral/mucosal lesions ■ Train caregivers, as necessary, to provide regular oral inspection and record observations
Trauma	■ Monitor patient for symptoms of abuse ■ Monitor/educate regarding potential for facial/oral trauma during a fall ■ Educate regarding protocols for oral injury emergency care
Xerostomia	■ Identify medications with a potential for causing xerostomia ■ Eliminate the use of oral products with alcohol, glycerin, or lemon ■ Educate regarding regular sips of water or ice chips to relieve dryness ■ Encourage use of over-the-counter saliva substitutes ■ Recommend use of nonsucrose-containing candies or gums
Inadequate nutritional intake	■ Identify oral pain or inadequate chewing function that may be affecting the patient's nutritional intake ■ Consult with staff nutritionist, if required in the patient's residential setting ■ Educate the patient or caregivers, as necessary, regarding oral status and potential for compromised nutritional status
Candidiasis (and other oral infections)	■ Educate regarding signs and symptoms of oral infections ■ Educate regarding effect of oral infections on systemic health ■ Train caregivers to provide oral inspection and record observations

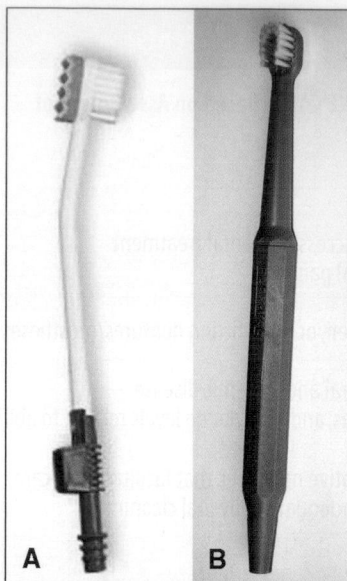

FIGURE 58-4 Commercial Suction Toothbrushes. Adapter on the hollow handle end attaches with tubing to portable or built-in hospital suction systems. **A:** Single-use suction toothbrush (Sage Products, Inc., Cary, IL). **B:** PlakVac suction toothbrush (Trademark Medical, St. Louis, MO).

B. Procedure for Use of Brush

▶ During caregiver training, procedure for use is demonstrated and included in an oral care procedures manual.

▶ An abbreviated outline of the basic steps is included in Box 58-5.

THE TERMINALLY ILL PATIENT

▶ The role of the dental hygienist is to:
- Provide comfort care for the patient
- Educate patients and caregivers about the importance of daily oral care
- Help develop standardized protocols for daily oral care

▶ Emphasis is on symptom relief and a clean oral environment, which can:
- Enhance the patient's sense of dignity
- Improve quality of life no matter how brief the life is to be.[16]

▶ Terminal illness is no excuse for neglect of oral cleanliness; daily personal oral hygiene care is essential.

▶ The major difference in providing dental hygiene care for a terminally ill patient is a focus on short-term palliative care rather than long-term preventive care.

I. Objectives of Care

▶ Provide oral care that emphasizes patient comfort more than preventive or restorative aspects of care.

BOX 58-5

Procedure for Use of Suction Toothbrush

▷ Prepare the patient
  ▷ Although not able to respond in a usual manner, the patient may be aware of what is going on.
  ▷ Tell patient that the teeth are going to be brushed, and thereafter maintain a one-way conversation despite patient's inability to respond verbally.
  ▷ Turn patient on the side and place a pillow at the back for support.
  ▷ Place a small towel behind the patient's head and an emesis basin under patient's chin.
▷ Follow routine infection control and personal protective equipment guidelines.
▷ Attach toothbrush to suction outlet and lay brush on towel near patient's mouth.
▷ Place a rubber bite block on one side of the patient's mouth between the posterior teeth. Floss tied to the bite block is fastened to patient's clothing with a safety pin.
▷ Dip brush in nonalcoholic, fluoridated mouthrinse or chlorhexidine; do not use toothpaste.
▷ Turn on suction.
▷ Gently retract lip and carefully apply the appropriate toothbrushing procedures; apply suction over each tooth surface with particular care at each interproximal area. Remoisten brush frequently.
▷ Move bite block to opposite side of mouth and continue brushing procedure.
▷ After brushing, place brush in cup of clear water and allow water to be sucked through to clear and clean the tube.
▷ Remove bite block, wipe patient's lips, and apply a water-based lubricant.
▷ Rinse and disinfect toothbrush; sterilize bite block.

▶ Provide relief of painful or aggravating symptoms of oral disease or lesions.

▶ Prevent aspiration of debris and oral microorganisms and reduce risk for pneumonia.

▶ Provide a "clean mouth" environment to reduce malodor and improve appearance and enhance personal interaction with caregivers and family members.

II. General Mouthcare Considerations

A. Cleanliness

▶ Gentle but thorough daily cleaning of teeth, tongue, and oral mucosa is necessary.

▶ Provide oral care in any way the patient will allow, using soft toothbrush, gauze, or cloth.

▶ Dentifrice or other oral products are not necessary, but can add a refreshing flavor that the patient may like.

B. Visual Inspection

Frequent inspection of the patient's mouth is necessary to identify oral lesions that can cause discomfort or lead to serious infection.

C. Oral Lesions

One study of terminally ill patients found mucosal soreness and ulceration, Candidiasis, glossitis, and xerostomia are frequently identified on clinical examination.[17]

► *Candidiasis infection*[17]

- Oral cultures of *Candida albicans* were found in as many as 79% of terminally ill patients.
- The infection can become life-threatening in immunocompromised individuals.
- Once recognized, Candidiasis infection is easily treated with antifungal medication.

► *Xerostomia*[17]

- Xerostomia is common among terminally ill individuals due to medications, dehydration, or mouthbreathing.
- Instruct patient or caregiver to moisten intraoral tissues and lips frequently using water, ice chips, or appropriate over-the-counter saliva substitute products.
- Avoid mouthrinses or other oral products that contain alcohol.
- Consider the use of a saliva substitute.

► *Changes in oral mucosa*[17]

- Approximately 75% of hospice patients examined in one study had evidence of pathologic changes in the oral mucosa, and 42% reported soreness of the oral mucosa.[17]
- Active oral lesions in the terminally ill may cause extreme discomfort when eating or talking as well as present an opportunity for development of secondary infections.

- Daily examination of tissues is needed with follow-up for immediate care of developing lesions.

► *Denture problems*[17]

- Because of severe weight loss, a denture may no longer fit. Chewing and talking are difficult. More than 70% of hospice patients who wore dentures reported having some kind of difficulty wearing their dentures.
- More serious concern are development of intraoral lesions due to denture movement and accumulation of biofilm organisms on an unclean denture.
- Denture-induced lesions are described in Chapter 54.
- Soft reline materials, combined with proper daily oral and denture cleansing, may solve the problem for the duration of the patient's life.

DOCUMENTATION

Key concepts for documenting dental hygiene care provided in alternative settings include:

► Description of location where treatment is provided.
► Description of the patient's current health status and functional ability, particularly related to ability to provide self-care.
► Notation of whether or not caregiver assistance is needed for daily oral care.
► Summary of oral health assessment data.
► Specific recommendations/instructions for oral care techniques and adjunct oral hygiene aids.
► Details of dental hygiene interventions/services provided.
► Recommendations for follow-up care and education.
► A sample documentation can be found in Box 58-6.

EVERYDAY ETHICS

Elena is 55 years old and is dying of esophageal cancer. She has been involved in an outpatient hospice program and receives all medical services in her home. Elena's daughter contacts the dental office of Dr. Gray and asks if someone can please come to the house and check her mother's teeth because they have not been able to help her brush every day and Elena's gums are bleeding.

Sandy, the dental hygienist in the practice, offers to go and provide whatever "comfort care" she can for Elena.

Questions for Consideration

1. What legal and ethical concerns need to be addressed before going to Elena's home since care will be limited?

2. Reviewing the principle of justice, if Elena's homebound status prevents her from accessing dental care, what options can the dental team offer to her at this time?

3. Describe several "Core Values" that can be exhibited by the dental team to benefit this patient.

BOX 58-6

Example Documentation: Bedside Oral Care for Patient in a Nursing Home

S –Routine nursing home visit for continuing care. The 89-year-old female patient is confined to a hospital bed, comfortable and alert; arm strength notably weakened since last visit and she is distressed that she can no longer support her own toothbrush for daily oral care. Nurse aide caregiver has been trying to assist but doesn't know how. Patient states: "Every time she tries to brush my teeth she chokes me or hurts my gums."

O–Excessive dental biofilm noted on facial surfaces of maxillary molars.

A–Patient can no longer engage independently causing increased risk for oral infection and subsequent increased risk for systemic effects. Caregiver needs training to provide efficient, effective, and comfortable intraoral brushing.

P–Discussed benefits of daily oral biofilm removal. Demonstrated effective oral care. Assured both patient and caregiver that oral care can be provided without discomfort. Demonstrated and supervised caregiver providing bedside oral care and biofilm removal with soft child-sized toothbrush.

Next steps: Follow-up visit scheduled with patient and caregiver in 2 weeks.

Signed _____, RDH

Date _____

Factors To Teach The Patient

▷ The contribution of good oral health to general health.
▷ How a clean mouth can contribute to wellness and quality-of-life factors.
▷ Need for prevention of dental caries by not using sugary snacks and sugar-sweetened beverages, especially between meals.

Factors To Teach The Caregiver

▷ How to care for the patient's natural teeth: toothbrushing, flossing, rinsing, and other personal needs.
▷ Removable denture care: cleaning daily, storage in a safe covered container when not in the mouth, changing solution for denture care daily.
▷ Selecting foods and snacks that are not cariogenic.
▷ How to use a suction toothbrush, power brush, or other device that can mean better oral care for the patient.

References

1. Gluzman R, Meeker H, Agarwal P, et al. Oral health status and needs of homebound elderly in an urban home-based primary care service. *Spec Care Dentist*. 2013;33(5):218–226.
2. American Dental Hygienists' Association. Advocacy: practice issues: direct access. https://www.adha.org/direct-access. Accessed April 14, 2014.
3. Smith BJ, Ghezzi EM, Manz MC, et al. Perceptions of oral health adequacy and access in Michigan nursing facilities. *Gerodontology*. 2008;25(2):89–98.
4. Strayer MS. Perceived barriers to oral health care among the homebound. *Spec Care Dentist*. 1995;15(3):113–118.
5. Rodriguez TE, Galka AL, Lacy ES, et al. Can Midlevel dental providers be a benefit to the American public? *J Health Care Poor Underserved*. 2013;24(2):892–906.
6. Edelstein BL. Training new dental health providers in the United States. *J Public Health Dent*. 2011;71 (Suppl 2):S3–S8.
7. U.S. Government Printing Office. Electronic code of federal regulations (Title 42: Public Health, Part 483—requirements for states and long term care facilities, Subpart B, Section 483.55, dental services). http://www.ecfr.gov/cgi-bin/text-idx?c=ecfr;sid=b97291f05d23f16ffa8e711922642bcc;rgn=div5;view=text;node=42%3A5.0.1.1.2;idno=42;cc=ecfr. Accessed April 14, 2014.
8. Medicaid.gov Website. Dental care. http://www.medicaid.gov/Medicaid-CHIP-Program-Information/By-Topics/Benefits/Dental-Care.html. Accessed April 14, 2014.
9. Smith BJ, Ghezzi EM, Manz MC, et al. Oral healthcare access and adequacy in alternative long-term care facilities. *Spec Care Dentist*. 2010;30(3):85–94.
10. Chen X, Clark JJ, Naorungroj S. Oral health in nursing home residents with different cognitive statuses. *Gerodontology*. 2013; 30(1):49–60.
11. Linden GJ, Lyons A, Scannapieco FA. Periodontal systemic associations: review of the evidence. *J Periodontol*. 2013;84(4, Suppl):S8–S19.
12. Organization for Safety, Asepsis and Prevention. Safe delivery of oral care outside the dental office. http://www.osap.org/?page=PortableMobile. Accessed April 14, 2014.
13. Shi Z, Xie H, Wang P, et al. Oral Hygiene care for critically ill patients to prevent ventilator-associated pneumonia. *Cochrane Database Syst Rev*. 2013;(8):CD008367.
14. Quinn B, Baker DL, Cohen S, et al. Basic nursing care to prevent nonventilator hospital-acquired pneumonia. *J Nurs Scholarsh*. 2014;46(1):11–19.
15. Meurman JH, Sorvari R, Peittari A, et al. Hospital mouth-cleaning aids may cause dental erosion. *Spec Care Dentist*. 1996;16(6):247–250.
16. Fischer DJ, Epstein JB, Yao Y, et al. Oral health conditions affect functional and social activities of terminally ill cancer patients. *Support Care Cancer*. 2014;22(3):803–810.
17. Aldred MJ, Addy M, Bagg J, et al. Oral health in the terminally ill: a cross-sectional pilot survey. *Spec Care Dentist*. 1991;11(2):59–62.

ENHANCE YOUR UNDERSTANDING

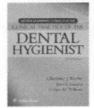

thePoint* **DIGITAL CONNECTIONS**
(see the inside front cover for access information)
- Audio glossary
- Quiz bank

SUPPORT FOR LEARNING
(available separately; visit lww.com)
- *Active Learning Workbook for Clinical Practice of the Dental Hygienist, 12th Edition*

prepU **INDIVIDUALIZED REVIEW**
(available separately; visit lww.com)
- Adaptive quizzing with *prepU for Wilkins' Clinical Practice of the Dental Hygienist*

59

The Patient with a Physical Impairment

Charlotte J. Wyche, RDH, MS

CHAPTER OUTLINE

LEARNING OBJECTIVES

After studying this chapter, the student will be able to:

1. Identify and define key terms and concepts related to physical impairment.

2. Describe the characteristics, complications, occurrence, and medical treatment of a variety of physical impairments.

3. Identify oral factors and findings related to physical impairments.

4. Describe modifications for dental hygiene care based on assessment of needs specific to a patient's physical impairment.

▶ Many conditions related to the neuromuscular system, joints, or connective tissue have as a symptom, or leave as a chronic after-effect, loss of function in the form of a physical impairment.

▶ Dental hygiene treatment modalities and oral care recommendations are adapted to the unique situations created by each disorder.

▶ General suggestions that may be adapted to a variety of patients with disabilities are described in Chapter 57.

▶ This chapter contains descriptions of selected diseases or conditions and describes modifications and adaptations needed by the patient during oral self-care, as well as by the dental hygienist during treatment appointments.

▶ Box 59-1 lists key words and definitions relating to physical impairments and disabilities.

NEUROLOGICAL DISORDERS ASSOCIATED WITH PHYSICAL DISABILITY

Most of the disabling conditions described in this chapter are considered neurological disorders.

▶ A characteristic of many neurological disorders is the death of nerve cells in the central nervous system.[1]

▶ Disruption of sensory or motor neuron signals is the cause of partial or complete paralysis associated with neurological disorders.

▶ Acute ischemia or traumatic injury to the brain or spinal cord causes necrotic (immediate) death of nerve cells in the most severely affected areas and immediate/complete destruction of transmission of neurological signals.

▶ Apoptotic cell death, a slower, biochemical or metabolic destruction of the nerve cell, occurs in chronic or degenerative neurologic conditions.

I. Acute Disorders

▶ Acute neurological disorders can be caused when one or more neurons are injured by trauma or biological assault or when there is disruption of blood flow to an area of the brain.

▶ Complete or partial loss of motor ability, sensory perception, or cognitive function can result.

▶ Acute neurological disorders discussed in more detail in this chapter include spinal cord injury (SCI), stroke, and Bell's palsy.

II. Degenerative Disorders

▶ Degenerative neural disorders are a result of progressive destruction of nerve cells.

▶ Patients with these disorders typically become increasingly disabled and dependent on caregivers to help them with everyday activities and personal care as their disease progresses over time.

▶ Degenerative neural disorders discussed in this chapter include multiple sclerosis (MS), amyotrophic lateral sclerosis (ALS), Parkinson's disease, postpolio syndrome (PPS).

III. Developmental Disorders

▶ Developmental impairments have their onset early in life, around the time of birth or before a child is 18 years old.

▶ Depending on the disorder, either a stable or a progressive impairment can result.

▶ Developmental disorders highlighted in this chapter include cerebral palsy, muscular dystrophies, and myelomeningocele.

OTHER CONDITIONS THAT LIMIT PHYSICAL ABILITY

▶ Joint and connective tissue diseases, such as arthritis, can affect a patient's ability to provide oral self-care and require adaptations during delivery of dental hygiene care.

▶ Autoimmune diseases, such as myasthenia gravis, scleroderma, and rheumatoid arthritis, which can limit physical ability, are discussed in sections of this chapter.

SPINAL CORD INJURY

▶ The spinal cord extends down the middle of the back and carries both motor and sensory nerves that branch to send messages between the brain and specific areas of the body.

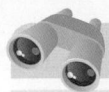 ## BOX 59-1 | KEY WORDS: Physical Impairments

Akinesia: absence or loss of power of voluntary motion.

Ankylosis: immobility due to direct union between parts.

   Bony ankylosis: union of bone with bone or bone with tooth resulting in complete immobility; the periodontal ligament of an ankylosed tooth is completely obliterated.

Aphasia: defect in, or loss of power of, expression by speech, writing, or signs, or of comprehension of spoken or written language.

Apoptosis: cell death activated by a biochemical reaction; sometimes referred to as "programmed cell death."

Ataxia: failure of muscular coordination; irregularity of muscle action.

Atrophy: wasting; decrease in size; occurs when muscle fibers are not used or are deprived of their blood supply, or when the nerve connection is interrupted.

Bradykinesia: abnormal slowness of movements.

Cerebrovascular accident (CVA): a focal neurologic disorder caused by destruction of brain substance because of intracerebral hemorrhage, thrombosis, embolism, or vascular insufficiency; also called stroke.

Decubitus ulcer: ulcer that usually occurs over a bony prominence as a result of prolonged, excessive pressure from body weight; also called pressure sore or bed sore.

Demyelinate: destruction/removal of the myelin sheath of a nerve.

Diplopia: double vision; perception of two images of a single object.

Dysarthria: impairment of oral, lingual, or pharyngeal muscles that causes verbal clumsiness or impairment.

Dysphagia: difficulty in swallowing.

Hypercholesterolemia: excess of cholesterol in the blood.

Hypertriglyceridema: raised triglyceride blood level.

Ischemia: deficiency of blood caused by functional constriction or actual obstruction of a blood vessel.

Kyphosis: abnormally increased convexity in the curvature of the thoracic spine (viewed from the side).

Microcephaly: head that is small in relation to the rest of the body; contrast with macrocephaly, head that is large in relation to the rest of the body.

Myopathy: any disease of muscle.

Orthosis: orthopedic appliance or apparatus used to support, align, prevent, or correct deformities or to improve the function of a movable part of the body.

Pallidotomy: surgical excision or destruction of part of the globus pallidus in the basal ganglia to prevent symptoms of Parkinsonism, including tremor, muscular rigidity, and bradykinesia.

Palsy: impaired ability to control movement.

Paralysis: a symptom of the loss or impairment of motor function in a body part caused by a lesion of the neural or muscular mechanism.

   Diplegia: paralysis of like parts on either side of the body.

   Hemiplegia: paralysis of one side of the body; usually caused by CVA or a brain lesion.

   Paraplegia: paralysis of the legs and in some cases the lower part of the body.

   Quadriplegia: paralysis of all four limbs from neck down; tetraplegia.

   Triplegia: paralysis of three limbs; hemiplegia with additional paralysis of one limb on the opposite side.

Paresis: slight or incomplete paralysis.

   Hemiparesis: slight or incomplete paralysis of one side of the body.

Paresthesia: abnormal sensation, such as burning, prickling, tingling.

Parkinsonism: a symptom complex comprising any combination of tremor, akinesia or bradykinesia, rigidity, loss of postural reflexes, and flexed posture. There are many causes of parkinsonism, one of which is Parkinson's disease.

Sclerosis: induration or hardening; especially hardening from inflammation and in disease of the interstitial substance.

Shunt: passage between two natural channels; to bypass or drain an area.

   Ventriculoatrial shunt: surgical creation of a communication between a cerebral ventricle and a cardiac atrium by means of a plastic tube; for relief of hydrocephalus.

   Ventriculoperitoneal shunt: communication between a cerebral ventricle and the peritoneum by means of a plastic tube; for relief of hydrocephalus.

Sialorrhea: excessive secretion of saliva.

Spinal shock: immediately after the injury, spinal shock causes a complete loss of reflex activity. The result is a flaccid paralysis below the level of injury that may last from several hours to several months.

TIA: transient ischemic attack; brief episode of cerebral ischemia that results in no permanent neurologic damage; symptoms are warning signals of impending CVA (stroke).

Visceral: pertaining to internal organs (digestive, respiratory, urogenital, endocrine, spleen, heart, and great vessels).

▶ External traumatic force can cause partial or complete loss of sensory and/or motor function related to the spinal cord level and the extent of the injury.

I. Occurrence[2]

▶ There are more than 200,000 people in the United States living with spinal cord injury (SCI); approximately 12,000 new cases each year.

▶ More than one-third of trauma cases result from motor vehicle accidents; other causes are falls, diving accidents, violence, and combat injuries.

▶ Nearly half of all injuries involve males between the ages of 16 and 30 years, but as the population ages, there has been an increase in average age of injury.

II. Characteristics/Effects of SCI

▶ The signs and symptoms of paralysis depend on the nature and level of injury to the spinal cord.

▶ There are 7 cervical (C), 12 thoracic (T), 5 lumbar (L), and 5 sacral (S) vertebrae, with paired spinal nerves extending from each; the areas of the body affected by injury at the different levels are illustrated in Figure 59-1.

  • *Complete lesion*: A complete transection or compression of the spinal cord leaves no sensation or motor function below the level of the lesion.

  • *Incomplete lesion*: Partial transection or injury of the spinal cord leaves some evidence of sensation or motor function below the level of the lesion. Some sensation and motor function may return within a few hours after injury, and maximum return may occur in 6–18 months.

▶ *Other possible effects*: Impairment of bladder and bowel control and sexual function; impairment of vasomotor and body temperature regulatory mechanisms.

III. Potential Secondary Complications

Patients with lesions at or above the T6 level are at greater risk for the complications described here.

A. Impaired Respiratory Function

▶ Pneumonia can significantly reduce life expectancy for a person with SCI.[2]

▶ Some quadriplegic patients are unable to elicit a functional cough and need assistance.

▶ By placing manual pressure over the abdomen, below the diaphragm, after the patient has inhaled, the patient may be assisted while an attempt to cough is made.[3]

B. Tendency for Decubitus Ulcers[4]

▶ A pressure sore (*decubitus ulcer*) results from tissue anoxia or ischemia caused by pressure exerted on the skin and subcutaneous tissues by bony prominences and the object on which they rest, such as a mattress.

▶ The cutaneous tissue becomes broken or destroyed, leading to destruction in the subcutaneous tissue.

▶ The ulcer that forms may become infected by secondary bacterial invasion and be slow to heal; anemia and poor nutrition may also contribute.

C. Spasticity

▶ As spinal shock subsides following a traumatic injury, muscle-reflex spasticity develops from a slight to a severe degree.

▶ Stimuli, such as decubitus ulcers, infections, and sensory irritation, may bring on a spasm.

D. Body Temperature

High-level quadriplegic patients are unable to regulate body temperature, requiring careful monitoring and intervention to warm or cool the patient as necessary.

E. Vulnerability to Infection

Complications related to elimination, urinary tract infections, renal stones, secondary infection of decubitus ulcers, and respiratory infections occur more commonly in this population.

F. Cardiovascular Instability

▶ Bradycardia and hypotension are common because of the loss of the sympathetic autonomic nervous system.

▶ Deep vein thrombosis is another potentially serious complication.

G. Neurogenic Bladder and Bowel

Complications related to dysfunctions in emptying bladder and bowels require planning to avoid the complications of autonomic dysreflexia.

H. Autonomic Dysreflexia[5]

▶ *Definition*

  • Autonomic dysreflexia, or hyperreflexia, is a life-threatening *emergency* condition in which the blood pressure increases sharply.

  • It may occur in patients with lesions at T6 or above.

  • A variety of stimuli may precipitate dysreflexia, including irritation to the bowel or bladder distension.

  • Patients who require manual bowel or bladder management techniques are more susceptible.[6]

▶ *Symptoms*

  • Increased blood pressure with slowed pulse rate. The blood pressure may rise to 300/160 mm Hg.

  • Pounding headache.

  • Flushing, chills, perspiration, stuffy nose.

  • Restlessness; increased spasticity.

▶ *Prevention*

  • Consult with physician when the patient has history of recurrent difficulties.

  • Avoid abrupt changes in body position and maintain a semi-upright chair position.

  • Monitor bladder outflow catheter tubing, outflow of urine into catheter bag, and bladder distention.

  • Schedule appointments that allow the patient to maintain the regular schedule for the bowel elimination program at home.

▶ *Emergency care*

  • Position chair upright gradually.

  • Do *not* recline the chair because increased blood pressure in the brain could result.

  • Check bladder distention and straighten catheter if clamped.

- Manually relieve bowel impaction if necessary.
- Monitor the blood pressure and vital signs using a medical emergency report form (Figure 8-1 in Chapter 8).
- Call for medical aid if blood pressure does not begin to drop within 2–3 minutes.

IV. Mouth-Held Implements

The patient with a high-level SCI who does not have strong function of hands and arms may use mouth-held appliances to perform many tasks and the teeth for holding

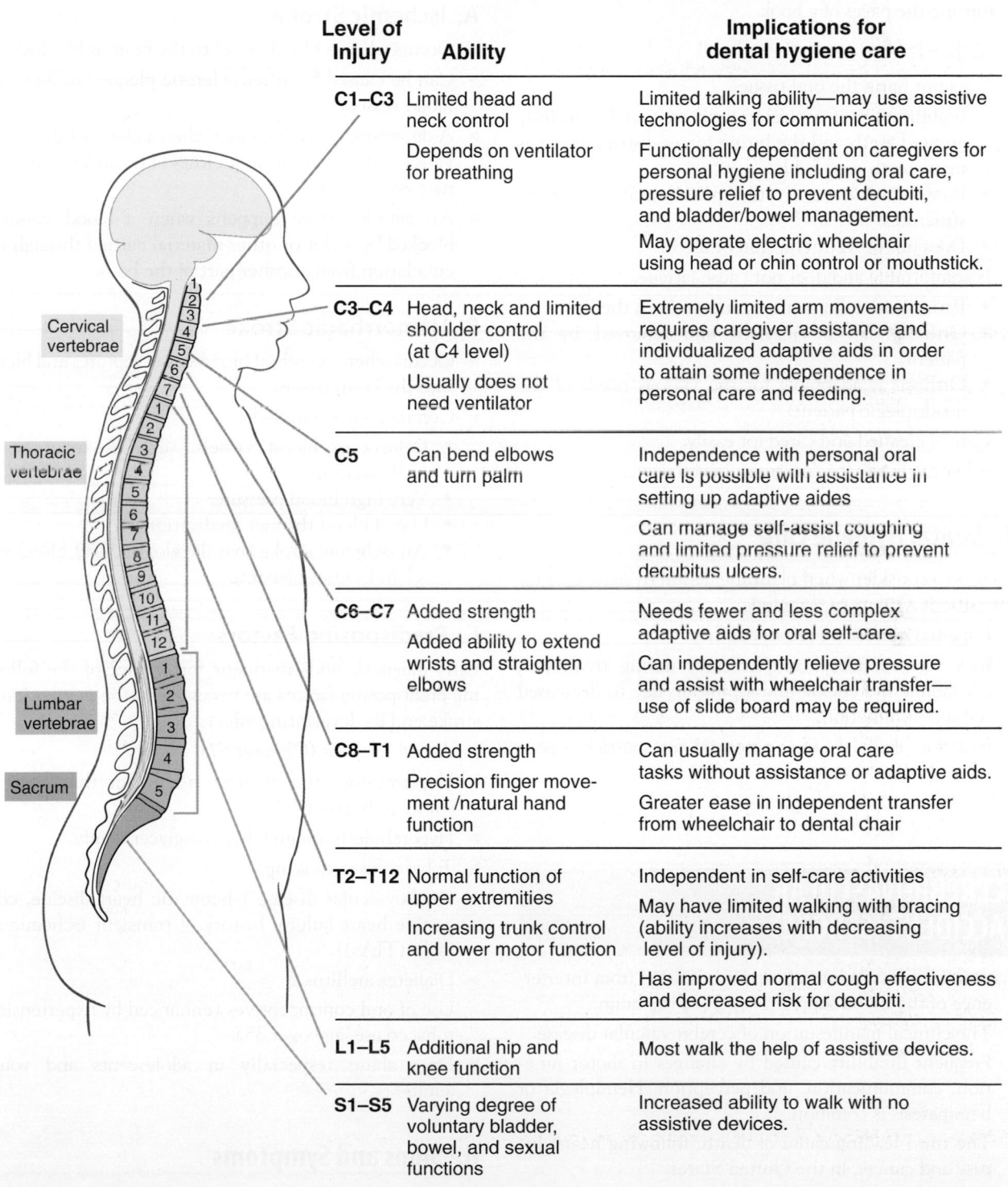

Level of Injury	Ability	Implications for dental hygiene care
C1–C3	Limited head and neck control	Limited talking ability—may use assistive technologies for communication.
	Depends on ventilator for breathing	Functionally dependent on caregivers for personal hygiene including oral care, pressure relief to prevent decubiti, and bladder/bowel management.
		May operate electric wheelchair using head or chin control or mouthstick.
C3–C4	Head, neck and limited shoulder control (at C4 level)	Extremely limited arm movements—requires caregiver assistance and individualized adaptive aids in order to attain some independence in personal care and feeding.
	Usually does not need ventilator	
C5	Can bend elbows and turn palm	Independence with personal oral care is possible with assistance in setting up adaptive aides
		Can manage self-assist coughing and limited pressure relief to prevent decubitus ulcers.
C6–C7	Added strength	Needs fewer and less complex adaptive aids for oral self-care.
	Added ability to extend wrists and straighten elbows	Can independently relieve pressure and assist with wheelchair transfer—use of slide board may be required.
C8–T1	Added strength	Can usually manage oral care tasks without assistance or adaptive aids.
	Precision finger movement /natural hand function	Greater ease in independent transfer from wheelchair to dental chair
T2–T12	Normal function of upper extremities	Independent in self-care activities
	Increasing trunk control and lower motor function	May have limited walking with bracing (ability increases with decreasing level of injury).
		Has improved normal cough effectiveness and decreased risk for decubiti.
L1–L5	Additional hip and knee function	Most walk the help of assistive devices.
S1–S5	Varying degree of voluntary bladder, bowel, and sexual functions	Increased ability to walk with no assistive devices.

FIGURE 59-1 Levels of SCI. On the left, the vertebrae are designated as C (cervical), T (thoracic), L (lumbar), and S (Sacral). The effects of SCI depend on the level of injury. (Source: The Spinal Cord Injury Information Network. *SCI Functional Goals for Specific Levels of Complete Injury.* Birmingham: University of Alabama at Birmingham—Spinal Cord Injury Model System (UAB-SCIMS); 2008. http://www.spinalcord.uab.edu/show.asp?durki=30166. Accessed August 6, 2010.)

objects. Optimum oral health and effective biofilm control has special significance because many functions cannot be accomplished by an edentulous mouth.

A. Uses

Fabrication of mouth-held appliances contributes to increased independence and makes possible such activities as operating an electric wheelchair, typing on a computer, or turning the pages of a book.

B. Criteria[7,8]

▶ Does not harm the oral tissues.
  • Stabilization of occlusion with contact for all fully erupted teeth and the biting forces distributed to as many teeth as possible.
  • Is not traumatic to the periodontal supporting structures.
  • Does not prevent eruption of teeth.
▶ Is comfortable and does not cause fatigue.
  • Patient can talk, swallow, and moisten the lips.
  • Orthosis can be inserted and removed by the patient.
  • Orthosis is adaptable for the various needs of the quadriplegic patient.
▶ Can be cleaned and cared for easily.
▶ Is relatively easy to construct; inexpensive.

V. Dental Hygiene Care

Factors to consider when planning dental hygiene care for the patient with an SCI include:

▶ Impaired motor and sensory ability.
▶ Risk for secondary complications during treatment; autonomic dysreflexia and aspiration due to decreased respiratory function.
▶ Risk for pressure sores, potential for spasticity, poor control of body temperature.
▶ Use of mouth-held implements.

CEREBROVASCULAR ACCIDENT (STROKE)

▶ A sudden loss of brain function resulting from interference of the blood supply to a part of the brain.
▶ The clinical manifestation of cerebrovascular disease.
▶ Frequent disability caused by changes in motor function, communication, and perception. Hemiplegia or hemiparesis is common.
▶ The third leading cause of death, following heart disease and cancer, in the United States.
▶ The stroke may be severe and death can occur within minutes; a less severe attack leaves the patient with residual and chronic effects.

I. Etiologic Factors

▶ The blood flow decreases to an area of the brain and shuts off the oxygen supply to the portion of the brain supplied by that vessel, resulting in cerebral infarction
▶ The two main causes or types of stroke are:[9]

A. Ischemic Stroke

▶ Occurs when a blood vessel to the brain is blocked.
▶ Can be caused by atherosclerotic plaque build-up in a blood vessel.
▶ A *thrombotic stroke* is caused when a clot within a blood vessel of the brain or neck closes or occludes an already narrowed vessel.
▶ An *embolic stroke* happens when a blood vessel is blocked by a clot or other material carried through the circulation from another part of the body.

B. Hemorrhagic Stroke

▶ Occurs when a cerebral blood vessel ruptures and bleeds into the brain tissues.
▶ Common causes include:
  • Defects in blood vessels, such as aneurysm or malformation.
  • Very high blood pressure.
  • Use of blood thinner medication.
  • An ischemic stroke that develops a burst blood vessel and causes bleeding.

C. Predisposing Factors

Early diagnosis and treatment for control of the following predisposing factors are necessary in the prevention of stroke and its devastating effects.

▶ Atherosclerosis (Chapter 67).
▶ Hypertension, the greatest risk factor that leads to stroke (Chapter 67).
▶ Hypercholesterolemia, hypertriglyceridemia.
▶ Tobacco use, smoking.
▶ Cardiovascular disease (rheumatic heart disease, congestive heart failure, history of transient ischemic attacks (TIAs)).
▶ Diabetes mellitus.
▶ Use of oral contraceptives (enhanced by hypertension, tobacco use, age over 35).
▶ Drug abuse (especially in adolescents and young adults).

II. Signs and Symptoms

The effects of a stroke depend on the location of the damage to the brain, as well as on the degree or extent of involvement.

A. TIA

- A brief event where the blood supply to a localized area of the brain is interrupted and the patient may have transient signs or symptoms of a stroke.
- These "little strokes" may last a few minutes to an hour and may leave no permanent damage.
- A history of transient attacks is a possible risk factor or warning for a stroke.

B. Acute Symptoms of a Stroke

Acute symptoms and emergency procedures are included in Table 8-3 in Chapter 8.

C. Residual or Chronic Effects

- Approximately two-thirds of those who survive have some degree of permanent disability.
- Temporary or permanent loss of thought, memory, speech, sensation, or motion results.
- The side of the face and body affected is opposite that of the brain injury (Figure 59-2).
- Persons with right hemiplegia have more difficulty with verbal communication and are more apt to be cautious, anxious, and disorganized.
- Patients with left hemiplegia have difficulty with action requiring physical coordination and may respond impulsively with overconfidence.
- Common signs and symptoms observed following a stroke are described in Box 59-2.

D. Disease Risk Detection

- Calcifications in the carotid artery are observable on a panoramic radiograph.[10,11] If present, the patient is referred for medical evaluation.

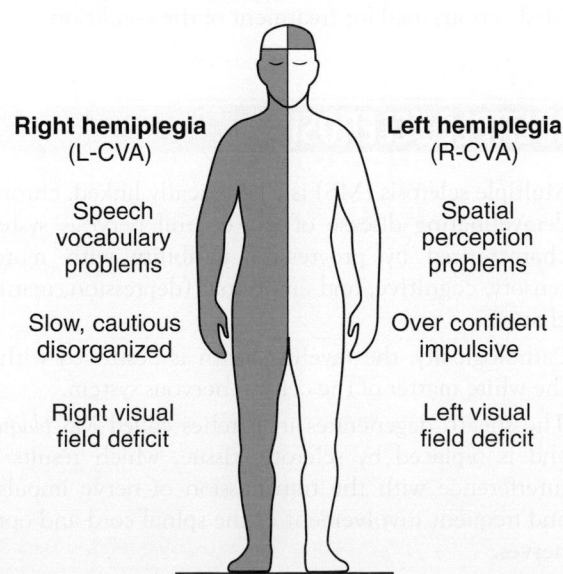

FIGURE 59-2 **Cerebrovascular Accident (Stroke).** Right hemiplegia is the result of left-sided brain damage; left hemiplegia results from right-sided brain damage.

BOX 59-2
Description of Signs and Symptoms Following Stroke

- **Paralysis:** hemiplegia (one side of the body) or portions, such as an arm, leg, or the face.
- **Articulation:** difficulty of speech, which may be caused by involvement of the tongue, mouth, or throat, as well as aphasia by brain damage related to the speech centers, and the patient may have difficulty finding the right word.
- **Salivation:** difficulty in control of saliva complicated by difficulty in swallowing; aspiration.
- **Sensory:** loss in affected parts may result in superficial anesthesia, or the opposite may occur with resultant increased sensitivity to pain and touch.
- **Visual impairment:** blurred vision, or diminished visual acuity.
- **Mental function:** may be unaffected, but slowness, poor memory, and loss of initiative are common. Brain deterioration may occur over a period of time.
- **Personal factors:** personality changes relate to emotional trauma, fear, discouragement, and dependency. Anxiety neuroses and periods of depression, which are common, may require assistance from a psychiatrist, psychologist, or social worker.

- Radiation therapy is associated with an accelerated form of atherosclerosis formation and risk of stroke.[12]

III. Medical Treatment

- Surgical correction of aneurysms, clots, or malformations may include removal of microscopic clots in the intracranial arteries or minute grafting to bypass blocked vessels and provide collateral circulation.
- Physical and occupational therapy and rehabilitation techniques are vital to the patient's recovery and functioning.
- Careful recording of the medical history includes the listing of medications. The patient who has experienced a stroke may be taking a variety of drugs for some or all of the purposes found in Box 59-3.

IV. Dental Hygiene Care

Particular factors to consider when planning dental hygiene care for the patient with a stroke-related disability:
- Impaired motor and/or cognitive ability.
- Hemiplegia; particularly if the dominant hand is affected. For example, the patient who wears dentures requires a suction cup brush, illustrated in Figure 57-6 in Chapter 57, to clean the dentures with one hand.
- Facial paralysis; decreased self-cleansing action of the tongue and lips; decreased control of saliva; risk for aerosol in eye during treatment.

► Medication for treatment of the condition: anticoagulant use is common following a stroke.

BELL'S PALSY (IDIOPATHIC TEMPORARY FACIAL PARALYSIS)

► Bell's palsy is paralysis of the facial muscles innervated by the facial or seventh cranial nerve.
► Although the cause is not known, various possible agents have been implicated, including:
  • Bacterial and viral infections; particularly herpes simplex
  • Injury, trauma from tooth removal or oral surgery such as the removal of a tumor in the parotid gland area.

I. Occurrence

► Although relatively rare, the incidence increases with each decade of life.
► In younger age groups, women are more frequently affected than are men.
► After age 50 years, the disorder is more common in men.

II. Characteristics[13]

A. Signs and Symptoms

Abrupt weakness or paralysis of facial muscles, usually without preceding pain, occurs on one side of the face.
► *Mouth:* The corner of the mouth droops, and salivation with drooling is uncontrollable.
► *Eye:* Eyelid on the affected side may not close; watering and drooping of the lower lid invites infection.
► When only the seventh nerve is affected, sensory responses are still intact.

B. Functional Problems

Speech and mastication may be impaired.

C. Prognosis

► A majority of patients experience a return to normal within a month with a spontaneous recovery.

► Others may have lasting residual effects or permanent paralysis.

III. Medical Treatment

A. Palliative

► Eye protection such as an eye patch during sleep and eye lubrication drops during waking hours.
► Hot compresses and massaging the involved muscles provides some relief.
► Analgesics may relieve pain.

B. Drugs

► Corticosteroids, administered within the first 72 hours, have been used to improve the prognosis.
► Antiviral drugs are prescribed sometimes, but the efficacy of such drugs is unclear.[14]
► Recent treatment protocols indicate combining corticosteroid and antiviral treatment may have added benefits for satisfactory recovery.[15]

C. Surgical

► Surgical procedures to relieve pressure on the nerve or reduce deformities have been used but are controversial and seldom recommended.[16]

IV. Dental Hygiene Care

Particular factors to consider when planning dental hygiene care for the patient with Bell's palsy:
► Facial paralysis; decreased self-cleansing action of the tongue and lips; decreased control of saliva; risk for aerosol in eye during treatment.
► Medications used for treatment of the condition.

MULTIPLE SCLEROSIS

► Multiple sclerosis (MS) is a genetically linked, chronic demyelinating disease of the central nervous system characterized by progressive disability with motor, sensory, cognitive, and emotional (depression, mania) changes.
► Pathologically, the myelin sheath is destroyed within the white matter of the central nervous system.
► The sheath degenerates in patches called MS *plaques* and is replaced by sclerotic tissue, which results in interference with the transmission of nerve impulses and frequent involvement of the spinal cord and optic nerves.
► The direct cause of MS is not known.

I. Occurrence

▶ Affects approximately 400,000 people in the United States (estimated 90 per 100,000 persons) and 2.5 million worldwide.[17]

▶ Usually adult onset; between 20 and 40 years of age, rarely before 15 or after 55 years.

▶ Prevalence higher among Caucasians than other ethnic groups.

▶ More prevalent in temperate climates.

II. Characteristics

A. Initial Symptoms

▶ Initial symptoms often fluctuate: transient difficulty in coordination, tremor, fatigue, or weakness.

▶ Transient tingling or paresthesia of the hands or feet.

▶ May have visual impairment with pain.

▶ May have a sudden onset with paralysis or marked weakness.

B. Course of Disease

▶ *Relapses and remissions*: An attack may last several days or weeks and be followed by a symptom-free period. The condition worsens with each relapse.

▶ *Longevity*: Close to normal life span; approximately 80% have functional limitations after 15 years.

C. Risk Factors

▶ Infection.
  • Various types of infection, systemic or local, can stimulate a relapse.
  • Oral infection is also a risk factor for relapse.

▶ Pregnancy.
  • Does not seem to affect the overall MS disease process.
  • Possible side effects of medications on the developing fetus are considered because certain medications used may have to be discontinued if they are teratogenic.

D. Physical Symptoms

MS can affect any area of the brain, optic nerve, or spinal cord and cause a wide variety of neurologic signs and symptoms.[17] Symptoms fluctuate, and several years may elapse between bouts of symptoms.

▶ Fatigue.

▶ Intermittent, unilateral facial numbness, pain, palsy or spasm.[17]

▶ Involuntary motion of eyes (nystagmus); the individual may later become partially or completely blind.

▶ Speech disorders; possible loss of speech in advanced stages.

▶ Changes in muscular coordination and gait; loss of balance; spasms.

▶ Paralysis of one or more extremities.

▶ Autonomic derangements, such as urinary frequency and urgency; later urinary incontinence.

▶ Susceptibility to infection, particularly upper respiratory.

III. Categories

▶ *Relapsing–remitting*: acute episodes worsening with recovery and a stable course between relapses.

▶ *Secondary progressive*: gradual neurologic deterioration with or without superimposed acute relapses in a patient who previously had relapsing–remitting MS.

▶ *Primary progressive*: gradual, nearly continuous neurologic deterioration from the onset of symptoms.

▶ *Progressive relapsing*: gradual neurologic deterioration from the onset of symptoms but with subsequent superimposed relapses (uncommon).

IV. Diagnosis and Treatment

▶ Diagnosis is based on history, clinical signs, and symptoms, supplemented by radiographic and laboratory test findings; there is no single diagnostic procedure specific for MS.

▶ Prompt diagnosis and early treatment within 6 months of onset is crucial to deter neurological damage.

▶ The goals of treatment are:
  • *Treat exacerbations*: prevent relapses and progressive worsening of the disease.
  • *Symptom relief*: provide palliative treatment to manage symptoms, improve function, and safety.
  • *Psychological support*: psychotherapy or medication to address depression or psychological problems may be indicated.

▶ General personal care; adequate nutrition, rest, avoidance of strain and stress, and prevention of infections and injury.

▶ Physical and occupational therapy; exercise, not strenuous exertion, is indicated.

▶ Medications used to treat neurological and other symptoms associated with MS are listed in Box 59-4.

V. Dental Hygiene Care

Particular factors to consider when planning dental hygiene care for the patient with MS include[18]:

▶ Orofacial manifestations, such as intermittent headaches, facial pain, numbness, palsy, and spasms.

▶ Visual disturbances.

▶ Impaired motor ability; changes to ability during relapses and remissions.

▶ Oral and systemic effects of medications used for treatment of the condition.

AMYOTROPHIC LATERAL SCLEROSIS

Amyotrophic lateral sclerosis (ALS, often referred to as Lou Gehrig's disease) is a progressive neurodegenerative disorder characterized by a progressive loss of motor neurons.

I. Occurrence[19]

▶ Prevalence is approximately 3.9 per 100,000 population; more than 12,000 people in the United States.

▶ Men more often affected than women; Caucasians more frequently than other ethnic groups.

▶ Onset usually occurs at middle age or later; prevalence highest in 60–69 years age group and lowest in age 18–39 or >80 age groups.

II. Diagnosis

▶ There are no diagnostic tests for ALS.

▶ Diagnosis is usually made after ruling out other disorders with similar symptoms.

▶ Clinically diagnosed with both upper and lower neuron dysfunction, although variants include a pure upper motor and pure lower motor syndrome.[20]

III. Etiology and Pathogenesis

▶ Unknown cause.

▶ About 90% of cases are sporadic.

▶ About 5%–10% are familial (predominantly autosomal dominant).

▶ Average life expectancy is 3–5 years; but the range is broad and some live much longer.

▶ Typically progressive degeneration of both upper and lower motor neurons with no periods of remission.

▶ More areas of the body are affected over time; nearly all systems eventually become involved.

▶ Respiratory failure is the usual cause of death.

IV. Two Forms of ALS[21]

▶ *Spinal form*
  • About two-third of patients.
  • Early symptoms include muscle weakness in upper and lower limbs and muscle wasting.

▶ *Bulbar onset form*
  • Initially presents with dysarthria.
  • Sometimes dysphasia for solids or liquids is initial symptom.
  • Facial weakness and wasting/spasticity of the tongue are common.
  • Limb symptoms may develop simultaneously; or can happen later as the disease progresses.
  • Sialorrhea (excessive secretion of saliva; drooling) develops in almost all who have the Bulbar onset form of the disease.

V. Symptoms[22]

▶ Cramps and spasticity

▶ Muscle weakness, particularly in extremities

▶ Increasing respiratory difficulty

▶ Difficulty swallowing and chewing

▶ Excessive saliva[23,24]

▶ Depression and anxiety

▶ Cognitive[25] and behavioral disorders that can affect compliance with recommendations.

VI. Treatment

▶ Only one current Food and Drug Administration approved treatment (rilusole); only extends survival about 2 months.[20]

▶ Palliative treatment is provided by interprofessional teams.[26]

▶ Treatment focused on progressive management of symptoms.

▶ Sialorrhea managed with medications, but in later stages treatment can include radiation or Botox injection into salivary glands.[20]

VII. Dental Hygiene Care

Factors to consider when planning dental hygiene care for the patient with ALS:

▶ Increased motor impairment over time.

▶ Need for body stabilization and support.

▶ Risk for respiratory difficulties.

▶ Effects of facial paralysis.

▶ Effects of treatment for sialorrhea.

PARKINSON'S DISEASE

▶ Progressive disorder of the central nervous system characterized by four primary symptoms[27]:
  • Tremor in hands, arms, legs, jaw, and face.
  • Rigidity of limbs and trunk.
  • Bradykinesia or slowness of movement.
  • Postural instability.

▶ It is also known as paralysis agitans and Parkinson's syndrome.

▶ Although the cause is not known, the basis for the specific group of symptoms is degeneration of certain neurons in the substantia nigra of the basal ganglia, where posture, support, and voluntary motion are controlled.

▶ In addition, a severe deficiency of dopamine, one of the substances that participates in nerve transmission, occurs.

I. Occurrence[28]

▶ Parkinson's disease affects as many as a million middle-aged and older persons in the United States.

▶ Incidence increases with age; only about 4% are diagnosed before age 50.

▶ Approximately 60,000 new cases are diagnosed each year.

▶ One and half times higher incidence in men than in women.

II. Characteristics

▶ The signs and symptoms center around tremor, rigidity, and loss or impairment of motor function (akinesia).

▶ These factors also occur in other conditions, which are differentiated by a physician when a diagnosis is made.

▶ The disease progresses through stages; from mild/early to severe/advanced with increasing impairment of motor function.

A. General Manifestations

▶ Body posture bent, with bent head and general stiffness.

▶ Motion and responses slowed; difficulty in keeping balance and turning.

▶ Gait slow and shuffling.

▶ Speech monotonous and slow.

▶ Resting tremor of one or both hands is common; the tremor can be reduced or stopped when the person engages in a purposeful action such as toothbrushing.

▶ The fingers may be involved in a "pill-rolling" motion in which the thumb and index finger are rubbed together in a circular movement.

▶ Nonmotor symptoms include variations in blood pressure, cardiac dysrhythmias, excessive sweating, bowel and bladder dysfunction, and sleep disorders.

▶ Cognitive ability is seldom affected except in the advanced stages.

▶ Eventually, after 10–20 years, the person may become incapacitated and may require complete care.

B. Face and Oral Cavity

▶ Expression is fixed and mask-like, with diminished eye blinking.

▶ Tremor or exaggerated movement in lips, tongue, and neck, and difficulty in swallowing.

▶ Excess salivation and drooling.

III. Treatment

▶ Although no known cure exists for Parkinson's disease, symptomatic control can be accomplished, in part, by replenishing the dopamine shortage with levodopa in combination with other medications; side effects can include dizziness and confusion.

▶ Maintenance of good general health is encouraged, including plenty of rest and nutritious meals.

▶ Professional physical therapy and occupational therapy have particular significance for a patient's well-being.

▶ Surgical relief for symptoms is sometimes accomplished by deep brain stimulation or pallidotomy (further defined in key words).

IV. Dental Hygiene Care

Particular factors to consider when planning dental hygiene care for the patient with Parkinson's disease include[29]:

▶ Increased motor impairment, tremor and rigidity over time, which interferes with daily activities.

▶ Rigid, uncontrolled facial muscles; poor control of eyes, lips, tongue, and swallowing muscles.

▶ Increased drooling of saliva.

▶ Need for short appointments.

▶ Potential for cognitive deficits over time.

▶ Adverse drug interactions and reactions.

▶ Need for caregiver education.

MYASTHENIA GRAVIS

▶ Myasthenia gravis is an autoimmune neuromuscular disease characterized by weakness and fatigability of symmetrical voluntary muscles.

▶ The patient with myasthenia gravis has a special significance for dental professionals because the cranial nerves involved affect facial and oral function.[30,31]

▶ It is caused by an autoimmune process that results in a defect in nerve impulse transmission at the neuromuscular junctions.

▶ In myasthenia gravis, the numbers of acetylcholine receptors in each neuromuscular junction are reduced markedly compared with the normal number of receptors.[32]

▶ Muscles of the eyes, facial expression, mastication, and swallowing are affected.

▶ In advanced severe forms of the disease, muscle involvement may be extensive and result in total paralysis.

I. Occurrence[32]

▶ Prevalence of individuals with the condition is around 36,000–60,000 cases, approximately 14–20 per 100,000 individuals in United States.

▶ Most common age of onset for women is 20–30 years of age; for men peak onset is 70 or older.

▶ Men are more frequently affected than women.

II. Signs and Symptoms

A. Early Signs

▶ Weakness of eye movements with double vision (diplopia) and drooping eyelids (ptosis) may be the initial indicators.

▶ In certain patients, the disease may not progress further.

B. Oral and Facial Problems

▶ As the disease progresses, involvement of muscles of the face, mastication, and tongue lead to swallowing difficulties (dysphagia) and a lack of facial expression.

▶ Disturbed speech and expression, with a weak voice that sounds tired and muffled, are typical.

▶ A patient may support the chin with one hand to help during talking.

▶ Because of the lack of facial expression, distress may be difficult for the patient to convey.

C. Progressive Involvement

▶ When the muscles that are used during breathing become involved, serious respiratory complications can result.

▶ Generalized fatigue is usually not so evident in the morning or immediately after rest. Weakness may increase as the day goes by, a factor pertinent to the time selected for dental and dental hygiene appointments.

D. Precipitating Factors

▶ Individual reactions vary, but the more common predisposing or aggravating factors affecting the severity of

muscular involvement include emotional excitement, surgical procedures, loss of sleep, alcoholic intake, and infections, including oral infection.

▶ Treatment with immunosuppressive drugs makes the patient vulnerable to infection.

▶ Myasthenic crisis is best avoided by elimination and prevention of infection and all precipitating factors.

III. Medical Treatment[33]

▶ Today, medical treatment can generally control myasthenia gravis.

▶ Anticholinesterase agents are used to improve neuromuscular transmission and increase muscle strength.

▶ Immunosuppressive medications include corticosteroids, azathioprine (when corticosteroids are contraindicated), and cyclosporin. Among the side effects of cyclosporin is gingival enlargement.

▶ Therapy for attempting to induce remission can include surgical removal of the thymus gland, particularly if a tumor of the gland develops, and drug therapy is ineffective.

IV. Potential Crises

A. Myasthenic Crisis[33]

▶ *Cause*
  • A myasthenic crisis may result from undermedication or increased severity of the disease, or it may be precipitated by one of the aggravating factors previously mentioned.
  • The relative deficiency of acetylcholine, which leads to the crisis symptoms, can usually be corrected by the administration of anticholinesterase by the physician.

▶ *Symptoms and signs*
  • The inability to swallow, speak, or maintain a patent airway is sudden.
  • Marked weakness of respiratory and pharyngeal muscles leads to depression of respiration and obstruction.
  • The patient may also have double vision and drooping eyelids.

▶ *Emergency care*
  • Suction.
  • Provide a patent airway.
  • Obtain medical assistance; transport to hospital emergency facility.

B. Cholinergic Crisis[34]

▶ *Cause*: The cholinergic crisis results from overmedication with anticholinesterase.

▶ *Symptoms and signs*: Increased muscle weakness occurs within 30–60 minutes of taking the medication. Excessive pulmonary secretion, cramps, and diarrhea also are characteristic.

▶ *Treatment:*
  • Anticholinesterase medication is discontinued.
  • Medical assistance is needed promptly.
  • When respiratory symptoms develop, urgent ventilation is required.

V. Dental Hygiene Care

Particular factors to consider when planning dental hygiene care for the patient with myasthenia gravis[30]:

▶ Early, progressive involvement of orofacial muscles.

▶ Increased difficulty chewing and swallowing, risk for choking, and compromised facial and head movement due to muscle weakness.

▶ Speech difficulties may compromise communication.

▶ Risk for myasthenic or cholinergic crisis.

POSTPOLIO SYNDROME

I. Description

▶ Condition that affects adults, years after recovery from an initial attack of the poliomyelitis virus when they were children.[35]

▶ Cause is unknown.

▶ Prevalence is currently unknown, but appears to be growing.

▶ Treatment focus is mainly palliative, with exercise often prescribed to strengthen specific muscle groups.

▶ Characterized by progressive muscle weakness, fatigue, muscle and joint pain, and potential muscle atrophy in muscles originally affected by the poliomyelitis as well as other muscles, including orofacial muscles.

II. Dental Hygiene Care

Particular factors to consider when planning dental hygiene care for the patient with postpolio syndrome:

▶ Impaired motor ability.

▶ Weakness in respiratory and swallowing muscles.

CEREBRAL PALSY

I. Description

▶ A group of disorders that involve a disorder of the cerebral cortex, the part of the brain that directs motor function.[36]

▶ Damage to the developing brain can occur such as:
  • During fetal development, usually (congenital)
  • Natally, or postnatally (acquired).

▶ In many cases the cause is unknown, but can be related to:

  • Abnormal development of the brain
  • Bleeding in the brain
  • Severe lack of oxygen

▶ Risk factors include[36]:
  • Maternal infections, thyroid abnormalities, or seizures during pregnancy.
  • Maternal exposure to toxic substances during pregnancy.
  • Blood type incompatibility between mother and child.
  • Complicated labor and delivery, breech position of baby during birth, or multiple births.
  • Infant jaundice, infection, or seizures after birth.
  • Severe head injury after birth.

▶ Symptoms usually can be observed during the first year after birth but if symptoms are mild may not be noticed for several years.

▶ Cerebral palsy is not progressive.

II. Classifications

Cerebral palsy is classified in four types according to associated motor impairment.[36]

A. Spastic Palsy

▶ Muscles have increased tone, tension; can be in one limb or all four; sometimes includes oral structures.

▶ Condition characterized by spasms (sudden, involuntary contractions of single muscles or groups of muscles) and stiff, rigid muscles resistant to movement.

▶ Complete or partial loss of ability to control muscular movement; therefore, movements are awkward and stiff with resistance to movement. Lack of control causes patient to fall easily.

B. Dyskinetic or Athetoid Palsy

▶ Characterized by constant, slow, involuntary writhing movements with frequent changes of muscle tone.

▶ Lack of ability to direct muscles in the motions desired.

▶ Grimacing, drooling, and speech defects are common.

▶ Factors influencing movements
  • Effort by patient to control muscle activity results in exaggerated muscle movement.
  • May be initiated and aggravated by stimuli outside body, such as sudden noises, bright lights, or quick movements by people or things in the area.
  • Intensity influenced by emotional factors. Patient is least in control in an emotionally charged environment, such as the dental office or clinic.

C. Ataxic Palsy

▶ Loss of equilibrium, balance, and depth perception; walk uncertain; has difficulty in sitting straight.

▶ Lack of coordination; needs time to execute changes.

► Involuntary muscle quivering may affect part or all of the body; placing gentle firm pressure on the affected muscles will help calm the tremor.

D. Combined Palsy

A combination of the three named types.

III. Accompanying Conditions

A. Primitive Reflexes and Abnormal Response to Stimuli

► *Asymmetric tonic neck reflex*: When head is turned, same side extremities extend and stiffen, while opposite side extremities flex.

► *Tonic labyrinthine reflex*: If neck is extended back, extremities also extend and back is arched.

► *Startle reflex*: Any surprising stimuli can trigger uncontrolled body movement.

B. Contractures

► Muscles fixed in abnormal positions.

► Increase in muscle spasticity and joint deformities.

C. Seizures

► As many as half have seizures and those with seizure disorder are more likely to have an intellectual disability.[36]

D. Sensory Disorders

► Visual impairments and hearing loss are common.

E. Speech and Language Disorders

► Speech may be slow and difficult to understand due to lack of control of mouth and throat muscles (dysarthria).

► Difficulty processing auditory information.

F. Cognitive Impairment

► Some individuals with cerebral palsy also have significant cognitive impairment.

► More than 50% *do not* have intellectual or cognitive disabilities; therefore, an inability to communicate does not necessarily mean lack of comprehension.

► Of the 50% who are not significantly intellectually impaired, some may learn more slowly because of sensory impairments, perceptive-cognitive deficiencies, and speech difficulties.

IV. Medical Treatment

► Interprofessional teams of healthcare providers caring for the individual with cerebral palsy can include medical, surgical, orthopedic and dental providers, as well as speech, physical, recreational, and occupational therapists.

► Orthotic devices to support the lower limbs and the use of cane, crutches, walker, or wheelchair may help to increase function.

► Surgery may be needed for addressing orthopedic deformities, correcting eye or ear difficulties, or severing nerves to relax muscles and reduce chronic pain.

► Oral medications may be used to reduce tension in affected muscles, aid in pain management, or control seizures.

V. Oral Characteristics

A. Disturbances of Musculature

► Facial grimacing, facial asymmetry, and abnormal function of muscles of mastication, swallowing, and speech are common.

► Spasticity of orofacial muscles can interfere with daily oral care.

► Inability to close lips contributes to increased drooling.

► Hyperactive bite and gag reflexes can present difficulties during dental and dental hygiene therapy, as well as during biofilm control at home.

B. Malocclusion

► The incidence of malocclusion is high; often a musculoskeletal abnormality rather than only misaligned teeth.[37]

► Oral habits of mouth breathing, tongue thrusting, and faulty swallowing contribute to open bite with protruding anterior teeth.[38]

C. Attrition and Erosion

► Severe, constant, involuntary bruxism is common and can severely wear down tooth structure and restorations.

► Gastroesophageal reflux can cause erosion of oral tissues.

D. Oral Injury

► Patients may fall frequently, which can damage and fracture teeth and jaws.

E. Dental Caries

► The rate of dental caries may be higher, but the risk factors for the patient with cerebral palsy are the same as the general population.

► Difficulties in maintaining biofilm control and problems of mastication can lead to the use of a soft diet, which increases risk for dental caries.

F. Periodontal Infections

► Periodontal or gingival infections are found in a high percentage of patients with cerebral palsy.[38]

► *Phenytoin-induced gingival overgrowth*: When phenytoin is used for the prevention of seizures, the patient is susceptible to gingival enlargement. The condition and its prevention are described in Chapter 63.

▶ *Risk factors for periodontal involvement*: Mechanical difficulties related to biofilm control, mouth breathing, and increased food retention because of ineffective self-cleansing all lead to increased periodontal involvement and biofilm collection.

▶ Many patients with cerebral palsy have heavy calculus deposits.

VI. Dental Hygiene Care

Particular factors to consider when planning dental hygiene care for the patient with cerebral palsy:

▶ Numerous associated oral characteristics and predisposing factors for oral disease.

▶ Impaired motor ability; uncontrolled movements, reflexive reactions.

▶ Compromised ventilatory capacity[39]

▶ Involvement of muscles in head and neck.

▶ Need for body stabilization and support due to joint contractures.

▶ Potential cognitive impairment and compromised communication.[39]

▶ Increased risk for seizure.

MUSCULAR DYSTROPHIES

▶ The muscular dystrophies are a group of more than 30 genetic myopathies characterized by progressive severe weakness and loss of use of groups of muscles.[40]

▶ The term *dystrophy* means degeneration and is associated with atrophy and dysfunction.

▶ The syndromes of muscular dystrophy have been separated by clinical and genetic means and range from mild (Becker type) with a later onset to more severe types (Duchenne, facioscapulohumeral).

▶ All types of muscular dystrophy are genetically inherited and the underlying pathologic processes do not differ.

▶ Generally, the diseases are limited to skeletal muscles, with cardiac muscle only rarely involved.

▶ In the United States, more than 50,000 children and adults are affected with some form of muscular dystrophy.[40]

I. Duchenne Muscular Dystrophy (Pseudohypertrophic)

A. Occurrence

▶ The Duchenne muscular dystrophy (DMD) type is primarily limited to males and transmitted by female carriers.

▶ Prevalence of approximately 1.3–1.8 males 5–24 years of age.[41]

B. Age of Onset

The condition is present at birth and becomes apparent during early childhood, usually diagnosed at an average age of 4.9 years.[41]

C. Characteristics

▶ *Musculature*: Enlargement (pseudohypertrophy) of certain muscles, particularly the calves, is present in early years.

▶ *Weakness of hips*: Child falls frequently, has increasing difficulty in standing erect.

▶ *Lordosis*: With an abdominal protuberance.

▶ *Waddling*: Either walks on toes or flat foot because of muscle contracture.

▶ *Precarious balance*: Patient arches back in attempt to find center of gravity; gait is slow because balance needs to be sustained during each step.

▶ *Progressive muscular wasting*:
  • Eventual involvement of thighs, shoulders, trunk; weakness of respiratory muscles.
  • Inactivity is detrimental and increases the individual's helplessness and dependency.

▶ *Intellectual impairment*: A mild degree of mental impairment is noted in some persons with DMD.

▶ *Cardiac abnormalities*: Arrhythmia and cardiomyopathy are common.

D. Prognosis

▶ Disablement severe by puberty; child is confined to a wheelchair.

▶ Patients rarely live to reach their third decade.

II. Facioscapulohumeral Muscular Dystrophy

A. Occurrence

▶ Males and females are equally affected.

▶ Incidence is approximately 1 in 20,000.[42]

B. Age of Onset

▶ Between 6 and 20 years, with an average at 13 years, after puberty.

▶ Mild symptoms may appear at later ages.

C. Characteristics

▶ Facial muscles involved, particularly involving the obicularis oris. The effect of gaping lips on oral tissues is similar to mouth breathing.

▶ Malocclusion and temporomandibular disorder problems have been noted.

▶ Scapulae prominent; shoulder muscles weak; difficulty in raising the arms.

- Difficulty in closing eyes completely.
- Cardiac involvement is rare.

D. Prognosis

- Progression is slower than that of the Duchenne type and progress may become arrested.
- Most patients live a normal life span and become incapacitated late in life.

III. Myotonic Muscular Distrophy (Steinert's Disease)

- Most common form in adults; can appear any time from early childhood to adulthood.
- Affects both men and women.
- Prolonged spasm of muscles after use; usually worse in cold temperatures.
- Also affects central nervous system, heart, gastrointestinal tract, eyes, and hormone-producing glands.

IV. Other Types of Muscular Dystrophy

Other less common types of muscular dystrophy include:[43]

- *Becker*: Similar to Duchenne type, but more benign with a later onset (5–15 years).
- *Emery–Dreifuss*: Onset between 5 and 30 years; generally benign, but severe cardiomyopathy and risk for sudden death is a feature.
- *Limb-girdle*: Most severely affects muscles of the hips and shoulders; manifests in late childhood/early adolescence and ranges from rapidly to slowly progressive.
- *Oculopharyngeal and myotonic dystrophies*: Each is relatively rare, has onset between 20 and 50 years of age, is slowly progressive, and features extensive involvement of orofacial muscles.

V. Medical Treatment

- Supportive treatments consist of:
  - Physical, occupational, and speech therapy
  - Respiratory therapy.
- Drug therapy includes[44]:
  - Corticosteroids
  - Anticonvulsants
  - Immunosuppressants
  - Antibiotics (for treating respiratory infections).
- Preventive treatment consists of prenatal diagnosis, carrier detection, and genetic counseling.

VI. Dental Hygiene Care

Particular factors to consider when planning dental hygiene care for the patient with muscular dystrophy:[43]

- Impaired motor ability.

- Potential need for body stabilization and support.
- Some types involve orofacial muscles.

MYELOMENINGOCELE

- *Spina bifida* is a congenital defect or opening in the spinal column. A portion of the spinal membranes may protrude through the opening with or without spinal cord tissue.
- When the spinal cord protrudes through the spina bifida, the condition is called *myelomeningocele*.
- Anticipatory guidance prior to conception includes the use of multivitamins containing recommended levels of *folic acid*. A reduced risk of offspring with spina bifida and other neural tube defects has been shown when mothers received folic acid.[45]
- Patients with spina bifida appear to be specifically at risk for latex hypersensitivity.[46] Precautions and management of latex hypersensitivity are discussed in Chapter 5.

I. Description

- Embryologically, a neural tube forms during the first month of pregnancy.
- From the neural tube, the brain, brain stem, and spinal cord arise, and, eventually, the vertebrae form and enclose the spinal cord.
- When a place in the spinal column fails to close, the result is an open defect in the spinal canal, which is called a spina bifida.

II. Types of Deformities[47]

A. Myelomeningocele

- A myelomeningocele is a protrusion or outpouching of the spinal cord and its covering (meninges) through an opening in the bony spinal column.
- Because part of the spinal cord and nerve roots protrude, flaccid paralysis of the legs and part of the trunk results, depending on the level of the protrusion (herniation).

B. Meningocele

- A meningocele is a protrusion of the meninges through a defect in the skull or spinal column.
- No neural elements are contained in the protrusion, but can cause minor disabilities.

C. Closed Neural Tube Defect

- Malformations in fat, bone, or meninges of spinal cord.
- Few or no symptom in most instances, sometimes causes incomplete paralysis with urinary and bowel dysfunction.

D. Spina Bifida Occulta

▶ Spina bifida occulta is a congenital cleft in the bony encasement of the spinal cord in which no outpouching of the meninges or spinal cord exists.

▶ Usually, spina bifida occulta has no symptoms.

III. Physical Characteristics

Depending on the level of the myelomeningocele, some or all of the following signs and physical characteristics may be found.[48]

A. Bony Deformities

Muscle imbalance from paralysis can cause dislocation of the hip, club foot, and spinal curvatures, such as humpback (kyphosis), curvature (scoliosis), or swayback (lordosis).

B. Loss of Sensation

Lack of skin sensitivity to pain, temperature, and other sensations can lead to problems of inadvertent an burn or trauma unrecognized by the patient or caregiver or to pressure sores. Frequent position changes are necessary during dental hygiene care.

C. Bladder and Bowel Paralysis

The nerve supplies to the bladder and bowel are usually affected. Lack of bowel and bladder control requires continual attention. Kidney infection with loss of kidney function is one cause of shorter life expectancy.

D. Hydrocephalus

▶ A high percentage of children with myelomeningocele have hydrocephalus. Hydrocephalus is a condition characterized by an excessive accumulation of fluid in the brain. The fluid dilates the cerebral ventricles, causes compression of brain tissues, and separates the cranial bones as the head enlarges (Figure 59-3).

▶ Development is slowed, and intellectual disability may be present.

▶ Many of these patients have seizures.

IV. Medical Treatment

Surgical, orthopedic, and urologic treatment as well as physical and occupational therapy may constitute a minimum of specialties involved in the care of a patient with myelomeningocele.

A. Neurosurgery

▶ *Closure of the myelomeningocele*: Surgical closure helps to prevent infections that may otherwise enter into the spinal cord. Paralysis is not lessened by surgery.

▶ *Treatment of the hydrocephalus*: Permanent drainage systems may be accomplished in the form of a

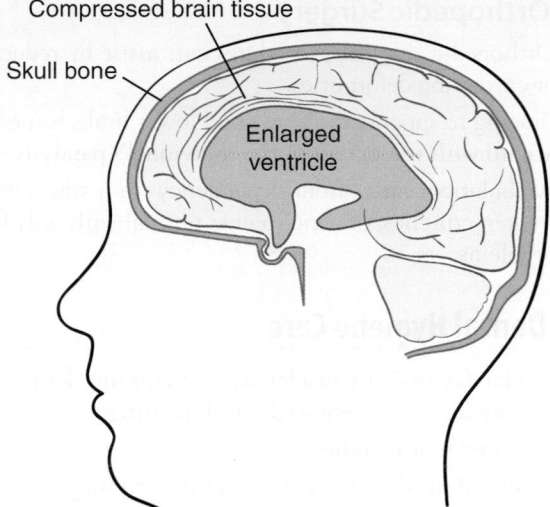

FIGURE 59-3 Hydrocephalus. The ventricle is enlarged because of the accumulation of fluid. Brain tissues are compressed.

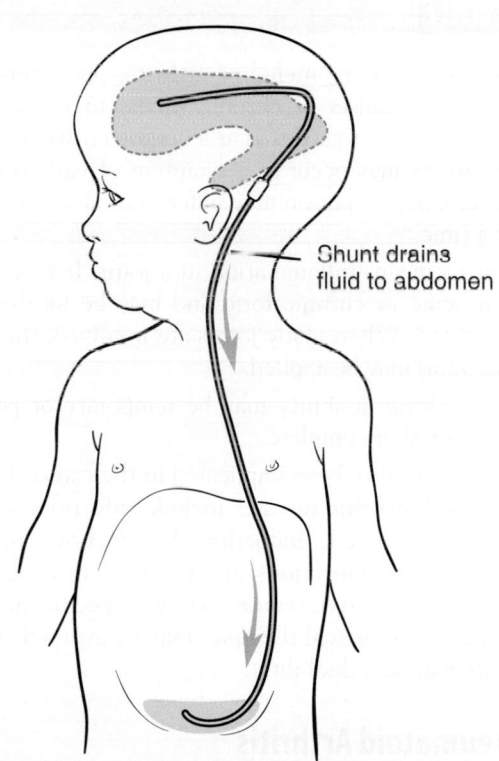

FIGURE 59-4 Shunt for Hydrocephalus Treatment. Fluid is drained by way of a ventriculoatrial or ventriculoperitoneal shunt.

ventriculoatrial shunt between the cerebral ventricle and the atrium of the heart. Sometimes, drainage by way of the abdomen in the form of a ventriculoperitoneal shunt is used (Figure 59-4).

▶ Individuals who have a cerebrospinal fluid shunt are at increased risk for transient infections. Need for premedication during dental treatment is established by medical consultation.[49]

B. Orthopedic Surgery

▶ Orthopedic surgical procedures can assist by reducing or correcting deformities.

▶ Bracing to support the trunk and lower limbs is used in accord with the extent of the individual's paralysis.

▶ Ambulation varies from dependency on a wheelchair, walker, crutches, or cane to near normal with only foot problems.

V. Dental Hygiene Care

Particular factors to consider when planning dental hygiene care for the patient with myelomeningoele:

▶ Impaired motor ability.

▶ Potential need for body stabilization and support.

▶ Increased risk for latex allergy and transient infections related to a cerebrospinal fluid shunt.

ARTHRITIS

Diseases of the joints, including arthritis, are among the most common causes of chronic illness in the United States. In addition to arthritis as a disease entity, arthritic manifestations may occur as a symptom of various other chronic diseases. A person may suffer from more than one type at a time.

▶ Arthritis means inflammation in a joint. It may occur in an acute or chronic form and may be localized or generalized. When many joints are involved, the term *polyarthritis* may be applied.

▶ The resulting disability may be temporary or permanent, partial or complete.

▶ Factors that have been implicated in the cause of rheumatic and arthritic diseases include infectious agents, traumatic disorders, endocrine abnormalities, tumors, allergy and drug reactions, and inherited or congenital conditions. When the cause is known, specific medical, physical, and surgical therapies may be available to alleviate pain and disability.

I. Rheumatoid Arthritis

▶ Chronic, systemic autoimmune disease in which inflammation of the joints occurs in exacerbations and remissions.[50]

▶ Cause is unknown, but believed to be the result of a faulty immune response.

▶ Progressive deformity, with limited motion and muscle atrophy in the severely involved joints.

A. Occurrence

▶ Usual onset between ages 20 and 40, although it may occur at any age.

▶ More women than men are affected.

B. Signs and Symptoms

▶ Pain, swelling, tenderness, redness, and warmth in symmetrical joints.

▶ Morning stiffness and stiffness after periods of inactivity.

▶ Weakness, fatigue and loss of energy, loss of appetite and weight, low-grade fever.

▶ Subcutaneous nodules in elbows, wrists, or fingers.

▶ Temporomandibular joint involvement may include

• Pain with jaw movements and difficulty in chewing.
• Ankylosis may develop but is not a common finding.

C. Medical Treatment

▶ Without a specifically known cause, therapy is limited to an individualized program involving pain relief, physical and occupational therapy, and overall health maintenance with adequate nutrition.

▶ Drugs commonly used in treatment include:[51]

• A wide variety of biologics and disease-modifying antirheumatic drugs
• Nonsteroidal anti-inflammatory drugs
• Corticosteroids
• Immunosuppressants.

D. Relationship to Periodontal Disease[52,53]

▶ Rheumatoid arthritis and periodontitis are both chronic inflammatory diseases that show evidence of common risk factors and pathologic processes.

▶ Literature suggests the extent and severity of periodontal disease and rheumatoid arthritis may be related.

II. Juvenile Rheumatoid Arthritis

▶ Autoimmune disease; occurs in children under 16 years of age.[54]

▶ Three types include:

• Pauciarticular: four or fewer joints involved; typically affects large joints such as knees.
• Polyarticular: five or more small and/or large joints involved including neck and jaw.
• Systemic: inflammation (joint swelling and redness) pain, fever, swollen glands and rash; least common form.

▶ Many patients have complete remissions, some have increasing disability, and others have mild arthritic symptoms that continue for years.

▶ The long-term treatment program includes activity to maintain function and drugs to relieve pain.

III. Degenerative Joint Disease (Osteoarthritis)

▶ Chronic condition related to breakdown and progressive loss of the hyaline cartilage cushion in the joints.[55]

▶ Eventually changes in underlying bone are noted.

▶ Inflammation is not a key symptom.

▶ Particularly affects the weight-bearing joints.

▶ No specific cause known, but predisposing risk factors may include:
  • Repeated trauma and mechanical stresses to the weight-bearing joints
  • Obesity
  • Age-related changes in the joint tissues
  • Genetic predisposition
  • Estrogen deficiency and high bone density may be factors.

A. Occurrence

▶ Affects approximately 14% of adults over 25 and more than one-third of those over 65.

▶ Incidence increases with age and levels off around age 80.

▶ Women, particularly those over 50, have higher rates than men.

B. Symptoms

▶ At first insidious, the eventual condition leads to much pain, deformity, and limitation of movement.

▶ Hips, knees, fingers, and vertebrae affected most frequently.

▶ Swelling and inflammation rare; ankylosis does not occur.

▶ Stiffness in the morning on rising and after periods of inactivity; diminishes with exercise.

▶ Pain aggravated by temperature changes, bearing body weight, and strenuous activity.

▶ Temporomandibular joint usually without pain or other clinical symptoms, although crepitation, clicking, or snapping may occur when the joints are exercised.

C. Medical Treatment

▶ Treatments to reduce symptoms include:
  • Physical therapy and regular, moderate exercise
  • Pain-relieving drug therapy
  • Weight reduction for obese patients.

▶ Total joint replacement has proved satisfactory for many patients.

IV. Dental Hygiene Care

Particular factors to consider when planning dental hygiene care for the patient with arthritis include:

▶ Joint pain contributes to impaired motor function and difficulty performing everyday activities of living (see Table 24-3 in Chapter 24).

▶ Affected areas, degree of impairment, and adaptations to provide for patient comfort are considered when planning care and providing instructions for oral self-care.

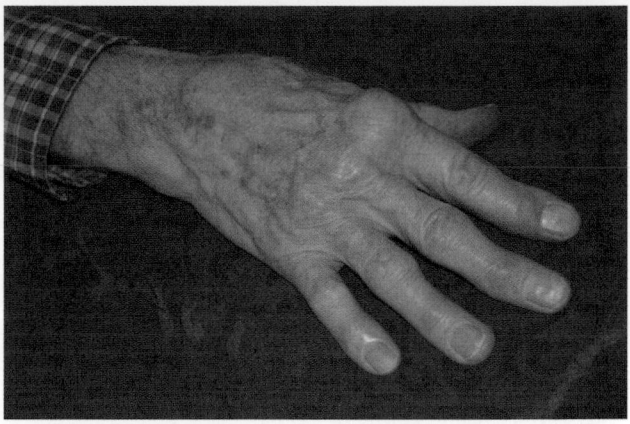

FIGURE 59-5 Adult Hand Compromised by Degenerative Joint Disease. Pain and lack of ability to grasp the small handle of a toothbrush affect ability to hold and maneuver oral self-care implements.

▶ The effect of osteoarthritis on the hands of an older patient is considered when planning for self-care procedures (see Figure 59-5).

SCLERODERMA (PROGRESSIVE SYSTEMIC SCLEROSIS)

▶ Scleroderma is an autoimmune disease of connective tissue in the body.[56]

▶ The most striking physical symptom is the immobility and rigidity of the skin, but inflammation and sclerosis occur throughout the body.

▶ Raynaud's phenomenon, color changes that occur in fingers or toes after exposure to cold, is often associated with the disease.

▶ The cause is not known, but collagen synthesis irregularities, associated immunologic disorders, and microvascular abnormalities have been implicated. Hereditary factors are not involved.

I. Occurrence

▶ Scleroderma usually has its onset between ages 30 and 50, but it may affect persons of any age, even infants.

▶ It may develop over months or years and is between 2 and 5 times more common in females.

II. Characteristics

▶ Scleroderma may be localized and involve only the skin, or it may be generalized and involve all body organs.

▶ The most notable changes are in the skin, gastrointestinal tract, kidneys, heart, muscles, and lungs.

▶ Eventual death results from renal failure, cardiac failure, pulmonary insufficiency, or intestinal malabsorption.

▶ Symptoms vary, and all individuals do not have all the symptoms and signs that follow.

A. General Manifestations

▶ *Joints*: pain, swelling, and stiffness of the fingers and knee joints.

▶ *Polyarthritis*: symmetrical polyarthritis, similar to rheumatoid arthritis.

▶ *Skin*: hard and fixed; ivory-white, yellow, or gray, sometimes with brown pigmentation in the late stages.

▶ *Face*: When affected, the face becomes masklike and expressionless.

▶ *Esophagus*: increasing dysmotility predisposes the patient to gastroesophageal reflux disease.

▶ Patients with scleroderma are sensitive to cold and dampness, stress, undue emotional tension, and fatigue.

B. Oral Characteristics[57,58]

▶ *Lips*: thin, rigid, with oral stricture (microstomia) with limited opening capacity as well as difficulty in opening and closing.

▶ *Mucosa*: thin, pale, tender, rigid, with poor healing capacity.

▶ *Gingiva*: pale and unusually firm.

▶ *Teeth*: increased mobility.

▶ *Radiographic findings*: marked widening of the periodontal ligament spaces. This finding is sometimes considered a diagnostic characteristic for scleroderma.

▶ *Mastication*: difficult; temporomandibular joint movement is limited.

▶ *Tongue*: may be immobile; speech difficult.

III. Medical Treatment

▶ Specific therapy is not known.

▶ Treatment, therefore, has been directed to
  • Reduce symptoms (dry, tight skin and stiff, painful joints)
  • Prevent systemic complications (gastrointestinal, lung, and heart problems)
  • Maintain normal physical activities.

IV. Dental Hygiene Care

Particular factors to consider when planning dental hygiene care for the patient with scleroderma:

▶ Joint pain contributes to impaired motor function; affected areas and degree of impairment are considered for planning care.

▶ Involvement of orafacial tissues and limited mouth opening complicates dental hygiene treatment and oral self-care regimens.

SUMMARY OF CONSIDERATIONS FOR DENTAL HYGIENE CARE

▶ High cost, dental anxiety, and physical barriers are three main reasons individuals with physical disabilities experience difficulty accessing dental care in traditional settings.[59]

▶ Not being aware of oral health needs is another important barrier to oral care.[60]

▶ Dental professionals are essential members of the interprofessional patient care team for a patient with a physical impairment.[61,62]

▶ Early dental hygiene intervention and regular preventive care will aid in optimizing oral health status and minimizing oral problems.

▶ Knowledge and understanding of the specifics of a patient's particular condition will help the clinician become confident in managing adaptations needed during the dental hygiene appointment.

▶ Communication to determine and support the patient's wishes in adapting patient care procedures is essential, particularly when the patient is unable to perform daily life activities independently and is dependent on others.

▶ Most patients with a physical impairment do not have an intellectual impairment.

▶ Information provided in Chapters 57 and 58 is useful for planning dental hygiene care for a patient with a physical impairment, either in a dental clinic or in an alternative practice setting.

▶ General suggestions for the older adult patient in Chapter 53 may also prove useful.

I. Preparation for Appointments

▶ Information for appointment scheduling and providing a barrier-free environment is found in Chapter 57.

▶ Communication with patient or caregiver prior to appointment to assess specific needs will help the clinician to identify and prepare for modifications necessary to provide care based on the individual patient's needs.

▶ Essential information, such as a completed health history and description of the patient's physical abilities and limitations, can be obtained by telephone.

▶ Ask specific questions about abilities and limitations in performing activities of everyday living.
  • Information about assistance needed from caregivers.
  • Adaptive aids the patient is currently using for oral self-care or other personal hygiene tasks.

▶ Determine factors related to the best time of day for dental appointments, for example:
  • Schedule of urinary/bowel management program for a patient with SCI.

- The time of day when symptoms associated with the particular condition are most likely to be relieved or diminished.
▶ Assess methods preferred by the patient to communicate with healthcare providers or caregiver.
▶ Determine adaptations needed for the patient's comfort or safety during the appointment.
  - Blankets or increased air circulation if body temperature control is compromised.
  - Positioning and padding needed for stabilization.
  - Procedures for stress reduction.
▶ Identify medications that may put the patient at risk for:
  - Xerostomia
  - Increased bleeding
  - Potential interactions with local anesthesia.

II. Additional Considerations During Clinical Care

▶ Frequent, short appointments in a warm, quiet, comfortable atmosphere lessen patient fatigue and emotional stress.
▶ Emergency care may be needed during the period of recovery, such as immediately following a stroke or traumatic spinal injury; nonemergency care is delayed until the patient is stabilized.
▶ When the patient's condition involves partial or complete paralysis of facial muscles:
  - Decreased self-cleaning action of the tongue increases potential for collecting dental biofilm on oral surfaces.
  - Rinsing may be difficult or impossible.
  - When anesthesia is used, the affected cheek and lip may be at higher risk for biting injury until the anesthesia has worn off.
  - If the eyelid lacks natural ability to close for protection, care is taken to ensure that calculus, polishing agent, or other foreign material does not splash into the eye by assuring that protective eyewear and suction are used during treatment.
▶ Potential effects from interactions with medications taken for many disorders and conditions require particular care when administering anesthetics.
  - For example, epinephrine interaction with levadopa, often prescribed for Parkinson's disease, may cause the patient to experience an exaggerated effect on blood pressure and heart rate.
▶ Dental hygiene care is complicated if the patient has a disorder that involves involuntary movement; for example, athetoid movements in a patient with cerebral palsy.
  - Involuntary movement is not interpreted as lack of cooperation.
  - Ask the patient or caregiver for suggestions about assistance or management.
  - Sedation through premedication may be possible.

III. Assistance for the Ambulatory Patient

Suggestions for how to aid patients who walk with one or more assistive aides such as braces, a cane, crutches, or a walker are found in Chapter 57.

IV. Wheelchair Transfer

▶ Most patients who use wheelchairs can be treated in a traditional clinical setting.
▶ Detailed information about wheelchair to dental chair transfer is available in Chapter 57.

V. Patient Positioning and Body Stabilization

▶ Danger for the patient and dental personnel can result from the uncontrolled movement of the patient.
▶ Communication with patient or caregiver prior to appointment to assess specific needs related to body positioning and use of specific measures such as padding, warm coverings, or other supportive devices will help enhance safety, patient comfort, and clinician efficiency.
▶ The patient is asked to provide direction for correct, individualized procedures.
▶ Slow and incremental adjustments of the patient chair during treatment will help maintain comfort and patient stability.
▶ Prevention of decubitus ulcers can be accomplished by:
  - Appropriate positioning of the dental chair
  - Use of padding
  - Periodic repositioning to prevent or reduce pressure.
▶ Before dental hygiene treatment, the patient is asked about susceptibility to spasms and to describe the procedure to follow should one occur.
▶ Suggestions for body stabilization and use of mouth props are found in Chapter 57.
▶ Chapter 58 provides ideas for treatment adaptations when the patient is bed-bound or if care is provided in a nonclinical setting.

VI. Four-Handed Dental Hygiene

▶ Continuous assistance when providing dental hygiene care for patients with a physical impairment is essential.
▶ Use of a dental hygiene assistant will:
  - Enhance the clinician's efficiency.
  - Ensure the patient's comfort and safety.

VII. Personal Factors that Affect Self-care

▶ Depression from limitations or discouragement from the pain and pressure of treatment and rehabilitation can affect attitude toward oral self-care practices for the patient who has a physical impairment.

▶ Daily oral care can become a part of the personal hygiene routine accomplished as independently as the patient's ability allows. Physical and occupational therapists provide self-care training to enable as much independence as possible for personal care.

▶ Paralysis or muscle contractions may make grasping and manipulating a toothbrush difficult or impossible.

▶ Adaptations that may assist in maintaining daily oral care include:
- Toothbrush handle modifications (Figures 57-2 and 57-3 in Chapter 57)
- A specially designed toothbrush (Figure 57-4 in chapter 57)[63]
- A lightweight power-driven toothbrush
- Instruction for the caregiver assistance, provided on the basis of patient ability and limitations.

▶ Hemiplegia, common after a stroke, can require the challenge of helping the patient develop dexterity in the nondominant hand in order to manipulate biofilm removal implements.

VIII. Residence-Based Delivery of Care

▶ People with physical disabilities may benefit from oral health service delivery models that provide care in their place of residence.

▶ Delivery of dental hygiene care in alternative settings is discussed in Chapter 58.

BOX 59-5

Example Documentation: Maintenance Appointment for Patient with a Physical Impairment

S –A 32-year-old female patient presents for routine 3 months maintenance appointment. Patient is ambulatory with a walker and prefers no assistance at this time, but padding under knees helps her relax and enhances her comfort during treatment.

O –Medical history includes diagnosis of MS 2 years ago. Update today indicates no changes in health history or medications. Decreased ability to grasp a regular toothbrush was noted during oral hygiene instruction. No changes in oral status. Biofilm scores <20%.

A –Routine 3 months maintenance care today with the use of padding for patient comfort and reassessment of daily self-care procedures are indicated.

P –Full-mouth scaling/root planing, polish, fluoride varnish application. Several options for modifying/enlarging a toothbrush handle to facilitate better grasp during oral care were discussed with patient. At patient request, instruction for using a power toothbrush was provided. The use of a floss holder was demonstrated and ideas for enlarging the handle were given to the patient.

Signed _____, RDH

Date _____

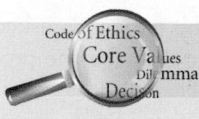

EVERYDAY ETHICS

John had an accident when diving into surf at the beach 2 years ago at age 18. He has a complete transection lesion at the C5 level. John came today for his biannual dental visit with his mother, who is his primary caregiver. Amy, the dental hygienist, was assisting in the wheelchair transfer into the dental chair. During the transfer, John's t-shirt was inadvertently lifted slightly, and Amy noticed obvious decubitus ulcers that showed signs of secondary infection. Amy continues to transfer him safely into the dental chair and then stops to consider what to do next. Dramatic images from a lecture in dental hygiene school flash through her mind. She will never forget those photographs of patients suffering from neglect.

Questions for Consideration

1. It is possible, although not clearly established in this scenario, that John is the victim of neglect. Is this an ethical issue or an ethical dilemma for Amy? What issues does Amy need to consider and what questions does she need to ask before she can proceed through the framework for making decisions about:
   - continuing today's appointment when she thinks that John's decubitus ulcers may be infected?
   - addressing the issue of potential neglect?

2. What does the core value of autonomy have to do with this scenario as Amy considers John's competency to make his own choices and treatment decisions versus his dependence on his mother for care?

3. What additional core values (Table II-1 in Section II, Introduction) come into play as Amy contemplates how she can best advocate for her patient's safety and well-being?

DOCUMENTATION

Documentation in the permanent record for each appointment with a physically impaired patient includes a minimum of the following factors:

▶ Description of the patient's impairment level and ability to provide oral self-care, with changes/updates noted for each dental hygiene visit, particularly if the patient has a degenerative condition.

▶ Recommendations for adaptive aids and modifications to daily oral care regimens.

▶ Description of oral hygiene care instructions provided to the caregiver.

▶ Description of patient position modifications and other adaptations during patient care.

▶ An example of documentation for an appointment with a patient with a physical disability is in Box 59-5.

Factors To Teach The Patient

▷ The need to communicate is key to successful dental treatment and oral health and is achieved by speaking openly about medical history, patient limitations, and adaptations needed for safe dental treatment and effective oral care.

▷ Daily, thorough biofilm removal is necessary to reduce the occurrence of oral disease.

▷ Regular maintenance appointments are needed to promote oral health.

▷ Why maintaining periodontal health can help maintain teeth that are necessary as abutments in order to tolerate a mouth-held adaptive aid.

▷ How to clean and maintain a mouth-held aid.

References

1. Friedlander RM. Apoptosis and caspases in neurodegenerative diseases. *N Engl J Med.* 2003;348(14):1365–1375.

2. National Spinal Cord Injury Statistical Center. *Spinal Cord Injury Facts and Figures at a Glance.* Birmingham, AL: National Spinal Cord Injury Statistical Center; 2013. https://www.nscisc.uab.edu/PublicDocuments/fact_figures_docs/Facts%202013.pdf. Accessed October 14, 2014.

3. Brown R, DiMarco A, Hoit J, et al. Respiratory dysfunction and management in spinal cord injury. *Respir Care.* 2006;51(8):853–868.

4. Remaley DT, Jaeblon T. Pressure ulcers in orthopaedics. *J Am Acad Orthop Surg.* 2010;18(9):568–575.

5. Stephenson RO, Berliner J. Autonomic dysreflexia in spinal cord injury. Medscape Website. http://emedicine.medscape.com/article/322809-overview. Accessed October 14, 2014.

6. Furusawa K, Tokuhiro A, Sugiyama H, et al. Incidence of symptomatic autonomic dysreflexia varies according to the bowel and bladder management techniques in patients with spinal cord injury. *Spinal Cord.* 2011;49(1):49–54.

7. Smith R. Mouth stick design for the client with spinal cord injury. *Am J Occup Ther.* 1989;43(4):251–255.

8. Ruff JC. Selection criteria for static and dynamic mouthsticks. *Gen Dent.* 1990;38(6):414–416.

9. U.S. National Library of Medicine, National Institutes of Health, Medline Plus. Stroke. http://www.nlm.nih.gov/medlineplus/ency/article/000726.htm. Accessed October 14, 2014.

10. Uthman A, Al-Saffar A. Prevalence in digital panoramic radiographs of carotid area calcification among iraqi individuals with stroke-related disease. *Oral Surg Oral Med Oral Pathol Oral Radiol Endod.* 2008;105(4):e68–e73.

11. Alves N, Deana NF, Garay I. Detection of common carotid artery calcifications on panoramic radiographs: prevalence and reliability. *Int J Clin Exp Med.* 2014;7(8):1931–1939.

12. Friedlander AH, Freymiller EG. Detection of radiation-accelerated atherosclerosis of the carotid artery by panoramic radiography. A new opportunity for dentists. *J Am Dent Assoc.* 2003;134(10):1361–1365.

13. Dawidjan B. Idiopathic facial paralysis: a review and case study. *J Dent Hyg.* 2001;75(4):316–321.

14. Hazin R, Azizzadeh B, Bhatti MT. Medical and surgical management of facial nerve palsy. *Curr Opin Ophthalmol.* 2009;20(6):440–450.

15. de Almeida JR, Al Khabori M, Guyatt GH, et al. Combined corticosteroid and antiviral treatment for bell palsy: a systematic review and meta-analysis. *JAMA.* 2009;302(9):985–993.

16. National Institute of Neurological Disorders and Stroke. Bell's Palsy Fact Sheet. http://www.ninds.nih.gov/disorders/bells/detail_bells.htm. Accessed October 14, 2014.

17. Hersh CM, Fox RJ. Multiple sclerosis. Cleveland Clinic Website. http://www.clevelandclinicmeded.com/medicalpubs/diseasemanagement/neurology/multiple_sclerosis/. Accessed October 14, 2014.

18. Fischer DJ, Epstein JB, Klasser G. Multiple sclerosis: an update for oral health care providers. *Oral Surg Oral Med Oral Pathol Oral Radiol Endod.* 2009;108(3):318–327.

19. Mehta P, Antao V, Kaye W, et al.; Division of Toxicology and Human Health Sciences, Agency for Toxic Substances and Disease Registry, Atlanta, Georgia; and Centers for Disease Control and Prevention (CDC). Prevalence of amyotrophic lateral sclerosis—United States, 2010–2011. *MMWR Surveill Summ.* 2014;63 (Suppl 7):1–14.

20. Lomen-Hoerth C. Amyotrophic lateral sclerosis from bench to bedside. *Semin Neurol.* 2008;28(2):205–211.

21. Wijesekera LC, Leigh PN. Amyotrophic lateral sclerosis. *Orphanet J Rare Dis.* 2009;4:3.

22. National Institute of Neurological Disorders and Stroke. Amyotrophic Lateral Sclerosis (ALS) Fact Sheets. NINDS/NIH Website. http://www.ninds.nih.gov/disorders/amyotrophiclateralsclerosis/detail_als.htm. Accessed October 14, 2014.

23. Asher RS, Alfred T. Dental management of long-term amyotrophic lateral sclerosis: case report. *Spec Care Dentist.* 1993;13(6):241–244.

24. Meningaud JP, Pitak-Arnnop P, Chikhani L, et al. Drooling of saliva: a review of the etiology and management options. *Oral Surg Oral Med Oral Pathol Oral Radiol Endod.* 2006;101(1):48–57.

25. Mitsumoto H, Rabkin JG. Palliative care for patients with amyotrophic lateral sclerosis: "prepare for the worst and hope for the best". *JAMA.* 2007;298(2):207–216.

26. Houde SC, Mangolds V. Amyotrophic lateral sclerosis: a team approach to primary care. *Clin Excell Nurse Pract.* 1999;3(6):337–345.

27. National Institute of Neurological Disorders and Stroke. NINDS Parkinson's Disease Information Page. NINDS/NIH Website. http://www.ninds.nih.gov/disorders/parkinsons_disease/parkinsons_disease.htm. Accessed October 14, 2014.

28. Parkinson's Disease Foundation. What is Parkinson's disease: statistics on Parkinson's. http://www.pdf.org/en/parkinson_statistics. Accessed October 14, 2014.

29. Friedlander AH, Mahler M, Norman KM, et al. Parkinson disease: systemic and orofacial manifestations, medical and dental management. *J Am Dent Assoc.* 2009;140(6):658–669.

30. Tolle L. Myasthenia gravis: a review for dental hygienists. *J Dent Hyg.* 2007;81(1):12.

31. Yarom N, Barnea E, Nissan J, et al. Dental management of patients with myasthenia gravis: a literature review. *Oral Surg Oral Med Oral Pathol Oral Radiol Endod.* 2005;100(2):158–163.

32. Howard JF, Jr. Myasthenia Gravis—a summary. Myasthenia Gravis Foundation of America, Inc. Website. http://www.myasthenia.org/HealthProfessionals/ClinicalOverviewofMG.aspx. Accessed October 14, 2014.

33. National Institute of Neurological Disorders and Stroke. Myasthenia Gravis fact sheet. NINDS/NIH Website. http://www.ninds.nih.gov/disorders/myasthenia_gravis/detail_myasthenia_gravis.htm#261083153. Accessed October 14, 2014.

34. Hetherington KA, Losek JD. Myasthenia gravis: myasthenia vs. cholinergic crisis. *Pediatr Emerg Care.* 2005;21(8):546–548; quiz 549–551.

35. National Institute of Neurological Disorders and Strokes. Post-Polio syndrome fact sheet. NINDS/NIH Website. http://www.ninds.nih.gov/disorders/post_polio/detail_post_polio.htm. Accessed October 14, 2014.

36. National Institute of Neurological Disorders and Stroke. Cerebral palsy: hope through research. NINDS/NIH Website. http://www.ninds.nih.gov/disorders/cerebral_palsy/detail_cerebral_palsy.htm. Accessed November 11, 2014.

37. National Institutes of Health, National Institute of Dental and Craniofacial Research. Practical oral care for people with Cerebral palsy. http://www.nidcr.nih.gov/oralhealth/Topics/DevelopmentalDisabilities/PracticalOralCarePeopleCerebralPalsy.htm. Accessed July 24, 2015.

38. Al-Allaq T, Debord TK, Liu H, et al. Oral health status of individuals with cerebral palsy at a nationally recognized rehabilitation center. *Spec Care Dentist.* 2015;35(1):15–21. doi:10.1111/scd.12071.

39. Dougherty NJ. A review of cerebral palsy for the oral health professional. *Dent Clin North Am.* 2009;53(2):329–338.

40. National Institute of Neurological Disorders and Stroke. NINDS muscular dystrophy information page. http://www.ninds.nih.gov/disorders/md/md.htm. Accessed November 11, 2014.

41. Centers for Disease Control and Prevention. Muscular dystrophy: data and statistics. http://www.cdc.gov/ncbddd/musculardystrophy/data.html. Accessed November 11, 2014.

42. U.S. National Library of Medicine, National Institutes of Health, Department of Health and Human Services: Genetics Home Reference Website. Facioscapulohumeral muscular dystrophy. http://ghr.nlm.nih.gov/condition/facioscapulohumeral-muscular-dystrophy. Accessed November 11, 2014.

43. Balasubramaniam R, Sollecito TP, Stoopler ET. Oral health considerations in muscular dystrophies. *Spec Care Dentist.* 2008;28(6):243–253.

44. National Institutes for Health, Eunice Kennedy Shriver National Institute of Child Health and Human Development. What are the treatments for muscular dystrophy? http://www.nichd.nih.gov/health/topics/musculardys/conditioninfo/pages/treatment.aspx. Accessed November 11, 2014.

45. Honein MA, Paulozzi LJ, Mathews TJ, et al. Impact of folic acid fortification of the US food supply on the occurrence of neural tube defects. *JAMA.* 2001;285(23):2981–2986.

46. Garg A, Utreja A, Singh SP, et al. Neural tube defects and their significance in clinical dentistry: a mini review. *J Investig Clin Dent.* 2013;4(1):3–8.

47. National Institute of Neurological Disorders and Stroke. Spina bifida fact sheet. NINDS/NIH Website. http://www.ninds.nih.gov/disorders/spina_bifida/detail_spina_bifida.htm#261973258. Accessed November 11, 2014.

48. U.S. National Library of Medicine, National Institutes of Health, MedlinePlus. Myelomeningocele. http://www.nlm.nih.gov/medlineplus/ency/article/001558.htm. Accessed November 11, 2014.

49. American Academy of Pediatric Dentistry, Clinical Affairs Committee. Guideline on antibiotic prophylaxis for dental patients at risk for infection. Reference Manual, Revised. 2014. http://www.aapd.org/media/Policies_Guidelines/G_AntibioticProphylaxis.pdf. Accessed November 11, 2014.

50. Centers for Disease Control and Prevention. Arthritis: rheumatoid arthritis. http://www.cdc.gov/arthritis/basics/rheumatoid.htm. Accessed November 11, 2010.

51. U.S. National Library of Medicine, PubMed Health. Arthritis. http://www.ncbi.nlm.nih.gov/pubmedhealth/PMH0002223/. Accessed November 11, 2014.

52. Kaur S, White S, Bartold PM. Periodontal disease and rheumatoid arthritis: a systematic review. *J Dent Res.* 2013;92(5):399–408.

53. Dissick A, Redman RS, Jones M, et al. Association of periodontitis with rheumatoid arthritis: a pilot study. *J Periodontol.* 2010;81(2):223–230.

54. U.S. National Library of Medicine, National Institutes of Health, MedlinePlus. Juvenile rheumatoid arthritis. http://www.nlm.nih.gov/medlineplus/juvenilerheumatoidarthritis.html. Accessed November 11, 2014.

55. Centers for Disease Control and Prevention. Osteoarthritis. http://www.cdc.gov/arthritis/basics/osteoarthritis.htm. Accessed November 11, 2014.

56. National Institutes of Health, National Institute of Arthritis and Musculoskeletal and Skin Diseases. Scleroderma. http://www.niams.nih.gov/Health_Info/Scleroderma/scleroderma_ff.asp. Accessed November 11, 2014.

57. Fischer DJ, Patton LL. Scleroderma: oral manifestations and treatment challenges. *Spec Care Dentist.* 2000;20(6):240–244.

58. Albilia JB, Lam DK, Blanas N, et al. Small mouths … big problems? A review of scleroderma and its oral health implications. *J Can Dent Assoc.* 2007;73(9):831–836.

59. Yuen HK, Wolf BJ, Bandyopadhyay D, et al. Factors that limit access to dental care for adults with spinal cord injury. *Spec Care Dentist.* 2010;30(4):151–156.

60. Sullivan AL. Perception of oral status as a barrier to oral care for people with spinal cord injuries. *J Dent Hyg.* 2012;86(2):111–119.

61. Greig V, Sweeney P. Special care dentistry for general dental practice. *Dent Update.* 2013;40(6):452–454, 456–458, 460.

62. American Academy on Pediatric Dentistry; and Council on Clinical Affairs. Guideline on management of dental patients with special health care needs. *Pediatr Dent.* 2008–2009;30(7, Suppl):107–111.

63. Yitzhak M, Sarnat H, Rakocz M, et al. The effect of toothbrush design on the ability of nurses to brush the teeth of institutionalized cerebral palsy patients. *Spec Care Dentist.* 2013;33(1):20–27.

ENHANCE YOUR UNDERSTANDING

the**Point**® **DIGITAL CONNECTIONS**
(see the inside front cover for access information)

- **Audio glossary**
- **Quiz bank**

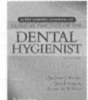

SUPPORT FOR LEARNING
(available separately; visit lww.com)

- *Active Learning Workbook for Clinical Practice of the Dental Hygienist, 12th Edition*

prepU **INDIVIDUALIZED REVIEW**
(available separately; visit lww.com)

- **Adaptive quizzing with *prepU for Wilkins' Clinical Practice of the Dental Hygienist***

60

The Patient with a Sensory Impairment

Robert D. Smethers, BASDH, RDH and Esther M. Wilkins, BS, RDH, DMD

CHAPTER OUTLINE

LEARNING OBJECTIVES

After studying this chapter, the student will be able to:

1. Describe the purpose of the Americans with Disabilities Act.

2. Explain the causes and types of visual and hearing impairment.

3. Identify different auxiliary aids that help the visually and hearing impairment.

4. Outline a plan for continuing care for the patient with visual or hearing impairment.

Successful management and treatment of patients depends largely on the interpersonal communication between the patient and the clinician.

▶ When a patient has either a vision or hearing impairment, communication assumes a different dimension.

▶ This chapter describes adaptations for patients with hearing or visual problems.

▶ Box 60-1 contains key words and definitions pertaining to sensory impairments.

AMERICANS WITH DISABILITIES ACT (ADA)

▶ *Purpose*

• The ADA is civil rights legislation enacted into law on July 26, 1990 to prohibit discrimination and ensure that people with disabilities have opportunities equal to everyone including employment opportunities, purchase of goods and services, and access to state and local government programs and services.[1]

▶ *Definition*

The ADA specifies that communications with individuals with hearing and vision impairments need to be as effective as communications with nonimpaired people, and appropriate auxiliary aids must be provided.

• Special skills used to counsel, motivate, and educate a patient with a sensory disability can be developed and practiced.

• Although visual modes of communication provide a primary method of communication with most individuals, audible and "touch" approaches are essential for the person with a visual impairment.

VISUAL IMPAIRMENT

▶ Limitations of sight cover a broad spectrum from the slightly affected to completely blind with no perception of light.

▶ Loss of sight is a major physical deprivation. In many persons, blindness is secondary to a primary condition that may have been the cause of the blindness and in itself may be disabling.

▶ "Legal blindness" is defined as having central vision (or acuity) of not more than 20/200 in the better eye with correction (glasses), or having peripheral fields (side vision) of no more than 20° diameter.[2]

▶ There are an estimated 285 million individuals who are visual impaired worldwide with 39 million blind and 246 million with low vision.[3]

▶ For the visually impaired, ADA requirements for facilities include things such as removal of physical barriers and the use of braille markers for elevators.

▶ Visually impaired individuals may use a cane to aid them while walking and for identification purposes.[4]

▶ Technology and assistive devices available for the visual impaired include:

• Computer screen readers that allow the individual to read the displayed data by a speech synthesizer.[2]

• Screen magnifiers are available to help the low-vision user by enlarging the text and graphics on the screen.[2]

• Wrist watches with braille and printers that print in braille.

I. Causes of Blindness

A. Age Related

▶ The leading causes of blindness are diabetic retinopathy, age-related macular degeneration, cataracts, glaucoma, trauma, and infections.[5]

▶ In individuals over the age of 60, the leading cause of blindness is macular degeneration. This disease affects the viewing of fine details, which interferes with reading, driving, and perform daily tasks.[5]

B. Children

▶ At least half of the blindness in children is of prenatal origin, resulting from maternal infections such as rubella, syphilis, toxoplasmosis.

▶ Other causes are injuries, neoplasms, and retinopathy of prematurity (formerly called retrolental fibroplasia).

▶ The incidence of retinopathy of prematurity has increased as more premature babies survive.

II. Personal Factors

▶ Consider each patient in relation to individual aptitudes, interests, abilities, and potentialities, with sight as one factor involved.

▶ The only common characteristic this group of patients has is visual impairment.

A. Patient History

▶ Assistance in completing the health history questionnaire may be needed.

▶ Specific details of the patient's limitations are recorded so that adaptations can be made during the current and future appointments.

B. Child

▶ *Learning ability*

• Sensory defects may mask a child's intellectual capacity because responses may differ from other children.[6]

• Blind children are deprived of the opportunity to learn by imitation.[6]

• Blind children may learn to speak later than sighted children and may start school later.

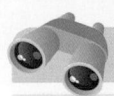 **BOX 60-1** | **KEY WORDS:** Sensory Disabilities

Vision

Astigmatism: impaired vision caused by irregularities in the curvature of the cornea or lens.

Audiotactile: use of touch and sound.

Blind spot: the area on the retina that marks the site of entrance of the optic nerve.

Blindness: no perception of visual stimuli; lack or loss of ability to see.

Legal blindness: less than 20/200 vision with corrective eyeglasses.

Braille: a system of writing and printing by means of raised points representing letters; enables people with a visual disability to read by touch.

Cataract: clouding or opacity of the lens of an eye.

Color blindness: inability to distinguish between certain colors; most common is red/green confusion; color vision is a function of the cones of the retina.

Computer screen reader: software programs that allow visually impaired individuals to read data displayed on a computer screen with a speech synthesizer.

Diplopia: double vision; perception of two images of a single object.

Glaucoma: group of diseases of the eye characterized by intraocular pressure from pathologic changes in the optic disc; person has visual-field defects.

Hyperopia: farsightedness; eyeball is shorter behind the retina; vision is better for distant objects than for near objects.

Myopia: nearsightedness; longer eyeball from front to back so the image is focused in front of the retina.

Nyctalopia: night blindness; may be hereditary or related to vitamin deficiency.

Ocular: pertaining to the eye.

Ophthalmologist: physician who specializes in diagnosing and prescribing treatment for defects, injuries, and diseases of the eye (obsolete term: oculist).

Ophthalmology: the branch of medicine that deals with the anatomy, diagnosis, pathology, and treatment of the eye.

Optician: technician who prepares and adapts lenses; fills prescriptions from an ophthalmologist.

Optometrist: a specialist in optometry, the measurement of visual acuity and the adaptation of lenses for correction of visual defects.

Retinitis: inflammation of the retina.

Retinopathy: noninflammatory disease of the retina; identified by the chronic disease of which it is a symptom; for example, diabetic retinopathy reflects the retinal manifestations of diabetes mellitus, including microaneurysms.

Retinopathy of prematurity: a condition peculiar to premature infants; characterized by opaque tissue behind the lens resulting from a high concentration of oxygen, which causes spasm of the retinal vessels, leads to retinal detachment, and arrests eye growth and development; prevented by keeping oxygen administration as low as possible and discontinuing the oxygen as soon as possible.

Tactile: sense by touch.

Visual impairment: an visual condition that impacts a person's abilities to succeed normal everyday activities during life.

Hearing

Audiogram: graphic record of the findings of an audiometer.

Audiologist: certified allied health worker, often with advanced degrees; trained in the identification, diagnosis, measurement, and rehabilitation of hearing impairment.

Audiometer: instrument used to determine degree and type of hearing ability.

Aural: pertaining to the ear.

Decibel: unit for expressing the relative loudness of a sound; abbreviation, dB.

Hearing: the sense by which sounds are perceived; conversion of sound waves into nerve impulses, which are then interpreted by the brain.

Hearing impairment: a full or partial reduction in the ability to understand or detect any sounds.

Otitis: inflammation of the ear.

Otitis media: inflammation of the middle ear.

Otologist: physician specialist in otology, the branch of medicine dealing with the anatomy, physiology, pathology, and treatment of the ear.

Speechreading: recognizing spoken words by watching the speaker's lips, face, and gestures.

Tinnitus: noise in the ears, as ringing, buzzing, or roaring.

TTY: Text telephone device.

Tuning fork: instrument used to test for hearing loss; vibrations of the fork produce sound waves that can be heard in both ears by a person with normal hearing when the stem is placed on top of the head; sound is heard louder in an ear affected by conductive loss and softer in an ear affected by sensorineural loss.

Tympanic membrane: ear drum; vibrates when sound waves strike; transmits waves to nerve endings by way of ossicles in the middle ear and to cochlea in the inner ear.

Vertigo: sensation of rotation or movement of one's self (subjective vertigo) or of one's surroundings (objective vertigo); a subtype of dizziness, but not a synonym.

- A blind child may take longer than does the sighted child to cover the same material; therefore, the educational level for the blind child may be different from that for the sighted child of the same chronologic age.

▶ *Personal factors*

- Environment influences the child's adjustment, and parental attitude affects the blind child as it does the sighted child.

- When the parent is overindulgent and protective, the child may be dependent, and emotionally less independent.

C. Adult

▶ A natural reaction for those who become blind in adulthood may be depression and feeling of helplessness.[7]

▶ Loss of vision may be gradual; the reactions of shock and upheaval usually are less with gradual loss of sight, but dread, worry, and anxiety may be experienced for years in anticipation.

▶ When the individual begins to accept the impairment, efforts for rehabilitation are made easier.

▶ Independence and self-confidence are needed to avoid feelings of helplessness.

III. Dental Hygiene Care: Totally Blind

A. Factors in Patient Care

▶ A person who is totally blind is more likely to accept a new experience if told about it in detail.

▶ Because of the visual impairment, the patient may tend to rely more on other senses such as touch and hearing.

▶ A totally blind person tries to be neat and orderly. One should avoid moving items belonging to a visually impaired person without alerting them.

▶ A totally blind person learns to interpret and rely on tone of voice more than do persons with sight who can watch facial expressions.

B. Patient Reception and Seating

▶ Lower the chair before seating the patient; move other dental equipment, such as the bracket tray and clinician's stool, from the path to the chair.

▶ Ask the older patient their preference for how to guide them to the dental chair. Many prefer to hold the clinicians arm and follow them (Figure 60-1).

▶ Provide forewarning of potential hazards in the way.

▶ The patient who has become familiar with the dental setting from previous appointments needs to be informed of changes to prevent embarrassment.

▶ *Protective eyewear*: The patient may prefer to wear the personal glasses regularly worn. Many wear dark glasses.

▶ When the dental hygienist leaves the treatment room during the appointment, explain absence to prevent embarrassment of the patient speaking to someone who is not there; speak when re-entering the room.

C. The Service or Guide Dog

▶ Do not distract a service or guide dog on duty by touching or speaking to it.[8]

▶ Do not walk on the dog's left side, which can distract the dog.

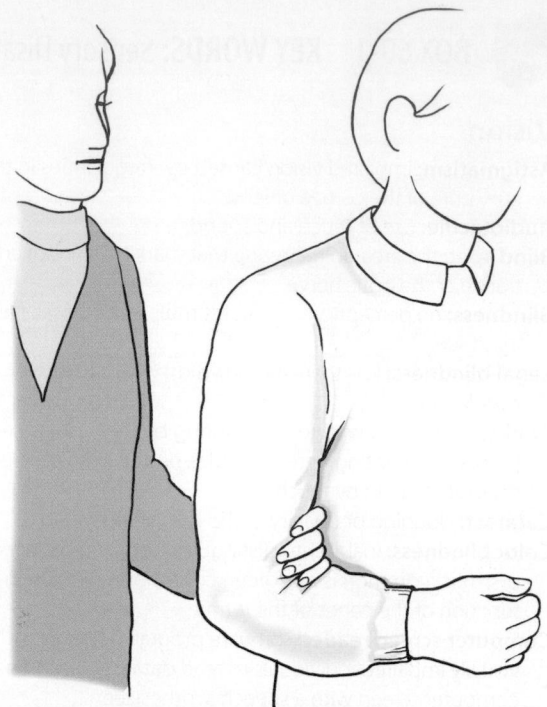

FIGURE 60-1 Escorting a Visually Impaired Individual. A visual impaired person holds the arm of the guide just above the elbow and walks beside and slightly behind. The guide verbally gives advance notice of approaching changes. The blind person can sense the body motion of the guide and anticipate changes.

▶ Do not lead or grab the patient while the dog is guiding.[8]

▶ Ask the patient where the best place would be for the dog to stay during the appointment.

- Service dogs are well-trained animals and usually lie quietly in a corner of the treatment room as directed by the patient.

D. Introduce Clinical Procedures

▶ *Child*

- Create a casual and relaxed environment.
- Introduce the child to the dental office by utilizing other senses.[9]
- Ask them permission prior to starting treatment.[9]
- Create unique ways to communicate during treatment explaining the procedure step-by-step, always face child when explaining the clinical procedures.[9]
- For a child patient who is not familiar with dental procedures, let them feel the mouth mirror.
- Allow child to hear the equipment, such as the saliva ejector, that will be used during the appointment.[10]
- Introduce unusual smells or taste utilized during the different treatment.[10]
- Apply rubber cup to child's finger so they can experience how polishing feels.

▶ *Additional instructions*

- Describe each step in detail before proceeding. Explain instruments, materials, and how each will be applied. Describe flavors.
- Permit patient to handle dull or blunted instruments if able to do so safely.
- Explain to patient the sound of the suction before turning it on for the procedure.
- Prepare patient for power-driven instruments; avoid surprise applications of compressed air, water from syringe, or power-driven instruments.
- Speak before touching the patient. By maintaining contact of a finger on a tooth or through retraction while changing instruments, repeated orientation can be avoided.

E. Instructions for Patient

▶ *Child*

- Demonstrate what will be done using the sense of touch (tactile method) to allow the patient to use other senses.
- Guide patient with hand-over-hand toothbrush technique to help with placement of the toothbrush in the mouth.[10]
- Novel music-aided toothbrushing instructions in a song format can be used to reinforce oral self-care instructions.[11]
- Audiotactile performance technique to utilize the sense of touch and hearing together helps to educate about oral self-care.[12]

▶ *Additional instructions*

- Give instructions clearly and concisely.
- Explain to the patient what biofilm feels like on the tooth surface.
- Allow the patient to feel the texture of the bristles on the toothbrush.
- Demonstrate toothbrushing in the patient's mouth and describe the feeling of the filament tips on and under the gingival margin and the feeling of clean teeth.
- Demonstrate dental flossing by explaining each step in detail.
  - Compare the length of floss needed by having the patient stretch the floss from the tip of the finger to the elbow.
  - Help the patient learn the correct technique to hold the floss by wrapping it around both of the patient's middle fingers.
  - Have the patient feel the floss placement underneath the gingival margin to the depth of the sulcus while wrapping around each tooth.
  - Explain the up and down motion and lateral pressure of the floss to remove the supragingival and subgingival biofilm.
  - Instruct the patient to unwrap the floss, from their fingers, when a clean thread of floss is needed.

IV. Dental Hygiene Care: Partially Sighted

Persons with sight often underestimate how useful a little vision can be. Patience is needed to help a patient make full use of available vision, without being oversolicitous. Although many of the procedures described for the totally blind person can be applied to the partially sighted person, a few additional hints are included in this section.

▶ Sight failure or lowered vision in a person of any age may be suspected from the patient's unusual squinting, blinking, or lack of continued attention.[13]

▶ Procedures can be adapted without mention of sight to the patient.

A. Patient Position

▶ Adjust for patient comfort.

B. Light

▶ Avoid directing the dental light in the patient's eyes.

▶ Sensitivity to light is characteristic of many eye conditions.[14]

C. Patient Instruction

▶ Position patient for best vision. For example, a patient with glaucoma has no peripheral vision; thus, instruction must be given directly from in front of the patient.[15]

▶ Do not expect a patient to see fine detail, such as that in a radiograph without enlargement.

▶ Work patiently and give instruction slowly. Patient may have slow visual accommodation.

- Respectfully, ask the patient to repeat their understanding of the instructions.

HEARING IMPAIRMENT

▶ When hearing is impaired to the extent that it has no practical value for the purpose of spoken communication, a person is considered *deaf*.[16]

▶ A person who cannot hear as well as someone with normal hearing is referred to have *hearing loss*.

- The hearing loss can be mild to severe or profound, and can be in one ear or both ears.
- It can lead to difficulty in hearing conversational speech and loud sounds.[16]

▶ Terminology is changing and reflects the ways in which people prefer to identify themselves.

▶ Assistive measures and devices for those with hearing impairment include: qualified interpreters, assistive listening headsets, text telephone devices for hearing impaired persons, readers, videotext displays, and closed caption.

I. Causes of Hearing Impairment

▶ The auditory system includes the anatomic parts from the outer ear to the termination of the auditory nerve in the brain.

▶ The cause of hearing loss may be associated with the outer, middle, or inner ear mechanisms, singly or in combinations. Many factors may contribute to deafness.
  • Congenital: Prenatal infection in the mother, especially rubella, and birth trauma are significant in the earliest years.[17]
  • Acquired: Chronic inner ear infections, infectious diseases (meningitis), trauma, and toxic effects of drugs have all been implicated.[17]

▶ *Newborn screening*: The spread of universal programs to identify hearing defects in newborns has been a significant contribution to healthcare.[18]

II. Types of Hearing Loss

A. Conductive Hearing Loss

Outer or middle ear involvement of the conduction pathways to the inner ear.[17]

B. Sensorineural Hearing Loss

Damage to the sensory hair cells of the inner ear or the nerves that supply the inner ear.[17]

C. Mixed Hearing Loss

Combination of conductive and sensorineural.[17]

D. Central Hearing Loss

Damage of the nerves or nuclei of the central nervous system in the brain or the pathways to the brain.[17]

III. Characteristics Suggesting Hearing Loss

▶ Partial deafness may not have been diagnosed, or certain patients, particularly elderly ones, may not admit hearing limitation. Clues to the identification of a hearing problem are suggested as follows:
  • Lack of attention; fails to respond to conversation.
  • Intentness; strained facial expression; stares at others.
  • Turns head to one side; hearing may be good on one side only.
  • Gives unexpected answer unrelated to question; does one thing when told to do another.
  • Frequently asks others to repeat what was said.
  • Unusual speech quality.

IV. Hearing Aids

▶ A hearing aid is an electronic device worn in or behind the ear and is used for people who have sensory cell damage in the inner ear.

• It amplifies and shapes sound waves that enter the external auditory canal.
• The hair cells detect the vibrations and convert them into neural signals that transfer to the brain.[19]

▶ Current hearing aids are more technically advanced and tend to be smaller and less visible.

▶ Standards for the manufacture and distribution of hearing aids are set by the United States Food and Drug Administration. A medical evaluation is required along with extensive audiological testing.

A. In-the-Ear Model

The units are practically invisible and lightweight. Used for mild-to-severe hearing loss.[19]

B. Behind-the-Ear Model

▶ This unit is an open-fit hearing aid that is small, fits behind the ear, and has a narrow tube that is inserted into the ear canal.

▶ This type of hearing aid might be a better choice for individuals who experience earwax buildup.[19]

▶ The person's perception of their voice does not sound "plugged up," referring to blockage from the earwax buildup.[19]

C. Canal Aid

This model fits entirely within the canal and is the most cosmetically acceptable of all types. It may take extra skill to remove and adjust.[19]

V. Cochlear Implants

▶ A small electronic device that helps provide a sense of sound to a child or an adult who is profoundly deaf or severely hard of hearing.[20]

▶ The implant consists of an external portion behind the ear and a second part surgically placed under the skin.[20]

▶ An implant does not restore normal hearing. It gives useful representations of sounds from the environment through a microphone and speech processor and sends them directly to the auditory nerve of the brain.[20]

VI. Modes of Communication

▶ A person with a hearing loss may learn a particular way of personal communication.
  • Choices include speaking, speechreading, writing, manual, or a combination.
  • Manual communication includes using sign language or "signing" and fingerspelling.

▶ *Always ask the patient which means of communication is preferred and how communication can be improved.*

A. American Sign Language (ASL)

The American manual alphabet is shown in Figure 60-2.[21] A few examples of signs are shown in Figure 60-3.[21]

▶ ASL is a visual/gestural language with a unique grammar and syntax.

▶ Many deaf people who prefer this mode of communication grew up using ASL and consider themselves part of a cultural group.

▶ Other individuals who have become deaf in later years may learn sign language and use the signs in English word order, meaning the subject comes before the verb and the verb comes before the object in a sentence structure.

▶ Some deaf people prefer to communicate using ASL in medical or dental situations. They can request the services of an ASL interpreter.

▶ Although a universal sign language has not been recognized, many countries have their own.

B. Fingerspelling

▶ Spelling "in the air" is often combined with sign language.

▶ When making an introduction, for example, the name may be fingerspelled.

▶ New words often do not have signs and are fingerspelled.

C. Oral Communication

Oral communication by a deaf person means a combination of some speech, residual hearing, and speechreading.

D. Speechreading

▶ Speechreading consists of recognizing spoken words by watching the lips, face, and gestures.

▶ Many of the mouth movements for spoken words have the same appearance as one or more other words, so speechreading may need to be combined with another method of communication.

▶ Speechreading is not a reliable means of communication for extended, complex discussions for most people with hearing loss.

▶ Speechreading is not a choice when clinician must wear a mask.

E. Writing

Writing may be an alternative when other methods are not satisfactory. Ensure to have a big writing pad available with pencils for communication purposes.

VII. Dental Hygiene Care

▶ Patients with hearing problems are of all ages; some have been deaf all their lives, and others lost their hearing later in life. Each has special challenges.

▶ Determination of the mode of communication is a critical first step. Always ask the patient. An interpreter may be required.

▶ When the patient's preferred mode of communication is sign language and the clinician does not know sign language, or when the patient lip-reads but cannot read the clinician's lips because the clinician is wearing a mask, writing on a pad of paper may be the first choice.

▶ Some deaf individuals may not be fluent in the English language and will need the services of an interpreter for extensive communication such as review of an involved medical history or treatment plan.

A. Patient with Hearing Aid

▶ Be careful not to touch a hearing aid when it is turned on.

▶ Adjust patient's head so ears are not compressed against the headrest or pillow, which can cause discomfort.

B. Patient with Partial Hearing Ability

▶ Speak clearly and distinctly.

▶ When it is necessary to talk, be sure to face the patient.
  • With the dental light is directed toward the patient's mouth, the clinician's face may be too difficult to see.

▶ Eliminate interfering noises from the street outside or from saliva ejector suction.

C. Speechreader

▶ Be sure patient is looking at your mouth; do not turn to the side; speak directly facing the patient.

▶ The speaker's face must be clearly visible so patient can read lips easily and the clinician needs to remove the mask when delivering information about treatment or education.

▶ Speak in a normal tone; do not exaggerate words; slow the pace of speech; pause more frequently than usual.

▶ Do not raise voice; raising the voice can distort lip movements and make lip reading more difficult.

▶ When the patient cannot understand, use alternate words to express the same thought; many letters and combinations of letters look the same on the lips; others are not visible at all.

▶ Keep calm; display of irritation or annoyance over difficulties in conversing can discourage or upset the patient.

▶ Write proper names or unusual words the patient fails to understand.

▶ When wearing a mask, certain gestures may be agreed upon in advance.

D. Sign Language

▶ All the points previously mentioned for the speechreader apply to the patient who uses sign language because lips are read along with signs.

▶ When a dental hygienist knows a few signs, a deaf patient will greatly appreciate them.

▶ Learning basic sign language and fingerspelling can provide healthcare workers with added skills and reduce stress for the deaf patient.

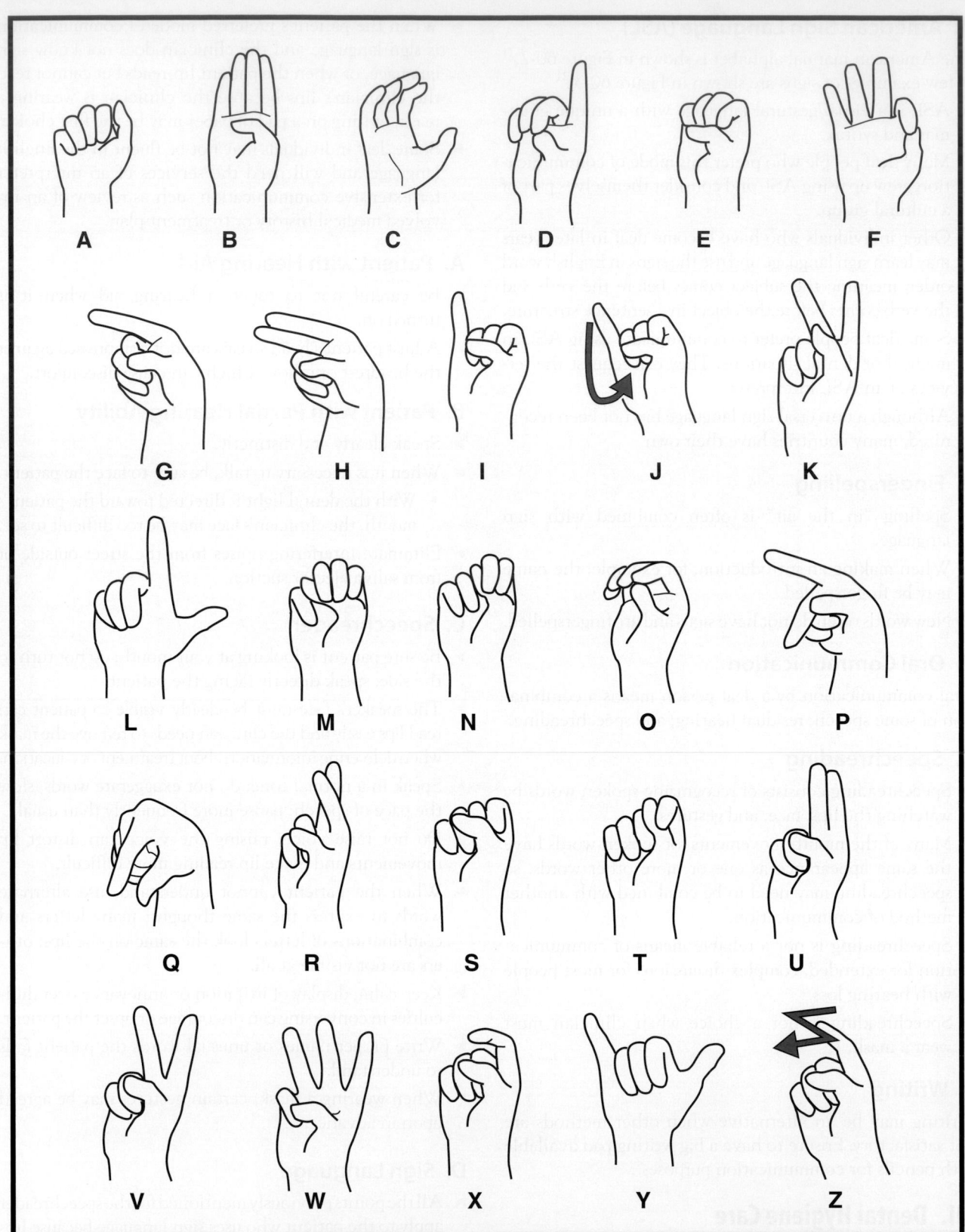

FIGURE 60-2 American Manual Alphabet. Fingerspelling is used in combination with signs and speechreading. (Reprinted with permission from Lane LG. *The Gallaudet Survival Guide to Signing.* Washington, DC: Gallaudet College for the Blind and Deaf and the University Press; 1990.)

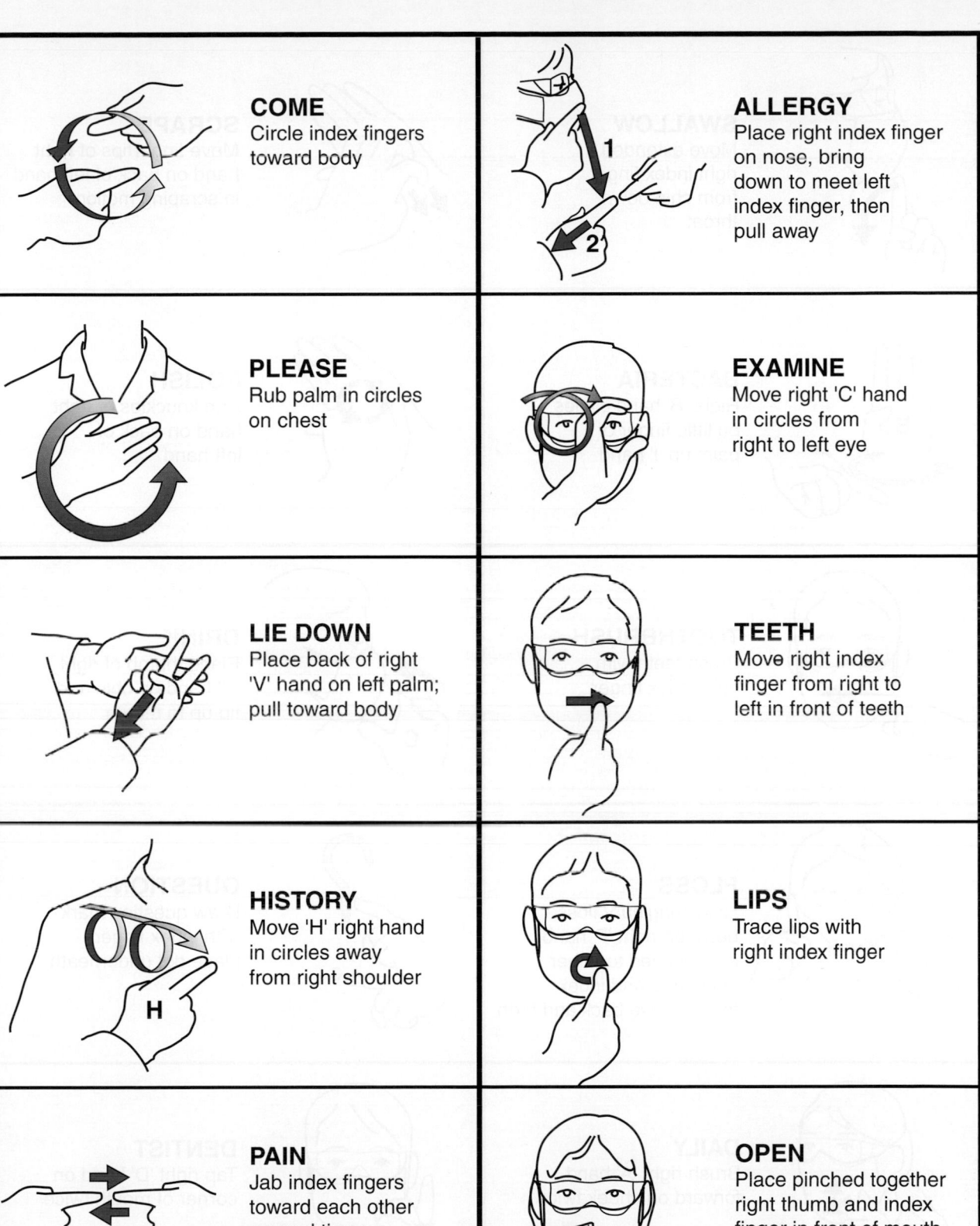

COME
Circle index fingers toward body

ALLERGY
Place right index finger on nose, bring down to meet left index finger, then pull away

PLEASE
Rub palm in circles on chest

EXAMINE
Move right 'C' hand in circles from right to left eye

LIE DOWN
Place back of right 'V' hand on left palm; pull toward body

TEETH
Move right index finger from right to left in front of teeth

HISTORY
Move 'H' right hand in circles away from right shoulder

LIPS
Trace lips with right index finger

PAIN
Jab index fingers toward each other several times

OPEN
Place pinched together right thumb and index finger in front of mouth, then separate

FIGURE 60-3 Examples of Signing. Selected words that may be used during a patient's dental appointment. (Adapted with permission from Lane LG. *The Gallaudet Survival Guide to Signing.* Washington, DC: Gallaudet College for the Blind and Deaf and the University Press; 1990.) (*continued*)

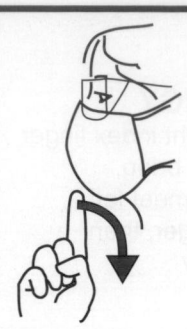

SWALLOW
Move extended right index finger from chin down throat

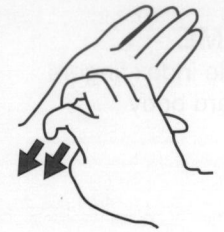

SCRAPE
Move fingertips of right hand on back of left hand in scraping motion

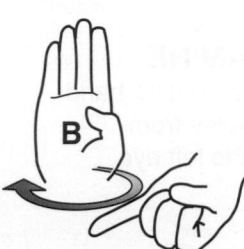

BACTERIA
Right 'B' hand circles on little finger of palm up 'I' hand

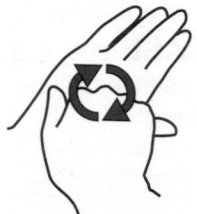

POLISH
Rub knuckles of right hand on back of left hand

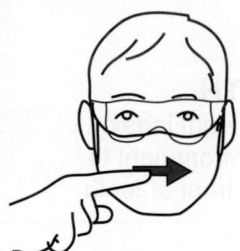

TOOTHBRUSH
Brush teeth with right index finger

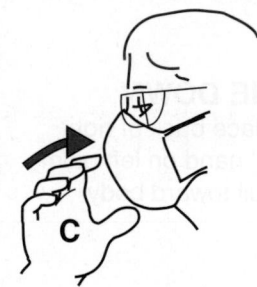

DRINK
Place thumb of right 'C' hand on chin and tip up to mouth

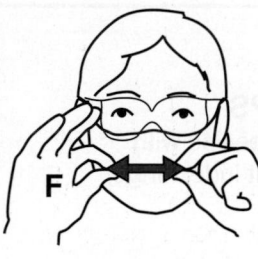

FLOSS
Hold imaginary floss between right 'F' hand and pinched together left thumb and index finger; move back and forth

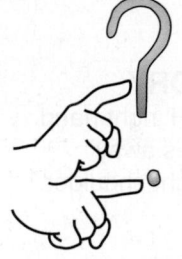

QUESTION
Draw question mark with index finger; place dot underneath

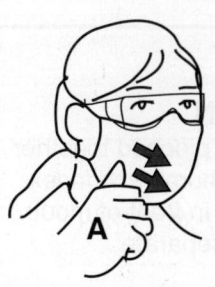

DAILY
Brush right 'A' hand forward on cheek twice

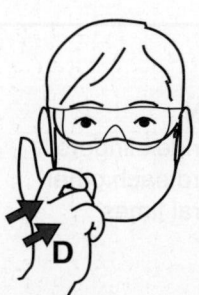

DENTIST
Tap right 'D' hand on corner of mouth twice

FIGURE 60-3 (*continued*)

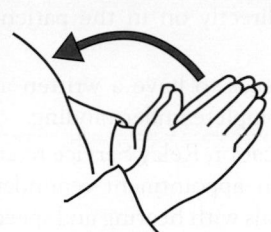

ASK
Place hands together
and arc toward body

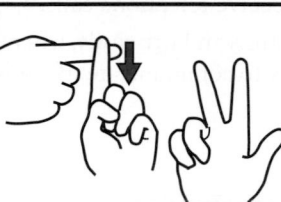

3 MONTHS
Slide back of right index
finger down back of left
index finger; then give
sign for number of months

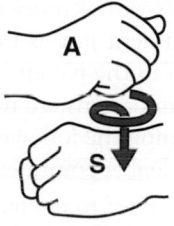

APPOINTMENT
Make circle with right
'A' hand then place on
left 'S' hand

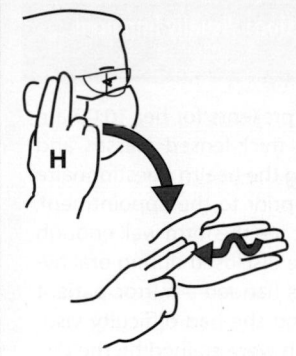

SECRETARY
Take imaginary pencil
from over ear with
'H' hand and write
across left palm

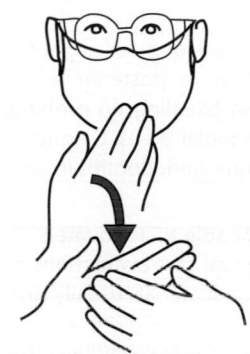

**GOOD
(PATIENT)**
Place right hand on chin
then drop to open
palm of left hand

FIGURE 60-3 (continued)

EVERYDAY ETHICS

Mr. Smith has been a patient with the practice for 5 years. Jane is a newly hired hygienist and just graduated from dental hygiene school. Mr. Smith always wants to get his cleaning completed fast so he can get out the door. Today, he was 15 minutes late, but Jane was patiently waiting for him at the door as he walked in. She noticed that Mr. Smith did not seem to respond to the questions she asked him and began to suspect he might not hear well. Even though she was not able to get a complete medical history update, she proceeded with the assessment. After completing the periodontal examination, she discovered that Mr. Smith has generalized moderate chronic periodontal disease and needs nonsurgical periodontal treatment. When Jane explained the condition to Mr. Smith, she again noticed that Mr. Smith did not seem to respond to the questions she asked him. She held out the signature pad so the patient could sign the treatment consent electronically. He signed, but Jane was not sure he understood what was proposed.

Questions for Consideration

1. Professionally and ethically, how would you describe the provider–dentist relationship in this scenario? Which of the dental hygiene core values (Table II-1, in Section II, Introduction) are illustrated here?

2. What ethical issues does Jane need to address? Did Jane handle the treatment consent appropriately Explain your rationale.

3. How can virtue ethics apply to a patient with special needs such as a hearing impairment or other loss of sensory functions? Go to Appendix II in the textbook (The Canadian Dental Hygienists' Code of Ethics) to read about "virtue ethics."

BOX 60-2

Example Documentation: Visually Impaired Patient

S–A new patient to the practice presents for her 10:00 am dental appointment wearing thick-lensed glasses and walking with a cane. Regarding the health questionnaire that had been mailed to her prior to the appointment, the patient stated, "I could not see the form well enough to fill it out." When teeth were disclosed during oral hygiene instruction and she was handed a mirror, patient said everything looked red and she had difficulty visualizing exactly where the teeth were stained by the disclosing solution and definitely could not see where the gingiva was red and inflamed.

O–Biofilm score: 90%. Gingiva revealed localized slight-to-moderate marginal inflammation in posterior areas. Pockets depths of 4–5 mm with bleeding on probing, subgingival calculus present in molar areas. Diagnosis: Localized early to moderate chronic periodontitis in posterior quadrants.

A–Patient has low vision and is not able to adequately visualize disclosed plaque during oral care instructions or read forms and patient education materials usually provided for patients.

P–Health history questionnaire completed verbally with the patient. Tooth brushing and flossing were reviewed using hand-over-hand demonstration and then practice by the patient. Techniques were discussed to help her adapt her self-care routine so she didn't have to rely on using a mirror to determine complete biofilm removal (the feel of correct placement of the toothbrush bristles, feel of biofilm-free, smooth tooth surfaces using her tongue). Gave patient an oral care handout that had been enlarged on the office copy machine.

Next appointment—Enlarge radiographs on the computer for patient's review.

Disclose to assess the patient's ability for biofilm removal and review oral self-care instructions as necessary. Initiate periodontal maintenance on maxillary and mandibular left quadrants with local anesthesia as needed.

Signed _____, RDH

Date: _____

E. General Suggestions

▶ For written messages, use a clipboard with a marker-type pen attached and large paper, at least 8½ × 11 inches. Write clearly.

▶ Ask the patient their preference for an appropriate signal to get their attention during the procedure.

▶ Plan in advance for a signal the patient can give to show reaction or discomfort.

▶ Teach by demonstration; use mirror and show dental biofilm removal methods directly on in the patient's mouth.

▶ Person with hearing loss needs to have a written appointment card to ensure complete understanding.

▶ Use the state Telecommunication Relay Service to call a deaf patient directly with appointment reminders. This service allows individuals with hearing and speech impairments to place and receive telephone calls.[22]

▶ Certain patients are under stress and tire easily, whereas others enjoy the opportunity to communicate. Be sensitive to the patient's needs.

DOCUMENTATION

The permanent records for patients with sensory disabilities are completed at each appointment just as the clinician does for all patients. Changes in the patient's health history, medications, and oral examinations are recorded. In addition, progress notes concerning the following need to be emphasized with each individual appointment:

▶ Special needs and adjustments related to the individual physical problems and how the disability affects attaining optimum oral health.

▶ Frequency of appointments to allow for extra assistance if necessary.

▶ Example documentation may be read in Box 60-2.

Factors To Teach The Patient

▷ Why accurate information is necessary when the medical history is reviewed.

▷ Instruction to use interproximal aids properly to avoid tissue trauma.

▷ If plaque biofilm removal is impaired, educate the patient in approaches to prevent dental caries, especially for children and teenagers with limited sight.

References

1. United States Department of Justice Civil Rights Division. Information and technical assistance on the Americans with disabilities act. http://www.ada.gov/ada_intro.htm. Updated 2011. Accessed May 25, 2014.

2. American Foundation for the Blind. Key definitions of statistical terms—visual terms. http://www.afb.org/info/blindness-statistics/key-definitions-of-statistical-terms/25. Updated 2008. Accessed May 25, 2014.

3. World Health Organization. Visual impairment and blindness. http://www.who.int/mediacentre/factsheets/fs282/en/. Updated 2013. Accessed June 19, 2014.

4. Department of Justice. Department of Justice ADA title III regulation: auxillary aids and services. http://www.ada.gov/reg3a.html#Anchor-97857. Updated 2010. Accessed May 30, 2014.

5. National Institute of Health. Leading causes of blindness. *NIH Medline Plus*. 2008;3(3):14–15.

6. Strickling C. Impact on visual impairment on development. http://www.tsbvi.edu/infants/3293-the-impact-of-visual-impairment-on-develop. Updated 2010. Accessed June 30, 2014.

7. Reinhardt J, Horowitz A, Sussman-Skalka CJ. Depression, visual loss and visual rehabilitation. http://www.lighthouse.org/services-and-assistance/social-services/depression-vision-loss-and-vision-rehabilitation/. Updated 2014. Accessed June 30, 2014.

8. Guide Dog Foundation. Etiquette and guide dogs. http://www.guidedog.org/Content.aspx?id=1416. Updated 2014. Accessed July 1, 2014.

9. The Association of State and Territorial Dental Directors; and The Oklahoma Association of Community Action Agencies. Oral health care for children with special health care needs: a guide for family members/caregivers and dental providers. http://www.okacaa.org/8.5%20x%2011%20Oral%20Health%20Care%20for%20Children%20with%20Special%20Health%20Care%20Needs.pdf. Updated 2008. Accessed August 28, 2014.

10. Brown D. An observation study of oral hygiene care for visually impaired children. http://dspace.gla.ac.uk:8080/bitstream/1905/775/3/. Updated 2008. Accessed August 28, 2014.

11. Shetty V, Hegde AM, Varghese E, et al. A novel music based tooth brushing system for blind children. *J Clin Pediatr Dent*. 2013;37(3):251–255.

12. Hebbal M, Ankola AV. Development of a new technique (ATP) for training visually impaired children in oral hygiene maintenance. *Eur Arch Paediatr Dent*. 2012;13(5):244–247.

13. Braille Institute of America. Facts about sight loss: symptoms and leading eye diseases. http://www.brailleinstitute.org/sight-loss-blog/395-facts-about-sight-loss-symptoms-leading-eye-diseases.html. Updated 2014. Accessed July 1, 2014.

14. American Foundation for the Blind. Glossary of eye conditions. http://www.afb.org/info/living-with-vision-loss/eye-conditions/12. Updated 2014. Accessed July 14, 2014.

15. Glaucoma Research Foundation. Symptoms of open-angle glaucoma. http://glaucoma.org/glaucoma/symptoms-of-primary-open-angle-glaucoma.php. Updated 2014. Accessed July 14, 2014.

16. World Health Organization. Deafness and hearing loss. http://www.who.int/mediacentre/factsheets/fs300/en/. Updated 2014. Accessed July 20, 2014.

17. National Dissemination Center for Children with Disabilities. Deafness and hearing loss. http://nichcy.org/disability/specific/hearingloss. Updated 2013. Accessed July 27, 2013.

18. Morton CC, Nance WE. Newborn hearing screening—a silent revolution. *N Engl J Med*. 2006;354(20):2151–2164.

19. National Institute on Deafness and Other Communication Disorders. Hearing aids. http://www.nidcd.nih.gov/health/hearing/pages/hearingaid.aspx. Updated 2013. Accessed July 15, 2014.

20. National Institute on Deafness and Other Communication Disorders. Cochlear implants. http://www.nidcd.nih.gov/health/hearing/pages/coch.aspx. Updated 2013. Accessed July 17, 2014.

21. Lane LG. *The Gallaudet Survival Guide to Signing*. 2nd ed. Washington, DC: Gallaudet University Press; 1990:218.

22. Federal Communications Commission. Telecommunications Relay Service (TRS). http://www.fcc.gov/guides/telecommunications-relay-service-trs. Updated 2014. Accessed July 29, 2014.

ENHANCE YOUR UNDERSTANDING

thePoint® DIGITAL CONNECTIONS
(see the inside front cover for access information)
- **Audio glossary**
- **Quiz bank**

SUPPORT FOR LEARNING
(available separately; visit lww.com)
- *Active Learning Workbook for Clinical Practice of the Dental Hygienist, 12th Edition*

prepU INDIVIDUALIZED REVIEW
(available separately; visit lww.com)
- **Adaptive quizzing with *prepU for Wilkins' Clinical Practice of the Dental Hygienist***

61

The Patient with a Neurodevelopmental Disorder

Charlotte J. Wyche, RDH, MS and Karen A. Raposa, RDH, MBA

CHAPTER OUTLINE

INTELLECTUAL DISORDERS
  I. Definition
  II. Dimensions of Intellectual Disorders
  III. Supportive Interventions
  IV. Classification of Intellectual Disorders
  V. Etiology
  VI. General Characteristics
  VII. Factors Significant for Dental Hygiene Care

DOWN SYNDROME
  I. Physical Characteristics
  II. Personal Characteristics

  III. Comorbidity and Health Considerations
  IV. Oral Findings

AUTISM SPECTRUM DISORDER (ASD)
  I. Characteristics
  II. Prevalence
  III. Etiology
  IV. Treatment Interventions
  V. Factors Significant for Dental Hygiene Care
  VI. D-Termined Program

DENTAL HYGIENE CARE
  I. Oral Health Problems
  II. Dental Staff Preparation

  III. Dental Hygiene Care Plan
  IV. Appointment Considerations
  V. Behavior Supports and Guidance

DOCUMENTATION
EVERYDAY ETHICS
FACTORS TO TEACH THE PATIENT
FACTORS TO TEACH THE CAREGIVER
REFERENCES

LEARNING OBJECTIVES

After studying this chapter, the student will be able to:

1. Define and describe neurodevelopmental disorders.

2. Give examples of the characteristics, oral findings, and health problems significant for providing dental hygiene care for patients with:

   • Intellectual disorder (ID)
   • Down syndrome
   • Autism spectrum disorder.

3. Recognize adaptations necessary for providing dental hygiene care for a patient with a neurodevelopmental disorder.

Neurodevelopmental disorders are a diverse group of chronic and potentially severe conditions that:

▶ Typically manifest in the early developmental period

▶ Usually last throughout a person's lifetime

▶ Lead to intellectual, social, and/or physical impairments

▶ Create problems with major life activities such as language, mobility, learning, self-help, and independent living.

Many people with neurodevelopmental disabilities seek dental care in private and community settings, where opportunities are available to contribute to the health and well-being of these individuals. Down syndrome and autism spectrum disorder (ASD) are two major categories of patients with neurodevelopmental disabilities that dental professionals encounter in standard dental settings. Box 61-1 provides descriptive terminology and other key words associated with IDs, and Box 61-2 lists the major diagnostic categories of neurodevelopmental disorders.

INTELLECTUAL DISORDERS

I. Definition[1]

Intellectual Disorders (IDs) are characterized by:

▶ Limitations in intellectual functioning.

▶ Limitations in adaptive functioning as expressed through conceptual, social, and practical skills.

▶ Origination and onset of symptoms during the developmental period, usually before the age of 18 years.

▶ Functional disability related to ID represents a more or less important symptom in well over 200 different conditions.

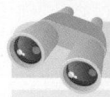

BOX 61-1   KEY WORDS: Intellectual Disorders

Adaptive behavior: conceptual, social, and practical skills learned by individuals to support the ability to function in everyday life.

Autism spectrum disorder: a developmental disorder, generally evident before age 3, affecting verbal and nonverbal communications and social interaction.

Brachycephalic: having a short, wide head.

Comorbid: existing simultaneously with and usually independently of another medical condition; coexisting or additional disease processes. Comorbidity may affect ability to function or survive.

Coprolalia: involuntary utterance of vulgar or obscene words.

Developmental disability: physical, behavioral, and/or ID that first manifests symptoms during developmental period (before age 21) and leads to intellectual, social, and/or physical impairment in everyday life activities.

Dysgenesis: defective development; malformation.

Dysmorphism: abnormality in morphologic development.

Echolalia: echo reaction; the involuntary repetition of a word or sentence just spoken by another person.

Epicanthus: a vertical fold of skin on either side of the nose, sometimes covering the inner canthus; a normal characteristic in persons of certain races.

Hyperactivity: abnormally increased activity.

Development hyperactivity (hyperkinesis): characterized by constant motion, fidgetiness, excitability, impulsiveness, and a short attention span.

Intelligence quotient (IQ): a score derived from one of several standardized tests used to assess intellectual ability.

Intellectual functioning: a broad term that takes adaptive behavior, mental health, opportunities to participate in life activities, and the context in which a life is lived into consideration.

Macroglossia: very large tongue.

Microcephalus: abnormally small head size in relation to the rest of the body.

Mutism: inability or refusal to speak; deafness may prevent learning to speak.

Selective mutism: consistent failure to speak in specific social situations despite speaking in other situations.

Pathognomonic: characteristic or indicative of a particular disease or syndrome; especially one or more typical symptoms.

Pervasive: throughout entire individual, entire development is severely and markedly impaired, as in ASD.

Pica: persistent craving/eating of nonnutritive substances or unnatural articles of food.

Rumination: repeated regurgitation of food in the absence of any associated gastrointestinal illness.

Self-injury: act of deliberate harm to one's own body. Also called self-abuse, self-directed aggression, self-harm, self-inflicted injury, self-mutilation.

Stereotypic movement disorder: repetitive, nonfunctional motor behavior that interferes with normal activities and may result in bodily injury.

Tic: an involuntary, sudden, rapid, recurrent, nonrhythmic, stereotyped motor movement or vocal sound.

Ultrasonography: the location, measurement, or delineation of deep structures by measuring the reflection or transmission of ultrasonic waves. Used in examination of fetus to determine birth defects.

An Overview of Neurodevelopmental Disorders[1]

Intellectual Developmental Disorders (ID) deficits in intellectual and adaptive functioning

▷ **Global developmental delay**: diagnosis used for individuals under 5 when assessment of reasons for not meeting developmental milestones is difficult.

▷ **Unspecified intellectual disability**: used in exceptional circumstances for individuals over 5 years old when diagnosis is impossible because of associated sensory deficits, physical impairments, severe behavioral problems, or mental disorders.

Communication Disorders

▷ **Language disorder:** Difficulty in acquisition and use of language, functional limitations in effective communication.

▷ **Speech sound disorder:** Persistent difficulty with sound production and speech intelligibility.

▷ **Childhood-onset fluency disorder (stuttering):** Disturbances in fluency, timing, and repetition patterns of speech.

Social (pragmatic) communication disorder: Difficulty using verbal and nonverbal communication in a manner that is appropriate for social context.

Autism spectrum disorder (ASD): Severity of the condition is based on the level of social communication impairment and restrictive, repetitive behavior patterns.

Attention-deficit/hyperactivity disorder (ADHD): Persistent inattention, hyperactivity, and impulsivity.

Specific learning disorder: Impairments in one or more academic domains (reading, writing, or mathematics).

Developmental coordination disorder: Characterized by clumsiness, slowness, and inaccuracy of expected performance level of motor skills.

Stereotypic movement disorder: Characterized by repetitive purposeless movements, with or without self-injurious behaviors.

Tic disorders: Characterized by sudden rapid motor movement or vocalizations.

▷ Tourette's disorder: Both motor and vocal tics.

▷ Persistent (chronic) motor or vocal tic disorder: Either motor or vocal tics, but not both that have persisted for more than 1 year.

▷ Provisional tic disorder: Motor and/or vocal tics present for less than 1 year since first onset.

II. Dimensions of ID

Five interrelated dimensions contribute to an individual's functioning ability as follows:[2]

▶ *Intellectual capability*:
  • Includes reasoning, planning, solving problems, thinking abstractly, comprehending complex ideas, learning quickly, and learning from experience.
  • Is represented by IQ scores.

▶ *Adaptive behavior*: a collection of skills in three domains learned and applied in order to function in everyday life.

• Conceptual skills (language, reading, self-direction).
• Social skills (responsibility, self-esteem, law abiding).
• Practical skills (daily living activities, occupational skills).

▶ Participation, interactions, and social roles
  • Participation (interaction with others in a social setting).
  • Social roles (age-specific activity).

▶ Health (physical health, mental health, etiology)
  • Physical and mental health and especially medications have definite influence on the assessment of intelligence and adaptive behavior.

▶ Context (environment, culture)
  • *Environmental*: residence and surroundings that provide for learning and development.
  • Fostering personal well-being, safety, in relation to all of the first four dimensions.

III. Supportive Interventions

▶ Supportive interventions are strategies and resources selected after assessment of individual level of ability and can help to improve the functioning of the individual with an intellectual disability.

▶ Purposes
  • To promote development, education, interests, and personal well-being
  • To improve individual functioning and functional capabilities.
  • To lessen the person's disorder by providing services and interventions that focus on prevention.
  • To enhance personal outcomes related to independence, community participation, and personal well-being.

▶ Types of supportive interventions
  • Supported learning and education.
  • Supported living.
  • Supported health services.
  • Supported employment.

▶ Application of supportive interventions
  • Needs of the individual determine necessary support.
  • Health deficiencies can influence improvements expected from other supports.

▶ Dental hygiene care provides support for the patient's:
  • Freedom from oral discomfort and pain.
  • Learning self-care for daily oral biofilm removal.
  • Improved quality of life.

IV. Classification of Intellectual Disorders

▶ The levels of intellectual functioning are designated as *mild*, *moderate*, *severe*, and *profound*.[1]

▶ Standardized intelligence tests are used to determine individual levels.

▶ The intelligence quotient (IQ) expresses the test results.

▶ A diagnostic category of "*unspecified*" is used when standard tests cannot be performed because of lack of cooperation, severe impairment, or infancy.

A. Mild

▶ IQ approximate range 50–69 (adult mental age from 9 to under 12 years).

▶ Adaptive behavior: child
   • In special classes for the educable, child advances to a level of third to sixth grade.
   • Practical skills can be learned.

▶ Adaptive behavior: adult
   • Individual cares for own personal hygiene and other necessities, with support.
   • Communication is good; attention span and memory are less than average.
   • Activities that do not require complicated planning or rapid implementation can be carried out satisfactorily.
   • Most individuals can engage in semi-skilled or simple skilled work with guidance, and so maintain themselves.

B. Moderate

▶ IQ approximate range 35–49 (adult mental age from 6 to under 9 years).

▶ Adaptive behavior: child
   • A marked developmental lag occurs in the early years; child can be trained in personal care and hygiene with support.
   • Attends classes and learns simple habits and skills; may not learn to read and write.
   • Speaks in short sentences; understands best when single-thought, short sentences are used.
   • Participates well in group activities.

▶ Adaptive behavior: adult
   • Attends to personal care, with support.
   • Has relatively short attention span and memory.
   • May have problems of coordination, but performs simple tasks and is conscientious about taking responsibility for errands and helpful duties.
   • Not completely capable of self-maintenance; many do unskilled work with supervision and support.

C. Severe

▶ IQ approximate range 20–34 (adult mental age from 3 to under 6 years).

▶ Adaptive behavior: child
   • Benefits from systematic habit training.
   • May make attempts at personal care and dressing with support.
   • Usually walks, uses some speech, and responds to directions.

▶ Adaptive behavior: adult
   • Conforms to daily routine.

• May help with household and other small tasks in spite of limited attention span.
• Likely to need continuous support.

D. Profound

▶ IQ under 20 (adult mental age below 3 years).

▶ Adaptive behavior: child
   • Delays occur in all phases of development.
   • Close supervision and care are necessary.

▶ Adaptive behavior: adult
   • Many remain inert and placid throughout early years; never learn to sit up.
   • Results in severe limitation in self-care, continence, communication, and mobility.

V. Etiology

Anything that interferes with normal brain development can result in intellectual disability. Examples include:[1]

▶ Genetic conditions such as Down syndrome or fragile X syndrome.

▶ Alcohol, drug use, or malnutrition during pregnancy.

▶ Pregnancy complications such as pre-eclampsia, premature birth, or depravation of oxygen during childbirth.

▶ Childhood illness such as meningitis, whooping cough, or measles.

▶ Childhood injury such as severe head injury, near drowning.

▶ Exposure to toxic substances such as lead.

▶ Nutritional or social deprivation.

▶ Diagnosis can be complicated; many cases can only be identified as of unknown origin.

A. Importance of Etiology

Understanding the cause of ID for each individual can:

▶ Provide information for future functional support needs.

▶ Facilitate genetic counseling and family planning.

▶ Assist the individual for life planning.

B. Risk Factors

▶ Risk factors for ID may be divided into:
   • Four domains: biomedical, social, behavioral, and educational.
   • Three time categories: occurring before birth, during birth, and after birth.

▶ Examples of risk factors for ID are listed in Table 61-1.

▶ Several risk factors may interact over time to result in impaired functioning of the individual.

VI. General Characteristics

A. Physical Features

Because most individuals with an ID are in the borderline and mild categories, unusual physical characteristics

TABLE 61-1	Examples of Risk Factors for Intellectual Disabilities			
	BIOMEDICAL	**SOCIAL**	**BEHAVIORAL**	**EDUCATIONAL**
Prenatal	■ Genetic or chromosome disorders ■ Metabolic disorders ■ Maternal illness or advanced age	■ Poverty ■ Lack of access to health care ■ Nutritional deficits ■ Violence	■ Maternal drug or alcohol intake ■ Maternal tobacco use	■ Parents not prepared for parenthood or with cognitive deficits ■ No parenting support system
Perinatal	■ Premature delivery ■ Birth injury or disorder	■ Lack of access to health care	■ Parental rejection or abandonment	■ lack of referral or access to support and medical services
Postnatal	■ Injury ■ Malnutrition ■ Neurodevelopmental disorders ■ Seizure disorders	■ Inadequate social interaction or stimulation ■ Poverty ■ Family chronic illness	■ Violence, abuse, or neglect ■ Difficult child behaviors leading to social deprivation	■ Delayed diagnosis and intervention ■ Lack of access to services ■ Inadequate parenting, family support

Source: American Association on Intellectual and Developmental Disabilities. *Intellectual Disabilities Definition, Classification, and Systems of Support*. 11th ed. Washington, DC: American Association on Intellectual and Developmental Disabilities; 2010:60.

may not be present. There may be delayed growth and development.

▶ Facial or other characteristics may be pathognomonic for a particular condition or syndrome; for example, Down syndrome, described in this chapter.

▶ Skull anomalies include microcephalus (smaller), hydrocephalus (larger, contains fluid), spherical, conical, or otherwise asymmetrical shapes.

▶ Dysmorphic features, such as asymmetries of the face, malformations of the outer ear, anomalies of the eyes, or unusual shape of the nose, may become apparent as the child develops.

B. Oral Findings

▶ A higher than average prevalence and severity of periodontal disease is common.[3]

▶ Dental caries
  • Caries rates are similar to the general population.
  • However, the rate of untreated caries is considerably higher.[3,4]
  • Level of function and soft diet intake are significant risk factors for dental caries.[5]

▶ A higher incidence of oral developmental malformations may be noted.

▶ Lips: increased thickness; lip biting is a self-injurious habit.

▶ Tooth anomalies: imperfect formation; delayed or irregular eruption patterns.

▶ Oral habits: increased clenching, bruxing, mouthbreathing, tongue thrusting.

VII. Factors Significant for Dental Hygiene Care

▶ Patients with ID often experience significant barriers to accessing dental care.[6]

▶ A patient with an ID may have physical, sensory, or systemic disease comorbidities[1]; therefore, information from various chapters in Section IX of this book may be applied.

▶ Patients and caregivers need basic dental hygiene care supports for the health of all oral tissues, consisting of:
  • Intensive daily personal biofilm removal
  • Frequent maintenance supervision.

▶ Patience for repetition of self-care instruction is needed.

▶ Training a care provider to provide assistance or monitoring of self care is necessary.

DOWN SYNDROME

▶ Unique group of individuals with intellectual disability caused by a chromosomal abnormality; also referred to as trisomy 21 syndrome.

▶ Prevalence is about 8 in 10,000 individuals in the United States.[7]

▶ Life expectancy has increased dramatically.

▶ Most live with family in private homes or settings such as group residential homes and expect to access oral healthcare services within their communities.

▶ People with mild-to-moderate disability can be successfully treated in a general practice dental setting.[8]

I. Physical Characteristics

Patients with Down syndrome have a combination of common characteristics.[9]

▶ Poor muscle tone and awkward, waddling gait.

▶ Stature: short with short neck.

▶ Flattened facial profile with short, underdeveloped nose.

▶ Eyes: oblique slant laterally.

  • Narrow opening between eyelids.
  • Epicanthic fold of skin continues from upper eyelid over the inner angle of the eye (Figure 61-1).
  • Nearsightedness, eyes crossing inward, and cataracts are common.
  • White spots (Brushfield spots) on the colored part of the eye.

▶ Hands

  • Fingers: stubby, short.
  • Palm: single, transverse palmar crease may be present (Figure 61-2).

II. Personal Characteristics

Typical characteristics listed here may suggest management approaches for dental and dental hygiene appointments.

▶ Common cognitive problems include:[9]

  • Short attention span
  • Impulsive behavior
  • Delayed language development.

▶ Many understand more than they can readily verbalize.

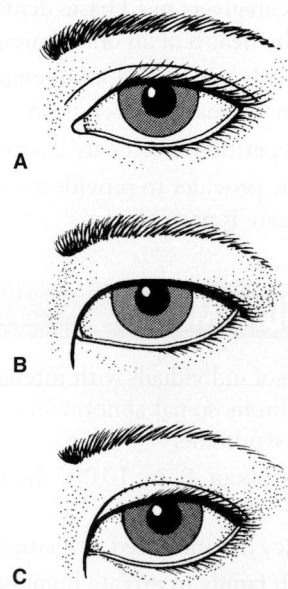

FIGURE 61-1 Down Syndrome: Eye Characteristics. A: Absence of an epicanthic fold. **B:** Epicanthic fold in oriental populations. **C:** Epicanthic fold of person with Down syndrome. (Source: Smith GF, Berg JM. *Down's Anomaly.* 2nd ed. Edinburgh: Churchill Livingstone; 1976.)

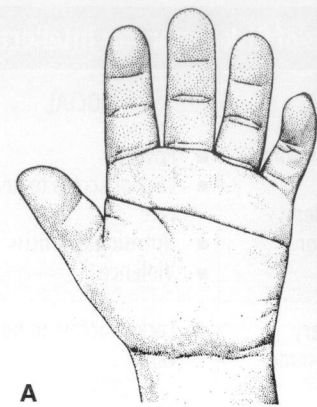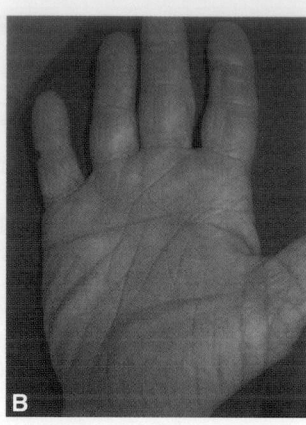

FIGURE 61-2 Down Syndrome: Hand. The artist's drawing (Source: Smith GF, Berg JM. *Down's Anomaly.* 2nd ed. Edinburgh: Churchill Livingstone; 1976.) and the photograph both illustrate characteristic short, stubby fingers with little finger curved inward and the single transverse palmar crease.

▶ Many are socially advanced and may appear to have higher intellectual function.

▶ Many enjoy music and have a good sense of rhythm. Background music in office may help in gaining rapport.

▶ Most like attention; require affection for feeling of security.

▶ Cheerful disposition; rarely irritable; easily amused.

▶ Sociable, observant; take initiative.

▶ Tendency to imitate; mischievous.

▶ Periods of stubbornness; obstinate and determined to have their own way. Parental discipline is necessary. In the dental hygiene appointment, the initial approach can be important to continued control and cooperation.

III. Comorbidity and Health Considerations

Although improvements in health care and immunizations have brought a longer life expectancy, many patients with Down syndrome also present with additional special needs and health concerns.[8,10] Common medical problems include:

▶ Congenital heart defects, mitrovalve prolapse, and diastolic dysfunction.

▶ Ear infections and hearing loss.

▶ Eye diseases and visual impairment, including cataracts.

▶ Seizures.

▶ Alzheimer's disease and other dementias.

▶ Compromised immune system.

▶ Obstructive airway problems.[11]

  • Contributing factors: congenital softening of the larynx tissues and obstructive sleep apnea, macroglossia, increased secretions, frequent respiratory infections, enlarged tonsils and adenoids.
  • Dental hygiene adaptations: chair position, fluid suctioning, gag reflex.

IV. Oral Findings

▶ Lips
  - Habitually, the child with Down syndrome holds the mouth open with the tongue protruded as illustrated in Figure 61-3.
  - Lips may be thickened, cracked, and dry, a result of bathing in saliva while the mouth is open.

▶ Mouth breathing is common.

▶ Tongue may be deeply fissured and appear large.

▶ Palate may be narrow and vaulted.

▶ Common tooth anomalies
  - Delayed or irregular sequence of eruption.
  - Congenitally missing teeth.
  - Irregularities in tooth formation: microdontia fused teeth.

▶ Occlusion
  - Angle's Class III and posterior crossbite are common and relate to the flat face and underdevelopment of the midfacial region.
  - Teeth may be spaced because certain anomalous teeth take less space.

▶ Trauma and injuries to mouth from falls and accidents are common.

▶ Periodontal infections are more prevalent and often more severe in people with Down syndrome. Risk factors include[8]:
  - Poor oral hygiene
  - Malocclusion
  - Bruxism
  - Conical shaped roots
  - Abnormal response because of compromised immune system.

▶ Children and young adults with Down syndrome often have fewer dental caries. Factors that may contribute include:
  - Delayed eruption
  - Smaller-sized teeth (with easier to clean spaces)
  - Diet supervision intended to reduce tendency toward obesity; limitation of cariogenic foods and beverages.

▶ Some adults have higher caries rates due to:
  - Poor dietary choices
  - Insufficient daily oral self care
  - Xerostomia, possibly related to medications
  - Hypotonia of oral tissues resulting in ineffective natural cleansing effect.

AUTISM SPECTRUM DISORDER (ASD)

Autism, first described by Dr. Leo Kanner in 1944, is a complex spectrum of developmental disorders marked by limitations in the ability to understand and communicate.[1]

▶ Usually appears during early childhood and persists throughout life, although many individuals with ASD can learn coping behaviors to enhance daily functioning.

▶ Manifests as a range of disorders, as listed in Box 61-3, rather than by the presence or absence of a single behavior or symptom.

▶ Comorbidity with other disabling and medical conditions is common.[1]

I. Characteristics

▶ Impairment in social interaction
  - Impairment in use of nonverbal behaviors (e.g., eye-to-eye gaze, facial expression, gestures)
  - Failure to develop peer relationships appropriate to developmental level
  - Lack of spontaneous seeking to share enjoyment, interests, or achievements with others
  - Lack of social or emotional reciprocity.

▶ Impairment in communication
  - Delay or total lack of spoken language
  - Individuals with adequate speech: impairment in conversational abilities
  - Repetitive use of language
  - Lack of spontaneous make-believe play.

▶ Restricted repetitive and stereotyped patterns of behavior
  - Preoccupation with stereotyped and restricted patterns of interest
  - Inflexible adherence to routines or rituals
  - Repetitive body movements and mannerisms
  - Persistent preoccupation with parts of objects.

▶ Delays or abnormal functioning before age 3 years in:
  - Social interaction
  - Language as used in social communication
  - Symbolic or imaginative play.

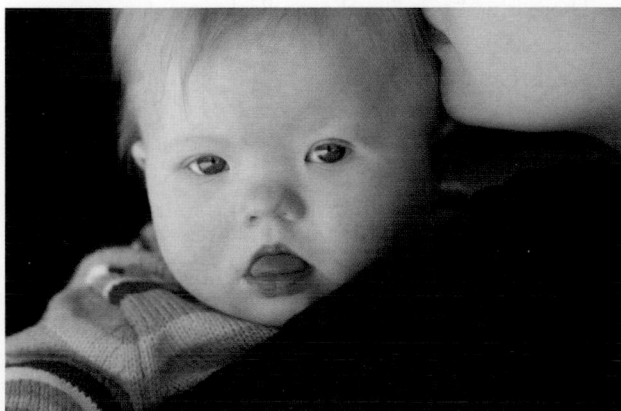

FIGURE 61-3 Child with Down Syndrome. Note the large, protruding tongue, thickened lower lip, and drool of saliva from the corner of the mouth. (Source: From Ricci SS, Essentials of Maternity, Newborn, and Women's Health Nursing, 3rd Edition. Philadelphia: Wolters Kluwer Health, 2012.)

Box 61-3

Autism Spectrum Disorders[1]

Autistic Disorder

▷ Impairments in verbal and nonverbal communication and social (aka: classic autism) interaction, and restrictive or repetitive patterns of behavior, interests, and activities.

▷ Symptoms are usually measurable by 18 months of age; formal diagnosis is usually made between ages 2 and 3, when delays in language development are apparent.

Asperger Disorder

▷ Three to four times more likely in boys.

▷ Characterized by impairments in social interactions and restricted interests and activities, without clinically significant delays in language, cognitive ability, or developmental age-appropriate skills.

Pervasive Developmental Disorder, not Otherwise Specified (PDD-NOS)

▷ Severe and pervasive impairment in specified behaviors, without meeting all of the criteria for a specific diagnosis (aka: atypical autism).

Rett Disorder

▷ An autism-like genetic disorder, which occurs only in girls, causing the development of autism-like symptoms after a period of seemingly normal development.

▷ Purposeful use of hands is lost and replaced by repetitive hand movements beginning between ages 1–4 years.

Childhood Disintegrative Disorder

▷ Rare autism-like disorder characterized by normal development for at least the first 2 years, followed by a significant loss of previously acquired skills.

Box 61-4

Autism Spectrum Disorders: Levels of Severity[1]

Level 3: Requires Very Substantial Support

▷ Severe verbal and nonverbal communication deficits

▷ Initiates social interactions only to meet immediate needs

▷ Limited intelligible speech

▷ Inflexible behavior, extreme difficulty coping with change or changing focus

▷ Repetitive behaviors markedly interferes with functioning

Level 2: Requires Substantial Support

▷ Limited initiation of social interactions; reduced response to overtures from others

▷ Deficits in nonverbal communication/behaviors

▷ Inflexible, difficulty in switching between activities

▷ Difficulty changing focus or action

Level 1

▷ Some difficulty initiating social interactions; atypical response to social overtures from others

▷ Inflexible behavior; difficulty switching between activities

▷ Problems with organization and planning

▶ Not all individuals diagnosed with ASD have the same degree of impairment; *any combination* of symptoms and behaviors *in any degree of severity* can be exhibited.

▶ Severity designation is based on level of communication impairments and behavior patterns (see Box 61-4).

▶ Comorbidity: ASD is commonly associated with other intellectual impairment, structural language disorder, attention deficit and hyperactivity disorders, learning disabilities, and seizure disorders.[1]

II. Prevalence

▶ Prevalence has increased in recent years, about 1 in 68 children have been identified with ASD.[12]

▶ Some increase in prevalence may be attributable to changes in diagnostic criteria.

▶ Occurs in all racial, ethnic, and social groups worldwide.

▶ Frequency of occurrence is almost five times greater in males than in females.

III. Etiology

▶ Exact cause is unknown.

▶ Risk factors include:
  • Perinatal and neonatal factors (such as birth trauma or injury, low birth weight)[13]
  • Genetic and physiological factors (heredity estimates are between 37% and 90%).[14]

IV. Treatment Interventions

▶ There is no "cure," in the medical sense, for autism.

▶ Interventions usually target behavioral issues and support behavioral adaptations.

A. Pharmacological

▶ Purpose: relief of negative behavioral symptoms (such as aggression, self-injury, and other more difficult behaviors).

▶ Types of drugs: stimulants (such as methylphenidate, *Ritalin*), antidepressants, opiate blockers, and tranquilizers.

▶ Strong evidence supports the use of *risperidone*, an atypical antipsychotic medication, to alleviate behavioral disturbances, aggression, and sleep disturbances common in children with autism.[15]

▶ Identification and medical management of comorbid, potentially treatable conditions (e.g., epilepsy seizures, allergies, gastrointestinal problems, or sleep disorders), can lead to quality-of-life improvements.

B. Cognitive-Behavioral Therapy

▶ A form of treatment that focuses on relationships between thoughts, feelings, and behaviors.

▶ Purpose: help people with autism lead more normal lives by decreasing anxiety and increasing their ability to respond to everyday stimuli with appropriate coping mechanisms.[16,17]

▶ No one behavior-based or educational approach is effective in alleviating symptoms in all cases of autism because of the spectrum nature of the condition and the many behavior combinations that can occur.

▶ Examples: special teachers in intensive structured programs directed toward individual instruction, applied behavior analysis, sensory integration, music therapy, occupational therapy, speech and language therapy, and auditory integration training.

C. Prognosis

▶ Life expectancy: normal.

▶ Social and communication deficits continue in some form throughout life; some of the negative behaviors may change or diminish over time with appropriate treatment.

V. Factors Significant for Dental Hygiene Care

▶ Except when a diagnosis of ASD has a comorbid diagnosis, no specific oral manifestation exists.

▶ Impairment in social interaction and difficulty in shifting focus of attention make traditional oral health education approaches difficult.

▶ Repetitive body movements and mannerisms may compromise patient safety and impact infection control protocols.

▶ Patience and a consistent approach to behavioral guidance can enhance the probability of a successful dental visit.

VI. D-Termined Program[18]

Dental Program of Repetitive Tasking and Familiarization in Dentistry

▶ A behavior guidance approach for dental professionals developed to use specifically for patients with ASD.

▶ D-Termined techniques have allowed many patients with ASD to receive appropriate dental treatment in standard practice environments without sedation.

▶ The D-Termined program involves:
 • Pretreatment assessment.
 • Familiarization visits.
 • Practicing and learning cooperation skills.

▶ Cooperation skills to be learned include:
 • Positioning oneself in the dental chair.
 • Sitting with legs straight and hands at side or on tummy.
 • Making eye contact as instructions are given.
 • Opening the mouth and remaining consistently open.
 • Allowing instrumentation, and responding appropriately to instructions.

▶ The five "D" steps for learning cooperation skills:
 • *Divide the skill into smaller parts*: the key for people with autism is to take each small step of a dental appointment one at a time, and master it before moving ahead.
 • *Demonstrate the skill*: use the tell–show–do technique.
 • *Drill the skill*: repeat/practice the skill many times until it becomes second nature.
 • *Delight the learner*: reward successful attainment of any small portion of the task with reinforcers.
 • *Delegate the repetition*: involve other members of the dental staff in reinforcing the skills, and have parents and caregivers rehearse/practice at home.

DENTAL HYGIENE CARE

▶ Appointments for medical or dental health care may be frightening, difficult experiences for some patients with a neurodevelopmental disorder, and most especially for patients with an ASD.

▶ Dental care may have been neglected due to problems with social interactions, language and communication problems, or difficult behaviors.

▶ Severity of symptoms dictates the appropriate setting for the delivery of dental care services for these patients.

▶ With some modifications to the treatment plan and implementation of appropriate behavior guidance techniques, patients with mild-to-moderate manifestations of the condition may be treated successfully in the general dental setting.[19]

▶ Patients with more severe symptoms may require sedation, general anesthesia, or immobilization in a specialized setting.

I. Oral Health Problems

Several factors can contribute to poor oral health for individuals with a neurodevelopmental disorder.

A. Previous Dental Care

▶ Dental care may have been a low priority.

▶ Caregivers may no longer seek dental services if they have not found services that are available or appropriate in the past.

▶ Reasons for dental neglect

- Parental fear of embarrassment over resistant or possible aggressive/impulsive behaviors.
- Fear of discomfort.
- Fear of injury.
- Satisfactory quality of previous services may not have been achievable.

B. Dental Caries

▶ Feeding problems can lead to offering foods that will be accepted, without regard for nutrient content or caries prevention.

▶ Dietary selection may have been limited by needs for sameness, with the possibility of serving an excess of cariogenic foods.

▶ Sweet food rewards for behavior modification/guidance, repeated frequently over time, promote dental caries development.

▶ Aversion to certain food textures can lead to extreme diets that result in either entirely soft food selections or entirely hard crunchy/crispy food selections.

▶ Foods used in therapy sessions to stimulate speech or help develop the muscles necessary for improved language are frequently cariogenic (i.e., chewy or sticky candy).

C. Oral Hygiene

▶ Daily oral care procedures may be inadequate for the uncooperative individual, even when delivered by an informed caregiver.

▶ Sensory issues may need to be overcome for the individual to be able to tolerate the mouth sensations that are a necessary part of routine home care.

II. Dental Staff Preparation

▶ Learn how to work with the patient.
- Review medical, dental, and personal histories with the caregiver by telephone appointment in advance of the first office appointment.
- Discuss information with parent/caregiver, physician, psychiatrist, teacher, or other persons associated with the patient.
- Gather specific information about appropriate motivators and rewards that are safe and effective reinforcers for the individual.

▶ Provide the individual with photos of the office and staff before the first appointment.

▶ Make recommendations for practice sessions that can be conducted at home before the first appointment.
- Touch the teeth for a count of 10.
- Place a plastic mirror and flashlight in and out of the mouth.
- Follow commands such as "Hands on your tummy".... "Feet out straight."

▶ Plan several short orientation and familiarization appointments initially with not more than a week between visits.

▶ Involve the same members of the dental team at each appointment to avoid distressing the patient and losing time for reorientation.

III. Dental Hygiene Care Plan

▶ Plan four-handed dental hygiene for the resistant patient.

▶ Frequent appointments to include all phases of prevention:
- Dental biofilm control for the patient and the caregiver.
- Scaling.
- Fluoride varnish therapy: simple easy to do procedure that can be especially helpful for patients unable to cooperate with biofilm control (refer to Chapter 36).
- Dental sealants (see Chapter 37).

IV. Appointment Considerations

▶ Provide a predictable and consistent experience.

▶ Create a quiet environment free from sensory stimuli; patients with autism may have sensitivity to light, sounds, touch, and smell.
- Avoid loud, inconsistent background music, noisy dental equipment, and irrelevant conversations.
- Avoid unnecessary touching during treatment.

▶ Desensitization/practice
- Begin with orientation to the setting and each part of the equipment.
- If patient is not ready, instrumentation may not be included at the first appointment.
- Instruction takes the form of "tell–show–do" repeated many times. Patience and firmness are necessary elements.
- Have caregiver help condition the patient by giving a plastic mouth mirror and a few dental films to take home for practice in the mouth each day.

▶ Use behavior guidance procedures when the patient is familiar with that method.
- Involve caregiver(s) while presenting preventive measures in a simple step-by-step manner.
- Provide reinforcing rewards immediately following each success.
- Use inedible rewards (stickers, picture cards, child-safe tokens, or toys) and explain rationale against cariogenic food rewards.

▶ Physical immobilization
- The least restrictive method of body stabilization is selected for each patient.

EVERYDAY ETHICS

At the Caring Community Dental Health Clinic, the first and third Mondays of each month are reserved for special needs patients referred by health professionals in the local area. Adults and children with Down syndrome, ASD, and other intellectual disabilities are scheduled frequently for dental hygiene appointments. With only one full-time and one part-time dental hygienist, more hygiene appointment time has been needed. Dental hygiene students from a nearby dental hygiene program have been invited to rotate through the clinic as a community practicum experience.

Questions for Consideration

1. Two days before a scheduled assignment, Ellie, a student, confides to her classmate, Julie, that she cannot participate in this field experience because she is too afraid of people with intellectual disabilities. Which core values are evident in this situation?

2. When arriving at the assignment, the students are greeted and oriented by the part-time hygienist, Ms. Gray. She advises the students, "Just get 'em in and get 'em out. They don't understand anything anyway and it's a waste of your time to try to talk to them for patient instruction." What are the ethical principles applicable to this situation?

3. How might the students handle these ethical issues using the "Steps in the Resolution of an Issue or Dilemma" Box 1-10 in Chapter 1 to determine an acceptable course of action?

- The use of physical immobilization techniques during routine clinical procedures is currently considered inappropriate.
- Various body stabilization techniques for use in limited situations are described in Chapter 57.
- Written informed parental/guardian consent and complete postprocedure documentation is provided when any types of physical body enclosure or body stabilization techniques are used during dental hygiene treatment.

V. Behavior Supports and Guidance

▶ Behavioral interventions are available to help patients who physically resist dental procedures learn to cooperate. Many resistant patients can learn to cooperate more, and can learn these cooperative behaviors more quickly when:

- At least two or more active behavioral interventions are used.
- Individualized tangible reinforcers are used and provided frequently.
- Patients can be actively involved in the behavior intervention and are provided with choices when appropriate.
- The behavior intervention is practiced repetitively.

DOCUMENTATION

Factors to document include:
▶ Chronological age versus developmental age.
▶ Communication strengths and weaknesses.
▶ Helpful behavioral supports and guidance techniques.
▶ Treatment that was accomplished and modifications to treatment that were helpful.

▶ Recommended home care oral hygiene and behavior practice skills.
▶ Box 61-5 contains example documentation for a patient with an ID.

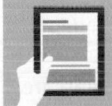

BOX 61-5
Example Documentation: Patient with an ID

S–Patient presented as a 10-year-old boy with a developmental age of approx. 4 years old. Used three-to-four word simple sentences and caregivers presented a picture board that showed the steps of the appointment. This helped the patient recognize how many more steps were needed until the end of the appointment. Patient needs to have his hands held to remind him not to touch and finds comfort in holding his favorite rubber tube toy that he brought from home. He also loves to hear quiet singing and counting throughout the appointment.

O–Mirror only examination performed. Biofilm score noted as roughly 50%. No visual decay found.

A–Dental hygiene diagnosis: biofilm-induced gingivitis.

P–Oral hygiene instruction with patient and caregiver. Rubber cup prophy completed. Flossing of entire mouth. Fluoride varnish applied to entire dentition. Caregivers congratulated on preparing the patient for the visit; patient congratulated on a successful visit.

Next steps: 3 months recall-examination with explorer and biofilm removal with toothbrush.

Signed _____, RDH

Date _____

Factors To Teach The Patient

When the patient is able to perform other self care skills independently and can expectorate, then proceed with instruction using language and methods appropriate to the intellectual level and abilities of each patient.

Explain:

▷ How to perform oral hygiene procedures at an appropriate skill level.

▷ What the disclosing agent shows and why the biofilm needs to be removed.

▷ Why assistance from others is a necessary supplement to the patient's own efforts.

▷ How to use and show their cooperation skills.

Factors To Teach The Caregiver

▷ Why complete oral examinations and oral hygiene care services at regular frequent intervals are necessary.

▷ Why a total preventive program is necessary; emphasize its significance.

▷ Individualized oral care techniques for each patient.

▷ Ways to provide assistance for patients with limited abilities, such as:

  ▷ How to stabilize the patient's head.

  ▷ How to retract the patient's lips to insert and adapt the toothbrush.

▷ How to incorporate behavior modification into oral care procedures.

▷ Emphasize the necessity of repeating tell–show–do instructions often.

References

1. American Psychiatric Association. Section II: Diagnostic criteria and codes: neurodevelopmental disorders. In: *Diagnostic and Statistical Manual of Mental Disorders*. 5th ed. Arlington, VA: American Psychiatric Association; 2013:31–86.

2. Buntinx WHE, Schalock RL. Models of disability, quality of life, and individualized supports: implications for professional practice in intellectual disability. *J Policy Pract Intellect Disabil*. 2010;7(4);283–294.

3. Anders PL, Davis EL. Oral health of patients with intellectual disabilities: a systematic review. *Spec Care Dentist*. 2010;30(3):110–117.

4. Morgan JP, Minihan PM, Stark PC, et al. The oral health status of 4,732 adults with intellectual and developmental disabilities. *J Am Dent Assoc*. 2012;143(8):838–846.

5. Bakry NS, Alaki SM. Risk factors associated with caries experience in children and adolescents with intellectual disabilities. *J Clin Pediatr Dent*. 2012;36(3):319–323.

6. Rouleau T, Harrington A, Brennan M, et al. Receipt of dental care and barriers encountered by persons with disabilities. *Spec Care Dentist*. 2011;31(2):63–67.

7. Presson AP, Partyka G, Jensen KM, et al. Current estimate of Down syndrome population prevalence in the United States. *J Pediatr*. 2013;163(4):1163–1168.

8. National Institute of Dental and Craniofacial Research. Practical oral care for people with Down syndrome. http://www.nidcr.nih.gov/OralHealth/Topics/DevelopmentalDisabilities/PracticalOralCarePeopleDownSyndrome.htm. Accessed July 15, 2014.

9. Eunice Kennedy Shriver National Institute of Child Health and Human Development. What are the common symptoms of Down syndrome? http://www.nichd.nih.gov/health/topics/down/conditioninfo/Pages/symptoms.aspx. Accessed July 15, 2014.

10. Määttä T, Määttä J, Tervo-Määttä T, et al. Healthcare and guidelines: a population-based survey of recorded medical problems and health surveillance for people with Down syndrome. *J Intellect Dev Disabil*. 2011;36(2):118–126.

11. Mitchell RB, Call E, Kelly J. Diagnosis and therapy for airway obstruction in children with Down syndrome. *Arch Otolaryngol Head Neck Surg*. 2003;129(6):642–645.

12. Centers for Disease Control and Prevention. Autism spectrum disorder (ASD): data & statistics. http://www.cdc.gov/ncbddd/autism/data.html. Accessed July 15, 2014.

13. Gardener H, Spiegelman D, Buka SL. Perinatal and neonatal risk factors for autism: a comprehensive meta-analysis. *Pediatrics*. 2011;128(2):344–355.

14. Geschwind DH. Genetics of autism spectrum disorders. *Trends Cogn Sci*. 2011;15(9):409–416.

15. Politte LC, Henry CA, McDougle CJ. Psychopharmacological interventions in autism spectrum disorder. *Harv Rev Psychiatry*. 2014;22(2):76–92.

16. Sukhodolsky DG, Bloch MH, Panza KE, et al. Cognitive-behavioral therapy for anxiety in children with high-functioning autism: a meta-analysis. *Pediatrics*. 2013;132(5):e1341–e1350.

17. Storch EA, Arnold EB, Lewin AB, et al. The effect of cognitive-behavioral therapy versus treatment as usual for anxiety in children with autism spectrum disorders: a randomized, controlled trial. *J Am Acad Child Adolesc Psychiatry*. 2013;52(2):132–142.

18. The Nancy Lurie Marks Family Foundation. D-Termined program of repetitive tasking and familiarization in dentistry. http://www.nlmfoundation.org/media/dental_clips.htm. Accessed July 15, 2014.

19. Raposa KA, Perlman SP. *Treating the Dental Patient with a Developmental Disability*. 1st ed. Ames, IA: Wiley; 2012:272.

 ENHANCE YOUR UNDERSTANDING

thePoint® DIGITAL CONNECTIONS
(see the inside front cover for access information)
- **Audio glossary**
- **Quiz bank**

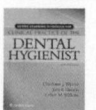 **SUPPORT FOR LEARNING**
(available separately; visit lww.com)
- *Active Learning Workbook for Clinical Practice of the Dental Hygienist, 12th Edition*

prepU INDIVIDUALIZED REVIEW
(available separately; visit lww.com)
- **Adaptive quizzing with *prepU* for Wilkins' *Clinical Practice of the Dental Hygienist***

62

Family Abuse and Neglect

Pamela S. Ridilla, RDH, MS

LEARNING OBJECTIVES

After studying this chapter, the student will be able to:

1. Describe the general, extraoral, and intraoral signs of child abuse and neglect.

2. Describe the general, physical, extraoral, and intraoral signs of elder abuse and neglect.

3. Discuss the signs and attitudes of the abused in an intimate partner abuse and violence situations.

4. Discuss the role of the dental hygienist in reporting suspected maltreatment of children, elders, and intimate partners.

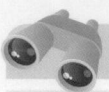

BOX 62-1 KEY WORDS: Family Abuse and Neglect

Acute primary herpetic gingivostomatitis: clinical presentation of an initial HSV infection from HSV1 (oral) or HSV2 (genital) that can appear as multiple ulcerations on both keratinizing and gland-bearing mucosa.

Alopecia: baldness.

    Traumatic alopecia: an area of baldness on the head caused by pulling out the hair at the roots.

Cachexia: ill health, malnutrition, wasting (emaciating).

Condyloma acuminatum: multiple papillary or focal sessile-based lesions caused by the human papilloma virus (HPV6 or HPV11).

Differential diagnosis: determining the probability of one disease or condition versus another by comparing and contrasting the symptoms.

Ecchymosis: discoloration on the skin that is blue-black with irregularly formed hemorrhagic areas. Color changes with time to yellow or greenish-brown.

Edema: swelling.

Forensic: pertaining to or used in legal proceedings.

Idiopathic thrombocytopenia purpura: hemorrhages on the skin caused by abnormal decrease in the number of blood platelets with unknown etiology.

Intimate relationship: marriage partners, partners living together, dating relationships, and former spouses, partners, and boyfriends/girlfriends.

Lichenification: area of skin that has thickened and hardened from continuous irritation.

Raccoon sign: bilateral periorbital ecchymosis, which can occur as a result of a basilar skull fracture.

Scale photography: a method of photography to record bite marks; the use of a metric scale placed directly above or below the injury to indicate scale; use of grid photographic film.

Domestic violence is the abuse by one individual of another in an intimate or family relationship. The entire dental health team needs to be aware of the problem of family abuse and neglect and prepared to identify and report suspected cases to authorities.

▶ Those most at risk for maltreatment are children, the elderly, persons with disabilities, and women.

▶ Family abuse may be categorized as physical violence, emotional abuse, sexual abuse, neglect, or financial exploitation.

▶ Abuse of women can include spousal abuse and dating violence.

▶ Table 62-1 summarizes the major types of family maltreatment.

▶ Abuse can be detected during the initial assessment of a patient, particularly during the extraoral and intraoral examination.

▶ Head and facial injuries, oral trauma, lesions, and abnormal pathology can lead to a suspicion of abuse and neglect.

▶ Patients may be seen in a dental office or clinic, whereas others may be taken to a hospital emergency department because serious bodily injuries have been inflicted.

▶ Key words associated with family abuse and neglect are defined in Box 62-1.

CHILD MALTREATMENT

▶ Any act or series of acts of abuse and neglect by a parent or other caregiver that results in harm, potential for harm, or threat of harm to a child under the age of 18.[1]

▶ Special needs children are more at risk to be victims of abuse and neglect.

▶ Several thousands of children a year die as a result of severe physical damage, and others suffer permanent brain damage or physical deformities as well as emotional trauma. As much as 50%–65% of child physical abuse involves injuries to the head, neck, or mouth.[2]

▶ Maltreatment is considered in the differential diagnosis for any injury involving a child.

TABLE 62-1	Major Types of Family Maltreatment
CATEGORY	**DESCRIPTION**
Physical violence	Nonaccidental injuries on family members by parents, caregivers, spouses, or siblings.
Physical neglect	Willful or unwillful failure of the caregiver or parents to provide necessities to individuals in their care; abandonment; medical, dental, and deprivation neglect.
Sexual violence	Non-consensual or exploitive sexual contact, including sexual intercourse, oral sex, fondling, or pornographic activities on one family member by another.
Emotional abuse	Mental anguish and despair caused by ridicule, intimidation, humiliation, name-calling, harassment, threats, and controlling behavior; isolation.

I. Definitions

▶ *Abuse*: The non-accidental physical, emotional (psychological), or sexual acts against a child.[1]

▶ *Neglect*: The intentional or unintentional failure to provide for a child's basic physical, emotional, educational, and medical/dental needs.[1]

▶ *Dental neglect*: The willful failure of a parent or guardian to seek and follow through with treatment necessary to ensure a level of oral health essential for adequate function and freedom from pain and infection.[3]

II. General Signs of Abuse and Neglect

Recognition of signs of suspected abuse is the first step toward protection of the child. As the child enters the treatment room, identifiable characteristics may be displayed that are suggestive of abuse or neglect.

A. Overall Appearance

▶ Clothing with long sleeves and long pants, even in warm weather, may suggest that bruises and lacerations are being covered.

▶ Uncleanliness and other signs of lack of care.

▶ Failure to thrive; malnutrition.

▶ Infestation of lice.
  • Live bugs on the scalp.
  • Bug bite marks on the scalp.
  • Nits or lice eggs on the shaft of the hair; appear as tiny silvery tears.
  • Drops that can be attached anywhere along the hair shaft from the scalp to the ends and that do not move or fall off.

B. Behavioral

In Table 62-2, categories of child abuse and neglect are separated into physical and behavioral indicators.

▶ May be very fearful and cry excessively or will show no fear at all.

▶ May appear unhappy and withdrawn.

▶ May not exhibit normal behavior consistent with the present age of the child.

▶ May act differently when the parent is present than when alone, which may provide clues to the type of relationship that exists.

▶ May exhibit evidence of developmental delays, including those of language or motor skills.

III. Extraoral Wounds and Signs of Trauma

▶ Abrasions and lacerations may be present at varying degrees of healing inconsistent with explanations given by the caregiver.

▶ Recognizing injuries to the head and neck and connecting them to suspected child maltreatment can save the lives of the children involved.

▶ Deliberate or inflicted injuries usually occur on both sides of the face, whereas accidental injuries usually occur only on one side.

▶ Common sites of deliberate injuries inflicted on children and accidental injuries on children are illustrated in Figure 62-1.
  • Skull injuries; edema, combined with ecchymosis of varying stages.
  • Bald spots (traumatic alopecia); caused by pulling the hair out by the roots.
  • Raccoon sign: bilateral periorbital ecchymosis.
  • Nose fractures or displacements.
  • Lip bruises and lacerations; angular bruising, lichenification, or scarring, which can be caused from gags applied to the mouth.
  • Marks on the skin that form a pattern of an object like a belt buckle or handprint.
  • Human bite marks.

▶ Table 62-3 lists possible conditions that can mimic lesions from child maltreatment.

IV. Intraoral Signs of Abuse

Care is given to the assessment of intraoral traumatic injuries. Many injuries of the mouth in children can also be caused by accidental means.

▶ Lacerations of the tongue, buccal mucosa, or palate.

▶ Lingual and labial frenal tears.

▶ Teeth that are fractured, displaced, avulsed, or nonvital.

▶ Radiographic evidence of fractures in different degrees of healing.

V. Signs of Sexual Abuse

▶ Bruising or petechiae of the palate can indicate forced oral sex.

▶ Sexually transmitted genital lesions found intraorally.
  • Condyloma acuminatum presents as a focal sessile-based lesion and also as a multiple papillary lesion. When present, it is necessary to look for other signs of oral sexual abuse because condyloma acuminatum can also occur with contact to verruca vulgaris or from self-inoculation.
  • Primary herpetic gingivostomatitis can occur as a primary infection of herpes simplex virus type 2 (HSV2), which is a genital infection transmitted through oral sex.

▶ Exhibits difficulty in walking or sitting.

▶ Extreme fear of the oral examination.

▶ Pregnancy, especially in the early adolescent years.

VI. Intraoral Signs of Neglect

Failure of the caregiver, who is responsible for the child, to seek dental care for that child can be considered

TABLE 62-2	Physical and Behavioral Indicators of Child Abuse and Neglect

TYPE OF CHILD ABUSE AND NEGLECT	PHYSICAL INDICATORS	BEHAVIORAL INDICATORS

Physical abuse	*Unexplained bruises and welts*
	■ face, lips, mouth
	■ torso, back, buttocks, thighs
	■ various stages of healing
	■ clustered, regular patterns
	■ reflecting shape of article used to inflict (e.g., buckle)
	■ on several different areas
	■ regular appearance after absence, weekend, vacation
	Unexplained burns
	■ cigarette, cigar burns, esp. on soles, palms, back, buttocks
	■ immersion burns (sock or glovelike, circular, on buttocks or genitalia)
	■ patterned: electric burner, iron
	■ rope burns on arms, legs, or torso
	Unexplained fractures
	■ skull, nose, facial structures
	■ in various stages of healing
	■ multiple or spiral fractures
	Unexplained laceration or abrasion
	■ to mouth, lips, gingiva, eyes
	■ to external genitalia
		■ Wary of adult contacts
		■ Apprehensive when others cry
		■ Behavioral extremes:
		  • Aggressive
		  • Withdrawn
		■ Frightened of parents
		■ Afraid to go home
		■ Reports injury by parents

Physical neglect	■ Constant hunger, poor hygiene, inappropriate dress ■ Consistent lack of supervision, esp. in dangerous situations or for long periods ■ Unattended physical problems or medical/dental needs ■ Abandonment	■ Begging, stealing food ■ Extended stays at school, early arrival, late departure ■ Constant fatigue, falling asleep in class ■ Alcohol or drug abuse ■ Delinquency (e.g., thefts) ■ Says there is no caretaker
Sexual abuse	■ Difficulty in walking or sitting ■ Torn, stained, bloody underwear ■ Pain or itching in genital area ■ Bruises or bleeding on external genitalia, vaginal, or anal areas ■ Venereal disease, esp. in preteen ■ Pregnancy	■ Unwilling to change for physical education ■ Withdrawal, fantasy or infantile behavior ■ Bizarre, sophisticated sexual knowledge or behavior ■ Poor peer relationship ■ Delinquency; runaways ■ Reports sexual assault by caretaker

Emotional maltreatment	■ Speech disorders
	■ Lags in physical development
	■ Failure to thrive
		■ Habit disorders (sucking, biting, rocking, etc.)
		■ Conduct disorders (antisocial, destructive)
		■ Neurotic traits (sleep disorders, inhibited play)
		■ Psychoneurotic behaviors (hysteria, phobia, obsession, compulsion, hypochondria)
		■ Behavioral extremes:
		  • Compliant, passive
		  • Aggressive, demanding
		■ Overly adaptive behavior:
		  • Inappropriately adult
		  • Inappropriately infantile
		■ Developmental lags (physical or mental)
		■ Attempted suicide

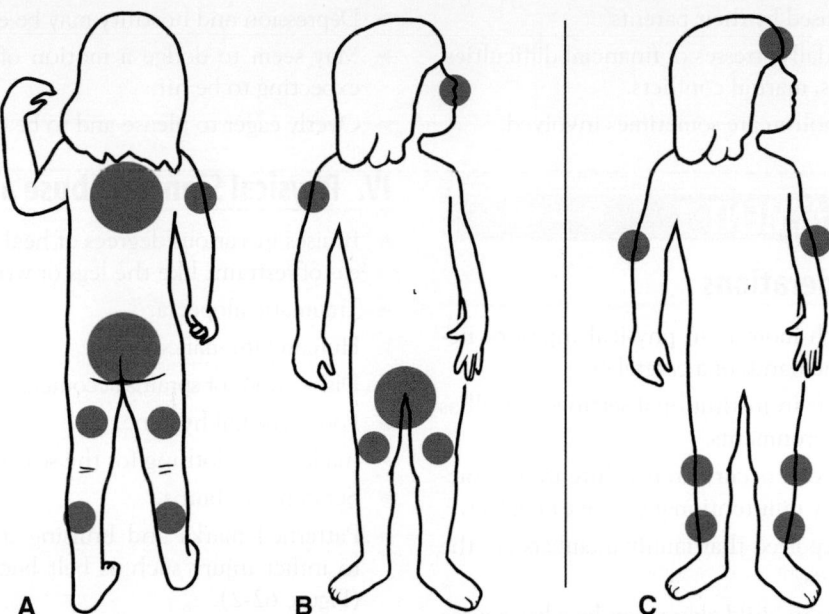

FIGURE 62-1 Common Sites of Children's Injuries. A and **B:** Common sites of inflicted or deliberate injuries. **C:** Common sites of accidental injuries.

TABLE 62-3	Conditions that can Mimic Abuse
APPEARANCE	**POSSIBLE CONDITIONS**
Bruising	Accidental injuries Idiopathic thrombocytopenia purpura Hemophilia
Burns/red lesions	Port-wine stain Accidental burns
Skin lesions	Bullous impetigo Birthmarks

intentional or unintentional neglect. Neglect becomes intentional when the caregiver is negligent in following through with the recommended treatment.

A. Signs of Oral Neglect

▶ Signs of lack of personal daily care.

▶ Untreated disease, including rampant dental caries, pain, gingival inflammation, and bleeding.

▶ Lack of regularity of dental care; appointments may have been made primarily for tooth or mouth pain.

B. Responsibilities of Dental Professionals

▶ Provide education to the caregivers and age-appropriate children in personal oral health care and disease prevention procedures.

▶ Inform the caregiver of the total treatment plan necessary to control oral diseases.

▶ Provide information about access to care, financial aid, and transportation, when needed.

VII. Parental Attitude

A. Reasons for Dental Neglect: Parental Factors Involved

▶ Oral health care considered a low priority.

▶ Lack of education concerning the significance of oral health care and the relation to general health.

▶ Limited finances.

▶ Family isolation: access to care.

▶ Religious beliefs.

B. General Attitudes of Abusers

▶ Disinterest or denial in relationship to the child; may be critical, scolding, or belittling in front of others, including dental personnel.

▶ Lack of interest in proposed dental and dental hygiene treatment plan, with a tendency to want only pain relief for the child. Such an attitude may not be shown toward other children in the family.

▶ Unavailable for consultation. Does not usually accompany the child for dental appointments, but sends the child with another sibling.

▶ Provides inconsistent information about the sources and causes of damaged teeth, bruises, or other signs of trauma.

C. Contributing Factors to Abusive Parents

▶ Immature and unprepared for accepting the responsibilities of parenthood.

- May have been abused by their parents.
- Unable to handle daily stresses of financial difficulties, work stress, job loss, marital conflicts.
- Drug use and alcoholism are sometimes involved.

ELDER MALTREATMENT

I. General Considerations

- Elder abuse is much more than physical injury or neglect inflicted at the hands of a caretaker.
- Mistreatment occurs in institutional settings as well as in family home environments.
- Harm to the elder can occur through intentional (active) infliction or by unintentional (passive) neglect.[4]
- It is consistently reported that family members are the primary elder abusers.[5]
- The dental team, as in child abuse, can be a key source for the gathering of information to prove or disprove abuse of the elder patient.

II. Definitions

- *Physical abuse*: The intentional use of force that results in bodily injury, pain, or anguish.
- *Physical neglect*: The failure to provide basic necessities such as food, clothing, water, shelter, medicine, dental care, and personal hygiene. This type of neglect can be intentional or unintentional due to the caregiver's lack of ability to provide such care.
- *Psychological abuse*: Mental anguish and despair caused by ridicule, name-calling, humiliation, harassment, manipulation, threats, and controlling behavior.
- *Psychological neglect*: Nonverbal anguish caused by the lack of communication and isolation.
- *Financial abuse*: Improper, illegal, or unethical exploitation of resources or assets.
- *Sexual abuse*: Sexual contact with an elder who is unable to consent or otherwise nonconsensual sexual contact or exploitation.
- *Self-neglect*: This can occur owing to depression from a loss of a loved one. The elder may feel unable to continue living.

III. General Signs of Abuse and Neglect

When assessing for the possibility of abuse, it is necessary to have a working knowledge of lesions related to aging, health problems, or medications. Taking a thorough history and comparing it with lesions present will help determine an appropriate differential diagnosis.

- Appears withdrawn, anxious, and shy and has low self-esteem.
- Gives an illogical explanation of how an injury occurred.

- Depression and hostility may be evident.
- May seem to dodge a motion of another person as if expecting to be hit.
- Overly eager to please and to be compliant.

IV. Physical Signs of Abuse and Neglect

- Bruises in various degrees of healing, particularly in areas of restraint like the legs or wrists.
- Traumatic alopecia.
- Human bite marks.
- Dislocations or sprains accompanied by fingertip pattern.
- Poor personal hygiene.
- Inadequate clothing for the season.
- Scratches or burns.
- Patterned marks and bruising indicating object used to inflict injury such as belt buckle, ropes, or a hand (Figure 62-2).
- Cachexia.

V. Extraoral Signs of Abuse and Neglect

- Lip trauma.
- Bruising of facial tissues.
- Eye injuries.
- Fractured or bruised mandible.
- Temporomandibular joint pain.

VI. Intraoral Signs of Abuse and Neglect

- Fractured, displaced, or avulsed teeth.
- Bruising of the edentulous ridge. May indicate forced oral sex.
- Sexually transmitted disease lesions such as condyloma acuminatum and primary herpetic gingivostomatitis.
- Lesions or sore areas in the mouth from ill-fitting dentures: epulis fissuratum, atrophic candidiasis.

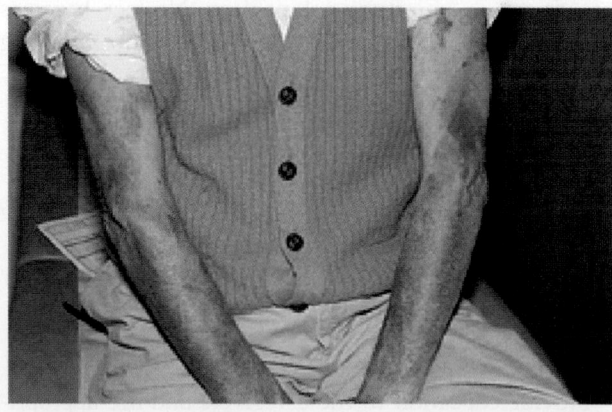

FIGURE 62-2 Hand and Finger-Shaped Bruises. Large and small bruises in various stages of healing on the upper arms of this elderly patient may trigger suspicions of abuse. (Source: From Weber JR, Kelley JH. Health Assessment in Nursing 2e. Philadelphia: Wolters Kluwer Health, 2006.)

(Lesions that occur under dentures are described in Chapter 54.)

▶ Fractured denture.

▶ Poor oral hygiene.

▶ Rampant dental caries.

▶ Untreated periodontal disease.

INTIMATE PARTNER ABUSE AND VIOLENCE

Spousal or partner abuse is another type of abuse that can be detected in the dental setting. The dental team is in a good position to examine and evaluate the oral areas of injury to a battered partner. The majority of intimate partner violence (IPV) cases have female victims. Such abuse often goes unreported.

I. Signs and Attitudes of the Abused

▶ Many of the same injuries listed for the elder person are also evident with partner abuse. They involve most frequently the face, eyes, and neck.

▶ Battered partner may be very reluctant to admit abuse because of threats of more serious harm.

▶ Abused may deny the abuse, defend the abuser, or provide excuses.

▶ Battering is a choice in order to gain power and control over another individual.[6]

▶ Types of abuse are physical, sexual, emotional, psychological, and economic deprivation.

II. Dental Hygienist's Approach

▶ Provide support; encourage open communication; be a source of reassurance.

▶ Discuss clinical findings in a nonjudgmental manner.

▶ Respect and maintain confidentiality; talk in a private setting (door closed to treatment room).

▶ Provide references for counseling; telephone numbers; community services.

▶ Respect patient's autonomy; ask about plans for future safety.

▶ Prepare to share your findings with authorities when called to provide evidence.

▶ When it is known that the interview will be used in a legal setting, a witness needs to be present.

▶ Document clinical findings, including extra/intraoral photographs of injuries.

REPORTING MALTREATMENT

I. Discussion of Findings

▶ A decision is be made by the dental team whether or not to discuss the suspicion of abuse with the caregiver.

▶ If the decision is made to confront the spouse, parent or caregiver, the professional never directly accuses anyone and refrains from being judgmental.

▶ The legal obligation to report a suspected case of abuse can be explained.

II. Proper Training

▶ Training in the recognition and reporting of abuse and neglect need to be implemented in every dental practice. Abusers may avoid the same physician but return to the same dentist.[7]

▶ Many state governing boards require completion of continuing education courses on abuse and neglect before licensure and relicensure to practice dentistry and dental hygiene.

▶ "Prevent Abuse and Neglect through Dental Awareness" (PANDA) is a program for training dental personnel.

  • The coalition, founded in 1992 by the Missouri Bureau of Dental Health and Delta Dental of Missouri, is a public–private partnership committed to the education of all dental professionals in the recognition and reporting of suspected cases of child abuse and neglect.

  • Since its inception, nearly all of the United States and several international coalitions have replicated the program.[8]

▶ "Ask, Validate, Document, Refer (AVDR) Tutorial for Dentists" is an interactive tutorial program that utilizes a case study to demonstrate the AVDR four-step process in response to domestic violence.

  • *Asking* the patient about the abuse

  • *Validating* messages that acknowledge battering is wrong

  • *Documenting* the signs, symptoms, and disclosures

  • *Referring* victims to specialists and community resources.[9]

▶ Project RADAR is a provider-focused initiative to promote the assessment and prevention of IPV in the healthcare setting.

▶ Project RADAR seeks to enable healthcare providers to recognize and respond to IPV by providing them access to:

  • "Best Practices" policies, guidelines, and assessment tools

  • Training programs and specialty-specific curricula

  • Awareness and educational materials

  • Information on the latest research/data related to IPV

▶ *Routinely* inquire about current and past violence; *Ask* direct questions; *Document* findings; *Assess* safety; and *Review* options and referrals.[10]

III. Reporting Laws

▶ Reporting laws vary from state to state.

▶ Each state has laws regarding the reporting of abuse and neglect to the proper authorities. It is imperative to research the laws for the state and have them available for reference in the office.

▶ Each dental practice needs a written protocol for the documentation and reporting of abuse and neglect.

IV. Reportable Required Information

▶ All states mandate healthcare workers to report suspected violence, abuse, and neglect of children to child protective services agencies.[11]

▶ When reporting suspected child maltreatment, it is necessary to have the following information available:
  • Name and address of the child and parents or other persons having custody of the child.
  • Child's age.
  • Names of siblings if there are any.
  • Nature of the child's condition, including evidence of previous injuries.
  • Any information that might be helpful in establishing the cause of abuse or neglect and the identity of the person believed to have caused such abuse or neglect.

▶ In most states, healthcare workers are legally required to report suspected maltreatment of elders and adults with disabilities.

▶ Healthcare workers are required by law to report suspected IPV in only a few states.

FORENSIC DENTISTRY

Forensic dentistry is that aspect of dental science that relates and applies dental facts to legal problems. Forensic dentistry encompasses dental identification, malpractice litigation, legislation, peer review, and dental licensure.

I. Use of Forensics in Abuse Cases

There are instances when it becomes necessary to request the aid of a forensic odontologist to determine if a particular injury, usually a bite mark, is a result of abuse by a particular suspect.

▶ Many times the abuser will state that the bite mark occurred from a sibling squabble, an animal bite, or the child biting himself or herself.

▶ When photographs have been obtained and the history of the injury does not match the location of the marks, a bite mark analysis can be requested of the forensic odontologist.

▶ Impressions and a bite registration are taken from the suspect/caregiver. A careful analysis will determine if the bite came from that suspect.

▶ The information can then be taken into the legal process involved with prosecuting a child abuser.

II. Other Uses of Forensics

▶ Forensic procedures are utilized in the identification of victims of a disaster.

▶ Forensic teams include dentists, dental hygienists, and assistants with special training in the process of identifying remains by comparing the dentition of the remains with dental records.

▶ Team members are assigned a task, and the team works together to check and double check results so the families of the victims can have closure regarding the loss of a loved one.

DOCUMENTATION

I. Purposes of Thorough and Accurate Documentation

▶ For future reference and comparison.

▶ To provide authorities meticulous information to support an investigation.

▶ To protect the abused patient from harmful circumstances or even death. A second person needs to be present to witness the examination and interview.

II. Content of the Record

▶ Obtain thorough histories of the injury from both the caregiver and the patient. Identify inconsistencies.

▶ Document the date, time, and place of the examination.

▶ Record all observable facts.

▶ Record questions asked of the abused patient and document all answers in the patient's exact words as closely as possible.

▶ Document all lesions, giving descriptive location, size, shape, and color. Pay close attention to ecchymoses of varying colors and injuries that appear bilaterally.

▶ Use diagrams showing the location, size, and description.

▶ Photographs and radiographs can also be used to supplement findings. Photographs can only be made with patient consent and could be released only with consent. There may be special provisions by law that allow the taking and releasing of photographs without consent when the healthcare provider is required by law to report suspected abuse.

▶ Scale photography would be necessary for bite marks so further analysis can be done.

▶ Use the words *suspected abuse* if the patient denies abuse.

▶ Box 62-2 provides a sample of documenting suspected abuse during a patient visit.

 **EVERYDAY ETHICS**

Sarah, a young, usually vivacious patient in Dr. Stuart's practice for about 2 years, presents for a maintenance appointment with Amy, the dental hygienist. Since her previous appointment, Sarah had had a big wedding. Amy was expecting to hear about it and maybe even see pictures.

When Sarah came into the treatment room, she seemed very quiet and avoided eye contact with Amy. On completion of Sarah's oral assessment, the following was noted: Class II mobility on teeth numbers 6, 7, and 8; distoincisal edge fractures on 7 and 8; a 4-mm scar on the vermilion border of the upper lip. Sarah explained that she slipped and fell on a wet kitchen floor. She could not remember how she got the scar, which was not present 6 months ago. Amy is not sure that Sarah is telling the truth. She suspects Sarah may be in an abusive relationship with her new husband. There is not enough time to have a long discussion with Sarah or with Dr. Stuart, who is in the middle of a crown preparation procedure.

Questions for Consideration

1. Which of the dental hygiene Core Values (Table II in the Section II, Introduction) have application in this case? Explain the relationship of each dental hygiene core value you select.

2. Is this an ethical issue or an ethical dilemma for Amy? Why? Using the four-step framework in making ethical decisions in Box 1-10 in Chapter 1, develop a course of action that would assist Amy in resolving the issue.

3. How would Amy incorporate her suspicions about Sarah into her discussion of the oral assessment with Dr. Stuart?

 **BOX 62-2**

Example Documentation: Patient Injury Related to Suspected Abuse

S A 23-year-old female presents for an emergency visit because of pain in mandibular right second premolar area. Patient complains of recent headaches and pain in right temporomandibular joint area. She states "my boyfriend slapped me recently, but he has been under a lot of pressure lately and he didn't mean to bruise me." Patient seems nervous and agitated.

O –Patient presents with multiple contusions on right side of face above inferior border of mandible and right buccal mucosa. Bruises are in various stages of healing; red, purple, and greenish yellow. Bruises are oval shaped about 2–5 cm in size. Intraoral and extraoral photographs were taken.

A –Panoramic radiograph revealed a simple fracture on the body of the mandible below right second premolar area. Patient confirmed that injuries are likely related to partner abuse.

P –Reassured patient that she did not deserve the abuse and provided her with the National Domestic Violence Hotline number. Patient was referred to oral surgeon for evaluation of fractured mandible.

Next step: Follow-up telephone call to patient after her scheduled appointment with the oral surgeon.

Signed _____, RDH

Date _____

 Factors To Teach The Patient

Factors to Teach the Abused or Neglected Child

▷ The value of oral hygiene with age-appropriate materials.

▷ What the dental biofilm is on teeth, using disclosing agent.

▷ How to use the new toothbrush the child just received from the dental hygienist.

▷ Why it is especially important to brush the teeth and tongue just before going to sleep.

Factors to Teach the Abused Elder or Intimate Partner

▷ Where help can be obtained: emergency assistance including phone numbers and referrals.

▷ The tendency for the maltreatment to increase in severity and frequency over time.

▷ Battering is a choice. It is used to gain power and control over another individual.

References

1. Leeb RT, Paulozzi LJ, Melanson C, et al. *Child Maltreatment Surveillance: Uniform Definitions for Public Health and Recommended Data Elements* (Version 1.0). Atlanta, GA: Center for Disease Control and Prevention, National Center for Injury Prevention and Control; 2008. http://www.cdc.gov/violenceprevention/pub/cmp-surveillance.html. Accessed September 30, 2013.

2. Senn DR, McDowell JD, Alder ME. Dentistry's role in the recognition and reporting of domestic violence, abuse, and neglect. *Dent Clin North Am.* 2001;45(2):343–363.

3. American Academy of Pediatric Dentistry. Guideline on oral and dental aspects of child abuse and neglect. *Pediatr Dent.* 2008–2009;30(7, Suppl):86–89.

4. Dong X. Advancing the field of elder abuse: future directions and policy implications. *J Am Geriatr Soc.* 2012;60(11):2151–2156.

5. Cowen HJ, Cowen PS. Elder mistreatment: dental assessment and intervention. *Spec Care Dentist.* 2002;22(1):23–32.

6. Gondolf EW. *Theoretical and Research Support for the Duluth Model: A Reply to Dutton and Corvo.* Indiana, PA: Indiana University of Pennsylvania, Mid-Atlantic Addiction Training Institute; 2007. http://www.theduluthmodel.org/about/research.html. Accessed September 30, 2013.

7. Nelms AP, Gutmann ME, Solomon ES, et al. What victims of domestic violence need from the dental profession. *J Dent Educ.* 2009;73(4):490–498.

8. Oertling KM. Prevent Abuse and Neglect through Dental Awareness (P.A.N.D.A.). *LDA J.* 2003;62(1):16–17.

9. Hsieh NK, Herzig K, Gansky SA, et al. Changing dentists' knowledge, attitudes and behavior regarding domestic violence through an interactive multimedia tutorial. *J Am Dent Assoc.* 2006;137(5):596–603.

10. Virginia Department of Health. *Project RADAR.* Richmond, VA: Virginia Department of Health, Division of Prevention and Health Promotion; 2013. http://www.projectradarVA.com. Updated September 10, 2013. Accessed September 30, 2013.

11. Katner D, Brown C. Mandatory reporting of oral injuries indicating possible child abuse. *J Am Dent Assoc.* 2012;143(10):1087–1092.

ENHANCE YOUR UNDERSTANDING

thePoint® DIGITAL CONNECTIONS
(see the inside front cover for access information)
- **Audio glossary**
- **Quiz bank**

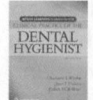

SUPPORT FOR LEARNING
(available separately; visit lww.com)
- *Active Learning Workbook for Clinical Practice of the Dental Hygienist, 12th Edition*

prepU INDIVIDUALIZED REVIEW
(available separately; visit lww.com)
- **Adaptive quizzing with *prepU for Wilkins' Clinical Practice of the Dental Hygienist***

63

The Patient with a Seizure Disorder

Katherine A. Woods, MPH, PhD, CRDH and Kathryn R. Davis, RDH, MS, DMD

CHAPTER OUTLINE

LEARNING OBJECTIVES

After studying this chapter, the student will be able to:

1. Define each of the terms associated with types of seizure disorders.

2. Describe the etiology of seizure disorders.

3. Discuss the clinical manifestations of seizure disorders.

4. Develop a dental hygiene care plan, including patient education prevention strategies, for working with patients who have seizure disorders.

5. Prepare a protocol for emergency care of a patient having a seizure.

A seizure is a paroxysmal event that results from abnormal brain activity. A seizure may involve loss of consciousness or awareness with or without convulsive movements or spasms. Epilepsy is a term to describe a group of functional disorders of the brain characterized by recurrent seizures. Seizures are a symptom of epilepsy.

▶ The patient's medical history may reveal a susceptibility to seizures. A complete evaluation is required in all cases.

▶ Treatment modalities of epilepsy and a seizure itself may affect the oral tissues and dental and dental hygiene treatment.

▶ Dental personnel need to be aware of the issues associated with seizures, know how to evaluate the patient, and how to apply emergency measures in and out of the dental office or clinic.

▶ Care of the oral cavity is necessary because of its relationship both to general health and to oral accidents that may occur during a seizure.

▶ All patients are advised by their physicians to live a moderate lifestyle and to pay strict attention to general health.

▶ Occupation and lifestyle may be limited for patients who have recurrent seizures. A person susceptible to seizures cannot participate in activities that may precipitate a seizure or provide hazards in the event of a seizure. Such limitations may lead to loss of driving privileges or loss of work and may lead to depression.

▶ According to the Center for Disease Control, there are 2.3 million adults and over 450,000 children in the United States who have recurrent seizures associated with epilepsy. The WHO estimates 50 million worldwide have epilepsy.[1,2]

- New cases are most common in children and in older adults.

▶ Box 63-1 contains key words used in this chapter.

SEIZURES

I. Seizure Definition

▶ A sudden paroxysmal electrical discharge of neurons in the brain.

▶ Results from a transient, uncontrolled alteration in brain function.

▶ Seizures are usually unprovoked, unpredictable, and involuntary.

▶ A seizure begins with an abrupt onset of symptoms that may be of a motor, sensory, cognitive, or emotional nature, depending on which brain cells are involved.

▶ As a seizure progresses, it may or may not cause loss of consciousness or awareness, tonic and/or clonic

movements, incontinence, saliva foaming, or tongue biting.

▶ Length of a seizure is uncontrollable.

▶ Other terms: convulsion, fit, spell, ictus.

II. Classification[3]

The syndromes associated with seizures are complex. The international classification of seizures is outlined in Box 63-2. Diagnosis of a seizure is made from the following:

▶ Clinical signs and symptoms

- A patient with a complex seizure disorder may exhibit a trancelike state with confusion that can last for a few minutes to hours.
- Consciousness is impaired to varying degrees.
- Patient may manifest purposeless movements or actions followed by confusion, incoherent speech, ill humor, unpleasant temper; does not remember what happened during the attack.

▶ History

▶ Electroencephalography

▶ Functional neuroimaging

▶ The syndromes have been classified by the following:

- Age-related onset
- Symptoms (vary with the type of seizure)
- Anatomic localization in the brain (temporal, frontal, parietal, or occipital lobes).

III. Types of Seizures

▶ The three basic types of seizures are *generalized*, *focal*, and those *of unknown origin*.

▶ A seizure of focal origin that involves only a part of the brain is called a partial seizure.

▶ A generalized seizure affects the entire brain at the same time.

A. Generalized Seizures

▶ Tonic–clonic

- Muscles of the chest and pharynx may contract at the same time, forcing air out and a sound known as the "epileptic cry."
- Loss of consciousness is sudden and complete; the patient becomes stiff and falls or may slide out of the dental chair.
- Musculature contraction: tonic phase tension with rigidity, clonic movements followed with intermittent muscular contraction and relaxation.
- Skin color turns pale to bluish, breathing is shallow or stops briefly.
- Possible loss of bladder, and rarely, bowel control.
- Tongue may be bitten.
- Incident usually lasts 1–3 minutes.
- Respiration returns.

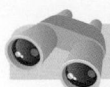

BOX 63-1 KEY WORDS: Seizure Disorders

Absence: a generalized seizure of sudden onset characterized by a brief period of unconsciousness. Formerly called *petit mal*.

Anticonvulsant: a drug that inhibits or suppresses convulsions.

Antiepileptic/antiseizure: a remedy for epilepsy and/or seizures.

Ataxia: failure of muscular coordination; irregularity of muscular action.

Atonic: relaxed; without normal tone or tension.

Aura: warning sensation felt by some people immediately preceding a seizure; may be flashes of light, dizziness, peculiar taste, or a sensation of prickling or tingling.

Automatism: involuntary motor activity, such as lip smacking or repeated swallowing.

Autonomic symptoms: pallor, flushing, sweating, pupillary dilation, cardiac arrhythmia, incontinence.

Clonic: alternate contraction and relaxation of muscle; *clonic phase* is the convulsion phase of a seizure.

Consciousness: degree of awareness and/or responsiveness of a person to externally applied stimuli.

Convulsion: violent spasm.

Cryptogenic: a disorder for which the cause is hidden or occult.

Diplopia: perception of two images of a single object; double vision.

Dyspepsia: impairment of the power or function of digestion.

Electroencephalography: the recording of changes in electric potentials in various areas of the brain by means of electrodes placed on the scalp or on/in the brain itself and connected to a computer, which records the brain's activity on a monitor or on paper as wavy lines; a clinical test used for partial diagnosis of epilepsy.

Epilepsy: brain disorder recognized after a patient has suffered two or more seizures.

Facies: expression or appearance of the face.

Grand mal: former name for a generalized or major seizure as contrasted with *petit mal*, a minor or relatively mild seizure.

Hirsutism: abnormal hairiness; excessive hair growth.

Hypertrichosis: excessive growth of hair.

Ictal: pertaining to or resulting from a stroke or a seizure.

Myoclonus: isolated or repetitive shocklike contractions of a muscle or group of muscles; adj., myoclonic.

Paresthesia: an abnormal sensation, such as burning, prickling, or tingling.

Paroxysm: sharp spasm or convulsion; sudden recurrence or intensification of symptoms.

Petit mal: attack or brief impairment of consciousness often associated with flickering of the eyelids and mild twitching of the mouth.

Postictal: is the altered state of consciousness experienced after a seizure.

Prodrome: a premonitory symptom; a symptom indicating the onset of a disease or condition; adj., prodromal.

Psychic: pertaining to the mind or psyche.

Refractory epilepsy: not readily yielding to basic treatment; usually with a single antiseizure drug.

Seizure: paroxysmal spell of transitory alteration in consciousness, motor activity, or sensory phenomenon; convulsion.

Spasm: sudden involuntary contraction of a muscle or group of muscles; may be tonic or clonic; may vary from small twitches to severe convulsions.

Status epilepticus: rapid succession of epileptic spasms without intervals of consciousness; life threatening; emergency care urgent.

Teratogenesis: production of deformity in the developing embryo.

Tonic: state of continuous, unremitting action of muscular contraction; patient appears stiff.

Tonic–clonic: in a seizure, a sudden sharp tonic contraction of muscles followed by clonic convulsive movements.

- Saliva, which previously could not be swallowed, may become mixed with air and appear as foam.
- Patient begins to recover, may be confused, tired, complain of muscle soreness or injury; may fall into a deep sleep.
- Phases of seizure may be called preictal, ictal, and postictal.
- Seizure may continue without recovery and progress to *status epilepticus*.

▶ Absence Seizure
- Loss of consciousness begins and ends abruptly in about 5–30 seconds.
- Most common in children, and might lead to learning difficulties if not identified.
- Patient has blank stare, usually does not fall, posture becomes fixed, may drop whatever is being held.

- May become pale.
- May have rhythmic twitching of eyelids, eyebrows, head, or chewing movements.
- Attack ends as abruptly as it begins. Patient quickly returns to full awareness, resumes activities, unaware of what occurred.

B. Focal Seizures

▶ Focal seizures involve only part of the brain.

C. Unknown Seizures

▶ Seizures of unknown origin include epileptic spasms.

IV. Etiology[3,4]

In addition to epilepsy, seizures can be a symptom of many different conditions. The causes can be genetic, structural/metabolic, or unknown.

BOX 63-2

International Classification of Seizures

Generalized

▷ Tonic–clonic (in any combination)
▷ Absence
  ▷ Typical
  ▷ Atypical
  ▷ Absence with special features
    • Myoclonic absence
    • Eyelid myoclonia
▷ Myoclonic
  ▷ Myoclonic
  ▷ Myoclonic atonic
  ▷ Myoclonic tonic
▷ Clonic
▷ Tonic
▷ Atonic

Focal Seizures

Unknown

▷ Epileptic spasms

Source: Reprinted with permission from International League Against Epilepsy, Commission on Classification and Terminology. Revised terminology and concepts for organization of seizures and epilepsies: report of the ILAE Commission on Classification and Terminology, 2005–2009. *Epilepsia.* 2010;51(4):676–685.

A. Genetic

Genetic predisposition to seizures or to other neurologic abnormalities for which seizure may be a symptom.

B. Structural/Metabolic

Seizures can arise during many neurologic and nonneurologic medical conditions, such as:

▶ Congenital conditions, such as maternal infection (rubella); toxemia of pregnancy
▶ Perinatal injuries
▶ Brain tumor
▶ Cerebrovascular disease (stroke)
▶ Trauma (head injury)
▶ Infection (meningitis, encephalitis, opportunistic infections of HIV)
▶ Degenerative brain disease
▶ Metabolic and toxic disorders, including lead exposure, alcoholism and other drug addictions; seizures are common during alcohol and/or drug withdrawal
▶ Complication of cancer.

C. Unknown Cause

▶ A neurological examination may diagnose the reason.

V. Prognosis[5]

▶ Prognosis for seizure control is good.
▶ Approximately 75% of patients become seizure free.
▶ Seizure disorders tend to be stable, and do not worsen over time.

VI. Implications

Owing to a possibility of severe injury, accidents, or embarrassment, patients who experience recurrent seizures may choose to avoid or be legally restricted from participating in certain activities. These may include:

▶ *Vocation*: occupations that involve use of machinery or require physical activity may not be an option.
▶ *Licenses*: certain licenses, such as driver's license, may be restricted until the patient is deemed to be seizure free.
▶ *Independent living*: living alone may not be advised due to health risks.

CLINICAL MANIFESTATIONS[6–8]

I. Precipitating Factors

A patient may have factors that precipitate a seizure. The patient or a caregiver may provide helpful information to prepare healthcare personnel to handle an emergency. Possible precipitating factors include the following:

▶ Psychological stress; apprehension
▶ Fatigue; sleep deprivation
▶ Sensory stimuli, such as flashing lights, noises, peculiar odors
▶ Use or withdrawal of alcohol or other addictive drugs
▶ Fever
▶ Noncompliance with anti-seizure medications
▶ Menstruation
▶ Physical exercise/physical trauma
▶ Neonatal conditions.

II. Aura

▶ The aura may be a special sensory stimulus, a sensation of numbness, tingling, twitching, or stiffness of certain muscles.
▶ Not all patients have a warning, or aura, before a seizure.
▶ A patient with a warning may seek a safe place to sit or lie down in privacy.
▶ In the dental environment, the patient can inform the personnel so that procedures can be terminated and brief preparations can be made.

III. Prevention of Seizures[9]

A patient may experience only one type of seizure or differing types. Seizures may be prevented through modification of behaviors that may include the following:

▶ Primary prevention of seizures involves avoiding brain injury through use of protective devices such as helmets.

▶ Secondary prevention involves early detection and compliance with recommended treatment.

▶ Tertiary prevention includes interventions that decrease precipitating factors that may trigger seizures encompassing education strategies for patients, caregivers, and healthcare practitioners.

TREATMENT[10–12]

I. Medications

Antiepileptic drug therapy is one method used to control seizures.

A. Choices

▶ Choice of therapy is related to type of seizure disorder and possibly to desired side effect or elimination of an undesirable side effect.

▶ Patients may be placed on one antiepileptic drug or a combination of several.

▶ Frequently prescribed medications are listed in Table 63-1.

B. Side Effects

▶ *Each* medication has side effects a patient may experience to varying degrees. It is necessary for patients to follow the directions for the use of antiseizure medications from the primary care provider.

▶ Side effects may include the following:

- Allergic reaction, rash
- Fatigue, drowsiness, weakness, ataxia, headache, slurred speech
- Nausea, vomiting
- Memory loss; behavioral and cognitive deficits
- Damage to liver, interactions of medications processed in liver
- Leukopenia: delayed healing and infection
- Thrombocytopenia or decreased platelet aggregation: increased bleeding, petechiae
- Osteoporosis
- Increased or unknown risk of birth defects
- Hirsutism; hypertrichosis
- Oral change of *gingival enlargement* most common with phenytoin
- Numerous drug interactions, including other antiepileptic drugs, acetaminophen, nonsteroidal anti-inflammatory drugs, erythromycins, and reduction in efficacy of *oral contraceptives*.

TABLE 63-1	Antiepileptic/Antiseizure Medications
GENERIC NAME	**BRAND NAME**
Older Medications	
Carbamazepine	Tegretol, carbatrol
Phenytoin	Dilantin
Valproic acid/valproate	Depakote
Phenobarbital	Luminal
Primidone	Mysoline
Ethosuximide	Zarontin
Clonazepam	Klonopin
Clorazepate	Tranxene
Newer Medications	
Felbamate	Felbatol
Gabapentin	Neurontin
Lamotrigine	Lamictal
Topiramate	Topamax
Tiagabine	Gabitril
Levetiracetam	Keppra
Oxcarbazepine	Trileptal
Zonisamide	Zonegran

▶ *Elderly and children*

- Both are more sensitive to side effects of weakness, unsteadiness, cognitive alterations.
- Elderly more likely to be on other medications with possible drug interactions and more likely to forget to take medications.

C. Precaution: Herbal Supplements[13]

▶ Certain over-the-counter herbal supplements are used as a self-medication to help prevent seizures. These supplements may interfere with the prescribed antiepileptic drug and cause serious complications.

▶ Patients are asked to inform their primary care provider and dental team when using.

▶ Herbal supplements such as ginkgo biloba, St. John's wart, and some essential oils may also affect dental treatment, for example, causing increased bleeding.

II. Surgery[14,15]

A variety of surgical interventions are available and indicated when epilepsy is refractory to traditional antiepileptic drug therapy. Surgical intervention has become more precise through the advances in identifying the epileptogenic area with magnetic resonance imaging, electroencephalographic studies, tomography, neuropsychological testing, and other analyses. Surgical options include:

▶ *Resection* of the epileptogenic area in the brain.

▶ If total resection leads to unacceptable deficits, *multiple subpial transections*, which are a series of small parallel slices, are removed.

▶ *Gamma-knife radiosurgery* involves delivery of a focused dose of radiation to the epileptogenic area in the brain. This technique reduces risk of infection, bleeding, and hospitalization.

▶ Vagus nerve stimulation utilizes a pacemaker-like device to deliver signals to the vagus nerve.
  • Research showed no adverse effects on patients with vagus nerve stimulators when using common electrical dental devices.[15]

III. Ketogenic Diet[16,17]

▶ The goal of the ketogenic diet is to induce fat metabolism and maintain ketosis through a diet high in fat and low in carbohydrates.

▶ The new diet is initiated after a starvation period, which induces fat metabolism and the production of ketones.

▶ The diet has been shown to be an effective treatment for patients with epilepsy, particularly children. However, care must be taken to make sure patients on a ketogenic diet are properly nourished.

ORAL FINDINGS[18]

▶ Seizures themselves produce no oral changes.

▶ Specific oral changes relate to:
  • Side effects of antiepileptic drugs or other therapy
  • Oral accidents during a seizure
  • Side effects of the epilepsy, such as depression leading to poor oral hygiene and neglect.

I. Traumatic Effects During Seizures

A. Scars of Lips and Tongue

▶ Oral tissues, particularly tongue, cheek, or lip, may be bitten.

▶ Scars may be observed during the extraoral/intraoral examination; cause may be differentiated from other types of healed wounds.

B. Fractured Teeth

▶ Teeth may be clamped and bruxing may be forceful enough to fracture teeth.

▶ Fractured teeth may be sharp and lacerate tissue and need to be smoothed or restored.

▶ Fractures may extend into pulp of a tooth, allowing bacterial infection; requires treatment with root canal therapy or extraction.

II. Gingival Overgrowth/Gingival Hyperplasia[19–21]

▶ Gingival overgrowth occurs in 25%–50% of persons using phenytoin for treatment.

▶ Other antiseizure drugs also induce gingival overgrowth less frequently.

▶ Phenytoin and the other antiseizure drugs have been used in the treatment of many conditions other than epilepsy, including stuttering, headaches, neuromuscular disturbances, and cardiac conditions; therefore, their use does not lead to an assumption that the patient has epilepsy.

▶ When related to phenytoin use, gingival enlargement may also be called Dilantin hyperplasia, diphenylhydantoin-induced hyperplasia, diphenylhydantoin gingival hyperplasia, Dilantin-induced gingival fibrosis, or phenytoin-induced hyperplasia.

A. Mechanism

▶ Phenytoin may cause fibroblasts and osteoblasts to deposit excessive extracellular matrix, causing gingival overgrowth.

▶ Tissue color and texture are generally within normal limits with lobular shape.

▶ Local irritants such as biofilm or ill-fitting appliances make response more excessive.

▶ Meticulous oral hygiene has been found to reduce the occurrence and severity of gingival overgrowth.

B. Occurrence

▶ Incidence is greater in younger patients than in older patients just beginning therapy.

▶ The gingiva may start to enlarge within a few weeks or even after a few years following the initial administration of the drug.

▶ The size of the dose and the length of treatment are not necessarily factors in the incidence or nature of the gingival enlargement.

▶ The anterior gingiva are usually more affected than are posterior, and maxillary more than mandibular.

▶ Facial and proximal areas: more affected than lingual and palatal areas.

▶ Although rare, an overgrowth of tissue may occur in an edentulous area and is usually associated with trauma, irritation from a denture, the presence of retained roots, or unerupted teeth.[22,23]

▶ Overgrowth of tissue surrounding dental implants can occur.[24]

C. Tissue Characteristics

▶ *Early clinical features*
- Overgrowth appears as a painless enlargement of interdental papillae with signs of inflammation.
- Eventually, the tissue becomes fibrotic, pink, and stippled, with a mulberry- or cauliflower-like appearance, as in Figure 63-1B.

▶ *Advanced lesion*
- Tissue increases in size, extends to include the marginal gingiva, and covers a large portion of the anatomic crown.
- Cleftlike grooves may occur between the lobules, as shown in Figure 63-1A.

▶ *Severe lesion*
- Large, bulbous gingiva may cover the enamel, tend to wedge the teeth apart, and interfere with mastication.
- Note the severe growth about the mandibular left canine to lateral incisor area in Figure 63-2.

▶ *Microscopic appearance*
- During therapy, phenytoin is present in the saliva, blood, gingival sulcus fluid, and dental biofilm.
- Number of fibroblasts and the amount of collagen in the connective tissue increases.
- Stratified squamous epithelium is thick, with long rete ridges.
- Inflammatory cells are in greatest abundance near the base of the pockets.

D. Effects[25]

▶ Poses dental biofilm control problem
▶ May affect mastication
▶ May alter tooth eruption
▶ May interfere with speech
▶ May cause serious esthetic concerns.

E. Complicating Factors

▶ Dental biofilm
- Biofilm appears to be the most significant determinant of the severity of phenytoin-induced gingival enlargement.[26]
- Adequate biofilm control, particularly if started before the administration of phenytoin, helps control the extent of gingival overgrowth.

▶ Contributing factors
- Mouth breathing.
- Overhanging and other defective restorations.

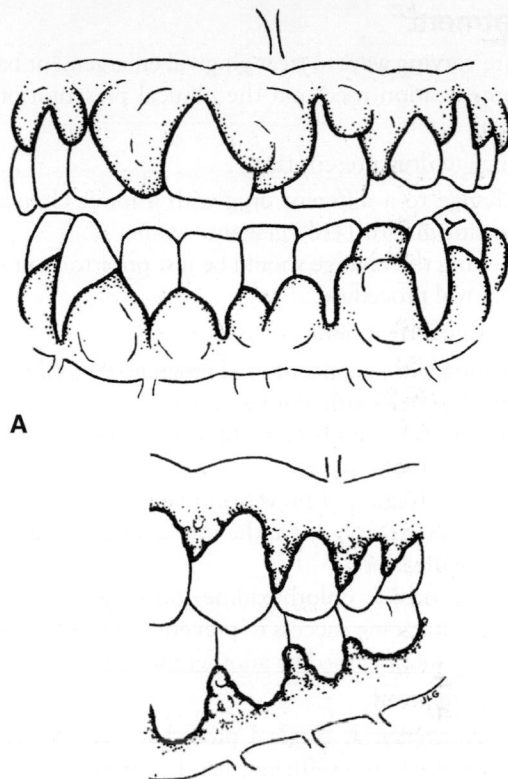

A

B

FIGURE 63-1 **Phenytoin-Induced Gingival Enlargement. A:** Papillary enlargement with cleftlike grooves. Note the effect of the pressure of the fibrotic tissue on the position of teeth. Maxillary incisors and the mandibular left canine have been wedged away from normal positions. **B:** Mulberrylike shape of interdental papillae.

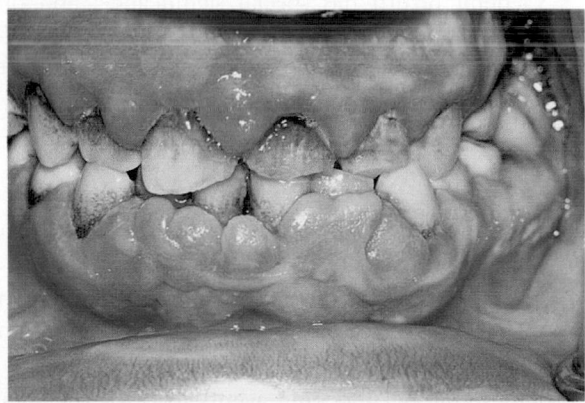

FIGURE 63-2 **Severe Phenytoin-Induced Gingival Enlargement.** Note extent of gingival overgrowth on lower left between canine and lateral incisor and presence of local irritants of biofilm, calculus, and stain. (Source: Reprinted with permission from Langlais RP, Miller CS. Section 5: Intraoral findings by color changes. In: *Color Atlas of Common Oral Diseases.* 3rd ed. Philadelphia, PA: Lippincott Williams & Wilkins; 2003:81.)

- Large carious lesions.
- Calculus and other biofilm-retaining factors encourage gingival overgrowth.
- Treatment must include removal of these factors by recontouring overhangs, placing or replacing restorations, and removing calculus.

F. Treatment[27]

There are varying ways to treat gingival enlargement based on the medication used and the clinical presentation of the lesion.

▶ Change in drug prescription
  • Change to a different drug with a lower chance of causing gingival enlargement.
  • Making the change should be just prior to a surgical removal procedure.
▶ Nonsurgical treatment
  • Scaling with a concentrated program of biofilm control may help early lesions regress.
  • Where tissue has become fibrotic, shrinkage cannot be expected.
  • Start a program of prevention and control prior to, or simultaneously with, the initial administration of the medication.
  • About 0.12% chlorhexidine gluconate rinses are used with some success to prevent return of gingival enlargement caused by another medication.[28,29]
▶ Surgical removal
  • *Gingivectomy*: A surgical procedure used for tissue removal when a sufficient band of attached gingiva exists.
  • A *periodontal flap procedure*: may be the choice for healing and esthetics.
  • Prior to surgery, a regulated program of biofilm control is introduced and continued after surgical dressings have been removed.
  • General health has special significance, and oral health contributes to general health.
  • Meticulous oral hygiene is required to minimize gingival overgrowth.

G. Differential Diagnosis of Medications Causing Gingival Enlargement[30]

Numerous medications may cause gingival enlargement, including:

▶ Antiseizure medications, especially phenytoin and to a lesser extent ethosuximide, valproic acid, and primidone.
▶ Calcium channel blocking agents used for the treatment of hypertension and other diseases.
▶ Immunosuppressant cyclosporin used frequently with organ transplant patients. Tacrolimus may be a substitute with less occurrence of gingival overgrowth.

DENTAL HYGIENE CARE PLAN[31]

▶ The majority of patients with epilepsy or a history of seizure can and need to receive the same level of dental care as the general population.
▶ The dental hygienist works in collaboration with the patient's other healthcare providers.

• The patient with a seizure disorder may be under the care of other specialists including a neurologist, social worker, and primary care physician.

I. Patient History

▶ Most patients with epilepsy have regular, thorough medical examinations.
▶ Contact the primary care provider when the patient is unable to provide needed information, is noncompliant, if seizure activity has increased or changed, or if treatment for epilepsy is impacting the patient's oral health.
▶ Patients with autism may present with social, communication, and/or behavioral problems, in addition to seizure disturbances.[32,33]
▶ A well-controlled patient with epilepsy may still be at risk to have a seizure.
▶ For seizure-prone patients: advise wearing medical alert jewelry.

II. Information to Obtain

Information to obtain from a patient with a history of seizures is listed in Box 63-3.

III. Patient Approach

▶ Provide a calm, reassuring atmosphere and treat with patience and empathy.
▶ Use a motivational interviewing approach to patient education, enabling patients to be partners in decision making (see Chapter 26).
▶ Encourage self-expression, particularly if the patient tends to be quiet and withdrawn and has narrowed interests.
▶ Recognize possible impairment of memory when reviewing personal oral care procedures.
▶ Help the patient develop an interest in caring for the mouth; commend all little successes.
▶ Drugs used in treatment tend to make the patient drowsy, and chronic illness sufferers tend to have more frequent health issues that interfere with appointments.
▶ Be understanding when the patient is late or misses an appointment; plan telephone reminders at opportune time; do not mistake drowsiness (effect of drugs) for inattentiveness.

IV. Care Plan: Instrumentation

▶ All patients need to be instructed and motivated to comply with an effective biofilm control program.
▶ Complete removal of all deposits on teeth, and thorough nonsurgical periodontal therapy is essential for patients who plan to or are taking an antiseizure medication such as phenytoin, which may cause gingival overgrowth.

BOX 63-3

Risk Assessment for Dental Hygiene Treatment: Information to Obtain from Patient With a History of a Seizure Disorder

Basic Information

▷ Thorough medical history review, including date of last physical examination, other medical conditions or risk factors present
▷ Physician: name and phone number
▷ Emergency contact person and phone number

Additional Factors

▷ Inquire about recent illness, stress, alcohol use, menstrual cycle, fatigue, or pain as factors that may provoke a seizure.
▷ General well-being; refer for evaluation for any signs or symptoms of other conditions such as depression.
▷ Ask if the patient had to change any aspect of their activities of daily living.

Treatment

▷ Medications, surgery, or diet
▷ Effectiveness of seizure control treatment
▷ Investigate each medication for possible interaction with proposed dental treatment and side effects
▷ Nonprescription, herbal supplement use
▷ Adherence to prescribed treatment; medications taken on schedule

About the Seizures

▷ Type of seizure(s) experienced, severity, and duration of episodes
▷ Age at onset
▷ The precipitating factors or cause of seizure if known
▷ Frequency of seizures
▷ Description of prodrome, aura if known
▷ Experience alteration or loss of consciousness
▷ Characteristic motor movements
▷ Urinary/fecal incontinence
▷ History of injuries, including oral injuries, broken teeth, tongue lacerations
▷ Postictal symptoms such as confusion

Suggestions

▷ Any other helpful information that may be provided by patient for comfort and management

A. Prior to and at the Start Appointments for Patients Treated with Phenytoin Therapy

▶ A rigorous biofilm control program and complete scaling are introduced in preparation for phenytoin therapy.
▶ The patient (and caregivers) can be helped to understand that, with controlled oral hygiene and emphasis on all phases of prevention, gingival overgrowth can be prevented to a large degree.

B. Initial Appointment Series for the Patient Treated with Phenytoin

Weekly appointments for complete biofilm control instruction and scaling are planned with the following objectives:

1. *Slight or mild gingival overgrowth*
   - Nonsurgical treatment, including frequent thorough scalings, can be expected to lead to tissue reduction, provided the patient cooperates in daily biofilm control.
   - Frequent continuing care appointments can contribute to function and comfort with minimum periodontal involvement.

2. *Moderate gingival overgrowth*
   - After the initial series of weekly biofilm instruction and scalings, re-evaluation of the tissue can determine whether further treatment is needed.
   - An optimum level of oral health may be attained by changing the medication to another antiseizure drug, using surgical removal of excess tissue, and frequent continuing care appointments.

3. *Severe fibrotic overgrowth*
   - Initial scaling and biofilm control are provided to prepare the mouth for surgical tissue removal.
   - Plans for changing the drug or altering the dose can be discussed with the patient's physician.

C. Continuing Care Intervals

▶ Frequent appointments on a 1-, 2-, or 3-month schedule are indicated, depending on the severity of the gingival enlargement and the ability and motivation of the patient to maintain the oral health.
▶ Most patients need continuing assistance and supervision.

V. Care Plan: Prevention

▶ Daily biofilm removal and fluoride therapy, the use of pit and fissure sealants, and dietary control.
▶ Initiation of preventive measures as soon as possible after the disorder has been diagnosed contributes to the overall health and well-being.

EMERGENCY CARE[34–36]

I. Objectives

A. Prevent body injury and accidents related to the oral structures, such as:
   - Tongue bite
   - Broken or dislocated teeth
   - Dislocated or fractured jaw
   - Broken fixed or removable dentures.
B. Ensure adequate ventilation.

II. Differential Diagnosis of Seizure[37]

▶ Syncope

▶ Migraine headache

▶ Transient ischemic attack

▶ Cerebrovascular accident, stroke

▶ Sleep disorder such as narcolepsy

▶ Movement disorders such as dyskinesia, common, for example, in patients with cerebral palsy or multiple sclerosis

▶ Overdose of local anesthetic

▶ Hypoglycemia or insulin overdose in a patient with diabetes

▶ Hyperventilation.

III. Preparation for Appointment

When the patient's medical history indicates susceptibility to seizures, advance preparation may prevent complications should a seizure occur.

▶ Place emergency materials in a convenient location.

▶ Have patient remove dentures for duration of appointment.

▶ Provide a calm and reassuring atmosphere.

▶ Have other dental personnel available in case of an emergency.

IV. Emergency Procedure

The dental clinic or office team has assigned responsibilities during any emergency. Initiation of procedures for seizure emergency follows preplanned routines.

▶ Make no attempt to stop the convulsion or restrain the patient.

▶ Terminate clinical procedure; call for assistance.

▶ Protect the patient from injury.

- Position patient: lower chair and tilt to supine; raise feet.
- Keep patient from falling out of dental chair.
- Push aside sharp objects, movable equipment, and instrument trays.
- Loosen tight belt, collar, necktie.
- Do *not* place (or force) anything between the teeth.
- Establish airway; check for breathing obstruction; provide basic life support when indicated. Place on side recovery position. Use high-speed suction with wide tip to remove vomit.
- Monitor vital signs.
- Stay beside the patient to prevent personal injury and reassure.
- Check for level of consciousness and determine if emergency medical assistance is required.
- When seizure is still occurring or has recurred within 5 minutes, activate emergency medical system.

BOX 63-4

Example Documentation: The Patient with a Seizure Disorder

S –Steve, a healthy appearing 55-year-old man presents for the first of four scheduled periodontal scaling appointments. He stated he recently had a seizure at work when he felt his arms and legs stiffen and he felt confused. When pressed for more information, he stated that he had seen a physician for the seizure. He also states that he will be losing his job in 1 month and has started looking for another.

O –Vitals normal (see medical profile). No chief complaint, other than being upset due to impending job loss. Reassessed medical profile—added Tegretol; no other medications are taken. Noticed rash on left side of patient's neck. Patient stated the rash began when antiseizure medication was added. Contacted physician for advice on patient care postseizure; physician recommended longer appointments to account for frequent breaks during treatment and for patient to call concerning rash. Intraoral assessment reveals generalized 4–5 mm pocketing on posterior teeth. No gingival enlargement found.

A –Increased risk for potential emergency situation during appointment until seizure disorder is stabilized. Need for use of stress-reduction protocols and extension of treatment time during patient visit. Potential for side effects of new medication, including current skin rash.

P –Patient Education—Discussed potential side effects of medications for treatment of seizures. Recommended patient check with medical provider about skin rash on neck. Provided patient with information from the Epilepsy Foundation, also on local stress-reduction and exercise classes.

Oral self-care—Discussed need for meticulous oral hygiene to avoid gingival enlargement. Showed patient how to perform an intraoral examination to check for gingival enlargement and possible areas of trauma should he experience another seizure.

Treatment provided—Asked patient to verbalize any discomfort or uneasiness he may have during treatment. Completed debridement with hand and ultrasonic instruments using high-speed evacuation on quadrant one with no adverse reaction to additional sounds or light. Patient tolerated treatment well but required frequent breaks to relax and reduce stress.

Next visit: Assess tissue response to quadrant one debridement; reassess plaque score and home care technique, modify as needed. Assess skin condition and determine whether patient contacted his physician. Monitor stress-reduction progress.

Signed _____, RDH

Date _____

EVERYDAY ETHICS

Lillian, the dental hygienist, just finished treating her last patient of the day. Diana, the patient, is a very pleasant woman with excellent oral health and a history of a car accident with concussion over a month ago. She has no other medical findings. While passing the window, Lillian notices that Diana has collapsed in the parking lot and is convulsing. She calls for assistance from the dentist and dental assistant, and they rush out to the parking lot. By the time they reach Diana, she is getting to her feet and says she just tripped and fell.

Individuals with seizures may have their driver's license revoked because of the potential for serious automobile accidents that may occur during a seizure. Diana is about to get into her car to drive home.

Questions for Consideration

1. Which of the dental hygiene ethical core values have application in this scenario?

2. Given the patient's medical history, will this information be documented in Diana's dental record, remain confidential, or be otherwise handled? To evaluate one's responsibilities towards self, one's patients, and others, read over, in the Codes of Ethics (Appendices I–IV) professional responsibilities to help Lillian decide the correct procedure.

3. Describe the rights of the patient and also the professional duties of the dental hygienist who witnessed the incident.

V. Postictal Phase

▶ Document the emergency situation as described in Figure 8-1 (Chapter 8).

▶ Allow the patient to rest.

▶ Talk to the patient in a quiet, reassuring tone. Ask onlookers to leave the patient in privacy.

▶ Check oral cavity for trauma to teeth or tissues. Palliative care can be administered. When a tooth is broken, the piece must be located so that aspiration is prevented.

▶ Contact the patient's family/friend to accompany the patient if requested.

VI. Status Epilepticus

▶ Status epilepticus is defined as one or more seizures lasting more than 30 minutes.

▶ The prolonged seizure may not end spontaneously; brain injury may occur and result in long-term morbidity or death.

▶ Generally, a seizure lasting more than 5 minutes should be considered to progress to status epilepticus unless emergency intervention is taken.

▶ Emergency medical assistance is sought immediately, and the patient is transported to an emergency department.

▶ Basic life support provided if necessary (see Chapter 8).

DOCUMENTATION

The patient who is subject to seizures will need complete permanent records that show the following:

▶ Complete health history, vital signs, radiographs, findings of the extra- and intraoral examination;

periodontal history, charting, and tissue description; dental caries history, charting, and current demineralization and carious lesions.

▶ Progress notes for each appointment with abbreviated history and current clinical findings.

▶ Information about the type of seizure; the treatment the patient is receiving; how to handle in an emergency.

▶ A sample progress note may be reviewed in Box 63-4.

Factors To Teach The Patient

▷ Relationship of systemic health to oral health.

▷ Importance of careful daily care of mouth.

▷ Need for providing complete medical history information for dental appointments.

▷ Antiseizure medication side effects, including gingival enlargement and how to minimize its growth.

▷ Seek immediate care if any oral change or injury is suspected.

References

1. Azanzini G, Beghi E, de Boer H, et al. Epilepsy. In: *Neurological Disorders: Public Health Challenges*. Geneva: World Health Organization; 2006:14. http://www.who.int/mental health/neurology/chapter 3 a neuro disorders public h challenges.pdf. Accessed July 29, 2013.

2. *Fact sheet: Epilepsy*. Geneva: World Health Organization; 2012. http://www.who.int/mediacentre/factsheets/fs999/en. Accessed July 29, 2013.

3. Berg AT, Berkovic SF, Brodie MJ, et al. Revised terminology and concepts for organization of seizures and epilepsies: report of the ILAE Commission on Classification and Terminology, 2005–2009. *Epilepsia*. 2010;51(4):676–685.

4. Centers for Disease Control and Prevention. Epilepsy in adults and access to care—United States, 2010. In: *Morbidity and Mortality Weekly Report*. Atlanta, GA: Centers for Disease Control and Prevention; 2012:5. http://www.cdc.gov/mmwr/preview/mmwrhtml/mm6145a2.htm?s cid=mm6145a2_w. Accessed July 28, 2013.

5. Brodie M, de Boer HM, Johannessen SI. Epidemiology. *Epilepsia*. 2003;44(6, Suppl):17.

6. Fattal-Valevski A, Nissan N, Kramer U, et al. Seizures as the clinical presenting symptom in children with brain tumors. *J Child Neurol*. 2012;28(3):292–296.

7. Nakken KO, Solaas MH, Kjeldsen MJ, et al. Which seizure-precipitating factors do patients with epilepsy most frequently report? *Epilepsy Behav*. 2006;6(1):85–89.

8. Balamurugan E, Aggarwal M, Lamba A, et al. Perceived trigger factors of seizures in persons with epilepsy. *Seizure*. 2013;22(9):743–747.

9. Dua T, Janca A, Kale R, et al. Public health principles and neurological disorders. In: *Neurological Disorders: Public Health Challenges*. Geneva: World Health Organization; 2006:20. http://www.who.int/mental_health/neurology/chapter1_neuro_disorders_public_h_challenges.pdf. Accessed July 29, 2013.

10. Schoenberg MR, Frontera AT, Bozorg A, et al. An update on epilepsy. *Expert Rev Neurother*. 2011;11(5):639–645.

11. Guncu G, Caglayan F, Dincel A, et al. Plasma and gingival crevicular fluid phenytoin concentrations as risk factors for gingival overgrowth. *J Periodontol*. 2006;77(12):2005–2010.

12. Burneo JG, McLachlan RS. When should surgery be considered for the treatment of epilepsy? *Can Med Assoc J*. 2005;172(9):1175–1177.

13. Li Q, Chen X, He L, et al. Traditional Chinese medicine for epilepsy. *Cochrane Database Syst Rev*. 2009;(3):CD006454.

14. Nguyen DK, Spencer SS. Recent advances in the treatment of epilepsy. *Arch Neurol*. 2003;60(7):929–935.

15. Roberts HW. The effect of electrical dental equipment on a vagus nerve stimulator's function. *J Am Dent Assoc*. 2002;133(12):1657–1664.

16. Guerrini R. Epilepsy in children. *Lancet*. 2006;367 (9509):499–524.

17. Keene DL. A systematic review of the use of the ketogenic diet in childhood epilepsy. *Pediatr Neurol*. 2006;35(1):1–5.

18. Pette GA, Siegel MA, Parker WB. Gingival enlargement. *J Am Dent Assoc*. 2011;142(11):1265–1268.

19. Angelopolous AP, Goaz PW. Incidence of diphenylhydantoin gingival hyperplasia. *Oral Surg Oral Med Oral Pathol*. 1972;34(6):898–906.

20. Rees TD, Levine RA. Systematic drugs as a risk factor for periodontal disease initiation and progression. *Compendium*. 1995;16(1):20, 22, 26 passim; quiz 42.

21. Hassell TM, ed. *Epilepsy and the Oral Manifestations of Phenytoin Therapy*. London: Karger; 1981:116–127. (Huysmans MC, Lussi A, Weber HP, eds. Monographs in Oral Science; vol 9).

22. Bredfeldt GW. Phenytoin-induced hyperplasia found in edentulous patients. *J Am Dent Assoc*. 1992;123(6):61–64.

23. McCord JF, Sloan P, Hussey DJ. Phenytoin hyperplasia occurring under complete dentures: a clinical report. *J Prosthet Dent*. 1992;68(4):569–572.

24. Chee WW, Jansen CE. Phenytoin hyperplasia occurring in relation to titanium implants: a clinical report. *Int J Oral Maxillofac Implants*. 1994;9(1):107–109.

25. Camargo PM, Melnick PR, Pirih FQ, et al. Treatment of drug-induced gingival enlargement: aesthetic and functional considerations. *Periodontol 2000*. 2001;27:131–138.

26. Majola MP, McFadyen ML, Connolly C, et al. Factors influencing phenytoin-induced gingival enlargement. *J Clin Periodontol*. 2000;27(7):506–512.

27. Mavrogiannis M, Ellis JS, Thomason JM, et al. The management of drug-induced gingival overgrowth. *J Clin Periodontol*. 2006;33(6):434–439.

28. Saravia ME, Svirsky JA, Friedman R. Chlorhexidine as an oral hygiene adjunct for cyclosporine-induced gingival hyperplasia. *ASDC J Dent Child*. 1990;57(5):366–370.

29. Pilatti GL, Sampaio JE. The influence of chlorhexidine on the severity of cyclosporin A—induced gingival overgrowth. *J Periodontol*. 1997;68(9):900–904.

30. Jaiarj N. Drug-induced gingival overgrowth. *J Mass Dent Soc*. 2003;52(3):16–20.

31. Mehmet Y, Senem O, Sülün T, et al. Management of epileptic patients in dentistry. *Surg Sci*. 2012;3:47–52.

32. Friedlander AH, Yagiela JA, Paterno VI, et al. The neuropathology, medical management and dental implications of autism. *J Am Dent Assoc*. 2006;137(11):1517–1527.

33. Rada RE. Controversial issues in treating the dental patient with autism. *J Am Dent Assoc*. 2010;141(8):947–953.

34. Malamed SF. Knowing your patients. *J Am Dent Assoc*. 2010;141 (Suppl 1):3S–7S.

35. Reed KL. Basic management of medical emergencies: recognizing a patient's distress. *J Am Dent Assoc*. 2010;141 (Suppl 1):20S–24S.

36. Panayiotis PN, Spanaki MV, Mirski MA. Status epilepticus: an update. *Curr Neurol Neurosci Rep*. 2013;13(7):1–9.

37. Shneker BF, Fountain NB. Epilepsy. *Dis Mon*. 2003;49(7):426–478.

ENHANCE YOUR UNDERSTANDING

thePoint° DIGITAL CONNECTIONS
(see the inside front cover for access information)
- Audio glossary
- Quiz bank

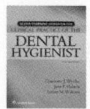

SUPPORT FOR LEARNING
(available separately; visit lww.com)
- *Active Learning Workbook for Clinical Practice of the Dental Hygienist, 12th Edition*

prepU INDIVIDUALIZED REVIEW
(available separately; visit lww.com)
- Adaptive quizzing with *prepU for Wilkins' Clinical Practice of the Dental Hygienist*

64

The Patient with a Mental Health Disorder

Linda D. Boyd, RDH, RD, EdD, Esther M. Wilkins, BS, RDH, DMD

CHAPTER OUTLINE

LEARNING OBJECTIVES

After studying this chapter, the student will be able to:

1. Describe the various types of mental health disorders and major symptoms.

2. Summarize the side effects of treatment for mental health disorders that may have oral health implications.

3. Explain dental hygiene treatment considerations for each major category of mental health disorder.

OVERVIEW OF MENTAL DISORDERS

A psychiatric or mental health disorder is a complex, clinically significant behavioral or psychological syndrome that may impact the individual's ability to engage in daily activities of living. The causes may be related to behavioral, psychologic, or biologic dysfunction in the individual.[1]

▶ The American Psychiatric Association has classified more than 200 types of mental disorders in the document *Diagnostic and Statistical Manual of Mental Disorders (DSM-5)*.[1]

▶ Each disorder has characteristic signs and symptoms.

▶ Terminology related to the disorders is listed and defined in Box 64-1.

▶ This chapter includes descriptions of common mental disorders including: anxiety, mood, and eating disorders along with schizophrenia.

• Additional disorders are described in other chapters, for example, alcoholism (see Chapter 65), Alzheimer's disease (see Chapter 53), autism spectrum disorder and attention deficit disorder (see Chapter 61), and dementia due to Parkinson's disease (see Chapter 59).

▶ With the current policies of deinstitutionalization, more individuals with mental disorders are seeking dental and dental hygiene care in dental offices and clinics.

▶ *Person first language* is used to refer to someone with a mental disorder, chronic disease, or disability.[2] The person is emphasized first and not the disorder, disease, or disability.

• For example, refer to the patient as "an individual with schizophrenia," not as "a schizophrenic."

I. Prevalence of Mental Disorders[3]

▶ In a meta-analysis of 175 studies in 63 countries, 1 in 5 respondents met the criteria for a common mental disorder in the previous year.

• About 29% of respondents had experienced a mental disorder during their lifetime.

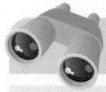

BOX 64-1   KEY WORDS: Mental Disorders

Affect: emotion or feeling; tone of reaction to persons and events.

Agitation: excessive motor activity, usually not purposeful and associated with internal tension.

Anxiolytic medication: ability to relieve anxiety or emotional tension, also called antianxiety agent.

Bradykinesia: abnormal slowness of movement; sluggish physical and mental responses.

Catatonia: no voluntary movement; physical rigidity; fixed position may be maintained for hours.

Cognitive: mental process of comprehension, judgment, memory.

Compensatory behavior: behavior meant to relieve guilt or anxiety over eating.

Decompensate: appearance or exacerbation of a mental disorder which may include hallucinations, delusion, violent or bizarre behavior.

Delusion: false belief firmly held, although contradicted by social reality.

Dementia: loss of cognitive and intellectual functions sufficiently severe to interfere with social and occupational functioning.

Dysarthria: impairment in uttering words due to diseases that affect oral and pharyngeal muscles.

Dysguesia: changes in sense of taste.

Electroconvulsive therapy (ECT): electroshock therapy; a form of somatic therapy in which an electric current is used to produce convulsions; primarily used to treat depression.

Euphoria: feeling of well-being; in psychiatry, abnormal or exaggerated sense of well-being.

Hallucination: false sensory perception in the absence of an actual external stimulus.

Illusion: a mental impression derived from misinterpretation of an actual sensory stimulus; a false perception.

Insomnia: wakefulness; inability to sleep in the absence of noise or other disturbance.

Lanugo: fine, downy hair.

Neurosis: a mental disorder that usually involves the use of unconscious defense mechanisms as a means of coping; individual is not out of touch with reality.

Noncompliance: failure to carry out prescribed healthcare plan, for example, failure to take medications as prescribed.

Paranoia: mental disorder characterized by delusions of persecution.

Perimylolysis: erosion of enamel and dentin as a result of chemical and mechanical effects.

Phobia: persistent, unrealistic pathologic fear or dread out of proportion to the stimulus from a particular object or situation.

Prodrome: a premonitory symptom; a symptom indicating the onset of disease.

Psychosis: a significant major mental disorder that so greatly impairs perception, thinking, emotional response, and/or personal orientation that the individual loses touch with reality.

Psychotherapy: treatment of emotional, behavioral, personality, and psychiatric disorders by means of individual or group verbal or nonverbal communication with the patient.

Psychotropic medication: a medication that alters the mind; the major categories are antipsychotic, antianxiety, antidepressant, and antimanic agents.

Tardive dyskinesia: involuntary movements of the mouth, lips, tongue, and jaws, usually associated with long-term use of antipsychotic medication.

- Women had higher rates of mood and anxiety disorders while men had higher rates of substance abuse disorders.
- English-speaking countries had the highest lifetime prevalence of mental disorders with North and South East Asia among the lowest reported prevalence.

ANXIETY DISORDERS

▶ Anxiety disorders are the most common class of mental disorders in the general population.
- Anxiety disorders are common with a global prevalence of around 7%.
- Euro/Anglo countries having prevalence over 10%, suggesting 1 in 10 people have an anxiety disorder.[4]

▶ Anxiety is a normal reaction to stress.
- In anxiety disorders, the anxiety is exaggerated resulting in excess worry and avoidance behavior that can impact day-to-day functioning.
- For formal diagnosis, the symptoms must be present for at least 6 months.[1]

▶ Some individuals may have secondary problems of alcohol and other substance abuse.
- The abuse may be the result of an attempt at self-medication.

▶ Individuals with anxiety disorders often have comorbid conditions including hypertension, gastrointestinal issues, thyroid disease, cardiovascular conditions, migraine headaches, allergies, and/or a respiratory disease.[5]

I. Types and Symptoms of Anxiety Disorders

A. Generalized Anxiety Disorder[6,7]

▶ Persistent, pervasive anxiety and excessive worry, but are not associated with life-threatening fears or "attacks."

▶ May be complicated by depression, alcohol abuse, or anxiety related to a general medical condition.

▶ Symptoms include:
- Startle easily
- Difficulty falling and staying asleep
- Difficulty concentrating
- Muscle tension

B. Obsessive-Compulsive Disorder (OCD)[8]

▶ Frequent upsetting thoughts (obsessions) and when the individual tries to control them there is an overwhelming urge (compulsion) to repeat routines or rituals over and over.

▶ Symptoms include:
- Spend at least 1 hour a day with obsessive thoughts and rituals that cause distress and interfere with normal daily functioning.

- Thoughts or obsessions might include fear of germs, dirt, or intruders.
- Rituals might include washing hands, locking and unlocking doors, keeping unneeded items (hoarding).

C. Panic Disorder[9]

▶ Panic disorder is characterized by sudden and repeated episodes of extreme fear (panic attacks).

▶ Symptoms center on panic attacks:
- A panic attack may be unexpected (uncued) or "situationally bound" (cued). A situationally bound panic attack invariably results from exposure to a specific trigger.
- Fear of being out of control during a panic attack.
- Physical symptoms during an attack may include: pounding or racing heart, sweating, difficulty breathing, chest pain, or dizziness (Box 64-2).

D. Posttraumatic Stress Disorder (PTSD)

▶ PTSD develops after a terrifying ordeal involving physical harm or threat of physical harm.[10]
- Onset may be triggered by destruction to the home or family or may result from a manmade disaster, such as war, imprisonment, torture, rape, physical or sexual abuse, or other exposure associated with intense fear or serious threat to life.

▶ Signs and symptoms include:
- Flashbacks of the traumatic experience and terror may be triggered by a stimulus that can be readily associated with the original event.
- Dreams or recollections may cause the individual to feel they are reliving the event.
- Avoidance of places, events, or objects that are reminders of the triggering event.

BOX 64-2

Symptoms of Panic Attack

▷ Shortness of breath
▷ Dizziness, unsteady feelings, or faintness
▷ Palpitations or accelerated heart rate
▷ Trembling or shaking
▷ Sweating (clammy hands)
▷ Choking
▷ Nausea or abdominal stress
▷ Parasthesia (numbness or tingling sensation)
▷ Flushes (hot flashes) or chills
▷ Chest pain or discomfort
▷ Fear of dying
▷ Fear of losing control

Source: American Psychiatric Association. *Diagnostic and Statistical Manual of Mental Disorders* (DSM-5). Washington, DC: American Psychiatric Association; 2013:214.

- Loss of interest in activities that were enjoyable in the past.
- Hyperarousal symptoms including: feeling tense, difficulty sleeping, angry outbursts, and may be easily startled.
- In children, symptoms may be slightly different and include: bedwetting, acting out the scary event during playtime, or being unusually clingy to a parent or other adult.

II. Treatment[5,7,11,12]

A. Basic Therapeutic Approach

▶ Lifestyle modifications include regular physical activity, adequate sleep, and avoidance of drugs and alcohol.
▶ Diagnose and treat other medical and psychiatric problems.

B. Pharmacologic Treatment

▶ *Antidepressants*: Antidepressants preferred as an initial treatment of anxiety disorders.
- Examples include: fluoxetine (Prozac), paroxetine (Paxel), and sertraline (Zoloft).
- Side effects: headache, weight gain, tremor, irritability, and xerostomia.
▶ *Anxiolytics*: These are used only short term because of the risk of dependency.
- Examples include: benzodiazipines (Valium, lorazepam). These are highly addictive and must be carefully monitored.
- Side effects: confusion, dizziness, muscle memory impairment, weakness, difficulty in speaking, skin rash, and xerostomia.
▶ *Atypical antipsychotics*: not a first choice for treatment.
- Examples include: risperidone (Risperdol).
- Side effects: weight gain, diabetes, sedative effects.
▶ Anticonvulsants:
- Examples: gabapentin and carbamazepine.
- Side effects: weight gain, tremor, sleep problems.

B. Psychotherapy

▶ Cognitive Behavioral Therapy (CBT)
- CBT is a combination of strategies to address the cognitive, behavioral, and emotional components of the anxiety disorder.
- May be conducted in individual or group sessions.
- Support groups are also helpful.

III. Dental Hygiene Care

A. Personal Factors

▶ Each anxiety disorder has its own characteristics.
▶ Relationships with other people can be strained.
▶ Physical complaints, such as rapid heartbeat, hyperventilation, tightness in the throat, and constant fatigue, are common.

B. Oral Implications

▶ Xerostomia related to medications put the patient at high risk for dental caries.
▶ Individuals with a diagnosis of an anxiety disorder are at 25% higher risk of tooth loss than individuals without an anxiety disorder.[13]
▶ The odds for periodontal disease in a patient with panic disorder is three times that of someone without the disorder.[14]
▶ A patient with OCD may perform such excessive, vigorous toothbrushing that gingival and dental abrasion may result.

C. Appointment Interventions

▶ Review medical history and medications carefully.
▶ Enhance the patient's sense of control.[15]
- One technique is to establish a "stop signal," which may consist of the patient raising the left hand when they are uncomfortable or need to stop treatment.
- Explain each step to the patient and keep communication as open as possible.
▶ Cognitive distraction involves encouraging the patient to think about something besides the dental treatment.
- Headphones for music and relaxation can help to reduce stress.
▶ Environmental changes can help to reduce anxiety.
- An example would be the smell of lavender in the waiting room to relax the patient, but this needs to be used in addition to the previously mentioned techniques.
▶ Nitrous oxide sedation may be helpful to relax the patient (see Chapter 38).
▶ Effective pain control is needed.
- Use local anesthesia for nonsurgical periodontal therapy (NSPT).
- Attention to technique to minimize discomfort is essential.
▶ Appointments are best scheduled in the morning; eliminate unnecessary waiting in the reception area; length of appointment can be minimized and planned to prevent stress.
▶ Be alert to symptoms of a panic attack (Box 64-2), such as sweating or hyperventilation. Allow the patient to sit up and enjoy short breaks.

DEPRESSIVE DISORDERS

Mood disorders that include depressive disorders are another common classification of mental disorder.

▶ The prevalence of mood disorders for adults is 7.1% in the previous 12 months with a lifetime prevalence of nearly 31% in the United States.[16]

- Women are more likely to experience mood disorders.
- Onset is usually in the mid-20s, but it can occur at any age.
- Depression is the leading cause of disability worldwide.[17]

I. Types of Depressive Disorders[18,19]

A. Major Depressive Disorder

▶ Transient depressed moods occur in the lives of most people.

- Sadness over unforeseen tragic events, illnesses, death, or disappointments in career or other life plans can cause depressed feelings.

▶ Major depressive disorder interferes with daily life.

▶ Some individuals experience only one episode of major depression in their lifetime, but it is more common to have multiple episodes.

B. Postpartum Depression

During the postpartum period, many physiologic and psychologic stresses are related to the changes taking place in the mother's life.

▶ A moderate-to-severe depression within the first month postpartum.

- The prevalence of postpartum depression is estimated to be 10%–15%.

▶ It is critical to identify women with postpartum depression because it can lead to negative mother–infant interactions that include maternal withdrawal, disengagement, and abuse.[20]

- The mother may be less likely to engage in preventive care and is less responsive to providing care to the infant; this may include engaging in appropriate feeding practices and oral health care for the infant/children.[21]
- The impact on development of the infant may include: excessive infant crying, sleep problems, and signs of stress.[21]

II. Signs and Symptoms

▶ Symptoms vary between individuals, but common symptoms include:

- Depressed mood or loss of interest or pleasure in activities present for at least 2 weeks.
- Feelings of hopelessness, worthlessness, or guilt.
- Fatigue and lack of energy.
- Difficulty with memory and concentration.
- Appetite disturbance.
- Insomnia, early-morning wakefulness.
- Thoughts of suicide.

III. Treatment[22]

In the case of depression, one of the first things assessed is suicide risk. Hospitalization may be indicated when potential danger of suicide or harm to others exists.

A. Basic Therapeutic Approach

▶ Lifestyle modifications include regular physical activity, adequate sleep, and avoidance of drugs and alcohol.

▶ Diagnose and treat other medical and psychiatric problems.

B. Pharmacotherapy[10–12]

Antidepressants are preferred as an initial treatment of depressive disorders.

▶ *Selective serotonin re-uptake inhibitors*

- Advantages: tolerability better than earlier drugs; better compliance; safety in overdose
- Examples: fluoxetine (Prozac), paroxetine (Paxel), and sertraline (Zoloft).

▶ *Serotonin and noradrenergic reuptake inhibitors*

- Examples: duloxetine (Cymbalta) and venlafaxine (Efflexor).

▶ *Dopamine norepinephrine reuptake inhibitor*

- Example: bupriopion (Wellbutrin).

▶ *Tricyclic and heterocyclic antidepressants*

- Not used for initial treatment; higher risk of overdose.
- Example: amitriptyline.

▶ *Monoamine oxidase inhibitors*

- Certain foods and other drugs to be avoided to prevent hypertensive crisis.
- Example: phenelzine and tranylcypromine.

C. Psychotherapy

Psychotherapy combined with pharmacotherapy is more effective than either one alone for treating depressive disorders.[22,23]

▶ Cognitive Behavioral Therapy (CBT)

▶ Problem-solving therapy

▶ Interpersonal psychotherapy.

D. Electroconvulsive Therapy (ECT)

▶ About 70%–90% of patients experience improvement following ECT.

▶ Patient may experience confusion for 30–60 minutes after treatment.

▶ May have cardiovascular side effect and is contraindicated in patients with a history of cardiac arrhythmia or recent myocardial infarction.

IV. Dental Hygiene Care

A. Personal Factors

▶ Self-care impairment and lack of motivation negatively impact oral health.[24]

▶ Symptoms not controlled by medication, such as difficulties with memory, may need to be considered when planning dental hygiene care.

- ▶ The medicated patient may experience side effects of medication.
- ▶ Individuals with depression may have diets higher in fatty and sweet foods: sweets, which increase the risk of dental caries.[24]
  - Poor nutrition can also impact healing following periodontal therapy.

B. Oral Health Implications[13]

- ▶ *Side effects of medications:* xerostomia along with poor dietary choices encourages growth of lactobacilli and increases the risk for enamel and root caries.[25]
- ▶ Omission of general health habits and neglect of oral care make the person susceptible to oral diseases.
  - Research shows adults with depression are less likely to have regular dental care.[13]
  - Adults with a lifetime diagnosis of depression are more likely to have at least one tooth extracted.[13]
  - Increases the risk of periodontal disease
- ▶ Loss of taste perception can contribute to a diet high in cariogenic foods with high levels of sucrose.

C. Appointment Interventions

- ▶ *Assessment*
  - Monitor the medical and medications histories closely; note side effects and contraindications related to new drug therapies.
  - Review consultations with medical/psychiatric specialists caring for the patient.
  - *Intraoral/extraoral examination:* check for signs of xerostomia.
- ▶ *Approach*
  - Provide positive reinforcement and reassurance. Avoid negative guilt-inducing words. Depressed patients may needlessly blame themselves.
  - Show genuine interest in the patient to build rapport.
- ▶ *Preventive instruction*
  - *Dental biofilm control:* Teach patient and caregivers the need for daily measures to preserve the teeth and periodontal tissues.
  - *Xerostomia:* Manage caries risk with dietary counseling, office and home fluorides, saliva substitutes, and xylitol gum between meals.
- ▶ *Implementation of care plan*
  - Adjust dental light carefully and provide tinted protective eyewear for the patient with photosensitivity, a side effect of certain medications.
  - Profound local anesthesia when needed for pain control.
  - In-office fluoride treatment after instrumentation.
  - Use care to prevent postural hypotension. Sit the patient up slowly from a reclined position and have the patient remain seated a few moments before standing.

BIPOLAR DISORDER[26]

- ▶ Bipolar disorder was formerly known as manic-depressive disorder and involves mood changes from extreme highs (mania) to extreme lows (depression).
  - The lifetime prevalence in the United States is approximately 4%.[14]
  - It is more prevalent in women and the average age of onset is mid-20s.
- ▶ Bipolar disorder is the most costly behavioral health issue in part because of high rates of comorbidities such as anxiety disorder, metabolic syndrome, substance abuse, and attention-deficit disorder.[27]

I. Signs and Symptoms

- ▶ Manic episode symptoms include behaviors that are not consistent with the patient's usual behavior including the following:
  - Inflated self-esteem.
  - Decreased need for sleep.
  - Irritable.
  - Attention gets focused on unimportant activities.
  - Excessive involvement in risky activities.
  - Extreme changes in energy, activity, sleep, and behavior based on the large swings in mood.
- ▶ Major depressive episode symptoms are the same as those described for depressive disorders.

II. Treatment

Both pharmacotherapy and psychotherapy are used during all phases of the disorder. Initially, hospitalization may be needed to protect the individual from harm to self or others.

A. Pharmacotherapy

- ▶ *Mood stabilizers*
  - Example: lithium
  - Side effects: xerostomia, restlessness, joint and muscle pain, salivary gland swelling, indigestion and bloating.
- ▶ *Anticonvulsants* are also used as mood stabilizers.
  - Examples: valproic acid (Depakote), lamotrigine (Lamictal), and gabapentin (Neurotin).
  - Some of these medications increase the risk for suicidal thoughts and need close monitoring.
  - Side effects: drowsiness, dizziness, headache, heartburn, and coldlike symptoms (stuffy or runny nose).
- ▶ *Atypical antipsychotics* are sometimes used in conjunction with antidepressants.
  - Examples: quetiapine (Seroquel), risperidone (Risperdal), olanzapine (Zyprexa), and aripiprazole (Abilify).
  - Side effects: dizziness, blurred vision, rapid heartbeat, skin rashes, and drowsiness.

► *Antidepressants* are usually taken with a mood stabilizer.
  • Example: fluoxetine (Prozac), paroxetine (Paxil), sertraline (Zoloft), and bupropion (Wellbutrin).

B. Psychotherapy

► Cognitive behavioral therapy helps patients to learn to change harmful or negative thought patterns and behaviors.

► Family-focused therapy improves communication and coping strategies to aid in early recognition of manic or depressive episodes.

III. Dental Hygiene Care

A. Personal Factors

► In a manic episode:
  • Many patients talk quickly, jump from thought to thought, and have a short attention span.
  • A tendency to argue and become irritable may be apparent.

► In a depressive episode:
  • The patient may not be interested in oral care and be unmotivated.

B. Oral Health Implications[28]

► Oral hygiene needs are often not a priority to the patient.

► Gingival tissues may appear abraded and lacerated because of over eager grandiose brushing motions.

► Side effects of medications with implications for oral health and dental care include:
  • Xerostomia.
  • Dysgeusia and impart a metallic taste in the mouth (lithium).
  • Stomatitis and glossitis.
  • Loss of taste acuity.
  • Dizziness.

C. Appointment Interventions

► Carefully review medical and medication history; consult with patient's physician/psychiatrist as needed.

► Simplify the surroundings; provide a comfortable, calm, and uncluttered environment.

► Patient instruction may be difficult due to a short attention span. Use direct, simple instructions.
  • When applicable, help the patient's caregiver to learn procedures for dental caries prevention and periodontal health.

► Manage caries and periodontal risk with saliva substitutes, office and home fluoride application, dietary counseling, and sugar-free xylitol gum or mints between meals.
  • Chlorhexidine gluconate mouthrinse may be prescribed for short intervals (1 week) to reduce caries risk and aid healing after NSPT.

► Three- to four-month continuing care appointments may be needed.

FEEDING AND EATING DISORDERS[29]

Feeding and eating disorders are serious disturbances in the amounts and types of foods consumed.

► Prevalence ranges from 0.4% for anorexia nervosa to 1%–1.5% for bulimia and binge-eating disorder.

► Prevalence of other feeding disorders such as pica and rumination disorder is unclear.

► Identification and referral of a patient suspected of having an eating disorder for medical evaluation may be lifesaving because serious medical problems may exist and psychiatric therapy is indicated.

► An interdisciplinary team approach for successful rehabilitation of an individual with an eating disorder involves, at the least, medical, psychiatric, nutritional, dental, and dental hygiene professionals.

I. Types and Symptoms of Feeding and Eating Disorders

A. Pica

► Consumption of nonfood items typically occurs in children, but it also common in adults particularly those with mental disorders and/or intellectual disabilities.

► Persistent eating of nonfood substances such as dirt, clay, starch, gum, or ice for at least 1 month.

► Consumption of nonfood items may replace healthy foods and lead to nutrient deficiencies that can impact immune response and healing.

B. Anorexia Nervosa

Anorexia nervosa is characterized by a refusal of the individual to maintain body weight over the minimal normal weight for age and height. The aversion to eating results in life-threatening weight loss.

► Anorexia nervosa has the highest mortality rate of any mental disorder.[30]

► Commonly begins in adolescence or young adulthood.

► Signs and symptoms (Box 64-3) include:
  • Restriction of energy intake resulting in severe weight loss with emaciation; "waiflike" appearance.
  • Intense fear of weight gain or becoming fat.
  • Body image distortion (Figure 64-1).
  • Purging by vomiting, laxatives, and excessive exercise.
  • Malnutrition that can have long-term impact on bone mineral density (osteopenia or osteoporosis).
  • *Vital signs:* low pulse rate, hypotension, decreased respiratory rate, and low body temperature.
  • *Metabolic changes:* gastrointestinal, cardiovascular, hematologic, and renal system disturbances.
  • Amenorrhea (missed menstrual periods).

> **BOX 64-3**
>
> ### Characteristics of Anorexia Nervosa
>
> ▷ Refusal to maintain body weight over a minimally normal weight for age and height
> ▷ Intense fear of gaining weight or becoming fat, even though underweight
> ▷ Disturbance in the way in which one's body weight or shape is experienced
> ▷ Denies the seriousness of the current low body weight
> ▷ In females, absence of menstrual cycles when otherwise expected to occur
>
> **Types**
>
> **Restricting type:** does not regularly engage in binge-eating or purging behavior (i.e., self-induced vomiting or misuse of laxatives, diuretics, or enemas).
>
> **Binge-eating/purging type:** regularly engages in binge-eating or purging behavior (i.e., self-induced vomiting or the misuse of laxatives, diuretics, or enemas).
>
> Source: American Psychiatric Association. Feeding and eating disorders. In: *Diagnostic and Statistical Manual of Mental Disorders* (5th ed., DSM-5). Washington, DC: American Psychiatric Association; 2013:329–354.

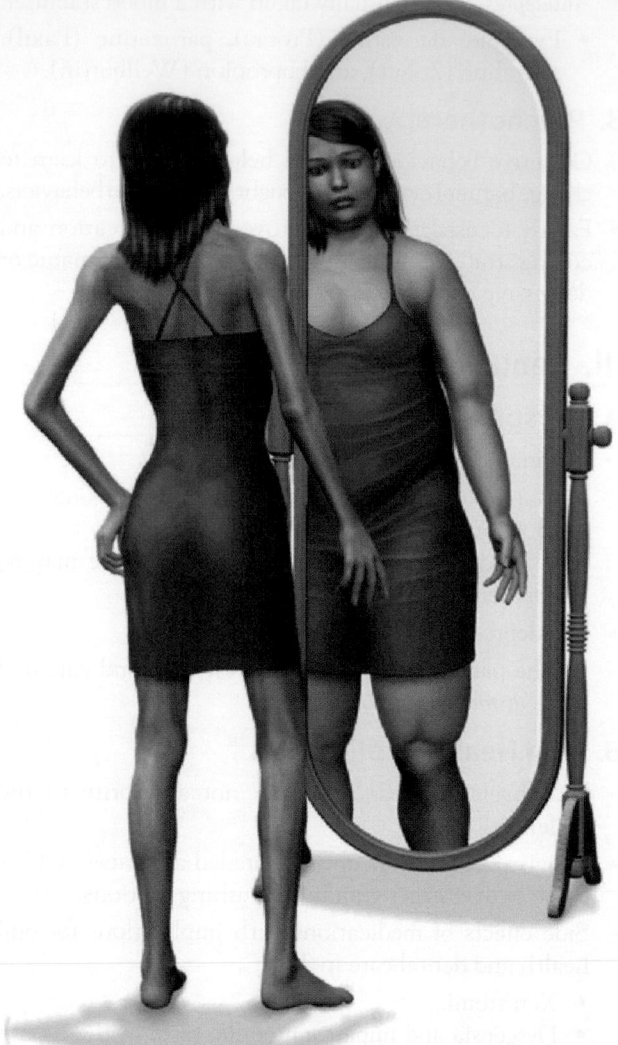

FIGURE 64-1 Anorexia Nervosa. The person with anorexia typically has a distorted body self-image. Although small and waiflike in real life, the mirror image appears as an overweight individual. (Reprinted from Werner R. Massage Therapist's Guide to Pathology. Philadelphia: Lippincott Williams & Wilkins; 2012.)

C. Bulimia Nervosa

▶ Bulimia nervosa is a mental disorder marked by recurrent episodes of uncontrollable binge eating that occurs an average of once a week for 3 months.[29]

▶ Two types of compensatory behaviors are seen in individuals with bulimia nervosa known as the purging type and the nonpurging type (Box 64-4).

- Because of the fear of becoming overweight, self-induced vomiting after eating or the use of laxatives or diuretics is characteristic of the purging type (Figure 64-2).
- The nonpurging type uses strict dieting, fasting, and/or vigorous exercise.

▶ Signs and symptoms include:

- Normal body weight or slightly overweight is typical, in contrast to the thin anorectic person.
- Comorbidity with other mental disorders is common especially depression and bipolar disorders.[29]
- Lifetime prevalence of alcohol or substance abuse is 30% for people.
- Food consumed during a binge include more simple carbohydrate cariogenic items.[31]

D. Binge-Eating Disorder

▶ Recurrent episodes of binge eating without compensatory behaviors seen in bulimia nervosa at least once a week for 3 months.

▶ Signs and symptoms include:

- Occurs in normal weight, overweight, and obese individuals.
- Binge eating is associated with feeling embarrassed or guilty about how much one is eating.
- The most common comorbid disorders are bipolar, depressive, and anxiety disorders.

II. Medical Complications

Medical complications are primarily associated with anorexia nervosa and people with bulimia who engage in purging behaviors.

▶ Problems include dehydration, electrolyte imbalance, protein malnutrition, and cardiac arrhythmia.

▶ Self-medications include abuse of laxatives and diuretics, which contribute to gastrointestinal disturbances.

▶ Esophageal tears.

▶ Amenorrhea or menstrual irregularities.

BOX 64-4

Characteristics of Bulimia Nervosa

▷ Recurrent episodes of binge eating. An episode of binge eating is characterized by both of the following:
  ▷ Eating, within any 2-hour period, an amount of food that is definitely larger than most people would eat in a similar period of time.
  ▷ A sense of lack of control over eating during the episode, for example, a feeling that one cannot stop eating or control what or how much one is eating.
▷ Recurrent inappropriate behavior to prevent weight gain, such as self-induced vomiting; misuse of laxatives, diuretics, enemas; fasting; or excessive exercise.
▷ Self-evaluation is unduly influenced by body shape and weight.

Types

Purging type: regularly engages in self-induced vomiting or the misuse of laxatives, diuretics, or enemas.

Nonpurging type: uses inappropriate compensatory behaviors such as fasting or excessive exercise, but does not engage in self-induced vomiting or the misuse of laxatives, diuretics, or enemas.

Source: American Psychiatric Association. Feeding and eating disorders. In: *Diagnostic and Statistical Manual of Mental Disorders* (5th ed., DSM-5). Washington, DC: American Psychiatric Association; 2013:329–354.

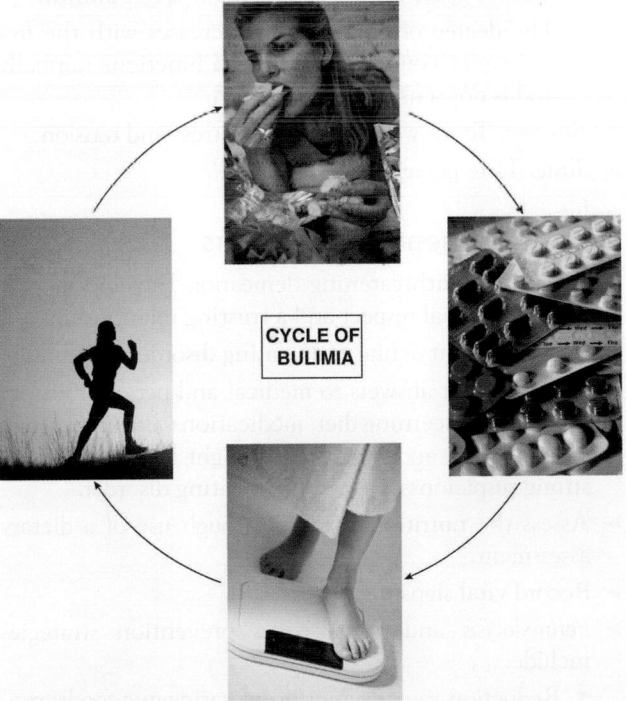

FIGURE 64-2 Bulimia Nervosa. The person with bulimia becomes trapped in recurring behaviors involving food and weight management. They ingest a vast number of calories at once and then take measures to purge themselves of their binge (e.g., abuse of laxatives, diet pills, and diuretics). They monitor their weight several times a day; some exercise obsessively to burn off the calories. (Reprinted from Mohr W. Psychiatric-Mental Health Nursing. Philadelphia: Lippincott Williams & Wilkins; 2012.)

III. Treatment[32]

Multidisciplinary team treatment for eating disorders is considered best practice, with hospitalization for the severely ill patient. The primary objectives are to promote weight gain and restore the nutritional status. Treatment may require months or even years.

A. Pharmacotherapy

▶ *Antidepressants (primarily in bulimia nervosa)*
  • Example: fluoxetine (Prozac)
  • Side effects: headache, weight gain, tremor, irritability, and xerostomia.

B. Psychotherapy

▶ Individual, group, and family-based therapies are used.
  • The goal of therapy is to help the individual discover underlying causes of the problems and source of the disordered eating behaviors.

C. Nutrition Therapy

  • Registered dietitians with advanced training in eating disorders work as part of the interprofessional team to conduct a full nutrition assessment, diagnosis, and individualize a plan for medical nutrition therapy in collaboration with the team.
  • This in-depth type of nutrition counseling is beyond the scope of practice for dental professionals.

IV. Dental Hygiene Care

A. Personal Factors

▶ Anorexia nervosa
  • Individuals with anorexia are frequently engaged in excessive exercise and preoccupied with food and weight loss.
  • Frequently the person is a high achiever and highly motivated scholastically, but may be socially isolated and withdrawn.
  • Suicide risk is elevated in anorexia.[29]
▶ Bulimia nervosa and binge-eating disorder
  • The patient is well aware the eating habits are abnormal, and as a result may suffer low self-esteem and guilt feelings.

B. Oral Implications[33]

▶ *Perimylolysis:* This is the chemical erosion of the tooth surfaces by acid from the regurgitation of stomach contents. After vomiting, acid is retained by the tongue papillae and provides longer contact with the palatal surfaces of maxillary teeth.
  • Because of perimylolysis, the earliest evidence of bulimia or binge-eating/purging type of anorexia may be on the smooth palatal surfaces of the teeth.
  • The lingual surfaces of the maxillary anterior teeth appear translucent and glasslike (Figure 64-3B).

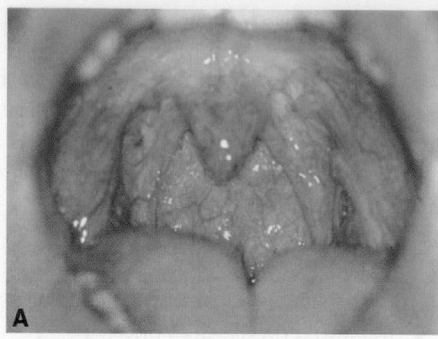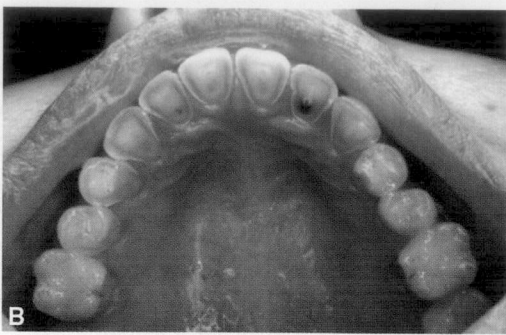

FIGURE 64-3 **Oral Manifestations of Purging Type Eating Disorders.** Signs of purging include (**A**) irritation and inflammation of the pharynx as well as the esophagus from chronic vomiting and (**B**) erosion of the lingual surface of the teeth, loss of dental enamel, periodontal disease, and extensive dental caries. (Reprinted from Timby B, Smith N. Introductory Medical-Surgical Nursing. Philadelphia: Lippincott Williams & Wilkins; 2013.)

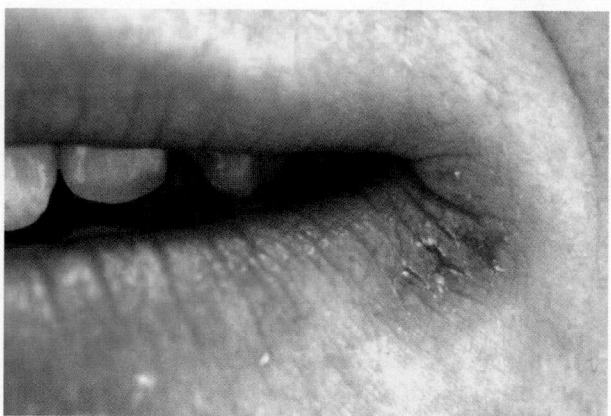

FIGURE 64-4 **Angular Chelitis.** Angular cheilitis may occur in vitamin B deficiencies, which can occur in patients with eating disorders. (Reprinted from Schalock P, Hsu J, Arndt K. Lippincott's Primary Care Dermatology. Philadelphia: Lippincott Williams & Wilkins; 2010.)

- With time, the erosion extends over the occlusal and incisal surfaces and chipping may be observed.[29]
- Restorations in posterior teeth may appear raised because of erosion of the enamel around the margins.

▶ *Dental caries*: An increase in caries incidence is found, particularly in cervical caries. Demineralization results from pH changes in the saliva, from xerostomia, and from the large quantities of cariogenic foods ingested during binges.

▶ *Mucosal lesions*: Nutrient deficiencies especially in the B vitamins may result in angular cheilitis (Figure 64-4), glossitis, inflammation of pharynx (Figure 64-3A), and a burning sensation.

▶ *Periodontal manifestations*: Nutritional deficiencies along with inadequate control of dental biofilm due to depression may predispose the patient to gingivitis.

▶ *Saliva*: The decrease in quantity, quality, and pH of the saliva limits its buffering and lubricating properties. Dehydration of the oral soft tissues occurs.

- Body fluid is lost from vomiting and the use of diuretics may result in xerostomia.
- Xerostomia is also a side effect of antidepressant medication prescribed for certain patients with bulimia and anorexia.

▶ *Hypersensitive teeth*: The loss of enamel and the exposure of dentin results in sensitivity, which can be especially noticeable for the maxillary anterior teeth.

▶ *Trauma*

- The soft palate can be traumatized by fingers, comb, pencils, or toothbrush used to induce vomiting. The same implement may injure the mouth at the commissures.
- Pharyngeal trauma is caused by a large food bolus that is swallowed or regurgitated.
- Callous formation or scars on fingers or knuckles used for self-induced vomiting may be observed.

▶ *Parotid gland*: Enlargement may occur for 2–6 days after a binge. A cause for the enlargement is not known.

- The degree of enlargement increases with the frequency of vomiting. The gland functions normally and is not sensitive to palpation.

▶ *Bruxism*: Tooth wear is related to stress and tension.

▶ *Taste*: Taste perception is impaired.

C. Appointment Interventions

▶ Present a nonthreatening demeanor. Develop rapport through mutual respect and a trusting relationship.

▶ Recognize that denial of an eating disorder is common.

▶ Be aware that answers to medical and personal history questions concerning diet, medications, use of laxatives and diuretics, and weight and weight loss may provide strong suspicions of a feeding or eating disorder.

▶ Assess the nutritional status through use of a dietary assessment.

▶ Record vital signs.

▶ *Perimylolysis* and *dental caries* prevention strategies include:

- Reduction in consumption of cariogenic foods; provide list of suggestions for substitutions.
- Improvement in oral self-care. Show use of appropriate brushing and flossing with additional interdental aids if required for biofilm removal. Clean the tongue (see Chapter 28).

- Avoidance of brushing after vomiting. Demineralization of the tooth surface by the acid from the stomach starts immediately on contact. Brushing may remove additional enamel/dentin.
- Remineralization after vomiting with an alkaline rinse of sodium bicarbonate solution to neutralize the acid.

▶ *Dental hypersensitivity* is managed as follows:
- Office application of fluoride varnish.
- Use fluoride dentifrice at least twice daily.
- Daily application of 1.1% neutral sodium fluoride toothpaste or gel.
- Avoid acidic foods and beverages.

▶ *Xerostomia* management includes:
- Advise sugar-free mints or chewing gum containing xylitol if patient uses them to stimulate saliva flow.
- Recommend saliva substitutes.
- To reduce problems caused by hypersensitive teeth: choose sugar substitute and acid-free foods and beverages.

SCHIZOPHRENIA[34,35]

▶ Schizophrenia is a complex, chronic mental disorder. Disturbances in feeling, thinking, and behavior significantly impair function to a level below normal for the individual.
▶ Prevalence of schizophrenia is 0.3%–0.7%
▶ The onset is usually between the ages of 16 and 30.
  - Men tend to develop symptoms at an earlier age than women.
▶ Genetic factors are strong contributors to risk for schizophrenia.
▶ Associated medical issues such as cardiovascular disease, obesity, diabetes, and metabolic syndrome reduce life expectancy.
▶ About 20% of people with schizophrenia attempt suicide and 5%–6% die as a result of suicide.

I. Signs and Symptoms

Symptoms fall into three categories: *positive symptoms*, *negative symptoms*, and *cognitive symptoms*.[34,35]

▶ *Positive symptoms* are those that reflect unusual, exaggerated behavior and include:
- Hallucinations that may include hearing voices.
- Delusions.
- Disorganized thinking characterized by the person having difficulty organizing thoughts or connecting them logically.
- Movement disorders such as agitated body movements.
- People with positive symptoms may "lose touch" with reality and the symptoms may come and go.

▶ *Negative symptoms* are associated with disruptions in normal emotions or behaviors and may be mistaken for depression. Symptoms include:
- The individual may have a "flat affect" meaning the person shows no emotion.
- Lack of pleasure in activities once enjoyed.
- Inability to start and carry out tasks.
- Little communication even when forced to interact.
- These individuals have difficulty with everyday tasks such as oral self-care.

▶ *Cognitive symptoms* are less obvious and may be difficult to recognize. Symptoms include:
- Poor executive functioning, meaning difficulty with understanding information and using it to make decisions.
- Difficulty paying attention.
- Challenges with working memory or the ability to use information immediately after it is learned.

▶ Rates of alcohol and other substance abuse are high among patients with schizophrenia.[34]
- Over 50% of patients with schizophrenia use tobacco.

II. Treatment

The response to initial treatment can be a predictor of the long-term prognosis. The prognosis has generally been considered guarded to poor. Evidence shows that although deterioration may occur during the early years, the condition may stabilize with treatment during middle age.

A. Pharmacotherapy[35]

▶ The objectives of treatment are to reduce or alleviate the delusions, hallucinations, and other symptoms and to enable the patient to function in daily living.
▶ The use of antipsychotic medications has improved the outcomes of treatment.
▶ *Typical antipsychotics* are used to block dopamine receptors and are effective against positive symptoms with less effect on negative symptoms.
- Examples: chlorpromazine (Thorazine), haloperidol (Haldol), and perphenazine (Etrafon, Trilafon).
- Side effects: xerostomia, persistent muscle spasms, tremors, restlessness, long-term use can lead to tardive dyskinesia (uncontrolled muscle movements), which commonly happens around the mouth.
▶ *Atypical antipsychotics* were developed in the 1990s and are second-generation antipsychotics:
- Examples: clozapine (Clozaril), quetiapine (Seroquel), risperidone (Risperdal), olanzapine (Zyprexa), and aripiprazole (Abilify).
- Side effects: xerostomia, dizziness, blurred vision, rapid heartbeat, skin rashes, and drowsiness.

TABLE 64-1	Effects of Antipsychotic Medication
SIDE EFFECTS	**IMPLICATIONS FOR DENTAL HYGIENE CARE**
Dystonia Muscle contractions	Laryngeal spasm; coughing Unable to turn head
Dysarthria Difficult speech	Communication difficulty
Parkinson-like syndrome Shuffling gait Muscular rigidity Resting tremor (pill rolling) Facial grimacing Bradykinesia	Cooperation may be difficult Patient positioning Instrument positioning; retraction
Akathisia Restlessness, pacing	Plan short appointments
Akinesia Loss of voluntary movement Lethargy, fatigue feelings	Adjust patient position
Tardive dyskinesia Involuntary mouth and jaw movements	Difficulty in instrumentation Wearing dentures difficult or impossible Muscle fatigue; may need mouth prop
Anticholinergic effects Xerostomia Blurred vision	Dental caries prevention Fluoride dentifrice; saliva substitute Difficulty seeing visual aids
Cardiovascular Postural hypotension Tachycardia, palpitations	Have patient sit up slowly and wait before standing Monitor vital signs
Sedation Drowsiness	Interfere with patient's daily routine Patient may be late; needs reminders
Blood Reduced leukocytes Agranulocytosis	Increased susceptibility to infection Oral candidiasis may be present

▶ Table 64-1 lists a few of the many side effects of antipsychotic medications, with suggestions for appointment adaptations.

B. Psychosocial Therapy

▶ Psychosocial therapy is utilized once the patient is stabilized on antipsychotic medication.

▶ Treatment is to help give general support in dealing with the challenges of the illness such as self-care, work, interpersonal relationships, and communication.

▶ Rehabilitation once stabilized includes social and vocational training so a person with schizophrenia can function in the community.

▶ Family education is also essential to help them learn coping strategies and problem-solving skills to support their loved one.

▶ Cognitive Behavioral Therapy (CBT) focuses on thinking and behavior and helps the person with schizophrenia manage symptoms that remain despite medication.

III. Dental Hygiene Care

A. Oral Implications[36]

▶ Overall degeneration of health factors may have occurred because of neglect of diet, exercise, sleep, general cleanliness, personal grooming, and oral care.

▶ Concurrent alcohol and/or other drug abuse, as well as smoking, can influence dental and periodontal health.

▶ Xerostomia can lead to an increase in rampant dental caries.

B. Appointment Planning

▶ Elective dental and dental hygiene treatment is not carried out until the schizophrenia is stabilized.

▶ If the patient decompensates, such as hallucinations or exhibits bizarre behavior, during a dental or dental hygiene appointment, immediate referral is needed.

▶ Telephone numbers of the patient's physicians are kept in an easily accessible location for quick referrals.

C. Appointment Interventions

▶ Because schizophrenia is often a lifelong disorder, planning for future oral health is essential.

▶ Review medical and medication history; analyze drugs for possible side effects that require appointment modifications (Table 64-1).

▶ Consult with the mental health provider relative to medications, alcohol or other substance use, and medicolegal competence for informed consent.
  • Negative symptoms are associated with poor oral health and a greater need for periodontal treatment.[36]

▶ Plan a simple routine. For a series of appointments and maintenance, use a familiar, organized routine that is comfortable for the patient.

▶ Decrease stimulation; create a restful atmosphere; if background music is present, keep it low and soft.

▶ Management of the risk for caries, periodontal, and oral cancer includes the following:
  • Oral self-care instruction to improve biofilm removal on a daily basis.
  • When applicable, evaluate the patient's personal caregiver for attitude and knowledge and provide information and instruction.
  • Diet assessment and counseling to assist patient in making noncariogenic food choices (see Chapter 35 for ideas).

- Encourage use of xylitol-containing gum or mints when cariogenic snacks or beverages are consumed between meals.
- Office and home fluorides (see Chapter 36).
- Tobacco cessation (see Chapter 34) may be more difficult for people with schizophrenia because nicotine withdrawal may cause psychotic symptoms to worsen so the dental professional must collaborate with the medical treatment team to closely monitor the patient.[35]

▶ Use a mouth prop to assist the patient with tardive dyskinesia. The patient who does not have control of mouth movements might appreciate the stability.

MENTAL HEALTH EMERGENCY

I. Psychiatric Emergency

A psychiatric emergency in a dental clinic or private dental practice would be rare. The most common causes of emergency include panic attack, atypical drug reaction, and schizophrenic or manic decompensation.

II. Patients at Risk for Emergencies

▶ Patient with a significant psychiatric history
▶ Patient with a known substance abuse history
▶ Patient new to the clinic or office; not known by the practitioners.

III. Prevention of Emergencies

▶ Prepare a complete history; collect as much information as possible; consult with the patient's physician and psychiatrist.

▶ Be alert to risks and characteristic symptoms of each disorder.
▶ Apply all the principles of stress management.
▶ Know the patient's medications and when they are taken.
  - Request that patient (or caregiver if accompanied) have readily available any necessary medication that may be effective in an emergency.
▶ Develop rapport with each patient; avoid confronting the patient and present a nonthreatening demeanor.

IV. Preparation for an Emergency

▶ Attend to surroundings, such as door access, objects in the room.
▶ Arrange for colleagues to be aware of the possible needs of a special patient appointment; plan for an assistant to participate in clinical procedures.
▶ Review characteristics of specific emergencies; have necessary equipment ready.
▶ Keep names of the patient's case worker, psychiatrist, and responsible family member in the record in a prominent position for ready reference.

V. Intervention

▶ Stay with the patient; request colleague to contact patient's case worker, psychiatrist, or other responsible person.
▶ Maintain a calm, serene manner; talk quietly but firmly.
▶ Move the patient to a quiet, less stimulating environment. The dental equipment and environment may have contributed to the patient's disturbance.

 **EVERYDAY ETHICS**

Samuel, age 28, suffers from panic disorder and generally requests short appointments because he becomes very anxious while receiving dental care. Even with a moderate amount of generalized deposits, Ginny, the dental hygienist, usually schedules two visits to complete the treatment.

During his visit today, Samuel appears in an almost dreamlike state. He was asked by the receptionist at the check-in about any new medications, but he stated that only a sleep aid was added to his pills, which he takes at night. Ginny suspects the patient may have taken his medication incorrectly and is concerned that Samuel is driving himself home after the appointment.

Questions for Consideration

1. Without breaching confidentiality, what ethical or other responsibility does Ginny have in verifying the type and amount of medication Samuel took and how does that influence the current day's dental hygiene appointment procedures?

2. Which of the dental hygiene core values (Table II-1, Section II Introduction) are evidenced in this scenario? Describe each in terms of the concern Ginny shows relative to Samuel's "competency" at driving himself home after the appointment as well as management during the appointment.

3. Is this an ethical dilemma or issue for Ginny? Using the questions in Table VI-1 in Section VI Introduction, suggest several alternative procedures that Ginny can follow during this appointment.

Example Documentation: Patient with a Mental Disorder

S –Mary is a 23-year-old. Sporadic dental care mainly for emergency root canals and extractions. She presents for an examination and "cleaning" because her physician recommended she seek dental care for obvious dental caries.

O–Medical history: She reports trouble sleeping and waking at 2 or 3 every morning and not being able to get back to sleep. Mary reports hallucination of neon people walking down the hallway. She said when she was at work she experienced high levels of anxiety. Her psychiatrist has diagnosed Mary as suffering from panic attacks. She also reported a previous history of being hospitalized for schizophrenia. She has smoked 1 pack of cigarettes/day since she was 13 years old. Medications: Risperidone (Risperdal). Dental examination: Caries noted MOD-#2, 14, 15, 18, 30; M & D #7–10 and #22–27. Leukoplakia noted in vestibule buccal to #28–29. Generalized pocket depths 4–5 mm with bleeding on probing indicating generalized moderate chronic periodontitis. Biofilm score: 95%. Generalized moderate supra- and subgingival calculus.

A–Patient education to include oral self-care along with strategies to manage risk factors for caries and periodontal disease. Consult with primary care provider to coordinate tobacco cessation based on her history of schizophrenia. Disease control treatment phase to include restoration of carious lesions and NSPT.

P –Disclosed biofilm and patient demonstrated oral self-care techniques. Mary seems to have good toothbrushing and flossing technique, but motivation seems to be her main problem. Suggested putting a sticky note on her bathroom mirror to remind her to perform oral self-care. Another suggestion was to make it a family affair and brush and floss with her children to be a role model to them. Mary was anxious at the beginning of the appointment, but seem calmer towards the end. Nutrition counseling focused on reducing the frequency of sugar-sweetened snacks and beverages with recommendations to use xylitol gum or mints when she snacks between meals and cannot brush. She was given a prescription for 1.1% sodium fluoride paste to begin using at home. There was not adequate time to begin NSPT at today's appointment.

Next visit: Review oral-self care. Follow-up on diet and tobacco cessation. NSPT maxillary and mandibular right quadrants with 2 carpules, 2% lidocaine with 1:100,000 epinephrine for Gow Gates, PSA, MSA, and GP injections.

Signed _____, RDH

Date _____

DOCUMENTATION

▶ The patient with a mental health disorder must complete a health history with details of the medical problem and medication history at the initial appointment.

▶ Follow-up with progress notes at each succeeding appointment to review all procedures and medications for changes.

▶ The following list suggests the minimum information to include in the permanent record:
- Resources for assistance in a convenient place in the event of need to contact: telephones, e-mails, and working addresses for physicians, psychiatrist, family, and emergency sources
- Progress notes for each appointment and other contacts to update all personal data and treatment
- Contacts and correspondence with specialists and others
- A sample progress note may be reviewed in Box 64-5.

Factors To Teach The Patient

▷ The significance of daily oral-self care of the oral cavity.
▷ How medications cause dry mouth and how it increases the risk for caries.
▷ The importance of minimizing sweets such as cake, candy, and sugar-sweetened drinks to prevent dental caries.
▷ The use of saliva substitutes to make a dry mouth more comfortable.
▷ For the patient with bulimia or the binge-eating/purging type of anorexia:
  ▷ The causes and effects of enamel erosion; the high acidity of the vomitus from the stomach.
  ▷ The importance of rinsing after vomiting but not brush immediately; demineralization begins promptly after the acid from the stomach reaches the teeth. Brushing can cause abrasion of the demineralizing enamel.
  ▷ The need for multiple fluoride applications through office and home fluoride containing dentifrice, rinse, and brush-on gel, as well as professional application of varnish at regular dental hygiene appointments.

References

1. American Psychiatric Association. *Diagnostic and Statistical Manual of Mental Disorders* (5th ed., text revision [DSM-5]). Washington, DC: American Psychiatric Association; 2013:19.
2. Centers for Disease Control and Prevention. Communicating with and about people with disabilities. 2014.

http://www.cdc.gov/ncbddd/disabilityandhealth/pdf/disability-poster_photos.pdf. Accessed November 30, 2014.

3. Steel Z, Marnane C, Iranpour C, et al. The global prevalence of common mental disorders: a systematic review and meta-analysis 1980–2013. *Int J Epidemiol*. 2014;43(2):476–493.

4. Baxter AJ, Scott KM, Vos T, et al. Global prevalence of anxiety disorders: a systematic review and meta-regression. *Psychol Med*. 2013;43(5):897–910.

5. Katzman MA, Bleau P, Blier P, et al. Canadian clinical practice guidelines for the management of anxiety, posttraumatic stress and obsessive-compulsive disorders. *BMC Psychiatry*. 2014;14 (Suppl 1):S1.

6. National Institute of Mental Health. Generalized anxiety disorder. http://www.nimh.nih.gov/health/topics/generalized-anxiety-disorder-gad/index.shtml. Accessed November 30, 2014.

7. American Psychiatric Association. Anxiety Disorders. In: *Diagnostic and Statistical Manual of Mental Disorders* (5th ed.). Washington, DC: American Psychiatric Association; 2013:189–223.

8. National Institute of Mental Health. Obsessive-compulsive disorder. http://www.nimh.nih.gov/health/topics/obsessive-compulsive-disorder-ocd/index.shtml. Accessed November 30, 2014.

9. National Institute of Mental Health. Panic disorder. http://www.nimh.nih.gov/health/topics/panic-disorder/index.shtml. Accessed November 30, 2014.

10. National Institute of Mental Health. Post-traumatic stress disorder. http://www.nimh.nih.gov/health/topics/post-traumatic-stress-disorder-ptsd/index.shtml. Accessed November 30, 2014.

11. National Institute of Mental Health. Anxiety disorders. http://www.nimh.nih.gov/health/topics/anxiety-disorders/index.shtml. Accessed November 30, 2014.

12. Sheldon LK, Swanson S, Dolce A, et al. Putting evidence into practice: evidence-based interventions for anxiety. *Clin J Oncol Nurs*. 2008;12(5):789–797.

13. Okoro CA, Strine TW, Eke PI, et al. The association between depression and anxiety and use of oral health services and tooth loss. *Community Dent Oral Epidemiol*. 2012;40(2):134–144.

14. Khambaty T, Stewart JC. Associations of depressive and anxiety disorders with periodontal disease prevalence in young adults: analysis of 1999–2004 National Health and Nutrition Examination Survey (NHANES) data. *Ann Behav Med*. 2013;45(3):393–397.

15. Newton T, Asimakopoulou K, Daly B, et al. The management of dental anxiety: time for a sense of proportion? *Br Dent J*. 2012;213(6):271–274.

16. Kessler RC, Petukhova M, Sampson NA, et al. Twelve-month and lifetime prevalence and lifetime morbid risk of anxiety and mood disorders in the United States. *Int J Methods Psychiatr Res*. 2012;21(3):169–184.

17. World Health Organization. Depression fact sheet. 2012. http://www.who.int/mediacentre/factsheets/fs369/en/. Accessed December 2, 2014.

18. American Psychiatric Association. Depressive Disorders. In: *Diagnostic and Statistical Manual of Mental Disorders* (5th ed., DSM-5). Washington, DC: American Psychiatric Association; 2013:155–188.

19. National Institute of Mental Health. Depression. http://www.nimh.nih.gov/health/topics/depression/index.shtml. Accessed December 2, 2014.

20. Pearlstein T, Howard M, Salisbury A, et al. Postpartum depression. *Am J Obstet Gynecol*. 2009;200(4):357–364.

21. Field T. Postpartum depression effects on early interactions, parenting, and safety practices: a review. *Infant Behav Dev*. 2010;33(1):1–6.

22. American Psychiatric Association. *Practice Guideline for the Treatment of Patients With Major Depressive Disorder*. 3rd ed. Washington, DC: American Psychiatric Association; 2010:1–152.

23. Cuijpers P, Sijbrandij M, Koole SL, et al. Adding psychotherapy to antidepressant medication in depression and anxiety disorders: a meta-analysis. *World Psychiatry*. 2014; 13(1):56–67.

24. Camilleri GM, Méjean C, Kesse-Guyot E, et al. Nothing to smile about. *Neuropsychiatr Dis Treat*. 2014;10: 1999–2008.

25. Bellisle F, Hercberg S, Péneau S. The associations between emotional eating and consumption of energy-dense snack foods are modified by sex and depressive symptomatology. *J Nutr*. 2014;144(8):1264–1273.

26. American Psychiatric Association. Bipolar and related disorders. In: *Diagnostic and Statistical Manual of Mental Disorders* (5th ed., DSM-5). Washington, DC: American Psychiatric Association; 2013:123–154.

27. Abdul Pari AA, Simon J, Wolstenholme J, et al. Economic evaluations in bipolar disorder: a systematic review and critical appraisal. *Bipolar Disord*. 2014;16(6): 557–582.

28. Clark DB. Dental care for the patient with bipolar disorder. *J Can Dent Assoc*. 2003;69(1):20–24.

29. American Psychiatric Association. Feeding and eating disorders. In: *Diagnostic and Statistical Manual of Mental Disorders* (5th ed., DSM-5). Washington, DC: American Psychiatric Association; 2013:329–354.

30. Smink FR, van Hoeken D, Hoek HW. Epidemiology of eating disorders: incidence, prevalence and mortality rates. *Curr Psychiatry Rep*. 2012;14(4):406–414.

31. Segura-García C, De Fazio P, Sinopoli F, et al. Food choice in disorders of eating behavior: correlations with the psychopathological aspects of the diseases. *Compr Psychiatry*. 2014;55(5):1203–1211.

32. National Institute of Mental Health. Eating disorders. http://www.nimh.nih.gov/health/publications/eating-disorders/index.shtml. Accessed December 23, 2014.

33. Lo Russo L, Campisi G, Di Fede O, et al. Oral manifestations of eating disorders: a critical review. *Oral Dis*. 2008;14(6):479–484.

34. American Psychiatric Association. Feeding and eating disorders. In: *Diagnostic and Statistical Manual of Mental Disorders* (5th ed., DSM-5). Washington, DC: American Psychiatric Association; 2013:87–122.

35. National Institute of Mental Health. Schizophrenia. http://www.nimh.nih.gov/health/topics/schizophrenia/index.shtml. Accessed December 23, 2014.

36. Arnaiz A, Zumárraga M, Díez-Altuna I, et al. Oral health and the symptoms of schizophrenia. *Psychiatry Res.* 2011; 188(1):24–28.

 ENHANCE YOUR UNDERSTANDING

thePoint® **[THEPOINT LOGO] DIGITAL CONNECTIONS**
(see the inside front cover for access information)
- **Audio glossary**
- **Quiz bank**

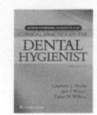 **[WORKBOOK COVER IMAGE] SUPPORT FOR LEARNING**
(available separately; visit lww.com)
- *Active Learning Workbook for Clinical Practice of the Dental Hygienist, 12th Edition*

prepU **[PREPU LOGO] INDIVIDUALIZED REVIEW**
(available separately; visit lww.com)
- **Adaptive quizzing with *prepU* for Wilkins' *Clinical Practice of the Dental Hygienist***

65

The Patient with a Substance-Related Disorder

Ernestine R. Daniels, RDH, BS

LEARNING OBJECTIVES

After studying this chapter, the student will be able to:

1. Explain key terms and concepts related to the metabolism, intoxication effects, and use patterns of alcohol.

2. Identify physical health hazards, medical effects, and oral manifestations associated with alcohol and other drug abuse.

3. List the names of the most commonly abused drugs and describe their intoxication effects and methods of use.

4. Describe methods for clinical assessment of potential substance abuse.

5. Recognize risk management principles to prevent prescription pad theft and abuse.

INTRODUCTION

▶ Drug and alcohol dependence often go hand in hand; people who are dependent on alcohol are more likely than the general population to use other drugs, and people with drug dependence are more likely to drink alcohol.[1]

▶ Substance abuse reflects a complex interaction between the individual, the abused drugs, and society.

▶ Drug use varies from recreational use to addiction; people from various stages of drug use appear as patients needing dental and dental hygiene care.

▶ Patients who use drugs recreationally may "premedicate" themselves when a stressful situation such as a dental appointment is anticipated; therefore, questions at each appointment are required to determine clinical procedure and prevent complications.

▶ There is no classic cultural, socioeconomic, or educational profile for a substance abuser.

▶ A patient's medical and dental history does not always provide the information necessary to determine whether the patient uses substances at all, or the level of dependency.

▶ It is a professional responsibility of the dental hygienist to:
  • View chemical dependency as an illness and to be aware of the characteristics that suggest possible substance use.
  • Address the issues of an appropriate dental hygiene care plan for the chemically dependent patient.

▶ Key words and terminology related to the use and abuse of drugs are defined in Box 65-1.

▶ Alcohol use is common in a large percentage of the population and varies from social drinking to alcoholism.

▶ Physical dependence and tolerance are both present in an individual suffering from alcoholism.

▶ Alcohol used for consumption purposes is ethyl alcohol or ethanol. Other alcohols are methyl, an industrial solvent, and isopropyl, used for rubbing alcohol.

ALCOHOL CONSUMPTION

I. Clinical Pattern of Alcohol Use

▶ Abstinence and low-risk use.

▶ Increased consumption.

▶ Moderate alcohol use: two drinks per day for men and one drink per day for women is not considered harmful for the average adult.[2] The individual is able to function appropriately in work, family, and social situations.

▶ Unhealthy alcohol use: early-stage problems such as hypertension, depression, insomnia, heartburn, and absenteeism develop.[3]

▶ Alcohol dependency and alcoholism develop after periods of unhealthy alcohol use followed by pathologic abuse.[4]

▶ The spectrum of alcohol use is illustrated by Figure 65-1.

▶ Volume and alcohol content in a standard drink of various alcoholic beverages is shown in Box 65-2.

A. Effects of Alcohol Intoxication[4]

▶ Behavioral changes: aggressiveness, mood instability, impaired judgment; impaired social or occupational functioning; impaired attention and memory; stupor or coma.

▶ Physical characteristics: slurred speech, lack of coordination, unsteady gait, and nystagmus.

▶ Complications: irresponsible actions in work and family settings.

▶ Accidents with resultant bruises, fractures, or brain trauma.

▶ Vehicular accidents.

▶ Suicide.

B. Consequences of Underage Drinking[5]

▶ Drinking and driving.

▶ Suicide.

▶ Sexual assault.

▶ High-risk sex.

▶ Alcohol-induced mental impairment.

C. Signs of Alcoholism[6]

Alcoholism, also known as alcohol dependence, includes four main symptoms:

▶ *Craving*: A strong need or compulsion to drink.

▶ *Loss of control*: The inability to limit one's drinking on any given occasion.

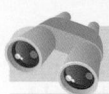 **BOX 65-1** | **KEY WORDS:** Alcoholism and Drug Abuse

Abstinence: refrain from use; complete abstinence from alcohol is the objective of a recovering alcoholic.

Abuse: substance abuse; with respect to alcohol abuse involves persistent patterns of heavy alcohol intake associated with health consequences and/or impairment in social functioning.

Acne rosacea: facial skin condition usually characterized by a flushed appearance; often accompanied by puffiness and a "spider-web" effect of broken capillaries.

Addiction: habitual psychologic and physiologic dependence on a substance or practice that is beyond voluntary control.

Alcohol intoxication: results from recent ingestion of excessive amounts of alcohol; characterized by behavioral changes that alter the usual behavior of the individual.

Alcoholism: a chronic progressive behavioral disorder characterized by a strong urge to consume ethanol and inability to limit the amount despite adverse consequences.

Amnesia: impairment of long- and/or short-term memory.

   Anterograde amnesia: difficulty in recalling new information.

   Retrograde amnesia: difficulty in remembering old information.

Amethystic agents: a class of substances capable of counteracting the acute effects of alcohol on the central nervous system.

Analgesia: loss of sensibility to pain without loss of consciousness.

Antabuse: brand name of the generic drug disulfiram; used to deter consumption of alcohol by persons being treated for alcohol dependency by inducing vomiting.

Blackout: temporary amnesia occurring during periods of intensive drinking; person is not unconscious.

DEA drug schedules: drugs, substances, and certain chemicals used to make drugs are classified by the U.S. Drug Enforcement Administration (DEA) into five (5) distinct categories or schedules depending upon the drug's acceptable medical use and the drug's abuse or dependency potential (see Box 65-5).

DEA registration number: assigned by DEA allowing health care providers to write prescriptions for controlled substances (drugs that have been assigned a DEA drug schedule category).

Delirium: extreme mental and usually motor excitement marked by a rapid succession of confused and unconnected ideas; often with illusions and hallucinations; may be accompanied by tremors.

Delirium tremens: "DTs"; a serious acute condition associated with the last stages of alcohol withdrawal.

Dementia: condition of deteriorated mentality characterized by a marked decline of intellectual functioning.

Dependence: drug or substance dependence; with respect to alcohol refers to a physical and psychological dependence on alcohol that results in impaired ability to control drinking behavior; dependence is differentiated from abuse by manifestations of craving tolerance and physical dependence, as well as an inability to exercise restraint over drinking.

Chemical dependence: the interaction between a drug and the individual when there is a compulsion to take the drug to obtain its effects and/or to avoid the discomforts of withdrawal.

Physical dependence: when a drug becomes necessary for continued body functioning. An altered physiologic state has developed from repeatedly increasing drug concentrations.

Polysubstance dependence: addiction to at least three categories of psychoactive substances (not including nicotine or caffeine) but in which no single psychoactive substance predominates.

Psychologic dependence: refers to the state of mind in which the individual believes the drug is required for maintaining well-being.

Detoxification: treatment designed to assist in recovery from the toxic effects of a drug; involves withdrawal and may include pharmacologic and/or nonpharmacologic treatment with psychotherapy and counseling.

Drug: a chemical substance used for diagnosis, prevention, or treatment of disease. Drugs are classified by biochemical action, physiological effect, or organ system involved.

Euphoria: feeling of well-being, elation; without fear or worry.

Hallucination: a sensory impression (sight, sound, touch, smell, or taste) that has no basis in external stimulation; may have psychological causes, or may result from the use of drugs, (including alcohol), a brain tumor, senility, or exhaustion.

Hyperthermia: body temperature higher than normal.

Illicit: illegal; not authorized, not sanctioned by law.

Micrognathia: abnormal smallness of the jaws, especially of the mandible.

Nystagmus: involuntary, rapid, rhythmic movements of the eyeball.

Opiate antagonist: examples include naltrexone and naloxone. These drugs have a high affinity for opiate receptors but do not activate them and block the effect of exogenously administered opioids (e.g., morphine, heroin, and methadone) or of endogenously released endorphins.

Opioid: synthetic narcotic that has opiatelike activities but is not derived from opium.

Psychotropic drug: a drug capable of modifying mental activity; used in the treatment of mental illness.

Recovering alcoholic: a person afflicted with the disease of alcoholism who is abstaining from the use of alcohol; recovering alcoholics prefer the term "recovering" to reformed, cured, or recovered because recovering implies an ongoing process.

Saddlenose deformity: a collapse of the nasal bridge.

Substance abuse: The regular use of a drug for other than its accepted medical purpose or in dosages greater than those that are considered appropriate.

Tolerance: ability to endure without effect or injury. Increased amount of the drug is needed to achieve the same effect.

   Drug tolerance: the need for higher and higher dosages of a drug to achieve the same effect.

Withdrawal syndrome: a group of signs and symptoms, both physiologic and psychologic, that occurs on abrupt discontinuation of drug use.

▶ *Physical dependence*: Withdrawal symptoms, such as nausea, sweating, shakiness, and anxiousness, when alcohol use is stopped after a period of heavy drinking.

▶ *Tolerance*: The need to drink greater amounts of alcohol in order to get intoxicated. Other signs include amnesia and binge drinking.

II. Etiology

A. Genetics

▶ The Collaborative Study on the Genetics of Alcoholism has successfully identified GABRA2 and CHRM2 as two genes involved in the predisposition to alcohol dependence.[7]

▶ A defective allele (variant) of the gene ALDH2 substantially (although not completely) protects carriers from developing alcoholism by making them ill after drinking alcohol.[2]

B. Biopsychosocial

▶ Alcohol-specific parenting is a distinct and influential predictor of adolescent alcohol use partially shaped by parents' own drinking experiences.

▶ Parental conversations about their own personal experiences with alcohol may not represent a form of parent–child communication about drinking that deters adolescent drinking.[8]

▶ Children of alcohol-dependent parents are exposed to a higher level of multiple risk factors that lead to alcohol-related problems:

- Mental and behavioral disorders and adverse family environments.
- Decreased sensitivity to intoxication effects of alcohol.

C. Environmental

▶ Psychological stress, family, peers, and social forces.

▶ Current lifestyle, culture, advertisements, and economics.

▶ Motivational factors: both emotional (stress reduction, mood enhancement, social rewards) and cognitive (conscious and unconscious beliefs about alcohol) may play a role in an individual's decision to drink.

METABOLISM OF ALCOHOL[2]

I. Ingestion and Absorption

▶ Upon intake, alcohol is absorbed promptly from the stomach and small intestine into the bloodstream.

▶ Transported to liver for metabolism.

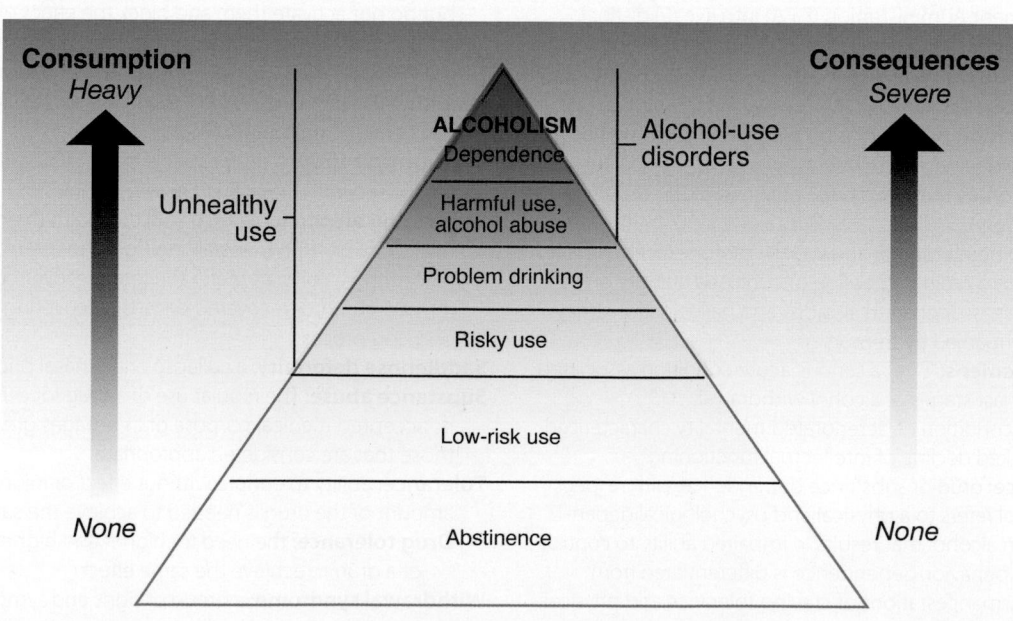

FIGURE 65-1 The Spectrum of Alcohol Use. As clinicians, the shaded categories in the upper portions of the pyramid are of primary concern while treating patients. These categories reflect unhealthy alcohol use. (Source: Saitz R. Clinical practice. Unhealthy alcohol use. *N Engl J Med*. 2005;352(6):596–607.)

II. Liver Metabolism

▶ More than 90% of ingested alcohol is converted into acetaldehyde, then acetone, and finally into carbon dioxide and water by action of various liver enzymes.

▶ High acetaldehyde levels and chronic alcohol consumption impair liver function and lead to liver damage.

III. Diffusion

▶ Within 5 minutes after ingestion, alcohol can be detected in the blood.

▶ Alcohol is quickly diffused into all cells and intercellular fluid of the body.

▶ Less than 10% is excreted directly through the lungs, skin, and kidney (breath, sweat, and urine).

▶ A person's alcohol level can be determined by several tests of the blood, urine, saliva, or water vapor in the breath.

IV. Blood Alcohol Concentration (BAC)[9]

▶ In the United States, law enforcement agencies primarily test the BAC of automobile drivers using the breath test. The results are then converted to equivalent BACs.

▶ A BAC of 0.08% has been established as the legal level of intoxication.

  • The amount of alcohol by weight, in a set volume of blood.

  • Measured in milligrams per deciliter (mg/dL).

  • A BAC of 0.10% is the equivalent of 0.10 g of alcohol per 100 mL of blood.

▶ The tolerance level varies among individuals. The inexperienced drinker may lose self-control and become nauseated with low levels of alcohol. The experienced drinker tolerates a higher level of alcohol without nausea.

▶ BAC measurement reflects a person's drinking rate and rate of metabolism.

▶ Alcohol is metabolized more slowly than it is absorbed. The BAC increases when alcohol is consumed faster than previous drinks are metabolized.

▶ The rate at which the body will absorb and metabolize alcohol is based on factors such as age, gender, percentage of fatty tissue in the body, and whether food is also being metabolized.

▶ Ethanol is a powerful depressant of the central nervous system; in low doses, alcohol can act as a disinhibitor and as a relaxant. Euphoria may be produced.

▶ In high doses, alcohol can produce analgesic effects with reduction of anxiety generally accompanied by reduced alertness and reduced judgment.

▶ The characteristic effects exhibited at various levels of blood alcohol can be seen in Table 65-1.

HEALTH HAZARDS OF ALCOHOL

Prolonged alcohol use causes many serious medical disorders. The alcohol-dependent person is most seriously afflicted, but even unhealthy alcohol use may have complications. Alcohol-related illnesses may involve any body system. A few are mentioned here.

I. Liver Disease

Chronic alcohol abuse is the most frequent cause of morbidity and mortality from liver diseases. Alcoholic liver disease (ALD) includes the following conditions[10]:

▶ Fatty liver with degeneration: early stages are reversible with abstinence.

TABLE 65-1	Effects of BACS at Various Levels
DOSE	**EFFECT**
50 mg/dL	Sedation, tranquility, fine motor coordination reduced, unsteadiness on standing.
50–100 mg/dL	Reduced anxiety, alertness, and critical judgment; enhanced self-esteem, slowed reaction time, and impulsive risk-taking behavior.
100–300 mg/dL	Slowed reaction time, slurred speech, staggering; mood swings, memory deficits, blackouts; increased aggressive behavior.
300–400 mg/dL	Labored breathing, nystagmus, lowered blood pressure and body temperature; loss of consciousness.
400–500 mg/dL	Depressed respiration, alcoholic coma, possibly fatal.

Source: National Institute on Alcohol Abuse and Alcoholism. *8th Special Report to the U.S. Congress on Alcohol and Health*. Rockville, MD: National Institute on Alcohol Abuse and Alcoholism; 1993:89.

▶ Alcoholic hepatitis: inflammation of the liver.

▶ Early fibrosis: healthy cells replaced by scar tissue.

▶ Cirrhosis: scarring of the liver with irreversible damage.

▶ Individuals with hepatitis C virus are more susceptible to ALD.[11]

II. Immunity and Infection

▶ Those who abuse alcohol have diminished immune response, suppression of immune system defense, and disturbed function of neutrophils.

▶ Risk for many bacterial infections is increased, particularly pulmonary diseases (pneumonia, tuberculosis) and viral infections (hepatitis B and C).

III. Digestive System

▶ Alcohol ingestion alters the stomach mucosa, stimulates gastric acid secretion, and affects gastric function.

▶ Lesions that bleed may develop with desquamation of the stomach lining (acute gastritis).

▶ Injury to small intestines: diarrhea, weight loss, and vitamin deficiencies.

IV. Nutritional Deficiencies

▶ Alcohol provides an excess of caloric intake. With the intake of large quantities of alcohol, the individual loses interest in regular mealtime nutritious food, which leads to many deficiencies.

▶ Deficiencies result from malabsorption of vitamins and essential nutrients.

▶ Secondary malnutrition develops from direct effects of alcohol on the gastrointestinal tract; malabsorption and maldigestion occur after cellular changes in the intestinal wall.

V. Cardiovascular Diseases

▶ Risk for cardiomyopathy, coronary artery disease, hypertension, arrhythmias, and hemorrhagic stroke.

▶ Decreased risk for heart attack and stroke is associated with light-to-moderate alcohol use.[2]

▶ Heavy consumption increases the death rate from cardiovascular disease.

▶ Associated with early coronary calcification in young adults.[12]

VI. Neoplasms

▶ Alcohol use increases the risk for many types of cancers, notably of the alimentary and respiratory tracts.[13]

▶ Alcohol combined with tobacco use has long been associated with increased neoplasms of the oral cavity, pharynx, and larynx.

VII. Nervous System

A. Central and Peripheral

▶ Early changes affect intellectual actions, judgment, and learning ability.

▶ Long-term alcohol abuse combined with malnutrition can lead to damage of both central and peripheral nervous systems.

▶ Prolonged and heavy alcohol consumption leads to chronic brain damage.

B. Wernicke–Korsakoff's Syndrome[14]

Brain disorder of the cerebellum is the result of a thiamine deficiency associated with chronic alcohol consumption. Two syndromes are involved as follows:

▶ *Wernicke's encephalopathy*: symptoms of mental confusion, ocular dysfunction, and gait disturbances.

▶ *Korsakoff's psychosis*: persistent knowledge and memory problems characterized by forgetfulness, easy frustration, lack of muscle coordination, and retrograde and anterograde amnesia.

VIII. Reproductive System

▶ Alcohol affects every branch of the endocrine system, directly and indirectly, through the body's organization of the endocrine hormones.

▶ Female: increased risk for menstrual disturbances, infertility, and miscarriage, stillbirth, or premature delivery.[15]

▶ Male: diminished testicular function and male hormone production resulting in increased risk for impotence, infertility, and reduction of secondary sex characteristics.[16]

FETAL ALCOHOL SPECTRUM DISORDERS (FASD)

▶ The significant incidence and prevalence of FASD highlights the need for dental professionals to recognize symptoms and characteristics.

▶ Patients with FASD have orofacial characteristics and various psychological and physical symptoms that may affect a dental hygiene treatment plan.

▶ The offspring of women who use alcohol to excess during pregnancy have an increased risk for developmental disorders that range from subtle to lifelong serious effects.[17]

I. Alcohol Use During Pregnancy

▶ There is no known safe amount of alcohol use during pregnancy.

• The amount of alcohol required to produce adverse fetal consequences varies among fetuses. When

BOX 65-3
FASD Terminology and Abbreviations

FAS: Fetal alcohol syndrome. A characteristic pattern of abnormal growth, minor facial anomalies, and abnormal central nervous system (CNS) development resulting from maternal consumption of alcohol during pregnancy.

PFAS: Partial fetal alcohol syndrome. FAS without the growth deficiency.

FASD: Fetal alcohol spectrum disorder. An umbrella term describing the range of effects that can occur in an individual whose mother drank alcohol while pregnant. Diagnoses that fall under the umbrella include FAS, PFAS, ARND, static encephalopathy/alcohol exposed (SE/AE), and neurobehavioral disorder alcohol exposed (ND/AE).

ARND: Alcohol-related neurodevelopment disorder. Individuals with ARND have confirmed prenatal alcohol exposure and present with significant structural and/or functional CNS abnormalities. They do not present with the FAS facial phenotype. Alternate terms used to define this outcome include SE/AE and ND/AE.

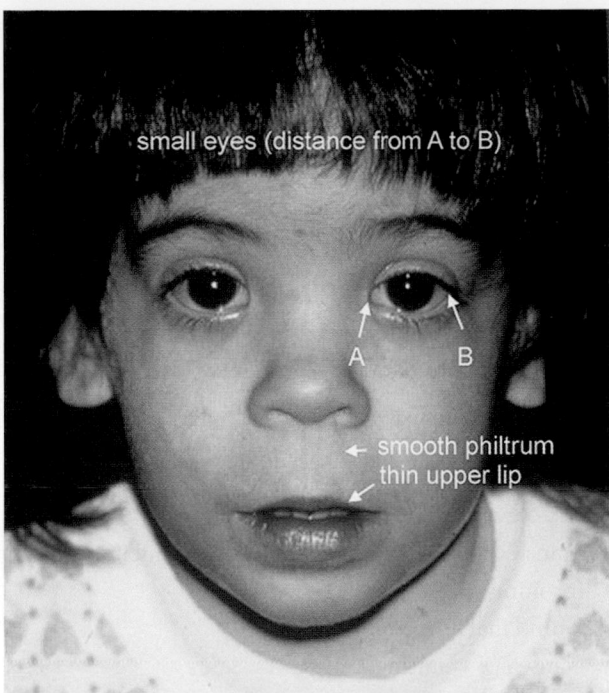

FIGURE 65-2 Facial Features of Fetal Alcohol Syndrome. Child presenting with the characteristic pattern of abnormal facial features diagnostic for FASD, including short palpebral fissure lengths (distance from A to B), smooth philtrum, and thin upper lip. (Photo courtesy of Susan Astley, PhD, University of Washington.)

genetically different twins are exposed to the same levels of alcohol, one twin can be born with FASD while the other twin is normally developed.[18]
- Complete abstinence during pregnancy is safest to prevent FASD.
▶ Prenatal alcohol exposure is cited as the leading preventable cause of birth defects and intellectual disability.
▶ Box 65-3 contains terminology and abbreviations for FASD.

A. No Placental Barrier
▶ Alcohol passes freely across the placenta.
▶ Increased incidence of spontaneous abortions and still-births associated with alcohol consumption.

B. Other Factors
▶ Other poor health habits often accompany the use of alcohol, including inadequate diet and use of tobacco.
▶ The use of prescription or illicit drugs with alcohol can increase risk of adverse outcomes.

II. Criteria for FASD Diagnosis[19]
▶ Facial dysmorphology as shown in Figure 65-2.
▶ Growth deficits.
▶ Central nervous system problems.

III. Characteristics of an Individual with FASD

Common characteristics of an individual with FASD are listed in Box 65-4.

Box 65-4
Common Characteristics of an Individual with FASD

Abnormal facial features, for example, small eyes, a smooth ridge between the nose and upper lip (ridge entitled the philtrum), and thick upper lip.
▷ Small head size; shorter-than-average height; low body weight
▷ Problems with the heart, kidneys, or bones
▷ Vision or hearing problems
▷ Poor coordination
▷ Hyperactive behavior
▷ Speech and language delays; learning difficulties (especially with math)
▷ Poor memory; difficulty paying attention
▷ Poor reasoning and judgment skills

Source: Centers for Disease Control and Prevention (CDC): Fetal Alcohol Spectrum Disorders (FASDs). Facts about FASDs. http://www.cdc.gov/ncbddd/fasd/facts.html. Accessed September 30, 2014.

ALCOHOL WITHDRAWAL SYNDROME[4]

▶ Withdrawal consists of the disturbances that occur after abrupt cessation of alcohol intake in the alcohol-dependent person.
▶ Withdrawal signs appear within a few hours after drinking has stopped.

▶ Even a relative decline in blood concentration can precipitate the syndrome.

I. Predisposing Factors

▶ Malnutrition, fatigue, depression, and physical illnesses aggravate withdrawal symptoms.

II. Signs and Symptoms

▶ Tremor of hands, tongue, and eyelids.
▶ Nervousness and irritation; anxiety.
▶ Malaise, weakness, and headache.
▶ Dry mouth.
▶ Autonomic hyperactivity: sweating, rapid pulse rate, and elevated blood pressure.
▶ Transient visual, tactile, or auditory hallucinations.
▶ Insomnia.
▶ Grand mal seizures.
▶ Nausea or vomiting.

III. Complications

A. Alcohol Withdrawal Delirium (Delirium Tremens)

▶ May occur within 1 week of cessation of heavy alcohol intake.
▶ Features: marked autonomic hyperactivity: rapid heartbeat and sweating.
▶ Vivid hallucinations (visual, auditory, tactile).
▶ Delusions and agitated behavior; tremor.
▶ Confusion and disorientation.

B. Alcohol Hallucinosis

▶ Auditory and visual hallucinations can develop within 48 hours after the abrupt stop or reduction of heavy alcohol intake of long-standing dependency.
▶ Symptoms: may last weeks or months.
▶ Impairment is severe with schizophrenic symptoms, although schizophrenia is not a predisposing factor.
▶ Delirium is not present.

TREATMENT FOR ALCOHOLISM

▶ The overall objective of treatment is to help the person achieve and maintain total abstinence.
▶ An alcohol-dependent person can never drink even small amounts of alcohol without an eventual return to dependency.
▶ Treatment includes a combination of medical and psychiatric therapy with self-help.
▶ Patients are encouraged not to take other psychoactive drugs, including minor tranquilizers and caffeine.

I. Early Intervention

When problem drinkers who are not yet dependent can be identified, counseling may help to reduce and perhaps eliminate the use of alcohol.

II. Detoxification

The term detoxification applies to the management of acute intoxication and the withdrawal syndrome. A variety of treatments may be involved.

A. Treatment for Immediate Emergencies

▶ Accident or medical emergency other than withdrawal symptoms.
▶ Fractures, head injury, internal bleeding, or other problems may require initial attention.
▶ Alcohol dependency may be revealed after hospital admittance for other causes.

B. Removal from Source of Alcohol: Abstinence

▶ Advantages of hospitalization:
  • Supervision is available.
  • No access to sources of alcohol.

C. Goals of Therapy

▶ Treat medical complications.
▶ Restore general physical health: rest, sleep, and exercise.
▶ Treat nutritional deficiencies: proper diet.

D. Relief from Acute Withdrawal Signs

▶ Tranquilizers may be prescribed for short-term use.
▶ Vitamins, particularly thiamine, are usually administered.

III. Pharmacotherapy[2]

A. Medications Used in Alcoholism Treatment

Agents for withdrawal management include:
▶ Alcohol-sensitizing agents (cause aversive reactions in combination with alcohol).
▶ Anticraving agents (decrease desire for and consumption of alcohol).
▶ Amethystic agents (reverse the acute intoxicating and depressant effects of alcohol).
▶ Medications for treatment of coexisting psychiatric disorders, such as depression and anxiety.

B. Disulfiram (Antabuse®): Alcohol-Sensitizing Agent

▶ Interferes with the metabolism of alcohol by acting on the enzyme that converts acetaldehyde to acetone in the liver.
▶ Effect: acetaldehyde accumulates in the tissues.

- Alcohol and disulfiram taken at the same time result in nausea, vomiting, and hypotension.
- Drug acts as a deterrent to provide an adjunct to comprehensive therapy in selected patients.

C. Naltrexone (Revia): Anticraving Agent
- Interferes with neurotransmitter systems that produce pleasurable effects.
- The effect of taking alcohol with an "opiate antagonist:" no experience of a rewarded high or feelings of euphoria.

D. Acamprosate
- Affects certain chemical messengers (neurotransmitters) in the brain.
- Reduces the risk of heavy drinking; doubles the likelihood that patients will achieve abstinence.

E. Toirimate (Anticonvulsant)
- May also be beneficial for cocaine dependence treatment.
- Other anticonvulsants, including carbamazepine and valproate, have also shown some effectiveness in the treatment of alcohol use disorders.

IV. Rehabilitation

A. Counseling and Education
- Patients need to recognize that alcoholism is a serious disease and be agreeable to accept help.
- Family and work associates may be recruited to cooperate with the program.
- Behavioral therapy and psychotherapy have been used.

B. Group Therapy
- *Alcoholics Anonymous*: a fellowship of men and women who help themselves and others to recover from alcoholism; can provide help for motivated individuals.
- Some patients prefer treatment through special clinics and centers.
- *Al-Anon*: a separate program for parents, adult children, siblings, and spouses, as well as other persons concerned with the alcoholic patient in recovery.
- *Alateen*: a program for teenage children.

C. Psychiatric Treatment
- An increased frequency of schizophrenia, psychoneurosis, sociopathy, and manic-depressive diseases is being recognized among alcohol-dependent people.

D. Aftercare Services
- Recovery takes a long time; extended treatment required.

- Relapse more likely when a recovering alcoholic leaves a treatment system too early.
- Typical follow-up includes weekly aftercare group meetings for 9–12 months.

ABUSE OF PRESCRIPTION AND STREET DRUGS
- Drug abuse: habitual use of drugs not needed for therapeutic purposes.
- Prescription drug abuse: taking prescription medication that is not prescribed for that person; using a prescription for reasons or in dosages other than prescribed.
- Street drug abuse: taking drugs or substances purchased illegally from nonmedical sources and/or for nonmedical reasons.
- Drugs interfere with the function of the brain and create long-term effects on brain metabolism and activity.
- Dependency develops after periods of drug use followed by pathologic abuse.
- An increase in the amount and frequency of a drug is needed to alleviate withdrawal responses; the withdrawal symptoms become more severe and require a greater intake of the drug.
- Brain circuitry becomes altered with this cyclic process and the voluntary use of drugs becomes drug addiction: a compulsive craving for drugs, seeking, and use.

RISK MANAGEMENT FOR LEGAL PRESCRIPTIONS
- A major problem facing health care is the diversion of prescription medications with a high potential for abuse.
- Substances are classified in the US Drug Enforcement Administration (DEA) drug schedule according to use and abuse potential as listed in Box 65-5.
- Prescription drugs may become a very valuable product for drug traffickers.
- The theft of prescription pads and medication occurs in a variety of ways.
- Healthcare professionals need to safeguard against becoming an easy target for drug diversion.
- To avoid prescription pad theft and abuse, certain risk management principles need to be strictly observed, including the following:[20]
  - Secure inventory of prescription pads in locked area.
  - Number the prescription pads; keep count of all prescription pads by having a staff member appointed to document a weekly inventory count.
  - Do not leave prescription pads in dental treatment rooms or at work stations.

- Omit the prescriber's DEA registration number on preprinted prescription pads.
- Do not give DEA registration number to anyone in the office or family members.
- Write out the quantity (in words not a number) of doses on the prescription and indicate "No Refills." Never add extra doses: only minimum number that may be needed.
- The provider cannot allow anyone besides her/himself to sign a prescription.
- Know employees; conduct a pre-employment criminal background investigation and pre-employment drug screening for potential employees; include a policy for random drug testing in the office policy manual.
- Dental hygienists, dental assistants, and front office staff can query prescription monitoring programs, which are statewide electronic databases of data about controlled substances dispensed.
- Establish an office policy to ensure all risk management principles are met and understood by the entire dental team, reviewed frequently, and included for instruction of all new employees.[21]

I. Dental Team Responsibilities

▶ All members of the dental team are responsible to:
- Educate the patient about how to safeguard prescription given for pain medication.
- Be mindful of the inherent abuse potential of opioids.
- Understand and comply with federal and state regulations regarding legitimate prescribing and administration of controlled substances.

▶ The ADA encourages dentists to[22]:
- Obtain continuing education to promote responsible prescribing practices.

- Ensure opioids are available only to the patients who need them.
- Implement policies to limit instances of abuse and diversion.

II. Prevention of Prescription Drug Abuse

▶ The ADA suggestions to help parents prevent medications from becoming a source of abuse are listed in Box 65-6.[23]

MOST COMMON DRUGS OF ABUSE

The most common drugs of abuse are alcohol and those found in the categories in this section.[24] Examples of the substance names in each category and the commercial and street names are listed in Table 65-2.

I. Cannabinoids (Marijuana)

▶ Organic substances present in the plants of *Cannabis sativa* that have a variety of pharmacologic properties.

▶ Upper leaves, tops, and stems are cut, dried, and rolled into cigarettes (*marijuana*).

TABLE 65-2	Most Commonly Abused Prescription Drugs		
DRUG CATEGORY AND DEA SCHEDULE[a]	**STREET NAMES AND *COMMERCIAL NAME***	**HOW ADMINISTERED**[b]	**INTOXICATION EFFECTS**
Depressants			
Barbiturates DEA schedule: II, III, V[a]	Barbs, reds, red birds, phennies, tooies, yellows, yellow jackets; *Amytal, Nembutal, Seconal, Phenobarbital*	Injected, swallowed	Reduced pain and anxiety; feeling of well-being; lowered inhibitions; slowed pulse, breathing; lowered blood pressure; poor concentration
Benzodiazepines (other than flunitrazepam) DEA schedule: IV[a]	Candy, downers, sleeping pills, tranks; *Ativan, Halcion, Librium, Valium, Xanax*	Swallowed	Sedation, drowsiness; also for barbiturates
Flunitrazepam[c,d] DEA schedule: IV[a]	Forget-me pill, Mexican Valium, R2, Roche, roofies, roofinol, rope, rophies; *Rohypnol*	Swallowed, snorted	Sedation, drowsiness/dizziness increased heart rate and blood pressure, impaired motor function/memory loss
Dissociative Anesthetics			
Ketamine DEA schedule: III[a]	cat Valium, K, Special K, vitamin K; *Ketalar SV*	Injected, snorted, smoked	At high doses, delirium, depression, respiratory depression and arrest pain relief, euphoria, drowsiness
Opioids and Morphine Derivatives			
Codeine DEA schedule: II, III, IV[a]	Captain Cody, Cody, schoolboy; (with glutethimide) doors & fours, loads, pancakes and syrup; *Empirin with Codeine, Fiorinal with Codeine, Robitussin A-C, Tylenol with Codeine*	Injected, swallowed	Less analgesia, sedation, and respiratory depression than morphine
Fentanyl DEA schedule: II[a]	Apache, China girl, China white, dance fever, friend, goodfella, jackpot, murder 8, TNT, Tango and Cash; *Actiq, Duragesic, Sublimaze*	Injected, smoked, snorted	
Morphine DEA schedule: II[a]	M, Miss Emma, monkey, white stuff; *Roxanol, Duramorph*	Injected, swallowed, smoked	
Opium DEA schedule: II, III[a]	big O, black stuff, block, gum, hop; *laudanum, paregoric;*	Swallowed, smoked	
Other opioid pain relievers (oxycodone, meperidine, Hydromorphone, Hydrocodone, Propoxyphene) DEA schedule: II, III, IV[a]	oxy 80s, oxycotton, oxycet, hillbilly heroin, percs; *Tylox, OxyContin, Percodan, Percocet* demmies, pain killer *Demerol, meperidine hydrochloride* juice, dillies *Dilaudid, Vicodin, Lortab, Lorcet; Darvon, Darvocet*	Swallowed, injected, suppositories, chewed, crushed, snorted	

(continued)

TABLE 65-2	Most Commonly Abused Prescription Drugs (Continued)		
DRUG CATEGORY AND DEA SCHEDULE[a]	**STREET NAMES AND *COMMERCIAL NAME***	**HOW ADMINISTERED**[b]	**INTOXICATION EFFECTS**
Stimulants			
Amphetamines DEA schedule: II[a]	Bennies, black beauties, crosses, hearts, LA turnaround, speed, truck drivers, uppers; *Biphetamine, Dexedrine*	Injected, swallowed, smoked, snorted	Increased heart rate, blood pressure, metabolism; feelings of exhilaration, energy, increased mental alertness
Cocaine DEA schedule: II[a]	Blow, bump, C, candy, Charlie, coke, crack, flake, rock, snow, toot; *Cocaine hydrochloride*	Injected, smoked, snorted	Rapid breathing; hallucinations; also, for amphetamines
Methamphetamine DEA schedule: II[a]	Chalk, crank, crystal, fire, glass, go fast, ice, meth, speed; *Desoxyn*	Injected, swallowed, smoked, snorted	Aggression, violence, psychotic behavior; also for methylphenidate
Methylphenidate DEA schedule: II[a]	JIF, MPH, R-ball, Skippy, the smart drug, vitamin R; *Ritalin*	Injected, swallowed, snorted	Increase or decrease in blood pressure, psychotic episodes
Other Compounds			
Anabolic steroids DEA schedule: III[a]	Roids, juice; *Anadrol, Oxandrin, Durabolin, Depo-Testosterone, Equipoise*	Injected, swallowed, applied to skin	No intoxication effects

[a]See Box 65-5 for explanation of DEA schedule classifications.
[b]Taking drugs by injection can increase the risk of infection through needle contamination with staphylococci, HIV, hepatitis, and other organisms.
[c]Associated with sexual assaults.
[d]Not available by prescription in the United States.
Source: National Institute on Drug Abuse: The Science of Drug Abuse and Addiction. Commonly abused drugs. http://www.drugabuse.gov/drugs-abuse/commonly-abused-drugs-charts-0. Accessed August 9, 2015.

▶ Dried exudate that seeps from the tops and undersides of cannabis leaves (*hashish oil*).

▶ Marijuana smoke, similar to tobacco smoke, is associated with increased risk of cancer, lung damage, and oral health disease, such as oral cancers, periodontitis, and dental caries.[25]

II. Depressants

▶ An agent (such as a sedative or anesthetic) that reduces nervous or functional activity.

▶ Examples are *downers, sleeping pills, ludes, rophies*.

III. Dissociative Anesthetics

▶ A form of general anesthesia that promotes dissociation from the environment but not necessarily complete unconsciousness. Sometimes used for short diagnostic or surgical procedures.

▶ Street names: *angel dust, Special K*.

IV. Hallucinogens

▶ Chemical substances that produce mind-altering or mental perception-altering properties.

▶ A popular example is *LSD* (lysergic acid diethylamide).

▶ A disorder associated with the use of these substances can produce hallucinogen persisting perception disorder, commonly known as "flashbacks."

▶ *MDMA* (3,4 dimethoxymethamphetamine) or *Ecstasy*, a popular drug among teens and young adults, widely used at nightclubs and bars (a club drug).

▶ *MDMA* is classified as a stimulant, but is known for its hallucinogenic effects.

V. Opioids and Morphine Derivatives

▶ Narcotic substances made from the Asian poppy or produced as synthetic drugs with the effects of opium: they result in analgesic and euphoric effects.

▶ Opioids are prescribed as analgesics, anesthetics, antidiarrheal agents, and cough suppressants.

▶ *Heroin* is one of the most commonly abused drugs of this class: it can be injected, smoked, or snorted.

▶ *Hydrocodone* is a schedule III drug and its potency is between codeine and oxycodone.

▶ *Oxycodone* is a schedule II drug, and codeine is a moderate opioid with genetic impact on metabolism.

VI. Stimulants

▶ A class of drugs that enhances brain activity.
- Stimulants cause an increase in mental alertness, attention, and energy; they improve motor skills and elicit a general sense of well-being.
- Stimulants increase cardiac and respiratory function and speed up metabolism.

▶ *Cocaine hydrochloride powder* can be "snorted" through the nostrils, or, when mixed with water, can be injected intravenously.
- *Crack cocaine* is a cocaine alkaloid in the form of a small rock.
- *Crack* is cocaine that has been processed from cocaine hydrochloride to a free base for smoking. It is easily vaporized and inhaled and exhibits an extremely rapid onset of effects.

▶ *Methamphetamine* (*meth, speed*) is taken orally, intranasally (snorting the powder), by intravenous injection, or by smoking. Meth users are resistant to local anesthesia.[26]

▶ *Ice,* a very pure form of methamphetamine (seen as crystals under a high magnification), produces an immediate and powerful stimulant when smoked.

VII. Other Compounds

A. Steroids

▶ Used to build muscles and increased performance.

▶ May produce a feeling of well-being or euphoria, followed by lack of energy and irritability.

▶ More severe symptoms include depression and liver disease.

B. Inhalants

▶ A breathable chemical vapor that produces psychoactive effects.

▶ Capable of producing intoxication, abuse, and dependence.

▶ Available in a wide variety of commercial products: paint thinners, gasoline, and glue.

▶ A substance-soaked cloth or substance placed in a paper or plastic bag is applied to the nose and mouth and vapors are breathed in.

▶ Intoxication is characterized by a mild euphoria and a change in perception of time.

▶ Causes relaxation of the smooth muscle and a decrease in oxygen-carrying capacity of the blood.

▶ Toxic reactions: vomiting, headache, hypotension, and dizziness.

MEDICAL EFFECTS OF DRUG ABUSE

I. Cardiovascular Effects

There is a connection between the abuse of most addictive drugs and adverse cardiovascular effects that may range from arrhythmias to heart attacks. Cocaine in particular can:

▶ Increase blood pressure.

▶ Cause vasoconstriction.

▶ Alter electroactivity of the heart.

▶ Promote a cardiac stimulant effect.

▶ Induce angina; precipitate myocardial infarction.

▶ Cause a variety of arrhythmias and palpitations including sudden cardiac death.[4]

▶ Contribute to early subclinical atherosclerotic cardiovascular disease.[27]

II. Neurological Effects

▶ Drug use can cause changes in the brain leading to:
- Memory lapses
- Decision-making or attention problems.
- Euphoric effects.
- Seizures, stroke, or intracerebral hemorrhage.[28,29]
- Depression, paranoia, aggression, or hallucinations.

▶ Substance-induced disorders can include:
- Amnesia, delirium, or dementia.
- Mood or anxiety disorders.
- Sleep disorders.

III. Gastrointestinal Effects

▶ Cocaine in particular has been associated with gastrointestinal complications and abdominal pain, including the possibility of life-threatening hemorrhage.[30,31]

▶ Cocaine that is ingested can cause severe bowel gangrene due to reduced blood flow.

▶ Many drugs of abuse have been known to cause nausea and vomiting soon after use.

IV. Kidney Damage

▶ Chronic drug use causes toxicity to several organs including the kidney.

▶ Drugs affect renal function either through the toxic effects of the drug or by a reduction in kidney function.

▶ Pain medications, alcohol, antibiotics, and illegal drugs can all cause kidney damage if not used properly.

▶ Toluene can affect the liver and kidneys severely.[32]

V. Liver Damage[2]

▶ The liver detoxifies drugs, chemicals, and alcohol that are ingested.

▶ Changes in liver function due to drug abuse decrease the metabolism of drugs: when not able to break down properly, the drug can remain at a toxic level.

▶ Chronic abuse of heroin, inhalants, and steroids may cause significant liver damage.

▶ The consumption of alcohol and cocaine together compound the danger each drug poses.

  • The liver combines cocaine and alcohol to form a third substance: cocaethylene.[33]

  • Cocaethylene intensifies cocaine's euphoric effects, potentially increases the risk of sudden death.

VI. Musculoskeletal Effects[2]

▶ When rising levels of testosterone and other sex hormones, which trigger the growth spurt during puberty, reach a certain level, they signal the bones to stop growing.

  • Steroid use during childhood or adolescence can result in artificially high hormone levels; bone growth culminates earlier than usual, which results in a short stature.

▶ Other drugs may cause severe muscle cramping and overall weakness.

VII. Respiratory Effects

▶ Drug abuse can lead to a variety of respiratory problems.

▶ The use of smoking tobacco, marijuana, and inhalants all damage sensitive lung tissue.

▶ A compromised respiratory system can result in a reduced respiration rate, asthma, bronchitis, emphysema, and lung cancer.

VIII. Prenatal Effects

▶ Prenatal drug abuse has been associated with:

  • Miscarriage.
  • Premature birth.
  • Low birth weight.

▶ Inhalant abuse by expectant women can result in fetal solvent syndrome with abnormalities similar to those occurring in FASD.[34]

IX. Infections[35]

▶ Drug users are at risk for acquiring a large range of infections.

▶ Common bacterial infections among drug users include:

  • Skin and soft tissue: abscesses and cellulitis located at injection sites.

  • Musculoskeletal infections, septic arthritis, and osteomyelitis, a local extension of soft tissue infection.

▶ Poor nutrition and human immunodeficiency virus (HIV) infection can result in immunosuppression and increase the risk for:

  • Infective endocarditis.
  • Pulmonary tuberculosis (increased in crowded living quarters, crack houses, and homeless shelters).
  • Respiratory tract infections, including community-acquired pneumonia.

▶ Role in disease transmission between drug users and their partners:

  • Major mode for transmission of HIV, other sexually transmitted diseases, and viral hepatitis.
  • Blood-borne diseases by way of shared needles and other paraphernalia.
  • Transmission through drugs, drug adulterants, or unique drug preparations.
  • Poor hygiene may exacerbate the risk of infection.

▶ Prevention

  • Eliminate drug use.
  • Utilize risk-reducing strategies.
  • Medically supervised injection facilities; needle exchange programs.
  • Street-based education programs aimed at the use of sterile injection practices.
  • Clean the injection site with alcohol and the drug paraphernalia with bleach.
  • Avoid contamination by never sharing needles.
  • Avoid the use of dangerous injection sites such as the neck and groin.
  • Avoid high-risk behavior such as unprotected sex and sex with multiple partners.
  • Vaccinations and routine screening for tuberculosis, HIV, and other sexually transmitted diseases help to reduce disease transmission and prevent bacterial infections.

TREATMENT METHODS

▶ Drug addiction is a treatable disorder.

▶ Treatment is tailored to the individual needs of the patient and may involve behavioral changes and medications.

▶ Medications help to suppress craving for drugs and withdrawal symptoms.

▶ The principles that characterize the most effective drug abuse treatment can be found in Box 65-7.

I. Behavioral Change Interventions

▶ Counseling
▶ Support groups

Box 65-7

Basic Principles of Effective Drug Addiction Treatment

▷ No single treatment is appropriate for all individuals.

▷ Medical detoxification is only the first stage of treatment.

▷ Treatment does not have to be voluntary to be effective.

▷ Remaining in treatment for an adequate period of time is essential.

▷ Recovery can be a long-term process and relapses can occur.

▷ Effective treatment includes:

  ▷ Individual, group counseling, and behavioral therapies

  ▷ Use of treatment medications

  ▷ integration treatment for any coexisting mental disorders

  ▷ Infectious disease assessment and counseling (HIV/AIDS, Hepatitis)

  ▷ Monitoring of possible drug use during treatment.

  ▷ Medical, social, vocational, legal and family counseling.

Source: National Institute on Drug Abuse. *Principles of Drug Addiction Treatment: A Research-Based Guide* (Rep 2000). Bethesda, MD: National Institute on Drug Abuse; 1999. NIH Publication No. 00-4180.

▶ Psychotherapy

▶ Family therapy

II. Drug Withdrawal Medications

▶ The primary medically assisted withdrawal method for narcotic addiction is to switch the patient to a comparable drug with milder withdrawal symptoms, and then gradually taper off the substitute medication.

▶ Some patients cannot continue to abstain from opiates and are therefore given a maintenance therapy.

▶ The following drugs are used in maintenance therapy:

A. Methadone

▶ Suppresses withdrawal symptoms and drug craving, associated with narcotic addiction.

▶ In methadone maintenance programs, a daily dose (usually a minimum of 60 mg) is administered.

B. LAAM (Levo-Alpha-Acetyl-Methadol)

▶ Suppresses withdrawal symptoms and drug cravings.

▶ Administered three times per week only.

C. Naltrexone

▶ Competes with opioids at the opioid receptor sites, therefore blocking the effects of heroin.

▶ Does not eliminate drug craving so is not the preferred treatment for those addicted.

▶ This drug works best with highly motivated patients.

D. Phenobarbital or Diazepam

▶ Longer-acting sedatives used to treat sedative withdrawal symptoms.

▶ The dose is reduced gradually until there are no signs of withdrawal.

DENTAL HYGIENE PROCESS OF CARE

▶ Millions of people in the United States meet the diagnostic criteria for alcoholism and drug abuse.

▶ Dental professionals often have the first opportunity to treat early signs and symptoms of oral complications for the substance abuser.

▶ It is necessary to recognize the characteristics of each patient before treatment since it is rare that a patient will disclose information about an addiction.[36]

▶ Many drug-dependent people continue to maintain home, work, and social relationships, at least initially, and even for a span of years.

▶ The spectrum of substance use found in dental and dental hygiene patients varies from abstinence to dependence.

▶ Many patients with an alcohol use disorder may use psychoactive drugs such as cocaine, heroin, amphetamines, marijuana, and assorted sedatives or hypnotics.

I. Assessment

A. Patient History

▶ Carefully prepared personal, medical, and dental histories are needed to provide information for comprehensive patient care.

▶ A reluctance of the patient to reveal symptoms of alcoholism presents a danger because of alcohol's effect on oral and systemic health and an enhanced risk of medically related adverse events and drug interactions.[2]

▶ Many patients with a drug abuse problem are in denial, which makes their medical history less reliable.

▶ The medical history is updated with an interview at each continuing care appointment.

▶ Patients that abuse drugs may have many general health-related problems.

▶ Precautions, modifications, or adaptations may be needed to prevent an emergency situation.

▶ Other conditions may be identified that require further diagnosis, treatment, or referral.

B. The Interview

▶ Practice a motivational interviewing approach (Chapter 26).

- Keep the lines of communication open; refrain from comments that place the patient on the defensive.
- Remain empathetic, respectful, and nonjudgmental; patients may be far more likely to respond to questions.
- Discuss the effects of drug use on physical, psychosocial, and economic well-being at a level appropriate for patient understanding.

▶ Obtain patient confidence

- Patients may hesitate to reveal personal information about substance use because of a social stigma attached to users.
- Patients need to understand the information is required as a health-safety measure.
- The patient needs to be assured that personal information will remain confidential.

C. Screening: The CAGE Questionnaire[37]

▶ Dental providers concerned about a patient's use of alcohol or other drugs can screen for potential abuse and/or dependence using the CAGE questionnaire as shown in Box 65-8.

▶ The questionnaire is most effective when used during a routine medical history.

▶ The patient's answers may not provide a positive diagnosis, but can alert the interviewer to a need for follow-up questions.

▶ One positive reply can be followed by additional questions as suggested in Box 65-9.

D. Screening: The Five A's

▶ The "Five A's" (Ask, Advise, Assess, Assist, Arrange): a screening intervention used in tobacco counseling also can be used in substance abuse screening (See Chapter 34).

E. The Older Adult Patient[38]

▶ The number of older adult alcohol consumers is increasing; some of these are addicted.

▶ Potential for substance abuse in the older adult is high because of the number and variety of medications used.

▶ Physiological changes associated with aging permit the harmful effects of alcohol consumption to occur at lower levels than with a younger person.

▶ Excessive use of alcohol exacerbates medical and emotional problems and predisposes the person to drug reactions with medications used to control other illnesses.

▶ Memory lapses can upset routine prescription drug use.

▶ Use of over-the-counter medications and alcohol, combined with prescribed medications, can increase potential health risks associated with substance abuse.

BOX 65-8

CAGE Questionnaire and Scoring

Questionnaire

C Have you ever felt you ought to **C**ut down on your drinking or drug use?

A Have people **A**nnoyed you by criticizing your drinking or drug use?

G Have you ever felt **G**uilty about your drinking or drug use?

E Have you ever had a drink or used drugs first thing in the morning (**E**ye-Opener) to steady your nerves or to get rid of a hangover or to get your day started?

Scoring

▷ Each positive response receives one point.

▷ A score of 2 or more is considered probable for alcoholism.

▷ The predictive value of two positive responses is 30%–60%.

▷ Three positive responses is 60%–75%.

▷ Four positive responses is higher than 90.[a]

---

[a]Refer all patients with test results that suggest alcohol dependence to their primary care physician for a more in-depth evaluation.
Source: Schorling JB, Buchsbaum DG. Screening for alcohol and drug abuse. *Med Clin North Am.* 1997;81:845–865.

BOX 65-9

Additional Information to Obtain from a Patient Suspected of Drug Use

▷ Last time patient drank alcohol or used drugs.

▷ Pattern of substance use: consumption, frequency, or amount in a given time period.

▷ Any instances of five or more drinks at one time.

▷ Systemic conditions related to substance abuse.

▷ Accidents or hospital admittances due to substance abuse.

▷ Use of medications including prescribed, over-the-counter, and illicit drugs.

▷ Prescription drugs from multiple doctors or dentists.

▷ Taking prescription medications for reasons other than prescribed.

▷ Taking or buying prescriptions intended for another person.

Source: Trachtenberg AI, Fleming MF. Diagnosis and treatment of drug abuse in family practice. National Institute on Drug Abuse Website. http://archives.drugabuse.gov/diagnosis-treatment/diagnosis.html. Accessed June 27, 2014.

F. Vital Signs

► Record in patient record.

► Blood pressure frequently is increased when alcohol and other drugs are used; fluctuations can be particularly significant.

G. Clinical Examination[39]

► Information in the patient history may not reveal accurately the extent of a patient's drug use.

► Clinical observations along with the medical history may provide a high degree of suspicion.

► Specific oral manifestations are associated with particular drugs.[40-49] Examples are found in Box 65-10.

H. Extraoral Examination

► Alcohol signs
  • *Breath and body odor of alcohol and of tobacco*: Many alcohol users are also heavy tobacco users.
  • *Tremor of hands, tongue, eyelids*: Signs of withdrawal.
  • *Skin*: Redness of forehead, cheeks, dilated blood vessels that produce spider petechiae on the nose; may worsen pre-existing acne rosacea.
  • *Face color*: Light yellowish brown may indicate jaundice from liver disease.
  • *Eyes*: Red, baggy eyes or puffy facial features; bloated appearance.
  • *Evidences of trauma*: Facial injuries related to falls when intoxicated. Alcohol abusers are especially prone to traumatic accidents.
  • *Lips*: Angular cheilitis related to poor nutrition.
  • *Parotid glands*: Swelling.

► Personal appearance
  • Lack of interest in proper dress and personal hygiene.
  • Wears long sleeves to cover needle marks.
  • Small blood stains on clothes from previous injections.
  • Dramatic weight loss.

► Eyes
  • Wears sunglasses to conceal dilated or constricted pupils and eye redness, or to avoid bright light because of eye sensitivity.
  • Pupils dilated (amphetamine, LSD, cocaine, marijuana).
  • Pupils constricted (heroin, morphine, methadone), as shown in Figure 65-3.
  • Red, inflamed, bloodshot (marijuana).

► Arms
  • Needle marks may be noted when determining blood pressure.

► Behavior
  • Sneezing, itching.
  • Tendency to gaze into space; moodiness.
  • Drowsiness, yawning; may sleep long hours.

BOX 65-10

Oral Manifestations of Particular Drugs

A. **"Meth mouth":** key ingredients used in meth manufacturing are corrosive.[40,41]
  ▷ Meth smoker swirls heated, vaporized substances in the mouth.
  ▷ Oral mucosa is irritated and burned, creating sores and leading to infection.
  ▷ Chronic meth smoker: teeth decayed to the gingiva.
  ▷ Snorting meth also causes chemical damage to teeth.
  ▷ Symptoms: xerostomia, dryness of the mouth from a lack of normal secretions.
  ▷ Rampant dental caries on proximal surfaces and at the gingival margin.
  ▷ Cracked teeth caused from grinding and clenching.
  ▷ Enamel erosion: corrosive acids in ingredients.
  ▷ Periodontal infection: reduced blood supply and tissue breakdown.

B. **Cocaine abuse**[42-45]
  ▷ Perforation of the nasal septum and/or perforation of the palate (Figure 65-4).
  ▷ Saddlenose deformity.
  ▷ Erosive carious lesions.
  ▷ Rapid gingival recession and mucosal ulcerations.
  ▷ Trismus.

C. **"Speed" and "ecstasy," amphetamine-based drugs**[46-48]
  ▷ Xerostomia
  ▷ Tooth wear associated with chewing and grinding.
  ▷ Temporomandibular joint tenderness.
  ▷ Bruxism leading to trismus.
  ▷ Rampant dental caries.

D. **Cannabis abusers generally have poorer oral health than nonabusers**[49]
  ▷ Increased dental caries.
  ▷ Increased periodontal infections.
  ▷ Dysplastic changes: a premalignant stage in cellular structures.
  ▷ Premalignant lesions of the oral mucosa.
  ▷ Leukoplakia.
  ▷ Increased oral infections due to immunosuppressive effects.

• Appearance of intoxication with or without the odor of alcohol.
• Slurred speech.
• Changes in habits, attitudes, and efficiency. Irregular attendance at appointments by one who was previously prompt.
• Possession of pills, capsules.
• Hallucinations or convulsions indicate need for immediate emergency care.

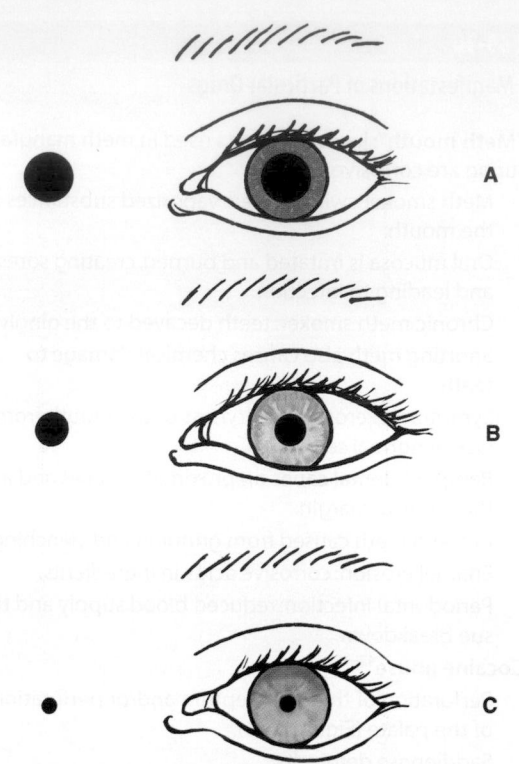

FIGURE 65-3 Examination of the Pupils. A: Dilated; occurs in shock, heart failure, other emergencies, and in the use of hallucinogens and amphetamines. **B:** Normal. **C:** Pinpoint; occurs in the use of morphine and related drugs, heroin, barbiturates. (*Source:* The American National Red Cross: Standard First Aid and Personal Safety.)

II. Intraoral Examination

▶ Mucosa, lips, tongue
  • Dry; drug-induced xerostomia, soft tissue abnormalities.
  • Tongue coated; glossitis related to nutritional deficiencies.
▶ Gingiva
  • Generalized poor oral hygiene; heavy biofilm not unusual.
  • Calculus deposits may be generalized, depending on patient neglect.
  • Moderate to severe gingival inflammation.
  • Gingiva that bleeds spontaneously or on probing.
  • Gingival lesions resulting from the direct application of cocaine.[50]
  • Higher incidence of periodontal infections than peers.
▶ Palate
  • Perforation of palate due to chronic cocaine snorting (Figure 65-4).
▶ Teeth
  • Chipped and fractured from falls and injuries; stained from tobacco use.
  • Attrition secondary to bruxism.
  • Erosion secondary to frequent vomiting, wine consumption,[51] and meth mouth.

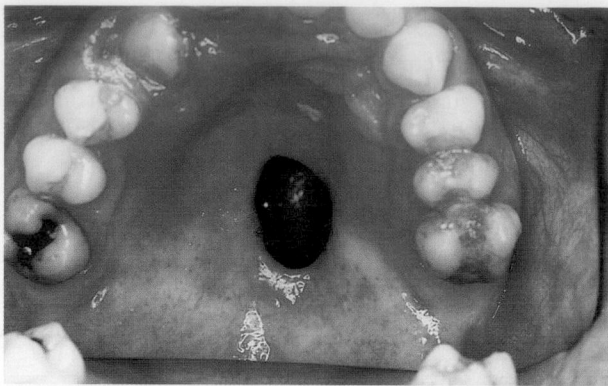

FIGURE 65-4 Nasopalatal Defect. The problems due to chronic cocaine snorting began to manifest themselves as nosebleeds followed by recurring sinus infections. Within 4 months, the patient discovered a pinhole in his palate. Each time he tried to swallow liquid it came out of his nose. (Photo courtesy of Peter Villa, DDS, FRDC.)

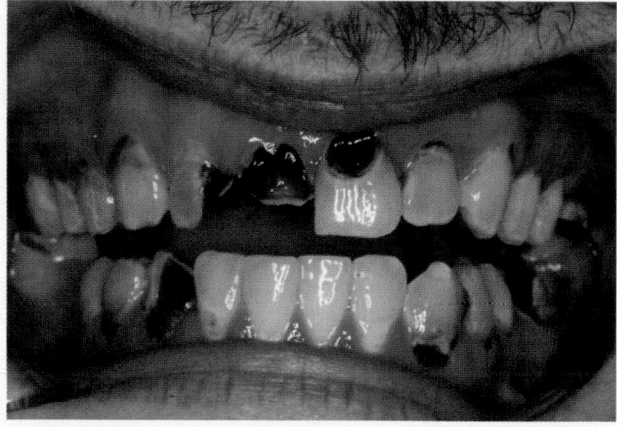

FIGURE 65-5 Rampant dental caries due to methamphetamine use in a 24-year-old patient who presented for treatment after serving time in prison and going to rehab; patient started using meth at age 16, initially snorting the powder and progressed to smoking the drug. Although some teeth could have been saved, the patient chose to have all remaining teeth extracted in order to receive full dentures. (Photo courtesy of Kessler BH, Dinnen M. Methamphetamine: oral effects and treatment. *Inside Dent.* 2010;6(2):44–46.)

  • Removable or fixed partial dentures: chipped or broken, may require frequent repairs.
▶ Dental caries
  • Increased risk factors: poor diet, lack of dental care, accumulation of biofilm, and xerostomia.
  • Diet high in cariogenic substances.
  • Root caries when gingival recession is evident.
  • Open rampant carious lesions: abuse of methamphetamine, diet of sweets, alcohol and sugar sweetened beverages as shown in Figure 65-5.[52]
  • Tooth loss.
▶ Minimal professional care
  • Substance abuse patients tend to delay dental and dental hygiene care.
  • Any available money is used in the purchase of drugs.

- Dental care is used on an emergency basis to alleviate any pain or discomfort, and to obtain prescriptions for drugs.

III. Dental Hygiene Diagnosis

Examples of dental hygiene diagnosis for drug users are suggested as follows:

▶ *Rampant caries* related to the changes in the addicted patient's lifestyle including:
  - Diet (multiple daily exposures to sucrose-containing foods and beverages).
  - Neglect of daily care of the oral cavity (lack of biofilm removal and use of fluoride dentifrice and other fluoride sources).

▶ *Periodontal infections* related to:
  - Changes resulting in infection due to reduced blood supply and tissue breakdown as a result of methamphetamine use.
  - Rapid gingival recession and mucosal ulcerations due to cocaine abuse.

▶ *Xerostomia* related to methamphetamine use (many drugs have dry mouth as a side effect).

IV. Planning

▶ Develop strategies to meet the individual needs of the patient as identified from the dental hygiene diagnosis.

▶ Priorities and goals are determined by the immediacy of the condition, severity of the problem.

▶ Examples of interventions to reduce, eliminate, or prevent rampant caries due to drug use:
  - Use of fluoride toothpaste and fluoride mouthrinse without alcohol.
  - Apply fluoride applications such as fluoride varnish in office and custom trays for home use if the patient will be compliant.
  - Do not administer local anesthetic for any procedure if unsure whether the patient has taken methamphetamine within the last 24 hours, as the patient may be resistant to local anesthesia.[26]

V. Implementation

The clinical procedures for dental hygiene care are greatly influenced by the many health problems that can result from drug use.

A. Preparation for Treatment

▶ Consult with patient's physician to determine whether prophylactic antibiotic premedication is indicated.

▶ Precaution is needed for potential drug interactions between specific drugs.

▶ Preprocedural rinse, antibacterial agents, and oral hygiene products that contain alcohol are to be avoided for all patients suffering from a past or current alcohol use problem. The smallest amount of alcohol ingested by a patient being treated with disulfiram can cause an emergency.

B. Scaling and Debridement

▶ Use of anesthesia: drug interactions, use of epinephrine, and choice of nitrous oxide/oxygen versus local

---

EVERYDAY ETHICS

Mr. Phillips is 20 minutes late for his continuing care appointment. The patient has previously missed two consecutive appointments. As he is being seated, he tells Christy, "Just hurry up and clean my teeth." He also tells her he can't eat because it is sore on the left side of his mouth. Mr. Phillips presents with an odor of smoke and appears quite agitated. The receptionist alerts Christy that the patient refused to update and sign his medical history; Christy begins to review the patient's medical history. Significant findings are (1) BP 160/110 (2) a cluster of ulcerated lesions on mandibular left buccal fold, (3) CAGE score of 3, (4) OHI-S index of 3. Christy consults with Dr. Franks who then examines the patient and questions Mr. Phillips about his medical history, including the CAGE questionnaire.

Dr. Franks is concerned about the patient's health and tells Mr. Phillips he is referring him for a complete physical examination and is recommending a mouthrinse with benzocaine to help reduce pain on the left side of his mouth. Dr. Franks requests that the patient stop by the receptionist to reschedule his appointment for further treatment. Mr. Phillips becomes very aggressive because no treatment was performed; he verbally abuses the staff before storming out of Dr. Franks' office without making a follow-up appointment. Dr. Franks and Christy both record Mr. Phillips' behavior in the patient chart.

Questions for Consideration

1. Does the decision to postpone treatment for today violate Mr. Phillip's rights? Why or why not?

2. If Dr. Frank decides to terminate his practitioner–client relationship with Mr. Phillips could this be considered "abandonment"? Answer the questions provided in the Questions to Ask column of Table VI-1 in the Section VI Introduction to determine at least one other ethical alternative action that Christy might recommend for Dr. Frank to take.

3. How might each of the professional issues listed in Table VII-1 in the Section VII Introduction apply to a decision whether or not to terminate the patient–client relationship with Mr. Phillips?

anesthesia is reviewed and discussed with the patient's physician.

▶ Contraindications for use of nitrous oxide/oxygen and medical considerations for local anesthesia with or without epinephrine are in Chapter 38.

C. Power-Driven Instruments

▶ Patients with respiratory problems, hepatitis, tuberculosis, HIV/AIDS, and diabetes may have increased risk for complications resulting from aerosols or contaminated water lines in power-driven instruments.

▶ Use ultrasonic scalers and air-powder stain-removal devices with caution to prevent inhalation of oral microorganisms by the patient.

▶ High-powered suction is essential.

▶ Patients with immunosuppression resulting from poor nutrition and HIV are more susceptible to lung infections caused by bacteria taken into the lungs from the oral cavity.

D. Response to Therapy

The usual oral tissue response expected following periodontal instrumentation may be limited by the changes in the patient's tissues such as:

▶ Prolonged bleeding time; impaired clotting mechanism from chronic liver disease.

▶ Resistance to local anesthetic.

▶ Impaired healing.

▶ Interference with collagen formation and deposition.

▶ Decreased immune system function.

▶ Increased susceptibility to postcare infection.

E. Dental Biofilm Control

▶ Maintaining oral health and cleanliness is essential for the prevention of infections.

▶ Motivation may be difficult because many patients with substance abuse problems are preoccupied with drugs and place less priority on personal hygiene.

▶ A preventive oral care program for a recovering substance abuse patient is a necessary part of the total rehabilitation process.

F. Diet and Nutrition

▶ Use of alcohol and abusive use drugs can affect nutrition intake.[53]

▶ Alcoholic beverages contain calories; a day's allotment of calories may be ingested when alcohol is used in excess and essential nutrients such as, minerals, proteins, and vitamins are lost.

▶ Deficiencies in proteins and vitamins, in particular vitamin A, may contribute to liver disease and other disorders related to drug use.

Instruction for the patient with a substance-related disorder includes:

• Review dietary assessment.
• Provide information about basic dietary needs.
• Encourage use of foods from the MyPlate Food Guidelines as shown in Chapter 35.

VI. Evaluation

▶ Develop continuing care program to prevent progression or reoccurrence of disease.

▶ Evaluate treatment plans and goals with patient.

▶ Make changes according to the patient's progress.

▶ Evaluate to determine the frequency of continuing care appointment.

DOCUMENTATION

▶ Patient record medical alert box for possible substance abuse alerts dental personnel to:

• Use a nonalcoholic mouthrinse.
• Review score of CAGE questionnaire.
• Avoid using local anesthetic with vasoconstrictors if patient is identified as an active user or has a positive CAGE score.
• Possible aggressive behavior.

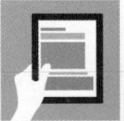

BOX 65-11

Example Documentation: Patient with Substance Abuse

S –A 35-year-old male patient presents for continuing care appointment. Patient commented, "Hurry up and clean my teeth." Patient states he cannot eat due to pain on the left side of his mouth

O –BP 160/100, pulse 98 bpm, CAGE score of 3, OHI-S index of 3, observed cluster of ulcerations on mandibular left buccal fold.

A –Possible hypertension; three positive responses on CAGE indicates 60%–75% possibility of alcoholism; score of 3 on OHI-S indicates soft debris covering more than two-thirds of exposed tooth surface. Ulcerated lesions contributing to patient's inability to consume solid foods.

P –Referred patient for medical consult to discuss possible hypertension and alcohol addiction. Recommended mouthrinse containing benzocaine to relieve pain of oral ulcerations. Reinforced biofilm removal. Reschedule in 2 weeks to evaluate the oral lesions. If medical clearance has been provided, provide continuing care treatment at this appointment.

Signed: _____, RDH

Date: _____

▶ Key concepts: documentation for sign/symptoms of early identification of substance abuse. Include in the permanent record:
- *Oral examination*: with attention to ulcerations, infections, and xerostomia.
- *Dental examination*: especially cervical dental caries.
- *Periodontal examination*: noticing rapid changes in periodontal status.
- *Patient education*: regarding relapse of previously good oral hygiene.
- *Psychological reactions and/or aggressive behavior.*

▶ Example of documentation for the patient with substance abuse is shown in Box 65-11.

Factors To Teach The Patient

▷ Drug abuse is a great risk to overall health.

▷ Risk of oral cancer is increased by the use of alcohol, tobacco, and marijuana.

▷ Need for routine oral screening at least twice a year for signs of early cancer.

▷ Drinking alcohol and using other drugs (prescription or over the counter) can lead to medical emergencies. Always check each drug and its actions before using it in combination with alcohol or in combination with another drug.

▷ Commercial antimicrobial and fluoride mouthrinse may contain up to 30% alcohol. Labels must be read carefully. Keep mouthrinse bottles out of reach of children.

▷ Alcohol and other drugs readily enter the breast milk and are transmitted to the infant during nursing.

▷ Illicit drug use during pregnancy can pose serious risks for unborn babies.

▷ Access *The Medicine Abuse Project* at http://medicineabuseproject.org/ to teach teenagers about falling victim to prescription drug abuse.

▷ Discard unused prescription pain medication that may be additive to young children or others within the household.

References

1. National Institute on Alcohol Abuse and Alcoholism. *Alcohol Alert Number 76: Alcohol and Other Drugs.* Bethesda, MD: U.S. Department of Health and Human Services; 2008.

2. United States Department of Health and Human Services; Secretary of Health and Human Services. *Alcohol and Health: 10th Special Report to the U.S. Congress on Alcohol and Health.* Rockville, MD: National Institute on Alcohol Abuse and Alcoholism; 2000:4, 169–190, 197–205, 240, 258–266, 334, 430, 451.

3. Saitz R. Unhealthy alcohol use. *N Engl J Med.* 2005; 352(6):596–607.

4. American Psychiatric Association. Substance-related disorders. In: *Diagnostic and Statistical Manual of Mental Disorders* (DSM-IV-TR). Washington, DC: American Psychiatric Association; 2000:497, 499–501, 502.

5. National Institute on Alcohol Abuse and Alcoholism. *Alcohol Alert Number 59: Underage Drinking: A Major Public Health Challenge.* Bethesda, MD: U.S. Department of Health and Human Services; 2003.

6. National Institute on Alcohol Abuse and Alcoholism. *Alcoholism, Getting the Facts.* Bethesda, MD: U.S. Department of Health and Human Services; 2004:2–4. NIH Publication No. 96-4153.

7. Dick DM, Jones K, Saccone N, et al. Endophenotypes successfully lead to gene identification: results from the collaborative study on the genetics of alcoholism. *Behav Genet.* 2006;36(1):112–126.

8. Handley, ED, Chassin, L. Alcohol-specific parenting as a mechanism of parental drinking and alcohol use disorder risk on adolescent alcohol use onset. *J Stud Alcohol Drugs.* 2013;74:684–693.

9. Hingson R, Winter M. Epidemiology and consequences of drinking and driving. *Alcohol Res Health.* 2003;27(1): 63–78.

10. National Institute on Alcohol Abuse and Alcoholism. *Alcohol Alert Number 64: Alcoholic Liver Disease.* Bethesda, MD: U.S. Department of Health and Human Services; 2005.

11. Schiff ER, Ozden N. Hepatitis C and alcohol. *Alcohol Res Health.* 2003;27(3):232–239.

12. Pletcher MJ, Varosy P, Kiefe CI, et al. Alcohol consumption, binge drinking and early coronary calcification: findings from the Coronary Artery Risk Development in Young Adults (CARDIA) Study. *Am J Epidemiol.* 2005;161(5):423–433.

13. Lieber CS. Medical disorders of alcoholism. *N Engl J Med.* 1995;333(16):1058–1065.

14. National Institute on Alcohol Abuse and Alcoholism. *Alcohol Alert Number 63: Alcohol's Damaging Effect on the Brain.* Bethesda, MD: U.S. Department of Health and Human Services; 2004:3.

15. Centers for Disease Control and Prevention (CDC): Alcohol and Public Health. Fact sheet—excessive alcohol use and risks to women's health. http://www.cdc.gov/alcohol/fact-sheets/womens-health.htm. Accessed September 30, 2014.

16. Centers for Disease Control and Prevention (CDC): Alcohol and Public Health. Fact sheet—excessive alcohol use and risks to men's health. http://www.cdc.gov/alcohol/fact-sheets/mens-health.htm. Accessed September 30, 2014.

17. Itthagarum A, Nair RG, Epstein JB, et al. Fetal alcohol syndrome: case report and review of the literature. *Oral Surg Oral Med Oral Pathol Oral Radiol Endod.* 2007; 103(3):e20–e25.

18. Astley, SJ. *Diagnostic Guide for Fetal Alcohol Spectrum Disorders: The 4-Digit Diagnostic Code.* 3rd ed. Seattle, WA: University of Washington Publication Services; 2004.

19. Astley SJ. Diagnosing fetal alcohol spectrum disorders (FASD). In: Adubato SA, Cohen DE, eds. *Prenatal Alcohol Use and Fetal Alcohol Spectrum Disorders; Diagnosis Assessment and New Directions in Research and Multimodal Treatment.* Oak Park, IL: Bentham Science Publishers Ltd., Bentham eBooks; 2011:3–29.

20. Rapp C. *Risk Management for the Medical Practice.* Jacksonville, FL: First Professionals Insurance Co; 2009.

21. Denisco RC, Kenna GA, O'Neil MG, et al. Prevention of prescription opioid abuse. The role of the dentist. *J Am Dent Assoc.* 2011;142(7):800–810.

22. American Dental Association. Statement on the use of opioids in the treatment of dental pain. http://www.ada.org/en/about-the-ada/ada-positions-policies-and-statements/statement-on-opioids-dental-pain. Accessed June 25, 2014.

23. American Dental Association, Mouth Healthy. Prescription drugs. http://www.mouthhealthy.org/en/az-topics/p/prescription-drugs. Accessed April 15, 2014.

24. U.S. National Institute on Drug Abuse. *Methamphetamine Abuse and Addiction* (Revised). Bethesda, MD: National Institute on Drug Abuse. NIH Publication Number 06-4210.

25. Ditmyer MM, Demopulos CA, Mobley C. Under the influence: an in-depth look at the association between tobacco and marijuana use and dental caries. *Dimens Dent Hyg.* 2013;11(7):41–43.

26. Kelsch NB. Methamphetamine abuse: oral implications and care. *RDH.* 2010;30(2):75.

27. Lai S, Lima JA, Lai H, et al. Human immunodeficiency virus 1 infection, cocaine, and coronary calcification. *Arch Intern Med.* 2005;165(6):690–695.

28. Ohta K, Mori M, Yoritaka A, et al. Delayed ischemic stroke associated with methamphetamine use. *J Emerg Med.* 2005;28(2):165–167.

29. McGee SM, McGee DN, McGee MB. Spontaneous intracerebral hemorrhage related to methamphetamine abuse: autopsy findings and clinical correlation. *Am J Forensic Med Pathol.* 2004;25(4):334–337.

30. Bellows CF, Raafat AM. The surgical abdomen associated with cocaine abuse. *J Emerg Med.* 2002;23(4):383–386.

31. Devitt E, Carroll R, Donnelly C, et al. An unusual cause of abdominal pain. *Ir Med J.* 2005;98(3):88–89.

32. Voss JU, Roller M, Brinkmann E, et al. Nephrotoxicity of organic solvents: biomarkers for early detection. *Int Arch Occup Environ Health.* 2005;78(6):475–485.

33. U.S. National Institute On Drug Abuse. *NIDA Infofacts: Cocaine.* Bethesda, MD: National Institute on Drug Abuse. Revised 2010:5.

34. Bowen SE, Hannigan JH. Developmental toxicity of prenatal exposure to toluene. *AAPS J.* 2006;8(2):E419–E424.

35. Gordon RJ, Lowy FD. Bacterial infections in drug users. *N Engl J Med.* 2005;353(18):1945–1954.

36. National Institute on Alcohol Abuse and Alcoholism. *Alcoholism, Getting the Facts.* Bethesda, MD: National Institute on Drug Abuse; 2004:2–4. NIH Publication No. 96-4153. http://www.drugabuse.gov/DrugPages/DrugsofAbuse.html. Accessed June 21, 2014.

37. Schorling JB, Buchsbaum DG. Screening for alcohol and drug abuse. *Med Clin North Am.* 1997;81:845–865.

38. Friedlander AH, Norman DC. Geriatric alcoholism: pathophysiology and dental implications. *J Am Dent Assoc.* 2006;137(3):330–338.

39. Friedlander AH, Marder SR, Pisegna JR, et al. Alcohol use and dependence: psychopathology, medical management, and dental implications. *J Am Dent Assoc.* 2003;134(6):731–740.

40. Rhodus NL, Little JW. Methamphetamine abuse and "meth mouth". *Northwest Dent.* 2005;84(5):29, 31, 33–37.

41. National Institute on Drug Abuse. The science of drug abuse and addiction: commonly abused drugs. http://www.drugabuse.gov/publications/media-guide/commonly-abused-drugs. Accessed September 13, 2014.

42. Vilela RJ, Langford C, McCullagh L, et al. Cocaine-induced oronasal fistulas with external nasal erosion but without palate involvement. *Ear Nose Throat J.* 2002;81(8):562–563.

43. Villa PD. Midfacial complications of prolonged cocaine snorting. *J Can Dent Assoc.* 1999;65(4):218–223.

44. Driscoll SE. A pattern of erosive carious lesions from cocaine use. *J Mass Dent Soc.* 2003;52(3):12–14.

45. Kapila YL, Kashani H. Cocaine-associated rapid gingival recession and dental erosion. A case report. *J Periodontol.* 1997;68(5):485–488.

46. Shaner JW. Caries associated with methamphetamine abuse. *J Mich Dent Assoc.* 2002;84(9):42–47.

47. Richards JR, Brofeldt BT. Patterns of tooth wear associated with methamphetamine use. *J Periodontol.* 2000;71(8):1371–1374.

48. McGrath C, Chan B. Oral health sensations associated with illicit drug abuse. *Br Dent J.* 2005;198(3):159–162.

49. Cho CM, Hirsh R, Johnstone S. General and oral health implications of cannabis use. *Aust Dent J.* 2005;50(2):70–74.

50. Yukna RA. Cocaine periodontitis. *Int J Periodontics Restorative Dent.* 1991;11(1):72–79.

51. Mandel L. Dental erosion due to wine consumption. *J Am Dent Assoc.* 2005;136(1):71–75.

52. Kessler BH, Dinnen M. Methamphetamine: oral effects and treatment. *Inside Dent.* 2010;6(2):44–46.

53. Lieber CS. Relationships between nutrition, alcohol use, and liver disease. *Alcohol Res Health.* 2003;27(3):220–231.

ENHANCE YOUR UNDERSTANDING

thePoint° DIGITAL CONNECTIONS
(see the inside front cover for access information)
- **Audio glossary**
- **Quiz bank**

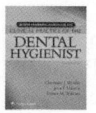

SUPPORT FOR LEARNING
(available separately; visit lww.com)
- *Active Learning Workbook for Clinical Practice of the Dental Hygienist, 12th Edition*

prepU INDIVIDUALIZED REVIEW
(available separately; visit lww.com)
- **Adaptive quizzing with *prepU for Wilkins' Clinical Practice of the Dental Hygienist***

The Patient with a Respiratory Disease

Katherine Yee, RDH, BSDH, MPH and Janet B. Selwitz- Segal, RDH, CDA, MS

CHAPTER OUTLINE

LEARNING OBJECTIVES

After studying the chapter, the student will be able to:

1. Identify and define key terms and concepts related to respiratory diseases.

2. Differentiate between upper/lower respiratory diseases.

3. Describe the etiology, symptoms, and management of respiratory diseases.

4. Plan and document dental hygiene care and oral hygiene instructions for patients with compromised respiratory function.

Patients with respiratory diseases have increased risks for complications due to decreased breathing function and treatment drug interactions.

▶ *Tobacco cessation:*
  - Many respiratory diseases are caused or aggravated by use of tobacco products.
  - Dental hygienists have a unique opportunity to educate their patients about this health hazard.

▶ *Emergency treatment:* Patients with respiratory distress may need emergency care, which dental hygienists are prepared to prevent or provide when necessary.
  - Signs and symptoms and medical emergency procedures for local anesthesia reactions, respiratory failure, airway obstruction, asthma attack, hyperventilation, anaphylaxis, and allergic reactions are found in Table 8-3 (Chapter 8).

▶ *Oral–systemic link:* Scientific evidence shows that dental biofilm and microorganisms from periodontal infections can contribute to the initiation and/or progression of certain infections in the respiratory system.[1] Dedication of the dental hygienist to the prevention and control of periodontal infections will have a major influence on the overall health of the patient.

▶ Box 66-1 defines key words related to respiration and respiratory diseases.

THE RESPIRATORY SYSTEM

I. Anatomy[2]

Structures: sinuses, nasal cavity, larynx, pharynx, trachea, bronchi, lungs, and pleura (Figure 66-1A).

II. Physiology

The respiratory tract from nasal cavity to lungs serves as a passageway for air exchange (Figure 66-1A).

▶ *Inhaled fresh air:* warmed and filtered in the nasal cavity, enters the lungs.

▶ *Exhaled air:* with carbon dioxide, leaves the body.

▶ *Gas exchange:* at the cellular level, occurs in the alveoli at the ends of the bronchioles, as shown in Figure 66-1B.

▶ *Cardiovascular system:* functions with the respiratory system to pump oxygenated blood from the lungs to every cell in the body and deoxygenated blood back to the lungs for exhalation.

III. Function of the Respiratory Mucosa

Figure 66-2 shows ciliated epithelial cells and mucus-secreting goblet cells that line the respiratory tract to make up the respiratory mucosa.

▶ Mucus secreted from goblet cells moistens inspired air, prevents delicate alveolar walls from becoming dry, and traps dust and other airborne particles.

▶ Cilia assist in removing foreign material and contaminated mucus by a constant beating and wavelike motion that propels this material back into the larger bronchi and trachea where it can be coughed up and expectorated or swallowed.

▶ Lack of function results when the inflammatory process of asthma and chronic bronchitis initiates an overabundance of mucus. Congestion is created and the cilia are prevented from assisting with normal breathing.

IV. Respiratory Assessment

Respiratory disease assessment includes several objective measures.

A. Vital Signs

▶ Determination of vital signs (body temperature, pulse, respiratory rate, blood pressure), and also smoking status is considered standard procedure in dental patient care.

▶ Methods determining vital signs are described in Chapter 11. Tobacco use is discussed in Chapter 34.

B. Spirometry

▶ Medical test that measures various aspects of breathing and lung function.

▶ Used to diagnose and monitor many lower respiratory tract diseases.

▶ Performed with a spirometer, a device that registers the amount of air a person inhales or exhales and the rate at which air is moved in and out of the lungs.

▶ Figure 66-3 shows the use of a spirometer to evaluate lung function.

C. Pulse Oximetry[3]

▶ Medical test that measures blood oxygen saturation levels.

▶ Performed with a pulse oximeter.
  - Color of blood varies depending upon the amount of oxygen it contains.
  - Pulse oximeter emits a light through the finger to calculate the percentage of oxygen.
  - Any finger (excluding the thumb) can be used. Nail polish or skin callous may interfere with reading.
  - Intended only as an adjunct in patient assessment along with other methods of assessing clinical signs and symptoms.
  - Healthy patients have an oxygen saturation of 97%–100%.
  - Saturation of 91% or below signifies poor oxygen exchange.

▶ Figure 66-4 shows the use of a pulse oximeter to measure blood oxygen saturation levels.

D. Chest Radiography (Imaging)

▶ Indicates presence of pathological density (radiopacity) in the lungs.

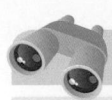

BOX 66-1 | KEY WORDS: Respiration and Respiratory Diseases

Acute: (of a disease or disease symptom) beginning abruptly with marked intensity or sharpness, then subsiding after a relatively short time; opposite of **chronic**.

Analgesic: relieving pain.

Allergen: see **antigen.**

Anaphylaxis: an exaggerated life-threatening hypersensitivity reaction to a previously encountered allergen.

Antigen: any substance that is capable of inducing a specific immune response and of reacting with the products of that response, that is, with specific antibody or specifically sensitized T-lymphocytes or both. When used to describe an allergic response, these antigens are called **allergens**.

Antipyretic: a substance or procedure that reduces fever.

Atopy: hereditary tendency to experience immediate allergic reactions (allergic asthma).
　Atopic: adj.

Bronchodilator: a drug that relaxes contractions of the smooth muscle of the bronchioles to improve ventilation of the lungs.

Chronic: (of a disease or disorder) developing slowly and persisting for a long period, often for the remainder of a person's lifetime; opposite of **acute.**

Comorbid: medical condition(s) existing simultaneously but independently with another condition.

Communicable disease: (contagious) any disease transmitted from one person or animal to another. *Direct:* from excreta or other bodily discharges. *Indirect:* from substances or inanimate objects (contaminated drinking glasses, water, insects, or toys).

Coryza: profuse discharge from mucous membrane of the nose.

Dysphagia: difficulty in swallowing. Do not confuse with **dysphasia:** loss of ability to understand language as a result of injury or disease to the brain.

Dyspnea: labored or difficult breathing.

Edema: abnormal accumulation of fluids in the intercellular spaces of tissues causing swelling.

Exacerbation: increase in severity of a disease or any of its symptoms.

Expiration: release of air from the lungs through the nose or mouth. See **inspiration**.

Gastroesophageal reflux: backflow of stomach contents into the esophagus where gastric juices produce a burning sensation.

Goblet cell: specialized epithelial cell that secretes mucus.

Hemoptysis: spitting of blood because of a lesion in the larynx, trachea, or lower respiratory tract.

Hyperventilation: greater rate and volume of breathing than metabolically necessary for pulmonary gas exchange; may lead to dizziness and possible syncope.

Hypoxia: diminished availability of oxygen to the body tissues characterized by tachycardia, hypertension, peripheral vasoconstriction, and mental confusion.

Inspiration: inhaling air into the lungs. See **expiration**.

Malaise: a vague uneasy feeling of body weakness, often marking the onset of, and persisting throughout, a disease.

Mast cell: constituent of connective tissue; releases substances in response to injury or infection.

Mediator: a substance that effects a change in a disease state.

Morbidity: relating to disease. See **comorbid**.

Mortality: relating to death.

Mucus: (n.) viscous, slippery secretion of mucous membranes and glands. Contains mucin, white blood cells, inorganic salts, and exfoliated cells.
　Mucous: adj.

Myalgia: muscle pain accompanied by malaise.

Mycoplasm: bacteria without a cell wall, more resistant to antibiotics.

Nosocomial: pertaining to, or originating in, a healthcare facility.

Nosocomial pneumonia: pneumonia contracted during confinement in a healthcare facility.

Orthopnea: ability to breathe easily only in an upright position.

Otalgia: pain in the ears.

Pathophysiology: disruption of bodily functions due to disease.

Pleura: delicate membrane enclosing the lungs.

Pleurisy: inflammation of the pleura; may be caused by infection, injury, or tumor, or a complication of lung diseases. Pleuritic: adj.

Pneumothorax: collection of air or gas causing the lungs to collapse.

Pulmonary hypertension: condition of abnormally high pressure within the pulmonary circulation.

Spirometer: instrument for measuring volume of air entering and leaving the lungs to determine lung function and breathing capacity.

Sputum: matter expectorated (coughed up) from the respiratory system, especially the lungs in a diseased state, composed chiefly of mucus and may contain pus, blood, or microorganisms.

Tachycardia: abnormally high heart rate (greater than 100 beats per minute) for an adult.

Tachypnea: abnormally high respiration rate (greater than 20 breaths per minute) for an adult.

Tracheostomy: direct opening into the trachea through the neck to facilitate breathing or removal of secretions.

Wheeze: breathe with difficulty, usually with a whistling sound.

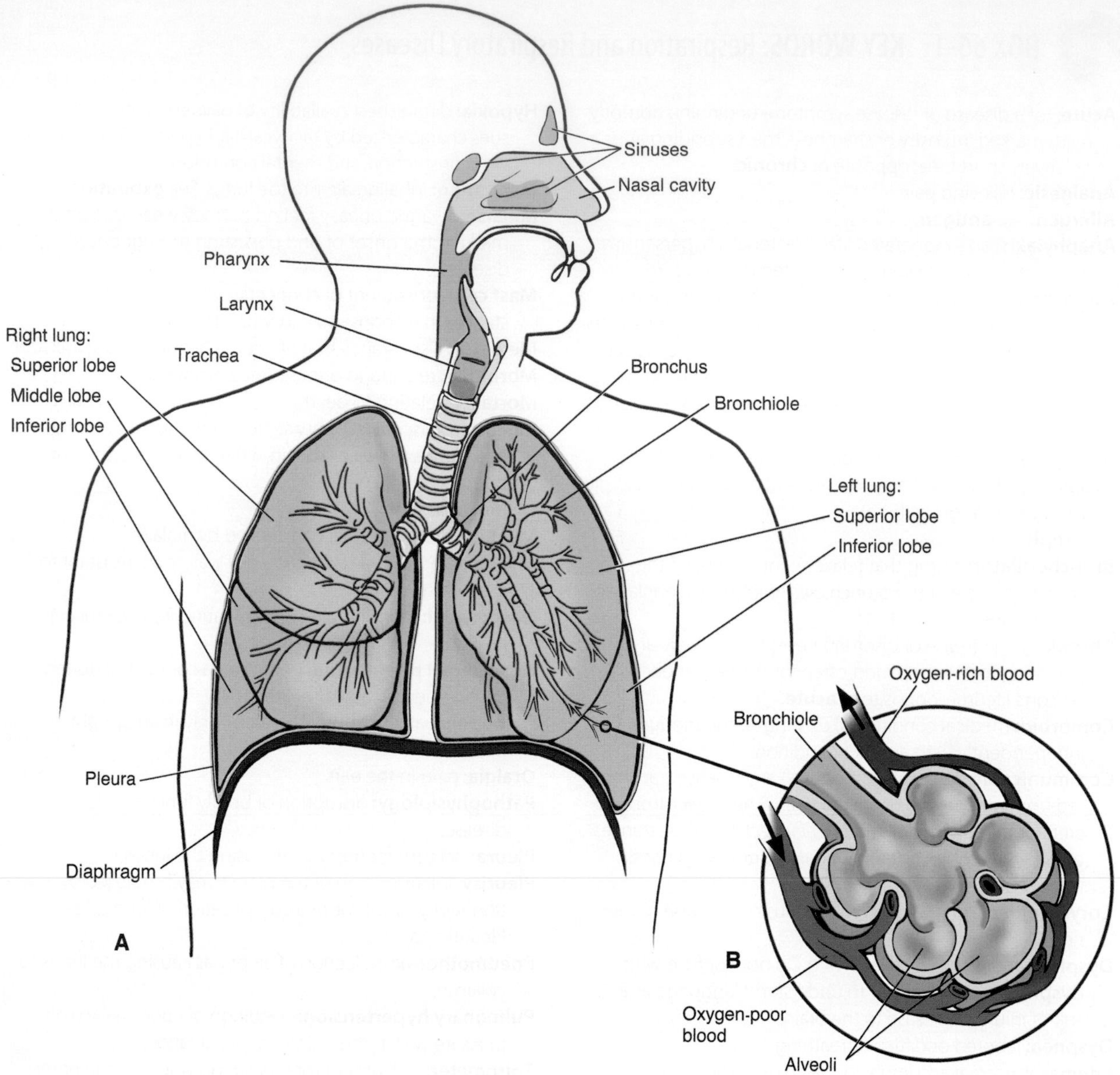

Sinuses

Nasal cavity

Pharynx

Larynx

Right lung:
Superior lobe
Middle lobe
Inferior lobe

Trachea

Bronchus

Bronchiole

Left lung:
Superior lobe
Inferior lobe

Pleura

Diaphragm

A

Oxygen-rich blood

Bronchiole

B

Oxygen-poor blood

Alveoli

FIGURE 66-1 Structures of the Respiratory System. A: Structures. The major anatomic structures of the respiratory system are shown. Each bronchus branches out to the bronchioles. **B:** Gas exchange. Exchange of oxygen and carbon dioxide occurs in the alveoli of the bronchioles.

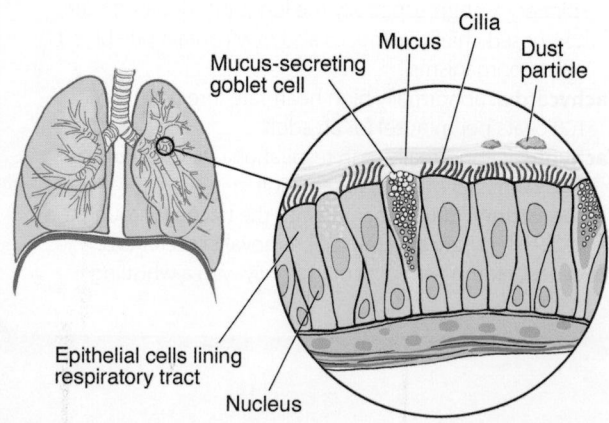

Cilia

Mucus

Mucus-secreting goblet cell

Dust particle

Epithelial cells lining respiratory tract

Nucleus

FIGURE 66-2 Lining of the Respiratory Mucosa. Ciliated epithelial cells and mucus secreted by goblet cells help to remove foreign objects (dust particles). The material is coughed up and either expectorated or swallowed.

- ▶ *Standard chest radiograph:* shows a two-dimensional view of lung tissues.
- ▶ *CAT or CT scan* (computed or computerized axial tomography radiograph): shows a three-dimensional cross section of lung tissues.

E. Blood Gas Analysis

- ▶ Blood test to determine acid/base balance, alveolar ventilation, arterial oxygen saturation, and carbon dioxide elimination.

F. Cytology (Body Cells and Fluids) and Hematology Evaluation

- ▶ Examination of body cells, blood, and other fluids to determine the presence of microorganisms that cause respiratory diseases.

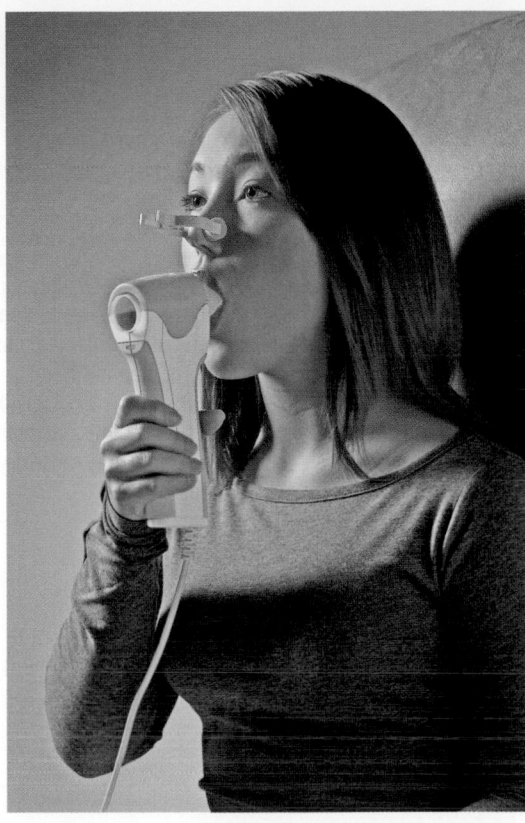

FIGURE 66-3 **Use of a Spirometer to Evaluate Lung Function.** Person being tested takes in a full breath, seals their lips over the mouthpiece of the spirometer, and then blows out as hard and as fast as possible for at least 6 seconds. Nose clips may be applied to ensure no air escapes through the nose. (Courtesy of Midmark Diagnostics, Versailles, Ohio.)

▶ Samples are taken from sputum, pleural cavity fluid, bronchial biopsy, or blood.

V. Classification

Classification of respiratory diseases is listed in Table 66-1.

UPPER RESPIRATORY TRACT DISEASES

The more common disorders of the upper respiratory tract are caused by infections or allergic reactions that result in inflammation.

▶ Signs and symptoms, etiology, medical treatment, and clinical evaluation assessment are summarized in Table 66-2.

I. Modes of Transmission[4]

▶ Inhalation of airborne droplets.
▶ Indirectly by contaminated hands or articles freshly soiled with discharge of nose or throat of infected person.

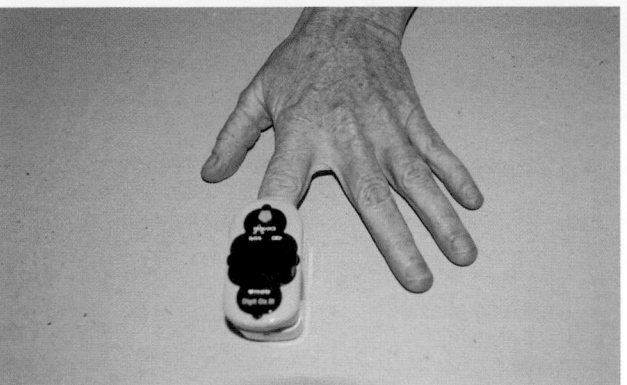

FIGURE 66-4 **Use of a Pulse Oximeter to Measure Blood Oxygen Saturation Level.** Color of blood varies depending on the amount of oxygen it contains. The pulse oximeter clips on any finger (except the thumb) and emits a light through the finger to calculate the percentage of oxygen in the blood. Nail polish and skin callous may interfere with reading.

TABLE 66-1	Classification of Respiratory Diseases	
LOCATION/ STRUCTURES	**ACUTE**	**CHRONIC**
Upper respiratory tract	Diseases of the nose, sinuses, pharynx, larynx Rhinitis (common cold) Sinusitis Pharyngitis/tonsillitis Influenza (flu) ▪ Seasonal ▪ Viral	Allergic rhinitis (hay fever)
Lower respiratory tract Diseases of the trachea, lungs	Acute bronchitis Pneumonia	TB Asthma COPD ▪ Chronic bronchitis ▪ Emphysema CF

Source: Centers for Disease Control and Prevention. *National Center for Immunization and Respiratory Diseases (NCIRD)*. Atlanta, GA: Centers for Disease Control and Prevention. http://www.cdc.gov/ncird/overview/websites.html. Updated May 20, 2014. Accessed July 9, 2014.

II. Dental Hygiene Care

A. Disease Prevention

▶ All healthcare professionals are expected to obtain immunizations for seasonal viral influenza.
▶ Observe standard precautions including respiratory hygiene and cough etiquette as listed in Table 66-3 to prevent transmission of pathogens from patient to clinician and to prevent healthcare-associated infections to the patient.[5]

			CLINICAL EVALUATION
TABLE 66-2	**Summary of Upper Respiratory Diseases: Signs/Symptoms, Etiology, Medical Management, and Dental Hygiene Care—Clinical Evaluation Assessment**		

SIGNS/SYMPTOMS	ETIOLOGY	MEDICAL MANAGEMENT	CLINICAL EVALUATION ASSESSMENT
Upper Respiratory Infections—Infectious Rhinitis (Common Cold)			
■ Sneezing ■ Nasal congestion ■ Nasal discharge (Coryza) ■ Headache ■ Watering of the eyes	■ Viral	■ Analgesic for sore throat, muscle ache ■ Anticholinergic agent to decrease nasal discharge ■ Oral decongestant to decrease nasal congestion ■ Antihistamine for itching, sneezing, "runny nose" ■ Fluids	■ May observe small round erythematous lesions on soft palate, enlarged tonsils, erythema multiforme, acute ulcerative gingivitis ■ Decongestants and mouth breathing may cause dry mouth
Allergic Rhinitis (Hay Fever)			
■ Watering, burning eyes ■ Sneezing ■ Nasal congestion	■ Seasonal triggers (grass, trees, pollen) or perennial triggers (dust mites, mold spores, animal dander) result in IgE-mediated hypersensitivity reactions	■ Avoidance of the allergen ■ Pharmacotherapy medication: antihistamines, decongestants ■ Immunotherapy: allergy injections increase tolerance to allergens and reduce symptoms	■ Dry mouth ■ Oral candidiasis from long-term use of topical corticosteroids
Sinusitis			
■ Nasal obstruction ■ Fever, chills ■ Constant mid-face head pain, more severe when lying down ■ Palpation over sinus area: tenderness, swelling	■ Bacterial infection of the epithelial lining of the sinus ■ Triggers include upper respiratory infections, dental infections, direct trauma	■ Antibiotics ■ Decongestants ■ Fluids	■ Dry mouth ■ Sinus congestion creates pressure on nearby maxillary molar roots and may cause symptoms of toothache; *important to determine if pain originates from tooth or sinus infection*
Pharyngitis/Tonsillitis			
■ Sore throat	■ Mostly viral ■ Rarely bacterial: Group A beta-hemolytic streptococcus infection	■ Viral: treat symptoms ■ Bacterial: antibiotics ■ Patient is no longer infective after 1 day on antibiotics	■ Enlarged tonsils ■ Erythematous tissues
Influenza (Flu)			
■ Chills, fever ■ Headache, coryza, ■ Sore throat ■ Nonproductive dry cough ■ Myalgia, malaise	■ Viral ■ Mode of transmission: airborne (coughing, sneezing) or direct (contact with contaminated surface) ■ Diagnostic testing is required to distinguish between types of influenza viruses.	■ Bed rest, fluids ■ Analgesics, antivirals (amantadine, rimantadine, zanamivir, oseltamivir) ■ Monitor for secondary bacterial infection ■ Prevent with vaccine ■ For information on infection control, vaccinations, prevention, treatment, and updates, see: www.cdc.gov/flu/professionals	■ Dry mouth

Source: Centers for Disease Control and Prevention. *Get Smart: Know When Antibiotics Work* (Treatment guidelines for upper respiratory tract infections). Atlanta, GA: Centers for Disease Control and Prevention. http://www.cdc.gov/getsmart/campaign-materials/treatment-guidelines.html. Updated June 30, 2009. Accessed July 9, 2014.

TABLE 66-3	Respiratory Hygiene and Cough Etiquette in Healthcare Settings[5]

To prevent transmission of *all* respiratory infections in healthcare settings, incorporate the following infection control practices as one component of standard precautions:

Visual alerts	■ Post visual alerts: symptoms of respiratory infection and respiratory hygiene and cough etiquette.
Respiratory hygiene and cough etiquette	■ Use tissue to cover coughs and sneezes and discard in no-touch receptacle. ■ Perform hand hygiene (handwashing with non-antimicrobial soap and water, alcohol-based rub, or antiseptic hand wash) after contact with respiratory secretions or contaminated objects.
Masking and separation of persons with respiratory symptoms	■ Offer masks to persons who are coughing and encourage coughing persons to sit at least three feet away from others in common waiting areas.
Droplet precautions	■ Observe droplet precautions (wearing a surgical or procedure mask for close contact) in addition to standard precautions when examining a patient with symptoms of a respiratory infection, particularly when a fever is present.

Source: Centers for Disease Control and Prevention. *Respiratory Hygiene/Cough Etiquette in Healthcare Settings*. Atlanta, GA: Centers for Disease Control and Prevention. http://www.cdc.gov/flu/professionals/infectioncontrol/resphygiene.htm. Updated February 27, 2012. Accessed July 9, 2014.

B. Appointment Management[6]

▶ Delay treatment until patient is no longer infectious.

▶ Noninfectivity is determined by temperature return to normal and regression of oral lesions such as erythematous lesions of the soft palate and erythema multiforme.

C. Bacterial Resistance to Antibiotics[7]

▶ Bacteria may become resistant to antibiotics within 14 days.

▶ For patients currently prescribed an antibiotic for a nondental condition (such as acute bacterial bronchitis or sinus infection): a different category of antibiotic will be necessary to treat an odontogenic (dental origin) infection.

LOWER RESPIRATORY TRACT DISEASES

▶ Considered to be a more serious infection.

▶ Diseases of the lower respiratory tract are listed in Table 66-1.

ACUTE BRONCHITIS[8]

▶ Acute bronchitis: an acute respiratory infection that involves large airways (trachea, bronchi).

▶ Primary symptom: cough with or without phlegm; may last up to 3 weeks.

▶ Lower respiratory tract disease symptoms: wheezing, shortness of breath, or chest tightness.

▶ Differentiated from pneumonia: no significant findings on chest radiography.

▶ A comparison of acute viral and bacterial bronchitis is listed in Table 66-4.

PNEUMONIA[9]

▶ Pneumonia, an infection and subsequent inflammation of the lungs, may be caused by either viruses, bacteria, fungi, mycoplasma, or parasites.

▶ The respiratory tract of a healthy person is able to defend against organisms aspirated into the lungs.

▶ With diminished salivary flow, decreased cough reflex, swallowing disorders, poor ability to perform good oral hygiene, or other physical disabilities, there is an increased risk of aspiration and respiratory infection.

I. Etiology

A. Viral and Bacterial

▶ Comparison of viral and bacterial pneumonias is listed in Table 66-5.

B. Fungal

▶ Etiologic agent of *pneumocystis* pneumonia is *Pneumocystis jirovecii* (yee-row-vetsee).

▶ Susceptibility is enhanced by chronic debilitating disease in which immune mechanisms are impaired, such as in HIV/AIDS.

TABLE 66-4	Comparison of Acute Viral and Bacterial Bronchitis	
ITEM	VIRAL	BACTERIAL
Occurrence	■ Most prevalent	■ Least prevalent
Medical treatment	■ Supportive: bed rest, fluids ■ May need inhaled bronchodilators and/or cough suppressant	■ Antibiotics: amoxicillin, macrolides, cephalosporin

Source: Centers for Disease Control and Prevention. *Get Smart: Know When Antibiotics Work* (Treatment guidelines for upper respiratory tract infections). Atlanta (GA): Centers for Disease Control and Prevention. http://www.cdc.gov/getsmart/campaign-materials/treatment-guidelines.html. Updated June 30, 2009. Accessed July 9, 2014.

TABLE 66-5	Comparison of Viral and Bacterial Pneumonias	
ITEM	VIRAL	BACTERIAL
Occurrence	■ Most prevalent	■ Least prevalent

Causative agent	■ Virus	Bacteria
		Nosocomial
		Aerobic gram-negative bacilli
		Example: *Pseudomonas aeruginosa Escherichia coli*
		    Klebsiella pneumoniae
		    Gram-positive cocci
		Example: *Staphylococcus aureus*
		    Methicillin-resistant
		    S. aureus
		Community acquired
		Gram-negative cocci
		Example: *Haemophilus influenzae*
		Gram-positive cocci
		Example: *Streptococcus pneumonia*

Signs and symptoms	■ Mild symptoms ■ Cough, sputum ■ Mild fever ■ Dyspnea	■ Sudden onset ■ Cough, purulent sputum ■ High fever ■ Dyspnea, tachypnea ■ Pleuritic chest pain
Diagnosis	■ Patient history ■ Physical findings ■ Chest radiography	■ Patient history ■ Physical findings ■ Chest radiography ■ Sputum sample
Medical treatment	■ Supportive: bed rest, fluids	■ Antibiotics

Source: American Lung Association. *Symptoms, Diagnosis and Treatment.* Chicago, IL: American Lung Association; 2014. http://www.lung.org/lung-disease/pneumonia/symptoms-diagnosis-and.html. Accessed July 9, 2014.

II. Symptoms

▶ Fever greater than 100.4°
▶ Productive cough
▶ Chest pain
▶ Shortness of breath
▶ Visible on chest X-ray.

III. Categories and Role of Oral Bacteria[1,9]

Pneumonia is often categorized by location and/or procedure.

A. Community-Acquired Pneumonia[10]

▶ Infection occurring in an individual in the community (not in a healthcare facility).
▶ Person-to-person transmission.

B. Healthcare-Associated (Nosocomial) Pneumonia

▶ Infection occurring 48–72 hours after admission to a healthcare facility.

▶ A major cause of death in hospitalized patients.

▶ Commonly multidrug resistant pathogens.

▶ More common in the very elderly >80 and those with comorbidities.

▶ Bacteria in periodontal pockets may serve as a reservoir for lung infection, especially in institutional settings.

▶ Bacteria from oral biofilm are released into saliva and can be aspirated into the lungs.

▶ Contributing factors:
 • Poor oral health, dependence on others to perform daily oral hygiene
 • Oral colonization of periodontal and respiratory pathogens
 • Influenced by periodontitis, are associated with nosocomial pneumonia.

▶ *Nursing home–acquired pneumonia*
 • Owing to dysphagia from decrease in saliva, cough reflex, and/or swallowing disorders.
 • Aspiration of saliva can be the main route of bacteria into the lungs and may lead to aspiration pneumonia.

▶ *Hospital-acquired pneumonia*
 • Ventilator-associated pneumonia: mechanically ventilated patients in the immediate care unit with no ability to clear oral secretions by swallowing or coughing.
 • Nonventilator-associated pneumonia: biofilm forms on endotracheal tubes, catheters.

IV. Medical Management

▶ *Viral*: supportive treatment of bed rest and fluids.
▶ *Bacterial*: antibiotic therapy.
▶ *Fungal*: sulfa drugs.

V. Dental Hygiene Care

Control of oral disease and periodontal disease for patients in nursing homes and hospitals will help prevent aspiration pneumonia.

▶ Use 0.12% chlorhexidine gluconate rinse prior to beginning treatment to reduce the bacterial load.[11]

▶ Avoid use of ultrasonic scalers due to production of aerosols.

TUBERCULOSIS (TB)[12]

▶ TB is a chronic, infectious, and communicable disease with worldwide public health significance as a cause of disability and death, especially in developing countries.

▶ Groups at high risk for exposure to TB include those who:[13]
 • Have close contact with people infected with TB.
 • Reside and work in institutional settings (prisons, nursing homes).
 • Are from countries that have a high TB incidence/prevalence.
 • Provide medical/dental care for any of the aforementioned high-risk groups.
 • People who abuse alcohol.
 • Patients with diabetes.
 • Malnourished.
 • Use of tobacco products.

▶ After locating and curing active TB cases, locating and treating contacts of TB patients (especially children, older adults, and those with HIV) is the highest public health priority.

▶ Box 66-2 lists key abbreviations related to TB.

I. Etiology

Mycobacterium tuberculosis, a rod-shaped bacterium (tubercle bacillus), is the most common causative agent.

II. Transmission

▶ Tubercle bacilli travel in airborne droplet nuclei in infected saliva or mucus from persons with pulmonary or laryngeal TB during forceful expirations (coughing, sneezing, talking, singing). A single cough can generate 3,000 droplets.[14]

▶ Inhalation and other modes of transmission are described in Chapter 4.

BOX 66-2

Key Abbreviations: Tuberculosis

AFB: acid-fast bacilli
HIV: human immunodeficiency virus
IGRA: interferon-gamma release assay
LTBI: latent tuberculosis infection

Medications:
▷ **EMB:** ethambutol
▷ **INH:** isoniazid
▷ **PZA:** pyrazinamide
▷ **RIF:** rifampin

Medication Resistance:
▷ **MDR-TB:** multidrug-resistant tuberculosis
▷ **XDR-TB:** extensively drug-resistant tuberculosis
PPD: purified protein derivative
TB: tuberculosis
TST: tuberculin skin test

III. Disease Development

► Inhaled tubercle bacilli travel to the lung alveoli where local infection begins.

► While TB can affect any organ or tissue, M. *tuberculosis* is an aerobe and survives best in an environment of high oxygen tension, such as the lungs.

► Latent tuberculosis infection (LTBI)

  • Within 2–10 weeks following exposure, immune response will limit further growth of M. *tuberculosis*, although not all bacilli will be eliminated.

  • At this stage, the infected person is categorized as having LTBI.

  • Approximately 5%–10% of people infected with M. *tuberculosis* and not treated for LTBI will develop TB disease during their lifetime.[14,15]

  • Comparison of LTBI and active TB disease including signs/symptoms, diagnosis, and medical treatment with TB drugs is listed in Table 66-6.

IV. Diagnosis

A. Latent tuberculosis infection (LTBI)

Two tests are available to determine exposure to M. *tuberculosis*.

► Tuberculin skin test (TST).

  • Also known as Mantoux test, purified protein derivative (PPD) test.

  • PPD is injected under the skin on the forearm. After 72 hours, the circumference of induration (hard swelling) is measured to determine exposure.

  • A negative TST does not exclude TB disease in a person with signs and symptoms of TB disease.

► Interferon-gamma release assay (IGRA).

  • Blood test to determine exposure to M. *tuberculosis*.

  • IGRA blood test, as with TST, cannot differentiate LTBI from active TB disease. Laboratory sputum smear and culture is required.

B. Active TB Disease

When tests to determine exposure to M. *tuberculosis* are positive, further examination is required to rule out active TB disease.

► Chest radiograph.

► Physical examination and evaluation of signs and symptoms.

► *Preliminary diagnosis*: Perform microscopic examination of sputum smears for acid-fast bacilli (AFB).

  • The waxy cell wall of tubercle bacilli does not absorb the traditional water-soluble Gram stain and cannot be identified.

  • However, when treated with an acid stain, the organisms appear pink, and are named AFB.

► *Definitive diagnosis*: When AFB are seen on a stained smear of sputum, or other clinical specimen, a diagnosis of TB disease is *suspected*. However, the diagnosis is *not confirmed* until a laboratory culture is grown and identified as M. *tuberculosis*.

V. Medical Management

A. Commonly Prescribed Drugs

Commonly prescribed TB drugs are included in Table 66-6.

B. Directly Observed Therapy

Observing the patient swallow anti-TB drugs is recommended for all LTBI and TB disease patients and will result in:

► High medication compliance.

► Prevention of multidrug-resistant bacterial development.

► Prevention of multidrug-resistant TB disease, which is more severe and difficult to treat.

C. Drug Resistance[12]

TB bacteria can become resistant (drugs are no longer effective in killing the bacteria).

► Types of resistance[16]

  • Primary resistance: individuals who have not been previously exposed to anti-TB drug treatments

  • Acquired resistance: individuals who have been previously exposed to anti-TB drug treatments. This is occurs frequently when a full course of anti-TB drug treatments is not completed.

► Multidrug-resistant TB (MDR-TB): TB bacterial resistance to at least two of the first-line (most preferred) drugs, isoniazid and rifampin.[17]

► Extensively drug-resistant TB (XDR-TB): TB bacterial resistance to isoniazid, rifampin, fluoroquinolone, and at least one of three injectable second-line drugs.

VI. Oral Manifestations[13]

► TB infrequently appears in the oral cavity from pulmonary organisms in infected sputum brought to the mouth by coughing.

► Classic mucosal lesion: painful, deep, irregular ulcer on dorsum of the tongue as seen in Figure 66-5.

► Lesions can also occur on palate, lips, buccal mucosa, and gingiva.

► A biopsy and laboratory culture of an oral lesion that reveals M. *tuberculosis* confirms a diagnosis of TB.

► Glandular swelling: cervical or submandibular lymph nodes infected with TB. Nodes may become enlarged.

TABLE 66-6	Comparison of LTBI and Active TB Disease: Signs/Symptoms, Diagnosis, and Medical Management with TB Drugs	

ITEM	LTBI	ACTIVE TB DISEASE
Signs and symptoms of pulmonary TB	None	*Early onset*: Low-grade fever Nonproductive cough lasting 3 wk or longer Fatigue Unexplained weight loss Sweating at night *Later onset*: Fever Chills Persistent cough with purulent sputum Hemoptysis Hoarseness (associated with pharyngeal TB) Chest pain Dyspnea
Wellness of patient	Does not feel sick	Usually feels sick
Infectivity	Does not infect others	May infect others
TST PPD, or Mantoux	Positive	May be positive
IGRA blood test	Positive	Positive
Sputum sample for AFB and culture	Negative	May be positive
Chest radiograph	Normal	Abnormal
Medical management for adults: commonly prescribed TB drugs	Isoniazid (INH) taken daily for 9 mo (twice weekly if directly observed therapy is available) OR Rifampin (RIF) taken daily for 4 mo	Various combinations of drugs taken daily for a minimum of 6 mo Drugs commonly prescribed: Isoniazid (INH) Rifampin (RIF) Ethambutol (EMB) Pyrazinamide (PZA) Therapy for multidrug-resistant TB Bedaquiline fumarate

Source: Centers for Disease Control and Prevention. *Extensively Drug-Resistant TB*. Atlanta, GA: Centers for Disease Control and Prevention. http://www.cdc.gov/tb/topic/drtb/xdrtb.htm. Updated January 17, 2012. Accessed July 9, 2014; Center for Disease Control and Prevention. *Morbidity and Mortality Weekly Report. Provisional CDC Guidelines for the Use and Safety Monitory of Bedaquiline Furmarate (Situro) for the Treatment of Multidrug Resistant Tuberculosis*. Atlanta, GA: Center for Disease Control and Prevention; 2013:12.

VII. Dental Hygiene Care

A. Implementation of Infection Control Measures

▶ Update medical history.

▶ Recognize signs and symptoms of TB as listed in Table 66-6.

▶ Follow CDC guidelines in Appendix V, for infection control and prevention of transmission of TB in healthcare settings.

▶ Create and routinely update written office/clinic protocols for:
  • Educating and training staff.
  • Instrument reprocessing and operatory cleanup.

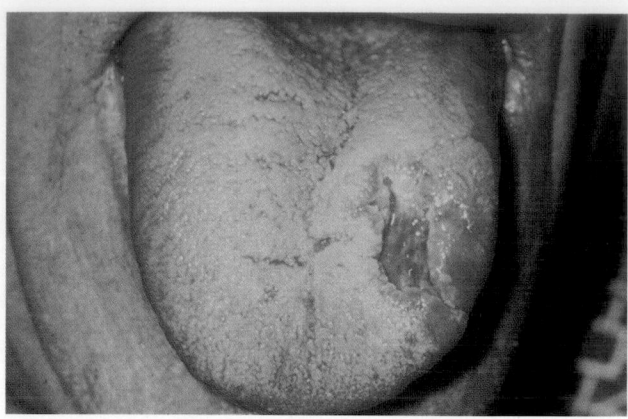

FIGURE 66-5 Oral Ulcer on Tongue Caused by *Mycobacterium tuberculosis.* The classic oral mucosal lesion is a painful, deep, irregular ulcer on the dorsum of the tongue. (Courtesy of the United States Department of Veteran's Affairs. From DeLong L and Burkhart N. *General and Oral Pathology for Dental Hygienists.* Baltimore, MD: Lippincott Williams & Wilkins; 2008.)

- Identifying, managing, and referring patients with active TB disease.
- Assessing, managing, and investigating dental staff with positive TST (PPD).

B. Management of Patients with Symptoms or History of TB[13]

Potential infectivity dictates decisions regarding whether to treat a patient or refer to a physician for medical clearance.

▶ Active TB disease and sputum-positive TB
- Do not treat in the dental office or any outpatient facility.
- Treatment needs to be performed in a hospital with appropriate isolation, sterilization, and engineering controls.

▶ History of TB
- Use caution, obtain history of disease, treatment duration, and discuss signs and symptoms of disease.
- Consult with physician before treatment.
- Also consult with physician if adequate treatment time/appropriate medical follow-up is unclear or patient presents with signs or symptoms of relapse.

▶ Recent conversion to positive TST or blood test. Treatment is permitted after:
- Patient is free of clinically active disease
- Evaluation by physician to rule out active TB disease
- Verification by physician of receiving isoniazid for 6 months to 1 year to prevent active TB disease.

▶ When the patient has signs and symptoms of TB, postpone non-emergency treatment and refer to physician.

ASTHMA[18]

Asthma is a chronic respiratory disease consisting of recurrent episodes of dyspnea, coughing, and wheezing leading to bronchial inflammation and muscle contraction.

I. Etiology

The exact cause of asthma is not completely understood. The following types are based on pathophysiology.

A. Extrinsic (Allergic or Atopic): Allergic Triggers from Outside the Body[19]

▶ Most common type of asthma.
▶ Exaggerated inflammatory response triggered by inhalation of an environmental allergen (dust, pollen, tobacco smoke, mold, dust mites, or animal dander).
▶ Allergic stimulus leads to activation of airway epithelial mast cells.
▶ Steps of an immunoglobulin E (IgE)-mediated hypersensitivity reaction are shown in Figure 66-6.

B. Intrinsic (Nonallergic): Nonallergic Triggers from Within the Body[20]

▶ Triggers: emotional stress, gastroesophageal reflux disease (GERD).
▶ Trigger may be unidentified.
▶ Obesity
▶ Usually seen in adults.

C. Drug- or Food-Induced (Nonallergenic, Nonatopic)

▶ Aspirin.

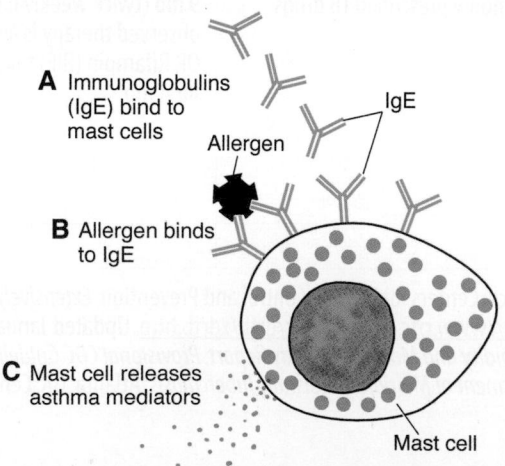

FIGURE 66-6 Steps of an IgE-mediated Hypersensitivity Reaction. A: Initial exposure. On initial exposure to an allergen (dust, pollen), immunoglobulins (IgE) are produced and bind to mast cells. **B:** Subsequent exposure. On subsequent exposures, allergen binds to IgE on the mast cell. **C:** Mast cells respond by releasing asthma mediators (histamines, leukotrienes, prostaglandins). The asthma mediators cause bronchoconstriction, vasodilation, and mucus production, resulting in coughing, wheezing, and dyspnea.

- Nonsteroidal anti-inflammatory drugs (NSAIDs).
- Beta-blockers.
- Food substances: nuts, shellfish, milk, strawberries.
- Tartrazine (yellow food dye).
- Metabisulfite preservative in food (wine, beer, shrimp, dried fruit).
- Metabisulfite preservative in drugs (local anesthetic with epinephrine).

D. Exercise Induced

- Vigorous physical activity: usually affects young people due to their level of activity.
- Thermal changes during inhalation of cold air may provoke mucosal irritation and airway hyperactivity.

E. Infection Induced

- Lung infections caused by viruses, bacteria, or fungi may provoke asthmatic symptoms.
- Treatment of the infection improves breathing.

II. Atopic (Allergic) Asthma

Atopic asthma is one type of IgE-mediated hypersensitivity reaction.

A. Immunoglobulin E

- One of the five types of antibodies produced by the body.
- Provides the primary defense against environmental allergens (pollen, tobacco smoke, and food substances).

B. Normal Inflammatory Reaction

- IgE breaks down the allergens and removes them from the body.
- Normally, such activity does not produce noticeable symptoms.

C. Asthmatic Hypersensitivity Reaction

- People with asthma are believed to "hyperreact" and produce more IgE antibodies than normal.
- The results can be symptoms of asthma: wheezing, coughing, dyspnea.

D. How Allergens Trigger Asthma

Steps in an IgE-mediated hypersensitivity reaction (Figure 66-6):

- On initial exposure to an allergen (dust, pollen, food), immunoglobulins (IgE) are produced and bind to mast cells (Figure 66-6A).
- On subsequent exposures, the antigen binds to the IgE on the mast cell (Figure 66-6B).
- Mast cells release asthma mediators such as histamines, leukotrienes, and prostaglandins (Figure 66-6C).

- Asthma mediators cause bronchoconstriction, vasodilation, and mucus production. The result is wheezing, coughing, and dyspnea.

E. Summary of IgE-Mediated Hypersensitivity Reactions

- Local anaphylaxis:
  - *Allergen binds to mast cell in nasal cavity*: results in allergic rhinitis (hay fever).
  - *Allergen binds to mast cell in bronchiole*: results in asthma.
- Systemic anaphylaxis: *Allergen (penicillin, bee venom, food substance) binds to mast cells throughout the body*: results in a reaction sometimes referred to as anaphylactic shock.

III. Asthma Attack

A. Recognize Signs and Symptoms of Severe or Worsening Asthma Attack

- Chest tightness, sense of suffocation.
- Ineffectiveness of bronchodilator to relieve dyspnea.
- Wheezing, cough.
- Flushed appearance, sweating.
- Confusion due to lack of oxygen.
- Dilated pupils.
- Inability to complete a sentence in one breath.
- Tachypnea.
- Tachycardia.

B. Prepare for Possible Emergency Care

- Recognize signs and symptoms.
- Stop dental hygiene treatment.
- Rule out foreign body obstruction.
- Assist with patient's own bronchodilator inhaler.
- Administer supplemental oxygen by nasal cannula.
- Assist with the administration of subcutaneous injection or inhalation of epinephrine.
- Monitor vital signs.
- Call emergency medical service and initiate emergency procedures described in Table 8-3, Chapter 8.

IV. Medical Management[18]

A. Diagnosis

Conduct physical examination and lung function assessment (spirometry).

B. Achieve and Maintain Asthma Control

- Assess and monitor asthma severity and asthma control.
- The National Asthma Education and Prevention Program classification is based on four levels of severity and frequency of symptoms as well as pulmonary function assessment (spirometry).[19]

- Intermittent.
- Persistent–mild.
- Persistent–moderate.
- Persistent–severe.

▶ Education: Patients are advised to have a written control plan from the physician explaining the process of disease, treatment options, and how to treat exacerbations (worsening of symptoms).

▶ Control of environmental factors (pollutants and allergens) and comorbid conditions that affect asthma (GERD, obesity, obstructive sleep apnea, rhinitis/sinusitis, stress/depression).

▶ Medications:
- There are two main types: Long-term control medications and quick-relief medications.

▶ Categories and examples of asthma medications are listed in Table 66-7.

- People with asthma are advised to get seasonal influenza vaccinations and may also benefit from immunotherapy (allergy injections).

▶ Asthma triggers: Potentially harmful drugs to avoid
- Aspirin-containing medications (use acetaminophen).
- Sulfite-containing local anesthetic solution, such as epinephrine.
- NSAIDs.

▶ Avoid drugs that decrease respiratory function such as narcotics and barbiturates.

▶ Avoid harmful drug-to-drug interactions
- Macrolide antibiotics (such as erythromycin) if patient takes theophylline.

TABLE 66-7	**Types, Categories, and Examples of Asthma Medications**
Long-Term Control: Used Daily for Persistent Asthma	
Corticosteroids ■ Anti-inflammatory ■ Decreases airway hyperresponsiveness. *Preferred:* inhaled corticosteroid for all levels of persistent asthma; oral systemic corticosteroid for severe, persistent asthma	Beclomethasone dipropionate (Vanceril) Prednisone
Mast cell stabilizers: for mild persistent asthma	Cromolyn sodium (Intal)
Immunomodulators: for severe persistent asthma with sensitivity to allergens ■ Prevents binding of IgE to basophils and mast cells	Omalizumab
Leukotriene receptor antagonist: also known as leukotriene modifiers ■ Interferes with leukotriene mediators that are released from mast cells, eosinophils, and basophils. *Alternative:* for mild persistent asthma	Montelukast (Singulair) (Zafirlukast)
Long-acting beta 2-agonists ■ Inhaled bronchodilator with 12-hr duration ■ Used in combination with other medications	Salmeterol, Formoterol
Methylxanthines: for mild persistent asthma ■ Bronchodilator to relax smooth muscle	Sustained-release theophylline (Theolair, Theo24)
Combination medication ■ Anti-inflammatory medication used in combination with bronchodilator medication	
Short-Term Control: Quick Relief Medication	
Short-acting beta 2-agonists (SABA): home use for relief of acute symptoms ■ Bronchodilator to relax smooth muscle	Albuterol (Ventolin, Levabuterol, Pirbuterol)
Anticholinergics ■ Used in hospital emergency room and in inhalers	
Systemic corticosteroids ■ For exacerbations used with SABAs to speed recovery and prevent reoccurrence of exacerbations	

Source: American Lung Association. *Understand Your Medication*. Chicago, IL: American Lung Association; 2014. http://www.lung.org/lung-disease/asthma/taking-control-of-asthma/understand-your-medication.html. Accessed July 9, 2014.

- Erythromycin inhibits metabolism of theophylline, which can result in an increase in serum level and possible overdose.
- Discontinue cimetidine 24 hours before intravenous sedation in patients taking theophylline.

V. Oral Manifestations

▶ Beta-2 agonist inhalers:
- Cause a decrease in salivary flow and dental biofilm pH.
- Are associated with xerostomia and a possible increase in caries and gingivitis in patients with less than ideal dental hygiene.
▶ Increase in GERD with use of beta-2 agonists and theophylline, which may contribute to enamel erosion.
▶ Oral candidiasis may occur with high dosage or frequency of inhaled corticosteroids.
- Occurrence may decrease with use of a "spacer" or aerosol-holding chamber attached to metered-dose inhaler.
- Rinse mouth with water after each use.

VI. Dental Hygiene Care

Table 66-8 summarizes dental hygiene care before, during, and after treatment.[19,20]

CHRONIC OBSTRUCTIVE PULMONARY DISEASE (COPD)[21]

▶ The term "COPD" is used to describe pulmonary disorders that obstruct airflow.
▶ Two of the most common diseases are chronic bronchitis and emphysema.
▶ Characterized as a progressive non-reversible disease.[22]
▶ The primary etiology is inhaling tobacco smoke with occupational and environmental pollutants as contributing factors.
▶ Tobacco use accounts for 80%–90% of COPD-related mortality in both men and women.[23]
▶ Motivating a patient with COPD to begin a tobacco cessation program can be one of the most rewarding aspects of dental hygiene practice.

I. Chronic Bronchitis

A. Etiology

Chronic bronchitis is defined as excessive respiratory tract mucus production sufficient to cause a cough with expectoration (coughing up mucus) for at least 3 months of the year for 2 or more years.

TABLE 66-8	Dental Hygiene Care for the Patient with Asthma
TIME	**DENTAL HYGIENE CARE**
Before treatment	■ Remind the patient to bring inhaler (rescue drug) and/or other medications. ■ Assess risk level: Review medical history, frequency/severity of acute episodes, and triggering agents. ■ Questions to ask: In the past 2 wk, how many times have you: • Had problems with coughing, wheezing, shortness of breath, or chest tightness during the day? • Awakened at night from sleep because of coughing or other asthma symptoms? • Awakened in the morning with asthma symptoms? • Had asthma symptoms that did not improve within 15 min of using inhaled medication? • Had symptoms while exercising or playing? ■ Evaluate current symptoms: Reappoint if symptoms are not well controlled. ■ Review current medications. See Table 66-7 for commonly prescribed asthma medications. ■ Ask if all prescription medication has been taken. ■ Schedule morning appointments for patients with nocturnal asthma (symptoms worsen at night). ■ Have bronchodilator and oxygen available. May use patient's bronchodilator as a preventive measure before the appointment. ■ Obtain a medical consultation for patients with unstable or severe acute asthma or if on corticosteroid to determine necessity of steroid replacement and/or antibiotics to prevent infection. ■ Provide a stress-free environment.
During treatment	■ Prevent triggering a hypersensitive airway by properly placing cotton rolls, fluoride trays, and suction tip. ■ Use local anesthetic without sulfites. ■ Fluoride treatment for all patients with asthma especially those using beta-2 agonists. ■ If asthma attack occurs, stop treatment, rule out foreign body obstruction, initiate emergency procedures shown in Chapter 8.
After treatment	■ Home care instructions: advise patient to rinse mouth with water after using inhaler to decrease oral candidiasis. ■ Analgesic drug of choice is acetaminophen (aspirin or NSAIDs may trigger attack).

▶ Obstruction caused by narrowing of small airways, increased sputum (phlegm), and mucus plugging.

▶ Difficulty breathing present on *inspiration* (breathing in) and *expiration* (breathing out).

B. Signs and Symptoms

▶ Chronic cough.

▶ Copious sputum.

▶ Chest radiograph abnormalities.

▶ Sedentary, overweight, cyanotic, edematous, breathless, leading to the term "blue bloater".

II. Emphysema

A. Etiology

Emphysema is defined as a distension (widening) of the air spaces distal to terminal bronchioles due to destruction of alveolar walls (septa).

▶ Smoke injures alveolar epithelium destroying alveolar walls and creating large air spaces.

▶ Difficulty breathing only on *expiration*.

B. Signs and Symptoms

▶ Difficulty in breathing on exertion.

▶ Minimal, nonproductive cough (dry, no mucus).

▶ Barrel chest (enlarged chest walls) due to increased use of respiratory chest muscles.

▶ Weight loss.

▶ Chest radiograph abnormalities.

▶ Purses lips to forcibly expel air, leading to the term "pink puffer."

III. Medical Management[19]

There is no cure for COPD. To decrease exacerbations, patients are encouraged to stop smoking, eliminate exposure to environmental pollutants, have adequate nutrition, drink water, and exercise regularly. Four medical intervention strategies are described below.[21]

A. Assess and Monitor Disease

▶ Confirm diagnosis with spirometry and determine severity.

▶ COPD is classified into five stages: at risk, mild, moderate, severe, and very severe.

• *At-risk* stage is defined by normal spirometry but patients have chronic symptoms of cough and sputum production.

• *Mild, moderate, and severe* COPD has evidence of increasing airway obstruction on spirometry in each progressive stage.

• *Very severe* COPD is defined by severe airway obstruction with chronic respiratory failure. At this stage, quality of life is significantly impaired and exacerbations may be life threatening.

B. Reduce Risk Factors

▶ Tobacco cessation.

▶ Reduction of exposure to environmental indoor/outdoor pollutants.

▶ Examples: Ozone and industrial air pollution, automobile emissions, household cleaning products.

▶ Periodontal infection, inadequate personal oral care, and lack of oral health knowledge are associated with increased risk of COPD.[22]

C. Manage Stable COPD

▶ Relief of symptoms: aerosol bronchodilators, inhaled corticosteroids, and other medications similar to those used to treat asthma.

▶ Pneumonia and seasonal influenza vaccinations.

▶ Antibiotics for infectious exacerbations.

▶ Pulmonary rehabilitation including a structured exercise program to relieve symptoms and improve quality of life.

▶ Surgery

• In severe emphysema, the removal of part of one or both lungs may result in more space for the remaining lungs to function.

• Lung transplant.

• Oxygen therapy: A patient who uses oxygen to improve breathing function may hold a portable unit during treatment as shown in Figure 66-7.

• Types: *Continuous flow*: oxygen flows at a determined rate of liters per minute.

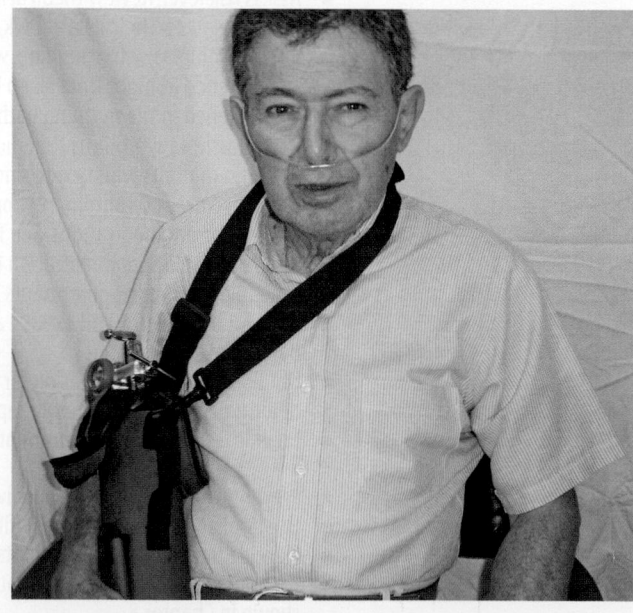

FIGURE 66-7 Use of a Portable Oxygen Tank. A patient who uses oxygen to improve breathing function may hold a portable unit during treatment. (Picture courtesy of Anne MacNeil Photography.)

- *On demand*: oxygen flows during inhalation only, extending the period of time between oxygen tank refills.
- Precautions: oxygen promotes rapid burning. Keep away from heat, flame, or other ignition source (cigarettes, Bunsen burner).

D. Prevent and Manage Exacerbations

▶ Infections, inhalation of irritants, and nonadherence to management programs lead to exacerbations.

IV. Oral Manifestations[24]

▶ Similar to patients with asthma.

▶ Patients who use any form of tobacco have an increased risk of the following oral conditions:
- Oral cancer.
- Nicotine stomatitis.
- Halitosis.
- Periodontal infections.
- Extrinsic tooth stain.

V. Dental Hygiene Care[24]

A. Before Treatment

▶ Precautions are needed when concurrent cardiovascular disease is present. Emergency procedures are outlined in Chapter 8.

▶ Assess severity of COPD and breathing difficulty.

▶ Treatment may be performed on stable patients with adequate breathing.

▶ Identify patients who may experience exacerbation of symptoms under emotional stress.

▶ Monitor blood pressure.

▶ Appointment length may need to be modified.

▶ Chair positioning: upright or semi-upright to facilitate breathing as shown in Chapter 7.

B. During Treatment

▶ Use antimicrobial preprocedural rinse.

▶ Avoid the use of power-driven scalers and air polishers.

▶ Administer local anesthesia without epinephrine.

▶ Nitrous oxide–oxygen inhalation sedation: avoid with severe COPD and emphysema.

C. Patient Education

▶ Encourage patients to stop smoking. Tobacco cessation strategies are described in Chapter 34.

▶ Promote oral care and oral health knowledge in prevention and treatment of COPD.

▶ Discuss oral–systemic link between periodontitis and COPD.

▶ Teach and promote oral cancer self-examination.

▶ Schedule frequent periodontal and maintenance visits.

CYSTIC FIBROSIS (CF)[25]

CF is an autosomal recessive gene disorder. Both parents must carry the genetic mutation for the disease to be transmitted to their children.

▶ CF is progressive and ultimately fatal.

▶ With improved multifaceted healthcare, many people now live beyond 30–40 years of age.

▶ Clinical signs and symptoms are shown in Box 66-3.

I. Disease Characteristics

The gene disorder affects the movement of salt and water in and out of epithelial cells in the respiratory tract and exocrine glands (respiratory, pancreas, gastrointestinal) and results in thickened secretions. Main systems affected are:

A. Respiratory Tract

Airways are filled with phlegm, similar to pus, leading to:

▶ Chronic sinusitis.

▶ Opportunistic bacterial lung infection.

  Both are difficult to eradicate, even with antibiotics, due to the ability of *Pseudomonas aeruginosa* to form biofilm.[25]

B. Pancreas and Intestinal Tract

▶ Thick mucus clogs pancreatic ducts.

BOX 66-3

Clinical Signs and Symptoms of Cystic Fibrosis (CF)

Early Stage

▷ In infancy, failure to thrive
▷ Persistent cough and wheezing
▷ Recurrent pneumonia
▷ Excessive appetite but poor weight gain
▷ Salty skin or sweat
▷ Bulky, foul-smelling stools (undigested lipids)

Late-Stage with Pulmonary Involvement

▷ Tachypnea (rapid breathing)
▷ Sustained chronic cough with mucus production and vomiting
▷ Barrel chest
▷ Cyanosis and digital (finger) clubbing
▷ Exertional dyspnea with decreased exercise capacity
▷ Pneumothorax
▷ Right heart failure secondary to pulmonary hypertension

Cystic Fibrosis Foundation. *What is Cystic Fibrosis*. Bethesda, MD: Cystic Fibrosis Foundation. http://www.cff.org/AboutCF/. Accessed July 9, 2014.

▶ Clogged ducts prevent the release of pancreatic enzymes into the intestinal tract.

▶ Without enzymes, food is not properly digested or absorbed.

II. Medical Management

Patients are encouraged to have regular physical activity and to adjust their diet to include pancreatic enzyme supplements, fat-soluble vitamins, liquids with high salt intake, and caloric supplementation. Comprehensive medical care includes[25]:

▶ Antibiotics including inhalation solution: Tobramycin sulfate nebulizer.

▶ Bronchodilators and anti-inflammatory agents.

▶ Chest physiotherapy.

  • Postural drainage: patient is placed in various body positions to allow mucus to drain from the airway.

  • Percussion (tapping): to loosen secretions.

III. Dental Hygiene Care

A. Oral Manifestations

▶ No specific oral lesions related to CF.

▶ Gingivitis associated with dry mouth.

B. To Facilitate Breathing

▶ Adapt chair positioning.

▶ Avoid use of rubber dam.

C. Summary Guidelines for Dental Hygiene Care

Summary guidelines for dental hygiene care for a patient with a respiratory disease are listed in Table 66-9.

SLEEP APNEA SYNDROME[26]

Sleep-related breathing disorders are usually due to chronic airway obstruction.

I. Etiology

▶ Repetitive narrowing and closure of the of upper airway during sleep

▶ Pharyngeal airway obstruction

▶ In children, the most common cause is tonsilar hypertrophy.[27]

II. Signs and Symptoms

▶ Interruption in sleep patterns

▶ Snoring may cause tissue inflammation

▶ Associated with comorbidities, motor vehicle accidents, and occupational accidents.

III. Medical Management[28]

▶ Continuous positive airway pressure (CPAP) machine (shown in Figure 66-8) increases air pressure in the throat so that the airway does not collapse when inhaling.

▶ Mandibular advancement device is shown in Figure 66-9. A splint that moves the mandible slightly forward which tightens the soft tissue and muscles of the upper airway to prevent obstruction of the airway during sleep.

▶ Weight loss.

▶ Positional therapy to prevent postural drainage.

▶ Surgery.

IV. Dental Hygiene Care

▶ Assessment of oral tissues at each maintenance visit

▶ Assessment of temporomandibular joint

▶ Recommend nonalcohol-based mouth moisturizer/rinse

▶ Bring mandibular advancement device to each continuing care appointment for evaluation.

DOCUMENTATION

Include in the patient's permanent record:

▶ Alerts for dental personnel to the possibility of disease transmission or a medical emergency due to medical condition or allergy.

▶ *Paper records*: to protect patient confidentiality, place the medical alert box inside front cover.

▶ *Electronic records*: insert in a prominent area.

▶ Box 66-4 shows an examples of a medical alert notifications.

▶ *Medical consultation*: file written reports and document telephone conversations.

▶ *Patient's current health status*: especially related to signs and symptoms of respiratory disease, known allergies, current medications.

▶ *Vital signs*: including pulse oximetry.

▶ *Oral examination*: with attention to oral cancer screening and periodontal evaluation.

▶ *Patient education*: especially issues about dry mouth, tobacco cessation, and medication compliance.

▶ *Changes in respiratory signs and symptoms during treatment and interventions performed.*

▶ A sample progress note for a patient with a positive TST is shown in Box 66-5.

TABLE 66-9	Summary Guidelines for Oral Hygiene Care for Patients with a Respiratory Disease
ITEM	**DENTAL HYGIENE CARE**
Medical consultation required when:	■ Signs or symptoms suggest respiratory disease. Examples: Cough/dyspnea at rest, hemoptysis, sputum, wheeze, chest pain, oxygen saturation level of 91% or lower as determined by pulse oximetry, or positive TB skin test (TST, PPD, Mantoux) ■ The clinician is uncertain of the patient's medical status, severity of disease, or level of control. ■ Patient with systemic conditions has not seen a primary care provider within the past year. ■ Patient has American Society of Anesthesiologists risk status class III or higher as shown in Chapter 24. ■ Patient has taken corticosteroids within the past 12 mo. ■ Patient unsure of medications and dosages.
Stress reduction protocol	■ Prevent asthma attack; helpful for patients with COPD. ■ Short morning appointments. ■ Avoid precipitating factors.
Chair position	■ Semi reclined or upright position may make breathing easier.
Anxiety and pain control	■ Local anesthetic: avoid epinephrine for patients with asthma/COPD. ■ Nitrous oxide–oxygen may be contraindicated: ■ For patients with upper respiratory infection or moderate/severe COPD. ■ With upper respiratory tract obstruction or infection if nose breathing would be difficult or breathing apparatus cannot be sterilized or replaced. ■ Be prepared to handle an emergency.
Analgesia	■ Avoid aspirin, aspirin-containing analgesics, and other NSAIDs as 10% of patients with asthma have aspirin-induced asthma.
Antibiotics	■ Patients with extrinsic asthma may have allergy to antibiotics.
Infection control	■ Standard precautions including respiratory hygiene and cough etiquette.
Emergency protocol	■ Recognize symptoms of respiratory distress. ■ Terminate treatment. ■ Emergency protocol is shown in Chapter 8.
Use of equipment that produces aerosols	■ Ultrasonic, sonic scalers, and polishing may be contraindicated. Septic material and microorganisms from biofilm and periodontal pockets can be aspirated into the lungs. For additional contraindications, see Chapter 41.

Source: Lozano AC, Perez MGS, Esteve CG. Dental Considerations in patients with respiratory problems. *J Clin Exp Dent.* 2011;3(3):e222-227. http://www.medicinaoral.com/odo/volumenes/v3i3/jcedv3i3p222.pdf. Accessed August 13, 2015.

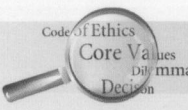

EVERYDAY ETHICS

On a beautiful spring day, Lana Thomas arrived for her 3-month continuing care visit. Vicki, the dental hygienist, noticed a labored breathing pattern as they walked down the hall to the dental hygiene treatment room. She rechecked the patient history before beginning the intraoral assessment but found the information unremarkable.

Lana stated that she was taking an over-the-counter product for seasonal allergies but it didn't seem to be helping with her nasal and chest congestion. The patient also requested that she should not be placed so far back in the dental chair because it was difficult for her to breathe. Vicki began to reconsider her plan to use the ultrasonic scaler given the patient's current condition.

Questions for Consideration

1. What are the ethical responsibilities of a primary health-care clinical dental hygienist when a patient presents with symptoms such as those of Lana Thomas?

2. How does each of the dental hygiene core values listed in Table II-1, Section II Introduction, have an application as Vicki prepares her care plan for the immediate appointment?

3. Take partners and plan a conversation between Vicki and Lana as Vicki explains:

   • Procedures they will follow for this appointment,

   • Need for medical clearance from Lana's physician for using anesthesia and other treatments, and

   • Special care Lana will need for her daily care because of the oral–systemic relationship that exists.

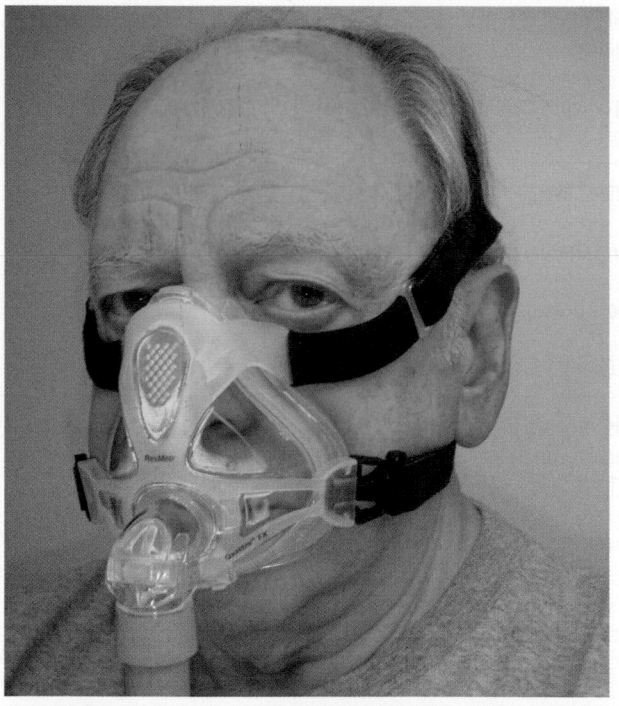

FIGURE 66-8 CPAP. This machine is attached by a hose to the nose mask which is held in place while sleeping by straps. The CPAP machine increases the air pressure in the throat so the airway does not collapse when inhaling. (Picture courtesy of Dennis Freeman, DDS.)

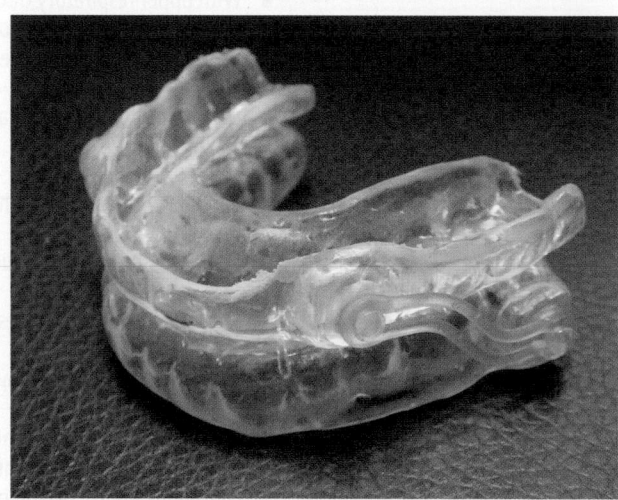

FIGURE 66-9 Mandibular Advancement Devise. A splint that moves the mandible slightly forward which tightens the soft tissue and muscles of the upper airway to prevent obstruction of the airway during sleep.

BOX 66-4

Examples of Medical Alert Notifications

Medical Alert Notifications should not be visible on the outside of the patient record.
Medical Alert: Asthma
Medical Alert: XDR-TB

BOX 66-5
Example Documentation: Patient with a Positive TST

S –A 36-year-old patient presents for new patient examination. Patient reports she had a positive TST test 1 year ago. She states that she was treated and is not contagious.

O –Called patient's physician (Dr Roberts). Spoke with nurse (Becky) who provided verbal summary and will also send written report to include in the patient's record. Patient successfully completed regime of isoniazid for 9 months. Latest medical examination Findings:
 ▷ Chest radiograph—negative
 ▷ Sputum smear and culture—negative
 ▷ Signs and symptoms—none

A –No signs of active TB disease; patient may receive any medical dental treatment without restriction.

P –Proceeded with patient assessment and dental prophylaxis.

Signed: _____, RDH

Date: _____

Factors To Teach The Patient

▷ Attention to respiratory hygiene and cough etiquette.

▷ The need for frequent hand washing to help prevent transmission of respiratory disease.

▷ The need for thorough daily cleaning and drying of toothbrushes to help prevent spread of infections.

▷ How using a new toothbrush and cleaning dentures/orthodontic appliances after bacterial infections can decrease possibility of reinfection.

▷ For elderly patients and those with chronic respiratory or cardiovascular disease, diabetes, or immunosuppressed conditions, the need for pneumonia and seasonal influenza immunization.

▷ To improve compliance in taking all prescribed medications, maintain a medication list and use pill containers that open easily and are labeled with large type.

▷ Options to combat medication-induced dry mouth.

▷ Educate the patient help avoid resistant bacteria by not requesting or taking antibiotics for a respiratory infection unless the infection has been determined by their physician to be bacterial rather than viral.[29,30]

References

1. Miyashita N, Kawai Y, Akaike H, et al. Clinical features and the role of atypical pathogens in nursing and health-care-associated pneumonia (NHCAP): differences between a teaching university hospital and a community hospital. *Intern Med.* 2012;51:585–594.

2. McLafferty E, Johnstone C, Hendry C, et al. Respiratory system part 1: pulmonary ventilation. *Nurs Stand.* 2013;27(22):40–47.

3. Hall MW, Jensen AM. The role of pulse oximetry in chiropractic practice: a rationale for its use. *J Chiropr Med.* 2012;11:127–133.

4. Seto WH, Conly JM, Pessoa-Silva CL, et al. Infection prevention and control measures for acute respiratory infections in healthcare settings: an update. *East Mediterr Health J.* 2013;19 (Suppl 1):S39–S47.

5. Centers for Disease Control and Prevention. *Respiratory Hygiene/Cough Etiquette in Healthcare Settings*. Atlanta, GA: Centers for Disease Control. http://www.cdc.gov/flu/professionals/infectioncontrol/resphygiene.htm. Updated February 27, 2012. Accessed September 4, 2013.

6. Agado BE, Crawford B, DeLaRosa J, et al. Effects of periodontal instrumentation on quality of life and illness in patients with chronic obstructive pulmonary disease: a pilot study. *J Dent Hyg.* 2012;86(3):204–214.

7. Davies J, Davies D. Origins and evolution of antibiotic resistance. *Microbiol Mol Biol Rev.* 2010;74(3):417–433.

8. Boujaoude ZC, Pratter MR. Clinical approach to acute cough. *Lung.* 2010;188 (Suppl 1):S41–S46.

9. Reyes S, Montull B, Martinez R, et al. Risk factors of A/H1N1 etiology in pneumonia and its impact on mortality. *Respir Med.* 2011;105:1404–1411.

10. Ewig S, Welte T, Chastre J, et al. Rethinking the concepts of community-acquired and health-care-associated pneumonia. *Lancet Infect Dis.* 2010;10(4):279–287.

11. Gupta G, Mitra D, Ashok KP, et al. Efficacy of preprocedural mouth rinsing in reducing aerosol contamination produced by ultrasonic scaler: a pilot study. *J Periodontol.* 2014;85:562–568.

12. Dye C, Williams BG. The population dynamics and control of tuberculosis. *Science.* 2010;328:856–861.

13. Pontali E, Matteelli A, Miglion GB. Drug-resistant tuberculosis. *Curr Opin Pulm Med.* 2013;19(3):266–272.

14. Cleveland JL, Robison VA, Panlilio AD. Tuberculosis epidemiology, diagnosis and infection control recommendations for dental settings. An update on the centers for disease control and prevention guidelines. *J Am Dent Assoc.* 2009;140(9):1092–1099.

15. Humphries C. A sleeping giant. *Nature.* 2013;502:S14–S15.

16. Lemos ACM, Matos ED. Multidrug-resistant tuberculosis. *Braz J Infect Dis.* 2013;17(2):239–246.

17. Center for Disease Control and Prevention. Morbidity and Mortality Weekly Report. Provisional CDC Guidelines for the Use and Safety Monitoring of Bedaquiline Furmarate (Sirturo) for the Treatment of Multidrug Resistant Tuberculosis. Atlanta, GA: Center for Disease control and Prevention; 2013:12.

18. U.S. Department of Health and Human Services; National Institutes of Health; National Heart, Lung, and Blood Institute. *Asthma Care Quick Reference Diagnosing and Managing Asthma.* Bethesda, MD: NHLBI Health Information Center; 2002. Revised 2012:12. NIH Publication No. 12-5075.

19. von Mutius E, Hartert T. Update in Asthma 2012. *Am J Respir Crit Care Med.* 2013;188(2):150–616.

20. U.S. Department of Health and Human Services; National Institutes of Health; National Heart, Lung, and Blood Institute. *Expert Panel Report 3: Guidelines for the Diagnosis and Management of Asthma. Full Report.* Bethesda, MD: NHLBI Health Information Center; 2007:417. NIH Publication No. 07-4051.

21. Rahman SS, Faruque M, Khan MHA, et al. Dental management of COPD patient. *Bang Med J.* 2011;44:21–24.

22. Kucukcoskun M, Baser U, Oztekin G, et al. Initial periodontal treatment for prevention of chronic obstructive pulmonary disease exacerbations. *J Periodontol.* 2013;84:863–870.

23. Dance A. Breathless. *Nature.* 2012;489:S1–S3.

24. Lozano AC, Perez MGS, Esteve CG. Dental considerations in patients with respiratory problems. *J Clin Exp Dent.* 2011;3(3):e222–e227.

25. Cystic Fibrosis Foundation. *Frequently Asked Questions.* Bethesda, MD: Cystic Fibrosis Foundation. http://www.cff.org/AboutCF/Faqs/. Updated May 8, 2011. Accessed September 26, 2013.

26. Maurer JT. Etiology of obstructive sleep apnea—the number of nerve fibers at the base of the uvula seems important. *Sleep Breath.* 2012;16:939–940.

27. Pinto JA, Kohler R, Wambier H, et al. Laryngeal pathologies as an etiologic factor of obstructive sleep apnea syndrome in children. *Int J Pediatr Ororhinolaryngol.* 2013;77:573–575.

28. Chen H, Lowe AA. Updates in oral appliance therapy for snoring and obstructive sleep apnea. *Sleep Breath.* 2013;17:473–486.

29. Fridkin S, Baggs J, Fagen R, et.al. Vital Signs: Improving Antibiotic Use Among Hospitalized Patients. MMWR. 2014;63(09):194-200. http://www.cdc.gov/mmwr/preview/mmwrhtml/mm6309a4.htm. Accessed August 12, 2015.

30. U.S. Dept. of Health and Human Services, Centers for Disease Control and Prevention. Antibiotic Resistance threats in the United States, 2013. Atlanta, GA: CDC;2013. http://www.cdc.gov/drugresistance/threat-report-2013/pdf/ar-threats-2013-508.pdf. Accessed August 12, 2015.

ENHANCE YOUR UNDERSTANDING

thePoint® DIGITAL CONNECTIONS
(see the inside front cover for access information)
- **Audio glossary**
- **Quiz bank**

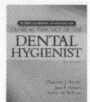

SUPPORT FOR LEARNING
(available separately; visit lww.com)
- *Active Learning Workbook for Clinical Practice of the Dental Hygienist, 12th Edition*

prepU INDIVIDUALIZED REVIEW
(available separately; visit lww.com)
- **Adaptive quizzing with *prepU for Wilkins' Clinical Practice of the Dental Hygienist***

The Patient with a Cardiovascular Disease

Dianne Smallidge, RDH, MDH and Esther M. Wilkins, BS, RDH, DMD

CHAPTER OUTLINE

LEARNING OBJECTIVES

After studying this chapter, the student will be able to:

1. Identify the cardiovascular conditions that may be encountered in patients seeking oral health care.

2. Discuss the etiology, symptoms and risk factors associated with cardiovascular conditions.

3. Discuss the impact of cardiovascular diseases on the oral cavity and their relationship to oral health.

4. Plan dental hygiene treatment modifications for the patient with cardiovascular disease.

Cardiovascular includes diseases of the heart and blood vessels.

▶ Patients with cardiovascular conditions are encountered frequently in a dental office or clinic and may be from any age group, although the highest incidence is among older people.

▶ Although a causal relationship between periodontal disease and coronary heart disease (CHD) has not been proven, current data suggest the presence of periodontal disease may be a marker for CHD risk.[1]

▶ Dental hygienists need to take responsibility to inform patients of the significant relationship between oral and systemic health and the related need for maintenance of healthy oral tissues and prevention of periodontal disease.

▶ The major cardiovascular diseases are included in this chapter with their principle symptoms and treatments as well as applications for dental hygiene care.

▶ Key words and terminology are defined in Box 67-1. Prefixes and suffixes to clarify the terminology are listed in Appendix VII.

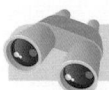 **BOX 67-1 KEY WORDS: Cardiovascular Diseases**

Aneurysm: sac formed by the localized dilatation of the wall of an artery, a vein, or the heart.

Angina: a condition marked by spasmodic suffocative attacks.

Angina pectoris: acute pain in the chest from decreased blood supply to the heart muscle.

Anoxia: absence of oxygen in the tissues; may be accompanied by deep respirations, cyanosis, increased pulse rate, and impairment of coordination.

Anticoagulant: a substance that suppresses, delays, or nullifies coagulation of the blood.

Apnea: temporary cessation of breathing.

Arrhythmia: variation from the normal rhythm, especially with reference to the heart.

Arthralgia: joint pain.

Arterial blood: oxygenated blood carried by an artery away from the heart to nourish the body tissues.

Arteriosclerosis: group of diseases characterized by thickening and loss of elasticity of the arterial wall.

Asphyxia: a condition in which there is a deficiency of oxygen in the blood and an increase in carbon dioxide.

Atheroma: lipid (cholesterol) deposit on the intima (lining) of an artery; also called atheromatous plaque.

Atherosclerosis: disease process caused by the deposit of atheromas on the inner lining of arteries that results in the obstruction of blood flow.

Bradycardia: slowness of heartbeat with slowing of pulse rate to less than 60 per minute.

Coronary heart disease: narrowing of the arteries that supply blood and oxygen to the heart caused by the buildup of plaque in the arteries.

Cyanosis: bluish discoloration of the skin and mucous membranes caused by excess concentration of reduced hemoglobin in the blood.

Diaphoresis: profuse perspiration.

Dyspnea: labored or difficult breathing.

Echocardiography: recording of the position and motion of the heart walls and internal structures of the heart and neighboring tissue by the echo obtained from beams of ultrasonic waves directed through the chest wall; used to show valvular and other structural deformities; the record produced is called an echocardiogram.

Edema: abnormal accumulation of fluid in the intercellular spaces of the body.

Electrocardiography: the graphic recording from the body surface of the potential of electric currents generated by the heart as a means of studying the action of the heart muscle; the record produced is called an electrocardiogram.

Embolism: the sudden blocking of an artery by a clot of foreign material, an embolus, that has been brought to its site of lodgment by the bloodstream; the embolus may be a blood clot (most frequently) or an air bubble, a clump of bacteria, or a fat globule.

Epistaxis: bleeding from the nose.

Heparin: anticoagulant; prevents platelet agglutination and thrombus formation.

Hypoxia: diminished availability of oxygen to blood tissues.

Infarct: localized area of ischemic necrosis produced by occlusion of the arterial supply or venous drainage of the part.

Ischemia: deficiency of blood to supply oxygen in part resulting from functional constriction or actual obstruction of a blood vessel.

Lumen: the cavity or channel within a tube or tubular organ, such as a blood vessel or the intestine.

Murmur: irregularity of heartbeat caused by a turbulent flow of blood through a valve that has failed to close.

Myocardium: the middle and thickest layer of the heart wall, composed of cardiac muscle.

Occlusion: blockage; state of being closed.

Prolapse: when an organ falls out of its normal position due to lack of support from ligaments and muscles.

Restenosis: recurrent stenosis.

Sclerosis: induration, hardening.

Shunt: abnormal communication between chambers or blood vessels; *verb*, to bypass, divert.

Stenosis: narrowing or contraction of a body passage or opening.

Tachycardia: abnormally rapid heart rate, usually taken to be over 100 beats per minute.

Tetralogy: a group or series of four.

Tetralogy of fallot: congenital, cyanotic malformation of the heart that includes pulmonary stenosis, ventricular septal defect, hypertrophy of the right ventricle, and dextroposition of the aorta.

Thrombus: blood clot attached to the intima of a blood vessel; may occlude the lumen; contrast with embolus, which is detached and carried by the bloodstream.

Venous blood: nonoxygenated blood from the tissues; blood pumped from the heart to the lungs for oxygenation.

CLASSIFICATION

▶ *Anatomic classification*
- Diseases of the heart: pericardium, myocardium, endocardium, heart valves
- Diseases of the blood vessels and peripheral circulation

▶ *Etiologic classification*
- Congenital anomalies
- Atherosclerosis, hypertension
- Infectious agents, immunologic mechanisms

INFECTIVE ENDOCARDITIS (IE)[2,3,4]

Infective Endocarditis (IE) is a microbial infection of the heart valves or endocardium with a high mortality rate.

I. Description

▶ IE is a serious disease, the prognosis of which depends on the degree of cardiac damage, the valves involved, the duration of the infection, and the treatment.

▶ IE is characterized by the formation of bacterial vegetations on the heart valves or surface of the heart lining (endocardium).

▶ When IE develops, it directly affects the function of the heart.

II. Etiology

▶ *Microorganisms*
- Streptococci and staphylococci are responsible for IE in most cases, with alpha-hemolytic streptococci being the most prevalent.
- As yeast, fungi, and viruses have been implicated, the choice of the name "infective" endocarditis is more inclusive than "bacterial" endocarditis.
- *Incidence related to dental procedures:* The majority of IE cases related to oral microflora are random bacteremias that are a result of routine daily activities. An exceedingly small number of cases are believed to result from dental procedures.

▶ *Risk factors*
- *Preexisting cardiac abnormalities:* Bacteria lodge on the endocardial (valvular) surface during bacteremia.
- *Prosthetic (artificial) heart valves:* There is an increased number of patients who have had valve replacement surgery who are susceptible. Patients who have had prosthetic valve replacements have a risk of developing prosthetic valve endocarditis.
- *History of previous endocarditis.*
- *Intravenous drug abuse.* Infected material is injected by contaminated needles directly into the bloodstream. Intravenous drug abusers are at high risk for endocarditis, which can initiate on previously normal valves.

▶ *Precipitating factors*
- *Self-induced bacteremia:* In the oral cavity, self-induced bacteremias may result from eating, bruxism, chewing gum, or any activity that can force bacteria through the wall of a diseased sulcus or pocket. Interdental aids for oral hygiene can also cause self-induced bacteremia.
- *Infection at portals of entry:* Infections at sites where microorganisms may enter the circulating blood provide a constant source of potential infectious microorganisms. In the oral cavity, organisms enter the blood by way of periodontal and gingival pockets, where multitudes of many species of microorganisms are harbored. An open area of infection, such as an ulcer caused by an ill-fitting denture, may also provide a site of entry. Patients are exposed daily to bacteremias.
- *Trauma to tissues by instrumentation:* Bacteremias are created during general or oral surgery, endodontic procedures, periodontal therapy, scaling, and any therapy that causes bleeding.

III. Disease Process[2]

▶ *Transient bacteremia initiated*
- Trauma to a mucosal surface such as the gingival sulcus during instrumentation releases bacteria into the bloodstream.
- Ease of entry of organisms directly relates to the severity of tissue trauma, quantity of bacterial biofilm, and the severity of inflammation or infection such as periodontitis.

▶ *Bacterial adherence*
- Circulating microorganisms attach to a damaged heart valve, prosthetic valve, or other susceptible area on the endocardium.

▶ *Proliferation of bacteria*
- Microorganisms proliferate to form vegetative lesions containing masses of plasma cells, fibrin, and bacteria.
- Heart valve becomes inflamed; function is diminished.
- Clumps of microorganisms (emboli) may break off and spread by way of the general circulation (embolism); complications result.

▶ *Clinical course*
- A small number of patients are symptomatic within 2 days, but usually symptoms appear within 2 weeks.
- Severe symptoms of fever, loss of appetite and weight loss, weakness, arthralgia, and heart murmurs require hospitalization. Diagnosis is based on symptoms, echocardiography, blood cell count, and positive blood cultures.
- Complications lead to eventual susceptibility to reinfection with IE, congestive heart failure, and cerebrovascular disease.

IV. Prevention

The basic areas for attention in dental and dental hygiene care that contribute to the prevention of IE are shown in Box 67-2.

▶ *Patient history*

- *Special content*: Specific questions need to be directed to elicit any history of congenital heart defects, cardiac transplant, presence of prosthetic valves, acquired valvular defects, or previous episode of IE.
- *Consultation with patient's physician*: Consultation can be assumed necessary for all patients with a history of heart defects, and any other condition suggesting the need for prophylactic antibiotic premedication.
- *Withhold instrumentation*: The use of a probe or explorer during assessment of the patient is withheld until the medical status is cleared.

▶ *Prophylactic antibiotic premedication*

- *Recommended regimens*: The current recommendations of the American Heart Association are followed.[3,4]
- Boxes 10-2 and 10-3 and Table 10-4 include the specific information in Chapter 10.
- When premedication is indicated, question the patient at the time of the appointment to verify the antibiotic was taken on schedule. In the patient record, document the name of the antibiotic, time, and dosage taken by the patient.

▶ *Dental hygiene care*

- *Oral health*: Maintenance of a high degree of oral health is necessary for each patient susceptible to IE.
- *Education*: Instruction in oral self-care such as brushing and flossing at initial appointments can be provided while the patient is under antibiotic coverage.
- *Sequence of treatment*: Biofilm removal instruction precedes instrumentation for scaling to bring the tissues to a healthy state. The more severe the gingival or periodontal inflammation, the higher the incidence of bacteremia during and following instrumentation.
- *Instrumentation*: Reduce the microbial population about the teeth and on the oral mucosa prior to instrumentation by having the patient brush, floss, and rinse thoroughly with an antimicrobial mouth rinse such as 0.12% chlorhexidine.

CONGENITAL HEART DISEASES[5,6]

I. The Normal Healthy Heart

▶ A diagram of the normal heart is shown in Figure 67-1 to provide a comparison with the anatomic changes that may appear in a defective heart.

▶ In the healthy heart, the blood flows in one direction as each chamber contracts, with the valves acting as trap doors that snap shut after each contraction to prevent backflow of blood.

▶ The right side of the heart contains deoxygenated blood from the body cells on its way to the lungs for reoxygenation. The left side of the heart contains oxygenated blood from the lungs being pumped out to the aorta on its way to the cells of the body. The septal wall divides the left and right sides of the heart.

II. Anomalies

▶ Anomalies of the anatomic structure of the heart or major blood vessels result following irregularities of development during the first 9 weeks in utero.

▶ The fetal heart is completely developed by the 9th week.

▶ Early diagnosis is necessary, but not all defects require treatment.

▶ Treatment usually involves surgical correction.

III. Etiology

Causes may be genetic, environmental, or a combination of both. Many are unknown.

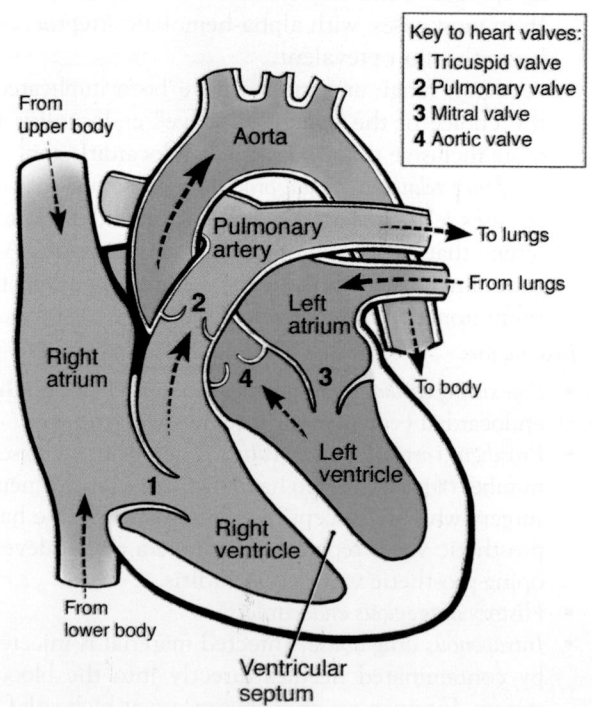

FIGURE 67-1 **The Normal Heart.** The major vessels and the location of the tricuspid, pulmonary, aortic, and mitral valves are shown.

- *Genetic*
  - Heredity is apparent in some types of defects.
  - An example of a chromosomal defect is Down syndrome, in which congenital heart anomalies occur frequently (described in Chapter 61).
- *Environmental*
  - Most congenital anomalies originate between the 5th and 8th weeks of fetal life, when the heart is developing.
  - Viral infections from the mother (rubella, cytomegalovirus).
  - Drugs (thalidomide; isotretinoin).
  - Drinking alcohol and use of cocaine.
  - Exposure to industrial chemical solvents.

IV. Types of Defects[4]

- The types of heart defects that occur most frequently are the ventricular septal defect, atrial septal defect, pulmonary stenosis, and patent ductus arteriosis.
- Defects (openings) in the septal wall cause a mixing of oxygenated and deoxygenated blood.
- Atrial and/or ventricular septal defects result in mixing of the blood from the left and right sides of the heart.
- Other defects include a passageway between the great arteries and veins, which also causes mixing of oxygenated and deoxygenated blood. Two of the more common congenital heart defects are described here.
- *Ventricular septal defect*
  - In this type of defect, the left and right ventricles exchange blood through an opening in their dividing wall (septum).
  - The oxygenated blood from the lung, which is normally pumped by the left ventricle to the aorta and then to the entire body, can pass across to the right ventricle through the septal defect, as shown in Figure 67-2.
  - The severity of symptoms is directly related to the specific location and size of the defect. Small defects may close without surgical correction.
- *Patent ductus arteriosus*
  - A patent ductus arteriosus means the passageway (shunt) is open between the two great arteries that arise from the heart, namely, the aorta and the pulmonary artery.
  - Normally, the opening closes during the first few weeks after birth.
  - When the opening does not close, blood from the aorta can pass back to the lungs, as shown in Figure 67-3.
  - The heart compensates in the attempt to provide the body with oxygenated blood and becomes overburdened.

V. Prevention[6]

- Vaccination with rubella for women of childbearing age is highly advised for those not vaccinated in childhood

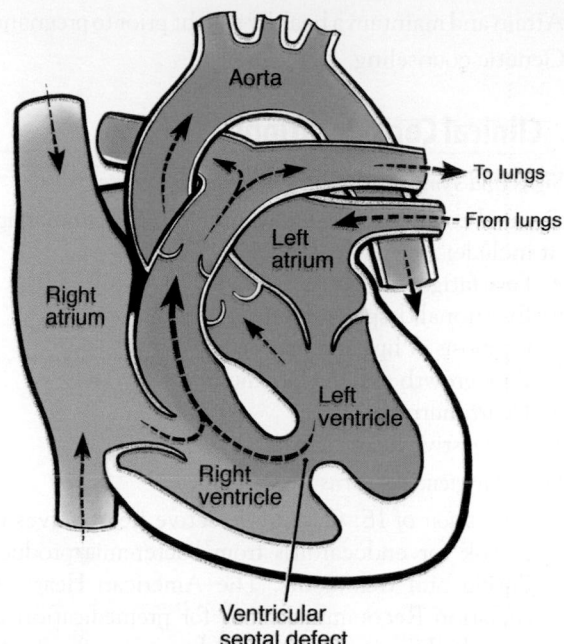

FIGURE 67-2 **Ventricular Septal Defect.** The right and left ventricles are connected by an opening that permits oxygenated blood from the left ventricle to shunt across to the right ventricle and then recirculate to the lungs. Compare with Figure 67-1, in which the septum separates the ventricles.

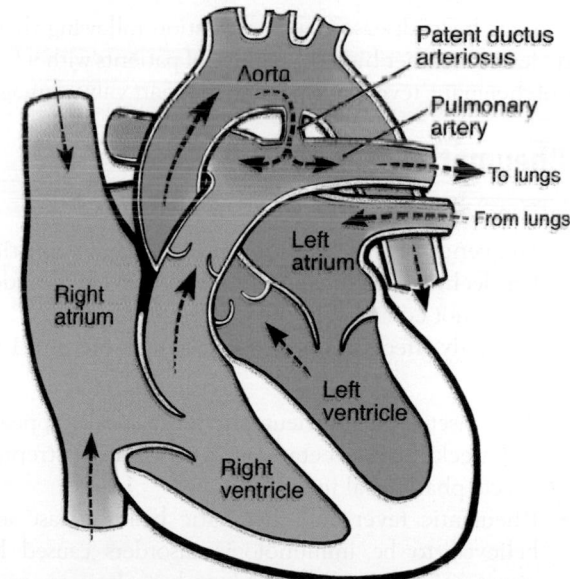

FIGURE 67-3 **Patent Ductus Arteriosus.** An open passageway between the aorta and the pulmonary artery permits oxygenated blood from the aorta to pass back into the lungs. Arrows show directions of flow through the patent ductus. Compare with normal anatomy in Figure 67-1.

or those without confirmation of immunity by a laboratory test.
- No medications, including over the counter and herbal medications, are to be taken during pregnancy without prior consultation with the physician.
- Avoid tobacco use at least 1 month before pregnancy and throughout the pregnancy.

▶ Attain and maintain a healthy weight prior to pregnancy.

▶ Genetic counseling.

VI. Clinical Considerations

▶ *Signs and symptoms of congenital heart disease*

General conditions that may influence patient management include:

- Easy fatigue
- Exertional dyspnea; fainting
- Cyanosis of lips and nail beds
- Poor growth and development
- Heart murmurs
- Congestive heart failure.

▶ *Dental hygiene concerns*

- *Prevention of IE*: Certain defective heart valves are at risk for endocarditis from bacteremia produced during oral treatments. The American Heart Association Recommendations for premedication are consulted for procedure with this group of patients.[2]
- *Elimination of oral disease*: Maintenance of a high level of oral health.

RHEUMATIC HEART DISEASE[7]

Rheumatic heart disease is a complication following rheumatic fever. A rather high percentage of patients with a history of rheumatic fever have permanent heart valve damage.

I. Rheumatic Fever

▶ *Incidence*

- Frequency of this condition in developed countries has declined significantly in the last several decades and is not common in the United States.
- Primarily effects children between ages of 5 and 15.

▶ *Etiology*

- The onset of acute rheumatic fever usually appears 2–3 weeks after a beta-hemolytic group A streptococcal pharyngeal infection.
- Rheumatic fever and rheumatic heart disease are believed to be immunologic disorders caused by sensitization to antigens of beta-hemolytic group A streptococci.

▶ *Prevention*

- The persistence and severity of the pharyngeal infection are significant factors in determining whether rheumatic fever follows.
- Early diagnosis and treatment of streptococcal throat and pharyngeal infections are necessary.

▶ *Symptoms of acute rheumatic fever*

- Low grade fever.
- Abdominal pain.
- Shortness of breath and chest pain related to cardiac issues.

- Joint pain with arthritis present in ankles, knees, elbows and wrists as well as joint swelling with redness and warmth.
- Nosebleeds.
- Skin rash on trunk and upper parts of the arms and legs or nodules on skin.
- Emotional instability.
- Muscle weakness with quick uncontrolled jerky movements affecting the face, feet, and hands.

II. The Course of Rheumatic Heart Disease

Following the acute stage of rheumatic fever, usually symptoms do not persist except the effects of the valvular deformity.

▶ *Symptoms*

- Stenosis or incompetence of valves; most commonly, the aortic and mitral valves.
- Heart murmur influenced by the amount of scarring of the valves and myocardium.
- Cardiac arrhythmias.
- Late symptoms include shortness of breath, murmur, angina pectoris, epistaxis, elevation of diastolic blood pressure, enlargement of the left ventricle, and increasing signs of congestive cardiac failure.

▶ *Practice applications*

- The American Heart Association no longer recommends antibiotic prophylaxis prior to dental treatment for patients with this condition due to their minimal risk of developing IE.[2]

MITRAL VALVE PROLAPSE[8]

I. Description

▶ The mitral valve is between the left atrium and the left ventricle (Figure 67-1).

▶ Oxygenated blood from the lungs passes from the pulmonary vein into the left ventricle, where it is pumped through the aortic valve and into the aorta for distribution to the body cells.

▶ When the mitral valve leaflets are damaged, the closure is imperfect and oxygenated blood can backflow or regurgitate.

▶ Mitral valve prolapse is the most common disorder of the valve that causes regurgitation.

▶ The mitral valve is prolapsed (becomes misaligned) backwards into the atrium during systole.

II. Symptoms

▶ Most patients with mitral valve prolapse are without symptoms.

▶ A small number of cases will have symptoms of palpitations, fatigue, atypical chest pain, and a late systolic murmur.

- When there is more severe involvement, an increase in frequency of palpitations and progressive mitral regurgitation is apparent along with a systolic click and murmur.
- Initial suspicion for diagnosis of valvular heart disease is the recognition of a heart murmur.
- The American Heart Association no longer recommends antibiotic prophylaxis during dental treatment for patients with this condition.[2]

HYPERTENSION[9,10]

Hypertension means an abnormal elevation of arterial blood pressure. It has been called the "silent killer," as one-third of people who have it do not have symptoms. It is a contributing risk factor in many vascular diseases, or it may be a result or an effect of underlying pathologic changes.

- Detection of blood pressure for dental and dental hygiene patients has become an essential step in patient assessment prior to treatment.
- Early detection, with referral for additional diagnosis and treatment when indicated, can prove to be lifesaving for certain people.
- Knowledge of the health problems of patients is needed to ensure treatment is safe and risk of emergencies.

I. Etiology

A. Primary or Essential Hypertension

- *Incidence*: Approximately 90% of all hypertension is primary or essential.
- *Predisposing or risk factors*: Combinations of the factors listed are more significant than any one alone. Risk factors for atherosclerosis are interrelated.
- *Tobacco use*
- *Heredity*
- *Overweight*
- *Race*: The incidence is higher among African-Americans than among white Americans, the illness is more severe, and the mortality rate is higher at a younger age.
- *Salt*: Particularly in excess in the diet.
- *Sex*: Men are more affected before age 45 years; women slightly more than men in later years.
- *Age*: General increase from birth to age 20 years; levels off until 40 years of age; then a slow increase into older age.
- *Environment*: Environmental conditions that increase stress factors.

B. Secondary Hypertension

About 10% of all hypertension is secondary to other underlying medical conditions. In secondary hypertension, usually both systolic and diastolic blood pressures are elevated. Examples of causes are:

- *Oral contraceptives*[8]
  - Oral contraceptives may elevate blood pressure and is more likely to occur in women who are overweight, have a history of hypertension during pregnancy, have a family history, or have mild kidney disease.
  - The combination of birth control pills and cigarette use may be especially dangerous for some women.
- *Renal disease*
  - Renal artery obstruction
  - Pyelonephritis
  - Renal failure
- *Endocrine disorders*
  - Hyperthyroidism
  - Diabetes
  - Cushing's syndrome
  - Thyroid or parathyroid disease
- *Medications*
  - Decongestants
  - Steroids

II. Blood Pressure Levels

- Blood pressure is documented in the patient's record as the systolic pressure reading over the diastolic pressure reading (systolic/diastolic).
- The *systolic* blood pressure is the pressure exerted against the arterial walls during the ventricular contraction. It is altered by the cardiac output, resistance of the capillary bed, and volume and viscosity of the blood.
- The *diastolic* blood pressure is the pressure exerted by the blood within the arteries during the total resting resistance after the contraction of the left ventricle.
- Diseases can have an effect on any of these factors, altering the blood pressure.
- Blood pressure fluctuates, so the baseline blood pressure needs to be measured two or three times and the average reading entered in the patient's record when hypertension is suspected.

A. Normal and High Blood Pressure[9]

Table 67-1 lists the normal readings for blood pressure and the stages of hypertension for adults 18 years and over.

B. Low Blood Pressure

- Many healthy people have a normal systolic pressure under 90 mm Hg, which may be considered "low blood pressure."
- Such a level is normal for that person, and no clinical problems are evident.

TABLE 67-1	Classification of Blood Pressure for Adults Aged 18 Years or Older	
BLOOD PRESSURE CATEGORY	**SYSTOLIC (mm Hg)**	**DIASTOLIC (mm Hg)**
Normal	<120	<80
Prehypertension	120–139	80–89
Stage 1 hypertension	140–159	90–99
Stage 2 hypertension	≥160	≥100

Data from National High Blood Pressure Education Program. *The Seventh Report of the Joint National Committee on Prevention, Detection, Evaluation, and Treatment of High Blood Pressure.* Bethesda, MD: U.S. National Heart, Lung, and Blood Institute; 2003. NIH Publication No. 03-5233.

▶ A marked sudden drop in blood pressure is usually associated with an emergency, such as severe blood loss, shock, myocardial infarction, sepsis, or other medical problem.

▶ Procedures to following during specific medical emergencies can be found in Table 8-4 in Chapter 8.

III. Clinical Symptoms of Hypertension

Essential hypertension is frequently recognized only by blood pressure readings. The condition may go unrecognized because of the lack of clinical symptoms.

▶ *High blood pressure*

Those who have early symptoms may describe them as:
- Occipital headaches
- Dizziness
- Visual disturbances
- Weakness
- Ringing in the ears
- Tingling of the hands and feet

▶ *Major sequela of long-standing elevation of blood pressure*
- The brain, eyes, heart, or kidney may undergo marked changes in function.
- Hypertensive heart disease; enlarged heart with eventual cardiac failure.
- Cerebral vascular accident (stroke, described in Chapter 59).
- Hypertensive renal disease.
- Ischemic heart disease.

▶ *Malignant hypertension*[11]
- Malignant hypertension is a life threatening that comes on suddenly with a diastolic reading often above 130 mm/Hg.
- This disorder affects about 1% of patients with hypertension and symptoms can include:

- Any of the early symptoms of high blood pressure.
- Blurring of vision; possible loss of sight.
- Severe dyspnea.
- Chest pains similar to angina pectoris.
- Mental confusion leading to stupor, coma, convulsions.
- *Activate emergency* procedures as the situation can be fatal if not treated immediately or may result in damage to multiple body systems.

IV. Treatment[9]

A. Goals

▶ *Primary hypertension*
- Achieve and maintain diastolic pressure level below 80 mm Hg.
- Lower the risk of serious complications and premature death.

▶ *Secondary hypertension*
- Medical treatment of underlying systemic disease is needed.

B. Lifestyle Changes (Box 67-3)

▶ *Weight and exercise*: Control weight and exercise daily.

▶ *Diet*: Sodium restriction, in those who are salt sensitive, and modest weight loss of 5%–10% of body weight may be all that are needed for the control of mild elevations of blood pressure.

▶ *Tobacco use*: All forms of tobacco must be eliminated.

▶ *Other risk factors*: In addition to factors listed in Box 67-3, life activity contributions to stress and tension need to be minimized.

V. Hypertension in Children[12]

▶ Children 3 years of age and older need to have blood pressure determinations made at least annually.

BOX 67-3

Lifestyle Modifications for Hypertension Control and/or Overall Cardiovascular Risk

▷ If overweight, lose weight 5%–10% of body weight.
▷ Limit alcohol intake to no more than 1 ounce of ethanol per day (24 ounces of beer, 8 ounces of wine, or 2 ounces of 100-proof whiskey).
▷ Exercise (aerobic) daily.
▷ Reduce sodium intake.
▷ Maintain adequate dietary potassium, calcium, and magnesium intake.
▷ Stop use of tobacco.
▷ Reduce dietary saturated fat and cholesterol intake for overall cardiovascular health. Reducing fat intake also helps to reduce caloric intake.

▶ If the BP of a child or adolescent is equal to or above the 90th percentile, the BP measurement is repeated during the visit to determine if the patient is hypertensive (see Chapter 11, Table 11-1 for blood pressure values for children and adolescents).

ISCHEMIC HEART DISEASE

Ischemic heart disease is the cardiac disability, acute and chronic, that arises from reduction or arrest of blood supply to the myocardium.

▶ The heart muscle (myocardium) is supplied through the coronary arteries, which are branches of the descending aorta.

▶ Because of the relationship to the coronary arteries, the disease is often referred to as CHD or coronary artery disease.

▶ Ischemia means oxygen deprivation in a local area from a reduced passage of fluid into the area.

▶ Ischemic heart disease is the result of an imbalance of the oxygen supply and demand of the myocardium resulting from a narrowing or blocking of the lumen of the coronary arteries.

I. Etiology

Other factors may be involved, but the principal cause of reduction of blood flow to the heart muscle is *atherosclerosis* of the vessel walls, which narrows the lumen, thus obstructing the flow of blood.

▶ *Definition of atherosclerosis*[13]

• Atherosclerosis is an inflammatory disease of medium and large arteries in which atheromas deposit and thicken the intimal layer of the involved blood vessel.

• An atheroma is a fibro-fatty deposit or plaque containing several lipids, especially cholesterol.

• With time, the plaques continue to thicken and, eventually, close the vessel (Figure 67-4).

• Some plaques calcify, whereas others may develop an overlying thrombus.

▶ Risk factors for atherosclerosis[13]

• Inflammation plays a significant role in the formation of atheromas. Low-grade chronic inflammation in other parts of the body, including chronic periodontitis, has been shown to have a relationship to adverse cardiovascular outcomes.

• Pathogenic microorganisms from these inflammatory processes have been associated with atheroma formation in the blood and the subsequent progression of atherosclerosis.

• Many risk factors for periodontal disease are also risk factors for atherosclerosis.[14]

• Each risk factor is significant alone. When these factors occur in combinations, the risk of atherosclerosis, and therefore that of ischemic heart disease, is increased.

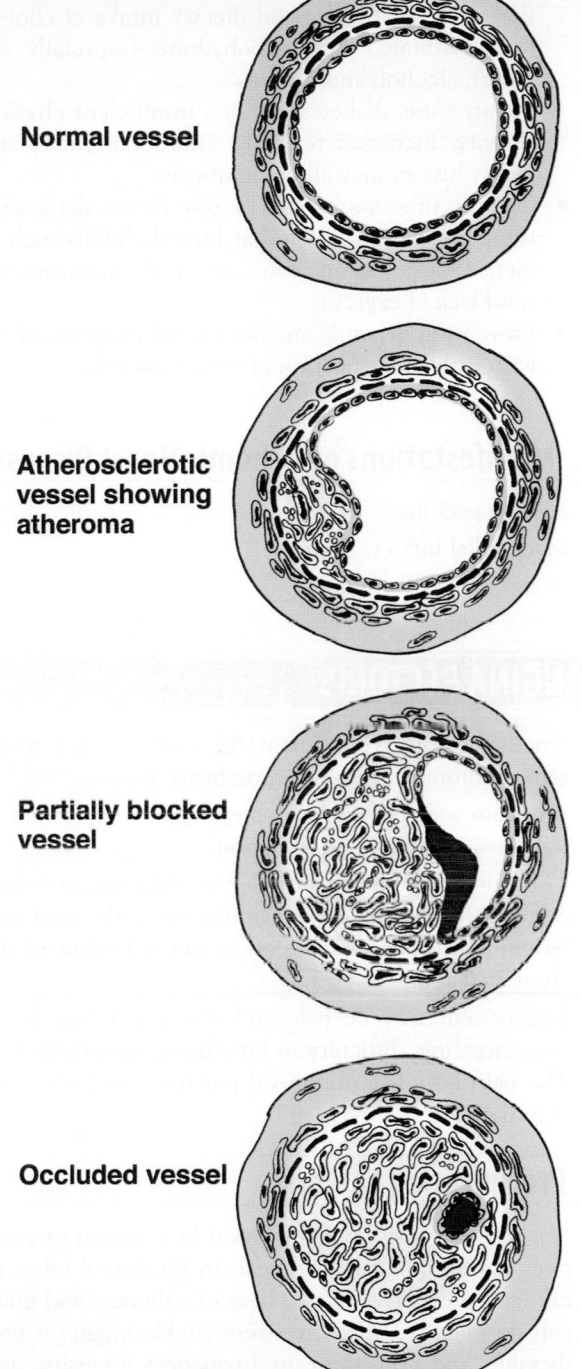

Normal vessel

Atherosclerotic vessel showing atheroma

Partially blocked vessel

Occluded vessel

FIGURE 67-4 Atherosclerosis. An atheroma develops within the lining of the normal blood vessel. The atheroma is made of a fatty deposit containing cholesterol. At first, the atheroma is small and no symptoms are apparent, but eventually it enlarges and completely blocks the vessel, thus depriving the area served by the vessel of oxygen. (Source: National Institute of Health. *Report of the Working Group on Arteriosclerosis of the National Heart, Lung, and Blood Institute, National Institutes of Health, United States Department of Health and Human Services.* Bethesda, MD: National Institute of Health; 1981. NIH Publication No. 81-2034.)

- Risk factors include: elevated levels of blood lipids, the result of an increased dietary intake of cholesterol, saturated fat, carbohydrate (especially sucrose), alcohol, and calories.
- Tobacco use, diabetes, obesity, insufficient physical activity, increased tensions, emotional stress, and family history may all be significant.
- Genetic inheritance can be one factor along with the perpetuation of familial lifestyle habits such as diet, tobacco habits, tensions, and tendencies toward lack of exercise.
- Prevention depends on educational programs along with early identification of persons at risk.

II. Manifestations of Ischemic Heart Disease

▶ Angina pectoris
▶ Myocardial infarction
▶ Congestive heart failure

ANGINA PECTORIS[15]

▶ Angina pectoris is chest pain, the most common symptom of coronary atherosclerotic heart disease.

▶ The pain is described as a heavy, squeezing pressure or tightness in the mid-chest region.

▶ The pain may radiate to the left or right arm and neck or even the mandible. On rare occasion, the pain may be limited to one of these areas and not occur in the chest area at all.

▶ The patient may be pale and also experience faintness, sweating, difficulty in breathing, anxiety, or fear. The pain lasts 1–5 minutes if precipitating factors are eliminated.

I. Precipitating Factors

▶ *Stable angina* may be precipitated by exertion or exercise, emotion, or a heavy meal. In the dental office or clinic, a preventive atmosphere of calmness and quiet can do much to alleviate stress. Stable angina is predictable and consistent in frequency, intensity, and duration.

▶ *Unstable angina* occurs without exertion or other precipitating factors. The pain may occur while the patient is at rest, and it may vary in intensity at each attack.

II. Treatment

▶ A vasodilator, usually nitroglycerin, is administered sublingually.

▶ Basic life support that includes supplemental oxygen is part of the treatment provided in a dental office or clinic.

III. Procedure During an Angina Attack

▶ *Terminate treatment*
- Stop the dental or dental hygiene procedure.
- Call for assistance and the emergency kit or cart.

▶ *Position patient*
- Return the patient chair to a comfortable position.
- Reassure the patient.

▶ *Administer vasodilator*
- Administer nitroglycerin sublingually.
- Use of the patient's own supply is preferable. Prior to starting the appointment procedures make sure the patient's supply is placed within reach.
- The patient can be asked when the nitroglycerin was purchased because the potency is lost after 6 months out of a sealed storage container.
- Patient with xerostomia may not have sufficient saliva to moisten the nitroglycerin. A few drops of water from the unit syringe can be placed on the tablet under the tongue.

▶ *Check patient response*
- Give additional vasodilator. Usually, the first tablet relieves the condition within minutes.
- When it is suspected that the patient's supply may not be fresh and the first tablet has been ineffective, use of a second tablet from the dental office emergency kit may be advisable.

▶ *Call for medical assistance*
- When the patient does not respond to the second dose of vasodilator, assume the attack to be a myocardial infarction.
- *Call emergency medical service (EMS).*
- Administer oxygen.

▶ *Record vital signs*
- Use the *Medical Emergency Report*, Figure 8-1, Chapter 8.
- Measure blood pressure, check pulse rate, and count respirations, as described in Chapter 11.

▶ *Observe recovery*
- For the patient who recovers without additional medical assistance, allow a rest period before dismissal.
- Record vital signs again.

▶ *Documentation*
Thoroughly document the events that occurred and assessment data collected in the patient's chart for future reference.

MYOCARDIAL INFARCTION[16]

▶ Myocardial infarction is the most extreme manifestation of ischemic heart disease.

▶ Other names: heart attack, coronary occlusion, or coronary thrombosis.

▶ The infarction results from a sudden reduction or arrest of coronary blood flow.

▶ The most common artery associated with a myocardial infarction is the anterior descending branch of the left coronary artery. That is also the most common site of advanced atherosclerosis.

I. Etiology

▶ Immediate cause: can be a thrombosis that blocks an artery already narrowed by atherosclerosis.

▶ The blockage creates an area of infarction, which leads to necrosis of the area.

▶ Necrosis of the area can occur within a few hours.

▶ A few patients die immediately or within a few hours. Sudden death may be caused by ventricular fibrillation.

II. Symptoms

▶ *Pain*

- *Location*: Pain symptoms may start under the sternum, with feelings of indigestion, or in the middle to upper sternum. Pain may last for extended periods, even hours.

- When the pain is severe, it gives a pressing or crushing heavy sensation and is not relieved by rest or nitroglycerin.

- *Onset*. The pain may have a sudden onset, sometimes during sleep or following exercise. The pain may be radial, similar to angina pectoris, which extends to the left or right arm, neck, and mandible.

▶ *Other symptoms*

- Cold sweat, weakness and faintness, shortness of breath, nausea, and vomiting may occur.

- Blood pressure falls below baseline.

- Women do not always present with symptoms similar to men and may not experience chest pain; fainting, pain in the upper back and lower abdomen, and extreme fatigue are chief symptoms.[17]

III. Management During an Attack[18]

▶ *Terminate treatment*

- Sit the patient up for comfortable breathing.

- Give nitroglycerin, and reassure the patient.

▶ *Summon medical assistance*

- When nitroglycerin does not reduce the anginalike pain within 3 minutes, prepare for basic life support (Table 8-3, Chapter 8).

- **Call EMT.** Administer oxygen.

- Use *Medical Emergency Report*, Figure 8-1, and record vital signs.

- Apply basic life support measures, if indicated, while waiting for medical assistance.

- Transport to hospital.

IV. Treatment After Acute Symptoms[19]

▶ *Medical supervision*

- Current medical care for heart attack calls for a shortened rest period with increased activity, in keeping with the strength and progress of the patient.

- Most patients experience extreme fatigue during their convalescence.

▶ *Lifestyle changes*

- Dietary changes and elimination of all forms of tobacco and stressful activities, as well as control of diseases that exacerbate ischemic heart disease, are essential.

- Periodontal health has particular significance.

- Many patients need considerable education, reassurance, and motivation.

▶ *Subsequent appointments*

- Elective dental appointments are postponed until the patient's physician has given consent.

HEART FAILURE[20]

▶ Heart failure, often referred to as Congestive Heart Failure (CHF), is a syndrome in which an abnormality of cardiac function is responsible for the inability or failure of the heart to pump blood at a rate necessary to meet the oxygen needs of the body tissues.

▶ Considered an end-stage heart condition, it results from many forms of cardiovascular diseases and can be related to a number of other systemic conditions.

I. Etiology

Examples of diseases that contribute to heart failure are:

▶ Coronary heart disease

▶ Hypertension

▶ Diabetes

▶ Arrhythmias

▶ Congenital heart disease

▶ Thyroid disorders

▶ Alcohol or illegal drug use such as cocaine

▶ HIV/AIDS.

II. Clinical Manifestations[21]

▶ The clinical manifestations coincide with the parts of the heart involved.

▶ Signs and symptoms are different, depending, in general, on whether the left or the right side of the heart or both are affected. The general effects are extreme weakness, fatigue, fear, and anxiety.

A. Left Heart Failure

▶ The left side of the heart receives oxygenated blood from the lungs and pumps the blood into the aorta to the rest of the body.

▶ A pathologic condition of the left ventricle or the mitral valve alters output, and causes respiratory difficulty because of the backup of serous fluid into the lungs.

▶ Most heart failure, and the conditions leading to it, are a result of left ventricular failure, which is followed by right ventricular failure.

▶ Clinical symptoms are more prominent at night. The patient rests better in a sitting or semisitting position with more than one pillow.

▶ Signs and symptoms of left heart failure include the following:
  • Weakness, fatigue
  • Dyspnea, particularly evident on exertion. Shortness of breath when lying supine, relieved when sitting up
  • Cough and expectoration
  • Nocturia
  • Pallor; sweating, cold skin
  • Diastolic blood pressure increased
  • Heart rate rapid
  • Anxiety, fear.

B. Right Heart Failure

▶ The right heart receives the venous blood from the vena cava and pumps it to the lungs for oxygenation.

▶ Right heart failure shows evidence of systemic venous congestion with peripheral edema.

▶ When left heart failure precedes right heart failure, the heart is already congested. Resistance to receiving the venous blood is an additional factor.

▶ Signs and symptoms of right heart failure include the following:
  • Weakness, fatigue
  • Swelling of the feet and/or ankles. The edema progresses to the thighs and abdomen (ascites) in advanced stages of heart failure
  • Cold hands and feet
  • Clubbing of fingers
  • Cyanosis of mucous membranes and nail beds
  • Prominent jugular veins
  • Congestion with edema in various organs: enlarged spleen and liver; gastrointestinal distress with nausea and vomiting; central nervous system involvement with headache and irritability
  • Anxiety, fear.

III. Treatment During Chronic Stages[20]

A patient with an appointment in a dental office or clinic may be receiving a variety of medical treatments. These are revealed by questioning during preparation of histories. Nearly all patients with heart failure complications have the following in their medical treatment plan:

▶ *Drug therapy*
  • Physicians may prescribe many different medications for patients with cardiovascular disease.

▶ *Dietary control*
  • Limited sodium intake to alleviate fluid retention
  • Limited fluid intake
  • Weight reduction.

▶ *Limitation of activity*
  • Activity is limited depending on the severity of the health problem and the advice of the physician.

IV. Emergency Care for Heart Failure and Acute Pulmonary Edema

A medical emergency that demands urgent attention may occur anywhere. The patient with heart failure or acute pulmonary edema is usually conscious.

▶ Position the patient upright for comfortable breathing (Table 8-3 in Chapter 8).

▶ **Call EMS.** Administer oxygen.

▶ Use the *Medical Emergency Report*, Figure 8-1, Chapter 8, and monitor vital signs (blood pressure, respiratory rate, and pulse).

▶ Reassure the patient.

LIFESTYLE MANAGEMENT FOR THE PATIENT WITH CARDIOVASCULAR DISEASE[22]

The recommendation for the following is appropriate for all patients with cardiovascular disease:

▶ *Education*: The patient is counseled to be reassured that lifestyle changes are necessary but a productive life can be led.

▶ *Lifestyle changes* (Box 67-3)
  • Reduction of blood pressure
  • Tobacco cessation
  • Reduction of low-density lipoprotein and total cholesterol
  • Increase physical activity
  • Eat a heart healthy diet, like the DASH (dietary approaches to stop hypertension), which is high in vegetables, fruits, whole grains, low-fat dairy, lean poultry and fish, legumes, and nuts with limited added sugar and red meats.[23]

▶ *Medications*: A variety of medications may be required depending on individual needs.

SURGICAL TREATMENT[19]

I. Coronary Dilation

▶ *Percutaneous transluminal coronary angioplasty*
- Widely used procedure to stretch the coronary blood vessel using fluoroscopic guidance allows various tools to be inserted.
- An inflatable balloon widens the narrowed lumen.
- An atherectomy may be used to remove atheromatous plaque from the vessel lining.

▶ *Coronary stent*
- The stent is placed to maintain the open vessel lumen. Stents are made of metal and become covered with endothelium.
- The coronary stent provides a semirigid scaffolding within the lumen, which helps prevent restenosis or renarrowing of the lumen.

II. Coronary Bypass

▶ *Coronary artery bypass grafting (CABG)*
- Coronary bypass is primarily for patients with significant obstruction.
- The purpose is to "jump-pass" over arteries that have been narrowed with atherosclerosis.
- The beneficial effects are relief from anginal pain, less workload for the heart, and an increase of oxygen and blood supply to the myocardium.
- Figure 67-5 shows the use of a saphenous vein graft and the internal mammary artery for bypasses.

III. Cardiac Pacemakers and Implantable Cardioverter Defibrillators (ICD)[24,25]

A. Cardiac Pacemakers

▶ The natural pacemaker, or center where the normal heartbeat is initiated, is the sinoatrial (S-A) node located in the right atrium.

▶ From that node, impulses are sent along the muscle walls to stimulate and regulate the contractions of the ventricles, which pump the blood throughout the body.

▶ When the natural pacemaker cells are not able to maintain a reliable rhythm, or when the impulses are interrupted because of heart block, cardiac arrest, various arrhythmias, or other disease conditions, treatment by a cardiologist may include the placement of an artificial pacemaker.

1. *Description*
- A cardiac pacemaker is an electronic stimulator used to send a specified electrical current to the myocardium to control or maintain a minimum heart rate.
- It may be single-chambered (to ventricle or atrium) or dual-chambered to sense and pace both heart chambers.

2. *Parts and power*
- A permanently implanted pacemaker has electrodes inserted transvenously to the endocardium. Less commonly, the leads may go to the pericardium of the external heart wall.

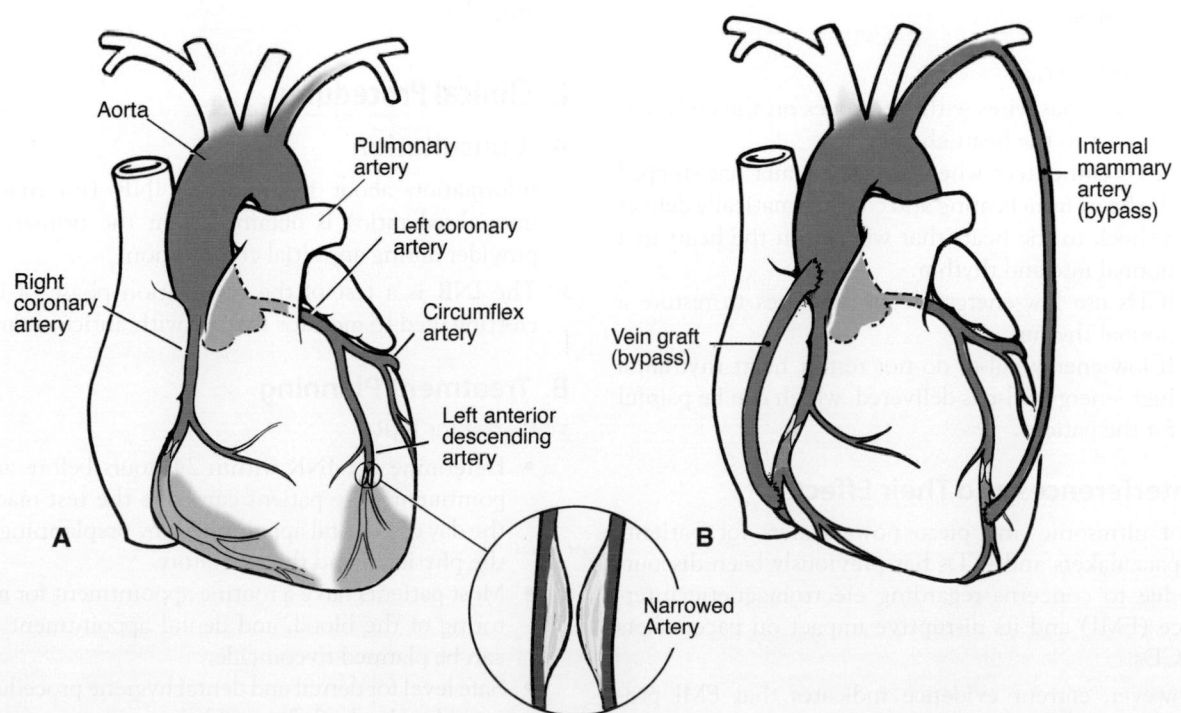

FIGURE 67-5 Coronary Bypass Surgery. A: Heart showing infarcted (shaded) areas created by coronary arteries narrowed by atherosclerosis. **B:** Vein graft from saphenous vein connected with aorta to bypass narrowed area of right coronary artery, and internal mammary artery used to bypass narrowed left anterior descending artery.

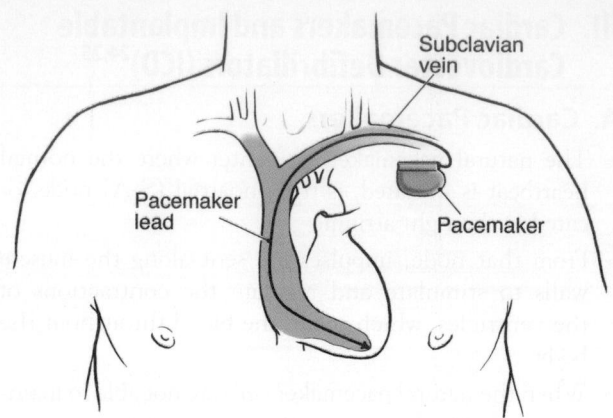

FIGURE 67-6 Cardiac Pacemaker. The pulse generator is implanted under the skin in the thorax or upper abdomen. The lead electrodes may go to the ventricle or to the atrium or both to provide the necessary stimulus for regulation of the heartbeat.

- The electrodes are connected to the power source, a plastic- or metal-encased, hermetically sealed pulse generator containing a lithium anode battery.
- The pulse generator is implanted under the skin in the thorax or upper abdomen. The area selected depends on the individual condition as determined by the cardiologist (Figure 67-6).

B. Implantable Cardioverter Defibrillator

1. *Description*
   - An ICD is a device that is surgically placed in the chest or abdomen to help treat cardiac arrhythmias.
   - Patients with cardiac arrhythmias can experience life-threatening events that can result in sudden cardiac arrest.

2. *Parts and power*
   - An ICD has wires with electrodes on the ends that connect to the heart chambers.
   - ICDs can detect when an arrhythmia has stopped the heart from beating and can automatically deliver a shock to the heart that will return the heart to a normal rate and rhythm.
   - ICDs use low-energy electrical pulses to restore a normal rhythm
   - If low-energy pulses do not restart heart rhythm, a high-energy pulse is delivered, which can be painful for the patient.

C. Interferences and Their Effects

Use of ultrasonic and piezo powerscalers for patients with pacemakers and ICDs has previously been discouraged due to concerns regarding electromagnetic interference (EMI) and its disruptive impact on pacemakers and ICDs.

- However, current evidence indicates that EMI produced from these technologies is not sufficient to disrupt the function of pacemakers and ICDs.[25–27]

D. Prophylactic Antibiotic Premedication[3,4]

- IE has occurred in patients with pacemakers and ICDs, and an increase in the incidence of infection following placement of these devices has prompted increased use of pre- and postantibiotic prophylaxis before and after implantation.
- Although evidence suggests the patient with a pacemaker is at low risk for endocarditis, the cardiologist may choose to use antibiotics to cover dental and dental hygiene procedures. Consultation with the patient's physician regarding the need for antibiotic prophylaxis is necessary prior to providing dental treatment for the patient with a pacemaker or ICD.

ANTICOAGULANT THERAPY[28]

- Anticoagulants are used in the treatment of many cardiovascular diseases to prevent embolus and thrombus formation.
- A prescribed drug may be continued indefinitely by the patient as a preventive measure.
- Drugs most commonly used to prevent or delay blood coagulation are heparin (hospital-administered intravenous) and coumarin derivatives.
- Although precautions are needed to prevent hemorrhage, discontinuing the drug may be more hazardous for the patient than performing dental and dental hygiene therapy with precautions.
- Consultation with the patient's physician must occur prior to proceeding with invasive oral surgical procedures.

I. Clinical Procedures

A. Consultation

- Information about the patient's INR (international normalized ratio) is obtained from the primary care provider during an initial consultation.
- The INR is a test of the coagulation phase of blood clotting used to monitor therapy with anticoagulants.

B. Treatment Planning

- Pretest for INR
  - Determine the INR within 24 hours before an appointment. The patient can have the test made on the day of a dental appointment by preplanning with the physician and the laboratory.
  - Most patients have a routine appointment for monitoring of the blood, and dental appointment dates can be planned to coincide.
  - Safe level for dental and dental hygiene procedures is considered to be 2–3, provided precautions are taken during instrumentation and postoperative care.

► Quadrant nonsurgical periodontal therapy
- Teach and emphasize daily dental biofilm control procedures in a series of appointments to prepare the gingival tissue for instrumentation. Healthy, healed tissue does not bleed as readily or as profusely.
- Complete treatment, including removal of all calculus and subgingival biofilm and other irritants, is necessary to contribute to the goal of healthy tissue that does not bleed.

C. Local Hemostatic Measures

► Instrumentation can be performed for most patients without complication, provided precautions are taken to minimize tissue trauma and control bleeding and not to dismiss the patient until bleeding has stopped.

► *Pressure*: Pressure with sponges or cotton pellets packed interdentally can aid in control.

II. Postprocedural Instructions

► The practice by oral surgeons of closely observing patients for 6–8 hours following a surgical procedure has application following selected dental procedures. At the least, a check that postcare instructions are being followed is advisable.

► The patient is advised to avoid vigorous toothbrushing and rinsing on a treated area for several hours or until the next day.

► The use of extraoral icepacks may be helpful.

► General postcare instructions on for the care of an area with a periodontal dressing can be found in Table 43-2 in Chapter 43.

► The use of a soft diet, cool rather than hot foods.

► Moderation of physical activity may be advisable.

► Long-term instruction must emphasize the maintenance of gingival health to prevent future bleeding problems.

CARDIAC SURGERY

► Patients in dental offices and clinics who have had or will have cardiac surgery such as CABG and heart transplantation are identified and need special procedures.

I. Presurgical

► Before elective cardiac surgery, the patient is brought to a state of optimum oral health, with all sources of infection removed.

► All restorations and other dental procedures are completed.

► Patients requiring cardiac surgery need information and motivation relative to the importance of oral health in eliminating a potential source of IE.

► Vigilance in a preventive program that includes biofilm control and self-applied fluorides is essential.

II. Postsurgical

A. Continuing Care Appointments

Frequent appointments are necessary for supervision and dental hygiene care.

B. Prophylactic Antibiotic[3,4]

► Antibiotic coverage for all dental and dental hygiene procedures for patients with prosthetic cardiac valves is essential. Because of the high susceptibility to infections, a special regimen for high-risk patients may be indicated.

► Patients with implanted vascular *autografts* generally do not need antibiotic premedication before dental and dental hygiene appointments. An example of an implanted vascular autograph is the use of a patient's own blood vessel to provide a coronary bypass (Figure 67-5).

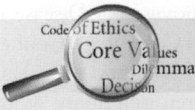

EVERYDAY ETHICS

Leo is a 68-year-old, obese, black male with a history of hypertension and hypercholesterolemia. He reminds Kerstin, the dental hygienist, that he has an extreme dislike of dental appointments as he grasps very tightly to the armrests of the dental chair.

During the medical history review, Leo admitted that he usually remembers to take his blood pressure medications but since he does not feel well after the cholesterol-lowering medication, he does not take it regularly. Kerstin takes his right arm blood pressure of 165/90 mm Hg. Leo then starts rubbing his left arm, and Kerstin asks him how he is feeling. Leo says he is having heartburn from a spicy dinner last night and his left arm is sore, probably from doing some yard work a couple of days ago.

Questions for Consideration

1. What medical, legal, and ethical questions come to mind to be taken into account when a dental hygienist has a patient like Leo with a complicated medical history that involves medications, patient symptoms, and is a nervous patient about any dental appointments?

2. Which of the dental hygiene core values has application in this scenario? How does each of the core values selected affect the appointment plan?

3. Using the questions in Table V-1 in Section V Introduction, prepare at least three possible procedure outlines that Kerstin could consider as she decides steps in Leo's treatment that day.

C. Immunosuppressive Therapy

▶ Principal drugs used for patients with transplants are cyclosporin, azathioprine, and prednisolone to prevent rejection of the transplant.

▶ Among the side effects, particularly of cyclosporin, is gingival enlargement.[27] Many patients may receive medication with the nifedipine group, also effective in causing gingival enlargement. Special periodontal care will be needed.

DOCUMENTATION

Documentation for a routine dental hygiene continuing care or periodontal maintenance appointment for a patient with a cardiovascular illness would need to include a minimum of the following items:

▶ Note and record the responses to health history review questions about visitations to the cardiologist, and in addition to the patient's report on the state of health, answers from the MD concerning changes that could influence procedures.

▶ Note, record, and compare all findings with previous findings: blood pressure determination, findings in the extraoral and intraoral examination, and the gingival and periodontal clinical examination with complete probing.

▶ An example documentation note may be reviewed in Box 67-4.

BOX 67-4

Example Documentation: Patient with Uncontrolled Hypertension

S –Forty-six year old African-American patient arrives in the dental office for a 3-month periodontal continuing care appointment. He reports he has been diagnosed with high blood pressure and is taking Procardia.

O –Vital signs: blood pressure: 180/100. Patient reports he cannot afford his medication so he takes it every other day. Contact his cardiologist and/or primary care provider to ensure it is safe to proceed with treatment. The providers gives permission, but recommends no vasoconstrictor in the local anesthetic until the blood pressure is under control.

A –A comprehensive periodontal and caries examination findings include localized moderate chronic periodontitis with bleeding on probing in molar areas along with recurrent caries MO-#14, MO-#15.

P –Oral self-care is reviewed with a focus on use of an interdental brush in posterior interproximal areas. Periodontal maintenance is completed except for in the area of #14–15 where localized nonsurgical periodontal therapy (NSPT) with local anesthesia is recommended. Patient to follow-up with his primary care provider and return for localized NSPT once BP is controlled. Office will follow-up in 2 weeks.

Signed: _____, RDH

Date: _____

Factors To Teach The Patient

▷ Encourage patients who have been diagnosed as hypertensive to continue their prescribed therapy.

Stress Reduction Procedures

▷ Select an appointment time that is optimum with respect to that time of the day when the patient is feeling best and may be less fatigued. Most anxious patients prefer a morning appointment.

▷ Get adequate sleep and rest, and engage in non-fatiguing activities during the 24 hours before the appointment.

▷ Use premedication as prescribed for sleeping the night before. A sedative may be prescribed to be taken 60 minutes before an appointment or at the dental office, if possible. When taken at home 1 hour before, it is not recommended for the patient to drive a car.

▷ Allow time to get to the dental office or clinic; bring own reading material, knitting or sewing, or other relaxing activity in the event that waiting is unavoidable.

▷ Eat breakfast, lunch, or other usual between-meal food and take usual medications on schedule.

▷ When other family members, especially children, have dental or dental hygiene appointments, do not add to their stress by relaying personal negative feelings.

References

1. Humphrey L, Fu R, Buckley D, et al. Periodontal Disease and coronary heart disease incidence: a systematic review and meta-analysis. *J Gen Intern Med.* 2008;23(12):2079–2086.

2. Glenny AM, Oliver R, Roberts GJ, et al. Antibiotics for the prophylaxis of bacterial endocarditis in dentistry. *Cochrane Database Syst Rev.* 2013;(10):CD003813.

3. Wilson W, Taubert KA, Gewitz M, et al. Prevention of infective endocarditis: guidelines from the American Heart Association Rheumatic Fever, Endocarditis, and Kawasaki Disease Committee, Council on Cardiovascular Disease in the Young, and the Council on Clinical Cardiology, Council on Cardiovascular Surgery and Anesthesia, and the Quality of Care and Outcomes Research Interdisciplinary Working Group. *Circulation.* 2007. http://circ.ahajournals.org/content/116/15/1736.full. Accessed August 2013.

4. Nishimura RA, Otto CM, Bonow RO, et al. American College of Cardiology/American Heart Association Task Force on Practice Guidelines. 2014 AHA/ACC guideline for the management of patients with valvular heart disease: executive summary: a report of the American College of Cardiology/American Heart Association Task Force on Practice Guidelines. *J Am Coll Cardiol.* 2014;63(22):2438–2488.

5. March of Dimes. Congenital heart defects. March of Dimes Foundation. 2008. http://www.marchofdimes.com/baby/congenital-heart-defects.aspx. Accessed August 2013.

6. Centers for Disease Control and Prevention. Facts about congenital heart defects. http://www.cdc.gov/ncbddd/heart-defects/facts.html. Updated July 18, 2014. Accessed August 20, 2015.

7. National Institutes of Health, National Library of Medicine, Medline Plus. Rheumatic fever. http://www.nlm.nih.gov/medlineplus/ency/article/003940.htm. Updated May 11, 2014. Accessed August 30, 2015.

8. National Institutes of Health, National Heart, Blood, and Lung Institute. What is mitral valve prolapse? http://www.nhlbi.nih.gov/health/health-topics/topics/mvp/. Updated July 1, 2011. Accessed August 30, 2015.

9. James PA, Oparil S, Carter BL, et al. 2014 evidence-based guideline for the management of high blood pressure in adults: report from the panel members appointed to the Eighth Joint National Committee (JNC 8). JAMA. 2014;311(5):507–520.

10. American Heart Association. High blood pressure. http://www.heart.org/HEARTORG/Conditions/HighBloodPressure/High-Blood-Pressure-or-Hypertension_UCM_002020_SubHomePage.jsp. Accessed June 30, 2014.

11. National Institutes of Health, National Library of Medicine, Medline Plus. Malignant hypertension. http://www.nlm.nih.gov/medlineplus/ency/article/000491.htm. Updated April 5, 2013. Accessed August 30, 2015.

12. Flynn JT, Daniels SR, Hayman LL, et al. American Heart Association Atherosclerosis, Hypertension and Obesity in Youth Committee of the Council on Cardiovascular Disease in the Young. Update: ambulatory blood pressure monitoring in children and adolescents: a scientific statement from the American Heart Association. Hypertension. 2014;63(5):1116–1135.

13. National Institutes of Health, National Heart, Lung, and Blood Institute. Atherosclerosis. http://www.nhlbi.nih.gov/health/health-topics/topics/atherosclerosis/atrisk.html. Updated August 4, 2014. Accessed August 30, 2015.

14. Lockhart PB, Bolger AF, Papapanou PN, et al. Periodontal disease and atherosclerotic vascular disease: does the evidence support an independent association?: a scientific statement from the American Heart Association. Circulation. 2012;125(20):2520–2544.

15. American Heart Association. Angina pectoris. http://www.heart.org/HEARTORG/Conditions/HeartAttack/SymptomsDiagnosisofHeartAttack/Angina-Pectoris-Chest-Pain_UCM_437515_Article.jsp. Updated May 15, 2015. Accessed August 30, 2015.

16. National Institutes of Health, National Library of Medicine, Medline Plus. Heart attack. https://www.nlm.nih.gov/medlineplus/ency/article/000195.htm. Updated August 12, 2014. Accessed August 30, 2015.

17. American Heart Association. Heart attack symptoms in women. http://www.heart.org/HEARTORG/Conditions/HeartAttack/WarningSignsofaHeartAttack/Heart-Attack-Symptoms-in-Women_UCM_436448_Article.jsp. Updated July 2015. Accessed August 30, 2015.

18. Reed KL. Basic management of medical emergencies: recognizing a patient's distress. J Am Dent Assoc. 2010;141 (Suppl 1):20S–24S.

19. American Heart Association. Prevention and treatment of heart attack. http://www.heart.org/HEARTORG/Conditions/HeartAttack/PreventionTreatmentofHeartAttack/Prevention-and-Treatment-of-Heart-Attack_UCM_002042_Article.jsp. Updated August 21, 2015. Accessed August 30, 2015.

20. National Institutes of Health, National Heart, Lung, and Blood Institute. What is heart failure? http://www.nhlbi.nih.gov/health/health-topics/topics/hf/. Updated March 27, 2014. Accessed August 30, 2015.

21. American Heart Association. Types of heart failure. http://www.heart.org/HEARTORG/Conditions/HeartFailure/AboutHeartFailure/Types-of-Heart-Failure_UCM_306323_Article.jsp. Updated June 1, 2015. Accessed August 30, 2015.

22. Eckel RH, Jakicic JM, Ard JD, et al. 2013 AHA/ACC guideline on lifestyle management to reduce cardiovascular risk: a report of the American College of Cardiology/American Heart Association Task Force on Practice Guidelines. Circulation. 2014;129(25, Suppl 2):S76–S99.

23. National Institutes of Health, National Heart, Lung, and Blood Institute. What is the DASH eating plan? http://www.nhlbi.nih.gov/health/health-topics/topics/dash/. Updated June 6, 2014. Accessed July 27, 2014.

24. Wilson BL, Broberg C, Baumgartner JC, et al. Safety of electronic apex locators and pulp testers in patients with implanted cardiac pacemakers or cardioverter/defibrillators. J Endod. 2006;32(9):847–852.

25. National Institutes of Health; National Heart, Lung and Blood Institute. What is a pacemaker? http://www.nhlbi.nih.gov/health/health-topics/topics/pace/. Updated February 28, 2012. Accessed August 20, 2015.

26. Gomez G, Duran-Sindreu F, Roig M, et al. The effects of six electronic apex locators on pacemaker function: an in vitro study. Int Endod J. 2013;46(5):399–405.

27. Uslan D, Gleva M, Poole J, et al. Cardiovascular implantable electronic device replacement infections and prevention: results from the REPLACE Registry. Pacing Clin Electrophysiol. 2012;35(1):81–87.

28. Douketis JD, Spyropoulos AC, Spencer FA, et al. Perioperative management of antithrombotic therapy: Antithrombotic Therapy and Prevention of Thrombosis, 9th ed: American College of Chest Physicians Evidence-Based Clinical Practice Guidelines. Chest. 2012;141(2, Suppl):e326S–e350S.

29. Dongari-Bagtzoglou A; and Research, Science and Therapy Committee, American Academy of Periodontology. Drug-associated gingival enlargement. J Periodontol. 2004;75(10):1424–1431.

ENHANCE YOUR UNDERSTANDING

thePoint® DIGITAL CONNECTIONS
(see the inside front cover for access information)
- **Audio glossary**
- **Quiz bank**

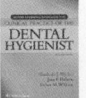 **SUPPORT FOR LEARNING**
(available separately; visit lww.com)
- *Active Learning Workbook for Clinical Practice of the Dental Hygienist, 12th Edition*

prepU INDIVIDUALIZED REVIEW
(available separately; visit lww.com)
- **Adaptive quizzing with *prepU for Wilkins' Clinical Practice of the Dental Hygienist***

68

The Patient with a Blood Disorder

Lisa Welch, RDH, MSDH and Barbara Dawidjan, RDH, MED

CHAPTER OUTLINE

LEARNING OBJECTIVES

After studying this chapter, the student will be able to:

1. Describe the major types of blood disorders.

2. Explain the general and oral signs and symptoms of the major types of blood disorders.

3. Identify clinical implications of selected blood values including the INR (international normalized ratio), platelet count, and neutrophil count.

4. Provide examples of dental hygiene treatment modifications necessary for the patient with a blood disorder.

Oral soft tissue changes, lowered resistance to infection, and bleeding tendencies are major factors to be considered for a patient with a blood disorder. Oral manifestations of blood disorders are generally exaggerated in the presence of dental biofilm and local predisposing factors.

Box 68-1 lists and defines terminology used to describe hematologic conditions.

NORMAL BLOOD[1]

I. Composition

▶ Blood is composed of 55% plasma fluid and 45% formed elements.
▶ The 45% formed elements consist of:
  • 44% erythrocytes (red blood cells or corpuscles)
  • 1% leukocytes (white blood cells).
▶ Figure 68-1 shows the cell forms and nuclei.
▶ Hematocrit, a test commonly used in health examinations, shows:
  • Percentage packed volume of blood cells
  • Normal values are listed in Table 68-1.
▶ Reference values for blood cells are also listed in Table 68-1, with examples of conditions in which increases and decreases in the normal values occur.

II. Origin of Blood Cells

▶ Adult blood cells originate in bone marrow.
▶ Hemocytoblast: the stem cell of origin.
▶ Erythrocytes and granulocytes leave the bone marrow as mature cells and enter the circulating blood.
▶ Agranulocytes (lymphocytes and monocytes) leave the bone marrow as immature cells and go to lymphoid tissues for maturing.
▶ Immature cell forms predominate in certain blood diseases and cancers.

PLASMA

▶ The constituents of the fluid portion of the blood are similar to the fluid constituents of the connective tissue.
▶ If plasma is allowed to clot, the remaining fluid is called serum.
▶ The plasma is composed of 90% water and 10% of the following:
▶ *Plasma proteins*
  • Albumin (functions to maintain tissue fluid balance within the vascular system).
  • Gamma globulins (circulating antibodies essential to the immune system).

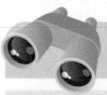

BOX 68-1   KEY WORDS: Bleeding Disorders

Chelation therapy: process to remove excess iron acquired from chronic blood transfusions.

Coagulation factor: factor essential to normal blood clotting contained within the blood plasma; designated by Roman numerals I–V and VII–XIII; their absence, diminution, or excess may lead to abnormality of clotting.

Differential cell count: record of the number of white blood cells, including determination of the percentage of each type of cell present; the "differential" is used in the diagnosis of various blood disorders, infections, and other abnormal conditions of the body.

Erythropoiesis: formation of red blood cells.

Glossitis: inflammation of the tongue.

Glossodynia: pain in the tongue.

Hemarthrosis: blood in a joint cavity.

Hematocrit: volume percentage of erythrocytes (red blood cells) in whole blood.

Hematopoiesis: the formation and development of blood cells, usually in bone marrow.

Hemoglobin: protein in the erythrocyte that transports molecular oxygen to body cells.

Hemolysis: rupture of erythrocytes with the release of hemoglobin into the plasma.

Hemolytic: destruction of blood cells, resulting in liberation of hemoglobin.

Hypoxia: diminished availability of oxygen to body tissues.

IF (Intrinsic Factor): produced by the parietal cells in the stomach; aids in vitamin B 12 absorption.

INR (International Normalized Ratio): ratio between actual blood coagulation time and the normal coagulation time.

Leukocytosis: increase in the total number of leukocytes.

Leukopenia: reduction in total number of leukocytes in the blood; count under 500 per mL.

Neutropenia: diminished number of neutrophils (polymorphonuclear leukocytes or PMNs).

Oxyhemoglobin: oxygenated arterial blood; bright red and about 97% saturated with oxygen; venous blood is a darker color and contains only 20%–70% oxygen.

Petechia: minute, pinpoint, round, nonraised, purplish-red spot in the skin or mucous membrane, caused by hemorrhage.

Phagocytosis: engulfing of microorganisms and foreign particles by phagocytes, such as macrophages.

Purpura: hemorrhage into the tissues, under the skin, and through the mucous membranes; produces petechiae and ecchymoses.

Vaso-occlusion: blood vessel blockage resulting in organ damage.

Vertigo: dizziness.

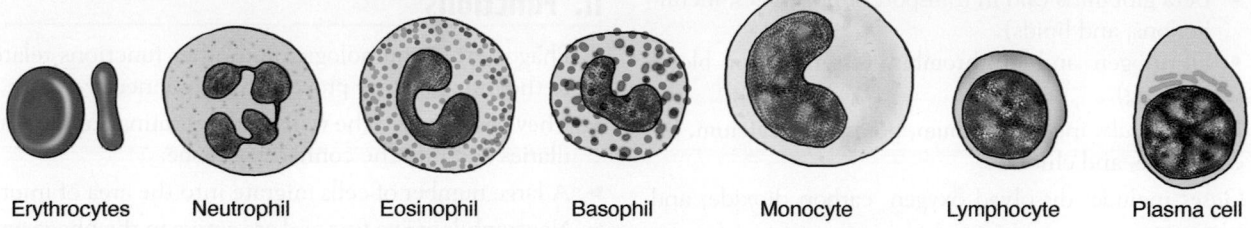

Erythrocytes Neutrophil Eosinophil Basophil Monocyte Lymphocyte Plasma cell

FIGURE 68-1 Red and White Blood Cells. Diagram shows normal cell forms drawn to scale for comparison of cell size. Note the shape of nuclei in each of the white blood cells. The erythrocyte or red blood cell does not have a nucleus; its biconcave disc shape is shown in the lateral view second from the left.

TABLE 68-1	Laboratory Values and Clinical Implications		
TEST	**NORMAL RANGE**[a]	**CLINICAL IMPLICATIONS**	**CAUSES OF DEVIATIONS**
PT (prothrombin time)	11–15 sec	Routine care can be performed when PT is <20 sec	Prolonged in: Prothrombin deficiency Anticoagulant therapy Vitamin K deficiency Liver diseases Aspirin use
INR	<2.5	Routine care can be performed when INR 2–3, MD consult when INR > 3.0	Prolonged in: Polycythemia vera (PV) Prothrombin deficiency Anticoagulant therapy Vitamin K deficiency Liver diseases Aspirin use
Activated partial thromboplastin time (aPTT)	25–35 sec	Routine care when aPTT is <1.5 × normal, MD consult when > 57 sec	Prolonged in: Hemophilia and von Willebrand's disease Anticoagulant therapy
Platelet count	140,000–400,000/mm^3	Routine care can be provided when values are >50,000/mm^3 MD consult needed when values <10,000/mm^3—potentially life threatening	Thrombocytopenia: <20,000 mm^3
Hemoglobin (g/dL)	Males: 13.6–17.2 g/100 mL Females: 12–15 g/100 mL	Delivers O_2 through circulation to body tissues and returns CO_2 from tissues to lungs	Increased in: Polycythemia Dehydration Decreased in: Anemias Hemorrhage Leukemias
Hematocrit (volume of packed red cells) (percentage)	Males: 39%–49% Females: 33%–43%	Indicates relative proportions of plasma and red blood cells	Increased in: Polycythemia Dehydration Decreased in: Anemias Hemorrhage leukemias
Absolute neutrophil count (ANC)	Normal ANC: 2,500–6,000	Measure of the number of infection fighting white blood cells. Routine care 50,000/mm^3 <500/mm^3—potentially life threatening	Decreased in: Anemias Chemotherapy

[a]Ranges vary among health facilities and laboratories. The reference ranges of the facility providing the results are used in interpreting the test result.

- Beta globulins (aid in transport of hormones, metallic ions, and lipids).
- Fibrinogen and prothrombin (essential for blood clotting).
▶ *Inorganic salts* include: sodium, potassium, calcium, bicarbonate, and chloride.
▶ *Gases* include: dissolved oxygen, carbon dioxide, and nitrogen.
▶ *Substances being transported* include: hormones, nutrients, waste products, and enzymes.

RED BLOOD CELLS (ERYTHROCYTES)

I. Description

▶ Although commonly called red blood cells, they are more properly termed corpuscles because they have no nuclei (Figure 68-1).
▶ Biconcave discs that contain hemoglobin.
▶ Sensitive and flexible; change shape readily as they pass through small capillaries.

II. Functions

▶ Transport hemoglobin.
▶ Carry oxygen to the body cells in the form of oxyhemoglobin.
▶ Carbon dioxide is transported from the cells.

III. Hemoglobin

▶ Measured in grams (g) per 100 milliliters (mL).
▶ Normal values range from 12 to 17.2 g per mL depending on gender (Table 68-1).
▶ Values reflect:
- Anemic state when hemoglobin is below normal.
- Pathologic conditions when hemoglobin increases over normal.

WHITE BLOOD CELLS (LEUKOCYTES)

I. Types of Leukocytes

▶ White blood cells are divided into two general groups, the granulocytes and the agranulocytes.
▶ Granulocytes have granules in their cytoplasm, whereas the agranulocytes do not.
▶ They are further subdivided into the following categories:
- *Granulocytes*: neutrophils, eosinophils, and basophils.
- *Agranulocytes*: lymphocytes, monocytes.

II. Functions

▶ Phagocytic, immunologic, and other functions related to the inflammatory process in the connective tissue.
▶ They pass through the walls at the terminal ends of capillaries and into the connective tissue.
▶ A large number of cells migrate into the area of injury.
▶ Neutrophils arrive first and are active in the phagocytosis of foreign material and microorganisms.
▶ Blood functions as a transport medium for the white cells as they pass to areas in the connective tissue where they are needed.
▶ Numbers and proportions in the blood maintain a constant level in health, as listed in Table 68-2.
▶ Differential cell count of the white blood cells is used in the detection and monitoring of disease states. Increases and decreases of each cell type can be associated with certain conditions.

III. Agranulocytes

▶ *Lymphocytes*
- Small round cells with a round nucleus that nearly fills the cell with a narrow rim of cytoplasm (Figure 68-1).
- Can move back and forth between the vessels and the extravascular tissues.
- Capable of reverting to blast-like cells of origin and then multiplying as the immunologic need arises.
▶ *Monocytes*
- Large cells with a bean-shaped or indented nucleus.
- Actively phagocytic.
- In connective tissue, monocytes differentiate into macrophages, which are important in immunologic processes.

IV. Granulocytes

▶ *Neutrophils*
- Also called polymorphonuclear leukocytes (PMNs).
- Most numerous of all the white blood cells.
- Nucleus has three to five lobes connected by thin chromatin threads.
- Cells are round in circulation.
- They are amoeboid (moving and changing shape) in the tissues and function in phagocytosis. Neutrophils are part of the first line of defense of the body.
▶ *Eosinophils*
- Two-lobed nucleus and larger, coarser granules than those of a neutrophil.
- Microscopically, the cells stain a distinct bright pink; are readily recognized.
- Few in number; increase markedly during allergic conditions.

TABLE 68-2	Blood Cells Reference Values

An examination of a blood smear (or film) may be requested by a physician in response to abnormality in blood counts.

CELL TYPE	NORMAL VALUE	CAUSES OF INCREASE	CAUSES OF DECREASE
Red blood cells (erythrocytes)	Males: 4.3–5.9 million per mm^3 Females: 3.5–5.0 million per mm^3	Polycythemia dehydration	Anemias Leukemias Hemorrhage
Platelets (thrombocytes) (cell fragments essential for the process of blood clotting)	150,000–400,000 per mm^3 Wintrobe method: 140,000–440,000 per mm^3	Polycythemia vera (PV) Chronic myelocytic leukemia Sickle cell anemia Rheumatic fever Hemolytic anemias Bone fractures	Acute severe infections Cirrhosis of the liver Thrombocytopenic purpura Acute leukemias Aplastic anemias Pernicious anemia
White blood cells (leukocytes)	5,000–10,000 per mm^3	Inflammation Overexertion Polycythemia vera (PV) Leukemia	Aplastic anemia Granulocytopenia Drug poisoning Thrombocytopenia Radiation Severe infections HIV/AIDS
Differential white cell count granulocytes • Neutrophils • Eosinophils • Basophils	 60%–70% 1%–3% 1%	Acute infections Myelogenous leukemia Poisoning Erythroblastosis Allergic diseases Dermatitis Hodgkin's disease Scarlet fever Certain chronic infections	Aplastic anemia Granulocytopenia Aplastic anemia Typhoid fever Aplastic anemia
Agranulocytes • Lymphocytes • Monocytes	 20%–35% 2%–6%	Lymphocytic leukemia Chronic infections Viral diseases Monocytic leukemias Tuberculosis Infective endocarditis Hodgkin's disease	Aplastic anemia Myelogenous leukemia Radiation Aplastic anemia

▶ *Basophils*
- Nucleus has a "U" or "S" form.
- Function is to increase vascular permeability during inflammation so that phagocytic cells can pass into the area.

PLATELETS (THROMBOCYTES)

▶ Small round or oval formed element without a nucleus
▶ Approximately one-fourth the size of a red blood cell.
▶ Active in the blood clotting mechanism.
▶ Essential in the maintenance of the integrity of blood capillaries by repairing them at the time of injury.
▶ Participate in clot dissolution after healing.

ANEMIA

▶ Anemia is a reduction in red blood cells to a level below a normal level for the individual.[2]
▶ Oxygen-carrying capacity to the cells is diminished.

I. Classification by Cause

A. Caused by Blood Loss

▶ *Acute:* Blood loss from trauma or disease
▶ *Chronic:* An internal lesion with constant slow bleeding, usually of gastrointestinal or gynecologic origin, can lead to a chronic loss of blood. *Iron-deficiency anemia* can result.

B. Caused by Increased Hemolysis

Hemolysis means the destruction of red blood cells; is also called "hemolytic anemia" because of cell destruction.

- Hereditary hemolytic disorders
  - *Sickle cell disease* (SCD), which belongs to the group of hereditary disorders called the hemoglobinopathies
- Acquired hemolytic disorders
  - Examples: drugs, infections, and certain physical and chemical agents may cause red cell destruction.
  - In the category of antibody-mediated anemia, *erythroblastosis fetalis* (also called hemolytic disease of the newborn) occurs when an expectant mother is Rh positive and the fetus is Rh negative.

C. Caused by Diminished Production of Red Blood Cells

- *Nutritional deficiency*
  - Inadequate dietary choices or inadequate intake.
  - Defective absorption from the gastrointestinal tract.
  - Examples: *pernicious anemia*, which results from a B_{12} vitamin absorption deficiency, *iron-deficiency anemia*, which may occur during pregnancy or during a growth spurt, and *celiac disease* (sprue), which results from sensitivity to dietary gluten.
  - Increased demand for nutrients such as in growth or pregnancy.
- *Bone marrow failure*
  - *Aplastic anemia* (which can be inherited) can occur without apparent cause or when the bone marrow is injured by medications, radiation, chemotherapy, or infection.
  - In aplastic anemia, a combination of anemia, neutropenia, and thrombocytopenia occurs, which leads to a quantitative decrease in all cells formed in the bone marrow.
  - Consult with physician to determine if antibiotic premedication would be indicated.

D. Anemia of Chronic Diseases[3]

- Second most prevalent anemia after iron-deficiency anemia.
- Many chronic systemic diseases are associated with anemia.

E. Caused by Genetic Blood Disorders

- *Thalassemia* is a diverse group of genetic blood disorders characterized by defects in synthesis of normal hemoglobin.[4]
- It typically affects people of Mediterranean, African, Middle Eastern, and Southeast Asian descent.
- The condition can range in severity from mild to life threatening.

- The most severe form is beta thalassemia major (Cooley's anemia).
- Blood counts are evaluated and monitored for delayed wound healing.
- Treatment[4]
  - May require periodic and lifelong blood transfusions and chelation therapy.
  - Folic acid supplements.
  - If performed during childhood, bone marrow transplant is a potential cure.
  - Hematopoietic (blood forming) stem-cell transplantation is the only available treatment for thalassemia.

II. Clinical Characteristics of Anemia[2]

When a patient's medical history shows the presence of anemia, certain general characteristics may be anticipated for which clinical adaptations may be needed. The general signs and symptoms are:

- Pale skin, nails, buccal mucosa
- Weakness, malaise, easy fatigability
- Dyspnea on slight exertion, faintness
- Brittle nails with loss of convexity referred to as spooning of the nails.

IRON-DEFICIENCY ANEMIA[5,6]

I. Characteristics

Iron-deficiency anemia is a hypochromic microcytic anemia, which means that:

- Hemoglobin content is deficient (hypochromic)
- Red blood cells are smaller than normal (microcytic)
- Occurs more in younger than older people and more in females than in males
- Diagnosis is by laboratory test that shows low hemoglobin and a reduced hematocrit value.

II. Causes

- Malnutrition, poor dietary intake, or malabsorption (e.g., celiac disease and Crohn's disease).
- Chronic infection.
- Bariatric surgery (gastric bypass).
- Increased body demand for iron over and above the daily intake. For example, during pregnancy.
- Acute or chronic blood loss due to:
  - Excessive menstrual flow.
  - Frequent blood donations.
- Internal bleeding due to:
  - Gastrointestinal diseases, such as ulcer and colon or stomach cancer.

- Drugs, notably aspirin.
- Hemorrhoids.
- Chronic alcoholism.

III. Signs and Symptoms

▶ *General*
- General weakness, pallor
- Fatigue on slight exertion
- Decreased immune function and increased risk for infection

▶ *Oral findings*
- Pallor of the mucosa and gingiva
- Tongue changes: atrophic glossitis with loss of filiform papillae. In moderate and severe anemia, when the hemoglobin is at 10 g/dL or below, the tongue is smooth and shiny. The patient may have burning, painful sensations (glossodynia).
- Secondary irritations to the thinned, atrophic mucosa may result from smoking, mechanical trauma, or hot, spicy foods.
- Angular cheilitis.
- Increased risk of candidiasis.

IV. Therapy

▶ Treatment of underlying cause to prevent further blood loss.

▶ Treated with oral ferrous iron tablets with vitamin C to aid absorption; to be taken on empty stomach for best absorption rates.

▶ Folic acid supplements may be indicated if there is an underlying folate deficiency.

▶ Nutritional counseling: recommend foods high in iron. Sources given in Chapter 35.

▶ Liquid preparations, which are sometimes used for children, may stain the teeth. Administering the medicine by way of a straw is advised.

MEGALOBLASTIC ANEMIA

Characterized by abnormally large (megalo-) red blood cells, many of which are oval shaped resulting from a deficiency of either vitamin B_{12} or folate, or both.

I. Pernicious Anemia[7–9]

▶ *Etiologic factors*
- Pernicious anemia is considered to be an autoimmune disease affecting the gastric mucosa so that it atrophies and fails to produce *intrinsic factor* (IF).
- IF is excreted by the stomach parietal cells and is necessary for absorption of vitamin B_{12}.

- Deficiency of vitamin B_{12} can also be caused by:
  1. Malabsorption of vitamin B_{12} due to gastrointestinal disorders such as celiac disease and Crohn's disease.
  2. Inadequate intake may occur in strict vegans (those who do not eat foods from animal sources, for example, dairy or meat).
  3. Chronic gastritis or surgical removal of part or all of the stomach (e.g., gastric bypass) can reduce or stop the production of IF.
  4. Long-term use of histamine (H_2) receptor antagonists, proton pump inhibitors, or metformin.

▶ *Age characteristics*
- Pernicious anemia is primarily a disease of adults and occurs with increasing frequency in those over age 60.

▶ *Signs and symptoms: general*
- Fatigue and weakness.
- Loss of appetite and weight loss.
- Poor memory.

▶ *Signs and symptoms: neurologic involvement*
- Sclerosis of the spinal cord.
- Polyneuritis (inflammation or degeneration of nerves causing pain).
- Numbness of hands and feet.
- Ataxia (loss of coordination).

▶ *Signs and symptoms: oral findings*
- Glossitis (Hunter's glossitis) slick or bald tongue, loss of filiform papillae, and burning sensation with certain foods.
- Sensitivity to hot or spicy foods.
- Gingiva and mucosa: pale, atrophic similar to vitamin B deficiency.

▶ *Treatment*
- For individuals with IF deficiency and/or malabsorption, vitamin B_{12} is administered by injection daily until the condition is controlled.
- Once controlled, administration will continue monthly for life or until the underlying condition causing the deficiency is managed.
- For patients with inadequate IF production, oral supplementation of vitamin B_{12} is the treatment of choice.
- Vitamin B_{12} is only found in foods from animal sources and fortified foods. Good dietary sources of vitamin B_{12} are meat, clams, liver, fortified breakfast cereals, fish, poultry, milk, cheese, and eggs.

II. Folate-Deficiency Anemia[10]

Folate-deficiency anemia has the same characteristics as pernicious anemia, except no clinical neurologic changes are evident.

▶ *Etiologic factors*
- Decreased intake.

- Inadequate intake: Severely restricted diets or diets influenced by such factors as poverty, food faddism, or alcoholism, when the use of alcohol takes precedence over food.
- Impaired absorption.

▶ *Individuals at risk of folate inadequacy*

- Women of childbearing age.
- Pregnant women.
- Patients with alcohol dependence.
- Individuals with malabsorption disorders, that is, postgastric surgery, celiac disease, and inflammatory bowel disease.
- Certain treatment regimens impair the utilization of folate, for example, cancer chemotherapy, rheumatoid arthritis, and medications, such as methotrexate and dilantin.

▶ *Dietary factors: sources*

- In 1998, the Food and Drug Administration required fortification of cereals, breads, flours, pastas, and other grain products with folate.
- Dietary sources can be found in Table 35-4 (Chapter 35).

▶ *Fetal development*

- Women with inadequate folic acid intake are at increased risk of having a baby with neural tube defects.
- Spina bifida (myelomeningocele): a severe condition affecting the formation of the nerves of the spinal cord, and resulting in infant paralysis. Spina bifida is described in Chapter 59.

SICKLE CELL DISEASE[11,12]

▶ (SCD) is a hereditary form of hemolytic anemia, resulting from a defective hemoglobin molecule.

▶ The name is derived from the crescent or "sickle" shape assumed by the erythrocytes when the defective hemoglobin loses oxygen (Figure 68-2).

▶ It is an autosomal recessive trait and approximately 10% of black Americans have sickle cell trait. Those with sickle cell trait demonstrate few symptoms unless placed under severe stress.

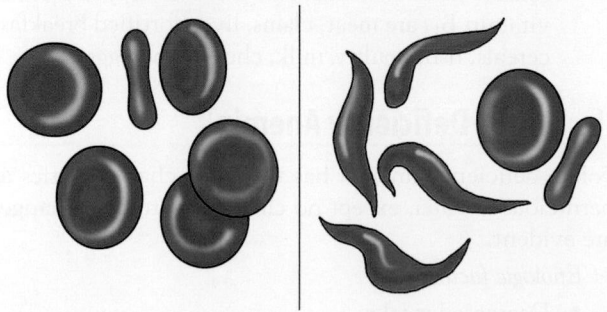

FIGURE 68-2 **Sickle Cell Disease.** Left, diagrammatic drawing of normal red blood cells. Right, sickle shapes of red blood cells of a patient with SCD.

I. Disease Process

Occurs primarily in the African-American population and in white populations of Mediterranean origin.

▶ *Diagnosis*

- Prenatal diagnosis can be made with 100% accuracy and genetic counseling provided for the parents.
- A simple blood test will detect SCD or sickle cell trait (parental carrier). Newborn screening is mandatory in most states in the United States.

II. Clinical Course[13]

▶ *Anemia*

- Life span of red blood cells is significantly reduced from a normal lifespan of approximately 90–120 days, to about 10–15 days.
- Anemia starts appearing within the first 6 months.
- Growth and development may be impaired during the early years.
- Increased susceptibility to infection and especially to pneumococcal infections.

▶ *Vaso-occlusion*

- Mortality is primarily from repeated episodes of vaso-occlusion (or blood vessel blockage) resulting in infarctions causing stroke and organ damage.
- There are progressive changes to blood vessels as a result of damage by the sickle-shaped red blood cells that result in the blood vessel blockage.
- Organ damage may be progressive and result in a shortened life expectancy, with most patients only living into their 30s.

▶ *Pain crises (sickle cell crisis)*

- Repeated episodes of acute pain that are highly unpredictable and result in hospitalization.
- Often preceded by a viral or bacterial infection.

▶ *Chronic organ damage*

Over time most sickle cell patients have damage to organs.

- Neurologic damage results in impaired cognition and hemorrhagic strokes.
- Cardiopulmonary damage impairs lung function and results in dilation of the left ventricle of the heart and heart murmurs.
- Hepatobiliary damage results in abnormal liver function and increases the likelihood of gallstones.
- Genitourinary damage may result in kidney failure.
- Skeletal damage may result in necrosis of the hips and shoulders with a need for joint replacement.
- Skin effects may result in chronic ulceration.
- Ocular damage in sickle cell anemia is the leading cause of blindness in patients of African ancestry.

III. Treatment and Disease Management

▶ *Supportive*

- Management of pain crises remains challenging.

- Oxygen is a mainstay of treatment to minimize hypoxia.
- Pain relief without depressing breathing.
- Avoid substance abuse.
- Fever
- Antibiotics for infectious diseases to avoid sepsis.
- *Prevention of sickling*
  - Pharmacologic therapy using a chemotherapy agent (Hydroxyurea) to increase hemoglobin F decreases the permanent formation of sickle cells.
  - Stem cell transplant may be an option.
  - Use of prophylactic penicillin to prevent pneumonia and meningococcal sepsis.
  - Regular blood transfusions.
  - Gene therapy shows promise in the future.

IV. Oral Implications[12,13]

- *Radiographic findings*
  - Coarse trabecular pattern appearing as horizontal rows between teeth ("step-ladder"), with large marrow spaces.
  - Osteoporotic changes.
- *Oral manifestations*[12,13]
  - Necrosis of the dental pulp.
  - Osteomyelitis of the mandible.
  - Enamel hypomineralization.
  - Overgrowth of the facial bones resulting in protrusion of the maxilla causing malocclusion.
  - Pallor of buccal mucosa.
  - Numb chin syndrome (mental nerve neuropathy).
  - Facial and dental pain.

V. Appointment Management

- Thoroughly review the comprehensive medical history. Gather information on the patient's:
  - Related complications specific to organ damage and other problems since birth.
  - Characteristics of pain control (frequency, duration, average number, date of last crisis).
  - Past and current medical treatment (surgeries, transfusions, medications, allergies).
  - Presence of venous access catheters and joint replacement.
  - Growth and development issues.
- Consultation with the patient's primary care provider to include the following:
  - Determine disease control including complete blood count.
  - Some patient's require the use of prophylactic antibiotics. For a patient so highly susceptible to infection, antibiotics may be considered routine, because any form of tissue manipulation creates a bacteremia.
- A stress reduction protocol is necessary to prevent precipitation of a sickle cell crisis.

- Implement a comprehensive preventive program to minimize oral infection and control oral disease risk factors.
- Avoid long complicated dental appointments by maintaining good oral health with frequent preventive care appointments with the dental hygienist.
- Use local anesthesia with low doses of vasoconstrictors to avoid intravascular occlusion of red blood cells.

POLYCYTHEMIAS

Polycythemia implies an increase in the number and concentration of red blood cells above the normal level. There are two categories of polycythemia: primary and secondary.

I. Polycythemia Vera (Primary Polycythemia)[14–16]

- *Cause*
  - Polycythemia vera (PV) is a neoplasm caused by a genetic mutation increasing the sensitivity of bone marrow cells to erythropoietin resulting in an increased production of red blood cells.[14,15]
  - Blood viscosity increases, affecting oxygen transport to tissues.
- *Clinical signs and symptoms*
  - Average age at diagnosis is 60.
  - Increased bleeding risk with spontaneous bleeding of the gingiva.
  - Bruise easily resulting in submucosal petechiae and hematoma formation.
  - Risk of fatal and nonfatal blood clot formation leading to heart attack, stroke, and pulmonary embolism.
  - Migraines.
  - Vertigo.
  - Fatigue.
  - Purplish or red areas on the oral mucosa, gingiva, lips or tongue.
- *Treatment*
  - Chemotherapy.
  - Phlebotomy, to reduce the total volume, and particularly the red cell volume, of the blood.
  - Low-dose aspirin (<100 mg/daily) as an antiplatelet.
- *Dental hygiene treatment considerations*
  - Thorough review of the medical history due to the increased risk of bleeding, bruising, cerebral vascular accident, and myocardial infarction.
  - Consult with the hematologist and/or primary care provider about disease management and patient's blood test results, especially hemoglobin and hematocrit.
  - Careful attention to oral self-care and preventive maintenance is required to maintain good oral health.

- Carefully monitor bleeding and monitor clotting during and following instrumentation.
- Provide careful postoperative instructions for early identification of bleeding that does not stop after applying pressure.

II. Secondary Polycythemia[15]

▶ Secondary polycythemia is also called erythrocytosis, which means an increase in the numbers of red blood cells.

▶ The increased red cell production can result from hypoxia like that experienced by residents of high altitudes, chronic obstructive pulmonary disease, cyanotic heart disease, emphysema, and tobacco smoking.

▶ Bleeding tendencies may be partially controlled with control of gingival irritants.

DISORDERS OF WHITE BLOOD CELLS

▶ Disorders of the white blood cells may occur because of a decrease (leukopenia) or an increase (leukocytosis) in cell numbers.

▶ The types of white blood cells are described in Table 68-2 and illustrated in Figure 68-1.

I. Neutropenia[17]

A decrease in the total number of neutrophils results when cell production cannot keep pace with the turnover rate or when an accelerated rate of removal of cells occurs, as in certain disease states.

A. Etiology

▶ Defects in myeloid cells that may be genetic.

▶ *Secondary neutropenia* may develop in the following conditions: alcohol abuse, autoimmune disease (e.g., HIV/AIDS), chemotherapy or radiation therapy, folate or vitamin B12 deficiency, infection, or bone marrow transplant.

B. Signs and Symptoms

▶ In neutropenias resulting from defects in myeloid cells, the patient may experience oral stomatitis and lymph node enlargement.

▶ Frequent, severe, or unusual infections such as pneumonia.

C. Diagnosis

▶ Moderate neutropenia (500–1,000/microliter µL of blood)

▶ Severe neutropenia (<500/µL)
  - When values drop below 500/µL, even normal microbial flora in the mouth can cause infection.

D. Dental Treatment Considerations

▶ Thorough review of the medical history is essential.

▶ Consultation with the primary care provider is necessary to determine if neutrophil count is at a safe level.

▶ Antibiotic prophylaxis may be needed.

II. Lymphocytopenia[17]

Abnormally low number of lymphocytes in the blood.

A. Etiology

▶ *Acquired lymphocytopenia* may be caused by protein–energy malnutrition, AIDS, chemotherapy, radiation therapy, or infectious disease such as hepatitis, influenza, and tuberculosis.

▶ *Hereditary lymphocytopenia* may be associated with inherited immunodeficiency disorders.

B. Signs and Symptoms

▶ Pallor

▶ Bruising (petechiae)

▶ Mouth ulcers

C. Dental Treatment Considerations

▶ The same as for neutropenia

III. Leukocytosis

Leukocytosis is an increase in the number of circulating white blood cells.

▶ Caused by inflammatory and infectious states, trauma, exertion, and other conditions listed in Table 68-2.

▶ The most extreme cause of leukocytosis is *leukemia*.[18]
  - Leukemias are malignant neoplasms of immature white blood cells that multiply uncontrollably.
  - Cancer cells are located within the circulating blood and in bone marrow; infiltrated into other body tissues and organs such as the spleen and lymph nodes.
  - Leukemias can be *acute* such as acute lymphocytic leukemia or *chronic* such as chronic lymphocytic leukemia.
  - Oral manifestations may include bruising and bleeding of the gingiva.

PLATELET DISORDERS[19]

Platelets function in the clotting system and disorders include abnormal increases or decreases in platelets or platelet dysfunction.

▶ When the number of platelets decreases, the risk for bleeding increases.
  - Risk of bleeding increases when platelet count is below 50,000/µL.

I. Thrombocytopenia

▶ A lower number of platelets may be caused by decreased production in the bone marrow.

▶ Bone marrow depression may be due to drugs, such as hydrochlorothiazide (used to treat high blood pressure), and acetaminophen, infections like HIV and hepatitis, or blood transfusions.

▶ If severe, a platelet transfusion may be necessary.

II. Platelet Dysfunction

▶ *Acquired platelet dysfunction*
  • Causes of acquired platelet dysfunction include cirrhosis, systemic lupus erythematosus, and certain drugs.

▶ *Hereditary platelet dysfunction*
  • Dysfunction may occur because of a disease such as von Willebrand's disease (a coagulation disorder).

BLEEDING OR COAGULATION DISORDERS

▶ Blood clotting or hemostasis is the body's mechanism for stopping injured blood vessels from forming clots, which can cause serious health problems.

▶ The three main processes of blood clotting include constriction of bleeding vessels, activity of platelets, and activity of blood clotting factors.

▶ A history or suspicion of a bleeding problem requires careful evaluation before treatment can be started.

▶ Spontaneous bleeding occurs as small hemorrhages into the skin or mucous membranes and other tissues, and appears as petechiae or purpura.

▶ Bleeding disorders have in common the tendencies to spontaneous bleeding and moderate to excessive bleeding following trauma, surgical procedure, or dental hygiene therapy, including nonsurgical instrumentation.

I. Oral Findings Suggestive of Bleeding Disorders

▶ Early signs of systemic conditions frequently appear in the oral soft tissues and clinical examination may identify these changes.

▶ Referral for medical examination may lead to diagnosis and treatment of a serious disease.

▶ In addition, the findings of a laboratory blood examination may provide essential information for safe and effective dental hygiene care.

▶ Oral soft tissue changes in patients with blood diseases are not necessarily exclusive to systemic blood disorders.

▶ It is necessary to recognize change in a previously healthy patient, or an apparently exaggerated response in a patient being examined at an initial appointment.

▶ Findings suggesting a blood disorder include the following:
  • Gingival bleeding, spontaneously or excessive bleeding on gentle probing.

  • History of difficulty in controlling bleeding by usual procedures.
  • History of bruising easily, with large ecchymoses.
  • Numerous petechiae.
  • Marked pallor of the mucous membranes.
  • Atrophy of the papillae of the tongue.
  • Persistent sore or painful tongue (glossodynia).
  • Acute or chronic infections, such as candidiasis, that do not respond to usual treatment.
  • Severe ulcerations associated with a lack of response to treatment.
  • Exaggerated gingival response to local irritants, sometimes with characteristics of necrotizing ulcerative gingivitis (ulceration, necrosis, bleeding, pseudomembrane).

II. Types of Disorders of Coagulation[20]

Vascular fragility is increased; petechial and purpuric hemorrhages appear in the skin or mucous membranes, including the gingiva.

A. Acquired Disorders

▶ Vitamin K deficiency
  • Vitamin K is essential in the synthesis of prothrombin and clotting factors VII, IX, and X.
  • Food sources of vitamin K may be found in Table 35-3. Vitamin K is also produced in the alimentary track by intestinal bacteria.
  • Excessive exposure to antibiotic therapy or prolonged gastrointestinal disturbances may affect vitamin K production.

▶ Liver disease: Nearly all the clotting factors are produced in the liver. When the liver is not functioning properly, the clotting factors may be altered.
  • May occur in cirrhosis.

▶ Anticoagulation drugs: Following are the examples of some common medications
  • Heparin
  • Coumadin (warfarin)
  • Aspirin and nonsteroidal anti-inflammatory drugs (NSAIDS).

B. Hereditary Disorders

At least 30 hereditary coagulation disorders exist, each resulting from a deficiency or abnormality of a plasma protein.

▶ *Hemophilia*

Hemophilias are the oldest known hereditary bleeding disorders caused by low levels or complete absence of a blood protein essential for clotting.
  • *Etiology*
    • Results from mutation or deletion affecting factor VIII or IX in the gene.

- Hemophilia is an X-linked recessive genetic disease. The defective gene is located on the X chromosome; thus, the disorder occurs primarily in males.
- *Treatment*
  - Most patients do well with proper medical management involving the administration of drugs to decrease bleeding or the infusion of platelets or plasma containing factors.
- *Effects and long-term complications*
  - Bleeding and bruising from minor trauma vary depending on the severity of the disease.
  - Bleeding into the soft tissue of joints (hemarthroses) of knees, ankles, and elbows begins in the very young with severe hemophilia.
  - Hemorrhage into the muscles (intramuscular hemorrhage) is accompanied by pain and limitation of motion.
  - Bleeding from the gingiva is common and more extensive when periodontal infection is more severe.
- *Management of uncontrolled bleeding*
  - When uncontrolled bleeding is observed, stop dental treatment.
  - If clotting does not occur within a few minutes, apply digital pressure to area with sterile gauze.
  - If needed, local hemostatic agents can be applied, such as absorbable gelatin sponge. Absorbs for 3–5 days.
  - Medical attention required if unsuccessful in stopping bleeding.

DENTAL HYGIENE CARE PLAN

- ▶ Although prevention and control of bleeding are the main issues when treating a patient with a blood clotting defect, other factors require attention.
- ▶ Patients with bleeding disorders have many emotional stresses related to the disease, its treatment, and medical expenses.
- ▶ As a result of internal and cerebral hemorrhages, a few patients may have a multitude of physical or cognitive disabilities.
- ▶ Because of the fear of bleeding, patients may neglect toothbrushing and flossing; doing so can lead to increased dental biofilm accumulation and inflammation.
- ▶ Suggestions for appointments from Chapter 57 may be useful for the patient with disability related to hemarthroses and orthopedic treatment.

I. Preparation for Clinical Appointment

- ▶ Certain blood tests may be needed on the same day as treatment.
  - For example, the patient taking coagulants is required to have a PT (prothrombin time) within 24 hours of

an appointment or report their most recent INR level to the oral health provider.
- ▶ Basic tests are listed in Table 68-1 with their ranges or values.
- ▶ Indications for screening and preappointment tests:
  - When the patient gives a history of a bleeding problem.
  - Clinical examination reveals signs of a bleeding disorder.
  - Patient is being treated with anticoagulation therapy.

II. Patient History

A. Medical History Review

The medical history needs to include information regarding the type, severity, medical treatment, medications, and family history of the blood clotting defect.
- ▶ Question patient specifically regarding bleeding after clinical and surgical procedures, such as tooth extractions.

B. Medication Review

A careful review of a patient's drug, supplements, and herb use is critical to determine potential oral and physiologic effects.
- ▶ The primary purpose of the drug and potential side effects needs careful review in a current drug reference guide.
- ▶ A variety of drugs and herbs may be factors in increased bleeding.
  - Herbs and supplements associated with increased bleeding are listed in Box 68-2.
  - It is recommended to discontinue these herbs and supplements 2 weeks prior to receiving invasive surgical procedures.[21]

BOX 68-2

Herbs and Supplements Associated With Increased Bleeding

Alfalfa	Cat's claw	Garlic
Allspice	Chamomile	Ginkgo
Angelica	Chondroitin	Ginger
Anise	Coenzyme Q10	Ginseng
Bilberry	Cranberry	Glucosamine
Blackhawk	Dong quai	Guggul
Bogbean	Evening primrose	Horse chestnut
Boldo	Fenugreek	Poplar
Bucho	Feverfew	Omega 3
Capsicum	Flax	Vitamin E
	Fish oil	White willow

Adapted from Alberto PL. Alternative medicine for the dental professional. 2009;23(1):20–24.

- Patients taking either Coumadin (for prevention of recurrent thrombosis), heparin (for short-term use following a total joint replacement procedure), or medication for long-term anticoagulation (such as aspirin) may need special consultation.
  - The most common side effect of both warfarin and heparin is hemorrhage.
  - Hemorrhages may present as gingival bleeding or submucosal bleeding with hematoma formation.
- Cancer chemotherapeutic agents may secondarily induce profound thrombocytopenia ($<20,000$ mm^3) or neutropenia (<500 mm^3).
- Antithrombotic agents such as aspirin and clopidogrel alter the ability of platelets to stick or clump together and form a clot.

C. Dental History Review

Discuss previous dental care and perceived treatment needs when developing the current care plan with the patient.

D. Risk Assessment

The patient with a bleeding disorder may be at high risk for dental caries and periodontal disease and the appropriate strategies to manage the risk are employed.

III. Consultation with Physician/ Hematologist

- Consultation with the primary care provider/hematologist is necessary to obtain complete and accurate information.
- The risk for intravascular clot formation is greater than the risk for hemorrhage.
- A joint policy advising healthcare providers who perform invasive or surgical procedures to contact the cardiologist and discuss patient management before discontinuing antiplatelet drugs has been developed by:[22]
  - The American Dental Association
  - The American Heart Association
  - The American College of Cardiology
  - The Society for Cardiovascular Angiography and Interventions
  - The American College of Surgeons.
- Consult primary care provider/hematologist to determine whether premedication is required during dental procedures to prevent infection in joint prostheses and/or indwelling catheter.[22]
- Many procedures require factor replacement therapy just prior to the dental appointment.[23]
- Request reports of current blood tests.

IV. Treatment

- Prevention of gingival infection and dental caries is an essential aspect of care for patients with a bleeding disorder.

- Preliminary tissue conditioning can help prevent severe bleeding during instrumentation. Teach daily personal biofilm removal at the initial appointment and reinforce at each session.
- Use a preprocedural chlorhexidine mouthrinse to reduce the bacterial load prior to beginning examination or treatment.
- Radiographic imaging: Films/sensor (infection control barriers) can cut and press on the mucous membranes. Care in placement is exercised to avoid bleeding and/or a hematoma.
- Encourage each patient to improve and maintain good oral health. Spontaneous oral bleeding problems can be partially controlled by the elimination of oral infections.[23]
  - Meticulous dental biofilm removal is practiced and repeated. A soft toothbrush is indicated. If patient indicates using a power brush, proper demonstration of technique is necessary.
  - Teach flossing carefully and correctly to prevent cutting the gingiva and inducing proximal bleeding.
  - Patients with limited manual dexterity can benefit from adaptive oral hygiene aids described in Chapter 57.
- Select age-appropriate preventive measures based on risk assessment including fluoride treatments, remineralizing agents, sealants, biofilm control, and professional dental supervision.
- A nutritional assessment and counseling is recommended for caries control and periodontal health to stress choosing foods that provide a healthy, well-balanced diet.
- Plan non-surgical periodontal therapy in sextants or quadrants.
- Local anesthesia administration: infiltration and intra-papillary injections do not require administration of clotting factors to prevent bleeding, but blocks like the inferior alveolar injection require clotting factor.[23]
- Postoperative: Monitor to ensure bleeding has stopped postoperatively.
  - Never recommend aspirin or NSAIDS for a patient with a bleeding disorder.
  - Bleeding tendency is greatly increased by a drug-induced platelet dysfunction caused by aspirin.
  - Ask the patient to call if bleeding occurs within first 24–48 hours and does not stop after applying pressure.[23]
- Impressions: Beading the rims of the trays protects the mucosa from pressure and damage from a hard, possibly rough surface, as described in Chapter 14.
- Evacuation: High-vacuum suction tips may be sharp. Caution in the use of suction is necessary to prevent pulling the sublingual or other mucosal tissues into the suction tip and causing hematomas.
- Stress reduction protocol: Prevention or reduction of stress begins before the appointment, is continued

throughout the treatment, and followed through into the postoperative period, when necessary.

▶ Frequency of continuing care: Frequent appointments can aid in keeping the oral tissues in an optimum state of health and help to prevent the need for complex or lengthy dental appointments.

DOCUMENTATION

Documentation in the permanent record for each appointment with a blood disorder includes a minimum of the following factors:

▶ Review or update medical history thoroughly. Document laboratory findings.

▶ Document extra- and intraoral examinations findings. Use written description and an intraoral picture when possible.

▶ Note treatment planning considerations such as shorter appointments, stress reduction protocols that need to be implemented, and oral hygiene considerations.

▶ Note consultations with other health professionals involved in the patient's care.

▶ Reference any difficulties with bleeding control during appointment.

▶ A sample progress notes is provided in Box 68-3.

BOX 68-3

Example Documentation: Patient with a Blood Disorder

S –A 70-year-old, white man presents for a new patient exam. He reports having a stroke a year ago and currently taking Coumadin (warfarin). Patient states that his INR last week was 2.8.

O –Oral cancer examination: all tissues appear normal. Full-mouth series of radiographs and caries examination reveal no new caries. Periodontal Examination: generalized 4–5 mm pocket depths with localized bleeding on probing. Plaque score: 50%.

A –Increased risk for oral bleeding following dental hygiene treatment.

P –Disclosed plaque biofilm and reviewed technique for oral hygiene aids. Stressed need for meticulous oral self-care to prevent infection and associated bleeding. Nonsurgical periodontal therapy completed maxillary and mandibular right quadrants with 2 carpules 2% xylocaine with 1:100,000 epinephrine for an inferior IA, LB, PSA, and palatal injections. Areas monitored to verify bleeding had stopped within 5 minutes following completion of instrumentation. Postoperation instructions provided to contact the office should he be unable to stop bleeding.

Next appointment: Complete NSPT with local anesthesia and apply fluoride varnish.

Signed: _____, RDH

Date: _____

EVERYDAY ETHICS

Just as Dena, the dental hygienist, begins to probe for recording the gingival examination for Mr. Bennett, a new patient in the practice, the receptionist interrupts to give Dena a medical clearance form that has been faxed from the patient's physician. As Dena reviews the information, she understands that the patient has a blood disorder but is unclear as to its extent from the laboratory values in the report. She briefly questions Mr. Bennett about any medical tests and he indicates that he was in the hospital 4 days the previous month.

As Dena continues the probing, she notices considerable bleeding with oozing around the gingival margins.

Questions for Consideration

1. What action, if any, does Dena need to take to ensure she is performing beneficently on behalf of this patient?

2. It appears that Mr. Bennett has not given sufficient information about his medical condition prior to this continuing care appointment. What obligation does a patient have to update the medical history at each appointment? And what obligation does the professional person have to help the patient understand this obligation?

3. While Dena quietly acknowledges to herself that she used to know the information about bleeding conditions, she is currently uncertain of the meaning of the laboratory values in this patient's report. Ethically, how can this realization be assessed? What is the immediate need? What can be done to prevent such a situation from occurring in the future?

Factors To Teach The Patient

▷ Meticulous oral hygiene techniques to practice daily: toothbrushing, flossing, and other appropriate oral hygiene aids.

▷ How to self-evaluate the oral cavity for deviations from normal. Watching for changes in size, shape, color, and contacting oral health professional when lesions last longer than 2 weeks.

▷ Selection of noncariogenic foods to prevent caries, and knowledge about the diet's relationship to health.

▷ Avoid use of salicylates (aspirin).

▷ Importance of informing the dental hygienist of any changes to the medical history, including drugs, herbs, supplements, and hospitalizations and providing recent laboratory values before beginning treatment.

References

1. Mesher AL. Blood. In: Mescher AL, ed. *Junqueira's Basic Histology: Text & Atlas*. 13 ed. New York, NY: McGraw-Hill; 2013.

2. Introduction to anemia and red cell disorders. In: Bunn H, Aster JC, eds. *Pathophysiology of Blood Disorders*. New York, NY: McGraw-Hill; 2011. http://accessmedicine.mhmedical.com/content.aspx?bookid=676&Sectionid=44827768. Accessed April 25, 2014.

3. Damon LE, Andreadis C. Blood disorders. In: Papadakis MA, McPhee SJ, Rabow MW, eds. *CURRENT Medical Diagnosis & Treatment 2014*. New York, NY: McGraw-Hill; 2014:chap 13.

4. Muncie HL Jr, Campbell J. Alpha and beta thalassemia. *Am Fam Physician*. 2009 15;80(4):339–344.

5. Goddard AF, James MW, McIntyre AS, et al. Guidelines for the management of iron deficiency anaemia. *Gut*. 2011;60(10):1309–1316.

6. Office of Dietary Supplements. *Iron: Dietary Supplement Fact Sheet*. National Institutes of Health. http://ods.od.nih.gov/factsheets/Iron-HealthProfessional/. Accessed January 19, 2014.

7. Andres E, Serraj K. Optimal management of pernicious anemia. *J Blood Med*. 2012;3:97–103.

8. Office of Dietary Supplements. *Vitamin B₁₂: Dietary Supplement Fact Sheet*. National Institutes of Health. http://ods.od.nih.gov/factsheets/VitaminB12-HealthProfessional/. Accessed January 19, 2014.

9. Medical Services Commission. *Cobalamin (vitamin B12) Deficiency—Investigation and Management*. Victoria, BC: British Columbia Medical Services Commission; 2012. http://www.guideline.gov/content.aspx?id=38881. Accessed January 19, 2014.

10. Office of Dietary Supplements. *Folate: Dietary Supplement Fact Sheet*. National Institutes of Health. http://ods.od.nih.gov/factsheets/Folate-HealthProfessional/. Accessed January 19, 2014.

11. Bunn H. Sickle cell disease. In: Bunn H, Aster JC, eds. *Pathophysiology of Blood Disorders*. New York, NY: McGraw-Hill; 2011:chap 9.

12. Sheth S, Licursi M, Bhatia M. Sickle cell disease: time for a closer look at treatment options? *Br J Haematol*. 2013;162(4):455–464.

13. Adeyemo TA, Adeyemo WL, Adediran A, et al. Orofacial manifestations of hematological disorders: anemia and hemostatic disorders. *Indian J Dent Res*. 2011;22: 454–461.

14. Squizzato A, Romualdi E, Passamonti F, et al. Antiplatelet drugs for polycythaemia vera and essential thrombocythaemia. *Cochrane Database Syst Rev* 2013;(4):CD006503.

15. College of Dental Hygienists of Ontario, CDHO Advisory Polycythemia. 2012. http://www.cdho.org/Advisories/CDHO Advisory Polycythemia.pdf. Accessed January 20, 2014.

16. National Cancer Institute. *PDQ⁻ Chronic Myeloproliferative Disorders Treatment*. Bethesda, MD: National Cancer Institute. http://cancer.gov/cancertopics/pdq/treatment/myeloproliferative/HealthProfessional. Accessed January 20, 2014.

17. Territo M. Overview of white blood cell disorders. *The Merck Manual—Professional Edition*. http://www.merckmanuals.com/home/blood-disorders/white-blood-cell-disorders/overview-of-white-blood-cell-disorders. Accessed June 29, 2015.

18. Rytting ME. Chronic myelogenous leukemia. *The Merck Manual—Professional Edition*. http://www.merckmanuals.com/professional/hematology-and-oncology/leukemias/chronic-myelogenous-leukemia-cml. Accessed June 29, 2015.

19. Kuter DJ. Overview of platelet disorders. *The Merck Manual—Professional Edition*. http://www.merckmanuals.com/professional/hematology and oncology/thrombocytopenia and platelet dysfunction/overview of platelet disorders.html. Accessed January 20, 2014.

20. Moake JL. Hemophilia. *The Merck Manual—Professional Edition*. http://www.merckmanuals.com/professional/hematology and oncology/coagulation disorders/hemophilia.html. Accessed January 25, 2014.

21. Andrews L, Spolarich AE. An examination of the bleeding complications associated with herbal supplements, antiplatelet and anticoagulant medications. *J Dent Educ*. 2007;81(3):2–14.

22. American Academy of Orthopaedic Surgeons, American Dental Association. *Prevention of Orthopaedic Implant Infection in Patients Undergoing Dental Procedures: Evidence-Based Guideline and Evidence Report*. Rosemont, IL: American Academy of Orthopaedic Surgeons; 2012. http://www.aaos.org/Research/guidelines/PUDP/PUDP guideline.pdf. Accessed January 25, 2014.

23. Dental Committee, Word Federation of Hemophilia. *Guidelines for Dental Treatment of Patients with Inherited Bleeding Disorders*. 2006. http://www1.wfh.org/publication/files/pdf-1190.pdf. Accessed January 25, 2014.

ENHANCE YOUR UNDERSTANDING

thePoint° DIGITAL CONNECTIONS
(see the inside front cover for access information)
- Audio glossary
- Quiz bank

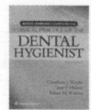

SUPPORT FOR LEARNING
(available separately; visit lww.com)
- *Active Learning Workbook for Clinical Practice of the Dental Hygienist, 12th Edition*

prepU INDIVIDUALIZED REVIEW
(available separately; visit lww.com)
- Adaptive quizzing with *prepU for Wilkins' Clinical Practice of the Dental Hygienist*

69

The Patient with Diabetes Mellitus

Linda D. Boyd, RDH, RD, EdD and Kathryn R. Davis, RDH, MS, DMD

CHAPTER OUTLINE

LEARNING OBJECTIVES

After studying this chapter, the student will be able to:

1. Describe the types of diabetes mellitus and major characteristics of each.

2. Explain current knowledge about the oral health–diabetes connection.

3. Describe risk factors and criteria used for diagnosis of diabetes.

4. Summarize lifestyle modifications and medications used to prevent and manage diabetes.

5. Identify key messages dental hygienist need to convey to patients with diabetes.

Dental professionals have a significant responsibility to:

▸ Recognize signs and symptoms of diabetes to promote early diagnosis, significantly reduce life-threatening complications of the disease, and improve quality of life.

▸ Assess the management and control of diabetes to determine the impact on treatment and oral health of the patient.

▸ Work with the patient and other healthcare professionals to provide preventive oral care aimed at

maintaining health and preventing infections and emergencies.

▸ Understand the presence of infection, including periodontitis, may make it more difficult to control the blood glucose levels in diabetes.

▸ Identify and treat acute emergencies.

Key words and abbreviations used in this chapter are found in Boxes 69-1 and 69-2, respectively.

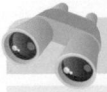

BOX 69-1 KEY WORDS: Diabetes Mellitus

Beta cells: insulin-producing cells of the islets of Langerhans in the pancreas.

Brittle diabetes: term formerly used to describe very unstable type 1 diabetes; characterized by unexplained oscillation between hypoglycemia and diabetic ketoacidosis (DKA).

Casual plasma glucose: blood glucose level at any time of day with no regard to time of eating.

Charcot's joints: a joint that is deprived of any pain or position sense due to severe osteoarthritis or as a result of disease such as diabetic neuropathy.

Exocrine: secreting externally via a duct.

Exogenous insulin: insulin from source outside patient.

Gastroparesis: delayed gastric emptying. Occurs when the vagus nerve is damaged or stops functioning normally and movement of food is slowed or stopped.

Gestational diabetes: diabetes that occurs during pregnancy.

Gluconeogenesis: synthesis of glucose from noncarbohydrate sources, such as amino acids and glycerol; can occur in the liver and kidneys when the carbohydrate intake is insufficient to meet the body's needs.

Glycated or glycosylated hemoglobin (HbA1c): the primary assay for assessing long-term glycemic control. Indicates blood glucose levels for the previous 2–3 months.

Glycemia: presence of glucose in blood.

Hyperglycemia: high blood glucose; opposite of hypoglycemia.

Hyperpnea: abnormal increase in depth and rate of respiration.

Hypogeusia: abnormally diminished acuteness of the sense of taste.

Hypoglycemia: an abnormally low level of glucose in the blood.

Insulin: a powerful hormone secreted by the beta cells in the islets of Langerhans of the pancreas; the major

fuel-regulating hormone; enters the blood in response to a rise in concentration of blood glucose and is transported immediately to bind with cell surface receptors throughout the body.

Ketoacidosis: diabetic coma; too little insulin; accumulation of ketone bodies in the blood. Occurs primarily in type 1 diabetes mellitus.

Ketone bodies: normal metabolic products of lipid (fat) within the liver; excess production leads to urinary excretion of these acidic chemicals.

Ketonuria: excess concentration of ketone bodies in the urine.

Oral glucose tolerance test: a test of the body's ability to utilize carbohydrates; aid to the diagnosis of diabetes mellitus. After ingestion of a specific amount of glucose solution, the fasting blood glucose rises promptly in a nondiabetic person, then falls to normal within an hour. In diabetes mellitus, the blood glucose rise is greater and the return to normal is prolonged.

Oral hypoglycemic agent: synthetic drug that lowers the blood sugar level; stimulates the synthesis and release of insulin from the beta cells of the islets of Langerhans in the pancreas; used to treat patients with type 2 diabetes mellitus.

Polydipsia: excessive thirst.

Polyphagia: excessive ingestion of food.

Polyuria: excessive excretion of urine.

Postprandial: after a meal.

Prediabetes: IFG (impaired fasting glucose) and IGT (impaired glucose tolerance) are risk factors for future diabetes and cardiovascular disease.

Pruritus: itching.

Retinopathy: noninflammatory degenerative disease of the retina; called diabetic retinopathy when it occurs with diabetes of long standing.

BOX 69-2

Key of Abbreviations: Diabetes Mellitus

A1c (A One C): common abbreviation for glycosylated hemoglobin (HbA1c)
DKA: Diabetes ketoacidosis
EMS: emergency medical service
FPG: fasting plasma glucose
GDM: gestational diabetes mellitus
HbA1c: glycosylated hemoglobin
HDL: high-density lipoprotein
IDDM: insulin-dependent diabetes mellitus
IFG: impaired fasting glucose
IGT: impaired glucose tolerance
LDL: low-density lipoprotein
NIDDM: noninsulin-dependent diabetes mellitus
OGTT: oral glucose tolerance test
PCOS: polycystic ovarian syndrome
PP: postprandial
SMBG: self-monitoring of blood glucose
WHO: World Health Organization

BOX 69-3

Symptoms of Low and High Blood Glucose

Hypoglycemia
▷ Mental confusion
▷ Sweating
▷ Irritability
▷ Palpitations
▷ Shakiness
▷ Pallor
▷ Headache
▷ Seizure
▷ Coma and death (if untreated)

Hyperglycemia
▷ Polyuria
▷ Polydipsia
▷ Weight loss
▷ Polyphagia
▷ Blurred vision
▷ Increased susceptibility to infections
▷ Impaired growth
▷ Ketoacidosis

DIABETES MELLITUS

I. Definition[1]

▶ Diabetes mellitus is a group of metabolic diseases associated with hyperglycemia (high blood glucose). Symptoms of hypo- and hyperglycemia are listed in Box 69-3.

▶ Hyperglycemia results from an insulin deficiency, resistance to insulin action, or both.

▶ People with poorly controlled diabetes mellitus are at risk of complications including:
 • Blindness
 • Kidney failure
 • Heart disease
 • Stroke
 • Amputation of toes, feet, and legs.

II. Diabetes Impact[2,3]

▶ In the United States, 29 million people (9.3% of the population) have diabetes. Approximately 8 million or 1 in 4 people with diabetes are undiagnosed.
 • Globally, 347 million adults (9.8% of men and 9.2% of women) have diabetes.[4]
 • In the United States, 86 million people, more than 1 in 3 adults, have prediabetes.

▶ As the population ages and with increases in obesity, diabetes has become more prevalent.

▶ Medical costs and lost work and wages for those with diabetes is 245 billion dollars annually in the United States.

▶ The risk of death is 50% higher for individuals with diabetes compared to those without diabetes.

ORAL HEALTH IMPLICATIONS OF DIABETES MELLITUS

▶ Infection that does not respond to treatment and/or healing may be signs of undiagnosed diabetes.

▶ The patient needs to be referred to a primary care provider for evaluation and diagnosis.

▶ Oral findings associated with diabetes can be found in Table 69-1.

I. Relationship Between Diabetes and Periodontal Disease[4]

▶ The association of diabetes mellitus with periodontal disease is hypothesized to be related to the inflammatory process involved in the pathogenesis of both diseases.

A. Diabetes as a Risk Factor for Periodontitis

▶ Systematic reviews suggest patients with diabetes are at a 2–4 times greater risk for more severe periodontal disease than individuals without diabetes.[4]

B. Effect of Periodontitis on Glycemic Control

▶ Evidence indicates individuals with diabetes had more severe periodontal disease and a higher A1c than healthy individuals.[4]

C. Effect of Periodontal Treatment on Diabetes

▶ Nonsurgical periodontal therapy and management of periodontal disease has resulted in an average decrease in A1c of 0.6%.
 • This is roughly equivalent to decreases seen in physical activity and weight loss intervention studies.

TABLE 69-1	Extraoral/Intraoral Findings Associated with Diabetes
LOCATION	**FINDINGS**
Gingiva	Increased gingival inflammation
Periodontium	Periodontitis: more frequent, severe, longer duration Attachment loss: more frequent, more extensive Probing depths: more teeth with deep pockets Alveolar bone loss: more Tooth mobility and migration: increased Healing: delayed, increased infection after surgery
Teeth	Poorly controlled diabetes: increased risk of caries related to decreased saliva, diet, and less successful resolution of endodontic therapy related to decreased resistance to infection Well-controlled diabetes: decreased caries related to low sugar, regular eating habits, dental maintenance appointments
Saliva	Glucose in sulcular fluid Xerostomia: contributes to opportunistic infection such as oral candidiasis
Mucosa	Edematous and red color Oral candidiasis Burning mouth and/or tongue, burning mouth syndrome Poor tolerance for removable prostheses Delayed healing May have increased prevalence of lichen planus and aphthous stomatitis
Taste	Hypogeusia, diminished taste perception
Neck	Acanthosis negricans is a skin condition that has a light brown to black appearance in the creases on the neck and in other areas.

- Management of periodontitis along with lifestyle changes may have an additive effect on lowering A1c.

II. Dental Caries[5]

▶ There is inadequate evidence for a direct relationship between diabetes and risk for coronal or root caries, but there is a reduction in salivary flow which puts the patient at risk for dental caries.

III. Endodontic Infections[6]

▶ Patients with diabetes have increased periodontal disease in teeth involved endodontically and have a

reduced likelihood of success of endodontic treatment in cases with preoperative periradicular lesions.

IV. Dental Implants[7]

▶ A meta-analysis found the failure rate for dental implants was similar between individuals with and without diabetes.
- Well-controlled diabetes is not a contraindication to placement of a dental implant.

BASICS ABOUT INSULIN

I. Definition

▶ Insulin is a hormone produced by the beta cells in the pancreas.
▶ Insulin directly or indirectly affects every organ in the body.

II. Description

▶ The beta cells of the pancreas are responsible for releasing insulin when stimulated by nutrients, primarily glucose.[8]
▶ Insulin acts like a key to unlock the cell to allow uptake of glucose to use as energy.
▶ Figure 69-1A shows the healthy pancreas and the action of insulin as it is taken up by the body cells.

III. Functions

The functions of insulin are listed in Box 69-4. Without insulin, glucose accumulates in the blood, resulting in hyperglycemia.

▶ Normal blood glucose levels in healthy individuals range from 60 to 100 mg/dL and the hemoglobin A1c is less than 5.7%.[1]

IV. Effects of Absolute Insulin Deficiency (Type 1 Diabetes)[9]

Glucose increases in the circulating blood (hyperglycemia) until a threshold is reached and glucose spills over into the urine (glycosuria).

▶ Increased glycosuria induces osmotic diuresis with excretion of large amounts of urine (polyuria). Water and electrolytes are lost.
▶ Fluid loss signals excessive thirst to the brain (polydipsia).
▶ Cells starving for glucose may cause the patient to increase food intake (polyphagia), but weight loss may still occur.
▶ Without glucose to use for energy, the body metabolizes fat for energy.

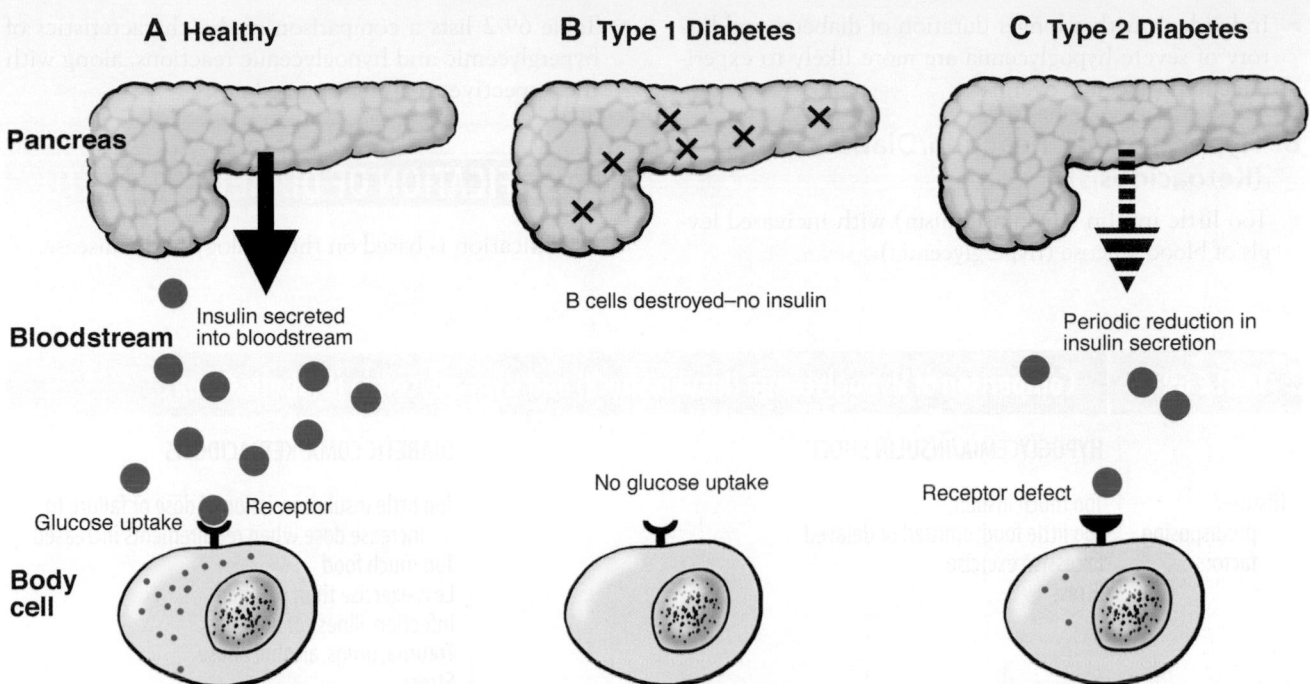

FIGURE 69-1 Pancreas and Action of Insulin on Body Cell in Health, and type 1 and 2 Diabetes. A: Healthy pancreas excretes insulin into bloodstream that enables glucose uptake by body cell. **B:** Type 1 diabetes shows no insulin produced by pancreas and no glucose uptake by cell. **C:** Type 2 diabetes shows normal, increased, or decreased insulin production by pancreas and the defective receptor on cell that hampers insulin uptake.

- End products of fat metabolism are harmful ketones that accumulate in the blood.
- Ketones are acidic, and when they accumulate, they are usually neutralized in the blood.
- When large quantities of ketones are present the neutralizing effect of the blood is depleted rapidly and an acidic condition (metabolic acidosis) results.
- Metabolic acidosis leads to diabetic coma (ketoacidosis) if not treated promptly.

▶ Figure 69-1B shows changes in pancreas function that occur in type 1 diabetes.

> **BOX 69-4**
>
> **Functions of Insulin**
>
> 1. Facilitates glucose uptake from blood into tissues, which lowers blood glucose level.
> 2. Speeds the oxidation of glucose within the cells to use for energy.
> 3. Speeds the conversion of glucose to glycogen to store in the liver and skeletal muscles and to prevent the conversion of glycogen back to glucose.
> 4. Facilitates conversion of glucose to fat in adipose tissue.

V. Effects of Impaired Secretion or Action of Insulin (Type 2 Diabetes)

▶ Deficient insulin action results from inadequate insulin secretion and/or diminished tissue responses to insulin.[1]

- Cell surface insulin receptors develop defects, and glucose cannot be transmitted into the cell.
- Blood glucose level increases as the insulin resistance of the cells increases. This stimulates more insulin to be released.

▶ Over time, insulin secretion may also decline and lead to both decrease of insulin in the blood as well as increased insulin resistance of cells.

▶ Figure 69-1C shows the effects of decreased insulin and action of insulin that can occur in type 2 diabetes. Note the defective receptor on the body cell.

VI. Insulin Complications

▶ Earlier diagnosis, improved treatment, and better informed patient, family, and friends have reduced the occurrence of emergency insulin complications.

▶ Constant verbal and visual contact is maintained with a patient to identify early behavioral and physical changes indicative of a developing crisis.

A. Hypoglycemia/Insulin Shock

▶ Too much insulin (hyperinsulinism), which lowers level of blood glucose (hypoglycemia).

▶ Hypoglycemia is the emergency more likely to occur in the dental setting. See Box 69-3 and Table 69-2 for symptoms of hypoglycemia.

► Individuals with a longer duration of diabetes and history of severe hypoglycemia are more likely to experience hypoglycemic events.[9]

B. Hyperglycemic Reaction/Diabetic Coma (Ketoacidosis)

► Too little insulin (hypoinsulinism) with increased levels of blood glucose (hyperglycemia).

► Table 69-2 lists a comparison of the characteristics of hyperglycemic and hypoglycemic reactions, along with the respective treatment procedures.

CLASSIFICATION OF DIABETES MELLITUS

► Classification is based on the etiology of the disease.

TABLE 69-2	Comparison of Hypoglycemia (Insulin Shock) and Hyperglycemia (Diabetic Coma)	
	HYPOGLYCEMIA/INSULIN SHOCK	**DIABETIC COMA/KETOACIDOSIS**
History/ predisposing factors	Too much insulin Too little food: omitted or delayed Excessive exercise Stress	Too little insulin: omission of dose or failure to increase dose when requirements increased Too much food Less exercise than planned Infection, illness of any sort Trauma, drugs, alcohol abuse Stress
Occurrence	More common complication than ketoacidosis, especially with less stable type 1 diabetes	Type I diabetes especially if poorly controlled, unstable
Onset	Sudden	Develops slowly over hours/days
Behavioral changes	Confusion, stupor Drowsy, restless Anxious, irritable, agitated Incoordination, weakness	Any hypoglycemia behavioral change
Physical findings	Skin: moist, sweaty, perspiration Hunger Headache Tremor, shakiness, weakness Pallor Dilated pupils, blurry vision Dizziness, staggering gait	Skin: flushed, dry Abdominal pain Nausea, vomiting Lack of appetite Dry mouth, thirst Fruity smelling breath Increased urination
Vital signs	Temperature: Normal or below Respiration: Normal Pulse: Fast, irregular Blood Pressure: Normal or slightly elevated	Temperature: Elevated when infection Respiration: Hyperpnea, rapid, and labored with acetone or fruity smelling breath Pulse: Rapid, weak Blood Pressure: Lowered, person may go into shock
If left untreated	Possible convulsions, eventual coma and death	Eventual coma and death
Treatment	Glucose gel (15–20 g) is the preferred treatment for the conscious individual with hypoglycemia After 15 min of treatment, if SMBG shows continued hypoglycemia, the treatment should be repeated. Once SMBG returns to normal, the individual should consume a meal or snack to prevent recurrence of hypoglycemia If unconscious/unresponsive: injection of glucagon or intravenous glucose	Immediate professional care Activate EMS, hospitalize Monitor vital signs Keep patient warm Fluids for conscious patient Insulin injection after medical assessment
Prevention	Monitoring and regulation of blood sugar and frequent blood glucose monitoring	Monitoring and regulation of blood sugar and frequent blood glucose monitoring

▶ The type of diabetes is based on the circumstances at the time of diagnosis, such as gestational diabetes during pregnancy.[1]

- Patients often do not fit into a single classification of diabetes so the focus needs to be on the pathogenesis and management of the hyperglycemia.[1]

▶ A comparison of type 1 and 2 diabetes is found in Table 69-3.

I. Type 1 Diabetes Mellitus[1]

A. Description

▶ Figure 69-1B illustrates the changes in type 1 diabetes.

▶ Results from the destruction of insulin-producing beta cells in the pancreas for one of the following reasons:

- Autoantibodies
- No known etiology.

▶ An absolute insulin deficiency requires exogenous insulin to sustain life.

▶ Patients are prone to ketoacidosis.

▶ Typically arises in childhood or adolescence.

▶ Individuals with other autoimmune disorders such as Graves' disease or Hashimoto's thyroiditis are prone to development of type 1 diabetes.

▶ Accounts for 5%–10% of those with diabetes.

TABLE 69-3	Comparison of Type I and Type 2 Diabetes Mellitus	
CHARACTERISTIC	**TYPE 1**	**TYPE 2**
Age of onset	Young, usually before or during puberty, but may appear later	Adult, usually after 30 years, but may occurring with increasing frequency in children and adolescents
Body weight	Normal or thin	Most are obese, body fat particularly in abdominal area
Ethnicity	More common in Caucasians	More common in African Americans, Asian Americans, Hispanics, Native Americans, Pacific Islanders
Hereditary	Yes, but less frequent occurrence than type 2	Much more frequent occurrence in families
Lifestyle	Restrictions very difficult for young patients	More frequent in sedentary individuals with high-fat diets
Onset of symptoms	Rapid, abrupt symptoms of hyperglycemia	Slow, insidious progression over years, frequently goes undiagnosed for years
Symptoms	Weight loss, weakness Polyuria Frequent/recurrent infections Polydipsia slow healing Polyphagia Tingling/numb extremities Blurred vision Fatigue Mimic flu Eye/kidney/cardiovascular problems	Any type 1 symptom
Severity	Severe, life threatening	Early mild but progressively serious
Complications	Acute hypoglycemic/hyperglycemic emergencies and chronic long-term complications common	Acute complications rare, chronic long-term complications common
Ketoacidosis	Common	Rare
Stability	Unstable, difficult and much effort to control	More stable, easier to manage
Insulin	No insulin production, exogenous insulin required	Insulin levels normal, elevated, or low; exogenous insulin needed by some
Prevention	None, due to multiple genetic predispositions and unclear environmental factors	May be possible to prevent or delay with lifestyle changes, increased activity, and weight loss

B. Former Names

Insulin-dependent diabetes mellitus (IDDM), juvenile diabetes, or juvenile-onset diabetes.

II. Type 2 Diabetes Mellitus[1]

A. Description

► Figure 69-1C shows changes that occur in Type 2 diabetes.

► Most prevalent type of diabetes, accounts for 90%–95% of all patients with diabetes.

► Pancreatic insulin secretion may be low, normal, or even higher than normal, but the patient exhibits an insulin resistance that impairs the use of insulin.

  • Insulin resistance is the inability of the peripheral tissues to respond to insulin.

► The risk increases with increased number of risk factors.

► Onset typical occurs in adulthood and the risk increases with age.

► However, incidence has increased dramatically in children and adolescents due to increases in sedentary lifestyle and obesity.[10]

  • In children the typical age at diagnosis is >10 years to late adolescence.

B. Screening[6]

► Type 1 diabetes is usually identified after acute symptoms of hyperglycemia (Box 69-3) prompt evaluation.

► Screening in asymptomatic adults is recommended for prediabetes and type 2 diabetes. Basic criteria for testing in healthcare setting:

  • Age 45 and above, repeated every 3 years or more frequently.

  • Screening begins earlier and more frequently if the patient is overweight or obese (body mass index (BMI) > 25 kg/m[2]) and has other risk factors.

  • When tests are normal, they are repeated at least every 3 years.

C. Former Names

► Noninsulin-dependent diabetes mellitus (NIDDM) or adult-onset diabetes.

III. Gestational Diabetes Mellitus (GDM)[6]

► The prevalence is as high as 9.2% of pregnancies in the United States and as high as 15% worldwide.[11,12]

► Defined as any degree of glucose intolerance first recognized during pregnancy.

► Onset is related to genetics, obesity, and hormones causing insulin resistance.

► Insulin adjustment, carefully supervised prenatal care, and improved obstetric practices have lessened much of the potential danger for the mother.

► Infants are larger; premature births more frequent; high incidence of congenital malformations and perinatal death; and lower rate with improved prenatal care.

► More than 50% of women with GDM go on to develop type 2 diabetes within 5–10 years.[11]

IV. Other Specific Types of Diabetes Mellitus[1]

Other types of diabetes result from genetic defects, diseases, endocrinopathies, surgery, drugs, malnutrition, infections, and injury.

► Genetic defects of the beta cell.

► Genetic defects in insulin action.

► Diseases of the pancreas that injure or destroy beta cells.

  • Include pancreatitis, trauma, pancreatectomy, carcinoma, cystic fibrosis.

► Endocrinopathies such as Cushing's syndrome cause an increase in hormones that antagonize insulin.

  • These hormones include growth hormone, cortisol, and glucagon.

► Drug or chemicals may impair insulin secretion, impair insulin action, or destroy beta cells, and precipitate diabetes.

  • These drugs include: glucocorticoids, thyroid hormone, dilantin, thiazides.

► Certain viruses are associated with destruction of beta cells.

  • These viruses include: congenital rubella, cytomegalovirus, and mumps.

► Uncommon forms of immune-mediated diabetes.

► Other genetic syndromes sometimes associated with diabetes include Down syndrome, Huntington's chorea, Prader–Willi syndrome.

DIAGNOSIS OF DIABETES

I. Diabetes Symptoms

Careful review of the medical history with follow-up questions is used to identify risk factors and symptoms (Table 69-3) of diabetes.

► The classic symptoms of diabetes include the 3 P's:

  • Polyphagia (excessive hunger)
  • Polydipsia (excessive thirst)
  • Polyuria (excessive urination)

II. Diagnostic Tests[1]

Criteria for diagnosis of diabetes include the following:

A. Glycated Hemoglobin Assay (HbA1c or A1c)

► The A1c measures the quantity of the end product of high glucose bound to a hemoglobin molecule (glycated hemoglobin).

▶ A1c value provides an average of blood glucose levels over a 2–3 months period.

▶ The HbA1c test is used to *diagnose* prediabetes and diabetes.
- Prediabetes is diagnosed with an A1c value from 5.7 to 6.4%.
- A1c > 6.5% is used to diagnose diabetes.

▶ The A1c is also used to *monitor* diabetes control.
- Testing is recommended twice per year for individuals with good glycemic control.
- Patients with unstable glycemic control may require testing every 3 months.

▶ A1c goal may vary slightly for an individual based on risk for hypoglycemia, but the goal for most nonpregnant adults is <7%.

B. Fasting Plasma Glucose (FPG)

Measurement taken after fasting at least 8 hours.

▶ FPG of 100 to 125 mg/dL is used to diagnose prediabetes.

▶ FPG > 126 mg/dL is the criterion used for diagnosis of diabetes.

▶ Repeat testing is recommended to confirm a diagnosis.

C. 2-hour Plasma Glucose ≥200 mg/dL

Typically taken during an oral glucose tolerance test (OGTT).

▶ Repeat testing is recommended to confirm a diagnosis.

IDENTIFICATION OF INDIVIDUALS AT RISK FOR DEVELOPMENT OF DIABETES[9]

I. Risk Factors

▶ Adults at risk for diabetes include those who are overweight with a BMI > 25kg/m² and have other risk factors such as:
- Physical inactivity.
- First degree relative with diabetes.
- High risk race/ethnicity such as African American, Hispanic, Native American, Asian, Pacific Islander.
- Women who have delivered a baby weight over 9 pounds or had gestational diabetes during pregnancy.
- Hypertension (>140/90 mm Hg) or taking antihypertensive medications.
- Women with polycystic ovarian syndrome (PCOS).
- History of cardiovascular disease.
- A1c > 5.7%, IGT (impaired glucose tolerance), or IFG (impaired fasting glucose).

▶ Dental visits provide an opportunity to screen patients for undiagnosed diabetes (see Figure 69-2).[13]
- A type 2 diabetes risk test is available on the American Diabetes Association website and could be used chairside in the dental office for screening.

- Screening may also include point-of-care A1c testing using fingersticks or gingival crevicular bleeding.[14–16]

II. Prediabetes

▶ Individuals who have blood glucose levels above normal, but do not meet the criteria for diagnosis of diabetes are considered to have prediabetes.
- Prediabetes means the individual is at high risk for developing diabetes.
- Lifestyle changes such as being physically active, achieving a healthy weight, and making healthy food choices are recommended.
- The most frequent medication used to manage the blood glucose level is metformin.

STANDARDS OF MEDICAL CARE FOR DIABETES MELLITUS[9]

▶ Medical management depends on the severity of the disease and on the individual.
- Consideration is given to individualized needs related to age, activities, vocation, lifestyle, knowledge, attitudes, personality, culture, emotional and psychological needs, as well as the health status and nutritional and weight issues of the patient.

I. Early Diagnosis

▶ Identify individuals with prediabetes and undiagnosed diabetes.

▶ Assess risk factors and refer for evaluation.

II. Management of Prediabetes

▶ The Diabetes Prevention Program demonstrated lifestyle changes including: physical activity, attaining and maintaining a healthy weight, and making wise food choices are effective in preventing or delaying the onset of diabetes.[17]

III. Diabetes Self-management Education

▶ The National Standards for Diabetes Education and Support guidelines indicate diabetes self-management education is essential for those at risk for developing diabetes as well as for those individuals who are newly diagnosed.[18]

▶ Maintain tight glycemic control to reduce the complications of diabetes through regular self-monitoring of blood glucose (SMBG) at home.
- *Glucose meter* (or *glucometer*) is used at home (and in the dental office). A fingerstick is used to obtain a drop of blood for measurement of blood glucose.

ARE YOU AT RISK FOR
TYPE 2 DIABETES?

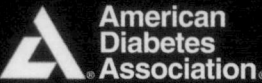 American Diabetes Association®

Diabetes Risk Test

1 How old are you?

Less than 40 years (0 points)

40–49 years (1 point)

50–59 years (2 points)

60 years or older (3 points)

Write your score in the box.

2 Are you a man or a woman?

Man (1 point)   Woman (0 points)

3 If you are a woman, have you ever been diagnosed with gestational diabetes?

Yes (1 point)   No (0 points)

4 Do you have a mother, father, sister, or brother with diabetes?

Yes (1 point)   No (0 points)

5 Have you ever been diagnosed with high blood pressure?

Yes (1 point)   No (0 points)

6 Are you physically active?

Yes (0 points)   No (1 point)

7 What is your weight status?
(see chart at right)

Height	Weight (lbs.)		
4′ 10″	119–142	143–190	191+
4′ 11″	124–147	148–197	198+
5′ 0″	128–152	153–203	204+
5′ 1″	132–157	158–210	211+
5′ 2″	136–163	164–217	218+
5′ 3″	141–168	169–224	225+
5′ 4″	145–173	174–231	232+
5′ 5″	150–179	180–239	240+
5′ 6″	155–185	186–246	247+
5′ 7″	159–190	191–254	255+
5′ 8″	164–196	197–261	262+
5′ 9″	169–202	203–269	270+
5′ 10″	174–208	209–277	278+
5′ 11″	179–214	215–285	286+
6′ 0″	184–220	221–293	294+
6′ 1″	189–226	227–301	302+
6′ 2″	194–232	233–310	311+
6′ 3″	200–239	240–318	319+
6′ 4″	205–245	246–327	328+
	(1 Point)	(2 Points)	(3 Points)

You weigh less than the amount in the left column
(0 points)

If you scored 5 or higher:

Add up your score.

You are at increased risk for having type 2 diabetes. However, only your doctor can tell for sure if you do have type 2 diabetes or prediabetes (a condition that precedes type 2 diabetes in which blood glucose levels are higher than normal). Talk to your doctor to see if additional testing is needed.

Type 2 diabetes is more common in African Americans, Hispanics/Latinos, American Indians, and Asian Americans and Pacific Islanders.

Higher body weights increase diabetes risk for everyone. Asian Americans are at increased diabetes risk at lower body weights than the rest of the general public (about 15 pounds lower).

For more information, visit us at diabetes.org/alert or call 1-800-DIABETES (1-800-342-2383)

Adapted from Bang et al., Ann Intern Med 151:775-783, 2009.
Original algorithm was validated without gestational diabetes as part of the model.

Lower Your Risk

The good news is that you can manage your risk for type 2 diabetes. Small steps make a big difference and can help you live a longer, healthier life.

If you are at high risk, your first step is to see your doctor to see if additional testing is needed.

Visit diabetes.org or call 1-800-DIABETES (1-800-342-2383) for information, tips on getting started, and ideas for simple, small steps you can take to help lower your risk.

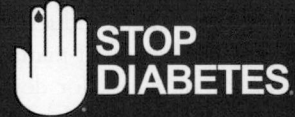 STOP DIABETES.

Special Thanks to our National Sponsor
Walgreens

FIGURE 69-2 Diabetes Risk Test. Are you at risk for type 2 diabetes screening tool. (Source: Copyright 2009 American Diabetes Association. From http://www.diabetes.org. Reprinted by permission of The American Diabetes Association.)

- Frequency and timing is individualized to patient needs, but is often recommended before breakfast, prior to meals, and prior to bedtime.
- More frequent monitoring is associated with better glycemic control and a lower A1c.

▶ Individuals with type 1 diabetes who are prone to diabetic ketoacidosis (DKA) may monitor for urinary ketones with test strips.

- Urinary ketone testing is used during illness, stress, and vigorous physical activity. It can be performed by patient at home or analyzed in a laboratory.

A. Interprofessional Healthcare Team

▶ Initial and ongoing individualized education is provided by the interprofessional team.

- Members include physicians, registered nurses, nurse practitioners, physician assistant, registered dietitian nutritionists, pharmacists, mental health professionals, dental professionals, and other specialists, such as endocrinologist, cardiologist, ophthalmologist, and podiatrist.

B. Educational Resources

▶ *Books and journals*: A number of excellent books, professional journals, and other printed materials have been prepared for the patient and for health professionals.

- Annually the American Diabetes Association publishes evidence-based Clinical Practice Recommendations in the *Diabetes Care* journal. These can be accessed free of charge on www.diabetes.org.

▶ *Internet*: Access to diabetes education and support resources continues to expand rapidly (review strategies to determine validity of information on websites in Chapter 2). In addition to static websites, the internet provides interactive resources that include the following[19]:

- Interactive behavior change programs.
- Peer support through blogs, email, chat rooms, and so on.

▶ *Technology*: Cell phone applications for tracking food intake, physical activity, weight, blood glucose, and blood pressure can be used to assist the individual with self-monitoring and can be shared with the healthcare team.[20]

IV. Medical Nutrition Therapy[9]

▶ Medical nutrition therapy is individualized to meet the needs of the patient to manage and control diabetes.

▶ The American Diabetes Associations recommends nutrition therapy be provided by a registered dietitian/nutritionist or certified diabetes educator.

▶ Goals for medical nutrition therapy include:

- Energy balance for modest weight loss (5–10 pounds) and weight maintenance.

- Carbohydrate intake needs to be balanced throughout the day and focus on vegetables, fruits, whole grains, beans, and low-fat dairy.
- Similar to the Dietary Guidelines for Americans, individuals with diabetes need to limit or avoid added sugar and refined carbohydrates.
- Limit intake of saturated fat, trans fat, and cholesterol.
- Recommendations for sodium intake are the same as for the general population (see section on Dietary Standards in Chapter 35).

V. Physical Activity

▶ Adults are encouraged to engage in 150 minutes per week of moderate-intensity physical activity spread over at least 3 days/week.

▶ Contributes to lowering insulin requirements by increasing the muscle sensitivity to insulin.

VI. Habits

A. Tobacco

▶ Patient must avoid all types of tobacco (see the section on Tobacco Cessation in Chapter 34).

- Tobacco use increases risk of heart disease, stroke, myocardial infarction, limb amputations, periodontal disease, and numerous other health problems.

B. Alcohol

▶ Avoid excessive alcohol; alcohol can raise blood pressure and contribute to other health problems.

PHARMACOLOGICAL THERAPY

I. Insulin Therapy

All patients with type 1 diabetes require exogenous insulin for survival. Type 2 patients may need to use insulin for control. Insulin available in the United States is manufactured in a laboratory.

A. Types of Insulin

Insulin is classified as rapid acting, regular or short acting, intermediate acting, or long acting based on the onset, peak, and duration of action. The types of insulin and range of peak action are found in Table 69-4.

B. Dosage

Depends on the individual.

▶ *Objective*: Attain optimum utilization of glucose throughout each 24 hours.

▶ *Factors affecting the need for insulin*: Food intake, illness, stress, variations in exercise, or infections.

▶ *"Sick Day Rules:"* Insulin dose is adjusted if there are any factors that are affecting the need for insulin.

TABLE 69-4	Types and Action of Insulin		
CLASS OF INSULIN	**TYPE/NAME**	**PEAK ACTION**	**DURATION**
Rapid acting	Lispro (Humalog), Aspart (NovoLog)	1 hr	2–4 hr
Regular or short acting	Humulin R, Novolin R	2–3 hr	3–6 hr
Intermediate acting	NPH (Humulin N, Novolin N)	4–12 hr	12–18 hr
Long acting	Detemir (Levemir), Glargine (Lantus)	24 hr	24 hr
Inhaled	Afrezza	15 min	

C. Methods for Insulin Administration

▶ *Subcutaneous injection with syringe*: A syringe is filled from vial of insulin. Injection sites are rotated usually on abdomen, thighs, or upper arm.

▶ *Insulin pen*: Prefilled cartridge of single type of insulin injected with attached needle. May be disposable or a reusable type.

▶ *Continuous subcutaneous insulin infusion with a battery-operated insulin pump*:

- The insulin pump delivers preprogrammed continuous basal rate of insulin and bolus doses when needed.
- Offers greater flexibility, smoother control of glycemia, but may increase the risk of hypoglycemia.
- The small cellphone-sized pump can be worn in a pocket or on a belt or waistband, as shown in Figure 69-3.

▶ *Inhalable insulin:*[21]

- Short-acting, "mealtime" insulin is taken through an inhaler.
- Side effects include lower lung function, cough, dry mouth, or chest discomfort.
- Brand name Afrezza.

▶ Future modes for insulin administration include an insulin patch, and implantable insulin pumps.

II. Oral Antidiabetic Medications

Oral medications are commonly used to treat type 2 diabetes in conjunction with diet, exercise, and possibly the injection of insulin.

▶ The medications, listed in Table 69-5, may be used individually or in combinations.

▶ The American Association of Clinical Endocrinologists (AACE) recommends the following in addition to lifestyle modifications[22]:

- The most common medications used in prediabetes is metformin.
- Monotherapy (one antidiabetic medication) for individuals with an A1c between 6.5% and 7.5%.

- Dual therapy (combination of two antidiabetic medications) for an A1c >7.5%.
- Triple therapy for an A1c >9%.

▶ The take away message for dental professionals is that when a patient is on multiple medications, it means the diabetes is not well controlled.

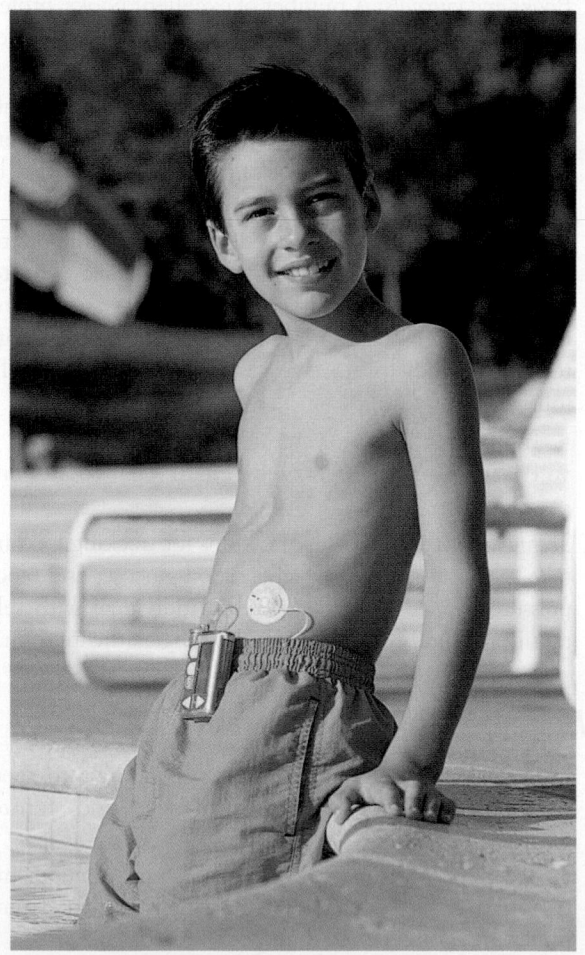

FIGURE 69-3 **Patient Wearing Insulin Pump.** Young boy with active lifestyle wearing an insulin pump. Photo courtesy of Minimed.

TABLE 69-5	Oral Hypoglycemic Agents Used for Treatment of Type 2 Diabetes	
AGENT	**EXAMPLE**	**ACTION/FUNCTION**
Biguanides	Metformin (Glucophage)	■ Prevents liver glycogen breakdown to glucose ■ Increases tissue sensitivity to insulin
Sulfonylureas	Glyburide (Diabeta, Mcronase) Glipizide (Glucotrol)	■ Stimulates pancreas to release more insulin after a meal ■ May cause hypoglycemia
Meglitinides	Repaglinide (Prandin) Nateglinide (Starlix)	■ Stimulates pancreas to release more insulin after a meal ■ May cause hypoglycemia
Thiazolidinediones	Pioglitazone (Actos)	■ Increases tissue sensitivity to insulin
Dipeptidyl peptidase-4 inhibitors	Sitagliptin (Januvia)	■ Improves insulin level after meals and lowers glucose production
Alpha-glucosidase inhibitors	Acarbose (Precose)	■ Slows digestion and absorption of glucose into bloodstream after eating

COMPLICATIONS OF DIABETES[9]

Patients with well-controlled blood glucose levels tend to develop fewer complications later in life than those whose diabetes is less well controlled.[23]

I. Infection

▶ Patients are more susceptible to infections and impaired healing, which can worsen prognosis.

▶ Presence of stress, trauma, and infection affects blood glucose levels.

▶ Failure to treat an infection intensifies the symptoms and increases severity of diabetes; can progress to life-threatening infections or precipitate diabetic coma.

▶ Insulin requirements may increase with fever, infection, inflammation, trauma, bleeding, pain, or stress. When the condition is eliminated, prescribed insulin may be reduced.

▶ Numerous factors are involved including impaired immune response, alterations in metabolism of carbohydrate and protein, vascular changes and impaired circulation, and altered nutritional state.

II. Neuropathy

▶ Neuropathy can cause pain, numbness, or tingling of mouth, face, and extremities.

A. Peripheral Neuropathy

▶ Symptoms vary based on the sensory nerve fibers affected and may result in loss of sensation in the feet, hands, and fingers.

▶ Numbness in the hands and fingers may make effective oral self-care difficult.

▶ As many as 50% of people with peripheral neuropathy may be asymptomatic and not recognize the loss of sensation which can put them at risk for injury and resulting infection.

▶ Leads to increased incidence of amputations and Charcot's joints.

B. Autonomic Neuropathy

▶ Manifestations include tachycardia, orthostatic hypotension, gastroparesis, and an hypoglycemic unawareness.

   • Cardiovascular autonomic neuropathy can be symptomatic other than changes in heart rate.
   • Gastroparesis is a slowing of digestion and motility of the gastrointestinal tract.
   • Hypoglycemic unawareness can quickly become an emergency situation because the patient is not able to recognize the usual symptoms of low blood glucose.

III. Nephropathy

▶ Diabetes is a leading cause of renal disease, and the most common cause of end-stage renal disease in the United States and Europe. Dialysis or kidney transplant is needed.

▶ Patients diagnosed with diabetes are screened for microalbuminuria (protein in the urine).

IV. Retinopathy

▶ Diabetes is a leading cause of blindness through the progression of diabetic retinopathy.

▶ Patients are more likely to have glaucoma and cataracts.

TABLE 69-6	Comparison of Average Blood Glucose and A1c[9]	
	Mean Plasma Glucose	
A1c (%)	**mg/dL**	**mmol/L**
6	126	7.0
7	154	8.6
8	183	10.1
9	212	111.8

V. Cardiovascular Disease

▶ Individuals with diabetes are at high risk for cardiovascular disease, a major cause of morbidity and mortality. Conditions common in people with diabetes include:
  • Hypertension.
  • Dyslipidemia (high total cholesterol and low-density lipoproteins).
  • Hypertriglyceridemia (high triglycerides).
▶ May lead to myocardial infarction and stroke.
▶ Owing to the excessive risk of coronary heart disease, aggressive treatment for dyslipidemia and hypertriglyceridemia is recommended.
▶ Low-dose aspirin therapy may be recommended for the prevention of cardiovascular disease in patients with diabetes. Daily aspirin intake may increase bleeding time.

VI. Amputation

Diabetes is a major cause of limb amputation (usually foot) from possible complications of neuropathy and vascular disease.

VII. Pregnancy Complications

Patients with diabetes are at higher risk for spontaneous miscarriages, having babies with birth defects, and increased weight.

VIII. Psychosocial Aspects

▶ Due to complications of diabetes, the daily life of the patient as well as those close to the patient is significantly affected.
▶ Treatment regimens may be challenging to cope with and lead to emotional and social problems, including depression.
▶ A suggestion for the patient to discuss psychosocial issues with the physician may improve patient's compliance with treatment and daily oral personal care.

DENTAL HYGIENE CARE PLAN

▶ The control of oral infection is vital. Infections can progress more quickly and can alter the management of diabetes.
▶ Frequent, thorough oral care requires the patient's utmost cooperation and motivation and regular professional care.
▶ The patient with diabetes is prone to life-threatening emergencies.
▶ Emergency practice drills can help the dental team prevent an emergency, identify early indications of a developing emergency, and act swiftly and appropriately.

I. Appointment Planning

Stress, including that created during a dental or dental hygiene appointment, can affect blood sugar levels. Appointment planning centers around many factors, including stress prevention.

A. Antibiotic Premedication

▶ *Well-controlled diabetes*: In general, the patient with well-controlled diabetes is treated the same as the patient without diabetes and requires no premedication related to diabetes.
▶ *Uncontrolled, unstable diabetes*: Routine dental treatment is deferred until diabetes is stabilized. Only emergency care is given to the uncontrolled patient. Consult patient's primary provider to determine if antibiotic premedication is needed.

B. Time

▶ Treat patient after a meal, preferably with protein and fat to slow carbohydrate absorption.
▶ Avoid peak insulin level noted in Table 69-4.
▶ Ideal time of appointment varies with individual patient's lifestyle and method of insulin intake.
▶ Preferred appointment may be morning, soon after the patient's normal breakfast and medication, during the ascending portion of the blood glucose level curve.

C. Precautions: Prevent/Prepare for Emergency

▶ Do not keep the patient waiting.
▶ Do not interfere with the patient's regular meal and between-meal eating schedule.
▶ Avoid long, stressful procedures; dental and dental hygiene care can be divided into short appointments appropriate to the individual's needs.
▶ Take additional precautions indicated for the patient with long-term diabetes with complications related to atherosclerosis and other cardiovascular diseases (see Chapter 67).
▶ Prevent and treat all infections promptly.

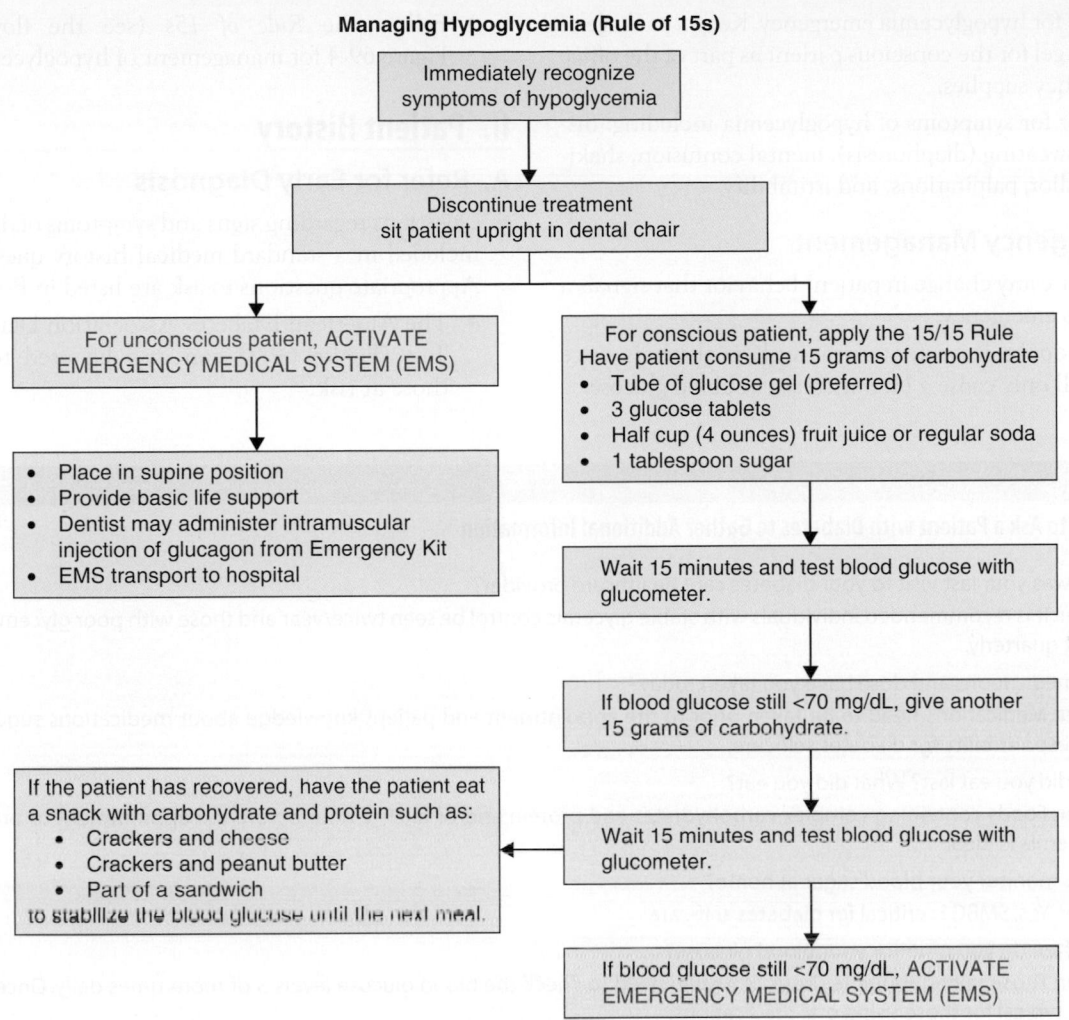

Managing Hypoglycemia (Rule of 15s)

Immediately recognize symptoms of hypoglycemia

↓

Discontinue treatment
sit patient upright in dental chair

For unconscious patient, ACTIVATE EMERGENCY MEDICAL SYSTEM (EMS)

↓

- Place in supine position
- Provide basic life support
- Dentist may administer intramuscular injection of glucagon from Emergency Kit
- EMS transport to hospital

For conscious patient, apply the 15/15 Rule
Have patient consume 15 grams of carbohydrate
- Tube of glucose gel (preferred)
- 3 glucose tablets
- Half cup (4 ounces) fruit juice or regular soda
- 1 tablespoon sugar

↓

Wait 15 minutes and test blood glucose with glucometer.

↓

If blood glucose still <70 mg/dL, give another 15 grams of carbohydrate.

↓

If the patient has recovered, have the patient eat a snack with carbohydrate and protein such as:
- Crackers and cheese
- Crackers and peanut butter
- Part of a sandwich
to stabilize the blood glucose until the next meal.

←

Wait 15 minutes and test blood glucose with glucometer.

↓

If blood glucose still <70 mg/dL, ACTIVATE EMERGENCY MEDICAL SYSTEM (EMS)

FIGURE 69-4 **Managing Hypoglycemia (Rule of 15s).** Flowchart to show steps to take when patient exhibits symptoms of hypoglycemia (insulin shock).

BOX 69-5

Common Medical History Questions to Screen for Diabetes

▷ Have you ever been diagnosed with prediabetes, borderline diabetes or diabetes? Yes No

▷ Have any members of your family ever been diagnosed with diabetes? Yes No

▷ Do you urinate frequently? How many times per day? Yes No

▷ Are you frequently thirsty? Yes No

▷ Does your mouth feel dry? Yes No

▷ Have you had any unexplained weight loss? Yes No

▷ Do you experience excessive hunger? Yes No

▷ Do you had recent blurred vision? Yes No

▷ Gather detailed information on all current prescribed and over-the-counter medications, including recommended dose.

▷ Gather information on vitamins, homeopathic, or herbal supplements.

▶ Prepare for hypoglycemia emergency. Keep a package of glucose gel for the conscious patient as part of the office emergency supplies.

▶ Monitor for symptoms of hypoglycemia including: dizziness, sweating (diaphoresis), mental confusion, shakiness, pallor, palpitations, and irritability.

D. Emergency Management

▶ Recognize any change in patient behavior that signals a diabetes emergency.

- • If in doubt, it is safer to treat for hypoglycemia since it will only cause a brief increase in blood glucose.

- • Follow the *Rule of 15s* (see the flowchart in Figure 69-4 for management of hypoglycemia).[9]

II. Patient History

A. Refer for Early Diagnosis

▶ Questions regarding signs and symptoms of diabetes are included in a standard medical history questionnaire. Appropriate questions to ask are listed in Box 69-5.

- • The American Diabetes Association Diabetes Risk Test (Figure 69-2) can also be used to identify those at risk.

BOX 69-6

Questions to Ask a Patient with Diabetes to Gather Additional Information

▷ When was your last visit to your diabetes care healthcare provider?
Answer: It is recommended individuals with stable glycemic control be seen twice/year and those with poor glycemic control at least quarterly.

▷ What medications and dose have you taken today?
Answer: Medications need to be taken prior to the appointment and patient knowledge about medications suggests personal responsibility for diabetes self-care.

▷ When did you eat last? What did you eat?
Answer: Foods containing complex carbohydrates and protein and/or fat 1–2 hour before the appointment to prevent hypoglycemia is ideal.

▷ Do you monitor your blood sugar at home?
Answer: Yes, SMBG is critical for diabetes self-care.

▷ How often do you monitor your blood glucose?
Answer: Those taking multiple doses of insulin need to check the blood glucose levels 3 or more times daily. Once or twice daily is typical for those using oral medications.

▷ What is your usual fasting blood sugar in the morning?
Answer: Glucose levels between 90 and 130 mg/dL premeal and below 180 mg/dL 2 hours postmeal.

▷ What is your hemoglobin A1c? How often does your primary care provider check the A1c?
Answer: About <7% and preferably <6.5%; A1c testing recommended twice/year in those with good glycemic control and quarterly in those with poor control.

▷ (If the patient reports poorly controlled diabetes) Are you experiencing frequent urination?
Answer: Response of "yes" may indicate hyperglycemia and poor diabetes control and requires referral. The patient will not heal and it is best to postpone treatment as healing will be suboptimal.

▷ Do you have frequent episodes of hypoglycemia (low blood sugar)? Can you tell when your blood sugar is getting low?
Answer: Response of "yes" to the first question and "no" to the second identifies a patient at risk for a medical emergency. Hypoglycemic unawareness occurs as a result of neuropathy and the patient is no longer able to identify when the blood sugar has dropped to dangerously low levels.

▷ (For those with a history of hypoglycemia, ask this question) What time of day does it usually happen and how do you treat it?
Answer: If the appointment is during a critical time of day for hypoglycemia, precautions need to be taken to prevent and treat it or the appointment can be rescheduled. Mid-afternoon is typically when some types of insulin and oral medications reach their peak action and glucose from the midday meal reaches a low resulting in a dangerous combination putting the patient at risk for hypoglycemia.

▷ Have you been hospitalized for hypoglycemia?
Answer: Response of "yes" indicates extreme risk and preparation needs to be made to rapidly treat hypoglycemia. Place a glucometer and glucose source near treatment area for quick access.

▷ Are you having problems with your eyes, feet, hands, or legs? If so, what kind of problems are you experiencing?
Answer: A patient experiencing complications may be poorly controlled and a medical consult is advised.

Adapted from Boyd LD. Commentary on survey of diabetes knowledge and practices of dental hygienists. *Access.* 2008;22(8):40–43.

▶ If an unexplained positive response is present suggesting symptoms of diabetes, the patient is referred to a primary care provider for evaluation.

B. Medical History

▶ Supplement the basic medical history with additional questions to obtain information about diabetes (suggested questions along with answers can be found in Box 69-6).

▶ Ask about exercise and tobacco use; review effect on health.

▶ Update medical history at each appointment.

▶ Identify health problems or complications of diabetes that may influence dental treatment. Refer to specialist when indicated.

III. Consultation with Primary Care Provider

▶ Consultation with the primary care provider to obtain A1c values can be initiated either prior to or at the first visit.
  • Table 69-6 provides a conversion for the A1c to average blood glucose levels.

▶ Further consultation may be necessary in more advanced periodontal disease to obtain clearance for treatment.

IV. Dental Hygiene Assessment and Treatment

A. Extraoral/Intraoral Examination

▶ Acanthosis negricans appears as a light brown to black discoloration of the skin in the creases of the neck and can indicate risk for diabetes (Figure 69-5).

B. Dental Biofilm Control Instruction

▶ Because of the impact of diabetes on periodontal health and the effect of oral infection on diabetes status, daily meticulous oral self-care is crucial.

▶ Disclosing the biofilm and individualized self-care measures for biofilm control are reviewed continuously.

C. Tobacco Cessation

▶ Refer to the information on Tobacco Cessation Programs in Chapter 34.

D. Instrumentation

▶ *Nonsurgical periodontal therapy*: Definitive nonsurgical periodontal therapy reduces the possibility of periodontal abscess formation. Allow several short appointments if needed for stress management.

▶ *Healing*: Avoid undue trauma to tissues to minimize the risk for complications associated with healing

E. Fluoride Application

▶ Fluoride treatments, varnishes, and home use of fluoride are encouraged, particularly with xerostomia.

▶ Methods for daily self-fluoride application are described in Chapter 36.

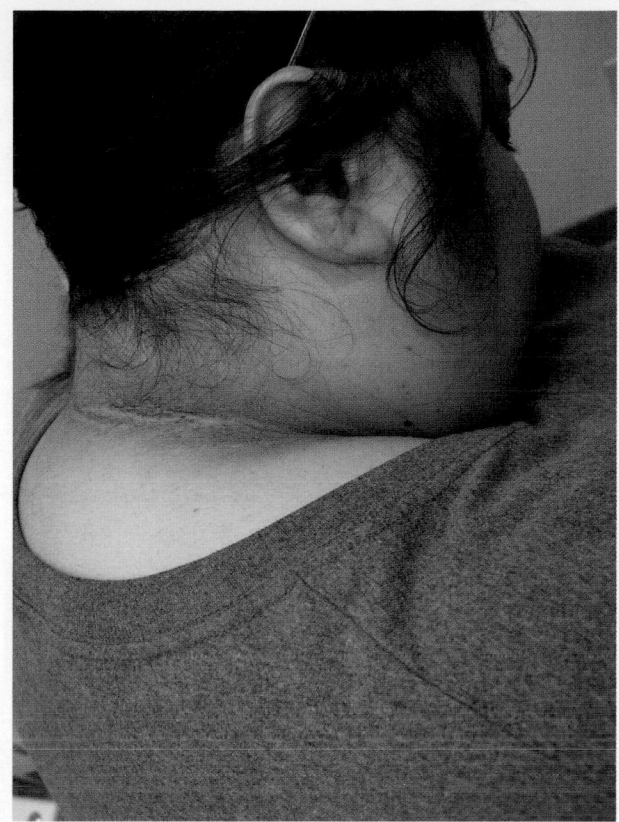

FIGURE 69-5 Acanthosis Negricans. This skin condition is seen in patients at risk for diabetes and typically appears on the creases in the neck as a light brown to black discoloration. (Reprinted from DeLong L, Burkhart N General and Oral Pathology for the Dental Hygienist. Philadelphia: Lippincott Williams & Wilkins; 2015. Courtesy of Dr. Frank Varon.)

V. Continuing Care

▶ Appointment for supervision and examination on regular 3- to 6-month basis as needed. Effectiveness of daily oral self-care is evaluated.

▶ Probe carefully to detect early bleeding on probing and evidence of pocket formation.

▶ Assess soft tissue with attention to areas of irritation related to fixed and removable prostheses.

▶ Identify any changes requiring consultation or referral to patient's primary care provider, dietitian, mental health professional, or other specialist.

▶ Check for dental biofilm control and review control with the patient at each appointment. Gingival health is of major importance. Keep the patient motivated.

DOCUMENTATION

▶ Record status of blood glucose control, including most recent HbA1c and other daily monitoring such as fasting blood glucose levels the patient has performed.

▶ Update current medications and doses.

▶ Confirm compliance of medication intake and food consumption.

EVERYDAY ETHICS

Ed, a 45-year-old restaurant owner, presents for an appointment with Susan, the dental hygienist. She has treated this patient before but he has not had an appointment for more than 2 years. The review of his medical history determines he is obese, complains of a dry mouth, has excessive thirst, gets up at night multiple times to urinate, and has not seen his primary care provider in several years. An intraoral examination reveals candidiasis on his hard palate. Susan suggests that he see his physician, but he refuses to even talk about it. He insists that he just wants "clean teeth" for his daughter's upcoming wedding.

Questions for Consideration

1. Describe how each of the dental hygiene ethical core values (Table II-1, Section II) apply to this scenario.

2. In what ways will Susan be violating the patient's rights if she agrees to Ed's request that she focus only on "cleaning" his teeth at this appointment? How may she be violating his rights if she refuses to clean his teeth unless he first has an examination with his primary care provider?

3. Explain choices or alternative actions Susan can consider as she decides how to continue treatment during Ed's appointment.

BOX 69-7

Example Documentation: Patient with Diabetes Mellitus

S –A 66-year-old Hispanic female who presents for a periodontal maintenance. She reports bleeding when she flosses for the last couple weeks. She was recently diagnosed with type 2 diabetes and is taking Metformin and Glipizide. Her initial HbA1c was 8.5 and she will have a follow-up test next month. She reports checking her blood glucose when she gets up in the morning and before dinner. Her fasting blood glucose this morning was 120. Patient reports taking her medications this morning.

O –Blood pressure: 131/79. Pulse: 88. Respirations 24. Risk assessment for caries was moderate, periodontal disease was high, and oral cancer was moderate. Periodontal examination reveals localized bleeding on probing and 1–2 mm pocket depth increases primarily in maxillary molar areas. Biofilm score: 30%. No new dental caries.

A –Moderate localized chronic periodontitis, complicated by poorly controlled diabetes mellitus.

P –Discussed the association of periodontal infection with diabetes and need for meticulous oral self-care and regular professional periodontal maintenance appointments. Reviewed use of interdental brushes for molar areas where biofilm was located. Patient had difficulty removing biofilm on the lingual line angles of the molars so careful wrapping of the floss was also reviewed. Complete periodontal debridement was performed. Applied 5% sodium fluoride varnish and provided a prescription for 0.12% chlorhexidine gluconate mouthrinse to use twice a day for 2 weeks to assist with healing.

Signed: _____, RDH

Date: _____

Factors To Teach The Patient

Factors to Teach Patients with Diabetes

▷ Importance of regular medical and dental care, eye examinations, blood pressure checks, blood tests for cholesterol, lipids, and kidney readings, and practice self-examination, particularly of feet, for nerve involvement or delayed healing visits to prevent complications.

▷ Connection between oral health and diabetes and need for meticulous oral self-care.

▷ The patient's role in self-management of diabetes with an emphasis on the need to be compliant with lifestyle modifications including healthy eating, physical activity, weight management, glucose monitoring, tobacco cessation, good oral self-care, limiting or avoiding alcohol, stress management, and use of prescribed medications.

▷ The value of seeking immediate medical attention for any signs of complications from diabetes.

Factors to Teach Patients Not Diagnosed with Diabetes

▷ Need for regular medical examinations and screening for diabetes.

▷ How to recognize the early warning signs of diabetes and seek medical consult.

▷ Factors that affect a healthy lifestyle, including healthy diet, daily exercise, no tobacco products, avoid alcohol, and maintain ideal weight.

▷ How to practice meticulous oral hygiene to prevent dental caries and periodontal disease.

▷ Stress reduction techniques.

► Record discussion about relationship between oral health status, oral hygiene status, risk factors, and diabetes.

► Box 69-7 contains an example progress note for a patient with diabetes.

References

1. American Diabetes Association. Diagnosis and classification of diabetes mellitus. *Diabetes Care.* 2014;37 (Suppl 1): S81–S90.

2. Centers for Disease Control and Prevention. *National Diabetes Statistics Report: Estimates of Diabetes and Its Burden in the*

United States, 2014. Atlanta, GA: US Department of Health and Human Services; 2014. http://www.cdc.gov//diabetes/pubs/statsreport14.htm. Accessed November 23, 2014.

3. Danaei G, Finucane MM, Lu Y, et al. National, regional, and global trends in fasting plasma glucose and diabetes prevalence since 1980: systematic analysis of health examination surveys and epidemiological studies with 370 country-years and 2.7 million participants. *Lancet.* 2011;378(9785):31–40.

4. Boyd LD, Giblin L, Chadbourne D. Bidirectional relationship between diabetes mellitus and periodontal disease: state of the evidence. *Can J Dent Hyg.* 2012;46(2):93–102.

5. Taylor GW, Manz MC, Borgnakke WS. Diabetes, periodontal diseases, dental caries, and tooth loss: a review of the literature. *Compend Contin Educ Dent.* 2004;25(3):179–184, 186–188, 190.

6. Fouad AF. Diabetes mellitus as a modulating factor of endodontic infections. *J Dent Educ.* 2003;67(4):459–467.

7. Chrcanovic BR, Albrektsson T, Wennerberg A. Diabetes and oral implant failure: a systematic review. *J Dent Res.* 2014;93(9):859–867.

8. Newsholme P, Cruzat V, Arfuso F, et al. Nutrient regulation of insulin secretion and action. *J Endocrinol.* 2014;221(3):R105–R120.

9. American Diabetes Association. Standards of medical care in diabetes—2014. *Diabetes Care.* 2014;37 (Suppl 1): S14–S80.

10. Reinehr T. Obesity and diabetes in young adults. *MMW Fortschr Med.* 2014;156(8):57–60.

11. DeSisto CL, Kim SY, Sharma AJ. Prevalence estimates of gestational diabetes mellitus in the united states, pregnancy risk assessment monitoring system (PRAMS), 2007–2010. *Prev Chronic Dis.* 2014;11:E104.

12. Linnenkamp U, IDF diabetes atlas reveals high burden of hyperglycaemia in pregnancy. *Diabetes Voice.* 2014;59:55–56.

13. American Diabetes Association. Type 2 diabetes risk test. http://www.diabetes.org/are-you-at-risk/diabetes-risk-test/. Accessed November 23, 2014.

14. Gupta A, Gupta N, Garg R, et al. Developing a chair side, safe and non-invasive procedure for assessment of blood glucose level using gingival crevicular bleeding in dental clinics. *J Nat Sci Biol Med.* 2014;5(2):329–332.

15. Strauss SM, Russell S, Wheeler A, et al. The dental office visit as a potential opportunity for diabetes screening: an analysis using NHANES 2003–2004 data. *J Public Health Dent.* 2010;70(2):156–162.

16. Strauss SM, Tuthill J, Singh G, et al. A novel intraoral diabetes screening approach in periodontal patients: results of a pilot study. *J Periodontol.* 2012;83(6):699–706.

17. The Diabetes Prevention Program Research Group. The 10-year cost-effectiveness of lifestyle intervention or metformin for diabetes prevention: an intent-to-treat analysis of the DPP/DPPOS. *Diabetes Care.* 2012;35(4):723–730.

18. Haas L, Maryniuk M, Beck J, et al. National standards for diabetes self-management education and support. *Diabetes Care.* 2014;37 (Suppl 1):S144–S153.

19. Brouwer W, Kroeze W, Crutzen R, et al. Which intervention characteristics are related to more exposure to internet-delivered healthy lifestyle promotion interventions? A systematic review. *J Med Internet Res.* 2011;13(1):e2.

20. Kaufman N. Internet and information technology use in treatment of diabetes. *Int J Clin Pract Suppl.* 2010;(166):41–46.

21. Liao ZH, Chen YL, Li FP, et al. Multicenter clinical study on the efficacy and safety of inhalable insulin aerosol in the treatment of type 2 diabetes. *Chin Med J (Engl).* 2008;121:1159–1164.

22. Garber AJ, Abrahamson MJ, Barzilay JI, et al. AACE comprehensive diabetes management algorithm 2013. *Endocr Pract.* 2013;19(2):327–336.

23. Nathan DM; and DCCT/EDIC Research Group. The diabetes control and complications trial/epidemiology of diabetes interventions and complications study at 30 years: overview. *Diabetes Care.* 2014;37(1):9–16.

ENHANCE YOUR UNDERSTANDING

thePoint® DIGITAL CONNECTIONS
(see the inside front cover for access information)
- **Audio glossary**
- **Quiz bank**

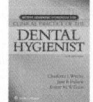

SUPPORT FOR LEARNING
(available separately; visit lww.com)
- *Active Learning Workbook for Clinical Practice of the Dental Hygienist, 12th Edition*

prepU INDIVIDUALIZED REVIEW
(available separately; visit lww.com)
- **Adaptive quizzing with *prepU* for Wilkins' *Clinical Practice of the Dental Hygienist***

Appendix I

American Dental Hygienists' Association Code of Ethics for Dental Hygienists*

PREAMBLE

As dental hygienists, we are a community of professionals devoted to the prevention of disease and the promotion and improvement of the public's health. We are preventive oral health professionals who provide educational, clinical, and therapeutic services to the public. We strive to live meaningful, productive, satisfying lives that simultaneously serve us, our profession, our society, and the world. Our actions, behaviors, and attitudes are consistent with our commitment to public service. We endorse and incorporate the Code into our daily lives.

PURPOSE

The purpose of a professional code of ethics is to achieve high levels of ethical consciousness, decision making, and practice by the members of the profession. Specific objectives of the Dental Hygiene Code of Ethics are:

► To increase our professional and ethical consciousness and sense of ethical responsibility.

► To lead us to recognize ethical issues and choices and to guide us in making more informed ethical decisions.

► To establish a standard for professional judgment and conduct.

► To provide a statement of the ethical behavior the public can expect from us.

The Dental Hygiene Code of Ethics is meant to influence us throughout our careers. It stimulates our continuing study of ethical issues and challenges us to explore our ethical responsibilities. The Code establishes concise standards of behavior to guide the public's expectations of our profession and supports existing dental hygiene practice, laws, and regulations. By holding ourselves accountable to meeting the standards stated in the Code, we enhance the public's trust on which our professional privilege and status are founded.

KEY CONCEPTS

Our beliefs, principles, values, and ethics are concepts reflected in the Code. They are the essential elements of our comprehensive and definitive code of ethics and are interrelated and mutually dependent.

BASIC BELIEFS

We recognize the importance of the following beliefs that guide our practice and provide context for our ethics:

► The services we provide contribute to the health and well-being of society.

► Our education and licensure qualify us to serve the public by preventing and treating oral disease and helping individuals achieve and maintain optimal health.

► Individuals have intrinsic worth, are responsible for their own health, and are entitled to make choices regarding their health.

► Dental hygiene care is an essential component of overall healthcare, and we function interdependently with other healthcare providers.

► All people should have access to healthcare, including oral healthcare.

► We are individually responsible for our actions and the quality of care we provide.

FUNDAMENTAL PRINCIPLES

These fundamental principles, universal concepts, and general laws of conduct provide the foundation for our ethics.

Universality

The principle of universality assumes that if one individual judges an action to be right or wrong in a given situation,

*Reprinted with permission from The American Dental Hygienists' Association. http://www.adha.org.

other people considering the same action in the same situation would make the same judgment.

Complementarity

The principle of complementarity assumes the existence of an obligation to justice and basic human rights. It requires us to act toward others in the same way they would act toward us if roles were reversed. In all relationships, it means considering the values and perspectives of others before making decisions or taking actions affecting them.

Ethics

Ethics are the general standards of right and wrong that guide behavior within society. As generally accepted actions, they can be judged by determining the extent to which they promote good and minimize harm. Ethics compel us to engage in health promotion/disease prevention activities.

Community

This principle expresses our concern for the bond between individuals, the community, and society in general. It leads us to preserve natural resources and inspires us to show concern for the global environment.

Responsibility

Responsibility is central to our ethics. We recognize there are guidelines for making ethical choices and accept responsibility for knowing and applying them. We accept the consequences of our actions or the failure to act and are willing to make ethical choices and publicly affirm them.

CORE VALUES

We acknowledge these values as general for our choices and actions.

Individual Autonomy and Respect for Human Beings

People have the right to be treated with respect. They have the right to informed consent prior to treatment, and they have the right to full disclosure of all relevant information so that they can make informed choices about their care.

Confidentiality

We respect the confidentiality of client information and relationships as a demonstration of the value we place on individual autonomy. We acknowledge our obligation to justify any violation of a confidence.

Societal Trust

We value client trust and understand that public trust in our profession is based on our actions and behavior.

Nonmaleficence

We accept our fundamental obligation to provide services in a manner that protects all clients and minimizes harm to them and others involved in their treatment.

Beneficence

We have a primary role in promoting the well-being of individuals and the public by engaging in health promotion/ disease prevention activities.

Justice and Fairness

We value justice and support the fair and equitable distribution of healthcare resources. We believe all people should have access to high-quality, affordable oral healthcare.

Veracity

We accept the obligation to tell the truth and assume that others will do the same. We value self-knowledge and seek truth and honesty in all relationships.

STANDARDS OF PROFESSIONAL RESPONSIBILITY

We are obligated to practice our profession in a manner that supports our purpose, beliefs, and values in accordance with the fundamental principles that support our ethics. We acknowledge the following responsibilities:

To Ourselves as Individuals

▶ Avoid self-deception, and continually strive for knowledge and personal growth.
▶ Establish and maintain a lifestyle that supports optimal health.
▶ Create a safe work environment.
▶ Assert our own interests in ways that are fair and equitable.
▶ Seek the advice and counsel of others when challenged with ethical dilemmas.
▶ Have realistic expectations of ourselves and recognize our limitations.

To Ourselves as Professionals

▶ Enhance professional competencies through continuous learning in order to practice according to high standards of care.

- Support dental hygiene peer-review systems and quality-assurance measures.
- Develop collaborative professional relationships and exchange knowledge to enhance our own lifelong professional development.

To Family and Friends

- Support the efforts of others to establish and maintain healthy lifestyles and respect the rights of friends and family.

To Clients

- Provide oral healthcare utilizing high levels of professional knowledge, judgment, and skill.
- Maintain a work environment that minimizes the risk of harm.
- Serve all clients without discrimination, and avoid action toward any individual or group that may be interpreted as discriminatory.
- Hold professional client relationships confidential.
- Communicate with clients in a respectful manner.
- Promote ethical behavior and high standards of care by all dental hygienists.
- Serve as an advocate for the welfare of clients.
- Provide clients with the information necessary to make informed decisions about their oral health and encourage their full participation in treatment decisions and goals.
- Refer clients to other healthcare providers when their needs are beyond our ability or scope of practice.
- Educate clients about high-quality oral healthcare.

To Colleagues

- Conduct professional activities and programs, and develop relationships in ways that are honest, responsible, and appropriately open and candid.
- Encourage a work environment that promotes individual professional growth and development.
- Collaborate with others to create a work environment that minimizes risk to the personal health and safety of our colleagues.
- Manage conflicts constructively.
- Support the efforts of other dental hygienists to communicate the dental hygiene philosophy and preventive oral care.
- Inform other healthcare professionals about the relationship between general and oral health.
- Promote human relationships that are mutually beneficial, including those with other healthcare professionals.

To Employees and Employers

- Conduct professional activities and programs and develop relationships in ways that are honest, responsible, open, and candid.
- Manage conflicts constructively.
- Support the right of our employees and employers to work in an environment that promotes wellness.
- Respect the employment rights of our employers and employees.

To the Dental Hygiene Profession

- Participate in the development and advancement of our profession.
- Avoid conflicts of interest and declare them when they occur.
- Seek opportunities to increase public awareness and understanding of oral health practices.
- Act in ways that bring credit to our profession while demonstrating appropriate respect for colleagues in other professions.
- Contribute time, talent, and financial resources to support and promote our profession.
- Promote a positive image for our profession.
- Promote a framework for professional education that develops dental hygiene competencies to meet the oral and overall health needs of the public.

To the Community and Society

- Recognize and uphold the laws and regulations governing our profession.
- Document and report inappropriate, inadequate, or substandard care and/or illegal activities by a healthcare provider to the responsible authorities.
- Use peer review as a mechanism for identifying inappropriate, inadequate, or substandard care provided by dental hygienists.
- Comply with local, state, and federal statutes that promote public health and safety.
- Develop support systems and quality-assurance programs in the workplace to assist dental hygienists in providing the appropriate standard of care.
- Promote access to dental hygiene services for all, supporting justice and fairness in the distribution of healthcare resources.
- Act consistently with the ethics of the global scientific community of which our profession is a part.
- Create a healthful workplace ecosystem to support a healthy environment.
- Recognize and uphold our obligation to provide pro bono service.

To Scientific Investigation

We accept responsibility for conducting research according to the fundamental principles underlying our ethical beliefs in compliance with universal codes, governmental standards, and professional guidelines for the care and management of experimental subjects. We acknowledge our ethical obligations to the scientific community:

▶ Conduct research that contributes knowledge that is valid and useful to our clients and society.

▶ Use research methods that meet accepted scientific standards.

▶ Use research resources appropriately.

▶ Systematically review and justify research in progress to ensure the most favorable benefit-to-risk ratio to research subjects.

▶ Submit all proposals involving human subjects to an appropriate human subject review committee.

▶ Secure appropriate institutional committee approval for the conduct of research involving animals.

▶ Obtain informed consent from human subjects participating in research that is based on specification published in Title 21 Code of Federal Regulations Part 46.

▶ Respect the confidentiality and privacy of data.

▶ Seek opportunities to advance dental hygiene knowledge through research by providing financial, human, and technical resources whenever possible. Report research results in a timely manner.

▶ Report research findings completely and honestly, drawing only those conclusions that are supported by the data presented.

▶ Report names of investigators fairly and accurately.

▶ Interpret the research and the research of others accurately and objectively, drawing conclusions that are supported by the data presented and seeking clarity when uncertain.

▶ Critically evaluate research methods and results before applying new theory and technology in practice.

▶ Be knowledgeable concerning currently accepted preventive and therapeutic methods, products, and technology and their application to our practice.

Appendix II

National Dental Hygienists' Association Code of Ethics*

PREAMBLE

We, the members of the National Dental Hygienists' Association, affirm our belief in dental health education for the prevention of dental disease and the importance of preventive treatment. We affirm and accept our responsibility to practice our profession according to the highest ethical standards. We hold ourselves, both individually and collectively, accountable for professional conduct in the dental hygiene profession according to the provision of this code.

Principle I: Commitment to the Patient

Our success is measured by the progress of each patient's achievement of maximum dental health. We work to motivate our patients to become aware of their individual state of dental health and engage in those practices that result in optimum dental health. To this end we will:

1. Address each patient with respect, giving consideration to the individual's needs.
2. Maintain each patient's confidentiality.
3. Maintain the highest level of mental, physical and spiritual health possible, to be a role model to our patients and the community.

Principle II: Commitment to the Community

In fulfilling our obligations to the community, we believe that cooperative relationships in the community will enhance the image of dental hygiene. As hygienists, we are accountable for participating in the development of education programs and policies. We are also accountable for interpreting this information for our patients.

Principle III: Commitment to the Profession

We believe that the quality of services the NDHA provides to its members directly influences the future of the profession and the patient population served by its members. We must exert every effort to raise performance standards to improve the skills of our members so that they can exercise the highest level of professional judgment. These actions should attract individuals who will make positive contributions to the practice of dental hygiene. We actively participate in the planning, development and learning of all members.

Principle IV: Commitment to the Student

We measure our success by the number of underrepresented minority students entering the dental hygiene profession and strive to increase the number of underrepresented minority dental hygienists by eliminating educational and social barriers. To accomplish this goal, the NDHA will provide educational and financial assistance to insure the continued success of underrepresented minorities in the profession of dental hygiene.

*Reprinted with permission from The National Dental Hygienists' Association Constitution and By-laws. 2012. http://www.ndhaonline.org.

Appendix III

Canadian Dental Hygienists Association: Dental Hygienists' Code of Ethics*

PREAMBLE

The CDHA Code of Ethics sets out the ethical principles and responsibilities which apply to all members of the dental hygiene profession across all practice areas including clinical care, education, research, administration and any other role related to the profession of dental hygiene.

Ethics is the study of moral values and moral reasoning. Ethical codes are formal statements that guide members of a profession in their obligations to clients, colleagues, the larger society, and to global health.

The Code of Ethics serves to:

1. Articulate the ethical principles and responsibilities by which dental hygienists are guided and under which they are accountable;

2. Provide a professional resource for education, reflection, self-evaluation, and peer review within dental hygiene and the broader health care community;

3. Inform the public about the ethical principles and responsibilities of the dental hygiene profession.

Dental hygienists' primary responsibility is to the client. In this document, "client" refers to a person or persons or a community with whom dental hygienists are engaged in a professional relationship. These relationships occur in all areas of dental hygiene practice including clinical services (e.g., private dental offices, independent practice, schools, community/public health clinics, acute and long term care, corporate environments); education, research, regulatory and policy roles; and administration/employment.

Dental hygienists work in an interprofessional collaborative environment. They are accountable to other codes of ethics/ethical guidelines including those of their provincial/territorial regulatory authority and their workplace. The CDHA Code of Ethics is a strong foundational document, effective on its own, and complementary to other ethical codes that address more specific situations and behaviours.

Dental hygienists use the Code of Ethics in conjunction with professional standards, workplace policies, and laws and regulations that guide practices and behaviours. In achieving these requirements, they fulfill their contract with society to meet a high standard of ethical practice.

ETHICAL PRINCIPLES AND RESPONSIBILITIES

The "Principles" depict the broad ideals to which dental hygienists aspire and which guide their practice. The "Responsibilities" outlined on the following pages are more precise and provide direction for behaviours in ethical situations.

Principle: Beneficence

Beneficence involves caring about and acting to promote the good of another. Dental hygienists use their knowledge and skills to assist clients to achieve and maintain optimal oral health and overall wellbeing, and to promote fair and reasonable access to quality oral health services as an integral part of the healthcare system.

Responsibilities for Beneficence

1. Dental hygienists put the needs, values, and interests of clients first.

2. Dental hygienists provide services to clients in a caring manner with respect for their individual needs, values, culture, safety, and life circumstances, and in recognition of their inherent dignity.

3. Dental hygienists regard informed choice as a precondition of intervention, and honour a client's informed choice including refusal of intervention.

4. Dental hygienists recommend or provide those services that they believe are necessary for promoting and maintaining a client's oral health and its effect on total body health and wellness, and which are consistent with the client's informed choice.

*Revised 2012. Reprinted with permission from The Canadian Dental Hygienists Association. http://www.cdha.ca/

5. Dental hygienists take appropriate action to ensure a client's safety and quality of care when they suspect unethical or incompetent care.

6. Dental hygienists seek to improve the quality of care, and advance knowledge in the field of oral health through advocacy and interprofessional practice.

Principle: Autonomy

Autonomy pertains to the right to make one's own choices. By communicating relevant information openly and truthfully, dental hygienists assist clients to make informed choices and to participate actively in achieving and maintaining their optimal oral health.

Responsibilities for Autonomy

1. Dental hygienists actively involve clients in their oral healthcare and promote informed choice by communicating relevant information openly, truthfully, and sensitively in recognition of their needs, values, and capacity to understand.

2. Dental hygienists involve and promote informed choice by substitute decision maker(s) in situations where clients lack the capacity for informed choice.

3. Dental hygienists, in the event of a substitute decision maker, involve clients to the extent of their capacity.

4. Dental hygienists recognize cultural differences, and assess and plan interventions with individuals and populations receiving their services relative to the cultural context.

Principle: Integrity

Integrity relates to consistency of actions, values, methods, expectations, and outcomes. It includes the promotion of fairness and social justice with consideration for those clients more vulnerable. It conveys a sense of wholeness and strength, and doing what is right with honesty and truthfulness.

Responsibilities for Integrity

1. Dental hygienists uphold the principles and standards of the profession with clients, colleagues and others with whom they are engaged in a professional relationship.

2. Dental hygienists maintain and advance their knowledge and skills in dental hygiene through lifelong learning.

3. Dental hygienists provide quality of interventions through ongoing self evaluation and quality assurance.

4. Dental hygienists promote conditions that enable social, economic, cultural values and institutions compatible with meeting basic human rights and dignity.

5. Dental hygienists collaborate with colleagues in a cooperative, constructive and respectful manner with the primary goal of providing safe, competent, fair and high quality interventions to individuals, families and communities.

6. Dental hygienists promote workplace practices and policies that facilitate professional practice in accordance with the principles, standards, laws and regulations under which they are accountable.

7. Dental hygienists communicate the nature and costs of professional services fairly and accurately, adhering to guidelines and/or regulations for advertising as outlined by their jurisdictional regulatory authority.

Principle: Accountability

Accountability pertains to taking responsibility for one's actions and omissions in light of relevant principles, standards, laws, and regulations. It includes the potential to self evaluate and be evaluated. It involves practising competently and accepting responsibility for behaviours and decisions in the professional context.

Responsibilities for Accountability

1. Dental hygienists accept responsibility for knowing and acting consistently with the principles, practice standards, laws and regulations under which they are accountable.

2. Dental hygienists practise within the bounds of their competence, scope of practice, personal and/or professional limitations.

3. Dental hygienists refer clients who require services outside their scope of practice to the appropriate professional.

4. Dental hygienists address issues in the practice environment that may hinder or impede the provision of care.

5. Dental hygienists inform their employers about the principles, standards, laws and regulations to which dental hygienists are accountable and determine whether employment conditions facilitate safe professional practice.

6. Dental hygienists inform their employers and/or appropriate regulatory authority of unethical practice by a colleague.

7. Dental hygienists inform the appropriate regulatory authority in the event of becoming unable to practise safely and competently.

Principle: Confidentiality

Confidentiality is the duty to hold secret any information acquired in the professional relationship. Dental hygienists respect a client's privacy and hold in confidence information disclosed to them except in certain narrowly defined exceptions.

Responsibilities for Confidentiality

1. Dental hygienists demonstrate respect for the privacy of clients.

2. Dental hygienists promote practices, policies and information systems that are designed to respect and protect clients' privacy and confidentiality.

3. Dental hygienists understand and respect the potential of compromising confidentiality when connecting with clients through social networks or other electronic media.

4. Dental hygienists hold confidential any information acquired in the professional relationship and do not use or disclose confidential information to others without a client's express consent. Exceptions include:
   - As required by law,
   - As required by the policy of the practice environment (e.g., quality assurance),
   - In an emergency situation,
   - In situations where disclosure is necessary to prevent serious harm to others,
   - To the client's guardian or substitute decision maker.

5. Dental hygienists inform clients in advance of treatment of how their information may be shared, in particular, around any uses or sharing that may occur without the client's express consent.

6. Dental hygienists obtain a client's consent to use or share information about his/her circumstances for the purpose of teaching or research.

Appendix IV

International Federation of Dental Hygienists Code of Ethics*

INTRODUCTION

The fundamental responsibility of dental hygienists is to promote and restore oral health.

Dental hygienists promote oral health by providing clinical, therapeutic remedies, and health education.

Dental hygienists serve the public as oral health professionals and thus contribute to the public's general health and well-being.

The need for dental hygiene services is universal and unrestricted by race, color, age, sex, language, religion, political or other opinion, national or social origin, property, birth or other status.

Dental hygienists are called upon to deliver care to the individual, the family and the community.

In a business relationship in which a dental hygienist is an employee the dental hygienist exhibits competence, loyalty and fair return of work for compensation. However, employee status does not minimize a dental hygienist's ethical responsibility to account for a patient's well-being. Nor does it lessen the dental hygienist's right to act competently, accountably and knowledgably on behalf of the patient.

Dental hygiene care is provided with integrity and respect and in collaboration with other health care professionals.

Values Embedded in the Code of Ethics

Dental hygienists value integrity and respect.

1. **Integrity:** moral soundness; uprightness; sincerity; freedom from corrupting influence or motive

   a. Dental hygienists value personal integrity and are honest, truthful, and respectful when interacting with other human beings.

   b. Dental hygienists value professional integrity and practice according to the profession's standards and values.

   c. Ethical practice requires both personal integrity and professional integrity.

2. **Respect:** to regard with special attention, to care for, to avoid violation of, or interference with. Dental hygienists value respect for *persons and personal dignity as human beings are unique, in their abilities, strengths, weaknesses and needs.*

   a. *Dental hygienists value respect for* truthfulness. Truthfulness is essential when assisting the patient to obtain relevant information about dental hygiene services, diagnosis, treatment and probable outcomes. Truthfulness builds trust.

   b. Dental hygienists value respect for *individual choice. Patients have choices and can decide which services to accept or decline.*

   c. *Dental hygienists value respect for* patient confidentiality. Confidentiality is preserved unless such confidentiality could pose substantial risk or serious harm and where that risk or harm is greater than the harm of breaking the confidentiality.

   d. Dental hygienists respect the natural *environment.*

These values are embedded in the four principle elements of the Code.

CODE OF ETHICS

The code of ethics has four principal elements that outline the standards of ethical conduct. This establishes the standards of behavior of dental hygienists and embodies integrity and respect.

1. Dental Hygienists and People/Society

2. Dental Hygienists and Practice

3. Dental Hygienists and Co-workers

4. Dental Hygienists and the Profession

Dental Hygienists and People/Society

▶ The dental hygienist strives to promote an environment in which the human rights, values, customs, and

*Reprinted with permission from The International Federation of Dental Hygienists. http://ifdh.org.

spiritual beliefs of the individual, family and community are respected.

▶ The dental hygienist endeavors to ensure that the individual receives sufficient and appropriate information on which to base consent for care and related dental hygiene treatment.

▶ The dental hygienist provides services consistent with the patient's needs and requests.

▶ The dental hygienist holds personal information confidential and uses professional reasoned judgment in sharing this information.

▶ The dental hygienist protects the environment by responsible disposal of all wastes in the dental hygiene practice.

▶ The dental hygienist's own personal interests, if in conflict with her/his professional obligation should be declared and resolved for the well-being of the client.

Dental Hygienists and Practice

▶ The dental hygienist has the qualifications, knowledge, training, skills, judgment and attitudes to practice safely.

▶ The dental hygienist has a thorough knowledge of the profession and its related laws.

▶ The dental hygienist at all times practices with integrity and adheres to the standards of practice and personal conduct of her/his legislative jurisdiction.

▶ The dental hygienist is personally responsible for remaining competent and current in her/his professional knowledge by continual education and training.

▶ The dental hygienist provides a choice of services within a range of safe affordable options consistent with the patient's needs.

▶ The dental hygienist provides timely competent care and charges reasonable fees for professional services.

▶ The dental hygienist, in providing care, ensures that use of technology and scientific advances are compatible with the safety, dignity and rights of people.

Dental Hygienist and Co-Workers

▶ The dental hygienist sustains a co-operative and collaborative relationship with co-workers in oral health and other fields.

▶ A dental hygienist recognizes particular skills and expertise of health care personnel working collaboratively in the patient's care.

▶ A dental hygienist advocates for the patient when another oral health provider is giving inappropriate or incompetent care, inconsistent with the patient's well-being.

Dental Hygienists and the Profession

▶ The dental hygienist adheres to and may exceed the standards of dental hygiene practice within the jurisdiction of the country of practice.

▶ The dental hygienist is active in developing and publishing a core of research based on the ongoing pursuit of professional knowledge.

▶ The dental hygienist, acting through the professional organization, participates in creating and maintaining equitable social and economic working conditions in oral health.

▶ The dental hygienist promotes respect for human beings ensuring the profession protects their right to health.

Appendix V

Guidelines for Infection Control in Dental Health Care Settings*

RECOMMENDATIONS

Each recommendation is categorized on the basis of existing scientific data, theoretical rationale, and applicability. Rankings are based on the system used by the Centers for Disease Control and Prevention (CDC) and the Healthcare Infection Control Practices Advisory Committee (HICPAC) to categorize recommendations:

Category IA: Strongly recommended for implementation and strongly supported by well-designed experimental, clinical, or epidemiologic studies.

Category IB: Strongly recommended for implementation and supported by experimental, clinical, or epidemiologic studies and a strong theoretical rationale.

Category IC: Required for implementation as mandated by federal or state regulation or standard. When IC is used, a second rating can be included to provide the basis of existing scientific data, theoretical rationale, and applicability. Because of state differences, the reader should not assume that the absence of an IC implies the absence of state regulations.

Category II: Suggested for implementation and supported by suggestive clinical or epidemiologic studies or a theoretical rationale.

Unresolved issue: No recommendation. Insufficient evidence or no consensus regarding efficacy exists.

I. Personnel Health Elements of an Infection-Control Program

A. General Recommendations

1. Develop a written health program for dental healthcare personnel (DHCP) that includes policies, procedures, and guidelines for education and training; immunizations; exposure prevention and postexposure management; medical conditions, work-related illness, and associated work restrictions; contact dermatitis and latex hypersensitivity; and maintenance of records, data management, and confidentiality (IB).[5,16–18,22]

2. Establish referral arrangements with qualified healthcare professionals to ensure prompt and appropriate provision of preventive services, occupationally related medical services, and postexposure management with medical follow-up (IB, IC).[5,13,19,22]

B. Education and Training

1. Provide DHCP (1) on initial employment, (2) when new tasks or procedures affect the employee's occupational exposure, and (3) at a minimum, annually, with education and training regarding occupational exposure to potentially infectious agents and infection-control procedures/protocols appropriate for and specific to their assigned duties (IB, IC).[5,11,13,14,16,19,22]

2. Provide educational information appropriate in content and vocabulary to the educational level, literacy and language of DHCP (IB, IC).[5,13]

C. Immunization Programs

1. Develop a written comprehensive policy regarding immunizing DHCP, including a list of all required and recommended immunizations (IB).[5,17,18]

2. Refer DHCP to a prearranged qualified healthcare professional or to their own health care professional to receive all appropriate immunizations based on the latest recommendations as well as their medical history and risk for occupational exposure (IB).[5,17]

D. Exposure Prevention and Postexposure Management

1. Develop a comprehensive postexposure management and medical follow-up program (IB, IC).[5,13,14,19]

   A. Include policies and procedures for prompt reporting, evaluation, counseling, treatment, and medical follow-up of occupational exposures.

---

*Excerpted from Centers for Disease Control and Prevention. Guidelines for Infection Control in Dental Health Care Settings, 2003. MMWR. 2003;52 (RR-17):1–61. http://www.cdc.gov/oralhealth/infectioncontrol/guidelines. Accessed August 31, 2015.

B. Establish mechanisms for referral to a qualified health-care professional for medical evaluation and follow-up.

C. Conduct a baseline tuberculin skin test (TST), preferably by using a two-step test, for all DHCP who might have contact with persons with suspected or confirmed infectious TB, regardless of the risk classification of the setting (IB).[20]

E. Medical Conditions, Work-Related Illness, and Work Restrictions

1. Develop and have readily available to all DHCP comprehensive written policies regarding work restriction and exclusion that include a statement of authority defining who can implement such policies (IB).[5,22]

2. Develop policies for work restriction and exclusion that encourage DHCP to seek appropriate preventive and curative care and report their illnesses, medical conditions, or treatments that can render them more susceptible to opportunistic infection or exposures; do not penalize DHCP with loss of wages, benefits, or job status (IB).[5,22]

3. Develop policies and procedures for evaluation, diagnosis, and management of DHCP with suspected or known occupational contact dermatitis (IB).[32]

4. Seek definitive diagnosis by a qualified healthcare professional for any DHCP with suspected latex allergy to carefully determine its specific etiology and appropriate treatment as well as work restrictions and accommodations (IB).[32]

F. Records Maintenance, Data Management, and Confidentiality

1. Establish and maintain confidential medical records (e.g., immunization records and documentation of tests received as a result of occupational exposure) for all DHCP (IB, IC).[5,13]

2. Ensure that the practice complies with all applicable federal, state, and local laws regarding medical record-keeping and confidentiality (IC).[13,34]

II. Preventing Transmission of Bloodborne Pathogens

A. HBV Vaccination

1. Offer the hepatitis B virus (HBV) vaccination series to all DHCP with potential occupational exposure to blood or other potentially infectious material (IA, IC).[2,13,14,19]

2. Always follow U.S. Public Health Service/CDC recommendations for hepatitis B vaccination, serologic testing, follow-up, and booster dosing (IA, IC).[13,14,19]

3. Test DHCP for hepatitis B surface antibody (anti-HBs) 1–2 months after completion of the 3-dose vaccination series (IA, IC).[14,19]

4. DHCP should complete a second 3-dose vaccine series or be evaluated to determine if they are hepatitis B surface antigen (HBsAg)-positive if no antibody response occurs to the primary vaccine series (IA, IC).[14,19]

5. Retest for anti-HBs at the completion of the second vaccine series. If no response to the second 3-dose series occurs, nonresponders should be tested for HBsAg (IC).[14,19]

6. Counsel nonresponders to vaccination who are HBsAg-negative regarding their susceptibility to HBV infection and precautions to take (IA, IC).[14,19]

7. Provide employees appropriate education regarding the risks of HBV transmission and the availability of the vaccine. Employees who decline the vaccination should sign a declination form to be kept on file with the employer (IC).[13]

B. Preventing Exposures to Blood and OPIM (Other Potentially Infectious Materials)

1. General recommendations

   a. Use standard precautions (Occupational Safety and Health Administration's [OSHA's]) blood-borne pathogen standard retains the term universal precautions) for all patient encounters (IA, IC).[11,13,19,53]

   b. Consider sharp items (e.g., needles, scalers, burs, lab knives, and wires) that are contaminated with patient blood and saliva as potentially infective and establish engineering controls and work practices to prevent injuries (IB, IC).[6,13,113]

   c. Implement a written, comprehensive program designed to minimize and manage DHCP exposures to blood and body fluids (IB, IC).[13,14,19,97]

2. Engineering and work-practice controls

   a. Identify, evaluate, and select devices with engineered safety features at least annually and as they become available on the market (e.g., safer anesthetic syringes, blunt suture needle, retractable scalpel, or needleless IV systems) (IC).[13,97,110–112]

   b. Place used disposable syringes and needles, scalpel blades, and other sharp items in appropriate puncture-resistant containers located as close as feasible to the area in which the items are used (IA, IC).[2,7,13,19,113,115]

   c. Do not recap used needles by using both hands or any other technique that involves directing the point of a needle toward any part of the body. Do not bend, break, or remove needles before disposal (IA, IC).[2,7,8,13,97,113]

   d. Use either a one-handed scoop technique or a mechanical device designed for holding the needle cap when recapping needles (e.g., between multiple injections and before removing from a nondisposable aspirating syringe) (IA, IC).[2,7,8,13,14,113]

3. Postexposure management and prophylaxis

   a. Follow CDC recommendations after percutaneous, mucous membrane, or nonintact skin exposure to blood or other potentially infectious material (IA, IC).[13,14,19]

III. Hand Hygiene

A. General Considerations

1. Perform hand hygiene with either a nonantimicrobial or antimicrobial soap and water when hands are visibly dirty or contaminated with blood or other potentially infectious material. If hands are not visibly soiled, an alcohol-based hand rub can also be used. Follow the manufacturer's instructions (IA).[123]

2. Indications for hand hygiene include
   a. when hands are visibly soiled (IA, IC);
   b. after bare-handed touching of inanimate objects likely to be contaminated by blood, saliva, or respiratory secretions (IA, IC);
   c. before and after treating each patient (IB);
   d. before donning gloves (IB); and
   e. immediately after removing gloves (IB, IC).[7–9, 11,13,113,120–123,125,126,138]

3. For oral surgical procedures, perform surgical hand antisepsis before donning sterile surgeon's gloves. Follow the manufacturer's instructions by using either an antimicrobial soap and water, or soap and water followed by drying hands and application of an alcohol-based surgical hand-scrub product with persistent activity (IB).[121–123,127–133,144,145]

4. Store liquid hand-care products in either disposable closed containers or closed containers that can be washed and dried before refilling. Do not add soap or lotion to (i.e., top off) a partially empty dispenser (IA).[9,120,122,149,150]

B. Special Considerations for Hand Hygiene and Glove Use

1. Use hand lotions to prevent skin dryness associated with handwashing (IA).[153,154]

2. Consider the compatibility of lotion and antiseptic products and the effect of petroleum or other oil emollients on the integrity of gloves during product selection and glove use (IB).[2,14,122,155]

3. Keep fingernails short with smooth, filed edges to allow thorough cleaning and prevent glove tears (II).[122,123,156]

4. Do not wear artificial fingernails or extenders when having direct contact with patients at high risk (e.g., those in intensive care units or operating rooms) (IA).[123,157–160]

5. Use of artificial fingernails is usually not recommended (II).[157–160]

6. Do not wear hand or nail jewelry if it makes donning gloves more difficult or compromises the fit and integrity of the glove (II).[123,142,143]

IV. PPE (Personal Protective Equipment)

A. Masks, Protective Eyewear, and Face Shields

1. Wear a surgical mask and eye protection with solid side shields or a face shield to protect mucous membranes of the eyes, nose, and mouth during procedures likely to generate splashing or spattering of blood or other body fluids (IB, IC).[1,2,7,8,11,13,137]

2. Change masks between patients or during patient treatment if the mask becomes wet (IB).[2]

3. Clean with soap and water, or if visibly soiled, clean and disinfect reusable facial protective equipment (e.g., clinician and patient protective eyewear or face shields) between patients (II).[2]

B. Protective Clothing

1. Wear protective clothing (e.g., reusable or disposable gown, laboratory coat, or uniform) that covers personal clothing and skin (e.g., forearms) likely to be soiled with blood, saliva, or OPIM (IB, IC).[7,8,11,13,137]

2. Change protective clothing if visibly soiled[134]; change immediately or as soon as feasible if penetrated by blood or other potentially infectious fluids (IB, IC).[13]

3. Remove barrier protection, including gloves, mask, eyewear, and gown before departing work area (e.g., dental patient care, instrument processing, or laboratory areas) (IC).[13]

C. Gloves

1. Wear medical gloves when a potential exists for contacting blood, saliva, OPIM, or mucous membranes (IB, IC).[1,2,7,8,13]

2. Wear a new pair of medical gloves for each patient, remove them promptly after use, and wash hands immediately to avoid transfer of microorganisms to other patients or environments (IB).[1,7,8,123]

3. Remove gloves that are torn, cut, or punctured as soon as feasible and wash hands before regloving (IB, IC).[13,210,211]

4. Do not wash surgeon's or patient examination gloves before use or wash, disinfect, or sterilize gloves for reuse (IB, IC).[13,138,177,212,213]

5. Ensure that appropriate gloves in the correct size are readily accessible (IC).[13]

6. Use appropriate gloves (e.g., puncture- and chemical-resistant utility gloves) when cleaning instruments and performing housekeeping tasks involving contact with blood or OPIM (IB, IC).[7,13,15]

7. Consult with glove manufacturers regarding the chemical compatibility of glove material and dental materials used (II).

D. Sterile Surgeon's Gloves and Double Gloving During Oral Surgical Procedures

1. Wear sterile surgeon's gloves when performing oral surgical procedures (IB).[2,8,137]

2. No recommendation is offered regarding the effectiveness of wearing two pairs of gloves to prevent disease transmission during oral surgical procedures. The majority of studies among health care personnel (HCP) and DHCP have demonstrated a lower frequency of inner glove perforation

and visible blood on the surgeon's hands when double gloves are worn; however, the effectiveness of wearing two pairs of gloves in preventing disease transmission has not been demonstrated (Unresolved issue).

V. Contact Dermatitis and Latex Hypersensitivity

A. General Recommendations

1. Educate DHCP regarding the signs, symptoms, and diagnoses of skin reactions associated with frequent hand hygiene and glove use (IB).[5,31,32]

2. Screen all patients for latex allergy (e.g., take health history and refer for medical consultation when latex allergy is suspected) (IB).[32]

3. Ensure a latex-safe environment for patients and DHCP with latex allergy (IB).[32]

4. Have emergency treatment kits with latex-free products available at all times (II).[32]

VI. Sterilization and Disinfection of Patient-Care Items

A. General Recommendations

1. Use only Food and Drug Administration (FDA)-cleared medical devices for sterilization and follow the manufacturer's instructions for correct use (IB).[248]

2. Clean and heat-sterilize critical dental instruments before each use (IA).[2,137,243,244,246,249,407]

3. Clean and heat-sterilize semicritical items before each use (IB).[2,249,260,407]

4. Allow packages to dry in the sterilizer before they are handled to avoid contamination (IB).[247]

5. Use of heat-stable semicritical alternatives is encouraged (IB).[2]

6. Reprocess heat-sensitive critical and semicritical instruments by using FDA-cleared sterilant/high-level disinfectants or an FDA-cleared low-temperature sterilization method (e.g., ethylene oxide). Follow manufacturer's instructions for use of chemical sterilants/high-level disinfectants (IB).[243]

7. Single-use disposable instruments are acceptable alternatives if they are used only once and disposed of correctly (IB, IC).[243,383]

8. Do not use liquid chemical sterilants/high-level disinfectants for environmental surface disinfection or as holding solutions (IB, IC).[243,245]

9. Ensure that noncritical patient-care items are barrier-protected or cleaned, or if visibly soiled, cleaned and disinfected after each use with a U.S. Environmental Protection Agency (EPA)-registered hospital disinfectant. If visibly contaminated with blood, use an EPA-registered hospital disinfectant with a tuberculocidal claim (i.e., intermediate level) (IB).[2,243,244]

10. Inform DHCP of all OSHA guidelines for exposure to chemical agents used for disinfection and sterilization. Using this report, identify areas and tasks that have potential for exposure (IC).[15]

B. Instrument Processing Area

1. Designate a central processing area. Divide the instrument processing area, physically or, at a minimum, spatially into distinct areas for (1) receiving, cleaning, and decontamination; (2) preparation and packaging; (3) sterilization; and (4) storage. Do not store instruments in an area where contaminated instruments are held or cleaned (II).[173,247,248]

2. Train DHCP to employ work practices that prevent contamination of clean areas (II).

C. Receiving, Cleaning, and Decontamination Work Area

1. Minimize handling of loose contaminated instruments during transport to the instrument processing area. Use work-practice controls (e.g., carry instruments in a covered container) to minimize exposure potential (II). Clean all visible blood and other contamination from dental instruments and devices before sterilization or disinfection procedures (IA).[243,249–252]

2. Use automated cleaning equipment (e.g., ultrasonic cleaner or washer-disinfector) to remove debris to improve cleaning effectiveness and decrease worker exposure to blood (IB).[2,253]

3. Use work-practice controls that minimize contact with sharp instruments if manual cleaning is necessary (e.g., long-handled brush) (IC).[14]

4. Wear puncture- and chemical-resistant/heavy-duty utility gloves for instrument cleaning and decontamination procedures (IB).[7]

5. Wear appropriate PPE (e.g., mask, protective eyewear, and gown) when splashing or spraying is anticipated during cleaning (IC).[13]

D. Preparation and Packaging

1. Use an internal chemical indicator in each package. If the internal indicator cannot be seen from outside the package, also use an external indicator (II).[243,254,257]

2. Use a container system or wrapping compatible with the type of sterilization process used and that has received FDA clearance (IB).[243,247,256]

3. Before sterilization of critical and semicritical instruments, inspect instruments for cleanliness, then wrap or place them in containers designed to maintain sterility during storage (e.g., cassettes and organizing trays) (IA).[2,247,255,256]

E. Sterilization of Unwrapped Instruments

1. Clean and dry instruments before the unwrapped sterilization cycle (IB).[248]

2. Use mechanical and chemical indicators for each unwrapped sterilization cycle (i.e., place an internal chemical indicator among the instruments or items to be sterilized) (IB).[243,258]

3. Allow unwrapped instruments to dry and cool in the sterilizer before they are handled to avoid contamination and thermal injury (II).[260]

4. Semicritical instruments that will be used immediately or within a short time can be sterilized unwrapped on a tray or in a container system, provided that the instruments are handled aseptically during removal from the sterilizer and transport to the point of use (II).

5. Critical instruments intended for immediate reuse can be sterilized unwrapped if the instruments are maintained sterile during removal from the sterilizer and transport to the point of use (e.g., transported in a sterile covered container) (IB).[258]

6. Do not sterilize implantable devices unwrapped (IB).[243,247]

7. Do not store critical instruments unwrapped (IB).[248]

F. Sterilization Monitoring

1. Use mechanical, chemical, and biological monitors according to the manufacturer's instructions to ensure the effectiveness of the sterilization process (IB).[248,278,279]

2. Monitor each load with mechanical (e.g., time, temperature, and pressure) and chemical indicators (II).[243,248]

3. Place a chemical indicator on the inside of each package. If the internal indicator is not visible from the outside, also place an exterior chemical indicator on the package (II).[243,254,257]

4. Place items/packages correctly and loosely into the sterilizer so as not to impede penetration of the sterilant (IB).[243]

5. Do not use instrument packs if mechanical or chemical indicators indicate inadequate processing (IB).[243,247,248]

6. Monitor sterilizers at least weekly by using a biological indicator with a matching control (i.e., biological indicator and control from same lot number) (IB).[2,9,243,247,278,279]

7. Use a biological indicator for every sterilizer load that contains an implantable device. Verify results before using the implantable device, whenever possible (IB).[243,248]

8. The following are recommended in the case of a positive spore test:
   a. Remove the sterilizer from service and review sterilization procedures (e.g., work practices and use of mechanical and chemical indicators) to determine whether operator error could be responsible (II).[8]
   b. Retest the sterilizer by using biological, mechanical, and chemical indicators after correcting any identified procedural problems (II).
   c. If the repeat spore test is negative, and mechanical and chemical indicators are within normal limits, put the sterilizer back in service (II).[9,243]

9. The following are recommended if the repeat spore test is positive:
   a. Do not use the sterilizer until it has been inspected or repaired or the exact reason for the positive test has been determined (II).[9,243]
   b. Recall, to the extent possible, and reprocess all items processed since the last negative spore test (II).[9,243,283]
   c. Before placing the sterilizer back in service, rechallenge the sterilizer with biological indicator tests in three consecutive empty chamber sterilization cycles after the cause of the sterilizer failure has been determined and corrected (II).[9,243,283]

10. Maintain sterilization records (i.e., mechanical, chemical, and biological) in compliance with state and local regulations (IB).[243]

G. Storage Area for Sterilized Items and Clean Dental Supplies

1. Implement practices on the basis of date- or event-related shelf-life for storage of wrapped, sterilized instruments and devices (IB).[243,284]

2. Even for event-related packaging, at a minimum, place the date of sterilization, and if multiple sterilizers are used in the facility, the sterilizer used, on the outside of the packaging material to facilitate the retrieval of processed items in the event of a sterilization failure (IB).[243,247]

3. Examine wrapped packages of sterilized instruments before opening them to ensure the barrier wrap has not been compromised during storage (II).[243,284]

4. Reclean, repack, and resterilize any instrument package that has been compromised (II).

5. Store sterile items and dental supplies in covered or closed cabinets, if possible (II).[285]

VII. Environmental Infection Control

A. General Recommendations

1. Follow the manufacturers' instructions for correct use of cleaning and EPA-registered hospital disinfecting products (IB, IC).[243–245]

2. Do not use liquid chemical sterilants/high-level disinfectants for disinfection of environmental surfaces (clinical contact or housekeeping) (IB, IC).[243–245]

3. Use PPE, as appropriate, when cleaning and disinfecting environmental surfaces. Such equipment might include gloves (e.g., puncture- and chemical-resistant utility), protective clothing (e.g., gown, jacket, or lab coat), and protective eyewear/face shield, and mask (IC).[13,15]

B. Clinical Contact Surfaces

1. Use surface barriers to protect clinical contact surfaces, particularly those that are difficult to clean (e.g., switches

on dental chairs) and change surface barriers between patients (II).[1,2,260,288]

2. Clean and disinfect clinical contact surfaces that are not barrier-protected, by using an EPA-registered hospital disinfectant with a low- (i.e., human immunodeficiency virus [HIV] and HBV label claims) to intermediate-level (i.e., tuberculocidal claim) activity after each patient. Use an intermediate-level disinfectant if visibly contaminated with blood (IB).[2,243,244]

C. Housekeeping Surfaces

1. Clean housekeeping surfaces (e.g., floors, walls, and sinks) with a detergent and water or an EPA-registered hospital disinfectant/detergent on a routine basis, depending on the nature of the surface and type and degree of contamination, and as appropriate, based on the location in the facility, and when visibly soiled (IB).[243,244]

2. Clean mops and cloths after use and allow to dry before reuse; or use single-use, disposable mop heads or cloths (II).[243,244]

3. Prepare fresh cleaning or EPA-registered disinfecting solutions daily and as instructed by the manufacturer (II).[243,244]

4. Clean walls, blinds, and window curtains in patient-care areas when they are visibly dusty or soiled (II).[9,244]

D. Spills of Blood and Body Substances

1. Clean spills of blood or OPIM and decontaminate surface with an EPA-registered hospital disinfectant with low-level (i.e., HBV and HIV label claims) to intermediate-level (i.e., tuberculocidal claim) activity, depending on size of spill and surface porosity (IB, IC).[13,113]

E. Carpet and Cloth Furnishings

1. Avoid using carpeting and cloth-upholstered furnishings in dental operatories, laboratories, and instrument processing areas (II).[9,293–295]

F. Regulated Medical Waste

1. General recommendations
   a. Develop a medical waste management program. Disposal of regulated medical waste must follow federal, state, and local regulations (IC).[13,301]
   b. Ensure that DHCP who handle and dispose of regulated medical waste are trained in appropriate handling and disposal methods and are informed of the possible health and safety hazards (IC).[13]

2. Management of regulated medical waste in dental health care facilities
   a. Use a color-coded or labeled container that prevents leakage (e.g., biohazard bag) to contain non-sharp regulated medical waste (IC).[13]
   b. Place sharp items (e.g., needles, scalpel blades, orthodontic bands, broken metal instruments, and burs) in an appropriate sharps container (e.g., puncture resistant, color-coded, and leakproof). Close container

immediately before removal or replacement to prevent spillage or protrusion of contents during handling, storage, transport, or shipping (IC).[2,8,13,113,115]
   c. Pour blood, suctioned fluids, or other liquid waste carefully into a drain connected to a sanitary sewer system, if local sewage discharge requirements are met and the state has declared this an acceptable method of disposal. Wear appropriate PPE while performing this task (IC).[7,9,13]

VIII. Dental Unit Waterlines, Biofilm, and Water Quality

A. General Recommendations

1. Use water that meets EPA regulatory standards for drinking water (i.e., ≤500 CFU/mL of heterotrophic water bacteria) for routine dental treatment output water (IB, IC).[341,342]

2. Consult with the dental unit manufacturer for appropriate methods and equipment to maintain the recommended quality of dental water (II).[339]

3. Follow recommendations for monitoring water quality provided by the manufacturer of the unit or waterline treatment product (II).

4. Discharge water and air for a minimum of 20–30 seconds after each patient, from any device connected to the dental water system that enters the patient's mouth (e.g., handpieces, ultrasonic scalers, and air/water syringes) (II).[2,311,344]

5. Consult with the dental unit manufacturer on the need for periodic maintenance of antiretraction mechanisms (IB).[2,311]

B. Boil-Water Advisories

1. The following apply while a boil-water advisory is in effect:
   a. Do not deliver water from the public water system to the patient through the dental operative unit, ultrasonic scaler, or other dental equipment that uses the public water system (IB, IC).[341,342,346,349,350]
   b. Do not use water from the public water system for dental treatment, patient rinsing, or handwashing (IB, IC).[341,342,346,349,350]
   c. For handwashing, use antimicrobial-containing products that do not require water for use (e.g., alcohol-based hand rubs). If hands are visibly contaminated, use bottled water, if available, and soap for handwashing or an antiseptic towelette (IB, IC).[13,122]

2. The following apply when the boil-water advisory is cancelled:
   a. Follow guidance given by the local water utility regarding adequate flushing of waterlines. If no guidance is provided, flush dental waterlines and faucets for 1–5 minutes before using for patient care (IC).[244,346,351,352]

b. Disinfect dental waterlines as recommended by the dental unit manufacturer (II).

IX. Special Considerations

A. Dental Handpieces and Other Devices Attached to Air and Waterlines

1. Clean and heat-sterilize handpieces and other intraoral instruments that can be removed from the air and waterlines of dental units between patients (IB, IC).[2,246,275,356,357,360,407]

2. Follow the manufacturer's instructions for cleaning, lubrication, and sterilization of handpieces and other intraoral instruments that can be removed from the air and waterlines of dental units (IB).[361–363]

3. Do not surface-disinfect, use liquid chemical sterilants, or ethylene oxide on handpieces and other intraoral instruments that can be removed from the air and waterlines of dental units (IC).[2,246,250,275]

4. Do not advise patients to close their lips tightly around the tip of the saliva ejector to evacuate oral fluids (II).[364–366]

B. Dental Radiology

1. Wear gloves when exposing radiographs and handling contaminated film packets. Use other PPE (e.g., protective eyewear, mask, and gown) as appropriate if spattering of blood or other body fluids is likely (IA, IC).[11,13]

2. Use heat-tolerant or disposable intraoral devices whenever possible (e.g., film-holding and positioning devices). Clean and heat-sterilize heat-tolerant devices between patients. At a minimum, high-level disinfect semicritical heat-sensitive devices, according to manufacturer's instructions (IB).[243]

3. Transport and handle exposed radiographs in an aseptic manner to prevent contamination of developing equipment (II).

4. The following apply for digital radiography sensors:
   a. Use FDA-cleared barriers (IB).[243]
   b. Clean and heat-sterilize, or high-level disinfect, between patients, barrier-protected semicritical items. If the item cannot tolerate these procedures, then, at a minimum, protect with an FDA-cleared barrier and clean and disinfect with an EPA-registered hospital disinfectant with intermediate-level (i.e., tuberculocidal claim) activity, between patients. Consult with the manufacturer for methods of disinfection and sterilization of digital radiology sensors and for protection of associated computer hardware (IB).[243]

C. Aseptic Technique for Parenteral Medications

1. Do not administer medication from a syringe to multiple patients, even if the needle on the syringe is changed (IA).[378]

2. Use single-dose vials for parenteral medications when possible (II).[376,377]

3. Do not combine the leftover contents of single use vials for later use (IA).[376,377]

4. The following apply if multidose vials are used:
   a. Cleanse the access diaphragm with 70% alcohol before inserting a device into the vial (IA).[380,381]
   b. Use a sterile device to access a multiple-dose vial and avoid touching the access diaphragm. Both the needle and syringe used to access the multidose vial should be sterile. Do not reuse a syringe even if the needle is changed (IA).[380,381]
   c. Keep multidose vials away from the immediate patient treatment area to prevent inadvertent contamination by spray or spatter (II).
   d. Discard the multidose vial if sterility is compromised (IA).[380,381]

5. Use fluid infusion and administration sets (i.e., IV bags, tubings, and connections) for one patient only and dispose of appropriately (IB).[378]

D. Single-Use (Disposable) Devices

1. Use single-use devices for one patient only and dispose of them appropriately (IC).[383]

E. Preprocedural Mouthrinses

1. No recommendation is offered regarding use of preprocedural antimicrobial mouthrinses to prevent clinical infections among DHCP or patients. Although studies have demonstrated that a preprocedural antimicrobial rinse (e.g., chlorhexidine gluconate, essential oils, or povidoneiodine) can reduce the level of oral microorganisms in aerosols and spatter generated during routine dental procedures and can decrease the number of microorganisms introduced in the patient's bloodstream during invasive dental procedures,[391–399] the scientific evidence is inconclusive that using these rinses prevents clinical infections among DHCP or patients (see discussion, Preprocedural Mouthrinses) (Unresolved issue).

F. Oral Surgical Procedures

1. The following apply when performing oral surgical procedures:
   a. Perform surgical hand antisepsis by using an antimicrobial product (e.g., antimicrobial soap and water, or soap and water followed by alcohol-based hand scrub with persistent activity) before donning sterile surgeon's gloves (IB).[127–132,137]
   b. Use sterile surgeon's gloves (IB).[2,7,121,123,137]
   c. Use sterile saline or sterile water as a coolant/irrigatant when performing oral surgical procedures.
   d. Use devices specifically designed for delivering sterile irrigating fluids (e.g., bulb syringe, single-use disposable products, and sterilizable tubing) (IB).[2,121]

G. Handling of Biopsy Specimens

1. During transport, place biopsy specimens in a sturdy, leakproof container labeled with the biohazard symbol (IC).[2,13,14]

2. If a biopsy specimen container is visibly contaminated, clean and disinfect the outside of a container or place it in an impervious bag labeled with the biohazard symbol, (IC).[2,13]

H. Handling of Extracted Teeth

1. Dispose of extracted teeth as regulated medical waste unless returned to the patient (IC).[13,14]

2. Do not dispose of extracted teeth containing amalgam in regulated medical waste intended for incineration (II).

3. Clean and place extracted teeth in a leakproof container, labeled with a biohazard symbol, and maintain hydration for transport to educational institutions or a dental laboratory (IC).[13,14]

4. Heat-sterilize teeth that do not contain amalgam before they are used for educational purposes (IB).[403,405,406]

I. Dental Laboratory

1. Use PPE when handling items received in the laboratory until they have been decontaminated (IA, IC).[2,7,11,13,113]

2. Before they are handled in the laboratory, clean, disinfect, and rinse all dental prostheses and prosthodontic materials (e.g., impressions, bite registrations, occlusal rims, and extracted teeth) by using an EPA-registered hospital disinfectant having at least an intermediate-level (i.e., tuberculocidal claim) activity (IB).[2,249,252,407]

3. Consult with manufacturers regarding the stability of specific materials (e.g., impression materials) relative to disinfection procedures (II).

4. Include specific information regarding disinfection techniques used (e.g., solution used and duration), when laboratory cases are sent off-site and on their return (II).[2,407,409]

5. Clean and heat-sterilize heat-tolerant items used in the mouth (e.g., metal impression trays and face-bow forks) (IB).[2,407]

6. Follow manufacturers' instructions for cleaning and sterilizing or disinfecting items that become contaminated but do not normally contact the patient (e.g., burs, polishing points, rag wheels, articulators, case pans, and lathes). If manufacturer instructions are unavailable, clean and heat-sterilize heat-tolerant items or clean and disinfect with an EPA-registered hospital disinfectant with low-level (HIV, HBV effectiveness claim) to intermediate-level (tuberculocidal claim) activity, depending on the degree of contamination (II).

J. Laser/Electrosurgery Plumes/Surgical Smoke

1. No recommendation is offered regarding practices to reduce DHCP exposure to laser plumes/surgical smoke when using lasers in dental practice. Practices to reduce HCP exposure to laser plumes/surgical smoke have been suggested, including use of (a) standard precautions (e.g., high-filtration surgical masks and possibly full face shields)[437]; (b) central room suction units with in-line filters to collect particulate matter from minimal plumes; and (c) dedicated mechanical smoke exhaust systems with a high-efficiency filter to remove substantial amounts of laser-plume particles. The effect of the exposure (e.g., disease transmission or adverse respiratory effects) on DHCP from dental applications of lasers has not been adequately evaluated (see previous discussion, Laser/Electrosurgery Plumes or Surgical Smoke) (Unresolved issue).

K. Mycobacterium Tuberculosis

1. General recommendations

   a. Educate all DHCP regarding the recognition of signs, symptoms, and transmission of tuberculosis (TB) (IB).[20,21]

   b. Conduct a baseline TST, preferably by using a two-step test, for all DHCP who might have contact with persons with suspected or confirmed active TB, regardless of the risk classification of the setting (IB).[20]

   c. Assess each patient for a history of TB as well as symptoms indicative of TB and document on the medical history form (IB).[20,21]

   d. Follow CDC recommendations for (1) developing, maintaining, and implementing a written TB infection-control plan; (2) managing a patient with suspected or active TB; (3) completing a community risk-assessment to guide employee TSTs and follow-up; and (4) managing DHCP with TB disease (IB).[2,21]

2. The following apply for patients known or suspected to have active *TB*:

   a. Evaluate the patient away from other patients and DHCP. When not being evaluated, the patient should wear a surgical mask or be instructed to cover mouth and nose when coughing or sneezing (IB).[20,21]

   b. Defer elective dental treatment until the patient is noninfectious (IB).[20,21]

   c. Refer patients requiring urgent dental treatment to a previously identified facility with TB engineering controls and a respiratory protection program (IB).[20,21]

L. Creutzfeldt-Jakob Disease (CJD) and Other Prion Diseases

1. No recommendation is offered regarding use of special precautions in addition to standard precautions when treating known CJD or vCJD patients. Potential infectivity of oral tissues in CJD or vCJD patients is an unresolved issue. Scientific data indicate the risk, if any, of sporadic CJD transmission during dental and oral surgical procedures is low to nil. Until additional information exists regarding the transmissibility of CJD or vCJD during dental procedures, special precautions

in addition to standard precautions might be indicated when treating known CJD or vCJD patients; a list of such precautions is provided for consideration without recommendation (see Creutzfeldt Jakob Disease and Other Prion Diseases) (Unresolved issue).

M. Program Evaluation

1. Establish routine evaluation of the infection-control program, including evaluation of performance indicators, at an established frequency (II).[470,471]

ACKNOWLEDGMENT

The Division of Oral Health thanks the working group as well as CDC and other federal and external reviewers for their efforts in developing and reviewing drafts of this report and acknowledges that all opinions of the reviewers might not be reflected in all of the recommendations.

Reference

A comprehensive list of references can be found in the original article: Centers for Disease Control and Prevention. Guidelines for Infection Control in Dental Health Care Settings, 2003. MMWR. 2003;52 (RR-17):1–61. http://www.cdc.gov/oralhealth/infectioncontrol/guidelines. Accessed October 2011.

Appendix VI

Average Measurements of Human Teeth

TABLE A-1	Average Measurements of the Primary Teeth (In Millimeters)				
		OVERALL LENGTH	LENGTH OF CROWN	LENGTH OF ROOT	WIDTH OF CROWN (MESIALDISTAL AT WIDEST POINT)
Maxillary	Central incisor	16.0	6.0	10.0	6.5
	Lateral incisor	15.8	5.6	11.4	5.1
	Canine	19.0	6.5	13.5	7.0
	First molar	15.2	5.1	10.0	7.3
	Second molar	17.5	5.7	11.7	8.2
Mandibular	Central incisor	14.0	5.0	9.0	4.2
	Lateral incisor	15.0	5.2	10.0	4.1
	Canine	17.5	6.0	11.5	5.0
	First molar	15.8	6.0	9.8	7.7
	Second molar	18.8	5.5	11.3	9.9

(Reprinted with permission from Black GV. *Descriptive Anatomy of the Human Teeth*. 4th ed. Philadelphia, PA: The S.S. White Dental Manufacturing Company; 1897, according to Ash MM. *Wheeler's Dental Anatomy, Physiology, and Occlusion*. 7th ed. Philadelphia, PA: W.B. Saunders, Co; 1993:58.)

TABLE A-2	Average Measurements of the Permanent Teeth (In Millimeters)			
		OVERALL LENGTH	**LENGTH OF CROWN**	**LENGTH OF ROOT**	**WIDTH OF CROWN (MESIALDISTAL AT WIDEST POINT)**

		OVERALL LENGTH	LENGTH OF CROWN	LENGTH OF ROOT	WIDTH OF CROWN (MESIALDISTAL AT WIDEST POINT)
Maxillary	Central incisor	23.5	10.5	13.0	8.5
	Lateral incisor	22.0	9.9	13.0	6.5
	Canine	27.0	10.0	17.0	7.5
	First premolar	22.5	8.5	14.0	7.0
	Second premolar	22.5	8.5	14.0	7.0
	First molar	B L 19.5 20.5	7.5	B L 12 13	10.0
	Second molar	B L 17.0 19.0	7.0	B L 11 12	9.0
	Third molar	17.5	6.5	11.0	8.5
Mandibular	Central incisor	21.5	9.0	12.5	5.0
	Lateral incisor	23.5	9.5	14.0	5.5
	Canine	27.0	11.0	16.0	7.0
	First premolar	22.5	8.5	14.0	7.0
	Second premolar	22.5	8.0	14.5	7.0
	First molar	21.5	7.5	14.0	11.0
	Second molar	20.0	7.0	13.0	10.5
	Third molar	18.0	7.0	11.0	10.0

B, buccal measurement; L, lingual measurement.
(Reprinted with permission from Ash MM. *Wheeler's Dental Anatomy, Physiology, and Occlusion*. 7th ed. Philadelphia, PA: W.B. Saunders, Co; 1993:15.)

Appendix VII

Prefixes, Suffixes, and Combining Forms

A

a-, an- absence, lack, without, e.g., *a*morphous

ab- from, away, e.g., *ab*normal

ad- (change d to c, f, g, p, s, or t before words beginning with those consonants) to, toward, e.g., *ad*hesion, *ac*cretion

adeno- gland, e.g., *adeno*fibroma

-algia pain, e.g., neur*algia*

ambi- all (both) sides, round, e.g., *ambi*dexterity

amelo- enamel, e.g., *amelo*genesis

amphi-, ampho- on both sides, double, e.g., *ampho*diplopia

ana- up, excessive, again, e.g., *ana*bolism

andro- masculine, male, e.g., *andro*gen

angio- vessel, e.g., *angio*ma

ante- before, e.g., *ante*febrile

anti- against, e.g., *anti*dote

aqu-, aqua- water, e.g., *aqu*eous

arthro-, arth- joints, e.g., *arth*ritis

-ase denotes an enzyme, e.g., dextrin*ase*

-asthenia weakness, e.g., my*asthenia* gravis

auto-, aut- self, e.g., *auto*transplant

B

bi- two, twice, double, e.g., *bi*furcation

bio-, bi- life, living, e.g., *bio*psy

-blast formative cell, e.g., osteo*blast*

-brachy- short, e.g., *brachy*dactylic

brady- slow, e.g., *brady*cardia

bucc- cheek, e.g., *bucc*inator

C

calc- stone, calcium, lime, e.g., *calc*ification

cardio-, cardi- heart, e.g., *cardio*vascular

cata- down, against, e.g., *cata*bolism

-cele swelling, protrusion, hernia, e.g., meningo*cele*

cephalo-, cephal- head, e.g., *cephalo*metry

cerebro-, cerebr- brain, e.g., *cerebr*al palsy

cheilo-, cheil- lip, e.g., *cheil*itis

chloro-, chlor- pale green, e.g., *chloro*phyll

chromo-, chromat- color, pigmentation, e.g., *chromo*genic

-cidal killing, e.g., bacteri*cidal*

-clast break up, divide into parts, e.g., osteo*clast*

-clus- shut, e.g., oc*clus*ion

co-, com-, con-, cor- with, together, e.g., *con*genital

coll- glue, e.g., *coll*oid

contra- opposite, e.g., *contra*lateral

cryo, cry- cold, freezing, e.g., *cryo*therapy

cuti- skin, e.g., *cuti*cle

cyan- blue, e.g., *cyan*otic

-cyto-, -cyt- cell, e.g., leuko*cyte*

D

-dactyl, dactylo- fingers, e.g., *dactyl*edema

de- down, away from, separation, e.g., *de*calcification

denti-, dent- tooth, e.g., *dent*ition

-derm-, derma- skin, e.g., hypo*derm*ic

dextr-, dextro- right, toward right, e.g., *dextro*cardia

di- twice, two, e.g., *di*plopia

dis- separation, opposite, taking apart, e.g., *dis*infect

disto-, dist- posterior, distant from center, e.g., *disto*buccal

-drome course, e.g., syn*drome*

dur- hard, e.g., in*dur*ation

dys- bad, ill, difficult, e.g., *dys*trophy

E

ecto-, ect- without, outer side, e.g., *ecto*derm

-ectomy surgical removal, e.g., gingiv*ectomy*

-emia (-aemia) blood condition, e.g., bacter*emia*

en- in, on, into, e.g., *en*demic

encephal-, encephalo- brain, e.g., *encephalo*meningitis

endo- inside, e.g., *endo*dontics

entero-, enter- intestine, e.g., *entero*toxin

epi- upon, after, in addition, e.g., *epi*dermis

erythro-, eryth- red, e.g., *eryth*ema

esthesio-, esthesia (-aesthesia) sensation, perception, e.g., an*esthesia*

ex- beyond, from, out of, e.g., *ex*udate

extra- outside of, beyond the scope of, e.g., *extra*cellular

F

faci- face, e.g., *faci*al

-facient causes or brings about, e.g., rube*facient*

-ferent carry, bear, e.g., af*ferent*

1207

fibro-, fibr- fibers, fibrous tissue, e.g., *fibroblast*
fract- break, e.g., *fractional*

G

galacto-, galact- milk, e.g., *galactose*
gastro-, gastr- stomach, e.g., *gastritis*
-gen- produced, e.g., glyco*gen*
genio- chin, lower jaw, e.g., *genioplasty*
germ- bud, early growth, e.g., *germinal*
gero- old age, e.g., *gerodontics*
glosso-, gloss- tongue, e.g., *glossitis*
gluco-, glue- glucose, e.g., *gluconeogenesis*
glyco-, glyc- sweet, e.g., *glycerin*
gnatho-, gnath- jaw, e.g., *gnathodynamometer*
-gnosis knowledge, e.g., pro*gnosis*
-gram, -graph write, draw, e.g., radio*graphic*
gran- grain, particle, e.g., *granuloma*
gyn-, gyne-, gynec- woman, e.g., *gynecology*

H

hemi- half, e.g., *hemisection*
hemo- (haemo-) blood, e.g., *hemorrhage*
hepato-, hepat- liver, e.g., *hepatitis*
hetero-, heter- other, different, e.g., *heterogeneous*
histo-, hist- tissue, e.g., *histology*
homo-, homeo- like, similar, e.g., *homeostasis*
hydro-, hydr- water, e.g., *hydrocephalic*
hygro-, hygr- moisture, e.g., *hygrophobia*
hyper- abnormal, excessive, e.g., *hypertrophy*
hypno-, hypn- sleep, e.g., *hypnotic*
hypo-, hyp- deficiency, lack, below, e.g., *hypotonic*
hystero-, hyster- uterus or hysteria, e.g., *hysterectomy*

I

-ia state or condition, e.g., glycosu*ria*
iatro- relation to medicine, a physician, dentist, or other health professional, e.g., *iatrogenic*
-ic of, pertaining to, e.g., gastr*ic*
idio- one's own, separate, distinct, e.g., *idiopathic*
in- not, without, e.g., *inactivate*
infra- beneath, below, e.g., *infraorbital*
inter- between, among, e.g., *intercellular*
intra- within, into, e.g., *intraoral*
ischo-, isch- suppression, stoppage, e.g., *ischemia*
iso- equality, similarity, e.g., *isotonic*
-ist one who practices, holds certain principles, e.g., hygien*ist*
-itis inflammation, e.g., dermat*itis*

J

-ject- throw, e.g., in*ject*ion
juxta- next to, near, e.g., *juxta*position

K

karyo-, kary- nucleus of a cell, e.g., *karyolysis*
kerato-, kerat- horny, keratinized tissue, e.g., *keratinization*
kin- move, e.g., *kinetic*

L

labio- lip, e.g., *labioversion*
lacto-, lact- milk, e.g., *lactation*
laryngo-, laryn- larynx, e.g., *laryngitis*
later- side, e.g., *lateroversion*
leuko-, leuk- white, e.g., *leukoplakia*
linguo, lingu- tongue, e.g., *lingual*
lipo-, lip- fat, fatty, e.g., *lipoma*
-logy doctrine, science, e.g., periodonto*logy*
lympho-, lymph- lymph, e.g., *lymphangioma*
-lysin, -lysis, -lytic dissolving, destructive, e.g., hemo*lysis*

M

macro-, macr- enlargement, elongated part, e.g., *macrodontia*
mal- bad, ill, e.g., *malnutrition*
mast-, mastro- breast, e.g., *mastectomy*
-megalo-, -megal- large, great, e.g., *megaloblast*
melano- dark-colored, relating to melanin, e.g., *melanogenesis*
meningo-, mening- meninges, e.g., *meningitis*
meno- month, e.g., *menopause*
mes-, medi, mesio- middle, intermediate, e.g., *mesoderm*
meta-, met- over, beyond, transformation, e.g., *metabolism*
metro-, metra- uterus, e.g., *metrofibroma*
-metry measure, e.g., cephalo*metry*
micro-, micr- small, e.g., *microorganism*
mono- one, single, e.g., *monosaccharide*
morpho-, morph- form, shape, e.g., *morphology*
muco-, muc- relating to mucous membrane, e.g., *mucogingival*
myel-, myelo- bone marrow, spinal cord, e.g., *myeloblast*
mylo- molar teeth or posterior portion of mandible, e.g., *mylohyoid*
myo-, my- muscle, e.g., *myocardium*

N

naso- nose, e.g., *nasopalatine*
necr- death, e.g., *necrotic*
neo-, ne- new, recent, e.g., *neoplasm*
nephro-, nephr- kidneys, e.g., *nephritis*
neuro-, neuri-, neur- pertaining to nerves, e.g., *neurasthenia*
nucleo-, nucle- pertaining to nucleus, e.g., *nucleoprotein*

O

ob- (change b to c before words beginning with c) against, toward, e.g., *occlusion*
odonto-, odont- tooth, e.g., *odontalgia*
-oid like, resembling, e.g., ameb*oid*
-olig-, oligo- a few, a little, e.g., *oligodontia*
-oma swelling, tumor, e.g., lip*oma*
-opia, -opy sight, eye defect, e.g., my*opia*
oro- mouth, oral, e.g., *oronasal*

ortho-, orth- straight, normal, e.g., *ortho*dontics
-osis condition, state, e.g., cyan*osis*
osteo-, oste- bone, e.g., *osteo*porosis
oto-, ot- ear, e.g., *oto*plasty
-ous full of, having, e.g., aque*ous*
ovi-, ovo-, ovu- egg, e.g., *ovu*lation

P

pan- all, every, general, e.g., *pan*acea
para- beyond, beside, near, e.g., *para*site
patho-, path- disease, e.g., *patho*gnomonic
pedia-, pedo- (paedo-) child, e.g., *pedo*dontics
-penia deficiency, e.g., leuk*openia*
per- throughout, completely, e.g., *per*cussion
peri- around, near, e.g., *peri*apical
phago- to eat, e.g., *phago*cytic
-phile, -phil- loving, e.g., hemo*philia*
phlebo-, phleb- vein, e.g., *phleb*itis
-phobe, -phobia fear, dread, e.g., photo*phobia*
pilo- hair, e.g., *pilo*erection
-plas- mold, shape, e.g., gingivo*plasty*
plasmo-, plasm form, e.g., cyto*plasm*
-plegia, -plexy paralysis, stroke, e.g., hemi*plegia*
pleo- more, e.g., *pleo*morphism
-pnea (-pnoea) breathing, e.g., dys*pnea*
pneumo- air, lung, e.g., *pneumo*thorax
-poiesis, -poietic production, e.g., erythro*poietic*
poly- many, much, e.g., *poly*saccharide
pont- bridge, e.g., *pont*ic
poro-, -por- opening, pore, duct, e.g., *por*ous
post- behind, after, e.g., *post*natal
pre- before, in front of, e.g., *pre*maxilla
pro- before, in front of, e.g., *pro*gnathic
proprio- one's own, e.g., *proprio*ceptive
proto- first, e.g., *proto*plasm
pseudo- false, deceptive, e.g., *pseudo*membrane
psycho-, psych- mind, mental processes, e.g., *psycho*somatic
pulmo- lung, e.g., *pulmo*nary
pur- pus, e.g., *pur*ulent
pyo- pus, e.g., *pyo*rrhea
pyro- fever, heat, e.g., *pyro*genic

R

re- back, again, e.g., *re*gurgitate
-renal kidney, e.g., ad*renal*

retro- back, backward, behind, e.g., *retro*molar
-rhage breaking, bursting forth, profuse flow, e.g., hemo*rrhage*
-rhea (-rhoea) flow, discharge, e.g., pyo*rrhea*
rhino-, rhin- nose, e.g., *rhin*itis
rube- red, e.g., *rube*facient

S

sarco- flesh, muscle, e.g., *sarco*ma
sclero- hard, e.g., *sclero*derma
-scopy examination, inspection, e.g., micro*scopy*
semi- half, partly, e.g., *semi*permeable
sero- serum, serous, e.g., *sero*purulent
sial-, sialo- saliva, e.g., *sialo*graphy
somat-, somato-, -some body, e.g., chromo*some*
-squam- scale, e.g., des*quam*ative
stomat- mouth, e.g., *stomat*itis
sub- beneath, under, deficient, e.g., *sub*acute
super- above, upon, excessive, e.g., *super*numerary tooth
supra- above, e.g., *supra*gingival calculus
syn- with, together, e.g., *syn*drome

T

tachy- swift, e.g., *tachy*cardia
tact- touch, e.g., *tact*ile
tera-, terato- monster, malformed fetus, e.g., *terato*genic
thermo- heat, e.g., *thermo*phile
thrombo-, thromb- clot, coagulation, e.g., *thromb*in
-thym-, thymo- mind, soul, emotions, e.g., dys*thym*ia
trans- beyond, through, across, e.g., *trans*plantation
tropho-, trophic nutrition, nourishment, e.g., hyper*trophic*
-tropic turning toward, changing, e.g., hydro*tropic*

U

-ule diminutive, small, e.g., tub*ule*
-uria urine, e.g., glucos*uria*

V

vaso- blood vessels, e.g., *vaso*dilation
vita- life, e.g., *vita*min

X

xero- dry, e.g., *xero*stomia

Appendix VIII

Charting Symbols and Standardized Abbreviations Useful for Documenting Dental Hygiene Care*

SELECTED SYMBOLS COMMONLY USED IN DENTAL CHARTING	
SYMBOL	MEANING
"X" or " = "	Missing tooth or pontic
≠	Fracture
‖	Open contact
↑	Increase
↓	Decrease
→ midline ←	Drifted mesially
← midline →	Drifted distally
↻	Rotated clockwise
↺	Rotated counterclockwise
C/	Complete upper denture
/C	Complete lower denture

STANDARDIZED ABBREVIATIONS	
ABBREVIATION	TERM
abn	abnormal
BOP	bleeding on probing
bp	blood pressure
brux	bruxism or bruxer
bw, bwx, or bwxr; pa or pax; pan or pano	bite wing radiograph; periapical radiograph; panoramic radiograph
CAL	clinical attachment level
Calc	calculus
CC	chief complaint
CEJ	cementoenamel junction
chk	check, observe
cm	centimeter
cons	consultation
debrd	debridement
decid	deciduous, primary
demo	demonstrate
dent hx	dental history
dup	duplicate
dx	diagnosis
emerg	emergency
esp	especially
eval	evaluate, evaluation
Ex, exam	examination
exf	exfoliate
ext	extraction
f/u	follow-up
F, fl, Ftx; APF; NaF; SnF	fluoride, fluoride treatment; acidulated phosphate fluoride; sodium fluoride, stannous fluoride

*Selected from the complete list available in: American Dental Association. *Dental Abbreviations, Symbols, and Acronyms.* 2nd ed. Chicago, IL; American Dental Association; 2008:5–20. Used with permission.

ABBREVIATION	TERM
fgm, GM	free gingival margin, gingival margin
food imp	food impaction
fur, furc	furcation
ging	gingival, gingival
H, hx, hist, h/o	history, history of
HH, med hx	health history, medical history
htn, hbp	hypertension, high blood pressure
hyg	dental hygiene
IC	informed consent
INS	insurance
LA; lido xylo; vaso	local anesthesia, Lidocaine; Xylocaine; vasoconstrictor
mand; max	mandibular; maxillary
mdl	midline
meds	medications
MGJ	mucogingival junction
n/a; n/c; n/d	not applicable; no change; not determined
N₂O	nitrous oxide
NKA; NKDA	no known allergies; no known drug allergies
NSPT	non surgical periodontal therapy
nv	next visit
occ, occl	occlusal or occlusion
OHI	oral hygiene instructions
OTC	over the counter
pk, pkt	pocket
PLD	partial lower denture
POI	post operative instructions
PFG	porcelain fused to gold
PFM	porcelain fused to metal
pol	polish
PPE	personal protective equipment

ABBREVIATION	TERM
pre op; post op	preoperative, postoperative
prev	prevention, preventive
prog, Px	prognosis
pt	patient
q4h	every 4 hours
q6h	every 6 hours
q1d	every day
qid	every day
qod	every other day
quad; LRQ; URQ	quadrant; lower right quadrant; upper right quadrant
reapp, reappt	reappoint(ment)
re-eval	re-evaluation
RMH	reviewed medical history
rp/sc, RPS, S&RP, SRP	scaling and root planing
Rx	prescription
S&Sx, S/S	signs and symptoms
S/D BP	systolic/diastolic blood pressure
SPT	supportive periodontal treatment
stat	immediately
sut	suture
sub, subggv, subgin	subgingival
supp	supperatio
Supra ggv	supragingival
tb	toothbrush
TID	three times per day
TMD	temporomandibular joint disorder
tmj	temporomandibular joint
Tx	treatment
unk	unknown
var	varnish
wnl	within normal limits

Index

Note: Page numbers followed by "*f*", "*t*" and "*b*" refer to figures, tables and boxes, respectively.